Blakiston's Pocket Medical Dictionary

Blakiston's Pocket Medical Dictionary

Fourth Edition

McGraw-Hill Book Company

New York   St. Louis   San Francisco   Auckland   Bogotá   Düsseldorf
Johannesburg   London   Madrid   Mexico   Montreal   New Delhi
Panama   Paris   São Paulo   Singapore   Sydney   Tokyo   Toronto

Library of Congress Cataloging in Publication Data
Main entry under title:

Blakiston's pocket medical dictionary.

    1. Medicine—Dictionaries. I. Igoe, Judith B.
II. Title: Pocket medical dictionary.
R121.B6 1979   610'.3   78-21926
ISBN 0-07-005715-X
ISBN 0-07-005714-1 pbk.

Blakiston's POCKET MEDICAL DICTIONARY

  234567890 DODO 7832109

The vocabulary portion of this book was set in Times Roman by
Rocappi, Inc. The appendix was set, also in Times Roman, by
York Graphic Services, Inc.
The editors were J. Dereck Jeffers and Richard S. Laufer;
the designer was Merrill Haber; and
the production Supervisor was Thomas J. LoPinto.
R. R. Donnelley & Sons Company was printer and binder.

CONTENTS

LIST OF CONTRIBUTORS

Don L. Allen, D.D.S.
Professor of Periodontics and
  Dean
University of Florida College of
  Dentistry
Gainesville, Florida

Tom P. Barden, M.D.
Professor of Obstetrics and
  Gynecology
University of Cincinnati College of
  Medicine
Cincinnati, Ohio

Alfred S. Berne, M.D.
Professor of Radiology
Upstate Medical Center
State University of New York,
  Syracuse
Attending Radiologist and Chief
Department of Radiology
Crouse-Irving Memorial Hospital
Syracuse, New York

Frederic W. Bruhn, M.D.
Chief, Pediatric Infectious
  Diseases
Walter Reed Army Medical Center
Washington, D.C.
Assistant Professor
Uniformed Services University of
  The Health Sciences
Bethesda, Maryland

Henry N. Claman, M.D.
Professor of Medicine and of
  Microbiology and Immunology
University of Colorado Medical
  School
Denver, Colorado

**Alastair M. Connell, M.D.,
  F.A.C.P., F.R.C.P.**
Mark Brown Professor of
  Medicine
Professor of Physiology and
Director, Division of Digestive
  Diseases
Department of Internal Medicine
University of Cincinnati Medical
  Center
Cincinnati, Ohio 45267

Lawrence R. DeChatelet, Ph.D.
Professor of Biochemistry,
Research Associate in Medicine
Bowman Gray School of Medicine
Winston-Salem, North Carolina

Ralph E. Fishkin, D.O.
Clinical Assistant Professor
  Psychiatry and Human Behavior
Thomas Jefferson University
Philadelphia, Pennsylvania

Warren W. Frost, D.V.M.
Director, Animal Care Facility
University of Colorado Medical
  Center
Denver, Colorado

Alfonso R. Gennaro, Ph.D.
Associate Dean for Science
Director, Department of
  Chemistry
Philadelphia College of Pharmacy
  and Science
Philadelphia, Pennsylvania

William Richard Green, M.D.
Professor of Ophthalmology and
Associate Professor of Pathology
Johns Hopkins University School
  of Medicine
Baltimore, Maryland

Paul A. Harper, M.D., M.P.H.
Professor Emeritus
Maternal and Child Health,
  Population Dynamics
Johns Hopkins School of Hygiene
  and Public Health
Baltimore, Maryland

Lawrence R. Hyman, M.D.
Assistant Professor
Pediatric Nephrology Division
Department of Pediatrics
Johns Hopkins University School
  of Medicine
Baltimore, Maryland

Judith B. Igoe, M.S.
Associate Professor
School of Nursing
Instructor, Department of Pediatrics
University of Colorado Medical
  Center
Denver, Colorado

David Jensen, Ph.D.
Physiologist and Author

Thomas H. Joyce, III, M.D.
Professor, Department of
  Anesthesiology
University of Cincinnati
Cincinnati, Ohio

Edward H. Miller, M.D.
Professor and Director of
  Orthopaedic Surgery
University of Cincinnati Medical
  Center
Cincinnati, Ohio

Hyman B. Muss, M.D.
Associate Professor of Medicine
Department of Medicine
Bowman Gray School of Medicine
Wake Forest University
Winston-Salem, North Carolina

Gerhard Nellhaus, M.D.
Pediatric Neurologist
Pacific State Hospital, State of
  California
Pomona, California

Audrey Hart Nora, M.P.H.
Director, Genetics
The Children's Hospital
Associate Clinical Professor of
Pediatrics
University of Colorado Medical
Center
Denver, Colorado

James J. Nora, M.D., M.P.H.
Professor of Pediatrics
Director of Pediatric Cardiology
University of Colorado Medical
Center
Denver, Colorado

Richard B. Odom, M.D.
Chief, Dermatology Service
Letterman Army Medical Center
Presidio of San Francisco,
California

Robert S. Pinals, M.D.
Professor, Department of Internal
Medicine
State University of New York
Upstate Medical Center
Syracuse, New York

Robert W. Prichard, M.D.
Professor and Chairman
Department of Pathology
Bowman Gray School of Medicine
Wake Forest University
Winston-Salem, North Carolina

Daniel D. Rabuzzi, M.D.
Professor, Department of
Otolaryngology and
Communication Sciences
State University of New York,
Upstate Medical Center
Syracuse, New York

Richard G. Sample, Ph.D.
Assistant Professor
Department of Pharmacology
Hahnemann Medical College and
Hospital of Philadelphia
Philadelphia, Pennsylvania

John J. Scocca, Ph.D.
Associate Professor
Department of Biochemistry
Johns Hopkins University School
of Hygiene and Public Health
Baltimore, Maryland

Richard W. Stander, M.D.
Director, Division of Education
The American College of
Obstetricians and Gynecologists
Chicago, Illinois

Richard George Wendel, M.D.
Assistant Clinical Professor of
Surgery (Urology)
University of Cincinnati College of
Medicine
Good Samaritan Hospital
Cincinnati, Ohio

Park Weed Willis, III, M.D.
Professor of Medicine (Cardiology)
Department of Internal Medicine
University of Michigan
Ann Arbor, Michigan

John H. Wulsin, M.D.
Professor of Surgery
University of Cincinnati Medical
  Center
Cincinnati, Ohio

John W. Vester, M.D.
Professor of Medicine
Professor of Clinical Biochemistry
University of Cincinnati
  College of Medicine
Director, Clinical Support
  Laboratory
Good Samaritan Hospital
Cincinnati, Ohio

Leon Weiss, M.D.
Professor of Cell Biology
Chairman, Department of Animal
  Biology
School of Veterinary Medicine
University of Pennsylvania

Maurice Victor, M.D.
Professor of Neurology
Case-Western Reserve University
School of Medicine
Director, Neurology Service
Metropolitan General Hospital
Cleveland, Ohio

PREFACE

As with past editions, this edition of *Blakiston's Pocket Medical Dictionary* is a shortened version of *Blakiston's Gould Medical Dictionary*. Past editions of this shorter work followed by at least a few months publication of the parent work. Through the marvels of computer composition and data processing, these two dictionaries are now published at the same time. From the publisher's perspective, that is progress.

As a computer-generated offspring, this dictionary is affected by the changes made in the parent. All the structural improvements in the parent, such as setting taxonomic genus and species entries in bold italic type, using small capital letters within definitions to signify preferred terms, refining the system of pronunciation guides (see Explanatory Notes), and adding pronunciations for proper names, are carried over into this shorter version. So it is also with the terms and definitions themselves; each one has been thoroughly reviewed and revised by the editors, contributors, and lexicographers in preparing the new edition of *The Gould,* and the files have been assiduously pruned of the obsolete (although obsolete terms of some historical interest are retained).

The culling of the computer files for this dictionary presents problems not shared with the parent. While we wish to maintain compactness, to do so at the expense of thoroughness would be fatuous. Our ambition is to provide an easy-to-use, handy albeit thorough dictionary that serves the needs of a varied audience in the health sciences. In this battle of mutually exclusive goals, size loses out. Indeed this edition contains over 30,000 entries. If it is deemed long, it is only because of the massive vocabulary of the health sciences and the manifold needs of the varied audience. We hope that we have achieved at least one of our goals, providing the fundamentals of this complex and immense lexicon.

Greek Alphabet with Transliterations

Greek letter		Name	Transliteration	Greek letter		Name	Transliteration
A	α	alpha	a	N	ν	nu	n
B	β	beta	b	Ξ	ξ	xi	x
Γ	γ	gamma	g; n before g, k, ch, x	O	o	omicron	o
Δ	δ	delta	d	Π	π	pi	p
E	ε	epsilon	e	P	ρ	rho	r, rh
Z	ζ	zeta	z	Σ	σ	sigma	s
H	η	eta	ē	T	τ	tau	t
Θ	θ	theta	th	Υ	υ	upsilon	y; u after vowel
I	ι	iota	i	Φ	φ	phi	ph
K	κ	kappa	k	X	χ	chi	ch
Λ	λ	lambda	l	Ψ	ψ	psi	ps
M	μ	mu	m	Ω	ω	omega	ō

EXPLANATORY NOTES

Arrangement of Entries

Alphabetical order The terms defined in this dictionary are set in boldface type and are arranged in one overall alphabetical order; that is, there are no subentries, and the spaces between words in phrases are disregarded. For example, phrases beginning with the word "methyl" are not all grouped together, but are interspersed with single words beginning with "methyl-," depending strictly on what the next letter is: **methyl alcohol** comes before **methylate,** which comes before **methyl chloride. Methyl red test** is not to be looked up under **test**—since there are no subentries—but is to be found between **methyl red** and **methyl-rosaniline chloride.**

Some of the "run-on" entries constitute an exception to this rule of strict alphabetization. These terms are not defined independently but are appended to the definitions of the terms they are derived from (or otherwise closely related to):

opac·i·fy (o·pas′i·fye) *v.* 1. to make opaque. 2. To become opaque.
—**opac·i·fi·ca·tion** (o·pas″i·fi·kay′shun) *n.*

A run-on entry is used only if its alphabetical place as an independent entry would be very close to the entry it is appended to.

Two other minor exceptions to the rule of strict alphabetical order are names beginning with Mc or M', which are alphabetized as if spelled Mac... , and those beginning with St., which are alphabetized as if spelled out: Saint.

Homographs Where there are entries for two or more terms spelled exactly alike, a superscript numeral is prefixed to each of them to alert the reader to this fact:

¹**mental,** *adj.* [L. *mentalis,* from *mens,* mind]. 1. Pertaining to the mind . . .
²**mental,** *adj.* [L. *ment*um, chin, + -*al*]. Pertaining to the chin.

On the other hand, differences involving typographic devices such as capital letters, italics, hyphens, and word spaces are regarded as differences in spelling, and entries so distinguished are not numbered:

Leishmania	**postmortem**	**keto-**
leishmania	post mortem	keto

In general, a term beginning with a capital letter precedes a similar term beginning with a small letter, and a term written as one word precedes a similar term written as two words. Sometimes, however, the more basic term precedes a secondary or derived version of it regardless of the way they are distinguished in punctuation or typography.

Nonalphabetical inclusions   Some terms incorporate symbols, such as numerals and Greek letters, that are disregarded in the alphabetical placement; these terms are to be looked up as if the symbol were not there: **2-OS interval** comes right after **os interparietale**, and **α-globulin** comes right after **globulin** (but when spelled out as **alpha globulin,** it comes at its own place in the a's). This rule applies also to chemical prefixes such as p-, o-, m-, d-, l-, D-, and L-; for example, **p-aminohippuric acid** is entered in the a's, but when spelled out as **para-aminohippuric acid,** it comes at its own place in the p's.

   Abbreviations and symbols in general—insofar as they consist of letters in the Roman alphabet—are entered at their own place in the alphabetical order.

The abbreviations and symbols used in the dictionary's own devices are:

accus.	accusative
adj.	adjective
adv.	adverb
com. n.	common noun (designating members of a biological taxonomic group having the corresponding proper name)
genit.	genitive
n.	noun
NA	Nomina Anatomica
nom.	nominative
obsol.	obsolete
pl.	plural
prep.	preposition
pron.	pronoun
sing., sg.	singular
syn.	synonym
v.	verb
=	which is equivalent to or a synonym of

Word Division

The centered dots in the boldface headwords are intended for one purpose only: to show where a word may be divided at the end of the line. Older systems of word division, still used in some dictionaries, purport to serve this function while at the same time marking all "syllable boundaries." Actually, not all syllable boundaries make acceptable division points, nor do all division points come at syllable boundaries.

The first or last letter of a word, for example, should not be split off even though it constitutes a syllable in itself: **ane·mia** (not **a·ne·mi·a**). In many cases this same principle applies within a complex word to the elements making it up: **poly·uria** (not **pol·y·u·ri·a**). In some cases, furthermore, the correct division comes between word elements in such a way that "syllable boundaries" are violated: **meth·yl·at·ed** (not **meth·y·la·ted**).

There are sometimes two or more acceptable ways of dividing a word, as for example **epi·neph·ri·ne·mia** or **epi·neph·rin·emia;** only one way, however, is shown for any entry.

In derivative terms that are not separately defined but are appended (run on) to main entries, center dots are usually inserted only from the point where the pronunciation (or the word division itself) departs from that of the main term (or from that of a preceding appended term): **nec·ro·bi·o·sis** (neck″ro·bye·o′sis) *n.* . . . . —**necrobi·ot·ic** (·ot′ick) *adj.* Similarly in the case of plurals and other inflectional forms: **psy·cho·sis** (sigh·ko′sis) *n.,* pl. **psycho·ses**(·seez) . . . .

In a series of homographs or of entries beginning with the same word, division points are shown only in the first entry:

¹**men·tal**	**ar·cu·ate**	**Joh·ne′s bacillus**
²**mental**	**arcuate artery**	**Johne′s disease**

Foreign word divisions   In Latin anatomical terms, the "native" Latin word divisions are shown: **zy·go·ma·ti·cus** (rather than **zy·go·mat·i·cus**), **pro·sta·ta** (rather than **pros·ta·ta**). This is the system used in Latin texts and also in the context of modern languages other than English. In an English context, however, it is also quite acceptable to divide the Latin words in the English way.

The division points shown for modern foreign names are generally those used in the language in question:

Al·ba·rrán (Spanish)	**Fa·vre** (French)
Bier·nac·ki (Polish)	**Mor·ga·gni** (Italian)

A few of the divisions allowable in the foreign language (especially in French) have been suppressed, however, as disconcerting or misleading in an English context: **Cal·mette** (rather than **Cal·met·te**).

Center dots in the parenthetic pronunciations have significance only for the phonetic spelling itself (see below), and do not necessarily coincide with the divisions shown in the boldface.

Pronunciation

In parentheses immediately after the boldface headwords, pronunciations are shown for single-word terms with the exception of (1) some of the ordinary words that any English-speaking person knows how to pronounce, (2) trademarks, and (3) alternate spellings and inflectional forms that are shown in the entry to which they are referred.

In a sequence of homographs that are pronounced alike, or of phrase entries involving one or more of the same words, the pronunciation of the repeated word is generally shown only in the first entry in which it occurs:

¹acrot·ic (a·krot′ick) *adj.*   **graaf·i·ian follicle** (graf′ee·un)
²acrotic, *adj.*   **graafian vessels**

    Lac·to·ba·cil·lus (lack″to·ba·sil′us) *n.*
    Lactobacillus ac·i·doph·i·lus (as″i·dof′i·lus)

The pronunciations are based as far as possible on actual usage rather than on theoretical considerations, but there are many terms, especially some of the rarer ones, for which no standard pronunciation can be determined; in such cases one must simply have recourse to criteria of consistency or analogy.

For many terms, several alternative pronunciations are given, though these do not always exhaust the possibilities.

We have attempted to maintain consistency in the pronunciation of the many Latin entries that are not firmly established in English use. Vowels and consonants are generally given their fully anglicized values, so that Latin $\bar{a}$ = "ay" (as in say), $\bar{i}$ = "eye," $\bar{e}$ and *ae* = "ee," *c* and *g* before *e* or *i* = "s" and "j," etc. Vowel length and accentuation, however, are modeled strictly on the Latin except where usage dictates otherwise. Thus Latin *intestīnum* is pronounced "in·tes·tye′num" and not, by analogy to the English, "in·tes′ti·num." On the other hand, it would be useless to insist that a word like *apex* be pronounced "ap′ecks" on the grounds that the *a* in Latin is short, since its pronunciation in English is already well established as "ay′pecks."

With varying degrees of consistency, many English speakers favor the "continental" or "school" pronunciation of Latin vowels, approximating the Italian (or German) values of the letters: Latin $\bar{a}$ = "ah," $\bar{e}$ = "ay," $\bar{i}$ = "ee," and *ae* = "eye" or "eh." These pronunciations are certainly more authentic and are better for purposes of international spoken communication, but they go against the norm established by a large body of uniformly anglicized pronunciations such as **nuclei:** "new′klee·eye" (not "nŏok′leh·ee") or **calcaneus:** "kal·kay′nee·us" (not "kal·kah′neh·ōōs"). To show both systems of pronunciation wherever variation might occur would increase the size and unwieldiness of thousands of Latin entries.

A different policy has been followed with the modern foreign names used in eponymic terms. Rather than give them broadly anglicized pronunciations we have used supplementary phonetic symbols for non-English sounds to show the authentic foreign pronunciations, as for example **Ehrlich** (e^yr′li^kh), **Quinquaud** (kæⁿ·ko′). Many of the better known foreign names, of course, have more or less familiar anglicized pronunciations, and to impose an exotic foreign pronunciation on them in English contexts would be regarded as an affectation. Thus in the entry **Gram's stain** we show the pronunciation (gra^hm′) so that anyone who is interested can consult the pronunciation key and perhaps get some idea of how the name is pronounced in Danish; it is not recommended for actual use in the English phrase "Gram's stain."

Some names—foreign, English, and (especially) American—have been left unphoneticized because at press time we had not been able to ascertain their correct pronunciation. Others are left unphoneticized because their pronunciations were judged to be obvious to any English speaker.

The system of "phonetic spelling" used in this dictionary is meant to be usually interpretable at a glance by anyone familiar with the elementary principles of English spelling. However—English spelling being what it is—no such system can be entirely foolproof. The key that follows should resolve anything that might be puzzling to the reader at first glance.

PRONUNCIATION KEY 1: ENGLISH

Phonetic Spelling   *Examples*

a (+ consonant)
    = ă, "short a"   **fat, cathode** (kath′ode), **manic**
                              (man′ick)

    Note: The phonetic spelling "a" before a center dot indicates an or-
    dinary "short a" in careful speech: **pathology** (pa·thol′uh·jee), but
    this may be reduced to an "uh" sound in more casual pronunciation:
    (puh·thol′uh·jee).

ă (before r) = "short a"   **carrot** (kăr′ut), **parasite**
                                   (păr′uh·site)

a...e = ā, "long a"   **same, face, vein** (vane), **hydrate**
                                   (high′drate)

ah = "broad a"   **father** (fah′thur), **quality**
                                   (kwahl′i·tee)
                                  far (fahr), **artery** (ahr′tur·ee)

ai = ā, "long a"   **nail, faint, abatement**
                                   (uh·bait′munt)
                                  dairy (dair′ee)

    Note: The phonetic spelling "air" often indicates a choice of pronun-
    ciations: **calcareous** (kal·kair′ee·us) (*or* kal·kerr′ee·us *or*
    kal·kăr′ee·us).

aɷw = "broad a" + "oo" *or*
      "short a" + "oo"   **now** (naɷw), **out** (aɷwt), **caoutchouc**
                                   (kaɷw′chook)

aw   **law, fall** (fawl), **daughter** (daw′tur)
ay = ā, "long a"   **say, daisy** (day′zee), **later** (lay′tur)

e (+ consonant)
    = ĕ, "short e"   **get, said** (sed), **merry** (merr′ee)

    Note: The phonetic spelling "e" before a center dot represents a choice
    of several sounds: **erythrocyte** (e·rith′ro·site) = (err·ith′ro·site *or*
    i·rith′ro·site *or* uh·rith′ro·site); **receptor** (re·sep′tur) = (ree·sep′tur *or*
    ri·sep′tur *or* ruh·sep′tur).

PRONUNCIATION KEY 1: ENGLISH (continued)

Phonetic Spelling   *Examples*

Note: A "silent e" is used (as in ordinary English spelling) after a consonant preceded by a, i, or o, to indicate the "long" sounds of these vowels. See a...e, i...e, o...e.

ee	= ē, "long e"	**see, ear** (eer), **fetal** (fee′tul), **machine** (muh·sheen′)
ew		**few, mute** (mewt), **beauty** (bew′tee) **new, duty** (dew′tee)

Note: After d, t, th, n, and l, the phonetic spelling "ew" represents a choice of pronunciations: **due** (dew) = (dyoo *or* doo).

eye	= ī, "long i"	**eye, island** (eye′lund)
g	"hard g" only	**get, give** (giv), **argue** (ahr′gew)

Note: See also ng and igh.

i	= ĭ, "short i"	**sit, physical** (fiz′i·kul) **irritate** (irr′i·tate)

Note: The phonetic spelling "i" in unaccented syllables often represents a reduced or obscure vowel approaching the "uh" sound rather than a clear short i: **hemolysis** (he·mol′i·sis), **polluted** (puh·lew′tid).

i...e	= ī, "long i"	**like, sign** (sine), **child** (chile′d)
igh	= ī, "long i"	**sigh, light, myositis** (migh″o·sigh′tis)
ng		**song, singer** (sing′ur)

Note: The "ng" sound in **singer** (sing′ur), **hangar** (hang′ur), is distinguished from the two-sound sequence in **finger** (fing′gur), **anger** (ang′gur), and from the still different sequence in **vanguard** (van′gahrd), **ungifted** (un·gif′tid).

PRONUNCIATION KEY 1: ENGLISH (continued)

Phonetic Spelling	*Examples*

o (+ consonant)
= ŏ, "short o"

not, lock, follicle (fol′i·kul) **foreign** (for′in), **coronary** (kor′uh·nerr·ee)

Note: In most kinds of American speech "short o" is pronounced the same as "broad a," so that **bother** rhymes with **father.** See ah.

o (end of syllable)
= ō, "long o"

go, low (lo), **motion** (mo′shun) **chlorine** (klo′reen)

Note: Before r, "long o" and "short o" are often interchangeable: **oral** (o′rul *or* or′ul).

o...e = ō, "long o"

bone, pore, roll (role), **yolk** (yoke)

oh = ō, "long o"

post (pohst), **methadone** (meth′uh·dohn)

oo

too, pool, lose (looz), **jejunum** (je·joo′num)

ŏŏ

look (lŏŏk), **pull** (pŏŏl), **sugar** (shŏŏg′ur)

s

miss (mis), **taste** (taist), **basic** (bay′sick)

Note: The phonetic spelling "s" never indicates the voiced ("z") sound: **music** (mew′zick), **plasma** (plaz′muh).

th (voiceless)

thin, teeth, arithmetic (uh·rith′me·tick)

~~th~~ (voiced)

this (~~th~~is), **teethe** (tee~~th~~), **rhythm** (rith′um)

u = ŭ, "short u"

nut, color (kul′ur), **stomach** (stum′uck) **burr** (bur), **worst** (wurst), **fertile** (fur′til)

PRONUNCIATION KEY 1: ENGLISH (continued)

Phonetic Spelling

u (in unaccented syllables)
uh

ue (used instead of "ew" in the syllable "sue")

uy (used instead of "ye" after g)
ye (after consonant and at end of syllable or before ')
    = ī, "long i"

zh

Examples

nature (nay'chur), **dorsal** (dor'sul)
America (uh·merr'i·kuh),
    psychology (sigh·kol'uh·jee)

pseudocyst (sue'do·sist = syoo'do·
    or soo'do·)
guiding (guy'ding)

dye, biceps (bye'seps), **pint** (pye'nt)
fusion (few'zhun), **measure**
    (mezh'ur), **rouge** (roozh)

Accents

A single accent (') follows the most heavily stressed syllables of a word and a double accent (") marks subordinate stresses: **hyperpigmentation** (high"pur·pig"men·tay'shun).

Note: Not all subordinate stresses are marked, since most of them are automatically determined either by the position of the main stress or by the sounds involved. In **parasite,** for example, the last syllable is pronounced with a subordinate stress, but the final accent mark (") is left out as unhelpful and visually cluttering: (păr'uh·site). Before a main accent, however, most subordinate stresses are shown, because they help to establish the rhythm of the word at a glance.

PRONUNCIATION KEY 2: FOREIGN

Phonetic Spelling

a = the same as aʰ (below): a sound between English "short a" and "broad a"

æ = a sound between English "short a" and "short e"

Examples

Cajal (ka·ᵏhal'), **Gehr·hardt**
    (gehr'hart)

Svedberg (sveʸd'bærʸ), **Einthoven**
    (æynt'ho·vun)

PRONUNCIATION KEY 2: FOREIGN (continued)

Phonetic Spelling   *Examples*

$æ^n$ = the same as æ but nasalized   **Marjolin** (mar·zho^h·læ$^{n'}$), **Guillain** (ghee·læ$^{n'}$)

a^h = a sound between English "short a" and "broad a"   **Pascal** (pa^{h}s·ka^{h}l'), **Mazzoni** (ma^{h}t·tso'nee), **Riga** (ree'ga^h),

ah^n = "broad a" nasalized   **Chamberland** (shah^n·be^{h}r·lah$^{n'}$), **Vincent** (væ^n·sah$^{n'}$)

aow^n = the same as aow but nasalized (see aow in English section)   **São Paulo** (saow^n paow'loo)

^{c}h = Used in some cases to show the palatal variant of ^{k}h. See ^{k}h (below)   **Böttcher** (bœt'^{c}hur)

^{e} (except after u; see u^e)
= a short obscure vowel, or syllabification of a following consonant; often the same as the short u or uh (see English key)   **Hyrtl** (hirr't^{e}l)

eh = a lengthened version of English "short e"   **Breda** (breh'da^h)

e^h = "short e"   **Fouchet** (foo·she$^{h'}$), **Huschke** (hoosh'ke^h), **Bernard** (be^{h}r·nahr')

Note: In French, the phonetic spelling e^h at the end of a syllable may also be pronounced like e^y (see below): **Fouchet** (foo·she$^{h'}$ = also foo·she$^{y'}$).

^{eh} See u^{eh}

e^y = a sound midway between eh and ee; comparable to the English "long a" (as in late) but not a diphthong, i.e., with no "ee" glide at the end   **Fede** (fe^y'de^h), **Barré** (ba·re$^{y'}$), **Swediaur** (sve^{y}d'yaowr)

gh = the same as g; used sometimes to avoid possible confusion with the j sound   **Guillain** (ghee·læ$^{n'}$)

PRONUNCIATION KEY 2: FOREIGN (continued)

Phonetic Spelling

		Examples

^{g}h = a velar fricative like ^{k}h (see below) but softer

van Bogaert (va^{h}n bo$'^g$hært)

^{h}, h Used in various combinations to modify the sound of a preceding letter (as in a^h, ^{c}h, e^h, gh, ^{g}h, i^h, ^{k}h, o^h). See these individual combinations.

hh Used after a vowel to show that an actual h sound is intended, not a modification of the vowel

Behçet (behh′chet)

i^h A retracted ee sound; like oo without rounded lips

Cyon (tsi^h·o^{h}n′)

^{k}h = A velar or palatal fricative; like k but without any stoppage of the air flow. In some types of Spanish pronunciation, it tends toward a simple h sound. In most pronunciations of German, it has a forward (palatal) quality after e or i and in certain other combinations—midway between the back ^{k}h as in *Bach* and an sh sound. (See also ^{c}h, above).

Gil (^{k}heel), **Cajal** (ka·^{k}hal′), **Gerlach** (ge^{h}r′la^{k}h), **Kocher** (ko^{k}h′ur), **Bekhterev** (be^{k}h′t^{y}e·r^{y}uf)

^{n} Used to indicate nasalization of the preceding vowel; not a separate sound. See æ^n, ah^n, aow^n, œ^n, oh^n.

œ = like the "short e" sound but with rounded lips

Loeffler (lœf′lur), **Farabeuf** (fa·ra·bœf′)

œh = like e^y but with rounded lips

Froelich (frœh′li^{k}h), **Dieulafoy** (dyœh·la·fwah′)

PRONUNCIATION KEY 2: FOREIGN (continued)

Phonetic Spelling	*Examples*

œ^n = like œ but nasalized

Brun (brœ^n)

o^h = a sound between o and aw, usually short. Somewhat like British o in *cot*, but in French it tends toward the u in American *cut*. In Italian at the end of a stressed syllable, it is long.

Golgi (go^{h}l′jee), **Gottlieb** (go^{h}t′leep), **Bonnevie** (bo^{h}n·vee′), **de Toni** (de^y·to^h′nee)

oh^n = a sound midway between o and o^h, nasalized

Londe (loh^{n}d), **Tenon** (tuh·noh^{n}′)

u^e = like ee but with rounded lips; in German before a consonant in the same syllable, like ''short i'' but rounded.

Dutemps (du^e·tah^{n}′), **Büdinger** (bu^e′ding·ur), **Büngner** (bu^{e}ng′nur)

u^{eh} = a sound midway between u^e and oo (in Swedish and Norwegian)

Guldberg (gu^{eh}l′bærg)

^{y} (except after e; see e^y)
 Indicates palatalization of a preceding consonant sound, i.e., modification of that sound by giving it a simultaneous ''y'' quality.

Morgagni (mor·gahn^y′ee)
 Sémélaigne (se^y·me^y·lehn^y′)
 Castañeda (ka^{h}s·ta^h·n^{y}e^h′tha^h)
 Bekhteref (be^{k}h′t^{y}e·r^{y}uf)
 Kultschitzky (kōōl^y·chit′skee)
 Szent-Györgyi (sen′d^{y}œr·d^{y}ee)
 Dupuis (du^e·pw^{y}ee′)

′ A glottal catch; a slight interruption of the air flow at the glottis as in the exclamation oh-oh! (o′′o). (Occurs in some Danish names.)

Faber (fah′′bur)

PRONUNCIATION KEY 2: FOREIGN (continued)

Phonetic Spelling   *Examples*

Many of the same phonetic spellings are used for the foreign names as for English, though in some cases the actual pronunciations differ considerably. For example:

ee	In a syllable closed by a consonant (and in French also finally) this sound is usually clipped short, not drawled or diphthongized as in English.	**Philippe** (fee·leep′), **Piccolo** (peek′ko·lo), **Petit** (puh·tee′), **Gil** (ᵏheel)
o, o...e, oh	A steady sound that does not vary in quality from beginning to end; not diphthongized like English long o; that is, it has no "w" glide at the end.	**Charcot** (shar·ko′), **Pautrier** (po·tree·eʸ′), **Roth** (rote), **Ghon** (gohn)
l	After a vowel (in French, German, Italian, Spanish) it has a "light" or "bright" quality, the same as before a vowel; as in English *lee,* not as in English *eel.*	**Gilles** (zheel), **Heschl** (hesh′ᵉl), **Held** (helt)
r	Varies widely in different languages. In Italian, Spanish, Russian, and many other languages, it is trilled on the tip of the tongue; in Spanish and Italian between vowels it gets a single tap if single and a multiple trill if doubled.	**Casares** (ka·sah′res), **Albarrán** (al·ba·rraʰn′)

Plurals and Other Inflectional Forms

Plurals formed on a Latin or Greek pattern are generally shown for the nouns that have them: **ovum** (o′vum) *n.*, pl. **ova** (o′vuh); **bron·chus** (bronk′us) *n.*, pl. **bron·chi** (·eye); **ba·sis** (bay′sis) *n.*, pl. **ba·ses** (·seez). When there is a regular English plural used as well as the Latin or Greek one, both are usually shown: **gan·gli·on** (gang′glee·un) *n.*, pl. **gan·glia** (·glee·uh), **ganglions.**

Plurals are not explicitly given for every noun with a Latin or Greek ending, because for some of them the plural is rarely if ever encountered, or is encountered too seldom for there to be any specific usage established. Note, however, the following regular patterns:

Singular ending	Plural ending	Examples
-sis	**-ses** (·seez)	diagnosis: diagnoses
		myiasis: myiases
		hemolysis: hemolyses
-itis	**-itides** (·it′i·deez)	arthritis: arthritides
		dermatitis: dermatitides
-oma	**-omas** or **-omata**	adenoma: adenomas *or* adenomata

Sometimes a Latin or Greek-pattern plural is used much more than the singular, and is chosen to serve as the main entry. In that case, the singular is shown for it in the same way that a plural is shown for a singular entry: **oto·co·nia** (o″to·ko′nee·uh) *n.*, sing. **otoco·ni·um** (·nee·um). If no singular is used, as in the case of higher biological taxa, then the entry is marked "*n.pl.*" (noun plural).

Genitive (possessive) forms of Latin nouns are used in many of the Latin phrases defined in the dictionary, for example, *dentis* in the term **corona dentis** "crown of a tooth." The more important of these genitives are shown at the entries of the terms to which they belong:

dens (denz) *n.*, genit. **den·tis** (den′tis), pl. **den·tes** (·teez), genit. pl. **den·ti·um** (den′tee·um, den′shee·um) . . . TOOTH.

For many nouns the genitive singular form is the same as the nominative plural, for example, *pili* "hairs" or "of a hair" (as in **arrector pili** "erector of a hair"), *vertebrae,* plural of *vertebra,* or genitive singular as in **arcus vertebrae** "arch of a vertebra, vertebral arch":

ver·te·bra (vur′te·bruh) *n.*, pl. & genit. sing. **verte·brae** (·bree)
pi·lus (pye′lus, pil′us) *n.*, pl. & genit. sing. **pi·li** (·lye)

For most Latin nouns ending in *-is*, the genitive singular coincides in form with the nominative singular, which is the headword form; these genitives are not explicitly indicated. Thus **ax·is** (ack'sis) *n.,* pl. **ax·es** (·seez), but in the phrase **dens axis,** for example, (''the dens of the axis''), *axis* is genitive.

Definitions: Preferred Terms and Synonyms

The terms entered fall into two broad categories: (1) the so-called preferred terms, for which full-fledged definitions are given, and (2) their synonyms, which are defined by the preferred term set in small capital letters:

(1)   **jaun·dice** . . . Yellowness of the skin, mucous membranes, and secretions; due to hyperbilirubinemia. Syn. *icterus.*

(2)   **ic·ter·us** . . . JAUNDICE.

With certain exceptions, there is only one preferred term in any set of synonyms, and—style and context permitting—only the preferred term is used in definitions. This principle is important in maintaining a dictionary's consistency and efficiency.

Ideally, the preferred term of a set of synonyms is the one that is judged by the editorial board to be the best choice for general use. Actually there are many cases in which no clear-cut superiority of one term over another exists, or in which one term is superior in certain contexts but not in others. In such cases the choice of a preferred term must be to some extent arbitrary.

Entries for terms that have more than one meaning are divided into separate, numbered definitions or ''senses'':

pars intermedia . . . 1. The posterior portion of the adenohypophysis, between the pars distalis and the neurohypophysis . . . 2. The nervus intermedius; the intermediate part of the facial nerve.

If such a term has synonyms in one or another of its senses and is preferred over them, the synonyms are referred to the relevant sense of the preferred term by means of the sense number in parentheses:

intermediate lobe of the hypophysis. PARS INTERMEDIA (1).

If the preferred term is a homograph, references to it from synonyms use the appropriate prefixed numeral:

¹im·plant (im·plant′) *v.* . . . . To embed, set in.

²im·plant (im′plant) *n.* 1. A small tube or needle which contains radioactive material, placed in a tissue or tumor to deliver therapeutic doses of radiation. 2. A tissue graft placed in depth.

implantation graft. ²IMPLANT (2).

The notation ''²IMPLANT (2)'' means that the second *implant* entry, in its second sense, is where the reader will find the meaning of *implantation graft*.

Blakiston's **Pocket Medical Dictionary**

A

A 1. *In chemistry,* a symbol for argon. 2. *In molecular biology,* a symbol for adenine. 3. *In radiology,* symbol for area of heart shadow. 4. *In physics,* an abbreviation for *angstrom.*

A₂ The aortic valve closure component of the second heart sound.

a. Abbreviation for (a) *accommodation;* (b) *ampere;* (c) *anode;* (d) *anterior;* (e) *aqua;* (f) *arteria.*

ā, āā Symbol meaning *the same quantity of each ingredient* in a prescription.

a-, ab-, abs- A prefix meaning (a) *away from, outside of;* (b) *deviating from.*

a-, an- A prefix meaning *un-, not, -less, lacking, lack of.*

A.A. Abbreviation for (a) *achievement age;* (b) *Alcoholics Anonymous.*

Aarane. Trademark for cromolyn sodium, a bronchial asthma inhibitor.

abac·te·ri·al (ay″back·teer′ee·ul) *adj.* Without bacteria.

Aba·die's sign (a·ba·dee′). 1. [J. *Abadie,* French neurologist, 1873–1946] Insensitivity to forceful pinching of the calcaneal tendon in tabes dorsalis. 2. [C. *Abadie,* French ophthalmologist, 1842–1932] Spasm of the levator palpebrae superioris muscle, occurring frequently in thyrotoxicosis but also seen normally, especially with tension and fatigue.

ab·alien·a·tion (ab·ay″lee·un·ay′shun) *n.* Mental deterioration or derangement.

A band The birefringent (doubly refractile) transverse band that forms the broad middle segment of each sarcomere in striated muscle fibrils, representing the zone occupied by thick myosin filaments interdigitated (except in the H zone) with the actin filaments.

aban·don·ment, *n. In medical jurisprudence,* the withdrawal of a physician from the care of a patient, without reasonable notice of such withdrawal or without discharge from the case by the patient.

ab·ap·i·cal (ab·ap′i·kul) *adj.* Away from or opposite the apex.

abar·og·no·sis (ay·băr″og·no′sis) *n.* Loss or lack of the ability to estimate weight. Syn. *baragnosis.*

ab·ar·tic·u·lar (ab″ahr·tick′yoo·lur) *adj.* Not connected with or situated near a joint.

ab·ar·tic·u·la·tion (ab″ahr·tick″yoo·lay′shun) *n.* 1. A diarthrodial joint. 2. A dislocation of a joint.

aba·sia (a·bay′zhuh, ·zee·uh) *n.* Inability to walk despite the preservation of strength, coordination, and sensation in the legs. **—aba·sic** (·sick, ·zick) *adj.*

ab·at·tage, ab·a·tage (ab″uh·tahzh′) *n.* 1. The slaughter of animals; specifically, the slaughter of diseased animals to prevent the infection of others. 2. The art of casting an animal preparatory to an operation.

ab·ax·i·al (ab·ack′see·ul) *adj.* Not situated in the line of the axis of a structure.

Ab·be condenser (aʰb′eh) A system of lenses, attached to a microscope, for concentrating light on the object being examined.

ab·do·men (ab·do′mun, ab′do·mun) *n.,* pl. **abdomens, abdom·i·na** (·dom′i·nuh) The large, inferior cavity of the trunk, extending from the brim of the pelvis to the diaphragm, bounded in front and at the sides by the lower ribs and abdominal muscles and behind by the vertebral column and the psoas and quadratus lumborum muscles.

abdomin-, abdomino-. A combining form meaning *abdomen, abdominal.*

abdominal angina. An acute attack of severe abdominal pain, commonly occurring after eating, and often recurrent and associated with weight loss, nausea, vomiting, and diarrhea. It is caused by narrowing or obstruction of the mesenteric arteries, primarily atherosclerotic in origin.

abdominal aorta. The abdominal continuation of the descending aorta.

abdominal apoplexy. Infarction of an abdominal organ, usually the small intestine, resulting from vascular stenosis or occlusion.

abdominal cavity. The space within the body between the diaphragm and the pelvic floor, containing the abdominal viscera.

abdominal epilepsy. A seizure equivalent in which abdominal pain, a sense of nausea, and often headache are the most prominent symptoms.

abdominal hysterectomy. Hysterectomy in which the removal is effected through an abdominal incision.

abdominal inguinal ring. DEEP INGUINAL RING.

abdominal migraine. Periodically recurring abdominal pain, nausea, vomiting, or diarrhea, replacing migraine headaches.

abdominal muscle deficiency syndrome. A congenital nonhereditary disorder characterized by partial or complete absence of abdominal muscles in association with anomalies of the gastrointestinal tract, urinary tract, and the extremities and cryptorchism. Syn. *prune-belly syndrome.*

abdominal paracentesis. Puncture of the abdominal wall with a trocar and cannula, usually for the relief of ascites.

abdominal respiration. Respiration caused by the contraction of the diaphragm and the elastic expansion and recoil of the abdominal walls.

abdominal seizure equivalent. ABDOMINAL EPILEPSY.

abdominal testis. A testis that is undescended and remains in the abdominal cavity.

ab·dom·i·no·cen·te·sis (ab-dom″i-no-sen·tee′sis) *n.,* pl. **abdominocente·ses** (-seez) ABDOMINAL PARACENTESIS.

ab·dom·i·no·hys·ter·ec·to·my (ab-dom″i-no-hiss-tur-eck′tuh-mee) *n.* ABDOMINAL HYSTERECTOMY.

ab·dom·i·no·hys·ter·ot·o·my (ab-dom″i-no-hiss-tur-ot′uh-mee) *n.* Hysterotomy through an abdominal incision.

ab·dom·i·no·per·i·ne·al (ab-dom″i-no-perr″i-nee′ul) *adj.* Pertaining to the abdominal and perineal regions.

ab·dom·i·no·pos·te·ri·or (ab-dom″i-no-pos-teer′ee-ur) *adj. Obsol. In obstetrics,* designating a fetal position in which the belly is toward the mother's back.

ab·dom·i·nos·co·py (ab-dom″i-nos′kuh-pee) *n.* Diagnostic examination of the abdomen, externally by physical methods and internally by endoscopic methods.

ab·dom·i·no·tho·rac·ic (ab-dom″i-no-tho-ras′ick) *adj.* Pertaining to the abdominal and thoracic regions.

ab·du·cens (ab-dew′sunz) *adj. & n.* 1. Of or pertaining to the abducens nerve. 2. ABDUCENS NERVE.

abducens nerve. The sixth cranial nerve, whose fibers arise from the nucleus in the dorsal portion of the pons near the internal genu of the facial nerve and run a long course to supply the lateral rectus muscle which rotates the eyeball outward.

ab·du·cent (ab-dew′sunt) *adj.* 1. Abducting. 2. ABDUCENS (1).

abducent nerve. ABDUCENS NERVE.

abducent paralysis. Paralysis of the lateral rectus muscle of the eye due to a lesion of the sixth cranial nerve or its nucleus. The eye cannot be abducted and is convergent.

ab·duct (ab-dukt′) *v.* To draw away from the median line or plane.

ab·duc·tion (ab-duck′shun) *n.* 1. A movement whereby one part is drawn away from the axis of the body or of an extremity. 2. *In ophthalmology,* (a) turning of one part outward from the central position by the lateral rectus muscles; (b) the turning of the eyes outward beyond parallelism under the artificial stimulus of base in prisms and expressed in terms of prism diopters, the measurement being the strongest prism power with which the eyes can maintain single vision at infinity.

abduction paralysis. ABDUCTOR PARALYSIS.

ab·duc·tor (ab-duck′tur) *n.* A muscle which, on contraction, draws a part away from the axis of the body or of an extremity.

Aberel. Trademark for tretinoin, a keratolytic.

ab·er·rant (uh-berr′unt) *adj.* Varying or deviating from the normal in form, structure, or course.

ab·er·ra·tion (ab″e·ray′shun) *n.* 1. A deviation from the normal or the standard. 2. Any mild mental disorder. 3. *In biology,* an abnormal part or individual. 4. *In optics,* any imperfection in the refraction or the focalization of a lens.

ab·er·rom·e·ter (ab″e·rom′e·tur) *n.* An instrument for measuring aberration (4).

abeta·lipo·pro·tein·emia, abeta·lipo·pro·tein·ae·mia (ay″bay″tuh·lip″o·pro·teen·ee′mee·uh) *n.* A disease entity due to almost total absence of β-lipoproteins, characterized by the presence in blood of acanthocytes, hypocholesterolemia, malabsorption of fat beginning in infancy, and later, ataxia, peripheral neuropathy, and frequent retinitis pigmentosa and muscular atrophy; an autosomal recessive hereditary trait. Syn. *Bassen-Kornzweig syndrome.*

abey·ance (a·bay′unce) *n.* 1. A cessation of activity or function. 2. A state of suspended animation.

ab·i·ent (ab′ee·unt) *adj.* Tending away from the source of a stimulus.

abietic acid. An acid, $C_{19}H_{29}COOH$, from the resin of various conifer species. The anhydride of the acid, or an isomeric form or modification of the anhydride, is the chief constituent of rosin.

A bile. Bile collected from the common bile duct.

abio- A combining form meaning (a) *nonliving;* (b) *nonviable.*

abio·gen·e·sis (ay″bye·o·jen′e·sis, ab″ee·o·) *n.* A theory that living organisms can originate from nonliving matter; spontaneous generation.

abi·o·sis (ay″bye·o′sis, ab″ee·) *n.* 1. Absence of life. 2. Nonviability. —**abi·ot·ic** (·ot′ick) *adj.*

abi·ot·ro·phy (ay″bye·ot′ruh·fee, ab″ee·) *n.* Loss of vitality such as to cause pathological deterioration and death of cells or tissue not associable with some mechanism such as infection or poisoning; or any condition presumed to be due to such a process, as baldness or Huntington's chorea; an old term introduced on the assumption that aging and degenerative disease represent the same defect of affected cells. —**abio·troph·ic** (ay″bye″o·trof′ick, ab″ee·o·trof′ick) adj.

ab·ir·ri·tant (ab·irr′i·tunt) adj. & n. 1. Tending to diminish irritation; soothing. 2. Pertaining to diminished sensitiveness. 3. An agent, such as a cream or powder, that relieves irritation. —**abirri·ta·tive** (·tuh·tiv) adj.; **abirri·tate** (·tate) v.

ab·lac·ta·tion (ab″lack·tay′shun) n. 1. The weaning of an infant. 2. The end of the period of mammary secretion.

ab·late (ab·late′) v. To remove, especially by cutting.

ab·la·tio (ab·lay′shee·o) n. Detachment; removal; ablation.

ab·la·tion (ab·lay′shun) n. The removal of a part, as a tumor, by amputation, excision, or other mechanical means. —**ab·la·tive** (ab′luh·tiv, ab·lay′tiv) adj.

able·phar·ia (ay″blef·ăr′ee·uh, ab″lef·) n. A congenital defect marked by partial or total absence of the eyelids. —**ableph·a·rous** (ay·blef′uh·rus) adj.

ablep·sia (a·blep′see·uh) n. Loss or absence of vision.

ab·lu·ent (ab′lew·unt) adj. & n. 1. Detergent; cleansing. 2. A cleansing or washing agent, as a soap.

ab·lu·tion (uh·blew′shun) n. The act of washing or cleansing the body.

ab·nor·mal psychology. A branch of psychology dealing with mental processes and phenomena as well as abnormal behavior in pathologic states in subnormal as well as superior individuals and with special mental conditions such as dreams and hypnosis.

ABO blood group. That genetically determined blood group system defined by the agglutination reaction of erythrocytes exposed to the naturally occurring isoantibodies anti-A and anti-B and to similar antiserums. The serum of normal individuals contains isoantibodies against the antigens lacking in their erythrocytes, giving the following arrangement of antigens (isoagglutinogens) and antibodies:

Group (Landsteiner)	Erythrocyte Antigen (Agglutinogen)	Serum Antibody (Agglutinin)
O	A & B absent	anti-A, anti-B
A	A	anti-B
B	B	anti-A
AB	A,B	none

Subgroups of A are recognized and designated by subscripts, as A_1, A_2, etc.

ab·oma·si·tis (ab″o·muh·sigh′tis) n. Inflammation of the abomasum.

ab·oma·sum (ab″o·may′sum) n., pl. **aboma·sa** (·suh) The true digestive or glandular stomach of ruminants. Syn. *fourth stomach.*

ab·orad (ab·o′rad) adv. & adj. Tending away from the mouth.

ab·oral (ab·o′rul) adj. Opposite to, or remote from, the mouth.

abort (uh·bort′) v. 1. To bring forth a nonviable fetus. 2. To terminate prematurely or stop in the early stages, as the course of a disease.

3. To check or fall short of maximal growth and development.

abort·er, n. One who has undergone abortion, especially habitual or spontaneous abortion.

abor·ti·cide (uh·bor′ti·side) n. 1. The killing of an unborn fetus. 2. An agent that destroys the fetus and produces abortion.

abor·ti·fa·cient (a·bor″ti·fay′shunt) adj. & n. 1. Causing or inducing abortion. 2. A drug or agent inducing abortion.

abor·tin (a·bor′tin) n. A broth filtrate of *Brucella abortus* used to elicit a reaction in patients with active brucellosis or in those who have recovered from the infection.

abor·tion (uh·bor′shun) n. 1. The spontaneous or artificially induced expulsion of an embryo or fetus before it is viable. 2. The prematurely expelled product of conception; ABORTUS. 3. The checking or arrest of a process or disease before its development.

abor·tion·ist, n. A person who performs abortions, especially, one who performs them illegally.

abor·tive (uh·bor′tiv) adj. 1. Prematurely born; undeveloped; immature; rudimentary. 2. Coming to an untimely end. 3. Checking the full development of a disease or cutting short its duration. 4. ABORTIFACIENT.

abortive poliomyelitis. A form of poliomyelitis characterized clinically by relatively mild symptoms which do not progress to central nervous system paralysis. Definite diagnosis rests upon isolation of the virus or serologic titer rise.

abor·tus (a·bor′tus) n., pl. **abortuses** An aborted fetus.

abra·chia (a·bray′kee·uh) n. Armlessness.

abra·chio·ceph·a·lia (a·bray″kee·o·se·fay′lee·uh) n. Congenital absence of the head and arms.

abra·chi·us (a·bray′kee·us) n. An armless individual.

abrade (uh·braid′) v. To rub or scrape away, to erode by friction.

abra·sion (uh·bray′zhun) n. 1. A spot denuded of skin, mucous membrane, or superficial epithelium by rubbing or scraping, as a corneal abrasion; an excoriation. 2. The mechanical wearing down of teeth, as from incorrect brushing, poorly fitting dental devices, or bruxism.

abra·sive (uh·bray′siv, ·ziv) adj. & n. 1. Tending to abrade. 2. An agent or mechanical device used to scrape or rub off the external layers of a part; specifically, a substance such as carborundum, diamond chips, or pumice, used for grinding or polishing dental tissues or appliances.

abra·sor (uh·bray′zur) n. Any file or instrument used in the abrasion of a surface; a rasp.

ab·re·ac·tion (ab″ree·ack′shun) n. *In psychoanalysis,* the mental process by which repressed emotionally charged memories and experiences are brought to consciousness and relived with appropriate release. It may also occur in hypnosis and narcoanalysis.

ab·ric (ab′rick) n. FLOWERS OF SULFUR.

abridged A. O. color vision test. Abridged version of American Optical Company's charts, a group of pseudoisochromatic plates designed to detect color-vision deficiency.

Abri·ko·sov's or **Abri·ko·soff's tumor** (ah-bree-koh'suf) GRANULAR-CELL MYOBLASTOMA.

abro·sia (a-bro'zhuh, -zee-uh) n. Abstinence from food; fasting.

ab·rup·tio (ab-rup'tee-o, -shee-o) n. Abruption; a tearing away.

abruptio pla·cen·tae (pla-sen'tee). Premature separation of the placenta prior to delivery of the infant.

ab·scis·sa (ab-sis'uh) n. 1. The horizontal of the two coordinates used in plotting the interrelationship of two sets of data. 2. In optics, the point where a ray of light crosses the principal axis.

ab·scis·sion (ab-sish'un, ab-sizh'un) n. Removal of a part by cutting.

ab·scop·al (ab'sko-pul, ab-skop'ul) adj. Occurring at a distance from the irradiated volume, but within the same organism; said of certain effects of radiation.

ab·sence, n. 1. Inattention to one's environment. 2. Temporary loss of consciousness, as in absence attacks or psychomotor seizures.

absence attack or **seizure.** A seizure characterized by a sudden transient lapse of consciousness, by a blank stare, as in a state of "suspended animation," sometimes accompanied by minor motor activities such as blinking of the eyes, smacking of lips, stereotyped hand movements and automatism, often occurring many times in succession; seen in petit mal epilepsy; associated with a typical three per second spike-and-wave pattern on the electroencephalogram. Syn. petit mal seizure.

absence status. Absence attacks persisting for many minutes or even hours with no interval of normal mental activity between attacks.

ab·so·lute, adj. 1. Simple; pure; free from admixture. 2. Unlimited and unqualified. 3. Complete; entire; real. 4. In physics, derived from basic data, not arbitrary. Abbreviated, A.

absolute accommodation or **adjustment.** Accommodation of each eye considered individually.

absolute alcohol. DEHYDRATED ALCOHOL.

absolute blood count. The total number of each different type of leukocyte per unit volume of blood.

absolute density. 1. The ratio of the mass of a substance to its volume. 2. The light-absorbing power of the silver image in photographic materials.

absolute glaucoma. The completed glaucomatous process when the eyeball is hard and totally blind.

absolute hyperopia. Manifest hyperopia that cannot be corrected completely by accommodation, so that there is indistinct vision even for distance without corrective lenses.

absolute scotoma. Scotoma with perception of light entirely absent.

absolute threshold. The lowest intensity, as measured under optimal experimental conditions, at which a stimulus is effective or perceived.

ab·sorb, v. 1. In physiology, to take up or assimi-

late through a membrane or into a tissue, as products of digestion through gastrointestinal mucosa, or medicinal agents into the skin. 2. In physics, radiology, and spectrophotometry, to retain by conversion to another form, as radiant energy by conversion to heat or to some other form of molecular energy.

ab·sorb·able, adj. Capable of being absorbed.

absorbable gelatin film. A sterile, non-antigenic, water-insoluble gelatin film prepared from a gelatin-formaldehyde; used both as a protective and as a temporary supportive structure in surgical membrane repair.

absorbable surgical suture. A sterile strand prepared from collagen derived from healthy mammals and capable of being absorbed by living tissue.

ab·sor·be·fa·cient (ab-sor''be-fay'shunt) adj. & n. 1. Causing or promoting absorption. 2. Any agent that promotes absorption.

ab·sorb·ent (ub-sor'bunt, ub-zor'bunt) adj. & n. 1. Capable of absorbing fluids, gases, or light waves. 2. A drug, application, or dressing that promotes absorption of diseased tissues.

absorbent cotton. Cotton deprived of fatty matter so that it readily absorbs water.

ab·sorp·tion (ub-sorp'shun, -zorp') n. The state or process of being absorbed or the process of absorbing, as assimilation through a membrane or retention of radiant energy in a tissue by conversion to heat.

absorption atelectasis. OBSTRUCTIVE ATELECTASIS.

ab·sorp·tive (ub-sorp'tiv) adj. Pertaining to absorption; absorbent.

ab·sti·nence (ab'sti-nunce) n. Voluntary self-denial of or forbearance from indulgence of appetites, especially from food, alcoholic drink, or sexual intercourse.

abstinence delirium. Delirium occurring on withdrawal of alcohol or of a drug from one addicted to it.

ab·strac·tion (ab-strack'shun) n. 1. Removal or separation of one or more ingredients from a compound, as an abstract from a crude drug. 2. Absorption of the mind; absent-mindedness; inattention to what goes on about oneself. 3. In psychology, isolation of a meaning or characteristic from a totality which is unique and inaccessible to comparison; may be performed by thinking, feeling, sensation, or intuition. 4. Bloodletting.

abu·lia (a-bew'lee-uh, a-boo'lee-uh) n. 1. In psychiatry, loss or defect of the ability to make decisions. 2. In neurology, failure in a conscious, alert, non-schizophrenic patient with intact motor capacity and understanding to respond adequately to internal or external stimuli by voluntary motor activity; in extreme cases may take the form of transient akinetic mutism; frequently associated with lesions of the frontal lobes. —**abu·lic** (-ick) adj.

abut·ment (uh-but'munt) n. A tooth used to support or stabilize a prosthetic appliance. —**abut,** v.

AC Abbreviation for (a) air conduction; (b) alternating current; (c) anodic closure; (d) acromioclavicular.

Ac 1. Symbol for actinium. 2. Abbreviation for *acetyl.*

ac, a.c., a–c Abbreviation for *alternating current.*

a.c. Abbreviation for *ante cibum;* before meals.

acacia, *n.* The dried gummy exudate from the stems and branches of *Acacia senegal* (Linné) Willdenow, or of some other African species of *Acacia,* occurring in translucent or somewhat opaque white to yellowish-white spheroidal tears; almost completely soluble in water. Consists of calcium, magnesium, and potassium salts of the polysaccharide arabic acid. Used as a suspending agent and, formerly, as a demulcent. Syn. *gum arabic, acacia gum.*

acal·ci·co·sis (ay-kal″si·ko′sis, uh·kal″) *n.* The condition resulting from a diet continuously low in calcium.

acal·cu·lia (ay″kal·kew′lee·uh) *n.* Inability to learn or to do even the simplest arithmetical problems.

acamp·sia (ay·kamp′see·uh, uh·kamp′) *n.* Inflexibility or rigidity of a joint or limb; ANKYLOSIS.

acanth-, acantho- A combining form meaning (a) *thorn, thorny;* (b) *spine, spiny;* (c) *prickle cell.*

acan·thes·the·sia, acan·thaes·the·sia (a·kanth″es·theezh′uh, ·theez′ee·uh) *n.* An abnormal sensation of being pricked with needles.

acan·tho·am·e·lo·blas·to·ma (uh·kan″tho·am″e·lo·blas·to′muh) *n.* An ameloblastoma in which the cells are of the squamous or prickle-cell type.

Acan·tho·ceph·a·la (uh·kan″tho·sef′uh·luh) *n.pl.* A phylum of thorny-headed worms; adults are intestinal parasites of vertebrates, rarely of man. —**acanthocepha·lan** (·lun) *adj.*

acan·tho·ceph·a·li·a·sis (uh·kan″tho·sef″uh·lye′uh·sis) *n.* Infection by worms of the phylum Acanthocephala.

acan·tho·cyte (uh·kan′tho·site) *n.* A malformed red blood cell characterized, in wet preparations, by projecting spines or spicules, giving the cell a thorny or burr-shaped appearance.

acan·tho·cy·to·sis (uh·kan″tho·sigh·to′sis) *n.* Large numbers of acanthocytes in the peripheral blood; characteristic of the congenital disorder abetalipoproteinemia.

acan·thoid (uh·kan′thoid) *adj.* Resembling a spine; spinous.

acan·tho·ker·a·to·ma (uh·kan″tho·kerr″uh·to′muh) *n.* KERATOACANTHOMA.

acan·thol·y·sis (ack″an·thol′i·sis, uh·kan″tho·lye′sis) *n.,* pl. **acantholy·ses** (·seez) Loss of cohesion between epidermal cells or adnexal keratocytes due to degeneration of the intercellular cement substance or faulty formation of the intercellular bridges. —**acan·tho·lyt·ic** (uh·kan″tho·lit′ick) *adj.*

ac·an·tho·ma (ack″an·tho′muh) *n.,* pl. **acantho·mas, acanthoma·ta** (·tuh) 1. Any mass composed of the prickle-cell type of squamous cells; it may be benign or malignant, hyperplastic or neoplastic. 2. Well-differentiated squamous cell carcinoma.

ac·an·tho·sis (ack″an·tho′sis) *n.,* pl. **acantho·ses** (·seez) Any abnormal condition of the prickle-cell layer of the epidermis, particularly hypertrophy. —**acan·thot·ic** (·thot′ick) *adj.*

acanthosis nig·ri·cans (nig′ri·kanz, nigh′gri·). Hyperpigmentation of the body folds, especially of the axillae, associated with verrucous skin lesions at such sites.

acap·nia (ay·kap′nee·uh) *n.* Subnormal concentration of carbon dioxide in the blood. Syn. *hypocapnia.* —**acap·ni·al** (·nee·ul) *adj.*

acap·su·lar (ay·kap′sue·lur) *adj. In biology,* without a capsule.

acar-, acari-, acaro- A combining form meaning (a) *mite;* (b) *itch.*

acar·dia (ay·kahr′dee·uh) *n.* Congenital absence of the heart, usually in omphalosites. —**acar·di·ac** (·dee·ack) *adj. & n.*

acar·dio·tro·phia (ay·kahr″dee·o·tro′fee·uh, a·kahr″) *n.* Atrophy of the heart.

ac·a·ri·a·sis (ack″uh·rye′uh·sis) *n.,* pl. **acaria·ses** (·seez). Any condition, usually a dermatitis, caused by an acarid or mite.

acar·i·cide (a·kăr′i·side) *n.* An agent that destroys acarids.

ac·a·rid (ack′uh·rid) *n.* A tick or mite. —**acar·i·dan** (a·kăr′i·dun), **ac·a·rid·i·an** (ack″uh·rid′ee·un) *adj. & n.*

Ac·a·ri·na (ack″uh·rye′nuh, ·ree′nuh) *n.pl.* An order of Arachnida comprising the ticks and mites. Many species are important vectors of bacterial, protozoan, rickettsial, and spirochetal diseases. In addition, severe reactions may result from their bites.

ac·a·ro·der·ma·ti·tis (ack″uh·ro·dur″muh·tye′tis) *n.* Any dermatitis caused by an acarid or mite.

acarodermatitis ur·ti·car·i·oi·des (ur″ti·kăr·ee·oy′deez). An urticarial and pruritic dermatitis resulting from contact with plant products infested with various species of mites.

ac·a·ro·pho·bia (ack″uh·ro·fo·bee·uh, a·kăr″o·) *n.* 1. Morbid fear of mites or of certain small animate or inanimate things, as worms or pins. 2. The delusion of being infested with parasites.

ac·a·ro·tox·ic (ack″uh·ro·tock′sick) *adj.* Poisonous or destructive to acarids.

Ac·a·rus (ack′uh·rus) *n.* A genus formerly including many kinds of mite, now limited to the cheese mites. —**acarus,** pl. **aca·ri** (·rye), *com. n.*

acat·a·la·se·mia, acat·a·la·sae·mia (ay·kat″uh·lay·see′mee·uh) *n.* Deficiency of the enzyme catalase in the blood.

acat·a·la·sia (ay″kat·uh·lay′zhuh, ·zee·uh) *n.* A congenital absence of the enzyme catalase, a rare disease occurring mostly in the Japanese.

acat·a·lep·sia (ay·kat″uh·lep′see·uh) *n.* 1. Abnormal inability to understand. 2. Uncertainty in diagnosis. —**acatalep·tic** (·tick) *adj. & n.*

acat·a·ma·the·sia (a·kat″uh·muh·theezh′uh, ·theez′ee·uh) *n. Obsol.* 1. Inability to understand conversation. 2. Pathologic blunting or deterioration of the senses, as in cortical deafness and blindness.

acat·a·pha·sia (ay·kat″uh·fay′zhuh, ·zee·uh) *n.* SYNTACTIC APHASIA.

ac·a·tas·ta·sia (ack″uh·tas·tay′zhuh, ·zee·uh) *n.* Irregularity; nonconformity to type; variation from the normal. —**acatas·tat·ic** (·tat'ick) *adj.*

ac·a·thex·ia (ack″uh·theck'see·uh) *n.* Failure or inability to retain bodily secretions and excretions. —**aca·thec·tic** (·theck'tick) *adj.*

ac·a·thex·is (ack″uh·theck'sis) *n. In psychiatry,* lack of affect toward some thing or idea which unconsciously is very important to the individual.

Acc. An abbreviation for *accommodation.*

ac·cel·er·a·tion, *n.* 1. Quickening, as of the pulse or the respiration. 2. Change of velocity (linear acceleration) or of direction of movement (centrifugal acceleration). 3. Advancement in physical growth beyond the norm for one's age and sex, applied particularly to bone age and height. 4. Advancement in intellectual growth or scholastic achievement beyond the average of one's age. 5. *In chemistry,* increase in the rate of a chemical reaction. —**ac·cel·er·ate,** *v.*

ac·cel·er·a·tor, *n.* 1. Any agent or part which quickens the speed of a function or process. 2. A machine, such as the betatron, cyclotron, linear accelerator, or synchrotron, that accelerates electrically charged atomic particles such as electrons, protons, deuterons, and alpha particles to nearly the speed of light. Syn. *atom smasher.* 3. CATALYST (2). —**ac·cel·er·a·to·ry** (ack·sel'ur·uh·tor″ee) *adj.*

acceleratory reflex. Any reflex originating in the labyrinth of the inner ear in response to an increase or decrease in the rate of movement of the head. Syn. *kinetic reflex.*

ac·cen·tu·a·tor (ack·sen'choo·ay″tur) *n.* A chemical substance which intensifies the action of a tissue stain.

ac·cep·tor (ack·sep'tur) *n.* A substance which accepts or combines with a product of a chemical reaction; applied especially to those substances which increase the rate of a reaction by acting as intermediaries in transferring another substance, such as hydrogen, from a reactant to the final product.

ac·ces·sion (ack·sesh'un) *n.* An addition, as to a set of something.

ac·ces·sion·al (ack·sesh'un·ul) *adj.* Pertaining to an accession; additional.

ac·ces·so·ry (ack·ses'uh·ree) *adj. & n.* Auxiliary, assisting; applied especially to a lesser organ or part which supplements a similar organ or part.

accessory chromosome. MONOSOME.

accessory nerve. The eleventh cranial nerve, a motor nerve having both a bulbar origin along the lateral aspect of the medulla oblongata and a spinal origin from the upper five or six cervical segments. The bulbar part (internal ramus) runs with the vagus, sending motor fibers to the striate muscles of the larynx and pharynx. The spinal portion (external ramus) innervates the trapezius and sternocleidomastoid muscles.

ac·ci·dent, *n.* 1. *In legal medicine,* an event occurring to an individual without his expectation, and without the possibility of his preventing it at the moment of its occurrence. 2. An intercurrent or complicating symptom or event,

not encountered in the regular course of a disease.

accidental albuminuria. FALSE PROTEINURIA.

accidental bursa. An inconstant bursa due to friction or pressure.

accident neurosis. TRAUMATIC NEUROSIS.

accident-prone, *adj.* Predisposed to accidents, due to psychological causes. —**accident-prone·ness,** *n.*

ac·cli·ma·tion (ack″li·may'shun) *n.* ACCLIMATIZATION. —**ac·cli·mate** (ack'li·mate) *v.*

ac·cli·ma·ti·za·tion (a·klye″muh·ti·zay'shun) *n.* The process of adjusting to a strange or foreign climate, soil, or water, applied to plants, animals, and people. —**ac·cli·ma·tize** (a·klye'muh·tize) *v.*

ac·com·mo·da·tion, *n. In ophthalmology,* adjustment of the eye to variations in distance; the changes in the ciliary muscle and lens whereby the focus of light rays on the retina is maintained. Abbreviated, a., Acc. —**ac·com·mo·da·tive** (a·kom'uh·day″tiv) *adj.*

accommodation paralysis. Paralysis of the ciliary muscle of the eye.

accommodation reflex. Constriction of the pupils, convergence of the eyes, and increased convexity of the lens when the eyes adjust for near vision. Syn. *near reflex.*

accordion graft. A full-thickness graft in which multiple slits are made so that the graft may be stretched to cover a large area.

ac·couche·ment (a·koosh·mahn″, uh·koosh'munt) *n.* PARTURITION.

accouchement for·cé (for·say′). Rapid delivery by manual dilation of the cervix followed by version or application of forceps and immediate extraction.

ac·cou·cheur (a·koo·shur′) *n.* Obstetrician; a professionally trained person attending women in childbirth.

accoucheur's hand. A spasmodic cone-shaped deformity of the hand; characteristically seen in tetany.

ac·cre·tion (a·kree'shun) *n.* 1. Growth characterized by addition to the periphery, as in crystalline and certain organic compounds. 2. Adherence of parts normally separate. 3. A growing together; adhesion. 4. An accumulation of foreign matter, as about a tooth or within any cavity. —**accre·tive** (·tiv) *adj.*

A.C.D. American College of Dentists.

ACD solution An anticoagulant acid citrate dextrose solution; used to prevent coagulation of blood in collection and storage of whole blood for indirect transfusions.

Ace bandage. Trademark for woven cotton elastic bandage, obtainable in various widths, used especially on the extremities to provide gentle uniform pressure.

acel·lu·lar (ay″sel'yoo·lur) *adj.* Without cells; not consisting of cells; not cellular.

ace·nes·the·sia, acoe·naes·the·sia (ay″see·nes·theezh'uh, ·theez'zee·uh, ay″sen·es·) *n.* Lack or loss of the normal awareness of one's own bodily parts or organs.

acen·o·cou·ma·rol (ay″sen·o·koo'muh·rol) *n.* 3-(α-Acetonyl-4-nitrobenzyl)-4-hydroxycoumarin, $C_{19}H_{15}NO_6$, an anticoagulant.

acen·tric (ay·sen'trick) *adj.* 1. Lacking a center. 2. Peripheral; eccentric. 3. Not arising centrally, as from a nerve center.

acentric chromosome. A chromosomal fragment without a centromere.

-aceous A suffix meaning *pertaining to or characterized by.*

ace·phal·ic (ay''se·fal'ick, as''e·) *adj.* ACEPHALOUS; headless or without a distinct head or headlike part.

aceph·a·lo·cyst (ay·sef'uh·lo·sist, a·sef') *n.* A sterile hydatid, without scolices or brood capsules, found in the human liver and other organs, representing aberrant development of the larval stage of *Echinococcus granulosus.*

aceph·a·lous (ay·sef'uh·lus) *adj.* Without a head; ACEPHALIC.

aceph·a·ly (ay·sef'uh·lee, a·sef') *n.* Absence of the head.

acer·bi·ty (a·sur'bi·tee) *n.* Acidity combined with astringency.

acer·bo·pho·bia (a·sur''bo·fo'bee·uh) *n.* Morbid fear of sourness.

Acerdol. A trademark for calcium permanganate.

aces·o·dyne (a·ses'o·dine) *n.* A pain-relieving agent; ANODYNE (2). **—ac·e·sod·y·nous** (as''e·sod'i·nus) *adj.*

acet-, aceto-. A combining form meaning *connection with or derivation from acetic acid or acetyl.*

acetabula. Plural of *acetabulum.*

ac·e·tab·u·lar (as''e·tab'yoo·lur) *adj.* Pertaining to the acetabulum.

acetabular fossa. A depression in the center of the acetabulum.

ac·e·tab·u·lec·to·my (as''e·tab''yoo·leck'tuh·mee) *n.* Excision of the acetabulum.

ac·e·tab·u·lo·plas·ty (as''e·tab'yoo·lo·plas''tee) *n.* Any plastic operation on the acetabulum, especially an operation aimed at restoring or enlarging the acetabular cavity.

ac·e·tab·u·lum (as''e·tab'yoo·lum) *n.,* pl. **acetabu·la** (·luh) 1. [NA] The cup-shaped depression on the outer aspect of the hipbone for the reception of the head of the femur. 2. The sucking cup of flukes.

ac·e·tal (as'e·tal'') *n.* 1. 1,1-Diethoxyethane, $CH_3CH(OC_2H_5)_2$, formerly used as a hypnotic. 2. Generic name for products of the interaction of aldehydes and alcohol characterized by the presence of the $=C(OR)_2$ group.

ac·et·al·de·hyde (as'e·tal'de·hide, a·seet''al·de·hide) *n.* $CH_3.CHO.$ A colorless liquid with a characteristic pungent odor. It results from the oxidation of ethyl alcohol or the reduction of acetic acid; a general narcotic. Syn. *acetic aldehyde, ethanal.*

ac·et·ami·no·phen (as''e·tuh·mee'no·fen) *n.* N-Acetyl-*p*-aminophenol, $CH_3CONH.$- $C_6H_4.OH$, an analgesic and antipyretic drug. Syn. *p-acetaminophenol.*

ac·et·an·i·lid (as''e·tan'i·lid) *n.* Acetylaniline, $C_6H_5NHCOCH_3$, an analgesic; prolonged use may lead to toxic symptoms.

ac·et·ar·sone (as''e·tahr'sone) *n.* 3-Acetylamino-4-hydroxyphenylarsonic acid, $C_8H_{10}AsNO_5$,

a white or yellowish powder, slightly soluble in water. Used in the treatment of amebiasis and also in prophylaxis and treatment in certain cases of syphilis. Syn. *acetarsol.*

ac·e·tate (as'e·tate) *n.* Any salt or ester of acetic acid.

acet·a·zol·amide (a·set''uh·zo'luh·mide) *n.* 2-Acetylamino-1,3,4-thiadiazole-5-sulfonamide, $C_4H_6N_4O_3S_2$, a renal carbonic anhydrase inhibitor; employed as a diuretic and in the treatment of epilepsy and glaucoma.

ace·tic (a·see'tick) *adj.* Pertaining to acetic acid.

acetic acid. 1. CH_3COOH, a colorless liquid with a pungent odor; the principal acid of vinegar. Syn. *ethanoic acid.* 2. An aqueous solution containing 36 to 37% CH_3COOH. It is occasionally used, when diluted, as an astringent and styptic.

acetic anhydride. The anhydride of acetic acid, $(CH_3CO)_2O$; a colorless, mobile liquid having the odor of acetic acid. Used industrially and in organic syntheses.

acetic fermentation. Any process of fermentation resulting in the formation of acetic acid.

ac·e·to·ace·tic acid (as''e·to·a·see'tick, a·see''to·a·see'tick). Acetylacetic acid, CH_3COC-H_2COOH, a ketone acid produced in small amounts as a normal product of fat metabolism, but excessively when hepatic oxidation of fatty acids is markedly accelerated as in diabetic ketosis or starvation. Syn. *diacetic acid.*

Ace·to·bac·ter (a·see'to·back''tur, as''e·to·back'tur) *n.* A genus of aerobic bacteria of the family Pseudomonadaceae, possessing high oxidative powers and acid tolerance and capable of oxidizing various organic compounds to organic acids and other products, as ethyl alcohol to acetic acid. Important industrially in the production of vinegar. *Acetobacter aceti* is the principal and typical species.

ac·e·to·me·naph·thone (a·see''to·me·naf'thone, as''e·to·) *n.* Menadiol diacetate or 2-methyl-1,4-naphthohydroquinone diacetate, $C_{15}H_{14}O_4$, a vitamin K analogue used in the prevention and treatment of hypoprothrombinemia caused by a deficiency of vitamin K.

ac·e·tom·e·ter (as''e·tom'e·tur) *n.* A device for determining the amount of acetic acid present in a solution, as in vinegar. **—ac·e·to·met·ric** (as''e·to·met'rick) *adj.*

ac·e·to·mor·phine (a·see''to·mor'feen, as''e·to·) *n.* HEROIN.

ac·e·ton·asth·ma (as''e·to·naz'muh) *n. Obsol.* Air hunger associated with ketonuria as in diabetic ketoacidosis.

ac·e·tone (as'e·tone) *n.* Dimethylketone or propanone, CH_3COCH_3; occurs normally in blood and urine in minute quantities which may become greatly increased in diabetics. Produced by synthesis for use as a solvent and industrial chemical.

acetone bodies. KETONE BODIES.

ac·e·ton·emia, ac·e·to·nae·mia (as''e·to·nee'mee·uh) *n.* KETONEMIA. **—aceton·emic** (·nee'mick) *adj.*

ac·e·ton·uria (as''e·to·new'ree·uh) *n.* KETONURIA.

ace·tous (a·see'tus, as'e·) *adj.* Pertaining to, resembling, forming, or containing vinegar or acetic acid.

ace·tyl (a·se'til, as'e·til, -teel) *n.* The univalent radical CH_3CO-, of acetic acid.

ac·e·tyl-beta-meth·yl·cho·line (as"e·til-bay"tuh-meth·il·ko'leen) *n.* METHACHOLINE CHLORIDE.

ac·e·tyl·cho·line (as"e·til·ko'leen, -lin, a·see"til·) *n.* The acetic acid ester of choline, $(CH_3)_3N(OH)CH_2CH_2OCOCH_3$, a normal constituent of many body tissues. It is the chemical mediator of cholinergic nerve impulses; removal of acetyl by enzymatic hydrolysis, producing choline, inactivates it. Has been used in the treatment of a variety of diseases, but its effects are transient and variable.

ac·e·tyl·cho·lin·es·ter·ase (as"e·til·ko"lin·es'tur·ace, -aze) *n.* Any enzyme, found in blood and various tissues, that catalyzes hydrolysis of acetylcholine but may also catalyze hydrolysis of noncholine esters.

acetyl coenzyme A. A compound in which an acetyl group is joined to coenzyme A by a thioester bond. It is an important metabolic intermediate, being an acetylating agent in a variety of reactions, providing energy for cell respiration, and also having other biochemical functions. Abbreviated, acetyl Co A. Syn. *active acetate.*

acet·y·lene (a·set'i·leen) *n.* A colorless gas, $CH\equiv CH$, with a characteristic, unpleasant odor; burns with a luminous, smoky flame. Has been used to determine cardiac output. Syn. *ethine, ethyne.*

ace·tyl·sal·i·cyl·ic acid (a·see"til·sal"i·sil'ick, as"e·til·) ASPIRIN.

acetyl sulfisoxazole. N^1-(Acetyl-3,4-dimethyl-5-isoxazolyl)sulfanilamide, a derivative of sulfisoxazole practically insoluble in water and, hence, tasteless; has the actions of sulfisoxazole.

ac·e·tyl·sul·fon·a·mide (as"e·til·sul·fon'uh·mide, -fo'nuh·mide) *n.* A sulfonamide in which the hydrogen atom of the NH_2 group, attached directly to the benzene ring, is replaced by an acetyl group; a conjugation which occurs in the liver of man and other species, except the canine. Harmful effects may be produced in the renal tubules and urinary tract by the precipitation of these compounds. This can be prevented if urine is kept alkaline.

ach·a·la·sia (ack"uh·lay'zhuh, -zee·uh) *n.* 1. Failure of relaxation of the lower esophagus at the cardiac sphincter with secondary dilatation of the upper esophagus. 2. *Obsol.* Generally, failure of relaxation of smooth muscle fibers in a tubular organ, for example at the cardiac or rectal sphincters in the intestinal tract, often resulting in dilatation of the tubular structure above (megaesophagus or megacolon).

ache (ake) *n. & v.* 1. A dull, persisting pain of fixed location and of more or less constant or throbbing intensity. 2. Of a body part or region: to be the locus of such a pain.

achei·lia, achi·lia (a·kigh'lee·uh) *n.* A condition marked by congenital absence of the lips.

achei·rus, achi·rus (a·kigh'rus) *n.* An individual without hands.

achieve·ment age. *In psychology,* accomplishment expressed as equivalent to the age in years of the average child showing similar attainments; determined by standard tests. Abbreviated, A.A.

achievement quotient. *In psychology,* the ratio between achievement age, or actual level of scholastic performance, and mental age, or expected level of performance for age. Abbreviated, AQ.

Achilles jerk or **reflex.** Plantar flexion of the foot, produced by contraction of the calf muscles and elicited by striking the tendon of the gastrocnemius and soleus muscles (calcaneal or Achilles tendon). Syn. *ankle jerk, triceps surae jerk.*

Achilles tendon CALCANEAL TENDON.

achil·lo·bur·si·tis (a·kil"o·bur·sigh'tis) *n.* Inflammation of the bursa of the calcaneal tendon.

achil·lo·dyn·ia (a·kil"o·din'ee·uh) *n.* Pain in the calcaneal tendon or its bursa.

ach·il·lor·rha·phy (ack"il·or'uh·fee) *n.* Any suturing operation to repair the calcaneal tendon.

achil·lo·te·not·o·my (a·kil"o·te·not'uh·mee) *n.* ACHILLOTOMY.

ach·il·lot·o·my (ack"il·lot'uh·mee) *n.* Surgical section of the calcaneal tendon.

ACH index An index of nutrition based on measurements of arm girth, chest depth, and hip width.

achlor·hy·dria (ay"klor·high'dree·uh, ack"lor·) *n.* The absence of hydrochloric acid in the stomach, even after stimulation with histamine. —**achlorhy·dric** (-drick) *adj.*

ach·luo·pho·bia (ack"loo·o·fo'bee·uh) *n.* Morbid fear of darkness.

acho·lia (ay·ko'lee·uh, a·ko') *n.* 1. Absence or suppression of biliary secretion. 2. Any condition obstructing the flow of bile into the small intestine. 3. A mild temperament. —**achol·ic** (ay·kol'ick), **ach·o·lous** (ack'o·lus) *adj.*

ach·o·lu·ria (ack"o·lew'ree·uh, ay"ko·) *n.* The absence of bilirubin in the urine. —**acholu·ric** (-rick) *adj.*

acholuric jaundice. Jaundice without demonstrable bilirubin in the urine.

achon·dro·pla·sia (a·kon"dro·play'zhuh, -zee·uh, ay·kon") *n.* Abnormal osteogenesis resulting in the typical congenital dwarf, with disproportionately short extremities, relatively large head, depressed nasal bridge, stubby trident hands, and thoracolumbar kyphosis; due to disordered chondrification and ossification of the ends of the long bones beginning early in intrauterine life, with membrane bones developing normally; autosomal dominant, with most cases due to fresh mutation, both parents being normal. Syn. *chondrodystrophia fetalis.* —**achondro·plas·tic,** *adj.*

achon·dro·plast (a·kon'dro·plast, ay·kon') *n. Informal.* ACHONDROPLASTIC DWARF.

achondroplastic dwarf. An individual affected with achondroplasia.

achor (ay'kor, ack'or) *n.* Inflammatory and pustular eruption of hairy parts.

Acho·ri·on (a·ko'ree·on) *n.* TRICHOPHYTON.

achres·tic (a·kres'tick) *adj.* Pertaining to failure of use, as of a principle in the body.

achrestic anemia. *Obsol.* A megaloblastic, macrocytic anemia morphologically similar to pernicious anemia but unresponsive to liver extract therapy, possibly due in at least some cases to folic acid deficiency.

achroa·cyte (ay·kro'uh·site, a·kro') *n.* LYMPHOCYTE.

achroi·o·cy·the·mia, achroi·o·cy·thae·mia (a·kroy"o·sigh·theem'ee·uh) *n. Obsol.* Achreocythemia (= HYPOCHROMIC ANEMIA).

achro·ma·cyte (ay·kro'muh·site, a·kro') *n.* A decolorized erythrocyte; a ghost or shadow corpuscle due to loss of hemoglobin.

achro·ma·sia (ack"ro·may'zhuh, ·zee·uh) *n.* 1. Any condition, such as albinism, leukoderma, or vitiligo, in which there is discernible loss of normal color, usually of melanin, in the skin or in the iris. 2. *In histopathology,* failure of tissue or elements thereof to take stains in usual intensity. Syn. *achromia, achromatosis.*

achromat-, achromato-. A combining form meaning *achromatic, colorless.*

achro·mat·ic (ay"kro·mat'ick) *adj.* 1. Without color. 2. Containing achromatin. 3. Not decomposing light into its constituent colors. 4. Staining with difficulty, as some cells or tissues.

achromatic fibrils. Fibrils of achromatic, nuclear, or cell substance forming lines which extend from pole to pole in a dividing nucleus, so as to form a spindle- or barrel-shaped figure.

achromatic figure. The spindle and asters in mitosis or meiosis.

achromatic lens. A double lens, each part made of such optical glass that the one neutralizes the dispersive effects of the other, without affecting the refraction.

achromatic objective. An objective corrected to bring two opposing colors to focus at the same point, by use of lens combinations containing glasses of differing refractive indices; they show moderate red and green fringes in oblique light.

achro·ma·tin (ay·kro'muh·tin, a·kro') *n.* The faintly staining substance of the cell nucleus including the nuclear sap and euchromatin. —**achro·ma·tin·ic** (ay·kro"muh·tin'ick) *adj.*

achro·ma·tism (ay·kro'muh·tiz·um, a·kro') *n.* 1. Absence of chromatic aberration. 2. Absence of color.

achro·ma·to·phil (ay·kro'muh·to·fil", ay"kro·mat'o·fil) *n. & adj.* Being or characterizing a microorganism or histologic element which does not stain readily.

achro·ma·top·sia (a·kro"muh·top'see·uh) *n.* Total color blindness due to disease or injury of the retina, optic nerve, or pathway.

achro·ma·to·sis (a·kro"muh·to'sis, ack"ro·) *n.,* pl. **achromato·ses** (·seez) ACHROMASIA.

achro·ma·tu·ria (a·kro"muh·tew'ree·uh) *n.* Lack of color in the urine.

achro·mia (a·kro'mee·uh, ay·) *n.* Absence of color.

achromia cutis. Absence of color in the skin.

achro·mic (ay·kro'mick, a·kro') *adj.* Deficient in color; nonpigmented.

achro·mo·trich·ia (a·kro"mo·trick'ee·uh) *n.* Loss or absence of pigment from hair; CANITIES.

Achromycin. A trademark for tetracycline, an antibiotic.

achyl·ane·mia, achyl·anae·mia (ay·kigh"luh·nee'mee·uh, a·kigh") *n.* Hypochromic microcytic anemia due to iron deficiency and associated with achlorhydria.

achy·lia (ay·kigh'lee·uh, a·kigh') *n.* Absence of chyle. —**achy·lic** (·lick), **achy·lous** (·lus) *adj.*

achylia gas·tri·ca (gas'tri·kuh). Absence of gastric secretion of proteolytic enzymes and of hydrochloric acid, even after stimulation with histamine; frequently associated with gastric atrophy.

achy·mia (ay·kigh'mee·uh, a·kigh') *n.* Deficient formation of chyme. —**achy·mous** (·mus) *adj.*

acic·u·lar (a·sick'yoo·lur) *adj.* Needlelike; shaped like a needle.

ac·id (as'id) *adj. & n.* 1. Sour. 2. A substance containing hydrogen replaceable by metals to form salts, and capable of dissociating in aqueous solution to form hydrogen ions (Arrhenius). 3. A substance, ionic or molecular, capable of yielding a proton to another substance (Brönsted and Lowry). This definition has the advantage over Arrhenius' in that it is applicable also to nonaqueous mediums. 4. A substance, ionic or molecular, capable of accepting a share in an electron pair, made available by a base, to form a coordinate covalent bond between the two substances (G. N. Lewis). This definition has the advantage over those of Arrhenius and of Brönsted and Lowry in being applicable also to substances which do not contain a proton (hydrogen ion). 5. Pertaining to or characteristic of an acid; ACIDIC (1). 6. *Slang.* LYSERGIC ACID DIETHYLAMIDE.

acid alcohol. Alcohol containing various percentages of acid. In histologic techniques, a common mixture is 0.1% hydrochloric acid in 95% alcohol.

ac·id·am·i·nu·ria (as"id·am"i·new'ree·uh) *n.* AMINOACIDURIA.

acid-ash diet. A diet the redissolved ashed residue of which has a pH lower than 7.0. Such diets tend to reduce the pH of the urine.

acid-base balance or **equilibrium.** The state of dynamic equilibrium of acids and bases maintained in the body by physiologic processes such as respiration, elimination, and manufacture of buffers which keep the pH of the body constant.

ac·i·de·mia, ac·i·dae·mia (as"i·dee'mee·uh) *n.* A decrease in blood pH below normal levels.

acid-fast, *adj.* Not decolorized by mineral acids after staining with aniline dyes; said of certain bacteria as well as some tissues and dyes.

acid-fast stains. Stains for certain bacteria (chiefly mycobacteria), hair cortex, ceroid and other lipofuscin pigments. Basic dyes and fluorochromes which resist decolorization by aqueous or alcoholic acid solutions are used.

acid-forming, *adj.* 1. Designating substances which produce acid in water. 2. *In nutrition,* designating those foods which yield an acid ash or residue when metabolized. Syn. *acidogenic.*

acid hematin method. A method for hemoglobin determination in which blood is diluted with 0.1 normal hydrochloric acid, and the color is compared with glass standards or with a standard hematin solution. Modifications of this are the Haden-Hausser method, the Wintrobe method, and the Sahli method.

acid·ic (a·sid'ick) *adj.* 1. Pertaining to or characteristic of an acid. 2. ACID-FORMING.

acid·i·fi·ca·tion (a·sid''i·fi·kay'shun) *n.* Conversion into an acid; process of becoming acid; addition of acid. **—acid·i·fy** (a·sid'i·figh) *v.;* **acid·i·fi·able** (a·sid'i·figh''uh·bul) *adj.*

acid·i·fi·er (a·sid'i·figh·ur) *n. In radiography and photography,* a weak organic acid, such as acetic acid, contained in or used prior to fixing solutions for the neutralization of developing solutions in order to arrest the developing process.

acid intoxication. A toxic condition of the body resulting from an excess of acids accumulated from within it or introduced from outside it.

acid·i·ty (a·sid'i·tee) *n.* 1. The quality of being acid; sourness. 2. The state of being excessively acid. 3. The acid content of any substance.

ac·i·do·cy·to·pe·nia (as''i·do·sigh''to·pee'nee·uh) *n. Obsol.* EOSINOPENIA.

ac·i·do·cy·to·sis (as''i·do·sigh·to'sis, a·sid''o·) *n. Obsol.* EOSINOPHILIA.

ac·i·do·gen·ic (as''i·do·jen'ick) *adj.* ACID-FORMING.

acid·o·phil (a·sid'o·fil) *adj. & n.* 1. ACIDOPHILIC. 2. An acidophilic cell, tissue element, or substance. 3. Specifically, an ALPHA CELL of the adenohypophysis.

acid·o·phil·ia (a·sid''o·fil'ee·uh) *n.* Affinity for acid stains. Syn. *oxyphilia.*

acidophilus milk. Milk inoculated with cultures of *Lactobacillus acidophilus;* has been used in various enteric disorders to provide a change of bacterial flora.

ac·i·do·re·sis·tant (as''i·do·re·zis'tunt) *adj.* Acid-resistant; not readily decolorized by acids; applied to certain microorganisms. **—acidoresis·tance** (·tunce) *n.*

ac·i·do·sis (as''i·do'sis) *n.,* pl. **acido·ses** (·seez) An abnormal state characterized by processes tending to increase the concentration of hydrogen ion in the body above the normal range or to increase the loss of base from the body. Physiological compensatory mechanisms act to return the lowered pH toward normal. **—aci·dot·ic** (·dot'ick) *adj.*

acid phosphate. A phosphate in which only one or two of the hydrogen atoms of phosphoric acid have been replaced by metals.

acid tide. A period of increased excretion of acid radicals by the kidney 1 to 2 hours after a meal.

acid·u·late (a·sid'yoo·late) *v.* To render sour or acid in reaction; to pour acid into; to acidify.

—acidu·lant (·lunt) *adj. & n.;* **acidu·lous** (·lus) *adj.*

Acidulin. Trademark for glutamic acid hydrochloride, a digestant.

ac·i·du·ria (as''i·dew'ree·uh) *n.* The condition in which the urine is acid.

¹**ac·i·du·ric** (as''i·dew'rick) *adj.* Exhibiting or pertaining to aciduria.

²**aciduric,** *adj. Obsol.* Of bacteria: able to grow in an acid medium; acid-tolerant.

ac·i·nar (as'i·nur, ·nahr) *adj.* Of or pertaining to an acinus.

acini. Plural of *acinus.*

acin·ic (a·sin'ick) *adj.* ACINAR.

ac·i·no·tu·bu·lar (as''i·no·tew'bew·lur) *adj.* Consisting of tubular acini.

ac·i·nous (as'i·nus) *adj.* Resembling, consisting of, or pertaining to acini.

ac·i·nus (as'i·nus) *n.,* pl. **ac·i·ni** (as'i·nigh) 1. A saccular terminal division of a compound gland having a narrow lumen, several of which combine to form a lobule. 2. The anatomic unit of the lung consisting of alveolar ducts and alveoli stemming from a terminal bronchiole.

A.C.L.A.M. American College of Laboratory Animal Medicine.

ac·la·sis (ack'luh·sis, a·klay'sis) *n.* The blending of abnormally developed tissue with normal tissue.

aclas·tic (a·clas'tick) *adj.* Not refracting.

acleis·to·car·dia (a·klye''sto·kahr'dee·uh, ay·klye''sto·) *n.* A condition in which the foramen ovale of the heart fails to close.

ac·me (ack'mee) *n.* 1. The highest point. 2. The crisis or critical stage of a disease.

ac·ne (ack'nee) *n.* An inflammatory condition of the sebaceous glands common in adolescence and young adulthood, characterized by comedones which often become inflamed and form papules, pustules, nodules, and cysts, usually on the face, chest, and back. Syn. *acne vulgaris.*

acne ar·ti·fi·ci·a·lis (ahr·ti·fish·ee·ay'lis). An acneform eruption caused by exposure to tars, waxes, grease, or chlorinated hydrocarbons.

acne ca·chec·ti·co·rum (ka·keck''ti·ko'rum). An acneform eruption seen in debilitated persons during long, wasting diseases, such as tuberculosis. The lesions occur on the trunk and legs, appearing as small, flat, dull-red papules and pustules.

acne co·ag·mi·na·ta (ko·ag''mi·nay'tuh). A pustular acneform eruption often seen after administering any of the halogens or their salts and among industrial workers exposed to hydrochloric acid, tar, tar vapor, oil, wax, or paraffin.

acne con·glo·ba·ta (kon·glo·bay'tuh). A severe and long-enduring form of acne, frequently affecting the lower part of the back, buttocks, and thighs in addition to the face and chest with abcesses, cysts, and sinuses as well as with the more common lesions of acne. Scarring, often hypertrophic and keloidal, is an inevitable consequence of healing.

acne cys·ti·ca (sis'ti·kuh). A form of acne in which the lesions are mainly cysts.

acne decalvans. FOLLICULITIS DECALVANS.

ac·ne·form (ack′ne·form) *adj.* Resembling acne.

acneform drug eruptions. Eruptions resembling acne and caused by certain drugs, principally iodides and bromides, but in some cases also caused by steroids.

ac·ne·gen (ack′ne·jen) *n.* A substance that promotes acne. —**ac·ne·gen·ic** (ack″ne·jen′ick) *adj.*

ac·ne·iform (ack·nee′i·form) *adj.* ACNEFORM.

acne in·du·ra·ta (in·dew·ray′tuh). A form of acne in which the lesions are mainly hard papules.

acne med·i·ca·men·to·sa (med″i·kuh·men·to′suh). An acneform drug eruption, caused by administration of certain drugs.

acne neo·na·to·rum. (nee″o·nay·to′rum). Acneform eruption in a newborn in the nature of a nevoid anomaly, acne medicamentosa as from iodides or bromides ingested by the mother, or truly precocious acne.

acne vul·ga·ris (vul·gair′is, ·gâr′). ACNE.

ac·ni·tis (ack·nigh′tis) *n. Obsol.* 1. PAPULONE-CROTIC TUBERCULID. 2. LUPUS MILIARIS DIS-SEMINATUS FACIEI.

aco·mous (ay·ko′mus, a·ko′) *adj.* Bald. —**aco·mia** (·mee·uh) *n.*

acon·a·tive (ay·kon′uh·tiv) *adj.* Having no wish or desire to make any physical or mental effort.

ac·o·nite (ack′o·nite) *n.* A very poisonous drug obtained from the roots of *Aconitum napellus.* It has a bitter, pungent taste and leaves a sensation of numbness and tingling on the lips and tongue. Physiologically, it is a cardiac, respiratory, and circulatory depressant and produces sensory paralysis. The principal alkaloid is aconitine. Has been used as a diaphoretic, antipyretic, and diuretic.

acon·i·tine (a·kon′i·teen, ·tin) *n.* An extremely poisonous alkaloid, $C_{34}H_{47}NO_{11}$, derived from *Aconitum napellus* and other species.

acon·ure·sis (a·kon″yoo·ree′sis) *n.* Involuntary urination.

acop·ro·sis (ay″kop·ro′sis, ack″o·pro′sis) *n.* A deficiency or absence of feces in the intestine.

ac·o·rea (ack″o·ree′uh) *n.* Absence of the pupil.

aco·ria, ako·ria (a·ko′ree·uh, ay·) *n.* A sensation of hunger not relieved even by a large meal, due to the absence of the feeling of satiety.

acos·tate (a·kos′tate, ay·) *adj.* Without ribs.

acou-, acouo- A combining form meaning *hearing.*

acou·sia (a·koo′zhuh, ·zee·uh) *n.* An involuntary act.

-acousia, -acusia A combining form meaning *condition of hearing.*

acous·ma (a·kooz′muh) *n.,* pl. **acousmas, acous·ma·ta** (·tuh) A simple auditory hallucination, as of buzzing or ringing.

acous·mat·ag·no·sis (a·kooz″muh·tag·no′sis) *n.* Inability to recognize sounds or understand spoken words; AUDITORY AGNOSIA.

acous·tic (uh·koos′tick) *adj.* Pertaining to sound or hearing.

acoustic aphasia. AUDITORY APHASIA.

acoustic meatus. See *external acoustic meatus, internal acoustic meatus.*

acoustic nerve. VESTIBULOCOCHLEAR NERVE.

acoustic neurilemmoma. A benign tumor of the sheath of the eighth cranial nerve, usually growing at one cerebellopontine angle. Syn. *schwannoma.*

acous·ti·co·fa·cial (uh·koos″ti·ko·fay′shul) *adj.* Pertaining jointly to the acoustic (vestibulo-cochlear) and facial nerves.

acous·ti·co·mo·tor (uh·koos″ti·ko·mo′tor) *adj.* Pertaining to motor activity in response to a sound stimulus.

acousticomotor epilepsy. A form of reflex epilepsy in which seizures occur in response to sound stimuli, usually loud sudden noises; AUDIOGENIC EPILEPSY.

acous·ti·co·pal·pe·bral (uh·koos″ti·ko·pal′pe·brul) *adj.* Pertaining jointly to the vestibulo-cochlear nerve and to the eyelids.

acousticopalpebral reflex. AUDITORY-PALPE-BRAL REFLEX.

acous·ti·co·pho·bia (uh·koos″ti·ko·fo′bee·uh) *n.* Morbid fear of sounds.

acous·tics (a·koos′ticks) *n.* The science of sound.

ac·quired, *adj.* Not present at birth but developed in an individual as a reaction to environment or through use or disuse.

acquired agammaglobulinemia. The depression of gamma globulin levels from previously normal to below 500 mg/dl which occurs equally in both sexes; may be primary without a clear underlying cause or secondary to a well-defined disease process leading to decreased synthesis or increased loss. In addition to greater susceptibility to bacterial infections, patients may develop symptoms of celiac syndrome and such diseases as systemic lupus erythematosus and other immunologic abnormalities.

acquired behavior. *In psychology,* the particular aspects of behavior that distinguish one individual from another or a child from an adult, ascribed primarily to experience rather than to heredity.

acquired drive. *In psychology,* a drive which is not part of the basic inherited makeup of the organism, but which was aroused and developed through experience.

acquired hemolytic anemia. Any anemia due to the action of an external agent or disease process upon normally constructed erythrocytes.

acquired immunity. The enhanced resistance of a host to disease as a result of naturally acquired or artificially induced experience.

acr-, acro- A combining form meaning (a) *extremity, tip, end;* (b) *height, promontory;* (c) *extreme, intense.*

ac·ral (ack′rul) *adj.* Pertaining to the limbs or extremities.

acra·nia (ay·kray′nee·uh, a·kra′) *n.* Partial or complete absence of the cranium at birth. —**acra·nial** (·nee·ul) *adj.:* **acra·ni·us** (·nee·us) *n.*

acra·sia (a·kray′zhuh, ·zee·uh) *n.* Intemperance; lack of self-control.

acra·tia (a·kray′shee·uh) *n.* Impotence, loss of power.

acrat·ure·sis (uh·krat″yoo·ree′sis) *n.* Inability to urinate due to atony of the urinary bladder.

-**acria** A combining form meaning *a condition of the extremities.*

ac·rid (ack'rid) *adj.* Pungent; irritating.

ac·ri·dine (ack'ri·deen, ·din) *n.* Dibenzo-[*b,e*]pyridine, $C_{13}H_9N$, a constituent of coal tar. It is employed in the synthesis of various dyes, certain of which (acriflavine, diflavine, proflavine) are used as antiseptics. Mutations produced by acridine dyes, by virtue of their intercalation into molecules of deoxyribonucleic acid, have been employed by Crick as evidence of the triplet nature of the genetic code.

ac·ri·fla·vine (ack"ri·flay'veen, ·vin, ·flav'een, ·in) *n.* 1. A mixture of 3,6-diamino-10-methylacridinium chloride and 3,6-diaminoacridine; a deep orange, granular powder, freely soluble in water. It is used chiefly as a local antiseptic, but has been administered intravenously in treating various infections. Syn. *neutral acriflavine.* 2. Basic acridine fluorochrome, C.I. No. 46000, used in a fluorescent Schiff reagent and as fluorochrome for elastic fibers.

acrit·i·cal (ay·krit'i·kul, a·krit') *adj.* 1. Without a crisis; not relating to a crisis. 2. Indeterminate, as regards prognosis.

acro-. See *acr-.*

ac·ro·ag·no·sis (ack"ro·ag·no'sis) *n.* 1. Absence of sense of position, weight, shape, or even existence of a limb or limbs. 2. Loss of sensation in a limb.

ac·ro·an·es·the·sia, ac·ro·an·aes·the·sia (ack"ro·an"es·theezh'uh) *n.* Anesthesia of the extremities, from disease or after an anesthetic.

ac·ro·ar·thri·tis (ack"ro·ahr·thrigh'tis) *n.* Arthritis of the extremities.

ac·ro·as·phyx·ia (ack"ro·as·fick'see·uh) *n.* Intermittent digital cyanosis and pallor, precipitated by cold or emotion, with subsequent reactive hyperemia on rewarming; a manifestation of Raynaud's phenomenon.

ac·ro·atax·ia (ack"ro·a·tack'see·uh) *n.* Incoordination of the muscles of the fingers and toes.

ac·ro·brachy·ceph·a·ly (ack"ro·brack"ee·sef'uh·lee) *n.* Congenital deformity of the skull, similar to oxycephaly, characterized by an abnormally high skull, greatly widened in the transverse diameter, and flattening of the head in the anteroposterior diameter.

ac·ro·cen·tric (ack"ro·sen'trick) *adj.* Of a chromosome: having the centromere closer to one end than to the center, resulting in one long and one very short arm.

ac·ro·ceph·a·lo·poly·syn·dac·ty·ly (ack"ro·sef"uh·lo·pol"ee·sin·dack'ti·lee) *n.* A syndrome of acrocephaly, brachysyndactyly of the fingers, preaxial polydactyly, and syndactyly of the toes; classified as either type I (Noack's syndrome), an autosomal dominant trait, or type II (Carpenter's syndrome), an autosomal recessive trait further characterized by mental retardation, obesity, and hypogenitalism.

ac·ro·ceph·a·lo·syn·dac·tyl·ia (ack"ro·sef"uh·lo·sin"dack·til'ee·uh) *n.* ACROCEPHALOSYNDACTYLY.

ac·ro·ceph·a·ly (ack"ro·sef'uh·lee) *n.* OXYCEPHALY.

ac·ro·chor·don (ack"ro·kor'don) *n.* A cutaneous tag or fibroma pendulum.

ac·ro·con·trac·ture (ack"ro·kun·track'chur) *n.* Contracture of the joints of the hands or feet.

ac·ro·cy·a·no·sis (ack"ro·sigh"uh·no'sis) *n.*, pl. **acrocyano·ses** (·seez). Symmetric mottled cyanosis of the hands and feet, associated with coldness and sweating; a vasospastic disorder accentuated by cold and emotion and relieved by warmth. Syn. *Crocq's disease.*

ac·ro·der·ma·ti·tis (ack"ro·dur"muh·tye'tis) *n.* Any inflammatory condition of the hands, arms, feet, or legs.

acrodermatitis chron·i·ca atroph·i·cans (kron"i·kuh a·trof'i·kanz). A characteristic, chronic, progressive inflammatory condition of the skin that tends to atrophy of the skin in a form that is likened to wrinkled cigarette paper.

acrodermatitis con·tin·ua (kon·tin'yoo·uh). A variant form of psoriasis resembling pustular psoriasis in all respects except that it arises without previous evidence of the disease. Syn. *Hallopeau's disease.*

acrodermatitis hi·e·ma·lis (high"e·may'lis). Inflammatory changes in the skin of the hands and feet, attributable to winter weather; chapping.

ac·ro·dol·i·cho·me·lia (ack"ro·dol"i·ko·mee'lee·uh) *n.* A condition in which the hands and feet grow disproportionately long or large.

ac·ro·dont (ack"ro·dont) *adj.* 1. Pertaining to a tooth which is ankylosed by its root to a bony eminence, and not inserted in a socket or alveolus. 2. Pertaining to an individual having teeth of this kind.

ac·ro·dyn·ia (ack"ro·din'ee·uh) *n.* A syndrome seen in infancy and occasionally in older childhood, of extreme irritability alternating with periods of apathy, anorexia, pink itching hands and feet, scarlet tip of nose and cheeks, photophobia, profuse sweating, tachycardia, hypertension, and hypotonia, and frequently desquamation of the skin of the hands and feet. This condition is associated with ingestion of or contact with mercury, but also with inflammatory changes of obscure origin in the central nervous system. Syn. *Feer's disease, pink disease.*

ac·ro·ede·ma, ac·ro·oe·de·ma (ack"ro·e·dee'muh) *n.* Persistent swelling of the hands or feet, due to any of numerous causes, such as peripheral neuropathy or trauma to the extremities.

ac·ro·es·the·sia, ac·ro·aes·the·sia (ack"ro·es·theezh'uh, ·theez'ee·uh) *n.* Paresthesia or dysesthesia in the hands or feet.

ac·ro·hy·per·hi·dro·sis (ack"ro·high"pur·hi·dro'sis) *n.* Excessive sweating of the hands or feet, or both.

ac·ro·hy·po·ther·my (ack"ro·high'po·thur"mee) *n.* Abnormal coldness of the extremities.

ac·ro·ker·a·to·sis (ack"ro·kerr"uh·to'sis) *n.* Hyperkeratosis of the extremities, particularly of the hands and feet.

acrokeratosis ver·ru·ci·for·mis (ve·roo"si·for'mis). A genodermatosis marked by development of wart-like excrescences on the hands and feet and sometimes on adjacent areas.

ac·ro·ki·ne·sis (ak″ro·ki·nee′sis) n. Excessive motion of the limbs, which may be the result of extrapyramidal motor disease or the side effect of psychotropic drugs.

acro·le·in (a·kro′lee·in) n. Acrylic aldehyde, CH_2=CHCHO, a liquid of pungent odor resulting from decomposition of glycerin. Syn. *acrylic aldehyde*.

ac·ro·ma·nia (ack″ro·may′nee·uh) n. A violent form of mania.

ac·ro·mas·ti·tis (ack″ro·mas·tye′tis) n. Inflammation of the nipple.

acro·me·gal·ic (ack″ro·me·gal′ick) adj. Pertaining to or exhibiting acromegaly.

acromegalic arthritis. A joint disease in acromegaly, characterized by initial hypertrophy and later degeneration of articular cartilage.

ac·ro·meg·a·loid (ack″ro·meg′uh·loid) adj. Resembling acromegaly.

ac·ro·meg·a·ly (ack″ro·meg′uh·lee) n. A chronic disease, usually of middle life, due to prolonged excessive secretion of adenohypophyseal growth hormone and characterized by overgrowth of bone, connective tissue, and viscera, especially enlargement of the acral parts of the body, as the hands, feet, face, head. May be due to an eosinophilic adenoma. Syn. *Marie's syndrome*.

ac·ro·meta·gen·e·sis (ack″ro·met″uh·jen′e·sis) n. Undue growth of the extremities.

acro·mi·al (a·kro′mee·ul) adj. Pertaining to the acromion.

ac·ro·mic·ria (ack″ro·mick′ree·uh, ·migh′kree·uh) n. Underdevelopment of the extremities and of the skull as contrasted with visceral development.

acro·mio·cla·vic·u·lar (a·kro″mee·o·kla·vick′yoo·lur) adj. Pertaining to the acromion and the clavicle.

acromioclavicular articulation or **joint.** The joint between the lateral end of the clavicle and the acromion of the scapula.

acro·mio·cor·a·coid (a·kro″mee·o·kor′uh·koid) adj. CORACOACROMIAL.

acro·mio·hu·mer·al (a·kro″mee·o·hew′mur·ul) adj. Pertaining to the acromion and the humerus.

acro·mi·on (a·kro′mee·on) n. The flat, somewhat triangular bony process formed by the lateral extension of the scapular spine, and situated just above the glenoid cavity. It articulates with the clavicle, and serves as a point of attachment for some of the fibers of the deltoid and trapezius muscles.

acro·mi·on·ec·to·my (a·kro″mee·on·eck′tuh·mee) n. Surgical removal of the acromion.

acromion process. ACROMION.

acro·mio·tho·rac·ic (a·kro″mee·o·tho·ras′ick) adj. Pertaining to the shoulder and thorax; thoracoacromial.

acrom·pha·lus (a·krom′fuh·lus) n. 1. The center of the umbilicus, where the cord attaches. 2. Unusual prominence of the navel, often the first sign of an umbilical hernia. 3. Remains of the umbilical cord attached to the child.

ac·ro·myo·to·nia (ack″ro·migh″o·to′nee·uh) n. Tonic muscular spasm of the hands or feet.

ac·ro·nar·cot·ic (ack″ro·nahr·kot′ick) adj. & n.

1. Combining a local irritant effect, by acting directly on the peripheral nerves, with a general obtunding effect, by affecting the brain and vital centers in the cord. 2. An agent that has these effects.

ac·ro·neu·rop·a·thy (ack″ro·new·rop′uth·ee) n. Any neuropathy most evident in the more distal parts of the extremities, usually seen in hereditary sensory neuropathies or as a result of an inflammatory process, diabetes, vitamin deficiency (as in alcoholism or beriberi), or poisoning with arsenic, lead, or mercury.

ac·ro·neu·ro·sis (ack″ro·new·ro′sis) n. Any neurosis affecting the hands or feet, usually vasomotor in nature.

ac·ro·nyx (ack′ro·nicks) n. An ingrowing nail.

ac·ro·os·te·ol·y·sis (ack″ro·os″tee·ol′i·sis) n. 1. Myelodysplasia with osseous lesions. 2. Loss of substance from the bones of the distal phalanges; may be familial or the result of occupational exposure to polyvinyl chloride.

ac·ro·pachy (ack′ro·pack″ee, a·krop′uh·kee) n. HYPERTROPHIC PULMONARY OSTEOARTHROPATHY.

ac·ro·pachy·der·ma (ack″ro·pack″ee·dur′muh) n. A syndrome characterized by abnormally small hands and feet with clubbing of the digits, and thickening of the skin over the face, scalp, and extremities, due to hypopituitarism.

ac·ro·pa·ral·y·sis (ack″ro·puh·ral′i·sis) n. Paralysis of the hands or feet.

ac·ro·par·es·the·sia, ac·ro·par·aes·the·sia (ack″ro·păr″es·theezh′uh, ·theez′ee·uh) n. A symptom complex associated with a variety of disorders of the peripheral nerves or posterior columns, characterized by tingling, pins-and-needles sensations, numbness or stiffness, and occasionally pain in the hands or feet or both.

ac·ro·pa·thol·o·gy (ack″ro·pa·thol′uh·jee) n. The pathology of the extremities, especially the morbid changes occurring in orthopedic diseases.

acrop·a·thy (a·krop′uth·ee) n. Any abnormal condition of the extremities. —**ac·ro·path·ic** (ack″ro·path′ick) adj.

ac·ro·pho·bia (ack″ro·fo′bee·uh) n. Morbid dread of being at a great height.

ac·ro·pig·men·ta·tion (ack″ro·pig″men·tay′shun) n. Increased melanin pigmentation of the distal parts of the extremities, particularly the knuckles.

ac·ro·pos·thi·tis (ack″ro·pos·thigh′tis) n. Inflammation of the prepuce.

ac·ro·scle·ro·der·ma (ack″ro·skleer·o·dur′muh) n. A condition in which the skin of arms, hands, legs, and feet is palpably indurated.

ac·ro·scle·ro·sis (ack″ro·skle·ro′sis) n. A form of scleroderma affecting the fingers, characterized by Raynaud's phenomenon and ulceration.

ac·ro·som·al (ack″ro·so′mul) adj. Of or pertaining to an acrosome.

ac·ro·some (ack′ro·sohm) n. A dense granule of varying size and shape developed during spermiogenesis; located at the anterior pole of the nucleus and enclosed by the head and cap.

ac·ros·te·al·gia (ack″ros·tee·al′jee·uh) *n.* Pain in one or more of the bones of an extremity.

ac·ro·ter·ic (ack″ro·terr′ick) *adj.* Pertaining to the periphery or most distal parts, as the tips of the toes, fingers, or nose. —**ac·ro·te·ria** (ack″ ro·teer′ee·uh) *n.pl.*

¹**acrot·ic** (a·krot′ick) *adj.* Pertaining to the surface or periphery; specifically, to the glands of the skin.

²**acrotic,** *adj.* Of the pulse, absent or imperceptible.

ac·ro·tism (ack′ro·tiz·um) *n.* Absence or imperceptibility of the pulse.

ac·ro·tro·pho·neu·ro·sis (ack″ro·tro″fo·new·ro′ sis) *n.* A trophic disturbance of the extremities caused by a nerve lesion.

acryl-, acrylo-. A combining form meaning *acrylic.*

acryl·ic (a·kril′ick) *adj. & n.* 1. Of or pertaining to acrylic acid or its derivatives, or to an acrylic (2). 2. Any of various thermoplastic substances prepared by reaction and polymerization of sodium cyanide, acetone, methyl alcohol, and acid. They resemble clear glass, but are lighter in weight and permit passage of ultraviolet rays; used in making dental prostheses and artificial intraocular lenses.

acrylic acid. Propenoic acid, $CH_2=CHCOOH$, used in the manufacture of plastics.

acrylic resin. A synthetic resin, usually a polymer of methyl methacrylate.

ac·ry·lo·ni·trile (ack″ri·lo·nigh′tril, ·treel, ·trile) *n.* Propene nitrile, $H_2C=CHCN$, used in the manufacture of synthetic rubber and plastics.

Actase. A trademark for a preparation of human fibrinolysin used intravenously to accelerate intravascular dissolution of clots.

ACTH Abbreviation for *adrenocorticotropic hormone.*

ACTH test. Any of a number of procedures employing a challenge dose of adrenocorticotropic hormone to assess adrenocortical response.

actin-, actino- A combining form meaning (a) *ray, radiant;* (b) *radiated structure.*

ac·tin (ack′tin) *n.* Protein constituent of the muscle fibril, occurring side by side with myosin and both participating in the muscle contractile mechanism. Actin can undergo a reversible transformation between a globular or monomeric (G-actin) and a fibrous or polymeric (F-actin) state.

acting out. 1. *In psychiatry,* the expression of anxiety, emotional conflict, or feelings of love or hostility through such behavior as sexual promiscuity, stealing, fire setting, or other destructive or socially disapproved acts rather than through words; mostly seen in individuals with character disorders who are not aware of the relationship between their behavior and their conflicts or feelings. 2. Dramatization as play therapy. —**act out,** *v.*

ac·tin·ic (ack·tin′ick) *adj.* Pertaining to or designating radiant energy, especially that in the visible and ultraviolet spectrum, which produces marked chemical change.

actinic carcinoma. A basal cell or squamous cell carcinoma of the face and other exposed surfaces of the body, seen in persons who spend prolonged periods of time in direct sunlight.

actinic dermatosis. A dermatosis due to exposure to sunlight. It may be urticarial, papular, or eczematous.

actinic keratoconjunctivitis. Inflammation of the conjunctiva and cornea with pain, photophobia, lacrimation, and smarting of the lids, caused by repeated flashes of bright light or ultraviolet radiation.

actinic keratosis. A premalignant hyperkeratosis, thought to be caused by chronic exposure to sunshine.

ac·tin·i·form (ack·tin′i·form) *adj.* Exhibiting radiate form or structure, such as the ray fungus or the sea anemone.

ac·ti·nism (ack′ti·niz·um) *n.* The production of chemical change by actinic radiation.

ac·tin·i·um (ack·tin′ee·um) *n.* Ac = 227. A radioactive element found in uranium ores, as pitchblende.

ac·ti·no·bac·il·lo·sis (ack″ti·no·bas″i·lo′sis) *n.,* pl. **actinobacillo·ses** (·seez) An actinomycosis-like disease of bovine and other domestic animals caused by *Actinobacillus lignieresii,* characterized by caseous abscesses in the tongue and cervical lymph nodes.

Ac·ti·no·ba·cil·lus (ack″ti·no·ba·sil′us) *n.* A genus of the family Brucellaceae, composed of small, slender, gram-negative, nonmotile, nonsporulating rods.

Actinobacillus mal·lei (mal′ee·eye). *Obsol.* PSEU-DOMONAS MALLEI.

ac·ti·no·chem·is·try (ack″ti·no·kem′is·tree) *n.* The branch of chemistry concerned with the reactions produced by actinic radiation.

ac·ti·no·der·ma·ti·tis (ack″ti·no·dur″muh·tye′tis) *n.* Dermatitis caused by exposure to sunlight, ultraviolet light, or x-rays.

ac·tino·gen (ack·tin′o·jen) *n.* Any substance producing radiation. —**ac·ti·no·gen·ic** (ack″ti·no· jen′ick) *adj.;* **actino·gen·e·sis** (·jen′e·sis) *n.;* **acti·no·gen·ics** (·jen′icks) *n.*

ac·ti·nom·e·ter (ack″ti·nom′e·tur) *n.* 1. An apparatus for determining the intensity of actinic rays. 2. A device which determines the degree of penetration of such rays. —**actinome·try** (·tree) *n.*

Ac·ti·no·my·ces (ack″ti·no·migh′seez) *n.* A genus of microaerophilic bacteria, formerly classified as fungi, characterized by delicate branching mycelia which tend to fragment. Several species are responsible for actinomycosis. In tissues, granules may form, presenting in stained preparations eosinophilic clubs surrounding a central basophilic mass.

Actinomyces bo·vis (bo′vis). The species of bacteria causing actinomycosis in cattle.

Actinomyces is·ra·e·lii (iz·ray·ee′lee·eye). The species of bacteria causing actinomycosis in man.

Ac·ti·no·my·ce·ta·ce·ae (ack″ti·no·migh″se·tay′ see·ee) *n.pl.* A family of the order Actinomycetales, including the genera *Nocardia* and *Actinomyces,* in which branching mycelium often fragments into shorter rod-shaped or spherical forms.

Ac·ti·no·my·ce·ta·les (ack″ti·no·migh″se·tay′

leez) *n.pl.* A large order of microorganisms which includes a family essentially lacking mycelium, the Mycobacteriaceae, and three families in which true mycelium is produced, the Actinomycetaceae, Streptomycetaceae, and Actinoplanaceae.

ac·ti·no·my·cete (ack″ti·no·migh′seet, ·migh·seet′) *n.* An organism of the family Actinomycetaceae.

ac·ti·no·my·ce·tin (ack″ti·no·migh·see′tin, ·migh′se·tin) *n.* An antibacterial substance synthesized by several strains of *Actinomyces*, and effective against certain gram-negative and gram-positive organisms.

ac·ti·no·my·cin (ack″ti·no·migh′sin) *n.* Any of an extensive family of polypeptide antibiotics, produced by various species of *Streptomyces*, believed to contain 3-amino-1,8-dimethylphenoxazonedicarboxylic acid as a common moiety. Specific members of the family are identified by roman numeral or letter designations, the latter often with numerical subscripts. Although toxicity limits general use of active members of this group of antibiotics, certain of them, as cactinomycin and dactinomycin, are of therapeutic interest because of antineoplastic activity.

ac·ti·no·my·co·ma (ack″ti·no·migh·ko′muh) *n.*, pl. **actinomycomas, actinomycoma·ta** (·tuh). A swelling produced by an organism of the genus *Actinomyces*.

ac·ti·no·my·co·sis (ack″ti·no·migh·ko′sis) *n.*, pl. **actinomyco·ses** (·seez). 1. A subacute or chronic granulomatous and suppurative infection of man, principally involving the orofacial, thoracic, and abdominal structures, chiefly caused by *Actinomyces israelii*. 2. A similar disease of animals such as cattle, caused by *Actinomyces bovis*, characterized by granulomatous lesions of the jaws.

ac·ti·no·my·cot·ic (ack″ti·no·migh·kot′ick) *adj.* Pertaining to or caused by actinomycosis.

ac·ti·no·my·co·tin (ack″ti·no·migh′ko·tin) *n.* An extract of cultures of *Actinomyces*, prepared like tuberculin and used in cases of actinomycosis.

ac·ti·non (ack′ti·non) *n.* Actinium emanation, a short-lived isotope of radon.

ac·ti·no·neu·ri·tis (ack″ti·no·new·rye′tis) *n.* Neuritis due to exposure to x-rays or radioactive substances.

ac·ti·no·phy·to·sis (ack″ti·no·figh·to′sis) *n.*, pl. **actinophyto·ses** (·seez) BOTRYOMYCOSIS.

ac·ti·no·ther·a·py (ack″ti·no·therr′uh·pee) *n.* Radiation therapy using light rays, most commonly ultraviolet. —**actino·ther·a·peu·tic** (·therr″uh·pew′tick) *adj.*

ac·tion current. The electric current accompanying membrane depolarization and repolarization in an excitable cell.

action potential. The complete cycle of electric changes in transmembrane potential occurring with depolarization and repolarization of an excitable cell as in nerve or muscle tissue.

activated charcoal. Charcoal that has been treated, as with steam and carbon dioxide or with other substances, to increase its adsorptive power. The medicinal grade is used to reduce hyperacidity, to adsorb toxins, and as an antidote against various poisons.

activated sleep. REM SLEEP.

ac·ti·va·tion, *n.* 1. The process of activating or rendering active. 2. Stimulation of general cellular activity by the use of nonspecific therapy; plasma activation. 3. Stimulation of the ovum by the sperm or other agents causing cell division. 4. *In chemistry,* the transformation of any substance into a more reactive form, including the renewal of activity of a catalyst. 5. *In nuclear science,* the process of making a material radioactive by bombardment with neutrons, protons, or other nuclear particles. —**ac·ti·vate,** *v.*; **acti·vat·ed,** *adj.*

activation analysis. A method of chemical analysis by which a small amount of an element, otherwise difficult to identify and quantitatively determine, is made radioactive by bombardment with neutrons or other activating particles, and then qualitatively identified by observing the half-life of one or more of its radioisotopes and the characteristics of its radiations. Quantitative analysis is achieved through similar treatment of reference material containing a known amount of the element found to be present.

ac·ti·va·tor, *n.* 1. An agent which is necessary to activate another substance as an agent, usually a metal ion, whose combination with a complete enzyme or its substrate activates the enzyme. 2. A substance which stimulates the development of an embryonic structure. Syn. *inductor, organizer.* 3. An apparatus which charges water with radium emanations. 4. CATALYST. 5. A substance capable of causing the breakdown of an initiator by chemical means, rather than by the application of heat, in the polymerization of synthetic resins. 6. A myofunctional appliance that acts as a passive transmitter of force to accomplish orthodontic movement.

ac·tive, *adj.* 1. Energetic, decisive, as active treatment. 2. Due to an intrinsic as distinguished from a passive force, as active hyperemia. 3. *In optics,* possessing the ability to rotate the plane of a polarized light beam. 4. *In psychoanalysis,* pertaining to masculine qualities in terms of the goal; also, pertaining to the endeavors of the analyst to influence the patient to produce material for analysis. 5. *In biochemistry,* pertaining to an actual or presumed derivative of a substance regarded as the participating form in biological reactions in which the parent compound itself does not exhibit full activity. 6. Causing or producing change.

active anaphylaxis. A state of immediate hypersensitivity produced by the reintroduction of the antigen, presumed to result from the interaction of antigen and antibody fixed to tissues releasing pharmacologically active substances.

active exercise. Exercise by voluntary effort of the patient.

active immunity. Immunity possessed by a host as the result of disease or unrecognized infection, or induced by immunization with microbes or their products or with other antigens.

active sleep. REM SLEEP.

active tuberculosis. A clinically significant form of the disease, which is undergoing clinical or roentgenographic change and causing or capable of causing symptoms or disability; tubercle bacilli can usually be isolated.

ac·to·my·o·sin (ack″to·migh′o·sin) n. A complex of the muscle proteins actin and myosin.

acu- A combining form meaning *needle*.

acu·i·ty (a·kew′i·tee) n. Sharpness; keenness of perception, as of vision or hearing.

acu·mi·nate (a·kew′mi·nut, ·nate) adj. Sharp-pointed; conical; tapering to a point.

acu·pres·sure (ack′yoo·presh″ur) n. 1. A procedure to stop hemorrhage by compressing the artery with a needle inserted into the tissues upon either side. 2. SHIATSU.

acu·punc·ture (ack′yoo·punk″chur) n. 1. A method originating in China, used for relief of pain, in which fine needles inserted at certain points and along certain meridians are twirled rapidly. 2. Puncture of an organ or tissue with multiple fine needle points; used in the multi-puncture method of smallpox vaccination.

acus (ay′kus) n. A surgical needle.

acu·sec·tor (ack″yoo·seck′tur) n. An electric needle, operating on a high-frequency current, which cuts tissues like a scalpel. —**acusec·tion** (·shun) n.

acus·ti·cus (a·koos′ti·kus) n. VESTIBULOCOCHLEAR NERVE.

acute (uh·kewt′) adj. 1. Sharp; severe. 2. Having a rapid onset, a short course, and pronounced symptoms. 3. Sensitive, perceptive.

acute abdomen. A pathologic condition within the abdomen, requiring prompt surgical intervention.

acute abscess. An abscess associated with acute inflammation of the part in which it is formed.

acute alcoholism. Inebriety; drunkenness; a transient disturbance of mental and bodily functioning due to excessive alcohol intake.

acute appendicitis. A severe and rapidly developing attack of appendicitis, characterized by abdominal pain and tenderness usually in the right lower quadrant, and often by nausea, vomiting, fever, and leukocytosis.

acute ascending myelitis. Inflammation of the spinal cord beginning in the lower segments and progressing cephalad; may occur in spinal poliomyelitis, postvaccinal or postexanthematous myelitis, and rarely in *Herpesvirus simiae* and rabies infections.

acute bacterial endocarditis. Fulminant, rapidly progressive endocarditis, usually associated with a significant systemic infection, often by *Staphylococcus aureus*.

acute bronchitis. Acute inflammation of the bronchi due to infectious or irritant agents, characterized by cough with variable sputum production, fever, substernal soreness, and lung rales.

acute cerebellar ataxia. A usually self-limited, benign cerebellar syndrome of sudden onset, with ataxia of stance and gait, dysmetria, intention tremor, dysarthria, nystagmus, adiadochokinesis, hypotonia, and occasionally fever, nausea, and vomiting, without evidence of an intracranial lesion or intoxication. Most common in childhood, may be related to a nonspecific respiratory or gastrointestinal illness or a viral infection.

acute disseminated encephalomyelitis. A demyelinating disorder of the brain and spinal cord with widespread, variable neurologic symptoms, course, and outcome. It may be postinfectious or postvaccinal and may represent an immune-allergic response of the nervous system.

acute duodenal ileus. Obstruction of the lumen of the duodenum following operations or resulting from external pressure. Syn. *arteriomesenteric ileus, gastromesenteric ileus.*

acute glomerulonephritis. An acute inflammatory disease involving the renal glomeruli, occurring principally as a sequel to infection with nephritogenic strains of group A beta-hemolytic streptococci, and variably characterized by hematuria, proteinuria, oliguria, azotemia, edema, hypertension, and hypocomplementemia occurring 7 to 14 days after infection; the mechanism is unknown but presumably involves glomerular deposits of immune complexes and activation of the complement system.

acute inflammation. Inflammation in which the onset is recent, progress is rapid, and the manifestations are pronounced.

acute intermittent porphyria. A metabolic disturbance of porphyrin metabolism, probably transmitted as a Mendelian dominant characteristic, affecting young adults or the middle-aged. Characterized clinically by periodic attacks of abdominal colic with nausea and vomiting, constipation, neurotic or psychotic behavior, and polyneuropathy. The urine contains excessive amounts of the porphyrin precursors δ-aminolevulinic acid and porphobilinogen.

acute leukemia. A form of leukemia with rapid onset and progress if untreated, characterized by severe anemia, hemorrhagic manifestations, and susceptibility to infection; the predominant cells in the bone marrow and peripheral blood are blast forms.

acute myelitis. Any acute inflammation of the spinal cord, including transverse myelitis and the Guillain-Barré disease.

acute necrotizing hemorrhagic encephalomyelitis. An acute disease mainly of children and young adults, usually preceded by a respiratory infection of indeterminate cause and characterized clinically by headache, fever, stiff neck, confusion, and signs of disease of one or both cerebral hemispheres and brainstem, and frequently by a fatal outcome; spinal fluid shows a polymorphonuclear pleocytosis and variable numbers of red cells, but normal glucose values. The destructive, hemorrhagic lesions of the brain are thought to represent the most fulminant form of demyelinative disease. Syn. *acute hemorrhagic leukoencephalitis of Weston Hurst.*

acute·ness (uh·kewt′nis) n. 1. The quality of

being acute or sharp, as in perception, learning, or feeling. 2. Suddenness, brevity, or severity of an illness as contrasted with insidiousness and chronicity. 3. *In ophthalmology and audiology,* acuity; keenness of vision or of hearing.

acute organic brain syndrome or **disorder.** ACUTE BRAIN SYNDROME.

acute peritonitis. Peritonitis with an abrupt onset and rapid course, characterized by abdominal pain, tenderness, vomiting, constipation, and fever; may be due to chemical irritation or bacterial infection, the latter being either primary or secondary.

acute pharyngitis. A form of pharyngitis due to temperature changes, to the action of irritant substances, or to certain infectious causes, and characterized by pain on swallowing, by dryness, later by moisture, and often by hyperemia of the mucous membrane.

acute-phase reactant. Any of various proteins, such as C-reactive protein or fibrinogen, which are not antibodies but which appear in, or are increased in amount in, plasma during acute trauma or inflammatory reaction.

acute renal failure. Rapid decline in renal function followed by physiologic and biochemical abnormalities, as in acute tubular necrosis; generally due to damage of renal parenchyma by intrinsic disease or extrinsic factors.

acute respiratory disease. 1. A respiratory infection due to adenovirus, particularly types 4 and 7, occurring especially among military personnel, and characterized by fever, sore throat, cough, and malaise. Abbreviated, ARD. 2. Any acute infectious disease of the respiratory tract.

acute rhinitis of the newborn. Rhinitis in premature and full-term neonates from a variety of causes including maternal drug ingestion, chemical irritation, and infectious agents.

acute schizophrenic episode. A form of undifferentiated schizophrenia marked by the acute onset of symptoms, often associated with confusion, emotional turmoil, ideas of reference, dissociation, depression, or fear. In many cases there is recovery, while in others the disorganization progresses and takes on the characteristics of the catatonic, hebephrenic, or paranoid types of schizophrenia.

acute toxic encephalopathy. A syndrome of obscure origin affecting children, characterized by sudden onset of stupor or coma, convulsions, fever, decorticate or decerebrate postures and impaired respiratory and cardiovascular function; the cerebrospinal fluid is usually under increased pressure but is otherwise normal, and the brain shows only edema unless hypoxic changes supervene.

acute traumatic subdural hygroma. Collection of cerebrospinal fluid with a small admixture of blood in the subdural space following trauma, apparently caused by tears in the arachnoid membrane near the villi.

acute tubular necrosis. A retrogressive change in the kidneys associated with crushing injuries and other conditions producing shock, and sometimes accompanied by necrosis of distal

and collecting tubules. Abbreviated, ATN. Syn. *lower nephron nephrosis.*

acute yellow atrophy. Rapid, massive destruction of the liver, usually as a result of viral hepatitis.

A.C.V.M. American College of Veterinary Microbiologists.

A.C.V.P. American College of Veterinary Pathologists.

acy·a·no·blep·sia (ay-sigh″uh-no-blep′see-uh, a-sigh″) *n.* ACYANOPSIA.

acy·a·nop·sia (ay-sigh″uh-nop′see-uh, a-sigh″) *n.* Inability to see blue colors.

acy·a·not·ic (ay-sigh″uh-not′ick) *adj.* Without cyanosis, as an acyanotic congenital cardiovascular defect.

acy·clia (ay-sigh′klee-uh, ay-sick′lee-uh) *n.* A state of arrested circulation of body fluids.

acy·clic (ay-sigh′klick, a-sick′lick) *adj.* 1. Not occurring in cycles; not characterized by a self-limited course; nonintermittent. 2. *In chemistry,* denoting organic compounds with an open-chain structure; ALIPHATIC. 3. *In botany,* not whorled.

ac·y·e·sis (as″ee-ee′sis, ay″sigh-ee′sis) *n.* 1. Sterility of the female. 2. Nonpregnancy. 3. Incapacity for natural delivery. —**acy·et·ic** (·et′ick) *adj.*

ac·yl (as′il, as′eel) *n.* An organic radical derived by removal of a hydroxyl group (OH) from an organic acid, as RCO— derived from RCOOH.

acys·tia (ay-sis′tee-uh, a·sis′) *n.* Absence of the urinary bladder.

A d Abbreviation for *anisotropic disk* (= A DISK).

a.d. Abbreviation for *auris dextra;* right ear.

ad- A prefix meaning (a) *to, toward;* (b) *near, beside;* (c) *addition to;* (d) *more intense.*

-ad *In anatomy and zoology,* an adverbial suffix meaning *-ward, toward.*

ADA American Dental Association; American Dietetic Association.

A.D.A.A. American Dental Assistants Association.

adac·rya (ay-dack′ree-uh, a-dack′) *n.* Absence or deficiency of tears.

adac·tyl·ia (ay″dack-til′ee-uh, a-dack·) *n.* Congenital absence of fingers or toes, or both.

adac·ty·lous (ay-dack′ti-lus) *adj.* Lacking fingers or toes.

Adalin. Trademark for carbromal, a sedative.

ad·a·man·tine (ad″uh-man′teen, ·tine) *adj.* 1. Pertaining to dental enamel. 2. Very hard.

ad·a·man·ti·no·car·ci·no·ma (ad″uh-man″ti·no-kahr″si·no′muh) *n.* A malignant ameloblastoma.

ad·a·man·ti·no·ma (ad″uh-man″ti·no′muh) *n.,* pl. **adamantinomas, adamantinoma·ta** (·tuh) AMELOBLASTOMA.

ad·a·man·ti·no·ma·toid craniopharyngioma (ad″uh-man·ti·no′muh·toid). A craniopharyngioma with a cellular pattern resembling ameloblastoma.

Ad·am's apple LARYNGEAL PROMINENCE.

Adams-Stokes syndrome or **disease** STOKES-ADAMS SYNDROME.

ad·ap·ta·tion, *n.* 1. *In biology,* any change in

structure, form, or habits of an organism enabling it to function adequately in a new or changed environment. 2. *In ophthalmology,* adjustment of the eye to varying intensities of light. 3. In reflex action, decline in the frequency of impulses when a receptor is stimulated repeatedly, or cessation of continuous discharge at the same frequency by most receptors when subjected to a constant stimulus. 4. *In dentistry,* proper fitting of a denture or accurate adjustment of bands to teeth; close approximation of filling material to the walls of a tooth cavity. 5. *In psychiatry,* The process of adjustment by an individual to intrapsychic, interpersonal, or social conditions.

adaptation disease. A biochemical or metabolic disorder due to physical or emotional stress, with a reversibility which may be effected spontaneously, therapeutically, or accidentally.

adapt·er, adap·tor, *n.* 1. A device which permits the fitting of one part of an instrument or apparatus to another, as a glass or rubber tube or metal collar. 2. An apparatus which converts the electric current to the form required in the various types of electrotherapy, or for a particular electrical appliance.

adap·tive, *adj.* 1. Capable of adapting. 2. Showing a tendency toward adaptation.

adaptive behavior. Any behavior that helps an organism adjust to its environment.

adaptive hypertrophy. An increase in size which acts as a compensatory mechanism to adapt an organ or other structure (as the heart or a skeletal muscle) to increased functional requirements.

ad·ap·tom·e·ter (ad″ap·tom′e·tur) *n.* An instrument for measuring the time taken for retinal adaptation or for regeneration of the rhodopsin (visual purple); used to determine the minimum light threshold and to diagnose night blindness.

adaptor. ADAPTER.

ad·ax·i·al (ad·ack′see·ul) *adj.* On the side of, or directed toward, the axis of a structure.

ADC Abbreviation for *anodic duration contraction.*

add. Abbreviation for *adde* or *additur* in prescription writing.

ad·de (ad′ee) Add; a direction used in prescription writing. Abbreviated, add.

¹**ad·dict** (ad′ikt) *n.* One who has become habituated to and dependent upon some practice, especially the use of alcohol or other drugs.

²**ad·dict** (uh·dikt′) *v.* To cause (an individual) to form an addiction. —**addict·ed,** *adj.*

ad·dic·tion (uh·dick′shun) *n.* Marked psychologic and physiological dependence upon a substance, such as alcohol or other drug, which has gone beyond voluntary control. —**addic·tive,** *adj.*

Addis count or **method** A technique for quantitative evaluation of the formed elements of urine, excluding squamous epithelial cells; the results are expressed as the numbers of a given element excreted per 24 hours.

Ad·di·so·ni·an (ad″i·so′nee·un) *adj.* Of or pertaining to Addison's disease or Addison's (pernicious) anemia.

Addisonian crisis. ADRENAL CRISIS.

Ad·di·son·ism (ad′i·sun·iz·um) *n.* 1. A syndrome sometimes present in pulmonary tuberculosis consisting of dark pigmentation of the skin, loss of weight and strength; somewhat resembles true Addison's disease. 2. ADDISON'S DISEASE (1).

Ad·di·son's anemia PERNICIOUS ANEMIA.

Addison's disease or **syndrome** 1. Primary adrenocortical insufficiency, characterized by weakness, skin and mucous membrane pigmentation or bronzing, emaciation, hypotension, and gastrointestinal symptoms; usually idiopathic, possibly due to an autoimmune mechanism, but known causes include tuberculosis and, more rarely, metastatic tumor, amyloidosis, and hemochromatosis. Syn. *asthenia pigmentosa, melanoma suprarenale.* 2. PERNICIOUS ANEMIA.

ad·di·tur (ad′i·tur, ·toor) Let there be added; a direction used in prescription writing. Abbreviated, add.

ad·du·cent (a·dew′sunt) *adj.* Adducting.

¹**ad·duct** (a·dukt′) *v.* 1. To draw toward the median line or plane of a body. 2. To turn the eyes inward from the central position.

²**ad·duct** (ad′ukt) *n.* A complex resulting from chemical addition of two compounds.

ad·duc·tion (a·duck′shun) *n.* 1. Any movement whereby one part is brought toward another or toward the median line or plane of the body or part. 2. *In ophthalmology,* turning of the eyes inward from the central position, through contraction of the medial rectus muscles. This action may be voluntary, but usually is subconscious, following the stimulus of accommodation.

ad·duc·tor (a·duck′tur) *n.* Any muscle that draws a part toward the median line of the body or of a part.

adductor canal. A triangular fascial tunnel in the anterior region of the thigh bounded by the sartorius, vastus medialis, and adductor muscles; it extends from the femoral triangle to the adductor hiatus and gives passage to the femoral vessels, saphenous nerve, and nerve to the vastus medialis muscle. Syn. *Hunter's canal, subsartorial canal.*

adductor hiatus. A gap in the insertion of the adductor magnus into the femur, the level of transition between the femoral and popliteal vessels.

adductor lon·gus (long′gus). The long adductor of the thigh.

adductor mag·nus (mag′nus). The large adductor of the thigh.

adductor reflex of the foot. Contraction of the posterior tibial muscle resulting in adduction, inversion, and slight plantar flexion of the foot on stroking its inner border from the great toe to the heel. Syn. *Hirschberg's reflex.*

adductor reflex of the thigh. Contraction of the adductors of the thigh, produced by tapping the tendon of the adductor magnus with the thigh in abduction.

adelph-, adelpho- A combining form meaning

(a) *sibling;* (b) *twin, double, multiple;* (c) *grouping of like units.*

aden-, adeno- A combining form meaning *gland, glandular.*

ad·e·nal·gia (ad″e·nal′jee·uh) *n.* A painful condition of a gland.

ad·e·nase (ad′e·nace, ·naze) *n.* A deaminating enzyme that converts adenine to hypoxanthine.

ad·e·nec·to·my (ad″e·neck′tuh·mee) *n.* The excision of a gland or lymph node.

aden·i·form (a·den′i·form) *adj.* Glandlike; shaped like a gland.

adenine arabinoside. 9-β-D-Arabinofuranosidoadenine, an antiviral agent possibly of value in the treatment of certain herpes virus infections. Syn. *ara-A, vidarabine.*

ad·e·ni·tis (ad″e·nigh′tis) *n.* Inflammation of a gland or lymph node.

ad·e·no·ac·an·tho·ma (ad″e·no·ack″an·tho′muh) *n.* An adenocarcinoma with foci of squamous cell differentiation, most commonly of endometrial origin.

ad·e·no·am·e·lo·blas·to·ma (ad″e·no·a·mel″o·blas·to′muh, ·am′e·lo·) *n.* An ameloblastoma in which the epithelium exhibits a glandular structure and arrangement.

ad·e·no·an·gio·sar·co·ma (ad″e·no·an″jee·o·sahr·ko′muh) *n.* A malignant mixed mesodermal tumor with foci of both glandular and vascular differentiation.

ad·e·no·car·ci·no·ma (ad″e·no·kahr″si·no′muh) *n.* 1. In histologic classification, a carcinoma in which the anaplastic parenchymal cells form glands. 2. In histogenetic classification, a carcinoma arising from the parenchyma of a gland.

ad·e·no·car·ci·no·ma·to·sis (ad″e·no·kahr″si·no″muh·to′sis) *n.* Widespread involvement of the body by an adenocarcinoma.

ad·e·no·cel·lu·li·tis (ad″e·no·sel″yoo·lye′tis) *n.* Inflammation of a gland and the surrounding tissue.

ad·e·no·chon·dro·ma (ad″e·no·kon·dro′muh) *n.* A tumor consisting of both glandular and cartilaginous tissue.

ad·e·no·cys·tic (ad″e·no·sis′tick) *adj.* Containing glands, some or all of which form cystic spaces.

adenocystic disease. CYSTIC DISEASE OF THE BREAST.

ad·e·no·cys·to·ma (ad″e·no·sis·to′muh) *n.* CYSTADENOMA.

adenocystoma lym·pho·ma·to·sum (lim·fo·muh·to′sum) WARTHIN'S TUMOR.

ad·e·no·fi·bro·ma (ad″e·no·figh·bro′muh) *n.* FIBROADENOMA.

ad·e·no·fi·bro·sis (ad″e·no·figh·bro′sis) *n.* 1. Fibrosis of a gland. 2. CYSTIC DISEASE OF THE BREAST.

ad·e·nog·e·nous (ad″e·noj′e·nus) *adj.* Originating from a gland.

ad·e·no·hy·poph·y·sis (ad″e·no·high·pof′i·sis) *n.* The anterior, glandular part of the hypophysis, developing from somatic ectoderm of the posterior nasopharynx and secreting the following important hormones: prolactin, growth hormone, adrenocorticotropic hormone (ACTH), melanocyte-stimulating hormone (MSH), thyroid-stimulating hormone (TSH), follicle-stimulating hormone (FSH), and luteinizing hormone (LH); consists of a main body (the pars distalis), a tuberal part (the pars tuberalis), which extends upward on the anterior surface of the infundibulum, and the pars intermedia, located between the pars distalis and the neurohypophysis and sometimes classified as part of the neurohypophysis. Syn. *anterior pituitary, anterior lobe of the hypophysis.* NA alt. *lobus anterior hypophyseos.* —**adeno·hy·poph·y·se·al** (·high·pof″i·see′ul, ·high″po·fiz′ee·ul), **adeno·hy·po·phys·i·al** (·high″po·fiz′ee·ul) *adj.*

ad·e·noid (ad′e·noid) *adj. & n.* 1. Glandlike or glandular; especially, lymphoid. 2. Pertaining to the adenoids. 3. Hyperplastic lymphoid tissue often present in the nasopharynx, especially in children. Syn. *pharyngeal tonsil.*

adenoid cystic carcinoma. A malignant tumor composed of nests and cords of small polygonal cells, often arranged in glandlike fashion around cores of mucoid material; found in the lower respiratory tract and salivary glands and occasionally in such other locations as the breast.

ad·e·noid·ec·to·my (ad″e·noy·deck′tuh·mee) *n.* Surgical removal of the adenoids.

adenoid facies. The characteristic open-mouthed and pinched-nose appearance associated with adenoid hypertrophy which interferes with nasal breathing.

ad·e·noid·ism (ad″e·noy·diz′um) *n.* A series of changes in respiration, facial contour, and tooth arrangement attributed to the presence of adenoids.

ad·e·noid·itis (ad″e·noy·dye′tis) *n.* Inflammation of the adenoids.

adenoid tissue. LYMPHATIC TISSUE.

ad·e·no·leio·my·o·ma (ad″e·no·lye″o·migh·o′muh) *n.* ADENOMYOMA.

ad·e·no·li·po·ma (ad″e·no·li·po′muh) *n.* A benign tumor with both glandular and adipose tissue elements.

ad·e·no·lym·pho·ma (ad″e·no·lim·fo′muh) *n.* Squamoid metaplasia of salivary gland tissue with hyperplasia of ectopic lymphoid tissue in the salivary gland.

ad·e·no·ma (ad″e·no′muh) *n.,* pl. **adenomas, adenoma·ta** (·tuh) A benign epithelial tumor whose parenchymal cells are similar to those composing the epithelium from which it arises; usually employed with tumors of the parenchyma of glands, but also applied to benign tumors of mucosal epithelium.

adenoma des·tru·ens (des′troo·enz). An adenoma with aggressive and destructive characteristics.

ad·e·no·ma·la·cia (ad″e·no·muh·lay′shuh, ·see·uh) *n.* Abnormal softening of a gland.

adenoma ma·lig·num (ma·lig′num). MALIGNANT ADENOMA.

adenoma sebaceum PRINGLE'S ADENOMA SEBACEUM.

ad·e·nom·a·toid (ad″e·nom′uh·toid, ·no′muh·toid) *adj.* Pertaining to or resembling an adenoma.

adenomatoid tumor. A rare, small, benign neoplasm of both male and female genital tracts, composed of varied stroma containing irregular spaces lined by cells which may resemble endothelium, epithelium, or mesothelium.

ad·e·no·ma·to·sis (ad″e·no″muh·to′sis) n., pl. **adenomato·ses** (·seez). The occurrence of adenomas at several sites within an organ, as in the lung, or in several related organs, as in the endocrine system.

ad·e·nom·a·tous (ad″e·nom′uh·tus) adj. Pertaining to an adenoma.

adenomatous goiter. Nodular hyperplasia of the thyroid. Syn. *nodular goiter, multiple colloid adenomatous goiter.*

ad·e·no·my·o·ma (ad″e·no·migh·o′muh) n. Endometriosis involving a leiomyoma, usually of the uterus. Syn. *adenoleiomyoma.*

ad·e·no·myo·sal·pin·gi·tis (ad″e·no·migh″o·sal′pin·jye′tis) n. ISTHMIC NODULAR SALPINGITIS.

ad·e·no·myo·sar·co·ma (ad″e·no·migh″o·sahr·ko′muh) n. A malignant mixed mesodermal tumor composed of muscular and glandular elements.

ad·e·no·my·o·sis (ad″e·no·migh·o′sis) n. 1. Endometriosis involving muscular tissues such as the uterine wall or the uterine tube. 2. Any abnormal growth of glands and muscle fibers.

ad·e·no·myxo·chon·dro·sar·co·ma (ad″e·no·mick″so·kon″dro·sahr·ko′muh) n. A malignant mixed mesodermal tumor containing glandular, myxoid, and cartilaginous elements.

ad·e·no·myx·o·ma (ad″e·no·mick·so′muh) n. A benign tumor containing glandular and myxoid elements, as mixed tumors of the salivary glands.

ad·e·no·myxo·sar·co·ma (ad″e·no·mick″so·sahr·ko′muh) n. A malignant mixed mesodermal tumor containing glandular and myxoid elements.

ad·e·nop·a·thy (ad″e·nop′uth·ee) n. Any glandular disease, especially one characterized by swelling and enlargement of lymph nodes.

ad·e·no·phar·yn·gi·tis (ad″e·no·făr″in·jye′tis) n. Inflammation of the tonsils and pharynx.

ad·e·no·sar·co·ma (ad″e·no·sahr·ko′muh) n. A malignant mixed mesodermal tumor with glandular and supportive tissue elements.

ad·e·nose (ad′e·noce, ·noze) adj. Glandular; abounding in glands; glandlike.

aden·o·sine (a·den′o·seen, ·sin) n. Adenine riboside, $C_{10}H_{13}N_5O_4$, a nucleoside composed of one molecule each of adenine and D-ribose; one of the four main riboside components of ribonucleic acid.

adenosine di·phos·phate (dye·fos′fate). $C_{10}H_{15}N_5O_{10}P_2$, a compound consisting of one molecule each of adenine and D-ribose and one molecule of pyrophosphoric acid. It is an intermediate in the production of energy by the cell. Abbreviated, ADP. Syn. *adenosinediphosphoric acid, adenosine pyrophosphate.*

adenosine mono·phos·phate (mon″o·fos′fate). $C_{10}H_{14}N_5O_7P$, an ester composed of one molecule each of adenine, D-ribose, and phosphoric acid. Adenosine 5′-monophosphate, or muscle adenylic acid, is an intermediate in the release of energy for muscular and other types of cellular work. Adenosine 3′-monophosphate (yeast adenylic acid) is found in yeast. Abbreviated, AMP. Syn. *adenosinemonophosphoric acid, adenylic acid.*

adenosine tri·phos·pha·tase (trye·fos′fuh·tace, ·taze). An enzyme that catalyzes hydrolysis of adenosine triphosphate, especially one by which adenosine diphosphate and phosphate ion are formed, whereby free chemical energy for various cellular activities, including muscular contraction, is released.

adenosine tri·phos·phate (trye·fos′fate). $C_{10}H_{16}N_5O_{13}P_3$, a compound consisting of one molecule each of adenine and D-ribose with three molecules of phosphoric acid. Hydrolysis of it to similar esters containing one or two molecules of phosphoric acid is accompanied by release of energy for muscular and other types of cellular activity. Abbreviated, ATP. Syn. *adenosinetriphosphoric acid, adenylpyrophosphoric acid, adenylpyrophosphate.*

aden·o·sine·tri·phos·pho·ric acid (a·den′o·seen·trye″fos·for′ick). ADENOSINE TRIPHOSPHATE.

ad·e·no·sis (ad″e·no′sis) n., pl. **adeno·ses** (·seez) 1. Development of an excessive number of glandular elements without tumor formation. 2. Any glandular disease, especially of the lymph nodes.

adenosis of the breast. A form of mammary dysplasia characterized by excessive ductular and acinar proliferation.

ad·e·no·tome (ad′e·no·tome) n. An instrument for removing the adenoids.

ad·e·not·o·my (ad″e·not′uh·mee) n. Incision of a gland.

ad·e·no·vi·rus (ad″e·no·vye′rus) n. A member of a large group of medium-sized, ether-resistant DNA viruses which may be pathogenic for the mucous membranes of the eye and the respiratory tract; associated with such syndromes as acute respiratory disease, pharyngoconjunctival fever, nonbacterial exudative pharyngitis, pneumonia, and sporadic and epidemic keratoconjunctivitis. Syn. *APC virus.*

ad·e·nyl·ic acid (ad″e·nil′ick). ADENOSINE MONOPHOSPHATE.

ad·eps (ad′eps) n., pl. **adi·pes** (ad′i·peez) 1. Lard, the purified omental fat of the hog; formerly used in ointments. 2. Animal fat.

ADH Abbreviation for (a) *antidiuretic hormone;* (b) *alcohol dehydrogenase.*

A.D.H.A. American Dental Hygienists Association.

ad·he·sion (ad·hee′zhun) n. 1. *In physics,* molecular force exerted between two surfaces in contact. 2. Abnormal fibrous union of an organ or part to another.

ad·he·si·ot·o·my (ad·hee″zee·ot′uh·mee) n. *In surgery,* cutting or division of adhesions.

ad·he·sive (ad·hee′ziv) adj. & n. 1. Sticky; tenacious; tending to cling or stick. 2. Resulting in or attended with adhesion. 3. An adhesive substance. 4. ADHESIVE PLASTER.

adhesive arachnoiditis. CHRONIC ADHESIVE ARACHNOIDITIS.

adhesive pericardiomediastinitis. Fibrous adhesions between the pericardium and the mediastinum.

adhesive pericarditis. A form of pericarditis in which the two layers of serous pericardium tend to adhere by means of fibrous adhesions, usually the result of the organization of acute exudate.

adhesive plaster or **tape.** A composition having pressure-sensitive adhesive properties, spread evenly upon fabric, the back of which may be coated with a water-repellent film.

adi·ad·o·cho·ki·ne·sis, adi·ad·o·ko·ki·ne·sis (ay"dye·ad"o·ko·ki·nee'sis, ad"ee·ad"o·ko·) n. Inability to perform rapidly alternating movements, such as pronation and supination of the hands; seen in cerebellar disease and, in a milder form, in children with the minimal brain dysfunction syndrome.

adi·a·pho·ret·ic (ay·dye"uh·fo·ret'ick) adj. & n. 1. Reducing, checking, or preventing perspiration; anhidrotic. 2. Any agent or drug that reduces, checks, or prevents perspiration. —**adiapho·re·sis** (·ree'sis) n.

a·di·as·to·le (ay"dye·as'tuh·lee, ad"eye·) n. Absence or imperceptibility of diastole.

Adie's pupil (ay'dee) An abnormality of the pupil characterized by very slow adaptation and accommodation. The myotonic pupil will contract or dilate only after prolonged stimulation but is unusually sensitive to a 2.5% Mecholyl salt solution, which will not constrict a normal pupil. Syn. *Adie's tonic pupil, pseudo Argyll Robertson pupil.*

Adie's syndrome Loss or impairment of pupillary constriction in reaction to light and slowness of constriction during accommodation, associated with loss of tendon reflexes in the legs.

adip-, adipo- A combining form meaning *fat, fats, fatty tissue.*

ad·i·pec·to·my (ad"i·peck'tuh·mee) n. Surgical removal of a mass of adipose tissue.

ad·i·phen·ine (ad"i·fen'een, a·dif'e·neen) n. 2-Diethylaminoethyl diphenylacetate, $C_{20}H_{25}NO_2$, an antispasmodic agent; used as the hydrochloride salt.

adip·ic (a·dip'ick) adj. Of or pertaining to fat.

ad·i·po·cele (ad"i·po·seel) n. A true hernia with a hernial sac, containing only fatty tissue. Syn. *lipocele.*

ad·i·po·cel·lu·lar (ad"i·po·sel'yoo·lur) adj. Made up of fat and connective tissue.

ad·i·po·cere (ad'i·po·seer) n. A wax-like substance formed during decomposition of dead animal tissues (corpses) in the presence of moisture and in the absence of air, as under earth or water. It consists chiefly of fatty acids and their salts. —**ad·i·po·cer·a·tous** (ad"i·po·serr'uh·tus) adj.

ad·i·po·ma (ad"i·po'muh) n. LIPOMA.

ad·i·po·ne·cro·sis (ad"i·po·ne·kro'sis) n. Necrosis of fatty tissue.

adiponecrosis neo·na·to·rum. (nee"o·nay·to'rum). Localized process of necrosis of fatty tissue occurring usually in large, well-nourished infants born after difficult labor, characterized by bluish-red lesions that become manifest 2 to 20 days after birth as deep subcutaneous indurations.

ad·i·pose (ad'i·poce) adj. Fatty, fatlike, fat.

adipose gynism. SIMPSON'S SYNDROME in girls.

adipose tissue. A form of connective tissue consisting of fat cells lodged in areolar tissue and arranged in lobules along the course of small blood vessels.

ad·i·po·sis (ad"i·po'sis) n. ADIPOSITY.

adiposis do·lo·ro·sa (do"luh·ro'suh). Extensive subcutaneous painful lipomas or diffuse accumulations of fat, occurring primarily during menopause. Syn. *Dercum's disease.*

ad·i·po·si·tis (ad"i·po·sigh'tis) n. Inflammation of the subcutaneous fatty tissue.

ad·i·pos·i·ty (ad"i·pos'i·tee) n. 1. Corpulence; obesity. 2. An excessive accumulation of fat in the body, localized or general; fatty infiltration. Syn. *adiposis.*

ad·i·po·so·gen·i·tal (ad"i·po"so·jen'i·tul) adj. Involving both adipose tissue and genitalia.

adiposogenital dystrophy. Adiposity, retarded development of gonads, and occasionally diabetes insipidus; results from impaired function of the pituitary and hypothalamus; may be caused by craniopharyngioma, tumors of the hypophysis or other structures adjacent to the hypothalamus, trauma, basilar meningitis, or encephalitis. Syn. *Froelich's syndrome.*

ad·i·po·su·ria (ad"i·po·sue'ree·uh) n. The presence of fat in the urine; LIPURIA.

adip·sia (ay·dip'see·uh, a·dip') n. Absence of thirst; avoidance of drinking.

adip·sy (ay·dip'see, a·dip'see, ad'ip·see) n. ADIPSIA.

A disk. The transverse segment of a myofibril (or of a whole muscle fiber) which appears longitudinally as an A band.

ad·i·tus (ad'i·tus, a·dit'us) n., pl. **aditus, adituses** In anatomy, an entrance or inlet.

aditus la·ryn·gis (la·rin'jis) [NA]. The entrance to the larynx, bounded anteriorly by the epiglottis, posteriorly by the upper ends of and the notch between the arytenoid and corniculate cartilages, and laterally by the aryepiglottic folds.

ad·just·ment. n. 1. *In biology,* changes undergone by a plant or animal better to adapt to its environment. 2. *In psychology,* the establishment of a relatively harmonious or functionally effective relationship between the individual, his inner self, and his environment. 3. The mechanism of a microscope which brings the objective into focus. 4. Chiropractic treatment aimed at reduction of subluxated vertebrae. 5. Modification of a completed dental restoration, appliance, or prosthesis.

adjustment reaction. A transient situational disturbance of personality occurring in reaction to some significant person, immediate event, or internal emotional conflict. The character of the reaction often varies with the age group.

adjuvant arthritis. Arthritis produced in rats by a single subcutaneous injection of Freund's adjuvant into the foot pad or tail; used as an experimental model for rheumatoid arthritis.

Ad·le·ri·an (ad·leer'ee·un) adj. Pertaining to the doctrines and followers of Alfred Adler, Austrian psychiatrist, 1870–1937, founder of the school of individual psychology.

ad·me·di·al (ad-mee'dee-ul) *adj.* Located near or approaching the median plane or central axis.

ad·mi·nic·u·lum (ad''mi·nick'yoo·lum) *n.*, pl. **ad·minicu·la** (·luh) 1. A supporting structure. 2. A triangular fibrous expansion which extends from the superior pubic ligament to the posterior surface of the linea alba.

ad·mix·ture (ad·micks'chur) *n.* 1. The act, process, or product of mixing. 2. A substance added by mixing.

ad·nate (ad'nate) *adj.* Congenitally attached or united.

ad nau·se·am (ad naw'zee·um, ·shee·um) To the point of producing nausea.

ad·nexa (ad·neck'suh) *n.*, sing. **adnex·um** Accessory parts or appendages of an organ. Syn. *annexa.* **—adnex·al** (·sul) *adj.*

adnexa ocu·li (ock'yoo·lye). Appendages of the eye, as the lids and the lacrimal apparatus.

adnexa ute·ri (yoo'tur·eye). The uterine tubes and ovaries.

ad·nex·i·tis (ad''neck·sigh'tis) *n.* Inflammation of the adnexa uteri; SALPINGO-OOPHORITIS.

ad·o·les·cence, *n.* The period of life extending from puberty to maturity. **—adoles·cent,** *adj. & n.*

adolescent crisis. IDENTITY CRISIS.

adolescent goiter. Diffuse enlargement of the thyroid of unknown cause, most frequently seen in girls during puberty.

ad·oral (ad·or'ul) *adj.* Situated near the mouth; toward the mouth. **—adoral·ly,** *adv.*

ad·or·bit·al (ad·or'bi·tul) *adj.* Situated near the orbit; toward the orbit.

ADP Abbreviation for *adenosine diphosphate.*

adren–, adreno–. A combining form meaning *adrenal.*

ad·re·nal (a·dree'nul) *adj. & n.* 1. Situated adjacent to the kidney. 2. Pertaining to the adrenal glands. 3. ADRENAL GLAND.

adrenal apoplexy. Hemorrhage into the adrenal glands, usually part of the Waterhouse-Friderichsen syndrome.

adrenal cortex. The cortical portion of the adrenal gland.

adrenal cortical insufficiency. An acute or chronic failure of adrenal cortical secretion of glucocorticoid and mineralocorticoid hormones; the primary form is due to adrenal cortical disease and the secondary form to insufficient pituitary adrenocorticotropic hormone.

adrenal crisis. Acute adrenal failure; severe acute exacerbation of Addison's disease. Syn. *Addisonian crisis.*

adre·nal·ec·to·my (a·dree''nul·eck'tuh·mee) *n.* Surgical removal of an adrenal gland. **—adrenalecto·mize,** *v.*

adrenal gland. An endocrine gland located immediately above the superior pole of each kidney. It consists of a medulla that produces epinephrine and norepinephrine, and a cortex that is the source of many steroidal hormones involved in electrolyte and fluid balance, or in carbohydrate and protein metabolism. Syn. *suprarenal gland.*

Adrenalin. A trademark for epinephrine, the adrenal medullary hormone.

adren·a·line (a·dren'uh·lin, ·leen) *n. British Pharmacopoeia and Amer. colloq.* EPINEPHRINE.

adren·a·lin·emia, adren·a·lin·ae·mia (a·dren''uh·li·nee'mee·uh) *n.* The presence of epinephrine in the blood.

adren·a·lin·uria (a·dren''uh·li·nyoor'ee·uh) *n.* The presence of epinephrine in the urine.

adre·nal·ism (a·dree'nul·iz·um, a·dren''ul·iz·um) *n.* A condition due to dysfunction of the adrenal glands.

adre·nal·itis (a·dree''nul·eye'tis) *n.* Inflammation of the adrenal glands.

adrenal medulla. The medulla of the adrenal gland.

adrenal virilism syndrome. ADRENOGENITAL SYNDROME.

ad·re·ner·gic (ad''re·nur'jick) *adj.* Of or pertaining to the type of chemical activity characteristic of epinephrine and epinephrine-like substances.

adrenergic blocking agent. Any compound that selectively inhibits certain responses to adrenergic nerve activity and to norepinephrine and other sympathomimetic amines. On the basis of selective inhibition of the responses, the compounds may be classified as alpha- or beta-adrenergic blocking agents. Syn. *adrenolytic agent, sympatholytic agent.*

adrenergic nerve fibers. Nerve fibers which, upon stimulation, liberate norepinephrine at their terminations; include most of the postganglionic fibers of the sympathetic nervous system.

adrenergic receptor. See *alpha-adrenergic receptor, beta-adrenergic receptor.*

adre·no·chrome (a·dree'no·krome) *n.* A quinone-type oxidation product, $C_9H_9NO_3$, of epinephrine; occurs as red crystals.

adre·no·cor·ti·cal (a·dree''no·kor'ti·kul) *adj.* Pertaining to or derived from the adrenal cortex.

adrenocortical hormone. Any of the biologically active steroid hormones which have been isolated from the adrenal cortex.

adrenocortical obesity. BUFFALO OBESITY.

adre·no·cor·ti·coid (a·dree''no·kor'ti·koid) *adj. & n.* 1. Pertaining to or resembling the adrenal cortex or the hormones secreted by it. 2. An adrenal cortical hormone.

adrenocorticoid adenoma of the ovary. One of a group of rare masculinizing tumors of the ovary, of cells resembling those of the adrenal cortex; characteristically causes defemination or virilism.

adre·no·cor·ti·co·mi·met·ic (a·dree''no·kor'ti·ko·migh·met'ick, ·mi·met'ick) *adj.* Similar in activity or effect to an adrenal cortical steroid.

adre·no·cor·ti·co·tro·phic (a·dree''no·kor''ti·ko·tro'fick, ·trof'ick) *adj. Erron.* ADRENOCORTICOTROPIC.

adrenocorticotropic hormone. The adenohypophyseal hormone which stimulates and maintains the growth and hormone-secretory function of the adrenal cortex. Abbreviated, ACTH. Syn. *adrenocorticotropin.*

adre·no·cor·ti·co·tro·pin (a·dree''no·kor''ti·ko·tro'pin) *n.* ADRENOCORTICOTROPIC HORMONE.

adrenogenital syndrome. A clinical condition associated with hypersecretion of androgenic hormones by adrenal cortical tissue or due to excess steroid hormone administration. It may be congenital or acquired; the acquired forms are due to adrenal hyperplasia or tumor. In the female, the congenital forms may result in pseudohermaphroditism and advanced physical growth, while the acquired forms may produce enlargement of the clitoris or virilism. In the male, the congenital forms manifest early enlargement of the penis and advanced somatic growth; in the acquired forms, these findings appear later; rarely, an adrenal tumor in the male produces feminization with gynecomastia.

adre·no·lyt·ic (a·dree″no·lit′ick) adj. Inhibiting the function of adrenergic nerves or the physiologic responses to the action of epinephrine or norepinephrine.

adre·no·med·ul·lary (a·dree″no·med′yoo·lerr·ee, ·me·dul′ur·ee) adj. Of or pertaining to the adrenal medulla.

adre·no·pause (a·dree′no·pawz) n. The hypothetical age at which production of certain adrenocortical hormones is reduced.

adre·no·sym·pa·thet·ic (a·dree″no·sim″puh·thet′ick) adj. Pertaining to the adrenal glands and the sympathetic nervous system.

adrenosympathetic syndrome. Episodes of paroxysmal hypertension, nervousness, tachycardia, palpitations, sweating, flushing or pallor, headache, nausea, vomiting, glycosuria, and chest and abdominal pain due to increased epinephrine and norepinephrine secretion, usually caused by pheochromocytoma, but at times by neuroblastoma or ganglioneuroma. Syn. *Page's syndrome.*

adre·no·tro·pic (a·dree″no·tro′pick) adj. Having or pertaining to an effect on the adrenal gland, particularly the cortex.

ad·re·not·ro·pism (ad″re·not′ro·piz·um, a·dree″ no·tro′piz·um) n. Dominance of the adrenal in the endocrine functions.

adro·mia (a·dro′mee·uh) n. Complete failure of impulse conduction in muscle or nerve.

ad·sorb (ad·sorb′) v. Of a substance: to attract and concentrate upon its surface, in a thin layer, molecules of a gas, liquid, or dissolved substance. —**adsorbed,** adj.

ad·sor·bate (ad·sor′bate, ad·zor′bate) n. Any substance that is adsorbed.

ad·sor·bent (ad·sor′bunt) adj. & n. 1. Adsorbing or having the capacity to adsorb. 2. Any adsorbent substance, such as activated charcoal or silica gel.

ad·sorp·tion (ad·sorp′shun) n. The process of adsorbing or of being adsorbed. —**adsorptive** (·tiv) adj.

ad·tor·sion (ad·tor′shun) n. A condition in which both eyes are turned toward the nose, and their vertical meridians converge above instead of being parallel.

adult, adj. & n. 1. Mature; having attained full size, strength, and reproductive ability. 2. In human society: having attained the ability to handle personal affairs; of full legal age. 3. A full-grown and mature individual. 4. Of or pertaining to adults.

adult celiac disease. CELIAC SYNDROME.

adul·ter·ant (a·dul′tur·unt) n. Any substance that adulterates.

adul·ter·a·tion (a·dul″tur·ay′shun) n. Admixture or substitution of inferior, impure, inert, or cheaper ingredients for gain, deception, or concealment. —**adul·ter·ate** (a·dul′tur·ate) v.

adult Fanconi syndrome A recessive heritable or acquired disorder of renal tubular function, beginning in adult life and characterized by any combination of proteinuria, aminoaciduria, renal glycosuria, hyperphosphaturia, hypophosphatemia, acidosis, and resultant severe osteomalacia. Cystinosis, however, does not occur.

adult Still's disease Obsol. FELTY'S SYNDROME.

adult-type tuberculosis. CHRONIC TUBERCULOSIS.

ad·vance, v. In ophthalmology and surgery, to perform an advancement.

ad·vance·ment, n. 1. A tenotomy followed by reattachment of the tendon at a more advanced point. 2. In ophthalmology, operative correction of strabismus, in which the muscle tendon opposite to the direction of the squint is removed at its insertion and sutured to the sclera anterior to the original attachment.

ad·ven·ti·tia (ad″ven·tish′ee·uh) n. 1. The external covering of an organ derived from adjacent connective tissue. 2. Specifically, the outermost of the three coats of a blood vessel, consisting of connective tissue and elastic fibers. —**adven·ti·tial** (·tish′ul) adj.

ad·ven·ti·tious (ad″ven·tish′us) adj. 1. Accidental, foreign, acquired, as opposed to natural or hereditary. 2. Occurring in unusual or abnormal places. 3. Pertaining to the adventitia.

adventitious albuminuria. Proteinuria without detectable renal disease.

adventitious bursa. ACCIDENTAL BURSA.

adverse drug reaction. As defined by the Food and Drug Administration: a reaction that is noxious, unintended, and occurs at doses normally used in man for prophylaxis, diagnosis, or therapy of disease.

ad·ver·sive (ad·vur′siv) adj. Turning to one side; pertaining to rotation of the eyes, head, or trunk.

adversive seizure. CONTRAVERSIVE SEIZURE.

ady·nam·ia (ay″di·nam′ee·uh, ad″i·nay′mee·uh) n. Loss of vital strength or muscular power; weakness; debility; ASTHENIA. —**ady·nam·ic** (·nam′ick) adj.

adynamia epi·sod·i·ca he·red·i·ta·ria (ep″i·sod′i·kuh he·red″i·tair′ee·uh). A form of periodic paralysis, usually with hyperkalemia and sometimes with minor degrees of myotonia. Syn. *Gamstorp's disease.*

adynamic ileus. General or regional failure of peristalsis due to inadequate intestinal muscular activity, resulting in intestinal obstruction.

Aë·des (ay·ee′deez) n. A genus of mosquitoes of the family Culicidae, of cosmopolitan distribution and including about 600 species, some of which are important vectors of human diseases, such as yellow fever, dengue, virus encephalitis, and certain filarial infections.

Aëdes ae·gyp·ti (ee·jip'tye). The principal vector of yellow fever and dengue. It breeds in urban areas.

ae·lu·ro·phil·ia (e·lew''ro·fil'ee·uh) *n.* GALEOPHILIA.

ae·lu·ro·pho·bia (e·lew''ro·fo'bee·uh) *n.* GALEOPHOBIA.

ae·lu·rop·sis (ee''lew·rop'sis, el''yoo·) *n.* Obliquity of the eye or of the palpebral fissure.

ae·quum (ee'kwum) *n. Obsol.* The caloric intake necessary to maintain weight with normal physical activity. It varies with the individual's size and the nature of his activity.

aer-, aero- A combining form meaning (a) *air, aerial;* (b) *gas, gases.*

aer·ate (ay'ur·ate, air'ate) *v.* To charge with air or gas; to oxygenate, carbonate; to arterialize. **—aer·at·ed** (·id) *adj.;* **aer·a·tor** (·ay·tur) *n.*

aer·a·tion (ay''ur·ay'shun, air''ay'shun) *n.* 1. Exposure to air. 2. Saturation of a fluid with air or a gas, as carbon dioxide. 3. The exchange of oxygen and carbon dioxide in the lungs.

aer·emia, aer·ae·mia (ay''ur·ee'mee·uh, air·) *n.* The presence of air in the blood.

aer·i·form (ay'ur·i·form, ay·eer') *adj.* Airlike; gaseous.

aero·at·e·lec·ta·sis (air''o·at''e·leck'tuh·sis, ay''ur·o·) *n.* A partial, reversible collapse of the lungs observed in aviators breathing 100% oxygen while flying at high altitudes.

Aero·bac·ter (ay''ur·o·back'tur, air'o·back''tur) *n.* ENTEROBACTER.

Aerobacter aerogenes. ENTEROBACTER AEROGENES.

aer·obe (ay'ur·obe, air''obe) *n.* A microorganism which requires air or oxygen for the maintenance of life. The final hydrogen acceptor is molecular oxygen.

aer·o·bic (ay''ur·o'bick, air·) *adj.* 1. Utilizing oxygen. 2. Requiring air or free oxygen in order to live. 3. Pertaining to or produced by aerobes.

aero·bi·ol·o·gy (ay''ur·o·bye·ol'uh·jee, air''o·) *n.* The science concerned with air-borne microbes, pollen, spores, dust, smoke, and other substances, as well as with their occurrence, characteristics, relation to human welfare, and control.

aero·bi·o·sis (ay''ur·o·bye·o'sis, air''o·) *n.* Life that requires the presence of air, or molecular oxygen. **—aerobi·ot·ic** (·ot'ick) *adj.*

aero·cele (ay'ur·o·seel, air'o·) *n.* A swelling caused by the escape of air into an adventitious pouch usually connected with the trachea (tracheocele) or larynx (laryngocele); hence its size may vary with respiration or straining.

aero·col·pos (ay''ur·o·kol'pos, air''o·) *n.* Distention of the vagina with air or gas.

aero·cys·tos·co·py (ay''ur·o·sis·tos'kuh·pee, air''o·) *n.* Examination of the interior of the urinary bladder with a cystoscope, the bladder being distended with air. **—aero·cys·to·scope** (·sis'tuh·skope) *n.*

aer·o·don·tal·gia (air''o·don·tal'jee·uh, ay''ur·o''don·) *n.* Pain occurring in the teeth of individuals exposed to decreased atmospheric pressure such as may occur from high-altitude ascent and in decompression chambers.

aero·duc·tor (ay''o·duck'tur, ay''ur·o·) *n.* An apparatus to prevent asphyxia of the fetus when the aftercoming head is retained; no longer in common clinical use.

aero·gen (air'o·jen, ay'ur·o·) *n.* Any gas-producing microorganism.

aer·o·gen·e·sis (air''o·jen'e·sis, ay''ur·o·) *n.* Gas formation. **—aerogen·ic** (·ick), **aer·og·e·nous** (ay''ur·oj'e·nus) *adj.*

aero·gram (air'o·gram, ay'ur·o·) *n.* An x-ray film of an organ inflated with air; PNEUMOGRAM

Aerohalor. Trademark for a device to insufflate drugs into the respiratory tract.

aer·om·e·ter (air·om'e·tur, ay''ur·) *n.* An instrument for determining the density of gases.

aero·neu·ro·sis (air''o·new·ro'sis, ay''ur·o·) *n.* A form of neurosis found in aviators, characterized by anxiety, restlessness, and various physical manifestations.

aero·oti·tis (air''o·o·tye'tis, ay''ur·o·) *n.* BAROTITIS.

aer·op·a·thy (ay''ur·op'uth·ee) *n.* Any pathologic condition brought about by changes in atmospheric pressure, as decompression sickness.

aero·peri·to·ne·um, aero·peri·to·nae·um (air''o·perr''i·tuh·nee'um, ay''ur·o·) *n.* PNEUMOPERITONEUM.

aero·pha·gia (ay''ur·o·fay'jee·uh, air''o·) *n.* Spasmodic swallowing of air followed by noisy eructations.

aer·oph·a·gy (ay''ur·off'uh·jee) *n.* AEROPHAGIA.

aer·o·phil (air'o·fil, ay'ur·o·) *adj.* 1. Loving the open air. 2. AEROBIC (2).

aero·pho·bia (air''o·fo'bee·uh, ay''ur·o·) *n.* Morbid fear of drafts or of fresh air.

aero·phore (air'o·for, ay'ur·o·) *n.* 1. A device for inflating the lungs with air in any case of asphyxia. 2. An apparatus which purifies air for rebreathing, used by firemen and others.

Aeroplast. Trademark for vibesate, a film-forming surgical dressing.

aer·o·scope (air'o·skope, ay'ur·o·) *n.* An instrument for the examination of air dust and for estimating the purity of the air.

aero·si·nus·itis (ay''ur·o·sigh''nuh·sigh'tis, air''o·) *n.* BAROSINUSITIS.

aer·o·sis (air·o'sis, ay'ur·) *n.* Formation of gas in any of the body tissues.

aero·sol (air'o·sol, ay'ur·o·) *n.* 1. Atomized particles suspended in the air. 2. Any solution or compressed gas containing an agent for the treatment of the air to remove or destroy insects or microorganisms. 3. *In chemistry,* a colloid in which a gas is the dispersion medium.

Aerosporin. A trademark for polymyxin B sulfate, an antibiotic substance.

aero·ther·a·peu·tics (air''o·therr''uh·pew'ticks, ay''ur·o·) *n.* A mode of treating disease by varying the pressure or the composition of the air breathed.

aerotitis media BAROTITIS MEDIA.

aer·ot·ro·pism (air·ot'ro·piz·um, ay''ur·) *n.* 1. The inherent tendency of an aerobic organism to be attracted to a supply of air (positive aerotropism), as when various bacteria and protozoa collect about an air bubble; or (negative aerotropism) to be repelled by a supply of air. 2. *In botany*, the deviation of plant structures, such as roots, from the normal growth patterns because of the presence of air. —**aero·trop·ic** (air″o·trop'ick, ay″ur·o·) *adj.*

aero·ure·thro·scope (air″o·yoo·ree'thruh·skope) *n.* A modified endoscope which permits viewing the urethra after it is inflated with air. —**aero·ure·thros·co·py** (·yoo″ree·thros'skuh·pee) *n.*

Aes·cu·la·pi·an (es″kew·lay'pee·un) *adj.* 1. Of or pertaining to the art of healing; medical; medicinal. 2. Specifically, pertaining to the practices of the Aesculapian sect of healers in ancient Greece and Asia Minor.

afe·brile (ay·feb'ril, ·feeb') *adj.* Without fever.

¹**af·fect** (af'ekt) *n.* 1. *In psychology*, the emotional aspect or feeling tone of a mental state, sensation, perception, or idea; affection as compared to cognition and conation in any mental process. 2. *In Freudian psychology*, the sum total of the various feelings which may be conscious or suppressed, accompanying or influencing a mental state or idea. 3. Psychic tension as manifested by certain bodily changes, such as perspiration, tachycardia, or blushing. 4. Class name for any emotion, feeling, mood, temperament. 5. A specific feeling or emotion, such as joy or sadness.

²**af·fect** (uh·fekt') *v.* 1. To produce an effect upon. 2. To make an impression, as on the mind or emotions.

af·fect·a·bil·i·ty *n.* The capacity for responding to stimulation.

af·fec·tion, *n.* 1. Any pathologic state or condition. 2. *In psychology*, the emotional factor in consciousness.

af·fec·tive (a·feck'tiv) *adj.* Pertaining to or involving affect or affection.

affective disorder or **psychosis.** Any major mental disorder which is characterized by episodes of extreme depression or elation, dominating the mental life of the patient and responsible for whatever loss of contact there is with the environment. The swings of mood are not precipitated by external events, and there is a strong hereditary component.

af·fec·tiv·i·ty (af″eck·tiv'i·tee) *n.* Susceptibility to emotional stimuli; emotionality.

af·fec·to·mo·tor (a·feck″to·mo'tur) *adj.* Exhibiting emotional disturbance and muscular activity.

af·fer·ent (af'ur·unt) *adj.* Carrying toward; centripetal.

afferent loop syndrome. Upper abdominal fullness and pain after meals, relieved by bilious vomiting; it is caused by impaired emptying of the proximal loop of a gastrojejunostomy.

afferent lymphatic. A vessel conveying lymph to a lymph node.

afferent nerve. A nerve that transmits impulses from the periphery to the central nervous system; a sensory nerve.

afferent neuron. A neuron that conducts impulses to a nerve center; in the peripheral nervous system, that neuron which conducts impulses to nuclei in the central nervous system.

af·fil·i·a·tion (a·fil″ee·ay'shun) *n. In legal medicine,* imputing or fixing the paternity of a child.

af·fi·nal (a·fighn'nul) *adj.* 1. Connected through marriage. 2. Having the same origin.

af·fin·i·ty, *n.* 1. An inherent relationship or selective tendency, often mutual, as an attraction, resemblance, kinship, or liking. 2. *In chemistry,* the force of attraction between atoms which causes them to enter into and maintain certain combinations. 3. *In immunology,* the attractive force between antigen and antibody. 4. *In biology,* the relationship between members of different species or more specialized groups which depends upon their resemblance in structure, implying a common origin.

af·fir·ma·tion, *n.* During autosuggestion, the stage in which the subject acquires a positive reactive tendency; facilitation of positive reaction tendency.

af·flux (af'lucks) *n.* A sudden flow of blood or other fluid to a part. —**af·flu·ent** (af'lew·unt) *adj.;* **afflu·ence** (·unce) *n.*

af·fu·sion (a·few'zhun) *n.* Pouring of water upon a part or upon the body, as in fever, to reduce temperature and calm nervous symptoms. Treating fevers by pouring cold water over the patient is called cold affusion.

afi·brin·o·gen·emia, afi·brin·o·gen·ae·mia (ay″figh·brin″o·jen·ee'mee·uh) *n.* Complete absence of fibrinogen in the blood.

af·la·tox·in (af″luh·tock'sin) *n.* Any of a group of toxic, carcinogenic substances, chiefly affecting the liver, which are produced by strains of *Aspergillus flavus* and *A. parasiticus* and which may contaminate improperly stored peanuts or other foodstuffs.

African lymphoma. BURKITT'S LYMPHOMA.

African trypanosomiasis. Any one of a number of trypanosomal infections of man and of animals occurring in Africa, including Gambian and Rhodesian trypanosomiasis (or sleeping sickness of man) and nagana of cattle.

af·ter·birth (af'tur·burth) *n.* The placenta and membranes expelled from the uterus following birth of the child. Syn. *secundines.*

af·ter·care, *n.* 1. Care or nursing of convalescents, especially that of mother and infant after childbirth or the postoperative treatment of surgical patients. 2. *In psychiatry,* the continuation of treatment and the rendering of other rehabilitative services in the community to a patient following a period of hospitalization in order to help him maintain and continue his adjustment.

af·ter·cat·a·ract, *n.* 1. A portion of lens substance or of lens capsule retained after the extraction of an extracapsular cataract. 2. Any membrane in the area of the pupil following removal or absorption of the lens.

af·ter·com·ing head. The head of the fetus in a breech presentation.

af·ter·damp, *n.* A poisonous mixture of gases, containing principally carbon dioxide and nitrogen, found in coal mines after an explosion of inflammable gases.

af·ter·dis·charge, *n.* The discharge of impulses, as of a ganglion cell or neural circuit after the initial stimulus has ceased.

af·ter·ef·fect, *n.* A delayed response to a stimulus or agent, appearing only after the subsidence of the primary response.

af·ter·hear·ing, *n.* A sensation of hearing a sound after the stimulus which produces it has ceased; may be a symptom of some neuroses.

af·ter·im·age, *n.* A retinal impression that continues after the stimulus of the light or image has ceased to act.

afterimage test. *In ophthalmology,* a measurement of abnormal retinal correspondence in strabismus. The patient looks at a horizontal luminous filament first with the straight eye and then at a vertical one with the squinting eye. If the afterimages cross, correspondence is normal and binocular vision probably can be restored following correction of the strabismus.

af·ter·nys·tag·mus, *n.* Nystagmus that persists for some time after the stimulus producing optokinetic nystagmus is removed.

af·ter·pains, *n.* Pains from uterine contractions following delivery.

af·ter·po·ten·tial, *n.* A small positive or negative wave that follows and is dependent on the main spike potential, seen in the oscillograph tracing of an action potential passing along a nerve.

af·ter·pres·sure, *n.* The sense of pressure that remains for a brief period after the removal of an object from the surface of the body.

af·ter·sen·sa·tion, *n.* A sensation continuing after the stimulus that produced it has ceased.

af·ter·taste, *n.* A gustatory sensation continuing for some time after the stimulus provoking immediate taste has been removed.

af·ter·touch, *n.* The sensation that persists for a short time after contact with an object has ceased.

af·ter·vi·sion, *n.* Perception of an afterimage.

afunc·tion·al (ay-funk'shun·ul) *adj.* Without function; unable to function normally; lacking normal function.

aga·lac·tia (ay''ga·lack'shee·uh, -tee·uh) *n.* Nonsecretion or imperfect secretion of milk after childbrith. **—agalac·tous** (-tus) *adj.*

agalactia con·ta·gi·o·sa (kon·tay'jee·o·suh). An epidemic, contagious disease of sheep and goats caused by *Mycoplasma agalactiae,* characterized by mammitis, fever, keratoconjunctivitis, and arthritis.

ag·a·lor·rhea, ag·a·lor·rhoea (ag''uh·lo·ree'uh, a·gal''o·) *n.* A cessation of the flow of milk.

agam·ete (ay·gam'eet, ag'a·meet) *n. In biology,* any unicellular organism which reproduces asexually.

agam·ic (ay·gam'ick) *adj. In biology,* asexual; reproducing without union of sexual cells.

agam·ma·glob·u·li·ne·mia (ay·gam''uh·glob''yoo·li·nee'mee·uh) *n.* 1. Markedly reduced serum concentration of immunoglobulins. 2. Antibody-deficiency syndromes: specifically, congenital agammaglobulinemia, transient hypogammaglobulinemia, and acquired agammaglobulinemia. **—agammaglobuline·mic** (-mick) *adj.*

aga·mo·gen·e·sis (ay·gam''o·jen'e·sis, ag''uh·mo·) *n.* 1. Asexual reproduction. 2. PARTHENOGENESIS. Syn. *agamogony, agamocytogony.* **—agamo·ge·net·ic** (-je·net'ick) *adj.*

agan·gli·on·ic (ay·gang''glee·on'ick) *adj.* Having no ganglions; referring especially to the absence of the myenteric plexus cells of the colon.

aganglionic megacolon. HIRSCHSPRUNG'S DISEASE.

agan·gli·on·o·sis (ay·gang''glee·un·o'sis) *n.* 1. Absence of ganglion cells. 2. Congenital absence of the myenteric plexus ganglion cells seen in Hirschsprung's disease.

agar (ay'gahr, ag'ahr, ah'gahr) *n.* A solidifying agent consisting of a complex carbohydrate extracted from certain marine algae, as of the genus *Gelidium,* widely used as a base for bacteriologic media, as a hydrophilic colloid laxative, as a suspending agent, and as the basic ingredient of reversible hydrocolloid dental impression materials.

ag·a·rose (ag'uh·roce, -roze) *n.* A polysaccharide obtained from agar used as a supporting medium for column chromatography and gel electrophoresis.

agar streak plate. Any agar plate on which microorganisms are streaked out for such determinations as purity or variation.

-age. A suffix meaning (a) *cumulative result;* (b) *rate;* (c) *action or process.*

agen·e·sis (ay·jen'e·sis) *n.* 1. Lack of complete and normal development. 2. Congenital absence of an organ or part. 3. *Erron.* AGENNESIS.

agen·i·tal·ism (ay·jen'i·tul·iz·um) *n.* A symptom complex due to a deficiency of sex hormones, found in persons who lack testes or ovaries.

agen·o·so·mia (ay·jen''o·so'mee·uh, a·jen'') *n.* Defective development of the genitals.

agent, *n.* A substance or force which, by its action, effects changes.

age·ra·sia (aj''e·ray'zee·uh) *n.* Vigorous, healthy old age.

ageu·sia (a·gew'zee·uh, ay·joo') *n.* Loss or impairment of the sense of taste. **—ageu·sic** (a·gew'zick) *adj.*

ageusic aphasia. Impairment in the ability to express in words thoughts related to the sense of taste.

ag·ger (ag'ur, aj'ur) *n. In anatomy,* a projection, eminence, or mound.

agger na·si (nay'zigh) [NA]. An oblique ridge on the inner surface of the nasal process of the maxilla; the anterior part of the ethmoid crest.

ag·glom·er·ate (a·glom'ur·ut) *adj.* Grouped or clustered into a mass. **—ag·glom·er·a·tion** (a·glom''ur·ay'shun) *n.*

ag·glu·ti·nate (a·gloo'ti·nate) *v.* 1. To fuse, cohere, adhere. 2. Of suspended particles or corpuscles: to aggregate, form clumps. 3. To cause to aggregate or form clumps. **—agglutina·tive** (-nuh·tiv) *adj.;* **aggluti·na·ble** (nuh·bul) *adj.;* **ag·glu·ti·na·tion** (a·gloo''ti·nay'shun) *n.*

agglutination test. 1. A test in which an agglomeration or clumping of particles produces masses which may be seen either with the unaided eye or with the aid of a microscope. The test may be used for the identification of bacteria. 2. A test for the presence of specific antibodies in the blood serum of infected individuals which will produce clumping of the specific bacteria causing the infection.

ag·glu·ti·nin (a·gloo'ti·nin) n. An antibody occurring in a normal or immune serum which, when added to a suspension of its homologous, particulate antigen, causes the antigen elements to adhere to one another, forming clumps.

ag·glu·ti·no·gen (ag"lew·tin'o·jen, a·gloo'tin·o·jen) n. An antigen which, when injected into the animal body, stimulates the formation of a specific agglutinin. This, in turn, has the capacity to agglutinate the antigen.

¹ag·gre·gate (ag're·gut) adj. & n. 1. Clumped, forming a group. 2. A clump, as the mass formed by certain antibodies and their homologous antigens.

²ag·gre·gate (ag're·gate) v. To gather into a mass; to clump.

aggregate follicles. An aggregation of lymph nodules situated in the mucous membrane of the lower part of the small intestine, opposite the mesenteric attachment. Syn. *Peyer's patches.*

ag·gre·ga·tion, n. Agmination; a massing together of materials; a congeries or collection of particles, parts, or bodies, usually of a similar nature.

ag·gres·sion, n. 1. *In psychiatry,* an act or attitude of hostility, commonly arising out of frustration or feelings of inferiority. 2. *In psychoanalysis,* an innate, independent, instinctual disposition in man; it may be self- or outwardly destructive, may revert to the opposite, or may, when sublimated, serve to foster constructive, self-protective forms of adaptation and progressive self-assertion. —**ag·gres·sive,** adj.

aggressive behavior disorder. MINIMAL BRAIN DYSFUNCTION SYNDROME.

aging pigment. LIPOFUSCIN.

agit. Abbreviation for L. *agita,* shake.

ag·i·tat·ed dementia. Dementia distinguished by great excitement, motor activity, and often continuous hallucinations.

agitated depression. A type of manic-depressive illness or involutional melancholia; characterized by marked restlessness, continual activity, despondency, and anxiety.

ag·i·to·graph·ia (aj''i·to·graf'ee·uh) n. A condition characterized by excessive speed in writing, with unconscious omissions of letters, syllables, or words.

ag·i·to·pha·sia (aj''i·to·fay'zhuh, ·zee·uh) n. A condition marked by excessive rapidity of speech, with sounds, syllables, or words unconsciously slurred, omitted, or distorted.

aglan·du·lar (ay·glan'dew·lur) adj. Having no glands; without glands.

aglo·mer·u·lar (ay''glom·err'yoo·lur, ag''lom·) adj. Without glomeruli.

aglos·sia (ay·glos'ee·uh, a·glos') n. 1. Congenital

absence of the tongue. 2. Loss of the ability to speak; mutism.

ag·lu·ti·tion (ag''lew·tish'un) n. DYSPHAGIA.

agly·cone (ay·glye'kone, a·glye'kone) n. The nonsugar portion of a glycoside.

agly·cos·uric (ay·glye''ko·sue'rick, a·glye''ko·) adj. Free from glycosuria; exhibiting no urinary sugar.

ag·mi·nate (ag'mi·nate) adj. AGMINATED.

ag·mi·nat·ed (ag'mi·nay·tid) adj. Gathered into clumps or clusters; aggregate. —**ag·mi·na·tion** (ag''mi·nay'shun) n.

ag·na·thia (ag·nayth'ee·uh) n. Absence or deficient development of the jaws. —**ag·na·thous** (ag'nuth·us) adj.

ag·na·tho·ceph·a·lus (ag·nay''tho·sef'uh·lus, ag''nuth·o·) n., pl. **agnathocepha·li** (·lye) A type of otocephalus in which the eyes are situated low on the face with approximation or fusion of the zygomas. —**agnatho·ce·pha·lia** (·se·fay'lee·uh), **agnathoceph·aly** (·uh·lee) n.

ag·nea, ag·noea (ag·nee'uh) n. AGNOSIA.

ag·no·gen·ic (ag''no·jen'ick) adj. Of unknown etiology.

agnogenic myeloid metaplasia. Extramedullary hemopoiesis of unknown cause, characterized by hepatosplenomegaly and immature but not anaplastic cells in the peripheral blood.

ag·no·sia (ag·no'see·uh) n. Loss or impairment of the ability to recognize features of the external world, as shapes, symbols, geometric relations, directions, or sounds, caused by lesion of the dominant cerebral hemisphere but not by any lesion affecting primary sensation or general intellectual function; in contrast to amorphosynthesis, agnosia affects equally the interpretation of stimuli received on either side of the body. Usually classified according to the sense or senses involved.

ag·nos·te·rol (ag·nos'te·rol, ·role) n. A complex terpene alcohol, $C_{30}H_{47}OH$, found in wool fat. Formerly considered to be a sterol but now shown not to possess the structure characteristic of this group of compounds.

ag·nos·tic (ag·nos'tick) adj. Pertaining to or characterized by agnosia.

agnostic alexia. Alexia caused by loss of the ability to recognize characters or their combinations.

ag·om·phi·a·sis (ag''om·figh'uh·sis) n. 1. Looseness of the teeth. 2. Absence of teeth.

agom·phi·ous (a·gom'fee·us) adj. Toothless.

ag·o·nal (ag'uh·nul) adj. Pertaining to the period immediately preceding death; usually a matter of minutes but occasionally indicating a period of several hours.

agonal intussusception. Single or multiple areas of intussusception without clinical or pathological evidence of destruction or inflammation, sometimes found in the small intestine at the time of death.

ag·o·nist (ag'uh·nist) n. 1. A contracting muscle engaged in the movement of a part and opposed by an antagonistic muscle. Syn. *protagonist.* 2. A substance capable of combining with an appropriate cellular receptor and producing a typical response for that particular substance.

ag·o·ny (ag'uh·nee) n. 1. Violent pain; extreme anguish, distress of mind. 2. The death struggle.

ag·o·ra·pho·bia (ag''o·ruh·fo'bee·uh) n. Morbid fear of open places or spaces.

agram·ma·tism (ay·gram'uh·tiz·um, a·gram') n. A type of aphasia in which the patient is unable to frame a grammatical sentence, and though able to utter words, uses them without relation to their proper sequence or inflection.

agran·u·lar (ay·gran'yoo·lur) adj. Not granular; without granules.

agranular cortex. Cortex of the cerebrum which lacks a definite fourth cell layer, typical of areas in the frontal lobe.

agran·u·lo·cyte (ay·gran'yoo·lo·site, a·gran') n. A nongranular leukocyte. —**agran·u·lo·cyt·ic** (ay·gran''yoo·lo·sit'ick, a·gran'') adj.

agranulocytic angina. AGRANULOCYTOSIS (2).

agran·u·lo·cy·to·sis (a·gran''yoo·lo·sigh·to'sis, ay·gran'') n. 1. A decrease in the number of granulocytic leukocytes in the peripheral blood. 2. An acute febrile syndrome accompanied by fever, mucous membrane ulcers, and a decrease in granulocytes in the peripheral blood, often related to drug administration.

agraph·es·the·sia (a·graf''es·theezh'uh, ay·) n. GRAPHANESTHESIA.

agraph·ia (ay·graf'ee·uh, a·graf') n. Loss of ability to write as a manifestation of aphasia.

A/G ratio. Abbreviation for albumin-globulin ratio.

ag·ro·ma·nia (ag''ro·may'nee·uh) n. An abnormal desire to live in the open country or in isolation.

agryp·nia (a·grip'nee·uh, ay·grip') n. Obsol. INSOMNIA.

agryp·not·ic (ag''rip·not'ick, ay''grip·) adj. & n. 1. Inducing, pertaining to, or characterized by insomnia. 2. AGRYPNODE.

ague (ay'gyoo) n. 1. An attack of chills and fever; especially, a chill. 2. Specifically, an attack of malaria.

ague cake spleen. The enlarged spleen of chronic malaria.

agy·ria (ay·jye'ree·uh, a·jye') n. Congenital absence of cerebral convolutions.

AHF Abbreviation for antihemophilic factor (= FACTOR VIII).

AHG Abbreviation for antihemophilic globulin (= FACTOR VIII).

aich·mo·pho·bia (ike''mo·fo'bee·uh) n. Morbid dread of sharp or pointed objects, or of being touched by them or by a finger.

ail·ment, n. A disease; sickness; complaint; bodily infirmity.

ai·lu·ro·phil·ia (ay·lew''ro·fil'ee·uh, eye·lew''ro·) n. GALEOPHILIA.

ai·lu·ro·pho·bia (ay·lew''ro·fo'bee·uh, eye·lew''ro·) n. GALEOPHOBIA.

ai·nhum (eye·nyooⁿ', eye'nyum) n. A tropical disease of unknown etiology, most common in blacks, in which a toe is slowly and spontaneously amputated by a fibrous ring.

air, n. 1. The mixture of gases that constitutes the earth's atmosphere, consisting of approximately 4 volumes of nitrogen and 1 volume of oxygen, with small amounts of carbon dioxide, ammonia, nitrates, organic matter, and the rare gases argon, neon, krypton, and xenon. By virtue of its oxygen content it is able to sustain respiration in aerobic organisms. The density of air at $0°C$ and standard sea-level pressure is roughly 1 kg/m³. 2. Obsol. Any gas.

air-borne infection. The transfer of infection from one individual to another without direct contact between them by means of droplets of moisture containing the causative agent. Syn. droplet infection.

air-bra·sive (air·bray'siv) adj. Pertaining to the technique of cutting tooth structure or of removing stain and calculus from tooth surfaces by use of a stream of abrasive powder, such as aluminum oxide or calcium magnesium carbonate, propelled at high speed through a fine nozzle by a compressed gas, such as carbon dioxide.

air cell. 1. Any anatomical compartment or cavity, often part of a partitioned larger space, which is filled with air, such as a pulmonary alveolus, a mastoid cell, or an ethmoid air cell. 2. PARANASAL SINUS. 3. (of the auditory tube:) See cellulae pneumaticae tubae auditivae.

air conditioning. The process of modifying air by the control of its temperature and humidity and the removal of particulate matter.

air conduction. Transmission of sound vibrations to the eardrum through the external auditory canal. Abbreviated, A.C.

air conduction audiometry. Quantitative evaluation of hearing by introducing the stimulus through the air column in the external auditory canal.

air conduction hearing aid. An electronic hearing aid, the transmitter of which fits into the external auditory canal.

air conduction test. A test for hearing utilizing the transmission of sound through air.

air-contrast examination. A roentgenologic technique for coating the mucosa of a hollow viscus with a positive contrast agent (usually barium) and also distending it with gas (usually air). Syn. double contrast examination.

air embolism. Air producing an obstruction in the heart or vascular system, usually resulting from surgery or trauma.

air-fluid level. A gas-fluid interface demonstrable by an x-ray beam parallel to it.

air hunger. The deep gasping respiration characteristic of severe diabetic acidosis and coma. Syn. Kussmaul's respiration.

air myelography. Radiographic examination of the spinal cord after injecting air into the subarachnoid space.

air passage. RESPIRATORY PASSAGE.

airplane splint. A special type of splint that holds the arm in abduction with the forearm midway in flexion; generally of wire with an axillary strut and frequently incorporated in a plaster body support.

air sac. A pulmonary alveolus; ALVEOLUS (2).

air sac disease. A severe inflammation of the pulmonary alveoli of poultry caused by Mycoplasma gallisepticum and complicated with coliform infection.

air·sick·ness, *n.* Motion sickness in aircraft flights.

air sinus. A cavity containing air within a bone; especially, a paranasal sinus.

air·way, *n.* 1. Any of several devices used to maintain a clear and unobstructed respiratory passage during general anesthesia. 2. RESPIRATORY PASSAGE.

ak·i·ne·sia (ack"i·nee'zhuh, ·zee·uh) *n.* 1. Slowness of movement and underactivity (poverty of movement); characteristic of Parkinson's disease. 2. Any condition involving or characterized by immobility.

ak·i·ne·sis (ack"i·nee'sis) *n.* Immobility; AKINESIA.

akin·es·the·sia, akin·aes·the·sia (ay·kin"es·theezh'uh, ·theez'ee·uh, a·kin'") *n.* Loss of perception of position and movement; loss of deep sensation or muscle sense.

aki·net·ic (ack"i·net'ick, ay"ki·) *adj.* 1. Characterized by or affected with akinesia. 2. AMITOTIC.

akinetic epilepsy. A form of epilepsy characterized by akinetic seizures.

akinetic mutism. 1. A state in which the appearance of the patient, particularly that of the eyes, suggests consciousness, but in which the patient is in fact unconscious. 2. Any state in which the patient is conscious and alert but makes no voluntary movement; especially, PSEUDOCOMA.

akinetic seizure. An epileptic seizure marked by sudden loss of consciousness and motor power resulting in head nodding, body slumping, and often, a violent fall. The seizure is usually brief, and there may be no postictal confusion, stupor, or sleep.

Al Symbol for aluminum.

¹-al An adjective-forming suffix signifying *of or pertaining to; having the character of; appropriate to.*

²-al A suffix indicating *the presence of the aldehyde group.*

ala (ay'luh) *n.,* pl. & genit. sing. **alae** (ay'lee) 1. A wing. 2. Any winglike process. 3. AXILLA.

ala ci·ne·rea (si·neer'ee·uh) The trigone of the vagus nerve: the area in the floor of the fourth ventricle overlying the dorsal motor nucleus of the vagus nerve. Syn. *trigonum nervi vagi* [NA], *trigonum vagi, vagal triangle.*

alae. Plural and genitive singular of *ala.*

ala·lia (a·lay'lee·uh) *n.* Impairment or loss of speech. —**alal·ic** (a·lal'ick) *adj.*

ala na·si (nay'zye) [NA]. The lower portion of the side of the nose; a wing of the nose.

al·a·nine (al'uh·neen, ·nin) *n.* α-Aminopropionic acid or 2-aminopropanoic acid, CH₃CH(NH₂)COOH. The L- form is a constituent of many proteins; it is classified as a nonessential amino acid.

alar (ay'lur) *adj.* 1. Of or pertaining to a wing or ala. 2. AXILLARY.

alarm reaction. The sum of all nonspecific phenomena elicited by sudden exposure to stimuli, which affect large portions of the body and to which the organism is quantitatively or qualitatively not adapted; the first stage of the general adaptation syndrome, in which there is increased secretory activity of the anterior pituitary (adenohypophysis).

ala·ryn·ge·al (ay"la·rin'jee·ul, ·jul) *adj.* Without a larynx; not involving the larynx.

alaryngeal speech. Speech developed after total laryngectomy, usually esophageal speech.

ala·tus (ay·lay'tus) *n.* An individual with marked backward projection of the scapulas.

alb-, albo- A combining form meaning *white, whitish.*

al·ba (al'buh) *n.* WHITE SUBSTANCE.

Albamycin. A trademark for novobiocin, an antibiotic.

Al·bers-Schön·berg's disease (al"bursshœhn'behrk) OSTEOPETROSIS.

Albert's stain A stain used in a test for diphtheria bacilli. The cells are treated with a solution of toluidine blue and methyl green, then with a solution of iodine and potassium iodide. Diphtheria bacilli are stained light green, the metachromatic granules bluish-black, and the bars dark green to black.

al·bi·cans (al'bi·kanz) *L. adj.,* pl. **al·bi·can·tia** (al'bi·kan"tee·uh) White; whitish.

al·bi·du·ria (al"bi·dew'ree·uh) *n.* 1. Passage of very pale, almost colorless urine, of low specific gravity. 2. CHYLURIA.

al·bi·nism (al'bi·niz·um) *n.* Hereditary absence of melanin pigment from the eyes or from the skin, hair, and eyes due to defective metabolism of the melanin precursor tyrosine; associated with several congenital ocular abnormalities and with visual defects and nystagmus.

al·bi·nis·mus (al"bi·niz'mus) *n.* ALBINISM.

al·bi·no (al·bye'no, al·bee'no) *n.* An individual affected with albinism. —**al·bi·not·ic** (al"bi·not'ick) *adj.*

Albright's syndrome The polyostotic form of fibrous dysplasia associated with large irregular melanotic macules arranged in a linear or segmental pattern tending to remain on one side of the midline of the body, and precocious puberty in females though only rarely in males. Syn. *Albright-McCune-Sternberg syndrome.*

al·bu·gin·ea (al"bew·jin'ee·uh) *n.* TUNICA ALBUGINEA.

al·bu·gin·e·ous (al"bew·jin'ee·us) *adj.* 1. Whitish. 2. Belonging to a tunica albuginea.

al·bu·gi·ni·tis (al·bew"ji·nigh'tis, al"bew·ji·) *n.* Inflammation of a tunica albuginea.

al·bu·go (al·bew'go) *n.* A white spot upon the cornea; a corneal opacity.

al·bu·men (al·bew'mun) *n.* 1. Egg white, consisting chiefly of albumin. 2. The stored food matter in a vegetable seed. 3. ALBUMIN.

al·bu·min (al·bew'min) *n.* One of a group of protein substances, the chief constituents of animal tissues. They are soluble in water, coagulable by heat, and composed of carbon, hydrogen, nitrogen, oxygen, and sulfur. Some varieties are named after their sources or characteristic reactions, such as acid albumin, alkali albumin, muscle albumin, ovum albumin, serum albumin, vegetable albumin. —**albu·mi·nous** (·mi·nus) *adj.*

albumin-globulin ratio. The ratio of the albumin to the globulin concentration in blood serum.

Normal value = 1.3 to 1.8. Values below 1.0 are said to be inverted and may be associated with various pathologic processes. Abbreviated, A/G ratio.

al·bu·mi·no·cy·to·log·ic (al·bew″mi·no·sigh·to·loj′ick) *adj.* Referring to both the protein and cells (usually leukocytes) of a fluid; usually used in connection with the cerebrospinal fluid.

albuminocytologic dissociation. Elevated protein in cerebrospinal fluid without a corresponding rise in cell count, characteristic of the Guillain-Barré syndrome.

al·bu·mi·noid (al·bew′mi·noid) *adj. & n.* 1. Resembling albumin; applied to certain protein derivatives having many of the characteristics of albumin. 2. SCLEROPROTEIN.

al·bu·mi·nom·e·ter (al·bew″mi·nom′e·tur) *n.* An instrument for the quantitative estimation of protein in a fluid, as in urine. —**albuminometry** (·tree) *n.*

al·bu·mi·nous (al·bew′mi·nus) *adj.* Resembling, pertaining to, or containing albumin or albumen.

albuminous degeneration. CLOUDY SWELLING.

al·bu·min·uria (al·bew″mi·new′ree·uh) *n.* The presence of albumin in the urine; may or may not be associated with renal parenchymal disease. —**albumin·uric** (·rick) *adj.*

al·bu·mo·su·ria (al″bew·mo·sue′ree·uh) *n.* The presence of Bence Jones protein in the urine.

Al·ca·lig·e·nes fae·ca·lis (al″kuh·lij′e·neez fee·kay′lis) An organism consisting of gram-negative motile rods belonging to the family Achromobacteraceae which turns litmus milk alkaline, does not attack carbohydrates, is commonly found in the intestinal tracts of vertebrates and in dairy products, and is only rarely pathogenic.

alcaptonuria. ALKAPTONURIA.

al·che·my (al′ke·mee) *n.* The chemical science of the Middle Ages, which attempted to transmute base metals into gold and to find a remedy for all diseases.

al·co·hol (al′kuh·hawl) *n.* 1. A derivative of an aliphatic hydrocarbon that contains a hydroxyl (OH) group. Alcohols are classified on the basis of the number of hydroxyl groups present in the molecule, i.e., monohydric, dihydric, trihydric; or on the basis of the presence of a —CH_2OH (primary alcohol), a =CHOH (secondary alcohol), or a ≡COH (tertiary alcohol) group. 2. Specifically, ETHYL ALCOHOL. 3. Ethyl alcohol in a concentration of not less than 92.3 percent by weight or 94.9 percent by volume at 15.56° C.; a pharmaceutical solvent (USP).

alcohol dehydrogenase. An enzyme capable of reversibly oxidizing ethanol to acetaldehyde. Nicotinamide adenine dinucleotide (NAD) is required, and other aliphatic alcohols of low molecular weight are likewise oxidized. Abbreviated, ADH. Syn. *alcoholase.*

al·co·hol·ic (al″ko·hol′ick) *adj. & n.* 1. Pertaining to, containing, or producing alcohol. 2. An individual whose consumption of alcoholic beverages or other substances with similar effects results in his or her becoming habituated, dependent, or addicted, or interferes, or threatens to interfere, with his or her health, interpersonal relationships, or means of livelihood.

alcoholic delirium. Delirium tremens associated with alcoholism.

alcoholic myopathy. Any of several nonspecific disorders of skeletal muscles associated with alcoholism, such as hypopotassemia with vacuolar necrosis of muscle, or painful, swollen muscles accompanied by hyperpotassemia, myoglobinuria and renal damage.

Alcoholics Anonymous. A fellowship of persons formerly addicted to alcohol who together through personal and group support seek to help other alcoholics to overcome their addiction. Abbreviated, A.A.

al·co·hol·ism (al′kuh·hol·iz·um) *n.* 1. ACUTE ALCOHOLISM. 2. CHRONIC ALCOHOLISM (1, 2, & 3).

al·co·hol·ize (al′ko·hol·ize) *v.* 1. To saturate or treat with alcohol. 2. To convert to alcohol. 3. [from ML. *alcohol*, fine powder, sublimate]. To convert to fine powder.

al·co·hol·om·e·ter (al″ko·hol·om′e·tur) *n.* A hydrometer or other instrument for determining the amount of alcohol in a liquid. —**alcoholome·try** (·tree) *n.*

al·co·hol·uria (al″ko·hol·yoo′ree·uh) *n.* The presence of alcohol in urine.

Aldactone. Trademark for spironolactone, a diuretic agent.

al·de·hyde (al′de·hide) *n.* A class of organic compounds intermediate between alcohols and acids, derived from their corresponding primary alcohols by oxidation and removal of two atoms of hydrogen, and converted into acids by the addition of an atom of oxygen. They contain the group —CHO.

Alder's anomaly or **phenomenon** Inclusions of deeply staining, azurophilic, toluidine-blue positive material in the cytoplasm of lymphocytes, granulocytes, and monocytes, often associated with mucopolysaccharidosis.

al·dol (al′dole, ·dol) *n.* 1. Beta-hydroxybutyric aldehyde, $CH_3CH(OH)CH_2CHO$, a condensation product of acetaldehyde. 2. One of a class of condensation products formed from an aldehyde.

al·dol·ase (al′do·lace, ·laze) *n.* An enzyme occurring in muscle and capable of splitting fructose 1,6-diphosphate into dihydroxyacetone phosphate and phosphoglyceraldehyde. Syn. *zymohexase.*

Aldomet. Trademark for methyldopa, an antihypertensive agent.

al·do·pen·tose (al″do·pen′toce) *n.* A pentose containing an aldehyde group, such as arabinose, ribose, or xylose.

al·dose (al′doce, al′doze) *n.* Any carbohydrate containing the aldehyde group —CHO.

al·do·ste·rone (al·dos′te·rone, al″do·ste·rone′, ·sterr′one, ·steer′one) *n.* 11β,21-Dihydroxy-3,20-diketo-4-pregnene-18-al, $C_{21}H_{28}O_5$, a potent adrenocortical hormone which, in very small amounts, maintains the life of adrenalectomized animals. It is a very potent regulator of the metabolism of sodium and potassium, many times more active than deoxycorticosterone in its effects on electrolyte metabolism, less effective in regulating carbohydrate metabolism.

al·do·ste·ron·ism (al·dos'te·ro·niz·um, al''do·sterr'o·niz·um, al''do·ste·ro'niz·um) n. HYPER-ALDOSTERONISM.

al·dox·ime (al·dock'sim, ·seem) n. 1. The product derived from an aldehyde when the oxygen of the —CHO group is replaced by =NOH, forming the —CHNOH group. 2. Acetaldoxime, CH_3CHNOH.

Al·drich syndrome WISKOTT-ALDRICH SYNDROME.

alec·i·thal (a·les'i·thul, ay·) adj. Having little or no yolk, as the eggs of placental mammals.

al·et·a·mine (al·et'uh·meen) n. α-Allylphenethylamine, $C_{11}H_{15}N$, an antidepressant; used as the hydrochloride salt.

aleu·ke·mia, aleu·kae·mia (al''yoo·kee'mee·uh) n. ALEUKEMIC LEUKEMIA. —**aleuke·mic, aleu·kae·mic** (·mick) adj.

aleukemic leukemia. A form of leukemia in which the total leukocyte count is normal or low, despite leukemic changes in the tissues and sometimes qualitative changes in the blood.

aleu·ko·cy·to·sis (ay·lew''ko·sigh·to'sis) n. Severe leukopenia.

Aleu·tian disease (uh·lew'shun). A disease of mink characterized by hypergammaglobulinemia, glomerulonephritis, necrotizing arteritis, and accumulation of plasma cells in several organs, which is thought to be caused by a pronounced antibody response to viral antigens and has been used as a model for human viral diseases with immunologically mediated lesions; discovered in the Aleutian mink, a dark blue mutant of ranch-raised mink.

Al·ex·an·der's disease A rare degenerative disease of the central nervous system with onset in early infancy and a course of a few years, characterized clinically by lack of development, progressive spasticity, megalocephaly, and seizures, and pathologically by leukodystrophy and eosinophilic hyaline bodies at the pial surface and in the perivascular tissue.

alex·ia (a·leck'see·uh, ay·) n. Loss or impairment of ability to recognize or comprehend written or printed words as a manifestation of aphasia. Syn. *word blindness.*

alex·i·phar·mac (a·leck''si·fahr'mack) n. An antidote or defensive remedy against poison, venom, or infection.

Al·gae (al'jee) n.pl. One of the major divisions of the Thallophyta or primitive plants, including numerous marine plants, such as the seaweeds, rockweeds, freshwater pond scums, the stoneworts, and others. Because the algae can synthesize food, they are separated from the fungi which are saprophytic or parasitic.

al·ge·don·ic (al''je·don'ick) adj. Pertaining to pleasure and pain, or to the pleasantness-unpleasantness of an experience. —**algedon·ics** (·icks) n.

al·ge·sia (al·jee'zee·uh) n. 1. Sensitivity to pain. 2. Excessive sensitivity to pain. —**alge·sic** (·sick) adj.

al·ge·sim·e·ter (al''je·sim'e·tur) n. An instrument

for determining the acuteness of the sense of pain by eliciting a measurable pain response. Syn. *algometer.*

al·gid (al'jid) adj. 1. Cold or chilly. 2. Characterized by cold skin and hypotension, as algid malaria.

algid stage. A condition occurring in cholera, falciparum malaria, and other diseases marked by extensive intestinal discharges, characterized by subnormal temperature, feeble flickering pulse, hypotension, and various neurologic symptoms.

al·gi·nate (al'ji·nate) n. A salt of alginic acid extracted from marine kelp, believed to be a polymer of D-mannuronic acid. Certain such salts form viscous sols in water and may then react with calcium compounds to form an elastic, insoluble gel.

al·gio·mo·tor (al''jee·o·mo'tur) adj. Causing pain on movement; causing painful spasm.

al·gio·mus·cu·lar (al''jee·o·mus'kew·lur) adj. Causing pain in the muscles.

al·go·gen·e·sis (al''go·jen'e·sis) n. The source or origin of pain.

¹al·go·gen·ic (al''go·jen'ick) adj. Lowering the body temperature; producing cold or chill.

²algogenic, adj. Producing pain.

al·go·lag·nia (al''go·lag'nee·uh) n. A sexual perversion in which the experiencing or inflicting of pain heightens sexual gratification or gives sexual pleasure without intercourse; masochism or sadism. —**algolag·nist** (·nist) n.

al·gom·e·ter (al·gom'e·tur) n. ALGESIMETER.

al·go·pho·bia (al''go·fo'bee·uh) n. Unreasonable or morbid dread of witnessing or of experiencing pain.

al·gor (al'gor) n. Chill, coldness.

algor mor·tis (mor'tis) Chill of death; the lowering of body temperature after death to the ambient temperature.

al·go·spasm (al'go·spaz·um) n. A painful spasm or cramp. —**al·go·spas·tic** (al''go·spas'tick) adj.

ali- A combining form meaning (a) *wing;* (b) *shaped like a wing,* as the side parts of certain organs or structures.

al·i·ble (al'i·bul) adj. Nutritive; absorbable and assimilable, as a food.

al·i·cy·clic (al''i·sigh'click, ·sick'lick) adj. Having the properties of both aliphatic (open-chain) and cyclic (closed-chain) compounds.

Alidase. A trademark for hyaluronidase.

alien·a·tion (ay''lee·uh·nay'shun) n. 1. *In forensic psychiatry,* mental derangement; insanity. 2. SELF-ALIENATION.

alien·ist (ail'yuh·nist, ay·lee·uh·nist) n. 1. A psychiatrist. 2. Especially, a physician qualified in a court of law as an expert witness in the field of psychiatry. —**alien·ism** (·iz·um) n.

al·i·ment (al'i·munt) n. Any food or nutritive substance.

al·i·men·ta·ry (al''i·men'tuh·ree) adj. 1. Nourishing, nutritious. 2. Of or pertaining to food and nutrition. 3. Pertaining to or caused by diet.

alimentary canal. The whole digestive tube from the mouth to the anus; the gastrointestinal tract.

alimentary glycosuria. Glycosuria due to excessive ingestion of carbohydrates.

alimentary lipemia. Lipemia due to the ingestion of a high-fat diet.

al·i·men·ta·tion (al"i-men-tay'shun) *n.* Feeding; nourishment.

al·i·men·to·ther·a·py (al"i-men"to-therr'uh-pee) *n.* The treatment of disease by systematic feeding; dietary treatment.

al·i·phat·ic (al"i-fat'ick) *adj.* 1. Pertaining to a fat. 2. Belonging to or derived from the open-chain series of organic compounds; ACYCLIC (2).

ali·sphe·noid (al"i-sfee'noid) *adj. & n.* 1. Pertaining to the great wing of the sphenoid bone. 2. The bone that in adult life forms the main portion of the great wing of the sphenoid bone.

al·ka·le·mia, al·ka·lae·mia (al"kuh-lee'mee-uh) *n.* An elevation of blood pH above normal levels.

al·ka·li (al'kuh-lye) *n.*, pl. **alka·lies, alka·lis** (·lize) 1. Essentially a hydroxide of an alkali metal. 2. A class of compounds that react with acids to form salts, turn red litmus blue, saponify fats, and form soluble carbonates. 3. Sometimes, a carbonate of alkali metals.

al·ka·lim·e·ter (al"kuh-lim'e-tur) *n.* An instrument for estimating the alkali in a substance. **—alka·li·met·ric** (·li-met'rick) *adj.*; **alka·lim·e·try** (·lim'e-tree) *n.*

al·ka·line (al'kuh-line, ·lin) *adj.* 1. Containing more hydroxyl than hydrogen ions. 2. Having the qualities of or pertaining to an alkali. Noun *alkalinity*.

alkaline-ash diet. A diet used to raise the pH of the urine.

alkaline-earth metals. The divalent elements calcium, strontium, and barium. Some include magnesium in the group.

alkaline earths. The oxides of calcium, strontium, and barium, and sometimes including magnesium oxide.

alkaline phosphatase. An enzyme liberating phosphate ions from various organic phosphates such as β-glycerophosphate with optimal activity in the pH range from 8.3 to 10.5.

al·ka·lin·i·ty (al"kuh-lin'i-tee) *n.* The quality of being alkaline.

al·ka·lin·ize (al'kuh-lin·ize) *v.* To render alkaline. **—al·ka·lin·iza·tion** (al"kuh-lin·i-zay'shun) *n.*

al·ka·loid (al'kuh-loid) *n.* A naturally occurring, basic, organic, nitrogenous compound, usually of plant origin; found generally as salts of organic acids, sometimes as free bases, esters, amides, or in glycosidic combination. Most are insoluble in water, soluble in organic solvents, and react with acids to form salts which are soluble in water and insoluble in organic solvents. Many alkaloids are medicinally valuable. **—al·ka·loi·dal** (al"kuh-loy'dul) *adj.*

al·ka·lo·sis (al"kuh-lo'sis) *n.*, pl. **alkalo·ses** (·seez) An abnormal state characterized by processes tending to decrease the concentration of hydrogen ion in the body below the normal range or to increase the loss of acid from the body; physiological compensatory mechanisms act to return the heightened pH toward normal. Syn. *baseosis.* **—alka·lot·ic** (·lot'ic) *adj.*

al·kane (al'kane) *n.* Any member of the paraffin series of hydrocarbons.

al·ka·net (al'kuh·net) *n.* The root of the herb *Alkanna tinctoria,* which yields a red dye.

al·kap·ton, al·cap·ton (al·kap'tun, ·tone) *n.* HOMOGENTISIC ACID.

al·kap·ton·uria, al·cap·ton·uria (al·kap"to-nyoo'ree-uh) *n.* A hereditary defect of tyrosine metabolism, due to failure to synthesize active homogentisic acid oxidase in the liver, resulting in excessive excretion of homogentisic acid in the urine; characterized in middle life by darkening of connective tissue (ochronosis) and degenerative changes in joints, cartilage, and intervertebral disks; apparently transmitted, in most cases at least, by an autosomal recessive gene.

al·ka·ver·vir (al"kuh-vur'virr) *n.* A fraction of the alkaloids of *Veratrum viride* obtained by a process involving selective extraction of the crude drug and selective precipitation of the alkaloids; used as a hypotensive.

al·kene (al'keen) *n.* Any member of the series of unsaturated aliphatic hydrocarbons (ethylene series) having one double bond and represented by the general formula C_nH_{2n}.

Alkeran. Trademark for melphalan, an antineoplastic drug.

al·kyl (al'kil, al'keel) *n.* Any one of the univalent saturated hydrocarbon radicals of the general formula C_nH_{2n+1}; as methyl (CH_3), ethyl (C_2H_5), propyl (C_3H_7).

al·kyl·amine (al"kil-uh-meen', al"kil-am'in) *n.* A substance having the constitution of ammonia in which an alkyl replaces hydrogen; one, two, or three alkyl atoms of the ammonia molecule may be replaced, yielding primary (monalkylamines), secondary (dialkylamines), and tertiary (trialkylamines) alkylamines, respectively.

al·kyl·ate (al'ki·late) *v.* To introduce one or more alkyl radicals into a compound.

al·kyl·a·tion (al"ki·lay'shun) *n.* The introduction of one or more alkyl groups into an organic compound.

al·kyne (al'kine) *n.* Any member of the series of unsaturated aliphatic hydrocarbons having a triple bond and represented by the general formula, C_nH_{2n-2}. Acetylene is the first hydrocarbon of the series, sometimes called the acetylene series.

all-, allo- A combining form meaning (a) *other, different;* (b) *variant, alternate;* (c) *modified, altered;* (d) *deviant, abnormal;* (e) in chemistry, *an isomer, close relative, or variety of a compound;* (f) *the more stable of two isomers.*

al·la·ches·the·sia, al·la·chaes·the·sia (al"uh-kes-theezh'uh, ·theez'ee-uh) *n.* ALLESTHESIA.

allant-, allanto-. A combining form meaning (a) *allantoic, allantoid, allantois;* (b) *derived from or related to allantoic acid or allantoin.*

al·lan·to·cho·ri·on (a-lan"to-ko'ree-on) *n.* The allantois and chorion fused together and thus forming a single structure; a chorion supplied by allantoic blood vessels. Syn. *chorion allantoideum.*

al·lan·to·ic (al″an·to′ick) *adj.* Pertaining to or contained in the allantois.

allantoic acid. An intermediate product, $C_4H_8N_4O_4$, in the degradation of purines, formed by the action of allantoinase on allantoin.

allantoic cyst. Cystic dilatation of the urachus.

al·lan·to·in (a·lan′to·in) *n.* 5-Ureidohydantoin, $C_4H_6N_4O_3$, a product of purine metabolism; found in allantoic fluid, amniotic fluid, fetal urine, and some plants. Used topically in suppurating wounds and ulcers to accelerate cell proliferation.

al·lan·to·is (al·lan′to·is, ·toice) *n.,* pl. **al·lan·to·i·des** (al″an·to′i·deez, ·toy′deez) An extraembryonic membrane arising as an outgrowth of the cloaca in amniotes. It functions as an organ of respiration and excretion in birds and reptiles and plays an important part in the development of the placenta in most mammals, its blood vessels forming the important pathways for the umbilical circulation.

al·le·go·ri·za·tion (al″e·gor″i·zay′shun) *n.* 1. *In psychiatry,* the formation of neologisms. 2. CONDENSATION (6).

al·lele (a·leel′) *n.* One of a pair, or of a series, of variants of a gene having the same locus on homologous chromosomes. —**al·le·lic** (a·lee′lick) *adj.*

allelo- A combining form meaning (a) *reciprocal, complementary;* (b) *alternate, alternative.*

al·lelo·cat·a·lyt·ic (a·lel″o·kat″uh·lit′ick) *adj.* 1. Denoting two substances, each decomposing in the presence of the other; mutually catalytic or destructive. 2. Promoting reproduction, as when two or more unicellular organisms are placed in a drop of culture medium, reproduction proceeds more rapidly than when one organism is present. —**allelo·ca·tal·y·sis** (·kuh·tal′i·sis) *n.*

al·le·lo·morph (a·lee′lo·morf, a·lel′o·) *n.* 1. ALLELE. 2. *In chemistry,* one of two or more isomorphic substances that contain the same atoms and of the same valences but differing in the manner of their linkage. 3. *In chemistry,* the first of a mixture of isomers in a solution to separate or crystallize. —**al·le·lo·mor·phic** (a·lee″lo·mor′fick) *adj.;* **allelo·mor·phism** (·mor′fiz·um) *n.*

al·ler·gen (al′ur·jen) *n.* A substance capable of inducing an allergy. —**al·ler·gen·ic** (al″ur·jen′ick) *adj.;* **allergen·ic·i·ty** (·is′i·tee) *n.*

al·ler·gic (a·lur′jick) *adj.* Pertaining to or having an allergy.

allergic conjunctivitis. Conjunctivitis usually characterized by inflammation and lacrimation as an immunologic reaction.

allergic contact dermatitis. Allergic dermatitis due to contact of an allergenic substance with the skin.

allergic purpura. 1. Any purpura, thrombocytopenic or nonthrombocytopenic, which results from a presumed allergic reaction. Syn. *anaphylactoid purpura.* 2. HENOCH'S PURPURA. 3. SCHÖNLEIN'S PURPURA.

allergic reaction. The response elicited by an allergen after an allergic state has been established. It may be urticarial, eczematous, or tuberculin-type (infiltrative).

allergic rhinitis. Rhinitis which may be caused by any effective allergen, usually an inhalant such as pollen.

allergic urticaria. Wheals caused by sensitization and reexposure to an allergenic substance, usually from ingestion, frequently from injection, rarely from inhalation or contact.

al·ler·gist (al′ur·jist) *n.* A physician skilled in the diagnosis and treatment of allergic diseases.

al·ler·gi·za·tion (al″ur·ji·zay′shun) *n.* The process of inducing an allergic transformation.

al·ler·gy (al′ur·jee) *n.* A condition of acquired, specific alteration in biologic reactivity, initiated by exposure to an allergen and, after an incubation period, characterized by evocation of the altered reactivity upon reexposure to the same or a closely related allergen.

Al·les·che·ria (al″es·keer′ee·uh) *n.* A genus of fungi of the class Ascomycetes.

Allescheria boyd·ii (boy′dee·eye). The species regarded as one of the causes of mycetoma; it produces white or yellowish white granules. It is the perfect stage of *Monosporium apiospermum.*

al·li·ga·tion (al″li·gay′shun) *n. In pharmacy,* the formula for solving problems concerning the mixing of solutions of different percentages; the rule of mixtures. If two substances when mixed retain the specific values of a property, the value of the mixture can be calculated from the equation $(aA + bB) / (a + b)$, where a and b are the proportions and A and B equal the respective values for the property.

al·li·ga·tor forceps. 1. A special type of forceps having long, slender angulated handles designed to be used with such instruments as an operating cystoscope or proctoscope. 2. A strong toothed forceps having a double lever, used in orthopedic surgery.

Al·lis's forceps A surgical forceps with fine, interlocking teeth which are adapted especially to securing and holding intestine, stomach wall, and other hollow viscera, without crushing them during surgical operations.

al·lit·er·a·tion (a·lit″ur·ay′shun) *n.* A form of dysphasia in which the patient chooses words with the same consonant sounds.

allocheiria. ALLOCHIRIA.

al·lo·che·zia (al″o·kee′zee·uh) *n.* 1. The passage of feces from the body through an abnormal opening. 2. The passing of nonfecal matter from the bowels.

al·loe·o·sis (al″ee·o′sis) *n.* 1. A change; alterative effect; recovery from illness. 2. A change or alteration in the character of a constitution or a disease. —**al·loe·ot·ic** (·ot′ick) *adj. & n.*

al·lo·er·o·tism (al″o·err′o·tiz·um) *n.* The tendency to seek sexual gratification from another.

al·lo·gen·ic (al″o·jen′ick) *adj.* Differing in genotype.

allogenic transformation. *In bacterial genetics,* reciprocal transformation of two mutants to the wild type by the action of a transforming principle obtained from the other.

al·lo·graft (al″o·graft) n. A tissue graft taken from a genetically nonidentical donor of the same species as the recipient. Syn. *homograft.*

al·lo·iso·leu·cine (al″o·eye″so·lew′seen) n. Either of the pair of stereoisomers, D-alloisoleucine and L-alloisoleucine, resulting from inversion of D- or L-isoleucine about one of the two asymmetric carbon atoms of the latter compounds. The L-form of alloisoleucine is found in the plasma of patients with maple syrup urine disease.

al·lom·e·try (a·lom′e·tree) n. Variations in the relative size of a part, either in the course of an organism's growth or within a series of related organisms, or the measurement and study of such variations. —**al·lo·met·ric** (al″o·met′rick) adj.

al·lo·mor·phism (al″o·mor′fiz·um) n. The property possessed by certain substances of assuming a different crystalline form while remaining unchanged in chemical constitution. —**allo·mor·phic** (·mor′fick), **allomor·phous** (·fus) adj.; **al·lo·morph** (al′o·morf) n.

al·lo·path (al′o·path) n. 1. A practitioner of allopathy (1). 2. As used by homeopaths: a regular medical practitioner.

al·lop·a·thy (a·lop′uth·ee) n. 1. A system of medical treatment using remedies that produce effects upon the body differing from those produced by disease; the opposite of the homeopathic system. 2. As used by homeopaths: the regular medical profession. —**al·lo·path·ic** (al″o·path′ick) adj.

al·lo·plas·ty (al′o·plas″tee) n. 1. A plastic operation in which material from outside the human body is utilized, such as stainless steel. 2. *In psychoanalysis,* the process whereby the libido of the growing individual directs its energies away from self and toward other individuals and objects as in acting out. —**al·lo·plas·tic** (al″o·plas′tick) adj.

al·lo·psy·chic (al″o·sigh′kick) adj. Pertaining to mental processes in their relation to the outside world.

al·lo·pu·ri·nol (al″o·pew′ri·nol) n. 1H-Pyrazolo[3,4-d]pyrimidin-4-ol, $C_5H_4N_4O$, a xanthine oxidase inhibitor which reduces the production of uric acid.

all-or-none law. The response of a single fiber of cardiac muscle, skeletal muscle, or nerve to an adequate stimulus is always maximal. The strength of response when a whole muscle or nerve trunk is stimulated depends upon the number of fibers stimulated.

al·lo·some (al′o·sohm) n. 1. Originally, any chromosome distinguished from ordinary chromosomes (autosomes) by certain peculiarities of form, size, and behavior; usually a sex chromosome. Syn. *heterochromosome.* 2. A cytoplasmic inclusion introduced from without.

al·lo·ster·ic (al″o·steer′ick, ·sterr′) adj. Pertaining to an alteration at one site that affects function at another site.

al·lo·therm (al′o·thurm) n. An organism whose temperature is directly dependent upon that of its environment. —**allother·my** (·ee) n.; **al·lo·ther·mic** (al″o·thurm′ick) adj.

allotri-, allotrio- A combining form meaning *strange, unusual, abnormal.*

al·lot·ri·o·don·tia (a·lot″ree·o·don′chee·uh) n. 1. The transplantation of teeth. 2. Occurrence of teeth in abnormal places, as in teratomas.

al·lot·rio·geu·sia (a·lot″ree·o·gew′zee·uh, ·joo′zee·uh) n. 1. A perverted sense of taste. 2. Abnormal appetite.

al·lot·ri·oph·a·gy (a·lot″ree·off′uh·jee) n. PICA.

al·lo·trope (al′o·trope) n. One of the forms in which an element capable of assuming different forms may appear.

al·lo·trop·ic (al″o·trop′ick) adj. 1. Pertaining to, or exhibiting, allotropy. 2. *In psychiatry,* characterizing a person who is preoccupied with what "other people" think, mean, or do.

al·lot·ro·py (a·lot′ruh·pee) n. 1. The occurrence of an element in two or more distinct forms with differences in physical properties, as carbon, phosphorus, and sulfur. 2. Appearance in an unusual or abnormal form. 3. An attraction or tropism between different cells or structures, as between sperms and ova. 4. The manifestation of an allotropic personality.

al·lo·type (al′o·tipe) n. A genetically determined variant demonstrable by isoimmunization.

al·lox·an (al′ock·san″, a·lock′sun) n. 2,4,5,6(1H,3H)-Pyrimidinetetrone, $C_4H_2N_2O_4$, obtainable by oxidation of uric acid. It has been found in the intestinal mucus during diarrhea and is used for the production of experimental diabetes through selective necrosis of the islets of Langerhans.

alloxan diabetes. Severe hyperglycemia and degeneration of the beta cells of the pancreas following the experimental administration of alloxan to animals.

al·lox·a·zine (a·lock′suh·zeen) n. 1. The three-ring heterocyclic compound pyrimido[4,5-b]quinoxaline-2,4(1H,3H)dione, $C_{10}H_6N_4O_2$. 2. Loosely, any derivative of alloxazine. 3. Sometimes, isoalloxazine and its derivatives.

allyl sulfide. $(C_3H_5)_2S$. A liquid of garlic-like odor, possibly present in garlic; has been used in cholera and tuberculosis.

al·mond (ah′mund, am′und, al′mund) n. The seed of *Prunus amygdalus,* a small tree widely cultivated in warm temperate regions of the world.

almond oil. The fixed oil from the kernels of varieties of *Prunus amygdalus (Amygdalus communis)*; used as an emollient, a demulcent, and a nutrient. Syn. *sweet almond oil.*

alo·bar (ay·lo′bur, ·bahr) adj. Not lobed; having no lobes.

Al·oe (al′o·ee) n. A genus of liliaceous plants.

al·oe (al′o, al′o·ee) n. The dried juice of the leaves of *Aloe perryi, A. barbadensis, A. ferox,* and hybrids of this species with *A. africana* and *A. spicata.* A cathartic, whose purgative properties are due to three pentosides (barbaloin, iso-barbaloin, and beta-barbaloin) and to a resin. Syn. *aloes.*

alo·gia (a·lo′jee·uh) n. 1. Psychological or aphasic inability to speak. 2. Stupid or senseless behavior.

al·o·in (al′o·in) *n.* A mixture of active principles, chiefly barbaloin and iso-barbaloin, obtained from aloe. Used as laxative and purgative.

al·o·pe·cia (al″o·pee′shee·uh, ·see·uh) *n.* Loss of hair, usually from the scalp; may be partial or total, congenital, premature, or senile; baldness; CALVITIES. —**alope·cic** (·sick) *adj.*

alopecia ar·e·a·ta (âr″ee·ay′tuh, air″ee·ay′tuh). Loss of hair in circumscribed patches with little or no inflammation. The scalp and beard areas are usually involved.

alopecia cic·a·tri·sa·ta (sick″uh·tri·say′tuh). Circular and irregular patches of alopecia due to closely set points of inflammation and atrophy of the skin, causing permanent baldness of the area affected, usually the vertex. Syn. *pseudopelade.*

alopecia con·gen·i·ta·lis (kon·jen″i·tay′lis). An uncommon form of baldness apparent from birth, due to absence of hair follicles.

alopecia mu·ci·no·sa (mew″si·no′suh). Circumscribed patches of loss of hair, particularly on the face, attended by mucinous degeneration of the structure of the hair follicle; may be primary or a complication of malignant lymphoma.

alopecia pre·ma·tu·ra (pree″ma·tew′ruh). Baldness which occurs between puberty and middle life and resembles the senile type. The hair gradually thins and falls out in the male pattern, i.e., in frontal recession or on the vertex.

alopecia se·ni·lis (se·nigh′lis). Baldness which occurs in old age in the form of gradual thinning of the hair.

alopecia syph·i·lit·i·ca (sif″i·lit′i·kuh). Transient baldness occurring in the second stage of syphilis in the form of a "moth-eaten" appearance in the temporoparietal regions.

alopecia to·ta·lis (to·tay′lis). Complete baldness of the scalp, an extension of alopecia areata.

alopecia uni·ver·sa·lis (yoo″ni·vur·say′lis). Loss of hair from all parts of the body, related to alopecia areata.

al·pha (al′fuh) *n.* The first of a series, or any particular member or subset of an arbitrarily ordered set; as in chemistry, often combined with the name of a compound to distinguish isomers or otherwise related substances. For many terms so designated, see under the specific noun. Symbol, *α*.

alpha-adrenergic, α-adrenergic. Of or pertaining to an alpha-adrenergic receptor.

alpha-adrenergic blocking agent, α-adrenergic blocking agent. Any agent, such as azapetine, phentolamine, and tolazoline, that combines with and causes blockade of the alpha-adrenergic receptor.

alpha-adrenergic receptor, α-adrenergic receptor. A postulated locus of action of adrenergic (sympathomimetic) agents at which primarily excitatory responses are elicited. Epinephrine is the most potent activator of this receptor.

alpha-blocking, α-blocking. Having the properties of an alpha-adrenergic blocking agent.

alpha cells. 1. Certain granular cells in the pancreatic islets. 2. Cells containing acidophil granules in the adenohypophysis.

alpha chain, α chain. The heavy chain of the IgA immunoglobulin molecule.

alpha globulin, α-globulin. Any of the group of serum globulins having the greatest mobility on electrophoresis, including globulins that function in the transport of lipids, carbohydrates, thyroid hormone, and copper.

alpha granules. 1. The acidophil granules in the alpha cells of the adenohypophysis. 2. The acidophil granules in the cells of the pancreatic islets.

alpha hemolysin, α-hemolysin. An exotoxin of *Staphylococcus aureus* that is hemolytic for rabbit red blood cells, dermonecrotic, and acutely lethal. Syn. *alpha lysin, necrotoxin.*

alpha hemolysis, α-hemolysis. Partial lysis of red cells on a blood agar medium, resulting in a green discoloration.

alpha-hemolytic, α-hemolytic. Causing alpha hemolysis; said of various bacteria, especially certain streptococci.

alpha-lobeline, *n.* An alkaloid, $C_{22}H_{27}NO_2$, from lobelia; has been used as a respiratory stimulant.

alpha particle. A charged particle emitted from the nucleus of a radioactive atom, strongly ionizing, but weakly penetrating; a helium nucleus consisting of two protons and two neutrons, with a double positive charge and a mass of 4.0028 atomic mass units.

alpha rays. Positively charged helium nuclei emitted from radioactive substances.

alpha rhythm. *In electroencephalography,* electrical oscillations or waves occurring at a rate of 8 to 13 per second.

alpha streptococci. A group of streptococci that causes alpha hemolysis.

alpha tocopherol, α-tocopherol. The most potent form of tocopherol.

al·ser·ox·y·lon (al″sur·ock′si·lon) *n.* A fat-soluble alkaloidal fraction from the root of *Rauwolfia serpentina;* has the sedative, antihypertensive, and bradycrotic actions of reserpine and other alkaloids of the root.

al·ter·a·tive (awl′tur·uh·tive) *adj. & n.* 1. Changing; reestablishing healthy nutritive processes. 2. Any medicine that alters the processes of nutrition, restoring, in some unknown way, the normal functions of an organ or of the system. Arsenic, iodine, the iodides, mercury, and gold formerly were classed as alteratives.

al·ter ego (awl″tur ee′go) An individual so close to one's own character as to seem a second self.

alternate hemiplegia. CROSSED PARALYSIS.

alternate host. INTERMEDIATE HOST.

alternating tremor. The involuntary rhythmic oscillations, averaging 4 hertz (cycles per second) with brief and equal pauses between cycles and an amplitude of 5 to 45°, produced by the regular sequential contractions of the agonistic and antagonistic muscles of a part (such as the head, hand, or a digit) and only in the waking state; due to a wide variety of lesions involving the basal ganglia, substantia nigra, and related pathways.

al·ter·na·tion, *n.* 1. The act or process of alternating or of performing alternately. 2. *In neu-*

rophysiology, the phenomenon whereby only every other impulse is carried over the eighth cranial (vestibulocochlear) nerve when the exciting impulse is from 900 to 1800 hertz (cycles per second). Because of the refractory period of nerve impulses, the maximum frequency that can be carried by a nerve is about 900 hertz.

al·thea (al·thee′uh) *n.* Marshmallow root. The peeled root of *Althaea officinalis*, a plant of the mallow family. It contains starch, gum, pectin, sugar, and asparagin. Has been used in the form of a decoction as a demulcent; also as a pill excipient.

al·ti·tude alkalosis. Respiratory alkalosis resulting from hyperventilation during acclimatization to high altitude.

altitude sickness. A symptom complex resulting from the hypoxia encountered at high altitudes. The acute type is characterized by breathlessness, hyperventilation, lightheadedness, headache, malaise, irritability, and rarely by acute pulmonary edema. The chronic type (Monge's disease) usually occurs with acclimatization to altitudes above 15,000 feet and is manifested by polycythemia, vascular occlusions, gastrointestinal ulceration, and cardiac failure.

Aludrox. Trademark for alumina and magnesia oral suspension.

al·um (al′um) *n.* 1. Any one of a class of double salts of general formula $M_2′SO_4·M_2′′′$ $(SO_4)_3·24H_2O$ or $M′M′′′(SO_4)_2·12H_2O$, in which $M′$ is a univalent metal or group, and $M′′′$ is a trivalent metal. 2. Ammonium alum, $AlNH_4(SO_4)_2·12H_2O$, or potassium alum, $AlK(SO_4)_2·12H_2O$, used as an astringent and emetic. 3. Exsiccated alum, a form deprived of most of its water of crystallization, used as an astringent.

alum hematoxylin. A dye lake of hematoxylin or hematein with potassium or ammonium aluminum sulfate, used in many formulas for the staining of nuclei and some other tissue elements.

alu·mi·num (a·lew′mi·num) *n.* Al = 26.9815. Valence, 3. A silver-white, light, ductile metal occurring abundantly in nature, chiefly in combination with silica and metallic oxides. It is soluble in acids and alkalies and, on exposure to air, takes on a coating of oxide. Because of its lightness (sp. gr. 2.7) and relative stability, it is used extensively for manufacturing and construction purposes. It readily forms alloys, some of which are of great importance. Powdered aluminum is variously used as a protective in treating ulcers and fissures, and has been used in treating silicosis.

aluminum acetate solution. A solution containing about 5.3% aluminum acetate, $Al(C_2H_3O_2)_3$; an astringent and antiseptic used after dilution with 10 to 40 parts of water as a gargle or a local application for ulcerative conditions. Syn. *Burow's solution.*

aluminum chloride. $AlCl_3·6H_2O$. A white or yellow-white, deliquescent, crystalline powder, easily soluble in water; used as an astringent and antiseptic, especially in hyperhidrosis, applied as a 25% solution.

aluminum hydroxide. $Al(OH)_3$. A white, bulky, amorphous powder insoluble in water; a protective and astringent.

aluminum hydroxide gel. A white, viscous suspension of aluminum hydroxide equivalent to 4% Al_2O_3, used as gastric antacid, especially in the treatment of peptic ulcers. A dried aluminum hydroxide gel is used similarly.

Alurate. A trademark for aprobarbital, a sedative and hypnotic.

alu·sia (a·lew′zee·uh) *n.* HALLUCINATION.

al·ve·at·ed (al′vee·ay·tid) *adj.* Honeycombed; channeled; vaulted.

alveol-, alveolo-. A combining form meaning *alveolus, alveolar.*

al·ve·o·lar (al·vee′uh·lur) *adj.* 1. Of or pertaining to an alveolus. 2. *In phonetics,* articulated with the tongue tip or blade touching, or forming a stricture at, the gums above the upper incisors, as the English consonant sounds t, d, n, s.

alveolar abscess. An abscess associated with an alveolar process and usually originating at the apex of a tooth or along a lateral surface of the root of a tooth.

alveolar air. The air contained in the pulmonary alveoli and alveolar sacs.

alveolar artery. Any of the arteries supplying the teeth; the inferior alveolar artery, which provides branches to the teeth of the mandible, the posterior superior alveolar artery, which supplies the molar and premolar teeth of the maxilla, or any of the anterior superior alveolar arteries, which supply the maxillary incisors and canines. Syn. *dental artery.*

alveolar canals. 1. (of the maxilla:) The canals in the maxilla which transmit the posterior superior alveolar vessels and nerves to the upper molar teeth. 2. The alveolar canals of the maxilla and the mandibular canal. Syn. *dental canals.*

alveolar cancer. 1. BRONCHIOLAR CARCINOMA. 2. A malignant tumor whose parenchymal cells form alveoli.

alveolar-capillary block syndrome. Arterial hypoxia due to alteration of the alveolar-capillary membrane by various disorders, hindering the diffusion of oxygen from the alveolar gas to capillary blood.

alveolar cell. 1. Any epithelial cell in the wall of a pulmonary alveolus. 2. Specifically, GREAT ALVEOLAR CELL.

alveolar (cell) carcinoma. BRONCHIOLAR CARCINOMA.

alveolar duct. Any of the air passages in the lung branching from respiratory bronchioles and leading to alveolar sacs.

alveolar macrophage. A vigorously phagocytic cell, found in and on the surface of the pulmonary alveolar wall, which ingests inhaled particulate matter and microorganisms. Syn. *alveolar phagocyte, dust cell.*

alveolar mucosa. The vestibular mucous membrane between the attached gingiva and the fornix of the vestibule of the mouth.

alveolar phagocyte. ALVEOLAR MACROPHAGE.

alveolar point. *In craniometry,* the midpoint on the anterior surface of the superior alveolar arch.

alveolar pore. One of the minute openings in the

walls of the pulmonary alveoli, affording communication between neighboring alveoli.

alveolar process. The ridge of bone, in each maxilla and in the mandible, containing the alveoli of the teeth; the alveolar process of the maxilla or the alveolar process of the mandible.

alveolar ridge. 1. In the edentulous state, the bony remains of the alveolar process of the maxilla or mandible that formerly contained the teeth. 2. ALVEOLAR PROCESS.

alveolar sacs. The terminal groups of pulmonary alveoli; the branches of an alveolar duct.

alveolar soft-part sarcoma. A poorly differentiated malignant tumor of the soft tissues whose component cells have an alveolar arrangement.

alveolar ventilation. Gas exchange between the inspired air and the blood in the alveoli of the lung; its rate per minute is calculated by the following equation: alveolar minute ventilation = (tidal volume − dead space) × respiratory rate.

al·ve·o·late (al'vee·o·late) *adj.* Pitted like a honeycomb. **—alveo·lat·ed** (·lay·tid) *adj.*

al·ve·o·lec·to·my (al''vee·o·leck'tuh·mee) *n.* Surgical removal of part of the alveolar process of the upper or lower jaw.

alveoli. Plural of *alveolus.*

al·ve·o·li·tis (al''vee·o·lye'tis) *n.* Inflammation of alveoli or an alveolus.

al·ve·o·lo·ba·sal (al·vee''uh·lo·bay'sul) *adj.* Pertaining to the alveolar portion of a jaw and to the denser basal portion of each jaw subjacent to the alveolar area which transmits pressure.

al·ve·o·lo·cap·il·lary (al·vee''uh·lo·kap'i·lerr·ee) *adj.* Of or pertaining to pulmonary alveoli and capillaries.

alveolocapillary membrane. The membrane, consisting of alveolar epithelium, capillary endothelium, and a basal lamina between them, that separates the pulmonary alveoli from the capillary lumina and through which respiratory gas exchange takes place.

al·ve·o·lo·cla·sia (al·vee''uh·lo·klay'zhuh, ·zee·uh) *n.* A nonspecific breaking down of an alveolar process, causing loosening of the teeth.

al·ve·o·lo·con·dyl·ean (al·vee''uh·lo·kon·dil'ee·un) *adj. In craniometry,* pertaining to the anterior portion of the maxillary alveolus and the occipital condyles.

al·ve·o·lo·den·tal (al·vee''uh·lo·den'tul) *adj.* Pertaining to the teeth and their sockets.

al·ve·o·lo·la·bi·al (al·vee''uh·lo·lay'bee·ul) *adj.* Pertaining to the alveolar processes and the lips, or to the labial aspect of the alveolar process.

al·ve·o·lo·lin·gual (al·vee''uh·lo·ling'gwul) *adj.* Pertaining to the lingual aspects of the alveolar processes.

al·ve·o·lo·na·sal (al·vee''uh·lo·nay'zul) *adj.* Pertaining to the alveolar point and the nasion.

al·ve·o·lo·plas·ty (al·vee''uh·lo·plas''tee) *n.* Surgical alteration of the shape or size of the alveolar ridge to aid in the construction of dental prostheses.

al·ve·o·lot·o·my (al''vee·o·lot'uh·mee) *n.* Incision into a dental alveolus.

al·ve·o·lus (al·vee'o·lus) *n.,* pl. **alveo·li** (·lye) A cavity, depression, pit, cell, or recess. Specifically: 1. A tooth socket; the cavity in which the root of a tooth is held in the alveolar process. NA (pl.) *alveoli dentales* (sing. *alveolus dentalis*). 2. An air cell of the lung; any of the numerous small pulmonary compartments in which the respiratory pathways terminate and through whose walls respiratory gases pass between air and blood. NA (pl.) *alveoli pulmonis* (sing. *alveolus pulmonis*). 3. A saclike termination of a racemose gland.

al·ve·us (al'vee·us) *n.,* pl. **al·vei** (·vee·eye) 1. A trough, tube, or canal, as ducts and vessels of the body. 2. A cavity or excavation.

alym·pho·cy·to·sis (ay·lim''fo·sigh·to'sis, a·lim'') *n.,* pl. **alymphocyto·ses** (·seez) 1. A marked decrease or an absence of lymphocytes in the blood. 2. SEVERE COMBINED IMMUNODEFICIENCY.

alys·mus (a·liz'mus) *n.* Anxiety and restlessness which accompany physical disease.

Alzheimer's disease A disease characterized by progressive dementia and diffuse cerebral cortical atrophy, and microscopically by the presence of argyrophil plaques, loss of neurons, and neurofibrillary tangles and granulovacuolar degeneration in the neurons that remain. These changes are also present in the basal ganglia.

Alzheimer's plaque ARGYROPHIL PLAQUE.

A.M.A. American Medical Association.

amal·gam (uh·mal'gum) *n.* An alloy of mercury with any other metal or metals; used for restoring teeth and for making dental dies.

amal·ga·mate (uh·mal'guh·mate) *v.* 1. To unite a metal in an alloy with mercury. 2. To unite two dissimilar substances. 3. To cover the zinc elements of a galvanic battery with mercury. **—amal·ga·ma·tion,** *n.*

Am·a·ni·ta (am''uh·nee'tah, ·nigh'tuh) *n.* A genus of mushrooms belonging to the Agaricaceae.

Amanita mus·ca·ria (mus·kair'ee·uh, ·kār'ee·uh) A common poisonous mushroom; FLY AGARIC.

Amanita phal·loi·des (fa·loy'deez). A very poisonous species of mushroom; the source of amanita toxin and amanita hemolysin.

aman·ta·dine (a·man'tuh·deen) *n.* 1-Adamantanamine, $C_{10}H_{17}N$, an antiviral compound often effective as a prophylactic agent against Asian influenza virus and of value in the treatment of parkinsonism; used as the water-soluble hydrochloride.

am·a·ranth (am'uh·ranth) *n.* 1. Any plant of the genus *Amaranthus.* An important cause of hay fever in North America west of Missouri and Iowa. 2. The trisodium salt of 1-(4-sulfo-1-naphthylazo)-2-naphthol-3,6-disulfonic acid, $C_{20}H_{11}N_2Na_3O_{10}S_3$, a dark red-brown powder used as a dye. Syn. *F.D. & C. Red No. 2.*

am·a·roid (am'uh·roid) *n.* Any distinctly bitter vegetable extractive of definite chemical composition other than an alkaloid or a glycoside. The names of specific amaroids end in *-in* or *-inum.*

am·a·se·sis (am''uh·see'sis) *n.* Inability to chew.

amas·tia (a·mas'tee·uh, ay·mas') n. Congenital absence of the breasts.

am·a·tho·pho·bia (am''uh·tho·fo'bee·uh) n. A morbid fear of dust.

am·au·ro·sis (am''aw·ro'sis) n., pl. **amauro·ses** (·seez) Partial or total blindness, especially the type not associated with gross change or injury to the eye, such as that resulting from degenerative disease of the retina or optic nerve.

amaurosis fu·gax (few'gacks) Temporary blindness resulting from sudden acceleration, as in aerial flight, or from transient occlusion of the retinal arterioles.

amaurosis par·ti·a·lis fu·gax (pahr·shee·ay'lis few'gacks). Partial blindness associated with headache, vertigo, and scotomas. It is usually sudden and transitory.

am·au·rot·ic (am''aw·rot'ick) adj. & n. 1. Of or pertaining to amaurosis. 2. An individual affected with amaurosis.

amaurotic familial idiocy. Any of the lipidoses affecting the nervous system exclusively, classified according to time of onset as infantile or early infantile (TAY-SACHS DISEASE and SAND-HOFF'S DISEASE), late infantile (BIELSCHOW-SKY-JANSKÝ DISEASE), juvenile (SPIELMEYER-VOGT DISEASE), and adult or late juvenile (KUF'S DISEASE); characterized by dementia, motor paralysis, and except in the adult form, blindness.

amaxo·pho·bia (a·mack''so·fo'bee·uh) n. Morbid dread of being in, riding upon, or meeting any vehicle.

amb-, ambi- A prefix meaning about, around.

am·ber (am'bur) n. A fossil resin found in alluvial soils and lignite beds in various parts of the world, especially along the southern shores of the Baltic Sea.

Amberlite. Trademark applied to a group of ion-exchange resins of the cation-exchange and anion-exchange type; certain of the purified resins are used medicinally.

ambi-, ambo- A combining form meaning both.

am·bi·dex·ter (am''bi·deck'stur) n. An individual who can use either hand with equal facility.

am·bi·dex·ter·i·ty (am''bi·decks·terr'i·tee) n. The ability to use both hands with equal facility.

am·bi·dex·trous (am''bi·decks'trus) adj. Able to use both hands equally well. —**ambidex·trism** (·triz·um), **ambi·dex·tral·i·ty** (·decks·tral'i·tee) n.

am·bi·ent (am'bee·unt) adj. 1. Moving about. 2. Surrounding, encompassing.

am·big·u·ous nucleus. AMBIGUUS NUCLEUS.

am·big·u·us (am·big'yoo·us) adj. Of or pertaining to the nucleus ambiguus.

ambiguus nucleus. A column of cells lying in the lateral half of the reticular formation whose cells give origin to efferent fibers of the glosso-pharyngeal, vagus, and accessory nerves. Syn. *nucleus ambiguus* [NA].

am·bi·lat·er·al (am''bee·lat'ur·ul) adj. Pertaining to or affecting both sides.

am·bi·le·vous, am·bi·lae·vous (am''bi·lee'vus) adj. Clumsy in the use of both hands. Syn. *ambisinister.*

am·bi·oc·u·lar·i·ty (am''bee·ock·yoo·lerr'i·tee) n. The ability to use both eyes equally well.

am·bi·sex·u·al (am''bee·seck'shoo·ul) adj. 1. Common to both sexes. 2. Of undetermined or indeterminate sex. —**ambi·sex·u·al·i·ty** (·seck''shoo·al'i·tee) n.

am·bi·ten·den·cy (am''bee·ten'din·see) n. The state in which a trend in human behavior is accompanied by a corresponding counter-trend, as a manic reaction arouses a depressive one.

am·biv·a·lence (am·biv'uh·lunce) n. 1. In psychiatry, the coexistence of two opposing drives, desires, attitudes, or emotions toward the same person, object, or goal. 2. Mixed feelings, such as love and hate, toward the same person; may be conscious, partly hidden from conscious awareness, or one side of the feelings may be unconscious. —**ambiv·a·lent** (·uh·lunt) adj.

am·bi·vert (am'bi·vurt) n. A personality type intermediate between extrovert and introvert.

ambly- A combining form meaning obtuse, dull, faint.

am·bly·acou·sia (am''blee·a·koo'zhuh, ·zee·uh) n. Defective hearing without any apparent organic basis.

am·bly·ope (am'blee·ope) n. An individual with amblyopia.

am·bly·o·pia (am''blee·o'pee·uh) n. Dimness of vision, especially that not due to refractive errors or organic disease of the eye. It may be congenital or acquired. —**ambly·op·ic** (·op'ick, ·o'pick) adj.

amblyopia ex anopsia. Amblyopia from disuse or from nonuse, usually of one eye, as a result of uncorrected esotropia.

am·bo·cep·tor (am'bo·sep''tur) n. 1. Obsol. According to Ehrlich, an antibody present in the blood of immunized animals which contains two specialized elements: a cytophil group that unites with a cellular antigen, and a complementophil group that joins with the complement. 2. The anti-erythrocyte antibody in the complex of antibody and sheep erythrocytes used for determination of free complement in complement-fixation tests.

Am·bro·sia (am·bro'zhuh, ·zee·uh) n. A genus of composite-flowered herbs. The common ragweed of North America, Ambrosia artemisiifolia, was used as a stimulant, tonic, antiperiodic, and astringent; properties of A. trifida are similar. The pollen of these two species is generally regarded as a frequent cause of hay fever.

am·bu·lance (am'bew·lunce) n. 1. The staff and equipment of an army medical unit in the field. 2. In the United States, a vehicle for the transportation of the sick or wounded.

am·bu·lant (am'bew·lunt) adj. Moving, shifting; ambulatory.

am·bu·la·to·ry (am'bew·luh·tor''ee) adj. 1. Walking; of or for walking. 2. Able to walk; up and about; not bedridden. 3. Characterizing or pertaining to the conditions and treatment of ambulatory patients or of outpatients.

ambulatory automatism. A condition in which an epileptic patient, during a psychomotor seizure, walks around and is able to carry out some functions without being clearly conscious of either himself or his environment.

ambulatory schizophrenia. A form of schizophrenia, usually of the simple but also of the schizoaffective type, in which the person so afflicted manages for the most part to avoid institutionalization.

ameb-, amebo-. A combining form meaning (a) *ameba, amebic;* (b) *ameboid.*

ame·ba, amoe·ba (uh-mee'buh) *n.,* pl. **amebas, amoebas, amoe·bae** (·bee) A protozoan belonging to the class Rhizopodea which moves by means of cytoplasmic extensions that are projected and retracted in response to external stimuli. Although many species are free-living, others are parasitic, principally in the intestinal tract of vertebrates and invertebrates.

ame·ba·cide (uh-mee'buh·side) *n.* AMEBICIDE.

am·e·bi·a·sis, am·oe·bi·a·sis (am''ee-bye'uh·sis) *n.* Infection, primarily colonic but also of the liver and other sites, with *Entamoeba histolytica.*

amebiasis cu·tis (kew'tis). Ulceration of the skin due to amebas, especially in association with visceral amebiasis.

ame·bic, amoe·bic (uh-mee'bick) *adj.* Of, pertaining to, or caused by an ameba.

amebic abscess. A focus of liquefaction necrosis resulting from the histolytic action of amebas, usually *Entamoeba histolytica,* and differing from a true abscess by the absence of suppuration; occurs most often in the liver and the brain.

amebic colitis. Ulceration of the colon due to infection with *Entamoeba histolytica.*

amebic dysentery. Severe amebiasis, characterized by diarrhea (often containing mucus and blood), abdominal cramping, and fever. It is due to ulceration of the large intestine produced by *Entamoeba histolytica.*

amebic gangrene. Extensive destruction of the skin surrounding a drainage wound, following removal of an amebic abscess of the liver.

amebic granuloma. A massive, usually focal, involvement of the colon by *Entamoeba histolytica,* resulting in chronic proliferative inflammation that may be clinically confused with carcinomas. Syn. *ameboma.*

amebic hepatitis. A diffuse inflammation of the liver secondary to amebic colitis.

ame·bi·cide, amoe·bi·cide (a-mee'bi·side) *n.* An agent fatal to amebas, especially to *Entamoeba histolytica.* **—ame·bi·ci·dal** (a-mee''bi·sigh'dul) *adj.*

ame·bo·cyte, amoe·bo·cyte (a-mee'bo·site) *n.* 1. Any ameboid cell. 2. A cell found in the coelomic fluid of echinoderms or among the tissues of various invertebrates. 3. LEUKOCYTE.

ame·boid, amoe·boid (a-mee'boid) *adj.* Resembling an ameba in form or in movement, as the leukocytes.

am·e·bo·ma, am·oe·bo·ma (am''ee-bo'muh) *n.* AMEBIC GRANULOMA.

ame·bu·la, amoe·bu·la (a-mee'bew·luh) *n.,* pl. **amebulas, amebu·lae** (·lee) Spores of protozoa

and other organisms which are motile because of pseudopodial action.

amel·a·not·ic (ay·mel''uh·not'ick) *adj.* Containing no melanin or very small amounts of it.

amelanotic melanoma. A malignant melanoma without pigment production.

amel·eia (a-mel'ee·uh, am''e·lye'uh) *n.* Apathy or indifference as part of a psychosis.

amel·ia (a-mel'ee·uh, ay-mee'lee·uh) *n.* Congenital absence of the extremities.

am·e·lo·blast (a-mel'o·blast, am'e·lo·) *n.* An enamel cell; one of the columnar cells of the enamel organ, from which dental enamel is formed. Syn. *adamantoblast, ganoblast.* **—am·e·lo·blas·tic** (a-mel''o·blas'tick, am''e·lo·) *adj.*

ameloblastic odontoma. A neoplasm of epithelial and mesenchymal odontogenic tissue.

am·e·lo·blas·to·ma (am''e·lo·blas·to'muh, a·mel''o·) *n.* A tumor, found usually in the mandible, whose parenchyma is composed of epithelial cells resembling those of the enamel organ; locally aggressive and prone to recur. Syn. *adamantinoma, adamantoma.*

am·e·lo·gen·e·sis (am''e·lo·jen'e·sis) *n.* Histogenesis of the dental enamel.

amelogenesis im·per·fec·ta (im''pur·feck'tuh). An inherited condition of severe hypocalcification or hypoplasia of dental enamel.

am·e·lus (am'e·lus, a·mee'lus) *n.,* pl. **ame·li** (·lye) An individual with congenital absence of all extremities.

ame·nia (a-mee'nee·uh) *n.* AMENORRHEA.

ameno·ma·nia, amoeno·ma·nia (a-men''o·may'nee·uh) *n.* The manic phase of manic-depressive illness.

amen·or·rhea, amen·or·rhoea (a-men''o·ree'uh) *n.* Absence of menstruation; characterized as primary if menarche has not occurred by 18 years of age; secondary if menstruation, once established, has not occurred for at least three months. **—amenor·rhe·al, amenor·rhoe·al** (·ree'ul) *adj.*

ament (ay'ment, am'ent) *n.* A person suffering from severe mental subnormality, usually congenital.

amen·tia (a-men'shee·uh, ay·men') *n.* Subnormal mental development; especially, congenital mental deficiency; classified as undifferentiated or primary, or according to the known cause.

American mucocutaneous leishmaniasis. A form of leishmaniasis due to *Leishmania braziliensis,* transmitted by sandflies of the genus *Phlebotomus,* and characterized by skin ulcers and ulceration and necrosis of the mucosa of the mouth and nose.

American Red Cross. A quasi-governmental agency and member of the International Red Cross, whose principal services are to the armed forces in peace and war, to the civilian population in disaster, and community services such as the teaching of first aid, life saving, maintenance of blood banks, and many other medically related volunteer services.

American spotted fever. ROCKY MOUNTAIN SPOTTED FEVER; an acute febrile illness caused by *Rickettsia rickettsii,* transmitted to man by ticks, with sudden onset of headache, chills, and fever; a characteristic exanthem occurs on the extremities and trunk.

am·er·i·ci·um (am″ur·ish′ee·um, ·ee′shee·um) *n.* The radioactive element number 95; produced artificially. Symbol, Am.

ame·tria (a·mee′tree·uh, a·met′ree·uh) *n.* Congenital absence of the uterus. **—ame·trous** (·trus) *adj.*

am·e·tro·pia (am″e·tro′pee·uh) *n.* Imperfect refractive ability due to defects of the media or the structures of the eye, which causes images to fail to focus directly upon the retina. **—ame·tro·pic** (·tro′pick, ·trop′ick) *adj.;* **am·e·trope** (am′e·trope) *n.*

am·i·an·thi·nop·sy (am″ee·an′thi·nop″see) *n.* Inability to see the color violet; inability to distinguish violet rays.

Amicar. Trademark for the antifibrinolytic agent 6-aminohexanoic acid, an aminocaproic acid.

ami·clor·al (am″i·klor′al) *n.* A trichlorohydroxyethylglucose copolymer with glucose used as a veterinary food additive.

ami·cro·bic (ay″migh·kro′bick, am″eye·) *adj.* Pertaining to or characterized by absence of microorganisms.

ami·cron (ay·migh′kron, ay·mick′ron) *n.* A colloid particle, measuring about 10^{-7} cm or less than 5 nanometers in diameter, barely visible through the light microscope.

ami·cy·cline (am″i·sigh′kleen) *n.* A tetracycline derivative of unspecified antibiotic action.

am·i·dase (am′i·dace, ·daze) *n.* Any enzyme catalyzing the hydrolysis of nonpeptide C=N linkages, generally with elimination of ammonia. Syn. *desamidase.*

am·ide (am′ide) *n.* 1. Any organic compound containing the univalent radical $RCONH_2$, $RCONHR$, or $RCONR_2$, where R indicates an alkyl or aryl group. 2. A compound formed by the replacement of a hydrogen of ammonia by a metal, such as sodamide, $NaNH_2$.

am·i·din (am′i·din) *n.* The part of starch that is soluble in water; soluble starch.

ami·do·py·rine (a·mee″do·pye′reen ·rin, am″i·do·) *n.* AMINOPYRINE.

Amigen. A trademark for certain preparations of protein hydrolysate.

amim·ia (a·mim′ee·uh, ay·mim′) *n.* Loss of the ability to imitate and to communicate by gestures or signs.

amine (a·meen′, am′in) *n.* Any member of the group of compounds formed by replacing one or more of the hydrogens of ammonia by one or more univalent hydrocarbon or other nonacidic organic radicals, such as RNH_2, $RNHR′$, and $RN(R′)R″$, where R, R′, and R″ may or may not represent the same radical. The amines are classified as primary, secondary, and tertiary depending on whether one, two, or three hydrogens are replaced.

amine oxidase. Monoamine oxidase, an enzyme which deaminates tyramine and tryptamine by oxidation to aldehyde, with liberation of ammonia.

amino-, amin- A combining form meaning *pertaining to or containing the group* NH_2 *united to a radical other than an acid radical.*

ami·no·ace·tic acid (a·mee″no·a·see′tick). Aminoethanoic acid, NH_2CH_2COOH, a nonessential amino acid. It is a constituent of many proteins from which it may be obtained by hydrolysis. Has been used for treatment of muscular dystrophy and myasthenia gravis. Syn. *glycine.*

ami·no acid (a·mee′no, am′i·no). Any one of a large group of organic compounds of the general formula $RCH(NH_2)COOH$, R representing hydrogen or any organic radical. Naturally occurring amino acids have the NH_2 group in α position, and are usually of L-configuration. These compounds are amphoteric in reaction and represent the end products of protein hydrolysis. From amino acids, the body synthesizes its proteins. Ten of them that are essential to life cannot be synthesized by the human organism and must therefore be available in the diet: arginine, histidine, isoleucine, leucine, lysine, methionine, phenylalanine, threonine, tryptophan, and valine.

ami·no·ac·i·dop·a·thy (am″i·no·as″i·dop′uth·ee, a·mee′no·) *n.* A specific defect in an enzymatic step in the metabolic pathway of one or more amino acids, or in a protein mediator necessary for the transport of certain amino acids into or out of cells.

ami·no·ac·id·uria (a·mee″no·as″i·dew′ree·uh) *n.* The presence of amino acids in the urine, especially in excess amounts, as in Fanconi syndrome.

ami·no·ac·ri·dine (a·mee″no·ack′ri·deen, ·din) *n.* AMINACRINE.

ami·no·ben·zene·sul·fon·a·mide (a·mee″no·ben″zeen·sul·fon′uh·mide) *n.* SULFANILAMIDE.

ami·no·ca·pro·ic acid (a·mee″no·ka·pro′ick) Hexanoic acid (caproic acid) with an amino substituent. 2-Aminohexanoic acid, also called α-aminocaproic acid, CH_3-$(CH_2)_3CHNH_2COOH$, is norleucine, an amino acid occurring in many proteins. 6-Aminohexanoic acid, often designated simply aminocaproic acid, $CH_2NH_2(CH_2)_4COOH$, is used as an antifibrinolytic agent in the treatment of excessive bleeding from systemic hyperfibrinolysis and urinary fibrinolysis.

ami·no·glu·cose (a·mee″no·gloo′koce) *n.* GLUCOSAMINE.

***p*-ami·no·hip·pu·ric acid** (păr″uh·a·mee″no·hi·pew′rick). *p*-Aminobenzoylaminoacetic acid, $NH_2C_6H_4CONHCH_2COOH$, used as the sodium salt in kidney function tests. Syn. *p-aminobenzoylglycine.*

ami·no·lip·id (a·mee″no·lip′id, am″i·no·) *n.* A fatty acid ester of an alcohol containing nitrogen in the amino form.

ami·no·met·ra·dine (a·mee″no·met′ruh·deen) *n.* 1-Allyl-3-ethyl-6-aminotetrahydropyrimidinedione, $C_9H_{13}N_3O_2$, an orally effective nonmercurial diuretic.

ami·no·pep·ti·dase (a·mee″no·pep′ti·dace, ·daze) *n.* An enzyme occurring in intestinal mucosa, yeast, and certain bacteria. It catalyzes hydrolysis of polypeptides at the end having a free amino group, producing an amino acid and a smaller peptide which may undergo further hydrolysis under the influence of the enzyme.

ami·no·phyl·line (a-mee"no-fil'een, am"i-nof'i-leen, -in) *n.* Theophylline ethylenediamine, $(C_7H_8N_4O_2)_2C_2H_4(NH_2)_2.xH_2O$, occurring as white or slightly yellowish granules or powder, soluble in water. It has the action and uses of theophylline, modifying blood flow, relaxing bronchial and other smooth musculature, and producing diuresis.

ami·no·pter·in (a-mee"no-terr'in, am"i-nop'te-rin) *n.* 4-Aminopteroylglutamic acid or 4-aminofolic acid, $C_{19}H_{20}N_8O_5$, a folic acid antagonist.

ami·no·pu·rine (a-mee"no-pew'reen, am"i-no·) *n.* A purine in which one or more hydrogens are replaced by amino groups, as in adenine (6-aminopurine) and in 2-aminopurine, which functions as a mutagen by acting as an adenine analogue.

ami·no·py·rine (a-mee"no-pye'reen ·rin) *n.* 4-Dimethylamino-2,3-dimethyl-1-phenyl-3-pyrazolin-5-one, $C_{13}H_{17}N_3O$, an antipyretic and analgesic that may cause agranulocytosis on continued use. Syn. *amidopyrine*.

ami·no·sal·i·cyl·ic acid (a-mee"no-sal"i-sil'ick). 1. An acid, $NH_2C_6H_3OHCOOH$, occurring as ortho-, meta-, and para-isomers. 2. PARA-AMINOSALICYLIC ACID.

ami·no·su·ria (a-mee"no-sue'ree-uh, am"i-no·) *n.* The presence of amines in the urine.

am·iso·met·ra·dine (am"eye-so-met'ruh-deen) *n.* 6-Amino-3-methyl-1-(2-methylallyl)uracil, $C_9H_{13}N_3O_2$, an orally effective nonmercurial diuretic.

am·i·thi·o·zone (am"i-thigh'o-zone) *n.* p-Formylacetanilid thiosemicarbazone or p-acetylaminobenzaldehyde thiosemicarbazone, $C_{10}H_{12}N_4OS$; has been employed for treatment of tuberculosis, leprosy, and lupus vulgaris. Syn. *thiacetazone*.

ami·to·sis (am"i·to'sis, ay"migh·to'sis) *n.* Aberrant reproduction; reproduction by direct nuclear cleavage or simple fission. —**ami·tot·ic** (·tot'ick) *adj.*

amm-, ammo- A combining form meaning *sand*.

am·me·ter (am'ee·tur, am'mee·tur) *n.* A type of galvanometer in which the electric current is measured directly in amperes.

am·mo·nia (uh·mo'nyuh) *n.* A colorless, pungent gas, NH_3, very soluble in water, a very small portion combining with it to form ammonium hydroxide. The ammonia of commerce is produced synthetically from nitrogen and hydrogen or obtained by the destructive distillation of nitrogenous organic matter. It is used as a detergent, a saponifying agent, in refrigeration, and for other industrial applications.

ammoniated mercury. Ammoniated mercuric chloride, $HgNH_2Cl$; a topically applied anti-infective agent. Syn. *white precipitate*.

ammonia water. A 10% solution of ammonia in water.

am·mo·ni·e·mia, am·mo·ni·ae·mia (a-mo"nee·ee'mee·uh) *n.* AMMONEMIA.

am·mo·ni·fi·ca·tion (a·mon"i·fi·kay'shun, a·mo"ni·) *n.* The production of ammonia by bacterial action.

am·mo·ni·um (a·mo'nee·um) *n.* The univalent radical NH_4^+. It exists only as an ion in combination with an anion.

ammonium carbonate. A compound of ammonium acid carbonate, NH_4HCO_3, and ammonium carbamate, NH_2COONH_4, in varying proportions. It is a stimulant expectorant and reflex stimulant.

ammonium chloride. NH_4Cl. Used as a saline expectorant, diuretic, and systemic and urinary acidifier.

ammonium hydroxide. NH_4OH. A weakly ionizing base formed to a slight extent when ammonia (NH_3) is dissolved in water. The term is frequently applied, not correctly, to aqueous solutions of ammonia.

ammonium iodide. NH_4I. Has been used in treating asthma and in chronic bronchitis when the exudate is fibrinous.

am·mo·ni·uria (a·mo"nee·yoo'ree·uh) *n.* An excess of ammonia in the urine.

Ammon's horn HIPPOCAMPUS.

am·mo·ther·a·py (am"o·therr'uh·pee) *n.* Sand baths in the treatment of disease; no longer in general use. Syn. *arenation*.

am·ne·mon·ic (am"ne·mon'ick) *adj.* Pertaining to impairment or loss of memory.

amnemonic agraphia. Inability to write connected or meaningful sentences, even though able to write letters and words.

am·ne·sia (am·nee'zhuh, ·zee·uh) *n.* Loss or impairment of retentive memory.

am·ne·sic (am·nee'zick, ·sick) *adj.* Of, pertaining to, or suffering from amnesia.

amnesic amimia. *Obsol.* A condition in which gestures or signs can be made but their proper meanings cannot be remembered.

amnesic amusia. *Obsol.* A form of aphasia in which a patient is able to recognize a tune but is unable to name it.

amnesic aphasia. A form of aphasia in which the patient is unable to find specific words, particularly to name or describe objects, resulting in hesitant and fragmentary speech.

am·nes·tic (am·nes'tick) *adj.* AMNESIC.

amnestic apraxia. *Obsol.* A form of apraxia in which actions can be imitated but not performed on command.

amnestic-confabulatory syndrome. A syndrome observed in organic brain syndromes, characterized by retro- and anterograde amnesia, defects in retention and recall of ideas or facts, disorientation, and confabulation, seen in varying degrees of severity, usually due to senile sclerosis, Korsakoff's syndrome, electroshock therapy, or bilateral prefrontal lobotomy.

amnia. A plural of *amnion*.

amnio-. A combining form meaning *amnion, amnionic*.

am·nio·cen·te·sis (am"nee·o·sen·te'sis) *n.* Puncture of the intrauterine amniotic sac through the abdominal wall with a trochar and cannula to obtain a sample of amniotic fluid; used in prenatal diagnosis of certain chromosomal disorders, such as Down's syndrome, and many hereditary metabolic diseases, and to study fetal maturation in late pregnancy.

am·nio·cho·ri·al (am″nee·o·ko′ree·ul) *adj.* Pertaining to the amnion and the chorion.

am·nio·em·bry·on·ic (am″nee·o·em″bree·on′ick) *adj.* Pertaining to the embryo and the amnion.

am·ni·og·ra·phy (am″nee·og′ruh·fee) *n.* Radiography of the uterine contents after injection of a radiopaque substance into the amniotic cavity. —**am·nio·gram** (am′nee·o·gram) *n.*

am·ni·on (am′nee·on) *n.*, pl. **amnions, am·nia** (·nee·uh) The innermost of the fetal membranes forming a fluid-filled sac for the protection of the embryo. Its thin, translucent wall is composed of an inner layer of ectoderm and an outer layer of mesoderm continuous with the embryonic somatopleure at the umbilicus. After the second month of development, it obliterates the extraembryonic coelom, forms a sheath about the umbilical cord, and fuses loosely with the chorionic mesoderm.

am·ni·on·ic (am′nee·on′ick) *adj.* AMNIOTIC.

am·ni·o·ni·tis (am′nee·o·nigh′tis) *n.* AMNIOTITIS.

am·ni·or·rhea, am·ni·or·rhoea (am′nee·o·ree′uh) *n.* The premature escape or discharge of the amniotic fluid.

Am·ni·o·ta (am′nee·o′tuh) *n.pl.* A group comprising those vertebrates with an amnion and allantois: mammals, birds, and reptiles. —**am·ni·ote** (am′nee·ote) *adj. & n.*

am·ni·ot·ic (am′nee·ot′ick) *adj.* Of or pertaining to the amnion.

amniotic adhesions. Collagenous adhesions between the amnion and the fetus, usually resulting in fetal malformation.

amniotic amputation. Amputation of a portion of the fetus, usually an extremity, supposedly due to constriction by an amniotic adhesion or band.

amniotic cyst. An accumulation of amniotic fluid between the amniotic folds as a result of adhesive folds or of traumatic dissection during parturition.

amniotic fluid. The transparent, almost colorless, fluid contained within the amniotic sac surrounding the fetus, composed of albumin, urea, creatinine, water, various salts, and cells.

amniotic fluid syndrome. Obstetric shock and frequently sudden death due to massive intravenous infusion of amniotic fluid causing pulmonary edema and pulmonary embolic changes. The major complication is hemorrhage due to disseminated intravascular coagulation.

amniotic fold. One of the folds of the blastoderm that unite over the embryo to form amnion and chorion in sauropsidans and many mammals.

amniotic sac. The fluid-filled sac formed by the amnion.

am·ni·o·ti·tis (am″nee·o·tye′tis) *n.* Inflammation of the amnion.

am·nio·tome (am′nee·o·tome) *n.* An instrument for puncturing the fetal membranes.

am·ni·ot·o·my (am″nee·ot′uh·mee) *n.* Rupture of the fetal membranes.

amo·bar·bi·tal (am″o·bahr′bi·tal, ·tol) *n.* 5-Eth-

yl-5-isoamylbarbituric acid, $C_{11}H_{18}N_2O_3$, a hypnotic and sedative, used as such and also as the sodium derivative, which is water-soluble.

amor (am′or) *n.* Love.

amor·phic (a·mor′fick) *adj.* AMORPHOUS.

amor·phous (a·mor′fus) *adj.* 1. Formless, shapeless. 2. *In biology,* without visible differentiation in structure. 3. *In chemistry,* not crystalline.

amo·tio (a·mo′shee·o, a·mo′tee·o) *n.* Detachment.

amotio ret·i·nae (ret′i·nee) *Obsol.* DETACHMENT OF THE RETINA.

amo·ti·va·tion·al (ay″mo·ti·vay′shun·ul) *adj.* Pertaining to lack of motivation.

amp An abbreviation for (a) *ampere;* (b) *amperage.*

am·per·age (am′peer″ij, am′pur·ij) *n.* The number of amperes passing in a given electric circuit. Abbreviated, amp.

am·pere (am′peer, am·peer′) *n.* The unit of electric current defined by the Conférence Génerale des Poids et Mesures as the steady current which when flowing in straight parallel wires, infinite in length and of negligible cross section, 1 meter apart in free space, will produce a force between the wires of 2×10^{-7} meter-kilogram-second (mks) unit (newton) per meter of length. It is equivalent to the current produced by one volt through a resistance of one ohm. Abbreviated, a., amp.

am·phet·a·mine (am·fet′uh·meen, ·min) *n.* 1. Racemic 1-phenyl-2-aminopropane, C_6H_5-$CH_2CHNH_2CH_3$, a colorless, volatile, mobile liquid. Formerly used as a nasal vasoconstrictor, by inhalation. Various salts have been used as central nervous system stimulants. 2. In common usage, amphetamine sulfate, dextroamphetamine sulfate, and methamphetamine hydrochloride, all of which act as central nervous system stimulants.

amphi-, amph- A prefix signifying (a) *both, of both kinds,* (b) *on both sides, about, around;* (c) in chemistry, *having substituents in the 2 and 6 positions of two symmetrical 6-membered fused rings.*

am·phi·ar·thro·sis (am″fee·ahr·thro′sis) *n.,* pl. **am·phi·ar·thro·ses** (·seez) [BNA]. An articulation of contiguous bony surfaces which are connected by either fibrocartilage or an interosseous ligament, and permitting only slight motion. —**amphiar·throt·ic** (·throt′ick) *adj.*

am·phi·as·ter (am′fee·as″tur) *n.* The achromatic figure in mitosis, consisting of two asters connected by a spindle.

am·phib·i·ous (am·fib′i·us) *adj.* Capable of living both on land and in water.

am·phi·cra·nia (am″fi·kray′nee·uh) *n.* Headache affecting both sides of the head.

am·phi·er·o·tism (am″fee·err′o·tiz·um) *n. Obsol.* 1. A condition in which one can conceive of one's self as being either male or female or both at the same time. 2. Sexual attraction to both males and females.

am·phi·gen·e·sis (am″fi·jen′e·sis) *n.* 1. Sexual reproduction. Syn. *amphigony.* 2. BISEXUALITY (1). —**amphi·ge·net·ic** (·je·net′ick) *adj.*

am·phig·o·ny (am-fig'uh·nee) *n*. Sexual reproduction.

am·phi·mix·is (am''fi·mick'sis) *n*., pl. **amphimixes** (-eez) 1. *In genetics*, interbreeding; heterozygosis. 2. *In psychoanalysis*, urethral, oral, and anal erotism combined.

am·phi·path (am'fi·path) *n*. AMPHIPHILE. —**amphi·path·ic** (am''fi·path'ick) *adj*.

ampho- A combining form meaning *both*.

am·pho·di·plo·pia (am''fo·di·plo'pee·uh) *n*. Double vision affecting each of the eyes.

Amphogel. Trademark for aluminum hydroxide gel, an antacid.

am·pho·phil (am'fo·fil) *adj*. & *n*. 1. AMPHOPHILIC. 2. A cell whose cytoplasm stains with both acidic and basic dyes.

am·pho·phil·ic (am''fo·fil'ick) *adj*. Having an affinity for both basic and acidic dyes.

am·pho·ric (am·fo'rick) *adj*. Resembling the sound produced by blowing across the mouth of an empty jar or bottle; used to describe respiration or resonance.

amphoric resonance. A low-pitched, hollow sound, resembling tympanitic resonance, obtained by auscultation over a pneumothorax or large pulmonary cavity.

amphoric respiration or **breathing.** Respiration characterized by amphoric resonance on auscultation.

am·pho·ter·ic (am''fo·terr'ick) *adj*. Having both acidic and basic properties; capable of behaving either as a weak acid or a weak base, as aluminum hydroxide, $Al(OH)_3 = H_3AlO_3$.

am·pho·ter·i·cin B (am''fo·terr'i·sin) *n*. An antibiotic substance, $C_{46}H_{73}NO_{20}$, produced by strains of *Streptomyces nodosus*; active against fungi. Used for treatment of deep-seated mycotic infections.

am·pi·cil·lin (am''pi·sil'in) *n*. α-Aminobenzyl penicillin, $C_{16}H_{19}N_3O_4S$, a semisynthetic penicillin that is well absorbed when taken orally and is acid resistant. It is more effective than penicillin G against certain gram-negative bacteria.

am·pli·fi·ca·tion, *n*. 1. *In microscopy*, the enlargement of the visual area, as amplification 200×, or 200 diameters. 2. The magnification of sound. 3. *In electricity*, the increase of electric current in either voltage or amperage, as of a transformer. —**am·pli·fy,** *v*.

am·pli·fi·er, *n*. 1. Any device that enlarges, magnifies, or increases the size, strength, or power of an object or force. 2. The concavo-convex lens between the objective and ocular of a microscope. 3. Any device that increases the amplitude or power level of an electrical signal by using one or more electron tubes or solid-state devices which derive energy from a power supply.

am·pli·tude, *n*. Range; extent, as of a vibration or oscillation, represented as the greatest value of a quantity which varies periodically.

am·pro·tro·pine (am''pro·tro'peen, -pin) *n*. 3-Diethylamino-2,2-dimethylpropyl tropate, $C_{18}H_{29}NO_3$, a parasympatholytic agent employed as an antispasmodic; used as the phosphate salt.

am·pul, am·pule (am'pul, am'pyool, am'pool) *n*.

1. A container, commonly made of glass and capable of being hermetically sealed, intended to hold sterile preparations usually intended for parenteral use. 2. Any of a class of preparations consisting of a sealed container holding a medicament. Such preparations are now more commonly known as injections.

am·pul·la (am·pul'uh, am·pool'uh) *n*., pl. **ampullae** (-lee) [NA]. The dilated extremity of a canal or duct, as of the mammary ducts and semicircular canals.

ampulla ca·na·li·cu·li la·cri·ma·lis (kan·uh·lick' yoo·lye lack·ri·may'lis) [NA]. AMPULLA OF THE LACRIMAL DUCT.

ampulla of the ductus deferens. The dilated distal end of the ductus deferens just before its junction with the duct of the seminal vesicle.

ampulla of the gallbladder. A dilatation sometimes present where the gallbladder empties into the cystic duct.

ampulla of the lacrimal duct. A slight dilatation of the lacrimal duct beyond the punctum.

ampulla of the vagina. The dilated upper end of the vagina, where it joins the cervix of the uterus.

ampulla of Va·ter (fah'tur) HEPATICOPANCREATIC AMPULLA.

ampulla ossea posterior [NA]. The posterior osseous ampulla. See *osseous ampullae*.

am·pul·lar (am·pul'ur, -pool', am'puh·lur) *adj*. Pertaining to or resembling an ampulla.

ampullar pregnancy. Gestation in the outer portion of the uterine tube.

am·pul·lary (am'pul·err''ee) *adj*. AMPULLAR.

ampullary aneurysm. A small saccular aneurysm; it is most common in the arteries of the brain.

am·pu·tate (am'pew·tate) *v*. To cut off all or part of an extremity, digit, organ, or projecting part of the body.

am·pu·ta·tion (am''pew·tay'shun) *n*. 1. Surgical removal of all or a part of a limb, a projecting part or process, or an organ of the body. 2. Traumatic or spontaneous loss of a limb, part, or organ.

amputation flap. A simple, broad-based flap which needs no advancement, and is shaped to provide proper contour of the part to be covered.

amputation neuroma. A benign, tumorlike mass of proliferating proximal nerve fibers and fibrous tissue, which sometimes occurs in the stump of a severed nerve.

amputation stump. The rounded and shaped distal portion of an amputated limb or organ.

am·pu·tee (am''pew·tee') *n*. One who has had major amputation of one or more limbs.

amuck (uh·muck') *adv*. In a state of frenzy, often with homicidal tendencies.

amu·sia (a·mew'zee·uh) *n*. Loss or impairment of the ability to produce or comprehend music or musical sounds, caused by lesion of the cerebrum but not by lesion affecting primary sensory, motor, or general intellectual function.

am·y·cho·pho·bia (am''i·ko·fo''bee·uh) *n*. Morbid fear of being lacerated, scratched, or clawed.

am·y·dri·a·sis (am″i·drye′uh·sis) *n.* Pupillary contraction.

amy·e·lia (am″eye·ee′lee·uh, ·el′ee·uh, ay″migh·) *n.* Congenital partial or complete absence of the spinal cord. —**amy·el·ic** (·el′ick, ·ee′lick) *adj.*

amy·e·lon·ic (a·migh″e·lon′ick, ay·migh″) *adj.* 1. Without bone marrow. 2. Without a spinal cord; amyelic.

amy·e·lus (a·migh′e·lus) *n.* An individual with partial or complete absence of the spinal cord. —**amye·lous**, *adj.*

amyg·da·la (a·mig′duh·luh) *n.*, pl. **amygda·lae** (·lee) AMYGDALOID BODY.

amyg·da·lin (a·mig′duh·lin) *n.* A glycoside, $C_{20}H_{27}NO_{11}$, of mandelonitrile and gentiobiose, occurring in bitter almond and almond sources. In the presence of water, the enzyme emulsin causes its hydrolysis into glucose, benzaldehyde, and hydrocyanic acid.

amyg·da·loid (a·mig′duh·loid) *adj.* Shaped like an almond.

amygdaloid body. An almond-shaped mass of gray matter situated in the lateral wall and roof of the inferior horn of the lateral ventricle.

amyg·da·loid·ec·to·my (a·mig″duh·loy·deck′tuh·mee) *n.* AMYGDALOTOMY.

amygdaloid nucleus. AMYGDALOID BODY.

amyg·da·lot·o·my (a·mig″duh·lot′uh·mee) *n.* Surgical destruction of the amygdaloid body.

am·yl (am′il, ay′mil) *n.* 1. PENTYL. 2. Any mixture of several pentyl radicals. 3. Any five-carbon chain of unknown structure. —**amyl·ic** (a·mil′ick) *adj.*

amyl-, amylo- A combining form meaning *starch.*

am·y·la·ceous (am″i·lay′shus) *adj.* Containing starch; starchlike.

am·y·lase (am″i·lace, ·laze) *n.* Any of two general types of enzymes that accelerate hydrolysis of starch and glycogen to produce different carbohydrate derivatives. α-Amylase (alpha amylase) occurs in malt, in certain molds and bacteria, and in saliva and pancreatic juice; it produces dextrins as hydrolysis products. A concentrated preparation of this enzyme, obtained from nonpathogenic bacteria, is used medicinally as an anti-inflammatory agent. β-Amylase (beta amylase) occurs in grains, in malt, and in vegetables; it produces maltose.

amyl nitrite. Isoamyl nitrite, $C_5H_{11}ONO$. A yellowish liquid, having an ethereal, fruity odor and a pungent, aromatic taste; used by inhalation to relax arterial spasms and of especial value in angina pectoris. Its action is immediate but fleeting.

am·y·lo·clast (am′i·lo·klast) *n.* An enzyme that catalyzes hydrolysis of starch. —**am·y·lo·clas·tic** (am″i·lo·klas′tick) *adj.*

am·y·lo·dex·trin (am″i·lo·decks′trin) *n.* SOLUBLE STARCH.

am·y·lo·dys·pep·sia (am″i·lo·dis·pep′see·uh) *n.* Inability to digest starchy foods.

am·y·loid (am′i·loid) *n.* A complex protein deposited in tissues, characterized physically by its hyaline gross structure and fibrillar ultrastructure, and chemically by special staining reactions. It is composed, in part, of proteins very similar to or identical with immunoglobulins or their fragments.

amyloid bodies. Microscopic, concentrically laminated, hyaline bodies occurring in the acini of the prostate, in the meninges, in diseased lungs, and occasionally in other sites; staining like amyloid with metachromatic aniline dyes. Syn. *corpora amylacea.*

amyloid degeneration. A retrogressive change characterized by the replacement or distortion of normal structures by material having the waxy appearance and staining properties of amyloid.

amyloidosis cu·tis (kew′tis). The presence of amyloid in the skin in the clinical form of pruritic papules or plaques; it is not necessarily associated with systemic amyloidosis.

amyloid tumor. A nonneoplastic nodule situated usually on a vocal fold, a few millimeters in diameter, spherical, and often pedunculated. Made up principally of a hyaline acidophilic substance which has staining reactions like primary amyloid. Less often found in the wall of the urinary bladder and rarely in other sites.

am·y·lol·y·sis (am″i·lol′i·sis) *n.* The digestion of starch, or its conversion into maltose. —**amy·lo·lyt·ic** (·lo·lit′ick) *adj.*

amylolytic enzyme. An enzyme that hydrolyzes starch to dextrin and maltose, as ptyalin or pancreatic amylase.

am·y·lo·pec·ti·no·sis (am″y·lo·peck″ti·no′sis) *n.* Glycogenosis caused by a defect of amylo-(1,4→1,6)-transglucosidase (branching enzyme), with storage of glycogen having branches longer than normal in the liver, kidney, heart, muscle, and reticuloendothelial system, and diminished response to glucagon and epinephrine. Syn. *Andersen's disease, brancher deficiency glycogenosis, type IV of Cori.*

am·y·lop·sin (am″i·lop′sin) *n.* PANCREATIC AMYLASE.

am·y·lose (am′i·loce, ·loze) *n.* The inner, relatively soluble, unbranched or linear polysaccharide of starch granules. It stains blue with iodine.

amylo- (1,4→1,6)-trans·glu·co·sy·lase (trans·gloo·ko′si·lace, ·gloo′ko·) *n.* An enzyme involved in the conversion of amylose to glycogen. Syn. *brancher enzyme.*

am·y·lum (am′i·lum) *n.* STARCH (1).

amy·lu·ria (am″i·lew′ree·uh) *n.* The presence of starch in the urine.

amyo·es·the·sia, amyo·aes·the·sia (ay·migh″o·es·theezh′uh, ·theez′ee·uh, a·migh″) *n.* State of being without muscle sense; lack of the sense of motion, weight, and position.

amyo·es·the·sis, amyo·aes·the·sis (ay·migh″o·es·thees′is, a·migh″) *n.* AMYOESTHESIA.

amyo·pla·sia (ay·migh″o·play′zhuh, ·zee·uh) *n.* Lack of muscle formation and development. —**amyo·plas·tic** (·plas′tick) *adj.*

amyoplasia con·gen·i·ta (kon·jen′i·tuh). Arthrogryposis multiplex due to congenital muscle deficiency.

amyo·sta·sia (ay·migh″o·stay′zhuh, ·zee·uh, a·migh″) *n.* A tremor of the muscles, causing difficulty in standing, often seen in diseases involving the basal ganglia. —**amyo·stat·ic** (·stat'ick) adj.

amyo·tax·ia (ay·migh"o·tack'see·uh, a·migh"o·) n. Ataxia or incoordination due to difficulties in controlling voluntary movements. —**amyo·tax·ic** (·sick) adj.

amyo·to·nia (ay·migh"o·to'nee·uh) n. Lack of muscular tone; floppiness.

amyotonia con·gen·i·ta (kon·jen'i·tuh) Obsol. Pronounced muscular flaccidity and weakness in infancy, due to a variety of causes.

amyo·tro·phia (ay·migh"o·tro'fee·uh, a·migh"o·) n. Amyotrophy (= MUSCULAR ATROPHY).

amyotrophia spi·na·lis pro·gres·si·va (spye·nay'lis pro·gre·sigh'vuh). 1. Progressive muscular atrophy secondary to loss of spinal innervation. 2. INFANTILE SPINAL MUSCULAR ATROPHY.

amyotrophic lateral sclerosis. An idiopathic degenerative disease of the upper and lower motor neurons, with onset chiefly in middle age, characterized by motor weakness and spastic limbs associated with muscular atrophy, fasciculations, and fibrillations, and with bulbar and pseudobulbar palsy. Pathologically, there is a loss of neurons in the anterior horns of the spinal cord and in the bulbar nuclei and degeneration of the corticospinal and corticobulbar tracts.

amy·ot·ro·phy (am"eye·ot'ruh·fee, ay"migh·) n. MUSCULAR ATROPHY. —**amyo·troph·ic** (ay·migh"o·trof'ick, ·tro'fick, a·migh"o·) adj.

Amytal. Trademark for amobarbital, a sedative and hypnotic.

amyx·ia (a·mick'see·uh, ay·mick') n. Absence or deficiency of mucous secretion.

An., an. Abbreviation for anode.

-an. In chemistry, a suffix that indicates a sugarlike substance, a glycoside, or a gum.

an-. See a-.

ANA Abbreviation for nuclear antibody.

A. N. A. 1. American Nurses Association. 2. American Neurological Association.

ana (an'uh) So much of each. Symbol, ā, āā.

ana- A prefix meaning (a) up, upward, upper; (b) back, backward; (c) again, anew; (d) in chemistry, having substituents in the 1 and 5 positions of two symmetrical 6-membered fused rings.

an·a·bi·ot·ic (an"uh·bye·ot'ick) adj. & n. 1. Apparently lifeless but capable of being revived. 2. Any agent used to effect restoration or revival. —**anabi·o·sis** (·o'sis) n.

anab·o·lism (a·nab'uh·liz·um) n. 1. Synthetic or constructive metabolism; especially, the conversion of simple nutritive compounds into complex living matter. —**an·a·bol·ic** (an"uh·bol'ick) adj.

an·ac·id·i·ty (an"uh·sid'i·tee) n. 1. The absence of normal acidity. 2. ACHLORHYDRIA.

anac·la·sis (a·nack'luh·sis) n. Reflection or refraction of light or sound. —**an·a·clas·tic** (an"uh·klas'tick) adj.

anac·li·sis (a·nack'li·sis) n. The state of being emotionally dependent upon others; specifically, in psychoanalysis, the state in which the satisfaction of the sex libido is conditioned by

some other instinct, such as hunger; used especially in reference to the dependence of an infant on a mother or mother surrogate for his sense of well-being. —**ana·clit·ic** (an"uh·klit'ick) adj.

anaclitic depression. In child psychiatry, an acute and striking impairment of an infant's physical, social, and intellectual development which sometimes occurs following a sudden separation from a loving parent figure.

an·ac·me·sis (an·ack'me·sis, an"ack·mee'sis) n. Maturation arrest in the granulocytic cells of the bone marrow.

an·acou·sia, an·acu·sia (an"uh·koo'zhuh, ·zee·uh) n. Complete deafness.

anac·ro·a·sia (an·ack"ro·ay'zee·uh, ·zhuh) n. AUDITORY APHASIA.

an·a·crot·ic (an"uh·krot'ick) adj. Pertaining to the upstroke or ascending limb of a pressure wave.

anacrotic pulse. A palpable twice-beating arterial pulse with both pulses occurring during systole before the second heart sound; the first impulse is due to accentuation of the normal anacrotic shoulder; seen best in the carotid artery in cases of aortic stenosis.

anacrotic shoulder. A pause or notch in the ascending limb of the arterial pulse-wave tracing at the time of maximal left ventricular ejection; it is prominent in cases of aortic stenosis.

anac·ro·tism (a·nack'ruh·tiz·um) n. The condition in which one or more notches or waves occur on the ascending limb of the arterial pulse tracing.

an·aer·obe (an'air·obe, an·air'obe, ·ay'ur·obe) n. A microorganism that will grow in the absence of molecular oxygen. The final hydrogen acceptors are such compounds as nitrates, sulfates, and carbonates (anaerobic respiration) or organic compounds (fermentation).

an·aer·o·bi·ase (an·air"o·bye'ace, ·aze) n. A proteolytic enzyme which acts under anaerobic conditions and is present in a number of anaerobes.

an·aer·o·bic (an"air·o'bick) adj. 1. Not utilizing oxygen. 2. Growing best in an oxygen-free atmosphere. 3. Of or pertaining to an anaerobe.

anaerobic metabolism. Metabolism carried on in the absence of molecular oxygen.

an·aero·bi·o·sis (an"air·o·bye·o'sis, an·ay"ur·o·) n. Life sustained in the absence of molecular oxygen. —**anaerobi·ot·ic** (·ot'ick) adj.

an·aero·gen·ic (an"air·o·jen'ick, an·ay"ur·o·) adj. Not gas-producing.

an·a·gog·ic (an"uh·goj'ick) adj. 1. Pertaining to spiritual, moral, or idealistic thoughts. 2. In psychoanalysis, pertaining to the efforts of the subconscious to achieve such thoughts; also, pertaining to dream material which expresses such ideas, as contrasted with that representing the sexual forces of the unconscious.

ana·kata·did·y·mus (an"uh·kat"uh·did'i·mus) n. Conjoined twins exhibiting both inferior and superior duplicity. —**anakatadidymous,** adj.

anal (ay'nul) adj. 1. Pertaining to or situated

near the anus. 2. *In psychoanalytic theory,* pertaining to the anal stage.

anal canal. The terminal portion of the large intestine extending from the rectum to the anus.

anal columns. Vertical folds of the mucous membrane of the anal canal. Syn. *rectal columns.*

anal crypt. One of the small cul-de-sacs between the anal columns. Syn. *anal sinus, rectal sinus.* NA (pl.) *sinus anales* (sing. *sinus analis*).

an·a·lep·tic (an″uh·lep′tick) *adj. & n.* 1. Stimulating the central nervous system. 2. Restorative; hastening convalescence. 3. A drug or other agent whose most prominent action is analeptic, such as one used to restore consciousness after fainting, anesthesia, or coma.

anal erotism. Localization of libido in the anal zone.

anal fissure. An elongated break in the anal mucosa, frequently causing itching, pain, and bleeding, that tends to persist because of repeated trauma from passage of hard feces, infection, and sphincter spasm. The lesion may be associated with a sentinel pile.

anal fistula. A sinus opening from the anorectal area into the connective tissue about the rectum or discharging externally.

an·al·ge·sia (an″al·jee′zee·uh) *n.* Insensibility to painful stimuli without loss of consciousness.

analgesia al·ge·ra (al′je·ruh, al·jeer′uh) Spontaneous pain in a part that is insensitive to painful stimuli.

an·al·ge·sic (an″al·jee′zick, ·jee′sick) *adj. & n.* 1. Relieving pain. 2. Not affected by pain. 3. A drug that relieves pain. —**an·al·ge·sist** (an″al·jee′zist) *n.;* **an·al·gize** (an′al·jize) *v.*

an·al·ler·gic (an″uh·lur′jick) *adj.* Not producing allergy, anaphylaxis, or hypersensitivity.

an·a·logue, an·a·log (an′uh·log) *n.* 1. An organ or part having the same function as another but differing in structure and origin, as the wing of an insect and the wing of a bird. 2. One of a group of compounds with similar electronic structure, but with different atoms, as an isologue. 3. A chemical compound which resembles a metabolically active substance structurally, but may differ functionally by being either inactive or opposite in effect. 4. (*In attributive use*) Functioning by the use of a similar object or structure as a model; specifically, of a computer: representing numerical values by physical quantities, such as lengths or voltages, so as to allow the manipulation of numerical data over a continuous range of values.

anal·o·gy (uh·nal′uh·jee) *n.* 1. Resemblance in two or more attributes between two things which differ in other respects. 2. *In biology,* a similarity in function without correspondence in structure and origin. —**analo·gous** (·gus) *adj.*

anal papilla. Any of the small elevations occasionally present on the free margins of the anal valves or at the bases of the anal columns. Syn. *papilla of Morgagni.*

anal reflex. Contraction of the external anal sphincter in response to stroking or pricking the skin or mucous membrane in the perianal region. Syn. *wink response.*

anal stage. *In psychoanalysis,* the stage of development, from 9 or 12 months of age to as late as 36 months, during which the child becomes concerned with his excreta.

anal valves. Valvelike folds in anal mucous membrane which join together the lower ends of the anal columns.

anal·y·sand (a·nal′i·sand) *n.* A person being psychoanalyzed.

anal·y·sis (a·nal′i·sis) *n.,* pl. **analy·ses** (·seez) 1. The determination of the nature, properties, or composition of a substance. 2. The resolution of a compound body into its constituent parts. 3. *In psychiatry,* PSYCHOANALYSIS. —**an·a·lyt·ic** (an″uh·lit′ick), **analyt·i·cal** (·i·kul) *adj.*

an·a·lyst (an′uh·list) *n.* 1. A person who performs analyses to determine the properties of a substance. 2. *In psychiatry,* one who analyzes the psyche; usually, one who adheres to Freudianism; a psychoanalyst.

analytic psychiatry. The school of psychiatry based on psychoanalytic theories originally developed by Sigmund Freud.

analytic psychology. The school of psychology that regards the libido not as an expression of the sex instinct, but of the will to live; the unconscious mind is thought to express certain archaic memories of race. Individuals are differentiated as extroverts and introverts, and the personality is said to be made up of an outer-directed persona and a soul or anima. Syn. *Jungian psychology.*

analytic rule. *In psychoanalysis,* a rule for patients in therapy requiring free associations to be voiced, unedited and unselected, in the order of their occurrence. Syn. *fundamental rule.*

an·a·lyz·er (an′uh·lye″zur) *n.* 1. An analyst. 2. Any apparatus or instrument for determining a given component, whether chemical, as in an autoanalyzer, or electrical frequency, as in electroencephalography. 3. A functional neurological unit consisting of an afferent nerve pathway and its central connections, allowing differentiation of stimuli. 4. In a polariscope, the Nicol prism which exhibits the properties of light after polarization. 5. An apparatus for recording the excursions of tremor movements.

an·am·ne·sis (an″am·nee′sis) *n.,* pl. **anamne·ses** (·seez) 1. Memory, recall. 2. Information gained from the patient and others regarding his medical history.

an·am·nes·tic (an″am·nes′tick) *adj.* 1. Of or pertaining to anamnesis. 2. Aiding memory. 3. Pertaining to a quickened immunologic response, as in an anamnestic reaction.

anamnestic reaction or **response.** The heightened immunologic response of an organism to a specific antigen to which the organism has previously responded.

An·am·ni·o·ta (an·am″nee·o′tuh) *n.pl.* A group of vertebrates having no amnion; includes the fishes and the amphibia.

ana·mor·pho·sis (an″uh·mor′fuh·sis, ·mor·fo′sis) *n.,* pl. **anamorpho·ses** (·seez) 1. The tendency toward increasing complication and differentiation of animate systems. 2. *In optics*, the process by which a distorted image is corrected by means of a curved mirror.

an·an·a·ba·sia (an·an″uh·bay′zhuh) *n.* Neurotic inability to ascend to heights.

an·an·a·sta·sia (an·an″uh·stay′zhuh, ·zee·uh) *n.* Neurotic inability to rise from a sitting posture, or stand up.

an·an·dria (an·an′dree·uh) *n.* Lack of virility; impotence.

an·an·gio·pla·sia (an·an″jee·o·play′zhuh, ·zee·uh) *n.* Congenital narrowing of the caliber of the blood vessels.

an·an·gio·plas·tic (an·an″jee·o·plas′tick) *adj.* Characterized by defective development of the vascular system.

an·an·kas·tia, an·an·cas·tia (an″un·kas′tee·uh, an″ang·) *n.* 1. OBSESSIVE-COMPULSIVE NEUROSIS. 2. Any psychopathologic condition in which the individual feels forced to act, think, or feel against his will. —**anankas·tic, anancas·tic** (·tick) *adj.*

an·a·pei·rat·ic (an″uh·pye·rat′ick) *adj.* Designating a condition which results from overuse of a muscle or group of muscles, as a cramp.

anapeiratic paralysis. A neurosis in which the subject believes he is paralyzed from excessive use of his limbs.

ana·phase (an′uh·faze) *n.* 1. The stage of mitosis between the metaphase and telophase, in which the daughter chromosomes move apart toward the poles of the spindle, to form the amphiaster. 2. A late stage of the first (anaphase I) or second (anaphase II) meiotic division.

an·a·phia (an·ay′fee·uh) *n.* Defective or absent sense of touch. *Adj. anaptic.*

an·a·pho·re·sis (an″uh·fo·ree′sis) *n.* 1. Diminished activity of the sweat glands. 2. IONTOPHORESIS. —**anapho·ret·ic** (·ret′ick) *adj.*

an·a·pho·ria (an″uh·for′ee·uh) *n.* A tendency toward upward turning of an eye and of its visual axis when the other eye is covered.

an·aph·ro·dis·ia (an·af″ro·diz′ee·uh) *n.* Reduction or impairment of sexual desire.

an·aph·ro·dis·i·ac (an·af″ro·diz′ee·ack) *adj. & n.* 1. Allaying sexual desire. 2. An agent that allays sexual desire.

ana·phy·lac·tic (an″uh·fi·lack′tick) *adj.* 1. Pertaining to the production or state of anaphylaxis. 2. Increasing sensitivity.

anaphylactic reaction. ANAPHYLAXIS (2).

anaphylactic shock. Shock occurring as all or part of a severe anaphylactic reaction; may be preceded by acute respiratory distress.

ana·phy·lac·toid (an″uh·fi·lack′toid) *adj.* Of, pertaining to, or resembling anaphylactoid shock.

anaphylactoid purpura. ALLERGIC PURPURA (1).

anaphylactoid shock, crisis, or **reaction.** A syndrome resembling anaphylactic shock but independent of antigen-antibody reactions and produced by the injection of a variety of substances, including certain colloids such as peptones, into the body.

ana·phy·lax·is (an″uh·fi·lack′sis) *n.,* pl. **anaphylax·es** (·seez) 1. A state of immediate hypersensitivity following sensitization to a foreign protein, drug, or other substance, usually through the parenteral route. The responsible antibody is almost always of the IgE class. 2. The clinical manifestation of such a state, occurring in immediate response to reintroduction of the specific antigen, variably characterized by pruritic urticaria, edema, respiratory distress (due to bronchial constriction), pulmonary hyperemia, and shock, and ranging in severity from mild to quickly fatal. *Adj. anaphylactic.*

an·a·pla·sia (an″uh·play′zhuh, ·zee·uh) *n.* The assumption by a cell of morphologic characteristics not indigenous in normal derivatives of the inner cell mass of the embryo and correlated with the appearance of the functional characteristics of cancer. Often equated with assumption of embryonal characteristics, but differing from embryonal cells both morphologically and functionally.

anap·la·sis (a·nap′luh·sis) *n. Obsol.* The stage of normal development and growth in an individual.

An·a·plas·ma (an″uh·plaz′muh) *n.* A genus of blood parasites (order Rickettsiales, family Anaplasmataceae) found in the erythrocytes of cattle and other ruminants; formerly thought to be protozoans.

an·a·plas·mo·sis (an″uh·plaz·mo′sis) *n.* A disease of cattle and other ruminants characterized by anemia and icterus, due to parasitization of the red blood cells by *Anaplasma.*

an·a·plas·tic (an″uh·plas′tick) *adj.* 1. Pertaining to or affected with anaplasia; cancerous. 2. Pertaining to anaplasty.

an·a·plas·ty (an′uh·plas″tee) *n.* Plastic surgery for the restoration of lost or absent parts.

ana·poph·y·sis (an″uh·pof′i·sis) *n.,* pl. **anapophy·ses** (·seez) An accessory process of a lumbar or thoracic vertebra, corresponding to the inferior tubercle of the transverse process of a typical thoracic vertebra.

an·a·rith·mia (an″uh·rith′mee·uh) *n.* Inability to count due to a parietal lobe lesion.

an·ar·thria (an·ahr′three·uh) *n.* Loss of speech due to a defect in articulation. —**anar·thric** (·thrick) *adj.*

anarthria cen·tra·lis (sen·tray′lis) *Obsol.* Partial aphasia due to a lesion in the central nervous system.

anarthria lit·e·ra·lis (lit·e·ray′lis). Stammering.

an·a·sar·ca (an″uh·sahr′kuh) *n.* Generalized edema; an accumulation of interstitial fluid in the subcutaneous connective tissue and the serous cavities of the body. —**anasar·cous** (·kus) *adj.*

anasarca hys·ter·i·cum (hi·sterr′i·kum). A transient swelling, generally of the abdomen, in a hysterical individual.

anasarcous sound. A moist bubbling sometimes heard on auscultation over edematous skin.

an·a·stal·sis (an″uh·stahl′sis, ·stal′sis) *n.* 1. REVERSED PERISTALSIS. 2. Styptic action. —**anastal·tic** (·tick) *adj.*

anas·ta·sis (a·nas′tuh·sis) *n.,* pl. **anasta·ses** (·seez) Recovery; convalescence. —**an·a·stat·ic** (an″uh·stat′ick) *adj.*

an·as·tig·mat·ic (an″uh·stig·mat′ick, an·as″tig′·) *adj.* Free from astigmatism; corrected for astigmatism, said especially of photographic objectives which are also corrected for spherical and chromatic aberration.

anas·to·mo·sis (a·nas″tuh·mo′sis) *n.*, pl. **anasto·mo·ses** (·seez) 1. An intercommunication of blood or lymph vessels by natural anatomic arrangement (as the arterial arches in the palm of the hand between the radial and ulnar arteries) or by collateral channels around a joint (as at an elbow) whereby pathways for the blood supply to a peripheral part are maintained after interruption to the chief arterial supply. Anastomoses between small peripheral vessels are constant. 2. A surgical communication made between the blood vessels (as between the portal vein and the inferior vena cava) or between two hollow organs or by two parts of the same organ (as between the jejunum and stomach, the hepatic duct and small intestine, or the ureter and colon). 3. An intermingling of fibers from two nerves, or from joining the cut ends of a nerve. —**anasto·mot·ic** (·mot′ick) *adj.*; **anas·to·mose** (a·nas″tuh·moze) *v.*

anastomotic aneurysm. CIRSOID ANEURYSM (2).

anastomotic ulcer. An ulcer at the suture line between the stomach and jejunum, usually following gastroenterostomy for peptic ulcer disease.

anat. Abbreviation for *anatomic, anatomical, anatomy.*

an·a·tom·ic (an″uh·tom′ick) *adj.* 1. Pertaining to anatomy. 2. Structural.

anatomic age. Age as judged by body development.

an·a·tom·i·cal (an″uh·tom′i·kul) *adj.* ANATOMIC.

anatomical dead space. The space in the trachea, bronchi, and air passages in general which contains air that does not reach the alveoli during respiration, the total volume of air in these conduits being about 140 ml.

anatomic position. *In human anatomy,* the attitude of a person standing erect with arms at the sides and palms forward; presupposed in anatomical discourse using directional terms based on posture, such as anterior, posterior.

anat·o·mist (uh·nat′uh·mist) *n.* A person who specializes or is skilled in anatomy.

anatomist's snuffbox. A hollow, triangular space on the dorsum of the hand at the base of the metacarpal of the thumb, when it is extended. It is formed on the sides by the tendons of the long and short extensor muscles of the thumb. Syn. *tabatiesre anatomique.*

anat·o·my (uh·nat′uh·mee) *n.* 1. The science or branch of morphology which treats of the structure of animals or plants and the relation of their parts. 2. The structure of an organism or of one of its parts. 3. Dissection of the various parts of a plant or animal.

ana·tox·in (an″uh·tock′sin) *n.* TOXOID.

¹an·atroph·ic (an″uh·trof′ick) *adj.* Correcting or preventing atrophy.

²ana·troph·ic (an″uh·trof′ick) *adj.* Nourishing.

ana·tro·pia (an″uh·tro′pee·uh) *n.* A tendency of the eyes to turn upward when at rest.

ana·ven·in (an″uh·ven′in) *n.* A venom which has been altered by physical or chemical agents that eliminate its toxic property but make little or no change in its antigenic qualities.

an·chor·age (ank′ur·ij) *n.* 1. The fixation of a floating or displaced viscus, whether by a natural process or by surgical means. 2. A tooth, the teeth, or an extraoral base used for resistance in applying an orthodontic force.

anchyl-, anchylo-. See *ankyl-.*

An·cy·los·to·ma (an″si·los′tuh·muh, ang″ki·) *n.* A genus of hookworms.

Ancylostoma amer·i·ca·num (a·merr″i·kay′num). NECATOR AMERICANUS.

Ancylostoma bra·zil·i·en·se (bra·zil″ee·en′see). A species of hookworm that infects cats and dogs; instances of human infestation, producing larva migrans or creeping eruption, have been reported in South America, Africa, and the Orient.

Ancylostoma ca·ni·num (ka·nigh′num). A common species of parasite of dogs and cats but rarely of man, found particularly in the Northern Hemisphere.

Ancylostoma du·o·de·na·le (dew″o·de·nay′lee). The species of nematode also known as the Old World hookworm; a major cause of hookworm infection, principally of man.

an·cy·lo·sto·mi·a·sis (an″si·lo·sto·migh′uh·sis, ang″ki·) *n.*, pl. **ancylostomia·ses** (·seez) Hookworm infection; more specifically infection by *Ancylostoma duodenale, A. braziliense,* or *A. caninum.* Syn. *hookworm disease.*

An·der·sen's disease 1. AMYLOPECTINOSIS. 2. CYSTIC FIBROSIS OF THE PANCREAS.

Andersen's syndrome CYSTIC FIBROSIS OF THE PANCREAS.

andr-, andro- A combining form signifying *man, male, masculine.*

andrei-, andreio- See *andr-.*

an·dri·at·rics (an″dree·at′ricks) *n.* A branch of medicine dealing with disorders peculiar to men, especially of the genitalia.

an·dro·blas·to·ma (an″dro·blas·to′muh) *n.* A testicular or ovarian tumor composed of stromal cells; it may be very primitive, or differentiated into Sertoli cells resembling those of the normal testis, and may be hormonally inactive or may produce feminization or masculinization.

an·dro·gen (an′dro·jin) *n.* A hormone that promotes the development and maintenance of male secondary sex characteristics and structures. —**an·dro·gen·ic** (an″dro·jen′ick) *adj.*

an·dro·gen·e·sis (an″dro·jen′e·sis) *n.* Activation of the egg by the sperm followed by development of the egg without the participation of the egg nucleus.

androgenic zone. The hypertrophic, inner zone of the fetal adrenal cortex, which involutes rapidly after birth. Syn. *boundary zone, fetal cortex, x zone.*

an·drog·e·nous (an·droj′e·nus) *adj.* Giving birth to males.

an·dro·gyne (an′dro·jine, ·jin) *n.* 1. A female pseudohermaphrodite. 2. A person exhibiting androgynoid characteristics. —**an·drog′y·nous** (an·droj′i·nus) *adj.*

an·drog·y·noid (an·droj'i·noid) *adj.* 1. Hermaphroditic; showing the characteristics of both sexes. 2. Of doubtful sex.

an·drog·y·ny (an·droj'i·nee) *n.* 1. HERMAPHRODITISM. 2. The condition of being an androgyne.

an·droid (an'droid) *adj.* 1. Resembling the male. 2. Specifically, of a pelvis: having a shape typical of that of the male, with a deeper cavity than is usual in the female and an inlet which is wedge-shaped, having a narrowed anterior portion.

an·drol·o·gy (an·drol'uh·jee) *n.* The science of diseases of the male sex, especially of those of the male reproductive organs.

an·dro·mor·phous (an''dro·mor'fus) *adj.* Having the form of a man.

an·dro·pho·bia (an''dro·fo'bee·uh) *n.* Pathologic fear or dislike of men.

an·dro·ster·one (an·dros'te·rone) *n.* 3α-Hydroxy-17-androstanone, $C_{19}H_{30}O_2$, an androgenic steroid isolated from male urine.

an·elec·trot·o·nus (an''e·leck·trot'uh·nus) *n.* The reduced irritability of a nerve or muscle at the positive pole during passage of an electric current, caused by hyperpolarization of the cell membrane. **—an·elec·tro·ton·ic** (·tro·ton'ick) *adj.*

ane·mia, anae·mia (uh·nee'mee·uh) *n.* A reduction below normal in erythrocytes, hemoglobin, or hematocrit.

ane·mic, anae·mic (uh·nee'mick) *adj.* Affected with, pertaining to, or characteristic of anemia.

anemic infarct. WHITE INFARCT.

anemic murmur. A hemic murmur, presumably due to an increased velocity of blood flow, that may be heard in patients with anemia.

anemic necrosis. Death of tissue following a decrease in blood flow or oxygen content below a critical level.

ane·mo·pho·bia (an''e·mo·fo'bee·uh, a·nee'mo·) *n.* Morbid dread of drafts or of winds.

an·en·ce·pha·lia (an·en''se·fay'lee·uh, an''en·) *n.* ANENCEPHALY. **—anence·phal·ic** (·fal'ick) *adj. & n.*

an·en·ceph·a·lus (an''en·sef'uh·lus) *n.,* pl. **anencepha·li** (·lye) A fetus showing partial or complete anencephaly. **—anenceph·a·lous,** *adj.*

an·en·ceph·a·ly (an''en·sef'uh·lee) *n.* Absence of the cerebrum, cerebellum, and flat bones of the skull in a fetus.

an·en·ter·ous (an·en'tur·us) *adj. In biology,* having no intestine, as a tapeworm.

aneph·ric (ay·nef'rick, a·) *adj.* 1. Lacking one or both kidneys as a congenital or acquired defect. 2. Having suffered complete and permanent loss of kidney function.

an·ep·ia (an·ep'ia) *n.* Inability to speak.

an·er·ga·sia (an''ur·gay'zhuh, ·zee·uh) *n.* 1. Lack of purposeful functioning. 2. ORGANIC BRAIN SYNDROME. **—aner·gas·tic** (·gas'tick) *adj.*

an·er·gic (an·ur'jick) *adj.* Pertaining to or exhibiting anergy.

an·er·gy (an'ur·jee) *n.* Absence of reaction to a specific antigen or allergen.

an·er·oid (an'ur·oid) *adj.* Working without a fluid, as an aneroid barometer.

an·eryth·rop·sia (an''e·rith·rop'see·uh, an·err''ith·) *n.* Impaired color perception of red; PROTANOPIA.

an·es·the·ki·ne·sis, an·aes·the·ki·ne·sis (an·es''thi·ki·nee'sis, ·kigh·nee') *n.* Sensory and motor paralysis, combined.

an·es·the·sia, an·aes·the·sia (an''es·theezh'uh, ·theez'ee·uh) *n.* 1. Insensibility, general or local, induced by anesthetic agents, hypnosis, or acupuncture. 2. Loss of sensation, of neurogenic or psychogenic origin.

an·es·the·sim·e·ter, an·aes·the·sim·e·ter (an·es''thi·zim'e·tur) *n.* 1. An instrument that measures the amount of an anesthetic administered in a given time. 2. An instrument that determines the amount of pressure necessary to produce a sensation of touch.

an·es·the·si·ol·o·gist, an·aes·the·si·ol·o·gist (an''es·theez''ee·ol'uh·jist) *n.* A physician who is a specialist in anesthesiology.

an·es·the·si·ol·o·gy, an·aes·the·si·ol·o·gy (an''es·theez''ee·ol'uh·jee) *n.* The art and science of administering local and general anesthesia to produce the various types of anesthesia.

an·es·thet·ic, an·aes·thet·ic (an''es·thet'ick) *adj. & n.* 1. Causing anesthesia. 2. Insensible to touch, pain, or other stimulation. 3. A drug that produces local or general loss of sensibility.

anesthetic leprosy. TUBERCULOID LEPROSY.

an·es·the·tist, an·aes·the·tist (an·es'thi·tist) *n.* A person, not necessarily a physician, who administers anesthetics.

an·es·the·tize, an·aes·the·tize (an·es'thi·tize) *v.* To place under the influence of an anesthetic; to induce anesthesia; to render anesthetic. **—an·es·the·ti·za·tion, an·aes·the·ti·za·tion** (an·es''thi·ti·zay'shun), **an·es·the·ti·zer, an·aes·the·ti·zer** (an·es'thi·tye''zur) *n.*

an·es·trus, an·oes·trus (an·es'trus) *n.* Cessation of ovarian function, transient or permanent, in female animals, depending on seasonal changes, pregnancy, lactation, age, or pathologic conditions. **—anestrous,** *adj.*

an·e·thole (an'e·thole) *n.* 1-Methoxy-4-propenylbenzene, $C_{10}H_{12}O$, the chief constituent of anise and fennel oils; used as a flavoring agent and carminative.

an·e·to·der·ma (an''e·to·dur'muh) *n.* Dermatosis of unknown cause that may start as inflamed macules that later become atrophied. In the Jadassohn type, the atrophy is marked by wrinkling and depression; in the Schweninger and Buzzi type, the atrophy is marked by protrusion. In both types, a sense of herniation is appreciated by palpation of the lesions.

an·eu·ploid (an'yoo·ploid, an·yoo'ploid) *adj.* Having an uneven multiple of the basic number of chromosomes. **—aneu·ploidy** (·ploy'dee) *n.*

aneu·ria (a·new'ree·uh) *n.* Lack of nervous energy. **—aneu·ric** (·rick) *adj.*

an·eu·rysm (an'yoo·riz·um) *n.* A localized, abnormal dilatation of an artery, or laterally communicating blood-filled sac, which typically progresses in size, manifests expansile pulsation, and has a bruit. It is often associated with pain, pressure symptoms, erosion of contiguous parts, and hemorrhage.

an·eu·rys·mal (an''yoo·riz'mul) *adj.* Of or pertaining to an aneurysm.

aneurysmal bone cyst. A subperiosteal tumor which bulges the periosteum, usually showing a rim of calcification.

aneurysmal varix. An arteriovenous aneurysm in which the blood flows directly into adjacent veins, causing them to be dilated, tortuous, and pulsating.

an·eu·rys·mec·to·my (an''yoo·riz·meck'tuh·mee) *n.* Excision of an aneurysm.

an·eu·rys·mo·plasty (an''yoo·riz'mo·plas''tee) *n.* Restoration of an artery in the treatment of aneurysm; reconstructive endoaneurysmorrhaphy.

an·eu·rys·mor·rha·phy (an''yoo·riz·mor'uh·fee) *n.* Repair of an aneurysm by means of obliterative suture of the sac.

an·eu·rys·mot·o·my (an''yoo·riz·mot'uh·mee) *n.* Incision of an aneurysm for the purpose of suturing or to promote granulation.

an·eu·tha·na·sia (an''yoo·thuh·nay'zhuh, ·zee·uh) *n.* A painful or difficult death.

An·ger camera A direct-viewing radiation imaging apparatus; the system locates the site of a gamma-ray interaction by comparison of pulses produced by an array of photomultiplier tubes looking at a scintillator.

angi-, angio- A combining form meaning *vessel, vascular.*

an·gi·ec·ta·sia (an''jee·eck·tay'zhuh, ·zee·uh) *n.* ANGIECTASIS.

an·gi·ec·ta·sis (an''jee·eck'tuh·sis) *n.*, **angiecta·ses** (·seez) Abnormal dilatation of a blood vessel. —**angi·ec·tat·ic** (·eck·tat'ick) *adj.*

an·gi·ec·to·my (an''jee·eck'tuh·mee) *n.* Excision of all or part of a blood vessel; an arteriectomy or a venectomy.

an·gi·itis (an''jee·eye'tis) *n.*, *pl.* **angi·it·i·des** (·it'i·deez) Inflammation of a blood or lymph vessel.

an·gi·na (an'ji·nuh, an·jye'nuh) *n.* 1. A spasmodic, cramplike, oppressive pain or attack. 2. Specifically, ANGINA PECTORIS. 3. Any of various diseases marked by attacks of choking or suffocation, especially an affection of the throat. 4. *Obsol.* Sore throat.

angina cor·dis (kor'dis). ANGINA PECTORIS.

angina pec·to·ris (peck'to·ris). Paroxysmal retrosternal or precordial pain, often radiating to the left shoulder and arm, due to inadequate blood and oxygen supply to the heart, characteristically precipitated by effort, cold, or emotion and relieved by nitroglycerin.

an·gi·no·pho·bia (an''ji·no·fo'bee·uh, an·jye''no·) *n.* Abnormal fear of angina pectoris.

an·gi·nose (an''ji·noce, ·noze) *adj.* Pertaining to angina or angina pectoris.

angio-. See *angi-.*

an·gio·blast (an'jee·o·blast) *n.* 1. Special primordium derived from extraembryonic endoderm, which gives rise to the blood cells and blood vessels in the early embryo. 2. That part of the mesenchyme, especially extraembryonic, from which the first blood cells and blood vessels arise. 3. A vasoformative cell of the mesenchyme. —**an·gio·blas·tic** (an''jee·o·blas'tick) *adj.*

angioblastic meningioma. A meningioma containing large numbers of blood vessels of differing size and shape.

an·gio·blas·to·ma (an''jee·o·blas·to'muh) *n.*, *pl.* **angioblastomas, angioblastoma·ta** (·tuh) 1. A blood-vessel tumor, usually described as invasive or malignant. 2. The development of blood-vessel-like spaces in a cellular tumor of mesodermal type.

an·gio·car·di·o·gram (an''jee·o·kahr'dee·o·gram) *n.* A radiograph of the heart and great vessels after the intravascular injection of a radiopaque medium.

an·gio·car·di·og·ra·phy (an''jee·o·kahr''dee·og'ruh·fee) *n.* Radiographic examination of the thoracic vessels and the heart chambers after the intravascular injection of radiopaque material. —**angiocar·dio·graph·ic** (·dee·o·graf'ick) *adj.*

an·gio·cav·er·no·ma (an''jee·o·kav''ur·no'muh) *n.* CAVERNOUS ANGIOMA.

an·gio·cav·ern·ous (an''jee·o·kav'ur·nus) *adj.* Pertaining to cavernous angioma.

an·gio·chei·lo·scope (an''jee·o·kigh'lo·scope) *n.* An instrument which magnifies the capillary circulation of the lips, permitting direct observation.

an·gio·chon·dro·ma (an''jee·o·kon·dro'muh) *n.* A benign tumor containing both vascular and cartilaginous elements; sometimes applied to certain hamartomas and sometimes to certain benign cartilaginous tumors with a prominent vascular stroma or capsule.

an·gio·der·ma·ti·tis (an''jee·o·dur''muh·tye'tis) *n.* Inflammation of the blood vessels of the skin.

an·gio·di·a·ther·my (an''jee·o·dye'uh·thur''mee) *n.* Obliteration of blood vessels by diathermy.

an·gio·dys·tro·phy (an''jee·o·dis'truh·fee) *n.* Defective nutrition of the blood vessels.

an·gio·ec·ta·sia (an''jee·o·eck·tay'zhuh, ·zee·uh) *n.* Varices or dilated tufts of capillaries in the skin; usually seen in older people as red or purplish areas on the skin of the trunk. Syn. *senile ectasia.*

an·gio·ede·ma (an''jee·o·e·dee'muh) *n.* An acute, transitory, localized, painless swelling of the subcutaneous tissue or submucosa of the face, hands, feet, genitalia, or viscera. It may be hereditary or caused by a food or drug allergy, an infection, or by emotional stress. Syn. *angioneurotic edema.*

an·gio·en·do·the·li·o·ma (an''jee·o·en''do·theel''ee·o'muh) *n.* 1. A tumor thought to arise from the endothelium of blood vessels rather than from reticuloendothelial cells. 2. EWING'S SARCOMA.

an·gio·fi·bro·blas·to·ma (an''jee·o·figh''bro·blas·to'muh) *n.* An angioma with fibroblastic tissue between the vascular structures.

an·gio·fi·bro·ma (an''jee·o·figh·bro'muh) *n.*, *pl.* **angiofibromas, angiofibroma·ta** (·tuh) A fibroma rich in blood vessels or lymphatics, usually forming a pedunculated skin tag.

an·gio·gen·e·sis (an''jee·o·jen'e·sis) *n.* The development of the blood vessels. —**angio·gen·ic** (·jen'ick) *adj.*

an·gio·gli·o·ma (an″jee·o·glye·o′muh) n. A glioma which is rich in blood vessels.

an·gio·gli·o·ma·to·sis (an″jee·o·glye·o″muh·to′sis) n. The presence of numerous foci of proliferating capillaries and neuroglia.

an·gio·gram (an′jee·o·gram) n. A radiographic visualization of a blood vessel or vessels after intravascular injection of a radiopaque medium.

an·gi·og·ra·phy (an″jee·og′ruh·fee) n. 1. Determination of the arrangement of blood or lymph vessels without dissection, as by capillaroscopy, fluoroscopy, or radiography. 2. *In radiology,* the visualization of blood vessels by injection of a nontoxic radiopaque substance.

an·gio·he·mo·phil·ia, an·gio·hae·mo·phil·ia (an″jee·o·hee″mo·fil′ee·uh) n. VASCULAR HEMOPHILIA.

an·gio·hy·per·to·nia (an″jee·o·high″pur·to′nee·uh) n. *Obsol.* VASOCONSTRICTION.

an·gio·hy·po·to·nia (an″jee·o·high″po·to′nee·uh) n. *Obsol.* VASODILATATION.

an·gi·oid (an′jee·oid) adj. 1. Linear. 2. Resembling a blood or lymph vessel.

angioid streaks. The brown, gray, black, or red flat serrated streaks radiating out from the optic disk in the ocular fundus, usually seen in patients with pseudoxanthoma elasticum and less commonly with Paget's disease.

an·gio·ker·a·to·ma (an″jee·o·kerr″uh·to′muh) n., pl. **angiokeratoma·ta** (·tuh) A small, vascular tumor topped by hyperkeratosis.

angiokeratoma cor·po·ris dif·fu·sum (kor′po·ris di·few′sum). ANGIOKERATOMA CORPORIS DIFFUSUM UNIVERSALE.

angiokeratoma corporis diffusum uni·ver·sa·le (yoo·ni·vur·say′lee). An inherited disorder of glycolipid metabolism, due to a deficiency of a ceramide-trihexosidase-cleaving enzyme; characterized clinically by a "critical phase" in childhood and adolescence of periodic fevers, pain, and acroparesthesia, transient proteinuria, and usually the appearance of the typical angiokeratomas over the trunk, buttocks, and genitalia; a "quiescent phase" during early maturity of asymptomatic proteinuria, hypohidrosis and anhidrosis, hypertension, and edema; and an "accelerated phase" with central nervous system disturbances and renal and cardiac failure in middle life; transmitted as a sex-linked recessive trait with full expression in the hemizygous male and occasionally partial penetrance in the heterozygous female. Abnormalities of the conjunctiva, cornea, lens, and retina may be observed. Syn. *Fabry's disease.*

angiokeratoma For·dyce (for′dice) A common characteristic condition of small, vascular tumors commonly situated on the scrotum. Hyperkeratosis is not particularly evident.

angiokeratoma Mi·bel·li (mee·bel′lee) A progressive condition, beginning at puberty, in which small, vascular, verrucous growths develop on the backs of the fingers and toes and over the knees.

an·gio·li·po·ma (an″jee·o·li·po′muh) n. A lipoma with prominent blood vessels.

an·gio·lith (an′jee·o·lith) n. A calculus in a blood vessel. **—an·gio·lith·ic** (an″jee·o·lith′ick) adj.

an·gi·ol·o·gy (an″jee·ol′uh·jee) n. 1. The scientific study and body of knowledge of the blood vessels and the lymphatic system. 2. The lymphatic and blood vessel systems.

an·gio·lu·poid (an″jee·o·lew′poid) n. A form of cutaneous sarcoidosis characterized by blue-red nodules and telangiectasia, usually on the nose or adjacent areas of the face.

an·gi·ol·y·sis (an″jee·ol′i·sis) n. Obliteration of a blood vessel during embryonal, fetal, or postnatal life; by progressive fibrosis, or by thrombosis followed by organization and cicatrization, as obliteration of the ductus arteriosus.

an·gi·o·ma (an″jee·o′muh) n., pl. **angiomas, angioma·ta** (·tuh) A hamartomatous tumor composed of blood vessels or lymphatic vessels; a hemangioma or lymphangioma. **—angi·om·a·tous** (·om′uh·tus) adj.

an·gio·ma·la·cia (an″jee·o·ma·lay′shuh, ·see·uh) n. Softening of the blood vessels.

angioma ser·pi·gi·no·sum (sur·pij·i·no′sum). A rare dysplasia of small blood vessels marked by a serpiginous progression of the condition.

an·gi·o·ma·to·sis (an″jee·o″muh·to′sis) n., pl. **angiomato·ses** (·seez) A pathologic state of the blood vessels marked by the formation of multiple angiomas.

an·gi·om·a·tous (an″jee·om′uh·tus) adj. Of, pertaining to, or resembling angiomas.

an·gio·meg·a·ly (an″jee·o·meg′uh·lee) n. Enlargement of the blood vessels, especially of the eyelids.

an·gi·om·e·ter (an″jee·om′e·tur) n. An instrument formerly used for measuring the diameter or tension of a blood vessel.

an·gio·myo·li·po·ma (an″jee·o·migh″o·li·po′muh) n. A benign hamartomatous tumor with muscular, vascular, and adipose tissue elements.

an·gio·my·op·a·thy (an″jee·o·migh·op′uth·ee) n. Any disorder involving the muscular portion of the blood vessels.

an·gio·myo·sar·co·ma (an″jee·o·migh″o·sahr·ko′muh) n. A sarcoma with differentiation into muscular cells and development of primitive vascular structures; a variety of malignant mixed mesodermal tumor.

an·gio·neu·ro·ma (an″jee·o·new·ro′muh) n. A benign tumor composed of vascular tissue and nerve fibers.

an·gio·neu·ro·my·o·ma (an″jee·o·new″ro·migh·o′muh) n. GLOMUS TUMOR.

an·gio·neu·ro·sis (an″jee·o·new·ro′sis) n., pl. **angioneuro·ses** (·seez) A disorder of the vasomotor nerves. **—angioneu·rot·ic** (·rot′ick) adj.

angioneurotic edema. ANGIOEDEMA.

an·gio·no·ma (an″jee·o·no′muh) n. Ulceration of a blood vessel.

an·gio·pa·ral·y·sis (an″jee·o·puh·ral′i·sis) n. VASOMOTOR PARALYSIS. **—angio·par·a·lyt·ic** (·păr″uh·lit′ick) adj.

an·gio·pa·re·sis (an″jee·o·pa·ree′sis, ·păr′e·sis) n. Partial vasomotor paralysis.

an·gi·op·a·thy (an″jee·op′uth·ee) n. Any disease of the vascular system.

an·gio·plas·ty (an′jee·o·plas″tee) n. Plastic surgery of injured or diseased blood vessels.

an·gio·poi·e·sis (an″jee·o·poy·ee′sis) *n.*, pl. **angiopoie·ses** (·seez) The formation of blood vessels in new tissue. **—angiopoi·et·ic** (·et′ick) *adj.*

an·gio·pres·sure (an′jee·o·presh″ur) *n.* The production of hemostasis without ligation, by angiotribe, hemostat, or other pressure.

an·gio·ret·i·nog·ra·phy (an″jee·o·ret′i·nog′ruh·fee) *n.* Visualization of the blood vessels of the retina after injection of a nontoxic radiopaque or fluorescing substance.

an·gi·or·rha·phy (an″jee·or′uh·fee) *n.* Suture of a blood vessel.

an·gi·or·rhex·is (an″jee·o·reck′sis) *n.*, pl. **angiorrhex·es** (·seez) Rupture of a blood vessel.

an·gio·sar·co·ma (an″jee·o·sahr·ko′muh) *n.* A sarcoma in which anaplastic cells form vascular spaces.

an·gio·scle·ro·sis (an″jee·o·skle·ro′sis) *n.* Hardening and thickening of the walls of the blood vessels. **—angioscle·rot·ic** (·rot′ick) *adj.*

an·gio·scope (an′jee·o·skope) *n.* An instrument, such as a specialized microscope, for examining capillary vessels.

an·gio·sco·to·ma (an″jee·o·sko·to′muh) *n.* A visual-field disturbance caused by entoptic shadows of retinal blood-vessels and other structures.

an·gio·spasm (an′jee·o·spaz·um) *n.* A localized, intermittent contracture of a blood vessel. **—an·gio·spas·tic** (an″jee·o·spas′tick) *adj.*

an·gio·ste·no·sis (an″jee·o·ste·no′sis) *n.* Narrowing of the lumen of a blood vessel.

an·gio·ten·sin (an″jee·o·ten′sin) *n.* An octapeptide, produced in circulating plasma by interaction of the enzyme renin and the alpha₂-globulin angiotensinogen. It appears to be the pressor-vasoconstrictor and aldosterone-stimulating component of the renal pressor system. Used as a pressor agent in hypotensive states. Sometimes called angiotensin II, to distinguish it from its physiologically inactive decapeptide precursor angiotensin I. The 2-8 heptapeptide fragment of angiotensin II, sometimes called angiotensin III, is also found in human and other plasma and is known to stimulate aldosterone secretion.

an·gi·ot·o·my (an″jee·ot′uh·mee) *n.* Incision into a blood vessel.

an·gio·tribe (an′jee·o·tribe) *n.* A clamp with powerful jaws for crushing arteries embedded in tissue.

an·gi·tis (an·jye′tis) *n.* ANGIITIS.

angle bisection technique. A technique for the roentgenographic exposure of intraoral films, by which the beam of radiation is directed at right angles to an imaginary plane which bisects the angle formed by the long axis of the tooth being examined and the plane of the film.

angle of convergence. The angle between the two visual axes when the eyes are turned inward.

angle of elevation. *In optics,* the angle made by the visual plane with its primary position when moved upward or downward.

angle of incidence. *In optics,* the acute angle between a ray, incident upon a surface, and the perpendicular to the surface at the point of incidence.

angle of inclination of the pelvis. 1. INCLINATION OF THE PELVIS. 2. The angle formed by the anterior wall of the pelvis with the antero-posterior diameter of the pelvic inlet. 3. The angle formed by the pelvis with the general line of the trunk or by the plane of the outlet of the pelvis with the horizon.

angle of reflection. The angle that a reflected ray of light makes with a line drawn perpendicular to the point of incidence.

angle of refraction. The angle formed by a refracted ray of light with the perpendicular at the point of refraction.

an·go·phra·sia (ang″go·fray′zhuh, ·zee·uh) *n. Obsol.* A halting, choking, and drawling type of speech occurring in general paralysis.

an·gor (ang′gor) *n.* 1. Extreme distress. 2. ANGINA (1).

angor an·i·mi (an′i·migh) A sense of imminent death.

ang·strom, ång·ström (ang′strum, awng′strem) *n.* 1. An angstrom unit; a unit of length equal to 10^{-8} cm ($1/100$ millionth of a centimeter); used for measuring wavelengths, as of visible light, x-rays, and radium radiation. Abbreviated, A, Å. 2. Sometimes defined as the wavelength of the red line of the cadmium spectrum divided by 6438.4696, and then called the international angstrom.

angstrom unit. ANGSTROM. Abbreviated, A.U., Å.U.

an·gu·lar (ang′gew·lur) *adj.* 1. Of, pertaining to, or forming an angle. 2. Pertaining to or situated near an angle. 3. Describing or pertaining to a type of chemical structure in which a component ring or group forms an angle rather than a straight alignment.

angular blepharitis. Blepharitis involving the medial angle of the eye with blocking of the puncta lacrimalia.

angular cheilosis. 1. Cheilosis affecting the angles of the lips. 2. Specifically, ANGULAR CHEILITIS.

angular gyrus. A cerebral convolution which forms the posterior portion of the inferior parietal lobule and arches over the posterior end of the superior temporal sulcus.

angular movement. The movement—backward or forward, inward or outward—that may take place between two bones.

an·gu·la·tion (ang″gew·lay′shun) *n.* 1. The formation of an abnormal angle in a hollow organ (as of the intestine or ureter), often becoming the site of an obstruction. 2. A deviation from the normal long axis, as in a fractured bone healed out of line. **—an·gu·late** (ang′gew·late) *v.*

an·he·do·nia (an″he·do′nee·uh) *n. In psychology,* overall or chronic absence of pleasure in acts which normally give pleasure.

an·he·ma·to·sis, an·hae·ma·to·sis (an″hee″muh·to′sis, an″hem″uh·) *n.* ANHEMATOPOIESIS.

an·he·mo·lyt·ic, an·hae·mo·lyt·ic (an″hee″mo·lit′ick, an″hem′o·) *adj.* Not hemolytic; not destructive of blood corpuscles.

an·he·mo·poi·e·sis, an·hae·mo·poi·e·sis (an·hee″

mo·poy·ee'sis) *n.* ANHEMATOPOIESIS. —**anhe-mopoi·et·ic** (·et'ick) *adj.*

an·hi·dro·sis (an''hi·dro'sis, an''high·) *n.*, pl. **an·hidro·ses** (·seez') Deficiency or absence of sweat secretion. —**anhi·drot·ic** (·drot'ick) *adj.*

anhydr-, anhydro- A combining form meaning (a) *waterless, lacking fluid*; (b) *an anhydride of a compound.*

an·hy·drase (an·high'drace, ·draze) *n.* Any enzyme catalyzing a reaction involving removal of water.

an·hy·dre·mia, an·hy·drae·mia (an''high·dree' mee·uh) *n.* A decreased amount of water in the blood plasma.

an·hy·dride (an·high'dride) *n.* A compound resulting from the abstraction of water from a substance.

anhydro-. See *anhydr-*.

an·hy·drous (an·high'drus) *adj. In chemistry*, characterized by absence of water, especially of water of crystallization.

an·hyp·no·sis (an''hip·no'sis) *n.* Sleeplessness; insomnia.

an·i·an·thi·nop·sy (an''ee·an'thi·nop''see, an'' eye·) *n.* Inability to recognize violet tints.

an·ic·ter·ic (an''ick·terr'ick) *adj.* Without jaundice.

an·id·e·us (a·nid'ee·us) *n.* The lowest form of omphalosite, in which the parasitic fetus is a shapeless mass of flesh covered with skin. Syn. *acardiacus amorphus, amorphus, amorphus globulus, holocardius amorphus.* —**anid·i·an, anid·e·an** (·ee·un), **an·i·dous** (an·eye'dus) *adj.*

an·i·ler·i·dine (an''i·lerr'i·deen) *n.* Ethyl 1-(4-aminophenethyl)-4-phenylisonipecotate, $C_{22}H_{28}N_2O_2$, an analgesic related to meperidine; used as the hydrochloride and phosphate salts.

an·i·line (an'i·leen, ·lin, ·line) *n.* Phenylamine or aminobenzene, $C_6H_5NH_2$, a colorless liquid with a faint, characteristic odor, obtained from coal tar and other nitrogenous substances or prepared by the reduction of nitrobenzene. It is slightly soluble in water, miscible with alcohol and ether, and forms soluble, crystallizable salts with acids. Various derivatives constitute the aniline dyes or coal tar colors.

ani·lin·gus (ay''ni·ling'gus) *n.* The erotic practice of applying the mouth to the anus.

anil·i·ty (a·nil'i·tee) *n.* 1. Senility; imbecility. 2. The state or condition of being like an old woman. —**an·ile** (an'ile) *adj.*

an·i·ma (an'i·muh) *n.* 1. The soul; the vital principle. 2. The active principle of a drug or medicine. 3. According to Jung, the inner personality or the soul, as opposed to the outer character or persona, which an individual presents to the world; also, the more feminine aspect of the inner self.

an·i·mal·cule (an''i·mal'kewl) *n.* A minute or microscopic animal; a protozoan.

animal magnetism. The hypothetical force or spiritlike effluvium emanating from certain men, as from certain metals, to others and capable of healing through mesmerism.

animal pole. 1. The formative pole of an ovum distinguished by having more cytoplasm and

pigment. 2. In the mammalian blastocyst, the pole containing the inner cell mass. Syn. *apical pole, germinal pole.*

an·i·mas·tic (an''i·mas'tick) *adj.* Pertaining to the psyche or soul.

an·i·mism (an'i·miz·um) *n.* 1. The belief that all animals, inanimate objects, and natural phenomena possess conscious souls; a characteristic of many primitive religions. 2. The theory that all the phenomena of nature are the product of an immaterial, activating soul or spirit, the anima mundi (soul of the world).

an·i·mus (an'i·mus) *n.* 1. A spirit or feeling of hatred or hostility. 2. According to Jung, the masculine as compared with the feminine aspect of the inner self.

an·ion (an'eye·on) *n.* An ion carrying one or more negative charges, and migrating to the anode on electrolysis, usually shown with negative superscript, as Cl^- (chloride), $SO_4{}^{2-}$ (sulfate), $PO_4{}^{3-}$ (phosphate). —**an·ion·ic** (an'' eye·on'ick) *adj.*

anion exchange resin. A highly polymerized synthetic organic compound containing amine groups; the basic form has the property of withdrawing acid from a liquid medium in which the resin is placed, and for this reason is utilized as a gastric antacid to control symptoms in simple hyperacidity and in peptic ulcer.

an·irid·ia (an''eye·rid'ee·uh, an''i·rid'ee·uh) *n.* Absence or defect of the iris; specifically, congenital hypoplasia of the iris, usually bilateral and transmitted as a dominant autosomal trait.

anis-, aniso- A combining form meaning *unequal, unsymmetrical, dissimilar.*

an·ise (an'is) *n.* The dried ripe fruit of *Pimpinella anisum*; has been used as a mild aromatic carminative. Syn. *anise seed, aniseed.* —**anis·ic** (a·nis'ick, a·nee'sick) *adj.*

an·is·ei·kom·e·ter (an''is·eye·kom'e·tur) *n.* A device for measuring the inequality of size when the two retinal images differ. Syn. *eikonometer.*

an·is·ei·ko·nia (an''is·eye·ko'nee·uh) *n.* A condition in which the image size seen by one eye is different from that seen by the other. —**ani·sei·kon·ic** (·kon'ick) *adj.*

an·iso·chro·ma·sia (an·eye''so·kro·may'zhuh, ·zee·uh, an''i·so·) *n.* Decreased staining of the inner portion of erythrocytes, associated with lack of hemoglobin.

an·iso·chro·mia (an·eye''so·kro'mee·uh, an''i·so·) *n.* Variation in the intensity of staining of erythrocytes due to differences in hemoglobin content. 2. HETEROCHROMIA. —**anisochro·mic** (·mick) *adj.*

an·iso·co·ria (an·eye''so·ko'ree·uh) *n.* Inequality in the diameter of the pupils.

an·iso·cy·to·sis (an·eye''so·sigh·to'sis, an''i·so·) *n.* Inequality in the size of erythrocytes.

an·iso·dac·ty·lous (an·eye''so·dack'ti·lus, an''i·so·) *adj.* Having digits of unequal length. —**anisodactylus,** *n.*

an·iso·dont (an·eye'so·dont) *adj.* Possessing irregular teeth of unequal length.

an·isog·na·thous (an''eye·sog'nuth·us) *adj.* Having jaws which do not match, one being considerably wider than the other, especially in the molar region.

an·iso·gyn·e·co·mas·tia (an″i·so·jin″e·ko·mas′ tee·uh) *n.* Unequal enlargement of the male breast due to unilateral glandular hyperplasia.

an·iso·kary·o·sis (an·eye″so·kär·ee·o′sis) *n.* Significant variation in nuclear size among cells of the same type.

an·iso·me·lia (an·eye″so·mee′lee·uh) *n.* An inequality between corresponding limbs. —**an·isom·e·lous** (an″eye·som′e·lus) *adj.*

an·iso·me·tro·pia (an·eye″so·me·tro′pee·uh) *n.* A difference in the refraction of the two eyes. —**anisome·trop·ic** (·trop′ick) *adj.*; **aniso·met·rope** (·met′rope) *n.*

an·iso·mor·phic (an·eye″so·mor′fick) *adj.* HETEROMORPHIC.

an·iso·nu·cle·o·sis (an·eye″so·new·klee·o′sis, an″ i·so·) *n.* Variation in nuclear size within a group of cells of the same general type.

an·iso·poi·kilo·cy·to·sis (an·eye″so·poy″ki·lo· sigh·to′sis) *n.* Variation of size and shape, especially in erythrocytes.

an·iso·sthen·ic (an″i·so·sthen′ick) *adj.* Not of equal power, said of pairs of muscles.

an·iso·ton·ic (an·eye″so·ton′ick) *adj.* Characterized by unequal osmotic pressure.

an·iso·trop·ic (an″eye″so·trop′ick) *adj.* 1. Having different values of a property (as refractive index, tensile strength, elasticity, electrical or heat conductivity, or rate of solution) in different directions, especially in a crystal. 2. *In biology,* responding differently to the same external stimulus in different parts of an organism. 3. In an ovum, possessing a predetermined axis or axes. Noun *anisotropy.*

anisotropic band. A BAND.

anisotropic disk. A DISK.

an·isot·ro·py (an″eye·sot′ruh·pee) *n.* The property or quality of being anisotropic.

ani·su·ria (an″i·sue′ree·uh) *n.* A condition characterized by alternate polyuria and oliguria.

Anitsch·kow cell or **myocyte** (ah·neech′kuf) A cardiac histiocyte having a characteristic bar of chromatin with fibrils radiating toward the nuclear membrane, normally present in connective tissue of the heart and coronary vessels; it proliferates in rheumatic inflammation and is seen in Aschoff nodules.

an·kle, *n.* 1. The region of juncture between the foot and leg. 2. The joint between the distal ends of the tibia and fibula proximally and the talus distally. It is a hinge joint or ginglymus.

ankle clonus. Clonic contractions of the calf muscles in response to sudden pressure against the sole of the foot, with the leg extended, or to tapping the calcaneal tendon; seen in corticospinal tract disorders.

ankle drop. DROPPED FOOT.

ankle jerk or **reflex.** ACHILLES JERK.

ankyl-, ankylo- A combining form meaning (a) *crooked, crookedness, bent;* (b) *adhesion, growing together of parts.*

an·ky·lo·bleph·a·ron (ank″i·lo·blef′uh·ron) *n.* The adhesion of the edges of the eyelids to each other.

an·ky·lo·chei·lia, an·ky·lo·chi·lia (ank″i·lo·kigh′ lee·uh) *n.* Adhesion of the lips to each other.

an·ky·lo·col·pos, an·ky·lo·kol·pos (ank″i·lo·kol′ pos) *n.* Atresia of the vagina or the vulva.

an·ky·lo·dac·tyl·ia (ank″i·lo·dack·til′ee·uh) *n.* A deformity resulting from the adhesion of fingers or toes to one another.

an·ky·lo·glos·sia (ank″i·lo·glos′ee·uh) *n.* TONGUE-TIE.

an·ky·losed (ank′i·loazd, ·loast) *adj.* 1. Stiff; firmly united; bound down with adhesions. 2. Designating a joint immobilized by some pathologic or operative process within or outside the capsule. —**an·ky·lose** (ank′i·loze, ·loce) *v.*

an·ky·lo·sis (ank″i·lo′sis) *n.,* pl. **ankylo·ses** (·sees) Stiffness or fixation of a joint.

an·ky·lo·tome (ank′i·lo·tome, ang·kil′o·) *n.* A knife for operating on tongue-tie.

an·ky·lot·o·my (ank″i·lot′uh·mee) *n.* An operation for the relief of tongue-tie.

an·la·ge (ahn′lah·guh) *n.,* pl. **anla·gen** (·gun) 1. The undifferentiated embryonic cells or tissue from which an organ or part develops; a rudiment. Syn. *primordium, blastema.* 2. *In genetics,* the hereditary predisposition for a given trait (such as a talent or disorder) or even for the entire genotype of an individual.

an·nat·to (ah·nah′to, a·nat′o) *n.* A coloring matter obtained from the pulp surrounding the seeds of the *Bixa orellana.*

an·neal (a·neel′) *v.* 1. To apply a regulated process of heating and cooling to glass or metal to relieve internal stress induced by manufacturing processes or heat. 2. *In dentistry,* to heat gold foil to render it cohesive.

an·nec·tent, an·nec·tant (a·neck′tunt) *adj.* Linking, joining, or binding together, as annectent convolutions.

an·ne·lid (a·ne′lid) *adj. & n.* 1. Of or pertaining to the phylum Annelida. 2. An annelid worm.

An·nel·i·da (a·nel′i·duh) *n.pl.* A phylum of segmented worms including the earthworms, marine and freshwater worms, and leeches.

an·nu·lar (an′yoo·lur) *adj.* Forming a ring; ring-shaped.

annular cataract. A peripheral ring-shaped lens opacity.

annular keratitis. MARGINAL KERATITIS.

annular pancreas. An anomalous form of the pancreas encircling the duodenum.

annular placenta. A placenta extending around the interior of the uterus in the form of a belt.

annular scleritis. Inflammation of the sclera at the limbus.

annular scotoma. A partial or complete area of blindness in the form of a ring. Syn. *ring scotoma.*

annular thrombus. A thrombus involving the whole circumference of a vessel but not occluding it.

an·nu·late (an′yoo·late) *adj. & n.* 1. Characterized by, made up of, or surrounded by, rings. 2. ANNELID.

an·nu·let (an′yoo·let) *n.* A narrow colored ring on the surface of or around some organs.

an·nu·lot·o·my (an″yoo·lot′uh·mee) *n.* Surgical division of a ring, usually an annulus of a cardiac valve.

an·nu·lus (an'yoo·lus) *n.*, pl. **annu·li** (·lye). ANU-
LUS; a ring or ringlike structure.

¹ano-. A combining form meaning *anus, anal.*

²ano- A combining form meaning *up, upper,
upward.*

an·o·chro·ma·sia (an"o·kro·may'zhuh, ·zee·uh)
n. 1. Concentration of hemoglobin about the
periphery of erythrocytes with the centers
pale; a condition noted in certain types of
anemia. 2. Absence of the usual staining reaction in a cell or tissue; ACHROMASIA (2).

ano·ci·as·so·ci·a·tion (a·no"see·uh·so"see·ay'
shun) *n.* An anesthetic procedure designed to
minimize surgical shock, fear, and postoperative neuroses by excluding most of the painful and harmful stimuli. Syn. *anocithesia.*

ano·ci·a·tion (a·no"see·ay'shun) *n.* ANOCIASSO-
CIATION.

ano·coc·cyg·e·al (ay"no·kock·sij'ee·ul) *adj.* Pertaining to the anus and the coccyx.

anococcygeal body. The intermingled mass of
muscular and fibrous tissue between the anal
canal and the coccyx.

ano·cu·ta·ne·ous (ay"no·kew·tay'nee·us) *adj.*
Pertaining to the anus and the skin.

anocutaneous line. The junction between skin
and mucous membrane at the anus.

an·ode (an'ode) *n.* The positive pole of a galvanic battery or other electric device. Abbreviated, A., a., An., an.

an·o·don·tia (an"o·don'chee·uh) *n.* Absence of
teeth; may be congenital or acquired.

an·o·dyne (an'o·dine) *adj. & n.* 1. Relieving pain.
2. A drug that eases or allays pain.

ano·gen·i·tal (ay"no·jen'i·tul) *adj.* Pertaining to
the anus and the genital organs.

anom·a·lad (a·nom'uh·lad) *n.* A pattern of development initiated by a single structural defect
which subsequently leads to associated secondary defects.

anom·a·lous (a·nom'uh·lus) *adj.* Abnormal, irregular.

anom·a·ly (a·nom'uh·lee) *n.* Any deviation from
the usual; any organ or part existing in an
abnormal form, structure, or location.

ano·mia (a·no'mee·uh) *n.* Loss of ability to name
objects; a type of amnesic aphasia. **—an·om·ic**
(a·nom'ick) *adj.*

anomic aphasia. ANOMIA.

an·onych·ia (an"o·nick'ee·uh) *n.* Absence of the
nails.

ano·op·sia (an"o·op'see·uh) *n.* Strabismus in
which the eye is turned upward; HYPER-
TROPIA; SUPRAVERGENCE.

ano·pel·vic (ay"no·pel'vick) *adj.* Pertaining to
the anus and the pelvis.

anopelvic version. *Obsol.* Manipulation of the
pelvis of the fetus with a finger in the mother's
rectum.

ano·per·i·ne·al (ay"no·perr"i·nee'ul) *adj.* Pertaining to the anus and the perineum.

Anoph·e·les (a·nof'e·leez) *n.* A genus of mosquitoes including the obligatory biologic vectors
of malaria, and vectors in filariasis and some
of the arbovirus encephalitides.

Anopheles quad·ri·mac·u·la·tus (kwah"dri·
mack·yoo·lay'tus). A species of mosquito that

is the chief vector of human malaria in the
United States.

anoph·e·li·cide (a·nof'e·li·side) *n.* An agent that
destroys mosquitoes of the genus *Anopheles.*

anoph·e·li·fuge (a·nof'e·li·fewj) *n.* An agent that
prevents the bite or attack of mosquitoes of
the genus *Anopheles.*

an·oph·thal·mia (an"off·thal'mee·uh) *n.* ANOPH-
THALMOS (1).

an·oph·thal·mos (an"off·thal'mos) *n.* 1. Congenital absence of one or both eyes. 2. An individual born without one or both eyes.

ano·plas·ty (ay'no·plas·tee) *n.* Plastic surgery or
repair of the anus or anal canal.

an·op·sia (an·op'see·uh) *n.* 1. Failure to use visual capacity. 2. ANOOPSIA.

an·or·chia (an·or'kee·uh) *n.* ANORCHISM.

an·or·chism (an·or'kiz·um, an'or·) *n.* Absence of
the testes. **—anor·chous** (·kus) *adj.*

ano·rec·tal (ay"no·reck'tul) *adj.* Pertaining to
the anus and the rectum. **—anorec·tum** (·tum)
n.

an·orec·tic (an"o·reck'tick) *adj. & n.* 1. Characterized by or causing anorexia. 2. Any agent
that causes anorexia.

ano·rec·to·plas·ty (ay"no·reck'to·plas"tee) *n. In
surgery*, repair or reconstruction of the anus
and rectum.

an·orex·ia (an"o·reck'see·uh) *n.* Absence of appetite. Adj. & n. *anorectic.*

anorexia ner·vo·sa (nur·vo'suh). A syndrome of
unknown cause characterized by profound
aversion to food, leading to emaciation and
sometimes serious nutritional deficiencies;
usually seen in young women.

an·orex·i·ant (an"o·reck'see·unt) *adj. & n.*
1. Causing depression of appetite. 2. An agent
that depresses appetite.

an·orex·i·gen·ic (an"o·reck"si·jen'ick) *adj.* Causing depression of appetite.

an·or·gas·my (an"or·gaz'mee) *n.* A condition,
usually psychic, in which there is a failure to
reach a climax during coitus.

an·or·thog·ra·phy (an"or·thog'ruh·fee) *n. Obsol.*
Inability to write correctly.

ano·scope (ay'no·skope) *n.* An instrument for
examining the lower rectum and anal canal.
—anos·copy (ay·nos'kuh·pee) *n.*

an·os·mia (an·oz'mee·uh) *n.* Absence of the
sense of smell due to organic or psychological
factors; organic forms are characterized as
afferent when due to loss of olfactory nerve
conductivity, central when due to cerebral
disease, obstructive when due to obstruction
of nasal fossae, and peripheral when due to
diseases of the peripheral ends of the olfactory
nerves.

an·os·mic (an·oz'mick) *adj.* Of or pertaining to
anosmia.

anosmic aphasia. Impairment in the ability to
express in words thoughts related to the sense
of smell.

ano·sog·no·sia (a·no"sog·no'zhuh, ·zee·uh) *n.*
Inability to recognize, or denial, on the part of
the patient that he is hemiplegic.

an·os·teo·pla·sia (an·os"tee·o·play'zhuh) *n.* CLEI-
DOCRANIAL DYSOSTOSIS.

an·o·tia (an·o'shuh, ·shee·uh) *n.* Congenital absence of the pinnae or external ears.

ano·tro·pia (an''o·tro'pee·uh) *n. In optometry.* HYPERTROPIA.

ano·ves·i·cal (ay''no·ves'i·kul) *adj.* Pertaining to the anus and the urinary bladder.

an·ovu·lar (an·o'vew·lur, ·ov'yoo·) *adj.* Not associated with ovulation.

anovular menstruation. Menstruation not preceded by the release of an ovum.

an·ovu·la·to·ry (an·o'vew·luh·to''ree) *adj.* 1. ANOVULAR. 2. Suppressing ovulation.

an·ox·emia, an·ox·ae·mia (an''ock·see'mee·uh) *n.* Subnormal blood oxygen content. —**anox·emic, anox·ae·mic** (·mick) *adj.*

anoxemic erythrocytosis. Secondary polycythemia due to hypoxia.

an·ox·ia (an·ock'see·uh) *n.* Extreme deficiency of oxygen in tissues; severe hypoxia. —**anox·ic** (·sick) *adj.*

an·sa (an'suh) *n.,* pl. & genit. sing. **an·sae** (·see) A loop.

ansa len·ti·cu·la·ris (len·tick''yoo·lair'is) [NA]. A bundle of efferent fibers from the globus pallidus, passing around the medial border of the internal capsule to join the fasciculus lenticularis.

an·ser·ine (an'sur·ine, ·in) *adj.* 1. Pertaining to or like a goose. 2. Designating an extremity with unduly prominent tendons because of muscle wasting.

an·si·form (an'si·form) *adj.* Loop-shaped; ANSATE.

ansiform lobule. A lobule of the posterior lobe of the cerebellum, extending from the superior surface of the hemisphere around the posterior border to the inferior surface; the inferior and superior semilunar lobules collectively. Syn. *lobulus ansiformis.*

Ansolysen Tartrate. Trademark for pentolinium tartrate.

ant-. See *anti-.*

Antabuse. Trademark for disulfiram, a substance used in the treatment of alcoholism.

ant·ac·id (ant·as'id) *n.* A substance that neutralizes acids or relieves acidity.

an·tag·o·nism (an·tag'uh·niz·um) *n.* Opposition; the mutually opposing or resisting action seen between organisms (antibiosis), muscles, functions, disease, and drugs; or between drugs and functions; or between drugs and disease. —**an·tag·o·nis·tic** (an·tag''uh·nis'tick) *adj.*

an·tag·o·nist (an·tag'uh·nist) *n.* 1. A drug that opposes the effects of another by physiological or chemical action or by a competitive mechanism for the same receptor sites. 2. ANTAGONISTIC MUSCLE. 3. ANTAGONISTIC TOOTH.

antagonistic muscle. A muscle acting in opposition to another (the agonist), as the triceps, which extends the elbow, in opposition to the biceps, which flexes the elbow.

antagonistic tooth. A tooth that meets another tooth or teeth of the opposite dental arch during mastication or in occlusion.

an·tag·o·nize (an·tag'uh·nize) *v.* 1. To neutralize the effects of a substance, such as a drug or chemical; to counteract. 2. To act in opposition to, as certain muscles.

ant·al·gic (ant·al'jick) *adj.* 1. Countering pain. 2. Pertaining to a position, attitude, or posture in order to avoid pain.

ant·al·ka·line (ant·al'ka·line, ·lin) *adj. & n.* 1. Neutralizing alkalies. 2. An agent that neutralizes alkalies.

ant·aph·ro·dis·i·ac (ant''af''ro·diz'ee·ack) *adj. & n.* ANAPHRODISIAC.

ante- A prefix meaning *before, preceding, in front of, prior to, anterior to.*

an·te·au·ral (an''te·aw'rul) *adj.* Situated in front of the ear.

an·te·bra·chi·al (an''te·bray'kee·ul) *adj.* Of or pertaining to the forearm or antebrachium.

an·te·bra·chi·um (an''te·bray'kee·um) *n.,* pl. **an·te·bra·chia** (·kee·uh) [NA]. FOREARM.

an·te ci·bum (an''te sib'um, see'bum) Before meals, used in prescription writing. Abbreviated, a.c.

an·te·cu·bi·tal (an''te·kew'bi·tul) *adj.* Situated in front of the elbow.

antecubital fossa. The depression in front of the elbow.

antecubital space. The triangular space in front of the elbow, often used as the site of venipuncture.

an·te·cur·va·ture (an''te·kur'vuh·chur) *n.* A forward curvature.

an·te·flex·ion (an''te·fleck'shun) *n.* A bending forward.

anteflexion of the uterus. A condition in which the fundus of the uterus is bent excessively forward on the cervix.

an·te·grade (an'te·grade) *adj.* ANTEROGRADE.

an·te·mor·tem (an''tee·mor'tum) *adj.* Before death.

antemortem thrombus. An intravascular blood clot that occurs before death.

an·te·na·tal (an''tee·nay'tul) *adj.* Occurring or existing before birth; prenatal.

an·te·pa·ri·e·tal (an''tee·puh·rye'e·tul) *adj.* In front of the parietal lobe of the brain.

ante par·tum (pahr'tum) *adv. phrase* Before delivery, as: 12 hrs ante partum.)

Antergan. Trademark for *N*-benzyl-*N*',*N*'-dimethyl-*N*-phenylethylenediamine, an antihistaminic substance used as the hydrochloride salt.

an·te·ri·ad (an·teer'ee·ad) *adv. In anatomy,* forward; in a posterior-to-anterior direction.

an·te·ri·or (an·teer'ee·ur) *adj. In anatomy* with reference to the human or animal body as poised for its usual manner of locomotion): fore, in front; situated or advanced relatively far in the direction of normal locomotion.

anterior adductor space. THENAR SPACE (2).

anterior asynclitism. Biparietal obliquity; the lateral inclination of the fetal head at the superior pelvic strait, which brings the sagittal suture nearer to the sacral promontory. Syn. *Naegele's obliquity.*

anterior chamber. The space between the cornea and the iris.

anterior chamber drainage angle. ANTERIOR CHAMBER ANGLE.

anterior clinoid process. A prominent process

that juts backward from the medial extremity of the lesser wing of the sphenoid bone behind the optic canal.

anterior column. A division of the longitudinal columns of gray matter in the spinal cord.

anterior cranial fossa. The most elevated in position of the three fossae into which the internal base of each side of the skull (right and left) is divided. It lodges the frontal lobe of the brain and is formed by the orbital part of the frontal bone, the cribriform plate of the ethmoid bone, and the lesser wing of the sphenoid bone.

anterior cubital region. The triangular area distal to the elbow, bounded above by a line joining the two humeral epicondyles, medially by the pronator teres muscle, and laterally by the brachioradialis muscle.

anterior embryotoxon. A congenital defect of the eye characterized by an opaque ring in the corneal stroma extending almost to the limbus and resembling an arcus senilis, but evident at or shortly after birth. It may be hereditary or occur in association with blue sclera syndrome, megalocornea, aniridia, or hypercholesterolemia. Syn. *arcus juvenilis.*

anterior ethmoid foramen. A canal between the ethmoid and frontal bones, giving passage to the nasal branch of the ophthalmic nerve and anterior ethmoid vessels.

anterior fontanel. The membranous area at the point of union of the frontal, sagittal, and coronal sutures, which closes usually during the second year.

anterior forceps. The U-shaped bundles from the radiation of the corpus callosum that are distributed to the frontal pole of the cerebral hemisphere.

anterior horn. The anterior column of gray matter as seen in a cross section of the spinal cord.

anterior horn cell. A large multipolar nerve cell in the anterior horn of the spinal cord whose axon constitutes an efferent fiber innervating a muscle. These cells are the most likely to be affected by the virus causing paralytic spinal poliomyelitis.

anterior mediastinum. The division of the mediastinum that contains the internal thoracic vessels, loose areolar tissue, lymphatic vessels, and a few lymph nodes.

anterior nuclei of the thalamus. Nuclear masses located in the anterior part of the thalamus.

anterior perforated substance. A depressed area of gray matter at the base of the brain, rostral to the optic tract, containing numerous small foramens transmitting arteries to the basal ganglions. Syn. *olfactory area.*

anterior pillar of the fauces. PALATOGLOSSAL ARCH.

anterior pituitary. ADENOHYPOPHYSIS.

anterior staphyloma. Thinning and ectasia of the cornea, with the iris adhering to the corneoscleral limbus.

anterior superior iliac spine. The projection formed by the anterior extremity of the iliac crest.

anterior synechia. Adhesion between the iris and the transparent cornea.

antero-. A combining form meaning *anterior, forward, from front to.*

an·tero·dor·sal (an″tur·o·dor′sul) *adj. In embryology,* pertaining to the dorsal aspect of the head region.

an·tero·ex·ter·nal (an″tur·o·ecks·tur′nul) *adj.* Situated in front to the outer side.

an·tero·grade (an′tur·o·grade) *adj.* 1. Proceeding forward. 2. Concerning events following the onset of the condition, as anterograde amnesia.

anterograde amnesia or **memory.** Loss of ability to form new memories or to learn.

an·tero·in·fe·ri·or (an″tur·o·in·feer′ee·ur) *adj.* Situated in front and below.

an·tero·in·te·ri·or (an″tur·o·in·teer′ee·ur) *adj.* Situated in front and internally.

an·tero·in·ter·nal (an″tur·o·in·tur′nul) *adj.* Situated in front to the inner side.

an·tero·lat·er·al (an″tur·o·lat′ur·ul) *adj.* In front and to one side; from the front to one side.

an·tero·me·di·al (an″tur·o·mee′dee·ul) *adj.* In front and toward the midline.

an·tero·me·di·an (an″tur·o·mee′dee·un) *adj.* In front and in the midline.

an·tero·pos·te·ri·or (an″tur·o·pos·teer′ee·ur) *adj.* Extending from before backward; pertaining to both front and back.

anteroposterior diameter. 1. In measuring the pelvic inlet, the line which joins the sacrovertebral angle and pubic symphysis. 2. In measuring the pelvic outlet, the distance between the lower margin of the symphysis pubis and the tip of the sacrum or the tip of the coccyx. Syn. *sacropubic diameter, coccygeopubic diameter.*

an·tero·su·pe·ri·or (an″tur·o·sue′peer′ee·ur) *adj.* Situated in front and above.

an·te·ver·sion (an″te·vur′zhun) *n.* A tipping, tilting, or displacement forward of an organ or part, especially of the uterus. —**ante·vert** (·vurt′) *v.; * **ante·vert·ed** (·vur′tid) *adj.*

anth-, antho- A combining form meaning *flower, floral, flowerlike.*

ant·he·lix (ant·hee′licks) *n.* [NA]. The curved ridge of the pinna just anterior to the helix and following through most of the course of the helix.

ant·hel·min·tic (ant″hel·min′tick, an″thel·) *adj.* & *n.* 1. Destructive or eliminative of intestinal worms. 2. A remedy for intestinal worms.

an·the·ma (an·theem′uh, anth′e·muh) *n.,* pl. **an·them·a·ta** (·tuh), **anthemas** 1. EXANTHEMA. 2. Any skin eruption.

an·the·mis (anth′e·mis) *n.* English or Roman camomile. The flower heads of *Anthemis nobilis;* have been used in coughs and spasmodic infantile complaints, and as a stomachic tonic.

Anthiomaline. Trademark for antimony lithium thiomalate, an antiprotozoal agent.

antho-. See *anth-.*

an·tho·cy·a·nin (an″tho·sigh′uh·nin) *n.* Any of a class of glycosides comprising the soluble coloring matter of blue, red, and violet flowers, and the reds and purples of autumn leaves.

an·tho·pho·bia (an″tho·fo′bee·uh) *n.* An abnormal dislike or fear of flowers.

anthr-, anthra-. A combining form denoting *the presence of the anthracene nucleus.*

anthrac-, anthraco-. A combining form meaning (a) *coal, charcoal, carbon;* (b) *anthrax.*

an·thra·ce·mia, an·thra·cae·mia (an''thruh-see'mee-uh) *n.* 1. Bacteremia or septicemia caused by *Bacillus anthracis.* 2. An increase in the level of carbon monoxide in the blood, due to carbon monoxide poisoning.

an·thra·cene (an'thruh-seen) *n.* $C_{14}H_{10}$, a tricyclic solid hydrocarbon obtained by distillation from coal tar and other carbon compounds.

an·thra·co·sil·i·co·sis (an''thruh-ko-sil-i-ko'sis) *n.* Pneumoconiosis characterized by deposition of carbon and silicon, the pathologic effects being those of silicon dioxide.

an·thra·co·sis (an''thruh-ko'sis) *n.,* Pigmentation, particularly of the lungs, by carbon particles; usually harmless. —**anthra·cot·ic** (·kot'ick) *adj.*

an·thra·lin (an'thruh-lin) *n.* 1,8-Dihydroxyanthranol, $C_{14}H_{10}O_3$, used externally for treatment of various skin diseases. Syn. *dithranol (Brit.).*

an·thra·qui·none (an''thruh-kwi·nohn', ·kwin' ohn) *n.* 9,10-Dioxoanthracene, $C_{14}H_8O_2$. Derivatives of it occur in aloe, cascara sagrada, rhubarb, and senna and are responsible for the cathartic action.

an·thrax (an'thraks) *n.,* pl. **an·thra·ces** (an'thruh-seez) 1. An acute infectious disease of cattle and sheep, transmissible to man and caused by *Bacillus anthracis.* 2. A carbuncle or malignant pustule.

anthrop-, anthropo- A combining form meaning *human being.*

an·thro·po·bi·ol·o·gy (an''thruh-po-bye-ol'uh-jee) *n.* The biologic study of man and the anthropoid apes.

an·thro·po·gen·e·sis (an''thruh-po-jen'e·sis) *n.,* pl. **anthropogen·ses** (·seez) 1. The evolution (phylogenesis) of the human species. 2. The development (ontogenesis) of the human organism. —**anthropo·ge·net·ic** (·je-net'ick) *adj.*

an·thro·poid (an'thruh-poid) *adj.* 1. Pertaining to the Anthropoidea. 2. Characteristic of anthropoid apes. 3. Specifically, of a pelvis: resembling that of the great apes, being long, narrow, and oval, with the anteroposterior diameter greater than the transverse.

An·thro·poi·dea (an''thro-poy'dee-uh) *n.pl.* The suborder of Primates that includes monkeys, apes, and humans.

anthropoid thinking. PRIMITIVE THINKING.

an·thro·pol·o·gy (an''thruh-pol'uh-jee) *n.* The scientific study of humanity. See *cultural anthropology, physical anthropology.*

an·thro·pom·e·ter (an''thro-pom'e-tur) *n.* A somatometric caliper used in taking the larger measurements of the human body.

an·thro·pom·e·try (an''thro-pom'e-tree) *n.* The scientific measurement of the human body, its various parts, and the skeleton; often used in serial and comparative studies and in systems of identification. —**anthro·po·met·ric** (·po-met'rick) *adj.;* **anthro·pom·e·trist** (·pom'e-trist) *n.*

an·thro·po·mor·phic (an''thruh-po-mor'fick) *adj.*

1. Manlike; having a human form. 2. Of or pertaining to anthropomorphism.

an·thro·poph·a·gy (an''thro-pof'uh-jee) *n.* 1. Cannibalism. 2. Sexual perversion leading to rape, mutilation, and cannibalism.

an·thro·po·pho·bia (an''thruh-po-fo'bee-uh) *n.* Pathologic fear of people or society.

an·thro·po·so·ma·tol·o·gy (an''thruh-po-so''muh-tol'uh-jee) *n.* The science of the development, structure, and functions of the human body.

ant·hyp·not·ic (ant''hip-not'ick) *adj. & n.* 1. Tending to induce wakefulness or prevent sleep. 2. An agent that tends to induce wakefulness or prevent sleep.

anti-, ant- A prefix meaning (a) *against, opposed to, counter;* (b) *combating, inhibiting, preventing, counteracting, neutralizing;* (c) *alleviating;* (d) *situated opposite;* (e) (italicized) in chemistry, *the stereoisomeric form of certain compounds* (as aldoximes) *in which substituent atoms or groups are in trans- relationship.*

an·ti·ad·re·ner·gic (an''tee-ad're·nur'jick) *adj.* Inhibiting, counteracting, or modifying adrenergic action.

an·ti·ag·glu·ti·nin (an''tee-uh-gloo'ti-nin) *n.* A substance having the power of neutralizing the corresponding agglutinin.

antianemia factor or **principle.** A substance counteracting or preventing anemia; usually the specific substance in liver (vitamin B_{12}) used in treating pernicious anemia.

an·ti·ane·mic, an·ti·anae·mic (an''tee-uh-nee'mick) *adj. & n.* 1. Preventing or correcting anemia. 2. A substance used in the treatment or prevention of anemia.

an·ti·an·ti·body (an''tee-an'ti-bod''ee) *n.* An antibody to an antibody.

an·ti·ar·rhyth·mic (an''tee-a-rith'mick) *adj.* Preventing or effective against arrhythmia.

an·ti·ar·thrit·ic (an''tee-ahr·thrit'ick) *adj. & n.* 1. Tending to relieve the symptoms of arthritis. 2. An agent that tends to relieve arthritic pain.

an·ti·asth·mat·ic (an''tee-az·mat'ick) *adj. & n.* 1. Preventing or relieving asthmatic attacks. 2. An agent that prevents or checks asthmatic attacks.

an·ti·bac·te·ri·al (an''tee-back·teer'ee·ul) *adj. & n.* 1. Preventing the growth of bacteria or destroying bacteria by physical and chemical agents. 2. An agent that prevents or hinders the growth of or destroys bacteria.

an·ti·bi·o·sis (an''tee-bye-o'sis) *n.* 1. An association between organisms of different species that is harmful to at least one of them; specifically, an association between organisms of ecologically competing species in which one party harms or inhibits the other, most typically by production of a chemical substance, as in the case of various microorganisms. 2. The field of therapy utilizing antibiotics.

an·ti·bi·ot·ic (an''tee-bye-ot'ick) *adj. & n.* 1. Pertaining to antibiosis. 2. Of or pertaining to the products of certain organisms (as penicillin) used against infections caused by other organisms. 3. An antibiotic substance.

antibiotic spectrum. The range of activity of an

antibiotic against different microorganisms. Syn. *antibacterial spectrum, antimicrobial spectrum.*

an·ti·body (an'ti·bod''ee) *n.* One of a class of substances, natural or induced by exposure to an antigen, which have the capacity to react with specific or closely related antigens. In the serum, they occur within the immunoglobulins. Abbreviated, Ab.

antibody-deficiency syndromes. The heterogeneous defects of production of antibody, usually associated with a diminution in the concentration in the serum of one or more immunoglobulins. Included in this grouping are transient hypogammaglobulinemia, congenital and acquired agammaglobulinemias, congenital and acquired dysgammaglobulinemias, and hereditary thymic aplasias.

an·ti·car·cin·o·gen (an''tee·kahr·sin'o·jen) *n.* An agent that opposes the action of carcinogens.

an·ti·ca·rio·gen·ic (an''tee·kăr''ee·o·jen'ick) *adj.* Having the quality of being able to prevent or inhibit decay, especially dental decay.

an·ti·cat·a·lyst (an''tee·kat'uh·list) *n.* Any substance that retards the action of a catalyst by acting directly upon it.

an·ti·ca·thex·is (an''tee·ka·theck'sis) *n.* A condition in which an emotional charge is released from one impulse and shifted to an impulse of an opposite nature, as when unconscious hate appears as conscious love. Syn. *counterinvestment.*

an·ti·cath·ode, an·ti·kath·ode (an''tee·kath'ode) *n.* The metal plate or target of a Crookes or x-ray tube. It is situated opposite the cathode and is struck by the cathode rays, giving rise to the x-rays.

an·ti·chei·rot·o·nus, an·ti·chi·rot·o·nus (an''ti·kigh·rot'uh·nus) *n.* Forcible and steady inflexion of the thumb, sometimes seen before or during an epileptic seizure.

an·ti·cho·les·ter·emic (an''tee·ko·les''tur·ee'mick) *adj.* Having an action that reduces the level of cholesterol in the blood.

an·ti·cho·lin·er·gic (an''tee·ko''lin·ur'jick, ·kol'in·) *adj.* Pertaining to, acting as, or caused by a cholinergic blocking agent.

an·ti·cho·lin·es·ter·ase (an''tee·ko''lin·es'tur·ace, ·aze) *n.* A substance which inhibits the enzyme activity of cholinesterase.

an·ti·co·ag·u·lant (an''tee·ko·ag'yoo·lunt) *adj. & n.* 1. Preventing or retarding coagulation, especially of blood. 2. A substance, such as heparin or bishydroxycoumarin, that prevents or retards clotting of blood. —**anticoagu·la·tive** (·luh·tiv) *adj.*

an·ti·co·ag·u·lat·ed blood (an''tee·ko·ag'yoo·lay·tid). Blood that has been kept fluid by the addition of an anticoagulant.

an·ti·co·don (an''tee·ko'don) *n.* The nucleotide triplet in a transfer ribonucleic acid molecule which pairs with a messenger ribonucleic acid codon during translation.

an·ti·com·ple·ment (an''tee·kom'ple·munt) *n.* A substance capable of neutralizing, inhibiting, or destroying a complement. Syn. *antialexin.* —**anti·com·ple·men·ta·ry** (·kom''ple·men'tuh·ree) *adj.*

an·ti·con·vul·sant (an''tee·kun·vul'sunt) *adj. & n.* 1. Tending to prevent or arrest seizures. 2. A therapeutic agent that prevents or arrests seizures.

anti·con·vul·sive (an''tee·kun·vul'siv) *adj.* Of or pertaining to an action or to a therapeutic agent that prevents or allays seizures.

an·ti·cus (an·tye'kus) *adj.* ANTERIOR; in front of.

an·ti·cu·tin (an''tee·kew'tin) *n.* Any substance capable of specifically inhibiting or reducing the capacity of an antigen to produce a reaction in the skin of a sensitized subject.

an·ti·de·pres·sant (an''tee·de·pres'unt) *adj. & n.* 1. Tending to prevent or alleviate depression. 2. Any drug used for the treatment of depression. Two classes of such drugs are of major importance: (a) certain dibenzazepine derivatives (tricyclic antidepressants), such as imipramine and amitriptyline; (b) monoamine oxidase inhibitors, such as isocarboxazid and tranylcypromine.

an·ti·di·a·bet·ic (an''tee·dye''uh·bet'ick) *adj. & n.* 1. Having an action that alleviates diabetes. 2. An agent used for treatment of diabetes.

antidiabetic hormone. INSULIN.

an·ti·di·ar·rhe·al, anti·di·ar·rhoe·al (an''tee·dye''uh·ree'ul) *adj.* Preventing or overcoming diarrhea.

an·ti·di·uret·ic (an''tee·dye'yoo·ret'ick) *adj. & n.* 1. Opposing, diminishing, or preventing the excretion of urine. 2. An agent that suppresses excretion of urine.

antidiuretic hormone. The pressor principle, a peptide hormone, of the posterior pituitary; used in medicine primarily for its antidiuretic effect. Abbreviated, ADH. Syn. *vasopressin, beta-hypophamine.*

an·ti·dote (an'ti·dote) *n.* Any agent administered to prevent or counteract the action of a poison. —**anti·dot·al** (·doat'ul) *adj.*

an·ti·drom·ic (an''ti·drom'ick) *adj.* Conducting nerve impulses in a direction opposite to the normal. —**antidrom·i·cal·ly,** *adv.*

an·ti·dys·en·ter·ic (an''tee·dis''in·terr'ick) *adj. & n.* 1. Tending to combat dysentery. 2. An agent for preventing, relieving, or curing dysentery.

an·ti·emet·ic (an''tee·e·met'ick) *adj. & n.* 1. Relieving or preventing nausea and vomiting. 2. An agent that prevents or relieves nausea and vomiting.

an·ti·en·zyme (an''tee·en'zime) *n.* 1. Any agent or substance that inhibits or prevents the action of an enzyme, such as an antibody or another enzyme. Syn. *antiferment.* 2. Specifically, an antibody formed in reaction to the injection of an enzyme.

an·ti·ep·i·lep·tic (an''tee·ep''i·lep'tick) *adj. & n.* 1. Suppressing or controlling epileptic seizures. 2. A therapeutic agent for suppression or control of epileptic seizures.

an·ti·es·tro·gen (an''tee·es'tro·jin) *adj. & n.* 1. Inhibiting or modifying estrogen action. 2. A compound that inhibits or modifies the action of an estrogen.

an·ti·fe·brile (an''tee·fee'bril, ·feb'ril) *adj. & n.* 1. Relieving or reducing fever. 2. An agent used to relieve or reduce fever.

an·ti·fer·ment (an″tee·fur′ment) *n.* 1. An agent that prevents fermentation. 2. ANTIENZYME. **—anti·fer·men·ta·tive** (·fur·men′tuh·tiv) *adj.*

an·ti·fi·bri·nol·y·sin (an″tee·figh″bri·nol′i·sin) *n.* Any substance that inhibits the proteolytic action of fibrinolysin. **—antifibri·no·lyt·ic** (·no·lit′ick) *adj.*

an·ti·fi·bro·ma·to·gen·ic (an″tee·figh·bro″muh·to·jen′ick) *adj.* Acting to prevent the formation of fibromas or fibrous connective tissue.

an·ti·fi·lar·i·al (an″tee·fi·lår′ee·ul) *adj. & n.* 1. Combating filaria. 2. Any drug or agent useful in treating infections caused by filaria.

an·ti·flat·u·lent (an″tee·flat′yoo·lunt) *adj. & n.* 1. Tending to prevent flatulence or gastric distress. 2. A drug or agent that prevents flatulence or gastric distress.

an·ti·fun·gal (an″tee·fung′gul) *adj. & n.* 1. Suppressing or destroying fungi, or effective against fungal infections. 2. Any agent useful in treating fungal infections. Syn. *antimycotic.*

an·ti·ga·lac·tic (an″tee·guh·lack′tick) *adj. & n.* 1. Lessening the flow of milk. 2. A drug or agent that lessens the flow of milk.

an·ti·gen (an′ti·jin) *n.* Any substance eliciting an immunologic response, such as the production of antibody specific for that substance. Abbreviated, Ag. **—anti·gen·ic** (·jen′ick) *adj.*

antigen–antibody reaction. The specific combination of an antigen and its antibody.

an·ti·ge·ne·mia (an″ti·je·nee′mee·uh) *n.* The presence of an antigen in the blood.

an·ti·ge·nic·i·ty (an″ti·je·nis′i·tee) *n.* The capacity to produce an immune response; the state or quality of being an antigen.

an·ti·glob·u·lin (an″tee·glob′yoo·lin) *n.* A naturally occurring or artificially induced antibody that reacts with globulin, usually gamma globulin.

antiglobulin serum. An immune serum containing antibodies to one or more globulins, usually immunoglobulins; used in the antiglobulin test.

antiglobulin test. A test originally developed for the detection of Rh antibodies. It depends on the fact that the antibodies coating the erythrocytes consist of human serum globulins. A potent precipitating rabbit anti-human serum is used. It will detect human globulin coating any particle (e.g., erythrocytes, brucella organisms). Syn. *Coombs′ test, direct developing test, Race-Coombs test.*

an·ti·grav·i·ty (an″tee·grav′i·tee) *adj.* Resisting or opposing the force of gravity.

antigravity muscles. Muscles, chiefly extensors, the contractions of which support the body against the force of gravity, as in standing.

antigravity reflexes. Reflexes which, through contraction of the extensor muscles, support the body against the force of gravity.

an·ti·he·lix (an″ti·hee′licks) *n.* ANTHELIX.

an·ti·he·mol·y·sin, anti·hae·mol·y·sin (an″tee·hee·mol′i·sin) *n.* A substance that prevents or inhibits hemolysis.

an·ti·he·mo·lyt·ic, anti·hae·mo·lyt·ic (an″ti·hee″mo·lit′ick, ·hem″o·) *adj.* 1. Pertaining to an antihemolysin. 2. Acting to prevent hemolysis.

an·ti·he·mo·phil·ic factor (an″tee·hee″mo·fil′ick) FACTOR VIII. Abbreviated, AHF.

antihemophilic globulin. FACTOR VIII. Abbreviated, AHG.

an·ti·hem·or·rhag·ic, an·ti·haem·or·rhag·ic (an″tee·hem″or·raj′ick) *adj. & n.* 1. Checking hemorrhage. 2. An agent that prevents or arrests hemorrhage.

an·ti·hem·or·rhoi·dal, anti·haem·or·rhoi·dal (an″tee·hem″uh·roy′dul) *adj. & n.* 1. Preventing or relieving hemorrhoids. 2. A drug or agent that prevents or relieves hemorrhoids.

anti·hi·drot·ic (an″tee·hi·drot′ick, ·high·drot′ick) *adj. & n.* 1. Diminishing or preventing the secretion of sweat. 2. A drug or agent that diminishes or prevents the secretion of sweat.

an·ti·his·ta·mine (an″tee·hiss′tuh·meen, ·min) *n.* A substance capable of preventing, counteracting, or diminishing the pharmacologic effects of histamine. **—anti·his·ta·min·ic** (·hiss″tuh·min′ick) *adj. & n.*

an·ti·hor·mone (an″tee·hor′mone) *n.* A substance formed in blood that antagonizes the action of a hormone, particularly a polypeptide or protein hormone which may have an antigenic action in producing the antihormone.

an·ti·hy·a·lu·ron·i·dase (an″tee·high″uh·lew·ron′i·dace, ·daze) *n.* An antienzyme that destroys hyaluronidase.

an·ti·hy·drop·ic (an″tee·high·drop′ick) *adj. & n.* 1. Relieving edematous or dropsical conditions. 2. A drug or agent that prevents or relieves edematous or dropsical conditions.

an·ti·hy·per·ten·sive (an″tee·high″pur·ten′siv) *adj. & n.* 1. Counteracting elevated blood pressure. 2. A drug that counteracts elevated blood pressure.

an·ti·hyp·not·ic (an″tee·hip·not′ick) *adj. & n.* 1. Tending to prevent sleep. 2. Any agent that tends to prevent sleep.

an·ti·in·fec·tive (an″tee·in·feck′tiv) *adj. & n.* 1. Tending to counteract or prevent infection. 2. A substance that counteracts infection.

an·ti·in·flam·ma·to·ry (an″tee·in·flam′uh·tor·ee) *adj. & n.* 1. Combating inflammation. 2. Any agent that combats inflammation.

an·ti·ke·to·gen·e·sis (an″tee·kee″to·jen′e·sis) *n.* Prevention of the production of ketone bodies, as by the utilization of carbohydrate rather than fatty acids. **—antiketogen·ic** (·ick) *adj.*

an·ti·leu·ke·mic, an·ti·leu·kae·mic (an″tee·lew·kee′mick) *adj.* Suppressing or controlling leukemia or its symptoms.

an·ti·li·pase (an″tee·lye′pace, ·paze, ·lip′ace, ·aze) *n.* A substance inhibiting or counteracting a lipase.

an·ti·lu·et·ic (an″tee·lew·et′ick) *adj. & n.* ANTISYPHILITIC.

an·ti·lym·pho·cyt·ic (an″tee·lim″fo·sit′ick) *adj.* Inhibiting or suppressing the proliferation of lymphocytes.

antilymphocytic globulin. Globulin removed from the serum of a subject immunized against the lymphocytes of the same species (homologous antilymphocytic globulin) or of a different species (heterologous antilymphocytic globulin).

an·ti·lym·pho·cyt·ic se·rum. A specially prepared serum containing antibodies against lymphocytes, used especially in prevention of rejections against transplanted organs.

an·ti·ly·sin (an″tee·lye′sin) *n.* Antibody to lysin which destroys the latter.

an·ti·ly·sis (an″tee·lye′sis) *n.*, pl. **antily·ses** (·seez) The process of destruction of a lysin by its antilysin.

an·ti·lyt·ic (an″tee·lit′ick) *adj. & n.* 1. Pertaining to an antilysin or to antilysis. 2. Destroying lysin or preventing its action. 3. A substance that destroys lysin or prevents its action.

an·ti·ma·lar·i·al (an″tee·muh·lār′ee·ul) *adj. & n.* 1. Preventing or suppressing malaria. 2. A drug that prevents or suppresses malaria.

an·ti·men·or·rhag·ic (an″tee·men·o·ray′jick, ·raj′ick) *adj. & n.* 1. Tending to reduce menstrual flow. 2. A medication or method for controlling profuse prolonged menstrual flow.

an·ti·mes·en·ter·ic (an″tee·mes″in·terr′ick) *adj.* Of or pertaining to the part of the intestine opposite the mesenteric attachment.

an·ti·me·tab·o·lite (an″tee·me·tab′o·lite) *n.* A substance having a molecular structure similar to an essential metabolite but inhibiting or opposing its action. The mechanism of antagonism is considered to be a competition between antimetabolite and metabolite for a specific enzyme in an organism.

an·ti·mi·cro·bi·al (an″tee·migh·kro′bee·ul) *adj. & n.* 1. Destroying microbes; inhibiting, suppressing, or preventing their growth. 2. An agent that destroys microbes or suppresses or prevents their growth.

an·ti·mo·ni·al (an″ti·mo′nee·ul) *adj. & n.* 1. Pertaining to or containing antimony. 2. A pharmacologic preparation containing antimony.

an·ti·mo·nous (an″ti·mo′nus) *adj.* Containing antimony in the trivalent state.

an·ti·mo·ny (an′ti·mo″nee) *n.* Sb = 121.75. A metallic, crystalline element possessing a bluish-white luster. Found native as the sulfide, Sb_2S_3, and the oxide; it is a constituent of many minerals. Used commercially chiefly for making alloys where its property of expanding on solidification is of considerable value. The actions of antimony compounds resemble those of arsenic, but they are less toxic. They produce nausea, emesis, enteritis, and nephritis. The nauseant action is used in expectorant and diaphoretic mixtures; they were formerly employed to produce circulatory depression in fever, and for catharsis and emesis. Certain complex antimony compounds are valuable antiprotozoan agents.

an·ti·mo·nyl (an″ti·mo·nil) *n.* SbO, the univalent radical of antimonous compounds.

antimony lithium thiomalate. Approximately $C_{12}H_9Li_6O_{12}S_3Sb.9H_2O$, used for treatment of filariasis, trypanosomiasis, lymphogranuloma, and schistosomiasis.

antimony potassium tartrate. $2KSbOC_4H_4O_6.$-H_2O, used as an antiprotozoal agent and, rarely, as an expectorant and emetic. Syn. *tartar emetic.*

antimony sodium tartrate. $NaSbOC_4H_4O_6$, used for the same purposes as antimony potassium tartrate but more soluble in water.

an·ti·my·cot·ic (an″tee·migh·kot′ick) *adj. & n.* ANTIFUNGAL.

an·ti·nar·cot·ic (an″tee·nahr·kot′ick) *adj. & n.* 1. Preventing narcosis. 2. Any antinarcotic substance, such as the morphine antagonists nalorphine and naloxone.

an·ti·nau·se·ant (an″tee·naw′zee·unt) *adj. & n.* 1. Tending to prevent or alleviate nausea. 2. An agent used to prevent or alleviate nausea.

an·ti·neo·plas·tic (an″tee·nee″o·plas′tick) *adj.* Inhibiting or destroying neoplastic cells or tumors.

an·ti·neu·rit·ic (an″tee·new·rit′ick) *adj. & n.* 1. Effective in relieving or preventing neuritis or neuropathy. 2. An agent or drug used to prevent or relieve neuritis or neuropathy, such as vitamin B_1 or thiamine.

an·ti·no·ci·cep·tive (an″tee·no″si·sep′tiv) *adj.* ANALGESIC.

an·ti·nu·cle·ar (an″tee·new′klee·ur) *adj.* Of an antibody: reacting with components of cell nuclei.

antinuclear antibody or **factor.** An antibody against DNA, nucleoprotein, or other components of cell nuclei; present in most cases of systemic lupus erythematosus.

an·ti·odon·tal·gic (an″tee·o·don·tal′jick) *adj.* Relieving or preventing toothache.

an·ti·ox·i·dant (an″tee·ock′si·dunt) *n.* Any substance that delays or prevents the process of oxidation.

an·ti·par·a·sit·ic (an″tee·pār″uh·sit′ick) *adj. & n.* 1. Inhibiting or destroying parasites. 2. An agent that destroys or inhibits parasites.

an·ti·per·i·stal·sis (an″tee·perr″i·stahl′sis, ·stal′sis) *n.* REVERSED PERISTALSIS. —**antiperistal·tic** (·tick) *adj.*

an·ti·phage (an′ti·faje) *adj.* Counteracting bacteriophages.

an·ti·phlo·gis·tic (an″tee·flo·jis′tick) *adj. & n.* 1. Counteracting, reducing, or preventing inflammation or fever. 2. An agent that subdues or reduces inflammation or fever.

an·ti·phone (an′ti·fone) *n.* A device worn in the auditory meatus, intended to protect the wearer from noise.

an·ti·plas·tic (an″tee·plas′tick) *adj.* 1. Unfavorable to granulation or to the healing process. 2. Preventing or checking plastic exudation.

an·ti·pneu·mo·coc·cic (an″tee·new″mo·kock′sick) *adj.* Inhibiting or destructive to *Streptococcus pneumoniae.*

an·tip·o·dal (an·tip′uh·dul) *adj.* Situated directly opposite.

an·ti·pro·throm·bin (an″tee·pro·throm′bin) *n.* A substance that directly or indirectly reduces prothrombin activity, such as bishydroxycoumarin or heparin.

an·ti·pru·rit·ic (an″tee·proo·rit′ick) *adj. & n.* 1. Relieving or preventing itching. 2. A medicinal agent that relieves or prevents itching.

an·ti·pyo·gen·ic (an″tee·pye″o·jen′ick) *adj.* Preventing or inhibiting suppuration.

an·ti·py·rine (an″ti·pye′rin, ·reen, ·pye·reen′) *n.*

2,3-Dimethyl-1-phenyl-3-pyrazolin-5-one, $C_{11}H_{12}N_2O$, an antipyretic and analgesic. Syn. *phenazone.*

an·ti·rab·ic (an″tee·rab′ick, ·ray′bick) *adj.* Preventing rabies, as the Pasteur treatment.

an·ti·ra·chit·ic (an″tee·ra·kit′ick) *adj. & n.* 1. Preventing or counteracting development of rickets. 2. An agent for the prevention or cure of rickets.

an·ti·re·tic·u·lar (an″tee·re·tick′yoo·lur) *adj.* Pertaining to a factor operating against the reticuloendothelial system.

an·ti·rheu·mat·ic (an″tee·roo·mat′ick) *adj. & n.* 1. Preventing or allaying rheumatism. 2. An agent that prevents or allays rheumatism.

anti-Rh serum. 1. A serum containing antibodies against one or more of the Rh antigens. 2. A serum containing antibodies against $Rh_o(D)$ antigens.

an·ti·sca·bet·ic (an″tee·ska·beet′ick, ·ska·bet′ick) *adj. & n.* 1. Effective against the *Sarcoptes scabiei,* which causes scabies. 2. An agent effective in the treatment of scabies.

an·ti·scor·bu·tic (an″tee·skor·bew′tick) *adj. & n.* 1. Preventing or curing scurvy. 2. An agent that prevents or cures scurvy.

an·ti·seb·or·rhe·ic (an″tee·seb″o·ree′ick) *adj. & n.* 1. Combating seborrhea. 2. An agent effective in the treatment of seborrhea.

an·ti·se·cre·to·ry (an″tee·se·kree′tuh·ree) *adj.* Inhibiting the action of secretory glands.

an·ti·sep·sis (an″ti·sep′sis) *n.* Prevention of sepsis or poisoning by the destruction of microorganisms or their exclusion from the body tissues and fluids, or by preventing or checking their growth and multiplication.

an·ti·sep·tic (an″ti·sep′tick) *adj. & n.* 1. Stopping or inhibiting growth of bacteria. 2. Any one of a large group of organic and inorganic compounds which stops or inhibits the growth of bacteria without necessarily killing them, thus checking putrefaction.

antiseptic surgery. The application of antiseptic methods in surgery and in the treatment of infected wounds.

antisera. A plural of *antiserum.*

an·ti·se·ro·to·nin (an″tee·see″ro·to′nin) *adj.* Inhibiting or modifying serotonin activity.

an·ti·se·rum (an′tee·seer″um, ·serr″um) *n.*, pl. **antiserums, antise·ra** (·uh). Any serum of man or animals containing antibodies, either natural or acquired, as by immunization or disease.

an·ti·si·al·ic (an″tee·sigh·al′ick) *adj. & n.* 1. Diminishing or checking salivation. 2. An agent that diminishes or checks salivation.

an·ti·so·cial (an″tee·so′shul) *adj.* Characterizing a sociopathic state marked by the refusal to accept the obligations and restraints imposed by society.—**anti·so·ci·al·i·ty** (·so″shee·al′i·tee) *n.*

antisocial personality. *In psychiatry,* an individual whose behavioral patterns are basically unsocialized, bringing him constantly into conflict with other people or society. Such a person feels no guilt, does not profit from experience or punishment, maintains no loyalties nor identifies with any authority or code, is frequently callous, hedonistic, emotionally immature, and irresponsible, and usually rationalizes this behavior so that it appears warranted and reasonable.

an·ti·spas·mod·ic (an″tee·spaz·mod′ick) *adj. & n.* 1. Relieving or preventing spasms of smooth muscle. 2. An agent that relieves or prevents spasms of smooth muscle. Syn. *spasmolytic.*

an·ti·spas·tic (an″tee·spas′tick) *adj. & n.* 1. Relieving or preventing spasms of skeletal muscle or spasticity. 2. An agent that relieves or prevents spasms of skeletal muscle or spasticity.

an·ti·spi·ro·che·tic, an·ti·spi·ro·chae·tic (an″tee·spye″ro·kee′tick, ·ket′ick) *adj. & n.* 1. Arresting the growth and development of spirochetes. 2. An agent that arrests the growth and development of spirochetes.

an·ti·strep·to·coc·cic (an″tee·strep″to·cock′sick) *adj.* Antagonistic to or preventing the growth of streptococci.

anti·strep·to·ki·nase (an″tee·strep″to·kigh′nace) *n.* An antibody present in the serum which prevents the activation of plasminogen by streptokinase. It may develop in serum following infection with hemolytic streptococci or by injections of streptokinase for therapeutic reasons.

an·ti·strep·tol·y·sin (an″tee·strep·tol′i·sin, ·strep″to·lye′sin) *n.* The specific antibody to streptolysin of group A hemolytic streptococci, useful in the diagnosis of recent streptococcal infection and such sequellae as rheumatic fever.

an·ti·su·dor·if·ic (an″tee·sue″duh·rif′ick) *adj. & n.* 1. Checking excretion of sweat. 2. An agent that checks excretion of sweat.

an·ti·syph·i·lit·ic (an″tee·sif″i·lit′ick) *adj. & n.* 1. Active against syphilis. 2. An agent effective in the treatment of syphilis.

an·ti·the·nar (an″ti·theen′ahr, ·ur) *n.* HYPOTHENAR.

an·ti·throm·bin (an″tee·throm′bin) *n.* A substance that inhibits the activity of thrombin; may be naturally occurring in blood, a chemical agent, or a physical agent.

an·ti·throm·bo·plas·tin (an″tee·throm″bo·plas′tin) *n.* A substance capable of inhibiting the clot-accelerating effect of thromboplastins.

an·ti·tox·in (an″tee·tock′sin) *n.* 1. An antibody elaborated in the body, capable of neutralizing a given toxin (bacterial, plant, or animal toxin). 2. A sterile solution of one or more antibodies for a specific toxin, generally prepared from blood serum or plasma of an animal or human immunized against the toxin; used to counteract the same toxin in humans or other animals.

an·ti·tra·gus (an″ti·tray′gus) *n.* [NA]. The projection of the pinna just opposite and posterior to the tragus. —**anti·trag·ic** (·traj′ick) *adj.*

an·ti·tris·mus (an″tee·triz′mus) *n.* A condition of tonic spasm in which the mouth is forced open and cannot be closed.

an·ti·tryp·sin (an″tee·trip′sin) *n.* An antibody inhibiting the action of trypsin.

an·ti·tu·ber·cu·lous (an″tee·tew·bur′kew·lus) *adj.* Directed or acting against tuberculosis.

an·ti·tus·sive (an″tee·tus′iv) *adj. & n.* 1. Decreasing or relieving the amount and severity of coughing. 2. An agent that reduces the amount and severity of coughing.

an·ti·ty·phoid (an″tee·tigh′foid) *adj. & n.* 1. Counteracting or preventing typhoid fever. 2. An antityphoid serum.

an·ti·ul·cer·a·tive (an″tee·ul′sur·uh·tiv) *adj. & n.* 1. Preventing or combating ulceration. 2. A substance used to prevent or combat ulceration.

an·ti·ve·ne·re·al (an″tee·ve·neer′ee·ul) *adj.* Preventing or curing venereal disease.

an·ti·ven·in (an″tee·ven′in) *n.* 1. An antitoxin to a venin. 2. An antitoxic serum prepared by immunizing animals against the venom of snakes, insects, or other animals.

Antivert. Trademark for meclizine hydrochloride, an antinauseant.

an·ti·vi·ral (an″tee·vye′rul) *adj.* Antagonistic to, weakening, or destroying a virus.

an·ti·vi·rus (an″tee·vye′rus, an′tee·vye″rus) *n.* Any substance, antibody or otherwise, capable of neutralizing the activity of a virus.

an·ti·vi·ta·min (an″tee·vye′tuh·min) *n.* Any substance that prevents the normal metabolic functioning of vitamins; a vitamin-destroying enzyme, or a chemical substance that renders the vitamin unabsorbable or ineffective.

an·ti·viv·i·sec·tion (an″tee·viv″i·seck′shun) *n. & adj.* Opposition to, or opposed to, vivisection or animal experimentation. —**antivivisection·ist,** *n.*

an·ti·zy·mot·ic (an″tee·zye·mot′ick) *adj. & n.* 1. Preventing or checking fermentation or enzymic action. 2. An agent that checks or prevents fermentation or enzymic action.

ant·lo·pho·bia (ant″lo·fo′bee·uh) *n.* A morbid fear of floods.

antr-, antro-. A combining form meaning *antrum, antral.*

an·tral (an′trul) *adj.* Pertaining to an antrum.

antral fistula. A fistula communicating with an antrum or cavity in bone.

an·trec·to·my (an·treck′tuh·mee) *n.* Surgical removal of an antrum or its walls, especially the pyloric antrum or the mastoid antrum.

an·tri·tis (an·trye′tis) *n.* 1. Inflammation of an antrum, for example, the pyloric antrum. 2. *Obsol.* Specifically, inflammation of the antrum of Highmore (= MAXILLARY SINUS); maxillary sinusitis.

an·tro·at·ti·cot·o·my (an″tro·at″i·kot′uh·mee) *n. In surgery,* the opening of the mastoid antrum and the attic of the tympanum.

an·tro·cele (an′tro·seel) *n.* A saclike accumulation of fluid in the maxillary sinus.

an·tro·na·sal (an″tro·nay′zul) *adj.* Pertaining to the maxillary sinus and the nasal cavity.

an·tro·scope (an′tro·skope) *n.* An instrument for examining the maxillary sinus. —**an·tros·co·py** (an·tros′kuh·pee) *n.*

an·tros·to·my (an·tros′tuh·mee) *n.* Surgical opening of an antrum for drainage.

an·tro·tym·pan·ic (an″tro·tim·pan′ick) *adj.* Pertaining to the mastoid antrum and the tympanic cavity.

an·trum (an′trum) *n.,* pl. **an·tra** (·truh) 1. Any of various anatomic cavities or dilatations, such as: mastoid antrum, cardiac antrum, pyloric antrum. 2. *Obsol.* Specifically, the antrum of Highmore (= MAXILLARY SINUS).

antrum of the ear. MASTOID ANTRUM.

antrum py·lo·ri·cum (pi·lor′i·kum) [NA]. PYLORIC ANTRUM.

antrum tym·pa·ni·cum (tim·pan′i·kum) [BNA]. Antrum mastoideum (= MASTOID ANTRUM).

ANTU. 1-(1-Naphthyl)-2-thiourea, $C_{11}H_{10}N_2S$, a rodenticide.

anu·cle·ar (ay·new′klee·ur, a·new′) *adj.* Without a nucleus; applied to an erythrocyte.

anu·lus (an′yoo·lus) *n.,* pl. **anu·li** (·lye) A ring of tissue about an opening.

an·ure·sis (an″yoo·ree′sis) *n.,* pl. **anure·ses** (·seez) ANURIA. —**anu·ret·ic** (·ret′ick) *adj.*

an·uria (an·yoo′ree·uh) *n.* Suppression or arrest of urinary output, resulting from impairment of renal function (secretory type) or from obstruction in the urinary tract (excretory type). —**anu·ric** (·rick) *adj.*

anus (ay′nus) *n.* [NA]. The termination of the rectum; the outlet of the alimentary canal. *Adj. anal.*

anx·i·e·ty (ang·zye′i·tee) *n.* A feeling of apprehension, uncertainty, or tension stemming from the anticipation of an imagined or unreal threat, sometimes manifested by tachycardia, palpitation, sweating, disturbed breathing, trembling, or even paralysis.

anxiety attack. A feeling of impending death or physical collapse, acute panic or crisis.

anxiety neurosis, reaction, or **state.** A psychoneurotic disorder characterized by diffuse anxious expectation not restricted to definite situations, persons, or objects; emotional instability; irritability; apprehensiveness and a sense of fatigue; caused by incomplete repression of emotional problems, and frequently associated with somatic symptoms.

AORN Association of Operating Room Nurses.

aort-, aorto-. A combining form meaning *aorta, aortic.*

aor·ta (ay·or′tuh) *n.,* L. pl. & genit. sing. **aor·tae** (·tee) [NA]. The large vessel arising from the left ventricle and distributing, by its branches, arterial blood to every part of the body. It ends by bifurcating into the common iliacs at the fourth lumbar vertebra. The portion extending from the heart to the third thoracic vertebra is divided into an ascending, an arch, or transverse part, and a descending part. The thoracic portion extends to the diaphragm; the abdominal, to the bifurcation.

aor·tal·gia (ay″or·tal′jee·uh) *n.* Pain in the region of the aorta, usually due to the pressure of an aneurysm against surrounding tissues.

aor·tic (ay·or′tick) *adj.* Of or pertaining to the aorta.

aortic aneurysm. An aneurysm of the aorta, which may cause severe pressure symptoms and eventually may rupture.

aortic arches. Six pairs of embryonic vascular arches encircling the pharynx in the visceral arches. In mammals, the left fourth arch becomes a part of the systemic circulatory system and the sixth pair becomes incorporated in the pulmonary circulation.

aortic arch syndrome or **arteritis.** Partial or total thrombotic obliteration of the major branches of the aortic arch secondary to inflammatory changes of varied etiology, usually encountered in young women. Pulses are impalpable in the head, neck, and arms, and there is evidence of cerebral, cardiac, and arm ischemia.

aortic atresia. An uncommon congenital anomaly of the aortic orifice associated with hypoplasia of the ascending aorta and the left ventricle; there is severe congestive heart failure and cyanosis; the prognosis is invariably poor.

aor·ti·co·pul·mo·nary (ay''or·ti·ko·pul'mo·nerr·ee) *adj.* Pertaining to the aorta and the pulmonary system.

aor·ti·co·pul·mon·ic (ay·or''ti·ko·pul·mon'ick) *adj.* Pertaining to the aorta and the pulmonary artery.

aor·ti·co·re·nal (ay·or''ti·ko·ree'nul) *adj.* Near the aorta and kidney.

aortic regurgitation. Backflow of blood from the aorta into the left ventricle through or around an abnormal or prosthetic aortic valve.

aortic sinus. One of the pouch-like dilatations of the aorta opposite the cusps of the semilunar valves. Syn. *aorta of Valsalva.*

aortic stenosis. A narrowing of the aortic valve orifice, the aortic outflow tract, or of the aorta itself.

aortic valve. A valve consisting of three semilunar cusps situated at the junction of the aorta and the left ventricle of the heart.

aortic window. A radiolucent area on the left anterior oblique and lateral roentgenogram of the chest, below the aortic arch and above and behind the cardiopericardial silhouette.

aor·ti·tis (ay''or·tye'tis) *n.* Inflammation of the aorta.

aor·to·ca·val (ay·or''to·kay'vul) *adj.* Pertaining to or involving the aorta and vena cava (as: aortocaval fistula).

aor·to·gram (ay·or'to·gram) *n.* The film made by aortography.

aor·tog·ra·phy (ay''or·tog'ruh·fee) *n.* Roentgenography of the aorta after the intravascular injection of radiopaque material. **—aor·to·graph·ic** (ay·or''to·graf'ick) *adj.*

aortoiliac steal syndrome. Mesenteric vascular insufficiency due to reflux redistribution of blood from the mesenteric to the iliofemoral system; seen with aortoiliac reconstructive surgical procedures or lumbar sympathectomy in patients with marginal mesenteric blood supply.

aor·tot·o·my (ay''or·tot'uh·mee) *n.* Cutting or opening the aorta.

A.O.T.A. American Occupational Therapy Association.

AP. An anteroposterior projection of x-rays, i.e., passing from front to back of an anatomic part.

ap-, aph-, apo- A prefix meaning (a) *away from, from;* (b) *deprived, separated;* (c) *derived from,*

related to (especially in names of chemical compounds).

A.P.A. American Physiotherapy Association; American Psychiatric Association.

apal·les·the·sia, apal·laes·the·sia (a·pal''es·theezh'uh, ·theez'ee·uh) *n.* Loss of the ability to perceive vibrations. Syn. *pallanesthesia.*

apan·crea (ay·pan'kree·uh, ay·pang') *n.* Absence of the pancreas. **—apan·cre·at·ic** (·kree·at'ick) *adj.*

ap·an·dria (ap·an'dree·uh) *n.* Pathologic dislike of the male sex.

apas·tia (a·pas'tee·uh) *n.* Abstinence from food; seen in mental disorders. **—apas·tic** (·tick) *adj.*

ap·a·thism (ap'uh·thiz·um) *n.* Slowness in reacting to any stimuli.

APC A therapeutic formulation of aspirin, phenacetin, and caffeine.

ape fissure. A fissure of the human brain which corresponds with that present in an ape as the lunate sulcus.

ape hand. A deformity of the hand such that the thumb is turned out and the hand flattened, caused by wasting of the abductor indicis, thenar and hypothenar, interossei and lumbrical muscles; seen in progressive spinal muscular atrophy or lesions of the median and ulnar nerve.

apei·ro·pho·bia (a·pye''ro·fo'bee·uh) *n.* A morbid fear of infinity.

apel·lous (a·pel'us) *adj.* 1. Skinless; not cicatrized, applied to wounds. 2. Without a prepuce; circumcised.

ape·ri·ent (a·peer'ee·unt) *adj. & n.* LAXATIVE.

ape·ri·od·ic (ay''peer''ee·od'ick, a·peer'') *adj.* Devoid of periodicity or rhythm.

aper·i·stal·sis (a·perr''i·stal'sis, ·stahl'sis, a·perr'') *n.* 1. Absence of peristalsis. 2. Specifically, ACHALASIA.

aper·i·tive (a·perr'i·tiv) *adj. & n.* 1. Stimulating the appetite; a stimulant to the appetite. 2. LAXATIVE.

aper·tu·ra (ap''ur·tew'ruh) *n.,* pl. **apertu·rae** (·ree) Aperture; opening.

ap·er·ture (ap'ur·chur) *n.* 1. An opening; orifice. 2. *In optics,* the diameter of the exposed portion of a lens, designated as the ratio of the focal length to this diameter, as f4, in which the aperture is 1 inch and the focal length is 4 inches.

apex (ay'pecks) *n.,* genit. **api·cis** (ap'i·sis), L. pl. **api·ces** (ap'i·seez) 1. The tip or top of anything; point or extremity of a cone. 2. *In optics,* the junction of the two refractive sides of a prism. 3. *In craniometry,* the highest point in the transverse vertical section of the vault of a skull oriented on the Frankfort horizontal plane, the plane of section passing through the poria. 4. The radicular end of a tooth.

apex beat. APEX IMPULSE.

apexcardiogram, apex cardiogram. A graphic recording of ultra-low-frequency precordial chest-wall movements. Abbreviated, ACG.

apex impulse. The point of maximum outward movement of the cardiac left ventricle during systole, normally localized in the fifth left intercostal space in the midclavicular line. Syn. *left ventricular thrust.*

apex murmur. A murmur heard best over the apex of the heart. Syn. *apical murmur.*

apex of the heart. The lowest and leftmost point of the heart represented by the left ventricle. It is usually described as being behind the fifth left intercostal space 8 to 9 cm (in the adult) from the midsternal line.

APF Abbreviation for *animal protein factor* (= VITAMIN B$_{12}$).

Ap·gar score or **rating** A quantitative estimate of the condition of an infant 1 to 5 minutes after birth, derived by assigning points to the quality of heart rate, respiratory effort, color, muscle tone, and reflexes; expressed as the sum of these points, the maximum or best score being 10.

A.P.H.A. American Public Health Association.

A.Ph.A. American Pharmaceutical Association.

apha·gia (a·fay'jee·uh) *n.* Inability to swallow, either of organic or psychic origin.

aphagia al·ge·ra (al·jeer'uh, al'je·ruh) Inability or refusal to swallow because of pain.

apha·kia (a·fay'kee·uh) *n.* The condition in which the lens is absent from the dioptric system. **—apha·kic** (·kick), **apha·ki·al** (·kee·ul) *adj.*

aphakic eye. An eye deprived of its crystalline lens.

apha·lan·gia (af''uh·lan'jee·uh, ay''fa·) *n.* Loss or absence of fingers or toes.

aph·al·ge·sia (af''al·jee'zee·uh) *n.* A hysterical state wherein pain is induced by contact with a harmless object that has symbolic significance for the patient.

apha·sia (a·fay'zhuh, a·fay'zhuh, ·zee·uh) *n.* Loss or impairment of the reception or use of language caused by lesion of the cerebrum but not by any lesion affecting primary sensation, motility of the vocal musculature or its subjection to voluntary control, or general intellectual function; includes alexia, the agnosias affecting linguistic abilities, the apraxias limited to spoken and written language, and other disorders.

apha·sic (a·fay'zick, a·fay'zick) *adj. & n.* 1. Of, pertaining to, or afflicted with aphasia. 2. A person afflicted with aphasia.

aphasic alexia. Alexia in which characters and their combinations can be recognized and classified but in which the language they represent is not fully understood.

aphasic seizure. Transient cessation of speech as a manifestation of an abnormal electrical discharge usually from the temporal lobe.

aphelx·ia (a·felk'see·uh) *n.* 1. Absentmindedness; inattention or indifference to external impressions. 2. Daydreaming.

aphe·mia (a·fee'mee·uh) *n.* PURE WORD MUTENESS.

aph·e·pho·bia (af''e·fo'bee·uh) *n.* Pathologic fear of physical contact with people or objects.

apho·nia (a·fo'nee·uh, ay·fo'nee·uh) *n.* 1. Loss of speech due to a peripheral lesion, as in laryngeal paralysis or vocal cord tumor. 2. Hysterical loss of the power of speech. 3. Voicelessness. **—aph·o·nous** (af'uh·nus), **aphon·ic** (a·fon'ick) *adj.*

aphose (ay'foze, a·foze', af'oze) *n.* A subjective dark spot or shadow in the field of vision.

aphra·sia (a·fray'zhuh, ·zee·uh) *n.* 1. Loss of ability to utter connected words or phrases. 2. Refusal to speak; APHONIA PARANOICA.

aph·ro·dis·i·ac (af''ro·diz'ee·ack) *adj. & n.* 1. Stimulating the sexual appetite; erotic. 2. An agent that stimulates, or is purported to stimulate, sexual passion or power.

aph·ro·dis·io·ma·nia (af''ro·diz'ee·o·may'nee·uh) *n.* Exaggerated sexual interest and excitement; EROTOMANIA (1).

aph·tha (af'thuh) *n.*, *pl.* **aph·thae** (af'thee) 1. A white painful oral ulcer of unknown cause. 2. APHTHOUS STOMATITIS.

aph·thous (af'thus) *adj.* Pertaining to, affected with, or resembling aphthae.

aphthous stomatitis. Inflammation of the oral mucosa, characterized by the presence of small, painful ulcerations.

aphthous ulcer. CANKER SORE.

api-, apio- A combining form meaning *bee.*

apic-, apici-, apico-. A combining form meaning *apex, apical.*

api·cal (ap'i·kul, ay'pi·kul) *adj.* 1. At or pertaining to the apex. 2. Situated relatively near the apex.

apical granuloma. PERIAPICAL GRANULOMA.

apical murmur. APEX MURMUR.

api·cec·to·my (ay''pi·seck'tuh·mee, ap''i·) *n.* 1. Removal of the apex of a tooth root. Syn. *apicoectomy.* 2. Exenteration of the air cells of the apex of the petrous pyramid.

apices. Plural of *apex.*

api·co·ec·to·my (ap''i·ko·eck'tuh·mee) *n.* Removal of the apex of a tooth root. Syn. *apicectomy.*

apio·pho·bia (ay''pee·o·fo'bee·uh, ap''ee·o·) *n.* APIPHOBIA.

api·pho·bia (ay''pi·fo'bee·uh, ap''i·) *n.* Morbid terror of bees and their sting.

apla·cen·tal (ay''pla·sen'tul, ap''luh·) *adj.* Without a placenta.

apla·sia (a·play'zhuh, ·zee·uh) *n.* 1. Defective development or production of a tissue or organ. 2. In the somatotype, a physique in which the whole body or a region of the body is poorly developed.

aplas·tic (ay·plas'tick, a·plas'tick) *adj.* 1. Structureless; formless. 2. Incapable of forming new tissue. 3. Of or pertaining to aplasia. 4. Designating an inflammation with little or no production of granulation tissue.

aplastic anemia. 1. Anemia resulting from failure of cell production in the bone marrow, associated with marrow hypoplasia, hyperplasia, or dysplasia. 2. A clinical syndrome characterized by decrease in all formed elements of the peripheral blood and all their bone-marrow precursors, with associated manifestations of anemia, bleeding, and infection.

ap·nea, ap·noea (ap'nee·uh, ap·nee'uh) *n.* The cessation or suspension of breathing. **—ap·ne·ic, ap·noe·ic** (ap·nee'ick) *adj.*

ap·neu·sis (ap·new'sis) *n.*, *pl.* **apneu·ses** (·seez) A state of maintained contraction of the inspiratory muscles due to prolonged tonic discharge of inspiratory medullary neurons.

apo·chro·mat·ic (ap″o·kro·mat′ick) adj. Without or free from chromatic and spherical aberration.

apo·clei·sis (ap″o·klye′sis) n. Aversion to eating.

apo·crine (ap′o·krin) adj. 1. Designating a type of secretion in which the secretion-filled free end of a gland cell is pinched off, leaving the nucleus and most of the cytoplasm to recover and repeat the process. Contr. *holocrine, merocrine.* 2. Of or pertaining to the apocrine glands.

apocrine carcinoma. A tumor composed of anaplastic cells resembling those of apocrine epithelium; the term is often applied to extramammary Paget's carcinoma.

apocrine glands. Glands producing sweat of a characteristic odor; larger and more deeply situated than the ordinary sweat glands, and found in the axillary, mammary, anal, and genital areas.

apoc·y·num (a·pos′i·num) n. The dried rhizome and roots of *Apocynum cannabinum* or of *A. androsaemifolium.* Contains cymarin, a glycoside closely related to many glycosides of the digitalis group. The physiologic actions of apocynum are similar to those of the digitalis. Syn. *black Indian hemp, Canada hemp.*

apo·dal (ap′o·dul) adj. Without feet; lacking feet.

apo·de·mi·al·gia (ap″o·dee″mee·al′jee·uh) n. An abnormal dislike of home life, with a desire for wandering; wanderlust.

apo·dia (ay·po′dee·uh, a·pod′) n. Congenital absence of feet.

apo·en·zyme (ap″o·en′zime, ·zim) n. The purely protein part of an enzyme which, with the coenzyme, forms the complete enzyme or holoenzyme.

apo·fer·ri·tin (ap″o·ferr′i·tin) n. A protein in the intestinal mucosa having the property of binding and storing iron as ferritin.

apog·a·my (a·pog′uh·mee) n. The asexual production of a sporophyte from a gametophyte.

ap·o·mix·is (ap″o·mick′sis) n., pl. **apomix·es** (·seez) Asexual reproduction, which may be vegetative (vegetative apomixis) or may involve seed production (agamospermy).

apo·mor·phine (ap″o·mor′feen, ·fin) n. An alkaloid, $C_{17}H_{17}NO_2$, derived from morphine by abstraction of a molecule of water. The hydrochloride salt is used as an emetic.

apo·neu·ro·sis (ap″o·new·ro′sis, a·pon″yoo·) n., pl. **aponeuro·ses** (·seez) [NA]. An expanded tendon consisting of a fibrous or membranous sheet, serving as a means of attachment for flat muscles at their origin or insertion, or as a fascia to enclose or bind a group of muscles. —**aponeu·rot·ic** (·rot′ick) adj.

apo·neu·ro·si·tis (ap″o·new″ro·sigh′tis) n. Inflammation of an aponeurosis.

apo·neu·rot·o·my (ap″o·new·rot′uh·mee) n. Incision of an aponeurosis.

apoph·y·se·al (a·pof″i·see′ul, ap″o·fiz′ee·ul) adj. Of or pertaining to an apophysis.

apoph·y·sis (a·pof′i·sis) n., pl. **apophy·ses** (·seez) [NA]. A process, outgrowth, or projection of some part or organ, as of a bone.

apoph·y·si·tis (a·pof″i·sigh′tis) n. Inflammation of an apophysis.

ap·o·plec·tic (ap″o·pleck′tick) adj. Of or pertaining to apoplexy.

ap·o·plec·ti·form (ap″o·pleck′ti·form) adj. Resembling apoplexy.

ap·o·plexy (ap′o·pleck″see) n. 1. CEREBROVASCULAR ACCIDENT. 2. Gross hemorrhage into or infarction of any organ. Adj. *apoplectic.*

apo·pnix·is (ap″o·pnick′sis) n. GLOBUS HYSTERICUS.

ap·or·rhip·sis (ap″o·rip′sis) n. The inappropriate discarding of clothing or throwing off of bedclothes; seen in delirium and in some mental disorders.

apo·sia (a·po′zhuh, ·zee·uh) n. ADIPSIA.

ap·o·si·tia (ap″o·sish′ee·uh, ·sit′ee·uh) n. Aversion to or loathing of food. —**apo·sit·ic** (·sit′ick) adj.

apos·ta·sis (a·pos′tuh·sis) n., pl. **aposta·ses** (·seez) 1. The end or crisis of an attack of disease; termination of a disease by crisis. 2. ABSCESS.

apos·thia (a·pos′thee·uh) n. Congenital absence of the prepuce.

apoth·e·caries' weight (a·poth′e·kair″eez). A system of weights and measures once used in compounding medicines. The troy pound of 5760 grains is the standard. It is subdivided into 12 ounces. The ounce is subdivided into 8 drachms, the drachm into 3 scruples, and the scruple into 20 grains. For fluid measure the quart of 32 fluidounces is subdivided into 2 pints, the pint into 16 fluidounces, the fluidounce into 8 fluidrachms, and the fluidrachm into 60 minims.

apoth·e·cary (a·poth′e·kerr″ee) n. 1. A pharmacist; one who prepares and distributes medicinal products, particularly those dispensed on the prescription of a licensed medical practitioner. 2. PHARMACY (2).

ap·pa·ra·tus (ap″uh·ray′tus, ·rat′us) n., pl. **apparatus** 1. A collection of instruments or devices used for a special purpose. 2. *In anatomy,* the system or group or organs or parts of organs performing a certain function; a physical mechanism.

append-, appendo-. See *appendic-, appendico-.*

ap·pend·age (uh·pen′dij) n. 1. Anything appended, usually of minor importance. 2. A limb or limblike structure.

ap·pen·dec·to·my (ap″en·deck′tuh·mee) n. 1. Excision of the vermiform appendix. 2. Excision of any accessible appendix or appendage.

ap·pen·di·ceal (ap″en·dis′ee·ul, ·dish′ee·ul, a·pen″di·see′ul) adj. Of or pertaining to the vermiform appendix.

appendiceal abscess. An abscess in the vermiform appendix and adjacent tissue, usually following acute suppurative appendicitis.

ap·pen·di·cec·to·my (a·pen″di·seck′tuh·mee) n. APPENDECTOMY.

appendices. Plural of *appendix.*

appendices epi·plo·i·cae (ep·i·plo′i·see) [NA]. Fatty projections of the serous coat of the large intestine.

ap·pen·di·ci·tis (a·pen″di·sigh′tis) n. Inflammation of the vermiform appendix.

ap·pen·di·clau·sis (a·pen″di·klaw′sis) n. Obstruction or obliteration of the vermiform appendix, producing the clinical features of acute appendicitis.

ap·pen·di·co·en·ter·os·to·my (a·pen''di·ko·en·tur·os'tuh·mee) n. The establishment of an artificial opening between the appendix and small intestine.

ap·pen·di·co·lith (a·pen'di·ko·lith'') n. A fecalith in the appendiceal lumen, usually calcified enough to be radiologically visible.

ap·pen·di·cos·to·my (a·pen''di·kos'tuh·mee) n. An operation to bring the vermiform appendix through the abdominal wall and cut off its tip, so as to provide for external drainage and irrigation of the bowel.

ap·pen·dic·u·lar (ap''en·dick'yoo·lur) adj. 1. Of or pertaining to an appendage. 2. APPENDICEAL.

appendix au·ri·cu·la·ris (aw·rick''yoo·lair'is). AURICLE (2).

appendix epi·di·dy·mi·dis (ep''ee·di·dim'i·dis) [NA]. A small appendage on the head of the epididymis consisting of vestigial mesonephric tubules or ducts.

appendix tes·tis (tes'tis) [NA]. A remnant of the cranial part of the paramesonephric duct, attached to the testis.

appendix ver·mi·for·mis (vur·mi·for'mis) [NA]. VERMIFORM APPENDIX.

ap·per·cep·tion (ap''ur·sep'shun) n. Consciousness of the relation of new events, situations, or sensations to the individual's own emotions, past experiences, and memories. —**ap·percep·tive** (·tiv) adj.

ap·per·son·i·fi·ca·tion (ap''ur·son''i·fi·kay'shun) n. In psychiatry, unconscious identification with another, sometimes famous, person in part or in whole.

ap·pe·tite (ap'e·tite) n. 1. Any natural desire or craving to satisfy a physical or psychic need. 2. Specifically, a desire for food, not necessarily prompted by hunger.

ap·pe·tiz·er (ap'e·tye''zur) n. A food, medicine, or aperitif taken before a meal to stimulate the appetite.

ap·pla·nate (ap'la·nate) adj. Horizontally flattened. —**ap·pla·na·tion** (ap''la·nay'shun) n.

applanation tonometry. A method of determining the intraocular pressure by measuring the force required to flatten a small area of cornea.

ap·pli·ca·tor (ap'li·kay''tur) n. An instrument used in making local applications.

ap·po·si·tion (ap''o·zish'un) n. 1. The act of fitting together; the state of being fitted together; juxtaposition. 2. The laying on of successive layers, as in bone or tooth formation.

ap·pre·hen·sion (ap''re·hen'shun) n. 1. The act of mentally grasping a fact; thus it lies somewhere between mere perception and full understanding or comprehension. 2. Suspicion or fear; a foreboding about a future event, usually an unfavorable one.

ap·proach, n. In surgery, the manner of securing access to a joint, cavity, part, or organ by a suitable incision through the overlying or neighboring structures.

ap·prox·i·mal (a·prock'si·mul) adj. Situated close or near; contiguous; next to each other.

¹**ap·prox·i·mate** (uh·prock'si·mut) adj. APPROXIMAL.

²**ap·prox·i·mate** (uh·prock'si·mate) v. To bring together, bring near. —**ap·prox·i·ma·tion,** n.

aprac·tag·no·sia (ay·prack''tag·no'see·uh, a·prack'') n. A perceptual disorder involving the visual and motor elements in the spatial disposition of an action, in which the patient is unable to arrange objects, figures, or lines according to a two-dimensional or three-dimensional plan.

aprac·tic (ay·prack'tick, a·prack') adj. Pertaining to or marked by apraxia.

apractic aphasia. MOTOR APHASIA.

aprax·ia (ay·prack'see·uh, a·prack') n. Loss or impairment of the ability to perform a learned motor act due to lesion of the cerebral hemispheres but not to any lesion affecting mobility or the patient's desire to perform the act, or causing involuntary movement; presumably represents a disconnection of the cortical motor areas from the cortical areas in which the decision to perform a motor act is made. —**ap·rax·ic** (·sick), **aprac·tic** (·prack'tick) adj.

Apresoline. Trademark for hydralazine.

ap·ro·bar·bi·tal (ap''ro·bahr'bi·tal, ·tol) n. 5-Allyl-5-isopropylbarbituric acid, $C_{10}H_{14}N_2O_3$, a sedative and hypnotic having an intermediate duration of action.

aproc·tia (ay·prock'shee·uh, a·prock') n. IMPERFORATE ANUS. —**aproc·tous** (·tus) adj.

apro·sex·ia (ap''ro·seck'see·uh, ay''pro·seck') n. A mental disturbance consisting in inability to fix attention upon a subject.

apro·so·pia (ap''ro·so'pee·uh, ay''pros·o'pee·uh) n. Congenital absence of part or all of the face. —**apros·o·pous** (ay·pros'o·pus) adj; **aprosopus,** n.

ap·sel·a·phe·sia (ap·sel''uh·fee'zhuh, ·zee·uh) n. Loss of the tactile sense.

ap·si·thy·ria (ap''si·thigh'ree·uh) n. HYSTERICAL APHONIA.

A.P.T.A. American Physical Therapy Association.

ap·ti·tude (ap'ti·tewd) n. A natural ability or inclination to learn or understand.

aptitude test. Any set of selected and standardized tests to provide an estimate of an individual's ability in a particular field or profession.

Apt test A test to differentiate maternal from fetal blood in a newborn child's stomach by exposing a hemolysate of the stomach content to a weakly alkaline solution; if it is fetal hemoglobin, the solution remains pink.

ap·ty·a·lism (ap·tye'u·liz·um, ay·tye') n. Deficiency or absence of saliva.

APUD cell. Acronym for a cell possessing the capability of amine precursor uptake and decarboxylation and of synthesizing and secreting polypeptide hormones. It originates in the neural crest and is found in diverse tissues.

APUD tumor. A benign or malignant tumor which is composed of APUD cells and which may cause secondary clinical effects by secreting polypeptide hormones. Syn. apudoma.

apus (ay'pus) n. An individual lacking feet or the entire lower extremities.

apy·rex·ia (ay''pye·reck'see·uh, ap''eye·) n. Absence of fever. —**apy·rex·i·al** (·see-ul), **apy·ret·ic** (·ret'ick) *adj.*

AQ Abbreviation for *achievement quotient.*

aq·ua (ack'wuh, ay'kwuh, ah'kwuh) *n.*, pl. **aq·uae** (·wee), **aquas** Water; especially medicated water, as aromatic waters, saturated solutions of volatile oils, or other volatile substances in water. Abbreviated, a., aq.

aq·ua·pho·bia (ack'wuh·fo'bee·uh) *n.* HYDROPHOBIA (2).

aq·ue·duct (ack'we·dukt) *n.* A canal for the passage of fluid; any canal. —**aq·ue·duc·tal** (ack'' we·duck'tul) *adj.*

aqueduct of Syl·vi·us (sil'vee·us) CEREBRAL AQUEDUCT.

aqueduct of the cochlea. A canal which establishes a communication between the perilymphatic space of the osseous labyrinth and the subarachnoid space and transmits a vein for the cochlea.

aqueduct of the vestibule. A canal of the vestibule of the ear, running from the vestibule and opening on the back of the petrous portion of the temporal bone and containing the endolymphatic duct and a small vein.

aque·ous (ay'kwee·us, ack'wee·us) *adj. & n.* 1. Watery; in, of, or with water. 2. AQUEOUS HUMOR.

aqueous flare. *In ophthalmology,* the Tyndall effect or light scattering as the light traverses the anterior chamber of the eye in inflammatory conditions, due to increased protein concentration in the aqueous humor caused by dilatation of blood vessels.

aqueous humor. A clear, watery secretion product of the ciliary epithelium. It fills the anterior and posterior chambers of the eye.

aquo- A combining form denoting (a) *presence of water in a complex ion,* called aquo ion; (b) *derivation from water,* as an aquo acid or aquo base.

ar-. In chemistry, a combining form meaning *aromatic.*

ar·a·bic acid (ăr'uh·bick, a·rab'ick). A polysaccharide; the chief constituent of acacia (gum arabic), in which it occurs in the form of calcium, magnesium, and potassium salts. Syn. *arabin.*

arab·i·nose (a·rab'i·noce, ăr'uh·bi·noce'') *n.* CHO(CHOH)$_3$CH$_2$OH; an aldopentose which exists in two structural configurations, differentiated as L-arabinose and D-arabinose. The L- sugar, also called pectinose, pectin sugar, gum sugar, is widely distributed in plants, usually as a component of a complex polysaccharide. D-Arabinose may be obtained by degradation of dextrose (D-glucose).

ar·a·chi·don·ic acid (a·rack''i·don'ick, a·ray''ki·, ăr''uh·ki·). 5,8,11,14-Eicosatetraenoic acid, C$_{20}$H$_{32}$O$_2$, an unsaturated fatty acid occurring in animal phosphatides and certain fats.

arachn-, arachno- A combining form meaning (a) *spider, spiderlike;* (b) *arachnoid.*

arach·ne·pho·bia (uh·rack''ne·fo'bee·uh) *n.* Morbid fear of spiders.

arach·nid (uh·rack'nid) *n.* A member of the class Arachnida.

Arach·ni·da (a·rack'ni·duh) *n.pl.* A large class of

the Arthropoda which includes scorpions, spiders, mites, and ticks. They are wingless, usually lack antennae, and, as adults, have four pairs of legs.

arach·nid·ism (uh·rack'nid·iz·um) *n.* A condition produced by the bite of a poisonous spider; spider venom poisoning.

ar·ach·ni·tis (ar''ack·nigh'tis) *n.* ARACHNOIDITIS.

arachno-. See *arachn-.*

arach·no·dac·ty·ly (uh·rack''no·dack'ti·lee) *n.* A condition in which the fingers, and sometimes the toes, are abnormally long and thin; seen in Marfan's syndrome and in homocystinuria. Syn. *spider fingers.*

arach·no·gas·tria (uh·rack''no·gas'tree·uh) *n.* The protuberant abdomen of an emaciated person with ascites. Syn. *spider belly.*

arach·noid (uh·rack'noid) *n.* The arachnoid membrane; the central of the three meninges covering the brain (arachnoidea encephali) and spinal cord (arachnoidea spinalis). It is very fine and delicate in structure, following the pia mater into each sulcus and around each convolution, but separated from it by the subarachnoid space. The two membranes are often considered as one, the piarachnoid. —**arachnoid, arach·noi·dal** (ăr''ack·noy'dul) *adj.*

arachnoidal granulations. ARACHNOID GRANULATIONS.

arach·noid·ism (uh·rack'noid·iz·um) *n.* ARACHNIDISM.

arach·noid·itis (uh·rack'noy·dye'tis) *n.* Inflammation of the piarachnoid of the spinal cord and brain.

Aralen. Trademark for chloroquine, an antimalarial and antiamebic.

Aramine. Trademark for metaraminol, a sympathomimetic amine used as the bitartrate salt.

Aran-Du·chenne disease or **syndrome** (a·rahn', du^c·shen') PROGRESSIVE SPINAL MUSCULAR ATROPHY.

ara·ne·ism (a·ray'nee·iz·um) *n.* ARACHNIDISM.

ara·ro·ba (ahr''uh·ro'buh, ăr''uh·ro'buh) *n.* An oxidation product of resin deposited in the wood of the trunk of *Andira araroba.* From it is obtained chrysarobin, a complex mixture of reduction products of chrysophanol. It has been used in skin affections. Syn. *Goa powder.*

ar·bo·res·cent (ahr''bo·res'unt) *adj.* Branched like a tree; resembling a tree in appearance.

ar·bo·ri·za·tion (ahr''bo·ri·zay'shun) *n.* 1. A conformation or arrangement resembling the branching of a tree. 2. DENDRITE. 3. FERNING. —**ar·bo·rize** (ahr'bo·rize) *v.*

arborization block. A delay in cardiac conduction in the terminal fibers of the Purkinje network.

ar·bor·vi·tae (ahr''bur·vye'tee) *n.* A tree or shrub of the genus *Thuja* or the related genus *Thujopsis.*

arbor vitae. 1. [BNA] ARBOR VITAE CEREBELLI. 2. A series of ridges and folds of the mucosa within the uterine cervix. 3. ARBORVITAE.

arbor vitae ce·re·bel·li (serr·e·bel'eye) [NA]. The arborescent appearance of the white substance in a sagittal section of the cerebellum.

ar·bo·vi·rus (ahr''bo·vye'rus) *n.* Any one of over 200 RNA viruses biologically transmitted between susceptible vertebrate hosts by bloodsucking arthropods.

arbovirus encephalitis. Any encephalitis or encephalomyelitis caused by an arbovirus, such as eastern equine encephalomyelitis and St. Louis encephalitis.

ar·code (ahr·kade') *n.* A series of arches; used especially of blood vessels.

ar·ca·num (ahr·kay'num) *n.*, pl. **arca·na** (·nuh) A medicine compounded from a secret formula.

arch, *n.* A structure or an anatomic part having a curved outline resembling that of an arc or a bow.

arch-, archi- A prefix meaning (a) *chief, first;* (b) in anatomy and biology, *primitive, original, ancestral.*

ar·cha·ic (ahr·kay'ick) *adj.* In psychiatry, designating elements, largely unconscious, in the psyche which are remnants of man's prehistoric past, and which reappear in dreams and other symbolic manifestations; used primarily in analytic psychology. —**ar·cha·ism** (ahr'kay·iz·um) *n.*

arch bar. ARCH WIRE.

arch·en·ter·on (ahr·ken'tur·on) *n.*, pl. **archen·tera** (·tur·uh) The embryonic alimentary cavity of the gastrula, lined by endoderm. Syn. *archigaster, coelenteron, gastrocoel, primitive gut.* —**arch·en·ter·ic** (ahr''ken·terr'ick) *adj.*

arches of the foot. See *longitudinal arch of the foot, transverse arch of the foot.*

ar·che·type (ahr'ke·tipe) *n.* 1. A basic model; prototype. 2. *In comparative anatomy,* an ideal, generalized structural pattern of one of the main kinds of organisms, assumed to be the form of the original ancestor of the group. 3. *In analytic and Jungian pyschology,* a mental remnant or primordial urge, largely unconscious, of man's prehistoric past, which reappears in symbolic form in dreams, works of art, various impulses, or symptomatic acts.

archi-. See *arch-.*

ar·chi·neph·ron (ahr''ki·nef'ron) *n.* PRONEPHROS. —**archineph·ric** (·rick) *adj.*

ar·chi·pal·li·um (ahr''ki·pal'ee·um) *n.* The olfactory pallium or the olfactory cerebral cortex; the rhinencephalon; the oldest part of the cerebral cortex. —**archipalli·al** (·ul) *adj.*

ar·chi·tec·ton·ic (ahr''ki·teck·ton'ick) *adj.* Pertaining to the structural arrangement or architectural construction of an organ or part. —**architecton·ics** (·icks) *n.*

archo- *Obsol.* A combining form meaning *rectal.*

arch of the aorta. The transverse portion of the aorta between its ascending and descending portions.

ar·chu·sia (ahr·kew'zee·uh, ·choo') *n.* A hypothetical cellular substance, possibly a vitamin B, which aids the migration, growth, and reproduction of cells.

arch wire. A wire that is fitted along either side of the dental arch for stabilization of the teeth or to provide a basis for orthodontic movement.

ar·ci·form (ahr'si·form) *adj.* ARCUATE.

arc·ta·tion (ahrk·tay'shun) *n.* Contracture of an opening or canal; STENOSIS.

ar·cu·ate (ahr'kew·ate) *adj.* Arched; curved; bow-shaped.

ar·cu·a·tion (ahr''kew·ay'shun) *n.* Curvature, especially of a bone.

ar·cus (ahr'kus) *n.*, pl. & genit. sing. **ar·cus** (ahr'koos) [L.]. 1. ARCH. 2. A discernible arc or ring, as corneal arcus.

arcus ju·ve·ni·lis (joo·ve·nigh'lis). A congenital opaque ring in the corneal stroma resembling an arcus senilis but evident at or shortly after birth; ANTERIOR EMBRYOTOXON.

arcus se·ni·lis (se·nigh'lis). An opaque ring at the edge of the cornea, seen in many individuals of middle age and especially old age; due to lipoid deposits in the stroma. Syn. *gerotoxon, arcus lipidus.*

arcus senilis len·tis (len'tis). An opaque ring in the equator of the crystalline lens; it sometimes occurs in the aged.

arcus tendineus fas·ci·ae pel·vis (fash'ee·ee pel'vis) [NA]. The tendinous arch of the pelvic fascia. See *tendinous arch.*

arc-welder's disease or **nodulation.** SIDEROSIS (2).

ARD Abbreviation for *acute respiratory disease.*

area (air'ee·uh, ār'ee·uh) *n.*, L. pl. & genit. sing. **are·ae** (air'ee·ee) 1. A limited extent of surface; a region. 2. A field or system of intellectual activity or study. 3. A structural or functional part of the cerebral cortex.

area acu·sti·ca (a·koos'ti·kuh) [BNA]. AREA VESTIBULARIS.

area pos·tre·ma (pos·tree'muh). A narrow zone on the lateral wall of the fourth ventricle, separated from the ala cinerea by the funiculus separans.

are·a·tus (air''ee·ay'tus) *adj.*, f. **area·ta** Occurring in patches.

area ves·ti·bu·la·ris (ves·tib''yoo·lair'is) [NA]. An area in the lateral angle of the floor of the fourth ventricle overlying the nuclei of the vestibular nerve.

are·co·line (a·ree'ko·leen, ·lin, a·reck'o·) *n.* Methyl 1,2,5,6-tetrahydro-1-methylnicotinate, $C_8H_{13}NO_2$, a liquid alkaloid from the seeds of *Areca catechu.* It is a parasympathomimetic agent; formerly used in human medicine but now used only as a veterinary anthelmintic and cathartic.

are·flex·ia (ay''re·fleck'see·uh) *n.* Absence of reflexes.

are·gen·er·a·tion (ay''re·jen''ur·ay'shun) *n.* Failure of tissue to regenerate after disease or injury. —**are·gen·er·a·tive** (ay''re·jen·ur·uh·tiv), **aregenera·to·ry** (·to'ree) *adj.*

ar·e·na·tion (ār''e·nay'shun) *n.* 1. A sand bath. 2. Sand baths in the treatment of disease; no longer in general use. Syn. *ammotherapy.*

are·o·la (a·ree'o·luh) *n.*, L. pl. **areo·lae** (·lee) 1. Any minute interstice or space in a tissue. 2. A colored or pigmented ring surrounding some central point or space, as a nipple or pustule. 3. The part of the iris enclosing the pupil. —**areo·lar** (·lur) *adj.*

areola mam·mae (mam'ee) [NA]. The pigmented area surrounding the nipple of the breast.

This enlarges during pregnancy, producing the second areola. Syn. *areola papillaris, mammary areola.*

areolar glands. Glands in the areola about the nipple in the female breast. They are intermediate in character between mammary glands and apocrine sweat glands.

areolar tissue. A form of loose connective tissue composed of cells and delicate collagenous and elastic fibers interlacing in all directions.

Arfonad camphorsulfonate. Trademark for trimethaphan camsylate.

ar·gam·bly·o·pia (ahr-gam″blee-o′pee-uh) *n. In optometry,* amblyopia from disuse or from nonuse, usually of one eye, as a result of uncorrected esotropia. Syn. *amblyopia ex anopsia.*

Ar·gas (ahr′gas) *n.* A genus of ticks of the Argasidae.

argent-, argento- A combining form meaning *silver, containing silver.*

ar·gen·taf·fin, ar·gen·taf·fine (ahr·jen′tuh-fin) *adj.* Reducing silver of its own innate capacity, without aid of light or subsequently applied developers or reducing agents.

argentaffin cells. Cells having an affinity for silver salts and therefore capable of being stained by them.

argentaffin fibers. RETICULAR FIBERS.

ar·gen·taf·fi·no·ma (ahr·jen″tuh·fi·no′muh, ahr″jen·taf″i·no′muh) *n.* CARCINOID.

ar·gen·tic (ahr·jen′tick) *adj.* Containing silver in its higher, bivalent state (Ag^{2+}).

ar·gen·to·phil, ar·gen·to·phile (ahr·jen′to-fil) *adj.* Stainable by impregnation with silver salts; ARGYROPHIL.

ar·gil·la·ceous (ahr″ji·lay′shus) *adj.* Claylike; composed of clay.

ar·gi·nase (ahr′ji·nace, ·naze) *n.* An enzyme, found in liver and other tissues, that catalyzes hydrolysis of L-arginine to ornithine and urea.

ar·gi·nine (ahr′ji·neen, ·nin) *n.* 1-Amino-4-guanidovaleric acid, $C_6H_{14}N_4O_2$, the L-form of which is an amino acid component of animal and vegetable proteins; while nitrogen equilibrium can be maintained in its absence for a short period, it appears to be a dietary essential for humans. The glutamate and hydrochloride salts are used therapeutically as ammonia detoxicants.

arginine glutamate. The L(+)-arginine salt of L(+)-glutamic acid, $C_{11}H_{23}N_5O_6$, used in the treatment of ammonia intoxication due to hepatic failure.

ar·gi·ni·no·suc·cin·ic acid (ahr″ji·nee′no·suck·sin′ick). An intermediate compound, $C_{10}H_{18}N_4O_6$, in the synthesis of arginine, formed by the enzymatic condensation of citrulline and aspartic acid.

ar·gi·ni·no·suc·cin·ic·ac·id·u·ria (ahr″ji·nee′no·suck·sin′ick as″i·dew′ree·uh) *n.* A recessively inherited metabolic disorder in which there is a deficiency of argininosuccinase with high concentration of argininosuccinic acid in blood, cerebrospinal fluid, and urine as well as ammonia intoxication; manifested clinically by mental retardation, friable and tufted hair,

ataxia, convulsions, vomiting, often a refusal to eat proteins, and hepatomegaly.

ar·gol (ahr′gol) *n.* The crust, consisting largely of crude potassium bitartrate (tartar), deposited on the inside of wine casks during fermentation.

ar·gon (ahr′gon) *n.* An inert gaseous element, atomic weight 39.948, present in the atmosphere. It may be obtained by fractionation of liquid air. Symbol, Ar.

Ar·gyll Rob·ert·son pupil or **sign** (ahr·gile′) A pupil which constricts on accommodation but not to light; usually bilateral and seen in syphilis of the central nervous system, in miosis, and occasionally in other diseases.

argyr-, argyro- A combining form meaning *silver.*

ar·gyr·ia (ahr·jirr′ee·uh, ahr·jye′ree·uh) *n.* A dusky-gray or bluish discoloration of the skin and mucous membranes produced by the prolonged administration or application of silver preparations. Syn. *argyrosis.* —**argyr·ic** (·ick) *adj.*

Argyrol. Trademark for a preparation somewhat similar to mild silver protein used as a nonirritating antiseptic in infections of the mucous membranes.

ar·gy·ro·len·tis (ahr·jye″ro·len′tis, ahr″ji·ro·) *n.* A condition of the lens of the eye seen rarely in prolonged silver intoxication, characterized by a golden sheen to the anterior lens capsule.

ar·gy·ro·phil, ar·gy·ro·phile (ahr·jye′ro-fil, ahr′ji·ro·) *adj.* Stainable by impregnation with silver salts, followed by light or photographic development or both.

ar·gy·ro·phil·ia (ahr·jye″ro·fil′ee·uh, ahr″ji·ro) *n.* The property of being argyrophil(ic).

argyrophil plaque. A microscopic, extracellular lesion of the cerebral gray matter, marking an area of active neuronal degeneration, staining readily with silver, and consisting of particles of neuronal debris surrounding a core of coagulation necrosis that frequently contains amyloid material; a major pathologic feature of Alzheimer's disease.

ar·gy·ro·sid·er·o·sis (ahr″ji·ro·sid″ur·o′sis) *n.* A form of pneumoconiosis caused by inhalation of iron oxide mixed with silver; seen in arc welders, silver polishers, and workers in iron and steel factories.

arhinencephalia. ARRHINENCEPHALIA.

arhinia. ARRHINIA.

Arias-Ste·lla cells (ar″yas·teh′l′yah, ar″yas·es·tey′yah) Endometrial columnar cells with hyperchromatic nuclei displaying both proliferative and secretory activity under the influence of trophoblastic tissue; an atypical pattern of endometrium associated with ectopic pregnancy.

ari·bo·fla·vin·o·sis (ay·rye″bo·flay·vi·no′sis) *n.* Dietary deficiency of riboflavin, associated with the syndrome of angular cheilosis and stomatitis, corneal vascularity, nasolabial seborrhea, and genitorectal dermatitis.

aristo- A combining form meaning *best.*

Aristocort. A trademark for the glucocorticoid triamcinolone and certain of its derivatives.

aris·to·gen·ics (a·ris″to·jen′icks) *n. Obsol.* EUGENics; specifically, positive eugenics. —**aristoge-nic,** *adj.*

Aristol. A trademark for thymol iodide, a topical antiseptic.

ar·ith·met·ic mean, (är″ith·met′ick). The result obtained by the addition of a series of quantities and division by the number of such quantities.

arith·mo·ma·nia (a·rith″mo·may′nee·uh) *n.* A morbid impulse to count objects; a preoccupation with numbers.

Ar·i·zo·na bacteria. Lactose-fermenting Enterobacteriaceae, biochemically and serologically related to the *Salmonella,* capable of producing illness in man, other mammals, and in fowl; frequently carried by reptiles.

Arlidin. Trademark for nylidrin.

arm, *n.* 1. *In anatomy,* the upper extremity from the shoulder to the elbow. 2. Popularly, the arm and the forearm. 3. That portion of the stand connecting the body or tube of a microscope with the pillar. 4. *In prosthodontics,* part of a clasp or other retaining or stabilizing device of a removable prosthesis.

ar·ma·men·tar·i·um (ahr″muh·men·tair′ee·um) *n.,* pl. **armamentar·ia** (·ee·uh), All the books, journals, medicines, instruments, and laboratory and therapeutic equipment possessed by a physician, surgeon, or medical institution to assist in the practice of medicine.

Ar·man·ni-Eb·stein lesion (ar·mahⁿn′nee, ep′shtine) Glycogen vacuolation of the terminal straight portion of the renal proximal convoluted tubules, seen in diabetic glomerulosclerosis.

Ar·mil·li·fer (ahr·mil′li·fur) *n.* A genus of pentastomes (tongue worms) normally parasitic of reptiles, whose larvae have been found in the liver, lungs, and spleen of man. The medically important species are *Armillifer armillatus* and *A. moniliformis.*

arm-lung time test. A test in which the time is measured from the injection of ether into a vein of the arm until the odor of ether appears in the breath; used as a measurement of the velocity of blood flow; a circulation time test.

arm·pit, *n.* AXILLA.

arm-tongue time test. A test in which the time is measured from the injection of a substance into an arm vein until the taste of it is noticed in the mouth; used as a measurement of the velocity of blood flow; a circulation time test.

Ar·neth's count or **classification** (ahr′net) A system of dividing peripheral blood granulocytes into five classes according to the number of nuclear lobes, the least mature cells being tabulated on the left, giving rise to the terms "shift to left" and "shift to right" as an indication of granulocytic immaturity or hypermaturity, respectively.

ar·ni·ca (ahr′ni·kuh) *n.* The dried flower heads of the *Arnica montana.* A counterirritant, arnica was formerly popularly used as a tincture for sprains, bruises, and surface wounds.

Ar·nold-Chia·ri syndrome or **malformation** (ahr′nohⁿlt, kyah′ree) A group of congenital anomalies at the base of the brain characteristically including an extension of the cerebellar tissue

and a displacement of the medulla and inferior part of the fourth ventricle into the cervical canal; may or may not be accompanied by a meningomyelocele. Syn. *cerebellomedullary malformation syndrome.*

Ar·noux's sign (ar·noo′) In twin pregnancy the double and quadruple rhythmic sounds of the two fetal hearts beating in and then out of unison.

ar·o·mat·ic (ar″o·mat′ick) *adj.* & *n.* 1. Having a spicy odor. 2. Characterized by a fragrant, spicy taste and odor, as cinnamon, ginger, or an essential oil. 3. Any aromatic plant or substance, as a medicine or drug. 4. Designating any carbon compound originating from benzene, C_6H_6, or containing at least one benzene ring or similar unsaturated heterocyclic ring, as pyridine. 5. Any aromatic organic compound.

aromatic acid. Any acid derived from benzene or containing a benzene or other aromatic ring.

aromatic alcohol. Any alcohol containing a benzene or other aromatic ring.

aromatic ammonia spirit. A flavored, hydroalcoholic solution of ammonia and ammonium carbonate having an aromatic, pungent odor; used as a reflex stimulant.

aromatic bitters. Medicinal preparations that combine the properties of aromatics with those of simple bitters.

aromatic elixir. A pleasant-tasting vehicle prepared from compound orange spirit, syrup, and alcohol.

aromatic series. The series of organic compounds derived from benzene and characterized by the presence of a number of carbon atoms arranged in the form of a closed chain with conjugate double bonds.

arous·al reaction (uh·row′zul). The electrical change from cerebral cortical rhythms characteristic of a sleeping or anesthetized animal to rhythms resembling those recorded during the waking condition, produced by stimulation of parts of the ascending reticular activating system, and leading to physical signs of arousal in the animal.

ar·rec·tor (a·reck′tur) *n.,* pl. **ar·rec·to·res** (ar″eck·to′reez) An erector muscle.

arrector pi·li (pye′lye), pl. **arrectores pi·lor·um** (pi·lo′rum). Any of the minute, fan-like, involuntary muscles attached to the hair follicles which, by contraction, erect the hair and cause so-called goose-flesh. Syn. *pilomotor muscle.* NA (pl.) *musculi arrectores pilorum.*

ar·rest (uh·rest′) *v.* & *n.* 1. To interrupt or check. 2. To render inactive. 3. An interruption or stoppage, as of a bodily, developmental, or pathological process.

arrhen-, arrheno- A combining form meaning *male.*

ar·rhe·no·blas·to·ma (ăr″e·no·blas·to′muh, a·ree′no·) *n.* An ovarian tumor, sometimes malignant, whose cells reproduce to varying degrees the appearance of immature testicular tubules, the less differentiated forms being masculinizing.

ar·rhin·en·ce·pha·lia, arhin·en·ce·pha·lia (ăr″in-en·se·fay'lee·uh, ay·rye''nen·) n. A form of partial anencephalia in which there is partial or total absence of the rhinencephalon and malformation of the nose.

ar·rhi·nia, arhi·nia (a·rin'ee·uh, a·rye'nee·uh) n. Congenital absence of the nose.—**arhi·nic** (·nick) adj.

ar·rhyth·mia, arhyth·mia (a·rith'mee·uh) n. An alteration or abnormality of normal cardiac rhythm. —**arrhyth·mic, arhyth·mic** (·mick) adj.

ar·row·root, n. A variety of starch derived from *Maranta arundinacea*, a plant of the West Indies and southern United States.

ar·sa·nil·ic acid (ahr''suh·nil'ick). *p*-Aminobenzenearsonic acid, $NH_2C_6H_4AsO(OH)_2$, the starting compound for the synthesis of many useful medicinal arsenicals.

arsen-, arseno-. A combining form designating (a) *a compound containing arsenic;* (b) *a compound containing the* —*As:As*— *group.*

ar·se·nate (ahr'se·nate) n. Any salt or ester of arsenic acid.

ar·se·nic (ahr'se·nick, ahrs'nick) n. As = 74.9216. 1. A brittle, usually steel-gray element of both metallic and nonmetallic properties. It exists in four allotropic modifications, the most important of which is the gray, or so-called metallic, arsenic. It sublimes readily, the vapor having a garlicky odor. Its salts have been used in medicine for their tonic effect, for ability to increase the hematinic effect of iron, in skin diseases, in certain pulmonary diseases, for destruction of protozoan parasites, and as caustics. 2. ARSENIC TRIOXIDE.

ar·sen·ic (ahr·sen'ick) adj. Of, pertaining to, or containing arsenic.

arsenic acid. Orthoarsenic acid, H_3AsO_4; used in the manufacture of medicinal and insecticidal arsenates.

ar·sen·i·cal (ahr·sen'i·kul) adj. & n. 1. Of, pertaining to, caused by, or containing arsenic. 2. A drug, fungicide, or insecticide the effect of which depends on its arsenic content.

arsenical carcinoma. A carcinoma of the skin following prolonged ingestion or exposure to arsenical compounds.

arsenical keratosis. Hyperkeratosis, usually of the palms and soles, due to arsenic in the body as a result of ingestion or injection.

arsenical paralysis. ARSENICAL POLYNEUROPATHY.

arsenical polyneuropathy. Polyneuropathy with paresthesia, sensory deficits, and muscle weakness seen in the later stages of arsenic poisoning, and often associated with hyperpigmentation of the skin, palmar and plantar hyperkeratosis, white transverse lines (Mees' lines) on the nails, and sometimes signs and symptoms of encephalopathy.

arsenical tremor. A tremor seen in arsenic poisoning.

arsenic trioxide. Arsenous oxide, As_2O_3, the principal form in which inorganic arsenic was used medicinally. Syn. *arsenous acid, white arsenic.*

ar·se·nide (ahr'se·nide) n. A compound of arsenic with another element in which the arsenic is negatively charged.

ar·se·nite (ahr'se·nite) n. A salt of arsenous acid.

ar·se·no·ther·a·py (ahr''se·no·therr'uh·pee) n. Treatment of disease by means of arsenical drugs.

ar·se·nous (ahr'se·nus, ahr·see'nous) adj. Containing arsenic in the positive trivalent form.

ar·sine (ahr·seen', ahr'seen, ahr'sin) n. Hydrogen arsenide, or arsenous hydride, AsH_3. A poisonous gas with a garlicky odor.

ars·phen·a·mine (ahrs·fen'uh·meen, ·min) n. Diaminodihydroxyarsenobenzene dihydrochloride, $C_{12}H_{12}As_2N_2O_2 \cdot 2HCl \cdot 2H_2O$. The antisyphilitic, effective also in other protozoal infections, first prepared by Ehrlich in 1909. It has been superseded by other organic arsenicals and by antibiotics. Syn. *Ehrlich's 606.*

ar·ter·e·nol (ahr·teer'e·nole, ahr''tur·en'ol) n. NOREPINEPHRINE.

arteri-, arterio-. A combining form meaning *artery, arterial.*

ar·te·ria (ahr·teer'ee·uh) n., pl. & genit. sing. **arte·ri·ae** (·ee·ee) ARTERY. Abbreviated a.

ar·te·ri·al (ahr·teer'ee·ul) adj. Of or pertaining to an artery.

arterial blood. The blood in the vascular system from the point of origin of the small venules in the lungs to the capillary beds in tissues where oxygen is released and carbon dioxide taken up; includes the blood in the pulmonary veins.

arterial bridge. A segment of vein or a synthetic graft used to bridge a gap in an injured or diseased artery.

arterial circle of the cerebrum. The arterial anastomosis at the base of the brain, formed in front by the anterior communicating artery joining together the anterior cerebral arteries; laterally by the internal carotid arteries and the posterior communicating arteries joining them with the posterior cerebral arteries; and behind by the posterior cerebral arteries branching from the basilar artery.

arterial hypertension. Abnormally elevated blood pressure in the arterial side of the circulatory system.

ar·te·ri·al·iza·tion (ahr·teer''ee·ul·i·zay'shun) n. 1. The process of making or becoming arterial; the change from venous blood into arterial. 2. VASCULARIZATION. —**ar·te·ri·al·ize** (ahr·teer'ee·uh·lize) v.

arterial murmur. A sound made by arterial blood flow.

arterial nephrosclerosis. Renal atrophy and scarring characterized by coarse granulation of the parenchymal surface and by glomerular, tubular, and interstitial alterations associated with arteriosclerotic changes in the large and medium-sized renal arteries. Syn. *benign nephrosclerosis, senile arteriosclerotic nephrosclerosis.*

arterial pressure. Hydrostatic pressure of the blood within an arterial lumen.

arterial systole. The highest phase of the arterial pressure pulse, consequent upon ejection of blood from the heart.

arterial transfusion. Transfusion of blood by intraarterial injection.

arterial ulcer. Ulceration due to arterial insufficiency or occlusion.

ar·te·ri·a·sis (ahr˝te·rye´uh·sis) n., pl. **arteria·ses** (·seez) Rare. Degeneration of an artery.

ar·te·ri·ec·ta·sis (ahr·teer˝ee·eck´tuh·sis) n. Arterial dilatation.

ar·te·ri·ec·to·my (ahr·teer˝ee·eck´tuh·mee) n. Excision of an artery or portion of an artery.

ar·te·ri·ec·to·pia (ahr·teer˝ee·eck·to´pee·uh) n. Displacement or abnormality of the course of an artery.

arterio-. See arteri-.

ar·te·ri·o·cap·il·lary (ahr·tee˝ree·o·kap´i·lār·ee) n. PRECAPILLARY.

arteriocapillary fibrosis. Fibrosis of small arteries and arterioles, with variable degrees of hyalinization and reduction in the size of the lumens, a manifestation of arteriolosclerosis.

ar·te·ri·o·fi·bro·sis (ahr·teer˝ee·o·figh·bro´sis) n. An increment of fibrous connective tissue in the walls of arteries; endarteritis obliterans.

ar·te·ri·o·gram (ahr·teer´ee·o·gram) n. 1. A roentgenogram of an artery after injection with a contrast material. 2. A tracing of the arterial pulse.

ar·te·ri·o·graph (ahr·teer´ee·o·graf) n. An instrument which graphically presents the pulse.

ar·te·ri·og·ra·phy (ahr·teer˝ee·og´ruh·fee) n. 1. Graphic presentation of the pulse; sphygmography. 2. Roentgenography of the arteries after the intravascular injection of a radiopaque substance. —**ar·te·ri·o·graph·ic** (ahr·teer˝ee·o·graf´ick) adj.

ar·te·ri·o·la (ahr·teer˝ee·o´luh, ahr˝te·rye·o´luh) n., pl. & genit. sing. **arterio·lae** (·lee) [NL.]. ARTERIOLE.

ar·te·ri·o·lar (ahr·teer˝ee·o´lur) adj. Of or pertaining to an arteriole.

arteriolar nephrosclerosis. Renal atrophy and scarring characterized by fine granulation of the parenchymal surface and by glomerular, tubular, and interstitial alterations associated with arteriosclerotic changes of the afferent arterioles.

ar·te·ri·ole (ahr·teer´ee·ole) n. Any of the minute, smallest arterial branches which, together with the precapillaries, comprise the intermediate vessels between the larger arteries and the capillaries; arterioles have a relatively thick muscular wall and are responsible in large part for peripheral resistance in the vasculature and the effects thereof on rate of blood flow.

ar·te·ri·o·li·tis (ahr·teer·ee·o·lye´tis) n. Inflammation of arterioles.

ar·te·ri·o·lo·ne·cro·sis (ahr·teer·ee·o˝lo·ne·kro´sis) n. Degeneration of the arterioles resulting in necrosis. —**arteriolo·ne·crot·ic** (·ne·krot´ick) adj.

ar·te·ri·o·lo·scle·ro·sis (ahr·teer·ee·o˝lo·skle·ro´sis) n., pl. **arteriolosclero·ses** (·seez) Thickening of arterioles, usually due to hyalinization or fibromuscular hyperplasia. —**arteriolosclerot·ic** (·rot´ick) adj.

ar·te·ri·o·ma·la·cia (ahr·teer˝ee·o·ma·lay´shee·uh) n. Softening of an arterial wall.

ar·te·ri·o·mes·en·ter·ic (ahr·teer˝ee·o·mes˝en·terr´ick) adj. Pertaining to the arteries in the mesentery.

ar·te·ri·o·ne·cro·sis (ahr·teer˝ee·o·ne·kro´sis) n. Necrosis of an artery or arteries.

ar·te·ri·op·a·thy (ahr·teer˝ee·op´uth·ee) n. Any diseased state of arteries.

ar·te·ri·o·plas·ty (ahr·teer˝ee·o·plas˝tee) n. An operation for aneurysm in which the artery is reconstructed by using the aneurysmal walls to restore its continuity. —**ar·te·ri·o·plas·tic** (ahr·teer˝ee·o·plas·tick) adj.

ar·te·ri·o·punc·ture (ahr·teer˝ee·o·punk˝chur) n. Insertion of a needle into an artery, or surgical division or opening of an artery, chiefly for the abstraction of blood.

ar·te·ri·or·rha·phy (ahr·teer˝ee·or´uh·fee) n. Suture of an artery.

ar·te·ri·or·rhex·is (ahr·teer˝ee·o·reck´sis) n., pl. **arteriorrhex·es** (·seez) Rupture of an artery.

ar·te·ri·o·scle·ro·sis (ahr·teer˝ee·o·skle·ro´sis) n., pl. **arteriosclero·ses** (·seez) Any of various proliferative and degenerative changes in arteries, not necessarily related to each other, resulting in thickening of the walls, loss of elasticity, and in some instances, calcium deposition. —**arteriosclerot·ic** (·rot´ick) adj.

arteriosclerosis oblit·er·ans (o·blit´ur·anz). Arteriosclerosis with proliferation of the intima to the extent of obstructing the lumen.

arteriosclerotic gangrene. A dry gangrene of the extremities, due to failure of the terminal circulation in persons afflicted with arteriosclerosis. Syn. senile gangrene.

arteriosclerotic psychosis. ARTERIOSCLEROTIC DEMENTIA.

ar·te·ri·o·spasm (ahr·teer˝ee·o·spaz´um) n. Spasm of an artery. —**ar·te·ri·o·spas·tic** (ahr·teer˝ee·o·spas´tick) adj.

ar·te·ri·o·ste·no·sis (ahr·teer˝ee·o·ste·no´sis) n., pl. **arteriosteno·ses** (·seez) Narrowing of the caliber of an artery.

ar·te·ri·os·to·sis (ahr·teer˝ee·os·to´sis) n. Calcification of an artery.

ar·te·ri·ot·o·my (ahr·teer˝ee·ot´uh·mee) n. Incision or opening of an artery.

ar·te·ri·o·ve·nous (ahr·teer˝ee·o·vee´nus) adj. Both arterial and venous; involving an artery and a vein or an arteriole and a venule.

arteriovenous anastomosis. A modified vessel which connects an arteriole and a venule without the intervention of capillaries. Such structures are numerous in the palm, the sole, and the pulp of terminal digital phalanges.

arteriovenous fistula or **aneurysm.** Abnormal direct communication, single or multiple, between an artery and a vein without interposition of capillaries; it may be congenital or acquired.

ar·te·ri·o·ver·sion (ahr·teer˝ee·o·vur´zhun) n. A method of arresting hemorrhage by turning arteries inside out.

ar·te·ri·o·vert·er (ahr·teer´ee·o·vur˝tur) n. An instrument used to perform arterioversion.

ar·te·ri·tis (ahr˝te·rye´tis) n. Inflammation of an artery.

ar·te·ry (ahr´tur·ee) n. A vessel conveying blood away from the heart. It is composed of three coats: the intima (interna), the media, and the adventitia (externa). In comparison to veins, arteries have a thick wall and small lumen.

For arteries listed by name, see Table of Arteries in the Appendix.

artery forceps. A forceps, usually self-locking and with scissors handles, used for seizing and compressing an artery.

arthr-, arthro- A combining form meaning *joint*.

ar·thral·gia (ahr·thral'jee·uh) *n.* Pain affecting a joint. —**arthral·gic** (·jick) *adj.*

ar·threc·to·my (ahr·threck'tuh·mee) *n.* Excision of a joint.

ar·thres·the·sia (ahr″thres·theezh'uh, ·theez'ee·uh) *n.* Sensory perception of movements of a joint.

ar·thrit·ic (ahr·thrit'ick) *adj. & n.* 1. Pertaining to or affected by arthritis. 2. An individual affected with arthritis.

ar·thri·tis (ahr·thrigh'tis) *n.,* pl. **ar·thrit·i·des** (·thrit'i·deez) Inflammation of a joint.

arthritis de·for·mans (de·for'manz). RHEUMATOID ARTHRITIS.

arthritis deformans juvenilis. OSTEOCHONDRITIS DEFORMANS JUVENILIS.

arthritis ure·thrit·i·ca (yoo″re·thrit'i·kuh). REITER'S SYNDROME.

arthro-. See *arthr-*.

ar·thro·cele (ahr'thro·seel) *n.* 1. Any swollen joint. 2. Hernia of the synovial membrane through a joint capsule.

ar·thro·cen·te·sis (ahr″thro·sen·tee'sis) *n.,* pl. **ar·throcente·ses** (·seez) Incision into or puncture through a joint capsule to relieve an effusion.

ar·thro·chon·dri·tis (ahr″thro·kon·drye'tis) *n.* Obsol. OSTEOCHONDRITIS (1).

ar·thro·cla·sia (ahr″thro·klay'zhuh, ·zee·uh) *n.* The breaking down of an ankylosis in order to produce free movement of a joint.

ar·thro·de·sis (ahr·thro·dee'sis, ahr·throd'e·sis) *n.,* pl. **arthrode·ses** (·seez) Fusion of a joint by removing the articular surfaces and securing bony union. Syn. *operative ankylosis.*

ar·thro·dia (ahr·thro·dee·uh) *n.,* pl. **arthro·di·ae** (·dee·ee) GLIDING JOINT. —**arthro·di·al** (·dee·ul) *adj.*

ar·thro·dyn·ia (ahr″thro·din'ee·uh) *n.* ARTHRALGIA. —**arthrodyn·ic** (·ick) *adj.*

ar·thro·dys·pla·sia (ahr″thro·dis·play'zhuh, ·zee·uh) *n.* A condition, usually inherited, in which the patellas are rudimentary, the heads of the radii dislocated, and the nails generally absent.

ar·thro·em·py·e·sis (ahr″thro·em·pye·ee'sis) *n.* PYARTHROSIS.

ar·thro·en·dos·co·py (ahr″thro·en·dos'kuh·pee) *n.* ARTHROSCOPY.

ar·thro·gram (ahr'thro·gram) *n.* A roentgenogram of a joint space after injection of contrast media.

ar·thro·ra·phy (ahr·throg'ruh·fee) *n.* Roentgenography of a joint space after the injection of positive or negative (or both positive and negative) contrast media.

ar·thro·gry·po·sis (ahr″thro·gri·po'sis) *n.* Retention of a joint in a fixed position due to muscular contraction or to extracapsular or intracapsular adhesions.

arthrogryposis mul·ti·plex con·gen·i·ta (mul'ti·plecks kon·jen'i·tuh). A syndrome, congenital in origin, characterized by deformity and an-

kylosis of joints, usually in flexion, with limitation of motion, muscular atrophy, and contractures; may be neurogenic or rarely myogenic.

ar·thro·ka·tad·y·sis (ahr″thro·ka·tad'i·sis) *n.* Intrapelvic protrusion of the acetabulum from thinning and eburnation of the pelvic wall; of undetermined etiology. Syn. *Otto's pelvis.*

ar·thro·lith (ahr'thro·lith) *n.* A calcareous or gouty deposit within a joint.

ar·thro·li·thi·a·sis (ahr″thro·li·thigh'uh·sis) *n.,* pl. **arthrolithia·ses** (·seez). GOUT.

ar·throl·y·sis (ahr·throl'i·sis) *n.* Surgical freeing of an ankylosed joint.

ar·throm·e·ter (ahr·throm'e·tur) *n.* An instrument for measuring and recording the extent of movement in a joint. —**arthrome·try** (·tree) *n.*

ar·thron·cus (ahr·thronk'us) *n.* 1. A joint tumor. 2. Swelling of a joint.

ar·thro·on·y·cho·dys·pla·sia (ahr″thro·on″i·ko·dis·play'zhuh, ·zee·uh) *n.* NAIL-PATELLA SYNDROME.

ar·thro·a·thy (ahr·throp'uth·ee) *n.* 1. Any joint disease. 2. CHARCOT'S JOINT. —**ar·thro·path·ic** (ahr″thro·path'ick) *adj.*

ar·thro·phyte (ahr'thro·fight) *n.* An abnormal growth occurring within a joint; a joint mouse.

ar·thro·plas·ty (ahr'thro·plas″tee) *n.* 1. Reconstruction, by natural modification or artificial replacement, of a diseased, damaged, or ankylosed joint. 2. The making of an artificial joint. —**ar·thro·plas·tic** (ahr″thro·plas'tick) *adj.*

ar·thro·pod (ahr'thro·pod) *n.* A member of the Arthropoda.

Ar·throp·o·da (ahr·throp'o·duh) *n.pl.* The largest phylum of the animal kingdom; includes the crustacea, insects, myriopods, arachnids, and related forms. The members are bilaterally symmetrical, having a limited number of segments, a chitinous exoskeleton, and jointed appendages. —**arthropo·dal, arthropo·dan,** *adj.*

ar·thror·rha·gia (ahr″thro·ray'jee·uh) *n.* Hemorrhage into a joint.

ar·thro·scle·ro·sis (ahr″thro·skle·ro'sis) *n.* The hardening or stiffening of a joint or joints.

ar·thro·scope (ahr'thro·skope) *n.* An instrument used for the visualization of the interior of a joint.

ar·thros·co·py (ahr·thros'kuh·pee) *n.* Examination of the interior of a joint with an arthroscope.

ar·thro·sis (ahr·thro'sis) *n.,* pl. **arthro·ses** (·seez) 1. An articulation or joint; a suture. 2. A degenerative process in a joint.

ar·thro·spore (ahr'thro·spore) *n.* A fungal spore formed by the segmentation of the hyphae, resulting in the formation of rectangular, thick-walled cells.

ar·thros·to·my (ahr·thros'tuh·mee) *n.* An incision into a joint, as for drainage.

ar·thro·tome (ahr'thro·tome) *n.* A stout knife used in joint surgery; a cartilage knife.

ar·throt·o·my (ahr·throt'uh·mee) *n.* An incision into a joint.

ar·thro·tro·pia (ahr″thro·tro'pee·uh) *n.* Torsion or twisted condition of a limb.

ar·throus (ahr'thrus) *adj.* Pertaining to a joint or joints; jointed.

Ar·thus' phenomenon or **reaction** (ar·tu⁸ss') A generalized or local anaphylactic reaction, the result of the union of antigen and antibody within the tissues, manifested by local edema and inflammation.

ar·tic·u·lar (ahr·tick'yoo·lur) *adj. & n.* 1. Pertaining to an articulation, or to a muscle or ligament associated with it. 2. A bone of the lower jaw of fishes, amphibians, and reptiles which articulates with the quadrate bone to form the mandibular joint. Its homologue in man is the malleus.

articular cartilage. Cartilage that covers the articular surfaces of bones.

articular disk. A disk of fibrocartilage, dividing the joint cavity of certain joints.

articular fracture. A fracture that also involves the articular surface of a bone.

articular tubercle. The projection upon the zygomatic process of the temporal bone which marks the anterior boundary of the mandibular fossa. Syn. *articular eminence.*

¹ar·tic·u·late (ahr·tick'yoo·lut) *adj.* 1. Divided into joints. 2. Expressed or expressing oneself in concatenations of discrete symbols, as in human speech. 3. Expressed or expressing oneself coherently and fluently.

²ar·tic·u·late (ahr·tick'yoo·late) *v.* 1. To unite by one or more joints. 2. To produce ordered and coordinated speech sounds; to enunciate. 3. To express (thoughts, feelings) in connected discourse. 4. *In dentistry,* to position or adjust artificial teeth.

ar·tic·u·la·tio (ahr·tick"yoo·lay'shee·o) *n.,* pl. **ar·tic·u·la·ti·o·nes** (·lay"shee·o'neez) 1. [NA] ARTICULATION. 2. [BNA, PNA] Junctura synovialis (= SYNOVIAL JOINT).

ar·tic·u·la·tion (ahr·tick"yoo·lay'shun) *n.* 1. The production of ordered and coordinated speech sounds. 2. The junction of two or more bones or skeletal parts. The articulations include the fibrous joints (syndesmoses, sutures, and gomphoses), cartilaginous joints (synchondroses and symphyses), and synovial joints (the movable joints). Syn. *joint.* 3. The positioning of artificial teeth. 4. OCCLUSION.

ar·tic·u·la·tor (ahr·tick'yoo·lay"tur) *n.* An instrument used in dentistry for holding casts of the jaws or teeth in proper relation during the construction of artificial dentures. It may be adjusted so as to duplicate the mandibular movements of the patient.

ar·tic·u·lus (ahr·tick'yoo·lus) *n.,* pl. **articu·li** (·lye) 1. A joint; a knuckle. 2. A segment; a part; a limb.

ar·ti·fact, ar·te·fact (ahr'ti·fakt) *n. In science and medicine,* an artificial or extraneous feature accidentally or unavoidably introduced into an object of observation and which may simulate a natural or relevant feature of that object.

ar·ti·fi·cial abortion. INDUCED ABORTION.

artificial antigen. Any laboratory-made or modified antigen, not occurring naturally; including conjugated antigens, such as azoproteins, antigens modified by other chemical or physical treatment, and specially synthesized polypeptides.

artificial anus. An opening made surgically from the lumen of the bowel to the external surface of the body to permit expulsion of feces.

artificial catalepsy. Catalepsy induced by hypnosis.

artificial crown. A metallic, porcelain, or plastic substitute that replaces all or most of the crown of a tooth.

artificial denture. A prosthesis that replaces missing natural teeth.

artificial eye. Glass, celluloid, rubber, or plastic made to resemble the front of the eye, and worn in the socket to replace a lost one, or over a blind eye for cosmetic effect.

artificial fecundation. Fertilization by artificial insemination.

artificial fever. Purposefully produced fever for therapeutic benefit, as by the induction of malaria, by the injection of foreign protein, or by means of a fever cabinet.

artificial insemination. The instrumental injection of semen into the vagina or uterus to induce pregnancy; insemination without coitus.

artificial pneumothorax. PNEUMOTHORAX (2).

artificial respiration. The maintenance of breathing by artificial ventilation, in the absence of normal spontaneous respiration. Most effective methods include mouth-to-mouth breathing for emergencies and the use of a respirator for prolonged application.

ar·tis·tic anatomy. That branch of anatomy which treats of the external form of man and animals, their osseous and muscular systems, and their relation to painting and sculpture.

ary·epi·glot·tic (ăr"ee·ep'i·glot'ick) *adj.* Pertaining to the arytenoid cartilage and the epiglottis.

aryepiglottic fold. A fold of mucous membrane in each lateral wall of the aditus laryngis, which extends from the arytenoid cartilage to the epiglottis.

ar·yl (ăr'il) *n.* An organic radical derived from an aromatic hydrocarbon by the removal of one hydrogen atom, as phenyl (C_6H_5—) from benzene.

ar·y·te·no·epi·glot·tic (ăr"i·tee"no·ep·i·glot'ick, a·rit"e·no·) *adj.* ARYEPIGLOTTIC.

ar·y·te·noid (ăr"i·tee'noid, a·rit'e·noid) *adj.* 1. Resembling the mouth of a pitcher. 2. Pertaining to the arytenoid cartilages and muscles.

arytenoid cartilage. One of two cartilages of the back of the larynx resting on the cricoid cartilage and regulating, by means of the attached muscles, the tension of the vocal folds.

ar·y·te·noid·ec·to·my (ăr·i·tee"noy·deck'tuh·mee) *n.* Removal of an arytenoid cartilage.

ar·y·te·noi·di·tis (ăr"i·tee"noy·dye'tis, a·rit"e·noy·) *n.* Inflammation of the arytenoid cartilages or muscles.

As Symbol for arsenic.

As. Abbreviation for *astigmatism; astigmatic.*

a.s. Abbreviation for *auris sinistra,* left ear.

as·a·fet·i·da, as·a·foet·i·da (as"uh·fet'i·duh) *n.* An oleo-gum-resin obtained from the rhizomes and roots of species of *Ferula*. It occurs as soft yellow-brown masses and has a bitter taste and a persistent offensive odor due to a volatile oil consisting largely of a mercaptan. It has been used as a carminative and psychic sedative.

asar·cia (a·sahr'shee·uh, ·see·uh) *n.* Emaciation; leanness.

as·a·rum (as'uh·rum, a·sǎr'um) *n.* The dried rhizome and roots of *Asarum canadense*, formerly used as a carminative and bitter aromatic flavor. Syn. *Canada snakeroot, wild ginger.*

as·bes·tos (as·bes'tus, az·) *n.* A calcium-magnesium silicate mineral of flexible or elastic fibers; the best nonconductor of heat.

asbestos bodies. Long, slender cylinders with a transparent capsule composed of protein and a core of altered asbestos fiber; found in the lungs, air passages, sputum, and feces of patients with asbestosis and of many apparently normal people.

as·bes·to·sis (as''bes·to'sis, az·) *n.*, pl. **asbesto·ses** (·seez) Diffuse interstitial pulmonary fibrosis due to the prolonged inhalation of asbestos dust.

asbestos transformation. A change in cartilage, especially of the hyaline type, often associated with advanced age, which leads to a softening of the tissue and to the formation of spaces in it.

as·ca·ri·a·sis (as''kuh·rye'uh·sis) *n.*, pl. **ascaria·ses** (·seez) 1. Infection by a nematode of the genus *Ascaris*. 2. Specifically, infection of the human intestine, with a short migratory phase, by *Ascaris lumbricoides*, with occasional involvement of other organs, as the stomach or liver; heavy infection may cause bronchopneumonia, abdominal pain, and, occasionally, intestinal obstruction.

as·ca·ri·cide (as·kǎr'i·side) *n.* A medicine that kills ascarids.

as·ca·rid (as'kuh·rid) *n.*, pl. **ascarids, as·car·i·des** (as·kǎr'i·deez). A worm of the family Ascaridae.

As·car·i·dae (as·kǎr'i·dee) *n.pl.* A family of nematode worms, which includes the genera *Ascaris* and *Toxocara*.

As·ca·ris (as'kuh·ris) *n.* A genus of intestinal nematodes of the family Ascaridae.

Ascaris lum·bri·coi·des (lum·bri·koy'deez). A species of roundworm causing ascariasis in man and (var. *suis*) in swine.

as·cend·ing. *adj.* 1. Taking an upward course; rising. 2. In the nervous system, AFFERENT; conducting impulses or progressing up the spinal cord or from peripheral to central.

ascending aorta. The first part of the aorta.

ascending colon. The portion of the colon that extends from the cecum to the hepatic flexure.

ascending degeneration. Secondary or wallerian degeneration of the myelin sheath and axons of sensory tracts progressing cranially from the point of injury in the spinal cord.

Asch·heim-Zon·dek reaction (ahsh'hime, tsohn'deck) Follicular growth and luteinization are produced by substances in the urine of pregnant women, whereas the urine following oophorectomy and the menopause contains only the follicle growth-stimulating substance.

Asch·off cell (ahsh'ohf) The characteristic cell of the Aschoff body in rheumatic fever; a large, elongated cell with one or more vesicular nuclei, having a central mass of chromatin from which fibrils radiate toward the nuclear membrane.

Aschoff's bodies or **nodules** A myocardial granuloma specific for the carditis associated with rheumatic fever, located in the vicinity of a blood vessel, consisting of a central eosinophilic zone surrounded by roughly parallel rows of Anitschkow cells, Aschoff cells, lymphocytes, plasma cells, neutrophils, mast cells, and fibrocytes.

as·ci·tes (a·sigh'teez) *n.*, pl. **ascites** The accumulation of serous fluid in the peritoneal cavity, most commonly encountered with heart failure and portal hypertension. Syn. *abdominal dropsy, hydroperitoneum.* —**as·cit·ic** (a·sit'ick) *adj.*

ascites ad·i·po·sus (ad·i·po'sus). Milky fluid in the peritoneal cavity due to lipid-containing cells, probably resulting from lymphatic obstruction, and usually associated with cancer or tuberculosis.

ascites chy·lo·sus (kigh·lo'sus). Chyle in the peritoneal cavity due to rupture of the lacteals. Syn. *chylous ascites.*

As·co·li test (ah'sko·lee) A precipitin test for the detection of soluble anthrax antigens in which a saline solution extract of suspected tissue is superimposed on anthrax antiserum; a precipitate forming at the junction of the liquids is a positive test.

As·co·my·ce·tes (as''ko·migh·see'teez) *n.pl.* One of the four large classes of fungi in which the ultimate reproductive spores are produced internally in an ascus. —**ascomyce·tous** (·tus) *adj.*

ascor·bate (uh·skor'bate) *n.* A salt of ascorbic acid.

ascor·bic acid (uh·skor'bick) The enol form of 3-oxo-L-gulofuranolactone, $C_6H_8O_6$, occurring in significant amounts in citrus fruits, the systemic lack of which eventually leads to scurvy. It is a white or slightly yellowish crystalline powder, fairly stable when dry, but in aqueous solution rapidly destroyed by the oxygen of the air. Ascorbic acid functions in various oxidation-reduction reactions of the tissues and is essential for normal metabolism. Syn. *vitamin C.* See Table of Chemical Constituents of Blood in the Appendix.

A.S.D.C. American Society of Dentistry for Children.

-ase A suffix which is attached to the name of a biochemical substance to designate an *enzyme* that catalyzes reactions with that substance.

asep·sis (ay·sep'sis, a·sep'sis) *n.* Exclusion of microorganisms. —**asep·tic** (·tick) *adj.*

aseptic meningitis. Meningeal inflammation produced by one of numerous agents, predominantly viral, characterized by meningeal irritation with cerebrospinal fluid showing an increase in white blood cells (usually mononuclear); normal glucose, usually normal protein, and bacteriologic sterility.

aseptic necrosis. Necrosis without infection.

aseptic peritonitis. CHEMICAL PERITONITIS.

aseptic surgery. Operative procedure in the absence of germs, everything coming in contact with the wound being sterile; a system of surgical techniques and practices designed to exclude all infectious microorganisms from the wound.

asex·u·al (ay·seck'shoo·ul, a·seck') *adj.* 1. Not involving the distinction between male and female. 2. Characterizing reproduction without sexual union. —**asexual·ly** (·lee) *adv.*

asexual dwarf. A dwarf with deficient sexual development.

asexual spore. A spore formed without previous fusion of nuclear material, as in fungi.

ash, *n.* The incombustible mineral residue that remains when a substance is incinerated.

asi·a·lia (ay"sigh·ay'lee·uh, ay"sigh·al'ee·uh) *n.* Deficiency or failure of the secretion of saliva.

Asian influenza virus. A subtype of influenza virus A, designated A_2, first recovered from an influenza epidemic in Hong Kong and Singapore in 1957.

asid·er·o·sis (ay·sid"ur·o'sis) *n.* An abnormal decrease in the iron reserves of the body. —**asider·ot·ic** (·ot'ick) *adj.*

asiderotic anemia. IRON-DEFICIENCY ANEMIA.

As·kle·pios (as·klee'pee·os). Greek god of healing; as Roman god of medicine, *Aesculapius.*

aso·cial (ay·so'shul) *adj.* 1. Withdrawn from, not interested in other people and their activities nor in the realities of one's environment. 2. Indifferent toward accepted social standards, customs, and rules. —**aso·ci·al·i·ty** (ay·so"shee·al'i·tee) *n.*

aso·nia (a·so'nee·uh) *n.* 1. TONE DEAFNESS. 2. A type of amusia in which the patient is no longer able to distinguish between one musical tone and another.

asp, *n.* 1. A small venomous snake, *Vipera aspis,* found in Africa and the Near East. 2. The horned viper, *Cerastes cornutus.*

as·par·a·gin·ase (as·pår''uh·ji·nace, ·naze) *n.* An enzyme, present in liver and other animal tissues as well as in plants, yeast, and bacteria, which catalyzes hydrolysis of asparagine to aspartic acid and ammonia; has antileukemic activity.

as·par·a·gine (as·pår'uh·jeen, ·jin) *n.* α-Aminosuccinamic acid, the β-amide of asparaginic or aspartic acid, $C_4H_8N_2O_3$, a nonessential amino acid occurring in many proteins. Syn. *asparamide, aminosuccinamic acid.*

as·par·tase (as·pahr'tace, ·taze) *n.* An enzyme, present in several bacteria, which catalyzes the conversion of aspartic acid to fumaric acid and ammonia.

as·par·tic acid (as·pahr'tick). Aminosuccinic acid, $COOHCH(NH_2)CH_2COOH$, a hydrolysis product of asparagine and of many proteins. Syn. *asparaginic acid.*

aspas·tic (ay·spas'tick) *adj.* Not spastic; not characterized by spasm.

aspe·cif·ic (ay"spe·sif'ick) *adj.* Nonspecific; not a specific.

as·pect, *n.* 1. The part or side that faces in a particular direction. 2. The particular appearance, as of a face.

As·per·gil·la·ce·ae (as"per·ji·lay'see·ee) *n.pl.* A family of fungi and molds which includes the genera *Aspergillus* and *Penicillium.*

as·per·gil·lic acid (as"per·jil'ick). 2-Hydroxy-3-isobutyl-6-(1-methylpropyl)pyrazine 1-oxide, $C_{12}H_{20}N_2O_2$, an antibiotic substance produced by *Aspergillus flavus.*

as·per·gil·lin (as"per·jil'in) *n.* A pigment obtained from the spores of *Aspergillus niger.*

as·per·gil·lo·sis (as"per·ji·lo'sis, as·pur") *n.,* Primary or secondary infection by any of various species of *Aspergillus,* especially *A. fumigatus.* The most common site of human infection is the lung where, after inhalation of spores, aspergillomas may form in preexisting cavities or bronchiectases, the fungus sometimes invading contiguous tissues or disseminating hematogenously to other organs.

As·per·gil·lus (as"per·jil'us) *n.* A genus of fungi of the family Aspergillaceae, in which the conidiophore is swollen into a head from which radiate numerous sterigmata bearing chains of conidia, and sometimes producing secondary sterigmata bearing in turn chains of conidia. Generally saprophytic, but plant and animal infections occur. The species *Aspergillus fumigatus* is the most common invader of plants and animals; *A. flavus* and *A. parasiticus* produce aflatoxins. —**aspergillus,** pl. **aspergilli** (·eye) *com. n.*

asper·ma·tism (ay·spur'muh·tiz·um, a·spur') *n.* 1. Nonemission of semen, whether owing to nonsecretion or to nonejaculation. 2. Defective secretion of semen or lack of formation of spermatozoa. —**asper·mat·ic** (ay"spur·mat'ick) *adj.*

asper·ma·to·gen·e·sis (ay·spur"ma·to·jen'e·sis) *n.* Failure of spermatozoa to mature.

asper·mia (ay·spur'mee·uh, a·spur') *n.* ASPERMATISM. —**asper·mous** (·mus) *adj.*

as·phyx·ia (as·fick'see·uh) *n.* Systemic oxygen deficiency and carbon dioxide accumulation, usually due to impaired respiration, leading to loss of consciousness. —**asphyx·i·al** (·see·ul) *adj.*

asphyxia liv·i·da (liv'i·duh). Asphyxia neonatorum associated with cyanotic skin, strong pulse, and active reflexes. Syn. *blue asphyxia.*

as·phyx·i·ant (as·fick'see·unt) *adj. & n.* 1. Producing asphyxia. 2. An agent capable of producing asphyxia. —**asphyxi·ate** (·ate) *v.*

asphyxia pal·li·da (pal'i·duh). Asphyxia neonatorum attended by a slow, weak pulse, abolished reflexes, and a very pale skin.

as·pid·i·um (as·pid'ee·um) *n.* The rhizome and stipes of European aspidium or male fern, *Dryopteris filix-mas,* or of American aspidium or marginal fern, *D. marginalis;* both are sources of aspidium oleoresin, used for expelling tapeworm.

as·pi·do·sper·ma (as"pi·do·spur'muh) *n.* The dried bark of *Aspidosperma quebracho-blanco* containing the alkaloids aspidospermine, quebrachine, and others; it has been used as a respiratory stimulant in asthmatic and cardiac dyspnea. Syn. *quebracho.*

as·pi·ra·tion (as″pi·ray′shun) *n.* 1. *Obsol.* Breathing, especially breathing in. 2. The drawing of foreign matter or other material in the upper respiratory tract into the lungs with the breath. 3. The withdrawal by suction of fluids or gases from a cavity, as with an aspirator. 4. In speech, the expulsion of breath as in the pronunciation of h or after an initial p or t in English. **—as·pi·rate** (as′pi·rate) *v.*

aspiration pneumonia. Pneumonia due to inhalation into the bronchi of a foreign body, gastric contents, or infected material from the upper respiratory tract, usually occurring during periods of depressed consciousness.

as·pi·ra·tor (as′pi·ray″tur) *n.* A negative pressure apparatus for withdrawing fluids from cavities.

as·pi·rin (as′pi·rin, as′prin) *n.* Acetylsalicylic acid, $C_6H_4O(COCH_3)COOH$, a white crystalline powder hydrolyzing in moist air to acetic and salicylic acids. An analgesic, antipyretic, and antirheumatic.

asple·nia (a·splee′nee·uh) *n.* Acquired or congenital absence of the spleen.

asplenia syndrome. IVEMARK SYNDROME.

aspo·ro·gen·ic (ay·spo″ro·jen′ick, as″po·ro·) *adj.* 1. Producing no spores. 2. Reproduced without spores.

aspo·rous (a·spo′rus, ay·spor′us) *adj.* Without spores; especially without the resistant phase, as in the case of many bacteria.

as·say (ass′ay, a·say′) *n. & v.* 1. The testing or analyzing of a substance to determine its potency or the proportion of one or more constituents. 2. The recorded result of an assay. 3. To perform an assay (on). 4. The substance to be assayed.

as·sim·i·la·tion (a·sim″i·lay′shun) *n.* 1. Absorption of a substance by tissues, cells, or organs. 2. Specifically, absorption of nutrients and other substances by the cells of the body after ingestion and digestion. 3. *Obsol.* ANABOLISM. 4. *In psychology,* mental reception of impressions, and their assignment by the consciousness to their proper place; mental assimilation. 5. A psychic process by which an unpleasant fact, having been faced, is integrated into a person's previous experience. 6. The abnormal fusion of bones, as the fusion of the transverse processes of the last lumbar vertebra with the lateral masses of the first sacral vertebra, or the atlas with the occipital bone. **—as·sim·i·late** (a·sim′i·late) *v.;* **as·sim·i·la·ble** (a·sim′i·luh·bul) *adj.*

as·so·ci·ate *n.* 1. *In psychology,* any item or phenomenon mentally linked with another. 2. A person with whom one is grouped by some common trait, experience, or interest. **—asso·ci·ate** (·ate) *v.*

associated movements. 1. Synergic, coincident, or consensual movements of muscles other than the leading ones, as swinging of the arms in walking. 2. In the normal infant, movements of one limb tending to be accompanied by similar involuntary movements of the opposite limb, a phenomenon which disappears as coordination and muscle power are increased. Persistence of such or similar movements, or return thereof in states of cortical dysfunction, is pathologic.

as·so·ci·a·tion *n.* 1. *In chemistry,* the correlation or aggregation of substances or functions. 2. *In psychology,* a mental linking, as that of objects, persons, or events with ideas, thoughts, or sensations.

association area. Any area of the cerebral cortex connected with the primary sensory and motor areas by association fibers, and usually homotypical in structure; concerned with the higher mental activities, such as the integration, interpretation, and memory storage of various stimuli, and the ability to carry out complex tasks, such as speaking, reading, or writing.

association fibers. Nerve fibers situated just beneath the cortical substance and connecting the adjacent cerebral gyri.

association of ideas. The mental link established between two similar ideas or two ideas of simultaneous occurrence.

association test. 1. *In psychology,* any test designed to determine the nature of the mental or emotional link between a stimulus and a response. 2. Commonly, a test used to determine the nature, or to measure the speed, of the response with a word given by a subject to a word offered him. The response is determined by previous experience and may reveal a great deal about the subject's past, personality, and attitudes.

association time. *In psychology,* the time required to establish a response to a given stimulus in an association test.

association word. The verbal stimulus or verbal response in an association test.

as·so·cia·tive (a·so′shee·uh·tiv, a·so′see·, ·ay″tiv) *adj.* Pertaining to or based upon association.

associative facilitation. *In psychology,* the effect of previous associations in making it easier to establish new ones.

associative inhibition or **interference.** 1. *In psychology,* the blocking or weakening of a mental link when one part of it is linked to a new association. 2. Difficulty in establishing a new association because of previous ones.

associative learning. *In psychology,* the principle that items experienced together are mentally linked, so that they tend to reinforce one another.

associative memory. 1. *In psychology,* the recalling of some item, thought, or event previously experienced by thinking of something linked with it, in order for the present idea to invoke the former associations. 2. The process of recalling by association.

associative thinking. 1. *In psychology,* the mental process whereby a subject brings to bear on a thought at hand all relevant present factors. 2. *In psychiatry,* FREE ASSOCIATION.

as·so·nance (as′uh·nunce) *n.* A pathologic tendency to employ alliteration.

as·sort·a·tive mating (a·sor′tuh·tiv). Nonrandom mating based on phenotypic similarity.

asta·sia (a·stay′zhuh, ·zee·uh) *n.* Inability to

stand despite the preservation of strength, coordination, and sensation in the legs. —**static** (a·stat′ick) adj.

astasia-abasia. Inability to walk or stand despite retained strength, coordination, and sensation in the legs; usually a symptom of hysteria, sometimes of bilateral frontal lobe disease.

as·ta·tine (as′tuh-teen, -tin) n. At = 210. Element number 85, prepared in 1940 by bombarding bismuth with alpha particles. It is radioactive and forms no stable isotopes.

aste·a·to·sis (a·stee′′uh-to′sis, as′′tee·) n. A dermatosis in which sebum is deficient in amount or quality, resulting in dryness, scaliness, or fissuring of the skin.

aster-, astero- A combining form meaning *star, star-shaped.*

as·ter (as′tur) n. The radiating structure made up of microtubules, surrounding the centriole of a cell, seen at the beginning of mitosis. —**astral** (·trul) adj.

aster·e·og·no·sis (a·steer′′ee·og·no′sis, ay·sterr′′) n., Inability to recognize the size, shape, or texture of objects, even though the primary senses (tactile, painful, thermal, vibratory) are intact or relatively intact. Syn. *tactile amnesia.*

as·te·rix·is (as′′te·rick′sis) n. A motor disturbance characterized by intermittent lapses of postural tone, producing flapping movements of the outstretched hands; seen with such conditions as hepatic coma, uremia, and respiratory acidosis. Syn. *flapping tremor.* —**asterictic** (·rick′tick) adj.

aster·nia (ay·stur′nee·uh, a·stur′) n. Absence of the sternum.

as·ter·oid (as′tur·oid) adj. Star-shaped.

asteroid body. Any star-shaped structure such as is found in the cytoplasm of giant cells in sarcoidosis or berylliosis or in a number of fungous infections, actinomycosis, and nocardiosis.

asteroid hyalitis. Inflammation of the vitreous body in which calcium soaps form, giving rise to crystalline opacities.

asthen-, astheno- A combining form meaning *weak, weakness.*

as·the·nia (as·theen′ee·uh) n. Absence or loss of strength; weakness; ADYNAMIA.

asthenia pig·men·to·sa (pig·men·to′suh). ADDISON′S DISEASE.

asthenia uni·ver·sa·lis con·gen·i·ta (yoo′′ni·vur·say′lis kon·jen′i·tuh). A psychophysiologic disorder characterized by many gastrointestinal as well as vasomotor disturbances.

as·then·ic (as·thenn′ick) adj. 1. Of or pertaining to asthenia. 2. See *asthenic type.*

asthenic personality. A personality disorder marked by chronic easy fatigability, low energy, lack of enthusiasm, inability to enjoy one′s self, and hypersensitivity to physical and emotional stress.

asthenic type. A physical type marked by a tall, slender, flat-chested, angular form, and poor muscular development.

as·the·no·co·ria (as′′thi·no·ko′ree·uh) n. A sluggish or slow pupillary reaction to light, seen in hypoadrenocorticism.

as·the·no·pia (as′′thi·no′pee·uh) n. Any of the symptoms dependent on fatigue of the ciliary or the extraocular muscles, such as pain around the eyes, headache, photophobia, dimness or blurring of vision, nausea, vertigo, and twitching of the eyelids; eyestrain. —**asthenopic** (·nop′ick) adj.; **as·the·nope** (as′thi·nope) n.

as·the·no·sper·mia (as′′thi·no·spur′mee·uh) n. Weakness or loss of vitality of the spermatozoa.

as·the·nox·ia (as′′thi·nock′see·uh) n. A condition of insufficient oxidation of waste products, as ketosis from insufficient oxidation of fatty acids.

asth·ma (az′muh) n. A disease characterized by an increased responsiveness of the trachea and bronchi to various stimuli (often allergens) and manifested by widespread airway narrowing that changes in severity either spontaneously or as a result of therapy; present as episodic dyspnea, cough, and wheezing.

asthma crystals. CHARCOT-LEYDEN CRYSTALS.

asth·mat·ic (az·mat′ick) adj. & n. 1. Pertaining to, caused by, or affected with asthma. 2. An individual chronically affected with asthma.

asthmatic bronchitis. Asthmatic signs and symptoms associated with apparent bronchial infection.

asthma weed. LOBELIA.

astig·ma·graph (a·stig′muh·graf) n. An instrument for detecting astigmatism.

as·tig·mat·ic (as′′tig·mat′ick) adj. 1. Of, pertaining to, or affected with astigmatism. 2. Pertaining to an apparatus for detecting astigmatism. 3. Pertaining to a means (as lenses) to correct astigmatism.

astigmatic band. In refraction, an apparent band of light seen under retinoscopy when one of the chief meridians is neutralized.

astig·ma·tism (a·stig′muh·tiz·um) n. A congenital or acquired defect of vision which results from irregularity in the curvature of one or more refractive surfaces (cornea, anterior and posterior surfaces of the lens) of the eye. When such a condition occurs, rays emanating from a point are not brought into focus at one point on the retina, but appear to spread as a line in various directions depending upon the curvature. Abbreviated, As.

as·tig·mom·e·ter (as′′tig·mom′e·tur) n. An instrument which measures the degree of astigmatism. —**astigmometry** (·tree) n.

astig·mo·scope (a·stig′muh·skope) n. An instrument for detecting and measuring astigmatism. —**as·tig·mos·copy** (as′′tig·mos′kuh·pee) n.

astom·a·tous (a·stom′uh·tus, ·sto′muh·) adj. 1. Without a mouth or stoma. 2. *In botany,* without stomas.

asto·mia (a·sto′mee·uh) n. Congenital absence of the mouth.

astr-, astro- A combining form meaning (a) *pertaining to the stars;* (b) *resembling a star.*

as·trag·a·lec·to·my (as·trag′′uh·leck′to·mee) n. Excision of the talus.

as·trag·a·lus (as·trag′a·lus) n., pl. **astraga·li** (·lye) TALUS. —**astraga·lar** (·lur) adj.

as·tra·pho·bia (as″truh·fo′bee·uh) n. ASTRAPO-PHOBIA.

as·tra·po·pho·bia (as″truh·po·fo′bee·uh) n. Morbid fear of lightning and thunderstorms.

as·trin·gent (a·strin′junt) adj. & n. 1. Producing contractions; capable of or tending to shrink or pucker tissues or mucous membranes. 2. An agent that produces contraction or shrinkage of organic tissues or that arrests hemorrhages, diarrhea, or other discharges. —**astrin·gen·cy** (·jun·see) n.

as·tro·blast (as′tro·blast) n. A primitive cell that develops into an astrocyte.

as·tro·blas·to·ma (as″tro·blas·to′muh) n. A glioma intermediate in differentiation between glioblastoma multiforme and astrocytoma.

as·tro·cyte (as′tro·site) n. A many-branched stellate neuroglial cell, attached to the blood vessels of the brain and spinal cord by perivascular feet. —**as·tro·cyt·ic** (as″tro·sit′ick) adj.

as·tro·cy·to·ma (as″tro·sigh·to′muh) n., pl. **astro-cytomas, astrocytoma·ta** (·tuh) A benign glial tumor made up of well-differentiated astrocytes.

astrocytoma gi·gan·to·cel·lu·la·re (jye·gan″to·sel″yoo·lair′ee). GLIOBLASTOMA MULTIFORME.

as·tro·cy·to·sis (as″tro·sigh·to′sis) n. An increase both in the number and the size of astrocytes.

as·trog·lia (as·trog′lee·uh) n. Neuroglia composed of astrocytes.

as·trog·li·o·ma (as·trog″lee·o′muh) n. ASTROCY-TOMA.

as·tro·gli·o·sis (as″tro·glye·o′sis) n. 1. ASTROCY-TOSIS. 2. Enlargement and excessive production of astrocytic fibers.

as·troid (as′troid) adj. Star-shaped.

as·tro·pho·bia (as″tro·fo′bee·uh) n. Morbid fear of the stars and celestial space.

as·tro·sphere (as′tro·sfeer) n. The collective radiations of fibrillar cytoplasm which extend from the centrosphere during cell division.

asyl·la·bia (as″i·lay′bee·uh, ay″si·) n. A form of motor aphasia in which individual letters are recognized, but the formation of syllables and words is difficult or impossible.

asy·lum (uh·sigh′lum) n. An institution for the support, safekeeping, cure, or education of those incapable of caring for themselves.

asym·bo·lia (as″im·bo′lee·uh) n. An aphasia in which there is an inability to understand or use acquired symbols, such as speech, writing, or gestures, as means of communication.

asym·met·ric (as″i·met′rick, ay″si·) adj. Pertaining to or exhibiting asymmetry.

asym·met·ri·cal (ay″si·met′rick·al, as″i·) adj. ASYMMETRIC.

asym·me·try (ay·sim′i·tree, a·sim′) n. 1. In anatomy and biology, lack of similarity or correspondence of the organs and parts on each side of an organism. 2. In chemistry, absence of symmetry in the arrangement of the atoms and radicals within a molecule.

asymp·to·mat·ic (ay″simp″tuh·mat′ick, a·simp″to·) adj. Symptomless; exhibiting or producing no symptoms.

asymptomatic neurosyphilis. Syphilitic infection of the central nervous system diagnosed by pathologic findings in the cerebrospinal fluid in an individual with no clinical symptoms or abnormal signs on neurologic examination. The newer serologic tests for syphilis are almost always positive.

as·ymp·tot·ic (as″im·tot′ick) adj. Of or pertaining to a straight line which an indefinitely extended curve continually approaches as a limit, that is, reaches only at infinity.

asymptotic wish fulfilment. 1. A psychological state wherein the patient has found the neurotic expression which would resolve his conflicts or compensate for them, but wherein his ego is strong enough to compel him to postpone indefinitely putting the neurotic solution into effect (Freud). 2. The gratification of a desire in a substitute, "almost-but-not-quite" way.

asyn·ap·sis (ay″si·nap′sis) n. Failure of homologous chromosome pairs to fuse during meiosis.

asyn·chro·nism (ay·sing′kro·niz·um, a·sing′) n. Absence of synchronism; disturbed coordination.

asyn·cli·tism (ay·sing′kli·tiz·um, a·sing′) n. A somewhat lateral tilting of the fetal head at the superior strait of the pelvis.

asyn·de·sis (a·sin·de·sis) n., pl. **asynde·ses** (·seez) 1. SYNTACTIC APHASIA. 2. SYNAPSIS. —**asyn·det·ic** (as″in·det′ick, ay″sin·) adj.

asyn·ech·ia (ay″si·neck′ee·uh, as″i·) n. Absence of continuity in structure.

asyn·er·gy (ay·sin′ur·jee, a·sin′) n. DYSSYNERGIA. —**asy·ner·gic** (ay″si·nur′jick, as″i·) adj.

asy·ne·sia (as″i·nee′zee·uh) n. Stupidity; loss or disorder of mental power. —**asy·net·ic** (·net′ick) adj.

asy·no·dia (as″i·no′dee·uh) n. Nonsimultaneous orgasm in sexual intercourse.

asys·tem·at·ic (ay·sis″te·mat′ick) adj. 1. ASYSTE-MIC. 2. Without a system or orderly arrangement.

asys·tem·ic (ay″sis·tem′ick, as″is·) adj. Diffuse or generalized; not restricted to a specific system or to one organ system.

asys·to·le (ay·sis′to·lee, a·sis′) n. Absence of contraction of the heart, especially of the ventricles. —**asys·tol·ic** (·tol′ick) adj.

A t, Ât In electrocardiography, symbol for the mean manifest direction and magnitude of repolarization of the myocardium determined algebraically and measured in degrees and microvolt seconds.

Atabrine. A trademark for quinacrine.

atac·tic (a·tack′tick) adj. Irregular; incoordinate; ataxic.

atac·ti·form (a·tack′ti·form) adj. Ataxialike; mildly ataxic.

at·a·rac·tic (at″uh·rack′tick) adj. & n. 1. Of or pertaining to ataraxy; tranquilizing. 2. A drug capable of promoting tranquility; a tranquilizer.

at·ar·al·ge·sia (at″ār·al·jee′zee·uh) n. A combination of sedation and analgesia.

Atarax. Trademark for hydroxyzine hydrochloride.

at·a·rax·ic (at″uh·rack′sick) adj. & n. 1. Promoting tranquility, tranquilizing. 2. A drug capable of promoting tranquility; a tranquilizer.

at·a·raxy (at'uh·rack''see) n. A state of complete equanimity, mental homeostasis, or peace of mind.

atav·ic (a·tav'ick, at'uh·vick) adj. Not resembling either parent, but similar to a grandparent or more remote ancestor.

at·a·vism (at'uh·viz·um) n. The reappearance of remote ancestral characteristics in an individual. —**ata·vis·tic** (at''uh·vis'tick) adj.

atax·apha·sia (a·tack''suh·fay'zhuh, ·zee·uh) n. SYNTACTIC APHASIA.

atax·ia (a·tack'see·uh) n. Incoordination of voluntary muscular action, particularly of the muscle groups used in activities such as walking or reaching for objects; due to any interference with the peripheral or central nervous system pathways involved in balancing muscle movements. —**atax·ic** (a·tack'sick) adj.

atax·i·a·graph (a·tack'si·uh·graf) n. A device for recording the degree of ataxia.

ataxi·apha·sia (a·tack''see·uh·fay'zhuh, ·zee·uh) n. SYNTACTIC APHASIA.

ataxia-telangiectasia. An inherited disorder characterized by onset of progressive cerebellar ataxia in infancy or childhood; oculocutaneous telangiectasia; frequently, recurrent infections of the lungs and sinuses; and often, defects in cellular immunity and in the immunoglobulin system; and a propensity for the development of malignant disease. Syn. *Louis-Bar syndrome.*

ataxic amimia. *Obsol.* Inability to make gestures because of loss of muscle power and coordination.

ataxic aphasia. *Obsol.* MOTOR APHASIA.

ataxic gait. A clumsy and uncertain gait in which the legs are far apart, and when taking a step, the leg is lifted abruptly and too high and then is brought down so that the whole sole of the foot strikes the ground at once; seen usually in patients with lesions of the posterior column of the spinal cord, as in tabes dorsalis.

ataxic paraplegia. SUBACUTE COMBINED DEGENERATION OF THE SPINAL CORD.

atax·io·pho·bia (a·tack''see·o·fo'bee·uh) n. A morbid fear of untidiness or disorder.

ataxo·phe·mia (a·tack''so·fee'mee·uh) n. Incoherence; faulty coordination of speech muscles.

ATCC Abbreviation for *American Type Culture Collection.*

atel-, atelo- A combining form meaning *imperfect or incomplete.*

at·e·lec·ta·sis (at''e·leck'tuh·sis) n., pl. **atelecta·ses** (·seez) A state of incomplete expansion of the lungs, because of their failure to expand at birth or the collapse of pulmonary alveoli soon after; collapse of a portion of a lung. —**ate·lec·tat·ic** (·leck·tat'ick) adj.

atelectasis of the newborn. Incomplete expansion of the lungs at birth and for the first few days of life.

atel·ei·o·sis (a·tel''eye·o'sis, at''e·lye·o'sis) n., pl. **ateleio·ses** (·seez) PITUITARY DWARFISM. —**ate·lei·ot·ic** (·ot'ick) adj.

at·el·en·ce·pha·lia (at''el·en·se·fay'lee·uh) n. Imperfect development of the brain.

ate·lia (a·tee'lee·uh) n. 1. Lack of, or deficiency in, development. 2. PITUITARY DWARFISM. —**ate·lic** (·lick) adj.

atel·i·o·sis (a·tel''ee·o'sis, ·eye·o'sis, a·tee''lee·) n., pl. **atelio·ses** (·seez) PITUITARY DWARFISM. —**ateli·ot·ic** (·ot'ick) adj.

at·e·lo·car·dia (at''e·lo·kahr'dee·uh) n. An imperfect or undeveloped state of the heart.

at·e·lo·ceph·a·lous (at''e·lo·sef'uh·lus) adj. Having the skull or head more or less imperfectly developed.

at·e·lo·chei·lia (at''e·lo·kigh'lee·uh) n. Defective development of the lip.

at·e·lo·chei·ria (at''e·lo·kigh'ree·uh) n. Defective development of the hand.

at·e·lo·en·ce·pha·lia (at''e·lo·en''se·fay'lee·uh) n. ATELENCEPHALIA.

at·e·lo·glos·sia (at''e·lo·glos'ee·uh) n. Congenital defect in the tongue.

at·e·lo·gna·thia (at''e·log·nath'ee·uh, ·nayth'ee·uh) n. Imperfect development of a jaw, especially of the lower jaw.

at·e·lo·ki·ne·sia (at''e·lo·kigh·nee'zhuh, ·zee·uh) n. TREMOR.

at·e·lo·my·e·lia (at''e·lo·migh·el'lee·uh) n. Congenital defect of the spinal cord.

at·e·lo·po·dia (at''e·lo·po'dee·uh) n. Defective development of the foot.

at·e·lo·pro·so·pia (at''e·lo·pro·so'pee·uh) n. Incomplete facial development.

at·e·lo·ra·chid·ia, at·e·lor·rha·chid·ia (at''e·lo·ra·kid'ee·uh) n. Imperfect development of the spinal column, as in spina bifida.

at·e·lo·sto·mia (at''e·lo·sto'mee·uh) n. Incomplete development of the mouth.

ate·pho·bia (at''e·fo'bee·uh) n. Morbid fear of catastrophe.

athe·lia (a·theel'ee·uh) n. Absence of the nipples.

athero- A combining form meaning (a) *fatty degeneration;* (b) *atheroma.*

ath·ero·gen·e·sis (ath''ur·o·jen'e·sis) n. The development of atherosclerosis. —**atherogen·ic** (·ick) adj.

ath·er·o·ma (ath''ur·o'muh) n., pl. **atheromas, atheroma·ta** (·tuh) 1. An atherosclerotic plaque in an artery. 2. SEBACEOUS CYST. —**ather·om·a·tous** (·om'uh·tus) adj.

ath·er·o·ma·to·sis (ath''ur·o''muh·to'sis) n., ATHEROSCLEROSIS.

atheromatous abscess. The pultaceous, poorly cellular material of an atherosclerotic plaque. Not a true abscess. Syn. *atherocheuma.*

atheromatous degeneration. A retrogressive change, with the deposition of lipids in the degenerated tissue.

ath·ero·scle·ro·gen·ic (ath''ur·o·sklerr''o·jen·ick) adj. 1. Produced by or due to atherosclerosis. 2. Producing atherosclerosis.

ath·ero·scle·ro·sis (ath''ur·o''skle·ro'sis) n., pl. **atherosclero·ses** (·seez) A variable combination of changes in the intima of arteries (as distinct from arterioles) consisting of the focal accumulation of lipids, complex carbohydrates, blood and blood products, fibrous tissue, and calcium deposits, and associated with medial changes.

ath·ero·scle·rot·ic (ath''ur·o·skle·rot'ick) adj. Of or pertaining to atherosclerosis.

ath·e·toid (ath'e·toid) *adj. & n.* 1. Pertaining to or resembling athetosis; affected with athetosis. 2. An individual with athetosis.

ath·e·to·sis (ath"e·to'sis) *n.*, pl. **athe·to·ses** (·seez) Involuntary movements characterized by recurrent, slow, wormlike, and more or less continual change of position of the fingers, toes, hands, feet, and other parts of the body; usually the result of one or more lesions of the basal ganglia, particularly their central connections and the putamen; seen chiefly in cerebral palsy and kernicterus, as well as after encephalitis, toxic encephalopathies, and cerebrovascular accidents.

athi·a·min·o·sis (ay·thigh"uh·mi·no'sis) *n.* Thiamine deficiency.

ath·lete's foot. TINEA PEDIS.

athlete's heart. Cardiac enlargement, without underlying heart disease, seen in trained athletes.

ath·let·ic type. A physique characterized by good muscular development, leanness, flat abdomen, and broad chest.

athrep·sia (a·threp'see·uh) *n.* 1. MARASMUS. 2. MALNUTRITION. 3. ATHREPTIC IMMUNITY. —**athrep·tic** (·tick) *adj.*

athreptic immunity. Immunity resulting from the failure of an infecting organism to find the necessary conditions for the production of infection.

athy·mic (ay·thigh'mick, a·) *adj.* 1. Lacking the thymus. 2. Without feeling.

athy·re·o·sis (ay·thigh"ree·o'sis, a·) *n.*, pl. **athy·reo·ses** (·seez) Inadequate or absent secretion of thyroid hormone, producing the clinical picture of cretinism in infancy and of myxedema in children and adults.

atlant-, atlanto- A combining form meaning *atlas, atlantal.*

at·lan·tal (at·lan'tul) *adj.* Pertaining to the atlas.

at·lan·to·ax·i·al (at·lan"to·ack'see·ul) *adj.* Pertaining to the atlas and the axis or epistropheus.

at·lan·to·oc·cip·i·tal (at·lan"to·ock·sip'i·tul) *adj.* Pertaining to the atlas and the occipital bone.

at·las (at'lus) *n.* [NA]. The first cervical vertebra, articulating with the occipital bone of the skull and with the axis.

atm Abbreviation for *atmosphere.*

at·mol·y·sis (at·mol'i·sis) *n.*, pl. **atmoly·ses** (·seez) A method of separating mixed gases or vapors by means of diffusion through a porous substance.

at·mom·e·ter (at·mom'e·tur) *n.* An instrument that measures the amount of water evaporated from a given surface in a given time, to determine the humidity of the atmosphere.

at·mo·sphere (at'muh·sfeer) *n.* 1. The gaseous envelope overlying the solid or liquid surface of a planet. 2. Any gaseous medium in relation to objects immersed in it or exposed to it. 3. A standard unit of gas pressure based on the average pressure of the earth's atmosphere at sea level, equal to 1.01325×10^5 newtons/m² (1013.250 mb), which is equivalent to 760 mmHg, 1.0332 kg/cm², or 14.696 lb/in². Abbreviated, atm. —**at·mo·spher·ic** (at"muh·sferr'ick, ·sfeer'ick) *adj.*

ATN Abbreviation for *acute tubular necrosis.*

at·om (at'um) *n.* The smallest particle of an element capable of existing individually or in combination with one or more atoms of the same or another element. It consists of a relatively heavy inner core, or nucleus, with a positive electric charge, and a number of lighter planetary particles, with negative charges, revolving or vibrating continuously around the nucleus in a vast empty space. The positive heavy particles in the nucleus are called protons, and the orbital particles are called electrons. The number of protons or of electrons in an electrically neutral atom is given by its atomic number. In addition to protons, the nucleus also contains neutrons, which are neutral particles resulting from the combination of a proton and an electron. The sum of protons and neutrons in the nucleus is called the mass number of the atom, or its mass or atomic weight. All atoms are constructed of these three fundamental building stones. —**atomic** (uh·tom'ick) *adj.*

atomic energy. Energy released in reactions involving the nucleus of an atom, as by fission of a heavy nucleus or fusion of light nuclei, hence more specifically called nuclear energy.

atomic mass. The mass of an element measured on an arbitrary scale and expressed relatively to mass 12 for carbon.

atomic weight. A number representing the relative weight of an atom of an element compared with the carbon isotope of mass 12 as standard. It is the mean value of the isotopic weights of an element. Abbreviated, at. wt.

at·om·iza·tion (at"um·i·zay'shun) *n.* The mechanical process of breaking up a liquid into a fine spray.

at·om·iz·er (at'uh·migh·zur) *n.* A device for converting a liquid into a fine spray; used in medicine for inhalation therapy. Syn. *vaporizer.*

ato·nia (a·to'nee·uh) *n.* Absence of tonus.

aton·ic (a·ton'ick) *adj.* Characterized by atonia.

atonic bladder. Markedly diminished or absent tonus of the detrusor muscle of the urinary bladder.

ato·nic·i·ty (a·to·nis'i·tee) *n.* 1. Lack of tone. 2. HYPOTONICITY.

atonic ulcer. An indolent or slow-healing ulcer.

at·o·ny (at'uh·nee) *n.* ATONIA.

ato·pen (at'o·pen) *n.* An antigen or allergen of the sort involved in atopic conditions such as seasonal rhinitis and asthma.

atop·ic (ay·top'ick, a·top'ick) *adj.* 1. Pertaining to atopy or to an atopen. 2. ECTOPIC.

atopic dermatitis or **eczema.** An intensely pruritic, frequently chronic, exematous dermatitis that occurs in persons of atopic constitution and characteristically involves the face and antecubital and popliteal fossae.

atop·og·no·sia (a·top"og·no'see·uh, ay·) *n.* Lack of ability to locate a sensation accurately.

at·o·py (at'uh·pee) *n.* A genetically determined disorder in which there is an increased capacity to form reagin antibodies and to acquire certain allergic diseases, especially asthma, hay fever, urticaria, and atopic dermatitis.

atox·ic (ay·tock'sick, a·tock'sick) *adj.* Not venomous; not poisonous.

ATP Abbreviation for *adenosine triphosphate.*

ATPase Abbreviation for *adenosine triphosphatase.*

atre·mia (a·tree'mee·uh) *n.* Hysterical inability to walk, stand, or sit without general discomfort and trembling, all movements being readily and smoothly executed in the recumbent position. Syn. *Neftel's disease.*

atre·sia (a·tree'zhuh, ·zee·uh) *n.* Closure, imperforation, or congenital absence of a normal opening or canal, as of the anus, vagina, auditory meatus, or pupil. *Adj. atresic, atretic.*

atresia ani vag·i·na·lis (ay'nye vaj''i·nay'lis). An anomaly in which there is imperforate anus, the rectum opening into the vagina. Syn. *anus vaginalis.*

atret-, atreto- A combining form meaning *imperforate, imperforation.*

atre·tic (a·tret'ick) *adj.* Pertaining to or characterized by atresia.

atretic follicle. An involuted or degenerated ovarian follicle. Syn. *corpus atreticum.*

atrial beat. A WAVE (2).

atrial septum. INTERATRIAL SEPTUM.

atrial tachycardia. A rapid regular tachycardia with a rate of 140 to 220 per minute, originating from an ectopic focus in the atrium. Episodes may be paroxysmal.

atrich·ia (a·trick'ee·uh) *n.* Any condition, congenital or acquired, in which hair is substantially gone.

atrichosis con·ge·ni·ta·lis (kon·jen·i·tay'lis). Absence or failure of development of hair from birth.

atrioventricular band. ATRIOVENTRICULAR BUNDLE.

atrioventricular block. A cardiac conduction abnormality in which transmission of the excitatory impulse from the cardiac atrium to the ventricle through the AV node is slowed or stopped. Three degrees of severity are recognized: first degree (prolonged atrioventricular conduction), second degree (partial atrioventricular block), and third degree (complete atrioventricular block). Syn. *heart block.*

atrioventricular bundle. A band of specialized conduction tissue of the heart which arises from the atrioventricular node. It divides into two branches which descend on either side of the interventricular septum and ramify among the muscle fibers of the ventricles, transmitting contraction impulses to the ventricles. Syn. *bundle of His.*

atrioventricular heart block. ATRIOVENTRICULAR BLOCK.

atrio·ven·tric·u·la·ris com·mu·nis (ay''tree·o·ven·trick·yoo·lair'is com·yoo'nis). A congenital malformation of the heart in which the atrial and ventricular septa and the endocardial cushions have failed to fuse; there is a single atrioventricular valve ring with deformity of the valve leaflets and large atrial and ventricular septal defects, resulting functionally in a two-chambered heart. Syn. *common atrioven-*

tricular canal, complete endocardial cushion defect.

atrioventricular valves. The mitral and tricuspid valves of the heart.

atri·um (ay'tree·um) *n.*, pl. **atria** (ay'tree·uh), genit. sing. **atrii** (ay'tree·eye) 1. The first chamber on either side of the heart, which receives the blood from the veins. 2. The part below the tympanic cavity of the ear below the head of the malleus. 3. The end of an alveolar duct.

Atromid-S. Trademark for clofibrate.

At·ro·pa (at'ro·puh) *n.* A genus of herbs of the Solanaceae; the source of belladonna and atropine.

atroph·ic (a·trof'ick, a·tro'fick) *adj.* Pertaining to or characterized by atrophy.

atrophic arthritis. RHEUMATOID ARTHRITIS.

atrophic cirrhosis. LAENNEC'S CIRRHOSIS.

atrophic glossitis. HUNTER'S GLOSSITIS.

atrophic pharyngitis. Chronic pharyngitis attended by atrophy of the mucous membrane.

atrophic rhinitis. 1. A disease of uncertain etiology affecting young swine, causing chronic atrophy of the turbinate bones and deformity of the face. 2. OZENA.

atrophic vaginitis. Inflammation of the mucous membrane of the vagina, usually occurring after the menopause.

at·ro·pho·der·ma (at''ruh·fo·dur'muh) *n.* Atrophy of the skin.

at·ro·phy (at'ruh·fee) *n. & v.* 1. An acquired local reduction in the size of a cell, tissue, organ, or region of the body, which may be physiologic or pathologic. 2. To undergo such reduction.

at·ro·pine (at'ro·peen, ·pin) *n. dl-*Hyosciamine or *dl-*tropyl tropate, $C_{17}H_{23}NO_3$, an alkaloid obtained from *Atropa belladonna* and other solanaceous plants. It is a parasympatholytic agent used principally for its spasmolytic effect on smooth muscle and for its action in diminishing secretions.

atropine sulfate. $(C_{17}H_{23}NO_3)_2 \cdot H_2SO_4 \cdot H_2O$. The most frequently used salt of atropine.

at·ro·pin·iza·tion (at''ro·pin·i·zay'shun) *n.* 1. The bringing under the influence of, or treating with, atropine. 2. The administration of belladonna or atropine until physiologic effects become manifest. —**at·ro·pin·ize** (at'ro·pi·nize) *v.*

attached gingiva. The portion of the gingiva firmly attached to the tooth and to the periosteum of the alveolar bone.

at·tach·ment *n.* 1. The place where one organ is fixed to another, such as the origin or the insertion of a muscle in a bone. 2. A component of a partial denture which retains and stabilizes it by frictional retention to a natural tooth or abutment. 3. Development of an interpersonal bond or commitment, as of a mother to her child.

at·tar (at'ur) *n.* Any of the fragrant volatile oils.

at·tend·ing nurse. 1. PUBLIC HEALTH NURSE. 2. A nurse responsible for the care of a patient or a group of patients for a given period of time or for specific activities.

attention hypothesis. *In psychology,* the hypothesis that attention tends to be selectively, automatically, and irresistibly drawn toward the area of greatest personal interest or concern and that therefore a person is selectively attracted to those whose character makeup most fits his own inner needs, whether healthy or neurotic.

attention span. 1. The period of time an individual can actively attend to or concentrate upon one thing; used particularly with respect to learning processes, active play, and work. 2. *In psychology,* the number of objects or impressions that can be reported after a brief period of observation, usually 0.1 second.

at·ten·u·at·ed virus. A virus whose disease-producing ability has been lessened by heat, chemicals, and other means.

at·ten·u·a·tion (a·ten″yoo·ay′shun) *n.* 1. A thinning, weakening, or diluting; especially a reduction of the virulence of a virus or pathogenic microorganism, as by successive culture, repeated inoculation, or exposure to light, heat, air, or a weakening agent. 2. *In radiology,* the process by which a beam of radiation is reduced in energy when passing through some material. **—at·ten·u·ate** (a·ten′yoo·ate) *v.*

at·tic (at′ick) *n.* Part of the tympanic cavity situated above the atrium of the ear. It contains the incus and the head of the malleus. Syn. *epitympanum.*

attic disease. Chronic suppurative inflammation of the attic of the tympanic cavity; often resulting from cholesteatoma.

at·tic·i·tis (at″ick·eye′tis) *n.* Inflammation of the lining membrane of the attic of the middle ear.

at·ti·co·an·trot·o·my (at″i·ko·an·trot′uh·mee) *n.* Surgical opening of the attic and mastoid air cells.

at·ti·co·mas·toid (at″i·ko·mas′toid) *adj.* Pertaining to the attic and the mastoid.

at·ti·cot·o·my (at″i·kot′uh·mee) *n.* Surgical opening of the attic of the tympanum.

at·ti·tude (at′i·tewd) *n.* 1. Posture; the position of the body and limbs. 2. A consistent predisposition, or readiness, which is acquired and generally characterized by its affective aspects, to respond to an object, idea, or person in a certain way.

at·ton·i·ty (a·ton′i·tee) *n.* A state of stupor with complete or partial immobility; occurs most frequently in the catatonic type of schizophrenia, but also in severe depressive illnesses.

at·tri·tion (a·trish′un) *n.* 1. An abrasion, rubbing, or chafing of the skin or any surface. 2. A functional wearing away by the forces of usage; as of tooth structure by mastication.

at. wt. Abbreviation for *atomic weight.*

atyp·ia (ay·tip′ee·uh) *n. In exfoliative cytology,* cellular variations from normal which fall short of anaplasia.

atyp·i·cal (ay·tip′i·kul) *adj.* Not typical; irregular.

atypical facial neuralgia. Persistent severe pain in the face, head, and neck for which no cause can be found; usually observed in young women and unresponsive to analgesic medications.

atypical lymphocyte. Any lymphocyte differing from the normal but not anaplastic; often

applied to cells seen in infectious mononucleosis and in other viral infections.

atypical pneumonia. PRIMARY ATYPICAL PNEUMONIA.

atypical verrucous endocarditis. LIBMAN-SACHS ENDOCARDITIS.

Au Symbol for gold.

A.U., Å.U. An abbreviation for *angstrom unit* (= ANGSTROM), sometimes written A.u., Å.u., a.u., å.u.

au·di·mut·ism (aw″dee·mew′tiz·um) *n.* Muteness not associated with deafness.

au·dio (aw′dee·o) *adj.* Pertaining to sound or to hearing.

audio- A combining form meaning (a) *auditory, hearing;* (b) *sound.*

audio frequency. Any one of the frequencies that fall within the normal range of human hearing.

au·dio·gen·ic (aw″dee·o·jen′ick) *adj.* Caused or induced by sound.

audiogenic epilepsy, seizure, or **convulsion.** A form of reflex epilepsy induced by sound, usually a loud, sudden noise. Syn. *acousticomotor epilepsy.*

au·dio·gram (aw′dee·o·gram) *n.* A graphic record showing the variations of auditory acuity of an individual over the normal frequency range, as indicated by an audiometer.

au·di·ol·o·gy (aw″dee·ol′uh·jee) *n.* The science of hearing.

au·di·om·e·ter (aw″dee·om′e·tur) *n.* An instrument, such as a pure tone audiometer or a speech or phonograph audiometer, for measuring hearing acuity. **—au·dio·met·ric** (aw″dee·o·met′rick) *adj.*

au·di·om·e·trist (aw″dee·om′e·trist) *n.* A person skilled in the use of an audiometer.

au·di·om·e·try (aw″dee·om′e·tree) *n.* The quantitative and qualitative evaluation of a person's hearing by the use of an audiometer.

audio-ocular reflex. Movement of the eyes toward the source of a sudden sound.

au·dio·vis·u·al (aw″dee·o·vizh′yoo·ul) *adj.* Of, pertaining to, or using both sound and sight, especially in teaching and learning methods.

au·di·tion (aw·dish′un) *n.* 1. The process of hearing. 2. The sense of hearing.

au·di·tive (aw′di·tiv) *adj.* AUDITORY.

au·di·tog·no·sis (aw″di·tog·no′sis) *n.,* pl. **auditogno·ses** (·seez) 1. The ability to perceive and interpret sounds. 2. In physical diagnosis, the use of percussion and auscultation.

au·di·to·psy·chic (aw″di·to·sigh′kick) *adj.* Pertaining to the auditory association area.

au·di·to·ry (aw′di·tor″ee) *adj.* Pertaining to the act or the organs of hearing.

auditory acuity test. The determination of the threshold of a person's hearing by the use of various instruments and techniques, such as an audiometer, recorded word list, or tuning forks.

auditory agnosia. Failure to recognize sounds in general in the absence of deafness.

auditory aphasia. A form of sensory or receptive impairment of language capacity with lack of comprehension of the spoken word in the absence of deafness.

auditory association area. The cortical association area just inferior to the auditory projection area, related to it anatomically and functionally by association fibers; Brodmann's area 42.

auditory aura. An acoustic sensation that sometimes ushers in an epileptic seizure, in particular any seizure originating in the temporal lobe.

auditory center. The auditory projection area and auditory association area together.

auditory meatus. Acoustic meatus. See *external acoustic meatus, internal acoustic meatus.*

auditory memory span. The number of unrelated speech sounds (syllables, numerals, words) a person is able to recall and to repeat in order after having heard them once at the rate of one per second.

auditory nerve. VESTIBULOCOCHLEAR NERVE.

auditory-palpebral reflex. Reflex closing of the eyes in response to a sudden loud noise; may be demonstrated on one side. Syn. *auropalpebral reflex, acousticopalpebral reflex.*

auditory percussion. AUSCULTATORY PERCUSSION.

auditory pit. The embryonic invagination of the auditory placode that later becomes the otocyst or auditory vesicle. Syn. *otic pit.*

auditory projection area. The cortical receptive center for auditory impulses, located in the transverse temporal gyri. Syn. *Brodmann's area 41, auditosensory area, auditory cortex.*

auditory radiation. ACOUSTIC RADIATION.

auditory receptive aphasia. AUDITORY APHASIA.

auditory receptive center. AUDITORY PROJECTION AREA.

auditory reflex. 1. Any reflex that involves an auditory mechanism. 2. Specifically, AUDITORY-PALPEBRAL REFLEX.

auditory threshold. The minimum perceptible sound, usually measured in decibels.

auditory tube. The canal, lined by mucous membrane, with partly bony, partly cartilaginous support, connecting the pharynx with the tympanic cavity on each side. Syn. *eustachian tube, pharyngotympanic tube.*

auditory verbal agnosia. Failure to recognize ordinary words in a spoken language with which the patient is familiar; the patient's reaction is like that of an individual listening to a foreign language with which he is very slightly familiar.

auditory vesicle. The vesicular anlage of the inner ear. Syn. *otocyst, otic vesicle.*

Au·er·bach's ganglia (ɒw′ur-bahᵏh) Nerve cell bodies in the myenteric plexus.

Auerbach's plexus MYENTERIC PLEXUS.

Auer bodies Large granules, globules, or slender rods of azurophilic substance, which are peroxidase-positive and give positive reactions for protein, found in the cytoplasm of myeloblasts, myelocytes, occasionally in older granulocytes, monoblasts, monocytes, and histiocytes in acute leukemia.

aug·men·ta·tion mammoplasty. A plastic surgical procedure in which the size and shape of the breasts are altered by implantation of autologous or artificial materials.

aug·men·tor (awg-men′tur) n. An agent that increases or accelerates the action of auxetics, though it is unable to initiate cell division when used alone.

aug·na·thus (awg-nayth′us) n. A rare anomaly in which a second lower jaw is parasitic on that of the host.

au·lo·pho·bia (aw″lo·fo′bee-uh) n. A morbid fear of flutes.

aur-, auri-, auro- A combining form meaning *the ear.*

au·ra (aw′ruh) n., pl. **auras, au·rae** (·ree) A premonitory sensation or warning experienced at the beginning of a seizure, which the patient remembers and which indicates the location of the discharging focus.

aura asth·mat·i·ca (az·mat′i·kuh). A sensation of tightness in the chest, or other subjective phenomena which forewarns the patient of an asthmatic attack.

aura hys·ter·i·ca (his·terr′i·kuh). Any warning sensation which supposedly occasionally introduces a hysterical attack.

au·ral (aw′rul) adj. Pertaining to the ear; AUDITORY.

aural calculus. Inspissated and sometimes calcified cerumen in the external acoustic meatus.

aural forceps. A dressing forceps used in aural surgery.

aural reflex. Any reflex that involves an auditory mechanism.

aural speculum. A small, hollow instrument with an expanded end inserted in the ear for examination of the external auditory meatus and the tympanic membrane.

aural syringe. A syringe for flushing out excessive cerumen from the external auditory meatus.

aur·an·ti·a·sis (aw″ran·tye′uh·sis) n. CAROTENOSIS.

aurantiasis cu·tis (kew′tis). Any condition in which the skin appears golden in color, usually caused by excessive ingestion of carotene.

Aureomycin. Trademark for chlortetracycline.

auri- A combining form designating (a) *gold;* (b) in chemistry, *the presence of gold in the trivalent or auric state.*

au·ric (aw′rick) adj. 1. Pertaining to or containing gold. 2. *In chemistry,* pertaining to compounds of trivalent gold.

au·ri·cle (aw′ri·kul) n. 1. The pinna of the ear; the projecting part of the external ear. 2. An appendage to an atrium of the heart; auricular appendage. 3. Any ear-shaped structure or appendage. 4. ATRIUM.

au·ri·cu·la (aw·rick′yoo·luh) n., pl. **auricu·lae** (·lee). AURICLE.

au·ric·u·lar (aw·rick′yoo·lur) adj. 1. Pertaining to or shaped like an auricle. 2. ATRIAL. 3. An auricular muscle.

auricular appendage or appendix. AURICLE (2).

au·ri·cu·la·ris (aw·rick″yoo·lair′is) n., pl. **auricula·res** (·reez) An auricular muscle.

au·ric·u·lo·pal·pe·bral (aw·rick″yoo·lo·pal′pe·brul, ·pal·pee′brul) adj. Pertaining to the auricle (1) and the eyelids.

auriculopalpebral reflex. Closure of the eyelids

in response to noxious stimuli applied to the top part of the auditory meatus.

au·ric·u·lo·tem·po·ral (aw·rick″yoo·lo·tem′puh·rul) *adj.* Pertaining to the auricle (1) and to the temporal region.

auriculotemporal syndrome. Local redness and sweating of the cheek with pain anterior to the tragus, produced during mastication of food or tasting; following a suppuration and fistulation of the parotid gland. Syn. *Frey's syndrome.*

au·ris (aw′ris) *n.*, pl. **au·res** (·reez), genit. pl. **au·ri·um** (aw′ree·um) [NA]. EAR.

auris ex·ter·na (ecks·tur′nuh) [NA]. EXTERNAL EAR.

auris in·ter·na (in·tur′nuh) [NA]. INTERNAL EAR.

auris me·di·a (mee′dee·uh) [NA]. MIDDLE EAR.

auris si·nis·tra (si·nis′truh). The left ear. Abbreviated, *al.*

auro- A combining form designating (a) *gold;* (b) in chemistry, *the presence of gold in the univalent or aurous state.*

au·ro·ra·pho·bi·a (aw·ro″ruh·fo′bee·uh) *n.* A morbid fear of northern lights.

au·ro·ther·a·py (aw″ro·therr′uh·pee) *n.* The administration of gold salts in the treatment of disease.

au·ro·thio·glu·cose (aw″ro·thigh″o·gloo′koce) *n.* A compound of gold with thioglucose, $C_6H_{11}AuO_5S$, used for the treatment of rheumatoid arthritis; administered in oil suspension.

au·rous (aw′rus) *adj.* 1. Pertaining to gold and its compounds. 2. *In chemistry,* pertaining to compounds of univalent gold.

au·rum (aw′rum) *n.* GOLD.

aus·cul·ta·tion (aws″kul·tay′shun) *n.* The perception and interpretation of sounds arising from various organs, especially the heart, lungs, and pleura, to aid in the determination of their physical condition. —**aus·cul·ta·to·ry** (aws·kul′tuh·to·ree) *adj.;* **aus·cult** (aws·kult′), **aus·cul·tate** (aws′kul·tate) *v.;* **aus·cult·able** (aws·kult′uh·bul) *adj.*

auscultatory percussion. Auscultation of the sounds produced by percussion. Syn. *auditory percussion.*

Aus·tra·lian antigen. HEPATITIS-ASSOCIATED ANTIGEN.

aut-, auto- A combining form meaning *self, one's own, spontaneous, independent.*

au·ta·coid (aw′tuh·koid) *n.* Any member of a group of substances of diverse chemical structure that occur normally in the body and have a wide range of intense pharmacological activities, such as serotonin, histamine, bradykinin, and angiotensin.

au·te·me·sia (aw·te·mee′shuh, ·see·uh) *n.* 1. Idiopathic vomiting. 2. Vomiting at will by certain psychiatric patients.

au·tism (aw′tiz·um) *n.* 1. A tendency in one's thinking where all material, including objective reality, is given meaning unduly influenced by personal desires or needs; an interest in daydreaming and fantasy. 2. A form of behavior and thinking observed in young children, in which the child seems to concentrate upon himself or herself without regard for reality; often appears as excessive shyness,

fearfulness, or aloofness and later as withdrawal and introspection. Intellect is not impaired. It may be an early manifestation or part of the childhood type of schizophrenia.

au·tis·tic (aw·tis′tick) *adj.* 1. Pertaining to or characterized by autism. 2. Descriptive of behavior, particularly seen in the autistic child, in which there is little or no attempt at verbal communication, disregard for other people and animate objects, excessive playing with one's body such as spinning about, and often a preoccupation with bright or pointed inanimate objects; sometimes also seen in children who are emotionally deprived, perceptually handicapped, or mentally retarded, or who lack sensory stimulation.

autistic child. A child who does not relate to his environment, especially not to people, and whose overall functioning is immature and often appears retarded.

autistic gesture. A muscular automatism involving more muscles than a tic.

autistic thinking. AUTISM.

auto-. See *aut-.*

au·to·ag·glu·ti·na·tion (aw″to·uh·gloo″ti·nay′shun) *n.* 1. Agglutination which occurs without the addition of a specific antiserum. 2. Agglutination of the blood cells of an individual by his own serum.

au·to·ag·glu·ti·nin (aw″to·uh·gloo′ti·nin) *n.* An agglutinin contained in the serum of an individual which causes an agglutination of his own cells.

au·to·al·ler·gi·za·tion (aw″to·al″ur·ji·zay′shun) *n.* AUTOSENSITIZATION.

au·to·am·pu·ta·tion (aw″to·am″pew·tay′shun) *n.* Spontaneous amputation, as of a diseased organ, growth, or appendage.

au·to·anal·y·sis (aw″to·uh·nal′i·sis) *n.,* pl. **auto·analy·ses** (·seez). Analysis of one's own mental disorder; employed as a psychotherapeutic method.

Autoanalyzer. Trademark for an instrument in which chemical and other analyses are done automatically as the fluid-borne unknown substance is mixed with reagents in a continuously-flowing stream which passes through appropriate environmental and analytical modules.

au·to·an·ti·body (aw″to·an′ti·bod″ee) *n.* 1. An antibody produced by an organism to its own tissues. 2. *In hematology,* an antibody contained in the serum of an individual that causes agglutination or lysis of his erythrocytes.

au·to·au·di·ble (aw″to·aw′di·bul) *adj.* Audible to one's self; applied to heart sounds or cephalic bruits.

au·to·ca·tal·y·sis (aw″to·ka·tal′i·sis) *n.,* pl. **auto·cataly·ses** (·seez) The process by which a chemical reaction is accelerated by one or more products of the reaction acting as catalysts. —**auto·cat·a·lyst** (·kat′uh·list) *n.;* **auto·cat·a·lyt·ic** (·kat″uh·lit′ick) *adj.*

au·to·ca·thar·sis (aw″to·ka·thahr′sis) *n.* Psychotherapy by encouraging the patient to write out or paint his experiences or impressions and thus rid himself of his mental complexes.

au·to·cho·le·cys·to·du·o·de·nos·to·my (aw"to-ko"le·sis"to·dew"o·de·nos'tuh·mee) n. The spontaneous formation of an opening between the gallbladder and duodenum, secondary to adhesions between the two organs; the opening may permit passage of gallstones into the duodenum.

au·to·cho·le·cys·to·trans·verse·co·los·to·my (aw"to·ko"le·sis"to·trans·vurs"ko·los'tuh·mee) n. The spontaneous formation of an opening between the gallbladder and the transverse colon, secondary to adhesions between the two organs; the opening may permit passage of gallstones into the transverse colon.

au·toch·tho·nous (aw·tock'thuh·nus) adj. 1. Formed or originating in the place where found, as a clot. 2. Native; aboriginal.

autochthonous idea. An idea originating in the unconscious, which to the patient seems literally to have come from the outside.

au·to·clave (aw'to·klave) n. & v. 1. An apparatus for sterilizing objects by steam under pressure. 2. To sterilize in an autoclave.

au·to·cy·to·tox·in (aw"to·sigh"to·tock'sin) n. A cell toxin produced against the cells of one's own body.

au·to·di·ges·tion (aw"to·di·jes'chun) n. Digestion of the stomach walls by gastric juice, as in disease of the stomach or after death.

au·to·echo·la·lia (aw"to·eck"o·lay'lee·uh) n. Stereotypy in which the patient continually repeats some word or phrase of his own and perseverates on words said meaningfully; seen in neuropathologic states such as Pick's disease.

au·to·echo·prax·ia (aw"to·eck"o·prack'see·uh) n. Stereotypy in which the patient continually repeats some action he has previously experienced; a form of perseveration.

au·to·erot·i·cism (aw"to·e·rot'i·siz·um) n. AUTO-EROTISM.

au·to·er·o·tism (aw"to·err'o·tiz·um) n. Self-gratification from sexual instinct, including satisfaction from masturbation and from the individual's own oral, anal, and visual sources and fantasies. —**auto·erot·ic** (·e·rot'ick) adj.

au·to·fel·la·tio (aw"to·fe·lay'shee·o) n. Fellatio practiced upon oneself.

au·tog·e·nous (aw·toj'e·nus) adj. 1. Self-generated. 2. Arising within the organism; applied to toxins, pathologic states, or vaccines.

autogenous graft. AUTOGRAFT.

autogenous vaccine. A vaccine made from a culture of microorganisms obtained from the patient himself.

au·to·graft (aw'to·graft) n. Any tissue removed from one part of an individual's body and applied to another part.

au·tog·ra·phism (aw·tog'ruh·fiz·um) n. DERMO-GRAPHIA.

au·to·hyp·no·sis (aw"to·hip·no'sis) n. Self-induced hypnosis. —**autohyp·not·ic** (·not'ick) adj.

au·to·hyp·no·tism (aw"to·hip'nuh·tiz·um) n. The practice of autohypnosis.

au·to·im·mu·ni·ty (aw"to·i·mew'ni·tee) n. A condition in which an immune response is directed against a constituent of an organism's own body. —**auto·im·mune** (·i·mewn') adj.

au·to·im·mu·ni·za·tion (aw"to·im"yoo·ni·zay'shun) n. The production or development of an autoimmunity.

au·to·in·fec·tion (aw"to·in·feck'shun) n. Infection by an organism existing within the body or transferred from one part of the body to another.

au·to·in·oc·u·la·tion (aw"to·i·nock"yoo·lay'shun) n. Inoculation in one part of the body by an organism present in another part; self-inoculation.

au·to·in·tox·i·ca·tion (aw"to·in·tock"si·kay'shun) n. Poisoning by metabolic products elaborated within the body; generally, toxemia of pathologic states.

au·to·ki·ne·sis (aw"to·ki·nee'sis) n. Voluntary movement. —**autoki·net·ic** (·net'ick) adj.

autokinetic perception or **phenomenon.** The illusion of movement of an object in space, usually vague and perceived differently by different observers; may be due to displacement of the eyes or head or to successive stimulation of adjacent retinal points by momentary stationary lights.

au·tol·o·gous (aw·tol'uh·gus) adj. Derived from, or from a part of, the same organism; autogenous.

au·tol·y·sate (aw·tol'i·sate) n. That which results from or is produced by autolysis.

au·tol·y·sis (aw·tol'i·sis) n. 1. Self-digestion of tissues within the living body. 2. The chemical splitting-up of the tissue of an organ by the action of an enzyme peculiar to it. 3. The hemolytic action of the blood serum or plasma of an animal upon its own cells. —**auto·lyt·ic** (aw"to·lit'ick) adj.; **auto·lyze** (aw'to·lize) v.

automat-, automato- A combining form meaning automatic, spontaneous, initiatory.

au·to·mat·ic (aw"to·mat'ick) adj. 1. Performed without the influence of the will; spontaneous. 2. Self-regulatory, self-propelled.

automatic writing. 1. In psychology, a dissociative phenomenon in which an individual writes material while his attention is distracted and consciously unaware of what he writes; used occasionally for experimental purposes, for testing the relative disassociative capacity of a patient, and as a means of access to unconscious data. 2. The writing that follows the suggestions made to a patient while he is in a hypnotic trance.

au·tom·a·tism (aw·tom'uh·tiz·um) n. 1. Performance of normally voluntary acts without apparent volition, as in somnambulism and in hysterical and epileptic states. 2. In biology, independent activity of cells and tissues, as the beating of a heart freed from its nervous connections.

au·tom·a·ton (aw·tom'uh·ton) n., pl. **automatons, automa·ta** (·tuh) 1. A person who acts in an involuntary or mechanical manner. 2. A robot or mechanism designed to follow programmed instructions.

au·to·ne·phrec·to·my (aw"to·ne·freck'tuh·mee) n. The complete or nearly complete loss of renal parenchyma and function secondary to complete ureteral obstruction or to an inflammatory disease such as tuberculosis.

au·to·nom·ic (aw″tuh·nom′ick) *adj.* Normally independent of volition; specifically, pertaining to the involuntary or autonomic nervous system.

autonomic center. Any center of the brain or spinal cord regulating visceral functions by way of the parasympathetic and thoracolumbar outflows.

autonomic epilepsy. CONVULSIVE EQUIVALENT.

autonomic imbalance. Absence of normal equilibrium between actions of the sympathetic and parasympathetic nervous systems.

autonomic nerve. A nerve of the autonomic nervous system.

autonomic nervous system. An aggregation of ganglions, nerves, and plexuses through which the viscera, heart, blood vessels, smooth muscles, and glands receive their motor innervation. It is divided into the craniosacral or parasympathetic system, and the thoracicolumbar or sympathetic system.

au·ton·o·mous (aw·ton′uh·mus) *adj.* Independent in origin, action, or function; self-governing.

autonomous bladder. A paralytic condition of the urinary bladder characterized by loss of voluntary and reflex micturition, seen in patients with destructive lesions of the lumbosacral spinal cord or of both sensory and motor roots of the sacral plexus.

au·to·pha·gia (aw″to·fay′jee·uh) *n.* 1. Self-consumption; emaciation. 2. The biting or eating of one's own flesh.

au·to·phil·ia (aw″to·fil′ee·uh) *n.* NARCISSISM.

au·to·pho·bia (aw″to·fo′bee·uh) *n.* A pathologic dread of one's self or of being alone.

au·to·phono·ma·nia (aw″to·fon″o·may′nee·uh, ·fo″no·) *n.* Suicidal mania.

au·toph·o·ny (aw·tof′o·nee) *n.* A condition in some middle ear and auditory tube diseases in which an individual's voice seems more resonant to himself.

au·to·plas·tic (aw″to·plas′tick) *adj.* 1. Of or pertaining to autoplasty or to an autograft. 2. *In psychiatry,* pertaining to the indirect internal modification and adaptation of impulses prior to their outward expression, as found in neuroses.

au·to·pro·throm·bin (aw″to·pro·throm′bin) *n.* Any one of a group of substances that may result from the conversion of prothrombin to thrombin under specific circumstances. Several autoprothrombins have been described, and some have clot-promoting activity. The exact relationship of the autoprothrombins to the clotting factors demonstrated by other methods is not clear.

au·top·sy (aw′top·see) *n.* A medical examination of the body after death to confirm or correct the clinical diagnosis, to ascertain the cause of death, to improve understanding of disease processes and aid medical teaching. Syn. *necropsy, postmortem.*

au·to·psy·cho·sis (aw″to·sigh·ko′sis) *n.* A mental derangement in which the patient's ideas about himself are distorted.

au·to·ra·dio·gram (aw″to·ray′dee·o·gram) *n.* RADIOAUTOGRAPH.

au·to·ra·di·og·ra·phy (aw″to·ray″dee·og′ruh·fee) *n.* RADIOAUTOGRAPHY.

au·to·reg·u·la·tion (aw″to·reg·yoo·lay′shun) *n.* The process of adjustments whereby a physiologic system, usually an organ or a vascular bed, is able to maintain its own normal state by varying some factor such as blood flow or nutrient concentration to match its needs in the face of internal or external changes and stresses.

au·to·sen·si·ti·za·tion (aw″to·sen″si·ti·zay′shun) *n.* Sensitization to a constituent of an organism's own body.

autosensitization dermatitis. An inflammatory condition of the skin, usually eczematous in form, and thought to be caused by products of an already damaged epidermis after sensitization to those products.

au·to·sex·ing (aw″to·seck′sing) *n.* The determination of sex in animals by such genetic traits as feather color and other characteristics at birth or hatching.

au·to·site (aw′to·site) *n.* That member of an unequal twin monster which is capable of independent existence, and which nourishes the other twin (the parasite). The latter may be a complete fetus or accessory body parts attached to the autosite or to the placenta. —**au·to·sit·ic** (aw″to·sit′ick) *adj.*

au·to·some (aw′to·sohm) *n.* A non-sex-determining chromosome; any chromosome other than the X and Y chromosomes. —**auto·so·mal** (aw″to·so′mul) *adj.*

au·to·sple·nec·to·my (aw″to·sple·neck′tuh·mee) *n.* Destruction of most or all of the splenic tissue by a disease process, usually sickle cell anemia.

au·to·sug·gest·ibil·i·ty (aw″to·sug·jes″ti·bil′i·tee) *n.* Susceptibility to autosuggestion.

au·to·sug·ges·tion (aw″to·sug·jes′chun) *n.* 1. The acceptance of a thought or idea, predominantly from within one's own mind, which induces some mental or physical action or change. 2. The persistence in consciousness of impressions gained while in a hypnotic state. Syn. *self-suggestion.*

au·to·syn·noia (aw″to·si·noy′uh) *n.* A state of introversion in which the subject is so concentrated in his thoughts or hallucinations that he loses all interest in the outside world.

au·to·tech·ni·con (aw″to·teck′ni·kon) *n.* An electrically timed machine for the automatic fixation, dehydration, and impregnation of tissue specimens, and for staining sections.

au·tot·o·my (aw·tot′uh·mee) *n.* 1. A mechanism by means of which many organisms are able to cast off parts of their body. 2. Self-division; FISSION (2). 3. A surgical operation performed on one's own body.

au·to·top·ag·no·sia (aw″to·top·ag·no′zhuh, ·zee·uh) *n.* Loss of ability to identify or orient parts of one's own body; a defect in appreciation or awareness of the body scheme, seen in lesions involving the angular gyrus or thalamoparietal pathways. Syn. *somatotopagnosia.*

au·to·trans·form·er (aw″to·trans·for′mur) *n.* A

step-down transformer used extensively in varying the voltage to the primary windings of a high-voltage x-ray transformer.

au·to·trans·plan·ta·tion (aw″to·trans″plan·tay′shun) *n.* The operation of transplanting to a part of the body tissue taken from another area in the same body. **—au·to·trans·plant** (·trans′plant) *n.*

au·to·troph (aw′to·trof, ·trofe) *n.* A bacterium able to grow in an inorganic environment by using carbon dioxide as its sole source of carbon for anabolic metabolism. **—au·to·tro·phic** (aw″to·tro′fick, ·trof′ick) *adj.*

au·to·vac·ci·na·tion (aw″to·vack″si·nay′shun) *n.* Revaccination of an individual, using vaccine obtained from his own body.

au·to·vac·cine (aw″to·vack′seen) *n.* AUTOGENOUS VACCINE.

aux-, auxo- A combining form meaning (a) *growth;* (b) *increase;* (c) in biochemistry, *accelerating or stimulating.*

auxano- A combining form meaning *growth.*

-auxe A combining form meaning *hypertrophy, enlargement.*

aux·e·sis (awk·see′sis) *n.,* pl. **auxe·ses** (·seez) 1. An increase in size or bulk; growth. 2. Growth in size by cell expansion without cell division; hypertrophy.

aux·et·ic (awk·set′ick) *adj. & n.* 1. Of or pertaining to auxesis. 2 Stimulating growth. 3. A hypothetical substance that excites cell reproduction; an agent that causes proliferation of human cells, especially leukocytes.

aux·il·i·a·ry (awg·zil″ee·ur·ee) *n.* ADMINICULUM.

aux·in (awk′sin) *n.* Indoleacetic acid, a plant growth hormone formed from tryptophan.

auxo-. See *aux-.*

auxo·bar·ic (awk″so·băr′ick) *adj.* Denoting increased pressure, especially relating to a rise in pressure in the cardiac ventricles during the isovolumetric and early ejection phases.

auxo·chrome (awk′so·krome) *n.* 1. That which increases color. 2. A chemical group which, added to a chromophore group, will produce a dye. 3. Increase or development of color. **—auxo·chro·mous** (awk″so·kro′mus) *adj.*

auxo·cyte (awk′so·site) *n.* A spermatocyte, oocyte, or sporocyte during its early growth period.

auxo·drome (awk′so·drome) *n.* A standard schedule of development.

aux·om·e·ter (awk·som′e·tur) *n.* A device for measuring the magnifying power of lenses.

auxo·ton·ic (awk″so·ton′ick) *adj.* Contracting against increasing tension or resistance.

Av. Abbreviation for *avoirdupois.*

aval·vu·lar (ay·val′vew·lur, a·val′) *adj.* Lacking any structure for temporarily closing a passage or an opening.

avas·cu·lar·ize (ay·vas′kew·lur·ize, a·vas′) *v.* To render a part bloodless, as by compression or bandaging. **—avas·cu·lar·iza·tion** (ay·vas″kew·lur·i·zay′shun) *n.*

avascular necrosis. Necrosis due to inadequate blood flow.

AV block. ATRIOVENTRICULAR BLOCK.

av·er·age, *n. & adj.* 1. The figure arrived at by adding together several quantities and dividing by the number of quantities; arithmetic mean. 2. Usual, typical; median.

average dose. A dose which may be expected ordinarily to produce the therapeutic effect for which the ingredient or preparation is most commonly employed.

average life. Mean radioactive life; the average of the individual lives of all the atoms of a radioactive substance (1.443 times the radioactive half-life).

aver·sion therapy (a·vur′zhun). *In psychiatry,* any form of treatment that involves applying some painful experience or punishment to a well-established behavior, inducing a motivational conflict between the desire for acting in a certain way and the fear of the unpleasant consequences; applied particularly to the treatment of alcoholism or sexual deviation; a form of conditioning.

Avertin. Trademark for tribromoethanol.

avi·an (ay′vee·un) *adj.* Of, pertaining to, or caused by birds.

avian malaria. Malaria of birds and poultry due to numerous species of the genus *Plasmodium.*

avian pox. A disease of birds caused by poxviruses of the fowl, turkey, pigeon, and canary subgroups, characterized by inflammation and hyperplasia of the epidermis followed by scab formation and desquamation, and diphtheritic membranes in the upper respiratory and digestive tracts.

avian pseudoplague. NEWCASTLE DISEASE.

avian tuberculosis. A form of tuberculosis affecting fowl, caused by *Mycobacterium tuberculosis* var. *avium,* characterized by tubercles composed primarily of epithelioid cells. Various mammals including, rarely, humans may be infected.

av·i·din (av′i·din) *n.* A biotin-inactivating protein in raw egg white.

avid·i·ty (a·vid′i·tee) *n.* 1. *In immunology,* the rate of neutralization of antigen, such as toxin, by antibody. 2. The firmness of union of antibody to antigen.

avir·u·lent (ay·virr′yoo·lunt, a·virr′) *adj.* Without virulence.

avi·ta·min·osis (ay·vye″tuh·mi·no′sis, a·vye″, ay″vi·tam″i·no′sis) *n.,* pl. **avitamin·oses** (·no′seez) Any disease resulting from deficiency of a vitamin.

Avo·ga·dro's number (ah″vo·gah′dro) The number of molecules of a substance in one gram-molecular weight; it is 6.06×10^{23}.

avoid·ance *n. In psychiatry,* a conscious or unconscious defense mechanism through which the individual seeks to escape anxiety, conflict, danger, fear, and pain. Efforts at avoidance may be physical as well as psychologic.

av·oir·du·pois (av″ur·duh·poiz′) *n.* The English system of weights and measures. Abbreviated, Av.

Avosyl. A trademark for mephenesin.

A-V patterns or **syndromes.** Significant alterations in the degree of either exotropia or esotropia when the patient looks up or down. An A pattern shows more divergence in down gaze or more convergence in up gaze; in the V pattern, the reverse holds, with more divergence in up gaze rather than in down gaze.

a wave. 1. The positive-pressure wave in the atrial or venous pulse, produced by atrial contraction. 2. The atrial wave of the apex cardiogram representing the outward motion of the cardiac apex which results from additional ventricular filling produced by atrial contraction. Syn. *atrial beat.*

ax-, axo-. A combining form denoting (a) *axis;* (b) *axon or axis cylinder.*

axen·ic (ay-zen'ick, ay-zee'nick) *adj.* 1. Not contaminated by any foreign organisms, hence a pure culture, as of protozoa. 2. Of or pertaining to germ-free animals.

axe-roph·thol (ay″ze-rof′thol, ack″se-rof′thol) *n.* VITAMIN A.

ax·i·al (ack'see-ul) *adj.* 1. Of or pertaining to an axis. 2. *In dentistry,* relating to or parallel with the long axis of a tooth. —**axial·ly** (·ee) *adv.*

axial current. The faster-moving current along the axis or center of a vascular lumen, carrying in the bloodstream, especially in the smaller arteries, a preponderance of erythrocytes over the slower, plasma-rich, outer current.

axial hyperopia. Hyperopia due to abnormal shortness of the anteroposterior diameter of the eye, the refractive power being normal.

axial tomography. Sectional radiography in which a series of cross-sectional images along an axis is combined to constitute a three-dimensional scan.

axial walls. Walls of a prepared cavity in a tooth, which are parallel with its long axis.

ax·il·la (ack-sil′uh) *n.,* pl. & genit. sing. **axil·lae** (·ee) The region between the arm and the thoracic wall, bounded anteriorly by the pectoralis major muscle, and posteriorly by the latissimus dorsi muscle; the armpit.

ax·il·lary (ack'si-lerr″ee) *adj.* Of or pertaining to the axilla.

axillary region. A region upon the lateral aspect of the thorax, extending from the axilla to a line drawn from the lower border of the mammary region to that of the scapular region.

axillary vein thrombosis. PAGET-SCHROETTER'S SYNDROME.

ax·io·buc·co·lin·gual (ack″see-o-buck″o-ling′ gwul) *adj.* Pertaining to the long axis and the buccal and lingual surfaces of a tooth.

ax·io·la·bio·lin·gual (ack″see-o-lay″bee-o-ling′ gwul) *adj.* Pertaining to the long axis and the labial and lingual surfaces of a tooth.

ax·is (ack'sis) *n.,* pl. **ax·es** (·seez) 1. An imaginary line passing through the center of a body; also the line about which a rotating body turns. 2. [NA] The second cervical vertebra. Syn. *epistropheus.*

axis cylinder. AXON.

axis-traction forceps. An obstetric forceps, the so-called high forceps instrument, equipped with a mechanism to permit rotation of the fetal head and traction in the line of the pelvic axis.

axo·fu·gal (ack″so-few′gul, ack-sof′yoo-gul) *adj.* Pertaining to nerve impulses transmitted from the cell body to the periphery.

ax·on (acks'on) *n.* The efferent process of a nerve cell. Syn. *neurit, axis cylinder process.* —**ax·o·nal** (ack'suh-nul) *adj.*

axonal reaction. The sequence of changes whereby a nerve cell body seeks to restore the integrity of its axon when it has been interrupted by injury or disease; best seen in the anterior horn cells of the spinal cord, the larger sensory neurons, and the motor nuclei of the cranial nerves, the changes include swelling of the nerve cell body, chromatolysis so that the Nissl granules are no longer stained by basic aniline dyes, and swelling and peripheral displacement of the nucleus. Syn. *primary degeneration of Nissl.*

ax·o·nom·e·ter (ack″so-nom′e-tur) *n.* An instrument used for locating the axis of astigmatism, or for determining the axis of a cylindrical lens.

ax·on·ot·me·sis (ack″suh-not-mee′sis) *n.* Injury to a nerve, as from severe compression which damages the nerve fibers, causing motor and sensory deficits without completely severing the nerve, so that recovery may occur.

axon reflex. A response occurring without involvement of a nerve cell body or a synapse (hence not a true reflex), which results from a stimulus applied to a terminal branch of a sensory nerve and gives rise to an impulse that ascends to a collateral branch of the same nerve fiber, down which it is conducted antidromically to an effector organ; believed to be important in the local regulation of blood vessel caliber, especially in the skin.

ax·op·e·tal (ack-sop′e-tul) *adj.* Pertaining to nerve impulses transmitted along an axon toward the cell body.

axo·plasm (ack'so-plaz-um) *n.* Undifferentiated cytoplasm, neuroplasm, of the axon in which neurofibrils are embedded.

Ayer·za's syndrome or **disease** (a-yerr′sah) Intense cyanosis, polycythemia, heart failure due to chronic pulmonary insufficiency, and sclerosis of the pulmonary vascular bed.

az-, aza-, azo- A combining form indicating *the presence of nitrogen in a compound.*

azap·e·tine (az-ap′uh-teen, ay-zap′) *n.* 6-Allyl-6,7-dihydro-5*H*-dibenz[*c,e*]azepine, $C_{17}H_{17}N$, an adrenergic blocking agent; used as the phosphate salt for treatment of certain peripheral vascular diseases.

az·a·thi·o·prine (az″uh-thigh′o-preen) *n.* 6-[(1-Methyl-4-nitroimidazol-5-yl)thio]purine, $C_9H_7N_7O_2S$, a derivative of mercaptopurine used experimentally in the treatment of leukemia and as a suppressive drug in diseases produced by altered immune mechanisms.

azi-. A prefix indicating *the presence of the group* N_2.

az·ide (az'ide, ·id, ay'zide) *n.* A compound containing the univalent —N_3 group.

azo (az'o, ay'zo) *adj. In chemistry,* of or pertaining to a compound containing the group — N:N— united to two hydrocarbon groups.

azo·ben·zene (az″o-ben′zeen, ay″zo-) *n.* Benzeneazobenzene, $C_6H_5N{:}NC_6H_5$; used in organic synthesis.

azo dyes. A group of synthetic organic dyes

derivable from azobenzene, containing the chromophore—N:N—.

azo·lit·min (az″o·lit′min, ay″zo·) *n.* A dark-red coloring matter obtained from litmus and used as an indicator, especially in routine bacteriologic work with milk.

azo·o·sper·mia (ay·zo″o·spur′mee·uh, az″o·) *n.* Absence of live spermatozoa in the semen.

azo·pro·tein (az″o·pro′tee·in, ·pro′teen, ay″zo·) *n.* One of a group of synthetic antigens formed by coupling proteins with diazonium compounds.

azot-, azoto- A combining form meaning *nitrogen, nitrogenous.*

azotemic osteodystrophy. Those bony alterations occurring as a complication of renal failure or Fanconi's syndrome; includes osteomalacia, osteosclerosis, and osteitis fibrosa cystica.

azotic acid. NITRIC ACID.

azot·i·fi·ca·tion (a·zot″i·fi·kay′shun) *n.* Fixation of atmospheric nitrogen.

az·o·tom·e·ter (az″o·tom′e·tur, ay″zo·) *n.* A device for gasometrically measuring the nitrogen content of compounds in solution. —**azotome·try** (·tree) *n.*

az·o·tor·rhea, az·o·tor·rhoea (az″uh·to·ree′uh, ay·zo″to·) *n.* Excessive amounts of nitrogenous material in the urine; or in the feces, as seen in malabsorption syndromes.

az·o·tu·ria (az″o·tew′ree·uh, ay″zo·) *n.* 1. An increase of the nitrogenous substances in the urine. 2. A disease of horses associated with necrosis of cramped skeletal muscle and myoglobinuria. Syn. *Monday morning disease of horses.* —**azo·tu·ric** (·tew′rick) *adj.*

azure (azh′ur, ay′zhur) *n.* A basic thiazine dye; used in blood and connective-tissue stains.

azu·ro·phil (a·zhoor′o·fil, azh′ur·o·) *adj.* Staining purplish red with Giemsa, Wright, Leishman, and similar blood stains, contrasting with the darker red-purple of nuclei and the light blue of cytoplasms; characteristic of certain cytoplasmic granules in leukocytes.

azu·ro·phil·ia (azh″ur·o·fil′ee·uh, a·zhoor″o·) *n.* The property of being azurophil. —**azurophil·ic** (·ick) *adj.*

az·y·gos (az′i·gos, a·zye′gos) *n.* An unpaired anatomic structure.

azygos lobe. A variable, partially separate portion of the upper medial part of the superior lobe of the right lung. When present, it is isolated from the main part of the lobe by a deep groove occupied by the azygos vein.

azygos uvu·lae (yoo′vew·lee). UVULAE; the muscle of the uvula.

azygos vein. An unpaired vein of the posterior body wall beginning in the right lumbar region, ascending in the right thoracic wall, and finally emptying into the superior vena cava.

az·y·gous (az′i·gus, a·zye′gus) *adj.* Unpaired.

azym·ia (a·zye′mee·uh, a·zym′ee·uh) *n.* The absence of an enzyme or ferment.

azym·ic (a·zye′mick, a·zym′ick) *adj.* 1. Not rising from a fermentation; unfermented. 2. Not containing enzymes.

B

B Symbol for boron.

Ba Symbol for barium.

Baastrup's disease. Mutual compression of the spinous processes of adjacent vertebrae.

Babcock's operation Extirpation of varicose segments of the saphenous vein by inserting a bulb-tipped probe or stripper and drawing the vein out.

Ba·be·sia (ba·bee'zhuh, ·zee·uh) *n.* A genus of intracellular, nonpigmented sporozoa which invade the red blood cells of cattle, sheep, horses, rodents, dogs, and monkeys but rarely of man. Members of this genus are oval or pear-shaped.

bab·e·si·a·sis (bab"e·sigh'uh·sis) *n.*, pl. **babesiases** (·seez) BABESIOSIS.

Ba·bin·ski-Froeh·lich disease (F. ba·bæn·skee', Pol. ba·bin'skee) ADIPOSOGENITAL DYSTROPHY.

Babinski phenomenon or **reflex** 1. BABINSKI SIGN (1). 2. BABINSKI'S PRONATION PHENOMENON. 3. TRUNK-THIGH SIGN OF BABINSKI.

Babinski sign 1. Extension of the great toe when the lateral aspect of the sole is stroked sharply. After infancy this reflex is abnormal and indicates disturbance of the corticospinal tract. Syn. *extensor plantar reflex or response.* 2. BABINSKI'S PLATYSMA SIGN. 3. BABINSKI'S REINFORCEMENT SIGN. 4. TRUNK-THIGH SIGN OF BABINSKI.

Babinski's platysma sign Failure of the platysma to contract on the paretic side, with an exaggerated contraction of the platysma on the unaffected side, when the mouth is opened against resistance; seen in hemiplegia involving the muscles of facial expression. Syn. *platysma phenomenon.*

Babinski's pronation phenomenon Pronation of the paretic arm occurs (a) if the palms of the hands are held in approximation with the thumbs upward and then are shaken or jarred; (b) if the arms are actively abducted with the forearms in supination; or (c) if the arms are passively abducted with the forearms in supination and then suddenly released.

Babinski's reinforcement sign In hemiplegia, when the patient sits so that his legs hang free, forceful pulling of the flexed fingers of one side against those of the other results in extension of the leg on the paretic side.

ba·by, *n.* An infant; a child up to about one year of age when walking and first words usually are achieved.

bac·ca·lau·re·ate nurse. In the United States, a nurse holding a bachelor's degree in nursing from a university or collegiate program accredited by the National League for Nursing.

bac·ci·form (back'si·form) *adj.* Berry-shaped.

bacill-, bacilli-, bacillo-. A combining form meaning *bacillus.*

Bac·il·la·ce·ae (bas"i·lay'see·ee) *n.pl.* A family of Eubacteriales comprising the genera *Bacillus* and *Clostridium.*

bac·il·lary (bas'i·lerr"ee) *adj.* 1. Pertaining to bacilli or to a bacillus. 2. Consisting of or containing rods.

bacillary dysentery. Any of a group of infectious diseases caused by invasion of the colon, primarily by pathogenic bacteria of the genus *Shigella,* characterized by the frequent passage of blood-stained stools or of exudate consisting of blood and mucus, and often accompanied by tenesmus, abdominal cramps, and fever. Syn. *shigellosis.*

bac·il·le·mia, bac·il·lae·mia (bas"i·lee'mee·uh) *n.* The presence of bacilli in the blood.

bacilli-. See *bacill-.*

ba·cil·li·form (ba·sil'i·form) *adj.* Having the shape or appearance of a bacillus; rod-shaped.

bacillo-. See *bacill-.*

ba·cil·lo·pho·bia (ba·sil"o·fo'bee·uh) *n.* BACTERIOPHOBIA.

bac·il·lu·ria (bas"i·lew'ree·uh) *n.* The presence of bacilli in the urine.

Ba·cil·lus (ba·sil'us) *n.* A genus of rod-shaped, gram-positive bacteria capable of producing endospores, belonging to the family Bacillaceae; *Bacillus subtilis* is a prototype.

bacillus, *n.,* pl. **bacil·li** (·eye) 1. Any rod-shaped bacterium. 2. *Obsol.* Any member of the class Schizomycetes.

Bacillus acidophilus. LACTOBACILLUS ACIDOPHI-
LUS.

Bacillus aer·og·e·nes cap·su·la·tus (ay·ur·oj'e·
neez kap·sue·lay'tus). CLOSTRIDIUM PERFRIN-
GENS.

Bacillus aert·rycke (ärt'rye·ke^h). SALMONELLA
TYPHIMURIUM.

Bacillus ag·ni (ag'nigh). CLOSTRIDIUM PERFRIN-
GENS B.

Bacillus an·thra·cis (an'thruh·sis). An aerobic
spore-forming species pathogenic to man, although in nature it is primarily a pathogen of
cattle and horses; the cause of anthrax.

Bacillus bot·u·li·nus (bot''yoo·lye'nus). CLOS-
TRIDIUM BOTULINUM.

bacillus Cal·mette-Gué·rin (kal·met', gey·ræn^r) A
strain of *Mycobacterium tuberculosis* var. *bovis*,
attenuated by extended cultivation on a medium containing bile; used in vaccines for
immunization against tuberculosis. Abbreviated, BCG.

Bacillus coli. ESCHERICHIA COLI.

Bacillus dysenteriae. SHIGELLA DYSENTERIAE.

Bacillus enteritidis. SALMONELLA ENTERITIDIS.

Bacillus influenzae. HEMOPHILUS INFLUENZAE.

Bacillus lac·tis aer·og·e·nes (lack'tis ay·ur·oj'e·
neez). ENTEROBACTER AEROGENES.

Bacillus leprae. MYCOBACTERIUM LEPRAE.

Bacillus mallei. PSEUDOMONAS MALLEI.

Bacillus oe·de·ma·ti·ens (ee''de·may'shee·enz).
CLOSTRIDIUM NOVYI.

Bacillus para·ty·pho·sus A (păr''uh·tye·fo'sus).
SALMONELLA PARATYPHI A.

Bacillus paratyphosus B. SALMONELLA SCHOTT-
MUELLERI.

Bacillus pertussis. BORDETELLA PERTUSSIS.

Bacillus pestis. YERSINIA PESTIS.

Bacillus proteus. PROTEUS VULGARIS.

Bacillus pyo·cy·a·ne·us (pye''o·sigh·ay'nee·us).
PSEUDOMONAS AERUGINOSA.

Bacillus sub·ti·lis (sub'ti·lis, sub·tye'lis). The type
species of the genus *Bacillus*, which infects
human beings only rarely; the source of sub-
tilin.

Bacillus tetani. CLOSTRIDIUM TETANI.

Bacillus tuberculosis. MYCOBACTERIUM TUBER-
CULOSIS.

bac·i·tra·cin (bas''i·tray'sin) *n.* A polypeptide
antibiotic produced by an organism belonging
to the *licheniformis* group of *Bacillus subtilis*. It
is active against many gram-positive organisms, as streptococci, staphylococci, and
pneumococci, and certain gram-negative cocci, as gonococci and meningococci, but ineffective against most gram-negative organisms.

back, *n.* 1. Dorsum; the posterior aspect. 2. The
posterior part of the trunk from the neck to
the pelvis.

back·ache, *n.* Pain in the lower lumbar or lumbosacral region of the back.

back·bone, *n.* VERTEBRAL COLUMN.

back·ground radiation. Radiation arising from a
source other than the one directly under consideration or study, such as cosmic rays, environmental radiation, or radioactive material
that may be in the vicinity.

back·scat·ter, *n.* Radiation that is deflected by a

scattering process at angles greater than 90° to
the original direction of the beam of radiation.

back·ward failure. Heart failure in which symptoms result predominantly from elevation of
venous pressure behind the failing ventricle,
e.g., engorgement of the lung due to failure of
the left ventricle.

back·ward·ness, *n.* 1. Retarded physical or mental development or both due to any extrinsic
cause, as general illness, social or sensory
deprivation. 2. Educational retardation not
due to intrinsic mental deficiency.

bac·ter·emia, bac·ter·ae·mia (back''te·ree'mee·
uh) *n.* The presence of living bacteria in the
blood.

bac·ter·emic, bac·ter·ae·mic (back''te·ree'mick)
adj. Pertaining to or having bacteremia.

bacteremic shock. 1. Any shock state occurring
during bacteremia. 2. The shock state occurring in the course of bacteremia caused by
gram-negative bacteria, characterized by severe hypotension and generalized circulatory
failure, and simulated in laboratory animals
by the injection of endotoxin derived from
gram-negative bacteria.

bacteri-, bacterio-. A combining form meaning
bacteria, bacterial.

bac·te·ri·um (back·teer'ee·uh) *n.*, sing. **bacte·ri·um**
(·ee·um) Microscopic unicellular prokaryotic
organisms which generally divide by transverse binary fission, possess rigid cell walls,
and exhibit three principal forms: round or
coccal, rodlike or bacillary, and spiral or spirochetal. Also included are *Mycoplasma* lacking cell walls and the Actinomycetales in
which some forms are filamentous and
branching. Genetic recombination occurs.
Bacteria may be partially or totally aerobic or
anaerobic; they may or may not be motile,
capsulated, or spore-forming. They may possess diverse biochemical and enzymatic activities, are widely prevalent in nature and in
relation to plants and animals, and may be
saprophytic or pathogenic.

Bac·te·ri·a·ce·ae (back·teer''ee·ay'see·ee) *n.pl.*
Obsol. SCHIZOMYCETES.

bac·te·ri·al (back·teer'ee·ul) *adj.* Pertaining to,
consisting of, or caused by bacteria.

bacterial antagonism. The adverse effect produced by one species of microorganism upon
the growth and development of another.

bacterial endocarditis. A prolonged, febrile,
grave bacterial infection of the endocardium
or the heart valves, or both, characterized by
fever, heart murmur, splenomegaly, embolic
phenomena, and bacteremia. Syn. *subacute
bacterial endocarditis*.

bacterial enzyme. An enzyme existing in, or
produced by, bacteria.

bacterial spectrum. ANTIBIOTIC SPECTRUM.

bacterial vaccine. An emulsion of bacteria,
killed, living, or attenuated, used for the purpose of stimulating the immune response of a
patient to infection by the same organism.

bac·te·ri·cide (back·teer'i·side) *n.* An agent that
destroys bacteria. —**bac·te·ri·cid·al** (back·teer''
i·sigh'dul) *adj.*

bac·te·ri·cid·in (back·teer''i·sigh'din) *n.* An antibody that in the presence of complement kills bacteria.

bac·ter·id (back'tur·id) *n.* A pustular eruption on the hands and feet believed to be caused by sensitization to bacterial products from a focus of infection.

bac·ter·in (back'tur·in) *n.* BACTERIAL VACCINE.

bacterio-. See *bacteri-*.

bac·te·ri·o·cid·in (back·teer''ee·o·side'in) *n.* BACTERICIDIN.

bac·te·ri·oc·la·sis (back·teer''ee·ok'luh·sis) *n.*, pl. **bacterioclases** (·seez) The destruction or fragmentation of bacteria, a phenomenon similar to bacteriolysis by bacteriophage.

bac·te·ri·o·gen·ic (back·teer''ee·o·jen'ick) *adj.* 1. Caused by bacteria. 2. Of bacterial origin.

bac·te·ri·o·he·mol·y·sin, bac·te·ri·o·hae·mol·y·sin (back·teer''ee·o·hee·mol'i·sin) *n.* Any bacterial product or toxin, such as staphylolysin, streptolysin, tetanolysin, or hemolysins of *Clostridium perfringens*, that releases hemoglobin from red blood cells in vitro, but that may or may not be active in vivo.

bac·te·ri·ol·o·gist (back·teer''ee·ol'uh·jist) *n.* A person who specializes in bacteriology.

bac·te·ri·ol·o·gy (back·teer''ee·ol'uh·jist) *n.* The science and study of bacteria. —**bac·te·ri·o·log·ic** (·ee·o·loj'ick), **bacteriolog·i·cal** (·i·kul) *adj.*

bac·te·ri·o·ly·sin (back·teer''ee·o·lye'sin) *n.* A specific antibody which, together with other substances, is capable of causing the dissolution of the homologous bacterium.

bac·te·ri·ol·y·sis (back·teer''ee·ol'i·sis) *n.*, pl. **bacterioly·ses** (·seez) The intracellular or extracellular dissolution of bacteria. —**bacte·rio·lyt·ic** (·ee·o·lit'ick) *adj.*

bac·te·ri·o·phage (back·teer''ee·o·faij, ·fahzh) *n.* One of a group of viruses infecting bacteria, sometimes resulting in lysis of the bacterial cell. —**bac·te·rio·phag·ic** (·back·teer''ee·o·faj'ick) *adj.*; **bacteri·oph·a·gy** (·off'uh·jee) *n.*

bac·te·ri·o·pho·bia (back·teer''ee·o·fo'bee·uh) *n.* A morbid dread of bacteria or other microorganisms.

bac·te·ri·o·pro·tein (back·teer''ee·o·pro'tee·in) *n.* Any one of a number of protein substances contained in bacteria.

bac·te·ri·op·so·nin (back·teer''ee·op'so·nin) *n.* An opsonin which acts upon bacteria, as distinguished from one affecting erythrocytes. —**bacteri·op·son·ic** (·op·son'ick) *adj.*

bac·te·ri·o·sis (back·teer''ee·o'sis) *n.* Any disease of bacterial origin.

bac·te·ri·os·ta·sis (back·teer''ee·os'tuh·sis, ·o·stay'sis) *n.*, pl. **bacteriosta·ses** (·seez) Arrest or hindrance of the growth of bacteria.

bac·te·ri·o·stat (back·teer''ee·o·stat) *n.* Any agent which arrests or hinders the growth of bacteria.

bac·te·ri·o·stat·ic (back·teer''ee·o·stat'ick) *adj.* Arresting or hindering the growth of bacteria.

bacteriostatic spectrum. ANTIBIOTIC SPECTRUM.

bac·te·ri·o·ther·a·py (back·teer''ee·o·therr'uh·pee) *n.* The treatment of disease by the introduction of bacteria or their products into the system. —**bacterio·ther·a·peu·tic** (·therr·uh·pew'tick) *adj.*

bac·te·ri·o·tox·in (back·teer''ee·o·tock'sin) *n.* 1. A toxin that destroys bacteria. 2. A toxin produced by bacteria. —**bacteriotox·ic** (·sick) *adj.*

bac·te·ri·o·trop·ic (back·teer''ee·o·trop'ick) *adj. Obsol.* Rendering bacteria susceptible to phagocytosis.

bac·te·ri·ot·ro·pin (back·teer''ee·ot'ro·pin) *n. Obsol.* An opsonin aiding the phagocytic action of certain cells, as leukocytes.

Bac·te·ri·um (back·teer''ee·um) *n. Obsol.* A genus of bacteria.

bacterium. Singular of *bacteria.*

Bacterium am·big·u·um (am·big'yoo·um). SHIGELLA AMBIGUA.

Bacterium coli. ESCHERICHIA COLI.

Bacterium dysenteriae. SHIGELLA DYSENTERIAE.

Bacterium enteritidis. SALMONELLA ENTERITIDIS.

Bacterium flexneri. SHIGELLA FLEXNERI.

Bacterium fried·län·de·ri (freed'len'duh·rye). KLEBSIELLA PNEUMONIAE.

Bacterium para·dys·en·ter·i·ae (păr''uh·dis·en·terr'ee·ee). SHIGELLA FLEXNERI.

Bacterium para·ty·pho·sum A (păr''uh·tigh·fo'sum). SALMONELLA PARATYPHI A.

Bacterium pneumoniae. KLEBSIELLA PNEUMONIAE.

Bacterium shi·gae (shee'ghee). SHIGELLA DYSENTERIAE.

Bacterium sonnei. SHIGELLA SONNEI.

Bacterium tu·la·ren·se (too''luh·ren'see). FRANCISELLA TULARENSIS.

Bacterium ty·pho·sum (tye·fo'sum). SALMONELLA TYPHOSA.

bac·te·ri·u·ria (back·teer''ee·yoo'ree·uh) *n.* The presence of bacteria in the urine.

bac·ter·oid (back'tur·oid) *adj. & n.* 1. Resembling a bacterium. 2. A bacterium modified in form or structure.

ba·gasse (ba·gas') *n.* The fibrous, dusty material in sugarcane after the juice has been extracted.

ba·gas·so·sis (ba''ga·so'sis) *n.*, pl. **bagasso·ses** (·seez) A pneumoconiosis due to inhalation of the dust of bagasse, characterized clinically by dyspnea, malaise, fever, and diffuse bronchopneumonia.

bag of waters. The fetal membranes and amniotic fluid which serve during pregnancy to protect the fetus.

Ba·hia ulcer (ba·ee'uh) A skin ulcer occurring in American mucocutaneous leishmaniasis.

Ba·ker's cyst 1. A synovial cyst in the popliteal space arising from the semimembranosus bursa or the knee joint and, in the latter case, frequently associated with intraarticular abnormality in the knee. 2. A herniation of synovial membrane from the joint.

baking soda. SODIUM BICARBONATE.

balan-, balano- A combining form meaning *glans, balanic.*

ba·lan·ic (ba·lan'ick) *adj.* Of or pertaining to the glans of the penis or of the clitoris.

bal·a·nit·ic (bal''uh·nit'ick) *adj.* 1. Of or pertaining to balanitis. 2. *Erron.* BALANIC.

bal·a·ni·tis (bal''uh·nigh'tis) *n.* 1. Inflammation of the glans penis or glans clitoridis. 2. BALANOCHLAMYDITIS.

balano-. See *balan-.*

bal·a·no·chlam·y·di·tis (bal''uh·no·klam''i·dye'

tis) *n.* Inflammation of the glans and prepuce of the clitoris.

bal·a·no·plas·ty (bal'uh·no·plas''tee) *n.* Plastic surgery of the glans penis.

bal·a·no·pos·thi·tis (bal''uh·no·pos·thigh'tis) *n.* Inflammation of the glans penis and of the prepuce.

bal·a·no·pre·pu·tial (bal''uh·no·pre·pew'shul) *adj.* Pertaining to the glans penis and the prepuce.

bal·a·nor·rha·gia (bal''uh·no·ray'juh, ·jee·uh) *n.* Hemorrhage from the glans penis.

bal·a·nor·rhea, bal·a·nor·rhoea (bal''uh·no·ree' uh) *n.* Purulent balanitis.

bal·an·tid·i·al (bal''an·tid'ee·ul) *adj.* Of or pertaining to protozoans of the genus *Balantidium.*

bal·an·ti·di·a·sis (bal''an·ti·dye'uh·sis) *n.,* pl. **bal·antidia·ses** (·seez) An infection of the large intestine with *Balantidium coli,* varying in severity from mild colitis to acute dysentery.

Bal·an·tid·i·um (bal''an·tid'ee·um) *n.* A genus of ciliated, parasitic protozoans.

Balantidium co·li (ko'lye). A common parasite of hogs; occasionally infects man, causing severe dysentery.

bal·a·nus (bal'uh·nus) *n.* The glans of the penis or of the clitoris.

Balarsen. Trademark for arsthinol, a trivalent organic arsenical employed in the treatment of intestinal amebiasis and yaws.

bald·ness, *n.* Absence of hair; ALOPECIA; CALVITIES.

Bald·win operation The formation of an artificial vagina by transplantation of a loop of intestine between the urinary bladder and rectum.

Bal·kan frame An overhead quadrilateral frame, supported by uprights fastened to the bedposts; used to suspend immobilized fractured limbs and to apply continuous traction by weights and pulleys; also used to facilitate mobility of patients under treatment for fracture.

ball, *n.* 1. *In anatomy,* any globular part. 2. *In veterinary medicine,* a pill or bolus.

ball-and-socket joint. A type of synovial joint, such as that of the hip or shoulder, in which the rounded head of one bone lodges in a concave surface on the other. Syn. *spheroid articulation.*

bal·lism (bal'iz·um) *n.* Jerky, swinging, or flinging movements of the arms and legs, as seen in extrapyramidal disorders such as Sydenham's chorea.

bal·lis·mus (ba·liz'mus) *n.* BALLISM.

bal·lis·tic (ba·lis'tick) *adj.* 1. Associated with or activated by a sudden physical impulse. 2. Pertaining to missiles or projectiles.

ballisto-. A combining form meaning *ballistic.*

bal·lis·to·car·di·o·gram (ba·lis''to·kahr'dee·o·gram) *n.* The record made by a ballistocardiograph, consisting of a series of consecutive waves termed H, I, J, K, L, M, N, etc. Abbreviated, BCG.

bal·lis·to·car·di·o·graph (ba·lis''to·kahr'dee·o·graf) *n.* An instrument that records the recoil movements of the body resulting from cardiac

contraction and the impact produced thereon by the ejection of blood from the ventricles.

bal·lis·to·pho·bia (ba·lis''to·fo'bee·uh) *n.* Morbid fear of projectiles or missiles.

bal·loon·ing, *n.* Surgical distention of any body cavity by air or other means for examination or therapeutic purposes.

bal·lotte·ment (ba·lot·mahn'', ba·lot'munt) *n.* A diagnostic maneuver used to palpate a floating object or deeply placed movable organ or tumor. By judicious pushing and rebound (direct ballottement), or by sudden counterpressure (indirect ballottement), the displaced object is made to impinge on the containing wall, the impact being felt by the palpating fingers or hand.

ball thrombus. A rounded thrombus found in the heart, especially in an atrium.

balm (bahm) *n.* 1. BALSAM. 2. Any substance which heals, relieves, or soothes pain.

bal·ne·ol·o·gy (bal''nee·ol'uh·jee) *n.* The science of baths and their therapeutic uses.

bal·neo·ther·a·py (bal''nee·o·therr'uh·pee) *n.* Therapeutic use of baths.

bal·sam (bawl'sum) *n.* 1. The resinous, aromatic, liquid, or semisolid substance obtained from certain trees by natural exudation or by artificial extraction and consisting chiefly of resins and volatile oils containing esters of cinnamic and benzoic acids. 2. Sometimes, a substance which is not a true balsam in that it contains no cinnamic or benzoic acid, as copaiba. —**bal·sam·ic** (bawl·sam'ick) *adj.*

band, *n.* 1. That which binds. 2. A stripe. 3. *In zoology,* a stripe. 3. *In anatomy,* a ligament or long slender bundle of fibers; also, a disk of a striated muscle fiber as seen in its longitudinal section. 4. *In dentistry,* a metal strip encircling and fitted to a tooth.

ban·dage (ban'dij) *n.* A strip of gauze, muslin, flannel, or other material, usually in the form of a roll, of various widths and lengths, but sometimes triangular or tailed, used to hold dressing in place, to apply pressure, to immobilize a part, to support a dependent or injured part, to obliterate tissue cavities, or to check hemorrhage.

band-box resonance. TYMPANITIC RESONANCE (2).

band cell. A developmental stage of a granular leukocyte, found in the circulating blood, intermediate between the metamyelocyte and the adult segmented form. The nucleus is bandlike and the cytoplasm and granules are those of the corresponding adult cell.

bank, *n.* A reserve stock of body fluids and parts usually maintained at a hospital or other medical facility.

Banthine bromide. Trademark for methanthelzine bromide, an anticholinergic drug.

Ban·ti's syndrome or **disease** (bahn'tee) 1. Portal hypertension, congestive splenomegaly, and hypersplenism due to an obstructive lesion in the splenic vein, portal vein, or intrahepatic veins. 2. Originally, a primary disease of the spleen.

¹bar, *n.* 1. A band or stripe. 2. A fetal or visceral arch. 3. That part of the horse's upper jaw which has no teeth. 4. That portion of the wall of a horse's hoof reflected sharply anteriorly onto the sole from each buttress. The two bars are separated by the frog. 5. A segment of metal connecting two or more components of a removable partial denture.

²bar, *n.* A unit of atmospheric pressure representing one megadyne per square centimeter.

bar-, baro- A combining form meaning (a) *weight, pressure;* (b) *atmospheric pressure.*

Bá·rány's pointing test (bah'rahny) The patient points with finger or toe at a fixed object alternately with eyes open and closed. Constant failure of the limb to return to the former position indicates a unilateral cerebellar lesion.

bar·ba (bahr'buh) *n.* The beard.

barb·al·o·in (bahr·bal'o·in) *n.* The pentoside chiefly responsible for the purgative action of aloe.

bar·ber's itch. Folliculitis of the beard.

bar·bi·tal (bahr'bi·tol, ·tal) *n.* 5,5-Diethylbarbituric acid or diethylmalonylurea, $C_8H_{12}N_2O_3$, a white crystalline powder; a long-acting hypnotic and sedative. Syn. *barbitone, diethylbarbituric acid.*

bar·bi·tu·rate (bahr·bitch'oo·rate, bahr'bi·tewr'ate) *n.* Any derivative of barbituric acid, $C_4H_4N_2O_3$ formed by the substitution of an aliphatic or aromatic group on a carbon or nitrogen atom in the acid. Barbiturates are used as hypnotic and sedative drugs. Modifications in their structure influence the power and rapidity of their effects. The depressant effects of these drugs are exerted upon the higher centers of the brain.

bar·bi·tu·rism (bahr'bi·tewr·iz·um, bahr·bitch'oor·iz·um) *n.* Physiologic, pathologic, and psychologic changes produced by ingestion of barbiturates in excess of therapeutic amounts; may be acute or chronic.

bar·be·tage (bahr·bo·tahzh') *n.* A method of spinal anesthesia in which part of the anesthetic solution is injected into the subarachnoid space; spinal fluid is then aspirated into the syringe and reinjected. This procedure may be repeated several times before the entire content of the syringe is finally injected. In this way, the anesthetic agent is more widely diffused, though the anesthesia is frequently spotty.

bar·es·the·sia, bar·aes·the·sia (bär''es·theezh'uh, ·theez'ee·uh) *n.* Perception of weight or pressure; PRESSURE SENSE.

bar·i·to·sis (bär''i·to'sis) *n.* A pneumoconiosis due to the inhalation of barium dust.

bar·i·um (bär'ee·um) *n.* Ba = 137.34. A metal belonging to the alkaline earths and occurring in nature only in the form of divalent compounds. All its soluble salts are poisonous.

barium chloride. $BaCl_2 \cdot 2H_2O$; a water-soluble salt used to precipitate sulfate ions. A violent stimulant of all smooth muscles; has been used to increase the force of cardiac contraction in atrioventricular dissociation (Stokes-Adams syndrome).

barium sulfate. $BaSO_4$; a water-insoluble salt,

employed as an opaque radiographic contrast medium.

bar·ley, *n.* Any cereal grass of the genus *Hordeum,* order Graminales; used as food, and also in the preparation of malt.

barley water. A decoction of pearl barley prepared by boiling with water; used as demulcent and food for children with diarrhea.

Barlow's syndrome An apical systolic murmur, systolic click, and an electrocardiogram of inferior ischemia, in association with mitral regurgitation due to mitral valve prolapse. Syn. *electrocardiographic-auscultatory syndrome.*

baro-. See **bar-.**

baro·cep·tor (bär''o·sep'tur) *n.* BARORECEPTOR.

bar of the bladder. The transverse ridge joining the openings of the ureters on the inner surface of the urinary bladder; it forms the posterior boundary of the trigone.

bar·og·no·sis (bär''og·no'sis) *n.,* pl. **barogno·ses** (·seez) The ability to estimate weight; the perception of weight.

baro·graph (bär'o·graf) *n.* A self-registering barometer.

baro·ma·crom·e·ter (bär''o·ma·krom'e·tur) *n.* An apparatus to measure the weight and length of infants.

ba·rom·e·ter (ba·rom'e·tur) *n.* An instrument that measures atmospheric pressure; commonly a capillary tube sealed at one end, filled with mercury, and inverted in a mercury reservoir. At sea level the height of the mercury column normally stands at 760 mm, or 30 inches, rising or falling directly as the atmospheric pressure. **—ba·rom·e·try** (ba·rom'e·tree) *n.*

baro·met·ric (bär·o·met'rick) *adj.* Of, pertaining to, or indicated by a barometer or barometry.

baro·pho·bia (bär''o·fo'bee·uh) *n.* A morbid fear of the pull of gravity.

baro·re·cep·tor (bär''o·re·sep'tur) *n.* 1. A nerve ending, located largely in the walls of the carotid sinus and of the aortic arch, sensitive to stretching induced by changes of blood pressure within the vessels or direct pressure from without. It generates afferent impulses conducted to medullary centers to cause reflex vasodilatation and fall of blood pressure, as by increase of systemic pressure and a reflex rise in systemic arterial pressure when blood pressure within the carotid sinus and aortic arch is suddenly raised. 2. Any peripheral receptor sensitive to mechanical deformation.

baro·scope (bär'o·skope) *n.* A sensitive barometer.

baro·si·nus·itis (bär''o·sigh''nus·eye'tis) *n.* Inflammation of the sinuses, characterized by edema and hemorrhage, caused by changes in atmospheric pressure.

bar·o·tal·gia (bär''o·tal'jee·uh) *n.* Pain arising in the middle ear caused by a difference of air pressure between the middle ear and the surrounding atmosphere.

bar·o·ti·tis (bär''o·tye'tis) *n.* Inflammation of the ear, or a part of it, caused by changes in atmospheric pressure.

barotitis me·dia (mee'dee·uh). Inflammation or

bleeding in the middle ear due to a difference between air pressure in the middle ear and external atmospheric pressure (as during airplane descent, in diving, or in a hyperbaric chamber), producing pain, tinnitus, and, occasionally, diminution in hearing and vertigo. Syn. *otic barotrauma, aerotitis media.*

baro·trau·ma (băr″o·traw′muh) *n.,* pl. **barotrau·ma·ta** (·tuh) Injury of certain organs, especially the auditory tube and the middle ear, due to a change in atmospheric pressure or water pressure.

Barr body SEX CHROMATIN.

bar·rel chest. A large thorax rounded in cross section, which may be normal in certain types of stocky build, or may indicate increased vital capacity as in certain peoples indigenous to high altitudes, or may be a sign of pulmonary emphysema.

Barré's syndrome GUILLAIN-BARRÉ DISEASE.

Bar·tho·lin cyst (bar′to·leen) A cyst resulting from chronic bartholinitis, containing a clear fluid which replaces the suppurative exudate.

bar·tho·lin·itis (bar″tho·li·nigh′tis) *n.* Inflammation of the major vestibular glands.

Bartholin's gland Either of the major vestibular glands. See *vestibular glands.*

Bar·ton·el·la (bahr″tun·el′uh) *n.* A genus of the Rickettsiales (family Bartonellaceae) which multiply in fixed tissue cells and parasitize erythrocytes, consisting of minute, pleomorphic rods and cocci which invade erythrocytes and endothelium in man. They occur without an intermediate host in man and in arthropod vectors are found only as *Bartonella bacilliformis,* the causative agent of bartonellosis.

bar·ton·el·lo·sis (bahr″tun·el·o′sis) *n.* An arthropod-borne infection caused by *Bartonella bacilliformis,* presenting two clinical types of disease: a severe form (Oroya fever), characterized by fever, a rapidly developing macrocytic anemia, and frequently by intercurrent infections with high mortality; and a benign form (verruga peruana), characterized by a verrucous eruption of hemangioma-like nodules and by negligible mortality.

bary- A combining form meaning (a) *heavy;* (b) *deep, low.*

bary·pho·nia (băr″i·fo′nee·uh) *n. Rare.* A heavy or deep quality of voice.

ba·sal (bay′sul) *adj.* 1. Fundamental; basic. 2. Indicating the lowest or least, as basal metabolic rate; deepest, as basal layer. 3. Pertaining to the initial unconscious state as induced by basal anesthesia.

basal anesthesia. A preliminary, usually incomplete anesthesia requiring supplementation. Thus, narcosis may be induced by injection of appropriate drugs, whereupon relatively small amounts of inhalation anesthetics are needed to produce surgical anesthesia.

basal angle. The angle between the sphenoid and clivus in the lateral projection.

basal body. A minute granule at the base of a cilium or flagellum, derived from the centriole and producing the cilium or flagellum.

basal cell. One of the cells of the deepest layer of a stratified epithelium.

basal cell carcinoma. A tumor composed of embryonal cells resembling those of the basal cell layer of the skin. It is locally invasive but rarely metastasizes.

basal cell layer. The deepest layer of cells in the germinative layer of a stratified epithelium.

basal ganglia. The caudate and lenticular nuclei, claustrum, subthalamic nucleus, and substantia nigra.

basal metabolic rate. The quantity of energy expended per unit of time under basal conditions; usually expressed as large calories (Cal) per square meter of body surface per hour. Abbreviated, B.M.R.

basal metabolism. The minimum amount of energy expenditure necessary to sustain life, measured when the subject is conscious and at complete rest in a warm atmosphere 12 to 18 hours after the intake of food.

ba·sal·oid (bay′sul·oid) *adj.* Resembling a basal cell of the skin.

basal ridge. A bandlike ridge of enamel on the lingual surface of an incisor or canine tooth, arising from the neck of the tooth toward its crown.

basal temperature. The temperature of the healthy body after a sufficient period of rest, usually obtained in the fasting state before arising after at least 8 hours of relaxed sleep.

basal vein. A vein located at the base of the brain.

bas·cu·la·tion (bas′kew·lay′shun) *n.* Replacing a retroverted uterus by pressing upward on the fundus and downward on the cervix.

base, *n.* 1. The lowest part of a body or any of its parts, or the foundation upon which anything rests. 2. The principal ingredient of a substance or compound. 3. *In chemistry,* (1) a compound which yields hydroxyl ions (OH⁻) in aqueous solution and which reacts with an acid to produce a salt and water; (2) a proton acceptor: a substance capable of taking up protons such as a purine or pyrimidine; or (3) a substance having an electron pair which may be shared by another substance which lacks such a pair, and is therefore called an acid, to form a coordinate covalent bond between the two substances.

Ba·se·dow's disease (bah′ze·do) GRAVES' DISEASE.

basement membrane. The delicate, noncellular layer on which an epithelium is seated. It may contain reticular fibers and can be selectively stained with silver stains.

base-plate, *n.* A form which is a negative reproduction of the edentulous jaw made by either adapting a material such as shellac to cast or fabricating an acrylic resin form to the edentulous cast; upon the baseplate, an occlusal wax rim is developed which is used to help establish jaw relationships and in which the artificial teeth are initially set.

basi-, basio-. A combining form meaning (a) *basion, basial;* (b) *base, basis, basilar;* (c) *basic.*

ba·si·al (bay′see·ul) *adj.* Of or relating to the basion.

ba·si·al·ve·o·lar (bay"see·al·vee'uh·lur) *adj.* Pertaining to the basion and the alveolar point.

ba·si·breg·mat·ic axis (bay"see·breg·mat'ick). The line connecting the basion and bregma.

ba·sic (bay'sick) *adj.* 1. Pertaining to the base or basis; fundamental. 2. *In chemistry,* of or pertaining to a base.

basic fuchsin. A mixture of rosaniline and pararosaniline hydrochlorides, dyes of the triphenylmethane group; available also as the acetate salts. Used as a germicide, as an ingredient of the antifungal preparation Castellani's paint, as a bacterial and histologic stain, and as a chemical reagent. Syn. *magenta.*

ba·si·chro·ma·tin (bay"see·kro'muh·tin) *n.* That portion of the chromatin stained by basic aniline dyes. It represents tightly coiled DNA, inactive in transcription of the genetic code. Syn. *heterochromatin.*

ba·sic·i·ty (ba·sis'i·tee, bay·) *n.* 1. The quality of being basic. 2. Of an acid: the fact of having a given number of replaceable hydrogen atoms, as monobasic, dibasic.

ba·si·cra·ni·al (bay"see·kray'nee·ul) *adj.* Pertaining to the base of the skull.

Ba·sid·io·my·ce·tes (ba·sid"ee·o·migh·see'teez) *n.pl.* A large class of fungi comprising genera which produce spores upon basidia. It includes the smuts, rusts, mushrooms, puffballs, and their allies.

ba·sid·io·spore (ba·sid'ee·o·spore) *n.* A spore of the Basidiomycetes, formed by a basidium.

ba·sid·i·um (ba·sid'ee·um) *n.*, pl. **basid·ia** (·ee·uh) *In botany,* the cell which produces basidiospores.

ba·si·fa·cial (bay"see·fay'shul) *adj.* Pertaining to the lower portion of the face.

bas·i·lar (bas'i·lur) *adj.* Of or pertaining to the base or basis of a structure or organ.

basilar meningitis. Inflammation of the meninges affecting chiefly the base of the brain, with collection of exudate predominantly in the basal cisterns.

basilar process. A strong, quadrilateral plate of bone forming the anterior portion of the occipital bone, in front of the foramen magnum.

ba·sil·ic vein (ba·sil'ick) The large superficial vein of the arm on the medial side of the biceps brachii muscle.

bas·i·lo·men·tal (bas"i·lo·men'tul, ba·sil"o·) *adj.* Pertaining to the base of the skull and to the chin.

ba·si·na·sal (bay"see·nay'zul) *adj.* Pertaining to the basion and nasion.

ba·si·oc·cip·i·tal (bay"see·ock·sip'i·tul) *adj.* Pertaining to the basilar part of the occipital bone.

basioccipital bone. 1. In many of the lower vertebrate animals and in embryonic mammals, the separate bone forming the median posterior part of the central axis of the skull. 2. In the human adult, the basilar part of the occipital bone.

ba·si·on (bay'see·on) *n.* In craniometry, the point on the anterior margin of the foramen magnum where the midsagittal plane of the skull intersects the plane of the foramen magnum.

ba·sio·trip·sy (bay'see·o·trip"see) *n.* Crushing or perforating the fetal head to facilitate delivery.

ba·si·pha·ryn·ge·al (bay"si·fa·rin'jee·ul) *adj.* Pertaining to the posterior part of the body of the sphenoid bone (base of the sphenoid) and to the pharynx.

ba·si·rhi·nal (bay"si·rye'nul) *adj.* Designating a cerebral fissure located at the base of the rhinencephalon.

ba·sis (bay'sis) *n.*, pl. **ba·ses** (·seez) A base, foundation, or fundamental part; the part opposite the apex.

basis cra·nii ex·ter·na (kray'nee·eye ecks·tur'nuh) [NA]. The external aspect of the base of the skull.

basis cranii in·ter·na (in·tur'nuh) [NA]. The internal aspect of the base of the skull.

basis pe·dun·cu·li ce·re·bri (pe·dunk'yoo·lye serr'e·brye) [BNA]. Crus cerebri (= CRUS OF THE CEREBRUM).

ba·si·sphe·noid (bay"see·sfee'noid) *n.* The lower part of the sphenoid bone, which embryonically developed as a separate bone.

basis pul·mo·nis (pul·mo'nis) [NA]. The base of a lung; the diaphragmatic surface.

ba·si·syl·vi·an (bay"see·sil'vee·un) *n.* The transverse basilar portion or stem of the lateral cerebral sulcus of the cerebral hemisphere.

ba·si·tem·po·ral (bay"see·tem'po·rul) *adj.* Pertaining to the lower part of the temporal bone.

ba·si·ver·te·bral (bay"see·vur'te·brul) *adj.* Pertaining to the centrum of a vertebra.

basket cells. The cells of the cerebellar cortex, the axons of which give off sprays of small branches, which enclose the somata of adjoining Purkinje cells as though in a series of baskets.

baso-. A combining form meaning (a) *base, basic;* (b) *basal.*

ba·so·phil (bay'so·fil) *adj. & n.* 1. BASOPHILIC. 2. A basophilic substance, cell, or tissue element. 3. Specifically, a beta cell of the adenohypophysis.

ba·so·phil·ia (bay"so·fil'ee·uh) *n.* 1. An increased number of basophils in the circulating blood. 2. Stippling of the red cells with basic staining granules, representing a degenerative condition as seen in severe anemia, leukemia, malaria, lead poisoning, and other toxic states. 3. An affinity for basic dyes.

ba·so·phil·ic (bay"so·fil'ick) *adj.* Susceptible to staining by basic rather than by acid dyes.

basophilic adenoma. An adenoma of the hypophysis made up of basophil cells.

basophilic normoblast. A nucleated red blood cell with coarse, condensed nuclear chromatin, no nucleoli, and a moderate amount of deep blue cytoplasm without hemoglobin.

basophil leukocyte. A leukocyte containing granules that contain histamine and heparin and stain deep purple (basic dye) with Wright's stain. The nucleus often shows no distinct lobulation.

ba·so·pho·bia (bay"so·fo'bee·uh, bas"o·) *n.* A morbid fear of walking or standing erect without muscular impairment.—**basopho·bic** (·bick) *adj.*; **basopho·bi·ac** (·bee·ack) *n.*

ba·so·squa·mous (bay"so·skway'mus) *adj.* Pertaining to or composed of basal and squamous cells.

bas·si·net (bas″i·net′) n. 1. An infant's crib or bed; a wicker basket with a hood at one end, used as a cradle. 2. An infant's crib or bed in a hospital as representative of the services and equipment needed to care for one infant in an obstetrical or pediatric unit.

Bas·si·ni operation (bah\ :sup:s·see′nee) A basic hernioplasty in which the inguinal ligament and conjoined tendon are sutured behind the spermatic cord.

bath, n. 1. A washing or immersion for cleansing purpose. 2. A bathing place or room. 3. Any yielding medium such as air, vapor, sand, or water, in which the body is wholly or partially immersed for therapeutic purposes. It may be designed to cleanse, soothe, stimulate, irritate, heat, or cool.

bath-, batho- A combining form meaning (a) depth; (b) downward, lower.

bath·es·the·sia, bath·aes·the·sia (bath″es·theezh′uh, ·theez′ee·uh) n. Deep sensation; muscle, tendon, and joint sensation and pressure sensibility.

bathing-trunk nevus. A congenital anomaly in the clinical form of pigmentation, papules, nodules, and hair in a conglomeration that resembles bathing trunks when located on the lower part of body. Histologically, the lesion consists of ordinary melanocytes.

batho·pho·bia (bath″o·fo′bee·uh) n. Morbid fear of depths.

bath·ro·ceph·a·ly (bath″ro·sef′uh·lee) n. A condition in which the skull has a shelflike projection at the squamosal suture of the occipital bone.

bathy·car·dia (bath″i·kahr′dee·uh) n. An anatomic variant in which the heart is in a lower position than usual within the thorax.

ba·tra·chi·an (ba·tray′kee·un) adj. Frog-like.

Bat·son's plexus. VERTEBRAL VENOUS SYSTEM.

bat·ta·rism (bat′uh·riz·um) n. Battarismus; stammering.

bat·ta·ris·mus (bat″uh·riz′mus) n. Stammering.

bat·tered-child syndrome. A clinical condition in young children due to serious physical abuse, generally from a parent or foster parent, and a significant cause of childhood disability and death.

bat·tery, n. 1. A device which converts chemical to electrical energy. 2. A series of two or more pieces of apparatus connected so as to augment their effects, as a battery of boilers, prisms, or galvanic cells. 3. A group or series of things or procedures used similarly or for common purpose, as tests given to a subject for the purpose of diagnosis of disease or of psychological analysis. 4. The unlawful beating of another.

·a·u·ru ulcer (bah·oo·roo′) A skin ulcer occurring in American mucocutaneous leishmaniasis.

baux·ite (bawk′site) n. A naturally occurring mixture of hydrous aluminum oxides and aluminum hydroxides; the principal source of aluminum.

bay·ber·ry (bay′bur·ee, ·ber·ee) n. The wax myrtle, Myrica cerifera or M. pennsylvanica. The dried bark of the root was formerly used as an astringent.

B cell. B LYMPHOCYTE.

BCG Abbreviation for (a) bacillus Calmette-Guérin; (b) ballistocardiogram or ballistocardiograph.

BCG vaccine A vaccine made from cultures of attenuated bovine tubercle bacilli, used to obtain immunity against tuberculosis.

b.d. Abbreviation for bis die, twice a day; used in prescriptions.

bead·ed, adj. 1. Having or formed into, beads. 2. In bacteriology, indicating the nonuniform appearance of certain organisms such as Corynebacterium diphtheriae when stained.

beading of the ribs. RACHITIC ROSARY.

beam, n. In radiology and radiobiology, a directed stream of particles, such as electrons or photons.

bear·ing down. 1. The feeling of weight or pressure in the pelvis in pregnancy and some diseases. 2. Contraction of abdominal muscles during labor, either as a reflex of uterine contractions or in a conscious effort to expel the fetus.

bearing-down pain. 1. A feeling of distress with a sensation of dragging of the pelvic organs; occurs in pelvic inflammatory disease. 2. (usually plural) Pains accompanying bearing down in labor.

beat, n. An impulse, throb, or pulsation, as of the heart and blood vessels.

be·bee·rine (be·bee′reen, ·rin) n. The d- form of an alkaloid, $C_{36}H_{38}N_2O_6$, from the root of Cissampelos pareira or from Ocotea rodioei (Nectandra). The l- form of the alkaloid is curine. Syn. chondodendrine, pelosine.

bed·bug, n. A blood-sucking wingless bug, Cimex lectularius, which lives and lays its eggs in the crevices of bedsteads, upholstered furniture, and walls. It is apparently not a vector of pathogenic organisms, although it has been suspected.

bed·fast, adj. BEDRIDDEN.

bed·pan, n. A shallow, suitably shaped receptacle, serving to receive the urine and feces of a person confined to bed.

bed·rid·den, adj. Confined to bed.

bed·sore, n. DECUBITUS ULCER.

bees·wax, n. Wax obtained from honeycombs.

be·hav·ior, be·hav·iour (be·hay′vyur) n. 1. The sum total of responses of an organism to internal and external stimuli; loosely, anything an organism does. 2. Observable activity directly correlated with psychic processes. —**behavior·al, behaviour·al** (·ul) adj.

be·hav·ior·ism, be·hav·iour·ism (be·hay′vyur·iz·um) n. A school of psychology, concerned with observable, tangible, and measurable data, such as behavior and human activities, but excluding ideas and emotions as purely subjective phenomena.

be·hav·ior·is·tic (be·hay″vyur·is′tick) *adj.* 1. Of or pertaining to behaviorism. 2. BEHAVIORAL.

behavior therapy. *In psychiatry,* an approach to the treatment of overt disturbed human behavior and emotions, regarded as evidence of faulty learning and as maladaptive and undesirable conditioned responses, by dealing with the symptoms themselves through extinguishing the undesirable conditioned responses and establishing desirable ones according to the principles of modern learning theory.

bej·el (bej′ul) *n.* An infectious nonvenereal treponemal disease, occurring principally in children in the Middle East; the infecting organism is undistinguishable from *Treponema pallidum.*

Bekh·te·rev-Men·del reflex (bekh′t³e·r³uf) 1. Plantar flexion of the toes in a patient with corticospinal tract disease, elicited by tapping or stroking the dorsum of the foot over the cuboid bone or the fourth or fifth metatarsals. A normal person exhibits slight dorsoflexion of the toes or no response. 2. CARPOPHALAN-GEAL REFLEX (1).

¹bel, *n.* A unit frequently used to measure the intensity of sound, commonly the intensity above the normal threshold of hearing.

²bel, *n.* The dried, half-ripe fruit of *Aegle marmelos,* or baelfruit of India. It has been used as a remedy for chronic diarrhea and dysentery. The ripe fruit is slightly laxative. Syn. *belae fructus,* Bengal quince.

bel·la·don·na (bel′uh·don′uh) *n.* Deadly nightshade. A perennial plant, *Atropa belladonna,* of the order Solanaceae, indigenous to southern Europe and Asia and cultivated in the United States. Its properties are due chiefly to its content of hyoscyamine, which under certain conditions is racemized to atropine. Both leaves and root are employed, in various dosage and application forms. It is used as an antispasmodic, as a cardiac and respiratory stimulant, to check secretions (such as sweat and milk), and as an anodyne.

bel·la·don·nine (bel′uh·don′een, ·in) *n.* An alkaloid, $C_{34}H_{42}N_2O_4$, found in solanaceous plants such as belladonna and hyoscyamus.

bel·lones (be·lohnz′) *n.* Partial nasal obstruction in horses due to polyps in the posterior nares and sometimes associated with roaring.

Bell's palsy or **paralysis** Peripheral paralysis or weakness of muscles innervated by the facial nerve, of unknown cause.

bel·ly, *n.* 1. The abdominal cavity or abdomen. 2. Of a muscle: the most prominent, fleshy, central portion.

belly of a muscle. The most prominent, fleshy, central portion of a muscle.

bel·o·ne·pho·bia (bel″o·ne·fo′bee·uh) *n.* A morbid dread of pins and needles, and of sharp-pointed objects in general.

Benadryl. Trademark for diphenhydramine, an antihistaminic agent used as the hydrochloride salt.

Bence Jones protein An abnormal protein, usually consisting of immunoglobulin light chains, found in the urine of some patients with myeloma.

bench surgery. Surgery performed on an organ (such as a kidney) that has been removed from the body, to be reimplanted immediately after the operation. Syn. *ex vivo surgery.*

Ben·der gestalt test A diagnostic and experimental psychological test in which the subject reproduces a series of nine simple designs. Deviations from the originals are interpreted in terms of gestalt laws of perception and organization; especially useful in the diagnosis of visual-motor deficits.

Bendopa. Trademark for levodopa, an antiparkinsonian agent.

Benedict's method 1. Glucose in the urine is estimated by titrating the urine with Benedict's quantitative reagent. 2. Sulfur in the urine is estimated by adding urine to Benedict's sulfur reagent. 3. A test for uric acid in which a tungstic acid blood filtrate is mixed with acid lithium chloride and silver nitrate.

Benedict's solution An easily reduced solution containing copper sulfate; used in urine tests for glucose and other reducing substances.

Benedict's test A qualitative test for glucose and other reducing sugars, the presence of which is established by reduction of a blue cupric salt in alkaline solution with formation of a green, yellow, or red precipitate. May also be performed quantitatively.

Be·ne·dikt's syndrome (bey′ne·dikt) Ipsilateral oculomotor paralysis and contralateral cerebellar ataxia, tremor, and corticospinal tract signs, caused by a lesion of the midbrain involving the oculomotor and red nuclei. Involvement of the cerebral peduncle causes contralateral hemiparesis, and extension to the medial lemniscus, contralateral loss of position and tactile sensation.

Benemid. Trademark for probenecid, a uricosuric agent.

be·nign (be·nine′) *adj.* Not malignant.

ben·ox·i·nate (ben·ock′si·nate) *n.* 2-Diethylaminoethyl 4-amino-3-butoxybenzoate $C_{17}H_{28}N_2O_3$, a surface anesthetic agent useful in ophthalmology; used as the hydrochloride salt.

ben·ton·ite (ben′tun·ite) *n.* A native, colloidal hydrated aluminum silicate. It swells in water and is useful in the preparation of pastes and lotions and as a suspending agent for insoluble medicaments in mixtures and emulsions.

benz-, benzo-. A combining form meaning (a) *benzene;* (b) *presence of the benzene ring.*

benz·al·de·hyde (ben·zal′de·hide) *n.* C_6H_5CHO A colorless liquid, used as a flavoring agent and in the synthesis of drugs or perfumes.

benz·al·ko·ni·um chloride (ben″zal·ko′nee·um) A mixture of alkyl dimethylbenzylammonium chlorides of the general formula $C_6H_5CH_2N(CH_3)_2RCl$, in which R represents a mixture of alkyl radicals from C_8H_{17} to $C_{18}H_{37}$. A white or yellowish white powder or in gelatinous pieces; soluble in water. It is an effective surface disinfectant which is germicidal for many pathogenic, nonsporulating bacteria and fungi.

benz·an·thra·cene (ben·zan′thruh·seen) *n.* 1,2

Benzanthracene, $C_{18}H_{12}$, a hydrocarbon occurring in coal tar which has carcinogenic activity.

ben·za·thine penicillin G (ben'zuh·theen). *N,N'-*Dibenzylethylenediamine dipenicillin G, a penicillin of low water solubility that yields effective blood levels of the antibiotic for a prolonged period after injection and is relatively stable in the stomach after oral administration.

Benzedrex. Trademark for propylhexedrine, a volatile sympathomimetic used by inhalation as a vasoconstrictor to relieve nasal congestion.

Benzedrine. A trademark for amphetamine, a central nervous system stimulant used mainly as the sulfate salt.

ben·zene (ben'zeen, ben·zeen') *n.* An aromatic hydrocarbon, C_6H_6, obtained chiefly as a by-product in the manufacture of coke. It is a clear, colorless, highly flammable liquid of characteristic odor, miscible with many organic liquids. It is extensively used as a solvent and in synthesis. Inhalation of its fumes may be toxic. Syn. *benzol.*

benzene hexachloride. The designation commonly, though incorrectly, applied to commerical mixtures of stereoisomers of 1,2,3,4,5,-6-hexachlorocyclohexane $(C_6H_6Cl_6)$, employed as insecticides. The gamma isomer, a purified grade of which is called lindane, is of greatest entomological and medical interest. Abbreviated, BHC.

benzene ring. The arrangement of atoms in benzene whereby six carbon atoms are joined in a hexagonal ring by a bonding structure which is a hybrid between single and double bonds.

ben·zes·trol (ben·zes'trol) *n.* 4,4'-(1,2-Diethyl-3-methyltrimethylene)diphenol, $C_{20}H_{26}O_2$, in the isomeric form having greatest estrogenic activity; orally effective as an estrogen.

ben·ze·tho·ni·um chloride (ben''ze·tho'nee·um). Benzyldimethyl {2-[2-(*p*-1,1,3,3-tetramethylbutylphenoxy)ethoxy]ethyl}ammonium chloride, $C_{27}H_{42}ClNO_2$, a local anti-infective cationic detergent employed as a germicide and antiseptic.

ben·zi·dine (ben'zi·deen) *n. p-*Diaminodiphenyl, $NH_2C_6H_4C_6H_4NH_2$, formerly used as a reagent for the detection of blood and in certain other tests depending on the presence of peroxidase. Generally replaced because of demonstrated carcinogenicity.

ben·zin, ben·zine (ben'zin, ben'zeen, ben·zeen') *n.* A mixture mainly of aliphatic hydrocarbons obtained in the fractional distillation of petroleum.

benzo-. See *benz-.*

ben·zo·ate (ben'zo·ate) *n.* Any salt or ester of benzoic acid, as sodium benzoate or ethyl benzoate.

ben·zo·caine (ben'zo·kane) *n.* ETHYL AMINOBENZOATE.

ben·zo·ic acid (ben·zo'ick). Benzenecarboxylic acid, C_6H_5COOH, white scales or needles; used as a preservative and mild antiseptic.

ben·zoin (ben'zoin, ·zo·in, ben·zo'in) *n.* A balsamic resin obtained from *Styrax benzoin, S. tonkinensis,* and other species of *Styrax.* It is used as a stimulating expectorant, as an inhalant in respiratory tract inflammations, and as an external antiseptic and protective. Syn. *gum benjamin, gum benzoin.* —**ben·zoi·nat·ed** (ben·zo'i·nay''tid) *adj.*

ben·zol, ben·zole (ben'zole) *n.* BENZENE.

ben·zo·yl (ben'zo·il, ·eel) *n.* The univalent radical C_6H_5CO, derived from benzoic acid.

benz·pyr·in·i·um bromide (benz''pye·rin'ee·um). 1-Benzyl-3-hydroxypyridinium bromide dimethylcarbamate, $C_{15}H_{17}BrN_2O_2$, a cholinergic agent having the actions and uses of neostigmine.

benz·tro·pine (benz·tro'peen) *n.* 3-Diphenylmethoxytropane, $C_{21}H_{25}NO$, a parasympatholytic drug with anticholinergic, antihistaminic, and local anesthetic activity; used as the mesylate (methanesulfonate) in the symptomatic treatment of parkinsonism.

benzyl alcohol. Phenylmethyl alcohol, $C_6H_5CH_2OH$, a colorless liquid; employed as a local anesthetic on mucous membranes and as a bacteriostatic agent. Syn. *phenylcarbinol.*

ber·ber·is (bur'bur·is) *n.* The dried rhizome and roots of various shrubs of the genus *Mahonia;* formerly used as a bitter tonic. The chief constituents are berberine and resin. Syn. *barberry.*

beri·beri (berr'ee·berr'ee) *n.* A disease of the heart and peripheral nerves, with or without edema (wet and dry forms); prevalent in the orient among people subsisting on a diet of polished rice and in the occident among alcoholics; due to nutritional deficiency, mainly of vitamin B_1 (thiamine).

Ber·ke·feld filter (behr'ke·felt) A filter, graded V (coarse), N (normal), and W (fine), of diatomaceous earth designed to retain bacteria and spores and to allow the recovery of viruses in the filtrate.

Bernard's granular layer The inner granular zone of the acinar cells of the pancreas.

Ber·noul·li's principle (Ger. behr·noo'lee, F. behr·noo·yee') The lateral pressure of a fluid passing through a tube of varying diameter is least at the most constricted part, where velocity is greatest, and is most at the widest part, where velocity is least.

berry aneurysm. A small, thin-walled aneurysm that protrudes from the arteries of the arterial circle of the cerebrum or its major branches, usually located at bifurcations and branches, and attributed to developmental defects in the media and elastica. Syn. *saccular aneurysm.*

Ber·til·lon system (behr·tee·yohn') A system for identifying persons by the use of selected measurements of various parts of the body; now largely superseded by the use of fingerprints.

be·ryl·li·o·sis (berr·il''ee·o'sis) *n.,* pl. **beryllio·ses**

(·seez) An acute pneumonia or a chronic granulomatous pneumoconiosis due to the inhalation of certain beryllium salts.

be·ryl·li·um (be·ril'ee·um) *n.* Be = 9.0122. A divalent metallic element occurring chiefly as beryllium aluminum silicate or beryl.

bes·ti·al·i·ty (bes''tee·al'i·tee) *n.* 1. Behavior resembling that of an animal. 2. Sexual relations between human beings and animals.

be·ta (bay'tuh, bee'tuh) *n.* The second of a series, or any particular member or subset of an arbitrarily ordered set; in chemistry, often combined with the name of a compound to indicate (1) the second of two isomers, or (2) the position of a substituent on the second carbon atom from a functional group. For many terms beginning with *beta-*, see under the specific noun. Symbol, β.

beta-adrenergic, β-adrenergic. Of or pertaining to a beta-adrenergic receptor.

beta-blocking, β-blocking. Having the properties of a beta-adrenergic blocking agent.

beta cells. 1. Cells in the pancreatic islets in which the cytoplasm contains alcohol-soluble granules. 2. Cells containing basophil granules in the adenohypophysis.

Betadine. Trademark for a complex of polyvinylpyrrolidone and iodine (povidone-iodine) used locally as an anti-infective agent.

beta globulin, β-globulin. Any of a group of serum globulins intermediate between alpha and gamma globulins in electrophoretic mobility, including globulins that function in the transport of lipids, carbohydrates, hormones, and iron, and a small fraction of antibodies or immunoglobulins.

beta hemolysis, β-hemolysis. Complete lysis of red blood cells around a colony on a blood agar medium, resulting in a clear zone around the colony.

beta-hemolytic, β-hemolytic. Causing beta hemolysis; said of various bacteria, especially certain streptococci.

beta-hemolytic streptococcal pharyngitis. Inflammation of the pharynx caused by *Streptococcus pyogenes*, Lancefield group A streptococci; a major cause of acute sore throat or exudative pharyngitis.

be·ta·ine (bay'tuh·een, ·in, be·tay'een, ·in) *n.* 1. Carboxymethyltrimethylammonium hydroxide anhydride, $(CH_3)_3NCH_2COO$; a crystalline substance occurring in sugar beets or prepared synthetically. It is an active methyl donor in the synthesis of choline and creatine, and may be useful in preventing hepatic cirrhosis; used as the hydrochloride salt. 2. Any one of a group of organic compounds in which the proton donor and acceptor sites are parts of the same molecule; considered as internal salts of quaternary ammonium bases. Syn. *lycine, oxyneurine, trimethylglycine.*

beta particle. In nuclear science, a radiation from certain radioactive materials, identical with the electron or its positively charged counterpart, the positron.

Betapen VK. A trademark for penicillin V potassium.

beta rays. Electrons emitted from certain radioactive elements.

beta streptococci. Streptococci belonging to 13 groups, A to O, each of which is distinguished by a specific carbohydrate, and which generally produce a complete hemolysis on blood agar. Group A streptococci are responsible for most streptococcal diseases of man.

be·ta·tron (bay'tuh·tron, bee'tuh·tron) *n.* An apparatus for accelerating electrons, by magnetic induction, to energies equivalent to millions of electron volts.

be·ta·zole (bay'tuh·zole) *n.* 3-(2-Aminoethyl)pyrazole, $C_5H_9N_3$, an analogue of histamine; used as the dihydrochloride salt in diagnostic tests of gastric secretion.

be·thane·chol chloride (be·thane'kole). Carbamylmethylcholine chloride, $C_7H_{17}ClN_2O_2$, a cholinergic drug not destroyed by cholinesterase.

be·tween·brain *n.* DIENCEPHALON.

Betz cell A giant pyramidal cell of the fifth layer of the motor cortex.

bev, BEV Abbreviation for *billion electron volts.*

bev·a·tron (bev'uh·tron) *n.* PROTON-SYNCHROTRON.

be·zoar (bee'zor, bee'zo·ur) *n.* A concretion found in the stomach or intestine of some animals, especially ruminants, most commonly composed of ingested hair; may form a cast of the stomach large enough to cause obstruction. Also found in some children and adults who pluck their own or a doll's hair and ingest it, usually a highly neurotic trait. Formerly believed to have magic medicinal properties.

bhang (bang, bahng) *n.* Stems and leaves of the hemp plant as used in India for infusion in beverages and for smoking; a form of cannabis comparable to marijuana.

Bi Symbol for bismuth.

bi- A prefix meaning (a) *two, twice, double;* (b) in anatomy, *connection with or relation to each o, two symmetrically paired parts;* (c) in chemistry, *presence of two atoms or equivalent (of a component) or presence (of thi component) in double the usual proportion or i double the proportion of the other componen*

biased sample. A sample that is no representative of its field.

bi·astig·ma·tism (bye''uh·stig'muh·tiz·um) *n.* A condition of the eye in which both corneal ane lenticular astigmatism exist, and are correcte separately by crossed cylinders.

bi·au·ric·u·lar (bye''aw·rick'yoo·lur) *adj.* Pertaining to both external ears.

bi·ax·i·al (bye·ack'see·ul) *adj.* Furnished wit two axes.

bi·bal·lism (bye·bal'iz·um) *n.* Ballism involvin the limbs on both sides, indicative of lesions i both subthalamic nuclei.

biblio- A combining form meaning *book.*

bib·li·o·klep·to·ma·nia (bib''lee·o·klep'to·ma nee·uh) *n.* A morbid desire to steal books.

bib·lio·ma·nia (bib''lee·o·may'nee·uh) *n.* A

abnormal or intense desire to collect books, especially curious and rare ones.

bib·lio·pho·bia (bib″lee·o·fo′bee·uh) n. A morbid fear or hatred of books.

bib·lio·ther·a·py (bib″lee·o·therr′uh·pee) n. 1. Reading, especially of books, in the treatment of mental disorders. 2. Generally, the reading of books for mental health.

bi·cap·i·tate (bye·kap′i·tate) adj. Having two heads; dicephalous.

bi·car·bon·ate (bye·kahr′buh·nate) n. A salt of carbonic acid characterized by the radical HCO_3.

bi·car·dio·gram (bye·kahr′dee·o·gram) n. The summated electrocardiogram yielded by the atria and ventricles beating normally; no longer in use.

bi·ceps (bye′seps) n., pl. **biceps·es** (·iz) A muscle having two heads, as the biceps brachii, the biceps femoris.

biceps jerk or reflex. Contraction of the biceps brachii muscle with flexion at the elbow when its tendon is struck.

bi·chlo·ride (bye·klo′ride) n. 1. Any compound containing two atoms of chlorine, especially a salt having two chloride atoms. 2. MERCURY BICHLORIDE.

bi·chro·mate (bye·kro′mate) n. DICHROMATE.

Bicillin. A trademark for benzathine penicillin G, an antibiotic.

bi·cip·i·tal (bye·sip′i·tul) adj. 1. Two-headed. 2. Pertaining to a muscle having two heads.

bi·con·cave (bye″kon′kave, ·kon·kave′) adj. Bounded by two concave surfaces.

bi·con·vex (bye″kon′vecks, ·kon·vecks′) adj. Bounded by two convex surfaces.

bi·cor·nu·ate (bye·kor′new·ate) adj. Having two horns.

bi·cus·pid (bye·kus′pid) adj. & n. 1. Having two cusps, as bicuspid teeth, or as the mitral valve of the heart. 2. A bicuspid tooth; in the human dentition, a premolar.

b.i.d. Abbreviation for bis in die; twice daily.

bi·dac·ty·ly (bye·dack′ti·lee) n. Congenital absence of all fingers or toes except the first and fifth. Syn. lobster-claw deformity.

Bielschowsky's sign In paresis of the superior oblique muscle of the eyeball, tilting the patient's head toward the side of the paralyzed eye produces hypertropia and increased vertical diplopia.

bi·fid (bye′fid) adj. Divided into two parts; cleft.

bifid uvula. CLEFT UVULA.

bi·fo·cal (bye·fo′kul) adj. Having two foci; applied to a system of lenses or spectacles.

bi·fo·cals, n. pl. 1. A pair of lenses for spectacles, each one having a part that corrects for distant vision and another that corrects for close vision. 2. The spectacles containing such lenses.

bi·fron·tal (bye·frun′tul) adj. Pertaining to both frontal bones, or both frontal lobes of the brain, or subdivisions thereof.

bi·fur·ca·tion (bye″fur·kay′shun) n. 1. Division into two branches. 2. The site of a division into two branches. —**bi·fur·cate** (bye′fur·kate) adj. & v.

bi·gem·i·nal (bye·jem′i·nul) adj. Occurring in pairs; double; twin.

bigeminal rhythm. An arrhythmia in which every alternate heartbeat occurs prematurely.

bi·gem·i·ny (bye·jem′i·nee) n. 1. The condition of occurring in pairs. 2. BIGEMINAL RHYTHM.

bi·is·chi·al (bye·is′kee·ul) adj. Pertaining to the two ischial tuberosities.

bi·labe (bye′labe) n. A surgical instrument for removing foreign bodies from the urinary bladder through the urethra.

bi·lam·i·nar (bye·lam′i·nur) adj. Formed of or having two layers.

bi·lat·er·al (bye·lat′ur·ul) adj. Pertaining to two sides; pertaining to or affecting both sides of the body. —**bilateral·ism** (·iz·um) n.; **bilateral·ly** (·ee) adv.

bilateral subtotal ablation of the frontal cortex. FRONTAL GYRECTOMY.

bile, n. A bitter, alkaline, greenish-yellow to golden-brown fluid, secreted by the liver and poured into the duodenum. It contains bile salts, cholesterol, lecithin, fat, various pigments, and mucin. Functionally, it aids in the emulsification, digestion, and absorption of fats and in the alkalinization of the intestines.

bile acid. Any one of the naturally occurring free acids of bile or those formed by the conjugation of glycine or taurine with a cholic acid, forming glycocholic and taurocholic acids, respectively.

bile duct. The cystic, hepatic, or common duct or any of the ducts of the liver connecting with the hepatic duct.

bile pigment. Any of the substances responsible for the color of bile, principally bilirubin and biliverdin, both derived from hemoglobin.

bil·har·zi·a·sis (bil″hahr·zye′uh·sis) n. SCHISTOSOMIASIS.

bili-. A combining form meaning (a) bile, biliary; (b) derived from bile.

bil·i·ary (bil′ee·air″ee) adj. 1. Of or pertaining to bile, or involving the bile duct or biliary tract. 2. Conveying bile.

biliary calculus. A solid mass formed within the biliary system, composed of bile salts, calcium, bilirubin, and cholesterol in various proportions.

biliary cirrhosis. Cirrhosis due to extrahepatic bile duct obstruction or chronic intrahepatic inflammatory disease with bile duct obstruction; clinical manifestations include jaundice, pruritus, hepatosplenomegaly, xanthomatosis, and steatorrhea.

biliary colic. Pain caused by the passage of a gallstone in the bile duct.

biliary stasis. Abnormal stagnation of bile flow in biliary capillaries and ducts.

biliary tract or tree. The entire hepatic duct system, including hepatic ducts, gallbladder, cystic duct, and common bile duct.

bil·i·cy·a·nin (bil″i·sigh′uh·nin) n. A blue pigment obtained by the interaction of an ammoniacal solution of bilirubin and zinc chloride.

bil·i·fla·vin (bil″i·flav′in, ·flay′vin, bye′li·) n. A

yellow coloring matter derivable from biliverdin.

bil·i·fus·cin (bil″i·fus′in) *n.* A normal fecal pigment (or possibly two isomeric substances) analogous to mesobilifuscin but having two vinyl groups in place of the two ethyl groups of mesobilifuscin.

bi·lig·u·late (bye·lig′yoo·late) *adj.* Formed like two tongues or having two tongue-like processes.

bil·i·hu·min (bil″i·hew′min) *n.* An insoluble residue left after treating gallstones with various solvents.

Bili-Labstix. A trademark for reagent strips employed in urinalysis.

bil·i·leu·kan (bil″i·lew′kan) *n.* A colorless precursor of bilifuscin.

bil·ious (bil′yus) *adj.* 1. Pertaining to bile. 2. Designating disorders arising from an excess of bile.

bil·ious·ness (bil′yus·nis) *n.* A symptom complex combining varying degrees of malaise, headache, bloating, and constipation; traditionally, but probably erroneously, attributed to disorders of biliary flow.

bil·i·pra·sin (bil″i·pray′sin) *n.* An intermediate bile pigment formed in the oxidation of bilirubin to biliverdin. Syn. *choleprasin.*

bil·i·pur·pu·rin (bil″i·pur′pew·rin) *n.* CHOLEHEMATIN.

bil·i·ru·bin (bil″i·roo′bin) *n.* $C_{33}H_{36}N_4O_6$. Orange-red crystals or powder. The principal pigment of bile, formed by reduction of biliverdin, normally present in feces and found in the urine in obstructive jaundice. It is insoluble in water.

bil·i·ru·bin·ate (bil″i·roo′bi·nate) *n.* A salt of bilirubin.

bil·i·ru·bi·ne·mia, bil·i·ru·bi·nae·mia (bil″i·roo″bi·nee′mee·uh) *n.* 1. The presence of bilirubin in the blood; jaundice. 2. HYPER-BILIRUBINEMIA.

bil·i·ru·bin·glo·bin (bil″i·roo′bin·glo″bin) *n.* A transitional stage in the production of bilirubin from hemoglobin. It is the substance which remains after the removal of iron from the hemoglobin.

bil·i·ru·bi·nu·ria (bil″i·roo·bi·new′ree·uh) *n.* The presence of bilirubin in the urine. Normally it occurs in small amounts and is increased in obstructive jaundice.

bil·i·uria (bil″i·yoo′ree·uh) *n.* The presence of bile salts in the urine.

bil·i·ver·din (bil″i·vur′din) *n.* $C_{33}H_{34}N_4O_6$; a dark-green bile pigment, formed in the body from hemoglobin, but largely reduced in the liver to bilirubin. Biliverdin may also be obtained by oxidizing bilirubin.

Billroth's operation 1. Pylorectomy with end-to-end anastomosis of the upper portion of the stomach to the duodenum. Syn. *Billroth I operation.* 2. Partial gastric resection, with closure of the duodenal stump and gastrojejunostomy. Syn. *Billroth II operation.*

bi·lo·bate (bye·lo′bate) *adj.* Having, or divided into, two lobes.

bi·lobed, *adj.* BILOBATE.

bi·loc·u·lar (bye·lock′yoo·lur) *adj.* Having two cells, compartments, or chambers.

bi·loc·u·late (bye·lock′yoo·late) *adj.* BILOCULAR.

bi·man·u·al (bye·man′yoo·ul) *adj.* Pertaining to or performed by both hands.

bimanual palpation. 1. Employment of two examining hands in physical examination. 2. *In gynecology,* the palpation of the pelvic organs with one hand on the lower abdomen and the fingers of the other hand inserted in the vagina or rectum.

bimanual version. Manipulation through the abdominal wall with one hand with the aid of one or more fingers of the other within the vagina.

bin- A combining form meaning (a) *two, two at a time;* (b) in chemistry, *bi-.*

bi·na·ry (bye′nuh·ree, bye′nerr·ee) *adj.* 1. Dichotomous; divided or dividing in two. 2. Containing or consisting of two components or things. 3. *In chemistry,* compounded of two elements. 4. *In anatomy,* separating into two branches or parts.

bi·na·sal (bye·nay′zul) *adj.* Pertaining to both nasal visual fields.

bin·au·ral (bin·aw′rul) *adj.* 1. Pertaining to or having two ears. 2. Involving the use of both ears.

bind, *v. In chemistry,* to unite with, as in the combination of two substances having affinity.

bind·er, *n.* 1. A wide bandage or girdle worn to support the abdomen or breasts after childbirth or operations, as an obstetric or abdominal binder. 2. A substance, such as gelatin or glucose, used to impart cohesiveness to the powdered ingredients of tablet formulations on compression.

Bi·net-Si·mon intelligence scale or test (bee·neh′ see·mohn″) A method of estimating the relative mental development of a child between 3 and 12 years of age and expressing it as an intelligence quotient, the mental age being divided by the chronological age. Originally devised for French children, it has been adapted to many cultures, such as the Stanford revision for the United States.

Bing-Neel syndrome Hyperglobulinemia and increased viscosity of the blood, with impairment of articulation through small cerebral and retinal vessels and manifestations of diffuse central nervous system disturbance.

bin·oc·u·lar (bi·nock′yoo·lur, bye·nock′) *adj. & n.* 1. Of or pertaining to both eyes or to the use of both eyes at once. 2. An instrument with two eyepieces for use with both eyes at once.

binocular accommodation. Simultaneous accommodation of both eyes.

binocular diplopia. The most common type of diplopia; due to a derangement of muscular balance of the two eyes; the images of an object are thrown upon noncorresponding points of the retina.

binocular loupe. A binocular magnifier consisting of a combination of lenses in an optical frame, worn like spectacles, providing depth perception.

bi·no·mi·al (bye-no'mee-ul) *n.* 1. A botanical or zoological name consisting of two terms, the first designating the genus, the second the species. 2. A mathematical expression consisting of two variable terms.

bi·nu·cle·at·ed (bye-new'klee-ay-tid) *adj.* Having two nuclei.

bio·acous·tics (bye"o-uh-koos'ticks) *n.* The scientific study of the sounds produced by and affecting living organisms, especially with regard to communicative function.

bio·as·say (bye"o-as'ay) *n.* A method of determining the potency of a substance by comparing its effects on living material quantitatively with those of a standard substance. Syn. *biological assay.*

bio·avail·abil·i·ty (bye"o-uh-vale"uh-bil'i-tee) *n.* PHYSIOLOGICAL AVAILABILITY.

bi·oc·cip·i·tal (bye-ock-sip'i-tul) *adj.* Pertaining to the right and left occipital lobes of the brain, or both occipital bones, or subdivisions thereof.

bio·chem·is·try (bye"o-kem'is-tree) *n.* The chemistry of living tissues or of life; physiological or biological chemistry. —**biochem·i·cal** (-i-kul) *adj.*

bio·cli·mat·ics (bye"o-klye-mat'icks) *n.* BIOCLIMATOLOGY.

bio·cli·ma·tol·o·gy (bye"o-klye"muh-tol'uh-jee) *n.* The study of the effect of climate on life.

bi·o·cy·tin (bye"o-sigh'tin) *n.* A complex of biotin and lysine occurring in yeast and possibly in other natural products.

bio·elec·tric·i·ty (bye"o-e-leck-tris'i-tee) *n.* Electric phenomena occurring in living tissues; effects of electric currents upon living tissues.

bio·en·er·get·ics (bye"o-en"ur-jet'icks) *n.* The science of the transformation of energy in biologic functions.

bio·eth·ics (bye"o-eth'icks, bye'o-eth-icks) *n.* The ethical principles, or the discipline formulating such principles, which govern the uses of biological and medical technology, especially as they bear directly on the treatment of human life.

bio·feed·back (bye"o-feed'back) *n.* The technique of providing an individual with ongoing sensory awareness of the state of one or more of his body processes, through such means as monitoring devices which produce visual displays or tones of varying pitch, in order to facilitate the exercise of conscious control over normally involuntary or unconscious body functions.

bio·fla·vo·noid (bye"o-flav'o-noid, -flay'vo-noid) *n.* Any flavone compound or derivative having biological or pharmacological activity, such as vitamin P.

bio·gen·e·sis (bye"o-jen'e-sis) *n.* 1. The doctrine that living things are produced only from living things. 2. Loosely, both ontogeny and phylogeny. —**bio·ge·net·ic** (-je-net'ick), **bi·og·e·nous** (bye-oj'e-nus) *adj.*

bio·haz·ard (bye'o-haz''urd) *n.* A biological hazard to life or health, especially one constituted by the presence of dangerous microorganisms, as in experimentation on genetic recombination.

bio·ki·net·ics (bye"o-ki-net'icks, -kigh-net'icks) *n.* The kinetics of life; the science of the movements of or within living organisms.

bi·o·log·ic (bye"uh-loj'ick) *adj. & n.* 1. Of or pertaining to biology or to living organisms and their products. 2. BIOLOGICAL (2).

bi·o·log·i·cal (bye"uh-loj'i-kul) *adj. & n.* 1. BIOLOGIC (1). 2. A product of biologic origin used in the diagnosis, prevention, or treatment of disease. Included are serums, vaccines, antitoxins, and antigens.

biological assay. BIOASSAY.

biological availability. The extent to which the active ingredient of a food, nutrient, or drug can be absorbed and made available to the body in a physiologic state. Syn. *physiologic availability.*

Biological Stain Commission. A nonprofit corporation organized by the several national scientific societies concerned with the quality of dyes available for staining and other biological purposes. The Commission's laboratory tests various dyes and issues certification labels authorized to be affixed to bottles containing dye from batches meeting Commission standards. Such dyes are designated as Certified or Commission Certified.

biological warfare. *In military medicine,* tactics and techniques of conducting warfare by use of biological agents.

biologic test. A precipitin test for blood, meat, and similar protein-containing substances.

bi·ol·o·gist (bye-ol'uh-jist) *n.* A person specializing in biology.

bi·ol·o·gy (bye-ol'uh-jee) *n.* The science of life, including microbiology, botany, zoology, and all their branches.

bio·lu·mi·nes·cence (bye"o-lew"mi-nes'unce) *n.* Luminescence caused by living organisms; PHOSPHORESCENCE (1).

bio·ma·te·ri·al (bye"o-muh-teer'ee-ul) *n.* 1. Any material employed in a prosthetic device, such as a skeletal component, heart valve, or pacemaker, which is implanted in or is otherwise in contact with the tissues of a living organism. 2. (pl. form, *biomaterials:*) The branch of applied science concerned with the selection and evaluation of such materials, especially from the standpoints of durability and degree of tolerance by host tissues.

bio·math·e·mat·ics (bye"o-math"e-mat'icks) *n.* Mathematics applied to or concerned with biologic phenomena.

bio·me·chan·ics (bye"o-me-kan'icks) *n.* 1. The mechanics of the living organism, especially of the levers and arches of the skeleton, and the forces applied to them by the muscles and by gravity. 2. The science in which physical and engineering principles are applied to biological systems such as the musculoskeletal, cardiovascular, or central nervous system.

bio·med·i·cal (bye"o-med'i-kul) *adj.* Pertaining to both biology and medicine.

biomedical engineering. The branch of

engineering that deals with the design of materials and machines used in medicine.

bi·o·met·rics (bye″o-met′ricks) n. BIOSTATISTICS.

bi·om·e·try (bye-om′e-tree) n. 1. BIOSTATISTICS. 2. Calculation of the expectancy of life, for life insurance purposes.

bio·mi·cros·co·py (bye″o-migh-kros′kuh-pee) n. Microscopic study of living cell structures. —**bio·mi·cro·scope** (·migh″kruh·scope) n.; **bio·mi·cro·scop·ic** (·migh″kro-skop′ick) adj.

bi·on·ics (bye-on′icks) n. The science concerned with developing electronic, mathematical, or physical models which simulate parallel phenomena found in living systems, as the vertebrate nervous system for cybernetic engineering.

bio·phar·ma·ceu·tics (bye″o-fahr-muh-sue′ticks) n. The study of the interrelationships of absorption, distribution, metabolism, storage, and excretion of drugs with the physicochemical properties of body tissues, drugs, and drug dosage forms.

bio·pho·tom·e·ter (bye″o-fo-tom′e-tur) n. An instrument designed to measure the rate and degree of dark adaptation.

bio·phys·ics (bye″o-fiz′icks) n. The physics of life processes. 2. Application of the methods of physics in biological studies.

bio·plasm (bye′o-plaz·um) n. Living protoplasmic substance, as distinguished from inclusions and by-products of protoplasmic activity. —**bio·plas·mic** (bye″o-plaz′mick) adj.

bi·op·sy (bye′op-see) n. & v. 1. The excision, for diagnostic study, of a piece of tissue from a living body. 2. The tissue so excised. 3. To perform a biopsy on.

bio·psy·chic (bye″o-sigh′kick) adj. Pertaining to mental phenomena as they apply to biology; pertaining or relating to the mind or thinking in life.

bi·or·bi·tal (bye-or′bi·tul) adj. Of or pertaining to both orbits.

bio·rhythm (bye′o-rith″um) n. Any regular, cyclic, biologically regulated pattern of change or fluctuation in an organism, such as the menstrual cycle or regular periodic variations in body temperature, blood pressure, or mood.

bi·ose (bye′oce) n. DISACCHARIDE.

-biosis A combining form meaning a (specified) way of life.

bio·sta·tis·tics (bye″o-sta-tis′ticks) n. 1. The application of statistical principles and methods in biology. 2. Specifically, statistical analysis of vital and demographic data.

bi·os·ter·ol (bye-os′tur·ol, -ole) n. VITAMIN A.

bio·syn·the·sis (bye″o-sin′thi-sis) n., pl. **biosynthe·ses** (·seez) 1. The synthesis of a substance in living matter. 2. The formative reactions which take place during metabolism, as of enzymes or amino acids. —**bio·syn·thet·ic** (·sin·thet′ick) adj.

bio·te·lem·e·try (bye″o-te·lem′e·tree) n. Telemetry in which the results of measurements of certain vital functions of a subject are transmitted electronically to a distant receiving station and there are indicated or recorded.

bi·o·tin (bye′o-tin, bye·ot′in) n. cis-Hexahydro-2-oxo-1H-thieno[3,4]imidazoline-4-valeric acid, $C_{10}H_{16}N_2O_3S$, a member of the vitamin B complex, present in small amounts in plant and animal tissues. It counteracts the injury syndrome caused by egg white; probably essential for man. Syn. vitamin H, coenzyme R, bios IIb.

bio·trans·for·ma·tion, n. The chemical changes that a compound, especially a drug, undergoes in a living system.

bio·type (bye′o-tipe) n. 1. A group of individuals all of which have the same genotype. 2. SOMATOTYPE. —**bio·typ·ic** (bye″o-tip′ick) adj.

bi·ovu·lar (bye-o′vyoo·lur) adj. Pertaining to or derived from two ova.

biovular twins. FRATERNAL TWINS.

bip·a·ra (bip′uh-ruh) n., pl. **biparas, bipa·rae** (·ree) A woman who has borne two children at different labors.

bi·pa·ri·etal (bye″puh-rye′e·tul) adj. 1. Pertaining to both parietal bones. 2. Pertaining to the right or left parietal lobes of the brain, or subdivisions thereof.

biparietal diameter. The distance from one parietal eminence to the other.

biparietal obliquity. ANTERIOR or POSTERIOR ASYNCLITISM.

bip·a·rous (bip′uh-rus) adj. 1. Producing two offspring at a birth. 2. Having given birth twice.

bi·par·tite (bye-pahr′tite) adj. Divided into, or consisting of, two parts or divisions.

bi·ped (bye′ped) n. An animal that normally walks and stands on two feet. —**bi·ped·al** (bye″ped′ul) adj.

bi·pen·nate (bye-pen′ate) adj. Having the appearance of a feather with barbs on both sides of the shaft, as certain muscles.

bi·po·lar (bye-po′lur) adj. 1. Having or involving two poles; specifically, having negative and positive poles or leads. 2. Pertaining to a neuron having an afferent and efferent process.

bi·po·lar·i·ty (bye″po-lăr′i·tee) n. 1. The condition of having two processes extending from opposite poles, as a nerve cell. 2. The use of two electrodes in stimulation of muscle or nerve, or in recording bioelectric potentials.

bipolar version. Manipulation of both the pelvis and the vertex of the fetus.

bipp, n. A dressing for wounds, composed of bismuth subnitrate 1 part, iodoform 2 parts, petrolatum 1 part. Syn. bismuth iodoform paste.

bird-breeder's lung. A pulmonary hypersensitivity reaction to antigens in bird excreta, characterized by cough, fever, dyspnea, and weight loss; seen usually in pigeon and parakeet (budgerigar) fanciers.

bird-headed dwarfism. A congenital disorder, possibly due to various causes, characterized by low birth weight, marked but proportionate shortness of stature, a proportionately small head, hypoplasia of the maxilla and mandible with beak-like protrusion of the nose, mental retardation, and a variety of other skeletal, cutaneous, and genital anomalies. Syn. *Seckel's syndrome.*

bi·re·frin·gence (bye″re·frin′junce) *n.* The property of having more than one refractive index, according to the direction of the traversing light. It is possessed by all except isometric crystals, by transparent substances that have undergone internal strains (e.g., glass), and by substances that have different structures in different directions (e.g., fibers). Syn. *double refraction.* —**birefrin·gent** (·junt) *adj.*

birth, *n.* In viviparous species, the offspring's emergence from the womb of the mother.

birth certificate. A legal form on which the date and place of birth, name and sex of child, names of parents, and other pertinent information are recorded.

birth control. Any means used to help control reproduction, such as methods of facilitating, timing, or preventing conception, sexual abstinence or alternatives, abortion, sterilization, and artificial insemination.

birth injury. Any injury suffered by a neonate during parturition, such as fracture of a bone, subluxation of a joint, injury to peripheral nerves, or intracranial hemorrhage.

birth·mark, *n.* A congenital skin lesion, usually either a vascular hamartoma or pigmented nevus, but possibly of another nature.

birth palsy or **paralysis.** 1. Any paralysis due to injury sustained during birth. 2. CEREBRAL PALSY. 3. BRACHIAL BIRTH PALSY.

birth rate. The proportion of births in a given year and area to the midyear population of that area, usually expressed as the number of live births per thousand of population.

birth registration area. The territory from which the United States Bureau of the Census collects birth records. Since 1933, this has been the entire United States.

birth trauma. 1. *In psychiatry,* the hypothesis which relates the development of anxiety and neurosis to the universal psychic shock of being born. 2. BIRTH INJURY.

bis- A prefix meaning (a) *twice, both;* (b) in chemistry, *the doubling of a complex expression.*

bi·sect (bye·sekt′) *v.* To cut into two roughly equal parts.

bi·sex·u·al (bye·seck′shoo·ul) *adj.* 1. Exhibiting both homosexual and heterosexual behavior, or attracted sexually to both males or females. 2. HERMAPHRODITIC.

bis·fer·i·ous (bis·ferr′ee·us, bis·feer′) *adj.* Having two peaks or beats.

bis·hy·droxy·cou·ma·rin (bis″high·drock″see· koo′muh·rin) *n.* 3,3′-Methylenebis(4-hydroxycoumarin), $C_{19}H_{12}O_6$, originally isolated from spoiled sweet clover, eating of which caused hemorrhagic disease in cattle. It occurs as a white crystalline powder, practically insoluble in water; used as an anticoagulant. Syn. *dicoumarin, dicoumarol, melitoxin.*

bis·muth (biz′muth) *n.* Bi = 208.980. A white, crystalline metal with a reddish tint. Its insoluble salts are employed chiefly because of their protective action on mucous membranes; the salts are also feebly antiseptic. Various compounds of bismuth, soluble and insoluble, have been employed for the treatment of syphilis.

bismuth and emetine iodide. A reddish-orange salt, practically insoluble in water; used in the treatment of amebic colitis.

bis·muth·o·sis (biz″muth·o′sis) *n.* Chronic bismuth poisoning.

bismuth potassium tartrate. A water-soluble salt containing 60 to 64% bismuth; has been used as an antisyphilitic, by intramuscular injection.

bismuth sodium tartrate. A water-soluble salt formerly used as an antisyphilitic.

bismuth subcarbonate. Approximately $2(BiO)_2CO_3.H_2O$; a white salt, insoluble in water; used as a protective in gastrointestinal diseases as well as for local application.

bismuth subgallate. Approximately $C_6H_2(OH)_3COOBi(OH)_2$; a bright yellow powder, practically insoluble in water. Has been used externally as a dusting powder, sometimes internally in treating enteritis. Syn. *dermatol.*

bismuth subnitrate. Approximately $4BiNO_3(OH)_2.BiO(OH)$; a white powder, practically insoluble in water. Used like bismuth subcarbonate but yields some nitrite ion in the intestines.

bismuth subsalicylate. Approximately $C_6H_4(OH)COOBiO$; a white powder, practically insoluble in water. Its antiseptic action is superior to that of other basic bismuth salts. Used in the treatment of enteritis, and has been used as an antisyphilitic.

bis·muth·yl (biz′muth·il, ·eel) *n.* The univalent radical BiO.

bi·spi·nous diameter (bye·spye′nus). The distance between the spines of the ischia.

bis·tou·ry (bis′too·ree) *n.* A long, narrow knife, either straight or curved and sharp-pointed or probe-pointed, designed for cutting from within outward; formerly used to open abscesses, enlarge sinuses or fistulas, or cut constrictions in strangulated hernias.

bi·sul·fide (bye·sul′fide, ·fid) *n.* A binary compound containing two atoms of sulfur. Syn. *disulfide.*

bi·sul·fite (bye·sul′fite) *n.* Any compound containing the radical HSO_3; an acid sulfite.

bi·tar·trate (bye·tahr′trate) *n.* A salt of tartaric acid characterized by the radical $HC_4H_4O_6$, representing tartaric acid wherein one hydrogen has been replaced. Syn. *acid tartrate.*

bite, *v. & n.* 1. To seize or grasp with the teeth or to puncture with the mouthparts. 2. The forcible closure of the lower against the upper teeth; the measure of force exerted by such closure as recorded in pounds by a gnathodynamometer. 3. A skin puncture produced by the teeth or mouth parts of an insect or animal. 4. INTEROCCLUSAL RECORD.

bite block. 1. A device used to hold the jaws open while operating in or through the oral cavity. 2. A device used to hold a film in position in intraoral radiography. 3. OCCLUSION RIM.

bite guard. An appliance worn on the teeth to relieve excessive occlusal forces; usually used in the treatment of bruxism or occlusal trauma.

bi·tem·po·ral (bye·tem'pur·ul) adj. 1. Pertaining to both temples. 2. Pertaining to both temporal lobes of the brain, or both temporal bones, or subdivisions thereof. 3. Pertaining to both temporal fields of vision.

bite plate. OCCLUSION RIM.

bite·wing, n. A type of dental x-ray film having a central fin or wing upon which the teeth can close to hold the film in place.

bi·thi·o·nol (bye·thigh'o·nol) n. 2,2'-Thiobis(4,6-dichlorophenol), $C_{12}H_6Cl_4O_2S$, a crystalline powder, insoluble in water. Has been used as bacteriostatic agent in soap formulations.

bit·ters, n. A medicinal substance used for its bitter taste, chiefly to increase appetite or as a tonic.

Bitt·ner milk factor. MILK FACTOR.

bi·tu·men (bi·tew'mun, bye·, bit'yoo·mun) n. Any one of a group of native solid or semisolid hydrocarbons.

bi·urate (bye·yoo'rate) n. An acid salt of uric acid.

bi·u·ret (bye''yoo·ret', bye'yoo·ret) n. Carbamylurea, $NH_2CONHCONH_2$, obtained by heating urea.

biuret reaction. A reaction given by compounds which contain acid amide groups in close proximity, as by biuret or by proteins. A red-violet to blue-violet color is produced on adding a cupric sulfate solution to an alkaline solution of the specimen.

bi·va·lent (bye·vay'lunt, biv'uh·lunt) adj. & n. 1. Able to combine with or displace two atoms of hydrogen or their equivalent; having a valence of 2. Syn. *divalent.* 2. Double or paired. 3. AMBIVALENT. 4. BIVALENT CHROMOSOME.

bivalent chromosome. A structure formed by the association of homologous chromosomes in the zygotene and pachytene stages of meiosis and serving as source of the tetrad in diplotene.

bi·valve (bye'valv) n. & v. 1. A mollusk with double shells, as a clam or oyster. 2. To section a solid organ incompletely, as if opening a clam or oyster. —**bi·val·vu·lar** (·val'vew·lur) adj.

bi·ven·ter (bye·ven'tur) n. & L adj. 1. DIGASTRIC MUSCLE. 2. Having two bellies, as a muscle; DIGASTRIC. —**bi·ven·tral,** adj.

bi·ven·tric·u·lar (bye''ven·trick'yoo·lur) adj. Involving both cardiac ventricles.

bi·zy·go·mat·ic (bye·zye''go·mat'ick) adj. Of or pertaining to the two zygomatic bones.

black cancer. A malignant melanoma.

black·damp, n. A mixture of carbon dioxide and other gases which collects in mines and deep shafts; it supports neither respiration nor combustion. Syn. *chokedamp.*

Black Death. BLACK PLAGUE.

black, hairy tongue. A tongue with a brown, furlike patch on the dorsum, due to hypertrophied filiform papillae and the presence of pigment.

black·head, n. 1. COMEDO. 2. HISTOMONIASIS, a disease of poultry sometimes marked by a cyanotic condition of the head.

black jaundice. An extreme degree of jaundice; specifically, septicemia with acute hemolytic anemia and hemoglobinuria of the newborn.

black·leg, n. A febrile, generally fatal, infectious disease of cattle and sheep, characterized by diffuse, crepitating swelling in the muscles of the back and legs, usually caused by *Clostridium chauvei,* but sometimes by *C. septicum* or *C. novyi.* Syn. *black quarter, emphysematous gangrene.*

black measles. HEMORRHAGIC MEASLES.

black·out, n. 1. Temporary loss or diminution of vision and consciousness produced by transient cerebral and retinal ischemia; in aviation, it usually results from strong acceleration in a plane parallel with the long axis of the body. 2. A period during which the patient demonstrates no memory upon detoxication.

black plague. A form of plague, epidemic in Europe and Asia in the 14th century; so called because of extensive skin hemorrhages.

black·tongue, n. A disease of dogs similar to pellagra, due to a deficiency of niacin.

black vomit. Dark vomited matter, consisting of digested blood and gastric contents.

black·wa·ter fever. A complication of falciparum malaria, characterized by intravascular hemolysis, hemoglobinuria, tachycardia, high fever, and a poor prognosis.

black widow. *Latrodectus mactans,* a poisonous black spider with some red or yellow markings, found in most warm parts of the world. Its bite has been fatal in about 5 per cent of the reported cases. The body of the female is about half an inch long and, in the usual North American varieties, has a red hourglass figure on the underside of its globose abdomen. The male is smaller and does not bite.

blad·der, n. 1. A membranous sac serving for the reception of fluids or gases, as the swim bladder of some fishes. 2. A hollow organ which serves as a reservoir for urine or bile, as the urinary bladder or gallbladder.

bladder bar. BAR OF THE BLADDER.

bladder diverticulum. A congenital or acquired outpouching of the urinary bladder wall, lacking a normal complement of bladder muscle.

bladder training. Establishing the control of urination as a habit during infancy or early childhood.

Blake·more's tube A specially designed, triple-lumened tube, with sausage-shaped balloon tip, used to control acute hemorrhage from esophageal varices by tamponage.

Blalock-Taussig operation A surgical anastomosis between the subclavian artery and pulmonary artery, designed to circumvent pulmonary stenosis and increase pulmonary blood flow; used primarily in palliation of tetralogy of Fallot.

bland, *adj.* 1. Smooth or soothing. 2. Not irritating. 3. Not infected.

bland diet. A diet free of roughage, spices, or other irritating ingredients.

bland infarct. An infarct free from infection.

blast-, blasto- A combining form meaning (a) *bud;* (b) *budding;* (c) *germ;* (d) *the early stages of the embryo.*

-blast A combining form meaning (a) *a sprout, shoot,* or *germ;* (b) in biology, *a formative cell, a germ layer,* or *a formative constituent of living matter.*

blast cell The least differentiated member of a line of blood-forming elements which can be clearly identified as a member of that line.

blas·te·ma (blas-tee'muh) *n.,* pl. **blastemas, blastema·ta** (·tuh) 1. The formative cellular matrix from which an organ, tissue, or part is derived; ANLAGE (1). 2. A small bud of competent cells from which begins the regeneration of an organ or appendage. 3. The budding or sprouting part of a plant. 4. The hypothetical formative lymph or fluid from which cells or organs are formed. **—blas·te·mal** (·mul), **blas·te·mat·ic** (·te-mat'ick), **blas·tem·ic** (blas·tem'ick) *adj.*

blast injury or **syndrome.** Trauma to the viscera and to the central nervous system caused by rapid changes in the environmental pressure, as in bomb explosions; usually manifested by pulmonary hemorrhage, intestinal rupture, rupture of the eardrums, and shock. The brain and meninges may show diffuse and focal hemorrhages.

blastocele. BLASTOCOELE.

blas·to·coele, blas·to·coel (blas'to-seel) *n.* The central cavity of the blastula or blastocyst.

blas·to·cyst (blas'to-sist) *n.* 1. BLASTULA. 2. The modified mammalian blastula consisting of trophoblast, inner cell mass, and blastocoele.

blas·to·derm (blas'to-durm) *n. In embryology:* 1. The cellular disk of blastomeres derived from the blastodisk of meroblastic ova. 2. The primitive germ layer or epithelium of a blastula or blastocyst from which the primary germ layers are formed. 3. By extension, the germinal membrane after the formation of the several germ layers. **—blas·to·der·mal** (blas''to-dur'mul), **blastoder·mic** (·mick) *adj.*

blas·to·disk, blas·to·disc (blas'to-disk) *n.* 1. The uncleaved cytoplasmic disk capping the embryonic pole of meroblastic ova. 2. The embryonic or germinal disk of mammals.

blas·to·gen·e·sis (blas''to-jen'e-sis) *n.,* pl. **blastogene·ses** (·seez) 1. The early development of the embryo during cleavage and the formation of the germ layers. 2. Weismann's theory of origin and development from germ plasm, in contradistinction to pangenesis, as postulated by Darwin. 3. Reproduction by budding. **—blastogen·ic** (·ick), **blasto·ge·net·ic** (·je·net' ick) *adj.*

blas·to·ma (blas-to'muh) *n.,* pl. **blastomas, blastoma·ta** (·tuh) A tumor whose parenchymal cells have certain embryonal characteristics, as fibroblastoma or

chondroma. **—blas·tom·a·tous** (·tom'uh·tus) *adj.*

blas·to·mere (blas'to-meer) *n.* Any one of the cells into which the fertilized ovum divides. Syn. *cleavage cell, segmentation cell.*

Blas·to·my·ces (blas''to-migh'seez) *n.* A genus of fungi pathogenic to man.

Blastomyces der·ma·ti·ti·dis (dur''ma·tit'i·dis). A species of fungus that is the causative agent of North American blastomycosis. The organism is spheroid and budding in tissues; it produces aerial hyphae in culture.

Blas·to·my·ce·tes (blas''to·migh·seet'eez) *n.pl.* A group of pathogenic fungi which includes the genus *Blastomyces.*

blas·to·my·co·sis (blas''to-migh·ko'sis) *n.,* pl. **blastomyco·ses** (·seez) Any disease caused by yeast-like fungi, especially species of *Blastomyces.*

blas·to·pore (blas'to-pore) *n.* The external opening of the archenteron in a gastrula. The avian and mammalian primitive streaks have been regarded by some as closed blastopores; hence the primitive pit, or the opening into the notochordal canal, may be considered a remnant of a blastopore. **—blas·to·por·ic** (blas''to·por'ick) *adj.*

blas·tu·la (blas'tew·luh) *n.,* pl. **blastulas, blastu·lae** (·lee) A spherical mass consisting of a central cavity surrounded by a single layer of cells produced by the cleavage of the ovum; frequently modified by the presence of yolk. **—blastu·lar** (·lur) *adj.;* **blas·tu·la·tion** (blas''tew·lay'shun) *n.*

Bla·tel·la (bla·tel'uh) *n.* A genus of cockroaches.

Blat·ta (blat'uh) *n.* A genus of cockroaches of the family Blattidae. The species *B. orientalis,* the oriental cockroach, has been incriminated as an intermediate host of *Hymenolepis diminuta.*

BLB mask. BOOTHBY-LOVELACE-BULBULIAN MASK.

bleb, *n.* A localized collection of fluid, as serum or blood, in the epidermis.

bleed, *v.* 1. To lose blood from a blood vessel, either to the outside or the inside of the body. 2. To draw blood from a person.

bleed·er, *n.* 1. A person subject to frequent hemorrhages, as a hemophiliac. 2. A blood vessel which has escaped closure by cautery or ligature during a surgical procedure. 3. A blood vessel from which there is persistent uncontrolled bleeding.

bleed·ing, *n.* 1. The escape of blood from the vessels. 2. PHLEBOTOMY.

bleeding time. The time required for bleeding to cease from a puncture wound, usually of the ear lobe or ball of the finger, under standardized conditions. The normal value varies with the method.

blenn-, blenno- A combining form meaning *mucus, mucous.*

blen·noph·thal·mia (blen''off·thal'mee·uh) *n.* CATARRHAL CONJUNCTIVITIS.

blen·nor·rha·gia (blen''o·ray'jee·uh) *n.* 1. An excessive mucous discharge. 2. GONORRHEA.

blen·nor·rhea, blen·nor·rhoea (blen''o·ree'uh) *n.* BLENNORRHAGIA. **—blennor·rhe·al, blen·nor·rhoe·al** (·ree'ul) *adj.*

blephar-, blepharo- A combining form meaning *eyelid*.

bleph·ar·ad·e·ni·tis (blef″ur·ad″e·nigh′tis) *n.* Inflammation of the tarsal glands.

bleph·a·ral (blef′uh·rul) *adj.* Pertaining to the eyelids.

bleph·a·rec·to·my (blef″uh·reck′tuh·mee) *n.* Excision of a part or the whole of an eyelid.

bleph·ar·ede·ma (blef″ur·e·dee′muh) *n.* Swelling or edema of the eyelids.

bleph·a·re·lo·sis (blef″uh·re·lo′sis) *n.*, *pl.* **blepharelo·ses** (·seez) ENTROPION.

bleph·a·rism (blef′uh·riz·um) *n.* Spasm of the eyelids causing rapid repetitive involuntary winking.

bleph·a·ri·tis (blef″uh·rye′tis) *n.*, *pl.* **blepha·rit·i·des** (·rit′i·deez) Inflammation of the eyelids.

blepharo-. *See blephar-.*

bleph·a·ro·ad·e·no·ma (blef″uh·ro·ad″e·no′muh) *n. Obsol.* An adenoma of the eyelid.

bleph·a·ro·ath·er·o·ma (blef″uh·ro·ath″ur·o′muh) *n.* A sebaceous, epidermal, or dermoid cyst of the eyelid.

bleph·a·ro·blen·nor·rhea, bleph·a·ro·blen·nor·rhoea (blef″uh·ro·blen′o·ree·uh) *n.* Conjunctivitis with a purulent discharge.

bleph·a·ro·chal·a·sis (blef″uh·ro·kal′uh·sis) *n.* A redundance of the skin of the eyelids, seen in both sexes under the age of 20. Starting with an intermittent, painless angioneurotic edema and redness, repeated attacks result in loss of skin elasticity, subcutaneous atrophy, and capillary proliferation.

bleph·a·ro·chrom·hi·dro·sis (blef″uh·ro·krome″hi·dro′sis) *n.* Colored sweat of the eyelids, usually of a bluish tint.

bleph·a·roc·lo·nus (blef″uh·rock′lo·nus) *n.* Intermittent spasm, often merely fasciculation, of the orbicularis oculi muscle, especially the lower lid.

bleph·a·ro·con·junc·ti·vi·tis (blef″uh·ro·kun·junk″ti·vye′tis) *n.* Inflammation of both the eyelids and the conjunctiva.

bleph·a·ro·di·as·ta·sis (blef″uh·ro·dye·as′tuh·sis) *n.* Excessive separation of the eyelids; inability to close the eyelids completely.

bleph·a·ron (blef′uh·ron) *n.*, *pl.* **blepha·ra** (·ruh) EYELID.

bleph·a·ron·cus (blef″uh·ronk′us) *n.* A tumor or swelling of the eyelid.

bleph·a·ro·pa·chyn·sis (blef″uh·ro·pa·kin′sis) *n.* Abnormal thickening of the eyelid.

bleph·a·ro·phi·mo·sis (blef″uh·ro·figh·mo′sis) *n.* A rare condition characterized by diminution of both dimensions of the palpebral fissure; may be congenital or acquired.

bleph·a·roph·ry·plas·ty (blef″uh·rof′ri·plas″tee) *n.* Plastic surgery of the eyebrow and eyelid. —**blepha·roph·ry·plas·tic** (·rof″ri·plas′tick) *adj.*

bleph·a·ro·plast (blef′uh·ro·plast) *n.* 1. A basal body from which a cilium or flagellum grows. 2. A centriole which forms such basal bodies.

bleph·a·ro·plas·ty (blef′uh·ro·plas″tee) *n.* An operation for the restoration of any part of the eyelid. —**bleph·a·ro·plas·tic** (·blef″uh·ro·plas′tick) *adj.*

bleph·a·ro·ple·gia (blef″uh·ro·plee′jee·uh) *n.* Paralysis of an eyelid.

bleph·a·rop·to·sis (blef″uh·rop·to′sis) *n.* Ptosis of the upper eyelid.

bleph·a·ro·py·or·rhea, bleph·a·ro·py·or·rhoea (blef″uh·ro·pye·o·ree′uh) *n.* A flow of pus from the eyelid.

bleph·a·ro·rrha·phy (blef″uh·ror′uh·fee) *n.* Repair by suturing of a cut or lacerated eyelid.

bleph·a·ro·spasm (blef′uh·ro·spaz·um) *n.* Spasm of the orbicularis oculi muscle; in particular, tonic or persistent spasm as is present with foreign bodies or inflammatory conditions of the eye; occasionally psychogenic.

bleph·a·ro·sphinc·ter·ec·to·my (blef″uh·ro·sfink″tur·eck′tuh·mee) *n.* An operation to lessen the pressure of the upper lid upon the cornea.

bleph·a·ro·stat (blef′uh·ro·stat) *n.* An instrument for holding the eyelids apart during operations upon the eyes or lids.

bleph·a·ro·ste·no·sis (blef″uh·ro·ste·no′sis) *n.* BLEPHAROPHIMOSIS.

bleph·a·ro·syn·ech·ia (blef″uh·ro·si·neck′ee·uh, ·si·nee′kee·uh, ·sin″e·kigh′uh) *n.*, *pl.* **blepharosynech·i·ae** (·ee·ee) Adhesion or growing together of the eyelids.

bleph·a·rot·o·my (blef″uh·rot′uh·mee) *n.* Incision into the eyelid.

-blepsia A combining form meaning *a condition of sight or vision.*

blight, *n.* A fungus disease of plants.

blind fistula. A type of fistula which has only one opening, externally on the skin or internally upon the mucosal surface.

blind gut. CECUM.

blind headache. MIGRAINE.

blind-loop syndrome. The existence of bypassed segments or diverticula in the small intestine, postsurgical or congenital in origin, resulting in stasis, abnormal bacterial flora, diarrhea, weight loss, multiple vitamin deficiency, and megaloblastic anemia.

blind·ness, *n.* Loss or absence of vision; inability to see.

blind spot. The physiologic scotoma in the visual field, temporal to the fixation point, representing the entrance of the optic nerve, where the rods and cones are absent. Syn. *Mariotte's blind spot, punctum cecum.*

blink *v. & n.* 1. To close and open the eyes quickly; may be voluntary, spontaneous, of central origin, or a reflex response. 2. A single quick closure and opening of the eyes.

blink reflex or response. Involuntary blinking of both eyes in response to almost any stimulus about the face that suddenly compresses the muscle or underlying bone.

blis·ter, *n. & v.* 1. A vesicle resulting from the exudation of serous fluid between the epidermis and dermis. 2. The agent by which the blister is produced. 3. To cause a blister to be formed.

blister gas. *In military medicine,* a gas or finely dispersed liquid used for casualty effect; it injures the eyes and lungs and blisters the skin.

bloat, *n.* 1. Puffiness; swelling; distention; edema; turgidity from any cause. 2. *In veterinary medicine,* an abnormal accumulation of gas in the stomach or intestines, resulting in distention of the abdomen. Syn. *wind colic, tympany.*

block, *n.* 1. Any obstruction of a passage or opening. 2. Any form of interference with the normal propagation of an impulse, as in heart or nerve block or regional anesthesia. 3. *In histology,* a paraffin or celloidin mass in which a slice of tissue is embedded to facilitate the cutting of thin sections by a microtome. 4. *In psychiatry,* BLOCKING.

block anesthesia. Anesthesia produced by injecting an anesthetic solution into the nerve trunks supplying the operative field, or infiltrating close to the nerves, or by a wall of anesthetic solution injected about the field so that painful impulses will not reach the brain.

block·ing, *n.* 1. Interference with the propagation of nerve currents in a given direction. 2. *In psychiatry,* a sudden difficulty in remembering or an interruption of a train of thought, sometimes followed by an abrupt change of subject; usually due to unconscious emotional factors. 3. The cutting of tissue and organ specimens into pieces of proper size for histologic study. 4. The fastening of embedded histologic specimens onto an apparatus for microtome processing.

blood, *n.* The fluid tissue which circulates through the heart, arteries, capillaries, and veins, supplies oxygen and nutrients to the other tissues of the body, and removes from them carbon dioxide and waste products of metabolism. It is made up of plasma and cellular elements. The latter consists of erythrocytes, leukocytes, and blood platelets. Comb. form *hem(o)-, hemat(o)-.*

blood agar. A solid culture medium containing agar and blood, used for growing certain organisms.

blood bank. An organization or facility which procures, and stores under refrigeration, whole blood kept fluid by anticoagulants. In addition, blood banks usually recruit blood donors, bleed them, test donor and recipient for immunologic compatibility, provide one or more components of blood, and in some cases, infuse blood.

blood blister. A blister that contains blood.

blood-brain barrier. The functional barrier between the brain capillaries and the brain tissue which allows some substances from the blood to enter the brain rapidly while other substances either enter slowly or not at all.

blood cell. Any of the cells or corpuscles that constitute elements of the circulating blood; an erythrocyte or a leukocyte.

blood clot. A semisolid gel resulting from polymerization of fibrin and which may contain other blood elements trapped in fibrin network.

blood-clotting factor. COAGULATION FACTOR.

blood count. The determination of the number of erythrocytes or leukocytes per cubic millimeter of blood.

blood culture. The inoculation of microbiologic media with blood for the isolation and identification of microorganisms.

blood dop·ing. The withdrawal, preservation, and subsequent infusion of one's own blood after the original loss has been made up by the body; occasionally done by athletes on the assumption that it will augment the oxygen-carrying capacity of the blood by increasing the red cell mass above normal.

blood dyscrasia. Any abnormal condition of the formed elements of blood or of the constituents required for clotting.

blood fluke. Any of various flukes that inhabit the circulatory system of man or animals.

blood grouping. Determination of an individual's blood group by laboratory tests; blood typing.

blood groups. Immunologically distinct, genetically determined classes of human erythrocytes, depending on specific antigens (agglutinogens) in the erythrocytes for which the groups are named, and antibodies (agglutinins) in the serum. When incompatible bloods are mixed, agglutination results, which may be followed by hemolysis. Blood groups are of great importance in blood transfusions, hemolytic disease of the newborn (erythroblastosis fetalis), in medicolegal problems, anthropology, and genetics. In a broader sense, may include immunological inherited differences in leukocytes, platelets, hemoglobins, haptoglobins, and Gm serum groups. In the Standard or Universal grouping (Landsteiner's), the isoagglutinogens, A and B, can be lacking, or one or both be present in a given individual; the serum contains those isoagglutinins (anti-A or α, anti-B or β antibodies) which react upon the isoagglutinogens not present in the individual's erythrocytes. Thus:

Antigens on cells	O	A	B	AB
Antibodies in serum	anti-A anti-B	anti-B	anti-A	

Group A has been split into various subgroups (A_1, A_2, etc.). Moss's groups IV, II, III, I, and Janský's I, II, III, IV are equivalent to the Standard grouping. Commonly involved in erythroblastosis fetalis and in transfusion reactions are the

Rh/Hr groups

Fischer-Race's nomenclature	Weiner's nomenclature
C	rh'
D	Rh_0
E	rh''
c	hr'
d (postulated)	Hr_0
e	hr''

Other groups include the following systems: MNSs, P, Lutheran, Kell, Lewis, Duffy, Kidd, Diego, Sutter, Xg, I, and others. New groups are still being determined. Blood groups have been found in other animal species.

bloodless operation. A surgical procedure performed with little or no significant loss of blood.

bloodless phlebotomy. PHLEBOSTASIS.

blood·let·ting, *n.* PHLEBOTOMY.

blood mole. A mass of coagulated blood and

retained fetal membranes and placenta, sometimes found in the uterus after an abortion. Syn. *carneous mole.*

blood plasma. The fluid portion of blood.

blood platelet. A spheroidal or ovoid light-gray body found in blood, about 1.0 to 2.5 μm in diameter, and numbering about 300,000 per cubic millimeter; an essential part of the hemostatic mechanism.

blood poisoning. SEPTICEMIA.

blood pressure. The pressure exerted by the circulating blood on the walls of the vessels or of the heart, especially the arterial pressure as measured by sphygmomanometry. Abbreviated, B.P.

blood pump. 1. A device for pumping blood rapidly into an artery or vein. 2. The apparatus for propelling the blood in an extracorporeal circulatory system.

blood-stream, *n.* The flow of blood in its circulation through the body.

blood substitute. A substance, or combination of substances, used in place of blood, such as dextran, polyvinylpyrrolidone, plasma, albumin, gelatin, or certain electrolyte solutions.

blood sugar. The carbohydrate of the blood, chiefly glucose.

blood type. The specific reaction pattern found when blood is tested by its reactions to antiserums for the various blood groups.

blood typing. BLOOD GROUPING.

blood urea nitrogen. Nitrogen in the form of urea found in whole blood or serum; normal range is 8 to 20 mg per 100 ml. Its content is used to evaluate kidney function. Abbreviated, BUN.

blow-fly, *n.* A fly belonging to the family Calliphoridae.

blue baby. A newborn child suffering from cyanosis due either to pulmonary disease and inadequate oxygenation of the blood, as in congenital atelectasis, or to a congenital malformation of the heart or great vessels with significant shunting of venous blood to the arterial side.

blue bloater. A patient with chronic bronchitis, alveolar hypoventilation, cyanosis, hypercapnia, and cor pulmonale.

blue-diaper syndrome. A familial condition seen in infants involving abnormal tryptophan metabolism, with resultant conversion to indican and other indole derivatives by the intestinal flora, causing blue discoloration of the diapers.

blue-dome cyst. A breast cyst occurring in mammary dysplasia and characterized by the blue color imparted to light passing through the exposed portion of the cyst.

blue nevus. A nevus composed of spindle-shaped pigmented melanocytes usually in the middle and lower two-thirds of the dermis.

blue-sclera syndrome. A congenital, often hereditary, condition of unknown cause in which the scleras are deep indigo blue, sometimes fading with age; often associated with osteogenesis imperfecta and deafness, but may occur in the absence of bone fragility.

blue-tongue, *n.* An epizootic disease of sheep characterized by acute inflammation of the gastrointestinal, respiratory, and muscular systems; the causative agent is an arthropod-borne double-stranded RNA virus.

Blu-mer's shelf A pathological finding observed on rectal examination, due to a thickening of the peritoneum of the rectouterine pouch which produces a shelflike projection into the rectum. The thickening may be due to an inflammatory or neoplastic process.

blunt dissection. *In surgery,* the exposure of structures or separation of tissues without cutting.

blunt hook. An instrument for exercising traction upon the fetus in an arrested breech presentation.

blunt retractor. A toothed retractor, with rounded teeth to avoid injury to tissues.

blush, *n.* A reddening of the skin, usually involuntary and caused by embarrassment or sudden emotion; FLUSH (1).

B lymphocyte A lymphocyte which originates as a stem cell from bone marrow, differentiating in the bursa of Fabricus in birds and at an analogous but unknown site in mammals, and which bears immunoglobin receptors for antigen on its surface. Stimulation of its surface by antigen triggers its further differentiation into the plasma cell, which is responsible for production of circulating antibody. Syn. *B cell.*

B. M. A. British Medical Association.

B.M.R. Abbreviation for *basal metabolic rate.*

board of health. An official board in a municipality, state, or province, responsible for maintaining public health through sanitation and providing a limited range of clinical and laboratory services.

Bodansky unit The amount of phosphatase required to liberate 1 mg of phosphorus as the phosphate ion from a sodium glycerophosphate substrate during the first hour of incubation at 37°C and pH 8.6.

body, *n.* 1. The animal frame with its organs. 2. The largest and primarily central part of an organ, as the body of the uterus. 3. A mass of matter. 4. A small organ, as the carotid body.

body image. In psychology, the conscious and unconscious concepts, which may differ from each other, each person has of his own physical self as an object in and bound by space, including body parts, shape, posture, and motion. Syn. *body schema.*

body louse. The louse *Pediculus humanus corporis,* a vector of disease and the cause of pediculosis corporis.

body-righting reflex. A righting reflex initiated by asymmetric stimulation of pressure receptors on the surface of the body. It may be a body-righting reflex acting on the head, which tends to keep the head orientated in relation to the surface with which the body is in contact, or it may be acting on the body, which ensures orientation of the body in space or in relation to the surface with which it is in contact.

body segment. A somite, or a division of the body derived from an embryonic somite.

body sense. Impressions from somatic structures which orient with regard to the body or its parts in space or which concern contacts or degrees of contact.

body snatching. Unauthorized removal of a corpse from the grave.

body surface area. The area covered by a person's skin expressed in square meters, calculated from the formula $S = 0.007184 \times W^{0.425} \times H^{0.725}$, where S = surface area in square meters, W = body weight in kilograms, and H = height in centimeters. Nomograms constructed from this formula are used clinically to estimate body surface area, as for fluid requirements and drug dosages. An average newborn has a surface area of about 0.2 m²; a child weighing 30 kg, about 1 m²; and an adult weighing 70 kg, about 1.76 m².

body type. SOMATOTYPE.

boil, n. FURUNCLE.

bol·do (bol'do, bul'do) n. The dried leaves of the boldu tree, *Peumus boldus,* formerly used as an aromatic stimulant and diuretic.

bo·lom·e·ter (bo·lom'e·tur) n. A device for measuring minute differences in radiant heat. Syn. *thermic balance.*

bo·lus (bo'lus) n. 1. A large pill. 2. The rounded mass of food prepared by the mouth for swallowing. Syn. *alimentary bolus.* 3. BOLE. 4. *In angiography,* a rapidly injected volume of radiographic contrast medium.

bond, n. The linkage or adhesive force between atoms, as in a compound, usually effected by the transfer of one or more electrons from one atom to another, or by the sharing, equally or unequally, of one or more pairs of electrons by two atoms.

bone, n. 1. A supportive rigid connective tissue consisting of an abundant matrix of collagen fibers impregnated with minerals which are chiefly calcium compounds, enclosing many much-branched cells, the osteocytes. The body of each osteocyte occupies an ovoid space, the lacuna; its branches lie in minute, branching tubules, the canaliculi. 2. An element or individual member of the skeleton, as the femur, the parietal bone. Comb. form *osse(o)-, ossi-, ost-, oste(o)-.* For bones listed by name, see Table of Bones in the Appendix. —**bony,** *adj.*

bone age. Age as judged roentgenologically from bone development; it is compared with the normal ossification for that chronologic age.

bone cell or **corpuscle.** A cell in a lacuna of bone. Syn. *osteocyte.*

bone conduction. Transmission of sound vibrations to the middle and internal ear via the bones of the skull.

bone conduction hearing aid. An electronic hearing aid, the transmitter of which is held against the skin over the mastoid process.

bone conduction test. The testing of hearing threshold by placing a tuning fork or audiometer oscillator directly against a bone of the skull, usually the mastoid process.

bone cyst. A cyst occurring in bone, as the result of a pathologic change.

bone graft. A graft composed of bone; may be cortical, cancellous, or medullary; used to repair bone defects, to afford support, or to supply osteogenic tissue.

bone inlay. A bone graft fitted into the two fragments and lying across a fracture or filling a gap between the fragments, to promote healing.

bone nippers. 1. RONGEUR. 2. A small bone-trimming forceps.

bone on·lay. A strip of transplanted bone laid across a fracture to encourage or strengthen union, and held in position by wires, pins, screws, or other devices.

bone wax. A waxy material used for packing bone, especially during skull operations, for the arrest of bone bleeding.

Bonine. Trademark for meclizine, an antinauseant drug used as the hydrochloride salt.

bony ankylosis. Complete fixation of a joint due to fusion of the bones.

bony labyrinth. OSSEOUS LABYRINTH.

booster dose. That portion of an immunizing agent given at a later period to stimulate effects of a previous dose of the same agent.

Booth-by-Love·lace-Bul·bul·ian mask. An apparatus used in the administration of oxygen; the mask is fitted with an inspiratory-expiratory valve and a rebreathing bag.

boot-shaped heart. *In radiology,* the abnormal cardiac configuration associated with the marked right ventricular hypertrophy seen in tetralogy of Fallot with left ventricular dilatation and hypertrophy usually secondary to aortic regurgitation.

bo·rate (bo'rate) n. Any salt of boric acid.

bo·rax (bo'racks) n. SODIUM BORATE.

bor·bo·ryg·mus (bor''bo·rig'mus) n., pl. **borboryg·mi** (·migh) The rumbling noise caused by flatus gurgling through fluid in the intestines.

Bor·deaux mixture (bor·do') A fungicide prepared from copper sulfate, calcium oxide, and water.

bor·der·line, *adj.* 1. Pertaining to any phenomenon or datum not easily classifiable in such categories as normal or abnormal. 2. Describing an individual whose mentality or emotional status is near the dividing line between normal and abnormal.

Bor·de·tel·la (bor·de·tel'uh) n. A genus of gram-negative bacteria, formerly included in the genus *Hemophilus.*

Bordetella per·tus·sis (pur·tuss'is) A gram-negative rod-shaped bacterium that is the cause of whooping cough. Syn. *Hemophilus pertussis.*

bo·ric acid (bo'rick). H₃BO₃. Colorless scales, crystals, or white crystalline powder, soluble in water. Used as a mild antiseptic on mucous membranes. Serious or fatal poisoning resulting from transcutaneous absorption may occur. Syn. *boracic acid, orthoboric acid.*

bo·ron (bo'ron, bor'on) *n.* B = 10.81. A nonmetallic element of the aluminum group; it is the characteristic element of boric acid, the borates, metaborates, and perborates.

Bor·rel·ia (bo·ree'lee·uh, bo·rel'ee·uh) *n.* A genus of large, coarsely coiled spirochetes, of many species, parasitic in man and other warm-blooded animals, and including the causative agents of relapsing fever.

Borrelia re·cur·ren·tis (ree"kur·en'tis). The spirochete that causes louse-borne relapsing fever.

boss, *n.* A rounded or knoblike protuberance, as on the side of a bone or tumor.

bos·se·lat·ed (bos'e·lay·tid) *adj.* With a knoblike protuberance, or boss.

bos·se·la·tion (bos"e·lay'shun) *n.* The condition of having bosses or of becoming bosselated.

boss·ing, *n.* BOSSELATION.

bot, *n.* The larva of a botfly, especially of the species infecting the horse and related animals. Bots infect the cavities of the facial bones, the stomach and intestine, and the subcutaneous connective tissue, causing severe damage.

bo·tan·ic (buh·tan'ick) *adj.* 1. Of or pertaining to plants. 2. Of or pertaining to botany. —**botan·i·cal** (·i·kul) *adj.*

bot·a·ny (bot'uh·nee) *n.* The branch of biology dealing with plants. —**bot·a·nist** (bot'uh·nist) *n.*

both·ri·oid (both'ree·oid) *adj.* Pitted; foveolated; covered with pitlike marks.

both·ri·um (both'ree·um) *n.,* pl. **both·ria** (·ree·uh) A grooved sucker, such as is seen on the head of the tapeworm *Diphyllobothrium latum.*

bo·tog·e·nin (bo·toj'e·nin) *n.* A steroidal sapogenin obtained from the Mexican yam *Dioscorea mexicana;* a possible source for synthesis of other steroids.

bot·ry·oid (bot'ree·oid) *adj.* Resembling in shape a bunch of grapes, due to many rounded prominences.

botryoid sarcoma or tumor. SARCOMA BOTRYOIDES.

bot·ryo·my·co·sis (bot"ree·o·migh·ko'sis) *n.,* pl. **botryomyco·ses** (·seez) 1. A bacterial infection, usually staphylococcal, in which the organisms as seen in tissues form groups resembling actinomycotic colonies. 2. Specifically, a chronic infectious disease of horses and, rarely, of cattle; characterized by dense fibrous tissue containing multiple suppurating foci of staphylococci. —**botryomy·cot·ic** (·kot'ick) *adj.*

bots, *n.* Infection with botfly larvae.

bottle nose. A nasal deformity resulting from acne rosacea.

bottle sound. AMPHORIC RESPIRATION.

bot·u·li·form (bot'yoo·li·form) *adj.* Sausage-shaped.

bot·u·lin (bot'yoo·lin) *n.* The neurotoxin produced by *Clostridium botulinum,* which causes botulism. —**bot·u·li·nal** (bot'yoo·lye'nul) *adj.*

bot·u·lism (bot'yoo·liz·um) *n.* Poisoning of man and animals by a group of immunologically distinct types of *Clostridium botulinum,*

acquired by man generally by the ingestion of improperly canned or preserved food. The clinical syndrome results from the action of a potent neurotoxin at the myoneural junction, and is characterized by diplopia, dysphagia, muscle weakness, and respiratory failure.

bou·gie (boo·zhee', boo'zhee) *n.* 1. A slender cylindrical instrument of rubber, waxed silk, or other material, for introduction into the body passages, as the urethra, anus, or other canal. It may be plain or tipped, angled or straight, being intended for use in exploration, in dilatation of strictures, as a guide for the passage of other instruments, or for the induction of labor. 2. A suppository, particularly for insertion into the urethra.

Bouin's fixative (bwaeⁿ) A 75:25:5 mixture of picric acid, formaldehyde, and acetic acid; used in histologic procedures.

bour·donne·ment (boor·dun·mahn') *n.* A buzzing or humming sound heard during auscultation, or heard subjectively from any cause. The former is thought to be due to the contraction of muscle fibrils.

Bour·ne·ville's disease (boor·nᵉ·veel') TUBEROUS SCLEROSIS.

bou·ton·neuse fever (boo·ton·uhz') The prototype of the tick-borne typhus fevers of Africa, widely distributed in Africa and the Mediterranean, Caspian, and Black Sea basins; in which infection caused by *Rickettsia conori* is transmitted by the bite of ixodid ticks, with dogs and rodents as animal hosts. Clinically, characterized by a necrotic initial lesion (tache noire), headache, fever, rash, and, generally, a favorable prognosis.

bou·ton·niere deformity (boo·ton·yair'). BUTTONHOLE DEFORMITY.

bo·vine (bo'vine) *adj.* 1. Cattlelike. 2. Relating to or derived from a cow or ox.

bowel training. The establishing of regular habits of defecation during early childhood.

Bow·en's disease or epithelioma 1. Intraepithelial squamous cell carcinoma of the skin, forming distinctive plaques. 2. A similar carcinoma occurring in mucous membranes.

bow·leg, *n.* Lateral curvature of the lower extremities.

Bowman's capsule GLOMERULAR CAPSULE.

box·er's ear. A hematoma of the external ear.

Boyle's law At any given temperature the volume of a given mass of gas varies in inverse proportion to the pressure exerted upon it.

B.P. Abbreviation for (a) *blood pressure* (b) *British Pharmacopoeia.*

Br Symbol for bromine.

brace, *n.* An apparatus that gives support to any movable part of the body, intended for permanent use, in contradistinction to a splint; may assist in locomotion, and is frequently attached to clothing, as to shoes; sometimes jointed to permit flexion.

brachi-, brachio- A combining form meaning (a) *arm;* (b) *brachial.*

bra·chi·al (bray'kee·ul) *adj.* Of or pertaining to an arm or a structure like an arm.

brachial artery. An artery which originates as a

continuation of the axillary artery and terminally branches into the radial and ulnar arteries, distributing blood to the various muscles of the arm, the shaft of the humerus, the elbow joint, the forearm, and the hand.

brachial birth palsy. Paralysis of the arm due to injury of the brachial plexus during birth.

bra·chi·al·gia (bray"kee·al'juh, ·jee·uh, brack" ee·) n. Pain in the arm often related to a lesion of the brachial plexus.

bra·chi·a·lis (bray"kee·ay'lis, brack"ee·) n. A muscle lying under the biceps brachii and covering the front of the elbow joint.

brachial plexus. A plexus of nerves located in the neck and axilla and composed of the anterior rami of the lower four cervical and first thoracic nerves.

bra·chi·form (bray'ki·form) adj. Arm-shaped.

bra·chio·ce·phal·ic (bray"kee·o·se·fal'ick) adj. Pertaining to the arm and the head.

brachiocephalic trunk. The largest branch of the arch of the aorta which divides into the right common carotid and right subclavian arteries; the innominate artery.

bra·chio·ra·di·a·lis (bray"kee·o·ray"dee·ay'lis) adj. & n. 1. Pertaining to the arm and radius. 2. The brachioradialis muscle.

brachioradialis reflex. A stretch reflex due to contraction of the brachioradialis muscle, with flexion and supination of the forearm and occasionally flexion of the fingers on percussion of the styloid process or lower third of the lateral surface of the radius while the forearm is held in semiflexion and semipronation. Syn. *periosteoradial reflex, radial reflex, supinator reflex.*

bra·chi·ot·o·my (bray"kee·ot'uh·mee) n. *In surgery and obstetrics*, the cutting or removal of an arm.

bra·chi·um (bray'kee·um, brack'ee·um) n., genit. **bra·chii** (·kee·eye), pl. **bra·chia** (·uh) 1. The arm, especially the upper arm. 2. Any armlike structure.

brachy- A combining form meaning *short.*

brachy·ce·pha·lia (brack"ee·se·fay'lee·uh) n. Shortness of the head, the cephalic index being 81.0 to 85.4. —**brachyce·phal·ic** (·fal'ick), **brachy·ceph·a·lous** (·sef'uh·lus) adj.

brachy·ceph·a·ly (brack"ee·sef'uh·lee) n. BRACHYCEPHALIA.

brachy·chei·lia, brachy·chi·lia (brack"ee·kigh' lee·uh) n. Abnormal shortness of the lip.

brachy·chi·rous, brachy·chei·rous (brack"ee· kigh'rus) adj. Having short hands. —**brachychi·ria** (·ree·uh), **brachychi·rism** (·riz· um) n.

brachy·dac·tyl·ia (brack"ee·dack·til'ee·uh) n. Abnormal shortness of the fingers or toes. —**brachydactyl·ic** (·ick), **brachy·dac·ty·lous** (·dack'ti·lus) adj.

brachy·dac·ty·ly (brack"ee·dack'ti·lee) n. BRACHYDACTYLIA.

brachy·glos·sal (brack"ee·glos'ul) adj. Having a short tongue.

brachy·glos·sia (brack"ee·glos'ee·uh) n. Abnormal shortness of the tongue.

brachy·gnath·ous (brack"ee·nath'us) adj. Having an abnormally short lower jaw. —**brachy·gna·thia** (·nayth'ee·uh), n.; **brachygnathus,** n.

brachy·ker·kic (brack"ee·kur'kick) adj. Pertaining to or having a forearm disproportionately shorter than the upper arm.

brachy·mor·phic (brack"ee·mor'fick) adj. Characterized by a stature shorter than usual.

brachy·pel·lic (brack"ee·pel'ick) adj. Pertaining to or having an oval type of pelvis in which the transverse diameter exceeds the anteroposterior diameter by not more than 3 cm.

brachy·pha·lan·gia (brack"ee·fa·lan'jee·uh) n. A condition in which the phalanges are abnormally short. —**brachypha·lan·gous** (·lang' gus) adj.

brachy·pro·sop·ic (brack"ee·pro·sop'ick, ·so' pick) adj. Having a short face.

brachy·rhin·ia (brack"ee·rin'ee·uh) n. Abnormal shortness of the nose.

brachy·skel·ic (brack"ee·skel'ick) adj. Characterized by abnormal shortness of the legs.

brachy·sta·sis (brack"ee·stay'sis) n. A process in which a muscle does not relax to its former length following a contraction and maintains its original degree of tension in its new state. —**brachy·stat·ic** (·stat'ick) adj.

brack·et, n. A metal lug soldered to an orthodontic band by means of which other parts of an appliance, such as an arch wire, rubber band, or ligature, may be attached to the band.

Brad·ford frame A canvas-covered, rectangular, gas-pipe frame, devised originally for handling children with tuberculous disease of the spine, but extended later to the care of joint disease and for immobilization after operations, in adults as well as in children.

brady- A combining form meaning *slow.*

brady·aux·e·sis (brad"ee·awk·see'sis) n. A type of relative growth in which a part grows at a slower rate than the whole organism or another part.

brady·car·dia (brad"ee·kahr'dee·uh) n. Slowness of the heartbeat; a heart rate of less than 60 per minute for a human adult or 120 per minute for a fetus.

brady·crot·ic (brad"ee·krot'ick) adj. Characterized by a slowness of the pulse.

brady·di·as·to·le (brad"ee·dye·as'to·lee) n. Prolongation of the diastolic interval beyond normal limits.

brady·glos·sia (brad"ee·glos'ee·uh) n. Slowness of speech, due to difficulty in tongue movement.

brady·ki·ne·sia (brad"ee·ki·nee'zhuh, ·zee·uh, ·kigh·nee') n. Slowness and poverty of movement, as in disorders affecting the extrapyramidal system and in the catatonic type of schizophrenia. —**bradyki·net·ic** (·net' ick) adj.

brady·ki·nin (brad"ee·kigh'nin, ·kin'in) n. A polypeptide containing 9 amino acid residues, released from the plasma alpha globulin bradykininogen (kallidinogen) by a kallikrein. It derives its name from its effect in slowly developing contraction of isolated guinea pig ileum. A potent vasodilator, it also increases capillary permeability and produces edema. Syn. *kallidin-9*.

brady·ki·nin·o·gen (brad″ee·ki·nin′o·jen, ·kigh‐nin′o·jen) *n.* An alpha globulin present in blood plasma which serves as the precursor for bradykinin and the substrate for kallikreins. Bradykininogen appears to be identical with kallidinogen.

brady·la·lia (brad″ee·lay′lee·uh) *n.* 1. Slow or labored speech due to central nervous system disturbance, as in Sydenham's chorea or other extrapyramidal motor disorders. 2. The slow speech observed in certain depressive illnesses.

brady·lex·ia (brad″ee·leck′see·uh) *n.* Abnormal slowness in reading, due to either a central nervous system disturbance or an inadequate reading ability.

brady·phre·nia (brad″ee·free′nee·uh) *n.* Sluggish mental activity; may be due to organic causes or symptomatic of a depressive illness or reaction.

brady·pnea (brad″ee·nee′ah) *n.* An abnormally slow rate of breathing.

brady·pra·gia (brad″ee·pray′jee·uh) *n.* Abnormally slow action, especially physical activity.

brady·rhyth·mia (brad″ee·rith′mee·uh) *n.* 1. Slowing of the heart or pulse rate; BRADYCARDIA. 2. *In electroencephalography,* slowing of the brain wave rate below that expected for age and normal physiologic state, as awake, asleep, or drowsy; often, delta rhythm and slow-wave complexes.

brady·sper·ma·tism (brad″ee·spur′muh·tiz·um) *n.* Slow or delayed ejaculation of semen during intercourse.

brady·tel·eo·ki·ne·sis (brad″ee·tel″ee·o·ki·nee′sis, ·teel″ee·o·) *n.* The type of incoordination in which a movement is halted before completion, then completed slowly and irregularly; seen in cerebellar disease.

braille (brail) *n.* A compact alphabet and set of numbers and scientific and musical symbols adapted for the blind, using raised dots or points arranged in two six-dot vertical columns.

brain, *n.* That part of the central nervous system contained in the cranial cavity, consisting of the cerebrum, cerebellum, pons, and medulla oblongata.

brain·case, *n.* The portion of the skull containing the brain; NEUROCRANIUM.

brain concussion. 1. Violent shaking or agitation of the brain and the transient paralysis of nervous function therefrom. 2. Immediate abolition of consciousness, transient in nature, usually due to a blunt, nonpenetrating injury which causes a change in the momentum of the head.

brain-damaged child. A child who sustained some injury or insult to his nervous system before, during, or after birth and who usually has some impairment of perception or intellect, behavioral difficulties (especially undirected hyperkinetic behavior), and clumsiness or deficits in fine motor coordination. Speech problems and mild to major neurological abnormalities may be present. Causes are multiple and include hypoxia, infections, physical trauma, and toxins.

brain death. An irreversible abolition of all brain function. The following requirements for brain death are generally agreed upon: unresponsiveness to all stimuli, absence of spontaneous respiration and of pupillary, oculocephalic, vestibuloocular, and gag reflexes, and an electroencephalogram recorded for 30 minutes or longer at 24-hour intervals, showing no electrical activity over two microvolts at maximum gain despite stimulation with sound and pain-producing stimuli.

brain·ed·ness (bray′nid·nis) *n.* CEREBRAL DOMINANCE.

brain injury. 1. Any form of trauma to the brain, whether of infectious, mechanical (metabolic and toxic), or vascular origin, and resulting in a variety of pathologic changes. The clinical manifestations are highly variable, depending on the nature, extent, site, and duration of the injury. 2. Any one of the forms of cerebral dysfunction due to injury sustained before, during, or shortly after birth.

brain sand. Psammoma bodies in the pineal body; corpora arenacea.

brain-stem, *n.* The portion of the brain remaining after the cerebral hemispheres and cerebellum have been removed.

brain syndrome. ORGANIC BRAIN SYNDROME.

brain·wash·ing, *n.* The systematic psychologic intervention into and perversion of an individual's thoughts and mental organization in order to break down his own standards of values and induce behavior radically different from that expected as a result of his earlier upbringing, but conforming to a pattern set forth by the person or organization practicing the psychologic attack.

brain wave. A fluctuation in the spontaneous electrical activity of the brain observed with amplification as in an electroencephalogram. Regular frequencies of brain waves are classified as alpha, beta, gamma, delta, or theta rhythms.

branchi-, branchio- A combining form meaning (a) gill; (b) *branchial.*

bran·chi·al (brang′kee·ul) *adj.* 1. Pertaining to the branchiae or gills. 2. By extension, pertaining to the embryonic visceral arches.

branchial arch. 1. One of the posthyoid gill arches in lower vertebrates. 2. Any of the visceral arches in embryos of higher vertebrates.

branchial cleft. 1. One of the slitlike openings between the gills, as in fishes. 2. VISCERAL CLEFT.

branchial cleft cyst. BRANCHIAL CYST.

branchial cyst. A cyst due to anomalous development of the embryonal visceral pouches or grooves.

branchial fistula. LATERAL FISTULA OF THE NECK.

bran·chio·gen·ic (brang″kee·o·jen′ick) *adj.* Produced or developed from a branchial or visceral cleft or arch.

branchiogenic carcinoma. A squamous cell carcinoma arising from the epithelium of a branchial cyst or other branchial apparatus remnants.

bran·chi·og·e·nous (brang"kee-oj'e-nus) *adj.* BRANCHIOGENIC.

bran·chi·o·ma (brang"kee-o-muh) *n.,* pl. **branchiomas, branchioma·ta** (·tuh) BRANCHIOGENIC CARCINOMA.

bran·chio·mere (brang'kee-o-meer) *n.* A segment of the visceral mesoderm which develops into a branchial or visceral arch.

bran·ny, *adj.* Resembling broken and separated coats of grain, such as wheat or oats; scaly.

brash, *n.* 1. PYROSIS. 2. Any eruption. 3. An attack of illness.

brawny, *adj.* 1. Fleshy; muscular. 2. Thick or hard, as brawny edema.

Brax·ton Hicks contraction Irregular and usually painless uterine contractions that occur with increasing frequency throughout pregnancy.

Braxton Hicks sign A sign of pregnancy after the third month in which intermittent uterine contractions can be detected.

Braxton Hicks version Manipulation by the bimanual method to bring the fetal head into the pelvis. This has been advocated in treatment of placenta previa and prolapsed cord.

breakage–fusion–bridge cycle. A chromosomal sequence found in the gametophyte and endosperm of corn, initiated by a chromosomal break and fusion of broken ends of the duplicated chromosome to give a dicentric, which in anaphase forms a bridge broken by subsequent cell division. The process then recurs at the next cell division.

break·bone fever. DENGUE.

breast, *n.* 1. The front of the chest. 2. One of the mammary glands.

breast·bone, *n.* STERNUM.

breath, *n.* 1. The air inhaled or exhaled during respiration. 2. A single act of respiration.

breath alcohol method. A method for rapidly measuring the concentration of alcohol in the expired air of an individual to determine whether or not he is intoxicated.

Breathalyzer. Trademark for an instrument used to determine whether or not a person is alcoholically intoxicated.

breathe, *v.* To inhale and exhale air alternately; RESPIRE (1).

breath-holding attack or spell. A benign nonepileptic phenomenon observed in children, usually between 6 months and 4 years of age, almost always precipitated by a slight injury, anger, frustration, fear, or the desire for attention, in which the child holds his breath, becoming hypoxic and cyanotic, and rarely pale, and then briefly opisthotonic and unconscious, after which breathing is resumed automatically. Occasionally the opisthotonic phase may be followed by a brief generalized seizure. Syn. *reflex hypoxic crisis.*

breath sounds. Respiratory sounds heard on auscultation of the lungs.

breech, *n.* BUTTOCKS.

breech presentation. The presentation of the

fetal buttocks and/or the feet first at the cervix.

breg·ma (breg'muh) *n.,* pl. **bregma·ta** (·tuh) *In craniometry,* the junction of the coronal and sagittal sutures. **—breg·mat·ic** (breg-mat'ick) *adj.*

brei (brye) *n.* Mush; soupy mixture; tissue ground to a pulp.

Bren·ner tumor A solid or cystic tumor of the ovaries, composed of cords or nests of polyhedral epithelial cells separated by an abundant connective-tissue stroma; generally benign and having no known endocrine activity.

brepho·plas·tic (bref"o·plas'tick) *adj.* Designating embryonic, fetal, or newborn tissues which are used for transplantation to fetal, young, or adult animals.

Breus's mole (broyce) A type of missed abortion in which the patient expels, or has removed surgically, a small chorionic vesicle surrounded by blood clot, placenta, and decidual tissue. Syn. *subchorial tuberous hematoma of the decidua.*

brevi- A combining form meaning *short.*

brev·i·col·lis (brev"i·kol'is) *n.* A deformity characterized by shortness of the neck and limitation of head movements and sometimes of the facial muscles.

brevi·lin·e·al (brev"i·lin'ee·ul) *adj.* Pertaining to a body type which is shorter and broader than normal.

brevi·ra·di·ate (brev"i·ray'dee·ut, ·ate) *adj.* Having short processes.

bridge·work, *n.* 1. An appliance made of artificial crowns of teeth to replace missing natural teeth. Such crowns are connected to natural teeth or roots for anchorage by means of a bridge. A fixed bridge is one which is permanently fastened to its abutments; a removable bridge is one which, though held firmly in place, may be removed by the wearer. 2. The technique of making bridges.

bri·dle, *n.* 1. A band or filament stretching across the lumen of a passage, or from side to side of an ulcer, scar, or abscess. 2. FRENUM.

bright·ness, *n.* The attribute of sensation by which an observer is aware of different luminances.

Bright's disease CHRONIC GLOMERU-LONEPHRITIS.

Brill's disease Recrudescent louse-borne typhus caused by *Rickettsia prowazekii* and characterized by headache, fever, malaise, and rash.

Brill-Sym·mers disease NODULAR LYMPHOMA.

brim·stone, *n.* Native sulfur.

British thermal unit. In general, the heat required to raise the temperature of one pound of water one degree Fahrenheit. Because of variation of the specific heat of water with temperature, the reference temperature must be specified. For the interval 60 to 61°F, a BTU is equivalent to 1054.54 joules. The international table BTU, which is independent of temperature, is equivalent to 1055.06 joules.

broach, *n.* Any one of a variety of finely tapered

instruments used in endodontics for removing the contents of the dental pulp chamber and canals and inserting treatment materials; the basic types are barbed and smooth.

broad ligament of the uterus. A fold of peritoneum which extends laterally from the uterus to the pelvic wall on each side.

Broca's area Brodmann's area 44, situated in the left hemisphere at the posterior end of the third (inferior) frontal convolution; responsible for the executive or motor aspects of speech in most persons.

Bro·ders' classification A system in which tumors are divided into four grades, the prognosis supposedly becoming less favorable as the grade increases. Grade I tumors are chiefly composed of cells resembling adult cells; grade IV tumors, of markedly anaplastic cells; and grades II and III tumors are intermediate in appearance.

Bro·die's abscess A chronic metaphyseal abscess, usually seen in the tibia of young adults.

Brod·mann's areas (brohd'mah'nn) Numbered regions of the cerebral cortex originally differentiated by histologic criteria, now used to identify cortical functions: *areas 1, 2, 3,* the somesthetic area; *area 4,* the motor area; *area 4S,* between areas 4 and 6, a lesion of which causes spasticity of the muscles innervated by it; *areas 5, 7,* the somesthetopsychic area; *area 6,* the premotor area; *area 8,* the adjacent superior part of the frontal cortex, a region involved with eye movement and pupillary change; *area 17,* the visual projection area; *areas 18, 19,* the visuopsychic area; *area 41,* the auditory projection area; *area 42,* the auditopsychic area; *area 44,* Broca's area.

brom-, bromo- A combining form meaning (a) *a bad smell;* (b) in chemistry, *the presence of bromine.*

bro·mate (bro'mate) *n.* A salt of bromic acid.

bro·ma·to·tox·in (bro''muh·to·tock'sin) *n.* Any poison generated in food by the growth of microorganisms.

bro·me·lin (bro'me·lin) *n.* A protein-digesting enzyme from pineapple.

brom·hi·dro·si·pho·bia (brome''hi·dro''si·fo'bee·uh) *n.* Morbid dread of offensive smells, with hallucinations as to the perception of them.

brom·hi·dro·sis (brome''hi·dro'sis, brom''hi·) *n.* Excretion of sweat with an unpleasant odor. Syn. *osmidrosis, fetid perspiration.*

bro·mide (bro'mide, -mid) *n.* Any binary salt in which univalent bromine is the anion, as sodium bromide, NaBr. The bromides are used medicinally to check the convulsions of epilepsy and tetanus, as analgesics, and as sedatives.

bro·mine (bro'meen, -min) *n.* Br = 79.904. A reddish-brown liquid which, at ordinary temperatures, gives off a heavy, suffocating vapor. It is a very active escharotic and disinfectant.

bro·mism (bro'miz·um) *n.* A disease state caused by the prolonged or excessive administration of bromide compounds; it is characterized by headache, drowsiness, lethargy, dysarthria,

often mania with psychotic behavior and acneform skin lesions.

bro·mo·crip·tine (bro''mo·krip'teen) *n.* 2-Bromoergocryptine, $C_{32}H_{40}BrN_5O_5$, a prolactin inhibitor.

bro·mo·der·ma (bro''mo·dur'muh) *n.* An eruption due to ingestion of bromides.

bro·mo·form (bro'mo·form) *n.* Tribromomethane, $CHBr_3$, a heavy colorless, mobile liquid, slightly soluble in water. Has been used as a sedative but is toxic.

bro·mo·hy·per·hi·dro·sis (bro''mo·high''pur·hi·dro'sis, ·high·dro'sis) *n.* The excessive secretion of malodorous sweat.

bro·mo·ma·nia (bro''mo·may'nee·uh) *n.* Psychosis from the excessive use of bromides.

bro·mop·nea, bro·mop·noea (bro''mop·nee'uh, bro''mo·nee'uh) *n.* HALITOSIS.

Bromsulphalein. Trademark for sodium sulfobromophthalein, a diagnostic aid for evaluation of liver function. Abbreviated, BSP.

Bromsulphalein test. A test based upon the ability of the liver to remove injected Bromsulphalein from the blood. Delayed removal indicates hepatic dysfunction.

bronch-, broncho-. A combining form meaning *bronchus, bronchial.*

bronch·ad·e·ni·tis (bronk·ad''e·nigh'tis) *n.* Inflammation of the bronchial lymph nodes.

bronchi-, bronchio-. A combining form meaning *bronchial.*

bronchi. Plural and genitive singular of *bronchus.*

bron·chi·al (bronk'ee·ul) *adj.* Of, pertaining to, or involving the bronchi or their branches.

bronchial asthma. ASTHMA.

bronchial breath sounds. The tubular, blowing, harsh sound of bronchial respiration.

bronchial cyst. BRONCHOGENIC CYST.

bronchial fistula. 1. An abnormal tract communicating between the pleural cavity and a bronchus, usually associated with empyema. 2. An abnormal tract leading from a bronchus to a cutaneous opening, the result of gangrene or abscess of the lung.

bronchial pneumonia. BRONCHOPNEUMONIA.

bronchial respiration. On auscultation, tubular blowing breath sounds normally heard over the larynx, trachea, and larger bronchi; heard over the lungs in any disease process producing pulmonary consolidation, sounds are louder, longer, and higher pitched in expiration than in inspiration.

bronchial septum. The carina of the trachea. See *carina.*

bronchial tree. The arborization of the bronchi of the lung, considered as a structural and functional unit.

bron·chi·ec·ta·sis (bronk''ee·eck'tuh·sis) *n.,* pl. **bronchiecta·ses** (·seez) Saccular or tubular dilatation of one or more bronchi, usually due to bronchial obstruction and infection, and accompanied by cough, mucopurulent sputum, hemoptysis, and recurrent pneumonia. —**bronchi·ec·tat·ic** (·eck·tat'ick) *adj.*

bron·chio·gen·ic (bronk''ee·o·jen'ick) *adj.* BRONCHOGENIC.

bronchiolar carcinoma. A well-differentiated adenocarcinoma of the lung, either focal or multicentric, and of disputed origin, characterized by tall columnar, mucus-producing cells which spread over the pulmonary alveoli.

bron·chi·ole (bronk″ee-ole) *n.* One of the small (1 mm or less in diameter) subdivisions of the bronchi. —**bron·chi·o·lar** (brong·kigh′o·lur) *adj.*

bron·chi·o·lec·ta·sis (bronk″ee-o·leck′tuh·sis) *n.,* pl. **bronchiolecta·ses** (·seez) Dilatation of bronchioles.

bron·chi·ol·i·tis (bronk″ee·o·lye′tis) *n.* Inflammation of the bronchioles; most often caused by respiratory syncytial virus in infants. Syn. *capillary bronchitis.*

bronchiolitis oblit·er·ans (o·blit′ur·anz). Bronchiolitis characterized by the organization of exudate in the bronchioles with fibrotic obliteration of the lumen; may be due to inhalation of nitrogen dioxide or other irritating fumes.

bron·chi·tis (bron·kigh′tis, brong·kigh′tis) *n.,* pl. **bron·chit·i·des** (·kit′i·deez) Inflammation of the mucous membrane of the bronchi. —**bron·chit·ic** (·kit′ick) *adj.*

broncho-. See *bronch-.*

bron·cho·bil·i·ary (bronk″o·bil′ee·air″ee) *adj.* Pertaining to a bronchus and the biliary tract.

bron·cho·can·di·di·a·sis (bronk″o·kan·di·dye′uh·sis) *n.* BRONCHOMONILIASIS.

bron·cho·cav·ern·ous (bronk″o·kav′ur·nus) *adj.* Bronchial and cavernous.

bron·cho·cele (bronk′o·seel) *n.* A localized dilatation of a bronchus.

bron·cho·col·ic (bronk″o·kol′ic, ·ko′lick) *adj.* Pertaining to a bronchus and the colon.

bronchocolic fistula. An abnormal communication between a bronchus and the colon, usually as a result of empyema or subphrenic abscess.

bron·cho·con·stric·tion (bronk″o·kun·strick′shun) *n.* Constriction of the pulmonary air passages. —**bronchoconstric·tive** (·tiv) *adj.*

bron·cho·con·stric·tor (bronk″o·kun·strik′tur) *n.* Any substance which decreases the caliber of the pulmonary air passages.

bron·cho·dil·a·ta·tion (bronk″o·dil″uh·tay′shun, ·dye″luh·tay′shun) *n.* The widening of the caliber of the pulmonary air passages by the use of drugs or surgical instruments.

bron·cho·di·la·tor (bronk″o·dye·lay′tur, ·di·lay′tur) *n.* 1. Any drug which has the property of increasing the caliber of the pulmonary air passages. 2. An instrument used for this purpose.

bron·cho·ede·ma (bronk″o·e·dee′muh) *n.* Swelling of the bronchial epithelium which may produce airway obstruction.

bron·cho·esoph·a·ge·al, bron·cho·oesoph·a·ge·al (bronk″o·e·sof″uh·jee′ul) *adj.* Pertaining to a bronchus and the esophagus.

bronchoesophageal fistula. An abnormal communication between a bronchus and the esophagus; may be congenital or acquired.

bron·cho·esoph·a·gol·o·gy (bronk″o·e·sof″uh·gol′uh·jee) *n.* The field of medicine specializing in disorders of the esophagus and bronchial tree.

bron·cho·esoph·a·gos·co·py, bron·cho·oesoph·a·gos·co·py (bronk″o·e·sof″uh·gos′kuh·pee) *n.* Visual examination of the interior of the larger tracheobronchial tubes and the esophagus with the aid of an instrument.

bron·cho·gen·ic (bronk″o·jen′ick) *adj.* 1. Arising in a bronchus or in the bronchi. 2. *In embryology,* capable of forming the bronchi.

bronchogenic carcinoma. Any of several cellular types of carcinoma arising from the bronchi; usually squamous-cell and found in the segmental bronchi, with adenocarcinoma and poorly differentiated carcinoma less common and of different distribution.

bronchogenic cyst. Cysts having the structure of bronchial walls, usually occurring in the superior mediastinum.

bronchogenic tuberculosis. Drainage of a caseous tuberculous lesion into the bronchial lumen with dissemination of tuberculosis to new areas of the lung.

bron·cho·gram (bronk′o·gram) *n.* Radiograph of the bronchial tree made after the introduction of a radiopaque substance.

bron·chog·ra·phy (brong·kog′ruh·fee) *n.* Radiographic visualization of the bronchial tree after the introduction of a radiopaque contrast material. —**bron·cho·graph·ic** (bronk″o·graf′ick) *adj.*

bron·cho·lith (bronk′o·lith) *n.* A calculus or concretion in the bronchial tree.

bron·cho·li·thi·a·sis (bronk″o·li·thigh′uh·sis) *n.,* pl. **broncholithia·ses** (·seez) A condition characterized by the formation of calculi in the bronchi.

bron·cho·mon·i·li·a·sis (bronk″o·mon·i·lye′uh·sis) *n.,* pl. **bronchomonilia·ses** (·seez) A bronchial disease caused by infection with species of *Candida,* usually *C. albicans.*

bron·cho·mo·tor (bronk″o·mo′tur) *adj.* Pertaining to the neuromuscular mechanisms which control the caliber of the pulmonary air passages.

bron·cho·my·co·sis (bronk″o·migh·ko′sis) *n.,* pl. **bronchomyco·ses** (·seez) A fungous disease of the bronchial tree.

bron·choph·o·ny (brong·kof′uh·nee) *n.* The clear resonant voice sounds normally heard on auscultation over a large bronchus; heard in disease over an area of pulmonary consolidation.

bron·cho·plas·ty (bronk′o·plas·tee) *n. In surgery,* repair of a bronchial defect.

bron·cho·pleu·ral (bronk″o·ploor′ul) *adj.* Pertaining to a bronchus and the pleural cavity, as bronchopleural fistula.

bron·cho·pneu·mo·nia (bronk″o·new·mo′nyuh) *n.* Pulmonary inflammation with exudation into the alveoli, concentrated about the bronchi, which are also involved; occurs principally in childhood and old age; due to a variety of causative organisms.

bron·cho·pneu·mo·ni·tis (bronk″o·new″mo·nigh′tis) *n.* BRONCHOPNEUMONIA.

bron·cho·pul·mo·nary (bronk″o·pul′mo·nerr″ee)

adj. Pertaining to both the bronchi and the lungs.

bronchopulmonary dysplasia. An apparently dose-related consequence of oxygen therapy in newborns with respiratory distress syndrome, identified during life by overinflated lungs, heavy linear and curvilinear densities mixed with areas of lobular emphysema distributed throughout the lungs on chest roentgenograms, excessive shedding of normal epithelial cells on exfoliative cytology, and marked bronchiolar and alveolar damage at autopsy.

bronchopulmonary segment. Any of the subdivisions of a pulmonary lobe, each bounded by connective-tissue septa and supplied by a segmental bronchus; named, according to location within the lobe, as follows: (of the superior lobe of the right lung:) apical, posterior, anterior; (of the superior lobe of the left lung:) apicoposterior, anterior, superior lingular, inferior lingular; (of the middle lobe of the right lung:) lateral, medial; (of the inferior lobe of the right or the left lung:) apical (or superior), subapical (or subsuperior), basal medial (or cardiac), basal anterior, basal lateral, basal posterior. NA (pl.) *segmenta bronchopulmonalia.*

bron·chor·rha·phy (brong·kor'uh·fee) *n.* The suturing of a bronchus.

bron·chor·rhea, bron·chor·rhoea (bronk″o·ree'uh) *n.* Excessive discharge of mucus from the bronchial mucous membranes. —**bronchor·rhe·al** (-ree'ul) *adj.*

bron·cho·scope (bronk'o·skope) *n. & v.* 1. An instrument for the visual examination of the interior of the bronchi. 2. To examine with a bronchoscope. —**bron·cho·scop·ic** (bronk″o·skop'ick) *adj.*; **bron·chos·co·py** (brong·kos'kuh·pee) *n.*

bron·cho·spasm (bronk'o·spaz·um) *n.* Temporary narrowing of the bronchi due to violent, involuntary contraction of the smooth muscle of the bronchi.

bron·cho·spi·ro·che·to·sis, bron·cho·spi·ro·chae·to·sis (bronk″o·spye″ro·kee·to'sis) *n.* Hemorrhagic chronic bronchitis, associated with spirochetal organisms. Syn. *Castellani's disease.*

bron·cho·spi·rog·ra·phy (bronk″o·spye·rog'ruh·fee) *n.* The graphic recording of the functional capacity of the lungs.

bron·cho·spi·rom·e·ter (bronk″o·spye·rom'e·tur) *n.* A spirometer connected to an intrabronchial catheter, designed to measure the functional capacity of a single lung or lung segment.

bron·cho·spi·rom·e·try (bronk″o·spye·rom'e·tree) *n.* The determination of various aspects of the functional capacity of the lungs, a single lung, or a lung segment.

bron·cho·ste·no·sis (bronk″o·ste·no'sis) *n.,* pl. **bronchosteno·ses** (·seez) Narrowing of the lumen of one or more bronchi.

bron·chos·to·my (brong·kos'tuh·mee) *n.* Fistulization of a bronchus through the chest wall.

bron·chot·o·my (brong·kot'uh·mee) *n.* Incision into a bronchus.

bron·cho·ve·sic·u·lar (bronk″o·ve·sick'yoo·lur) *adj.* Pertaining to the bronchi and the pulmonary alveoli.

bronchovesicular respiration. A form of respiration intermediate between bronchial and vesicular; heard over areas of patchy pulmonary consolidation; inspiration and expiration are equal in duration.

bron·chus (bronk'us) *n.,* pl. & genit. sing. **bron·chi** (·eye) 1. [NA] One of the primary branches of the trachea or such of its branches within the lung as contain cartilage in their walls. 2. [BNA] Bronchus principalis (= PRIMARY BRONCHUS).

bron·to·pho·bia (bron″to·fo'bee·uh) *n.* A morbid fear of thunder.

bronze diabetes. HEMOCHROMATOSIS.

brood capsule or **cyst.** A stalked vesicle that develops from the germinative epithelium of an echinococcus cyst. Brood capsules may detach from the mother cyst, become enlarged, and produce brood capsules and scolices within themselves to form daughter cysts.

Brooke's tumor or **epithelioma.** TRICHOEPITHELIOMA.

broth, *n.* A liquid nutritive medium for the culture of microorganisms, prepared from finely chopped lean meat or dehydrated meat extract.

brow, *n.* 1. The upper anterior portion of the head; FOREHEAD. 2. SUPRAORBITAL RIDGE; EYEBROW (1).

brown atrophy. A form of atrophy in which the atrophic organ is of a deeper brown than normal because of an increase of pigment; observed in the heart, skeletal muscles, and liver.

Brown·ian motion or **movement** The ceaseless erratic motion of very small particles suspended in a liquid or gas, caused by unequal impact of the surrounding molecules of liquid or gas on the suspended particles. Syn. *pedesis.*

brown induration. Pulmonary hemosiderosis and fibrosis resulting from chronic, passive hyperemia of the lung, usually the result of left ventricular failure or mitral stenosis.

brown mixture. COMPOUND OPIUM AND GLYCYRRHIZA MIXTURE.

brown recluse. A poisonous spider, *Loxosceles reclusa,* of south central United States.

Brown-Sé·quard's syndrome or **paralysis** (broon sey·kwar', sey·kar') Contralateral loss of pain and thermal sensation and ipsilateral affection of proprioception and corticospinal tract function; due to a lesion confined to one-half of the spinal cord.

brown-tail caterpillar rash or **dermatitis.** BROWN-TAIL RASH.

brown-tail rash. A common form of dermatitis caused by the brown-tail moth, *Euproctis chrysorrhea.*

brow presentation. Presentation of the brow of the fetus at the cervix.

Bru·cel·la (broo·sel'uh) *n.* A genus of small,

gram-negative, nonmotile, short bacilli or coccobacilli which are not acid-fast and do not form endospores; the cause of brucellosis, infectious abortion in cattle, and other animal diseases. —**brucella**, pl. **brucel·lae** (-ee) com. n.; **brucel·lar** (-ur) adj.

Brucella abor·tus (a·bor'tus). The causative agent of infectious abortion in cattle; can also affect other species including humans.

Brucella mel·i·ten·sis (mel''i·ten'sis). A causative agent of brucellosis in goats, sheep, and cattle, which can be transmitted to man.

Brucella su·is (sue'is). The causative agent of infectious abortion in hogs; can also affect other species including humans.

Brucellin. Trademark for a culture filtrate from species of *Brucella*; used in the diagnosis, prophylaxis, and treatment of brucellosis.

bru·cel·lo·sis (broo''se·lo'sis) n., pl. **brucello·ses** (-seez) An infectious disease due to organisms of the genus *Brucella*, transmitted to man from other species. The acute illness is characterized by fever, sweating, weakness, and aching without localizing findings; the same manifestations may persist for months or years in the chronic illness.

Bruch's membrane (brŏŏᵏh) BASAL MEMBRANE.

bruc·ine (broo'seen, ·sin) n. $C_{23}H_{26}N_2O_4$. A poisonous alkaloid found in various species of *Strychnos*; a white crystalline powder with a bitter taste. Has been used chiefly as a simple bitter; appears to be depressant to peripheral motor and sensory nerves.

Bru·dzin·ski's cheek sign (broo·j'in'skee) A sign of meningeal irritation in which pressure on both cheeks just below the zygomatic arch causes flexion of both elbows and rapid lifting of the arms.

Brudzinski's contralateral leg signs Signs of meningeal irritation in which (a) passive flexion of one thigh is accompanied by flexion of the opposite hip and knee; and (b) when one leg and thigh are flexed and the other extended, lowering of the flexed limb is followed by flexion of the contralateral one.

Brudzinski's neck sign A sign of meningeal irritation in which passive flexion of the head is followed by flexion of both thighs and legs.

Brudzinski's symphysis sign A sign of meningeal irritation in which pressure on the symphysis pubis is followed by flexion of both lower extremities.

Brug·ia (brŏŏg'ee·uh, broo'jee·uh) n. A genus of filarial nematodes.

Brugia ma·la·yi (may·lay'eye, ·ee). A species of filaria infecting man by mosquito bite, endemic in the Far East.

bruis·a·bil·i·ty (brooz''uh·bil'i·tee) n. The readiness with which bruising occurs in response to trauma.

bruise (brooz) n. & v. 1. An injury producing capillary hemorrhage below an unbroken skin; contusion. 2. To inflict a bruise or bruises on a person or a part; to contuse. 3. To hurt or wound psychologically.

bruit (broo·ee') n. 1. Formerly, any abnormal noise in the body heard on auscultation. 2. Specifically, a murmur or other sound related to the circulation, heard over a part, such as arteriovenous bruit, carotid bruit, cephalic bruit, systolic bruit, or thyroid bruit.

Brun·schwig's operation 1. DUODENO-PANCREATECTOMY. 2. Complete pelvic exenteration for advanced pelvic cancer. 3. Radical hysterectomy and pelvic lymph node excision for cancer of the cervix.

Brushfield's spots Speckled white or very light yellow, clearly defined pinpoints seen on the irides of children with Down's syndrome, which disappear if later the color of the iris changes to brown; rarely seen in normal infants, but their absence may serve to rule out suspected cases of mongolism.

brux·ism (bruck'sizum) n. Grinding or gnashing of the teeth; an unconscious habit often occurring in sleep, but sometimes during mental or physical concentration or strain, or in disturbed or retarded children.

bry·o·nia (brigh·o'nee·uh) n. The root of the bryony plant, *Bryonia alba* or *B. dioica*, which contains the glycosides bryonin and bryonidin. Has been used as an irritant emetic, drastic cathartic, and vesicant.

bry·on·i·din (brigh·on'i·din) n. A glycoside from the plant *Bryonia alba*.

bry·o·nin (brigh'o·nin) n. A glycoside from *Bryonia alba*.

BSP, B.S.P. Abbreviation for *Bromsulphalein*, a trademark for sulfobromophthalein sodium.

Btu, BTU Abbreviation for *British thermal unit*.

bubonic plague. Plague characterized by lymph-node swelling, caused by *Yersinia pestis* infection.

buc·ca (buck'uh) n., pl. **buc·cae** (-ee, -see) [NA]. CHEEK. —**buc·cal** (-ul) adj.

buccal nerve. The sensory branch of the mandibular nerve to the cheek.

buccal occlusion. Occlusion occurring when a premolar or a molar tooth is situated lateral to the line of occlusion.

buc·ci·na·tor (buck'si·nay''tur) n. The muscular foundation of the cheek.

bucco-. A combining form meaning *cheek, buccal.*

buc·co·ax·i·al (buck''o·ack'see·ul) adj. Pertaining to the buccal and axial walls of a dental cavity.

buc·co·cer·vi·cal (buck''o·sur'vi·kul) adj. 1. Pertaining to the cheek and the neck. 2. Pertaining to the buccal surface and neck of a tooth.

buc·co·dis·tal (buck''o·dis'tul) adj. Pertaining to the buccal and distal walls of a dental cavity.

buc·co·fa·cial (buck''o·fay'shul) adj. Pertaining to the outer surface of the cheek.

buc·co·gin·gi·val (buck''o·jin'ji·vul, ·jin·jye'vul) adj. Pertaining to the cheek and the gums.

buc·co·la·bi·al (buck''o·lay'bee·ul) adj. Pertaining to the cheek and the lip.

buc·co·lin·gual (buck''o·ling'gwul) adj. Pertaining to the cheek and the tongue.

buc·co·me·si·al (buck''o·mee'zee·ul, ·mes'ee·ul) adj. Pertaining to the buccal and mesial walls of a dental cavity.

buc·co·na·sal (buck''o·nay'zul) adj. Pertaining to the cheek and nose.

buc·co·oc·clu·sal (buck"o·uh·kloo′zul) *adj.*
Pertaining to the buccal and occlusal surfaces
of a tooth.

buc·co·pha·ryn·ge·al (buck"o·fa·rin′jee·ul) *adj.*
Pertaining to the cheek and the pharynx.

buc·co·pulp·al (buck"o·pulp′ul) *adj.* Pertaining
to the buccal and pulpal walls of a dental
cavity.

buc·co·ver·sion (buck"o·vur′zhun) *n.* The
condition of a tooth being out of the line of
normal occlusion in the buccal direction.

buc·cu·la (buck′yoo·luh) *n.,* pl. **buccu·lae** (·lee)
The fleshy fold beneath the chin which forms
what is called a double chin.

bu·chu (bew′kew, boo′koo) *n.* The leaves of
several species of *Barosma,* which contain a
volatile oil. Formerly used as a diuretic.

Buck's extension Traction by means of adhesive
straps applied to the skin of the lower
extremity.

Buck's fascia The deep fascia of the penis.

buck tooth. A protruding front tooth.

Bucky diaphragm (book′ee) A radiographic
device that reduces the amount of scattered
radiation reaching the film, consisting of a
moving grid of thin parallel strips of lead
alternating with radiolucent material
arranged on the radius of curvature of a
cylinder whose center is at the focal spot of the
x-ray tube.

buc·ne·mia (buck·nee′mee·uh) *n.* Any diffuse,
tense swelling of the leg, as elephantiasis or
phlegmasia alba dolens.

bud, *n.* 1. *In embryology,* a protuberance or
outgrowth which is the primordium of an
appendage or an organ. 2. *In anatomy,* an
organ or structure shaped like the bud of a
plant. 3. *In mycology,* GEMMA; a cell arising by
extrusion, as in yeasts.

Budd-Chia·ri syndrome (kyah′ree) Hepatic vein
occlusion due to idiopathic thrombosis,
tumor, or other causes, resulting in
hepatosplenomegaly, jaundice, ascites, and
portal hypertension.

bud·ding, *n. In biology,* a form of asexual
reproduction occurring in the lower animals
and plants, in which the parent organism
develops projections which develop into new
individuals.

buffalo obesity. The obesity usually seen in
Cushing's syndrome, confined chiefly to the
trunk, face, and neck.

buf·fer, *n. & v.* 1. A substance which, when
present in a solution or added to it, resists
change of hydrogen-ion concentration when
either acid or alkali is added. 2. To treat with
a buffer.

buffer solution. A solution prepared from a
weak acid and a salt of the weak acid, or a
weak base and a salt of the weak base, which
resists any appreciable change in pH on the
addition of small amounts of acid or alkali or
by dilution with water.

buffy coat. The layer of white cells and platelets
which forms between the erythrocytes and
plasma when fluid blood is centrifuged.

bu·fo·ten·in, bu·fo·ten·ine (bew′fo·ten′in, ·een)
n. 5-Hydroxy-*N,N*-dimethyltryptamine,

$C_{12}H_{16}N_2O$, a component of the secretion of
the skin glands of the toad *Bufo vulgaris.* It
causes hypertension and strong and lasting
vasoconstriction.

bug, *n.* 1. An insect of the order Hemiptera or
suborder Heteroptera. 2. Loosely, any insect
or other small arthropod.

bug·gery (bug′ur·ee) *n.* SODOMY.

bulb, *n.* 1. An oval or circular expansion of a
cylinder or tube. 2. MEDULLA OBLONGATA.

bul·bar (bul′bur, bul′bahr) *adj.* 1. Of or
pertaining to a bulb, or a bulb-shaped
structure or part. 2. Pertaining to or involving
the medulla oblongata. 3. Of or pertaining to
the eyeball.

bulbar apoplexy. A cerebrovascular accident
involving the substance of the medulla
oblongata or pons, causing a variety of
neurologic disturbances depending upon the
extent of the lesion, and including paralysis of
one or both sides of the body, inability to
swallow, talk, move the tongue or lips, and
dyspnea.

bulbar conjunctiva. The mucous membrane
covering the anterior third of the eyeball, from
the junction with the eyelids to the margin of
the cornea.

bulbar poliomyelitis. PARALYTIC BULBAR
POLIOMYELITIS.

bulbar speech. The thick slurred speech
occurring when the nuclei of the medulla
concerned with speech are damaged or when
there is injury to both corticobulbar tracts.

bulbi. Plural and genitive singular of *bulbus.*

bulbo-. A combining form meaning *bulb, bulbar.*

bul·bo·atri·al (bul″bo·ay′tree·ul) *adj.* Pertaining
to the bulb of the heart and atrium of the
heart.

bul·bo·cav·er·no·sus (bul″bo·kav·ur·no′sus) *n.,*
pl. **bulbocaverno·si** (·sigh) BULBOSPONGIOSUS.

bulbocavernosus reflex. PENILE REFLEX.

bulb of the heart. The anterior division of the
embryonic heart within the pericardial cavity.
Its proximal part is incorporated into the right
ventricle; its distal part forms the aortic and
pulmonary valve region of the heart.

bulb of the penis. The expanded proximal
portion of the corpus spongiosum of the penis.

bul·bo·mem·bra·nous (bul″bo·mem′bruh·nus)
adj. Pertaining to the bulbar and membranous
portion of the urethra.

bul·bo·nu·cle·ar (bul″bo·new′klee·ur) *adj.*
Pertaining to the medulla oblongata and its
nerve nuclei.

bul·bo·spi·nal (bul″bo·spye′nul) *adj.* Pertaining
to the medulla oblongata and the spinal cord.

bulbospinal poliomyelitis. PARALYTIC BULBAR
POLIOMYELITIS and PARALYTIC SPINAL
POLIOMYELITIS.

bul·bo·spon·gi·o·sus (bul″bo·spon″jee·o′sus) *n.,*
pl. & genit. sing. **bulbospongio·si** (·sigh)
muscle encircling the bulb and adjacent
proximal parts of the penis in the male and
encircling the orifice of the vagina in the
female and covering the lateral parts of the vestibular
bulbs in the female. Syn. *bulbocavernosus.*
musculus bulbospongiosus.

bul·bo·ure·thral (bul″bo·yoo·ree′thrul) *adj.*

Pertaining to the bulb of the penis and the urethra.

bul·bo·ure·thral gland. Either of the compound tubular glands situated in the urogenital diaphragm, anterior to the prostate gland.

bul·bous (bul'bus) *adj.* Having or containing bulbs; bulb-shaped; swollen; terminating in a bulb.

bul·bo·ven·tric·u·lar (bul''bo·ven·trick'yoo·lur) *adj.* Pertaining to the bulb of the heart and the ventricle of the heart.

bul·bus (bul'bus) *n.*, pl. & genit. sing. **bul·bi** (·bye) BULB.

bu·le·sis (bew·lee'sis) *n.* The will, or an act of the will.

bu·lim·ia (bew·lim'ee·uh, boo·) *n.* An insatiable appetite and excessive food intake; seen in psychotic states and in the Kleine-Levin syndrome and with bilateral ablation of the temporal lobes.

Bu·li·nus (bew·lye'nus) *n.* A genus of freshwater snails, whose species serve as the intermediate hosts for *Schistosoma haematobium.*

bul·la (bool'uh, bul'uh) *n.*, pl. **bul·lae** (·ee) 1. A large bleb or blister either within or beneath the epidermis and filled with lymph or serum. 2. *In anatomy,* a rounded, thin-walled bony prominence.

bul·la eth·moi·da·lis ca·vi na·si (eth·moy·day'lis kay'vye nay'zye) [NA]. A rounded prominence in the lateral wall of the middle nasal meatus, overlying large ethmoid air cells.

bul·late (bool'ate, bul'ate) *adj.* 1. Blistered; marked by bullae. 2. Inflated, bladderlike, vesiculate. —**bul·la·tion** (bool·ay'shun, bul·) *n.*

bul·la tym·pan·i·ca (tim·pan'i·kuh). TYMPANIC BULLA.

bull·dog forceps. A short spring forceps used to occlude or compress a blood vessel temporarily.

bul·lec·to·my (bul·eck'tuh·mee) *n.* Excision of a bulla, especially bullae of the lungs.

bullet forceps. An instrument for extracting bullets.

bul·lous (bool'us, bul') *adj.* Pertaining to or characterized by bullae.

bullous dermatosis. A condition of the skin marked by bullae, as in erythema multiforme, dermatitis herpetiformis, and pemphigus vulgaris.

bullous emphysema. An obstructive type of pulmonary emphysema, characterized by replacement of normal lung tissue by large, air-containing, cystlike structures.

bullous impetigo. A type of impetigo caused by *Staphylococcus aureus* and characterized by bullae, seen usually in children. The lesions develop particularly in the axillae, groins, intergluteal areas, and in the creases of fat.

bullous pemphigoid. A chronic skin disease characterized by large bullae occurring over a wide area and having a tendency to heal without scarring; may represent an autoimmune disease.

UN Abbreviation for *blood urea nitrogen.*

un·dle, *n. In biology,* a fascicular grouping of elementary tissues, as nerve fibers or muscle fibers.

bundle branch block. Delay or block of conduction through either of the branches of the bundle of His, causing one ventricle to be activated and contract before the other.

bundle of His ATRIOVENTRICULAR BUNDLE.

bun·ion (bun'yun) *n.* A swelling of a bursa of the foot, especially of the metatarsophalangeal joint of the great toe; associated with a thickening of the adjacent skin and a forcing of the great toe into adduction (hallux valgus).

bun·ion·ec·to·my (bun''yun·eck'tuh·mee) *n.* Excision of a bunion; plastic repair of the first metatarsophalangeal joint.

bun·ion·ette (bun''yun·et') *n.* Enlargement of the metatarsophalangeal joint of the little toe in a fashion resembling a small bunion.

Bun·sen absorption coefficient (boon'zun) A quantitative expression of gas solubility; the ratio of the volume which would be occupied by the dissolved gas at standard conditions to the volume of the solvent under the experimental conditions.

buph·thal·mos, buph·thal·mus (bewf·thal'mus) *n.* BUPHTHALMIA.

bur, burr, *n.* 1. *In botany,* a rough, prickly shell or case. 2. EAR LOBE. 3. A rotary cutting instrument in any one of various shapes and having numerous fine cutting blades; used in the dental handpiece in the preparation of teeth for restoration. 4. *In surgery,* an instrument similar in form to a dental bur, but larger, designed for surgical operations upon the bones.

burbot liver oil. The oil, containing vitamins A and D, extracted from the liver of the burbot, *Lota maculosa.*

bu·ret, bu·rette (bew·ret') *n.* A graduated glass tube, commonly having a stopcock, used in volumetric analysis for measuring volumes of liquids.

Bur·kitt's lymphoma or **tumor** A malignant lymphoma usually occurring in children, typically involving the retroperitoneal area and the mandible, but sparing the peripheral lymph nodes, bone marrow, and spleen.

burn, *v.* & *n.* 1. To oxidize or be oxidized by fire or equivalent means. 2. To cause, or to be the locus of, a sensation of heat. 3. The tissue reaction or injury resulting from application of heat, extreme cold, caustics, radiation, friction, or electricity; classified as simple hyperemic (first degree), vesicant (second degree), destructive of skin and underlying tissues (third degree).

bur·nish·er, *n.* An instrument for condensing and smoothing and polishing the surface of a dental filling or inlay.

Bu·row's solution (boo'ro) ALUMINUM ACETATE SOLUTION; used topically as an astringent.

burr. BUR.

bur·row, *n.* A cuniculus, passage, gallery, or tunnel in the skin that houses a metazoal parasite, particularly the mite that causes scabies.

bur·sa (bur'suh) *n.*, L.pl. & genit. sing. **bur·sae** (·see) 1. A small sac lined with synovial membrane and filled with fluid interposed between parts that move upon each other. 2. A diverticulum of the abdominal cavity.

bur·sec·to·my (bur·seck'tuh·mee) *n.* Surgical removal of a bursa.

bur·si·tis (bur·sigh'tis) *n.* Inflammation of a bursa.

bur·so·lith (bur'so·lith) *n.* A calculus formed within a bursa.

bu·sul·fan (bew·sul'fan) *n.* 1,4-Butanediol dimethanesulfonate, $C_6H_{14}O_6S_2$, a neoplastic suppressant used in the treatment of chronic granulocytic leukemia.

but-, buto-. A combining form meaning *a substance or compound containing a group of four carbon atoms.*

bu·ta·bar·bi·tal (bew''tuh·bahr'bi·tol, ·tal) *n.* 5-Ethyl-5-*sec*-butylbarbituric acid, $C_{10}H_{16}N_2O_3$, a sedative and hypnotic of intermediate duration of action; used as the sodium derivative.

bu·ta·caine (bew'tuh·kane) *n.* 3-Di-*n*-butylaminopropyl-*p*-aminobenzoate, $C_{18}H_{30}N_2O_2$, a local anesthetic used as the sulfate salt.

bu·ta·di·ene (bew''tuh·dye'een) *n.* 1,3-Butadiene, $CH_2=CHCH=CH_2$, a gaseous hydrocarbon derived from petroleum and used in the manufacture of synthetic rubber and many other substances.

bu·ta·no·ic acid (bew''tuh·no'nick). BUTYRIC ACID.

bu·te·thal (bew'te·thal) *n.* 5-*n*-Butyl-5-ethylbarbituric acid, $C_{10}H_{16}N_2O_3$, a sedative and hypnotic of intermediate duration of action.

bu·teth·amine (bew·teth'uh·meen) *n.* 2-Isobutylaminoethyl *p*-aminobenzoate, $C_{13}H_{20}N_2O_2$, a local anesthetic; used as the formate and hydrochloride salts.

Butisol. A trademark for butabarbital, a sedative and hypnotic used as the sodium derivative.

butt, *v.* 1. *In prosthodontics,* to place directly against the tissues covering the alveolar ridge. 2. To bring any two square-ended surfaces into contact.

but·ter, *n.* 1. The fatty part of milk, obtained by rupturing the fat globules by churning or mechanical agitation. 2. Various vegetable fats having the consistency of butter. 3. Certain anhydrous chlorides having the appearance or consistency of butter.

but·ter·fly, *n.* 1. An adhesive dressing used to hold wound edges together in place of a suture. 2. A piece of paper so arranged over the air passages of an anesthetized patient that it will indicate whether or not he is breathing. 3. A type of intravenous needle with wings.

but·tock (but'uck) *n.* One of the two fleshy parts of the body posterior to the hip joints.

but·ton·hole, *n. In surgery,* a small, straight opening into an organ or part.

buttonhole deformity or **dislocation.** A protrusion or partial protrusion of the joint of a finger through a defect in the extensor aponeurosis. Syn. *boutonniere deformity.*

but·tress, *n.* 1. A support or prop. 2. A thickening of the sole of a horse's hoof between the frog and the posterior end of the bar.

bu·tyl (bew'til) *n.* The univalent hydrocarbon radical, C_4H_9. It occurs as normal butyl, $CH_3CH_2CH_2CH_2—$, abbreviated *n*-butyl; iso-butyl, $(CH_3)_2CHCH_2—$, abbreviated *i*-butyl; secondary butyl, $CH_3CH_2(CH_3)CH—$, abbreviated *sec*-butyl; and tertiary butyl, $(CH_3)_3C$, abbreviated *tert*-butyl.

Butyn. A trademark for butacaine, a local anesthetic; used as the sulfate salt.

butyr-, butyro-. A combining form meaning *butyric.*

bu·tyr·a·ceous (bew''ti·ray'shus) *adj.* Resembling butter; containing or yielding butterlike substances.

bu·tyr·ic (bew·tirr'ick) *adj.* Pertaining to, or derived from, butter.

butyric acid. Butanoic acid, $CH_3CH_2CH_2COOH$, a viscid liquid having a rancid smell. It occurs in butter as a glyceride and is found also in various plant and animal tissues.

bu·tyr·in (bew'ti·rin) *n.* Glyceryl tributyrate, $(C_3H_7COO)_3C_3H_5$, a constituent of butterfat. Syn. *tributyrin.*

bu·tyr·in·ase (bew'ti·ri·nace) *n.* An enzyme that hydrolyzes butyrin, found in the blood serum.

bu·tyr·oid (bew''ti·roid) *adj.* Buttery; having the consistency of butter.

bux·ine (buck'seen, ·sin) *n.* An alkaloid $C_{19}H_{21}NO_3$, from the leaves of the boxwood, *Buxus sempervirens.*

B virus. HERPESVIRUS SIMIAE.

by·pass, *n.* A surgically created detour between two points in a physiologic pathway, as in the vascular or gastrointestinal systems, often to circumvent obstruction or to place the circumvented portion at rest.

bys·si·no·sis (bis''i·no'sis) *n.,* pl. **byssino·ses** (·seez) A pneumoconiosis due to inhalation of high concentrations of the dust of cotton, linen, or other plant fibers used industrially; wheezing and dyspnea are most prominent when the patient returns to work on Monday after a Sunday holiday. The essentially irreversible chronic stage, occurring most frequently in long-time textile workers, is characterized by severe airway obstruction and impaired elastic recoil due to chronic bronchitis and emphysema. Syn. *Monday morning fever.*

C

¢ *In chemistry,* a symbol for carbon. *In molecular biology,* a symbol for cytosine.

c Abbreviation for (a) *complement;* (b) formerly, *curie.*

c., c. Abbreviation for (a) *calorie;* (b) *cathode;* (c) *centigrade;* (d) *centimeter;* (e) *congius;* (f) *hundredweight.*

¢' Symbol for complement.

c Abbreviation for (a) *cum,* with; (b) *centum,* one hundred; (c) *cuspid* or *canine* of the primary dentition.

CA Abbreviation for *chronological age.*

Ca 1. Symbol for calcium. 2. Abbreviation for *cancer.*

CABG (kab'ij). Acronym for coronary artery bypass graft, a surgical procedure for blockage of a coronary artery.

cable graft. *In neurosurgery,* the placing together of several sections of nerve to be transplanted, to bridge a gap in a nerve larger than the sections available for the grafting.

Cabot's rings RING BODIES.

cac-, caco- A combining form meaning *bad, diseased, defective, deformed, vitiated.*

cace A combining form meaning *a bad, diseased, deformed, or vitiated condition.*

cac·es·the·sia, cac·aes·the·sia (kack''es·theezh' uh, ·theez'ee·uh) *n.* Any disagreeable sensation. —**caces·the·sic, cacaes·the·sic** (·theez'ick) *adj.*

ca·chec·tic (ka·keck'tik) *adj.* Pertaining to or characterized by cachexia.

cachectic aphthae. Ulcerous lesions appearing beneath the tongue, along the inner cheeks and palates; seen in debilitated, severely undernourished individuals, particularly children, with poor oral hygiene. Syn. *Riga's aphthae.*

cachectic infantilism. Infantilism, or dwarfism, due to chronic malnutrition, infection, or emotional deprivation.

ca·chet (ka·shay', kash'ay) *n.* Two circles of wafer (rice paper) sealed together and enclosing medication; the resulting dosage form may be swallowed after moistening with water.

ca·chex·ia (ka·keck'see·uh) *n.* Severe general-

ized weakness, malnutrition, and emaciation. Adj. *cachectic.*

cachexia ex·oph·thal·mi·ca (eck''sof·thal'mi·kuh). Cachexia associated with thyrotoxicosis.

cachexia hy·po·phys·i·o·pri·va (high''po·fiz''ee·o·prye'vuh). 1. Cachexia associated with hypopituitarism. 2. SIMMONDS' DISEASE.

cachexia stru·mi·pri·va (stroo''mi·prye'vuh). POSTOPERATIVE MYXEDEMA.

cachexia thy·ro·pri·va (thigh''ro·prye'vuh). POSTOPERATIVE MYXEDEMA.

cach·in·na·tion (kack''i·nay'shun) *n.* Immoderate laughter, as in hysteria or certain psychoses.

ca·chou (kah·shoo') *n.* An aromatic pill or tablet for deodorizing the breath.

caco-. See *cac-.*

caco·de·mo·no·ma·nia (kack''o·dee''muh·no·may'nee·uh, ·de·mo''no·) *n.* CACODEMONIA.

cac·o·dyl (kack'o·dil) *n.* 1. The organic arsenical radical As—. 2. Tetramethyldiarsenic, $(CH_3)_2As=As(CH_3)_2$, a liquid with an extremely offensive odor.

cac·o·dyl·ate (kack''o·dil'ate) *n.* A salt of cacodylic acid. The sodium, calcium, and iron salts have been used in medicine.

cac·o·dyl·ic acid (kack''o·dil'ick). DIMETHYLARSINIC ACID.

cac·o·geu·sia (kack''o·gyoo'see·uh, ·joo'see·uh) *n.* A bad taste not due to food, drugs, or other matter; frequently a part of the aura in psychomotor epilepsy.

ca·coph·o·ny (ka·kof'uh·nee) *n.* An abnormally harsh or discordant voice or sound. —**caco·phon·ic** (kack·o·fon'ick) *adj.*

ca·cos·mia (ka·koz'mee·uh) *n.* Unpleasant, imaginary odors, particularly putrefactive odors; commonly reported as the aura in uncinate epilepsy.

cac·ti·no·my·cin (kack''ti·no·migh'sin) *n.* A mixture of antibiotics, now rarely used, produced by *Streptomyces chrysomallus,* that consists mainly of actinomycin C_2 and actinomycin C_3 with some dactinomycin, and that has antineoplastic activity. Syn. *actinomycin C.*

ca·dav·er (kuh·dav'ur) *n.* A dead body, especially that of a human being; a corpse. —**cadaver·ic** (-ick) *adj.*

cadaveric lividity. LIVOR MORTIS.

cadaveric reaction. *In electromyography,* the total loss of electrical response in the affected muscles, as in the acute stage of periodic paralysis.

cadaveric rigidity. RIGOR MORTIS.

cadaveric spasm. Early or, at times, immediate appearance of rigor mortis; seen after death from certain causes. The muscle spasm actually causes movements of the limbs.

ca·dav·er·ous (kuh-dav'ur·us) *adj.* Resembling a cadaver; of a deathly pallor.

cad·dy stools (kad'ee). Feces that resemble fine, dark, sandy mud; seen with yellow fever.

cad·mi·um (kad'mee·um) *n.* Cd = 112.40. A bluish-white metal used as a constituent of alloys and in electroplating.

ca·du·ce·us (ka·dew'see·us) *n.* 1. The symbol or insignia of medicine, consisting of the staff of Asclepius about which a single serpent is coiled. 2. In the Medical Corps of the United States Army, a symbol consisting of a staff with two formal wings at the top and two serpents entwined about the remainder.

Caes·al·pin·ia (sez''al·pin'ee·uh, ses''al·) *n.* A genus of tropical trees of the family Leguminosae. Several species have been used medicinally.

caesarean. CESAREAN.

café au lait spots (ka·fay'o lay') Light brown patches of the skin, seen especially in neurofibromatosis and in polyostotic fibrous dysplasia.

caf·feine (kaf'ee·in, ka·feen') *n.* An alkaloid, $C_8H_{10}N_4O_2$, chemically 1,3,7-trimethylxanthine, found in the leaves and beans of the coffee tree, in tea, and in guarana, the roasted pulp of the fruit of *Paullinia sorbilis,* or prepared synthetically. Occurs as long needles, slightly soluble in cold water. It is a cerebral, circulatory, and renal stimulant.

caffeine and sodium benzoate. A mixture of approximately equal parts of caffeine and sodium benzoate. It is a form of caffeine especially suited for subcutaneous injection.

caf·fein·ism (kaf'een·iz·um) *n.* A toxic condition due to the excessive ingestion of coffee or other caffeine-containing substances.

Caf·fey's disease or **syndrome** INFANTILE CORTICAL HYPEROSTOSIS.

caged-ball prosthesis. An artificial cardiac valve consisting of a plastic or metal ball within a cage formed of metal struts.

caged-lens prosthesis. A prosthetic cardiac valve consisting of a freely floating lens-shaped disk in the valve cage.

-caine A combining form designating *a local anesthetic compound or substance.*

cai·no·pho·bia (kigh''no·fo'bee·uh, kay''no·) *n.* NEOPHOBIA.

cais·son disease (kay'sun). DECOMPRESSION SICKNESS.

caked, *adj.* Compressed, tense, or hardened, due to engorgement or induration.

caked bag. In cows, inflammation of an udder.

cake kidney. A form of crossed renal ectopia in which there is congenital fusion of both kid-

neys into a solid, irregularly lobate mass. Th ureter of the displaced kidney crosses th midline before draining distally. Syn. *clum kidney, lump kidney.*

Cal Abbreviation for *Calorie* (= KILOCALORIE

cal Abbreviation for *calorie.*

Calabar swellings Edematous, painful, subcuta neous swellings occurring in different parts the body of natives of Calabar and other par of West Africa, probably due to an allergi reaction to *Loa loa* infection.

cal·a·mine (kal'uh·mine, ·min) *n.* 1. Native zin carbonate. 2. Prepared calamine: zinc oxid with a small amount of ferric oxide; a pin powder, insoluble in water, used as a loca application in the treatment of skin disease It is also used to impart a "flesh color" t ointments, washes, and powders.

calc-, calci-, calco- A combining form meanin (a) *calcium;* (b) *calcium salts.*

calcane-, calcaneo-. A combining form meanin *calcaneus, calcaneal.*

cal·ca·ne·al (kal·kay'nee·ul) *adj.* Pertaining t the heel or to the calcaneus.

calcaneal spur. Calcific healing of a chron avulsion injury of the plantar fascia from th calcaneus.

calcaneal tendon. The common tendon of th gastrocnemius and soleus muscles inserte into the heel.

cal·ca·neo·ca·vus (kal·kay''nee·o·kay'vus) TALIPES CALCANEOCAVUS.

cal·ca·neo·cu·boid (kal·kay''nee·o·kew'boid) *ad* Pertaining to the calcaneus and the cuboi

cal·ca·neo·dyn·ia (kal·kay''nee·o·din'ee·uh) Pain in the heel, or calcaneus.

cal·ca·neo·val·gus (kal·kay''nee·o·val'gus) TALIPES CALCANEOVALGUS.

cal·ca·ne·us (kal·kay'nee·us) *n.,* pl. & genit. sin **calca·nei** (·nee·eye) 1. [NA] The heel bone. N alt. *os calcis.* See Table of Bones in the Appe dix. 2. TALIPES CALCANEUS.

calcaneus apophysitis. Epiphysitis of the he bone, or calcaneus.

cal·car (kal'kahr) *n.,* pl. **cal·car·ia** (kal·kär'ee·u Any spur or spurlike point. —**cal·ca·rate** (ka kuh·rate) *adj.*

cal·car·e·ous (kal·kair'ee·us) *adj.* 1. Pertaining or of the nature of limestone. 2. Having chalky appearance or consistency. 3. Contai ing calcium.

cal·ca·rine (kal'kuh·rin, ·reen) *adj.* Pertaining or like a calcar.

calcarine fissure. CALCARINE SULCUS.

calcarine sulcus. A sulcus on the medial aspe of the occipital lobe of the cerebrum, betwee the lingual gyrus and the cuneus.

cal·car·i·uria (kal·kair''ee·yoo'ree·uh) *n.* Th presence of calcium salts in the urine.

cal·ce·mia, cal·cae·mia (kal·see'mee·uh) *n.* H PERCALCEMIA.

cal·ci·bil·ia (kal''si·bil'ee·uh) *n.* Calcium in th bile.

cal·ci·co·sis (kal''si·ko'sis) *n.,* pl. **calcico·ses** (·see A form of pneumoconiosis due to the inhal tion of marble (calcium carbonate) dust.

cal·cif·er·ol (kal·sif'ur·ol) *n.* Vitamin D_2, o tained by irradiation of ergosterol; 1 mg repr sents 40,000 units of vitamin D activity.

cal·cif·er·ous (kal·sif'ur·us) *adj.* Containing calcium carbonate.

cal·cif·ic (kal·sif'ick) *adj.* Forming, causing, or involving deposition of a calcium salt.

cal·ci·fi·ca·tion (kal''si·fi·kay'shun) *n.* The deposit of calcareous matter within the tissues of the body.

calcified fetus. LITHOPEDION.

cal·ci·fy (kal'si·figh) *v.* To deposit mineral salts as in calcification. —**calci·fied** (·fide) *adj.*

calcifying epithelioma of Mal·herbe (mal·eʰrb') PILOMATRICOMA.

cal·cig·er·ous (kal·sij'ur·us) *adj.* Containing a calcium salt.

cal·cim·e·ter (kal·sim'e·tur) *n.* An apparatus for determining the amount of calcium in the blood.

cal·ci·na·tion (kal''si·nay'shun) *n.* The process of expelling volatile matter by heating, especially carbon dioxide and water from inorganic compounds, but in some cases involving also the combustion of organic matter. —**cal·cine** (kal'sine) *v.; ***cal·cined** (kal'sine'd) *adj.*

cal·ci·nol (kal'si·nole) *n.* CALCIUM GLUCONATE.

cal·ci·no·sis (kal''si·no'sis) *n., pl.* **calcino·ses** (·seez) 1. The deposition of calcium salts in tissues. 2. Sometimes specifically, CALCINOSIS CUTIS.

calcinosis cu·tis (kew'tis). The deposition of calcium salts in the skin and subcutaneous tissues without detectable injury of the affected parts or without hypercalcemia.

calcinosis cutis cir·cum·scrip·ta (sur''kum·skrip'tuh). Nodular calcification in the skin and subcutaneous tissues; seen frequently in the extremities, particularly the hands, in scleroderma.

calcinosis uni·ver·sa·lis (yoo''ni·vur·say'lis). Widespread calcified plaques that tend to ulcerate and heal slowly, and involve subcutaneous tissues, muscles, tendons, and nerve sheaths; seen especially in children and young adults and associated with such disorders as dermatomyositis, scleroderma, and Raynaud's disease. Etiology is unknown, but serum calcium, phosphorus, and alkaline phosphatase levels are normal.

cal·ci·pe·ni·a (kal''si·pee'nee·uh) *n.* Calcium deficiency.

cal·ci·phy·lax·is (kal''si·fi·lack'sis) *n.* A type of experimentally induced calcification in which a hypersensitive state is induced by certain substances (e.g., parathyroid hormone), followed after a critical period by administration of a challenging substance (e.g., metal salts).

cal·ci·to·nin (kal''si·to'nin) *n.* A single-chain polypeptide hormone consisting of 32 amino acids, apparently existing as several active fractions; secreted by the parafollicular cells of the thyroid gland in mammals and by the ultimobranchial bodies in birds, reptiles, amphibians and fish. The hormone lowers both plasma calcium and phosphate by inhibiting bone resorption without augmenting calcium accretion. It also causes increased renal excretion of phosphate, calcium, chloride, sodium, and magnesium. Syn. *thyrocalcitonin.*

cal·ci·um (kal'see·um) *n.* Ca = 40.08. A brilliant, silver-white metal, characterized by strong affinity for oxygen. It is an abundant and widely distributed element.

calcium acetate. A white, amorphous powder, $Ca(C_2H_3O_2)_2$, soluble in water; has been used medicinally as a source of calcium.

calcium acetylsalicylate. A white powder, $(CH_3COOC_6H_4COO)_2Ca.2H_2O$, readily soluble in water; used as an antirheumatic and analgesic.

calcium bromide. A white granular salt, $CaBr_2$, very deliquescent and very soluble in water; has been employed as a sedative and antiepileptic.

calcium carbide. A gray, crystalline solid, CaC_2, decomposed by water to yield acetylene.

calcium carbonate. Any of the forms of $CaCO_3$, including chalk, marble, and whiting. Used as an antacid.

calcium chloride. $CaCl_2.2H_2O$. White, deliquescent fragments or granules, soluble in water; used medicinally for the effects of calcium ion.

calcium creosotate. A mixture of the calcium compounds of creosote, representing about 50% creosote; has been used as an expectorant and intestinal antiseptic.

calcium cyanamide. CaNCN. Gray lumps or powder. Reacts with water to produce ammonia. Used in fertilizers.

calcium disodium ede·tate (ed'e·tate). Calcium disodium (ethylenedinitrilo) tetraacetate or calcium disodium ethylenediaminetetraacetate, $C_{10}H_{12}CaN_2Na_2O_8.xH_2O$, a white, crystalline powder, freely soluble in water. A metal complexing agent used for diagnosis and treatment of lead poisoning.

calcium EDTA (ee·dee·tee·ay). CALCIUM DISODIUM EDETATE.

Calcium folinate SF. A trademark for leucovorin calcium.

calcium glu·bi·o·nate (gloo·bye'uh·nate). Calcium D-gluconate lactobionate, monohydrate, $C_{18}H_{32}CaO_{19}.H_2O$, a calcium replenishing agent.

calcium gluconate. A white crystalline or granular powder, $[CH_2OH(CHOH)_4COO]_2Ca.H_2O$, soluble in water; used medicinally for the effects of calcium.

calcium glycerophosphate. $CaC_3H_5(OH)_2PO_4$. A white crystalline powder, soluble in water; used as a calcium and phosphate dietary supplement.

calcium hydroxide. Slaked lime, $Ca(OH)_2$, the active ingredient of lime water.

calcium hypochlorite. $Ca(ClO)_2$. A principal ingredient of chlorinated lime; used as an antiseptic, disinfectant, and bleaching agent.

calcium lactate. A white powder, $Ca(C_3H_5O_3)_2.5H_2O$, soluble in water; used medicinally for the effects of calcium ion.

calcium mandelate. A white powder, $Ca(C_6H_5CHOHCOO)_2$, slightly soluble in water. Used medicinally for the effect of mandelic acid as a urinary antiseptic.

calcium oxalate. CaC_2O_4; a white, crystalline powder, practically insoluble in water. A form in which calcium is precipitated in certain pathological conditions and in analyses for the element.

calcium oxide. CaO. Lime; quicklime; burnt

lime. Used industrially but not medicinally.

calcium phenolsulfonate. A water-soluble powder, $Ca(C_6H_4OHSO_3)_2$; has been used as an intestinal antiseptic and astringent.

calcium phosphate. Any one of three salts, differing in the proportion of calcium and phosphate: monobasic calcium phosphate, $CaH_4(PO_4)_2.H_2O$, a deliquescent and strongly acid powder; dibasic calcium phosphate, $CaHPO_4.2H_2O$, used as a calcium and phosphorus dietary supplement; tribasic calcium phosphate, $Ca_3(PO_4)_2$, used as an antacid.

calcium sulfate. $CaSO_4$, occurring naturally as the dihydrate gypsum which, when partially or completely dehydrated (calcined) by heating, constitutes plaster of Paris.

cal·ci·uria (kal″see-yoo'ree-uh) *n.* 1. Calcium in the urine. 2. HYPERCALCINURIA.

cal·co·glob·u·lin (kal″ko-glob'yoo-lin) *n.* A combination of calcium with protein such as is found in calcospherites, probably representing an early stage in the process of laying down calcium salts in teeth and bone.

cal·co·sphe·rite, cal·co·sphae·rite (kal″ko-sfeer'ite) *n.* One of the granules or globules formed in tissues like bone and shell by a loose combination of protein and blood-borne calcium salts.

cal·cu·lary (kal'kew-lerr-ee) *adj.* Of or pertaining to a calculus or to calculi.

cal·cu·lo·gen·e·sis (kal″kew-lo-jen'e-sis) *n.,* pl. **calculogene·ses** (·seez) The origin or development of calculi.

cal·cu·lo·sis (kal″kew-lo'sis) *n.* The presence of a calculus or an abnormal concretion.

cal·cu·lus (kal'kew-lus) *n.,* pl. **calcu·li** (·lye) A solid concretion composed chiefly of mineral substances and salts found in ducts, passages, hollow organs, cysts, and on the surfaces of teeth. Organic materials such as cells and mucus may form a centrum or nidus and may be dispersed as a matrix for the mineral deposits, as salts of calcium, of uric acid, or of bile acids. —**calculous,** *adj.*

Caldecort. A trademark for calcium undecylenate, an antifungal agent.

cal·e·fa·cient (kal″e-fay'shunt) *adj. & n.* 1. Warming; causing a sensation of warmth. 2. A medicine, externally applied, that causes a sensation of warmth.

calf (kaf) *n.,* pl. **calves** (kavz) The thick, fleshy part of the back of the leg, formed by the gastrocnemius and soleus muscles and overlying tissues.

cal·i·ber, cal·i·bre (kal'i-bur) *n.* The diameter of a cylindrical or round body, as an artery.

cal·i·bra·tion (kal″i-bray'shun) *n.* 1. The specification and measurements of the properties or performance of a device, so that it may be used for subsequent measuring procedures. 2. The measurement of the caliber of a tube, or the determination or rectification of the graduations on a tube, pipet, or balance weights. —**cal·i·bra·tor** (kal'i-bray-tur) *n.;* **cal·i·brate** (kal'i-brate) *v.*

cal·i·ce·al (kal″i-see'ul) *adj.* Of or pertaining to a calix.

caliceal diverticulum. A congenital or acquired outpouching or sac arising from a renal calix.

cal·i·cec·ta·sis (kal″i-seck'tuh-sis, kay″li-) *n.,* pl. **calicecta·ses** (·seez) Dilatation of a renal calix.

calices. Plural of *calix.*

ca·lic·i·form (ka-lis'i-form) *adj.* Shaped like a calix.

ca·lic·u·lus (ka-lick'yoo-lus) *n.,* pl. **calicu·li** (·lye) A small cuplike structure.

caliculus gu·sta·to·ri·us (gus″tuh-tor'ee-us), pl. **caliculi gustato·rii** (·ee-eye) [NA]. TASTE BUD.

cal·i·for·ni·um (kal″i-for'nee-um) *n.* Cf = 249. A radioactive element discovered by bombarding an isotope of curium with alpha particles.

cal·i·per (kal'i-pur) *n.* 1. A curved and hinged instrument with adjustable legs or jaws for measuring the thickness and the outside or inside diameters of objects. 2. Any type of such an instrument, as a micrometer caliper.

cal·is·then·ics (kal″iss-then'icks) *n.* A system of or the practice of, light gymnastics by various rhythmic movements of the body; intended to develop the muscles and graceful carriage.

ca·lix (kay'licks, kal'icks) *n.,* pl. **ca·li·ces** (kal'i-seez, kay'li-seez) 1. A cuplike structure. 2. Specifically, RENAL CALIX. 3. (Of an ovum:) The wall of the graafian follicle from which the ovum has escaped.

Cal·kins method Delay of placental delivery until the uterus assumes a globular shape indicative of placental detachment from the uterine lining.

Cal·lan·der's amputation Amputation at the knee joint preserving long anterior and posterior flaps; the patella is removed, and the resulting fossa receives the femoral stump.

Call-Ex·ner bodies Minute rosettelike groupings of cells occurring in the granulosa membrane of the ovarian follicle either before or after formation; also sometimes seen in granulosa cell tumors.

cal·li·pe·dia (kal″i-pee'dee-uh) *n.* 1. The desire to give birth to a beautiful child. 2. The superstition that if a pregnant woman concentrates upon having a beautiful child or looks a representations of one, her baby will be beautiful.

Cal·li·phor·i·dae (kal″i-for'i-dee) *n.pl.* A family of the Diptera which includes many large blue green, or copper-colored species, commonly called bluebottle, greenbottle, and blowflies They normally deposit their eggs or larvae in the decaying flesh of dead animals but may be secondary invaders of neglected wounds and sores. —**cal·liph·o·rid** (ka-lif'uh-rid) *adj. & n.*

cal·lo·ma·nia (kal″o-may'nee-uh) *n.* A delusional state characterized by a belief in one's own beauty.

cal·lo·sal (ka-lo'sul) *adj.* Pertaining to the corpus callosum.

callosal sulcus. The groove separating the corpus callosum from the overlying cingulate gyrus.

cal·los·i·ty (ka-los'i-tee) *n.* A circumscribed area of skin thickened by hypertrophy of the horny layer of the epidermis, caused by friction or pressure. Syn. *callus.*

cal·lo·sum (ka-lo'sum) *n.,* pl. **callo·sa** (·suh). CORPUS CALLOSUM.

cal·lus (kal'us) *n.* 1. A callosity, especially of the palm or sole. 2. New growth of incompletely organized bony tissue surrounding the bone ends in fracture; a part of the reparative process. —**callous**, *adj.*

calm·a·tive (kahl'muh·tiv) *adj. & n.* SEDATIVE.

cal·o·mel (kal'o·mel) *n.* Mercurous chloride, HgCl. A white powder, insoluble in water; formerly used as a cathartic and diuretic, now used, in ointment form, as a local antibacterial.

cal·or (kal'or, kay'lor) *n.* Heat; one of the four classic signs of inflammation: calor, rubor, tumor, dolor.

cal·o·res·cence (kal''o·res'unce) *n.* The conversion of invisible heat rays into luminous heat rays.

calori- A combining form meaning *heat.*

ca·lo·ric (ka·lo'rick) *adj.* Pertaining to a calorie, calories, or to heat.

caloric test. With the patient's head tilted 30° forward from the horizontal, the external auditory meatuses are irrigated in turn for 30 seconds with water at 30°C and 44°C, with a pause of at least 5 minutes between irrigations. In normal persons, cold water induces a slight tonic deviation to the side being irrigated, followed, after about 20 seconds by nystagmus with the fast component to the opposite side. Irrigation with warm water induces nystagmus to the same side. If the vestibular nerve or labyrinth is destroyed as the result of disease, no nystagmus is produced upon testing the diseased side.

Cal·o·rie, Cal·o·ry (kal'uh·ree) *n.* KILOCALORIE.

cal·o·rie, cal·o·ry, *n.* Any one of several heat units that represent the quantity of heat required to raise the temperature of 1 g water by 1°C but that differ slightly from each other in the specific 1° interval of temperature selected. The units are also defined in equivalent mechanical energy units, the equivalents for one calorie ranging from 4.1816 to 4.2045 joules. Syn. *small calorie, gram calorie.*

cal·o·rif·ic (kal''o·rif'ick) *adj.* Heat-producing; pertaining to heat or calories.

ca·lo·ri·ge·net·ic (ka·lor''i·je·net'ick) *adj.* CALORIGENIC.

ca·lo·ri·gen·ic (ka·lor''i·jen'ick, kal''or·i·) *adj.* Heat-producing; applied to certain foods and hormones.

cal·o·rim·e·ter (kal''o·rim'e·tur) *n.* An instrument for measuring the heat production of an individual or a physical system under standard conditions.

cal·o·rim·e·try (kal''o·rim'e·tree) *n.* The determination of the total heat produced or released by an individual or a physical system by use of a calorimeter. —**cal·o·ri·met·ric** (kal''o·ri·met'rick) *adj.*

cal·var·ia (kal·vair'ee·uh) *n.*, pl. & genit. sing.

cal·var·i·ae (·ee·ee) The upper part of the skull; the skullcap. —**calvar·i·al** (·ee·ul) *adj.*

cal·var·i·um (kal·vair'ee·um) *n.* CALVARIA.

cal·vi·ti·es (kal·vish'ee·eez) *n.* Loss of hair, especially on the crown of the head; alopecia, baldness.

calyceal. CALICEAL.

calycectasis. CALICECTASIS.

calycectomy. CALICECTOMY.

calyces. A plural of *calyx.*

calyciform. CALICIFORM.

ca·ly·cine (kay'li·seen, kal'i·) *adj.* Pertaining to or resembling a calyx.

Ca·lym·ma·to·bac·te·ri·um gran·u·lo·ma·tis (ka·lim''uh·to·back·teer'ee·um gran·yoo·lo'muh·tis). A gram-negative coccobacillus that is responsible for the venereal disease granuloma inguinale. Syn. *Donovania granulomatis, Klebsiella granulomatis.*

ca·lyx (kay'licks, kal'icks) *n.*, pl. **calyxes, caly·ces** (kal'i·seez, kay'li·) 1. The outer sheath of a flower or bud, formed by the sepals. 2. CALIX.

ca·me·ra (kam'e·ruh) *L. n.*, pl. & genit. sing. **came·rae** (·ree). *In anatomy*, a chamber or compartment.

camera lu·ci·da (lew'si·duh). An optical device used to project onto paper the image of an object so that an accurate drawing can be made.

cam·i·sole (kam'i·sole) *n.* A canvas shirt with very long sleeves; used as a straitjacket.

Cam·per's fascia (kahᵐ'pur) The superficial, loose, fat-containing layer of the superficial fascia of the anterior abdominal wall.

camph-, campho-. A combining form meaning *camphor.*

cam·phor (kam'fur) *n.* A ketone, $C_{10}H_{16}O$, obtained from the volatile oil of *Cinnamomum camphora*, a tree indigenous to eastern Asia, or produced synthetically. It is a mild irritant and antiseptic and has been used as a carminative and stimulant. —**camphor·at·ed** (·ay·tid), **camphor·ic** (kam·for'ick) *adj.*

camphorated oil. CAMPHOR LINIMENT.

camphorated opium tincture. A hydroalcoholic solution of opium containing also anise oil, benzoic acid, camphor, and glycerin; used as an antiperistaltic drug in treating diarrheas. Syn. *paregoric.*

camphor liniment. A solution of camphor in cottonseed oil; a counterirritant embrocation.

camphor oil. A volatile oil obtained from the camphor tree, *Cinnamomum camphora*; has been used as a rubefacient.

cam·pim·e·ter (kam·pim'e·tur) *n.* An instrument for measuring the field of vision. —**campime·try** (·tree) *n.*

camp·to·cor·mia (kamp''to·kor'mee·uh) *n.* A static deformity of hysterical origin characterized by a forward flexion of the trunk.

camp·to·dac·ty·ly (kamp''to·dack'ti·lee) *n.* A condition in which one or more fingers are constantly flexed at one or both phalangeal joints.

Canada-Cronkhite syndrome. CRONKHITE-CANADA SYNDROME.

Ca·na·dian crutch. A lightweight crutch so constructed that the weight of the body is transmitted to it through the extended arm and palm of the hand that grasps the horizontal handle.

can·a·dine (kan'uh·deen, ·din) *n.* Tetrahydroberberine, $C_{20}H_{21}NO_4$, a colorless alkaloid from the plant *Hydrastis canadensis.*

ca·nal (kuh·nal') *n.* Any tubular channel; DUCT.

can·a·lic·u·lar (kan''uh·lick'yoo·lur) *adj.* Of or pertaining to a canaliculus.

canalicular scissors. Delicate scissors, one blade

of which is probe-pointed; used for slitting the lacrimal canaliculus.

canaliculi. Plural of *canaliculus.*

can·a·lic·u·lo·plas·ty (kan-uh-lick'yoo-lo-plas"tee) *n.* Plastic repair of a canaliculus, especially that leading from the punctum to the lacrimal sac.

can·a·lic·u·lus (kan"uh-lick'yoo-lus) *n.,* pl. **canaliculi** (·lye) 1. A small canal; especially that leading from the lacrimal punctum to the lacrimal sac of the eye. 2. Any one of the minute canals opening into the lacunas of bone. —**canaliculation** (·lick"yoo-lay'shun), **canaliculization** (·li-zay'shun) *n.*

ca·na·lis (ka-nay'lis) *n.,* pl. **cana·les** (·leez) CANAL.

canalis op·ti·cus (op'ti·kus) [NA]. OPTIC CANAL.

ca·nal·iza·tion (ka·nal"i·zay'shun, kan"ul·i·zay'shun, ·eye·zay'shun) *n.* 1. The formation of new channels in tissues, as the formation of new blood vessels in a thrombus. 2. A system of wound drainage without tubes. —**ca·nal·ize** (ka·nal'ize, kan'ul·ize) *v.*

canal of Corti TUNNEL OF CORTI.

canal of Nuck In the female, the vaginal process of peritoneum passing into the inguinal canal.

canal of the cervix of the uterus. The portion of the uterine cavity situated in the cervix, extending from the isthmus to the ostium of the uterus. Syn. *cervical canal.*

Can·a·van's disease or **spongy degeneration** (kan"uh·vun) SPONGY DEGENERATION OF INFANCY.

can·cel·lous (kan'se·lus) *adj.* Characterized by reticulated or latticed structure, as the spongy tissue of bones or, in botany, certain leaves consisting largely of veins. —**can·cel·la·tion** (kan·se·lay'shun) *n.*

cancellous bone. A form of bone in which the matrix is arranged in a network of rods, plates, or tubes (the trabeculae), with spaces between filled with marrow.

can·cer (kan'sur) *n.* 1. A malignant tumor. 2. Any disease characterized by malignant tumor formation or proliferation of anaplastic cells.

cancer en cui·rasse (ahn kwi·ras'). 1. Widely infiltrating carcinoma of the skin of the thorax, usually arising in mammary carcinoma. 2. Widespread carcinoma of the pleura.

can·cer·i·ci·dal (kan"sur·i·sigh'dul) *adj.* Able to kill the cells of a malignant tumor.

can·cer·i·gen·ic (kan"sur·i·jen'ick) *adj.* CARCINOGENIC.

can·cer·ol·o·gy (kan"sur·ol'uh·jee) *n.* Obsol. The study and science of cancer. —**cancerolo·gist,** *n.*

can·cero·pho·bia (kan"sur·o·fo'bee·uh) *n.* CARCINOPHOBIA.

can·cer·ous (kan'sur·us) *adj.* Of or pertaining to a cancer; like a cancer.

can·cer·pho·bia (kan"sur·fo'bee·uh) *n.* CARCINOPHOBIA.

can·croid (kang'kroid) *n. & adj.* 1. SQUAMOUS CELL CARCINOMA. 2. Of or pertaining to squamous cell carcinoma.

can·crum oris (kang'krum or'is). Noma of the mouth.

can·de·la (kan·dee'luh) *n.* The new unit of luminous intensity, of such magnitude that a black-body radiator at the temperature at which pure platinum solidifies has a luminous intensity of 60 candelas per square centimeter. Abbreviated, cd.

Can·di·da (kan'di·duh) *n.* A genus of yeastlike, opportunistically pathogenic fungi. Syn. *Monilia.* —**can·di·dal** (·dul) *adj.*

can·di·di·a·sis (kan"di·dye'uh·sis) *n.,* pl. **candidia·ses** (·seez) A condition produced by infection with a fungus of the genus *Candida,* usually *C. albicans;* involving various parts of the body, as skin, mucous membrane, nails, bronchi, lungs, heart, vagina, and gastrointestinal tract, and rarely, occurrence of septicemia.

can·di·did (kan'di·did) *n.* A sterile grouped vesicular lesion of the hands or body resulting from hypersensitivity to a focus of *Candida* infection.

ca·nel·la (ka·nel'uh) *n.* The bark of the tree, *Canella winterana,* native to the West Indies, dried and without the cork layer; popularly used as an aromatic tonic. Syn. *white cinnamon.*

ca·nic·o·la fever (ka·nick'o·luh). The form of leptospirosis in man caused by infection with *Leptospira canicola.*

ca·nine (kay'nine) *adj. & n.* 1. Pertaining to or resembling dogs. 2. A member of the dog family. 3. Pertaining to a canine tooth. 4. CANINE TOOTH.

canine distemper. A pantropic virus disease occurring among animals of the family Canidae and certain other carnivores such as mink and racoons; may be characterized by respiratory, enteric, or neurological symptoms.

canine fossa. A depression on the external surface of the maxilla, above and to the outer side of the socket of the canine tooth.

canine teeth. Sharp tearing teeth of mammals, located between the incisors and premolars. In the human dentition.

ca·ni·ti·es (ka·nish'ee·eez) *n.* Grayness or whiteness of the hair. Syn. *poliosis.*

can·ker (kang'kur) *n.* 1. An ulceration, especially one of the mouth and lips; also a gangrenous ulcer or gangrenous stomatitis. 2. APHTHOUS STOMATITIS; THRUSH. 3. A disease of the horn-forming membrane of horse's hoofs, leading to destruction of the cells and loss of the horn-secreting function. 4. Granulomatous inflammation of the external ears, particularly of dogs and rabbits.

canker sore. A small ulceration of the mucous membrane of the mouth.

can·na·bi·nol (ka·nab'i·nol) *n.* A substance, $C_{21}H_{26}O_2$, resulting from spontaneous dehydrogenation of tetrahydrocannabinol in cannabis. Though commonly considered physiologically inactive, cannabinol has some of the characteristic activity of cannabis.

can·na·bis (kan'uh·bis) *n.* The flowering or fruiting tops of the pistillate hemp plant, *Cannabis sativa,* of which there are two varieties, Indian and American, the former being the more potent. The active constituents have been shown to be tetrahydrocannabinols. Cannabis is classified as a hallucinogen. In large doses it produces mental exaltation, intoxication, and a sensation of double consciousness in some individuals. It is important as an intoxicant, but has no rational therapeutic use. Bhang, ganga, charas, kif, hashish, and marijuana are among the various names by which the drug and certain preparations of it are known.

can·na·bism (kan'uh·biz·um) n. Poisoning resulting from excessive or habitual use of cannabis.

can·ni·bal·ism (kan'i·bul·iz·um) n. 1. The eating of one's own kind, frequently observed in the postpartum rabbit or rat. 2. Specifically, the eating of human flesh by human beings. —**can·ni·bal·is·tic** adj.

can·non·ball, n. In radiology, a sharply defined, round, homogeneous, dense shadow in the lung, commonly produced by metastatic carcinoma or by a granuloma.

can·nu·la (kan'yoo·luh) n., pl. **cannulas, cannu·lae** (·lee) An artificial tube of various sizes and shapes often fitted with a trocar for insertion into a tube or cavity of the body, as an artery or the trachea. —**cannu·lar** (·lur), **cannu·late** (·late) adj.

can·nu·late (kan'yoo·late) v. To insert a cannula into a body cavity or hollow organ. —**can·nu·la·tion** (kan'yoo·lay'shun) n.

canth-, cantho-. A combining form meaning canthus, canthal.

can·thal (kan'thul) adj. Of or pertaining to a canthus.

can·thar·i·des (kan·thăr'i·deez) n. pl. The dried insects, Cantharis vesicatoria, yielding cantharidin; has been used externally as a rubefacient and vesicant.

can·thar·i·din (kan·thăr'i·din) n. The active principle, $C_{10}H_{12}O_4$, of cantharides and other insects; formerly used topically as a counterirritant.

can·tha·ris (kan'thuh·ris). Singular of cantharides.

can·thec·to·my (kan·theck'tuh·mee) n. Excision of a canthus.

canthi. Plural of canthus.

can·thi·tis (kan·thigh'tis) n. Inflammation of a canthus.

can·thol·y·sis (kan·thol'i·sis) n., pl. **cantholy·ses** (·seez) Canthotomy with section of the lateral palpebral ligament.

can·tho·plas·ty (kan'tho·plas''tee) n. 1. Increasing the length of the palpebral fissure by slitting the outer canthus. 2. Any plastic restoration of a canthal defect.

can·thor·rha·phy (kan·thor'uh·fee) n. In plastic surgery, shortening of the palpebral fissure by suture of the canthus.

can·thot·o·my (kan·thot'uh·mee) n. Surgical division of a canthus.

can·thus (kanth'us) n., pl. **can·thi** (·eye) Either of the two angles formed by the junction of the eyelids, designated outer or lateral, and inner or medial. Syn. palpebral angle.

cap. Abbreviation for (a) capiat; let him take; (b) capsula; a capsule.

cap, n. A covering or coverlike structure; a tegmen.

ca·pac·i·tance (ka·pas'i·tunce) n. The quantity of electricity which a condenser (capacitor) or other structure can hold per volt of electric pressure applied.

ca·pac·i·tor (ka·pas'i·tur) n. An instrument for holding or storing charges of electricity; CONDENSER (3).

Capastat. A trademark for capreomycin, an antibiotic.

Cape aloe. Aloe obtained from the plant Aloe ferox, and hybrids of this species with A. africana and A. spicata.

cap·il·lar·ec·ta·sia (kap''i·lăr''eck·tay'zee·uh, ·zhuh) n. Dilatation of the capillaries.

cap·il·lar·i·tis (kap''i·lăr·eye'tis) n. A progressive pigmentary disorder of skin with dilatation, but not inflammation, of superficial capillaries, not associated with any systemic complications and running a benign self-limited course.

cap·il·lar·i·ty (kap''i·lăr'i·tee) n. 1. CAPILLARY ATTRACTION. 2. Elevation or depression of liquids in capillary tubes due to the surface tension of the liquid.

cap·il·la·ros·co·py (kap''i·lăr·os'kuh·pee) n. Microscopical examination of the cutaneous capillaries for diagnosis.

cap·il·lary (kap'i·lair''ee) adj. & n. 1. Of or pertaining to a hair, to a hairlike filament, or to a tube with a minute bore. 2. A minute blood vessel connecting the smallest ramifications of the arteries with those of the veins or one of the smallest lymph vessels.

capillary angioma. An angioma whose vessels are of capillary size and structure.

capillary attraction. The surface force which draws aqueous liquids into and along the lumen of a capillary tube.

capillary bed. The capillaries, collectively, of a given area or organ.

capillary bronchitis. BRONCHIOLITIS.

capillary drain. A drain of horsehair or silkworm gut used to keep a wound open for a short period.

capillary hemangioma. A benign vascular tumor composed largely of capillaries.

capillary pulse. Pulsation sometimes observable at the arterial end of skin capillaries, best seen as alternate blanching and flushing of the nailbeds; occurs in aortic regurgitation and high-cardiac-output states.

capillary tube. A tube with a minute lumen.

cap·il·lo·ve·nous (kap''i·lo·vee'nus) adj. 1. Pertaining to a junctional vessel between a capillary and a venule. 2. Pertaining to the capillaries and first subpapillary venous plexus of the skin.

ca·pil·lus (ka·pil'us) n., pl. **capil·li** (·eye) A hair; specifically, a hair of the head.

cap·i·tate (kap'i·tate) adj. In biology, having a head or a headlike termination; head-shaped.

capitate bone. The largest of the carpal bones.

cap·i·ta·tum (kap''i·tay'tum) n., pl. **capita·ta** (·tuh) CAPITATE BONE.

cap·i·tel·lum (kap''i·tel'um) n., pl. **capitel·la** (·uh) A small head or rounded process of bone. —**capitel·lar** (·ur) adj.

ca·pit·u·lum (ka·pit'yoo·lum) n., genit. sing. **capi·tu·li** (·lye), pl. **capitu·la** (·luh) The small eminence on the distal end of the humerus, which articulates with the radius. —**capitu·lar** (·lur) adj.

Cap·lan's syndrome Massive anthracosilicotic

nodular fibrosis of the lung in patients with rheumatoid arthritis.

-capnia A combining form signifying *the presence of carbon dioxide.*

cap·o·ben·ic acid (kap·o·ben′ick). 6-(3,4,5-Trimethoxybenzamido)hexanoic acid, $C_{16}H_{23}NO_6$, an antiarrhythmic agent.

cap·ric acid (kap′rick). Decanoic acid, $CH_3(CH_2)_8COOH$, a solid fatty acid occurring as a glyceride in butter and other animal fats.

Caprocid. A trademark for aminocaproic acid, an antifibrinolytic agent.

Caprocin. A trademark for capreomycin sulfate.

ca·pro·ic acid (ka·pro′ick). Hexanoic acid, $CH_3(CH_2)_4COOH$, a liquid fatty acid occurring as a glyceride in butter and other animal fats.

ca·pryl·ic acid (ka·pril′ick). Octanoic acid, $CH_3(CH_2)_6COOH$, a solid fatty acid occurring in butter, coconut oil, and other fats and oils.

cap·si·cum (kap′si·kum) n. The dried fruit of *Capsicum frutescens* (bush red pepper) or of several other varieties (tabasco or Louisiana long or short peppers). Its characteristic pungent constituent is capsaicin. Various preparations of capsicum have been used for local counterirritant action and, internally, for tonic and carminative effects.

cap·sid (kap′sid) n. The protein coat surrounding the nucleic acid of viruses, formed in a helical or icosahedral shape by a regular arrangement of capsomers.

capsul-, capsulo-. A combining form meaning *capsule.*

cap·su·lar (kap′sue·lur) adj. Pertaining to, resembling, or within a capsule.

capsular ankylosis. An ankylosis due to cicatricial thickening or shortening of the joint capsule.

capsular cataract. Cataract due to opacity of the lens capsule or capsular remnants following surgery or trauma.

capsular hemiplegia or paralysis. Hemiplegia without aphasia or sensory or emotional disturbances, due to a lesion in the contralateral internal capsule.

cap·sule (kap′sool, ·syool) n. 1. A membranous investment of a part. 2. An envelope surrounding certain organisms. 3. A soluble shell, usually made of gelatin, for administering medicines. 4. *In physiology,* an instrument used for the optical recording of pressure changes or vibrations, as pressure pulses or heart sounds. It consists of a cylindrical chamber closed on one end by a thin membrane to which is glued a small mirror. Pressure changes cause movement of the membrane and deflections of a beam of light which is reflected to a photokymograph.

cap·su·lec·to·my (kap″sue·leck′tuh·mee) n. Excision of a capsule.

capsule of the lens. A transparent, structureless membrane enclosing the lens of the eye.

cap·su·li·tis (kap″sue·ligh′tis) n. Inflammation of a capsule, as that of the liver (perihepatitis), a joint (knee or ankle), or the labyrinth (otosclerosis).

capsulo-. See *capsul-.*

cap·su·lo·len·tic·u·lar (kap″sue·lo·len·tick′yoo·lur) adj. Pertaining to the capsule and the lens of the eye.

capsulolenticular cataract. A cataract involving the lens nucleus or cortex and capsule.

cap·su·lo·plas·ty (kap′sue·lo·plas″tee) n. An operation for plastic repair of a joint capsule.

cap·su·lor·rha·phy (kap″sue·lor′uh·fee) n. Suture of a capsule; especially suture of a joint capsule to repair a rent or to prevent dislocation.

cap·su·lo·tha·lam·ic (kap″sue·lo·thuh·lam′ick) adj. Pertaining to or involving the internal capsule and the thalamus.

cap·su·lot·o·my (kap″sue·lot′uh·mee) n. 1. Incision into a joint capsule. 2. Incision of the lens capsule or lens capsular remnants.

cap·ta·tion (kap·tay′shun) n. The first or light stage of hypnotism.

ca·put (kap′ut) n., genit. **ca·pi·tis** (kap′i·tis), pl. **capi·ta** (·tuh) HEAD.

caput me·du·sae (me·dew′see). Dilatation of the periumbilical venous plexus, with blood flowing away from the umbilicus; seen with portal hypertension.

caput ob·sti·pum (ob′sti·pum). TORTICOLLIS.

caput qua·dra·tum (kwah·dray′tum). A deformity of the head in rickets, manifested by a flattened top and sides, with projecting occiput and prominent frontal bosses.

caput suc·ce·da·ne·um (suck″se·day′nee·um). Swelling of the presenting part of the head of the fetus, produced during labor, and resulting in edema and varying degrees of hemorrhage of the scalp.

car·am·i·phen (kahr·am′i·fen) n. 1-Phenylcyclopentanecarboxylic acid 2-diethylaminoethyl ester, $C_{18}H_{27}NO_2$, a parasympatholytic drug; used as the hydrochloride salt in the treatment of parkinsonism.

ca·ra·te (ka·rah′teh) n. PINTA.

carb-, carbo- A combining form meaning (a) *carbon;* (b) *carbonic;* (c) *carboxyl.*

car·ba·chol (kahr′buh·kole, ·kol) n. Carbamoylcholine chloride, $C_6H_{15}ClN_2O_2$, a choline ester with potent parasympathomimetic action; now employed primarily as a miotic in the local treatment of glaucoma.

car·ba·mate (kahr′buh·mate, kahr·bam′ate) n. A salt of carbamic acid; it contains the univalent radical NH_2COO.

car·bam·ic acid (kahr·bam′ick). Aminoformic acid, NH_2COOH, the monoamide of carbonic acid; occurs only in the form of salts and esters; the latter are known as urethanes.

car·bam·ide (kahr·bam′ide, kahr′buh·mide) n. UREA.

car·bar·sone (kahr·bahr′sone) n. *p*-Ureidobenzenearsonic acid, $C_7H_9AsN_2O_4$, a pentavalent arsenical formerly used in the treatment of intestinal amebiasis and *Trichomonas* vaginitis.

car·ba·sus (kahr′buh·sus) n. Gauze; thin muslin used in surgery.

car·be·nox·o·lone (kahr·be·nock′suh·lone) n. 3β-Hydroxy-11-oxoolean-12-en-30-oic acid hydrogen succinate, $C_{34}H_{50}O_7$, an antibacterial usually used as the disodium salt.

car·be·ta·pen·tane (kahr·bay″tuh·pen′tane) n. 2-

(Diethylaminoethoxy)ethyl 1-phenylcyclopentyl-1-carboxylate, $C_{20}H_{31}NO_3$, an antitussive drug; used as the citrate salt.

car·bi·do·pa (kahr·bi·do'puh) n. (−)-L-α-Hydrazino-3,4-dihydroxy-α-methylhydrocinnamic acid monohydrate, $C_{10}H_{14}N_2O_4 \cdot H_2O$, an antihypertensive agent.

car·bi·nol (kahr'bi·nol) n. METHYL ALCOHOL.

Carbitol. 1. Trademark for diethylene glycol monoethyl ether, $C_6H_{14}O_3$, used principally as a solvent. 2. Trademark for various ethers of diethylene glycol, the specific ether being indicated by a qualifying adjective, such as methyl or butyl.

Carbocaine. Trademark for mepivacaine, a local anesthetic; used as the hydrochloride salt.

car·bo·cy·clic (kahr"bo·sigh'click, ·sick'lick) adj. *In chemistry,* pertaining to compounds of the closed-chain type in which all the ring atoms are carbon.

car·bo·hy·drase (kahr"bo·high'drace, ·draze) n. An enzyme capable of converting higher carbohydrates into simple sugars.

car·bo·hy·drate (kahr"bo·high'drate) n. An organic substance belonging to the class of compounds represented by the sugars, dextrins, starches, and celluloses; it contains carbon, hydrogen, and oxygen. Formerly it was believed that hydrogen and oxygen were always present in the proportion found in water; but this is not always the case. The carbohydrates form a large class of organic compounds; they may be further classified into monosaccharides, disaccharides, trisaccharides, oligosaccharides, and polysaccharides.

carbohydrate-induced hyperlipemia. 1. FAMILIAL HYPERBETA- AND HYPERPREBETALIPOPROTEINEMIA. 2. FAMILIAL HYPERPREBETALIPOPROTEINEMIA.

carbohydrate-induced hypertriglyceridemia. CARBOHYDRATE-INDUCED HYPERLIPEMIA.

car·bo·hy·dra·tu·ria (kahr·bo·high"dray·tew'ree·uh) n. The presence of an abnormally large proportion of carbohydrates in the urine; glycosuria.

carbol-. A combining form meaning *phenol.*

car·bo·late (kahr'bo·late) n. & v. 1. PHENATE. 2. To impregnate with phenol.

carbol-fuchsin solution. A solution of phenol, basic fuchsin, and resorcinol in a solvent medium of acetone, alcohol, and water; used topically as an antifungal preparation. Syn. *Castellani's paint.*

car·bol·ic acid (kahr·bol'ick). PHENOL.

car·bo·lize (kahr'bo·lize) v. CARBOLATE (2).

car·bo·lu·ria (kahr"bo·lew'ree·uh) n. The presence of phenol in the urine, producing a dark discoloration.

car·bo·my·cin (kahr"bo·migh'sin) n. An antibiotic substance, $C_{42}H_{67}NO_{16}$, produced by selected strains of *Streptomyces halstedii.* Possesses inhibitory activity especially against gram-positive bacteria, but is also active against certain rickettsiae and large viruses. It has been used to treat patients who have become resistant to penicillin and other antibiotics.

car·bon (kahr'bun) n. C = 12.011. A nonmetallic element widely distributed in nature. Its three allotropic forms are exemplified by the diamond, graphite, and charcoal. It occurs in all organic compounds; the ability of its atoms to link to each other affords an innumerable variety of combinations.

¹car·bon·ate (kahr'buh·nate, ·nut) n. The divalent radical CO_3; any salt or ester containing this radical, as salts or esters of carbonic acid.

²car·bon·ate (kahr'buh·nate) v. To charge with carbon dioxide.

carbon dioxide. CO_2, an odorless, colorless, noncombustible gas; a waste product of aerobic metabolism excreted via the blood in the pulmonary capillaries into the lung alveoli. It is an essential component of the blood buffer system and the prime physiologic stimulant of the respiratory center in the medulla oblongata.

carbon dioxide snow. Solid carbon dioxide used medicinally as an escharotic and commercially as a refrigerant. Syn. *dry ice.*

carbon dioxide therapy. 1. *In psychiatry,* a form of shock treatment in which carbon dioxide is administered by inhalation until profound physiologic changes, including convulsions, occur. 2. *In dermatology,* the application of solid carbon dioxide to lesions for purposes of extirpation by deep freezing.

car·bon·ic acid (kahr·bon'ick). A feebly ionizing acid, H_2CO_3, formed when carbon dioxide is dissolved in water.

carbonic anhydrase. An enzyme containing zinc, found in erythrocytes and in tissues, which catalyzes the reaction $H_2O + CO_2 \rightleftharpoons H_2CO_3$. In the transport of CO_2 in the body, the reaction proceeds to the right in the tissues and to the left in the lungs, and in each instance is catalyzed by carbonic anhydrase.

car·bon·iza·tion (kahr"bun·i·zay'shun) n. 1. Decomposition of organic compounds by heat in the absence of air, driving off the volatile matter and leaving the carbon. 2. Charring. —**car·bon·ize** (kahr'bun·ize) v.

carbon monoxide. A colorless, odorless, poisonous gas, CO, resulting from the combustion of carbonaceous compounds in an insufficient supply of oxygen. It combines firmly with hemoglobin, preventing subsequent union with oxygen.

car·bon·om·e·ter (kahr"bun·om'e·tur) n. An apparatus for measuring the amount of carbon dioxide in a room or in exhaled breath. —**car·bonom·e·try** (·tree) n.

carbon tetrachloride. Tetrachloromethane, CCl_4, a colorless, nonflammable liquid, active as an anthelmintic, especially against hookworm. Used as a fire extinguisher, a solvent, and an insecticide.

car·bon·uria (kahr"buh·new'ree·uh) n. The presence of carbon compounds in the urine, particularly carbon dioxide.

car·bon·yl (kahr'bon·il, ·eel) n. The divalent organic radical CO.

Carbowax. Trademark for certain polyethylene glycols, of the general formula $HOCH_2$-$(CH_2OCH_2)_xCH_2OH$, having a molecular weight above 1000. They are waxlike solids, soluble in water and in many organic solvents; employed in some ointment bases, also for embedding and sectioning of tissue for certain histologic studies.

Carboxide. Trademark for a mixture of ethylene oxide and carbon dioxide used as a fumigant.

car·boxy·he·mo·glo·bin, car·boxy·hae·mo·glo·bin (kahr·bock″see·hee′mo·glo″bin, ·hem′o·glo″bin) n. The compound formed when hemoglobin by carbon monoxide in the blood. The hemoglobin thus bound is unavailable for oxygen transport because its reaction with carbon monoxide is reversible only at an extremely slow rate.

car·boxy·he·mo·glo·bi·ne·mia, car·boxy·hae·mo·glo·bi·nae·mia (kahr·bock″see·hee′mo·glo″bi·nee′mee·uh) n. The presence in the blood of carboxyhemoglobin, or of excessive carboxyhemoglobin, with or without clinical evidence of poisoning.

car·box·yl (kahr·bock′sil) n. The group COOH characteristic of organic acids. The hydrogen can be replaced by metals, forming salts.

car·boxy·lase (kahr·bock′sil·ace, ·aze) n. 1. Any of a group of enzymes catalyzing the addition of CO_2 to appropriate acceptors; nearly all have biotin as a prothetic group. 2. Formerly, DECARBOXYLASE.

car·box·yl·ic acid (kahr″bock·sil′ick). An acid containing the COOH group.

Carboxymethocel. Trademark for the sodium salt of carboxymethylcellulose.

car·boxy·meth·yl·cel·lu·lose (kahr·bock″see·meth″il·sel′yoo·loce) n. A polycarboxymethyl ether of cellulose, available as the sodium salt, a white powder dispersible in water to form viscous solutions useful for their thickening, suspending, and stabilizing properties; when in the form of a negatively charged resin, it is used as a cation exchanger in ion-exchange chromatography. Abbreviated, CM-cellulose.

car·boxy·pep·ti·dase (kahr·bock″see·pep′ti·dace, ·daze) n. An enzyme, widely distributed but found especially in pancreatic juice, capable of catalyzing hydrolysis of polypeptides at the terminus having a free carboxyl group, producing an amino acid and a smaller peptide which may undergo further hydrolysis under the influence of the enzyme.

car·bro·mal (kahr′bro·mal, kahr·bro′mul) n. Bromodiethylacetylurea, $C_7H_{13}BrN_2O_2$, a white, crystalline powder, very slightly soluble in water; used as a sedative and mild hypnotic.

car·bun·cle (kahr′bunk·ul) n. An extensive, deep-seated, spreading, stubborn infection, usually staphylococcal, of skin and underlying tissues, usually situated on the back of the neck or on the back, with numerous irregular intercommunicating and coalescing abscesses, some of which discharge through multiple external openings. —**car·bun·cu·lar** (kahr·bunk′yoo·lur) adj.

car·bun·cu·lo·sis (kahr·bunk″yoo·lo′sis) n. A condition characterized by the formation of carbuncles in rapid succession or simultaneously.

carcin-, carcino- A combining form meaning cancer.

car·ci·no·gen (kahr′si·no·jen, kahr·sin′o·jen) n. Any agent or substance which produces cancer, accelerates the development of cancer, or acts upon a population to change its total frequency of cancer in terms of numbers of tumors or distribution by site and age. —**car·ci·no·gen·ic** (kahr″si·no·jen′ick) adj.; **carcino·ge·nic·i·ty** (·je·nis′i·tee) n.

car·ci·no·gen·e·sis (kahr″si·no·jen′e·sis) n. Origin or production of cancer. —**carcino·ge·net·ic** (·je·net′ick) adj.

car·ci·noid (kahr′si·noid) n. A tumor arising from the argentaffin cells of the gastrointestinal tract or sometimes from a bronchus, which occasionally metastasizes, producing the carcinoid syndrome.

carcinoid syndrome. Skin flushing, diarrhea, wheezing, and fibrosis of the right-sided cardiac structures; resulting from metastasis of a carcinoid tumor to the liver, and high levels of blood serotonin. Syn. carcinoidosis.

car·ci·no·ma (kahr″si·no′muh) n., pl. **carcinomas, carcinoma·ta** (·tuh) A malignant tumor whose parenchyma is composed of anaplastic epithelial cells.

carcinoma in situ. A growth disturbance of epithelial surfaces in which normal cells are replaced by anaplastic cells that show no behavioral characteristics of cancer, such as invasion and metastasis.

carcinoma oc·cul·ta (o·kul′tuh). A carcinoma which remains unsuspected until metastases occur.

carcinoma sim·plex (sim′plecks). A carcinoma in which differentiation is absent or poor; usually a cylindrical-cell carcinoma, but may be derived from epidermis or other lining epithelium.

car·ci·nom·a·toid (kahr″si·nom′uh·toid, ·no′muh·toid) adj. & n. 1. Resembling a carcinoma. 2. In experimental oncology, epithelial proliferation in induced papillomas without invasion of adjacent tissue.

car·ci·no·ma·to·sis (kahr″si·no′muh·to′sis) n. Widespread dissemination of carcinoma throughout the body.

car·ci·nom·a·tous (kahr″si·nom′uh·tus) adj. Pertaining to or having the characteristics of a carcinoma.

carcinomatous dermatitis. Reddening of the skin, usually of the breast, associated with a carcinoma.

carcinomatous mastitis. A variety of breast cancer which clinically resembles inflammation.

carcinomatous neuropathy or **polyneuropathy.** A subacute or chronic sensory or sensorimotor polyneuropathy, occurring as a remote effect of carcinoma and characterized pathologically by a noninflammatory degeneration of the peripheral nerves and dorsal root ganglia and roots and by an elevation of cerebrospinal fluid protein.

car·ci·no·pho·bia (kahr″si·no·fo′bee·uh) n. Obsessive or hypochondriacal fear of cancer.

car·ci·no·sar·co·ma (kahr″si·no·sahr·ko′muh) n. A tumor having the characteristics of carcinoma and sarcoma; a malignant mixed mesodermal tumor.

car·ci·no·sis (kahr″si·no′sis) n., pl. **carcino·ses** (·seez) CARCINOMATOSIS.

cardi-, cardio- A combining form meaning (a) *heart, cardiac;* (b) *cardial.*

car·di·a (kahr′dee-uh) *n.,* pl. **car·di·ae** (-dee-ee), **cardias** The esophageal orifice and adjacent area of the stomach. Adj. *cardiac, cardial.*

car·di·ac (kahr′dee-ack) *adj. & n.* 1. Of or pertaining to the heart. 2. Of or pertaining to the cardia of the stomach. 3. A person with heart disease.

cardiac aneurysm. Ballooning of a weakened portion of the heart wall, sometimes occurring after coronary occlusion.

cardiac angina. ANGINA PECTORIS.

cardiac arrest. The cessation of cardiac output and effective circulation either because of ventricular asystole or of ventricular fibrillation.

cardiac asthma. Paroxysmal dyspnea and wheezing, often during sleep, due to left ventricular cardiac failure.

cardiac catheter. A long flexible tube of inert material designed to be inserted into the heart, usually by way of a peripheral artery or vein, for diagnostic or therapeutic purposes.

cardiac cirrhosis. Progressive fibrosis of hepatic central lobular structures as well as of portal spaces, the result of chronic congestive heart failure.

cardiac cycle. The complete series of events occurring in the heart during systole and diastole.

cardiac diuretic. A substance, such as digitalis, which produces diuresis by increasing the efficiency of the heart in patients with cardiac edema.

cardiac edema. Edema due to the increased capillary and venous pressure of cardiac failure; it is most marked in the dependent parts of the body, particularly the ankles upon standing.

cardiac failure. HEART FAILURE.

cardiac ganglia. Ganglia of the superficial cardiac plexus, located between the aortic arch and the bifurcation of the pulmonary artery.

cardiac glands. 1. The glands of the cardia of the stomach. 2. Glands occurring in the esophagus which clearly resemble the glands seen in the cardia of the stomach.

cardiac glycogen storage disease. POMPE'S DISEASE.

cardiac index. The volume per minute of cardiac output per square meter of body surface area. The normal resting value is 2.2 liters.

cardiac massage. Rhythmic compression of the heart, either directly or through the closed chest, in the effort to maintain an effective circulation in cardiac asystole or ventricular fibrillation.

cardiac murmur. Any adventitious sounds or noises heard in the region of the heart, generally classified according to their area of origin and time of occurrence in the cardiac cycle.

cardiac neurosis. NEUROCIRCULATORY ASTHENIA.

cardiac orifice. The opening between the esophagus and the stomach.

cardiac output. The blood volume in liters ejected per minute by the left ventricle.

cardiac plexus. A network of visceral nerves situated at the base of the heart. The superficial part lies beneath the arch of the aorta just anterior to the right pulmonary artery. The deep part of the cardiac plexus lies anterior to the bifurcation of the trachea between it and the arch of the aorta. Each portion contains nerve fibers of both sympathetic and vagal origin.

cardiac reserve. The ability of the heart to increase its output in the face of increased physiologic demands, as during exercise.

cardiac resuscitation. Restoration of heartbeat after cardiac arrest or fibrillation, by the prompt employment of such measures as cardiac massage, artificial respiration, stimulating drugs, or (when indicated) defibrillation.

cardiac souffle. CARDIAC MURMUR.

cardiac sphincter. The area of high tone in the lower esophagus; an important component of the mechanism of gastroesophageal continence.

cardiac standstill. CARDIAC ARREST.

cardiac tamponade. Compression of the heart by fluid within the pericardium, which hinders venous return, restricts the heart's ability to fill, and produces increased systemic and pulmonary venous pressure and decreased cardiac output.

car·di·al (kahr′dee-ul) *adj.* Of or pertaining to the cardia.

car·di·al·gia (kahr″dee-al′jee-uh) *n.* 1. Pain in the region of the heart. 2. HEARTBURN.

car·di·am·e·ter (kahr″dee-am′e-tur) *n.* An apparatus for determining the position of the cardiac orifice of the stomach.

Cardidigin. A trademark for digitoxin, a cardiac stimulant.

car·di·ec·ta·sis (kahr″dee-eck′tuh-sis) *n.,* pl. **car·diecta·ses** (-seez) Dilatation of the heart.

car·di·ec·to·my (kahr″dee-eck′tuh-mee) *n. Rare.* Excision of the cardiac end of the stomach.

Cardilate. A trademark for erythrityl tetranitrate, a vasodilator and antihypertensive.

car·di·nal eye movements. The eight principal movements of the eye from the primary position gazing straight ahead: to the left, to the right, up, and up and to the right or left, down, and down to the right or left.

cardinal flower. A common name for several species of *Lobelia,* chiefly *L. cardinalis.*

cardinal ligament. The lower portion of the broad ligament which is firmly united to the supravaginal portion of the cervix.

cardinal vein. Any one of the common cardinal veins.

car·di·o·ac·cel·er·a·tor (kahr″dee-o-ack·sel′uh·ray″tur) *adj. & n.* 1. Quickening the action of the heart. 2. An agent which quickens the action of the heart. —**cardioac·cel·er·a·tion** (-sel″ur·ay′shun) *n.*

car·di·o·ac·tive (kahr″dee-o-ack′tiv) *adj.* Affecting the heart.

car·di·o·an·gi·ol·o·gy (kahr″dee-o-an″jee·ol′uh·jee) *n.* The branch of medicine that is concerned with the heart and blood vessels.

cardioarterial interval. The interval between the apex impulse and the arterial pulsation, measuring the speed of propagation of the pulse wave.

cardioauditory syndrome. A recessively inherited defect characterized by sensory deafness, mutism, prolonged QT interval on the electrocardiogram, recurrent syncope, and sudden death, the latter two usually due to ventricular arrhythmia. Syn. *Jervell and Lange-Nielson's syndrome, surdocardiac syndrome.*

car·di·o·cele (kahr′dee·o·seel) n. Hernia of the heart.

car·dio·cen·te·sis (kahr″dee·o·sen·tee′sis) n., pl. **cardiocente·ses** (·seez) Puncture of a chamber of the heart for diagnosis or therapy.

car·dio·cir·rho·sis (kahr″dee·o·sirr·o′sis) n. CARDIAC CIRRHOSIS.

car·di·oc·la·sis (kahr″dee·ock′lah·sis) n., pl. **cardiocla·ses** (·seez) CARDIORRHEXIS.

car·dio·di·la·tor (kahr″dee·o·dye·lay′tur) n. An instrument for dilating the esophageal opening of the stomach.

car·dio·esoph·a·ge·al (kahr″dee·o·e·sof′uh·jee′ul) adj. Pertaining to the stomach and the esophagus, usually to their junction.

car·dio·gen·ic (kahr″dee·o·jen′ick) adj. 1. Pertaining to the development of the heart. 2. Having origin in the heart or produced by the heart.

cardiogenic shock. Shock due to impairment of cardiac output, associated with inadequate peripheral circulatory compensatory response.

car·dio·gram (kahr′dee·o·gram) n. 1. ELECTROCARDIOGRAM. 2. A record of cardiac pulsation made by a cardiograph.

car·dio·graph (kahr′dee·o·graf) n. 1. ELECTROCARDIOGRAPH. 2. An instrument which records cardiac pulsation and movement as transmitted through the chest wall. —**car·dio·graph·ic** (kahr″dee·o·graf′ick) adj.

car·di·og·ra·phy (kahr″dee·og′ruh·fee) n. Analysis of cardiac action by instrumental means, especially by tracings which record its movements.

Cardio-green. A trademark for indocyanine green, a diagnostic aid.

car·dio·he·pat·ic (kahr″dee·o·he·pat′ick) adj. Pertaining to the heart and the liver.

car·dio·in·hib·i·to·ry (kahr″dee·o·in·hib′i·tor·ee) adj. Diminishing, restraining, or suppressing the heart's action, as the cardioinhibitory fibers which pass to the heart through the vagus nerves.

cardioinhibitory center. The dorsal motor nucleus of the vagus nerve from which arise inhibitory fibers to the heart.

car·dio·ki·net·ic (kahr″dee·o·ki·net′ick) adj. & n. 1. Stimulating the action of the heart. 2. An agent that stimulates the action of the heart.

car·dio·ky·mog·ra·phy (kahr″dee·o·kigh·mog′ruh·fee) n. A method for recording changes in the size of the heart by kymographic means.

car·dio·lip·in (kahr″dee·o·lip′in) n. A phospholipid composed of two molecules of phosphatidic acid esterified to a single glycerol molecule. Essential for the reactivity of beef heart antigens in the serologic test for syphilis.

car·di·ol·o·gist (kahr″dee·ol′uh·jist) n. A specialist in the diagnosis and treatment of disorders of the heart.

car·di·ol·o·gy (kahr″dee·ol′uh·jee) n. The study of the heart and its functions.

car·di·ol·y·sis (kahr″dee·ol′i·sis) n., pl. **cardioly·ses** (·seez) 1. Resection of the precordial ribs and sternum to free the heart and its adherent pericardium from the anterior chest wall, to which they are bound by adhesions, as in adhesive mediastinopericarditis. 2. Cardiac degeneration or destruction.

car·dio·ma·la·cia (kahr″dee·o·ma·lay′shee·uh) n. Pathologic softening of the heart musculature.

car·dio·meg·a·ly (kahr″dee·o·meg′uh·lee) n. Enlargement of the heart.

car·di·o·men·to·pexy (kahr″dee·o·men′to·peck″see) n. The operation of bringing vascular omentum through the diaphragm and attaching it to the heart for improving cardiac vascularization.

car·di·om·e·ter (kahr″dee·om′e·tur) n. An experimental apparatus which envelops the ventricles of a heart, recording their changes in volume, hence force of contraction, during a cardiac cycle.

car·di·om·e·try (kahr″dee·om′e·tree) n. The measurement of the size of the heart, or of the force exerted with each contraction.

car·dio·my·op·a·thy (kahr″dee·o·migh·op′uth·ee) n. Any disease of the myocardium; myocardiopathy.

car·dio·myo·pex·y (kahr″dee·o·migh′o·peck″see) n. The operation of suturing living muscular tissue, generally from the pectoral region to the abraded surface of the heart, to provide improved vascularization of the heart.

car·dio·my·ot·o·my (kahr″dee·o·migh·ot′uh·mee) n. An operation for stenosis of the cardiac sphincter; consists of freeing the esophagus from the diaphragm and pulling it into the abdominal cavity, where the constricting muscle is divided anteriorly and posteriorly without dividing the mucous coat.

car·dio·neph·ric (kahr″dee·o·nef′rick) adj. Pertaining to the heart and the kidneys.

car·dio·neu·ral (kahr″dee·o·new′rul) adj. Pertaining to the innervation of the heart.

car·dio·path (kahr′dee·o·path) n. A person with heart disease; CARDIAC (3). —**car·dio·path·ic** (kahr″dee·o·path′ick) adj.

car·di·op·a·thy (kahr″dee·op′uth·ee) n. Any disease or disorder of the heart.

car·dio·peri·car·dio·pexy (kahr″dee·o·perr″i·kahr′dee·o·peck″see) n. An operation for coronary artery disease, designed to increase collateral circulation and blood flow of the myocardium by the production of adhesive pericarditis.

car·dio·peri·car·di·tis (kahr″dee·o·perr″i·kahr·dye′tis) n. Rare. MYOPERICARDITIS.

car·dio·pho·bia (kahr″dee·o·fo′bee·uh) n. Abnormal fear of heart disease.

car·dio·phone (kahr′dee·o·fone) n. An instrument which makes the heart sounds audible.

car·dio·plas·ty (kahr′dee·o·plas″tee) n. Plastic surgery of the cardiac sphincter, as for cardiospasm.

car·dio·pneu·mat·ic (kahr″dee·o·new·mat′ick) adj. Pertaining to bodily events in which both the cardiovascular and the pulmonary systems participate.

car·di·o·pneu·mo·graph (kahr″dee·o·new″mo·graf′) n. An instrument designed for graphically recording cardiopneumatic movements. —**cardio·pneu·mog·ra·phy** (·new·mog′ruh·fee) n.

car·di·op·to·sis (kahr″dee·op·to′sis, kahr″dee·o·to′sis) n., pl. **cardiopto·ses** (·seez) Downward displacement of the heart; prolapse of the heart.

car·dio·pul·mo·nary (kahr″dee·o·pool′muh·nerr·ree) adj. Pertaining to the heart and lungs.

cardiopulmonary murmur. A murmur produced by the impact of the heart against the lungs, or in airways intermittently narrowed and compressed by the beating heart.

cardiopulmonary-obesity syndrome. PICKWICKIAN SYNDROME.

cardiopulmonary resuscitation. A prescribed sequence of steps including the establishment of a clear open airway, closed-chest cardiac massage, and drug treatments designed to reestablish normal breathing following cardiac arrest. Abbreviated, CPR.

car·di·o·pul·mon·ic (kahr″dee·o·pool·mon′ick) adj. CARDIOPULMONARY.

car·dio·punc·ture (kahr″dee·o·punk′chur) n. CARDIOCENTESIS.

car·dio·re·nal (kahr″dee·o·ree′nul) adj. Pertaining to the heart and kidneys.

car·dio·re·spi·ra·to·ry (kahr″dee·o·res′pi·ruh·tor″ee, ·re·spye′ruh·tor″ee) adj. Of or pertaining to the heart and the respiratory system.

cardiorespiratory murmur. CARDIOPULMONARY MURMUR.

car·di·or·rha·phy (kahr″dee·or′uh·fee) n. Suturing of the heart muscle.

car·di·or·rhex·is (kahr″dee·o·reck′sis) n., pl. **car·diorrhex·es** (·seez) Rupture of the heart.

car·di·os·chi·sis (kahr″dee·os′ki·sis) n., pl. **car·dioschi·ses** (·seez) Division of adhesions between the heart and the chest wall in adhesive pericarditis.

car·dio·scope (kahr″dee·o·skope) n. 1. An instrument for the examination or visualization of the interior of the cardiac chambers. 2. An instrument which, by means of a cathode-ray oscillograph, projects an electrocardiographic or a phonocardiographic record on a luminous screen.

car·dio·spasm (kahr′dee·o·spaz·um) n. ACHALASIA (1).

car·dio·ste·no·sis (kahr″dee·o·ste·no′sis) n. 1. Constriction of the heart, especially of the conus arteriosus pulmonalis. 2. The development of such a constriction.

car·dio·sym·phy·sis (kahr″dee·o·sim′fi·sis) n., pl. **cardiosymphy·ses** (·seez) ADHESIVE PERICARDIOMEDIASTINITIS.

car·dio·ta·chom·e·ter (kahr″dee·o·ta·kom′e·tur) n. 1. An instrument that counts the total number of heartbeats over long periods of time. 2. An instrument that continuously computes and displays the heart rate of an individual in beats per minute.

car·dio·ther·a·py (kahr″dee·o·therr′uh·pee) n. Treatment of heart disease.

car·di·ot·o·my (kahr″dee·ot′uh·mee) n. Dissec-

tion or incision of the heart or the cardiac end of the stomach.

car·dio·ton·ic (kahr″dee·o·ton′ick) adj. & n. 1. Increasing the contractility of the cardiac muscle; generally applied to the effect of digitalis and related drugs. 2. An agent that increases the contractility of the cardiac muscle.

car·dio·tox·ic (kahr″dee·o·tock′sick) adj. Having a poisonous effect on the heart.

car·dio·vas·cu·lar (kahr″dee·o·vas′kew·lur) adj. Pertaining to the heart and blood vessels. Abbreviated, CV.

cardiovascular syphilis. One of the complications of late syphilis, characterized primarily by aortitis, with aortic dilatation and aneurysm; aortic valvulitis producing aortic regurgitation; coronary ostial stenosis and rarely myocarditis.

cardiovascular system. The complex circuit of chambers and channels, including the heart, arteries, capillaries, and veins, by which the blood is propelled and conveyed throughout the body.

car·dio·ver·sion (kahr″dee·o·vur′zhun) n. Electrical reversion of cardiac arrhythmias to normal sinus rhythm, formerly using alternating current, but now employing direct current.

car·di·tis (kahr·dye′tis) n. Inflammation of the heart.

-cardium A combining form designating a structural layer of the heart or a membrane associated with the heart.

car·e·bar·ia (kăr″e·băr′ee·uh) n. Unpleasant head sensations, such as pressure or heaviness.

Carfusin. A trademark for carbol-fuchsin solution.

Carica pa·pa·ya (pa·pah′yuh). The papaw tree of tropical America; contains in its leaves and fruit the proteolytic enzyme papain (papayotin) and other enzymes, and the alkaloid carpaine; the leaves also contain the glycoside carposide. The dried latex and leaves are used as a digestant.

car·ies (kair′eez) n. A molecular death of bone or teeth, corresponding to ulceration in the soft tissues.

caries of the spine. Tuberculous osteitis of the bodies of the vertebrae and intervertebral fibrocartilages, producing curvature of the spine.

caries sic·ca (sick′uh). A form of tuberculous caries characterized by absence of suppuration, obliteration of the cavity of a joint, and sclerosis and concentric atrophy of the articular extremities of the bones.

ca·ri·na (ka·ree′nuh, ka·rye′nuh) n., L. pl. & genit. sing. **cari·nae** (·nee) 1. Any keel-like structure. 2. (of the trachea:) The anteroposterior cartilaginous ridge in the bifurcation of the two primary bronchi. —**cari·nal** (·nul), **car·i·nate** (kăr′in·ate) adj.

Carinamide. A trademark for p-(benzylsulfonamido)benzoic acid, $C_{14}H_{13}NO_4S$, which inhibits tubular excretion of penicillin and has been used in conjunction with the antibiotic to maintain therapeutic blood levels of the latter.

carinate abdomen. A keel-shaped belly, prominent in the middle and receding at the sides, with a sharply convex contour.

carinate breast. PIGEON BREAST.

carina tra·che·ae (tray'kee-ee) [NA]. The carina of the trachea; CARINA (2).

car·io·gen·ic (kār''ee·o·jen'ick) adj. Conducive to the development of dental caries.

car·io·stat·ic (kār''ee·o·stat'ick) adj. Having the quality of preventing or inhibiting carious activity.

car·i·ous (kair'ee·us) adj. 1. Pertaining to or affected with caries of the teeth. 2. Rotting or decaying.

Carls·bad salt A mineral salt mixture from the Carlsbad springs, whose waters have been used for their supposed curative properties, or a similar synthetic salt.

Carmethose. A trademark for sodium carboxymethylcellulose, a synthetic colloid.

car·min·a·tive (kahr'min'uh·tiv) adj. & n. 1. Having the power to relieve flatulence and colic. 2. A substance, usually an aromatic drug, used as a carminative agent.

car·mine (kahr'min, ·mine) n. 1. CARMINE DYE. 2. The color of carmine dye. —**car·min·ic** (kahr·min'ick) adj.

carmine dye. A bright-red coloring matter prepared from cochineal, the active staining principle being carminic acid; of use in staining in toto, for staining tissues in bulk which are later sectioned; used as a specific stain for glycogen and for mucus and as a counterstain for blue vital dyes.

carminic acid. The red coloring principle of cochineal.

car·nau·ba (kahr·naw'buh) n. The root of Copernicia cerifera, a wax-producing palm tree of tropical America; has been used as an alterative.

car·ne·ous (kahr'nee·us) adj. Of, pertaining to, or resembling flesh.

carneous mole. BLOOD MOLE.

car·ni·da·zole (kahr·nigh'duh·zole) n. Methyl [2-(2-methyl-5-nitroimidazol-1-yl)-ethyl]thiocarbamate, $C_8H_{12}N_4O_3S$, an antiprotozoal.

car·ni·fi·ca·tion (kahr''ni·fi·kay'shun) n. Alteration of tissue so that it resembles flesh (i.e., skeletal muscle); often used in reference to lung tissue alteration.

Car·niv·o·ra (kahr·niv'uh·ruh) n.pl. [NL.]. An order of mainly carnivorous and predatory mammals comprising the Canidae (dog family), Ursidae (bears), Procyonidae (raccoons, kinkajous, pandas), Mustelidae (weasels, skunks, badgers, otters), Viverridae (civets, genets, mongooses), Hyaenidae (hyenas), and Felidae (cat family).

car·ni·vore (kahr'ni·vore) n. A member of the order Carnivora.

car·niv·o·rous (kahr·niv'uh·rus) adj. Entirely or primarily meat-eating; subsisting on animal flesh, especially that of vertebrates.

car·no·sine (kahr'no·seen, ·sin) n. β-Alanylhistidine, $C_9H_{14}N_4O_3$, a dipeptide component of muscle tissue.

car·no·sin·emia (kahr''no·si·nee'mee·uh) n. An inborn error of amino acid metabolism in which there are abnormally high levels of carnosine in serum and urine, even when sources of this dipeptide are excluded from the diet, as well as high concentrations of homocarnosine in cerebrospinal fluid; manifested clinically by progressive neurologic deficit with severe mental retardation and seizures.

Ca·ro·li's disease (ka·roh'·lee') Multiple communicating cysts of the biliary tree.

car·o·tene (kār'o·teen) n. Any of three isomeric hydrocarbons, of the formula $C_{40}H_{56}$, distinguished by the prefixed symbols α-, β-, and γ-. All are synthesized by plants, the α- and β-isomers being the more abundant. When pure they are red or purple crystalline solids, the color being due to the presence of a series of conjugated ethylenic linkages. The carotenes are precursors of vitamin A, β-carotene yielding two molecules of vitamin A, the others one molecule.

car·o·ten·emia, car·o·te·nae·mia (kār''o·te·nee'mee·uh) n. The presence of carotene in the circulating blood. Syn. hypercarotenemia.

ca·rot·e·noid, ca·rot·i·noid (ka·rot'i·noid) n. & adj. 1. One of a group of plant pigments occurring in carrots, tomatoes, and other vegetables, and in fruits and flowers. Chemically, carotenoids are unsaturated hydrocarbons of high molecular weight containing a series of conjugated ethylenic linkages or derivatives of such hydrocarbons. 2. Pertaining to or characteristic of a carotenoid.

car·o·te·no·sis, car·o·ti·no·sis (kār''o·ti·no'sis) n., pl. **carotino·ses** (·seez) Pigmentation of the skin due to carotene and carotenoids in the tissues.

ca·rot·ic (ka·rot'ick) adj. Characterized by or pertaining to stupor or coma.

ca·rot·i·co·cli·noid (ka·rot''i·ko·klye'noid) adj. Pertaining to an internal carotid artery and a clinoid process of the sphenoid bone.

ca·rot·i·co·tym·pan·ic (ka·rot''i·ko·tim·pan'ick) adj. Pertaining to the carotid canal and the tympanum.

caroticotympanic nerves. See Table of Nerves in the Appendix.

ca·rot·id (ka·rot'id) adj. & n. 1. Pertaining to a carotid artery or nerve. 2. CAROTID ARTERY.

carotid arteriography. Radiography of the carotid artery after the injection of radiopaque material.

carotid artery. 1. The common carotid artery or either of its branches, the external and internal carotid arteries. 2. Specifically, the common carotid artery, the principal artery on either side of the neck.

carotid artery insufficiency syndrome. Contralateral weakness and numbness, aphasia, and ipsilateral monocular blindness due to atherosclerosis or other lesion causing obstruction of an internal carotid artery or one of its major branches.

carotid body. Any one of several irregular epithelioid masses situated at or near the bifurcation of the carotid artery, and innervated by the intercarotid or sinus branch of the glossopharyngeal nerve.

carotid-body reflex. A reflex initiated by changes in blood oxygen content, acting on chemoreceptors in the carotid body; marked hypoxia increases respiratory rate, blood pressure, and heart rate.

carotid-body tumor. A benign tumor, sometimes locally invasive, at the bifurcation of the common carotid artery, composed of nests of ovoid or polygonal cells having a rich cytoplasm and small vesicular or dense nuclei, in a vascular fibrous stroma duplicating the histologic structure of the carotid body.

carotid nerves. Sympathetic nerves, from the superior cervical ganglion, which innervate the smooth muscles and glands of the head.

carotid plexus. 1. Any of the networks of sympathetic nerve fibers surrounding the carotid arteries. 2. Specifically, INTERNAL CAROTID PLEXUS.

carotid sheath. The fibrous sheath about the carotid arteries and associated structures.

carotid sinus. 1. A slight dilatation of the common carotid artery at its bifurcation, the walls of which are innervated by the intercarotid or sinus branch of the glossopharyngeal nerve. It is concerned with the regulation of systemic blood pressure. 2. An extension of the cavernous sinus into the carotid canal.

carotid sinus hypersensitivity. Susceptibility to carotid sinus syncope.

carotid sinus reflex. A neural reflex arising from stimulation of pressure-sensitive mechanoreceptors in the carotid sinus. Carotid sinus hypotension, with decreased stretch of these receptors, results in vasoconstriction, venoconstriction, bradycardia, and increased cardiac contractility.

carotid sinus syncope or **syndrome.** Profound hypotension and bradycardia following carotid sinus stimulation, with resultant dizziness, fainting or convulsions, and occasionally other neurologic symptoms.

ca·ro·tin (kăr'o·tin) *n.* CAROTENE.

ca·rot·o·dyn·ia (ka·rot″o·din'ee·uh) *n.* Cervicofacial pain or migraine or both associated with pain and tenderness of the carotid artery at its bifurcation and swelling of the overlying tissues.

carp-, carpo-. A combining form meaning *carpus, carpal.*

car·pal (kahr'pul) *adj. & n.* 1. Pertaining to the wrist or carpus. 2. CARPAL BONE.

carpal bone. Any of the eight wrist bones between the metacarpals and the radius and ulna. ossa carpi.

carpal tunnel. The space between the flexor retinaculum of the wrist and the carpal bones, through which pass the tendons of the long flexors of the fingers and the long flexor of the thumb and the median nerve.

carpal tunnel syndrome. A symptom complex due to compression of the median nerve within the carpal tunnel, characterized by disturbances of sensation in the area of the skin supplied by the median nerve, pain on sharp flexion of the wrist, edema of the fingers, tense and shiny skin, and atrophy of the thenar muscles.

car·pec·to·my (kahr·peck'tuh·mee) *n.* Excision of a carpal bone or bones.

car·phol·o·gy (kahr·fol″uh·jee) *n.* Aimless picking and plucking at bedclothes, seen in delirious states, fevers, and exhaustion. Syn. *floccillation.*

car·po·meta·car·pal (kahr″po·met·uh·kahr′pul) *adj.* Pertaining to the carpal and the metacarpal bones.

carpometacarpal articulation. 1. Any of the joints between the distal row of carpal bones (trapezium, trapezoid, capitate, hamate) and the bases of the metacarpals. 2. (of the fingers:) Any of the joints between the distal row of carpal bones and the bases of the four medial metacarpals. NA (pl.) *articulationes carpometacarpeae.* 3. (of the thumb:) The saddle joint between the trapezium and the base of the first metacarpal.

carpometacarpal ligament. Any of the ligaments of the carpometacarpal articulations of the fingers, including the dorsal carpometacarpal ligaments (NA pl.) *ligamenta carpometacarpea dorsalia*), connecting the trapezium, trapezoid, and hamate to the base of the second metacarpal, the capitate to the third metacarpal, the hamate and capitate to the fourth, and the capitate to the fifth; the palmar carpometacarpal ligaments (NA pl.) *ligamenta carpometacarpea palmaria*), connecting the trapezium to the second metacarpal, the trapezium, capitate, and hamate to the third, and the hamate to the fourth and fifth; and the interosseous carpometacarpal ligaments, connecting the contiguous angles of the capitate and hamate to the third and fourth metacarpals.

carpometacarpal reflex. CARPOPHALANGEAL REFLEX.

car·po·ped·al (kahr′po·ped′ul) *adj.* Affecting the wrists and feet, or the fingers and toes.

carpopedal spasm. A spasm of the hands and feet, or of the thumbs and great toes; associated with tetany.

car·po·pha·lan·ge·al (kahr″po·fa·lan′jee·ul, ·fa·lan·jee′ul) *adj.* Pertaining to the wrist and the phalanges.

carpophalangeal reflex. 1. Percussion of the dorsal aspect of the carpal and metacarpal areas is followed by flexion of the fingers; a variation of the finger flexor reflex. 2. Percussion of the extensor tendons of the flexed wrist is followed by its reflex extension.

car·pro·fen (kahr′pro·fen) *n.* (±)-6-Chloro-α-methyl-9H-carbazole-2-acetic acid, $C_{15}H_{12}ClNO_2$, an anti-inflammatory agent.

car·pus (kahr′pus) *n.*, pl. & genit. sing. **car·pi** (·pye) 1. The group of eight bones between the metacarpals and the radius and ulna. 2. The part of the upper limb containing the eight carpal bones; WRIST (1). Adj. *carpal.*

car·ra·geen (kăr′uh·jeen) *n.* See *Chondrus crispus.*

Carrel flask A vessel with a slanting or horizontal neck, used in tissue culture.

car·ri·er, *n.* 1. A well person or one convalescing from an infectious disease who shows no signs or symptoms of the disease but who harbors and eliminates the microorganism, and so spreads the disease. 2. An individual who bears a mutant gene without manifesting its phenotypic expression, usually applied to those heterozygous for a severe recessive gene. 3. A quantity of a naturally occurring element added to a minute amount of pure isotope, especially one that is radioactive, to facilitate chemical handling of the isotope. **4.** A compound capable of reversible oxidation-reduction, which thus acts as a hydrogen carrier. **5.** A device, as an instrument, for holding something while it is being carried or is being used.

car·rier-free, *adj. In radiochemistry,* pertaining to or characterizing a radioactive isotope in which none of the stable forms of the isotope is present.

car·ri·on (kăr'ee·un) *n.* The putrefying flesh of animal carcasses.

Ca·rrion's disease (ka·rryoʰn') BARTONELLOSIS.

car·ron oil (kăr'un). A mixture of equal parts of linseed oil and lime water; used in the treatment of burns.

carrying angle. The angle between the longitudinal axis of the forearm and that of the arm when the forearm is extended.

car sickness. Motion sickness from riding in an automobile or similar road vehicle.

car·taz·o·late (kahr·taz'o·late) *n.* Ethyl 4-(butylamino)-1-ethyl-1*H*-pyrazolo[3,4-*b*]pyridine-5-carboxylate, $C_{15}H_{22}N_4O_2$, an antidepressant.

Cartesian diver method. Any method that measures pressure changes at a gas-liquid interface by determining the variations in position of a gas-filled tube floating in the liquid.

car·ti·lage (kahr'ti·lij) *n.* Gristle; a white, semi-opaque, nonvascular connective tissue composed of a highly resilient matrix containing nucleated cells which lie in cavities or lacunas of the matrix. When boiled, cartilage yields chondrin.

cartilage graft. A cartilage autograft or homograft, commonly used for replacing damaged or destroyed cartilage, or to replace bone loss.

cartilage-hair hypoplasia. A genetic disorder, reported among certain Amish people in the United States and Canada, characterized by dwarfism due to hypoplasia of cartilage and abnormally short, thin, and sparse hair; inherited as an autosomal recessive with reduced penetrance.

car·ti·la·gin·i·fi·ca·tion (kahr''ti·la·jin''i·fi·kay'shun) A change into cartilage; chondrification.

car·ti·lag·i·nous (kahr''ti·laj'i·nus) *adj.* Pertaining to or consisting of cartilage.

car·un·cle (kăr'ung·kul, ka·runk'ul) *n.* **1.** Any small, fleshy, red mass or nodule. **2.** Specifically, LACRIMAL CARUNCLE. **—ca·run·cu·lar** (ka·runk'yoo·lur), **caruncu·late** (·late), **caruncu·la·ted** (·lay·tid) *adj.*

ca·rus (kair'us) *n. Obsol.* Profound lethargy, stupor, or coma.

Car·val·lo's sign. A sign of tricuspid regurgitation in which the systolic murmur is augmented by inspiration.

car·vone (kahr'vone) *n.* A terpene ketone, $C_{10}H_{14}O$, found in the volatile oils of caraway, dill, fennel, and spearmint; used as a flavor.

CAS Chemical Abstracts Service.

cas·cade (kas·kade') *v. & n.* **1.** To spill over, usually rapidly, as over terraces. **2.** To be built up in stages, as an electrical process. **3.** A

structure or a process involving such spilling over or building up.

cascade stomach. *In radiology,* a variant of the normal gastric contour, in which the upper posterior wall is pushed forward, giving the stomach the appearance of a glass retort; the cardia fills first, with subsequent spilling over into the pyloric segment.

cas·cara (kas·kăr'uh) *n.* CASCARA SAGRADA.

cascara sa·gra·da (sah·grah'duh). The bark of *Rhamnus purshiana,* the chief constituents of which are anthraquinone derivatives; an irritant cathartic.

cas·ca·ril·la (kas''kuh·ril'uh) *n.* The bark of *Croton eluteria,* native to the Bahama Islands; an aromatic bitter.

cas·ca·ril·lin (kas''kuh·ril'in) *n.* The bitter principle, $C_{12}H_{18}O_4$, of cascarilla.

cas·ca·rin (kas'kuh·rin) *n.* A glycosidal cathartic fraction isolated from cascara sagrada.

case-, A combining form meaning (a) *casein;* (b) *caseous.*

¹**ca·se·ate** (kay'see·ate) *n.* **1.** LACTATE. **2.** CASEINATE.

²**caseate,** *v.* To undergo caseation necrosis.

ca·se·a·tion (kay''see·ay'shun) *n.* **1.** The precipitation of casein during the coagulation of milk. **2.** CASEATION NECROSIS.

caseation necrosis. A type of tissue death resulting in loss of all cellular outlines and the gross appearance of crumbly cheeselike material; seen typically in tuberculosis.

case fatality rate. The proportion of fatal cases of a specific disease, usually expressed as the number of deaths from the disease per 100 persons affected.

ca·se·i·form (kay'see·i·form) *adj.* Like cheese or casein.

ca·sein (kay'seen, ·sē·in) *n.* A protein obtained from milk by the action of rennin or acids.

ca·sein·ate (kay·see'nate, ·sē·i'nate) *n.* A compound of casein and a metal.

ca·sein·o·gen (kay·seen'o·jen, kay''see·in'o·jen) *n.* A compound protein of milk, yielding casein when acted upon by digestive enzymes; the precursor of casein, analogous to fibrinogen and myosinogen (myogen).

ca·seo·cal·cif·ic (kay''see·o·kal·sif'ick) *adj.* Possessing areas both of caseation and of calcification.

ca·se·ous (kay'see·us) *adj.* **1.** Resembling, or having the nature or consistency of, cheese. **2.** Characterized by caseation necrosis.

case·work, *n.* The task of professional social workers or psychiatric social workers who, through personal counseling and the aid of various social agencies, seek to help individuals and their families with their personal and social problems.

cas·sa·va, ca·sa·va (ka·sah'vuh) *n.* **1.** Any of several plants of the genus *Manihot.* **2.** The starch obtained from rhizomes of *M. esculenta* and *M. aipi;* a nutrient and the source of tapioca.

Cas·sia (cash'uh, cash'ee·uh) *n.* A genus of the Leguminosae, several species of which provide senna.

cast, *n. & v.* **1.** A mass of fibrous material, protein coagulum, or exudate that has taken the form of some cavity in which it has been molded; classified according to the source, as bronchial, intestinal, nasal, esophageal, renal, tracheal, urethral, or vaginal. 2. An accurate reproduction in form of an object, structure, or part in some plastic substance which has taken form in an impression or mold. 3. PLASTER OF PARIS CAST. 4. *Colloq.* Of the eye: STRABISMUS. 5. To produce a specific form by pouring metal or plaster into a prepared mold. 6. *In veterinary medicine,* to throw an animal on its side for restraint.

Ca·stel·la·ni's disease (kah'' stel·lah'nee) BRONCHOSPIROCHETOSIS.

Castellani's paint CARBOL-FUCHSIN SOLUTION.

cas·tile soap (kas·teel') A hard soap usually prepared from sodium hydroxide and olive oil. Much commercial castile soap contains coconut oil soap to increase its lathering quality.

cast·ing, *n.* 1. *In dentistry,* the act of forcing molten metal into a suitable mold. 2. The object or product formed by the casting. 3. *In veterinary medicine,* the act of throwing an animal on its side for restraint.

castor bean. The seed of *Ricinus communis,* from which castor oil is obtained.

castor oil. The fixed oil obtained from the seed of *Ricinus communis;* the oil contains glycerides of ricinoleic acid which impart cathartic activity.

cas·tra·tion (kas·tray'shun) *n.* ORCHIECTOMY; the excision of one or both testes or ovaries; taken as evidence of hypersecretion of follicle-stimulating or luteinizing hormone. —**cas·trat·ed** (kas'tray·tid) *adj.;* **cas·trate** (kas'trate) *n.* & *v.*

castration anxiety. 1. Anxiety due to the fantasied fear of loss of the genitals or injury to them; may be provoked by events which have symbolic significance, such as loss of a tooth, an object, or a job, or a humiliating experience. 2. Fear of a young boy that he will lose his penis.

castration cells. Enlarged beta cells of the pars distalis of the hypophysis, showing vacuolization and eccentric displacement of the nucleus following castration.

castration complex. 1. Castration anxiety occurring after childhood, associated primarily with fear of loss of the genital, especially the male, organ. 2. The symptoms of the fear of the loss of any pleasure-giving body part (or excretion) or of even the fear that every pleasure will be followed by loss and pain. 3. In the female, the fantasy of once having had a penis but of having lost it.

cas·tro·phre·nia (kas'tro·free'nee·uh) *n.* A morbid fear or delusion, occasional in schizophrenic patients, that their thoughts are being sucked out of their brains by enemies.

cas·u·is·tics (kazh''oo·is'ticks, kaz''yoo·) *n.* The study of individual cases as a means of arriving at the general history of a disease.

CAT Abbreviation for (a) *Children's Apperception Test;* (b) *computed axial tomography* or *computer-assisted tomography.*

cat-, cata-, cath- A prefix meaning (a) *downward;* (b) *in accordance with;* (c) *against, back;* (d) *completely.*

ca·tab·o·lism (ka·tab'uh·liz·um) *n.* The degradative or destructive phase of metabolism concerned with the breaking down by the body of complex compounds, often with liberation of energy. —**cat·a·bol·ic** (kat·uh·bol'ick) *adj.*

ca·tab·o·lite (ka·tab'o·lite) *n.* Any product of catabolism.

cat·a·clei·sis (kat''uh·klye'sis) *n.,* pl. **cataclei·ses** (·seez) *Obsol.* Closure of the eyelids by adhesion or by spasm.

cata·clo·nus (kat''uh·klo'nus) *n. Obsol.* Rhythmic convulsive movements which are of functional or hysterical nature rather than expressions of true epilepsy. —**cata·clon·ic** (·klon'ick) *adj.*

cat·ac·ro·tism (ka·tack'ro·tiz·um) *n.* A condition in which the descending, or catacrotic, limb of the arterial pulse wave is characterized by a notch, wave, or irregularity.

cat·a·gelo·pho·bia (kat''uh·jel''o·fo'bee·uh) *n.* Abnormal fear of ridicule.

cat·a·lase (kat'uh·laze, ·laze) *n.* An enzyme found in tissues, capable of decomposing hydrogen peroxide to water and molecular oxygen.

cat·a·lep·sy (kat'uh·lep''see) *n.* A state of markedly diminished responsiveness, usually trancelike, in which there is a loss of voluntary motion and a peculiar plastic rigidity of the muscles, by reason of which they retain for an exceedingly long time any position in which they are placed. The condition may occur in organic or psychologic disorders, especially in hysteria and in schizophrenia, and under hypnosis. —**ca·ta·lep·tic** (kat''uh·lep'tick) *adj.* & *n.*

cat·a·lep·toid (kat''uh·lep'toid) *adj.* Resembling catalepsy.

ca·tal·y·sis (ka·tal'i·sis) *n.,* pl. **cataly·ses** (·seez) The process of change in the velocity of a chemical reaction through the presence of a substance which apparently remains chemically unaltered throughout the reaction. The velocity may be increased, in which case the process is described as positive catalysis, or it may be decreased, in which case the process is described as negative catalysis.

cat·a·lyst (kat'uh·list) *n.* 1. A substance having the power to produce catalysis. 2. A substance which alters the velocity of a chemical reaction. Its concentration at the beginning of the reaction is equal to its concentration at the end. —**cat·a·lyt·ic** (kat''uh·lit'ick) *adj.*

cat·a·lyze (kat'uh·lize) *v.* 1. To act as a catalyst. 2. To influence a chemical reaction by means of a catalyst. —**cat·a·ly·za·tion** (kat''uh·li·zay'shun) *n.*

cat·a·me·nia (kat''uh·mee'nee·uh) *n.* MENSTRUATION. —**catame·ni·al** (·nee·ul) *adj.*

cat·am·ne·sis (kat''am·nee'sis) *n.,* pl. **catamne·ses** (·seez) The follow-up medical history of a patient after an initial examination or an illness. —**catam·nes·tic** (·nes'tick) *adj.*

cata·pha·sia (kat''uh·fay'zhuh, ·zee·uh) *n.* A form of stereotypy in which the patient keeps repeating the same word or series of words.

ca·taph·o·ra (ka·taf'o·ruh) *n. Obsol.* 1. Marked

somnolence with periods of partial wakefulness. 2. SEMICOMA.

cata·pho·re·sis (kat''uh·fo·ree'sis, ·for'e·sis) n. ELECTROPHORESIS. —**catapho·ret·ic** (·ret'ick) adj.

cata·pho·ria (kat''uh·for'ee·uh) n. A tendency of the visual axes of both eyes to incline below the horizontal plane.

cata·phy·lax·is (kat''uh·fi·lack'sis) n. 1. Movement and transportation of leukocytes and antibodies to the site of an infection. 2. The overcoming of bodily resistance to infection. —**cata·phy·lac·tic** (·fi·lack'tick) adj.

cata·pla·sia (kat''uh·play'zhuh, ·zee·uh) n. 1. The stage of decline of life. 2. Degenerative changes affecting cells and tissues, especially reversion to an earlier or embryonic type of cell or tissue. 3. Application of a plaster or coating.

ca·tap·la·sis (ka·tap'luh·sis) n., pl. **cata·pla·ses** (·seez) CATAPLASIA.

cat·a·plasm (kat'uh·plaz·um) n. A poultice, of various substances and usually applied when hot.

cat·a·plexy (kat'uh·pleck''see) n. Temporary paralysis of the cranial and somatic musculature brought on by bouts of laughter, anger, or other emotional states; part of the clinical tetrad of narcolepsy, cataplexy, sleep paralyses, and hypnagogic hallucinations.—**cata·plec·tic** (kat'uh·pleck'tick) adj.

Catapres. A trademark for clonidine hydrochloride, an antihypertensive.

cat·a·ract (kat'uh·rakt) n. Partial or complete opacity of the crystalline lens or its capsule. —**cat·a·rac·tous** (kat'uh·rack'tus) adj.

cataract needle. A needle used for operating upon a cataract or its capsule.

cataract spoon. A small spoon-shaped instrument used to remove the lens in cataract operations.

ca·tarrh (ka·tahr') n. Inflammation of mucous membranes, especially those of the air passages, associated with mucoid exudate. —**ca·tarrh·al** (·ul) adj.

catarrhal conjunctivitis. A usually acute inflammation of the conjunctiva with smarting of the eyes, heaviness of the lids, photophobia, and excessive mucous or mucopurulent secretion, due to a variety of contagious organisms such as those of the genera *Hemophilus* and *Staphylococcus*, but sometimes becoming chronic as a sequela of the acute form or because of irritation from polluted atmosphere or allergic factors. Syn. *pinkeye.*

catarrhal jaundice. INFECTIOUS HEPATITIS.

catarrhal otitis media. SEROUS OTITIS MEDIA.

cat·a·stal·sis (kat''uh·stal'sis, ·stahl'sis) n. A downward-moving wave of contraction occurring in the gastrointestinal tract during digestion. There is no preceding wave of inhibition.

cata·thy·mia (kat''uh·thigh'mee·uh) n. The existence of a complex in the unconscious mind which is heavily charged with affect or feeling so as to produce a pronounced effect in consciousness.

cata·to·nia (kat''uh·to'nee·uh) n. A phase or type of schizophrenia in which the patient seems to lack the will to talk or move and stands or sits in one position, assumes fixed postures, and resists attempts to activate motion or speech. A benign stupor which frequently may be punctuated by violent outbursts, hallucinosis, and panic. —**cata·ton·ic** (kat''uh·ton'ick) adj. & n.

catatonic type of schizophrenia. A form of schizophrenia characterized by disturbances in motor behavior, one type marked chiefly by withdrawal and generalized inhibition (stupor, mutism, negativism, and waxy flexibility) and the other by excitement and frenzied motor activity.

catch·ment area. A geographic area for whose inhabitants a health facility, such as a hospital or mental health center, has the responsibility.

cat·e·chol·a·mine (kat''i·kol'uh·meen, ·min) n. Any one of a group of sympathomimetic amines containing a catechol moiety, including especially epinephrine, norepinephrine (levarterenol), and dopamine.

cat·elec·trot·o·nus (kat''e·leck·trot'uh·nus) n. The increased irritability of a nerve or muscle at the negative pole during passage of an electric current, caused by partial depolarization of the resting transmembrane potential of the irritable tissue. —**catelec·tro·ton·ic** (·tro·ton'ick) adj.

cat·e·nat·ing (kat'e·nay·ting) adj. Connected with a group or series of other signs and symptoms.

cat·er·pil·lar dermatitis, rash, or **urticaria.** An eruption due to the highly irritating or sensitizing substances on hairs of the larvae of certain Lepidoptera, characterized first by erythematous macules and then by wheals.

cat·gut, n. A suture and ligature material made from the submucosa of sheep's intestine, cleansed, treated, and twisted. Sterilized and put up aseptically in glass tubes, in sizes from 00000 to 8. Varieties are: plain (untreated), chromicized (treated with chromic trioxide), and iodized (immersed in a solution of iodine and potassium iodide).

ca·thar·sis (ka·thahr'sis) n., pl. **cathar·ses** (·seez) 1. PURGATION. 2. *In psychoanalysis,* the healthful and therapeutic release of tension and anxiety by "talking out" and emotionally reliving repressed incidents and honestly facing the cause of the difficulty.

ca·thar·tic (ka·thahr'tick) adj. & n. 1. Producing catharsis; causing evacuation of the bowels. 2. A medicine used to produce evacuations of the bowels; is purgative.

ca·thect (ka·thekt') v. *In psychiatry,* to charge ideas with affect or feeling.

ca·thep·sin (ka·thep'sin) n. Any one of several proteolytic enzymes present in tissue, catalyzing the hydrolysis of high molecular weight proteins to proteoses and peptones, and having an optimum pH between 4 and 5. It is believed that after death the tissues become acid, and cathepsin produces autolysis (proteolysis).

ca·ther·e·sis (ka·therr'e·sis, ka·theer', kath''e·ree'sis) n. *Obsol.* 1. Prostration or weakness induced by medication. 2. A mild caustic action.

cath·e·ret·ic (kath″e-ret′ick) *adj. & n. Obsol.*
1. Reducing; weakening; prostrating.
2. Mildly caustic. 3. A mild caustic.

cath·e·ter (kath′e·tur) *n.* A hollow tube of metal, glass, hard or soft rubber, silicone, rubberized silk, or plastic for introduction into a cavity through a narrow canal, for the purpose of discharging the fluid contents of a cavity or for establishing the patency of a canal; specifically, one intended to be passed into the bladder through the urethra for the relief of urinary retention.

catheter·ize (kath′e·tur·ize) *v.* 1. To insert a catheter. 2. To withdraw urine by means of a urethral catheter. —**catheter·iza·tion** (·i·zay′shun) *n.*

ca·thex·is (ka·theck′sis) *n., pl.* **cathex·es** (·seez) *In psychoanalysis,* the conscious or unconscious investment of an object or idea with psychic energy, i.e., with feelings and meanings. It may be qualitatively defined by terms, such as ego, object, libidinal, instinctual, or erotic. *Adj. cathectic.*

cath·ode (kath′ode) *n.* The negative electrode or pole of an electric circuit. Abbreviated, C., ca., K., ka.

cathode ray. Streams of electrons emitted from the cathode in low-pressure electrical discharge tubes, such as a Crookes tube or cathode-ray tube, and accelerated by a potential applied at the anode. Beams of cathode rays may be deflected by electric or magnetic fields; when they impinge on a suitable screen, they produce fluorescence, as in an oscilloscope.

cathode-ray oscillograph. An instrument in which a pencil of electrons, striking a fluorescent screen, will trace a graph of any two variables that have been converted into electric equivalents. Its virtue is absence of mechanical inertia, and hence the ability to record changes of extreme rapidity with absolute accuracy. Abbreviated, CRO.

ca·thod·ic (ka·thod′ick) *adj.* 1. Pertaining to a cathode; electronegative. 2. Proceeding downward; efferent or centrifugal, as a nerve current or nerve impulse.

cat·ion (kat′eye·on) *n.* A positive ion moving toward, or being evolved at, the cathode in electrolytic cells or discharge tubes. —**cation·ic** (kat″eye·on′ick) *adj.*

cation exchange resin. 1. A highly polymerized synthetic organic compound consisting of a large nondiffusible anion and a simple diffusible cation, which latter can be exchanged for a cation in the medium in which the resin is placed. 2. *In medicine,* such a resin, often modified to avoid disturbance in the balance of other physiologically important ions; used to remove sodium ions from the body in treating conditions resulting from abnormal retention of sodium.

ca·top·trics (ka·top′tricks) *n.* The branch of physics dealing with the principles of reflected light.

CAT scan. A radiographic scan by computed (axial) tomography.

cat-scratch disease or **fever.** A usually self-limited disease clinically manifested by fever, regional or generalized lymphadenitis, and occasionally aseptic meningoencephalitis; probably due to a virus transmitted by a scratch from an animal with sheathed claws, most often a cat.

Cau·ca·sian (kaw·kay′zhun) *n.* A member of a white-skinned race of people.

caud-, caudo-. A combining form meaning *caudal, tail.*

cau·da (kaw′duh) *n., pl. & genit. sing.* **cau·dae** (·dee) 1. TAIL. 2. A structure resembling or analogous to a tail; a tail-like appendage.

cau·dad (kaw′dad) *adv.* Toward the tail; caudally; in human anatomy, downward.

cauda equi·na (e·kwye′nuh) [NA]. The roots of the sacral and coccygeal nerves, collectively; so called because of their resemblance to a horse's tail.

cauda equina syndrome. Pain, combined variously with sphincteric disturbances and an asymmetric, atrophic, areflexic paralysis and sensory loss in the distribution of the lumbosacral roots; due to compression of the cauda equina.

cau·dal (kaw′dul) *adj.* 1. Of, pertaining to, or involving the cauda. 2. Directed toward the tail or cauda; in human anatomy, inferior.

caudal anesthesia. Anesthesia induced by intermittent or continuous injection of the anesthetic into the sacral canal.

cau·date (kaw′date) *adj.* Having a tail or a tail-like appendage. —**cau·da·tion** (kaw·day′shun) *n.*

caudate lobe. The tailed lobe of the liver that separates the right extremity of the transverse fissure from the commencement of the fissure for the inferior vena cava.

caudate nucleus. An elongated arched gray mass which projects into and forms part of the lateral wall of the lateral ventricle; part of the corpus striatum.

cau·do·ceph·al·ad (kaw″do·sef′ul·ad) *adv.* In the direction from the tail toward the head.

caul, *n.* 1. A portion or all of the fetal membranes covering the head and carried out in advance of it in labor. 2. GREATER OMENTUM.

caul-, cauli-, caulo- A combining form meaning *stem.*

cau·li·flow·er ear. Thickening and irregularity of the auricle following repeated blows; seen in pugilists.

cau·lo·phyl·lum (kaw″lo·fil′um) *n.* The dried rhizome and roots of *Caulophyllum thalictroides,* containing the alkaloid caulophylline, glycosides, and saponins. It produces intermittent contractions of the gravid uterus and is also said to possess diuretic and anthelmintic properties.

cau·mes·the·sia, cau·maes·the·sia (kaw″mes·theezh′uh, ·theez′ee·uh) *n.* The sensation of burning up with heat, when the temperature of neither the patient nor the environment is high.

cau·sal·gia (kaw·sal′jee·uh) *n.* 1. A syndrome, described by Weir Mitchell, which develops after penetrating wounds with partial injury of the medial, ulnar, or sciatic nerve. It is characterized by a sensation of severe burning pain in the hand or foot, the skin of which becomes smooth and shiny, or scaly and discolored, accompanied by profuse sweating of the involved part, particularly under conditions of emotional stress. 2. Any burning pain in the affected part following a nerve injury.—**causal·gic** (·jick) *adj.*

causalgia syndrome or **causalgic syndrome.** CAUSALGIA (1).

caus·tic (kaws'tick) *adj. & n.* 1. Very irritant; burning; capable of destroying tissue. 2. A substance that destroys tissue. 3. *In optics,* a curve to which the rays of light reflected or refracted by another curve are tangent.

cau·ter·ant (kaw'tur·unt) *adj. & n.* CAUSTIC; ESCHAROTIC.

cau·ter·ize (kaw'tur·ize) *v.* 1. To apply a cautery or a caustic to. 2. To destroy (tissue) by the application of a cauterizing agent or by cautery.—**cau·ter·i·za·tion** (kaw'tur·i·zay'shun) *n.*

cau·tery (kaw'tur·ee) *n.* A device to coagulate or destroy tissue by a chemical or by heat.

ca·va (kay'vuh, kav'uh) *adj. & n.,* pl. **ca·vae** (·vee) 1. Feminine of L. *cavus,* hollow. 2. Plural of L. *cavum,* cavity. 3. VENA CAVA. —**ca·val** (·vul) *adj.*

caval mesentery or **fold.** An embryonic mesentery, separated from the primitive mesentery of the stomach by the mesenteric recess, in which develops a part of the inferior vena cava and the caudate lobe of the liver.

cav·a·scope (kav'uh·skope) *n.* An instrument for examining a body cavity.

cav·ern, *n.* A cavity or hollow, specifically: 1. A pathologic cavity in the lung due to necrosis of its tissues. 2. The cavity of a dilated bronchus.

cav·er·ni·tis (kav''ur·nigh'tis) *n.* Inflammation of the corpora cavernosa.

cav·er·no·ma (kav''ur·no'muh) *n.,* pl. **cavernomas, cavernoma·ta** (·tuh) A benign cavernous tumor; CAVERNOUS HEMANGIOMA.

cav·er·no·si·tis (kav''ur·no·sigh'tis) *n.* CAVERNITIS.

cav·er·nos·to·my (kav''ur·nos'tuh·mee) *n.* The drainage of a pulmonary abscess or cavity through the chest wall.

cav·er·no·sum (kav''ur·no'sum) *n.,* pl. **caverno·sa** (·suh) CORPUS CAVERNOSUM.

cav·ern·ous (kav'ur·nus) *adj.* Having hollow spaces.

cavernous angioma. An angioma in which the vascular spaces are large or cystic, like the erectile tissue of the penis.

cavernous hemangioma. A benign vascular tumor made up of large, thin-walled vascular channels.

cavernous lymphangioma. HYGROMA.

cavernous rale. A hollow, metallic sound heard in advanced tuberculosis, caused by the expansion and contraction of a pulmonary cavity during respiration.

cavernous sinus. An irregularly shaped sinus of the dura mater, located on the side of the body of the sphenoid bone, and extending from the superior orbital fissure in front to the apex of the petrous bone behind.

cavernous sinus syndrome. Proptosis, edema of the conjunctiva and eyelids, and palsy of the muscles supplied by the third, fourth, and sixth cranial nerves, due to partial or total occlusion of the cavernous sinus by thrombus, tumor, or arteriovenous aneurysm.

cavernous sinus thrombosis. Inflammation of a cavernous sinus with thrombus formation.

cav·i·tary (kav'i·terr·ee) *adj.* 1. Of or pertaining to a cavity. 2. Characterized by cavitation.

cav·i·tate (kav'i·tate) *v.* 1. To form a cavity. 2. To produce cavitation.

cav·i·ta·tion (kav''i·tay'shun) *n.* 1. The formation of a cavity or cavities in an organ or tissue, usually as a result of disease. 2. The process of amnion formation in man and certain mammals. 3. Reduction of the hydrodynamic pressure within a liquid, as by subjecting it to ultrasonic vibration, to a value below the vapor pressure, so that spaces or cavities form in it momentarily.

cav·i·ty (kav'i·tee) *n.* 1. A hole or hollow space. 2. The lesion produced by dental caries.

ca·vo·gram (kay'vo·gram) *n.* A radiographic depiction of the vena cava, inferior or superior.

ca·vog·ra·phy (kay·vog'ruh·fee) *n.* Radiographic demonstration of the vena cava, either superior or inferior.

ca·vo·sur·face (kay''vo·sur'fus) *adj.* Of, pertaining to, or designating the wall of a cavity and the surface of a tooth.

ca·vo·val·gus (kay''vo·val'gus) *n.* Talipes calcaneocavus combined with talipes valgus.

ca·vum (kay'vum) *n.,* genit. **ca·vi** (kay'vye), pl. **ca·va** (·vuh) *In anatomy,* a cavity or chamber.

ca·vus (kay'vus) *adj. & n.* 1. Hollow, concave. 2. PES CAVUS or TALIPES CAVUS.

cayenne-pepper spot. PAPILLARY VARIX.

Ca·ze·nave's disease (kah[z·nahv') PEMPHIGUS FOLIACEUS.

CBC Complete blood count.

CB lead. *In electrocardiography,* a precordial exploring electrode placed at the cardiac apex, paired with an indifferent electrode in the back near the angle of the scapula; a bipolar lead.

CBS Abbreviation for *chronic brain syndrome.*

C. C. Commission Certified; indicating that a sample of the dye so marked has been submitted to the Biological Stain Commission and has been found by the Commission to meet its standards for the dye.

cc An abbreviation for *cubic centimeter* (= c^3).

C carbohydrate. A carbohydrate found in pneumococci.

CCU Coronary care unit or cardiac care unit.

Cd Symbol for cadmium.

CDC Abbreviation for *Center for Disease Control* (formerly: *Communicable Disease Center*).

Ce Symbol for cerium.

ce·bo·ce·pha·lia (see''bo·se·fay'lee·uh) *n.* A condition, related to incipient cyclopia, in which there is absence or marked defect of the nose, with, however, two orbital cavities and two eyes, the region between the eyes being narrow and flat.

ce·cal, cae·cal (see'kul) *adj.* Of or resembling a cecum.

cecal appendage. VERMIFORM APPENDIX.

ce·cec·to·my, cae·cec·to·my (see·seck'tuh·mee) *n.* Excision of the cecum.

ce·ci·tis, cae·ci·tis (see·sigh'tis) *n.* Inflammation of the cecum.

ce·co·cele, cae·co·cele (see′ko·seel) n. Herniation of the cecum.

ce·co·co·lic, cae·co·co·lic (see″ko·ko′lick, ·kol′ick) adj. Pertaining to the cecum and the colon.

ce·co·co·los·to·my, cae·co·co·los·to·my (see″ko·ko·los′tuh·mee) n. The formation of an anastomosis between the cecum and some part of the colon.

ce·co·il·e·os·to·my, cae·co·il·e·os·to·my (see″ko·il″ee·os′tuh·mee) n. The formation of an anastomosis between the cecum and the ileum.

Cecon. A trademark for ascorbic acid.

ce·co·pexy, cae·co·pexy (see′ko·peck″see) n. Fixation of the cecum by a surgical operation.

ce·co·pli·ca·tion, cae·co·pli·ca·tion (see″ko·pli·kay′shun) n. An operation for the relief of dilated cecum, consisting in taking tucks or folds in the wall.

ce·cop·to·sis, cae·cop·to·sis (see″kop·to′sis) n., pl. cecopto·ses, caecopto·ses (·seez) Downward displacement of the cecum.

ce·cor·rha·phy, cae·cor·rha·phy (see·kor′uh·fee) n. Suture of the cecum.

ce·co·sig·moid·os·to·my, cae·co·sig·moid·os·to·my (see″ko·sig′moid·os′tuh·mee) n. The establishment of an anastomosis between the cecum and sigmoid colon.

ce·cos·to·my, cae·cos·to·my (see·kos′tuh·mee) n. The establishment of a permanent artificial opening into the cecum.

ce·cot·o·my, cae·cot·o·my (see·kot′uh·mee) n. Incision into the cecum.

ce·cum, cae·cum (see′kum) n., pl. ce·ca, cae·ca (·kuh) 1. [NA] The large blind pouch or cul-de-sac in which the large intestine begins. 2. The blind end of any of various tubular structures.

cedar oil. A transparent oil obtained from the red cedar, Juniperus virginiana; used as clearing agent in histology and with oil-immersion lenses.

Cedilanid. Trademark for crystalline lanatoside C, a cardioactive glycoside from Digitalis lanata.

cef·a·man·dole (sef″uh·man′dole) n. $C_{18}H_{18}N_6O_5S_2$, an antibiotic of the cephalosporin type.

ce·faz·o·lin (se·faz′o·lin) n. $C_{14}H_{14}N_8O_4S_3$, an antibiotic of the cephalosporin type, usually used as the sodium salt.

ce·fox·i·tin (se·fock′si·tin) n. $C_{16}H_{17}N_3O_7S_2$, an antibiotic of the cephalosporin type.

-cele A combining form meaning (a) tumor; (b) hernia; (c) pathologic swelling.

celi-, coeli-, celio-, coelio- A combining form meaning abdomen or belly.

ce·li·ac, coe·li·ac (see′lee·ack) adj. Abdominal; pertaining to the abdomen.

celiac artery. CELIAC TRUNK.

celiac axis. CELIAC TRUNK.

celiac disease. CELIAC SYNDROME.

celiac plexus. A large nerve plexus lying in front of the aorta around the origin of the celiac trunk. It is formed by fibers from the splanchnic and vagus nerves and is distributed to the abdominal viscera.

celiac syndrome or disease. One of the malabsorption syndromes characterized by malnutrition, abnormal stools, and varying degrees of edema, skeletal disorders, peripheral neuropathy, and anemia. Abnormalities of the small intestinal villi and the response to a gluten-free diet are diagnostic.

celiac trunk. The short, thick artery arising from the anterior (ventral) aspect of the abdominal aorta between the two crura of the diaphragm. It usually divides into the hepatic, splenic, and left gastric arteries.

ce·li·ec·ta·sia, coe·li·ec·ta·sia (see″lee·eck·tay′zhuh, ·zee·uh) n. Abnormal distention of the abdominal cavity.

celio-. See celi-.

ce·lio·col·pot·o·my, coe·lio·col·pot·o·my (see″lee·o·kol·pot′uh·mee) n. The opening of the abdomen through the vagina, for the removal of a tumor or other body.

ce·lio·en·ter·ot·o·my, coe·lio·en·ter·ot·o·my (see″lee·o·en″tur·ot′uh·mee) n. The opening of the intestine through an incision in the abdominal wall.

ce·lio·gas·trot·o·my, coe·lio·gas·trot·o·my (see″lee·o·gas·trot′uh·mee) n. The opening of the stomach through an abdominal incision.

ce·lio·my·o·mec·to·my, coe·lio·my·o·mec·to·my (see″lee·o·migh″o·meck′tuh·mee) n. The removal of a myoma (of the uterus) through an abdominal incision.

ce·lio·para·cen·te·sis, coe·lio·para·cen·te·sis (see″lee·o·păr″uh·sen·tee′sis) n., Tapping, or paracentesis, of the abdomen.

ce·li·or·rha·phy, coe·li·or·rha·phy (see″lee·or′uh·fee) n. Suture of the abdominal wall.

ce·li·os·co·py, coe·li·os·co·py (see″lee·os′kuh·pee) n. PERITONEOSCOPY.

ce·li·ot·o·my, coe·li·ot·o·my (see″lee·ot′uh·mee) n. In surgery, the opening of the abdominal cavity.

ce·li·tis, coe·li·tis (see·lye′tis) n. Any inflammatory condition of the abdomen.

cell-, cello-. A combining form meaning cellulose.

cell, n. 1. A highly integrated, constantly changing system that is the structural and functional unit of the living organism, and that has the ability to assimilate, grow, reproduce, and respond to stimuli. 2. An apparatus, consisting of electrodes and an electrolyte solution, for converting chemical into electrical energy or the reverse. 3. A compartment; particularly, a hollow space in a bone.

cel·la (sel′uh) n., pl. cel·lae (·ee) The central part of the lateral ventricle of the brain, extending from the interventricular foramen to the splenium of the corpus callosum.

cel·la·bu·rate (sel″uh·bew′rate) n. Cellulose acetate butyrate employed as an enteric coating for tablets.

Cel·la·no blood group At first thought to be a distinct blood group, but now recognized as belonging to the Kell blood group.

cell body. The portion of a neuron that contains the nucleus and its surrounding cytoplasm and from which the axon and dendrites extend.

cell-color ratio. The ratio between the percentage of erythrocytes in blood and the percentage of hemoglobin.

cell division. A biological process by which two or more cells are formed from one, usually by mitosis, meiosis, or amitosis.

cell-mediated immunity. Immunity which is maintained primarily by T lymphocytes rather than by the freely circulating antibody characteristic of humoral immunity; seen in immune response to viruses, fungi, and certain bacterial infections, in rejection of foreign tissue and of tumors, and in delayed hypersensitivity.

cell membrane. PLASMA MEMBRANE.

cel·lo·bi·ose (sel″o·bye′oce, ·oze) n. A disaccharide, $C_{12}H_{22}O_{11}$, formed by the partial hydrolysis of cellulose. On hydrolysis it yields two molecules of glucose.

cell of origin. A nerve cell body of the ganglion or nucleus from which a nerve fiber originates.

cell of termination. A nerve cell whose dendrites receive impulses from the axon of another cell or cells.

cel·loi·din (se·loy′din) n. One of many cellulose nitrates or cellulose acetates; used for embedding tissues in histologic technique.

Cellosize. A trademark for hydroxyethyl cellulose, a thickener and suspending agent for pharmaceutical preparations.

cells of Kul·tschitz·sky (kŏŏl′·chits′kee) The argentaffin cells of the intestinal glands.

cells of Pa·neth (pah′net) PANETH CELLS.

cell theory. The theory that the cell is the unit of organic structure and that cell formation is the essential process of life and its phenomena.

cellul-, celluli-, cellulo-. A combining form meaning cell, cellular.

cel·lu·lar (sel′yoo·lur) adj. Pertaining to or consisting of cells.

cellular immunology. The study of the cells which mediate immune responses, such as lymphocytes and macrophages.

cellular infiltration. 1. Passage of cells into tissues in the course of acute, subacute, or chronic inflammation. 2. Migration or invasion of cells of neoplasms.

cel·lu·lase (sel′yoo·lace, ·laze) n. 1. Any of several enzymes, found in bacteria and other lower organisms, capable of catalyzing the hydrolysis of cellulose to cellobiose. 2. A concentrate of cellulose-splitting enzymes, derived from Aspergillus niger, used as an inflammation counteractant.

cel·lule (sel′yool) n. 1. A small cell. 2. CELL.

cel·lu·lin (sel′yoo·lin) n. CELLULOSE.

cel·lu·li·tis (sel″yoo·lye′tis) n. A diffuse inflammation of connective tissue, especially of subcutaneous tissue.

Celluloid. Trademark for a tough, flammable synthetic thermoplastic composed of cellulose nitrate and camphor or other plasticizer; formerly used in surgery and dentistry.

cel·lu·lose (sel′yoo·loce) n. $(C_6H_{10}O_5)_n$. The principal carbohydrate constituent of the cell membranes of all plants. Absorbent cotton is one of the purest forms of cellulose; commercially, wood is the principal source of it. Pure cellulose is a white, amorphous mass, insoluble in most of the common solvents.

cell wall. In bacteria, fungi, most algae, and all higher plants, the more or less rigid envelope, exterior to the plasma membrane, which encloses and shapes the cell.

celomic. COELOMIC.

ce·lo·so·ma, coe·lo·so·ma (see″lo·so′muh) n. A congenital body cleft, with eventration; associated with various anomalies of the extremities, of the genitourinary apparatus, of the intestinal tract, and even of the whole trunk. Syn. abdominal fissure.

Cel·si·us (sel′see·us) adj. Pertaining to or designating the centigrade temperature scale in which 0° is set at the freezing point of water and 100° at the boiling point. Abbreviated, C.

ce·ment (se·ment′) n. 1. Any plastic material capable of becoming hard and of binding together the objects that are contiguous to it. 2. Any material used for filling cavities in teeth, seating crowns or inlays, or for protecting the dental pulp from harmful stimuli. 3. CEMENTUM.

ce·ment·i·cle (se·men′ti·kul) n. A calcified body found free in the connective tissue of the periodontal membrane, or fused with the cementum of a tooth.

ce·ment·i·fi·ca·tion (se·men″ti·fi·kay′shun) n. CEMENTOGENESIS.

cement line. The optically demonstrable interface between older bone matrix and more recently formed matrix.

ce·men·to·blast (se·men′to·blast) n. A cell that takes part in the formation of the dental cementum.

ce·men·to·blas·to·ma (se·men″to·blas·to′muh) n. A cementoma with prominent cellular components.

ce·men·to·den·ti·nal (se·men″to·den′ti·nul) adj. Pertaining to the cementum and dentin of a tooth.

ce·men·to·enam·el (se·men″to·e·nam′ul) adj. Pertaining to the cementum and enamel of a tooth.

ce·men·to·gen·e·sis (se·men″to·jen′e·sis) n. Formation of the cementum.

ce·men·to·ma (see″men·to′muh, sem″en·) n., pl. **cementomas, cementoma·ta** (·tuh) A benign dysontogenetic tumor composed of odontogenic, cementum-producing connective tissue.

ce·men·to·path·ia (se·men″to·path′ee·uh) n. Pathologic degeneration of the cementum surrounding a tooth; formerly thought to account for noninflammatory periodontal destruction (periodontosis).

ce·men·to·sis (see″men·to′sis) n., pl. **cementoses** (·seez) HYPERCEMENTOSIS.

ce·men·tum (se·men′tum) n., pl. **cemen·ta** (·tuh) The bony tissue that covers the root of a tooth, in man, and may cover parts of the crown of a tooth in certain animals, such as the ungulates.

¹cen-, caen-, ceno-, caeno- A combining form meaning new, recent.

²cen-, coen-, ceno-, coeno- A combining form meaning (a) general; (b) common.

Cendevax. A trademark for live rubella virus vaccine.

ce·nes·the·sia, coe·naes·the·sia (see″nes·theezh′uh, ·theez′ee·uh, sen″es·) n. The general sense of bodily existence, the sum of the multiple stimuli coming from the various parts of the body, and hence the basis for feelings of health or sickness. —**cen·es·thet·ic, coen·aes·thet·ic** (·thet'ick) *adj.*

ce·nes·thop·a·thy (see"nes·thop'uth·ee) *n.* The general feeling of discomfort or fatigue in illness as a result of multiple stimuli from various parts of the body; it may be accompanied by a mild form of depersonalization.

cen·sor, *In psychoanalysis,* that part of the unconscious self, composed of the superego and parts of the ego, which acts as a guard, as in dreams, to keep repressed material from emerging into consciousness.

cen·sor·ship, *n. In psychoanalysis,* the restrictions imposed upon a pure instinctual impulse by counterforces in the unconscious and conscious levels of the mind before it discharges itself upon the environment.

cen·tau·ry (sen'taw·ree) *n.* 1. A popular name for various plants of the genus *Centaurium.* 2. The dried flowering plant of *Centaurium umbellatum.* Centaury possesses the bitter properties of the gentians and has been used as a stomachic.

cen·ter, cen·tre, *n.* 1. The midpoint of any surface or body. 2. A nucleus or collection of nuclei, or even a relatively imprecisely defined anatomic region in the brain, brainstem, or spinal cord subserving a particular function.

Center for Disease Control. An agency of the United States government, located in Atlanta, Georgia, which plans, conducts, coordinates, supports, and evaluates national programs for the prevention and control of communicable and vector-borne diseases and other preventable conditions, including those related to malnutrition. Abbreviated, CDC.

cen·ter·ing, cen·tring (sen'tur·ing) *n.* 1. *In microscopy,* arrangement of an object or an accessory so that its center coincides with the optical axis of the microscope. 2. *In optics,* placing of the lens before the eye or in a spectacle frame so that the visual axis passes through the optical center of the lens. The decentering of the lens produces a prism effect. —**cen·ter, cen·tre,** *n. & v.*

cen·te·sis (sen·tee'sis) *n.,* pl. **cente·ses** (·seez) Puncture; perforation.

centi- A combining form meaning (a) *hundredth part;* (b) *hundred.*

cen·ti·bar (sen'ti·bahr) *n.* One one-hundredth of a bar; a unit of atmospheric pressure.

cen·ti·grade (sen'ti·grade) *adj.* Designating a temperature scale based on a given interval divided into 100 degrees; specifically, CELSIUS.

cen·ti·gram (sen'ti·gram) *n.* The hundredth part of a gram, equal to 0.1543 grain. Abbreviated, cg.

cen·ti·li·ter, cen·ti·li·tre (sen'ti·lee"tur) *n.* The hundredth part of a liter, equal to 0.6102 cubic inch. Abbreviated, cl.

cen·ti·me·ter, cen·ti·me·tre (sen'ti·mee"tur, son' ti·) *n.* The hundredth part of a meter, equal to 0.3937 (about ⅖) inch. Abbreviated, cm.

cen·ti·nor·mal (sen"ti·nor'mul) *adj.* Having one one-hundredth of the normal strength, said of

a solution containing one one-hundredth of a gram equivalent of the solute in 1 liter of solution.

cen·ti·pede (sen'ti·peed) *n.* Any myriapod of the class Chilopoda, with a pair of legs on each segment of the body except the last two. The claws of the first body segment have openings at the tips for expulsion of neurotoxic venom. The bite of centipedes of temperate climates seldom produces more than mild, local symptoms in man; that of tropical species causes necrotic lesions as well as general symptoms of lymphangitis, vomiting, fever, and headache.

centr-, centro-. A combining form meaning *center, central.*

¹cen·trad (sen'trad) *n.* An angular measure, one one-hundredth of a radian; about 0.57°.

²centrad, *adv.* Toward the center, or toward the median line.

cen·tral (sen'trul) *adj.* 1. Situated at or near the center. 2. Basic, fundamental. 3. Of or pertaining to the central nervous system. 4. Of or pertaining to the centrum (2).

central ageusia. Loss or impairment of taste due to a lesion in the cerebral centers for taste.

central anesthesia. Anesthesia due to a lesion of the central nervous system.

central aphasia. CONDUCTION APHASIA.

central canal of the spinal cord. The small tube, containing cerebrospinal fluid and lined by ependyma, that extends through the center of the spinal cord from the conus medullaris to the lower part of the fourth ventricle. It represents the embryonic neural tube.

central deafness. Deafness due to a lesion involving the auditory pathways or auditory centers of the brain.

central fovea. FOVEA CENTRALIS.

central inhibitory state. A relatively prolonged state in which inhibitory influences overbalance excitatory ones in the spinal cord, possibly due to reverberating circuits or prolonged effects of synaptic mediators.

central lobule. A lobule of the superior vermis of the cerebellum.

central necrosis. 1. Necrosis of the liver around the central vein. 2. Death of tissue in the middle of a mass of cells.

central nervous system. The structures of the nervous system supported by astrocytes and oligodendroglia rather than by fibroblasts and enclosed by the piarachnoid; includes the brain, spinal cord, olfactory bulb, and optic nerve. Abbreviated, CNS.

central paralysis. Paralysis due to a lesion or lesions of the brain or spinal cord.

central scotoma. Blindness in the central area of the visual field, or involving the normal point of fixation, caused by a lesion and dysfunction of the macular region of the eye.

central serous retinopathy. A condition characterized by edema and hyperemia of the retina, occurring in adult life and more often in men, in which there is an abrupt onset of blurred vision and central scotoma. Funduscopic examination reveals a wet-appearing raised macula with a surrounding ring-shaped reflex and slight hyperpigmentation, usually only in one eye. Etiology is unknown, but multiple factors, including allergies, may play a role. Although self-limited, the condition is often recurrent.

central sulcus. 1. A groove situated about the middle of the lateral surface of the cerebral hemisphere, separating the frontal from the parietal lobe. 2. (of the insula:) A deep groove crossing backward and upward on the surface of the insula, dividing it into a larger, anterior portion, occupied by the short gyri of the insula, and a smaller, posterior portion, occupied by the long gyrus of the insula.

central venous pressure. The pressure representative of the filling pressure of the right ventricle, measured peripherally or centrally, corrected for the hydrostatic pressure between the heart and the point of measurement; used to monitor fluid replacement, as in shock or severe burns. Abbreviated, CVP.

central vision. Vision with the eye turned directly toward the object so that the image falls upon the macula lutea, providing the most acute vision. Syn. *direct vision, macular vision.*

cen·tra·phose (sen′truh·foze) *n.* A subjective sensation of darkness originating in the visual center.

cen·tren·ce·phal·ic (sen″tren·se·fal′ick) *adj.* Pertaining to or designating the neuron systems that are symmetrically connected with both cerebral hemispheres and that serve to coordinate their functions. These circuits are located in the higher brainstem and include the thalamus with the diencephalon, mesencephalon, and rhombencephalon.

cen·tric (sen′trick) *adj.* Pertaining to a center, as opposed to peripheral.

-centric. A combining form meaning (a) *with a center or centers* (of a specified kind or number); (b) *with* (something) *at its center.*

centric occlusion. The maximum, unstrained, occlusal contact relationship of the teeth; associated with centric relation of the mandible to the maxilla.

cen·trif·u·gal (sen·trif′yoo·gul) *adj.* 1. Acting or proceeding in a direction away from a center or axis. 2. Efferent; moving outward from a nerve center.

cen·trif·u·ga·tion (sen·trif″yoo·gay′shun) *n.* Separation of a substance, e.g., a suspension of particulate matter, into components of different densities by means of a centrifuge.

cen·tri·fuge (sen′tri·fewj) *n. & v.* 1. An apparatus for separating substances of different densities by centrifugal force. 2. To separate into components of different densities by means of a centrifuge.

cen·tri·lob·u·lar (sen″tri·lob′yoo·lur) *adj.* In the central portion of a lobule, usually of the liver.

centrilobular emphysema. Emphysema involving primarily the central portion of the secondary lobule of the lung.

cen·tri·ole (sen′tree·ole) *n.* A minute oval composed of microtubules, representing a nucleation center of microtubule formation; usually found in the centrosome and frequently considered to be the division center of the cell.

cen·trip·e·tal (sen·trip′e·tul) *adj.* 1. Acting or proceeding toward the center from the periphery. 2. Afferent; moving toward a nerve center.

cen·tro·ac·i·nar (sen″tro·as′i·nur) *adj.* Of or pertaining to the specialized cells in the central part of pancreatic acini.

cen·tro·cyte (sen′tro·site) *n.* A cell containing single and double granules of various sizes.

cen·tro·don·tous (sen″tro·don′tus) *adj.* Furnished with sharp-pointed teeth.

cen·tro·dor·sal (sen″tro·dor′sul) *adj.* Central and dorsal.

cen·tro·me·di·an (sen″tro·mee′dee·un) *adj.* Central and median.

cen·tro·mere (sen′tro·meer) *n.* The constriction in a chromosome where it is attached to a spindle fiber. Syn. *kinetochore.*

cen·tro·phose (sen′tro·foze) *n.* A subjective sensation of light originating in the visual centers.

cen·tro·some (sen′tro·sohm) *n.* The centrosphere together with the centriole or centrioles.

cen·tro·sphere (sen′tro·sfeer) *n.* The specialized area of the cytoplasm in which the centriole is located and from which the astral fibers (astrospheres) extend during cell division; the Golgi apparatus often surrounds it.

cen·trum (sen′trum) *n.,* pl. **centrums, cen·tra** (·truh) 1. The center or middle part. 2. The body of a vertebra, exclusive of the bases of the arches.

Cepacol. A trademark for cetylpyridinium chloride.

cephal-, cephalo- A combining form meaning *head.*

ceph·a·lad (sef′ul·ad) *adv.* Toward the head.

ceph·a·lal·gia (sef″uh·lal′jee·uh) *n.* Headache. —**cephalal·gic** (·jick) *adj.*

ce·phal·gia (se·fal′jee·uh) *n.* CEPHALALGIA.

ceph·al·he·ma·to·ma (sef″ul·hee·muh·to′muh) *n.* A collection of blood beneath the pericranium, forming a tumorlike swelling.

ceph·al·hy·dro·cele (sef″ul·high′dro·seel) *n.* Effusion of cerebrospinal fluid beneath the scalp in fractures of the skull.

ce·phal·ic (se·fal′ick) *adj.* Pertaining to the head.

cephalic index. The ratio of the greatest width of the head, taken wherever it may be found in a horizontal plane perpendicular to the sagittal plane, × 100, to the greatest length, taken in the sagittal plane between glabella and opisthocranion. Its values are classified as:

dolichocephalic	x-75.9
mesocephalic	76.0-80.9
brachycephalic	81.0-85.4
hyperbrachycephalic	85.5-x

cephalic vein. A superficial vein located on the lateral side of the arm which drains blood from the radial side of the hand and forearm into the axillary vein.

cephalic version. Turning of the fetus to establish a cephalic presentation.

ceph·a·lin (sef′uh·lin) *n.* A phospholipid in which phosphatidic acid is esterified to an ethanolamine base. Syn. *phosphatidyl ethanolamine.*

cephalin–cholesterol flocculation test. A test for liver function which measures the capacity of serum of persons with hepatic disease to flocculate a colloidal suspension of cephalin cholesterol-complex. The result is expressed from 0 to 4 plus.

ceph·a·lo·cau·dal (sef''uh·lo·kaw'dul) *adj. In anatomy,* relating to the long axis of the body, head to tail.

ceph·a·lo·cele (sef'uh·lo·seel) *n.* Hernia of the brain; protrusion of a mass of the cranial contents.

ceph·a·lo·cen·te·sis (sef''uh·lo·sen·tee'sis) *n.,* pl. **cephalocente·ses** (·seez) *In surgery,* puncture of the cranium.

ceph·a·lo·dyn·ia (sef''uh·lo·din'ee·uh) *n.* Headache.

ceph·a·lo·gen·e·sis (sef''uh·lo·jen'e·sis) *n.,* pl. **cephalogene·ses** (·seez) The origin and development of the primordia of the head.

ceph·a·lo·graph (sef'uh·lo·graf) *n.* An instrument for diagrammatically recording the size and form of the head.

ceph·a·lo·gy·ric (sef''uh·lo·jye'rick) *adj.* Pertaining to or causing rotation of the head.

ceph·a·lo·hem·a·to·cele, ceph·a·lo·haem·a·to·cele (sef''uh·lo·hem'uh·to·seel'') *n.* A hematocele beneath the scalp, communicating with a dural sinus.

ceph·a·loid (sef'uh·loid) *adj.* Resembling the head; head-shaped.

ceph·a·lo·me·nia (sef''uh·lo·mee'nee·uh) *n.* Vicarious menstruation through the nose.

ceph·a·lo·men·in·gi·tis (sef''uh·lo·men''in·jye'tis) *n.* Inflammation of the meninges of the brain.

ceph·a·lom·e·ter (sef''uh·lom'e·tur) *n. In craniometry,* an instrument for measuring the head.

ceph·a·lom·e·try (sef''uh·lom'e·tree) *n.* 1. *In plastic surgery,* use of the cephalometer for comparison with casts in facial reconstruction. 2. *In orthodontics,* a procedure utilizing anatomical tracings of lateral head plates identifying anatomical points, planes, and angles to assay the patient's growth or evaluate treatment. —**ceph·a·lo·met·ric** (·lo·met'rick) *adj.*

ceph·a·lo·or·bi·tal (sef''uh·lo·or'bi·tul) *adj.* Pertaining to the cranium and orbits.

ceph·a·lop·a·thy (sef''uh·lop'uth·ee) *n.* ENCEPHALOPATHY.

ceph·a·lo·pel·vic (sef''uh·lo·pel'vick) *adj.* Pertaining to the head of the fetus and the pelvis of the mother.

cephalopelvic disproportion. A disparity between the size of the head of the fetus and the opening in the maternal pelvis; usually, excessive size of the fetal head in relation to the maternal pelvis. Abbreviated, CPD.

ceph·a·lo·pha·ryn·ge·us (sef''uh·lo·fa·rin'jee·us) *L. adj.* Of or pertaining to the cranium and pharynx.

ceph·a·lo·ple·gia (sef''uh·lo·plee'jee·uh) *n.* Paralysis of the muscles about the head and face.

ceph·a·lor·i·dine (sef''uh·lor'i·deen) *n.* A semisynthetic antibiotic, $C_{19}H_{17}N_3O_4S_2$, that differs from cephalothin in having a pyridine substituent in place of an acetoxy group, and in being more soluble in water; the antibacterial spectrum is similar to that of cephalothin but cephaloridine causes less pain on intramuscular injection.

ceph·a·lo·spor·in (sef''uh·lo·spor'in) *n.* Any one group of diverse antibiotic substances, produced by certain species of *Cephalosporium.*

Cephalosporin C, structurally related to the penicillins, has moderate antibacterial activity; its semisynthetic derivatives cephalothin, cephaloridine, and cephaloglycin are more active. Cephalosporin N is identical with penicillin N and synnematin B. Cephalosporins P_1 to P_5 are steroid derivatives.

ceph·a·lo·thin (sef''uh·lo·thin) *n.* Sodium 7-(thiophene-2-acetamido)cephalosporanate, $C_{16}H_{15}N_2NaO_6S_2$, a bactericidal antibiotic which is active against many gram-positive and gram-negative organisms.

ceph·a·lo·tho·rac·ic (sef''uh·lo·tho·ras'ick) *adj.* 1. Pertaining to the head and thorax. 2. Designating those arthropods having the head joined to the thorax.

cephalothoracopagus di·sym·me·tros (dye·sim'e·tros). Conjoined twins in which the single head exhibits two equal opposite faces.

ceph·a·lo·tome (sef''uh·lo·tome) *n.* An instrument for performing cephalotomy on a fetus.

ceph·a·lot·o·my (sef''uh·lot'uh·mee) *n.* The opening or division of the head of a fetus to facilitate delivery.

ceph·a·lo·trac·tor (sef''uh·lo·track'tur) *n.* OBSTETRIC FORCEPS.

ceph·a·lo·tribe (sef'uh·lo·tribe) *n.* An instrument for crushing the head of a fetus.

ceph·a·lo·trip·sy (sef'uh·lo·trip''see) *n. In obstetrics,* the crushing of the fetal head when delivery is otherwise impossible.

-cephalus A combining form designating (a) an individual with a specified *abnormality of the head,* or the abnormality itself; (b) in biological taxonomy, an organism with a specified *kind of head.*

-cephaly A combining form designating a *condition* or *characteristic of the head.*

cer-, cero- A combining form meaning (a) *wax;* (b) *resembling wax.*

ce·ra (seer'uh, serr'uh) *n.* Wax obtained from plants or made by insects; consists of monohydric, high molecular weight alcohols and/or their esters, fatty acids, hydrocarbons, and possibly other substances, depending on the source. —**ce·ra·ceous** (se·ray'shus) *adj.*

cer·a·sin (serr'uh·sin) *n.* 1. A resin from the bark of cherry, peach, and plum trees. 2. CERASINOSE. 3. KERASIN.

cer·a·si·nose (serr'uh·si·noce, se·ras'i·noce) *n.* A carbohydrate found in the gum of the cherry tree.

cerat-, cerato- A combining form meaning *horn, horny.*

ce·rate (seer'ate, serr'ate) *n. In pharmacy,* an unctuous preparation consisting of wax mixed with oils, fatty substances, or resins, and of such a consistency that at ordinary temperatures it can be spread readily on linen or muslin, and yet so firm that it will not melt or run when applied to the skin. —**ce·rat·ed** (seer'ay·tid, serr') *adj.*

Cer·a·to·phyl·lus (serr''uh·to·fil'us) *n.* A genus of fleas.

Ceratophyllus fas·ci·a·tus (fash·ee·ay'tus). The common rat flea of the United States and Europe; a vector of typhus fever and a host of *Hymenolepis diminuta.*

cer·car·ia (sur·kār'ee·uh) *n.,* pl. **cercari·ae** (·ee·ee)

Any trematode worm in its second stage of larval life. —**cercar·i·al** (·ee-ul) *adj.*; **cercari·an** (·un) *adj. & n.*

cercarial dermatitis. SCHISTOSOME DERMATITIS.

cer·clage (sair·klahzh′) *n. In orthopedics,* application of wire or metal band encircling a bone; a method of osteosynthesis in oblique and certain comminuted fractures.

cerebell-, cerebelli-, cerebello-. A combining form meaning *cerebellum, cerebellar.*

cer·e·bel·lar (serr″e·bel′ur) *adj.* Pertaining to or involving the cerebellum.

cerebellar ataxia. 1. Muscular incoordination due to disease of the cerebellum or its central connections. 2. Any of the degenerative cerebellar ataxias of genetic or uncertain origin, which may include olivopontocerebellar ataxia, Marie's hereditary cerebellar ataxia, dyssynergia cerebellaris progressiva, and other uncommon forms.

cerebellar epilepsy or **fit.** BRAINSTEM EPILEPSY.

cerebellar gait. A wide-based, unsteady, irregular, lateral reeling gait due to disease or dysfunction of the cerebellum or cerebellar pathways.

cerebellar pressure cone. The downward displacement of the inferior mesial parts of the cerebellar hemispheres (ventral paraflocculi or tonsillae) through the foramen magnum, the result of a sharp pressure gradient between intracranial and intraspinal pressures, as in posterior fossa tumors or general brain swelling, and frequently causing death from medullary compression.

cerebellar rigidity. The opisthotonic position sometimes observed in patients with large midline cerebellar lesions and probably due to compression of the brainstem.

cerebellar speech. The slow, slurred, and jerky speech seen in cerebellar disorders; may be intermittent and explosive or syllabic and singsong in character.

cerebellar tonsil. The tonsilla of the cerebellum. See *tonsilla* (1).

cer·e·bel·lif·u·gal (serr″e·be·lif′yoo·gul) *adj.* Tending away from the cerebellum.

cer·e·bel·lip·e·tal (serr″e·be·lip′i·tul) *adj.* Tending toward the cerebellum.

cer·e·bel·li·tis (serr″e·be·lye′tis) *n.* Inflammation of the cerebellum.

cer·e·bel·lo·bul·bar (serr″e·bel″o·bul′bur) *adj.* Pertaining to or involving the cerebellum and the medulla oblongata.

cer·e·bel·lof·u·gal (serr″e·be·lof′yoo·gul) *adj.* CEREBELLIFUGAL.

cer·e·bel·lo·med·ul·lary (serr″e·bel″o·med′yoo·lair-ee) *adj.* Pertaining to or involving the cerebellum and the medulla oblongata.

cerebellomedullary cistern. A large subarachnoid space formed by the arachnoid stretching across from the inferior surface of the cerebellum to the dorsal surface of the medulla oblongata.

cer·e·bel·lo·pon·tine (serr″e·bel″o·pon′teen) *adj.* Pertaining to or involving the cerebellum and the pons.

cerebellopontine angle. A region bounded laterally by the petrous portion of the temporal bone, medially by the cerebellum and brainstem, below by the floor of the posterior fossa of the skull, and above by the tentorium cerebelli. An area in which tumors frequently occur.

cerebellopontine angle tumor. An acoustic neurilemmoma occupying its usual site in one cerebellopontine angle.

cerebellopontine-angle tumor syndrome. Tinnitus, impairment and loss of hearing, ipsilateral paralysis of the sixth and seventh cranial nerves, involvement of the trigeminal (fifth cranial) nerve, vertigo and nystagmus, and signs of cerebellar disturbances, such as vomiting and ataxia due to a neurilemmoma or other tumor in the area of the cerebellopontine angle.

cer·e·bel·lo·ret·i·nal (serr″e·bel″o·ret′i·nul) *adj.* Pertaining to the cerebellum and the retina.

cer·e·bel·lo·ru·bral (serr″e·bel″o·roo′brul) *adj.* Pertaining to the tract of the superior cerebellar peduncle running from the dentate nucleus to the red nucleus.

cer·e·bel·lo·ru·bro·spi·nal (serr″e·bel″o·roo″bro·spye′nul) *adj.* Pertaining to the cerebellum, the red nucleus, and the spinal cord.

cer·e·bel·lo·spi·nal (serr″e·bel″o·spye′nul) *adj.* Pertaining to the cerebellum and the spinal cord, a descending fiber tract.

cer·e·bel·lo·tha·lam·ic (serr″e·bel″o·tha·lam′ick) *adj.* Pertaining to the cerebellum and the thalamus.

cer·e·bel·lo·ves·tib·u·lar (serr″e·bel″o·ves·tib′yoo·lur) *adj.* Pertaining to the cerebellum and the vestibular nuclei.

cer·e·bel·lum (serr″e·bel′um) *n.,* genit. sing. **cere·bel·li** (·eye), pl. **cerebel·la** (·luh) The inferior part of the brain lying below the cerebrum and above the pons and medulla oblongata, consisting of two lateral lobes and a middle lobe.

cerebr-, cerebri-, cerebro-. A combining form meaning *cerebrum, cerebral, brain.*

cer·e·bral (serr′e·brul, se·ree′brul) *adj.* Pertaining to or involving the cerebrum.

cerebral allergy. Symptoms of cerebral disturbances associated with a definitively established allergy.

cerebral aqueduct. The elongated, slender cavity of the midbrain which connects the third and fourth ventricles.

cerebral blast concussion or **syndrome.** Blast injury causing no external skull trauma, but rendering the patient unconscious, due to diffuse or focal cerebral and meningeal hemorrhages; observed chiefly in soldiers exposed to nearby explosions.

cerebral blindness. CORTICAL BLINDNESS.

cerebral blood flow. The rate, in milliliters per minute, at which blood flows through the brain, measured by the rate of diffusion of inert gases (nitrous oxide, krypton) into the brain. Approximate value of cerebral blood flow in normal persons is 750 ml per minute.

cerebral concussion. BRAIN CONCUSSION.

cerebral cortex. The cortex of the cerebrum. See *cortex* (3, 4).

cerebral deafness. CENTRAL DEAFNESS.

cerebral death. BRAIN DEATH.

cerebral dominance. The normal tendency for one cerebral hemisphere, usually the left, to be better developed in certain functions, especially speech and handedness.

cerebral dysrhythmia. Any abnormal electrical rhythm of the brain as revealed by the electroencephalogram. The brain waves may be too fast, too slow, or may alternate between the two types. Dysrhythmia is frequently associated with an epileptiform condition.

cerebral hemiplegia. Paralysis of one side of the body resulting from a lesion on the opposite side of the brain.

cerebral localization. 1. Assignment or determination of a certain area of the brain as the region exercising control over a given physiologic act or faculty. 2. Assignment or determination of an area of the brain as the site of a lesion.

cerebral palsy. Popularly, any of a group of congenital diseases, usually nonprogressive and dating from infancy or early childhood, characterized by a major disorder of motor function.

cerebral paraplegia. Paralysis of both legs due to a bilateral cerebral lesion, as in such conditions as meningioma of the falx or thrombosis of the superior sagittal sinus.

cerebral peduncle. One of two large bands of white matter containing descending axons of upper motor neurons which emerge from the underside of the cerebral hemispheres to approach each other as they enter the rostral border of the pons. Between the peduncles, which form the ventral part of the mesencephalon, lies the interpeduncular fossa.

cerebral thrombosis. 1. Thrombosis occurring in a cerebral blood vessel. 2. Cerebral infarction secondary to thrombotic occlusion of a cerebral blood vessel.

cerebral ventricles. VENTRICLES OF THE BRAIN.

cerebral vertigo. Vertigo that has its origin in the cerebral cortex, and more specifically in the temporoparietal cortex bordering the Sylvian fissure.

cerebral vesicles. The paired lateral outpouchings of the telencephalon which become the cerebral hemispheres.

cer·e·bra·tion (serr″e·bray'shun) *n.* Mental activity; thinking.

cer·e·bric acid (serr′e·brick, se·reb'rick). A fatty acid from brain tissue.

ce·re·bri·form (se·ree'bri·form) *adj.* Resembling the brain.

cer·e·brif·u·gal (serr″e·brif'yoo·gul) *adj.* Of nerve fibers or impulses: efferent with respect to the cerebral cortex; transmitting or transmitted from the brain to the periphery.

cer·e·brip·e·tal (serr″e·brip'e·tul) *adj.* Of nerve fibers or impulses: afferent with respect to the cerebral cortex; transmitting or transmitted from the periphery to the brain.

cer·e·bri·tis (serr″e·brye'tis) *n.* 1. ENCEPHALITIS. 2. Inflammation of the cerebrum.

cer·e·bro·cer·e·bel·lar (serr″e·bro·serr″e·bel'ur) *adj.* Pertaining to the cerebrum and the cerebellum.

cerebrocerebellar atrophy. Any degenerative disease of the central nervous system characterized by cerebellar signs in combination with such cerebral disturbances as loss of intellect, seizures, extrapyramidal signs, or loss of vision or hearing.

cer·e·bro·cor·ti·cal (serr″e·bro·kor'ti·kul) *adj.* Pertaining to or involving the cerebral cortex.

cer·e·broid (serr′e·broid) *adj.* Brainlike.

cer·e·bro·mac·u·lar (serr″e·bro·mack'yoo·lur) *adj.* Pertaining to or involving the brain and the macula of the eye.

cerebromacular degeneration. CEREBRORETINAL DEGENERATION.

cer·e·bro·ma·la·cia (serr″e·bro·ma·lay'shuh, ·see·uh) *n.* ENCEPHALOMALACIA.

cer·e·bro·med·ul·lary (serr″e·bro·med'yoo·lerr″ee) *adj.* Pertaining to the brain and spinal cord.

cer·e·bro·pon·tine (serr″e·bro·pon'tine) *adj.* Pertaining to the cerebrum and the pons.

cer·e·bro·ret·i·nal (serr″e·bro·ret'i·nul) *adj.* Of, pertaining to, or involving the brain and the retina.

cerebroretinal degeneration. Any of a group of hereditary degenerative diseases affecting chiefly the ganglion cells of brain, retina, and intestine, and manifested by progressive dementia and retinal changes. The principal forms are the infantile, late infantile, juvenile, and late juvenile forms of amaurotic familial idiocy, the infantile form of Gaucher's disease, and Niemann-Pick disease.

cer·e·bro·scle·ro·sis (serr″e·bro·skle·ro'sis) *n.* Sclerosis of cerebral tissue.

cer·e·bro·side (serr″e·bro·side) *n.* Any lipid, found in brain and other tissues, containing one molecule each of sphingosine, galactose (or occasionally glucose), and a fatty acid as the structural components. Syn. *galactolipid, glycolipid, glycosphingoside.*

cerebroside lipidosis. GAUCHER'S DISEASE.

cer·e·bro·spi·nal (serr″e·bro·spye'nul) *adj.* Pertaining to the brain and the spinal cord.

cerebrospinal axis. CENTRAL NERVOUS SYSTEM.

cerebrospinal fluid. The fluid within the cerebral ventricles and between the arachnoid membrane and pia mater of the brain and spinal cord. Abbreviated, CSF.

cerebrospinal otorrhea. Drainage of cerebrospinal fluid from the ear, usually the result of a posterior fossa basilar skull fracture, rarely from erosion of the petrous portion of the temporal bone caused by tumor.

cerebrospinal rhinorrhea. Leakage of cerebrospinal fluid from the nose, usually the result of a fracture of the frontal bone with associated tearing of the dura mater and arachnoid.

cer·e·bro·ten·di·nous (serr″e·bro·ten'di·nus) *adj.* Pertaining to the brain and the tendons.

cerebrotendinous xanthomatosis. A familial degenerative disease characterized clinically by cataracts, xanthomas of the Achilles tendon, and a neurologic disorder involving pathways in the spinal cord, brainstem, and cerebellum; pathologically xanthomatous lesions have been found not only in the tendons and white matter of the cerebellum, but also in the lungs; thought to be transmitted as an autosomal recessive trait.

cer·e·bro·to·nia (serr″e·bro·to'nee·uh) *n.* The behavioral counterpart of component III (ectomorphy) of the somatotype, manifested predominantly by extreme awareness of the external environment as well as of the internal self, with tendencies toward inhibition of bodily enjoyment and activity (the viscerotonic and somatotonic expressions).

cer·e·bro·vas·cu·lar (serr″e·bro·vas′kew·lur) adj. Pertaining to the blood vessels or blood supply of the brain.

cerebrovascular accident. A symptom complex resulting from cerebral hemorrhage or from embolism or thrombosis of the cerebral vessels, characterized by alterations in consciousness, seizures, and development of focal neurologic deficits. Syn. *stroke (informal)*.

cer·e·brum (serr′e·brum, se·ree′brum) n., genit. sing. **cere·bri** (·brye), pl. **cere·bra** (·bruh) The largest portion of the brain, occupying the whole upper part of the cranium, and consisting of the right and left hemispheres; the endbrain; telencephalon.

cer·e·lose (serr′e·loce, ·loze) n. DEXTROSE.

cer·e·sin (serr′e·sin, seer′e·sin) n. A naturally occurring solid mixture of hydrocarbons somewhat resembling white beeswax; used as an impression compound.

cer·e·sine (serr′e·seen, seer′e·seen, ·sin) n. CERESIN.

Cerespan. A trademark for papaverine.

ce·ri·um (seer′ee·um) n. Ce = 140.12. One of the rare-earth metals. It forms two series of salts, cerous and ceric.

ce·roid (seer′oid) n. Any of a variety of yellow to brown acid-fast pigments, insoluble in lipid solvents, representing end products of peroxidation of unsaturated fatty acids; they occur in many tissues, and in a variety of physiologic and pathologic states.

cer·ti·fi·a·ble (sur″ti·figh′uh·bul) adj. In law and medicine, indicating a person who by reason of a mental disorder needs guardianship, or requires commitment to a mental hospital or institution.

cer·ti·fi·ca·tion (sur″ti·fi·kay′shun) n. 1. The issuing of a guarantee by a person or organization authorized to do so. 2. A statement by an officially recognized and legally constituted body, such as a medical board, that a person or institution has met or complied with certain standards of excellence. 3. The issuance upon a prescribed form by a licensed medical practitioner as to the occurrence and cause of death. 4. The legal process whereby a judicial authority acting on factual and medical evidence declares a person legally insane. —**cer·ti·fy**, v.

certified color. In the United States, any coloring agent which is officially certified to meet specifications for use in foods, drugs, and cosmetics as determined by federal statute.

ce·ru·lean (se·roo′lee·un) adj. Sky-blue; azure.

ce·ru·lo·plas·min, cae·ru·lo·plas·min (se·roo″lo·plaz′min, seer″oo·lo·) n. A plasma protein (alpha$_2$-globulin) that contains eight atoms of copper, probably in covalent linkage. It represents at least 90% of the copper normally in plasma, and is estimated by its oxidase ability; blood values range from about 32 to 38 mg per 100 ml, but are usually markedly decreased in hepatolenticular degeneration.

ce·ru·men (se·roo′mun) n. A secretion of specialized glands of the external auditory meatus; earwax. —**ceru·mi·nous** (·mi·nus) adj.

Cerumenex. A trademark for a solution of polyethylene glycol and a surfactant, used to facilitate removal of ear wax by irrigation.

ce·ru·mi·no·sis (se·roo″mi·no′sis) n. An excessive secretion of cerumen.

ceruminous glands. The specialized glands of the external auditory meatus which secrete the watery component of the cerumen.

cervic-, cervico-. A combining form meaning neck, cervix, cervical.

cer·vi·cal (sur′vi·kul) adj. 1. Of or pertaining to the neck or the neck region of the body. 2. Pertaining to the cervix or neck of a part or organ, as of a tooth or of the uterus.

cervical adenitis. Inflammation of lymph nodes in the neck.

cervical enlargement. A thickening of the spinal cord from the level of the third cervical to the second thoracic vertebra, maximal at the sixth cervical vertebra, the level of attachment of the nerves of the brachial plexus.

cervical fissure. A congenital fissure of the neck.

cervical flexure. A flexure of the embryonic brain, concave ventrally, occurring at the junction of hindbrain and spinal cord.

cervical glands. The lymph nodes of the neck.

cervical intumescence. CERVICAL ENLARGEMENT.

cervical line. The line about the neck of a tooth at the junction of enamel and cementum.

cervical myalgic headache. MUSCLE-CONTRACTION HEADACHE.

cervical ribs. Occasional riblike processes of the cervical vertebrae.

cervical rib syndrome. Sensory, motor, or vascular symptoms in one or both upper extremities due to compression of the brachial plexus and subclavian artery in the neck by a rudimentary or fully developed cervical rib or an anomalous first thoracic rib.

cer·vi·cec·to·my (sur″vi·seck′tuh·mee) n. Excision of the cervix of the uterus.

cer·vi·ci·tis (sur″vi·sigh′tis) n. Inflammation of the cervix of the uterus.

cer·vi·co·au·ral (sur″vi·ko·aw′rul) adj. CERVICOAURICULAR.

cer·vi·co·au·ric·u·lar (sur″vi·ko·aw·rick′yoo·lur) adj. Pertaining to the neck and the ear.

cer·vi·co·ax·il·lary (sur″vi·ko·ack″si·lerr·ee) adj. Pertaining to the neck and the axilla.

cer·vi·co·bra·chi·al (sur″vi·ko·bray′kee·ul, ·brack′ee·ul) adj. Pertaining to the neck and the upper extremity or member.

cer·vi·co·bra·chi·al·gia (sur″vi·ko·bray″kee·al′jee·uh, ·brack′ee·) n. A neuralgia in which pain extends from the cervical region to the arms or fingers.

cer·vi·co·buc·cal (sur″vi·ko·buck′ul) adj. Pertaining to the buccal surface of the neck of a molar or premolar tooth.

cer·vi·co·col·pi·tis (sur″vi·ko·kol·pye′tis) n. Inflammation of the uterine cervix and the vagina.

cer·vi·co·dyn·ia (sur″vi·ko·din′ee·uh) n. Pain or neuralgia of the neck.

cer·vi·co·fa·cial (sur″vi·ko·fay′shul) adj. Pertaining to both the neck and the face.

cer·vi·co·la·bi·al (sur″vi·ko·lay′bee·ul) *adj.* Pertaining to the cervical portion of the labial surface of an incisor or canine tooth.

cer·vi·co·lin·gual (sur″vi·ko·ling′gwul) *adj.* Pertaining to the lingual surface of a tooth at or near the cervix.

cer·vi·co·pu·bic (sur″vi·ko·pew′bick) *adj.* Pertaining to the cervix of the uterus and the pubic bone.

cer·vi·co·rec·tal (sur″vi·ko·reck′tul) *adj.* Pertaining to the cervix of the uterus and the rectum.

cer·vi·co·tho·ra·cic (sur″vi·ko·tho·ras′ick) *adj.* Pertaining to the neck and the thorax.

cervicothoracic outlet syndrome. SCALENUS ANTERIOR SYNDROME.

cer·vi·co·uter·ine (sur″vi·ko·yoo′tur·ine) *adj.* Of or pertaining to the cervix of the uterus.

cer·vi·co·va·gi·nal (sur″vi·ko·va·jye′nul, ·vaj′i·nul) *adj.* Pertaining to the cervix of the uterus and to the vagina.

cer·vi·co·vag·i·ni·tis (sur″vi·ko·vaj″i·nigh′tis) *n.* Inflammation of the cervix of the uterus and the vagina.

cer·vi·co·ves·i·cal (sur″vi·ko·ves′i·kul) *adj.* Pertaining to the cervix of the uterus and urinary bladder.

cer·vix (sur′vicks) *n.*, genit. sing. cer·vi·cis (sur′vi·sis), pl. cer·vi·ces (sur′vi·seez) A constricted portion or neck.

cervix of the uterus. The cylindrical lower portion of the uterus between the isthmus and the ostium.

cervix ute·ri (yoo′tur·eye) [NA]. CERVIX OF THE UTERUS.

ce·sar·e·an, cae·sar·e·an (se·zair′ee·un) *adj.* Pertaining to a cesarean section.

cesarean hysterectomy. A hysterectomy performed immediately after a cesarean section.

cesarean section. Delivery of the fetus through an abdominal and uterine incision.

ce·si·um (see′zee·um) *n.* Cs = 132.905. A member of the alkali group of elements, which includes sodium, potassium, lithium, and rubidium. Cesium forms a number of salts in which its valence is 1. The physiologic actions of cesium are similar to those of potassium. Several of its salts have been used medicinally, largely experimentally.

Ces·to·da (ses·to′duh) *n. pl.* A subclass of Platyhelminthes that includes the tapeworms.

ces·tode (ses′tode) *adj. & n.* 1. Of or pertaining to the Cestoda. 2. One of the Cestoda.

ces·to·di·a·sis (ses″to·dye′uh·sis) *n.*, pl. cestodia·ses (·seez) Infection with tapeworms.

ce·ta·ce·um (se·tay′shee·um, ·see·um) *n.* SPERMACETI.

ce·tin (see′tin) *n.* Cetyl palmitate or cetyl cetylate, $C_{32}H_{64}O_2$, the chief constituent of spermaceti. —ce·tic (·tick), ce·tin·ic (se·tin′ick) *adj.*

ce·tyl (see′til, see′il) *n.* The univalent radical $C_{16}H_{33}$, compounds of which occur in beeswax, spermaceti, and other waxes. Syn. *hexadecyl.*

cetyl alcohol. Hexadecanol, $C_{16}H_{33}OH$; white, waxy crystals, insoluble in water. Used as an ingredient of washable ointment bases.

ce·tyl·pyr·i·din·i·um chloride (see″til·pirr″i·din′ee·um). A quaternary ammonium compound, $C_{21}H_{40}ClNO$; used as a topical antiseptic and detergent.

cev·a·dine (sev′uh·deen) *n.* An alkaloid, $C_{32}H_{49}NO_9$, from the sabadilla seed and veratrum viride. Syn. *veratrine.*

ce·vi·tam·ic acid (sev′i·tam′ick, see′vi·). ASCORBIC ACID.

CF lead. *In electrocardiography,* a precordial exploring electrode paired with an indifferent electrode on the left leg.

CGD Abbreviation for *chronic granulomatous disease.*

CGS Abbreviation for centimeter-gram-second, a system of measurement based on the centimeter as the unit of length, the gram as the unit of mass, and the second as the unit of time.

Chad·dock's reflex or sign 1. A great-toe reflex elicited by scratching the skin around the lateral malleolus, seen in pyramidal tract lesions. 2. Flexion of the wrist and extension and fanning of the fingers caused by irritation of the ulnar aspect of the lower forearm in hemiplegia.

chafe, *v.* To irritate the skin, usually by friction.

Chagas' disease A disease caused by the hemoflagellate *Trypanosoma cruzi,* transmitted by various bugs of the family Reduviidae. It occurs in the Western Hemisphere, especially in South and Central America, and affects mainly children and young adults. The acute disease is characterized by fever, edema, exanthemas, lymphadenopathy, and occasionally meningoencephalitis; chronic manifestations are cardiomyopathy with heart failure and arrhythmia, megaesophagus, and megacolon. Syn. *American trypanosomiasis.*

chain reaction. 1. *In chemistry,* a reaction that once initiated propagates itself by interactions of the reactants with active intermediate products such as atoms or free radicals. 2. *In nuclear science,* a reaction that stimulates its own repetition, as when a fissionable nucleus absorbs a neutron and fissions, releasing more than one additional neutron; the neutrons in turn can be absorbed by other fissionable nuclei, releasing more neutrons.

chain reflex. A series of consecutive reflexes, each of which is initiated by the preceding one, resulting in an integrated action.

chain-stitch suture. A suture made with the sewing machine stitch.

cha·la·sia (ka·lay′zee·uh) *n.* 1. Relaxation of a sphincter, as of the cardiac sphincter of the esophagus. 2. Specifically, a condition of unknown cause, frequently occurring in infants, rarely in adults, characterized by regurgitation immediately after feeding when supine. Barium examination reveals free reflux from the stomach into the esophagus with absence or decrease in esophageal peristalsis. It may be associated with esophagitis and hiatus hernia.

cha·la·zi·on (ka·lay′zee·on, kay·lay′) *n.*, pl. chalazia (·zee·uh) A chronic granulomatous inflammation of the eyelid occurring as the result of blockage of a tarsal gland.

chalc-, chalco- A combining form meaning (a) *copper;* (b) *brass.*

chal·co·sis (kal·ko'sis) *n.* A deposit of copper particles in the lungs or in other tissues.

chal·i·co·sis (kal''i·ko'sis) *n.*, pl. **chalico·ses** (·seez) A pneumoconiosis common among stonecutters, caused by inhalation of dust.

chalk (chawk) *n.* CaCO₃. An impure, native form of calcium carbonate. —**chalky** (chaw' kee) *adj.*

chalk·stone, *n.* A gouty deposit of sodium urate in the hands or feet; TOPHUS.

chal·lenge, *n. & v.* 1. The administration of a substance for the purpose of evoking and assessing the response; specifically, the administration of an antigen for the purpose of evoking an immune response, usually a secondary response. 2. To administer such an antigen or other substance.

cha·lone (kay'lone, kal'ohn) *n.* Any of various tissue-specific substances of uncertain composition, present in various tissues, that inhibit mitosis and may be a factor in maintaining balance between cell production and cell loss in tissues.

cha·lyb·e·ate (ka·lib'ee·it) *adj. & n.* 1. Containing iron; having the color or taste of iron. 2. A medicinal preparation containing iron.

cham·ber (chaim'bur) *n.* 1. *In anatomy,* a small cavity or space, as of an eye or the heart. 2. An apparatus in which material to be investigated is enclosed.

chame-, chamae- A combining form meaning *low.*

cham·fer (cham'fur) *n.* A form of gingival marginal finish given to the preparation of a tooth for a crown restoration; it is a shallow curve from an axial wall to the cavosurface; a cove-like margination.

chan·cre (shank'ur) *n.* A lesion, usually an ulcer, formed at the site of primary inoculation; generally, the initial lesion of syphilis or chancroid, or of such diseases as sporotrichosis and tularemia.

chan·croid (shank'roid) *n.* An acute localized venereal disease caused by *Haemophilus ducreyi,* characterized by ulceration at the site of inoculation and by painful enlargement and suppuration of regional lymph nodes. —**chancroi·dal** (shang·kroy'dul) *adj.*

chapped, *adj.* Designating areas of skin cracked, roughened, and sometimes reddened by exposure to cold. —**chap,** *v.*

char·ac·ter, *n. In biology,* any structural or functional property of an organism.

character disorder. A pattern of behavior and emotional response, such as acting out, that is socially disapproved or unacceptable with little evidence of anxiety or other symptoms seen in neuroses.

character neurosis. Disturbed behavioral patterns and emotional responses similar to those seen in a character disorder, except that the neurotic conflicts are expressed in socially acceptable though exaggerated ways not easily recognized as symptoms.

char·ac·ter·ol·o·gy (kār''uck·tur·ol'uh·jee) *n.* The study and defining of personality based on such physical attributes as the shape and color of body parts and the distribution of fat.

char·coal, *n.* The residue, largely amorphous carbon, obtained by incomplete combustion (destructive distillation) of animal or vegetable matter.

Charcot-Leyden crystals Colorless, pointed, often needlelike crystals occurring in the sputum in bronchial asthma and in the feces in amebic colitis and other ulcerative diseases of the colon.

Charcot-Marie-Tooth disease PERONEAL MUSCULAR ATROPHY.

Charcot's disease 1. CHARCOT'S JOINT. 2. PERONEAL MUSCULAR ATROPHY. 3. AMYOTROPHIC LATERAL SCLEROSIS.

Charcot's joint A neuropathic arthropathy in which articular cartilage and subjacent bone degenerate while hypertrophic changes occur at the joint edges and present an irregular deformity with instability of the joint. Most commonly seen in diabetic polyneuritis, syringomyelia, and tabes dorsalis.

Charcot triad Nystagmus, intention tremor, and staccato speech, occurring in multiple sclerosis due to brainstem involvement.

char·la·tan (shahr'luh·tun) *n.* 1. One who claims to have more knowledge or skill than he really has. 2. *In medicine,* a quack. —**charlatan·ism** (·iz·um) *n.*

char·ley horse. A contused or severely strained muscle, particularly the quadriceps, in athletes.

char·ta (kahr'tuh) *n.,* pl. **char·tae** (·tee) 1. A strip of paper impregnated, or coated, with a medicinal substance, applied externally. 2. A paper, suitably folded, containing a single dose or portion of medicinal powder to be used internally or externally.

char·tu·la (kahr'tew·luh) *n.,* pl. **chartu·lae** (·lee) A small paper, suitably folded, containing a single dose of a medicinal powder.

Chauf·fard-Min·kow·ski syndrome (sho·fahr'·ming·kohf'skee) HEREDITARY SPHEROCYTOSIS

chaul·moo·gra oil (chol·moo'gruh) A yellow oil expressed from the seeds of *Taraktogenos kurzii, Hydnocarpus wightiana* or *H. anthelmintica,* trees of Burma and India. It contains chaulmoogric, gynocardic, and hydnocarpic acids; used in the treatment of leprosy.

CHD Congenital heart disease; coronary heart disease.

check bite. A plastic impression of the teeth serving as a guide for alignment in an articulator; used in orthodontics and dental prosthetics. It consists of bites taken in hard wax or soft modeling compound, which record centric, eccentric, and protrusive occlusion.

check·up, *n.* A medical examination; may be general physical examination or involve specific organ or system, such as vision, hearing, or the cardiovascular system.

cheek, *n.* The side of the face; composed of skin, mucous membrane, and the fat, connective tissue, and muscles intervening.

cheek·bone, *n.* ZYGOMATIC BONE.

cheesy (cheez'ee) *adj.* Of the nature of cheese; CASEOUS.

cheil-, cheilo- A combining form meaning *lip.*

chei·lal·gia (kigh·lal'juh, ·jee·uh) *n.* Pain in the lips.

chei·lec·to·my (kigh·leck'tuh·mee) *n.* Excision of a portion of the lip.

cheil·ec·tro·pi·on (kyle''eck·tro'pee·on) *n.* Eversion of the lips.

chei·li·tis, chi·li·tis (kigh·lye'tis) *n.* Inflammation of the lips.

cheilitis ac·tin·i·ca (ack·tin'i·kuh). A form of cheilitis in which the lips are irritated by sunlight; usually seen in persons whose skin is sensitive to light.

cheilitis ex·fo·li·a·ti·va (ecks·fo''lee·uh·tye'vuh). Persistent peeling of the lips.

cheilitis ven·e·na·ta (ven''e·nay'tuh). Contact dermatitis of the lips, often caused by sensitization to allergens in lipsticks, toothpastes, or woodwind instruments.

chei·lo·gnatho·pal·a·tos·chi·sis (kigh''lo·nath''o·pal·uh·tos'ki·sis) *n.* Unilateral or bilateral cleft of the upper lip, alveolar process, and palate.

chei·lo·gnatho·pros·o·pos·chi·sis (kigh''lo·nath''o·pros·o·pos'ki·sis) *n.* Oblique facial cleft involving also the upper lip and upper jaw.

chei·lo·gnatho·ura·nos·chi·sis (kigh''lo·nath''o·yoor''uh·nos'ki·sis) *n.* A cleft which involves the upper lip, alveolar process, and palate.

chei·lo·plas·ty (kigh'lo·plas''tee) *n.* Any plastic operation upon the lip.

chei·lor·rha·phy (kigh·lor'uh·fee) *n.* Suture of a cut or lacerated lip.

chei·los·chi·sis (kigh·los'ki·sis) *n.,* pl. **cheiloschi·ses** (·seez) HARELIP.

chei·lo·sis (kigh·lo'sis) *n.,* pl. **cheilo·ses** (·seez) A disorder of the lips often due to a deficiency of riboflavin, characterized by fissures, especially at the angles of the lips.

chei·lo·sto·ma·to·plas·ty (kigh''lo·sto'ma·to·plas''tee) *n.* Plastic repair of the lips and mouth.

chei·lot·o·my (kigh·lot'uh·mee) *n.* Excision of a part of the lip.

chei·ma·pho·bia (kigh''muh·fo'bee·uh) *n.* Abnormal fear of cold or winter.

cheir-, cheiro- A combining form meaning *hand.*

chei·rag·ra, chi·rag·ra (kigh·rag'ruh) *n.* 1. Gout of the hand associated with twisting and deformity of the fingers. 2. Any painful condition of the hand.

chei·ral·gia, chi·ral·gia (kigh·ral'juh, ·jee·uh) *n.* Pain in the hand.

chei·rol·o·gy, chi·rol·o·gy (kigh·rol'uh·jee) *n.* 1. A method of communicating with deafmutes by means of the hands. 2. The study of the hand.

chei·ro·meg·a·ly, chi·ro·meg·a·ly (kigh''ro·meg'uh·lee) *n.* Enlargement of one or both hands, not due to disease of the hypophysis.

chei·ro·plas·ty, chi·ro·plas·ty (kigh'ro·plas''tee) *n.* Plastic operation on the hand.

chei·ro·pom·pho·lyx (kigh''ro·pom'fo·licks) *n.* An ill-defined, inflammatory, pruritic skin disease confined to the hands and feet, characterized by vesicles or blebs on the palms and sides of the fingers.

che·late (kee'late) *adj., n.,* & *v.* 1. Having the ring-type structure formed in chelation. 2. A compound formed by chelation. 3. To bind (a metal ion) with a chelating agent. —**che·lat·ed,** *adj.*

che·lat·ing agent. Any compound, usually organic, having two or more points of attachment at which an atom of a metal may be joined or coordinated in such a manner as to form a ring-type structure.

che·la·tion (ke·lay'shun) *n.* 1. A type of interaction between an organic compound (having two or more points at which it may coordinate with a metal) and the metal so as to form a ring-type structure. 2. A type of interaction, shown by organic compounds having both a carbonyl (CO) group and a hydroxyl (OH) group, in which by hydrogen bond formation involving generally two such molecules, but sometimes only one, a ring-type structure is produced.

chem-, chemi-, chemico-, chemio-, chemo- A combining form meaning *chemical, chemistry.*

chem·i·cal (kem'i·kul) *adj.* & *n.* 1. Of or pertaining to chemistry. 2. A substance of determinate chemical composition, especially such as may be produced or used in laboratory or industrial processes.

chemical action. The molecular change produced in any substance through the action of heat, light, electricity, or another chemical.

chemical antidote. An antidote that converts a poison to an insoluble compound or to some other harmless derivative.

chemical meningitis. Aseptic meningitis, usually resulting from subarachnoid injection of foreign materials such as gases or chemical compounds.

chemical peritonitis. Inflammation of the peritoneum due primarily to the irritating effects of a variety of chemical substances, either introduced from without or present as a result of disease or trauma. It occurs in both acute and chronic forms.

chemical reflex. A reflex initiated by hormones or other chemical substances in the blood. Syn. *humoral reflex.*

chemical warfare. The use in war of toxic gases, incendiary mixtures, and other chemicals, for defensive or offensive purposes.

chemical warfare agent. Any agent used in chemical warfare, especially toxic gas.

chemico-. See *chem-.*

chem·i·co·cau·tery (kem''i·ko·kaw'tur·ee) *n.* Cauterization by means of chemical agents.

chemi·lu·mi·nes·cence (kem''i·lew·mi·nes'unce) *n.* Light produced by means of a chemical reaction and entirely independent of any heat involved. Syn. *cold light.*

chem·ist (kem'ist) *n.* A person skilled in chemistry.

chem·is·try (kem'is·tree) *n.* The science of the structure of matter and the composition of substances, their properties, transformation, analysis, synthesis, and manufacture.

che·mo·co·ag·u·la·tion (kee''mo·ko·ag''yoo·lay'shun, kem''o·) *n.* The precipitation of proteins or colloids in a jellylike, soft mass by means of chemical agents.

che·mo·dec·to·ma (kee''mo·deck·to'muh, kem''o·) *n.,* pl. **chemodectomas, chemodectoma·ta** (·tuh) Any tumor whose parenchymal cells resemble those of chemoreceptor organs, such as the carotid body, and form cell balls.

che·mo·nu·cle·ol·y·sis (kee''mo·new''klee·ol'i·sis,

kem″o·) n. The dissolution of extruded nucleus pulposus by injection of a proteolytic enzyme, such as chymopapain.

che·mo·pal·li·dec·to·my (kee″mo·pal″i·deck′tuh·mee, kem″o·) n. The destruction of the globus pallidus by a chemical substance, usually ethyl alcohol, in the treatment of movement disorders.

che·mo·pro·phy·lax·is (kee″mo·pro″fi·lack′sis, kem″o·) n., pl. **chemoprophylax·es** (·seez) Prevention of disease by the administration of a chemotherapeutic agent.

che·mo·re·cep·tor (kee″mo·re·sep′tur, kem″o·) n. 1. One of the side chains or receptors of molecules in a living cell, presumed to have the power of fixing chemical substances in the same way that bacterial toxins are fixed. 2. A sensory end organ capable of reacting to a chemical stimulus.

che·mo·sis (ke·mo′sis) n., pl. **chemo·ses** (·seez) Swelling of the conjunctiva. —**che·mot·ic** (·mot′ick) adj.

che·mo·sur·gery (kee″mo·sur′jur·ee, kem″o·) n. 1. Removal of diseased or unwanted tissue by the application of chemicals. 2. The fixation in situ of malignant, gangrenous, infected, or other tissue by chemical means to facilitate the use of frozen sections in maintaining microscopic control over the extent of an excision.

che·mo·syn·the·sis (kee″mo·sin′thuh·sis, kem″o·) n. Chemical synthesis utilizing energy supplied by the reacting substances, as opposed to photosynthesis, in which radiant energy is utilized. —**chemo·syn·thet·ic** (·sin·thet′ick) adj.

che·mo·tax·is (kee″mo·tack′sis, kem″o·) n., pl. **chemotax·es** (·seez) 1. The response of organisms to chemical stimuli; attraction toward a substance is positive and repulsion is negative chemotaxis. 2. CHEMOTROPISM. —**chemo·tac·tic** (·tack′tick) adj.

che·mo·thal·a·mot·o·my (kee″mo·thal″uh·mot′uh·mee, kem″o·) n. The destruction of a portion of the thalamus, usually the ventral nucleus, by a chemical substance such as ethyl alcohol, in the treatment of movement disorders.

che·mo·ther·a·peu·tic (kee″mo·therr″uh·pew′tick, kem″o·) adj. Of or pertaining to chemotherapy.

chemotherapeutic index. The relationship existing between the toxicity of a compound for the body and the toxicity for parasites. Kolmer represents it as follows:

$$C.I. = \frac{\text{maximal tolerated dose per kg body wt}}{\text{minimal curative dose per kg body wt}}$$

che·mo·ther·a·py (kee″mo·therr′uh·pee, kem″o·) n. Prevention or treatment of disease by chemical agents.

che·mot·ro·pism (ke·mot′ro·piz·um) n. 1. Attraction of cells by chemical substances. 2. In immunology, the positive attraction of phagocytes to microorganisms, cellular debris, and areas of inflammation.

Che·no·po·di·um (kee″no·po′dee·um) n. A genus of herbs of the family Chenopodiaceae.

che·ro·pho·bia (kerr″o·fo′bee·uh, keer″o·) n. A morbid fear of gaiety or happiness.

cher·ry, n. The fruit of any of a number of species of the genus Prunus, trees having typical globose drupes; family, Rosaceae.

Cher·ry and Cran·dall's test. A test for lipase in which pancreatic lipase in serum is allowed to act on a substrate of olive oil, lipase then being determined by the amount of fatty acid liberated.

cherry-red spot. A bright red area seen in the macular region in such conditions as the infantile and juvenile forms of amaurotic familial idiocy, Niemann-Pick disease, and Gaucher's disease, as a result of the accumulation of metabolic products within the ganglion cells; the foveola is free of ganglion cells thus allowing visualization of the redness of the choroid.

cher·ub·ism (cherr′ub·iz·um, cherr′yoo·biz·um) n. The characteristic facies of familial multilocular cystic disease or familial fibrous swelling of the jaws, marked by protuberance of the cheeks and jaws with upturned eyes.

chest, n. The front of the thorax.

Cheyne-Stokes respiration (chain) Periodic breathing characterized by intervals of hyperpnea which alternate with intervals of apnea; rhythmic waxing and waning of respiration; occurs most commonly in older patients with heart failure and cerebrovascular disease.

CHF Abbreviation for congestive heart failure.

Chia·ri-From·mel syndrome or **disease** (kyah′ree) Postpartum galactorrhea with low levels of urinary gonadotropin associated with pituitary adenoma, with or without acromegaly.

Chiari's network Fine fibers stretching across the right atrium, and attaching to the openings of the vena cava and coronary sinus, and the crista terminalis.

Chiari's syndrome 1. ARNOLD-CHIARI SYNDROME. 2. BUDD-CHIARI SYNDROME. 3. CHIARI-FROMMEL SYNDROME.

chi·asm (kigh′az·um) n. CHIASMA.

chi·as·ma (kigh·az′muh) n., pl. **chiasma·ta** (·tuh). **chiasmas** (kigh·az′muh) n., pl. **chiasma·ta** (·tuh). 1. OPTIC CHIASMA. 2. In genetics, the crossing of two chromatids in meiotic prophase, thought to be a physical manifestation of genetic crossing-over. —**chias·mal** (·mul) adj.

chiasma syndrome or **chiasmal syndrome.** A group of symptoms due to a lesion in the optic chiasma and marked by impaired vision, headache, vertigo, and limitation of the visual field.

chi·as·mat·ic (kigh″az·mat′ick) adj. Pertaining to or resembling a chiasma.

chicken-fat clot. A blood clot formed after death consisting of a light-yellow upper portion and an accumulation of erythrocytes in its dependent portion.

chick·en·pox, n. An acute, contagious disease principally of childhood, caused by the varicella virus, characterized by a superficial eruption of macular transparent vesicles which appear in successive crops on different parts of the body.

chief cell. 1. The predominant, slightly basophilic pyramidal, granular cell of the gastric glands in the fundic region of the stomach. Zymogen granules, consisting of pepsinogen, are present. Occasionally, these cells are present in the cardiac portion of the stomach. Syn. *adelomorphous cell, central cell, peptic cell.* 2. CHROMOPHOBE CELL. 3. The principal cell of the parathyroid gland, often divided into dark chief cells and light chief cells.

chig·ger (chig'ur) *n.* A larval mite of the genus *Trombicula* or *Eutrombicula;* the attachment of the common chigger to the skin causes severe inflammatory lesions in warm-blooded animals, including man.

chig·oe, chig·o (chig'o) *n.* A flea of the species *Tunga penetrans.*

chi·kun·gu·nya (chick''ōōng·gōōn'yuh) *n.* A dengue-like disease caused by a group A togavirus, characterized especially by high fever, headache, rigor, and severe arthralgia.

Chi·lai·di·ti's syndrome. The presence in an x-ray film of interposed bowel loops between the liver and diaphragm when the patient is upright. There are usually no clinical signs or symptoms, but the condition has sometimes been associated with abdominal pain, distention, and nocturnal vomiting, with absent liver dullness or liver mass in the midabdomen or in the right lower quadrant.

chil·blain, *n.* Hyperemia and swelling of the skin, due to cold, and followed by severe itching or burning; vesicles and bullae may form, and these may lead to ulceration.

child, *n.* 1. An individual who has not reached the age of puberty. 2. An individual between the toddling stage and adolescence.

child abuse. Treatment of a child by a parent or guardian characterized by intentional acts that result in physical injury, toleration of conditions that injure the child or threaten the child's health, or illegal sexual acts upon the child. Legal definitions vary from state to state.

child-abuse syndrome. BATTERED-CHILD SYNDROME.

child·bed, *n.* The condition of a woman in labor; PARTURITION.

childbed fever. PUERPERAL FEVER.

child·birth, *n.* Giving birth to a child; human parturition.

child health associate. A physician's assistant with a baccalaureate degree specializing in pediatrics.

childhood type of schizophrenia. A condition characterized by schizophrenic or schizophrenic-like symptoms, occurring before puberty, which may vary from the more differentiated forms because of the immaturity of the patient. It may be manifested by grossly immature behavior, failure to develop a separate identity from the mother, marked withdrawal, and introspection, and may include infantile autism.

chill, *n.* 1. A sensation of cold accompanied by involuntary shivering or shaking and skin pallor. 2. A respiratory illness due to exposure to cold or damp.

chilo-. See *cheil-.*

Chi·lo·mas·tix (kigh''lo·mas'ticks) *n.* A genus of flagellates parasitic in man and other animals.

Chilomastix mes·nili (mes·nil'eye). The species of *Chilomastix* found in the intestine of man.

chi·me·ra, chi·mae·ra (kigh·meer'uh, ki·meer' uh) *n.* 1. A plant composed of two genetically distinct types of tissue resulting from somatic mutation, segregation, or from artificial fusion, as in graft hybrids; mosaic. 2. A compound embryo produced by grafting approximately equal halves of two embryos, usually of different species or strains. 3. An animal rendered immunologically tolerant to tissue of another species by prior viable cell transplants from that species. 4. *In genetics,* an individual whose tissues are composed of two genetically different cell lines derived from different zygotes, as, for example, is usually found for the blood cells of dizygotic cattle twins.

chi·mer·ism (ki·meer'iz·um, kigh'mur·iz·um) *n.* The presence of two distinct cell types in a given individual, each of which is derived from a different zygote.

chin-, chino- A combining form meaning *quinine.*

chin, *n.* The lower part of the face, at or near the symphysis of the lower jaw. Comb. form *geni(o)-, mento-.*

Chinacrin. A trademark for quinacrine, an antimalarial used as the hydrochloride salt.

Chinese restaurant syndrome. Sensation of burning, pressure about the face and chest, and often headache, produced in susceptible individuals by the ingestion of monosodium L-glutamate, often used in Chinese and other food to enhance flavors.

chi·ni·o·fon (ki·nigh'o·fon, kin'ee·o·fon) *n.* A mixture of 7-iodo-8-hydroxyquinoline-5-sulfonic acid, its sodium salt, and sodium bicarbonate; a canary yellow powder, soluble in water. Formerly used as an amebicide in the treatment of dysentery.

Chinosol. A trademark for the bactericide 8-hydroxyquinoline sulfate (oxyquinoline sulfate).

chi·on·ablep·sia (kye''on·a·blep'see·uh) *n.* SNOW BLINDNESS.

chip fracture. A minor fracture involving a bony process.

chir-, chiro-. See *cheir-. cheiro-.*

chi·ral (kigh'rul) *adj.* Being right- or left-handed; said of an asymmetrical molecule or crystal. **—chi·ral·i·ty** (kigh·ral'i·tee) *n.*

chi·rap·sia (kigh·rap'see·uh) *n.* Friction with the hand; MASSAGE.

chi·ris·mus (kigh·riz'mus) *n.* 1. Spasm of the hand. 2. A form of massage.

chi·rop·o·dist (kigh·rop'o·dist, ki·rop') *n.* PODIATRIST.

chi·rop·o·dy (kigh·rop'o·dee, ki·rop') *n.* PODIATRY.

chi·ro·prac·tic (kigh''ro·prack'tick) *n.* A system of therapeutics based upon the theory that disease is caused by abnormal function of the nervous system; attempts to restore normal function are made through manipulation and treatment of the structures of the body, especially those of the spinal column. **—chi·ro·prac·tor** (kigh''ro·prack'tur) *n.*

chi·ro·prac·tor (kigh'ro·prack"tur) n. A practitioner of chiropractic.

chi-square test. A test used to determine whether an observed series of frequencies differ between themselves, or from a series of frequencies expected according to some hypothesis, to a greater degree than may be expected to occur by chance.

chi·tin (kigh'tin) n. The structural material of skeletons of arthropods, with few exceptions occurring only in invertebrates. It is a condensation product of acetylglucosamine molecules, as cellulose is a condensation product of glucose molecules. —**chitin·ous** (·us) adj.

Chla·myd·ia (kla·mid'ee·uh) n. A genus of gram-negative bacteria (family Chlamydiaceae), readily filtrable, obligate intracellular parasites which are the causative agents of the psittacosis-lymphogranuloma-trachoma group of infections. Formerly called Bedsonia. —**chlamydia**, pl. **chlamyd·i·ae** (·ee·ee), com. n.; **chlamyd·i·al** (·ee·ul) adj.

Chla·myd·i·a·ce·ae (kla·mid"ee·ay'see·ee) n. pl. A family of obligate intracellular parasites, intermediate between true viruses and the rickettsiae and gram-negative bacteria, which includes the single genus Chlamydia. Formerly called Chlamydozoaceae.

Chlamydia psit·ta·ci (sit'uh·sigh). The species of Chlamydia which causes psittacosis in man and many clinical and subclinical diseases in other animals and in birds. Formerly called Chlamydozoon psittaci, Miyagawanella psittaci.

Chlamydia tra·cho·ma·tis (tra·ko'muh·tis). The species of Chlamydia that includes the causative agents of trachoma, inclusion conjunctivitis, lymphogranuloma venereum, and a large proportion of nongonococcal urethritis in man, and pneumonitis in laboratory mice.

chlo·as·ma (klo·az'muh) n., pl. **chloasma·ta** (·tuh) 1. Patchy hyperpigmentation located chiefly on the forehead, temples, cheeks, nipples, and median line of the abdomen. The condition may become marked during pregnancy, menstruation, functional derangements of the uterus, or in ovarian disorders and tumors. 2. Obsol. Patchy tan-brown-black hyperpigmentation, especially on the brow and cheeks; of unknown cause, but may be due to the action of sunshine upon perfume or to endocrinopathy.

chloasma ute·ri·num (yoo'te·rye'num). CHLOASMA (1).

chlor-, chloro- A combining form meaning (a) green, pale green; (b) chlorine; (c) in chemistry, having chlorine as a substitute for hydrogen.

chlor·ac·ne (klor·ack'nee) n. An acneform eruption caused by chlorinated hydrocarbons.

chlo·ral (klo'ral, klor'ul) n. 1. Trichloroacetaldehyde, CCl_3CHO, a colorless, caustic liquid of pungent odor. 2. CHLORAL HYDRATE.

chlo·ral·am·ide (klor"ul·am'ide, ·id) n. CHLORAL-FORMAMIDE.

chlo·ral·form·am·ide (klor"ul·form·am'ide, ·id, ·form'uh·mide, ·mid) n. A crystalline solid, $C_3H_4Cl_3NO_2$; has been used as a hypnotic.

chloral hydrate. 2,2,2-Trichloro-1,1-ethanediol, $CCl_3CH(OH)_2$, colorless or white crystals which are very soluble in water; used as a rapid somnifacient, an anticonvulsant, and as an ingredient of anodyne liniments.

chlor·am·bu·cil (klor·am'bew·sil) n. 4-{ p-[Bis(2-chloroethyl)amino]phenyl}butyric acid, $C_{14}H_{19}Cl_2NO_2$, a nitrogen mustard derivative used as an antineoplastic drug.

chloramine-T. Sodium p-toluenesulfonchloramide, $CH_3C_6H_4SO_2N(Na)Cl.3H_2O$. A white or faintly yellow crystalline powder, unstable in air; a topical antiseptic.

chlor·am·phen·i·col (klor"am·fen'i·kol) n. D(−)-threo-2,2-Dichloro-N-[β-hydroxy-α-(hydroxymethyl)-p-nitrophenethyl] acetamide, $C_{11}H_{12}Cl_2N_2O_5$, an antibiotic substance produced by Streptomyces venezuelae Burkholder, and also synthetically. It is effective against a variety of gram-positive and gram-negative organisms, such as Mycoplasma and Rickettsia; it may produce serious blood dyscrasias.

chlor·ane·mia, chlor·anae·mia (klor"uh·nee'mee·uh) n. CHLOROSIS (1).

chlo·rate (klo'rate, klor'ate) n. A salt of chloric acid; the radical ClO_3^-.

Chlorazene. A trademark for the antiseptic substance chloramine-T.

chlor·bu·ta·nol (klor·bew'tuh·nol) n. CHLOROBUTANOL.

chlor·cy·cli·zine (klor·sigh'kli·zeen) n. 1-(p-Chloro-α-phenylbenzyl)-4-methylpiperazine, $C_{18}H_{21}ClN_2$, an antihistaminic agent; used as the hydrochloride salt.

chlor·dane (klor'dane) n. 1,2,4,5,6,7,8,8-Octachloro-2,3,3a,4,7,7a-hexahydro-4,7-methanoindene, $C_{10}H_6Cl_8$, an insecticide.

chlor·di·az·ep·ox·ide (klor"dye·az·ep·ock'side) n. 7-Chloro-2-(methylamino)-5-phenyl-3H-1,4-benzodiazepine 4-oxide, $C_{16}H_{14}ClN_3O$, a tranquilizer; used as the hydrochloride salt.

chlor·e·mia, chlor·ae·mia (klor·ee'mee·uh) n. 1. CHLOROSIS (1). 2. An excess of chlorides in the blood.

Chloretone. A trademark for chlorobutanol, an antibacterial preservative.

chlor·hy·dria (klor·high'dree·uh) n. The presence of hydrochloric acid in the stomach.

Chlorhydrol. A trademark for aluminum chlorhydroxide, an antiperspirant.

chlo·ride (klo'ride, klor'ide) n. A salt of hydrochloric acid; a binary compound containing Cl^-.

chloride shift. The reversible exchange of chloride and bicarbonate ions between erythrocytes and plasma to effect transport of carbon dioxide and maintain ionic equilibrium during respiration.

chlo·rid·uria (klo"ri·dew'ree·uh) n. An excess of chlorides in the urine.

chlo·ri·nate (klo'ri·nate, klor'i·) v. 1. To treat or combine with chlorine, as for disinfecting sewage or drinking water. 2. To introduce chlorine atoms into (molecules of a compound). —**chlo·ri·nat·ed** (klo'ri·nay·tid) adj. **chlo·ri·na·tion** (·nay'shun) n.

chlo·rine (klo'reen, ·rin, klor'een) n. Cl = 35.453. A greenish yellow gas of suffocating odor and very irritant. A powerful germicide in the presence of moisture with which it forms hypochlorous and hydrochloric acids, the former decomposing with the liberation of nascent oxygen. It has been used by inhalation in the treatment of acute coryza.

chlor·i·son·da·mine chloride (klor″i·son′duh·meen). 4,5,6,7-Tetrachloro-2-(2-dimethylaminoethyl)isoindoline dimethylchloride, $C_{14}H_{20}Cl_6N_2$, a ganglionic blocking agent used for management of hypertension.

chlo·rite (klo′rite, klor′ite) n. A salt containing the radical ClO_2^-, derived from chlorous acid.

chlor·mer·o·drin (klor·merr′o·drin) n. 3-(Chloromercuri)-2-methoxypropylurea, $C_5H_{11}ClHgN_2O_2$, an orally effective mercurial diuretic.

chlormerodrin Hg 197. Chlormerodrin in which the mercury atom has been replaced by radioactive Hg-197, used as a diagnostic aid in renal function determination.

chlormerodrin Hg 203. Chlormerodrin in which the mercury atom has been replaced by radioactive Hg-203, used as a diagnostic aid in renal function determination.

chlo·ro·bu·ta·nol (klor″o·bew′ta·nol) n. 1,1,1-Trichloro-2-methyl-2-propanol, $C_4H_7Cl_3O$, white crystals, slightly soluble in water. Formerly used as a sedative and hypnotic, and externally as a local anesthetic and antiseptic. Now used as an antibacterial preservative in various solutions. Syn. *chlorbutol, acetone-chloroform.*

chlo·ro·cre·sol (klor″o·kree′sol) n. Parachlorometacresol, C_7H_7ClO, colorless crystals, slightly soluble in water; used for the sterilization and preservation of injections and, to some extent, as a surgical antiseptic.

chlo·ro·form (klor′uh·form) n. Trichloromethane, $CHCl_3$, heavy, colorless liquid having a characteristic ethereal odor. The commercial article contains up to 2% by volume of alcohol. It is used as an organic solvent and, medicinally, as an anesthetic, anodyne, and antispasmodic. Externally it is irritant. —**chlo·ro·form·ic** (klor″uh·form′ick) adj.

chlo·ro·form·ism (klor′uh·form·iz·um) n. 1. Habitual use of chloroform for its narcotic effect. 2. Symptoms produced by this use of the drug.

chlo·ro·form·i·za·tion (klor″uh·for·mi·zay′shun) n. 1. The act of administering chloroform as an anesthetic. 2. The anesthetic effect from the inhalation of chloroform.

chlo·ro·gua·nide (klor″o·gwah′nide) n. 1-(p-Chlorophenyl)-5-isopropylbiguanide, $C_{11}H_{16}ClN_5$, an antimalarial drug; used as the hydrochloride salt. Syn. *proguanil.*

chlo·ro·leu·ke·mia (klor″o·lew·kee′mee·uh) n. Obsol. GRANULOCYTIC SARCOMA.

chlo·ro·ma (klo·ro′muh) n., pl. **chloromas, chloroma·ta** (-tuh) GRANULOCYTIC SARCOMA.

Chloromycetin. Trademark for the antibiotic substance chloramphenicol.

chlo·ro·per·cha (klor″o·pur′chuh) n. Solution of gutta-percha in chloroform; used in dentistry for nonconducting cavity linings, pulp cappings, and for filling the roots of pulpless teeth.

chlo·ro·phe·nol (klor″o·fee′nol) n. Monochlorophenol, HOC_6H_4Cl. The o- variety is a colorless liquid; the m- and p-isomers are crystalline. p-Chlorophenol is used as a topical antiseptic.

chlo·ro·phen·o·thane (klor″o·fen′o·thane) n. 1,1,1-Trichloro-2,2-bis(p-chlorophenyl)ethane, $C_{14}H_9Cl_5$, white powder or crystals, insoluble in water; an insecticide. Used medicinally as a pediculicide. Commonly known as DDT. Syn. *dicophane.*

chlo·ro·phyll, chlo·ro·phyl (klor′uh·fil) n. The green coloring matter responsible for photosynthesis in plants. It consists of chlorophyll a, $C_{55}H_{72}MgN_4O_5$, and chlorophyll b, $C_{55}H_{70}MgN_4O_6$. Used as a coloring agent and, medicinally, in the treatment of various lesions, and as a deodorant.

chlo·ro·phyl·lase (klor″o·fil′ace, ·aze) n. An enzyme that splits or hydrolyzes chlorophyll.

chlo·ro·plast (klor′o·plast) n. An organelle bearing the chlorophyll of plant cells.

chlo·rop·sia (klo·rop′see·uh) n. A defect of vision in which all objects appear green. It occurs occasionally in digitalis poisoning.

chlo·ro·pu·rine (klor″o·pew′reen, ·rin) n. 6-Chloropurine, $C_5H_3ClN_4$, the chlorine analogue of 6-aminopurine or adenine. It inhibits experimental sarcoma, possibly through ability to block a metabolic step in conversion of adenine to guanine.

chlo·ro·quine (klor′o·kween) n. 7-Chloro-4-(4-diethylamino-1-methylbutylamino)quinoline, $C_{18}H_{26}ClN_3$, principally an antimalarial and antiamebic; used as the diphosphate salt.

chlo·ro·sar·co·ma (klor″o·sahr·ko′muh) n. GRANULOCYTIC SARCOMA.

chlo·ro·sis (klo·ro′sis) n., pl. **chloro·ses** (-seez) 1. A form of hypochromic microcytic anemia, most common in young women, characterized by a marked reduction of hemoglobin in the blood, with but a slight diminution in number of red cells. 2. In zoology, green tissue pigmentation in frogs and other lower vertebrates due to accumulation of biliverdin.

chlo·ro·then (klo′ro·then) n. 2-[(5-Chloro-2-thenyl)(2-dimethylaminoethyl)amino]pyridine, $C_{14}H_{18}ClN_3S$, an antihistaminic drug; used as the citrate or hydrochloride salt.

chlo·ro·thi·a·zide (klor″o·thigh′uh·zide) n. 6-Chloro-2H-1,2,4-benzothiadiazine-7-sulfonamide 1,1-dioxide, $C_7H_6ClN_3O_4S_2$, an orally effective diuretic and antihypertensive drug. Also used intravenously as the sodium salt.

chlo·ro·thy·mol (klor″o·thigh′mol) n. Monochlorothymol, $C_{10}H_{13}ClO$, a white, crystalline powder, almost insoluble in water; used as a germicide.

chlo·rot·ic (klo·rot′ick) adj. Affected by or pertaining to chlorosis.

chlo·ro·vi·nyl·di·chlo·ro·ar·sine (klor″o·vye″nil·dye″klor·o·ahr′seen) n. $ClCH=CHAsCl_2$, Lewisite; a potent lacrimator, lung irritant, and vesicant, developed for use as a chemical warfare agent. It is systemically toxic because of its arsenic content.

chlo·ro·xy·le·nol (klor″o·zye′le·nole, ·nol) n. 2-Chloro-5-hydroxy-1,3-dimethylbenzene, C_8H_9ClO; a creamy-white, crystalline powder used as an antiseptic in ointment form or in oil solution.

chlor·phen·ir·amine (klor″fen·irr′a·meen) n. 2-

[*p*-Chloro-α-(2-dimethylaminoethyl)benzyl]
pyridine, $C_{16}H_{19}ClN_2$, an antihistaminic
drug; used as the maleate salt.

chlor·prom·a·zine (klor·prom'uh·zeen) *n.* 2-
Chloro-10-(3-dimethylaminopropyl)pheno-
thiazine, $C_{17}H_{19}ClN_2S$, an antipsychotic
agent with sedative and antiemetic effects;
used chiefly as the hydrochloride salt.

chlor·pro·thix·ene (klor''pro·thick'seen) *n.* 2-
Chloro-9-(3-dimethylaminopropylidene)thia-
xanthene, $C_{18}H_{18}ClNS$, an antipsychotic
agent with antiemetic activity.

chlor·quin·al·dol (klor''kwin·al'dol) *n.* 5,7-Di-
chloro-8-hydroxyquinaldine, $C_{10}H_7Cl_2NO$, a
topically applied keratoplastic, antibacterial,
and antifungal drug.

chlor·tet·ra·cy·cline (klor''tet·ruh·sigh'kleen) *n.*
An antibiotic substance, $C_{22}H_{23}ClN_2O_8$, bio-
synthesized by the actinomycete *Streptomyces
aureofaciens;* a yellow, crystalline powder. It is
a broad-spectrum antibiotic, acting against
many gram-positive and gram-negative bacteria and also against rickettsiae and certain
viruses. Used mainly as the hydrochloride
salt.

Chlor-Trimeton. Trademark for chlorpheni-
amine, an antihistaminic drug used as the
maleate salt.

cho·a·na (ko·ay'nuh, ko·ah'nuh) *n., pl.* **choa·nae**
(·nee) 1. A funnel-like opening. 2. Either of
the posterior nasal orifices. —**choa·nal** (·nul)
adj.

chocolate cyst. 1. Any cyst filled with degenerated blood. 2. The ovarian lesion characteristic of endometriosis.

choke, *v.* 1. To prevent access of air to the lungs
by compression or obstruction of the trachea
or larynx. 2. To suffer partial or complete
suffocation from mechanical obstruction by a
foreign body or external pressure, or from
laryngeal spasm caused by an irritating gas or
liquid.

choke·damp, *n.* BLACKDAMP.

choked disk. PAPILLEDEMA.

chokes, *n.* A clinical manifestation of decompression sickness caused by free gas bubbles
lodged in the pulmonary capillaries, and characterized by severe dyspnia, a nonproductive
paroxysmal cough, and deep substernal pain
precipitated by deep inspiration or by inhalation of tobacco smoke.

chol-, chola-, cholo- A combining form meaning
bile or *gall.*

cho·la·gog·ue, cho·la·gog (ko'luh·gog, kol'uh·) *n.*
Any agent that promotes the flow of bile.

cho·lane (ko'lane, kol'ane) *n.* A tetracyclic hydrocarbon, $C_{24}H_{42}$, which may be considered
as the parent substance of sterols, hormones,
bile acids, and digitalis aglycones.

chol·an·e·re·sis (ko·lan''e·ree'sis, ko''lan·err'e-
sis) *n.* An increase in the output or elimination
of cholic acid, its conjugates and their salts,
such as sodium taurocholate and sodium glycocholate.

cholangi-, cholango- A combining form meaning *bile duct, biliary passage.*

chol·an·gi·ec·ta·sis (ko·lan''jee·eck'tuh·sis) *n., pl.*
cholangiecta·ses (·seez) A dilatation of extrahepatic or intrahepatic biliary passages.

cholangio-. See *cholangi-.*

chol·an·gio·car·ci·no·ma (ko·lan''jee·o·kahr''si-
no'muh) *n.* Carcinoma of the bile ducts.

chol·an·gio·en·ter·os·to·my (ko·lan''jee·o·en''tur-
os'tuh·mee) *n. In surgery,* an anastomosis between a bile duct and the intestine.

chol·an·gio·gas·tros·to·my (ko·lan''jee·o·gas-
tros'tuh·mee) *n. In surgery,* the formation of an
anastomosis between a bile duct and the stomach.

chol·an·gio·gen·e·sis (ko·lan''jee·o·jen'e·sis) *n.*
Bile duct formation.

chol·an·gio·gram (ko·lan'jee·o·gram) *n.* The x-
ray film produced by means of cholangiography.

chol·an·gi·og·ra·phy (ko·lan''jee·og'ruh·fee) *n.*
Radiography of the bile ducts.

chol·an·gi·ole (ko·lan'jee·ole) *n.* A small intrahepatic bile duct.

chol·an·gio·lit·ic (ko·lan''jee·o·lit'ick) *adj.* Pertaining to inflammation of the bile ducts, especially the small branches.

cholangiolitic cirrhosis. Biliary cirrhosis in
which the smallest bile radicles are the principal seat of disease.

cholangiolitic hepatitis. CHOLESTATIC HEPATITIS.

chol·an·gi·o·li·tis (ko·lan''jee·o·lye'tis) *n., pl.* **cho-
langio·lit·i·des** (·lit'i·deez) Inflammation of the
bile ducts within the liver.

chol·an·gi·o·ma (ko·lan''jee·o'muh) *n., pl.* **cho-
langiomas, cholangioma·ta** (·tuh) CHOLANGIO-
CARCINOMA.

chol·an·gi·os·to·my (ko·lan''jee·os'tuh·mee) *n. In
surgery,* the drainage of any of the bile ducts by
means of abdominal incision and penetration
into the hepatic, cystic, or common bile duct.

chol·an·gi·ot·o·my (ko·lan''jee·ot'uh·mee) *n.* Incision into any of the bile ducts, usually for
removal of a calculus.

cholangitic cirrhosis. A form of biliary cirrhosis
involving the larger intrahepatic bile ducts,
accompanied by fibrosis and inflammation.

chol·an·gi·tis (kol''an·jye'tis, ko''lan·) *n., pl.* **chol-
an·git·i·des** Inflammation of the biliary ducts.
—**cholan·git·ic** (·jit'ick) *adj.*

cho·lan·ic acid (ko·lan'ick). The hydroxyl-free,
steroid parent substance, $C_{24}H_{40}O_2$, of the
unconjugated bile acids, the most important of
which are cholic acid (1) and deoxycholic
acid.

cho·late (ko'late) *n.* Any salt of cholic acid.

chole-. See *chol-.*

cho·le·bil·i·ru·bin (kol''e·bil''i·roo'bin, ko''le·) *n.*
1. Bilirubin after passage through the hepatic
cells. 2. The form of bilirubin present in bile
and blood in hepatocellular or obstructive
jaundice, giving a positive reaction to the
direct van den Bergh test.

cho·le·cal·cif·er·ol (kol''e·kal·sif'ur·ol, ko''le·) *n.*
Vitamin D_3, prepared from 7-dehydrocholes-
terol. Syn. *activated 7-dehydrocholesterol.*

cho·le·chro·mo·poi·e·sis (kol''e·kro''mo·poy·ee'-
sis, ·ko''le·) *n.* The synthesis of bile pigments.

cho·le·cyst (kol'e·sist, ko'le·) *n.* GALLBLADDER.
—**chole·cys·tic** (·sis'tick) *adj.*

cho·le·cys·ta·gogue (kol''e·sist'uh·gog, ko''le·) *n.*
An agent or agency that causes or promotes
the evacuation of the gallbladder, by stimulating contraction of its musculature, or by relax-

ation of the sphincter of Oddi; a cholecystokinetic agent.

cho·le·cys·tal·gia (kol"e·sis·tal'juh, -jee·uh, ko"le·) *n.* BILIARY COLIC.

cho·le·cys·tec·to·my (kol"e·sis·teck'tuh·mee, ko"le·) *n.* Excision of the gallbladder and cystic duct.

cho·le·cyst·en·ter·or·rha·phy (kol"e·sist·en"tur·or'uh·fee, ko"le·) *n.* The suturing of the gallbladder to the small intestine.

cho·le·cyst·en·ter·os·to·my (kol"e·sist·en"tur·os'tuh·mee) *n. In surgery,* the formation of an anastomosis between the gallbladder and the small intestine.

cho·le·cys·ti·tis (ko"le·sis·tye'tis, kol"e·) *n.,* pl. **cholecys·tit·i·des** (·tit'i·deez) Inflammation of the gallbladder.

cho·le·cys·to·co·lon·ic (kol"e·sis"to·ko·lon'ick, ko"le·) *adj.* Pertaining to the gallbladder and the colon.

cho·le·cys·to·co·los·to·my (kol"e·sis"to·ko·los'tuh·mee) *n. In surgery,* the formation of an anastomosis between the gallbladder and some portion of the upper colon.

cho·le·cys·to·cu·ta·ne·ous (kol"e·sis"to·kew·tay'nee·us) *adj.* Pertaining to the gallbladder and skin, usually to a fistula connecting them.

cho·le·cys·to·du·o·de·nal (kol"e·sis"to·dew"o·dee'nul, ·dew·od'e·nul) *adj.* Pertaining to the gallbladder and duodenum.

cho·le·cys·to·du·o·de·no·col·ic (ko"le·sis"to·dew·od'e·no·ko'lick) *adj.* Pertaining to the gallbladder, duodenum, and colon.

cho·le·cys·to·du·o·de·nos·to·my (kol"e·sis"to·dew"o·de·nos'tuh·mee) *n. In surgery,* the formation of an anastomosis between the gallbladder and the duodenum.

cho·le·cys·to·elec·tro·co·ag·u·lec·to·my (kol"e·sis"to·e·leck"tro·ko·ag·yoo·leck'tuh·mee) *n.* Electrosurgical obliteration of the gallbladder.

cho·le·cys·to·en·ter·os·to·my (kol"e·sis"to·en"tur·os'tuh·mee) *n.* The surgical creation of a connection between the gallbladder and the small intestine.

cho·le·cys·to·gas·tric (kol"e·sis"to·gas'trick) *adj.* Pertaining to the gallbladder and stomach, usually to a fistula between these organs.

cho·le·cys·to·gas·tros·to·my (kol"e·sis"to·gas·tros'tuh·mee) *n. In surgery,* formation of an anastomosis between the gallbladder and the stomach.

cho·le·cys·to·gram (kol"e·sis"to·gram, ko"le·) *n.* A radiograph of the gallbladder.

cho·le·cys·tog·ra·phy (kol"e·sis·tog'ruh·fee, ko"le·) *n.* Radiography of the gallbladder after ingestion or intravenous injection of a radiopaque substance excreted in bile. —**cho·le·cys·to·graph·ic** (·sis"to·graf'ick) *adj.*

cho·le·cys·to·il·e·os·to·my (kol"e·sis"to·il·ee·os'tuh·mee) *n. In surgery,* the formation of an anastomosis between the gallbladder and the ileum.

cho·le·cys·to·je·ju·nos·to·my (kol"e·sis"to·jee"joo·nos'tuh·mee) *n. In surgery,* the formation of an anastomosis between the gallbladder and the jejunum.

cho·le·cys·to·ki·net·ic (kol"e·sis"to·ki·net'ick) *adj.* Possessing the property of causing or promoting gallbladder contraction.

cho·le·cys·to·ki·nin (kol"e·sis"to·kigh'nin, ko"le·) *n.* A hormone, produced by the upper intestinal mucosa, which causes contraction of the gallbladder and secretion of pancreatic enzymes; now known to be identical with the substance formerly called pancreozymin. Abbreviated, CCK.

cho·le·cys·to·li·thi·a·sis (kol"e·sis"to·li·thigh'uh·sis, ko"le·) *n.* The presence of one or more gallstones in the gallbladder.

cho·le·cys·to·li·thot·o·my (ko"le·sis"to·li·thot'uh·mee, ko"le·) *n. In surgery,* removal of gallstones from the gallbladder.

cho·le·cys·to·pexy (kol"e·sis'to·peck"see, ko"le·) *n.* Suture of the gallbladder to the abdominal wall.

cho·le·cys·tor·rha·phy (kol"e·sis·tor'uh·fee, ko"le·) *n.* Suture of the gallbladder, especially to the abdominal wall.

cho·le·cys·tos·to·my (kol"e·sis·tos'tuh·mee, ko"le·) *n. In surgery,* the establishment of an opening into the gallbladder, usually for external drainage of its contents.

cho·le·cys·tot·o·my (kol"e·sis·tot'uh·mee, ko"le·) *n.* Incision into the gallbladder to remove gallstones.

cho·le·doch (ko'le·dock) *adj.* CHOLEDOCHAL.

cho·le·doch·al (ko·led'uh·kul, ko·le·dock'ul) *adj.* Pertaining to the common bile duct.

choledochal cyst. CHOLEDOCHUS CYST.

cho·led·o·chec·ta·sia (ko·led"o·keck·tay'zhuh, ·zee·uh) *n.* Dilatation of the common bile duct.

cho·led·o·chec·to·my (ko·led"o·keck'tuh·mee) *n.* Excision of a part of the common bile duct.

choledochi. Plural and genitive singular of *choledochus.*

cho·led·o·chi·tis (ko·led"o·kigh'tis) *n.* Inflammation of the common bile duct.

cho·led·o·cho·cu·ta·ne·ous (ko·led"uh·ko·kew·tay'nee·us) *adj.* Pertaining to the gallbladder and skin, usually to a fistula between them.

cho·led·o·cho·cys·tos·to·my (ko·led"uh·ko·sis·tos'tuh·mee) *n. In surgery,* an anastomosis between the common bile duct and the gallbladder.

cho·led·o·cho·do·chor·rha·phy (ko·led"uh·ko·do·kor'uh·fee) *n. In surgery,* uniting the ends of a divided common bile duct, usually over an indwelling catheter.

cho·led·o·cho·du·o·de·nos·to·my (ko·led"uh·ko·dew"o·de·nos'tuh·mee) *n. In surgery,* the establishment of a passage between the common bile duct and the duodenum.

cho·led·o·cho·en·ter·os·to·my (ko·led"uh·ko·en"tur·os'tuh·mee) *n. In surgery,* the establishment of a passage between the common bile duct and the small intestine.

cho·led·o·cho·gas·tros·to·my (ko·led"uh·ko·gas·tros'tuh·mee) *n. In surgery,* the formation of an anastomosis between the common bile duct and the stomach.

cho·led·o·cho·je·ju·nos·to·my (ko·led"uh·ko·jee"joo·nos'tuh·mee) *n. In surgery,* an anastomosis between the common bile duct and the jejunum.

cho·led·o·cho·li·thi·a·sis (ko·led"uh·ko·li·thigh'

uh·sis) *n.* The presence of calculi in the common bile duct.

cho·led·o·cho·li·thot·o·my (ko·led″uh·ko·li·thot′uh·mee) *n. In surgery,* removal of a calculus by incision of the common bile duct.

cho·led·o·cho·litho·trip·sy (ko·led″uh·ko·lith′o·trip″see) *n. In surgery,* the crushing of a gallstone in the common bile duct without opening the duct.

cho·led·o·cho·plas·ty (ko·led′uh·ko·plas″tee) *n.* A plastic operation upon the common bile duct.

cho·led·o·chor·rha·phy (ko·led″o·kor′uh·fee) *n. In surgery,* the repair of the divided common bile duct.

cho·led·o·chos·to·my (ko·led″o·kos′tuh·mee) *n. In surgery,* the draining of the common bile duct through the abdominal wall.

cho·led·o·chot·o·my (ko·led″o·kot′uh·mee) *n.* An incision into the common bile duct.

cho·led·o·chus (ko·led′o·kus) *n.,* pl. & genit. sing. **choledo·chi** (·kye) COMMON BILE DUCT.

choledochus cyst. Congenital cystic dilatation of the common bile duct, usually due to its constriction close to the hepaticopancreatic ampulla, clinically manifested at times varying from shortly after birth to later in childhood by pain, abdominal tumor, hepatic enlargement, cirrhosis, and jaundice. Exacerbations and remissions are common. Syn. *bile cyst.*

Choledyl. Trademark for oxtriphylline, a drug with actions characteristic of theophylline.

cho·le·glo·bin (kol″e·glo′bin, ko″le·) *n.* Combined native protein (globin) and open-ring iron-porphyrin, which is bile pigment hemoglobin; a precursor of biliverdin. Syn. *verdoglobin.*

cho·le·hem·a·tin, cho·le·haem·a·tin (ko″le·heem′uh·tin, ko″le·) *n.* Pigment found in the bile and biliary concretions of ruminants; identical with phylloerythrin.

cho·le·ic (ko·lay′ick, ko·lee′ick) *adj.* Pertaining to bile.

cho·le·lith (ko′le·lith, kol″e·) *n.* BILIARY CALCULUS; GALLSTONE. —**cho·le·lith·ic** (ko″le·lith′ick) *adj.*

cho·le·li·thi·a·sis (ko″le·li·thigh′uh·sis, kol″e·) *n.,* pl. **cholelithia·ses** (·seez) The presence of, or a condition associated with, calculi in the gallbladder or in a bile duct.

cho·le·li·thot·o·my (ko″le·li·thot′uh·mee, kol″e·) *n.* Incision for the removal of gallstones.

cho·lem·e·sis (ko·lem′e·sis) *n.,* pl. **choleme·ses** (·seez) Vomiting of bile.

cho·le·mia, cho·lae·mia (ko·lee′mee·uh) *n.* 1. HEPATIC ENCEPHALOPATHY. 2. HEPATIC COMA. 3. The presence of bile in the blood.

cho·le·mic, cho·lae·mic (ko·lee′mick, ·lem′ick) *adj.* Pertaining to, resulting from, or caused by cholemia.

cho·le·poi·e·sis (kol″e·poy·ee′sis, ko″le·) *n.* The process of formation of bile by the liver.

cho·le·poi·et·ic (kol″e·poy·et′ick, ko″le·) *adj. & n.* 1. Stimulating the processes or a process concerned in the formation of bile. 2. A cholepoietic agent.

cho·le·pyr·rhin (ko″le·pirr′in, kol″e·) *n.* BILIRUBIN.

chol·era (kol′ur·uh) *n.* 1. A specific infectious disease of man caused by *Vibrio cholerae.* A soluble toxin produced in the intestinal tract by the vibrio alters the permeability of the mucosa and causes a profuse, watery diarrhea with fluid and electrolyte depletion; occurs endemically and epidemically in Asia. 2. *Obsol.* Any of various conditions characterized by profuse vomiting and diarrhea.

chol·er·a·ic (kol″ur·ay′ick) *adj.* Pertaining to, resembling, or having characteristics of cholera.

cholera mor·bus (mor′bus). *Obsol.* Any acute severe gastroenteritis.

cho·le·re·sis (ko″le·ree′sis, kol″e·) *n.,* pl. **cholere·ses** (·seez) Increased secretion of bile by the liver.

choleretic diarrhea. Diarrhea due to excess bile in the colon, usually resulting from resection or disease of the terminal ileum.

chol·er·ic (kol′ur·ick) *adj.* Easily angered; irritable.

chol·er·i·form (kol′ur·i·form) *adj.* Resembling cholera.

choler·oid (kol′ur·oid) *adj.* CHOLERIFORM.

chol·er·o·ma·nia (kol″ur·o·may′nee·uh) *n.* 1. The acute organic brain disorder seen during the course of cholera. 2. CHOLEROPHOBIA.

chol·er·o·pho·bia (kol″ur·o·fo′bee·uh) *n.* Abnormal fear of cholera.

chol·er·rha·gia (kol″e·ray′jee·uh, ·ko″le·) *n.* A copious flow of bile.

cho·les·tane (kol′es·tane, ko·les′) *n.* $C_{27}H_{48}$; a fully saturated hydrocarbon derivative of cyclopentanophenanthrene containing in addition two methyl groups (at carbon atoms 10 and 13) and a C_8H_{17} aliphatic group (at carbon atom 17). It may be considered a parent hydrocarbon from which many sterols, including cholesterol, are derived.

cho·les·ta·nol (kol′es·tuh·nol, ·nol) *n.* 1. Cholestan-3β-ol, or 3β-hydroxycholestane, $C_{27}H_{47}OH$, occurring in various tissues; it represents cholesterol in which the double bond is saturated. Syn. *dihydrocholesterol.* 2. Any hydroxyl derivative of cholestane of the general formula $C_{27}H_{47}OH$.

cho·le·sta·sis (ko″le·stay′sis) *n.* Stoppage or slowing of flow in biliary channels, especially in the small intrahepatic branches. —**chole·stat·ic** (·stat′ick) *adj.*

cholestatic cirrhosis. Cirrhosis secondary to biliary obstruction.

cholestatic hepatitis. Hepatitis due to obstruction of the small intrahepatic bile channels by bile of altered and presumably more viscous composition.

cho·les·te·a·to·ma (ko·les″tee·uh·to′muh) *n.,* pl. **cholesteatomas, cholesteatoma·ta** (·tuh) An epidermal inclusion cyst of the middle ear or mastoid bone, sometimes in the external ear canal, brain, or spinal cord. True cholesteatoma is rare and of congenital origin. Syn. *pearly tumor.* —**cholestea·tom·a·tous** (·tom′uh·tus) *adj.*

cho·les·te·a·to·sis (ko·les″tee·uh·to′sis) *n.,* pl. **cholesteato·ses** (·seez) The presence of an abundance of cholesterol or its esters in a focus of degeneration or necrosis, usually the intima of the aorta.

cho·les·tene (kol'es·teen, ko·les'teen) *n.* Any of several hydrocarbons of the formula $C_{27}H_{46}$, resulting from introduction of a double bond in cholestane; the position of the double bond characterizes specific cholestenes. Cholest-5-ene is the immediate parent hydrocarbon of cholesterol.

cho·les·ter·ase (ko·les'tur·ace) *n.* An enzyme, present in blood and other tissues, that hydrolyzes cholesterol esters to form cholesterol and fatty acids.

cho·les·ter·in (ko·les'tur·in) *n.* CHOLESTEROL.

cho·les·ter·in·uria (ko·les"tur·i·new'ree·uh) *n.* The presence of cholesterol in the urine.

cho·les·ter·ol (ko·les'tur·ol) *n.* 1. Cholest-5-en-3β-ol, $C_{27}H_{45}OH$, an unsaturated monohydric alcohol of the class of sterols; a constituent of all animal fats and oils, of bile, gallstones, nervous tissue, egg yolk, and blood, and sometimes found in foci of fatty degeneration. It is a white, crystalline substance, insoluble in water. It is important in metabolism and a derivative can be activated to form a vitamin D.

cho·les·ter·ol·emia, cho·les·ter·ol·ae·mia (ko·les"tur·ol·ee'mee·uh) *n.* 1. The presence of cholesterol in the blood. 2. HYPERCHOLESTEROLEMIA.

cho·les·ter·ol·er·e·sis (ko·les"tur·ol·err'e·sis) *n.* An increased elimination of cholesterol in the bile.

cho·les·ter·ol·o·poi·e·sis (ko·les"tur·ol·o·poy·ee'sis) *n.* The synthesis of cholesterol.

cho·les·ter·ol·o·sis (ko·les"tur·ol·o'sis) *n.* A condition marked by an abnormal deposition of cholesterol, as in mucosa of the gallbladder.

cho·les·ter·o·sis (ko·les"tur·o'sis) *n.* CHOLESTEROLOSIS.

cho·les·ter·yl (ko·les'tur·il) *n.* $C_{27}H_{45}$. The radical of cholesterol.

cho·les·tyr·a·mine (ko·les'ti·ruh·meen) *n.* A strongly basic anion exchange resin having a demonstrated affinity for bile acids; used in adjunctive therapy in the management of patients with elevated cholesterol levels.

cho·lic (kol'lick, kol'ick) *adj.* CHOLIC.

cholic acid. 1. 3,7,12-Trihydroxycholanic acid, $C_{24}H_{40}O_5$, one of the unconjugated bile acids. In bile it occurs as the sodium salt of the conjugated taurocholic or glycocholic acid. Syn. *cholalic acid.* 2. Any one of the several unconjugated bile acids which are hydroxy derivatives of cholanic acid.

cho·line (ko'leen, ·lin, kol'een, ·in) *n.* (β-Hydroxyethyl)trimethylammonium hydroxide, $(CH_3)_3N(OH)CH_2CH_2OH$, a liquid base widely distributed in nature as a component of lecithin and other phospholipids. An insufficient supply of choline or other lipotropic factors in the diet may result in accumulation of fat in the liver and other body dysfunctions. As a drug, choline has an effect similar to that of parasympathetic stimulation. Various salts of choline are used as lipotropic agents.

cho·lin·er·gic (ko"lin·ur'jick, kol'in·) *adj.* Pertaining to or designating the type of chemical activity characteristic of acetylcholine or of agents which mimic the actions of acetylcholine.

cholinergic blocking agent. Any agent which blocks the action of acetylcholine or acetylcholine-like substances, i.e., which blocks the action of cholinergic nerves.

cholinergic nerves. Those nerves which, upon stimulation, release a cholinergic substance (acetylcholine) at their terminations; they include all autonomic preganglionic nerves (sympathetic and parasympathetic), postganglionic parasympathetic nerves, somatic motor nerves to skeletal muscles, and fibers to sweat glands and certain blood vessels.

cholinergic urticaria. Small, relatively nonpruritic wheals, provoked by heat generated by exercise or emotion. Thought to be caused by acetycholine or a metabolic abnormality.

cho·lin·es·ter·ase (ko"li·nes'tur·ace, ·aze) *n.* Any enzyme found in blood and in various other tissues that catalyzes hydrolysis of choline esters, including acetylcholine. Abbreviated, ChE.

cho·li·no·lyt·ic (ko"li·no·lit'ick) *adj.* ANTICHOLINERGIC.

cho·li·no·mi·met·ic (ko"li·no·mi·met'ick) *adj.* Having an action similar to that of acetylcholine.

Cholografin. Trademark for iodipamide, a roentgenographic contrast medium for intravenous cholangiography and cholecystography used as the methylglucamine (meglumine) or sodium salt.

cho·lo·lith (kol'o·lith, ko'luh·) *n.* GALLSTONE. —**cho·lo·lith·ic** (ko"lo·lith'ick, ko'lo·) *adj.*

chol·or·rhea (kol·o·ree'uh, ko"luh·) *n.* Profuse secretion of bile.

cho·lo·tho·rax (ko"lo·tho'racks, kol'o·) *n.* Bile in the pleural cavities.

chol·uria (ko·lew'ree·uh) *n.* The presence of bile in the urine.

chondr-, chondri-, chondro- A combining form meaning *cartilage, cartilaginous.*

chon·dral (kon'drul) *adj.* Cartilaginous; pertaining to cartilage.

chon·drec·to·my (kon·dreck'tuh·mee) *n. In surgery,* the excision of cartilage.

chon·dri·fy (kon'dri·figh) *v.* To convert into cartilage; to become cartilage or cartilaginous. —**chon·dri·fi·ca·tion** (kon"dri·fi·kay'shun) *n.*

chon·dri·gen (kon'dri·jen) *n.* The protein of cartilage which is converted by boiling into chondrin; similar to collagen.

chon·drin (kon'drin) *n.* A protein material obtained by boiling cartilage; primarily gelatin obtained from the collagen component of the cartilage.

chondrio- A combining form meaning *chondriosome, mitochondrion.*

chon·dri·some (kon'dree·o·sohm) *n.* A general term for all forms of mitochondria and other cytoplasmic bodies of the same nature. —**chon·dri·som·al** (kon"dree·o·so'mul) *adj.*

chon·dri·tis (kon·dry'tis) *n.* Inflammation of a cartilage.

chon·dro·blast (kon'dro·blast) *n.* A cartilage-forming cell.

chon·dro·blas·to·ma (kon"dro·blas·to'muh) *n.* A rare chondrocytic tumor of young males, usually involving the epiphyses; it is locally aggressive but does not metastasize.

chon·dro·cal·ci·no·sis (kon″dro·kal″si·no′sis) *n.*
1. Deposition of calcium salts in cartilaginous
tissues. 2. PSEUDOGOUT SYNDROME.

chon·dro·cal·syn·o·vi·tis (kon″dro·kal·sin″o·vye′
tis) *n.* 1. Deposition of calcium salts in cartilage and synovial tissues. 2. PSEUDOGOUT SYN-
DROME.

chon·dro·cla·sis (kon″dro·klay′sis) *n.*, pl. **chon-
drocla·ses** (·seez) 1. Crushing of a cartilage.
2. Resorption of cartilage.

chon·dro·clast (kon′dro·klast) *n.* A cell concerned in the resorption of cartilage.

chon·dro·cos·tal (kon″dro·kos′tul) *adj.* Pertaining to the ribs and their cartilages.

chon·dro·cra·ni·um (kon″dro·kray′nee·um) *n.*
The embryonic cartilaginous cranium.

chon·dro·cyte (kon′dro·site) *n.* A cartilage cell.
—**chon·dro·cyt·ic** (kon″dro·sit′ick) *adj.*

chon·dro·der·ma·ti·tis (kon″dro·dur″muh·tye′
tis) *n.* Inflammation of cartilage and overlying
skin.

chondrodermatitis no·du·la·ris he·li·cis (nod·yoo·
lair′is hel′i·sis). Painful nodules of the ear,
usually seen on the rim of the ear in men.
Frostbite has often preceded their occurrence.

chon·dro·dys·pla·sia (kon″dro·dis·play′zhuh,
·zee·uh) *n.* ENCHONDROMATOSIS.

chondrodysplasia punc·ta·ta (punk·tay′tuh, ·tah′
tuh). CHONDRODYSTROPHIA CALCIFICANS CON-
GENITA.

chondrodystrophia cal·cif·i·cans con·gen·i·ta
(kal·sif′i·kanz kon·jen′i·tuh). An inherited (autosomal recessive) disease characterized by
shortness of the neck and limbs, kyphoscoliosis, flat nose and widely separated eyes, and
sometimes associated with cataracts and mental retardation. Syn. *Conradi's disease.*

chondrodystrophia fe·ta·lis (fee·tay′lis). ACHON-
DROPLASIA.

chondrodystrophia fetalis hy·po·plas·ti·ca
(high″po·plas′ti·kuh). CHONDRODYSTROPHIA
CALCIFICANS CONGENITA.

chondrodystrophia hy·per·plas·ti·ca (high·pur·
plas′ti·kuh). MULTIPLE HEREDITARY EXOSTO-
SES.

chon·dro·dys·tro·phy (kon″dro·dis′truh·fee) *n.*
One of a group of disorders characterized by a
defect in the formation of bone from cartilage,
congenital in origin. —**chon·dro·dys·tro·phic**
(·dis·tro′fick) *adj.*

chon·dro·ec·to·der·mal (kon″dro·eck″to·dur′
mul) *adj.* Pertaining to cartilage developed
from ectoderm, as certain branchial arch cartilages from the neural crest.

chondroectodermal dysplasia. A rare congenital
disorder characterized by enchondromatosis,
ectodermal dysplasia, bilateral polydactyly,
polymetacarpalism, dental dysplasia, and
sometimes congenital heart disease. Syn. *El-
lis-van Creveld syndrome.*

chon·dro·fi·bro·ma (kon″dro·figh·bro′muh) *n.* A
fibroma containing cartilaginous tissue.

chon·dro·fi·bro·sar·co·ma (kon″dro·figh″bro·
sahr·ko′muh) *n.* A type of malignant mixed
mesodermal tumor containing fibrosarcomatous and chondrosarcomatous components.

chon·dro·gen·e·sis (kon″dro·jen′uh·sis) *n.* Formation of cartilage. —**chondro·ge·net·ic** (·je·net′
ick), **chondro·gen·ic** (·jen′ick) *adj.*

chon·droid (kon′droid) *adj.* Resembling cartilage.

chon·dro·i·tin (kon·dro′i·tin) *n.* A complex nitrogenous substance which, in the form of
chondroitin sulfate, occurs combined with
protein as chondromucoid, a constituent of
cartilage.

chondroitin sulfate. A compound which on hydrolysis yields sulfuric acid, acetic acid,
chondrosamine, and glucuronic acid; the
prosthetic group of the glycoprotein chondromucoid; heparin has a similar chemical structure. Syn. *chondroitic acid, chondroitin sulfuric
acid.*

chon·dro·i·tin·sul·fu·ric acid (kon·dro″i·tin·sul·
few′rick). CHONDROITIN SULFATE.

chon·dro·lipo·sar·co·ma (kon″dro·lip″o·sahr·ko′
muh) *n.* A malignant mixed mesodermal tumor composed of liposarcomatous and chondrosarcomatous elements.

chon·dro·ma (kon·dro′muh) *n.*, pl. **chondromas,
chondroma·ta** (·tuh) A benign tumor composed
of cartilage (either hyaline cartilage or fibrocartilage); may grow from bone, cartilage, or
other tissue.

chon·dro·ma·la·cia (kon″dro·ma·lay′shuh, ·see·
uh) *n.* Softening of a cartilage.

chon·dro·ma·to·sis (kon″dro·ma·to′sis) *n.* The
presence of multiple chondromas.

chon·drom·a·tous (kon·drom′uh·tus) *adj.* 1. Of
or pertaining to a chondroma. 2. *Erron.* CARTI-
LAGINOUS.

chon·dro·mu·coid (kon″dro·mew′koid) *n.* A mucoid found in cartilage; a glycoprotein in
which chondroitin sulfate is the prosthetic
group.

chon·dro·myx·oid (kon″dro·mick′soid) *adj.*
Composed of cartilaginous and myxoid elements.

chon·dro·myx·o·ma (kon″dro·mick·so′muh) *n.*
A benign connective-tissue tumor with cartilaginous and mucinous compounds.

chon·dro·myxo·sar·co·ma (kon″dro·mick″so·
sahr·ko′muh) *n.* A sarcoma whose parenchyma is composed of anaplastic myxoid and
chondroid elements.

chon·dro·os·teo·dys·tro·phy (kon″dro·os″tee·o·
dis′truh·fee) *n.* MORQUIO'S SYNDROME.

chon·dro·os·te·o·ma (kon″dro·os″tee·o′muh) *n.*
1. OSTEOCHONDROMA. 2. EXOSTOSIS CARTILA-
GINEA.

chon·drop·a·thy (kon·drop′uth·ee) *n.* Any disease involving cartilage.

chon·dro·phyte (kon′dro·fite) *n.* A hypertrophic
cartilaginous outgrowth.

chon·dro·plas·ty (kon′dro·plas″tee) *n.* A plastic
operation on cartilage.

chon·dro·sar·co·ma (kon″dro·sahr·ko′muh) *n.* A
malignant tumor composed of anaplastic
chondrocytes; it may occur as a central or
peripheral tumor of bone. —**chondrosar·co·ma·
tous** (·ko′muh·tus) *adj.*

chon·dro·sis (kon·dro′sis) *n.*, pl. **chondro·ses**
(·seez) Formation of cartilage.

chon·dro·ster·nal (kon″dro·stur′nul) *adj.* Pertaining to the costal cartilages and to the
sternum.

chon·dro·tome (kon′dro·tome) *n.* An instrument
for cutting cartilage.

chon·drot·o·my (kon·drot'uh·mee) *n. In surgery*, the division of a cartilage.

Chon·drus (kon'drus) *n.* A small genus of red algae of the Gigartinaceae.

Chondrus cris·pus (kris'pus). A species of red algae; the dried bleached plant, called carrageen or Irish moss, yields carrageenin, a mucilaginous principle, proteins, and salts of iodine, chlorine, and bromine. It is demulcent and somewhat nutrient; used as an emulsifying agent.

cho·ne·chon·dro·ster·non (ko''nee·kon·dro·stur'non) *n.* FUNNEL CHEST.

Cho·part's amputation (shoʰ·pahr') An amputation of the foot consisting of a disarticulation of the tarsal bones, leaving only the talus and calcaneus.

Choranid. A trademark for chorionic gonadotropin.

chord-, chordo- A combining form meaning (a) *cord*; (b) *notochord*.

chor·da (kor'duh) *n., pl. & genit. sing.* **chor·dae** (·dee) 1. A cord, tendon, or nerve trunk. 2. The chorda dorsalis (= NOTOCHORD). —**chor·dal** (·dul), **chor·date** (·date) *adj.*

chorda dor·sa·lis (dor·say'lis). NOTOCHORD.

chordae ten·di·ne·ae (ten·din'ee·ee) [NA]. TENDINOUS CORDS.

chor·da·meso·derm (kor''duh·mez'o·durm, ·mee'so·durm) *n.* The embryonic area in a blastula or early gastrula destined to form the notochord and mesoderm. It occupies the region of the dorsal blastoporic lip and is thus the organizer.

Chor·da·ta (kor·day'tuh, ·dah'tuh) *n.pl.* A phylum of the animal kingdom whose members are characterized by having at some stage in their development a notochord, a tubular central nervous system lying dorsal to the notochord, and lateral clefts in the walls of the pharynx.

chor·date (kor'date) *adj. & n.* 1. Possessing a notochord; belonging or pertaining to the phylum Chordata. 2. A member of the phylum Chordata.

chorda tym·pa·ni (tim'puh·nigh) [NA]. A nerve that originates from the facial nerve, traverses the tympanic cavity, and joins the lingual branch of the mandibular nerve.

chor·dee (kor·dee') *n.* A curvature of the penis with concavity downward; an accompaniment of hypospadias, occasionally caused by scar tissue resulting from urethral infection or trauma. —**chor·de·ic** (·dee'ick) *adj.*

chor·di·tis (kor·dye'tis) *n.* 1. Inflammation of a spermatic cord. 2. Inflammation of a vocal fold.

chor·do·ma (kor·do'muh) *n., pl.* **chordomas, chordoma·ta** (·tuh) A locally aggressive tumor composed of embryonal notochordal cells and large (physaliphorous) and small vacuolated cells. It occurs anywhere along the vertebral column, usually in the sacrococcygeal region or the base of the skull.

chor·dot·o·my (kor·dot'uh·mee) *n.* Surgical division of certain tracts of the spinal cord, e.g., the lateral spinothalamic tract for relief of pain.

cho·rea (ko·ree'uh) *n.* 1. Widespread, arrhyth-mic, involuntary movements of a forcible, rapid, jerky type and of brief duration; seen in Sydenham's and Huntington's chorea.—**chore·al** (·ul), **chore·ic** (·ick), **cho·re·at·ic** (ko''ree·at'ick) *adj.*

chorea grav·i·da·rum (grav·i·dair'um). Sydenham's chorea occurring during or aggravated by pregnancy.

chorea minor. SYDENHAM'S CHOREA.

cho·re·i·form (ko·ree'i·form) *adj.* Resembling chorea.

cho·reo·ath·e·toid (ko''ree·o·ath'e·toid) *adj.* Pertaining to choreoathetosis.

cho·reo·ath·e·to·sis (ko''ree·o·ath''e·to'sis) *n.* A condition characterized by both choreiform and athetoid movements.

chori-, chorio-. A combining form meaning (a) *chorion*; (b) *choroid.*

cho·rio·ad·e·no·ma (ko''ree·o·ad·e·no'muh) *n.* A tumor intermediate in malignancy between hydatidiform mole and choriocarcinoma.

cho·rio·al·lan·to·ic (ko''ree·o·al''an·to'ick) *adj.* Pertaining to the chorion and to the allantois or to the chorioallantois.

cho·rio·al·lan·to·is (ko''ree·o·a·lan'to·is, ·a·lan'toice) *n.* The membrane formed by the union of chorion and allantois in birds and certain mammals and vascularized by the allantoic blood vessels. That of chicks is used for the culture of viruses in the preparation of vaccines.

cho·rio·am·ni·on·ic (ko''ree·o·am''nee·on'ick) *adj.* Pertaining to the chorion and the amnion.

cho·rio·am·nio·ni·tis (ko''ree·o·am''nee·o·nigh'tis) *n.* Inflammation of the fetal membranes.

cho·rio·an·gi·o·ma (ko''ree·o·an·jee·o'muh) *n.* The most common tumor of the placenta, composed of fetal blood vessels, connective tissue, and trophoblast; it is benign.

cho·rio·cele (ko·ree·o·seel) *n.* A hernial protrusion of the choroid coat of the eye.

cho·rio·ep·i·the·li·o·ma (ko''ree·o·ep''i·theel·ee·o'muh) *n.* CHORIOCARCINOMA.

cho·rio·gen·e·sis (ko''ree·o·jen'e·sis) *n., pl.* **cho·rio·gene·ses** (·seez) The development of the chorion.

cho·ri·o·ma (ko''ree·o'muh) *n., pl.* **choriomas, chorioma·ta** (·tuh) 1. Any benign tumor of chorionic elements. 2. CHORIOCARCINOMA.

cho·rio·men·in·gi·tis (ko''ree·o·men''in·jye'tis) *n.* LYMPHOCYTIC CHORIOMENINGITIS.

cho·ri·on (ko'ree·on) *n.* The outermost of the fetal membranes, consisting of an outer trophoblastic epithelium lined internally by extraembryonic mesoderm. Its villous portion, vascularized by allantoic blood vessels, forms the fetal part of the placenta.

cho·ri·on·ic (ko''ree·on'ick) *adj.* Of or pertaining to the chorion.

chorionic cyst. An uncommon cyst of the placenta, arising in the chorionic plate, usually near the umbilical cord bulging toward the fetus. Histologically, it is lined by cells of trophoblastic origin.

chorionic gonadotropin. The water-soluble gonadotropic substance, originating in chorionic tissue, obtained from the urine of pregnant women. It is also secreted by choriocarcinomas.

chorionic plate. The chorionic membrane of the placental region, formed externally by the trophoblastic layer and internally by a fibrous lining layer of mesoderm.

chorionic vesicle. The gestation sac covered by chorionic villi and containing the embryo.

cho·ri·o·ni·tis (kor″ee·o·nigh′tis) *n.* 1. Placental inflammation. 2. *Obsol.* SCLERODERMA.

chorion lae·ve (lee′vee) The smooth membranous part of the chorion devoid of prominent villi.

cho·rio·ret·i·nal (ko″ree·o·ret′i·nul) *adj.* Pertaining to the choroid and retina.

cho·rio·ret·i·ni·tis (ko″ree·o·ret″i·nigh′tis) *n.* Inflammation of the choroid and retina.

cho·rio·ret·i·nop·a·thy (ko″ree·o·ret″i·nop′uth·ee) *n.* Disease involving both the choroid and retina.

chor·i·sis (kor′i·sis) *n.*, pl. **chori·ses** (·seez) *In botany,* the splitting of an organ into parts, each of which forms a perfect organ.

chorist-, choristo- A combining form meaning *separated, misplaced.*

cho·ris·to·ma (kor″i·sto′muh) *n.*, pl. **choristomas, choristoma·ta** (·tuh) A benign tumor composed of elements foreign to the tissue where the tumor is found; it may arise through developmental displacement of tissue from one place to another, or from metaplasia; e.g., a mass of normal bone marrow cells in the adrenal gland.

cho·roid (kor′oid, ko′roid) *adj. & n.* 1. Designating or pertaining to a delicate vascular membrane or structure. 2. The pigmented vascular tunic of the eye, continuous with the ciliary body anteriorly, and lying between the sclera and the retina; the choroid membrane.

choroid-, choroido-. A combining form meaning *choroid.*

cho·roid·e·re·mia (ko″roid·e·ree′mee·uh) *n.* Atrophy of the choroid; transmitted as an autosomal recessive trait.

cho·roid·itis (ko″roy·dye′tis) *n.* Inflammation of the choroid of the eye.

choroid membrane or **coat.** CHOROID (2).

cho·roi·do·cy·cli·tis (ko·roy″do·sick·ligh′tis, ·sigh·klight′is) *n.* Inflammation of the choroid and ciliary body.

cho·roi·do·iri·tis (ko·roy″do·eye·rye′tis, ·i·rye′tis) *n.* Inflammation of the choroid and iris.

cho·roi·do·ret·i·ni·tis (ko·roy″do·ret″i·nigh′tis) *n.* CHORIORETINITIS.

choroid plexus. One of the longitudinal, lobulated, invaginated processes, consisting of a vascular plexus and a covering of ependyma, which project into each of the ventricles of the brain; specifically, the choroid plexus of the third ventricle, the choroid plexus of the fourth ventricle, or the choroid plexus of either lateral ventricle.

chre·ma·to·pho·bia (kree″muh·to·fo′bee·uh) *n.* Abnormal fear of money.

Christian Science. A religious sect and system of healing through prayer and the triumph of mind over matter.

Christian Science practitioner. One who practices the spiritual healing of illnesses according to the teachings of Mary Baker Eddy.

Christ·mas disease A hemophilioid disease resulting from a hereditary deficiency of the procoagulant factor IX. Syn. *hemophilia B.*

Christmas factor FACTOR IX.

chrom-, chromo- A combining form meaning (a) *color, colored;* (b) *pigment, pigmented;* (c) *chromium.*

chro·maf·fin (kro′muh·fin, kro·maf′in) *adj.* Describing or pertaining to the reaction of certain tissue constituents, as catecholamines and some other phenolic substances, in being oxidized to a yellow or brown compound on fixation with a dichromate. Certain cells of the adrenal medulla, of paraganglions, and of some other tissues react positively.

chromaffin bodies. Small chromaffin cell masses on either side of the abdominal aorta.

chromaffin cells. Cells of tissues, such as the adrenal medulla, that give a positive chromaffin reaction.

chro·maf·fi·no·ma (kro″muh·fi·no′muh, kro·maf″i·) *n.* PHEOCHROMOCYTOMA.

chro·ma·sia (kro·may′zhuh, ·zee·uh) *n.* Color effect produced by chromatic aberration in the functioning of lenses.

-chromasia A combining form designating *a condition or property involving color or color perception.*

chromat-, chromato- A combining form meaning (a) *color;* (b) *pigment, pigmentation;* (c) *chromatin.*

chro·mate (kro′mate) *n.* Any salt of chromic acid.

chro·ma·te·lop·sia (kro″mat·e·lop′see·uh) *n.* COLOR BLINDNESS.

chro·ma·te·lop·sis (kro″mat·e·lop′sis) *n.* COLOR BLINDNESS.

chro·mat·ic (kro·mat′ick) *adj.* 1. Of or pertaining to color, especially to hue, or to hue and saturation together. 2. Readily stainable; pertaining to readily stainable constituents in cells.

chromatic aberration. Unequal refraction of different parts of the spectrum, producing indistinct images surrounded by a halo of colors.

chro·ma·tid (kro′muh·tid) *n.* One of the two bodies, sister chromosomes, resulting from the longitudinal splitting of a chromosome, in preparation for mitosis; especially, one of the four parts of a tetrad, formed by the longitudinal splitting of synaptic mates, in preparation for meiosis.

chro·ma·tin (kro′muh·tin) *n.* The chromosomal DNA-containing material in a nucleus that readily stains with nuclear stains, as in the Feulgen reaction.

chromatin bodies. CHROMOSOMES.

chromatin-negative, *adj.* Lacking a sex chromatin body, as in gonial cells in both sexes and in somatic cells of individuals with only one X chromosome.

chromatin-positive, *adj.* Possessing a sex chromatin body in the nucleus of somatic cells, and therefore having more than one X chromosome, as in the normal female type and in the Klinefelter syndrome.

chro·ma·tism (kro′muh·tiz·um) *n.* 1. A hallucination in which colored lights are seen. 2. Abnormal pigment deposits.

chromato-. See *chromat-*.

chro·ma·to·der·ma·to·sis (kro″muh·to·dur″muh·to′sis) *n.*, pl. **chromatodermato·ses** (·seez) Any condition of the skin marked by a lasting change of color.

chro·ma·to·dys·o·pia (kro″muh·to·dis·o′pee·uh) *n.* COLOR BLINDNESS.

chro·ma·tog·e·nous (kro″muh·toj′e·nus) *adj.* Producing color.

chro·ma·to·gram (kro·mat′o·gram, kro′muh·to·) *n. In chromatography,* the porous solid matrix (column, paper, thin layer) after the separation procedure has been applied and the matrix treated with a suitable developing agent to indicate the location of the separated components of the mixture submitted to chromatographic treatment.

chro·ma·tog·ra·phy (kro″muh·tog′ruh·fee) *n.* The procedure by which a mixture of substances is separated by fractional extraction or adsorption or ion exchange on a porous solid (as a column of aluminum oxide, or cellulose) by means of one or more flowing liquid or gaseous solvents, especially by the process of partition chromatography. The principal types of chromatography are: column, gas, paper, liquid, and thin-layer. —**chro·ma·to·graph** (kro·mat′o·graf, kro′muh·to·) *v.;* **chro·mato·graph·ic** (kro·mat″o·graf′ick, kro″muh·to·) *adj.*

chro·ma·toid (kro′muh·toid) *adj.* Pertaining to or resembling chromatin.

chromatoid bodies. Hematoxylin-staining spicules and irregular masses, having a negative Feulgen reaction, found in amebic cysts.

chro·ma·tol·y·sis (kro″muh·tol′i·sis) *n.*, pl. **chro·matoly·ses** (·seez) Dissolution of the cytoplasmic Nissl substance of the body of a neuron; usually occurs as part of the axonal reaction.—**chro·ma·to·lyt·ic** (·to·lit′ick) *adj.*

chro·ma·to·mere (kro·mat′o·meer, kro′muh·to·) *n.* The part or parts of a platelet colored brightly with stains of the Romanovsky type.

chro·ma·tom·e·try (kro″muh·tom′e·tree) *n.* The measurement of degree of color or of color perception.

chro·ma·top·a·thy (kro″muh·top′uth·ee) *n.* Any abnormality of color of skin.

chro·ma·to·phore (kro·mat′o·fore, kro′muh·to·) *n.* 1. *In botany,* a colored plastid. 2. *In zoology,* a pigmented, branched connective-tissue cell.

chro·ma·to·pseu·dop·sis (kro″muh·to·sue·dop′sis) *n.* COLOR BLINDNESS.

chro·ma·top·sia (kro″muh·top′see·uh) *n.* A disorder of visual sensation in which color impressions are disturbed or arise subjectively, with objects appearing colored unnaturally or colorless objects as colored; may be due to disturbance of the optic centers, to psychic disturbances, or to drugs.

chro·ma·to·sis (kro″muh·to′sis) *n.*, pl. **chromato·ses** (·seez) 1. PIGMENTATION. 2. A pathologic process or pigmentary disease characterized by a deposit of coloring matter in a locality where it is usually not present, or in excessive quantity in regions where pigment normally exists.

chro·ma·tu·ria (kro″muh·tew′ree·uh) *n.* Abnormal coloration of the urine.

-chrome A combining form meaning *colored*.

chrome (krome) *n.* Chromium or one of its ores or compounds.

chrom·es·the·sia, chrom·aes·the·sia (kro″mes·theezh′uh, ·theez′ee·uh) *n.* The association or perception of colors together with the sensation of hearing, especially of certain words, and of smell, taste, or touch.

chrome ulcer. An ulcer due to the action of chrome salts; seen in tanners and others who work with chromium.

chrom·hi·dro·sis (krome″hi·dro′sis, ·high·dro′sis) *n.* The secretion of colored sweat.

-chromia A combining form designating (a) *a state of pigmentation;* (b) *a state involving color perception.*

chro·mic (kro′mick) *adj.* 1. Of or pertaining to chromium. 2. Designating compounds containing the trivalent form of chromium.

chro·mi·um (kro′mee·um) *n.* Cr = 51.996. A hard, bright, silvery metal; largely used as a protective plating for other metals and in the manufacture of alloys characterized by strength and resistance to corrosion. It forms chromous and chromic salts.

chromium release test. A method of assessing the ability in vitro of antiserum or cells to lyse target cells, which are labeled with radioactive ^{51}Cr; release of ^{51}Cr after addition of serum or cells is taken as a measure of their cytotoxicity.

chromo-. See *chrom-*.

chro·mo·blas·to·my·co·sis (kro″mo·blas″to·migh·ko′sis) *n.*, pl. **chromoblastomyco·ses** (·seez) An infection of the skin characterized principally by the development of verrucous lesions, caused by various fungi, including *Hormodendrum pedrosoi, H. compactum, H. dermatitidis, Cladosporium carrionii,* and *Phialophora verrucosa.*

chro·mo·crin·ia (kro·mo·krin′ee·uh) *n.* The secretion or excretion of colored material.

chro·mo·cys·tos·co·py (kro″mo·sis·tos′kuh·pee) *n.* Cystoscopy and inspection of the orifices of the ureters after the administration of a substance that will stain the urine.

chro·mo·cyte (kro′mo·site) *n.* Any colored cell.

chro·mo·gen (kro′mo·jen) *n.* Any substance which, under suitable conditions, is capable of producing color.

chro·mo·mere (kro′mo·meer) *n.* 1. One of the beadlike chromatin granules arranged in a linear series in a chromosome. 2. CHROMATO-MERE.

chro·mo·my·co·sis (kro″mo·migh·ko′sis) *n.*, pl. **chromomyco·ses** (·seez) CHROMOBLASTOMYCO-SIS.

chrom·onych·ia (kro″mo·nick′ee·uh) *n.* Abnormal coloration of a nail or nails.

chro·mo·phil (kro′mo·fil) *adj. & n.* 1. Taking a deep stain. 2. A cell that takes a deep stain. —**chro·mo·phil·ic** (kro′mo·fil′ick), **chro·moph·i·lous** (kro·mof′i·lus) *adj.*

chromophil cells. The alpha and beta cells of the adenohypophysis.

chromophil granules. Small basophilic granules in nerve cells. Syn. *Nissl bodies.*

chro·mo·phobe (kro′mo·fobe) *adj. & n.* 1. Not

staining easily. 2. A cell that does not stain easily. 3. Specifically, CHROMOPHOBE CELL.

chromophobe adenoma or **tumor.** An adenoma of the adenohypophysis made up of chromophobe cells, neither basophilic nor acidophilic.

chromophobe cell. One of the faintly staining cells of the adenohypophysis, thought to give rise to alpha cells and beta cells.

chro·mo·pho·bia (kro″mo·fo′bee·uh) n. 1. Abnormal fear or dislike of colors or of certain colors. 2. *In histology*, staining little or not at all, said of intracellular granules or of certain cells.

chro·mo·phore (kro′mo·fore) n. 1. An atom or group of atoms or electrons in a molecule which is chiefly responsible for a spectral absorption band. 2. CHROMATOPHORE.

chro·mo·phor·ic (kro″mo·for′ick) adj. 1. Pertaining to cells, such as bacteria or hemoglobin, which produce pigments and retain them within the cell. 2. Of or pertaining to a chromophore.

chro·moph·o·rous (kro·mof′uh·rus) adj. CHROMOPHORIC.

chro·mo·phy·to·sis (kro″mo·figh·to′sis) n. TINEA VERSICOLOR.

chro·mo·pro·tein (kro″mo·pro′tee·in) n. Any protein containing a chromophoric group, such as hematin.

chrom·op·tom·e·ter (kro″mop·tom′e·tur) n. An instrument for determining the extent of development of color vision. —**chromoptome·try** (·tree) n.

chro·mo·some (kro′muh·sohm) n. Any one of the separate, deeply staining bodies, commonly rod-, J- (or L-), or V-shaped, which arise from the nuclear network during mitosis and meiosis. They carry the hereditary factors (genes), and are present in constant number in each species. In man, there are 46 in each cell, except in the mature ovum and sperm where the number is halved. A complete set of 23 is inherited from each parent. —**chro·mo·so·mal** (kro″muh·so′mul) adj.

chromosome mapping. The process of locating genes on chromosomes.

chro·mo·tricho·my·co·sis (kro″mo·trick″o·migh·ko′sis) n. TRICHOMYCOSIS AXILLARIS.

chro·mo·trope (kro′mo·trope) n. 1. A tissue component that stains metachromatically when treated with a metachromatic dye. 2. Any of several dyes, differentiated by numerical suffixes.

chron–, chrono– A combining form meaning *time*.

chro·nax·ie, chro·naxy (kro′nack·see) n. The duration of time that a current of twice the rheobasic (galvanic threshold) intensity must flow in order to excite the tissue being tested. Chronaxie is related to irritability and is used in testing for irritability changes in nerve and muscle.

chron·ic (kron′ick) adj. Long-continued; of long duration or frequent recurrence. —**chro·nic·i·ty** (kro·nis′i·tee) n.

chronic adhesive arachnoiditis. Local or generalized thickening of the arachnoid due to inflammation from infection, noxious agents, or

hemorrhage, trauma, or congenital anomalies. Commonly involved are the spinal cord, posterior fossa around the cerebellum, and the optic chiasma. Symptoms and signs vary with the site and extent of the adhesions.

chronic alcoholism. 1. Chronic excessive use of alcoholic drinks such as to interfere with the drinker's health, interpersonal relations, or means of livelihood. 2. Addiction to alcohol. 3. Medical and psychiatric diseases caused by chronic excessive use of alcohol.

chronic brain syndrome. *In psychiatry*, any chronic cerebral disorder presumed to have a structural basis.

chronic bronchitis. A clinical disorder characterized by excessive mucous secretion in the bronchial tree and manifested by chronic productive cough.

chronic cystic mastitis. CYSTIC DISEASE OF THE BREAST.

chronic dental fluorosis. Hypoplasia and discoloration of the teeth, resulting from the continued use, during the formative period of the tooth, of water containing large amounts of fluorine. Syn. *mottled enamel*.

chronic desquamative gingivitis. A chronic, basically degenerative, condition of the gingivae characterized by a diffuse atrophy of the epithelium.

chronic discoid lupus erythematosus. A chronic skin disease characterized by well-defined erythematous patches, often resulting in scarring, chiefly on the areas of the face where flushing commonly occurs; systemic symptoms are absent and the LE test is negative.

chronic glomerulonephritis. Glomerulonephritis characterized clinically by variable duration and progressive renal insufficiency. Pathologically there is progressive interstitial fibrosis with chronic inflammatory cells, tubular atrophy, and glomerulosclerosis. Syn. *Bright's disease*.

chronic granulomatous disease. A disorder, thought to be X-linked, in which phagocytic ingestion of bacteria is normal but bactericidal action is impaired; characterized by lymphadenopathy, hepatosplenomegaly, rash, pneumonia, anemia, leukocytosis, and hypergammaglobulinemia. Abbreviated, CGD.

chronic leukemia. A form of leukemia in which the expected duration of life is 1 to 20 years or more. The cell types are usually the more mature forms of the specific blood series (granulocytic, lymphocytic, or monocytic). The onset is usually insidious, with few early symptoms.

chronic organic brain disorder. CHRONIC BRAIN SYNDROME.

chronic pharyngitis. A form of pharyngitis that is generally the result of repeated acute attacks and is associated with hypertrophic pharyngitis or atrophic pharyngitis.

chronic rhinitis. Rhinitis usually due to repeated attacks of acute rhinitis, producing in the early stages hypertrophic rhinitis and in the later stages atrophic rhinitis, and the presence of dark, offensive-smelling crusts (ozena).

chronic tuberculosis. Tuberculosis resulting

from progression of the primary lesion or reactivation of previously dormant foci, and rarely from exogenous reinfection. Syn. *adult-type tuberculosis.*

chrono·graph (kron'o·graf) *n.* An instrument for recording small intervals of time in physiologic and psychophysical experiments.

chron·o·log·ic (kron''uh·loj'ick) *adj.* 1. Arranged in time sequence. 2. Reckoned in terms of dates (years, months, days).

chronological age. The actual time elapsed since the birth of a living individual, as distinguished from anatomic, physiologic, developmental, or mental age. Abbreviated, CA.

chro·nom·e·try (kro·nom'e·tree) *n.* The measuring of time.

chrono·pho·bia (kron''o·fo'bee·uh) *n.* An abnormal fear of time.

chrono·tro·pic (kron''o·trop'ick, tro'pick) *adj.* Having an effect on or influencing the cardiac rate.

chrys-, chryso- A combining form meaning *gold, golden yellow,* or *yellow.*

chrys·a·ro·bin (kris''uh·ro'bin) *n.* A substance obtained from Goa powder, deposited in the wood of *Andira araroba,* a Brazilian tree. It is a brown to orange-yellow powder; chemically, it is largely a complex mixture of reduction products of chrysophanic acid, emodin, and the methyl ether of the latter. Used in the treatment of skin diseases.

chrys·i·a·sis (kri·sigh'uh·sis) *n.,* pl. **chrysia·ses** (·seez) A permanent pigmentation of the skin caused by the parenteral use of gold preparations; may be reticular in type, but is usually patchy, exaggerated by exposure to sunlight.

chryso-. See *chrys-.*

chryso·cy·a·no·sis (kris''o·sigh''uh·no'sis) *n.,* pl. **chrysocyano·ses** (·seez) A bluish discoloration of the skin caused by intracutaneous deposition of some gold salts.

chryso·der·ma (kris''o·dur'muh) *n.* CHRYSIASIS.

chry·soph·a·nol (kri·sof'uh·nol) *n.* 1,8-Dihydroxy-3-methylanthraquinone, $C_{15}H_{10}O_4$, a constituent of rhubarb, aloes, cascara, of species of *Rhamnus,* and of chrysarobin.

Chry·sops (krye'sops) *n.* A genus of small tabanid, biting flies, abundant in temperate and tropical America and Africa; certain species transmit diseases to man and animals. *Chrysops discalis,* the western deer fly, transfers *Pasteurella tularensis,* which causes tularemia. *C. silacea* and *C. dimidiata* are intermediate hosts of *Loa loa.*

chryso·ther·a·py (kris''o·therr'uh·pee) *n.* The use of gold compounds in the treatment of disease.

Chvos·tek's sign (khvos'teck) A sign of facial nerve hyperirritability in which tapping of the face in front of the ear produces spasm of the ipsilateral facial muscles; an important sign in tetany and hypocalcemic states, and seen in other conditions, including anxiety states.

chyl-, chyli-, chylo-. A combining form meaning *chyle.*

chyl·an·gi·o·ma (kigh·lan''jee·o'muh) *n.* 1. Retention of chyle in lymphatic vessels with dilatation of the latter. 2. A lymphangioma containing chyle.

chyle (kile) *n.* A milk-white emulsion of fat globules in lymph formed in the small intestine during digestion. **—chy·lous** (kigh'lus) *adj.*

chy·le·mia, chy·lae·mia (kigh·lee'mee·uh) *n.* The presence of chyle in the blood.

chylo-. See *chyl-.*

chy·lo·cele (kigh'lo·seel) *n.* Accumulation of chyle in the tunica vaginalis of the testis.

chy·lo·me·di·as·ti·num (kigh''lo·mee''dee·as·tye'num) *n.* The presence of chyle in the mediastinum.

chy·lor·rhea, chy·lor·rhoea (kigh''lo·ree'uh) *n.* 1. An excessive flow of chyle. 2. Diarrhea characterized by a milky color of the feces due to the rupture of small intestinal lymphatics. 3. Release of chyle from rupture or other injury of the thoracic duct.

chy·lo·sis (kigh·lo'sis) *n.,* pl. **chy·lo·ses** (·seez) The conversion of food into chyle, followed by absorption of the chyle.

chy·lo·tho·rax (kigh''lo·tho'racks) *n.* An accumulation of chyle in the thoracic cavity.

chy·lous (kigh'lus) *adj.* Pertaining to or involving chyle.

chylous ascites. ASCITES CHYLOSUS.

chy·lu·ria (kigh·lew'ree·uh) *n.* The presence of chyle or lymph in the urine, usually due to a fistulous communication between the urinary and lymphatic tracts or to lymphatic obstruction.

chyme (kime) *n.* 1. Strictly: the viscid, fluid contents of the stomach consisting of food that has undergone gastric digestion, and has not yet passed into the duodenum. 2. Loosely: any digesta in the stomach or small intestine. **—chy·mous** (kigh'mus) *adj.*

chy·mo·sin·o·gen (kigh''mo·sin'o·jen) *n.* The precursor of chymosin or rennin.

chy·mo·tryp·sin (kigh''mo·trip'sin) *n.* A proteolytic enzyme found in the intestine and formed from the chymotrypsinogen of the pancreatic juice by the action of trypsin. It acts simultaneously with trypsin to hydrolyze proteins and protein digestion products to polypeptides and amino acids. Chymotrypsin of bovine origin, obtainable in α-, β-, and γ-forms, differs in solubility and other properties. The enzyme is used to reduce soft-tissue inflammation and edema; the α- form is employed in zonulysis.

chy·mo·tryp·sin·o·gen (kigh''mo·trip·sin'o·jen) *n.* The precursor, occurring in pancreatic juice, of the enzyme chymotrypsin.

C. I. Abbreviation for (a) *color index;* (b) *chemotherapeutic index.*

ci·bo·pho·bia (sigh''bo·fo'bee·uh) *n.* Abnormal aversion to food, or to eating.

cic·a·tri·cial (sick''uh·trish'ul) *adj.* Pertaining to or like a scar.

cic·a·trix (sick'uh·tricks) *n.,* pl. **cic·a·tri·ces** (sick''uh·trye'seez), **cicatrixes** The fibrous connective tissue which follows healing of a wound or loss of substance due to infection. Typically soft and red when new, it tends to become avascular, hard, and contracted when old; SCAR.

ci·clo·pro·fen (sigh''klo·pro'fen) *n.* α-Methylfluorene-2-acetic acid, $C_{16}H_{14}O_2$, an anti-inflammatory agent.

-cide A combining form meaning (a) *killer;* (b) *killing.*

ci·dox·e·pin (sigh·dock'se·pin) *n.* 3-Dibenz[*b,e*]oxepin-11(6*H*)-ylidene-*N,N*-dimethyl-1-propanamine, $C_{19}H_{21}NO$, an antidepressant.

cig·a·rette drain. A drain of gauze surrounded by rubber tissue, rubber dam, or split rubber tubing.

ci·gua·te·ra (see''gwuh·terr'uh) *n.* A serious and sometimes fatal disease caused by ingestion of a variety of tropical marine fishes.

cili-, cilio- A combining form meaning (a) *cilia;* (b) *ciliary.*

cil·ia (sil'ee·uh) *n. pl.,* sing. **cil·i·um** (·ee·um) 1. [NA] EYELASHES. 2. The threadlike cytoplasmic processes of cells which beat rhythmically, thereby causing the locomotion of certain aquatic organisms or propelling fluids over surfaces covered by ciliated cells.

cil·i·ary (sil'ee·uh·ree, ·err''ee) *adj.* 1. Pertaining to or resembling an eyelid or eyelash. 2. Pertaining to the ciliary body or its component structures. 3. Pertaining to or resembling cilia.

ciliary artery. Any of the many branches of the ophthalmic and lacrimal arteries which supply the choroid, the ciliary body, and the iris. The posterior ciliary arteries arise from the ophthalmic artery and pass through the sclera near the optic nerve, with the several short posterior ciliary arteries supplying the choroid and the two long posterior ciliary arteries passing between the sclera and the choroid to the ciliary body, where they anastomose with the anterior ciliary arteries. The several anterior ciliary arteries derive from the lacrimal artery and the ophthalmic artery, give off episcleral and conjunctival branches, pierce the sclera near the cornea, and anastomose with the long posterior ciliary arteries in the greater arterial circle of the iris, which supplies the ciliary body and the iris.

ciliary blepharitis. MARGINAL BLEPHARITIS.

ciliary body. A wedge-shaped thickening in the middle layer (vascular tunic) of the eyeball, anterior to the choroid and posterior to the iris, consisting of the ciliary ring, the ciliary muscle, and, on the internal surface, the ciliary crown, which bears the ciliary processes.

ciliary glands. Modified sweat glands of the eyelids.

ciliary muscle. The muscular band which is located in the anterior outer portion of the ciliary body overlying the ciliary crown and whose contraction effects accommodation for near vision by relaxing the zonular fibers attached to the ciliary processes, thus allowing the lens to become more convex.

ciliary zonule. The suspensory structure for the lens of the eye, consisting of filaments (zonular fibers) attached to the capsule of the lens in the region of the equator and radiating outward to the ciliary body. Syn. *zonule of Zinn.*

Cil·i·a·ta (sil''ee·ay'tuh) *n. pl.* A class of Protozoa characterized by the presence of cilia. The only important human ciliate is the intestinal parasite *Balantidium coli.*

cil·io·cy·to·pho·ria (sil''ee·o·sigh''to·for'ee·uh) *n.* Massive destruction of the ciliated bronchial epithelium associated with certain infections, especially virus pneumonia.

cil·io·scle·ral (sil''ee·o·skleer'ul) *adj.* Pertaining to the ciliary body and the sclera of the eye.

cil·io·spi·nal (sil''ee·o·spye'nul) *adj.* Pertaining to the ciliary body and the spinal cord.

ciliospinal reflex. Dilatation of the ipsilateral pupil on pinching the skin on one side of the neck.

cilium. Singular of *cilia;* EYELASH.

cil·lo·sis (si·lo'sis) *n.* A spasmodic trembling of the eyelid. —**cil·lot·ic** (·lot'ick) *adj.*

Ci·mex (sigh'mecks) *n.* A genus of bedbugs and similar insects of the family Cimicidae, species of which are parasitic to man and vectors of disease.

Cimex lec·tu·la·rius (leck''tew·lair'ee·us) The common bedbug.

cin·cho·na (sing·ko'nuh) *n.* The dried bark of the stem or root of *Cinchona succirubra* or its hybrids, known as red cinchona, or of *C. ledgeriana, C. calisaya,* or hybrids of these with other species of *Cinchona,* known as calisaya bark or yellow cinchona. The trees are natives of South America. Cinchona contains more than 20 alkaloids, the most important being quinine, quinidine, cinchonine, and cinchonidine. Cinchona has the physiologic action and therapeutic uses of its chief alkaloid, quinine. It is also an astringent, bitter, and stomachic tonic. Syn. *Peruvian bark, Jesuits' bark.* —**cin·chon·ic** (sing·kon'ick) *adj.;* **cin·chon·i·za·tion** (sing·kon''i·zay'shun) *n.;* **cin·chon·ize** (sing'kon·ize) *v.*

cin·chon·a·mine (sing·kon·am'een, ·in, sing·kon'uh·meen, ·min) *n.* An alkaloid, $C_{19}H_{24}N_2O$, of cuprea bark.

cin·chon·i·dine (sing·kon'i·deen, ·din) *n.* An alkaloid, $C_{19}H_{22}N_2O$, from cinchona; it resembles quinine in its actions.

cin·cho·nine (sing'ko·neen, ·nin) *n.* An alkaloid, $C_{19}H_{22}N_2O$, derived from cinchona. It is similar to quinine in therapeutic effects, but less active.

cin·cho·nism (sing'ko·niz·um) *n.* The adverse systemic effect of cinchona or its alkaloids when given in full doses or the toxic effects of excessive use of these drugs. The symptoms include anorexia, nausea, vomiting, diarrhea, vertigo, tinnitus, headache, and visual disturbances.

cin·cho·phen (sing'ko·fen) *n.* 2-Phenylcinchoninic acid, $C_{16}H_{11}NO_2$, a white powder, almost insoluble in water. It has been used as a uricosuric agent, but it may cause severe toxic effects, including hepatitis.

cinc·ture (sink'chur) *n.* A girdle or belt.

cincture sensation. A sensation of constriction around the body.

cine- A combining form meaning *motion picture.*

cine (sin'ee) *adj.* Motion-picture, cinematic.

cine·an·gio·car·dio·gram (sin''ee·an''jee·o·kahr''dee·o·gram) *n.* An angiocardiogram recorded with x-ray motion-picture technique.

cine·an·gio·car·di·og·ra·phy (sin''ee·an''jee·o·kahr''dee·og'ruh·fee) *n.* The use of a motion-picture camera to record fluoroscopic images of the heart and great vessels after injection of radiopaque contrast material.

cine–angiogram, n. An angiogram recorded with x-ray motion-picture technique.

cine·esoph·a·go·gram (sin″ee·e·sof′uh·go·gram) n. An esophagogram recorded by x-ray motion-picture technique.

cine·flu·o·rog·ra·phy (sin″e·floo″ur·og′ruh·fee) n. The motion-picture recording of fluoroscopic images.

cin·e·plas·tic (sin″e·plas′tick) adj. KINEPLASTIC.

ci·ne·rea (si·neer′ee·uh) n. The gray substance of the brain or spinal cord.

cine·roent·gen·og·ra·phy (sin″e·rent″gen·og′ruh·fee) n. The depiction of the anatomic structure of an organ, usually in motion, by x-ray motion-picture technique.

cin·gu·late (sing′gew·late, ·lut) adj. 1. Of or pertaining to a cingulum. 2. Having a zone or girdle, usually of transverse bands or marks.

cingulate gyrus. The convolution that lies immediately above the corpus callosum on the medial aspect of each cerebral hemisphere. Syn. *gyrus cinguli [NA]. callosal gyrus.*

cin·gu·lec·to·my (sing″gew·leck′tuh·mee) n. Surgical removal under direct vision of a portion of the cingulate gyrus, usually Brodmann's area 24 and immediately adjacent tissue.

cin·gu·lot·o·my (sing″gew·lot′uh·mee) n. The interruption of fibers of the white matter of the cingulate gyrus by means of stereotactic application of heat or cold.

cin·gu·lo·trac·to·my (sing″gew·lo·track′tuh·mee) n. The surgical incision of the projections of the cingulate gyrus to the thalamus. It is used rarely, in control of psychotic disorders.

cin·gu·lum (sing′gew·lum) n., genit. **cingu·li** (·lye), pl. **cingu·la** (·luh) 1. A girdle or zone. 2. *Obsol.* HERPES ZOSTER. 3. [NA] A bundle of association fibers running in the cingulate gyrus of the brain from the anterior perforated substance to the hippocampal gyrus. 4. [NA] BASAL RIDGE.

cin·na·mal·de·hyde (sin″uh·mal′de·hide) n. Cinnamic aldehyde, $C_6H_5CH=CHCHO$, the chief constituent of cinnamon oil and prepared synthetically. A flavoring agent.

cin·nam·e·in (si·nam′ee·in, sin″uh·mee′in) n. Benzyl cinnamate, $C_{16}H_{14}O_2$, a constituent of Peruvian and tolu balsams.

cin·nam·ic acid (si·nam′ick). 3-Phenylpropenoic acid, $C_6H_5CH=CHCOOH$, occurring in Peruvian and tolu balsams, storax, and some benzoin resins. It has been used in treating tuberculosis.

cin·na·mon (sin′uh·mun) n. The dried bark of several species of *Cinnamomum,* native to Ceylon and China, the latter variety being known in commerce under the name of cassia. *Cinnamomum loureirii,* Saigon cinnamon, and *C. zeylanicum,* Ceylon cinnamon, are commonly used. It contains a volatile oil, and is used as a carminative and aromatic stimulant, and as a spice.

cinnamon oil. The volatile oil obtained from the leaves and twigs of *Cinnamomum cassia.* Its chief constituent is cinnamaldehyde. Syn. *cassia oil.*

cir·ca·di·an (sur·kay′dee·un) adj. Manifested or recurring in cycles of about 24 hours.

cir·ci·nate (sur′si·nate) adj. Having a circular outline or a ring formation.

circinate retinopathy. A lesion seen in a number of conditions in which vascular inadequacy is present, characterized by a complete or incomplete ring of lipids deposited in the deeper layers of the retina, usually in the area centralis.

cir·cle, n. 1. A ring; a line, every point on which is equidistant from a point called the center. 2. A ringlike anastomosis of arteries or veins.

circle of diffusion. The imperfect image formed by incomplete focalization, the position of the true focus not having been reached by some of the rays of light, or else having been passed.

circle of Wil·lis ARTERIAL CIRCLE OF THE CEREBRUM.

cir·cuit (sur′kit) n. A path or course which, when not interrupted, returns upon itself, such as the path of a circulating fluid in a system of tubes, or the path of nerve impulses in reflex arcs.

cir·cu·lar (sur′kew·lur) adj. 1. Ring-shaped. 2. Pertaining to a circle. 3. Marked by alternations of despondency and excitation, as in a manic-depressive illness.

circular amputation. An operation performed with the use of a flap by circular sweeps or incisions around the limb vertical to the long axis of the bone.

circular insanity or **dementia.** Manic-depressive illness of the circular type.

circular sinus. A sinus consisting of the two cavernous sinuses and their communications across the median line by means of the anterior and posterior intercavernous sinuses, all of which surround the hypophysis.

cir·cu·la·tion (sur″kew·lay′shun) n. Passage in a circuit, as the circulation of the blood. —**cir·cu·la·to·ry** (sur′kew·luh·tor″ee) adj.

circulation time. The rate of blood flow; the time required for blood to flow from one part of the body to another, as from arm to lung or arm to tongue, or to pass through the whole circulatory system.

circulatory failure. Inadequacy of the cardiovascular system to fulfill its function of providing transport of nutritive and other substance to and from the tissue cells; it may be caused by cardiac or peripheral conditions.

circum- A prefix meaning *around, about, on all sides, surrounding.*

cir·cum·anal (sur″kum·ay′nul) adj. Periproctal; surrounding the anus.

circumanal glands. The sebaceous and apocrine glands in the skin about the anus.

cir·cum·ar·tic·u·lar (sur″kum·ahr·tick′yoo·lur) adj. Around a joint.

cir·cum·ci·sion (sur″kum·sizh′un) n. The removal of the foreskin; excision of the prepuce. —**cir·cum·cise** (sur′kum·size) v.

cir·cum·cor·ne·al (sur″kum·kor′nee·ul) adj. Around or about the cornea.

cir·cum·duc·tion (sur″kum·duck′shun) n. The movement of a limb in such a manner that its distal part describes a circle, the proximal end being fixed.

cir·cum·fer·en·tial (sur·kum″fur·en′shul) adj. Pertaining to the circumference; encircling.

cir·cum·flex (sur′kum·flecks) adj. Bending

around; designating a number of arteries having a winding course.

cir·cum·in·su·lar (sur″kum·in′sue′lur) *adj.* Surrounding the insula of the cerebral cortex.

cir·cum·len·tal (sur″kum·len′tul) *adj.* Surrounding a lens.

cir·cum·lin·ear (sur″kum·lin′ee·ur) *adj.* Around a line.

cir·cum·lo·cu·tion (sur″kum·lo·kew′shun) *n.* A roundabout way of speaking; the use of several words to express the idea of a single one; may be volitional or due to partial aphasia. —**circum·loc·u·to·ry** (·lock′yoo.to·ree) *adj.*

cir·cum·nu·cle·ar (sur″kum·new′klee·ur) *adj.* Surrounding a nucleus; PERINUCLEAR.

cir·cum·oral (sur″kum·or′ul) *adj.* Surrounding the mouth.

cir·cum·pulp·ar (sur″kum·pulp′ur) *adj.* Surrounding the pulp of a tooth.

cir·cum·scribed (sur″kum·skrye′bd) *adj.* Enclosed within narrow limits by an encircling boundary.

circumscribed myxedema. Circumscribed deposition of mucinous material in the pretibial skin, occurring during thyrotoxicosis or treatment for thyrotoxicosis. Syn. *pretibial myxedema.*

cir·cum·stan·ti·al·i·ty (sur″kum·stan″shee·al′i·tee) *n. In psychiatry,* indulging in many irrelevant and unnecessary details when answering a simple question because of too little selective suppression.

cir·cum·ton·sil·lar (sur″kum·ton′si·lur) *adj.* PERITONSILLAR.

cir·cum·val·late (sur″kum·val′ate) *adj.* Surrounded by a trench, as the vallate papillae of the tongue.

circumvallate papilla. VALLATE PAPILLA.

circumvallate placenta. A placenta in which an overgrowth of decidua parietalis separates the placental margin from the chorionic membranous plate, resulting in the formation of a thick white ring about the circumference of the placenta and reduction in distribution of fetal blood vessels to the placental periphery.

cir·cus (sur′kus) *adj.* Characterized by circular movements.

circus movement. 1. Rapid, circular movements or somersaults, produced by injury on one side to some part of the posture-controlling mechanisms of the nervous system, as the vestibular apparatus or the cerebral peduncles. 2. A rolling gait with circumduction as seen in certain basal ganglion disorders. 3. A theory of the mechanism of atrial flutter and fibrillation in which a circular unidirectional excitation wave travels around and around the atrium and reenters the same pathway to initiate another contraction cycle, because the atrial tissue is no longer refractory to stimulation when the original impulse reaches its starting point.

cir·rho·sis (si·ro′sis) *n.,* pl. **cirrho·ses** (·seez) 1. Any diffuse fibrosis which destroys the normal lobular architecture of the liver with destruction and regeneration of hepatic parenchymal cells. 2. Interstitial inflammation of any tissue or organ. —**cir·rhot·ic** (si·rot′ick) *adj.*

cir·sec·to·my (sur·seck′tuh·mee) *n.* Excision of a varix or a portion thereof.

cir·soid (sur′soid) *adj.* Resembling a varix or dilated vein.

cirsoid aneurysm. 1. A tortuous lengthening and dilatation of a part of an artery. Syn. *racemose aneurysm.* 2. A dilatation of a group of vessels (arteries, veins, and capillaries), the whole forming a pulsating subcutaneous tumor, occurring most often in the scalp. Syn. *anastomotic aneurysm.*

cis- A prefix meaning (a) *on this side, on the same side;* (b) *in chemistry,* having certain atoms or groups of atoms on the same side of a molecule; usually restricted to cyclic compounds with two stereogenic atoms.

cis·tern (sis′turn) *n.* 1. A reservoir. 2. A large subarachnoid space.

cis·ter·na (sis·tur′nuh) *n.,* pl. **cister·nae** (·nee) 1. CISTERN. 2. CISTERNA CHYLI.

cisterna chy·li (kigh′lye) [NA]. The saclike beginning of the thoracic duct, located between the crura of the diaphragm at the level of the last thoracic vertebra.

cisternae sub·arach·noi·da·les (sub″uh·rack″noy·day′leez) [BNA]. CISTERNAE SUBARACHNOIDEALES.

cis·ter·nal (sis·tur′nul) *adj.* Of or pertaining to a cistern or cisterna.

cisternal puncture. Puncture of the cisterna magna with a hollow needle, for diagnostic or therapeutic purposes.

cisterna mag·na (mag′nuh). CEREBELLOMEDULLARY CISTERN.

cis·tern·og·ra·phy (sis″tur·nog′ruh·fee) *n. In radiology,* the visualization of the subarachnoid cisterns of the posterior fossa by means of special contrast media.

cis-trans effect (sis tranz). *In genetics,* a phenomenon whereby two separate mutant genes produce a phenotypic effect when located on homologous chromosomes (trans) but not when located on the same chromosome (cis), indicating that they belong to the same functional unit (cistron) and are allelic.

cis·tron (sis′tron) *n.* The portion of genetic material (DNA) that codes, and is responsible for the synthesis of, a protein or a polypeptide chain; classified according to their genetic response in the cis-trans effect.

cis·ves·ti·tism (sis·ves′ti·tiz·um) *n.* The practice of dressing in clothes suitable to the sex, but not the age, occupation, or position of the wearer, as in the case of a civilian impersonating a military person.

cit·ral (sit′al) *n.* 3,7-Dimethyl-2,6-octadienal, $C_{10}H_{16}O$, an aldehyde in oils of lemon, orange, and lemon grass; occurs as a mixture of two geometric isomers, known as geranial and neral. A yellow liquid of strong lemon odor; used as a flavor.

cit·rate (sit′rate, sigh″trate) *n. & v.* 1. Any salt or ester of citric acid. 2. To treat with a citrate or citric acid.

citrate synthase. An enzyme, present in large variety of animal, plant, and bacterial cells, that catalyzes condensation of acetyl coenzyme A with oxaloacetate to form citrate, in the first step of the citric acid cycle. Syn. *citric* *synthase, citrate condensing enzyme, citric condensing enzyme, citrogenase, condensing enzyme, oxaloacetate transacetase.*

cit·ric acid (sit'rick). 2-Hydroxy-1,2,3-propanetricarboxylic acid, $C_6H_8O_7$, widely distributed in plant and animal tissues; may be obtained from citrus fruits. White crystals or powder; very soluble in water. Used as an acidulant in pharmaceutical preparations, beverages, and confectionery. In the body, it is oxidized to carbon dioxide and water.

cit·rin (sit'rin) *n.* A crystalline substance, said to be a mixture of hesperidin, quercitrin, and eriodictyol glycoside, isolated from lemon juice. It combats the increased permeability of capillary walls, such as occurs in scurvy and certain other diseases.

cit·ro·gen·ase (sit''ro·jen'ace, ·aze, si·troj'en·ace, ·aze) *n.* CITRATE SYNTHASE.

cit·ron (sit'run) *n.* The tree, *Citrus medica*, or its fruit. The fruit rind is used in conserves.

cit·ro·nel·lal (sit''ro·nel'al) *n.* A mixture of stereoisomeric aldehydes, of the formula $C_{10}H_{18}O$, in citronella oil and other volatile oils.

cit·ro·nel·la oil (sit''ruh·nel'uh). A yellowish-green volatile oil obtained chiefly from the sweet-scented citronella grass. It consists largely of geraniol and citronellal; an insect repellant.

ci·tro·vo·rum factor (si·tro'vo·rum). A growth factor for *Leuconostoc citrovorum*, found in liver and green vegetables; member of the vitamin B complex closely related, if not identical, to folinic acid (2).

ci·trul·line (sit'rul·een, si·trul') *n.* δ-Ureidonorvaline, $C_6H_{13}N_3O_3$, an amino acid, first isolated from watermelon, involved in the formation, in the liver, of urea from ammonia and carbon dioxide; it is an intermediate between ornithine and arginine, two other amino acids involved in producing urea.

ci·trul·lin·emia, ci·trul·lin·ae·mia (sit''rul·in·ee'mee·uh, si·trul'') *n.* An inborn error of amino acid metabolism in which there is a deficiency in argininosuccinic acid synthetase in the liver, an excessive amount of citrulline in blood, urine, and cerebrospinal fluid, and ammonia intoxication; manifested clinically by failure to thrive, vomiting, irritability, seizures, mental retardation, cortical atrophy, and disturbances of liver function.

Cit·rus (sit'rus) *n.* A genus of trees of the Rutaceae. From this genus come the orange, lemon, citron, lime, and bergamot.

cit·to·sis (si·to'sis) *n.* PICA.

Cl Symbol for chlorine.

cl Abbreviation for *centiliter*.

Cl. Abbreviation for *Clostridium*.

Clad·o·spo·ri·um (klad''o·spo'ree·um) *n.* A genus of darkly pigmented fungi, including saprophytic and pathogenic species, in which conidiophores produce conidia in branched chains, called the Cladosporium type of sporulation (formerly called Hormodendrum type). *Cladosporium carrioni* is one of the fungi causing chromoblastomycosis; *C. mansonii* causes tinea nigra in Asia, and *C. werneckii*, in the Americas. *Cladosporium trichoides* (*C. bantianum*) causes brain and lung abscesses.

clair·voy·ance (klair·voy'unce) *n.* The direct awareness, with no help from sense impressions, of events taking place in the outside world.

clamp, *n.* An instrument for holding and compressing vessels or hollow organs to prevent hemorrhage or the escape of contents during the progress of an operation.

clang association Association of words or of ideas with words because of their similarity in sound; seen in psychoses, particularly in manic-depressive illness and schizophrenia.

clap, *n.* GONORRHEA.

clap·ping, *n. In massage,* percussion movements in which the cupped palms are brought down alternately in a rapid succession of blows. The movement of the hands is chiefly from the wrist.

clar·i·ficant (kla·rif'i·kunt) *n.* An agent used to clarify turbid liquids.

clar·i·fy (klăr'i·fye) *v.* To remove the turbidity of a liquid or a naturally transparent substance by allowing the suspended matter to subside, by adding a clarificant or substance that precipitates suspended matter, or by moderate heating. —**clar·i·fy·ing,** *adj.;* **clar·i·fi·ca·tion** (klăr''i·fi·kay'shun) *n.*

Clarke's column THORACIC NUCLEUS.

Clark's body area rule A rule to determine dosage of medicine for children; specifically, dose = body surface area of child, multiplied by adult dose, divided by body surface area of adult (or 1.7 m²).

Clark's rule A rule to determine dosage of medicine for children; specifically, dose = child's weight in pounds, multiplied by adult dose, divided by 150.

-clasis A combining form meaning *breaking, breaking up.*

clas·ma·to·cyte (klaz·mat'o·site, klaz'muh·to·) *n.* A macrophage of connective tissue. —**clasmato·cyt·ic** (klaz·mat''o·sit'ick, klaz''muh·to·) *adj.*

clas·mo·cy·to·ma (klaz''mo·sigh·to'muh) *n.* RETICULUM-CELL SARCOMA.

clasp-knife phenomenon, rigidity, or **spasticity.** A form of the stretch reflex in which resistance of a muscle to passive extension is followed by sudden relaxation, like the snapping of a clasp-knife blade; seen especially in spastic hemiparesis.

-clast A combining form meaning *something* (as an instrument) *that breaks.*

clas·tic (klas'tick) *adj.* Breaking up into fragments; causing division.

clas·to·thrix (klas'to·thricks) *n.* TRICHORRHEXIS NODOSA.

-clasty A combining form meaning *breaking, breaking up.*

clau·di·ca·tion (klaw·di·kay'shun) *n.* 1. Lameness or limping. 2. Specifically, INTERMITTENT CLAUDICATION.

claus·tro·phil·ia (klaws''tro·fil'ee·uh) *n.* An abnormal desire to shut doors and windows and be shut up in a confined space.

claus·tro·pho·bia (klaws''tro·fo'bee·uh) *n.* An abnormal fear of being in a small room or in a confined space, such as a railway compartment.

claus·trum (klaws'trum) *n.*, pl. **claus·tra** (·truh) 1. A barrier, as a membrane partially closing an opening, or one bearing a resemblance to a barrier. 2. [NA] The layer of gray matter between the insula of the cerebral cortex and the lenticular nucleus. —**claus·tral** (·trul) *adj.*

cla·va (klay'vuh) *n.*, pl. **cla·vae** (·vee) One of the two ovoid eminences in the caudal end of the fourth ventricle, representing continuations of the fasciculus gracilis. Subjacent to the clava is the gracilis nucleus. —**cla·val** (·vul) *adj.*

clav·a·cin (klav'uh·sin) *n.* An antibiotic substance, $C_7H_6O_4$, produced in cultures of several different fungi. Syn. *clavatin, claviformin, patulin.*

cla·vate (klay'vate) *adj.* Club-shaped.

Clav·i·ceps (klav'i·seps) *n.* A genus of fungi. The sclerotium of *Claviceps purpurea*, developed on plants of rye, *Secale cereale*, is the source of ergot.

clav·i·cle (klav'i·kul) *n.* A bone of the shoulder girdle articulating medially with the sternum and laterally with the acromion of the scapula; the collarbone. —**cla·vic·u·lar** (kla·vick'yoo·lur) *adj.*

cla·vic·u·lec·to·my (kla·vick"yoo·leck'tuh·mee) *n. In surgery,* removal of the clavicle, performed in some cases of thyroid cancer or other tumors, osteomyelitis of the clavicle, and limitation of arm motion where the shoulder joint has become fused.

clavi·pec·to·ral (klav"i·peck'tuh·rul) *adj.* Pertaining to the clavicle and the chest.

cla·vus (klay'vus) *n.*, pl. **cla·vi** (·vye) 1. A corn; a cone-shaped, circumscribed hyperplasia of the horny layer of the epidermis, in which there is an ingrowth as well as an outgrowth of horny substance forming epidermal thickenings, chiefly about the toes; caused by friction or pressure. 2. A severe headache described as the sensation of a nail being driven into the head.

claw foot. TALIPES CAVUS.

claw hand. A deformity, resulting from paralysis of the ulnar and/or median nerve, in which there is hyperextension of the proximal phalanges of the fingers and flexion of the terminal two phalanges, abduction of the fifth finger, and flattening of the hand. It is also seen as an end result of Volkmann's contracture.

clear·ance, *n.* The removal of a substance from the blood by the kidneys.

clearance test. 1. A test of the excretory efficiency of the kidneys based upon the amount of blood cleared of a substance in 1 minute as determined by the ratio of the substance in the blood to the amount excreted in the urine during a fixed time. 2. A test for liver function based on the ability of the liver to remove a substance from the blood.

clear·ing, *n.* 1. The displacement of alcohol or other dehydrating agent from tissue blocks by a paraffin solvent, preparatory to paraffin infiltration and embedding of histologic specimens. 2. The displacement of dehydrating agent from a stained section by an essential oil, xylene, or other liquid, to increase the clarity and transparency and prepare the section for mounting in a resinous mounting medium.

cleav·age (klee'vij) *n.* 1. The linear clefts in the skin indicating the general direction of the fibers and to a certain extent governing the arrangement of lesions in skin diseases. 2. An early stage of the process of development between fertilization and the blastula, when the embryo consists of a mass of dividing cells, the blastomeres. 3. The process or act of splitting or producing a cleft.

cleavage lines. Lines plotted on the skin to indicate the direction of tension. These lines lie in the direction in which the skin stretches least and are perpendicular to the direction of greatest stretch. Thus, linear scars following the direction of skin tension usually spread little, whereas scars crossing cleavage lines have an opposite tendency.

cleavage plane. 1. The area in a cell or developing ovum where cell division takes place. 2. Any plane in the body along which organs or structures may be separated with minimal damage.

cleft, *adj. & n.* 1. Divided. 2. A fissure; especially one of embryonic origin.

cleft lip. HARELIP.

cleft palate. A congenital defect due to failure of fusion of embryonic facial processes resulting in a fissure through the palate. This may be complete, extending through both hard and soft palates into the nose, or any degree of incomplete, or partial, cleft. Often associated with harelip.

cleft uvula. A congenital condition in which the uvula is split into two halves because of the failure of the posterior palatine folds to unite.

cleid-, cleido- A combining form meaning *clavicle, clavicular.*

clei·do·cos·tal (klye"do·kos'tul) *adj.* Pertaining to the ribs and the clavicle.

clei·do·cra·ni·al (klye"do·kray'nee·ul) *adj.* Pertaining to the clavicle and the cranium.

cleidocranial dysostosis, dysplasia, or **dystrophia.** A congenital complex consisting of poor tooth formation, incomplete ossification of the skull, malformation of the palatine arch, and more or less aplasia of the clavicles. Other bones may also be involved. The head is often large and brachicephalic, and there is shortness without dwarfism; may be due to a dominant genetic factor.

clei·do·hu·mer·al (klye"do·hew'mur·ul) *adj.* Pertaining to the clavicle and the humerus.

clei·do·ic (klye·do'ick, klye·do·ick) *adj.* Isolated from the environment; self-contained.

clei·do·mas·toid (klye"do·mas'toid) *adj.* Pertaining to the clavicle and the mastoid process.

clei·do·scap·u·lar (klye"do·skap'yoo·lur) *adj.* Pertaining to the clavicle and the scapula.

clei·do·ster·nal (klye"do·stur'nul) *adj.* Pertaining to the clavicle and the sternum.

clei·dot·o·my (klye·dot'uh·mee) *n. In obstetrics,* section of the clavicles when the shoulders of the fetus are too broad to pass; an operation performed when the head is delivered, and the child dead.

-cleisis A combining form meaning *closure, occlusion.*

cleist-, cleisto-, clist-, clisto- A combining form meaning *closed.*

clei·thro·pho·bia (klye"thro·fo'bee·uh) *n.* CLAUSTROPHOBIA.

clem·as·tine (klem'us·teen) *n.* (+)-2-[2-[(*p*-Chloro-α-methyl-α-phenylbenzyl)oxy]ethyl]-1-methylpyrrolidine, $C_{21}H_{26}ClNO$, an antihistaminic drug.

cli·ma·co·pho·bia (klye"muh·ko·fo'bee·uh) *n.* An abnormal fear of steps or staircases.

cli·mac·ter·ic (klye·mack'tur·ick, klye"mack·terr'ick) *n. & adj.* **1.** A period of life at which the bodily system is believed to undergo marked changes, usually between the ages of 40 to 50; the period in which menopause occurs. **2.** Of or pertaining to this period of life.

climacteric insanity, melancholia, or **psychosis.** An involutional psychotic disorder occurring at the menopause or at the corresponding age period in men.

cli·mac·te·ri·um (klye"mack·tirr'ee·um) *n.,* pl. **climacte·ria** (·ee·uh) [NL.]. CLIMACTERIC.

cli·mat·ic bubo. LYMPHOGRANULOMA VENEREUM.

cli·ma·tol·o·gy (klye"muh·tol'uh·jee) *n. In medicine,* the study of climate in relation to health and disease.

cli·max, *n.* **1.** The height of a disease; the period of greatest intensity. **2.** ORGASM.

clin-, clino- A combining form meaning (a) *inclination;* (b) *declination;* (c) *clinoid.*

clin·ic (klin'ick) *n.* **1.** Medical instruction given at the bedside or in the presence of the patient whose symptoms are studied and whose treatment is considered. **2.** A place where such instruction is given. **3.** A gathering of instructors, students, and patients for the study and treatment of disease. **4.** A place where medical care is given to ambulant patients who live at home. **5.** A form of group practice in which several physicians work in cooperative association.

clin·i·cal (klin'i·kul) *adj.* **1.** Pertaining to bedside treatment or to a clinic. **2.** Pertaining to the symptoms and course of a disease as observed by the physician, in opposition to the anatomic changes found by the pathologist, or to a theoretical or experimental approach.

clinical chemistry. The science and practice of the chemical analysis of body tissues to diagnose disease.

clinical equivalents. Those chemical equivalents which provide the same therapeutic effects when administered in equal amounts.

clinical immunology. The study of immunological processes and immunologically mediated diseases in patients.

clinical medicine. **1.** The study of disease of the living patient. **2.** The instruction of medical students from living patients.

clinical nurse specialist. A professional nurse with highly developed knowledge and skills in the care of patients within some specialty; ordinarily holds a master's degree in the nursing specialty.

clinical oncology. The study of naturally occurring tumors in patients.

clinical-pathological conference. A teaching exercise in which a selected example of a disease process is presented by a clinician who does not know the diagnosis, but attempts to make one from the clinical record, while detailing his reasoning to the audience. A pathologist then presents the examination either of autopsy material or of tissue removed at surgery, usually making a definitive diagnosis. Another discussion of interesting points in differential diagnosis, pathogenesis, or treatment follows. Abbreviated, CPC.

clinical pathology. The diagnosis of disease by laboratory methods.

clinical pharmacy. The division of pharmacy concerned principally with the appropriate use of drugs by patients whether prescribed by the physician or self-administered. It involves drug selection and surveillance, and is concerned with patient response, adverse reactions, and the avoidance of undesirable drug interactions in the patient.

clinical psychologist. A psychologist with a graduate degree, usually a Ph.D. who has had additional supervised postdoctoral training, who specializes in clinical psychology.

clinical psychology. A branch of applied psychology which specializes, often in collaboration with physicians and psychiatrists in a medical or mental health setting, in the evaluation and treatment of mental, behavioral, and neurologic disorders, as well as research into psychological aspects of such disorders.

clinical record. A group of forms used by a physician, clinic, or hospital to record a patient's medical history. It covers the results of physical examination, laboratory findings, admission diagnosis, progress of the disease, medications used, consultations, operations performed, and final diagnosis and disposition.

clinical surgery. Surgery on patients, as opposed to experimental or animal surgery; the application of surgical knowledge to the care of patients.

cli·ni·cian (kli·nish'un) *n.* **1.** A physician whose opinions, teachings, and treatment are based upon experience with living patients. **2.** A clinical instructor. **3.** One who practices medicine.

clinico-. A combining form meaning *clinical.*

Clinitest reagent tablet. A trademark for a reagent tablet used to determine the quantity of reducing sugars in urine.

clino-. See *clin-.*

cli·no·ceph·a·ly (klye"no·sef'uh·lee) *n.* A congenital defect of the skull in which the upper surface is concave or saddle-shaped. **—clino·ce·phal·ic** (·se·fal'ick), **clino·ceph·a·lous** (·sef'uh·lus) *adj.*

cli·no·dac·tyl·ism (klye"no·dack'til·iz·um) *n.* A congenital defect consisting of abnormal bending of fingers or toes. **—clinodacty·lous** (·us) *adj.*

cli·noid (klye'noid) *adj.* Resembling a bed.

clinoid process. See *anterior clinoid process, middle clinoid process, posterior clinoid process.*

clip, *n.* A device or appliance used in surgery to grip skin or other tissue to secure apposition, to control hemorrhage, or to assist in localization by radiography.

clit·o·ral·gia (klit″o·ral′juh, ·jee·uh, klye″to·) *n.* Pain referred to the clitoris.

clitorid-, clitorido- A combining form meaning *clitoris.*

clit·o·ri·dec·to·my (klit″o·ri·deck′tuh·mee) *n.* Excision of the clitoris.

clit·o·ri·di·tis (klit″o·ri·dye′tis) *n.* Inflammation of the clitoris.

clit·o·ri·dot·o·my (klit″o·ri·dot′uh·mee) *n.* Incision of the clitoris.

clit·o·ris (klit′o·ris, klye′to·ris) *n.,* genit. sing. **cli·to·ri·dis** (kli·to′ri·dis), L. pl. **cli·to·ri·des** (kli·to′ri·deez) A small erectile organ of the female external genitalia measuring about 2 cm in length and located at the anterior junction of the labia minora; homologous to the penis in the male, but lacking a corpus spongiosum and urethral passage. Adj. **clitoral.**

clit·o·rism (klit′o·riz·um, klye′to·) *n.* 1. Enlargement or hypertrophy of the clitoris. 2. TRIBADISM. 3. A condition of painful and persistent erection of the clitoris; analogous to priapism in the male.

clit·o·ri·tis (klit″o·rye′tis, klye″to·) *n.* Inflammation of the clitoris.

clit·o·ro·meg·a·ly (klit″uh·ro·meg′uh·lee) *n.* A pathologically large clitoris.

cli·vus (klye′vus) *n.,* pl. **cli·vi** (·vye) 1. A slope. 2. [NA] The slanting dorsal surface of the body of the sphenoid bone between the sella turcica and the basilar process of the occipital bone.

clo (klo) *n.* An arbitrary quantitative unit of the thermal insulation value of clothing. *In aviation medicine,* 1 clo is the amount of clothing required to maintain in comfort a resting-sitting human adult male whose metabolic rate is approximately 50 kilogram calories per square meter of body surface per hour, when the environmental temperature is 70° F (21.1° C), and humidity is less than 50%. In terms of absolute thermal insulation units, 1 clo is 0.18° C per square meter per kilogram calorie per hour.

clo·a·ca (klo·ay′kuh) *n.,* pl. **cloa·cae** (·see) 1. In the early embryo, the entodermal chamber common to the hindgut and allantois; later to the hindgut and urogenital duct or sinus. 2. In Anamniota, Sauropsida, and aplacental mammals, a common chamber for the rectum and urogenital orifices. —**cloa·cal** (·kul) *adj.*

cloacal membrane. A delicate membrane of ectoderm and endoderm separating the embryonic hindgut from the external or ectodermal cloaca.

clo·dan·o·lene (klo·dan′o·leen) *n.* 1-[[5-(3,4-Dichlorophenyl)furfurylidene]amino]hydantoin, $C_{14}H_9Cl_2N_3O_3$, a skeletal muscle relaxant.

clo·fi·brate (klo·figh′brate) *n.* Ethyl 2-(*p*-chlorophenoxy)-2-methylpropionate, $C_{12}H_{15}ClO_3$, an anticholesteremic drug.

Clomid. Trademark for clomiphene, a drug that induces ovulation.

clo·mi·phene (klo′mi·feen) *n.* 2-[*p*-(2-Chloro-1,2-diphenylvinyl)phenoxy]triethylamine, $C_{26}H_{28}ClNO$, a drug that induces ovulation and is used, as the citrate salt, for the treatment of infertility associated with anovulation.

clone, *n.* A group of individuals of like genetic constitution obtained by asexual reproduction from a single original individual. Reproduction may occur by continued fission, as in bacteria or protozoa; by continued budding, as in hydras; or by propagation from cuttings, as in plants. 2. A group of cells derived from a single cell by repeated mitoses. —**clo·nal** (klo′nal) *adj.*

clo·nic (klo′nick, klon′ick) *adj.* Pertaining to clonus; characterized by rapid involuntary alternate muscular contractions and relaxations, applied especially to generalized seizures.

clo·nix·in (klo·nick′sin) *n.* 2-(3-Chloro-*o*-toluidino)nicotinic acid, $C_{13}H_{11}ClN_2O_2$, an analgesic.

clo·nor·chi·a·sis (klo″nor·kigh′uh·sis) *n.* An infection caused by *Clonorchis sinensis,* characterized by hepatic lesions produced by adult worms in the biliary passages.

Clo·nor·chis (klo·nor′kis, klon·or′kis) *n.* A genus of flukes indigenous to the Orient.

Clonorchis si·nen·sis (si·nen′sis). The most common of the liver flukes, having as definitive hosts man or other mammals.

clo·nus (klo′nus) *n.* A series of rapid rhythmic contractions of a muscle occurring in response to maintained passive stretch of the muscle, as ankle clonus, patellar clonus. Adj. *clonic.* —**clo·nic·i·ty** (klo·nis′i·tee) *n.*

Clopane. Trademark for cyclopentamine, a sympathomimetic amine used as the hydrochloride salt.

Clorarsen. A trademark for dichlorophenarsine hydrochloride.

closed-chain, *adj.* Pertaining to or designating an organic compound in which the carbon (or substituent) atoms are bonded so as to form a closed ring.

closed-chest cardiac massage. Cardiac massage in the unopened chest by rhythmic compression of the heart between the sternum and vertebral column.

closed-circuit anesthesia. Anesthesia produced by an anesthetizing apparatus in which explosive agents used in anesthesia are prevented from coming in contact with sparks or flames.

closed fracture. SIMPLE FRACTURE.

closed pneumothorax. A pneumothorax which does not communicate with the lung and has no opening through the chest wall.

closed reduction. Reduction of a fractured bone, performed without making a surgical incision.

Clos·trid·i·um (klos·trid′ee·um, klo·strid′) *n.* A genus of anaerobic spore-bearing bacteria of ovoid, spindle, or club shape; widely distributed in nature. —**clostridium,** pl. **clostrid·ia,** *com. n.*; **clostridi·al,** *adj.*

Clostridium bot·u·li·num (bot″yoo·lye′num). A species of *Clostridium* that produces a very powerful toxin in food which when ingested may cause toxemia. The species includes types A, B, E, and F, the principal causes of human botulism; type C*β*, the cause of forage poisoning of cattle in Australia; and type D, the cause of lamzietke in cattle in Africa.

Clostridium botulinum **A.** A type of the species that produces botulism in man and limberneck in chickens, found predominantly in the Rocky Mountain and Pacific Coast states and in English soils.

Clostridium botulinum B. A type that produces botulism in man and limberneck in chickens, found most commonly in the Mississippi Valley, Great Lakes region, and Atlantic Coast states.

Clostridium no·vyi (no′vee-eye). A species of *Clostridium* that includes a type A found in gas gangrene, and types B and C which produce a strong soluble toxin.

Clostridium per·frin·gens (pur-frin′jenz). A species of plump, nonmotile, gram-positive rod, occurring in chains and singly, that produces a variety of toxins and is the most important cause of gas gangrene as well as the cause of dysentery of sheep. The species includes type A, the principal cause of gas gangrene in man; type B, the cause of lamb dysentery; type C, the cause of struck in sheep; types D and E, the cause of enterotoxemia of sheep.

Clostridium sep·ti·cum (sep′ti·kum). A species of *Clostridium* sometimes found in gas gangrene, in braxy of sheep, malignant edema of cattle, and also in some cases of blackleg in cattle.

Clostridium tet·a·ni (tet′uh·nigh). A species of *Clostridium* that causes tetanus and is present in soil and in human and animal intestines; characterized by spherical terminal spores and the production of tetanus toxin, a potent exotoxin.

Clostridium wel·chii (wel′chee-eye). CLOSTRIDIUM PERFRINGENS.

clo·sure, n. 1. The act of completing or closing an electric circuit. Abbreviated, C. 2. The closing of a wound by suture.

clot, n. & v. 1. The semisolid mass that forms as the result of coagulation, as of blood or lymph. Syn. *coagulum.* 2. To form a clot; to coagulate.

clot retraction. The contraction or shrinkage of a blood clot resulting in the extrusion of serum. A function of blood platelets within the fibrin network.

clot-retraction time. The length of time required under standard conditions, for the appearance or completion of clot retraction.

clo·trim·a·zole (klo-trim′uh-zole) n. 1-[(2-Chlorophenyl)diphenylmethyl]-1*H*-imidazole, $C_{22}H_{17}ClN_2$, a broad-spectrum antifungal agent demonstrating activity against dermatophytes.

clot·ting time. The length of time required, under standard conditions, for shed blood to coagulate.

cloudy swelling. A retrogressive change in the cytoplasm of parenchymatous cells, whereby the cell enlarges and the outline becomes irregular. These changes lead to gross swelling of the organ and obscuring of its usual features.

clove, n. The dried flower bud of *Eugenia caryophyllata*; contains volatile oil and caryophyllin, a lactone. Clove is stimulant; it has been used in nausea and vomiting and to correct flatulence.

clove oil. The volatile oil from clove; contains eugenol. It is a local anesthetic, a powerful germicide, and a local irritant.

clo·ver·leaf deformity. Roentgenologically, a disfigured duodenal bulb, having roughly the appearance of a three-leaf clover; due to contraction of scar tissue following, or associated with, chronic duodenal ulcer.

cloverleaf nail. An intramedullary nail which in cross section is shaped like a clover leaf; used particularly for internal fixation of fractures of the femur.

cloverleaf skull deformity syndrome. Intrauterine synostosis of the coronal and lambdoidal sutures associated with hydrocephalus, possibly secondary to platybasia. There is a grotesque trilobed skull, downward displacement of the ears, exophthalmos, secondary corneal damage, beak nose, prognathism, and frequently other associated skeletal deformities.

clox·y·quin (klock′si-kwin) n. 5-Chloro-8-quinolinol, C_9H_6ClNO, an antibacterial agent.

clo·za·pine (klo′zuh-peen) n. 8-Chloro-11-(4-methyl-1-piperazinyl)-5*H*-dibenzol[*b,e*][1,4]diazepine, $C_{18}H_{19}ClN_4$, a sedative.

CLSH Abbreviation for *corpus luteum-stimulating hormone* (= LUTEINIZING HORMONE).

clubbed, adj. Characterizing an extremity or structure that is gnarled, misshapen, or bulbous.

clubbed finger. A finger with bulbous enlargement of the terminal phalanx, a curved nail, and with or without osseous change.

club·bing, n. The condition of having a clubbed part or structure.

club·foot, n. A congenital malformation, either single or bilateral, in which the forefoot is inverted and rotated, accompanied by shortening of the calcaneal tendon and contracture of the plantar fascia.

club·hand, n. A congenital deformity of the hand characterized by one of the following distortions: (a) palmar displacement with or without radial or ulnar deviation; (b) dorsal displacement with or without radial or ulnar deviation. The deformity may be due to contracture of ligaments and muscles, or it may be caused by defective development of the radius, ulna, or carpal bones. The most common form of clubhand is caused by defective development of the radius, producing radial and palmar distortion.

clumsy child syndrome. MINIMAL BRAIN DYSFUNCTION SYNDROME.

clu·ne·al (kloo′nee-ul) adj. Pertaining to the buttocks.

clu·pe·ine (kloo′pee-een, -in) n. A protamine, having a molecular weight of approximately 4400, obtained from herring roe.

clus·ter, n. A number of similar things considered as a group because of their relation to each other or simultaneity of occurrence.

cluster headache. A type of headache that occurs predominantly in males, characterized by intense, unilateral orbital pain, lasting 30 to 60 minutes and recurring, usually nightly, for several weeks, followed by complete freedom for months or years; formerly attributed to release of histamine. Syn. *paroxysmal nocturnal cephalgia, migrainous neuralgia, Horton's headache.*

Clut·ton's joints Symmetrical bilateral hydrarthrosis of the knees occurring in congenital syphilis.

cly·sis (klye'sis) *n.*, pl. **cly·ses** (-seez) 1. Administration of an enema; cleansing by means of an enema. 2. Subcutaneous or intravenous administration of fluids.

clys·ter (klis'tur) *n.* ENEMA.

Cm Symbol for curium.

cm Abbreviation for *centimeter.*

CNS Abbreviation for *central nervous system.*

Co Symbol for cobalt.

co- A prefix meaning (a) *with, together, jointly, mutual;* (b) *to the same degree.*

CoA Abbreviation for *coenzyme A.*

co·ac·er·vate (ko·as'ur·vate, ko''a·sur'vate) *n.* The product formed when two hydrophilic colloids of opposite sign are mixed and form a stable particle which may form a separate phase. —**co·ac·er·va·tion** (ko·as''ur·vay'shun) *n.*

coagula. Plural of *coagulum.*

co·ag·u·la·ble (ko·ag'yoo·luh·bul) *adj.* Capable of coagulating or being coagulated. —**co·ag·u·la·bil·i·ty** (ko·ag''yoo·luh·bil'i·tee) *n.*

co·ag·u·lant (ko·ag'yoo·lunt) *adj. & n.* 1. Causing the formation of a clot or coagulum. 2. An agent that causes formation of a clot or coagulum.

co·ag·u·lase (ko·ag'yoo·lace, ·laze) *n.* A protein elaborated by cultures of *Staphylococcus aureus* which reacts with prothrombin or a closely related substance of plasma (the coagulase reacting factor) to cause plasma coagulation by converting fibrinogen to fibrin.

coagulase test. A test to determine the potential pathogenicity of staphylococci. Cultures of *Staphylococcus aureus* elaborate a protein, coagulase, which clots human or rabbit plasma in the presence of anticoagulants, but cultures of *Staphylococcus epidermidis* do not.

co·ag·u·late (ko·ag'yoo·late) *v.* To change, or cause to change, from a fluid to a gelatinous or semisolid state, especially by agglutination of colloidal particles.

co·ag·u·la·tion (ko·ag''yoo·lay'shun) *n.* The change from a fluid to a gelatinous or semisolid state, especially by agglutination of colloidal particles.

coagulation factor. Any factor in the blood or plasma that contributes to the coagulation of blood.

coagulation necrosis. A variety of necrosis characterized by cell death in situ with preservation of cell form and arrangement; most frequent in infarction.

coagulation time. CLOTTING TIME.

co·ag·u·lop·a·thy (ko·ag''yoo·lop'·uh·thee) *n.* Any disorder of blood coagulation.

co·ag·u·lum (ko·ag'yoo·lum) *n.*, pl. **coagu·la** (·luh) The semisolid mass that forms as the result of coagulation. Syn. *clot.*

co·a·lesce (ko·uh·less') *v.* 1. To unite or bring together previously separate parts or things. 2. To grow together or unite by growth.

co·a·les·cence (ko''uh·les'unce) *n.* The union of two or more parts or things previously separate. —**coales·cent** (·unt) *adj.*

coal min·er's disease. ANTHRACOSILICOSIS.

coal oil. KEROSENE OIL.

coal tar. A by-product in the destructive distillation of coal; a black, viscid fluid. Among the products obtained from coal tar by distillation are anthracene, benzene, naphtha, creosote, phenol, and pitch. From the basic oil of coal tar are manufactured the aniline or coal-tar colors or dyes. Preparations of coal tar are employed locally to relieve itching and in the treatment of certain skin diseases.

co·ap·ta·tion (ko''ap·tay'shun) *n.* The proper union or adjustment of displaced parts, such as the ends of a fractured bone or the lips of a wound. —**co·apt** (ko·apt') *v.; **coapt·ing,** adj.*

coaptation splint. A series of narrow splints of uniform size placed parallel to one another and held by adhesive plaster or leather, used to envlop a limb, such as the upper arm or thigh, where uniform and complete support is desired in the area covered.

coapting suture. A suture that brings the divided skin edges accurately together.

co·arct (ko·ahrkt') *v.* To narrow or constrict (especially, the lumen of a blood vessel). —**coarct·ed,** *adj.*

co·arc·ta·tion (ko''ahrk·tay'shun) *n.* Narrowing or stricture of a vessel, as the aorta, or of a canal.

coarse, *adj.* Involving movement through a relatively wide range. Said of tremors and other involuntary oscillatory movement of skeletal muscle.

coat·ing, *n.* A covering or layer of a substance, as of a wound or the tongue, or of a capsule or tablet.

Coats's disease RETINITIS EXUDATIVA.

co·bal·a·min (ko·bawl'uh·min) *n.* 1. Generic name for members of the vitamin B_{12} family, as cyanocobalamin and hydroxocobalamin. 2. The portion of the molecule of crystalline vitamin B_{12} (cyanocobalamin), exclusive of the cyano group, occurring in all vitamin B_{12} analogues.

co·balt (ko'bawlt) *n.* Co = 58.9332. A hard, gray, ductile metal used in alloys. It is a component of cyanocobalamin; lack of the element may result in anemia. It appears to other more complete utilization of iron in hemoglobin synthesis. Polycythemia has been produced in animals by administration of cobalt. Larger doses of soluble salts are emetic, due to local irritant effect.

cobalt 60. A radioactive isotope of cobalt, the radiation from which is employed in the treatment of cancer. This isotope, of atomic weight 60, has a half-life of 5.27 years and emits beta and gamma rays.

cob·ble·stone nevus. An anomaly of dermal connective tissue that produces a clinical appearance of cobbled paving stones on the overlying cutaneous surface.

co·bra·ly·sin (ko''bruh·lye'sin, ko·bral'i·sin) *n.* The hemolytic toxin of cobra venom. It is a lecithinase destroyed by heat and neutralized by antivenin.

co·ca (ko'kuh) *n.* The leaves of the shrubs *Erythroxylon coca, E. truxillense,* or *E. novogranatense,* containing cocaine and other alkaloids.

co·caine (ko·kane') *n.* Methylbenzoylecgonine, $C_{17}H_{21}NO_4$, an alkaloid obtained from the leaves of *Erythroxylon coca* and other species of *Erythroxylon;* occurs as colorless to white crystals, or white, crystalline powder; slightly soluble in water. For most purposes the hydrochloride is preferred to the base. The base is used in ointments and oily solution because of its greater solubility in fatty vehicles. **—cocain·ist** (·ist) *n.;* **cocain·ize** (·ize) *v.*

cocaine hydrochloride. The hydrochloride of the alkaloid cocaine; occurs as colorless crystals, or as white, crystalline powder; very soluble in water. Locally cocaine is a paralyzant to the peripheral ends of the sensory nerves, to a lesser degree to the motor nerves, and stimulating to the muscular coats of blood vessels. Systemically it is stimulant to all parts of the central nervous system. The most important use of cocaine is as a local application to mucous membranes, either for the purpose of contracting blood vessels or of lessening sensation. Continued use internally causes addiction.

co·cain·ism (ko-kain'iz-um, ko-kay'in-iz-um) *n.*
1. The habitual use of or addiction to cocaine.
2. The mental and systemic disturbances resulting from the habitual use of cocaine.

co·car·box·yl·ase (ko″kahr-bock'sil·ace, ·aze) *n.* Thiamine pyrophosphate, the coenzyme or prosthetic component of carboxylase; catalyzes decarboxylation of various α-keto acids, as pyruvic and α-ketoglutaric.

co·car·ci·no·gen (ko″kahr'si·no·jen, ·kahr·sin'o·) *n.* A noncarcinogenic agent which augments the carcinogenic process.

co·car·ci·no·gen·e·sis (ko″kahr″si·no·jen·e·sis) *n.* The induction of a tumor with the participation of a cocarcinogen.

cocc-, cocci-, cocco-. A combining form meaning (a) *grain, seed;* (b) *coccus.*

coc·cal (kock'ul) *adj.* Pertaining to or caused by a coccus.

cocci. Plural of *coccus.*

coccidi-, coccidio-. A combining form meaning *coccidium, coccidia.*

coccidia. Plural of *coccidium.*

Coc·cid·ia (kock·sid'ee·uh) *n. pl.* An order or group of cell parasites of the class Sporozoa; common in many vertebrates and invertebrates but rare in man.

coc·cid·i·oi·dal (kock·sid″i·oy'dul) *adj.* Pertaining to, or caused by fungi of the genus *Coccidioides.*

Coc·cid·i·oi·des (kock·sid″ee·oy'deez) *n.* A genus of parasitic fungi found in soil and pathogenic for many animals, characterized by branching mycelia with arthrospores on artificial cultivation and by endosporulating spherules in tissues.

Coccidioides im·mi·tis (i·migh'tis). The causative agent of coccidioidomycosis. The organism is spheroid, nonbudding, and endosporulating in the tissues; it produces branching, septate, aerial hyphae and arthrospores in culture.

coc·cid·i·oi·din (kock·sid″ee·oy'din) *n.* The sterile filtrate of cultures of *Coccidioides immitis* grown on a synthetic medium, used as a skin-testing material for the detection of delayed hypersensitivity to the infection and as the antigen in complement-fixation and precipitin tests.

coc·cid·i·oi·do·my·co·sis (kock·sid″ee·oy″do·migh·ko'sis) *n.* An infection or disease endemic in southwestern United States, Mexico, and some areas of South America, generally acquired by inhalation of the spores of *Coccidioides immitis.*

coc·cid·i·oi·do·sis (kock·sid″ee·oy·do'sis) *n.*, COC·CIDIOIDOMYCOSIS.

coc·cid·i·o·sis (kock·sid″ee·o'sis) *n.* A usually self-limited intestinal infection by a coccidium, *Isospora hominis* or *I. belli,* characterized by watery, mucoid diarrhea; most common in the tropics.

coc·cid·io·stat (kock·sid'ee·o·stat) *n.* Any agent that arrests or hinders the growth of a pathogenic coccidium to a degree sufficient for prophylactic or therapeutic treatment of disease caused by the organism.

coc·cid·i·um (kock·sid'ee·um) *n.,* pl. **coccid·ia** (·uh) Any organism of the order Coccidia.

coc·co·ba·cil·lary (kock″o·bas'i·lerr·ee) *adj.* Of or pertaining to a coccobacillus.

coc·co·ba·cil·lus (kock″o·ba·sil'us) *n.,* pl. **coccobacil·li** (·eye). A short, thick, oval bacillus; in appearance, midway between the coccus and the bacillus.

coc·coid (kock'oid) *adj.* Pertaining to or resembling a coccus.

coc·cus (kock'us) *n.,* pl. **coc·ci** (·sigh, ·eye) A bacterium whose greatest diameter is not more than twice its shortest.

coccy-. A combining form meaning *coccyx.*

coc·cy·al·gia (kock″see·al'juh, ·jee·uh) *n.* COCCYGODYNIA.

coc·cy·dyn·ia (kock″si·din'ee·uh) *n.* COCCYGODYNIA.

coc·cyg·e·al (kock·sij'ee·ul) *adj.* Pertaining to or involving the coccyx.

coccygeal ganglion. The terminal ganglion formed by the fusion of the caudal ends of the sympathetic trunks of both sides, situated in front of the coccyx.

coccygeal glabella. A minute hairless area located in the coccygeal region at the vertex of the hair whorls. It may become a small pit, the coccygeal foveola.

coccygeal nerve. Either of the last pair of spinal nerves, supplying the skin in the region of the coccyx.

coccygeal plexus. A plexus formed by the union of the anterior branches of the coccygeal nerve and the fifth sacral nerve with a communicating filament from the fourth sacral nerve.

coc·cy·gec·to·my (kock″si·jeck'tuh·mee) *n.* Surgical excision of the coccyx.

coccygeo-. A combining form meaning (a) *coccygeal;* (b) *coccygeus.*

coc·cy·geo·pu·bic (kock·sij″ee·o·pew'bick) *adj.* Pertaining to the coccyx and the pubes.

coc·cy·ge·us (kock·sij'ee·us) *n.,* pl. **coccyg·ei** (·ee·eye). One of the muscles of the pelvic diaphragm.

coc·cy·go·dyn·ia (kock″si·go·din'ee·uh) *n.* Pain in the region of the coccyx.

coc·cyx (kock'sicks) *n.,* genit. sing. **coccy·gis** (·jis), L. pl. **coc·cy·ges** (kock'si·jees, kock·sigh'jeez). The last bone of the vertebral column, formed by the union of four rudimentary vertebrae.

coch·i·neal (kotch″i·neel′, kotch′i·neen) *n.* The dried female insects, *Coccus cacti,* enclosing the young larvae. On extracting the insects with an aqueous solution of alum, a dark purplish solution representing an aluminum lake of the coloring principle carminic acid is obtained; the solution has been used for coloring medicinal preparations.

coch·lea (kock′lee·uh) *n.,* L. pl. & genit. sing. **coch·le·ae** (·lee·ee) The portion of the petrous part of the temporal bone which houses the membranous and osseous labyrinths, i.e., the essential organs of hearing. It describes 2½ turns about a central pillar called the modiolus or columella, thus forming the spiral canal of the cochlea, which is about 1½ inches in length. Projecting outward from the modiolus there is a thin, bony plate, the osseous spiral lamina, which divides the canal into the scala vestibuli and the scala tympani. —**coch·le·ar** (kock′lee·ur) *adj.*

coch·le·ar·i·form (kock″lee·ār′i·form) *adj.* Shaped like the shell of a snail.

cochlear nerve. The cochlear part of the vestibulocochlear nerve.

cochlear window. A round opening in the medial wall of the middle ear, closed by the secondary tympanic membrane. Syn. *round window.*

coch·le·or·bic·u·lar (kock″lee·o·or·bick′yoo·lur) *adj.* Pertaining to the cochlea and the orbicular muscles.

coch·leo·pal·pe·bral (kock′lee·o·pal′pe·brul) *adj.* Pertaining to the cochlea and the palpebral muscles.

cochleopalpebral reflex. AUDITORY·PALPEBRAL REFLEX.

coch·leo·ves·tib·u·lar (kock″lee·o·ves·tib′yoo·lur) *adj.* Pertaining to the cochlea and the vestibule of the ear.

co·cil·la·na (ko″si·lay′nuh, ·lan′uh) *n.* The bark of the tree *Guarea rusbyi.* Used as a nauseating expectorant.

Cock·ayne's syndrome Dwarfism, retinal atrophy, deafness, photosensitive dermatitis, beaklike nasal deformity, microcephaly and retardation, and slowly progressive signs of upper motor neuron and cerebellar dysfunction, probably an autosomal recessive trait.

cock·roach, *n.* An insect of the genus *Blatella, Blatta,* or *Periplaneta.*

cock·up splint. A splint for immobilizing the hand in hyperextension during healing of a wound or fracture.

cocoa butter. THEOBROMA OIL.

co·con·scious (ko·kon′shus) *n. & adj.* 1. *In psychiatry,* a dissociated mental state coexisting with a person's consciousness, but without his awareness, though it is psychodynamically active and may account for various normal and abnormal mental phenomena. 2. In or of such a state. —**coconscious·ness,** *n.*

co·co·nut oil. The fixed oil in the fruit of the coconut palm, *Cocos nucifera.* Used chiefly in soap manufacture for its high lathering quality.

cocto- A combining form meaning *boiled. modified by heat, at boiling point.*

coc·to·la·bile (kock″to·lay′bil, ·bile) *adj.* Destroyed or altered by heating to 100° C.

coc·to·sta·bile (kock″to·stay′bil, ·bile) *adj.* Able to withstand the temperature of boiling water without change.

co·de·hy·dro·gen·ase I (ko″dee·high′dro·je·nace, ·naze) NICOTINAMIDE ADENINE DINUCLEOTIDE.

co·deine (ko′deen, ko′dee·een, ko·dee′in) *n.* Methylmorphine, $C_{18}H_{21}NO_3$, an alkaloid of opium, resembling morphine in action, but weaker; an analgesic, antitussive, and antidiarrheal.

codeine phosphate. $C_{18}H_{21}NO_3.H_3PO_4.1\frac{1}{2}·H_2O$, the codeine salt most soluble in water (1 g in 2.5 ml).

codeine sulfate. $(C_{18}H_{21}NO_3)_2.H_2SO_4.5H_2O$; 1 g dissolves in 30 ml of water.

cod-liver oil. 1. The partially destearinated fixed oil obtained from fresh livers of *Gadus morrhua* and other species of the family Gadidae. Contains vitamins A and D, for the effects of which the oil is used medicinally. 2. A nondestearinated cod-liver oil of the same vitamin potency as cod-liver oil; used chiefly for administration to animals.

Cod·man's triangle The little trumpet-shaped cuff of reactive periosteal bone which surrounds the upper limit of a bone tumor or infection and which appears in an x-ray as a triangular space beneath the uplifted periosteal edge. This signifies subperiosteal, extracortical involvement.

Codman's tumor CHONDROBLASTOMA.

co·don (ko′don) *n.* An informational unit of genetic material composed of three nucleotides of DNA or RNA.

co·ef·fi·cient (ko″e·fish′unt) *n.* 1. Multiplier. 2. A figure indicating the degree of physical or chemical alteration characteristic of a given substance under stated conditions.

coefficient of correlation. A measure of the degree of association between two characteristics in a series of observations. Its value ranges from −1, representing perfect negative correlation, to +1, representing perfect positive correlation.

coefficient of solubility of a gas. The amount of a gas which is dissolved at a given temperature in 1 ml of a liquid, when the pressure of gas on the liquid is 760 mm Hg.

coefficient of variation. The standard deviation of a series of observations expressed as a per cent of the mean of the series.

-coele A combining form designating *a chamber, a ventricle, or a normal cavity of the body.*

Coe·len·ter·a·ta (se·len″ter·ay′tuh) *n. pl.* A phylum of primitive metazoans, including hydras, jellyfishes, corals, and sea anemones, which are radially symmetrical and whose only internal space is a digestive cavity; typified by alternate generations of asexual polyps and sexual medusae. Syn. *Cnidaria.* —**coe·len·ter·ate** (se·len′tur·ut, ·ate) *n. & adj.*

coe·lom, ce·lum (see′lum) *n., pl.* **coeloms, coe·lo·ma·ta** (se·lo′muh·tuh, se·lom′uh·tuh) The embryonic body cavity formed in the lateral mesoderm, which subsequently becomes divided into pericardial, pleural, and peritoneal cavities in developing mammals. —**coe·lom·ic, ce·lom·ic** (se·lom'ick) *adj.*

coelosoma. CELOSOMA.

coenesthesia. CENESTHESIA.

co·en·zyme (ko·en'zime) *n.* A nonprotein substance which, in combination with an apoenzyme, forms a complete enzyme, or holoenzyme; prosthetic group of an enzyme. Syn. *cofactor.*

coenzyme I. NICOTINAMIDE ADENINE DINUCLEOTIDE.

coenzyme II. NICOTINAMIDE ADENINE DINUCLEOTIDE PHOSPHATE.

coenzyme A. A nucleotide composed of adenylic acid, pantothenic acid, 2-mercaptoethylamine, and phosphoric acid which in the presence of a suitable enzyme can transfer an acyl group, as acetyl, from one substance to another. Abbreviated, CoA.

co·fac·tor (ko'fack·tur) *n.* 1. Any factor operating in conjunction with a principal factor. 2. COENZYME.

cof·fee, *n.* The dried and roasted ripe seeds of various species of *Coffea,* including *C. arabica, C. liberica,* and *C. robusta.* An infusion is stimulant because of its content of caffeine and, possibly, a volatile oil, caffeol.

cof·fee·ber·ry, *n.* CASCARA SAGRADA.

coffee-grounds vomit. Vomit consisting of altered blood in the contents of the stomach.

Co·gan's syndrome. 1. Vertigo, tinnitus, progressive bilateral deafness, pain in the eyes, photophobia and impaired vision, usually in young adults; associated with interstitial keratitis not due to syphilis, but possibly a form of vasculitis. 2. The congenital form of ocular motor apraxia.

Cogentin. Trademark for benztropine, a parasympatholytic drug used as the mesylate (methanesulfonate) salt in the symptomatic treatment of paralysis agitans.

cog·ni·tion (kog·nish'un) *n. In psychology,* the conscious faculty or process of knowing, of becoming, or being aware of thoughts or perceptions, including understanding and reasoning. —**cog·ni·tive** (kog'ni·tiv) *adj.*

cogwheel respiration. INTERRUPTED RESPIRATION.

cogwheel rigidity. A special type of extrapyramidal rigidity in which passive stretching of muscle, as for instance in the dorsiflexion of the hand, yields a rhythmically jerky resistance, as though the limb were being pulled over a ratchet; probably this represents a tremor which is masked by rigidity in an attitude of repose, but emerges during manipulation.

co·hab·i·ta·tion (ko·hab''i·tay'shun) *n.* The living together as, or as if, husband and wife.

co·here (ko·heer') *v.* To stick together. —**co·her·ent,** *adj.*

co·her·ence (ko·heer'unce) *n.* Reasonable connectedness of thought shown in speech, writing, or other activities.

co·he·sion (ko·hee'zhun) *n.* The attractive force between the same kind of molecules, i.e., the force which holds the molecules of a substance together. —**cohe·sive** (·siv') *adj.*

co·hort (ko'hort) *n. In statistics,* a group of individuals sharing some common characteristic, often age and sex.

coin lesion. A discrete spherical mass shadow on radiographs of the lung.

coin sound. In pneumothorax, a clear ringing note produced by striking a coin, placed flat upon the chest, with the edge of another coin.

co·i·tion (ko·ish'un) *n.* COITUS.

co·i·to·pho·bia (ko''i·to·fo'bee·uh) *n.* Abnormal dread or aversion to coitus.

co·i·tus (ko'i·tus) *n.* The act of sexual union; copulation. —**coi·tal** (·tul) *adj.*

coitus in·ter·rup·tus (in·tur·up'tus). Sexual intercourse in which the penis is withdrawn and the semen discharged outside the vagina.

coitus res·er·va·tus (rez''ur·vay'tus). Deliberately prolonged coitus without discharge of semen.

col-, coli-, colo-. A combining form meaning *colon.*

col (kol) *n.* A valleylike depression between the facial and lingual gingival papillae; it conforms to the shape of the interproximal surface of the tooth.

Colace. A trademark for dioctyl sodium sulfosuccinate.

co·la·tion (ko·lay'shun) *n.* The act of filtering or straining.

col·a·to·ri·um (kol''uh·tor'ee·um) *n.,* pl. **colato·ria** (·ee·uh) *In pharmacy,* a sieve, colander, or strainer.

col·a·ture (kol'uh·choor) *n.* 1. *In pharmacy,* a liquid that has been subjected to colation. 2. COLATION.

col·chi·cine (kol'chi·seen, ·sin, kol'ki·) *n.* An alkaloid, $C_{22}H_{25}NO_6$, of colchicum; a pale yellow, exceedingly bitter powder, freely soluble in water. Employed in the treatment of gout. It speeds up the evolutionary processes in plants by doubling chromosome numbers.

col·chi·cum (kol'chi·kum, kol'ki·kum) *n.* The corm and seed of the plant *Colchicum autumnale,* the properties of which are due to the alkaloid colchicine. It has been used in the treatment of acute gout and some forms of rheumatism.

cold, *n.* 1. The comparative lack of heat. 2. The COMMON COLD: a mild, acute, contagious, upper respiratory viral infection of short duration, characterized by coryza, watering of the eyes, cough, and occasionally, fever.

cold abscess. An abscess not associated with the usual signs of inflammation, such as redness, swelling, and heat.

cold agglutination phenomenon. The agglutination of human group O erythrocytes at 0 to 4°C, but not at body temperature, due to the adsorption on the surface of the red cells of 19S gamma globulins, and occurring in primary atypical pneumonia, certain viral disease, acquired hemolytic anemia, trypanosomiasis, blackwater fever, and other unidentifiable states.

cold agglutinin. An agglutinin in serum which produces maximum clumping of erythrocytes at 4°C and none at 37°C.

cold-blood·ed, *adj.* Poikilothermic; without ability to regulate the body temperature; said of fishes, reptiles, and amphibians whose temperatures remain close to that of the environment.

cold cautery. Cauterization by extreme cold, as by carbon dioxide snow.

cold cream. A type of cosmetic cream of varying composition.

cold freckle. LENTIGO.

cold hemolysin. A hemolysin active at temperatures lower than 37°C, usually most active at 4°C.

cold injury. Trauma to the body resulting from exposure to very low temperatures; may be a freezing or nonfreezing injury.

cold light. CHEMILUMINESCENCE.

cold pressor test. A rise in blood pressure is observed after the immersion of one hand in ice water for 1 minute. Individuals showing an excessive rise in blood pressure or an unusual delay in return to normal blood pressure are thought likely to develop essential hypertension.

cold sore. HERPES FACIALIS.

cold urticaria. A form of physical allergy elicitable by exposure to cold.

cole-, coleo- A combining form meaning (a) *sheath;* (b) *vagina.*

co·lec·to·my (ko·leck'tuh·mee) *n.* Excision of all or a portion of the colon.

co·leo·cele (ko'lee·o·seel", kol'ee·o·) *n.* A vaginal tumor or hernia.

co·leo·cys·ti·tis (ko"lee·o·sis·tye'tis) *n.* Inflammation of the vagina and urinary bladder.

Co·le·op·te·ra (ko"lee·op'tur·uh, kol"ee·) *n. pl.* The order of insects that comprises the beetles. —**coleopter·ous** (·us) *adj.*

co·le·op·to·sis (ko"lee·op·to'sis) *n.,* pl. **coleoptoses** (·seez) Prolapse of the vaginal wall.

co·li·bac·il·le·mia, coli·bac·il·lae·mia (ko"lee·bas"i·lee'mee·uh) *n.* The presence of *Escherichia coli* in the blood.

co·li·bac·il·lo·sis (ko"lee·bas"i·lo'sis) *n.* Infection with *Escherichia coli.*

co·li·bac·il·lu·ria (ko"lee·bas"i·lew'ree·uh) *n.* The presence of *Escherichia coli* in the urine.

co·li·ba·cil·lus (ko"lee·ba·sil'us) *n.,* pl. **colibacil·li** (·eye). The colon bacillus, *Escherichia coli.*

¹**col·ic** (kol'ick) *n.* 1. Acute paroxysmal abdominal pain usually due to smooth muscle contraction, obstruction, or twisting. 2. In early infancy paroxysms of pain, crying, and irritability, due to such causes as swallowing air, overfeeding, intestinal allergy, and emotional factors. Adj. *colicky.*

²**co·lic** (ko'lick) *adj.* Of or pertaining to the colon.

co·li·cin (ko'li·sin, kol'i·) *n.* Any of various bacteriocins active against particular strains of *Escherichia coli* or of other Enterobacteriaceae.

colic intussusception. Intussusception involving the colon only.

col·icky (kol'i·kee) *adj.* 1. Of, pertaining to, resembling, or causing colic. 2. Suffering from or caused by colic.

co·li·form (ko'li·form) *adj.* 1. Pertaining to or resembling the colon-aerogenes group.

co·li group (ko'lye). COLON-AEROGENES GROUP.

co·lis·ti·meth·ate sodium (ko·lis"ti·meth'ate).

Pentasodium colistinmethanesulfonate, $C_{58}H_{105}N_{16}Na_5O_{28}S_5$; a water-soluble derivative of colistin suitable for intramuscular injection.

co·lis·tin (ko·lis'tin, kol'is·tin) *n.* A basic polypeptide antibiotic obtained from *Bacillus colistinus;* closely related chemically and in antibacterial range to polymyxin B. It has largely been replaced by other antibiotics with less toxicity.

co·li·tis (ko·lye'tis) *n.* Inflammation of the colon.

coll-, colla-, collo- A combining form meaning (a) *collagen;* (b) *colloid.*

col·la·gen (kol'uh·jin) *n.* The albuminoid substance of the white fibers of connective tissues, cartilage, and bone. It is converted into gelatin by boiling. —**col·la·gen·ic** (kol"uh·jen'ick), **col·lag·e·nous** (kuh·laj'e·nus) *adj.*

col·la·gen·ase (kol'uh·je·nace, ·naze) *n.* A proteolytic enzyme which hydrolyzes collagen; one of the major exotoxins of *Clostridium perfringens* type A. It attacks the collagen of subcutaneous tissues and muscles and thus may contribute to the spread of gas gangrene. Syn. *kappa toxin.*

collagen disease. Any of various clinical syndromes characterized by widespread alterations of connective tissue, including inflammation and fibrinoid degeneration, as in rheumatic fever, rheumatoid arthritis, polyarteritis, systemic lupus erythematosus, generalized scleroderma, or dermatomyositis.

col·la·gen·iza·tion (kol"uh·je·nye·zay'shun, kol·aj"e·) *n.* The replacement of normal elements of a given area by collagenous connective tissue.

col·la·gen·o·sis (kol"uh·je·no'sis, kol·aj"e·no'sis) *n.,* pl. **collageno·ses** (·seez) 1. An African cardiopathy characterized by heart failure and visceral infarction with endocardial fibrosis and sclerosis, and mural thrombosis. 2. COLLAGEN DISEASE.

collagenous fibers. The flexible, fibrillar, nonelastic, connective-tissue fibers which are the commonest type. They make up the main mass of such structures as the corium, fasciae, tendons, ligaments, aponeuroses, periostea, and capsules of organs, and form also the fibrillar component of the intercellular substance (matrix) of bone and cartilage.

col·lapse, *v. & n.* 1. To cave in or be deflated. 2. To cause to cave in or be deflated. 3. Extreme depression, exhaustion, or prostration from physical or psychogenic causes. 4. SHOCK. 5. An abnormal sagging of an organ or the obliteration of its cavity.

collapse therapy. The treatment of pulmonary tuberculosis by any surgical procedure designed to decrease lung volume, such as artificial pneumothorax, extrapleural thoracoplasty, or interruption of the phrenic nerve.

col·lar·bone, *n.* CLAVICLE.

col·lar·ette (kol"ur·et') *n.* A ring or collar of scales following stimulation of some blisters.

col·lat·er·al (kuh·lat'ur·ul) *adj. & n.* Accessory or secondary; not direct or immediate. 2. A side branch, as of a vessel or a nerve fiber.

collateral artery. Any of the four branches of the brachial and deep brachial arteries which descend through a portion of the upper arm and terminate by anastomosis near the elbow joint.

collateral circulation. The circulation established for an organ or a part through anastomotic communicating channels, when the original direct blood supply is obstructed or abolished.

collateral eminence. A ridge on the floor of the lateral ventricle, corresponding to the depth of the collateral sulcus of the temporal lobe.

collateral sulcus. A furrow on the medial aspect of the cerebrum, between the subcalcarine and subcollateral gyri, corresponding to the collateral eminence.

col·lect·ing tubules. The ducts conveying the urine from the renal tubules (nephrons) to the minor calices of the renal pelvis.

col·lec·tive unconscious. *In analytic psychology,* the portion of the unconscious which theoretically is inherited and common to mankind.

Colles' fracture A fracture of the radius and ulna about 1 inch above the wrist with dorsal displacement of the distal fragment, creating a silver-fork deformity.

col·lic·u·li·tis (kol·ick″yoo·lye′tis) *n.* Inflammation of the colliculus seminalis.

col·lic·u·lo·ru·bral (kol·ick″yoo·lo·roo′brul) *adj.* Pertaining to the superior colliculus and the red nucleus.

col·lic·u·lus (kol·ick′yoo·lus) *n.,* pl. & genit. sing. **collic·u·li** (·lye) A small eminence.

col·li·ma·tor (kol′i·may″tur) *n.* 1. The diaphragm of a spectroscope, the purpose of which is to provide a beam of parallel rays of light by means of a small slit at the focus of its lens. 2. A fixed telescope for adjusting the optical axis of an instrument, as a photomicrographic camera. 3. A diaphragm or system of diaphragms made of an absorbing material, designed to define the dimensions and direction of a beam of radiation.

col·li·qua·tion (kol″i·kway′shun) *n.* The breakdown of tissue, usually necrotic, so that it becomes liquefied.

col·liq·ua·tive (kol·ick′wuh·tiv, kol′i·kway″tiv) *adj.* Marked by profuse or excessive fluid discharges.

col·li·sion *n. In obstetrics,* a complication which occurs occasionally when twins are small and when their presenting parts attempt to enter the superior strait at the same time.

collision tumor. A tumor in which a sarcoma is thought to invade a carcinoma, or vice versa.

col·lo·di·on (kol·o′dee·on) *n.* A dressing for wounds made by dissolving pyroxylin in ether and alcohol.

col·loid (kol′oid) *n.* 1. A state of subdivision of matter in which the individual particles are of submicroscopic size and consist either of single large molecules, as of proteins, or aggregates of smaller molecules; such particles, collectively referred to as the dispersed phase, occur more or less uniformly distributed in a dispersion medium. The dimension of a colloid particle, arbitrarily fixed, is between 1 and 100 nanometers. 2. A substance in the colloid state. 3. The clear, gelatinous, eosinophilic, stored secretion of the thyroid gland;

also other collections of gelatinous material, as the secretion of the intermediate lobe of the hypophysis. —**col·loi·dal** (kuh·loy′dul, kol·oy′dul) *adj.*

colloidal gold test. The precipitation by abnormal cerebrospinal fluid of colloidal gold from suspensions of various concentrations; formerly used in the diagnosis of neurosyphilis and other central nervous system diseases.

colloidal osmotic pressure. ONCOTIC PRESSURE.

colloid carcinoma. MUCINOUS CARCINOMA.

colloid cyst. A cyst containing gelatinous material whose consistency approaches that of thyroid gland colloid.

colloid goiter. A diffuse, lumpy goiter in which many of the follicles are abnormally distended with colloid; often associated with iodine deficiency.

colloid milium. A rare skin disease characterized by the presence, especially on the face and hands, of minute, shining, flat or slightly raised lesions of a pale lemon or bright lemon color. It is a form of colloid degeneration of the skin, affecting persons of middle or advanced age.

col·loi·do·cla·sia (kuh·loy″do·klay′zee·uh, ·zhuh) *n.* A breaking up of the physical equilibrium of the colloids in the living body, producing anaphylactoid shock; attributed to entrance into the bloodstream of unchanged (undigested) colloids. —**colloido·clas·tic** (·klas′tick) *adj.*

col·loid·oph·a·gy (kol″oy·dof′uh·jee) *n.* Invasion and ingestion of colloid by macrophages, as in the thyroid gland.

col·lum (kol′um) *L. n.,* genit. sing. **col·li** (·eye), pl. **col·la** (·luh) [NA]. NECK.

col·lu·nar·i·um (kol″yoo·nar′ee·um) *n.,* pl. **collu·nar·ia** (·ee·uh) A solution intended to be used in the nose.

col·lu·to·ri·um (kol″yoo·to′ree·um) *n.,* pl. **colluto·ria** (·ree·uh) A mouthwash.

col·lyr·i·um (kuh·lirr′ee·um) *n.,* pl. **collyr·ia** (·ee·uh), **collyriums** A preparation for local application to the eye, usually a wash or lotion.

colo-. See **col-.**

col·o·bo·ma (kol″uh·bo′muh) *n.,* pl. **coloboma·ta** (·tuh), **colobomas** 1. Any congenital, pathologic, or operative defect, especially of the eye; occurring most commonly in the iris, ciliary body, or choroid, usually as a cleft placed inferiorly. 2. One or more congenital fissures of the eyelid or eyelids, usually the upper. —**coloboma·tous** (·tus) *adj.*

co·lo·co·los·to·my (ko″lo·ko·los′tuh·mee) *n.* An anastomosis between two noncontinuous segments of the colon in order to short-circuit the lumen around inoperable obstructing tumors or to prepare for later resection.

co·lo·cys·to·plas·ty (ko″lo·sis′to·plas·tee) *n.* An operation in which a segment of the colon is sutured to the urinary bladder to increase bladder capacity.

co·lon (ko′lun) *n.* The part of the large intestine beginning at the cecum and terminating at the end of the sigmoid flexure. In the various parts of its course it is known as ascending colon, transverse colon, descending colon, and sigmoid colon; the last is sometimes divided into the iliac colon and the pelvic colon.

colon-aerogenes group. A group of non-spore-forming gram-negative aerobic bacilli of the genera *Escherichia* and *Aerobacter*, which when found in water is evidence of fecal contamination.

colon as·cen·dens (a·sen'denz) [NA]. ASCENDING COLON.

colon bacillus. *ESCHERICHIA COLI.*

colon des·cen·dens (de·sen'denz) [NA]. DESCENDING COLON.

co·lon·ic (ko·lon'ick) *adj.* Of or pertaining to the colon.

colon sig·moi·de·um (sig·moy'dee·um) [NA]. SIGMOID COLON.

colon trans·ver·sum (trans·vur'sum) [NA]. TRANSVERSE COLON.

col·o·ny (kol'uh·nee) *n.* 1. *In bacteriology,* a group or mass of microorganisms in a culture, derived from a single cell. Variations in bacterial structure or antigenic composition are often expressed in the form of the colony, as smooth, rough, dwarf. 2. *In cell biology,* a group of cells in culture or in certain experimental tissues, as spleen colony, a cluster of hematopoietic cells derived from stem cells administered to an irradiated animal.

colony counter. A device for counting bacterial colonies; usually consists of an illuminated transparent plate, divided into spaces of known area, over which a petri dish containing the colonies is placed.

co·lo·pexy (kol'o·peck"see, ko'lo·) *n.* The suturing of the sigmoid flexure to the abdominal wall.

co·lo·proc·tos·to·my (ko"lo·prock·tos'tuh·mee) *n.* The formation of a new passage between the colon and the rectum.

co·lop·to·sis (ko"lop·to'sis) *n.,* pl. **colopto·ses** (·seez) Prolapse or displacement of the colon.

Col·o·ra·do tick fever. A nonexanthematous acute viral disease of man occurring in the western United States and transmitted by a bite of the tick *Dermacentor andersoni;* characterized by short course, intermittent fever, leukopenia, and occasionally meningoencephalitis.

color blindness. Inability to perceive one or more, or rarely all, colors. —**color-blind,** *adj.*

color gustation. A form of synesthesia in which color sensations accompany the sensation of taste.

col·or·im·e·ter (kul"ur·im'e·tur) *n.* An instrument for determining color intensity, as for measuring the hemoglobin in blood.

col·or·i·met·ric (kul"ur·i·met'rick) *adj.* Of or pertaining to a colorimeter or to colorimetry. —**colorimet·ri·cal·ly** (·ri·kuh·lee) *adv.*

col·or·im·e·try (kul"ur·im'e·tree) *n.* 1. The science of determining colors. 2. Chemical analysis by the use of a colorimeter.

color index. The amount of hemoglobin per erythrocyte relative to normal, obtained by the following formula: C.I. = (percent normal hemoglobin concentration/percent normal erythrocyte count. Different laboratories use different normal values in this formula.

co·lo·sig·moid·os·to·my (ko"lo·sig"moid·os'tuh·mee) *n.* An anastomosis between the sigmoid and some other part of the colon.

co·los·to·my (ko·los'tuh·mee) *n.* The formation of an artificial anus in the anterior abdominal wall or loin. The opening into the colon may be anywhere depending on the location of the diseased condition, as cecostomy or sigmoidostomy.

colostomy bag. A rubber bag worn as a belt, especially constructed to receive the intestinal excreta from a colostomy opening.

col·os·tra·tion (kol"us·tray'shun) *n.* Any disorder of infants caused by colostrum, such as a diarrheal reaction.

co·los·trum (ko·los'trum) *n.* The first milk from the mother's breasts after the birth of the child. It is laxative, and assists in the expulsion of the meconium. Contains greater quantities of lactalbumin and lactoprotein than later milk.

co·lot·o·my (ko·lot'uh·mee) *n.* Incision of the colon; may be abdominal, lateral, lumbar, or iliac, according to the region of entrance.

colp-, colpo- A combining form meaning *vagina, vaginal.*

col·pal·gia (kol·pal'jee·uh) *n.* Pain in the vagina.

col·pa·tre·sia (kol"pa·tree'zhuh, ·zee·uh) *n.* Occlusion or atresia of the vagina.

col·pec·ta·sia (kol"peck·tay'zhuh, ·zee·uh) *n.* Dilatation of the vagina.

col·pec·to·my (kol·peck'tuh·mee) *n.* Excision of the vagina.

col·pi·tis (kol·pye'tis) *n.* Inflammation of the vagina.

col·po·cele (kol'po·seel) *n.* A hernia in the vagina.

col·po·clei·sis (kol"po·klye'sis) *n.,* pl. **colpoclei·ses** (·seez) Closure of the vagina by suturing.

col·po·per·i·neo·plas·ty (kol"po·perr"i·nee·o·plas"tee) *n.* Plastic surgery of the perineum and vagina.

col·po·per·i·ne·or·rha·phy (kol"po·perr"i·nee·or'uh·fee) *n.* Suture of a cut or lacerated vagina and perineum.

col·po·pexy (kol'po·peck"see) *n.* Fixation of the vagina by suturing it to a surrounding structure.

col·po·plas·ty (kol'po·plas"tee) *n.* Plastic repair of the vagina.

col·por·rha·phy (kol·por'uh·fee) *n.* Suture of the vagina for repair.

-colpos A combining form meaning *vagina.*

col·po·scope (kol'po·skope) *n.* An instrument for the visual examination of the vagina and cervix; a vaginal speculum. —**col·po·scop·ic** (kol"po·skop'ick) *adj.;* **col·pos·co·py** (kol·pos'kuh·pee) *n.*

col·pot·o·my (kol·pot'uh·mee) *n.* Incision of the vagina.

Columbia-SK virus. A strain of virus belonging to the picornavirus group and responsible for encephalomyocarditis, with the natural reservoir in rodents, but capable of infecting a wide range of hosts, including man.

co·lum·bi·um (ko·lum'bee·um) *n.* NIOBIUM.

col·u·mel·la (kol"yo·mel'uh) *n.,* pl. **columel·lae** (·lee) 1. The septum of the nasal vestibule, the medial boundary of the nostrils. 2. The modiolus or central axis of the cochlea of the human ear. 3. A bone in land Amphibia, many reptiles, and birds which takes the place of the ossicles of the ear in man.

col·umn (kol'um) *n. & v.* 1. A supporting pillar; a pillar-shaped structure. 2. To place tampons in the vagina to support a prolapsed uterus. —**co·lum·nar** (ko·lum'nur) *adj.*

columnar cell. An epithelial cell in which the height is markedly greater than the width.

columnar-cell carcinoma. ADENOCARCINOMA.

columnar epithelium. Epithelium that is distinguished by elongated, prismatic, or columnar cells.

column chromatography. Chromatography in which the porous solid is packed into a tube and separation is achieved either by adsorption, using a single solvent or a mixture of miscible solvents, or by partition, using two immiscible solvents.

co·lum·ni·za·tion (kol·um''ni·zay'shun, kol''um·ni·) *n. Obsol.* Placement of tampons in the vagina to support a prolapsed uterus.

columns of the gray matter. Divisions of the longitudinal column of gray matter in the spinal cord: the anterior column, the lateral column, and the posterior column.

Coly-Mycin M. A trademark for colistimethate sodium, an antibacterial.

com-, con-, cor- A prefix meaning *with, jointly, together.*

¹**co·ma** (ko'muh) *n.* A state in which the patient is incapable of sensing or responding, either to external stimuli or to inner needs.

²**coma** *In optics and ophthalmology,* a blurred part of an image resulting from spherical aberration.

com·a·tose (kom'uh·toce, ·toze, ko'muh·) *adj.* In a condition of coma; resembling coma.

combat fatigue, exhaustion, or **neurosis.** WAR NEUROSIS.

comb disease. FAVUS OF FOWLS.

combined anesthesia. 1. Anesthesia produced by a combination of anesthetics, such as chloroform, ether, and nitrous oxide, or by a combination of methods. 2. Anesthesia produced by anesthetics plus somnifacient drugs.

combined aphasia. The presence of two or more types of aphasia in the same individual.

combined sclerosis. SUBACUTE COMBINED DEGENERATION OF THE SPINAL CORD.

combined system disease. Any intrinsic disease of the spinal cord affecting the posterior and lateral columns.

combined version. BIMANUAL VERSION.

comb·ing (ko'ming) *n.* The radial arrangement of elongated cells around vessels or vascular spaces, seen particularly in spindle-cell sarcomas.

com·e·do (kom'e·do, ko·mee') *n., pl.* **com·e·do·nes** (kom''e·do'neez) A collection of sebaceous material and keratin retained in the hair follicle and excretory duct of the sebaceous gland, the surface covered with a black dot due to oxidation of sebum at the follicular orifice. It is the primary lesion of acne vulgaris; usually found on the face, chest, and back, and more commonly occurring during adolescence.

com·e·do·car·ci·no·ma (kom''e·do·kahr''si·no'muh) *n.* A type of adenocarcinoma of the breast in which the ducts are filled with cells,

which, when expressed from the cut surface, resemble comedos.

comedones. Plural of *comedo.*

com·men·sal·ism (kuh·men'sul·iz·um) *n.* A more or less intimate association between organisms of different species, without injury to either organism and with some benefit, such as nourishment and protection, to one; as the association of the small crab and the oyster in whose mantle cavity it lives. —**commensal,** *n. & adj.*

com·mi·nute (kom'i·newt) *v. & adj.* 1. *In chemistry,* to pulverize; to divide into fine particles. 2. *In surgery,* to fracture a bone so that it is shattered into several pieces. 3. Shattered, pulverized. —**comminut·ed** (·id) *adj.;* **com·mi·nu·tion** (kom''i·new'shun) *n.*

comminuted fracture. A fracture in which there is splintering or fragmentation of the bone.

com·mis·sur·al (kom·ish'ur·ul, kom''i·shoor'ul) *adj.* Pertaining to or having the properties of a commissure.

commissural fibers. Fibers joining an area of the cortex of one cerebral hemisphere to a similar area of the other.

com·mis·sure (kom'i·shur, ·syoor) *n.* 1. Strands of nerve fibers uniting like structures in the two sides of the brain or spinal cord. 2. The region of union of such structures as the lips, eyelids, labia majora, or cardiac valves.

commissure of the fornix. The transverse part of the fornix, uniting the crura.

com·mis·su·ro·spi·nal (kom·ish''oo·ro·spye'nul) *adj.* Pertaining to the posterior commissure of the spinal cord and the spinal cord.

com·mis·sur·ot·o·my (com''i·shur·ot'uh·mee) *n.* 1. Surgical destruction of a commissure, usually the anterior commissure, particularly in the treatment of certain psychiatric disorders. 2. Surgical division of a stenosed cardiac valve.

com·mit·ment, *n. In legal medicine,* the obligatory hospitalization or institutionalization of a patient in need of treatment, particularly for a mental disorder.

common bile duct. The duct formed by the union of the cystic and the hepatic ducts.

common cardinal veins. Paired primary veins located in the septum transversum, connecting the anterior and posterior cardinal veins with the sinus venosus. Syn. *ducts of Cuvier.*

common carotid artery. An artery that originates on the right from the brachiocephalic trunk and on the left from the arch of the aorta, and has external and internal carotid, rarely superior thyroid, ascending pharyngeal, and even vertebral branches. It distributes blood to the region of the neck and head.

common carotid plexus. A network of sympathetic nerve fibers surrounding the common carotid artery, formed by branches of the superior cervical ganglion.

common cold. A mild, acute, contagious upper respiratory viral infection of short duration, characterized by coryza, watering of the eyes, cough, and, occasionally, fever.

common hepatic artery. The hepatic artery to the point just distal to the branching off of the right gastric and gastroduodenal arteries.

common hepatic duct. The common duct formed by the union of the left hepatic duct, which drains the left and caudate lobes of the liver, and the right hepatic duct, which drains the right and quadrate lobes of the liver.

com·mo·tio (kuh·mo'shee·o) n. A concussion; shock.

commotio cer·e·bri (serr'i·brye). BRAIN CONCUSSION.

commotio ret·i·nae (ret'i·nee). Dysfunction of the retina from a blow on or near the eye; characterized by sudden blindness, but little or no ophthalmoscopic evidence of any lesion. The sight is usually regained, and its loss is supposedly due to disturbance of the retinal elements.

communicable disease. 1. An infectious disease transmissible from one source (either an animal or a person) to another, directly or indirectly (as via a vector). 2. Often, CONTAGIOUS DISEASE.

com·mu·ni·cans (kom·yoo'ni·kanz) L. adj. Communicating; connecting.

com·mu·ni·cate, v. In anatomy, to join or to form an unbroken passage from one place to another; ANASTOMOSE. —**com·mu·ni·ca·tion,** n.

communicating hydrocele. Hydrocele in which the fluid-filled tunica vaginalis is patent, connecting directly with the peritoneal cavity.

communicating hydrocephalus. A form of hydrocephalus in which there is communication between the ventricles and the spinal subarachnoid space; usually caused by obliteration of the cerebral subarachnoid space, the result of meningitis or subarachnoid hemorrhage.

com·pac·ta (kom·pack'tuh) n. Substantia compacta (= COMPACT BONE).

compact bone. Osseous tissue in which marrow spaces are replaced by cylindrical, concentrically laminated haversian systems, each with an axial vascular channel, the haversian canal.

companionate marriage. A form of marriage for sexual companionship without legal obligation, economic responsibility, or desire for children.

com·par·a·scope (kum·pâr'uh·scope) n. An apparatus attached to two microscopes for the simultaneous comparison of two different specimens.

com·par·a·tive anatomy. Investigation and comparison of the anatomy of different orders of animals or of plants, one with another.

comparative embryology. Investigation and comparison of the embryology of different orders of animals or of plants, one with another.

comparative pathology. Investigation and comparison of disease in various animals, including man, to arrive at resemblances and differences which may clarify disease as a phenomenon of nature.

comparative physiology. The comparative study of the physiology of different animals and plants, or the comparison of analogous physiologic mechanisms in different species.

com·pa·ra·tor (kom'puh·ray''tur, kum·pâr'uh·tur) n. A type of colorimeter in which a place is provided for a standard solution or solutions to be visually compared with an unknown solution under similar lighting conditions.

com·pat·i·bil·i·ty, n. 1. Congruity; the power of a drug or a drug substance in a medicine to mix with another without deleterious chemical change or loss of therapeutic power. 2. In blood grouping, (a) in vitro, no interaction between two bloods; (b) in vivo, no reaction whatsoever from the injection of a blood found to be compatible by laboratory tests. 3. HISTOCOMPATIBILITY. 4. The ability to exist together in harmony. —**com·pat·i·ble,** adj.

compatibility testing. CROSS MATCHING.

Compazine. Trademark for prochlorperazine, an antiemetic and tranquilizing drug used as the base and the edisylate (ethanedisulfonate) and maleate salts.

com·pen·sate, v. To correct a function that has been adversely affected. —**com·pen·sat·ing,** adj.

compensated acidosis. Acidosis in which the physiologic compensatory mechanisms are able to restore a normal pH of about 7.4.

compensated alkalosis. Alkalosis in which the physiologic compensatory mechanisms are able to restore a normal pH of about 7.4.

com·pen·sa·tion, n. 1. The process of counterbalancing a lack or a defect of a bodily or physiologic function.

com·pen·sa·to·ry (kum·pen'suh·to''ree) adj. Making up for a loss, counteracting an extreme.

compensatory curvature. In spinal curvature, a secondary curve, occurring as the result of the efforts of the trunk to maintain its upright position.

compensatory emphysema. Simple nonobstructive overdistention of lung segments or an entire lung in adaptation to collapse, destruction, or removal of lung tissue.

compensatory hypertrophy. 1. Hypertrophy in response to destruction or injury in the opposite paired organ or in another part of the same organ. 2. Hypertrophy, as of skeletal or cardiac muscles, in response to habitual vigorous exercise.

compensatory pause. In cardiology, a long interval immediately following a premature beat, compensating by its length for the prematurity of the beat; caused by a second impulse arriving when the previously excited myocardial tissue is still in a refractory state.

com·pe·tence, n. 1. In legal medicine, the possession of qualifications, capacity, soundness of mind, or other legally acceptable standards to perform certain acts and to take responsibility for them. 2. In genetics, the property whereby a cell is able to be transformed by a molecule of transforming DNA.

com·plaint, n. A disease or ailment.

com·ple·ment (kom'ple·munt) n. Any one of a group of at least nine factors, designated C1, C2, etc., that occurs in the serum of normal animals that enters into various immunologic reactions, is generally absorbed by combinations of antigen and antibody, and with the appropriate antibody, may lyse erythrocytes, kill or lyse bacteria, enhance phagocytosis and immune adherence, and exert other effects. Complement activity is destroyed by heating the serum at 56°C for 30 minutes. Abbreviated, C.

complemental air. The amount of air that can still be inhaled after a normal inspiration. Syn. *inspiratory reserve volume.*

complement fixation. The entering of complement into combination with an antigen-antibody aggregate so that it is not available for subsequent reaction in the indicator systems of hemolysis or bacteriolysis. The basis of the Wassermann test and other serologic tests.

complement-fixation test. A test based on the complement-fixation reaction in which antigen uniting with its antibody combines with the complement and thus inactivates or fixes it. Abbreviated, CFT.

com·ple·men·to·phil (kom"ple·men'to·fil) *n.* According to Ehrlich, the haptophore group of the antibody (amboceptor) by means of which it combines with the complement.

complete abortion. Abortion in which all the products of conception are shed or expelled, including fetus, placenta, and (if not already removed at curettage) decidua.

complete antibody. An antibody that is detectable by standard serologic procedures, saline active, such as agglutination or precipitation.

complete heart block. Complete atrioventricular block. See *atrioventricular block.*

com·plex (kom'pleks) *n.* 1. *In psychoanalysis,* a group of associated ideas with strong emotional tone, which have been transferred by the conscious mind into the unconscious, and which influence the personality. 2. A combination of signs and symptoms or related factors; a symptom complex. 3. *In electrocardiography,* a deflection corresponding to a phase of the cardiac cycle.

com·pli·ance (kom·pli'ans) *n.* 1. The extension or displacement of a substance under unit load. 2. Specifically, the volume change produced in the lungs by a given change in pressure, measured at the peak of tidal volume when there is no air flow. 3. The degree of distensibility of elastic structures, such as blood vessels, the heart, or lungs, with low compliance equivalent to stiffness, and high compliance to marked distensibility.

com·pli·ca·tion (kom"pli·kay'shun) *n.* An accidental condition or second disease occurring in the course of a primary process.

Compocillin-V. Trademark for hydrabamine phenoxymethyl penicillin or hydrabamine penicillin V.

com·po·si·tion, *n.* 1. The constitution of a mixture. 2. The kind and number of atoms contained in the molecule of a compound.

com·pound, *adj. & n.* 1. Composed of parts that are entities in their own right. 2. Complicated; multiple. 3. A substance composed of two or more elements chemically combined in definite proportion.

compound benzoin tincture. A tincture prepared from benzoin, aloe, storax, tolu balsam, and alcohol; used as an inhalant in bronchitis by steam vaporization; as an antiseptic and protective application to chapped hands, minor

wounds; and occasionally as a stimulating expectorant in chronic bronchitis. Syn. *Turlington's balsam.*

compound C (Kendall's). Allopregnane-3α,11β,17α,21-tetrol-20-one, a steroidal constituent of the adrenal cortex.

compound D (Kendall's). Allopregnane-3β,11β,17α,20β,21-pentol, a steroidal constituent of the adrenal cortex.

compound dislocation. A dislocation in which there is a communication with the joint from inside or outside, through a wound.

compound E (Kendall's). CORTISONE.

compound F (Kendall's). HYDROCORTISONE.

compound fracture. A fracture in which the point of fracture is in contact with the external surface of the body.

compound G-11. HEXACHLOROPHENE.

compound gland. A gland which has a branching system of ducts.

compound granule cell. A rounded phagocytic microglial cell with cytoplasm distended by globules of lipid and other debris.

compound microscope. A microscope that consists of two or more lenses or lens systems, of which one, the objective lens, placed near the object, gives a large and inverted real image; the other, the ocular lens, acting like a simple microscope, gives an enlarged virtual image of the real image.

compound nevus. A common pigmented mole consisting of areas of melanocytes in both the dermoepidermal and the intracutaneous zones.

compound opium and glycyrrhiza mixture. A preparation containing camphorated opium tincture, glycyrrhiza fluidextract, antimony potassium tartrate, alcohol, glycerin, and water. A nauseating expectorant. Syn. *brown mixture.*

compound tincture of camphor. PAREGORIC.

com·press (kom'press) *n.* A folded cloth or pad of other soft material, wet or dry, hot or cold, applied firmly to a part.

com·pres·sion (kum·presh'un) *n.* 1. The state of being compressed. 2. The act of pressing or squeezing together.

compression atelectasis. Collapse of part or all of a lung due to pressure by extrinsic factors such as pleural effusion or tumor.

compression atrophy. PRESSURE ATROPHY.

compression cone. A device that applies external pressure to the body during radiography; usually used in conjunction with fluoroscopy to compress a barium-filled viscus to demonstrate the mucosal pattern of a local portion of the gastrointestinal tract.

compression fracture. A fracture in which a surface of a bone is driven toward another bony surface; commonly found in vertebral bodies.

compression paralysis. Paralysis caused by pressure on a nerve.

com·pres·sor (kum·pres'ur) *n.* 1. An instrument for compressing an artery or other part. 2. A muscle having a compressing function.

com·pul·sion, *n.* 1. An irresistible impulse. 2. *In psychiatry,* an impulse to do something against the conscious will of the individual at the time it is done, and usually stemming from an obsession. 3. An unwanted, insistent, repetitive, and intrusive urge to carry out an act which is against the conscious wishes or standards of the individual, and representative of hidden, wholly unacceptable wishes or ideas. Failure to perform the act brings out overt anxiety.

compulsion neurosis. OBSESSIVE-COMPULSIVE NEUROSIS.

com·pul·sive, *adj.* Pertaining to, caused by, or characteristic of a compulsion. —**compulsiveness,** *n.;* **compulsive·ly,** *adv.*

compulsive laughter. Laughter that is without cause and mirthless as seen in certain psychoses, especially schizophrenia; the patient usually does not know he is laughing.

compulsive ritual. *In psychiatry,* a series of acts performed repetitively under compulsion; failure to carry out the acts results in tension and anxiety.

com·put·ed axial tomography. COMPUTED TOMOGRAPHY. Abbreviated, CAT.

computed tomography. A method of imaging in which a computer is used to reconstruct the anatomic features registered by axial tomography. Abbreviated, CT.

com·put·er-assisted tomography. COMPUTED TOMOGRAPHY. Abbreviated, CAT.

com·put·er·ized tomography. COMPUTED TOMOGRAPHY.

co·mus (ko'mus) *n.* A crescentic patch of yellow near the optic disk; seen in high myopia.

co·na·tion (ko-nay'shun) *n.* The exertive power of the mind, including will and desire, as expressed in a conscious tendency to act. —**co·na·tive** (kon'uh-tiv, ko'nuh-tiv) *adj.*

Con·ca·to's disease (kohng-kah'to) POLYSEROSITIS.

con·cave (kon'kave, kon·kave') *adj.* Possessing a curved, depressed surface. —**con·cav·i·ty** (kon·kav'i·tee) *n.*

con·ca·vo-con·vex (kon·kay''vo-kon'vecks, ·kon·vecks') *adj.* Bounded by a concave surface on one side and a convex surface on the other.

con·ceive, *v.* To become pregnant.

con·cen·tra·tion, *n.* 1. The bringing together, or collection within a limited area, of some entity, as of certain cells in a brain center or nucleus. 2. The fixing and limiting of a person's attention of an object, idea, field of endeavor, or aspect thereof. 3. The process of increasing the strength of a solution by evaporating the solvent, or of increasing the potency of a pharmacologically active substance by eliminating inactive constituents. 4. The relative content, variously expressed, of a component of a solution or other mixture of two or more substances.

concentration test. A test of kidney function based upon the normal ability of the kidneys to concentrate or dilute urine.

con·cen·tric (kun·sen'trick) *adj.* Having a common center.

concentric atrophy. Atrophy, as of an organ or a structure, beginning on the outside and proceeding inward.

concentric lamella. One of the plates of bone

making up the haversian systems in compact bone.

concentric sclerosis. A form of cerebral demyelinative disease, characterized by the occurrence of alternating bands of destruction and preservation of myelin in a series of concentric rings; probably a variant of Schilder's disease. Syn. *Baló's encephalitis periaxialis concentrica.*

con·cept, *n. In psychology,* the image or notion formed by the mind of an action or object. —**con·cep·tu·al,** *adj.*

con·cep·tion, *n.* 1. *In biology,* the fertilization of the ovum by the spermatozoon, occurring in the human female usually about the twelfth to fifteenth day after the first day of menstrual flow. 2. *In psychology,* the act of mentally forming ideas, especially abstract ideas; the process of conceiving ideas and of forming concepts. —**conception·al, concep·tive,** *adj.*

con·cep·tus (kon·sep'tus) *n.,* pl. **conceptuses** That which is conceived; an embryo or fetus.

con·cha (kong'kuh) *n.,* pl. & genit. sing. **con·chae** (·kee) A shell; a shell-like organ, as the hollow part of the external ear.

con·chi·tis (kong·kigh'tis) *n.* Inflammation of a concha.

con·cho·tome (kong'ko·tome) *n.* An instrument for the surgical removal of the conchae.

con·com·i·tant (kon·kom'i·tunt) *adj.* Accompanying.

con·cor·dance (kun·kor'dunce) *n. In genetics,* a similarity of the members of a twin pair with respect to a particular trait.

con·cre·ment (kong'kre·munt) *n.* CONCRETION.

con·cres·cence (kon·kres'unce) *n.* 1. A growing together of the roots of two teeth. 2. A process by which the formative embryonic cells of the germ ring converge and fuse at the blastopore to form the axial part of the embryo during gastrulation.

concrete thinking. *In psychology and psychiatry,* mental processes characterized by literalness and the tendency to be bound to the most immediate and obvious sense impressions, as well as a lack of generalization and abstraction. Thus, an individual who is asked in what way a pear and a banana are alike may answer concretely, "they are both yellow," or "soft," instead of "they are both fruits."

con·cre·tion (kon·kree'shun) *n.* 1. Solidification, calculus formation. 2. A calculus or deposit. 3. Parts normally separate, as the fingers.

con·cus·sion (kun·kush'un) *n.* 1. The state of being shaken; a severe shaking or jarring of a part, as by an explosion, or a violent blow. 2. The morbid state resulting from such a jarring. 3. BRAIN CONCUSSION.

con·den·sa·tion (kon''den·say'shun) *n.* 1. The act of making more compact or dense. 2. The changing of a gaseous substance to a liquid, or a liquid to a solid. 3. *In chemistry,* the union of two or more molecules by the linking of carbon chains and the formation of more complex carbon chains, usually with elimination of small molecules such as NH_3, H_2O. 4. The pathologic hardening, with or without contraction, of a soft organ or tissue. 5. The act of condensing a mass of amalgam or gold foil in the insertion of dental restorations in order to achieve accurate adaptation to cavity walls, to express excess mercury from amalgam, and to secure a more solid filling. 6. *In psychopathology*, a psychic mechanism whereby one idea becomes the symbolic expression of many incompatible, repressed ideas; the meaning of this symbol may not be clear to the conscious mind or to others. —**con·dense**, *v.*

con·dens·er, *n.* 1. A lens or combination of lenses used in microscopy for gathering and concentrating rays of light. 2. An apparatus for condensing gases or vapors. 3. An apparatus for the accumulation of electricity. 4. One of a number of instruments with a blunt end, usually serrated; used to condense amalgam or gold-foil filling material into a dental cavity.

con·di·tion, *v.* To establish, by training or re-peated exposure, a specific response to a particular stimulus.

conditioned avoidance response. *In psychology,* a conditioned reflex that prevents the occurrence of a painful or unpleasant stimulus. Abbreviated, CAR.

conditioned reflex or response. An automatic response to a stimulus which did not previously evoke the response; produced by repeatedly pairing a stimulus which normally does not produce a natural physiologic response with a second stimulus which normally produces a specific and innate response.

conditioned stimulus. A stimulus to which a conditioned reflex has been developed. Abbreviated, CS.

con·di·tion·ing, *n.* 1. *In psychology,* the process of attaching a new stimulus to an old response or a new response to an old stimulus; the process of establishing one or more conditioned reflexes. 2. The development of better physiologic condition through physical exercise.

con·dom (kon'dum) *n.* A sheath of thin rubber, plastic, or skin worn over the penis during copulation for preventing conception or infection.

con·duc·tance (kun·duck'tunce) *n.* The ability to conduct electrical or thermal energy; in electrical measurements the reciprocal of resistance.

con·duc·ti·bil·i·ty, *n.* 1. The capacity for being conducted. 2. CONDUCTIVITY; conducting power.

con·duct·ing artery. An artery of large caliber and elastic walls, as the aorta, common carotid artery, or subclavian artery.

con·duc·tion, *n.* The passage or transfer of electrons, heat, sound, or any form of mass or energy through suitable media, or of nerve and muscle impulses through those tissues. —**con·duc·tiv·i·ty,** *n.*

conduction aphasia. Aphasia due to interruption of association fibers connecting cortical centers, a concept prominent in nineteenth and early twentieth century schemes for classification of the aphasias, in which it included the syndromes of transcortical motor, transcortical sensory, subcortical motor, and subcortical sensory aphasia.

con·duc·tor, *n.* 1. A body or substance that transmits energy by direct molecular transfer; ap-

plied to carriers of heat, electric currents, and sound. 2. An instrument serving as a guide for the surgeon's knife.

condyl-, condylo-. A combining form meaning *condyle.*

con·dy·lar (kon'di·lur) *adj.* Pertaining to or associated with a condyle.

condylar joint. A form of synovial joint in which an ovoid articular surface or condyle of one bone is received into an elliptical articular surface.

con·dy·lar·thro·sis (kon''di·lahr·thro'sis) *n.,* pl. **condylarthro·ses** (·seez) CONDYLAR JOINT.

con·dyle (kon'dile, ·dil) *n.* Any rounded eminence such as occurs in the joints of many of the bones, especially the femur, humerus, and mandible.

con·dy·lec·to·my (kon''di·leck'tuh·mee) *n.* Excision of a condyle.

con·dy·loid (kon'di·loid) *adj.* CONDYLAR.

con·dy·lo·ma (kon''di·lo'muh) *n.,* pl. **condylomas, condyloma·ta** (·tuh) A wartlike growth or tumor, usually near the anus or pudendum. —**condy·lom·a·tous** (·lom'uh·tus, ·lo'muh·tus) *adj.*

condyloma acu·mi·na·tum (a·kew''mi·nay'tum), *pl.* **condyloma·ta acumina·ta.** A soft, warty nodule occurring on the mucosal surfaces of the female genitals, the glans penis, or around the anus; it is of viral origin.

condyloma la·tum (lay'tum). A syphilitic papule characteristic of secondary syphilis, where two surfaces of skin come into opposition; often warty and vegetative, very infectious, and usually teeming with *Treponema pallidum.*

con·dy·lot·o·my (kon''di·lot'uh·mee) *n.* OSTEOTOMY; especially, a division through the condyles of a bone.

cone, *n. & v.* 1. A solid body having a circle for its base and terminating in a point. 2. The mechanical element of the tooth crown; a term used by physical anthropologists in relation to the evolutionary development of teeth. 3. One of the light-receptive, flask-shaped cells which, with the associated rods, forms an outer layer, the neuroepithelial layer of the retina. 4. To make cone-shaped. 5. To cut and remove tissue in a rotary movement.

con·fab·u·la·tion (kon·fab''yoo·lay'shun) *n.* The fabrication of ready answers and fluent recitals of fictitious experiences in compensation for actual gaps in memory; seen primarily as a component of the amnestic syndrome.

con·fec·tion, *n. In pharmacy,* a soft mass of a vegetable drug mixed with sugar, syrup, or honey.

con·fi·den·ti·al·i·ty, *n. In medicine,* the relationship between a patient and his physician or any other member of a health care team, based on the assumption that all information will remain private and will be used only for his treatment and given out only with the patient's consent.

con·fig·u·ra·tion, *n.* Arrangement in space of atoms or groups of atoms of a molecule that can be changed only by breaking and making bonds. —**configuration·al,** *adj.*

con·fine·ment, *n.* 1. Restraint. 2. Lying-in, childbirth; parturition.

con·flict, *n. In psychiatry,* the clash of pure instinct with various psychic forces in its attempt to discharge its energies without modification, or between opposing forces within the psyche, as wishes.

con·flu·ence (kon′floo-unce) *n.* 1. A flowing together or merging of streams. 2. A uniting, as of neighboring lesions like vesicles and pustules.

con·flu·ens si·nu·um (kon′floo-enz sin′yoo-um) [NA]. Confluence of the sinuses; the dilated junction of the superior sagittal, the straight, the occipital, and the transverse sinuses of the dura mater.

con·flu·ent (kon′floo-unt) *adj.* 1. Running together; merged. 2. *In anatomy,* coalesced or blended; applied to two or more bones originally separate, but subsequently formed into one.

con·fo·cal (kon-fo′kul) *adj.* Having the same focus.

con·for·ma·tion (kon″for-may′shun) *n.* Any arrangement in space of atoms or groups of atoms of a molecule that can arise by rotation about a single bond and that is capable of finite existence. —**conformation·al,** *adj.*

con·fron·ta·tion, *n.* 1. Any method for approximating the visual fields without special equipment, commonly by bringing an object from the periphery into the patient's field of vision, and the patient indicating when he first sees the object. 2. The bringing together of a patient with another person, or confronting a patient with certain facts, for diagnostic or therapeutic purposes.

con·fu·sion, *n.* 1. A state of mental bewilderment. 2. *In neurology,* disorientation as to time, place, or person; sometimes accompanied by disturbed consciousness. 3. A mixing or confounding. —**confusion·al** *adj.*

confusion colors. A set of colors so chosen that they cannot be distinguished by one who is color-blind.

confusion letters. In testing vision, type letters, such as C, G, O, or F, P, T, liable to be mistaken for one another.

con·ge·la·tion (kon″je·lay′shun) *n.* 1. The effect of intense cold on the animal economy or any organ or part. 2. COAGULATION.

con·ge·ner (kon′je·nur) *n.* 1. An organism, structure, or substance allied by origin, nature, or function to another. 2. A species of organism belonging to the same genus as another. —**con·gen·er·ous** (kon·jen′ur·us), **con·ge·ner·ic** (kon″je·nerr′ick) *adj.*

con·gen·i·tal (kun·jen′i·tul) *adj.* Existing before or at birth, though not necessarily detected at that time.

congenital agammaglobulinemia. A congenital deficiency (in serum) of immunoglobulins, characterized clinically by increased susceptibility to bacterial infections; may be (a) a sex-linked recessive trait, affecting male infants, resulting in a failure to produce antibodies with undue susceptibility to bacterial infections usually in the second half-year of life, but with delayed hypersensitivity relatively intact and a tendency to develop symptoms similar to those seen in collagen diseases; (b) sporadic, affecting both sexes, with immunoglobulin levels somewhat higher than those seen in the sex-linked form; or (c) a part of combined immune deficiency.

congenital amaurotic familial idiocy. Tay-Sachs disease manifest at birth, formerly distinguished from Tay-Sachs disease by some writers.

congenital amputation. An amputation that occurs in the uterus as the result of some pathologic or accidental process; thought most often to be related to amniotic bonds or adhesions.

congenital aneurysm. An aneurysm due to a developmental defect.

congenital atelectasis. ATELECTASIS OF THE NEWBORN.

congenital disease. Any disorder present at birth; may be hereditary or acquired in utero.

congenital dislocation (of the hip). A potentially crippling abnormality, commonly involving one or both hip joints. Though present at birth, it is often discovered only after the child starts to walk.

congenital diverticulum. An outpouching of a hollow organ or viscus present at birth, as an esophageal diverticulum, an intestinal diverticulum, or a diverticulum ilei.

congenital fibrous ankylosis. Fibrosis affecting many of the joints; due to a variety of causes manifested as clubfoot and extension of knees and ankles.

congenital glaucoma. Glaucoma occurring in infants and children, usually transmitted as an autosomal recessive trait, resulting from incomplete or faulty development of the anterior chamber angle structures. May also occur as a primary or secondary glaucoma in association with numerous conditions such as oculocerebrorenal syndrome, rubella syndrome, neurofibromatosis, Sturge-Weber disease, aniridia, and Axenfeld's syndrome.

congenital harelip. Congenital fissure of the upper lip, due to failure of fusion of embryonic facial processes, often associated with cleft palate. The fissure may be of varying degrees, from a notch at the vermilion border to complete separation between the median nasal process and the maxillary process, the cleft extending into the nostril.

congenital hernia. A hernia present in fetal life and existing at birth, as an inguinal hernia in which the processus vaginalis remains patent, leading to the early descent of intestine into the scrotum, or a diaphragmatic hernia in which abdominal organs have passed into the thoracic cavity.

congenital hydrocele. The presence at birth of excessive fluid in the tunica vaginalis surrounding the testis, causing abnormal swelling.

congenital hydrocephalus. Hydrocephalus present at or shortly after birth; may be of the obstructive or communicating type and due to various causes.

congenital laryngeal stridor. Noisy, hoarse, or crowing respiratory sounds in newborns and infants, usually on inspiration; may be present transiently or persist due to a flabby epiglottis or malformations or tumors of the larynx or trachea.

congenital myasthenia. A frequently familial form of myasthenia, with onset in infancy or early childhood, usually with ptosis and extraocular muscle palsies, and a progressive course similar to the myasthenia seen in adults.

congenital polycystic disease. A hereditary disease in which the parenchyma of the kidney and less frequently that of the liver and pancreas are replaced to a variable extent by multiple cysts.

congenital porphyria. ERYTHROPOIETIC PORPHYRIA.

congenital rubella syndrome. RUBELLA SYNDROME.

congenital syphilis. Infection of a fetus with *Treponema pallidum* by placental transfer from the mother, usually after the fourth month of pregnancy.

congenital torticollis. Shortening and fibrosis of the sternomastoid muscle beginning in the first months of life, resulting in inclination of the head to one side.

con·ge·ries (kon'je·reez) *n.* Aggregation; agglomeration.

con·ges·tion, *n.* 1. An abnormal accumulation of fluid within the vessels of an organ or part; usually blood, but occasionally bile or mucus. 2. HYPEREMIA. —**con·gest·ed, conges·tive,** *adj.*

congestive heart failure. A state in which circulatory congestion exists as a result of heart failure.

con·gi·us (kon'jee·us) *n.*, *pl.* **con·gii** (kon'jee·eye) An apothecaries' measure equal to a gallon. Abbreviated, C., c., cong.

con·glo·bate (kon·glo'bate) *adj.* Forming a rounded mass.

²con·glom·er·ate (kon·glom'uh·rut) *adj.* 1. Massed together; aggregated. 2. A mass or aggregate of heterogeneous composition. — **con·glom·er·a·tion** (kun·glom''uh·ray'shun) *n.*

con·glu·tin (kon·gloo'tin) *n.* A simple protein of the globulin type; found in lupines, almonds, beans, and seeds of various leguminous plants.

con·glu·ti·nant (kon·gloo'ti·nunt) *adj.* Adhesive; promoting union, as of the edges of a wound.

con·glu·ti·na·tion (kon·gloo''ti·nay'shun) *n.* Abnormal union of two contiguous surfaces or bodies.

con·glu·ti·nin (kon·gloo'ti·nin) *n.* A nonspecific substance in the serums of certain animal species; it causes or aids in the agglomeration or lysis of certain cells or particles previously sensitized with antiserum and complement. Commonly found in bovine serums.

Con·go (kong'go). *n.* CONGO RED.

Congo red. Sodium diphenyldiazo-bis-α-naphthylamine sulfonate, $C_{32}H_{22}N_6Na_2O_6S_2$, a dye used as a pH indicator, as a test for amyloidosis, for determination of blood volume, as a histologic stain, and for other diagnostic tests.

Congo red test. A test for amyloidosis in which Congo red is injected intravenously. In normal persons, 30% of the dye disappears from the blood within an hour, but in amyloid disease 40 to 100% disappears.

con·gru·ence (kon·groo'unce) *n.* The quality or state of agreement or coinciding in some limited aspect of two or more otherwise different objects or data. —**congru·ent** (·unt) *adj.*

coni-, conio-, koni-, konio- A combining form meaning *dust.*

con·i·cal (kon'i·kul) *adj.* Resembling or shaped like a cone.

co·nid·io·phore (ko·nid'ee·o·fore) *n.* The mycelial structure of a fungus which bears conidia.

co·nid·i·um (ko·nid'ee·um) *n.*, *pl.* **conid·ia** (·ee·uh) An asexual spore cut from a fungus filament. —**conidi·al** (·ul) *adj.*

co·ni·ine (ko'nee·een, ·in, ko'neen) *n.* 2-Propylpiperidine, $C_8H_{17}N$, an alkaloid of conium.

co·ni·o·sis (ko''nee·o'sis) *n.*, *pl.* **conio·ses** (·seez) A disease or morbid condition due to inhalation of dust.

co·nio·spo·ri·o·sis (ko''nee·o·spo''ree·o'sis) *n.*, *pl.* **coniosporio·ses** (·seez). Acute pneumonitis from inhalation of spores of the fungus *Coniosporium corticale;* occurring among lumbermen stripping maple bark.

co·ni·um (ko·nigh'um, ko'nee·um) *n.* Poison hemlock, *Conium maculatum,* the fruit and leaves of which were formerly used medicinally in the treatment of spasmodic disorders. The activity of the plant is due to alkaloids which produce motor paralysis.

con·i·za·tion (kon''i·zay'shun) *n.* Excision of a cone of tissue, or a reaming out, as of a diseased endocervix.

con·joined, *adj.* Coming or brought together.

conjoined twins. Equal or unequal uniovular twins, united.

con·joint, *adj.* 1. Conjoined. 2. Pertaining to or done by two or more things in combination.

con·ju·gal (kon'juh·gul) *adj.* Of or pertaining to marriage or to husband and wife.

conjugata ve·ra (veer'uh) The distance from the middle of the sacral promontory to the posterior surface of the symphysis pubis.

con·ju·gate (kon'joo·gut, kon'juh·gate) *adj.* & *n.* 1. Coupled, conjoint, acting together. 2. Joined together but opposite in some characteristic, as a conjugate acid and base so related that when the acid loses a proton it is thereby converted to the base. 3. A substance formed by the union of two compounds. 4. CONJUGATE DIAMETER.

conjugate deviation. 1. The movement of both eyes in parallel, or the turning of the eyes in such a way that their visual axes remain parallel. 2. The forced and persistent turning of the eyes and head toward one side, usually toward the side of the lesion; observed with some disorders of the central nervous system.

conjugate diameter. Any of a number of diameters of the pelvis; especially, ANTEROPOSTERIOR DIAMETER (1).

conjugate gaze. The act of looking with the eyes coordinated in the same direction.

conjugate gaze paralysis, palsy, or **defect.** Lack of coordinate movements of the eyes, such as inability of both eyes to track concomitantly a moving object laterally or vertically.

con·ju·ga·tion, *n.* 1. The process in lower organisms, analogous to fertilization, involving the fusion of gametes, or the temporary union of individuals with exchange of nuclear material. 2. *In chemistry,* a specific structure in organic compounds exhibited by alternating single and double bonds between successive carbons atoms. 3. *In biochemistry,* the reaction by which an organic compound foreign to the body combines with a substance naturally available in the body to produce the elimination form of the foreign compound.

con·junc·ti·va (kon''junk·tye'vuh) *n.,* pl. & genit. sing. **conjuncti·vae** (·vee) The mucous membrane covering the anterior portion of the eyeball, reflected upon the lids and extending to their free edges. —**conjuncti·val** (·vul) *adj.*

conjunctival reflex. Closure of the eyelids induced by touching the conjunctiva. Syn. *lid reflex.*

conjunctival sac. The potential space between the bulbar and palpebral layers of conjunctiva.

con·junc·ti·vi·tis (kun·junk''ti·vye'tis) *n.* Inflammation of the conjunctiva.

con·junc·ti·vo·plas·ty (kon''junk·tye'vo·plas·tee) *n.* Plastic surgery of the conjunctiva.

con·nec·tive tissue. Any of the tissues of the body that support the specialized elements or parenchyma; particularly adipose, areolar, osseous, cartilaginous, elastic, fibrous connective, and lymphatic tissues.

con·nec·tor, *n.* The part of a dental bridge or prosthetic appliance that unites two or more components.

Conn's syndrome Hyperaldosteronism due to an adrenal tumor. Syn. *primary aldosteronism.*

cono-, con- A combining form meaning *cone.*

co·noid (ko'noid) *adj.* Conelike.

con·san·guin·i·ty (kon''sang·gwin'i·tee) *n.* 1. The relationship arising from common close ancestors; blood relationship. 2. INBREEDING; consanguineous mating. —**consanguin·e·ous** (·ee·us) *adj.*

con·science (kon'shunce) *n.* 1. The moral, self-critical part of one's self wherein have developed and reside standards of behavior and performance and value judgments. 2. The conscious superego.

con·scious (kon'shus) *adj. & n.* 1. Aware of one's own existence, of one's own mental states, and of the impressions made upon one's senses; able to take cognizance of sensations. 2. *In psychiatry,* the part of the psyche which is the object of immediate attention or awareness, as opposed to the subconscious and the unconscious.

con·sen·su·al (kun·sen'shoo·ul, kon·sens'yoo·ul) *adj.* 1. Of or pertaining to involuntary excitation by stimulation of another part. 2. Pertaining to or caused by involuntary movement accompanying voluntary movements.

consensual light reflex. The concurrent contraction of the shaded pupil when the other one is exposed to a bright light.

con·sent, *n.* An implicit or explicit acquiescence in a proposed course of medical action by a patient or one who can legally bind him. In emergencies, consent is implied by law.

con·ser·va·tive, *adj.* 1. Aiming at the preservation and restoration of injured parts. 2. Aiming at treatment by careful observation, limited or well-established therapy; not radical, experimental, or innovative.

con·sis·ten·cy, *n.* 1. The degree of density, firmness, viscosity, or resistance to movement of matter. 2. Agreement, constancy, or compatibility of a patient's history, signs, or symptoms of a disease.

con·sol·i·da·tion, *n.* The process of becoming firm or solid, as a lung in pneumonia. —**con·sol·i·date,** *v.*

con·so·nat·ing (kon'so·nay''ting) *adj.* Loud, clear, and resonant, as though reinforced by sympathetic vibrations.

consonating rale. A moderately coarse rale which sounds unusually loud and clear, being reinforced by transmission through an area of consolidated lung.

con·stant, *n.* 1. *In physics,* a property which remains numerically the same, and which may serve as a unit of measurement. 2. *In mathematics,* a quantity, having a definite and fixed value in a certain stage of investigation.

con·stel·la·tion (kon''ste·lay'shun) *n. In psychiatry,* a group of allied thoughts held together by a common emotional experience around a nuclear idea.

con·sti·pa·tion (kon''sti·pay'shun) *n.* A condition in which the bowels are evacuated at long intervals or with difficulty; costiveness. —**con·sti·pate** (kon'sti·pate) *v.*

con·sti·tu·tion, *n.* 1. GENOTYPE. 2. The total individuality of the person, including his inherited qualities and the cumulative effects of his reactions to all the environmental factors which influenced his physical and emotional development. 3. *In chemistry,* the arrangement of atoms to form a molecule. —**con·sti·tute,** *v.*

con·sti·tu·tion·al (kon''sti·tew'shun·ul) *adj.* 1. Having to do with or inherent in the structure of body or mind. 2. Forming the composition of something.

constitutional disease. 1. An inherent disease, owing to the individual's inherited genotypic characteristics. 2. A disease involving the entire body, as contrasted to a disease confined to one part.

constitutional reaction. 1. Any general, systemic, nonlocal reaction to a stimulus. 2. Any immediate or delayed systemic response to administration of a substance, as anaphylactic shock and serum sickness resulting from immunization, or the aftereffect of a histamine releaser.

con·sti·tu·tive enzyme. An enzyme whose concentration in a cell is constant and is not influenced by substrate concentration.

con·stric·tion, *n.* A contraction or narrowing.

con·stric·tive, *adj.* Tending to constrict; causing constriction.

constrictive pericarditis. Pericardial inflammation and fibrosis which results in squeezing of the heart and restriction of return blood flow as well as cardiac contraction. Syn. *Pick's disease.*

con·stric·tor, *n.* Any muscle that contracts or tightens any part of the body.

constructional apraxia. APRACTAGNOSIA.

con·sult, *v.* To hold a consultation; to confer, as with a consultant or an expert.

con·sul·tant, *n. In medicine,* a consulting physician; one summoned by the physician in attendance to give counsel in a case; usually, a specialist.

con·sul·ta·tion, *n. In medicine,* a deliberation between two or more physicians concerning the diagnosis and the proper method of treatment in a case.

con·sump·tion *n.* 1. Using up; depletion. 2. TUBERCULOSIS. **—consump·tive** (·tiv) *adj.*

consumption coagulopathy. DISSEMINATED INTRAVASCULAR COAGULATION.

con·tact, *n.* 1. Direct or indirect exposure to a source of infection, usually to a person affected with a contagious disease. 2. A person who has been exposed to a contagious disease. 3. A touching or connection. **—con·tac·tile** (kon·tack'til), **contac·tu·al** (·choo·ul) *adj.*

con·tac·tant (kon·tack'tunt) *n.* An allergen that induces sensitization and evokes the response of that sensitization by direct contact with the skin or mucous membranes.

contact areas. The areas on the proximal surfaces of teeth which touch adjacent teeth.

contact cancer. A cancer occurring on a surface, as on a lip, that has been in contact with a cancer of the opposing surface.

contact dermatitis. A dermatitis resulting either from the primary irritant effect of a substance or from sensitization to a substance coming in contact with the skin.

contact inhibition. The restraint in cell growth and division which normally follows contact between animal tissue cells, but which is lacking in cancer cells.

contact lens. A lens for the correction of refractive errors, consisting of a plastic shell, the concavity of which is in contact with the globe of the eye; a layer of liquid is interposed between the lens and the cornea.

contact radiation therapy. *In radiology,* relatively low-voltage, superficial therapy, delivered by an x-ray tube having an extremely short target-skin distance and capable of delivering large doses per minute.

contact ulcer. Superficial ulceration on the edge of the cartilaginous portion of the vocal folds; often caused by abuse of the voice or chronic aspiration.

contagious disease. 1. An infectious disease communicable by contact with one suffering from it, with his bodily discharge, or with an object touched by him. 2. Often, COMMUNICABLE DISEASE.

con·tam·i·na·tion, 1. Soiling with infectious or other harmful agents. 2. *In psychiatry,* the fusion of words, resulting in a neologism; often the first step in the process of condensation (6). 3. *In radiobiology,* the presence of radioactive material in an area where it is unwanted or harmful. **—con·tam·i·nate,** *v.;* **contami·nant,** *n.*

con·tent (kon'tent) *n.* 1. That which is contained; especially in psychology. 2. The amount or proportion (as of an element or substance) present or yielded.

con·ti·nence (kon'ti·nunce) *n.* 1. Self-restraint, especially in regard to sexual intercourse. 2. Control of bladder or bowel function.

3. The proper functioning of any sphincter or other structure of the gastrointestinal tract so as to prevent regurgitation or premature emptying. **—conti·nent** (·nunt) *adj.*

con·tin·gen·cy table. A two-way frequency table showing the frequency of occurrence of classifications of one variable for specified classification of the other variable.

continuous caudal anesthesia or **analgesia.** The maintaining of anesthesia by the insertion of a caudal needle or plastic catheter through the caudal hiatus into the sacrum for serial intermittent injections of the anesthetic agent.

continuous drainage. Constant emptying of a viscus, usually the urinary bladder by a retained catheter or tube.

continuous medium or **phase.** DISPERSION MEDIUM.

continuous spinal anesthesia. The maintaining of anesthesia by means of a spinal needle that is left in place so that the anesthetic drug can be administered periodically as needed.

continuous suture. A suturing in which the suture material is continued from one end of the wound to the other; may be of several types.

con·tour, *n.* 1. The line or surface that bounds, defines, or terminates a figure. 2. The surface shape of a dental restoration designed to restore functional anatomy of the tooth.

contra- A prefix meaning (a) *against, contrary;* (b) *opposite.*

con·tra·cep·tion (kon"truh·sep'shun) *n.* Prevention of conception, as a means of birth control.

con·tra·cep·tive (kon"truh·sep'tiv) *adj. & n.* 1. Preventing or tending to prevent conception. 2. An agent which prevents conception, such as medicated jelly in the vagina, a condom, a cervical pessary or diaphragm, or a systemically acting steroid that inhibits ovulation.

con·tract (kun·trakt') *v.* 1. To draw the parts together; shrink. 2. To acquire by contagion or infection.

contracted kidney. The shriveled condition of a kidney at the end stage of chronic glomerulonephritis, nephrosclerosis, or chronic pyelonephritis.

contracted pelvis. A pelvis having one or more major diameters reduced in size, interfering with parturition.

con·trac·tile (kon·track'til, ·tile) *adj.* Having the power or tendency to contract.

con·trac·til·i·ty (kon"track·til'i·tee) *n.* The property of shortening upon the application of a stimulus.

con·trac·tion (kun·track'shun) *n.* Shortening, especially of the fibers of muscle tissue.

con·trac·ture (kun·track'chur) *n.* 1. Shortening, as of muscle or scar tissue, producing distortion or deformity or abnormal limitation of movement of a joint. 2. Retarded relaxation of muscle, as when it is injected with veratrine.

con·tra·in·di·ca·tion (kon"truh·in"di·kay'shun) *n.* A symptom, indication, or condition in which a remedy or a method of treatment is inadvisable or improper. **—contra·in·di·cate** (·in·di·kate) *v.*

con·tra·lat·er·al (kon"truh·lat·ur·ul) *adj.* Situated on, affecting, or pertaining to the opposite side of the body.

con·trast, *n.* The visual differentiation of variations in photographic or film densities produced on a radiograph by structural composition of the object or objects radiographed.

contrast medium. A substance that, due to a difference in its absorption of x-rays from all or local surrounding tissues, permits radiographic demonstration of a space or organ.

con·tra·ver·sion (kon″truh-vur′zhun) *n.* A turning away from or in the opposite direction. —**contraver·sive** (·siv) *adj.*

con·tre·coup (kohn″truh-koo′) *n.* Injury of a part opposite to that struck, due to transmission of the shock, especially when the force is exerted against an organ or part containing fluid, as the skull, stomach, intestine, or urinary bladder.

con·trec·ta·tion (kon″treck·tay′shun) *n.* 1. The impulse to approach and caress a person of the opposite sex. 2. Foreplay preparatory to coition.

con·trol, *n.* 1. A standard by which to check observations, and insure the validity of their results. 2. A patient or subject, human or animal, or a group of patients or subjects, selected to participate in an experimental situation, as the trial of a drug, under the same experimental conditions as a similar individual or group except for omission or exclusion of the variable, e.g., drug, being investigated.

control experiment. An experiment used to check or verify other experiments, using conditions identical except for one factor.

con·tu·sion (kon·tew′zhun) *n.* 1. An injury usually caused by a blow in which the skin is not broken; BRUISE. —**con·tuse** (kon·tewz′) *v.; con·tused* (·tewzd′) *adj.*

co·nus (ko′nus) *n.,* pl. & genit. sing. **co·ni** (·nigh) 1. CONE. 2. A crescentic patch of atrophic choroid tissue near the optic disk, most common in myopia.

conus ar·te·ri·o·sus (ahr·teer″ee·o′sus) The cone-shaped eminence of the right ventricle of the heart from which the pulmonary trunk arises.

conus arteriosus pul·mo·na·lis (pul·mo·nay′lis). CONUS ARTERIOSUS.

con·va·les·cence (kon″vuh·les′unce) *n.* 1. The stage of gradual recovery of strength and health after an illness or injury. 2. The period of time spent in recovery. —**convales·cent** (·unt) *adj. & n.*

convalescent serum. The serum of the blood a patient recovering from an infectious disease; may be injected for prophylaxis of a particular infection in a susceptible individual, or used in diagnosis of a particular infection when the serum shows an appropriate titer rise.

con·val·lar·ia (kon″va·lair′ee·uh) *n.* The dried rhizome and roots of *Convallaria majalis,* the lily of the valley. It contains several cardioactive glycosides of variable activity.

con·vec·tion (kun·veck′shun) *n.* A transmission or carrying, as of heat.

con·ver·gence (kun·vur′junce) *n.* 1. Inclination or direction toward a common point, center, or focus, as of the axes of vision upon the near point. 2. CONCRESCENCE. 3. The coming to-

gether of a group of afferent nerves upon a motoneuron of the ventral horn of the spinal cord. —**conver·gent** (·junt) *adj.*

convergence defect, insufficiency, or **paralysis.** Inability to direct the visual axes of the two eyes toward each other, due to weakness of the extraocular muscles involved; usually of central nervous system origin, but sometimes precipitated by fatigue.

convergent strabismus. ESOTROPIA.

con·ver·sion (kun·vur′zhun) *n.* 1. *In psychiatry,* a defense mechanism whereby unconscious emotional conflict is transformed into physical disability, the affected part always having symbolic meaning pertinent to the nature of the conflict. 2. *In obstetrics,* an alteration in the presentation of the fetus to facilitate delivery.

conversion hysteria. 1. CONVERSION TYPE OF HYSTERICAL NEUROSIS. 2. DISSOCIATIVE TYPE OF HYSTERICAL NEUROSIS.

conversion reaction. CONVERSION TYPE OF HYSTERICAL NEUROSIS.

conversion type of hysterical neurosis. The form of hysterical neurosis in which the impulse causing anxiety is converted into functional symptoms of the special senses or voluntary nervous system, and may include anesthesia (anosmia, blindness, or deafness), paralysis (paresis, aphonia, monoplegia, or hemiplegia), or dyskinesias (tic, tremor, akinesia) and ataxia. The patient often shows a lack of concern (belle indifférence) for his deficits, which may provide him with secondary gains by the attention and sympathy obtained or by relieving him of responsibilities.

con·vex (kon′veks, kun·veks′) *adj.* Rounded, as a swelling of round or spherical form on the external surface; gibbous. —**con·vex·i·ty** (kon·veck′si·tee) *n.*

convexo-concave lens. A lens having a convex and a concave surface, which would not meet if continued. Its properties are those of a convex lens of the same focal distance.

con·vo·lut·ed (kon″vo·lew′tid) *adj.* Folded in curves or contorted windings; coiled, as tubules.

convoluted tubules. 1. The contorted tubules of the testis. 2. The parts of the renal tubule which lie in the cortex, as the proximal and distal convoluted portions of the nephron.

con·vo·lu·tion (kon″vo·lew′shun) *n.* A fold, twist, or coil of any organ, especially any one of the prominent convex parts of the brain, separated from each other by depressions or sulci. —**convolution·al,** *adj.*

convolutional atrophy. 1. Degeneration or atrophy primarily of the gray or white matter (or both) of the cerebral convolutions. 2. Shrinkage of the cerebral gyri and deepening of the sulci obvious on gross inspection of the outside of a brain, not necessarily representing atrophy primarily of the convolutions.

convolutional impressions or **markings.** Areas of decreased bone density in the shape of the subjacent cerebral convolutions, observed on the inner surface of the cranium, usually in cases of chronic abnormally high intracranial pressure. Syn. *digital markings or impressions.*

con·vul·sant (kun·vul'sunt) *n.* A medicine that causes convulsions.

con·vul·sion (kun·vul'shun) *n.* An involuntary general paroxysm of muscular contraction, which may be tonic or clonic or tonic followed by clonic. —**convul·sive**, *adj.*

convulsive equivalent. A form of epilepsy, especially in children, characterized by recurrent paroxysms of autonomic and sometimes behavioral disturbances, usually without specific systemic or intracranial disease, but with frequent abnormalities on the electroencephalogram, and responding to adequate anticonvulsant therapy. Common symptoms include headache, abdominal pain, nausea, vomiting, pallor, flushing, dizziness, faintness, sweating, fever, chills, and temper outbursts; postictal drowsiness and sleep of varying duration may follow. Other forms of epilepsy may be present. Syn. *seizure equivalent.*

Coo·ley's anemia or **disease** Thalassemia major. See *thalassemia.*

Cooley's trait Thalassemia minor. See *thalassemia.*

Coombs serum ANTIGLOBULIN SERUM.

Coombs' test ANTIGLOBULIN TEST.

Cooper's fascia CREMASTERIC FASCIA.

Cooper's hernia RETROPERITONEAL HERNIA.

Cooper's ligament 1. A fold of the transversalis fascia attached to the iliopectineal eminence and pubic spine. 2. A group of arching fibers connecting the base of the olecranon with the coronoid process on the medial aspect of the elbow joint.

co·or·di·na·tion (ko·or''di·nay'shun) *n.* 1. The harmonious activity and proper sequential action of those parts which cooperate in the performance of any function. 2. *In neurology,* the combination of nervous impulses in motor centers to ensure cooperation of the appropriate muscles in a reaction or reflex. 3. *In chemistry,* the joining of an ion or molecule to a metal ion by a nonionic valence bond to form a complex ion or molecule.

coot·ie (koo'tee) *n. Slang.* BODY LOUSE.

co·pai·ba (ko·pay'buh, ko·pye'buh) *n.* The oleoresin obtained from trees of *Copaifera* species (Leguminosae), native to South America. Has been used as stimulant, diuretic, diaphoretic, and expectorant; formerly was used in gonorrhea.

co·pe·pod (ko'pe·pod) *n.* Any of various small freshwater or saltwater crustaceans, some of which are intermediate hosts to worms parasitic in man.

cop·ing (ko'ping) *n.* A thin metal cap fitted to a prepared tooth to provide retention and support for an artificial crown.

Cop·lin jar A boxlike glass vessel with perpendicular grooves for holding microscopical slides apart during staining.

cop·per, *n.* Cu = 63.546. A reddish-brown, malleable metal, various salts of which have been used as astringents in inflammation of mucous membranes, as emetics, and, externally, as caustics. In certain nutritional anemias, particularly in infants, copper appears to enhance absorption of iron.

cop·per·as (kop'ur·us) *n.* FERROUS SULFATE.

copper sulfate. $CuSO_4.5H_2O$. Cupric sulfate, blue crystals or powder, soluble in water, used as an emetic, tonic, and astringent.

copr-, copro- A combining form meaning *feces, dung.*

co·pre·cip·i·ta·tion (ko''pre·sip''i·tay'shun) *n.* Precipitation of a contaminant with a desired precipitate even though the solubility constant of the contaminant has not been exceeded. This phenomenon is usually due to adsorption. —**co·pre·cip·i·tate** (ko''pre·sip'i·tate) *v.*

cop·rem·e·sis (kop·rem'i·sis) *n., pl.* **copreme·ses** (·seez) Vomiting of fecal matter.

cop·ro·an·ti·body (kop''ro·an'ti·bod·ee) *n.* Intestinal antibody found in the stool.

cop·roc·tic (kop·rock'tick) *adj.* Relating to feces; fecal.

cop·ro·lag·nia (kop''ro·lag'nee·uh) *n.* Sexual perversion in which pleasure is obtained from the idea, sight, or handling of feces.

cop·ro·la·lia (kop''ro·lay'lee·uh, ·lal'ee·uh) *n.* The repetitious, usually involuntary utterance of obscene words, primarily those referring to feces and fecal subjects, and to coitus; a symptom of such psychotic disorders as the Gilles de la Tourette syndrome and certain organic brain syndromes.

cop·ro·lith (kop'ro·lith) *n.* 1. A hard mass of fecal matter in the bowels. 2. Fossilized feces.

cop·roph·a·gy (kop·rof'uh·jee) *n.* Eating of feces. —**coropha·gous** (·gus) *adj.*

cop·ro·phil·ia (kop''ro·fil'ee·uh) *n.* An abnormal interest in fecal matter, seen in certain psychoses.

cop·roph·i·lous (kop·rof'i·lus) *adj.* Growing upon fecal matter; said of certain bacteria.

cop·ro·pho·bia (kop''ro·fo'bee·uh) *n.* 1. An abnormal fear of fecal matter. 2. The fear of or aversion to bowel movements.

cop·ro·por·phy·rin (kop''ro·por'fi·rin) *n.* Any of four isomeric, metal-free porphyrins, characterized by having four methyl groups and four propionic acid residues ($-CH_2CH_2COOH$) as substituent groups; first isolated from feces in congenital porphyria. One or more coproporphyrins occur also in normal urine, in larger amounts in urine in certain diseased states, and also following administration of certain drugs.

cop·ro·por·phy·rin·uria (kop''ro·por''fi·ri·new'ree·uh) *n.* The excretion of an abnormal amount of coproporphyrin in urine.

cop·ro·stane (kop'ro·stane) *n.* A steroid hydrocarbon, $C_{27}H_{48}$, isomeric with cholestane, differing from the latter in the manner of juncture of two of the component rings (the A and B rings). Syn. *pseudocholestane.*

co·pros·ter·ol (ko·pros'tur·ol) *n.* A sterol, $C_{27}H_{48}O$, excreted in feces; apparently derived from cholesterol, but structurally related to coprostane rather than to cholestane.

cop·ro·zo·ic (kop''ro·zo'ick) *adj.* Living in feces, as protozoans found in fecal matter.

Cop·tis, *n.* A genus of herbs of the Ranunculaceae, the crowfoot family. *Coptis groenlandica,* or goldthread, has been used as a simple bitter tonic.

cop·u·la·tion (kop''yoo·lay'shun) *n.* COITUS.

cor, *n.,* genit. **cor·dis** (kor'dis) HEART.

cor-, core-, coro- A combining form meaning *pupil* (of the eye).

coraco-. A combining form meaning *coracoid, coracoid process.*

cor·a·co·acro·mi·al (kor''uh·ko·a·kro'mee·ul) *adj.* Of, pertaining to, or involving the coracoid and the acromion processes.

cor·a·co·bra·chi·a·lis (kor''uh·ko·bray'kee·ay'lis, ·brack''ee·ay'lis) *n.* A muscle of the upper and medial part of the arm, arising from the coracoid process of the scapula.

cor·a·co·cla·vic·u·lar (kor''uh·ko·kla·vick'yoo·lur) *adj.* Pertaining to the coracoid process of the scapula and the clavicle.

cor·a·co·hu·mer·al (kor''uh·ko·hew'mur·ul) *adj.* Pertaining to the coracoid process of the scapula and the humerus.

cor·a·coid (kor'uh·koid) *adj. & n.* 1. Having the shape of a crow's beak. 2. CORACOID PROCESS.

coracoid process. A beak-shaped process of the scapula.

Coramine. A trademark for nikethamide, a respiratory stimulant.

cor bi·au·ric·u·la·re (bye''aw·rick''yoo·lair'ee). COR TRILOCULARE BIATRIUM.

cor bi·loc·u·la·re (bye·lock''yoo·lair'ee). A congenital malformation of the heart in which there is only one atrium and one ventricle, with a common atrioventricular valve, due to failure of development of the interatrial and interventricular septums. Syn. *bilocular heart.*

cor bi·ven·tric·u·la·re (bye''ven·trick''yoo·lair'ee). COR TRILOCULARE BIVENTRICULARE.

cor bo·vi·num (bo·vye'num) A greatly enlarged heart, particularly referring to the left ventricular hypertrophy associated with aortic regurgitation.

cord, *n.* 1. Any stringlike body. 2. A column of cells.

cor·date (kor'date) *adj.* Heart-shaped.

cord bladder. Dysfunction of the urinary bladder, due to a lesion in the spinal cord.

cord blood. Blood obtained from the umbilical cord.

cor·dec·to·my (kor·deck'tuh·mee) *n.* Excision of a cord, as removal of a vocal fold.

cor·di·form (kor'di·form) *adj.* Cordate; shaped like a heart.

cor·di·tis (kor·dye'tis) *n.* Inflammation of the spermatic cord; FUNICULITIS.

cor·do·pexy (kor'do·peck''see) *n.* The suturing of a vocal fold to a new support to relieve the stenosis resulting from bilateral abduction paralysis.

cordotomy. CHORDOTOMY.

core-. See *cor-.*

cor·e·cli·sis (kor''e·klye'sis) *n.,* pl. **cor·ecli·ses** (·seez) Pathologic closure or obliteration of the pupil.

cor·ec·ta·sis (kor·eck'tuh·sis) *n.,* pl. **corecta·ses** (·seez) Dilatation of the pupil.

cor·ec·to·pia (kor''eck·to'pee·uh) *n.* Displacement of the pupil; an abnormality in which the pupil is not in the center of the iris.

cor·e·di·al·y·sis (kor''e·dye·al'i·sis) *n.,* pl. **coredialy·ses** (·seez) Production of an artificial pupil at the ciliary border of the iris.

cor·el·y·sis (ko·rel'i·sis) *n.,* pl. **corely·ses** (·seez)

The detachment of iritic adhesions to the lens or cornea.

cor·eo·plas·ty (kor'ee·o·plas''tee) *n.* Any operation for forming an artificial pupil.

co·ri·an·der (ko''ree·an'dur) *n.* The dried ripe fruit of *Coriandrum sativum* (Umbelliferae). Aromatic, carminative, and stimulant, but used mainly to give flavor to certain medicinal preparations.

Cori cycle (kor'ee) A series of enzymatic reactions which purport to show the mode of conversion of lactic acid (formed during muscular activity from glycogen) to glucose in the liver, and its subsequent anabolism to glycogen in muscle.

co·ri·um (ko'ree·um) *n.* DERMIS.

corn, *n.* CLAVUS (1).

corne-, corneo-. A combining form meaning (a) *corneum, corneous;* (b) *cornea, corneal.*

cor·nea (kor'nee·uh) *n.* The transparent anterior portion of the eyeball, its area occupying about one-sixth the circumference of the globe. It is continuous with the sclera, and is nourished from the looped blood vessels at its peripheral border. —**cor·ne·al** (·nee·ul) *adj.*

cornea gut·ta·ta (guh·tay'tuh). A degenerative condition of the posterior surface of the cornea with wartlike thickenings of Descemet's membrane, resembling Hassall-Henle bodies but larger and axially as well as peripherally located; may progress to Fuch's dystrophy.

corneal arcus. An opaque ring in the corneal stroma; ARCUS JUVENILIS or ARCUS SENILIS.

corneal graft or **transplant.** Corneal tissue, usually human, transplanted into a defective cornea to provide a clear window.

corneal microscope. A high-power lens used to examine the cornea and iris in the living patient.

corneal pannus. Extension of vessels into the cornea from the limbus.

corneal reflex. Reflex closure of the eyelids when the cornea is touched.

Cor·ne·lia de Lange's syndrome (lahng'uh) 1. A complex of congenital malformations characterized by microbrachycephalia; peculiar facies; anomalies of the limbs, ranging from mild syndactyly to gross micromelia with or without phocomelia, hirsutism, and other abnormalities; and mild to usually severe mental and physical retardation. The cause is obscure, but abnormal dermatoglyphic and chromosomal patterns have been reported. 2. A complex of congenitally large muscles, giving the infant the appearance of a midget wrestler, together with mental retardation and, sometimes, spasticity or extrapyramidal disturbances.

Cornell Medical Index A medical history form, which can be checked by clerks, designed to save the physician's time; useful for large-volume work.

cor·neo·bleph·a·ron (kor''neo·o·blef'uh·ron) *n.* Adhesion of the surface of the eyelid to the cornea.

cor·neo·man·dib·u·lar (kor''nee·o·man·dib'yoo·lur) *adj.* Pertaining to the cornea and the mandible.

corneomandibular reflex. Deflection of the lower jaw to one side when, with the subject's mouth open, the cornea of the opposite eye is irritated.

cor·neo·oc·u·lo·gy·ric (kor″nee-o-ock″yoo-lo-jye′rick) *adj.* Pertaining to movements of the eye as a consequence of stimulation of the cornea.

corneooculogyric reflex. A variant of the conjunctival reflex, consisting of a contralateral or upward deviation of the eyes in response to stimulation of the conjunctiva or cornea, with associated contraction of the orbicularis oculi.

cor·neo·scle·ra (kor″nee-o-skleer′uh) *n.* The sclera and the cornea considered as forming one tunic. —**comeoscle·ral** (·ul) *adj.*

cor·ne·ous (kor′nee·us) *adj.* Horny or hornlike.

cor·nic·u·late (kor·nick′yoo·lut) *adj.* Furnished with horns or horn-shaped appendages.

cor·ni·fi·ca·tion (kor″ni·fi·kay′shun) *n.* The degenerative process by which the cells of a stratified squamous epithelium are converted into dead, horny squames as in the epidermis and such epidermal derivatives as hair, nails, feathers. —**cor·ni·fied** (kor′ni·fide) *adj.*

cor·noid (kor′noid) *adj.* Resembling horn.

cornoid lamella. A horn plug penetrating the epidermis and having a central column of parakeratotic cells, microscopically diagnostic of porokeratosis.

corn oil. The fixed oil from the embryo of the seed of *Zea mays.* Used as a therapeutic nutrient and as a solvent and vehicle for injectable medicaments, especially hormones.

cor·nu (kor′new) *n.,* genit. **cor·nus** (kor′noos, ·nus), pl. **cor·nua** (·new·uh) A horn; a horn-shaped process or excrescence. —**cornu·al** (·ul) *adj.*

cornual pregnancy. 1. Gestation occurring in one horn of a uterus bicornis. 2. INTERSTITIAL PREGNANCY.

cornu an·te·ri·us me·dul·lae spi·na·lis (an·teer′ee·us me·dul′ee spye·nay′lis) [NA]. ANTERIOR HORN; the anterior column of gray matter as seen in a cross section of the spinal cord.

cornua of the hyoid bone. Segments of the hyoid bone: the greater cornu projects backward from the lateral border of the body; the lesser cornu.

co·ro·na (ko·ro′nuh) *n.,* pl. & genit. sing. **coro·nae** (·nee) 1. A crown. 2. CORONA RADIATA.

corona ca·pi·tis (kap′i·tis). The crown of the head; the top of the head.

corona den·tis (den′tis) [NA]. CROWN OF A TOOTH.

corona glan·dis pe·nis (glan′dis pee′nis) [NA]. The posterior border of the glans penis.

cor·o·nal (kor′o·nul, ko·ro′nul) *adj.* 1. Of or pertaining to a corona or crown, especially the crown of the head, as: coronal suture. 2. Of or pertaining to the coronal suture, as: coronal plane. 3. Situated relatively near the crown, especially the crown of a tooth.

coronal plane. FRONTAL PLANE (1), especially one in the head.

coronal section. A section in a vertical and frontal plane making a 90° angle with the sagittal plane of the head.

coronal suture. The union of the frontal with the parietal bones transversely across the vertex of the skull.

corona ra·di·a·ta (ray″dee·ay′tuh) [NA]. 1. A radiating mass of white nerve fibers extending from the internal capsule to the cerebral cortex. 2. A zone of granulosa cells surrounding the zona pellucida of the ovum, which persists for some time after ovulation.

cor·o·nary (kor′uh·nerr″ee) *adj. & n.* 1. Of or pertaining to vessels, nerves, or attachments that encircle a part or an organ. 2. Pertaining to or involving the coronary arteries. 3. *Colloq.* A coronary thrombosis or occlusion with myocardial infarction; a "heart attack."

coronary cataract. A cataract which may be congenital or develop in early life, in which club-shaped opacities are arranged like a wreath or crown in the periphery of the cortex near the equator of the lens. Vision is usually not affected.

coronary insufficiency or **failure.** Prolonged precordial pain or discomfort without conventional evidence of myocardial infarction; subendocardial ischemia due to a disparity between coronary blood flow and myocardial needs.

coronary ligament 1. (of the liver:) A reflection of the peritoneum between the liver and the diaphragm surrounding the bare area of the liver. 2. (of the knee:) A thick inner portion of the capsule of the knee joint which attaches the medial and lateral menisci to the tibia.

coronary occlusion. Complete blockage of a branch of the arterial system that supplies blood to the heart muscle.

coronary sinus. A venous sinus that drains most of the cardiac veins, opens into the right atrium, and is located in the lower part of the coronary sulcus of the heart. It is derived from the transverse portion of the embryonic sinus venosus.

coronary thrombosis. Formation of a thrombus in a coronary artery of the heart.

cor·o·ner (kor′uh·nur) *n.* A legal officer, now usually a physician, of a municipality or county whose duty is to hold inquests regarding sudden, violent, or unexplained deaths.

cor·o·net (kor′o·net, kor·o·net′) *n.* 1. *In biology,* a crowning circle of hairs. 2. The lowest part of the pastern at its junction with a horse's hoof.

cor·o·ni·tis (kor″o·nigh′tis) *n.* Inflammation of the coronet of a horse's hoof.

co·ro·no·fa·cial (kuh·ro″no·fay′shul, kor″uh·no·) *adj.* Of or pertaining to the crown of the head and to the face.

cor·o·noid (kor′o·noid) *adj.* Curved like a beak, as the coronoid process of the ulna or of the mandible.

coronoid process. 1. A thin, flattened process projecting from the anterior portion of the upper border of the ramus of the mandible and serving for the insertion of the temporal muscle. 2. A triangular projection from the upper end of the ulna, forming the lower part of the radial notch.

corpora. Plural of *corpus.*

corpora albicantia. Plural of *corpus albicans.*

corpora amy·la·cea (am·i·lay′see·uh) AMYLOID BODIES.

corpora are·na·cea (ăr·e·nay′see·uh). Psammoma bodies in the pineal body; brain sand.

corpora ca·ver·no·sa (kav·ur·no'suh). Plural of *corpus cavernosum.*

corpora he·mor·rha·gi·ca (hem·o·raj'i·kuh). Plural of *corpus hemorrhagicum.*

corpora qua·dri·ge·mi·na (kwah·dri·jem'i·nuh). The inferior and superior colliculi collectively.

cor pul·mo·na·le (pul''mo·nay'lee). Acute right heart strain or chronic right ventricular hypertrophy with or without heart failure resulting from disease states which affect the function and/or structure of the lungs and cause pulmonary hypertension. Syn. *pulmonary heart disease.*

cor·pus (kor'pus) *n.,* genit. **cor·po·ris** (kor'po·ris), pl. **cor·po·ra** (kor'po·ruh) BODY.

corpus al·bi·cans (al'bi·kanz), pl. **cor·po·ra al·bi·can·tia** (kor'po·ruh al·bi·kan'tee·uh, ·chee·uh) [NA]. The white, fibrous scar in an ovary; produced by the involution of a corpus luteum.

corpus albicans cyst. A cystic corpus luteum remnant.

corpus cal·lo·sum (ka·lo'sum) [NA]. The great transverse commissure connecting the cerebral hemispheres; a broad, arched band of white matter at the bottom of the longitudinal fissure of the cerebrum.

corpus ca·ver·no·sum (kav''ur·no'sum) pl. **cor·po·ra ca·ver·no·sa** (kor'po·ruh kav·ur·no'suh). Either of the two cylinders of erectile tissue, right and left, separated proximally to form the crura and united distally, which constitute the greater part of the penis in the male and of the clitoris in the female .

corpus cavernosum cli·to·ri·dis (kli·tor'i·dis) [NA]. The corpus cavernosum of the clitoris.

corpus cavernosum penis (pee'nis) [NA]. The corpus cavernosum of the penis.

cor·pus·cle (kor'pus·ul) *n.* 1. A small rounded body. 2. An encapsulated sensory nerve end organ. 3. A cell, especially a blood cell.

corpus coc·cy·ge·um (kock·sij'ee·um) [NA]. A small arteriovenous anastomotic body associated with the median sacral artery.

corpuscula. Plural of *corpusculum.*

corpus he·mor·rha·gi·cum (hem''o·raj'i·kum). A collapsed graafian follicle containing blood; an early phase of a corpus luteum.

corpus lu·te·um (lew'tee·um) pl. **corpora lu·tea** [NA]. The yellow endocrine body formed in the ovary in the site of a ruptured graafian follicle. The large pale corpus luteum of pregnancy is called a true corpus luteum; the smaller dark corpus luteum of menstruation is called a false corpus luteum.

corpus luteum cyst. Cystic distention of a corpus luteum.

corpus luteum–stimulating hormone. LUTEINIZING HORMONE. Abbreviated, CLSH.

corpus spon·gi·o·sum pe·nis (spon''jee·o'sum pee'nis) [NA]. The cylinder of erectile tissue surrounding the penile urethra.

corpus stri·a·tum (strye·ay'tum) [NA]. The caudate and lenticular nuclei together with the internal capsule which separates them.

corpus ute·ri (yoo'tur·eye) [NA]. The body of the uterus, the portion between the cervix and the fundus.

cor·rect·ed transposition of the great arteries or **vessels.** A form of congenital heart disease in which the aorta occupies the anterior position usually occupied by the pulmonary artery, while the pulmonary artery lies behind it. The aorta, however, arises from a right ventricle which carries arterial blood and the pulmonary artery from a left ventricle carrying venous blood.

cor·rec·tive (ko·reck'tiv) *adj. & n.* 1. Intended or designed to correct or to modify favorably. 2. A substance used to modify or make more pleasant the action of the principal ingredients of a prescription.

corrective therapy. 1. *In physical medicine,* a medically supervised program of physical exercise and activities for the purpose of improving or maintaining the health of the patient through individual or group participation. 2. Specifically, techniques designed to conserve and increase neuromuscular strength and skill, to reestablish or improve ambulation, to improve habits of personal health, and to promote relaxation by adjustment to physical and mental stresses.

cor·re·la·tion (kor''e·lay'shun) *n. In biometry,* the degree of association between two characteristics in a series of observations, usually expressed as the coefficient of correlation. —**cor·re·late** (kor'e·late) *v.;* **cor·rel·a·tive** (ko·rel'uh·tiv) *adj.*

Cor·ri·gan's pulse A pulse characterized by a rapid forceful ascent (water-hammer quality) and rapid downstroke or descent (collapsing quality); seen with aortic regurgitation and hyperkinetic circulatory states.

cor·ro·sive, *adj. & n.* 1. Tending to eat or wear away, especially by chemical action. 2. A substance that destroys organic tissue either by direct chemical means or by causing inflammation and suppuration.

corrosive sublimate. MERCURY BICHLORIDE.

cor·set, *n. In surgery,* a removable appliance embracing the trunk from pelvis to chest; used for correction of deformities, for support of injured bones and muscles of the spine or thorax, or in control of ventral hernia.

corset liver. A liver with a fibrotic groove on the anterior surface at the costal margin, said to be produced by compression of the liver by a rib from tight corset stays.

Cortef. A trademark for hydrocortisone, an anti-inflammatory glucocorticoid.

cor·tex (kor'tecks) *n.,* pl. **cor·ti·ces** (·ti·seez) 1. The bark of an exogenous plant. 2. [NA] The peripheral portion of an organ, situated just beneath the capsule. 3. *In neuroanatomy,* the external gray layer of the brain, as: cerebral cortex, cerebellar cortex. 4. *In neurology,* a functional area of the cerebral cortex, as: auditory cortex, motor cortex. Comb. form *cortic(o)-.*

cortex re·nis (ree'nis) [NA]. The cortex of a kidney.

cortic-, cortico-. A combining form meaning *cortex, cortical.*

cor·ti·cal (kor'ti·kul) *adj.* Of or pertaining to a cortex.

cortical adenoma. A benign neoplasm composed principally of cells resembling those of the adrenal cortex, but with little or no tendency to form acini.

cortical blindness. Loss of visual sensation, including light and dark, together with loss of reflex blinking to bright illumination or threatening gestures, but with intact pupillary reflexes, normal ocular motility, and normal retinoscopy; due to disturbances of cerebral visual centers.

cortical bone. The compact bone next to the surface of a bone.

cortical cords. The secondary cordlike invaginations of the germinal epithelium of the embryonic gonad that differentiate into primary follicles and oogonia.

cortical deafness. Deafness due to bilateral lesions of Heschl's gyri.

cortical degeneration. 1. Any degenerative disease of the central nervous system involving primarily gray matter. 2. GENERAL PARALYSIS. 3. The degeneration of the cortex of any organ.

cortical hormone. ADRENOCORTICAL HORMONE.

cortices. Plural of *cortex*.

cor·ti·cif·u·gal (kor'ti·sif'yoo·gul) *adj.* Conducting away from the cortex.

cor·ti·cip·e·tal (kor'ti·sip'e·tul) *adj.* Conducting toward the cortex.

cortico-. See *cortic-*.

cor·ti·co·bul·bar (kor''ti·ko·bul'bur) *adj.* Pertaining to the cerebral cortex and the medulla oblongata.

corticobulbar tract. Fibers of the pyramidal system that originate in the motor cortex, pass through the internal capsule, and terminate in the motor nuclei of the cranial nerves.

cor·ti·co·col·lic·u·lar (kor''ti·ko·kol·ick'yoo·lur) *adj.* Pertaining to the cerebral cortex and a colliculus.

cor·ti·co·ge·nic·u·late (kor''ti·ko·je·nick'yoo·lut) *adj.* Pertaining to the cerebral cortex and a geniculate body.

cor·ti·co·hy·po·thal·am·ic (kor''ti·ko·high''po·thuh·lam'ick) *adj.* Pertaining to the cerebral cortex and the hypothalamus.

cor·ti·coid (kor'ti·koid) *n.* CORTICOSTEROID.

cor·ti·co·med·ul·lary (kor''ti·ko·med'yoo·lerr·ee) *adj.* Pertaining to the cortex and the medulla of an organ, as those of the kidney, or to the cerebral cortex and the medulla oblongata.

cor·ti·co·ni·gral (kor''ti·ko·nigh'grul) *adj.* Pertaining to the cerebral cortex and the substantia nigra.

cor·ti·co·nu·cle·ar (kor''ti·ko·new'klee·ur) *adj.* Pertaining to the cerebral cortex and the motor nuclei of the cranial nerves.

cor·ti·co·pal·li·dal (kor''ti·ko·pal'i·dul) *adj.* Pertaining to the cerebral cortex and the globus pallidus.

cor·ti·co·pon·tine (kor''ti·ko·pon'teen) *adj.* Pertaining to the cerebral cortex and the pons.

cor·ti·co·pon·to·cer·e·bel·lar (kor''ti·ko·pon''to·serr·e·bel'ur) *adj.* 1. Connecting the cerebral cortex with the cerebellum by way of the pons, as: corticopontocerebellar pathway.

2. Pertaining to any neurologic function or disorder involving this connection pathway.

cor·ti·co·ru·bral (kor''ti·ko·roo'brul) *adj.* Pertaining to the cerebral cortex and the red nucleus.

cor·ti·co·spi·nal (kor''ti·ko·spye'nul) *adj.* Pertaining to the brain cortex and the spinal cord.

corticospinal tracts. Efferent tracts that descend from the motor cortex through the internal capsule, cerebral peduncles, pons, and medulla, where they undergo incomplete decussation to form the lateral and anterior corticospinal tracts. They are concerned in finely coordinated voluntary movements.

cor·ti·co·ste·roid (kor''ti·ko·steer'oid, ·sterr'oid, kor''ti·kos'tur·oid) *n.* Any steroid which has certain chemical or biological properties characteristic of the hormones secreted by the adrenal cortex. Syn. *corticoide*.

cor·ti·cos·ter·one (kor''ti·kos'tur·ohn) *n.* 4-Pregnene-11,21-diol-3,20-dione, $C_{21}H_{30}O_4$, a steroid hormone occurring in the adrenal cortex. It influences carbohydrate and electrolyte metabolism and muscular efficiency and protects against stress.

cor·ti·co·stri·ate (kor''ti·ko·strye'ate) *adj.* Pertaining to nerve fibers arising in the cerebral cortex and terminating in the corpus striatum.

cor·ti·co·stri·a·to·spi·nal (kor''ti·ko·strye''uh·to·spye'nul) *adj.* Pertaining to nervous pathways involving the cerebral cortex, corpus striatum, and spinal cord.

cor·ti·co·strio·ni·gral (kor''ti·ko·strye''o·nigh'grul) *adj.* Pertaining to the cerebral cortex, the corpus striatum, and substantia nigra.

cor·ti·co·tha·lam·ic (kor''ti·ko·thuh·lam'ick) *adj.* Pertaining to the cerebral cortex and the thalamus.

corticotropic hormone. ADRENOCORTICOTROPIC HORMONE.

cor·ti·co·tro·pin (kor''ti·ko·tro'pin) *n.* A hormonal preparation having adrenocorticotropic activity derived from the adenohypophysis of certain domesticated animals. —**cortico·tro·pic** (·trop'ick, ·tro'pick) *adj.*

cor·tin (kor'tin) *n.* An extract of adrenal cortex that contains several hormones; has been used in treating adrenal cortical hypofunction.

cor·ti·sol (kor'ti·sol) *n.* HYDROCORTISONE.

cor·ti·sone (kor'ti·sone) *n.* 17-Hydroxy-11-dehydrocorticosterone, $C_{21}H_{28}O_5$, a glucogenic adrenocortical steroid produced commercially by synthesis; used, as the acetate, chiefly for substitution therapy in adrenal insufficiency, and in acute infections, in shock, in allergic states, and in the collagen diseases. Syn. *Kendall's compound E, Wintersteiner's compound F, Reichstein's substance Fa.*

cor tri·a·tri·a·tum (trye·ay''tree·ay'tum). A congenital cardiac anomaly assuming one of several types, with the shared feature of having three chambers preceding the ventricles: (a) division of the left atrium by a septum separating the mitral valve from the pulmonary vein openings; (b) three atria, the left receiving the pulmonary veins, the middle receiving the superior vena cava, the right receiving the inferior vena cava; (c) a third atrium lying between the septum primum and septum secundum, receiving the left superior vena cava and emptying into the coronary sinus.

cor tri·au·ri·cu·la·re (trye"aw·rick"yoo·lair'ee). A congenital cardiac anomaly in which failure of resorption of the common pulmonary vein leads to the formation of an appendage projecting into the left atrium to take a position close to the mitral valve.

Cortril. A trademark for hydrocortisone, an anti-inflammatory glucocorticoid.

cor tri·lo·cu·la·re (trye·lock"yoo·lair'ee). A three-chambered heart; in humans, a congenital anomaly in which there is either a single atrium or a single ventricle. Syn. *trilocular heart.*

cor triloculare bi·atri·um (bye·ay'tree·um). A congenital cardiac anomaly consisting of absence of the ventricular septum; the two atria communicate with a common single ventricle.

cor triloculare bi·ven·tri·cu·la·re (bye"ven·trick'yoo·lair'ee). A congenital cardiac anomaly due to failure of development of the interatrial septum; the heart is composed of a single atrium and two ventricles.

cor triloculare mon·atri·a·tum (mon·ay"tree·ay'tum). COR TRILOCULARE BIVENTRICULARE.

cor·us·ca·tion (kor"us·kay'shun) n. The subjective sensation of light flashes.

cor vil·lo·sum (vi·lo'sum). Fibrinous pericarditis in which fibrin projects from the pericardial surface in villous processes.

co·ryd·a·lis (ko·rid'uh·lis) n. The tuber of *Dicentra canadensis,* squirrel corn, or of *D. cucullaria,* Dutchman's-breeches, containing several alkaloids, including corydaline, isocorydine, and protopine; has been used as a tonic and alterative.

Cor·y·ne·bac·te·ri·um (kor"i·ne·back·teer'ee·um, ko·rye"ne·) n. A genus of slender, aerobic, nonmotile, non-spore-forming, gram-positive bacteria of which *Corynebacterium diphtheriae* is the type species; varying from slightly curved to club-shaped and branching forms; showing irregular staining. This genus includes a large group of diphtheroid bacilli, such as *C. acnes, C. pyogenes,* mainly saprophytic and morphologically similar to *C. diphtheriae;* found in normal tissues and secretions as well as in pathologic conditions; probably not causative. **—corynebacterium,** pl. **co·ryne·bac·te·ria,** *com. n.*

Corynebacterium diph·the·ri·ae (dif·theer'ee·ee). The causative organism of diphtheria; the varieties *gravis, mitis,* and *intermedius* have been described; produces a potent exotoxin. Syn. *Bacillus diphtheriae.*

co·ry·za (ko·rye'zuh) n. Inflammation of the mucous membranes of the nose, usually marked by sneezing, nasal airway congestion, and discharge of watery mucus; acute rhinitis.

cosm-, cosmo- A combining form meaning (a) *universe, universal;* (b) *pertaining to outer space.*

cos·met·ic (koz·met'ick) *adj. & n.* 1. Serving or intended to improve appearance. 2. A preparation applied to the skin or its appendages to alter its appearance, to protect it, to beautify, or to promote attractiveness.

cos·mic ray. A very penetrating radiation originating outside the earth's atmosphere, capable of producing ionization in passing through air or other matter. Primary cosmic rays probably consist of atomic nuclei, mainly protons, having energies up to 10^{15} electron volts; they are absorbed in the upper atmosphere. Secondary cosmic rays are produced when primary rays interact with nuclei and electrons in the earth's atmosphere; these consist mainly of mesons, protons, neutrons, electrons, and photons.

cost-, costi-, costo-. A combining form meaning *rib, costal.*

cos·ta (kos'tuh) n., pl. & genit. sing. **cos·tae** (·tee) RIB. **—cos·tal** (·tul) *adj.*

costal angle. The angle formed by the right and left costal cartilages at the xiphoid process.

costal cartilage. The cartilage occupying the interval between the ribs and the sternum or adjacent cartilages.

cos·tal·gia (kos·tal'jee·uh) n. Intercostal neuralgia; pain in the ribs.

costal respiration. Respiration effected primarily by intercostal muscles moving the thoracic cage.

cos·tec·to·my (kos·teck'tuh·mee) n. Excision of a rib or a part of one.

Cos·ten's syndrome Malfunction of the temporomandibular joint, originally thought to be secondary to dental malocclusion with associated neuralgia and ear symptoms; now considered part of the myofacial pain-dysfunction syndrome.

cos·ti·form (kos'ti·form) *adj.* Rib-shaped.

cos·tive (kos'tiv) *adj. & n.* 1. Causing, pertaining to, or characterized by constipation. 2. An agent that decreases intestinal motility. **—cos·tive·ness** (·nus) n.

cos·to·car·ti·lage (kos"to·kahr'ti·lij) n. COSTAL CARTILAGE.

cos·to·cer·vi·cal (kos"to·sur'vi·kul) *adj.* Pertaining to the ribs and the neck.

cos·to·chon·dral (kos"to·kon'drul) *adj.* Pertaining to the ribs and their cartilages.

cos·to·chon·dri·tis (kos"to·kon·drye'tis) n. Inflammation of a costal cartilage.

cos·to·cla·vic·u·lar (kos"to·kla·vick'yoo·lur) *adj.* Pertaining to the ribs and the clavicle.

cos·to·cor·a·coid (kos"to·kor'uh·koid) *adj.* Pertaining to the ribs and the coracoid process.

cos·to·me·di·as·ti·nal (kos"to·mee"dee·uh·stye'nul) *adj.* Pertaining to the ribs and the mediastinum.

cos·to·phren·ic (kos"to·fren'ick) *adj.* Pertaining to the ribs and the diaphragm.

costophrenic angle. The angle formed by the ribs and diaphragm.

cos·to·scap·u·lar (kos"to·skap'yoo·lur) *adj.* Of or pertaining to the ribs and the scapula; scapulocostal.

cos·to·ster·nal (kos"to·stur'nul) *adj.* Pertaining to a rib and the sternum.

cos·to·tome (kos'tuh·tome) n. Heavy curved shears or forceps with a hooked limb against which the knife blade acts; used for rib resection.

cos·tot·o·my (kos·tot'uh·mee) n. *In surgery,* the division of a rib.

cos·to·trans·ver·sec·to·my (kos"to·trans"vur-seck'tuh·mee) *n.* Excision of part of a rib and a transverse process of a vertebra.

cos·to·ver·te·bral (kos"to·vur'te·brul) *adj.* Pertaining to a rib and the vertebral column; applied to the joints between them.

cos·to·xiph·oid (kos"to·zif'oid) *adj.* Pertaining to the ribs and the xiphoid cartilage.

cot, *n.* FINGER COT.

co·tar·nine (ko·tahr'neen, ·nin) *n.* An alkaloid, $C_{12}H_{15}NO_4$, obtained by oxidation of narcotine. Cotarnine chloride has been used as a hemostatic in uterine hemorrhage and hemoptysis.

co·to (ko'to) *n.* Coto bark; the bark of a tree native to Bolivia, *Aniba coto.* It has been used in treatment of diarrhea and for the night sweats of pulmonary tuberculosis.

co·trans·am·i·nase (ko"trans·am'i·nace, ·naze) *n.* Pyridoxal phosphate, the prosthetic component of certain transaminating enzymes, as well as of the enzyme carboxylase which catalyzes decarboxylation of L-amino acids, in which latter case it is commonly referred to as codecarboxylase.

cot·ton, *n.* The hairs of the seed of cultivated varieties of *Gossypium herbaceum* or of other species of *Gossypium.*

cottonseed oil. The fixed oil from the seed of cultivated species of *Gossypium.*

cotton-wool exudates. Fluffy, white, superficial lesions in the retina from microinfarction of the nerve fiber layer; seen in hypertensive retinopathy and collagen vascular diseases.

cot·y·le·don (kot"i·lee'don) *n.* 1. Any one of the groups of villi separated by smooth chorion characteristic of the ruminant semiplacenta. 2. Any one of the rounded lobules bounded by placental septums into which the uterine surface of a discoid placenta is divided. 3. The primary or seed leaf in the phanerogamic embryo. —**coty·le·don·ary** (·lee'duh·nerr"ee) *adj.*

cough (kof) *v. & n.* 1. To expel air suddenly and violently from the lungs after deep inspiration and closure of the glottis; a protective reflex caused by irritation of the laryngeal, tracheal, or bronchial mucosa. 2. A single instance of such an expulsion of air. 3. A condition, transient or chronic, in which persistent irritation of respiratory mucosa gives rise to episodes of coughing.

cough plates. A dish of nutrient medium intended for inoculation by having the patient cough directly onto the medium; chiefly used in the diagnosis of whooping cough.

cough syncope. Fainting following a severe episode of coughing.

cou·lomb (koo·lom', koo'lom) *n.* 1. The unit of electric quantity; the quantity of electricity transferred by a current of 1 ampere in 1 second. 2. The unit of charge in the meter-kilogram-second (mks) system, being the charge that accumulates in a capacitor if a current of 1 ampere flows into the capacitor for 1 second.

Coumadin. Trademark for warfarin, an anticoagulant used as the sodium derivative.

cou·ma·rin (koo'muh·rin) *n.* 1,2-Benzopyrone, $C_9H_6O_2$, widely distributed in the vegetable kingdom, including the tonka bean. Has been used for its odorous quality, as in imitation vanilla extracts, and for concealing odors, but as continued ingestion may produce hemorrhage its use as a food flavor has been prohibited.

Coun·cil·man bodies or **cells** Oxyphilic inclusion bodies occurring in the cytoplasm of liver cells in yellow fever and certain other viral diseases, presumably zones of cytoplasmic coagulation necrosis surrounding virus particles.

count, *n.* The number obtained by reckoning the units of a series or collection, as blood count, the number of blood cells per unit volume of blood.

counter- A prefix meaning (a) *against, opposing;* (b) *opposite;* (c) *offsetting, counteracting;* (d) *contrastive, complementary;* (e) *reactive, retaliatory.*

count·er, *n.* An apparatus designed to facilitate counting.

coun·ter·ac·tion (kæwn"tur·ack'shun) *n.* The action of a drug or agent opposed to that of some other drug or agent.

coun·ter·die (kæwn'tur·dye) *n.* The opposite or reverse image of a die, made of metal or other substance of suitable hardness; used together with the die to form or swage some material in the fabrication of a dental restoration.

coun·ter·ex·ten·sion (kæwn"tur·ecks·ten'shun) *n.* Traction made in a direction opposite to that in which traction is made by another force.

coun·ter·ir·ri·tant (kæwn"tur·irr'i·tunt) *n.* An agent that produces inflammation of the skin for the relief of a more deep-seated inflammation. —**counter·ir·ri·ta·tion** (·irr"i·tay'shun) *n.;* **counter·ir·ri·tate** (·irr'i·tate) *v.*

coun·ter·open·ing (kæwn'tur·o"pun·ing) *n.* A second incision into an abscess or cavity, made opposite to the first, for purposes of drainage.

coun·ter·pho·bia (kæwn"tur·fo'bee·uh) *n.* The seeking out or preference for the same situation of which a phobic person was, or still is, afraid, as a result of the pleasure derived from having conquered or conquering the anxiety produced by that situation. —**counterpho·bic** (·bick) *adj.*

coun·ter·pres·sure (kæwn"tur·presh'ur) *n.* Manipulation to counterbalance pressure by exercising force in the opposite direction.

coun·ter·shock (kæwn'tur·shock") *n.* 1. A phase of the alarm reaction or first phase of the general adaptation syndrome. 2. An electric shock administered through two electrodes on the chest, to convert the cardiac rhythm from atrial or ventricular fibrillation to normal sinus rhythm.

coun·ter·stain (kæwn'tur·stain") *n.* 1. A second general stain applied before or after the principal stain, to afford better contrast and to color other tissue elements beside the one demonstrated by the principal stain. 2. To apply a counterstain.

coun·ter·trac·tion (kæwn"tur·track"shun) *n. In surgery,* a traction which offsets another, as in reducing fractures.

coun·ter·trans·fer·ence (kown″tur·trans′fur·unce) *n. In psychiatry,* the conscious or unconscious emotional reaction of the therapist to the patient, which may interfere with psychotherapy.

coup-con·tre·coup injury (koo′ kohn″truh·koo″) Bruising of the surface of the brain beneath the point of impact (coup injury) and the more extensive lacerations and contusions on the opposite side of the brain (contrecoup injury).

cou·pling (kup′ling) *n.* The phase of gene linkage in which two different mutant genes are located on the same chromosome and therefore are inclined to be inherited either together or not at all in the next generation.

court plaster. A solution of isinglass made with alcohol, glycerin, and hot water spread on silk and allowed to dry; used to hide blemishes or to close small wounds.

Cou·ve·laire uterus (koo·vᵉ·lair′) A pregnant uterus with a bluish, purplish, coppery coloration, and woody consistency due to premature separation of the placenta with interstitial myometrial hemorrhage.

Cour·voi·sier's law (koor·vwah²z·ye²ʸ) In jaundice due to obstruction of the common bile duct by gallstones, the gallbladder is often contracted; a distended gallbladder suggests obstruction from other causes, e.g., carcinoma of the pancreas.

cov·er glass. *In microscopy,* the thin slip of glass covering the object mounted on the slide.

cover slip. COVER GLASS.

cover test. *In ophthalmology,* a test for extraocular muscle defects in which the patient fixates on a target in different directions of gaze while one eye is covered; the position of that eye is noted on removal of the cover. If, on uncovering, an eye shifts outward, for example, its position under cover was inward.

cover-uncover test. *In ophthalmology,* a test for the evaluation of visual acuity in individuals, such as infants or mental retardates, for whom testing with a Snellen chart using pictures is not feasible, in which one eye is covered while the other is fixed on some target. If an eye moves consistently under covering the other, poor alignment or amblyopia may exist.

cow·per·i·tis (kow″pur·eye′tis, koo′pur·) *n.* Inflammation of the bulbourethral glands.

Cow·per's cyst (koo′pur, kow′pur) A retention cyst of the bulbourethral glands.

Cowper's glands BULBOURETHRAL GLANDS.

Cowper's ligament The part of the fascia lata attached to the pubic crest.

cow·pox, *n.* VACCINIA.

coxa (kock′suh) *n.,* pl. & genit. sing. **cox·ae** (·see) HIP. **—cox·al** (·sul) *adj.*

cox·al·gia (kock·sal′jee·uh) *n.* Pain in the hip joint; especially, disease of the hip. **—coxal·gic** (·jick) *adj.*

cox·ar·thro·lis·thet·ic pelvis (kocks·ahr″thro·lis·thet′ick) A unilateral or bilateral transversely contracted pelvis, resulting from softening about the acetabulum with projection of the head of the femur into the pelvic cavity.

coxa val·ga (val′guh). A condition, the reverse of coxa vara, in which the angle between the neck and the shaft of the femur is increased above 140°.

coxa va·ra (vair′uh). A condition in which the neck of the femur is bent downward sufficiently to cause symptoms; this bending may reach such an extent that the neck forms, with the shaft, a right angle or less, instead of the normal angle of 120 to 140°.

Cox·i·el·la (kock″see·el′uh) *n.* A genus of the family Rickettsiaceae, which includes the causative agent of Q fever.

Coxiella bur·ne·tii (bur·net′ee·eye). The species of *Coxiella* which is the etiologic agent of Q fever.

cox·i·tis (kock·sigh′tis) *n.,* pl. **cox·it·i·des** (kock·sit′i·deez) Inflammation of the hip joint.

Cox·sack·ie disease (kok·sak′ee, kuk·) A variety of clinical syndromes resulting from infection with the Coxsackie viruses. The clinical entities include herpangina, exanthematous febrile diseases, aseptic meningitis, a disease mimicking poliomyelitis, myocarditis, pericarditis, and pleurodynia.

Coxsackie virus. Any of a group of antigenically distinct picornaviruses; the cause of Coxsackie disease in humans and found experimentally to induce destruction of striated muscle, paralysis, and death in infant mice.

C.P. Chemically pure.

CPC Abbreviation for *clinical-pathological conference.*

Cr Symbol for chromium.

crab louse. PHTHIRIUS PUBIS.

cracked-pot resonance, note, or sound. A characteristic clinking sound, elicited by percussion over a pulmonary cavity communicating with a bronchus, especially when the percussion is forcible and the patient's mouth is open.

crackling rale. SUBCREPITANT RALE.

cra·dle, *n.* 1. A small bed for a baby. 2. A frame of wicker, wood or wire, used to prevent the bedclothes from coming in contact with a fractured or injured part.

cradle cap. Heavy, greasy crusts on the scalp of an infant; seborrheic dermatitis of infants.

cramp, *n.* 1. Painful, involuntary contraction of a muscle, such as occurs at night in normal individuals in a foot or leg, or in swimmers. 2. Any cramplike pain, as of the intestine. 3. Spasm of certain muscles, which may be intermittent, as in tetany, or occupational, resulting from their excessive use. 4. *Colloq.* (usually pl.) DYSMENORRHEA.

crani-, cranio- A combining form meaning *cranium, cranial.*

-crania A combining form designating (a specified) *kind or condition of the skull or head.*

cra·ni·ad (kray′nee·ad) *adv.* Toward the cranium or head.

cra·ni·al (kray′nee·ul) *adj.* 1. Of or pertaining to the cranium or the skull. 2. Directed toward the head; in human anatomy, superior.

cranial cracked-pot sound. The change in sound on percussion of the skull where there is widening of the sutures; a diagnostic sign after early infancy, of increased intracranial pressure.

cranial nerve palsy or **paralysis.** Paralysis of the

parts of the body controlled by the cranial nerves, usually caused by, and accompanying, some other disorder.

cranial nerves. Nerves arising directly from the brainstem and making their exit to the periphery via openings in the skull: I, olfactory; II, optic; III, oculomotor; IV, trochlear; V, trigeminal; VI, abducent; VII, facial (including nervus intermedius); VIII, vestibulocochlear (cochlear and vestibular); IX, glossopharyngeal; X, vagus; XI, accessory; XII, hypoglossal. Usually described and numbered as 12 pairs, the first two are not true nerves but nerve-fiber tracts of the brain; the caudal 10 pairs originate from nuclei in the brainstem, except for that part of XI which has a spinal root.

cranial sutures. The sutures between the bones of the cranium.

cra·ni·ec·to·my (kray″nee-eck′tuh-mee) *n. In surgery,* removal of strips or pieces of the cranial bones.

cranio-. See *crani-.*

cra·nio·buc·cal (kray″nee-o-buck′ul) *adj.* Pertaining to the cranium and the buccal cavity.

craniobuccal pouch. In the embryo, a diverticulum from the buccal cavity from which the anterior lobe of the hypophysis is developed. Syn. *Rathke's pouch.*

cra·nio·cele (kray′nee-o-seel) *n.* ENCEPHALOCELE.

cra·nio·cer·vi·cal (kray″nee-o-sur′vi-kul) *adj.* Of or pertaining to the cranium and the neck.

cra·ni·oc·la·sis (kray″nee-ock′luh-sis) *n.,* pl. **cra·nioc·la·ses** (-seez) The operation of breaking the fetal head by means of the cranioclast.

cra·nio·clast (kray′nee-o-klast) *n.* Heavy forceps for crushing the fetal head.

cra·nio·clei·do·dys·os·to·sis (kray″nee-o-klye″do-dis″os-to′sis) *n.* CLEIDOCRANIAL DYSOSTOSIS.

cra·nio·did·y·mus (kray″nee-o-did′i-mus) *n.,* pl. **craniodidy·mi** (-migh) CRANIOPAGUS.

cra·nio·fa·cial (kray″nee-o-fay′shul) *adj.* Of or pertaining to the cranium and the face.

craniofacial dysostosis. A malformation inherited as an autosomal dominant trait and characterized by premature closure of the coronal and/or sagittal sutures, leading to associated anomalies such as malformed auditory canals and ears, high narrow palate, crowded maligned upper teeth, and moderate mental retardation. Syn. *Crouzon's disease.*

cra·nio·fe·nes·tria (kray″nee-o-fe-nes′tree-uh) *n.* A congenital bony defect involving the total thickness of the skull.

cra·ni·og·ra·phy (kray″nee-og′ruh-fee) *n.* The part of craniology that describes the skull and its parts.

cra·nio·la·cu·nia (kray″nee-o-la-kew′nee-uh) *n.* Incomplete ossification of the inner table of the vault of the skull in infants, giving the appearance of dense bony ridges separated by radiolucent areas; often associated with spina bifida, meningoceles, meningoencephaloceles, and increased intracranial pressure. Syn. *lacuna skull.*

cra·ni·ol·o·gy (kray″nee-ol′uh-jee) *n.* The scientific study of the cranium, comprising craniography and craniometry.

cra·ni·om·e·ter (kray″nee-om′e-tur) *n.* A caliper used for measuring the dimensions of the skull.

cra·ni·om·e·try (kray″nee-om′e-tree) *n.* The science and technique of measuring the skull in order to establish exact, comparable, metric records for use in the comparative study of physical types, variation, and individual peculiarities in the skulls of man and other primates.

cra·ni·op·a·gus (kray″nee-op′uh-gus) *n.,* pl. **crani·opa·gi** (-guy, -jye) Conjoined twins united by their heads. Syn. *cephalopagus, craniodidymus.* **—craniopagous,** *adj;* **craniopa·gy** (-jee, -ghee) *n.*

cra·ni·op·a·thy (kray″nee-op′uth-ee) *n.* Any disease of the head, especially of the skull bones.

cra·nio·pha·ryn·ge·al (kray″nee-o-fa-rin′jee-ul, -făr″in-jee′ul) *adj.* Of or pertaining to the cranium and the pharynx.

craniopharyngeal canal. A fetal canal in the sphenoid bone formed by the growth of the bone about the stalk of the craniobuccal pouch.

cra·nio·pha·ryn·gi·o·ma (kray″nee-o-fa-rin″jee-o′muh) *n.,* pl. **craniopharyngiomas, craniopharyngioma·ta** (-tuh) A benign, but infiltrative tumor, usually occurring in children, derived from the epithelium of the embryonal craniopharyngeal canal. The intrasellar type arises from cells dispersed in the adenohypophysis; the suprasellar type, from cells in the infundibulum above the sella turcica.

cra·nio·plas·ty (kray′nee-o-plas″tee) *n. In surgery,* correction of defects in the cranial bones, usually by implants of metal, plastic material, or bone.

cra·nio·ra·chis·chi·sis, cra·ni·or·rha·chis·chi·sis (kray″nee-o-ra-kis′ki-sis) *n.* Congenital fissure of the cranium and vertebral column.

cra·nio·sa·cral (kray″nee-o-say′krul) *adj.* Pertaining to the cranium and the sacrum.

craniosacral system. PARASYMPATHETIC NERVOUS SYSTEM.

cra·ni·os·chi·sis (kray″nee-os′ki-sis) *n.,* pl. **cra·nioschi·ses** (-seez) Congenital fissure of the cranium.

cra·nio·spi·nal (kray″nee-o-spye′nul) *adj.* Of or pertaining to the cranium and the vertebral column.

cra·nio·ste·no·sis (kray″nee-o-ste-no′sis) *n.,* pl. **craniosteno·ses** (-seez) CRANIOSYNOSTOSIS.

cra·nio·syn·os·to·sis (kray″nee-o-sin″os-to′sis) *n.,* pl. **craniosynosto·ses** (-seez) Premature closure of the sutures of cranial bones, usually present at or shortly after birth, or due to idiopathic hypercalcemia. The resulting head shape and absence or presence of symptoms depend on the sutures involved.

cra·nio·ta·bes (kray″nee-o-tay′beez) *n.* An acquired change of the cranial bones occurring in infancy, with the formation of small, shallow, conical pits in the bone substance, as seen in rickets and other disease states, and in some newborn infants as localized softening of the parietal bones at the vertex of the skull. **—cra·nio·ta·bet·ic** (-ta-bet′ick) *adj.*

cra·nio·tome (kray′nee-o-tome) *n.* An instrument used in craniotomy.

cra·ni·ot·o·my (kray″nee-ot′uh-mee) *n.* 1. Any

operation on the skull. 2. An operation reducing the size of the fetal head by cutting or breaking when delivery is otherwise impossible.

cra·ni·o·ver·te·bral (kray″nee·o·vur′te·brul) *adj.* Of or pertaining to the cranium and the vertebrae.

cra·ni·um (kray′nee·um) *n.*, genit. **cra·nii** (·nee·eye), L. pl. **cra·nia** (·nee·uh) 1. The skull exclusive of the mandible. 2. SKULL. 3. BRAINCASE.

cranium bi·fi·dum (bif′i·dum). A congenital fissure of the cranium, usually midline, often associated with a meningocele or meningoencephalocele.

crap·u·lent (krap′yoo·lunt) *adj.* Marked by excess in eating and drinking.

cra·que·lé (krack·lay′) *adj. In dermatology,* scaling, with cracks such as appear in old china or ceramic tile.

-crasia A combining form designating (results of) *mixing of different humors or substances in the body.*

cra·ter·i·form (kray·terr′i·form) *adj.* 1. Shaped like a crater or bowl. 2. Conical.

cra·ter·i·za·tion (kray″tur·i·zay′shun) *n.* The removal of part of a bone, leaving a crater, as in operations for osteomyelitis.

cra·vat (kruh·vat′) *n.* A triangular bandage folded to form a band, used as a temporary dressing for a wound or fracture.

C-reactive protein. A globulin capable of precipitating the C carbohydrate in pneumococcal bodies; found in the serum of patients with inflammation and necrosis, and tests for this protein are used in the diagnosis of rheumatic fever.

cream, *n.* 1. The part of milk rich in butterfat. 2. A solid emulsion for external application, which may contain solutions or suspensions of medicinal agents.

cream of tartar. Potassium bitartrate, $KHC_4H_4O_4$, used as a saline cathartic.

creat-, creato- A combining form meaning (a) *meat, flesh;* (b) *creatine.*

cre·a·tine (kree′uh·teen, ·tin) *n.* (α-Methylguanido)acetic acid or *N*-methyl-*N*-guanylglycine, $C_4H_9N_3O_2$, an amino acid present in animal tissues, particularly muscle. Creatine reversibly combines with phosphate to form phosphocreatine, an important compound in the anaerobic phase of muscular contraction.

cre·at·i·nine (kree·at′i·neen, ·nin) *n.* 1-Methylhydantoin-2-imide or 1-methylglycocyamidine, $C_4H_7N_3O$, end product of creatine metabolism, excreted in the urine at a constant rate.

creatinine clearance. An index of the glomerular filtration rate, calculated by multiplying the concentration of creatinine in a timed volume of excreted urine by the milliliters of urine produced per minute and dividing the product by the plasma creatinine content. Normal values, when corrected to 1.73 sq m, are greater than 110 ml per minute for males and 100 ml per minute for females.

creatinine coefficient. The value obtained when the number of milligrams of creatinine in the 24-hour urine output is divided by the body weight expressed in kilograms.

cre·a·tin·uria (kree″uh·ti·new′ree·uh) *n.* 1. The

occurrence of creatine in the urine. 2. An increase in the amount of creatine in the urine.

creep·ing eruption. LARVA MIGRANS.

creeping pneumonia. MIGRATORY PNEUMONIA.

creeping ulcer. SERPIGINOUS ULCER.

cre·mas·ter (kre·mas′tur) *n.* CREMASTER MUSCLE. —**cre·mas·ter·ic** (krem″as·terr′ick) *adj.*

cremasteric fascia. Connective tissue surrounding the cremaster muscle; the middle spermatic fascia covering the spermatic cord and testis.

cremasteric reflex. Retraction of the testis on the same side induced by stimulation of the skin on the front and inner surface of one thigh.

cremaster muscle. An extension of the internal oblique abdominal muscle over the spermatic cord and testis. There is a similar muscle in the female which is very poorly developed.

cre·ma·tion (kree·may′shun) *n.* Destruction of a dead body by burning. —**cre·mate** (kree′mate) *v.*

cre·ma·to·ry (kree′muh·tor″ee) *n.* 1. An establishment for burning the bodies of the dead. 2. An incinerator.

crem·no·pho·bia (krem″no·fo′bee·uh) *n.* An abnormal fear of precipices or steep places.

cre·nate (kree′nate) *adj.* 1. Notched or scalloped. 2. *In botany,* having rounded scalloped edges, as certain leaves. —**cre·nat·ed** (·nay·tid) *adj.*

cre·na·tion (kre·nay′shun) *n.* 1. A notched or cogwheel-like appearance of shrunken erythrocytes; seen when they are exposed to hypertonic solutions. 2. The indentation markings on the tongue caused by a tooth.

cre·o·sol (kree′o·sol) *n.* 2-Methoxy-4-methylphenol, $C_8H_{10}O_2$, one of the principal phenols contained in creosote.

cre·o·sote (kree′o·sote) *n.* A mixture of phenols obtained by the distillation of wood tar, preferably that from the beech, *Fagus sylvatica;* a flammable, oily liquid. Creosote is antiseptic, astringent, styptic, anesthetic, and escharotic. Has been used in the treatment of pulmonary tuberculosis.

crep·i·tant (krep′i·tunt) *adj.* Producing or having a crackling or rattling sound. —**crepi·tance** (·tunce) *n.*

crepitant rale. A fine, dry, crackling rale simulated by the rubbing together of hairs, produced by fluid in the terminal bronchioles; transiently heard at the normal lung base during initial forced inspiration.

crep·i·tate (krep′i·tate) *v.* To make sharp repeated crackling sounds, as heard in crepitation.

crep·i·ta·tion (krep″i·tay′shun) *n.* 1. The grating of fractured bones. 2. The crackling of the joints. 3. The noise produced by pressure upon tissues containing an abnormal amount of air or gas, as in cellular emphysema. 4. The sound heard at the end of inspiration in the first stage of croupous pneumonia. It closely resembles the sound produced by rubbing the hair between the fingers held close to the ear.

crep·i·tus (krep′i·tus) *n.* 1. CREPITATION. 2. Discharge of intestinal flatus.

cres·cent (kres′unt) *n.* 1. Anything shaped like, or suggestive of, a new moon or a sickle. The

2. The curved gametocyte of *Plasmodium falciparum*, infectious for *Anopheles* mosquitoes and the most characteristic diagnostic form of the falciparum malarial parasite. —**cres·cen·tic** (kre·sen'tick) *adj.*

cre·sol (kree'sol) *n.* A mixture of *o*-, *m*-, and *p*-cresol, $CH_3C_6H_4OH$, obtained from coal tar. A colorless, brownish, or pinkish liquid of phenol-like odor; soluble in 50 volumes of water. Used chiefly as a surgical disinfectant, usually in the form of saponated cresol solution which contains 50% cresol. It is superior to phenol both as an antiseptic and as a germicide.

cre·sot·ic acid (kre·sot'ick, ·so'tick). Homosalicylic acid, *o*-, *m*-, and *p*-, $CH_3C_6H_3(OH)$-COOH, the sodium salts of which have been used medicinally like the salicylates.

crest, *n.* A ridge or linear prominence, especially of bone.

cres·yl (kres'il) *n.* TOLYL.

cres·yl·ate (kres'il·ate) *n.* Any compound of cresol with a metallic radical.

cre·syl·ic acid (kre·sil'ick). In commerce, a mixture of phenols from coal tar.

cre·ta (kree'tuh) *n.* Chalk; native calcium carbonate. —**cre·ta·ceous** (kre·tay'shus) *adj.*

cre·tin (kree'tin) *n.* An individual afflicted with cretinism.

cre·tin·ism (kree'tin·iz·um) *n.* The congenital and most common form of infantile hypothyroidism with severe deficiency of thyroid hormone; may be due to aplasia, hypoplasia or failure of the thyroid to descend to its normal adult site or locus in the neck resulting from an embryonic developmental defect, the administration of radioiodine to the mother during pregnancy, an autoimmune disease, defective synthesis of thyroid hormone (nonendemic goitrous cretinism), maternal ingestion of medications suppressing thyroid activity, or iodide deficiency (endemic cretinism). Clinically, the infant is characterized, before treatment, by a large protruding tongue, thickened subcutaneous tissues, dry skin, protruding abdomen, mental retardation, and dwarfed stature. Poor muscle tone, depressed tendon reflexes, constipation, and hoarse cry are also common. —**cretin·ous** (·us) *adj.*; **cretin·oid** (·oid) *adj. & n.*

Creutz·feldt-Ja·kob disease (kroits'felt, yah'kohp) 1. A chronic degenerative disorder of the nervous system described by H. G. Creutzfeldt and identified by W. Spielmeyer with one described by A. M. Jakob. The clinical descriptions included a slowly progressive dementia and signs of corticospinal and extrapyramidal disease; a diffuse loss of neurons in the cerebral cortex, basal ganglia, brainstem nuclei, and sometimes the anterior horns of the spinal cord, was observed pathologically. Identification of this disorder with subacute spongiform encephalopathy is extremely doubtful. Syn. *corticostriatospinal degeneration.* 2. SUBACUTE SPONGIFORM ENCEPHALOPATHY.

crev·ice (krev'is) *n.* A narrow opening caused by a fissure or crack.

cre·vic·u·lar (kre·vick'yoo·lur) *adj.* Pertaining to or having a crevice, especially of the gingiva.

crib·bing, *n.* 1. Air swallowing; AEROPHAGIA. 2. The repeated biting of the crib or manger by horses, resulting in a peculiar wearing of the incisor teeth.

crib death. See sudden infant death syndrome.

crib·ri·form (krib'ri·form) *adj.* Perforated like a sieve.

crick, *n. Colloq.* Any painful spasmodic affection, as of the back or neck.

cri·co·ar·y·te·noid (krye''ko·ăr''i·tee'noid, ·a·rit'e·noid) *adj. & n.* 1. Pertaining to the cricoid and arytenoid cartilages. 2. One of two muscles attached to the cricoid and arytenoid cartilages, the posterior and lateral cricoarytenoid muscles.

cri·co·esoph·a·ge·al (krye''ko·e·sof''uh·jee'ul) *adj.* Of or pertaining to the cricoid cartilage and the esophagus.

cri·coid (krye'koid) *adj. & n.* 1. Ring-shaped. 2. CRICOID CARTILAGE.

cricoid cartilage. The ring-shaped cartilage of the larynx.

cri·coi·dec·to·my (krye''koy·deck'tuh·mee) *n.* The excision of the cricoid cartilage.

cri·co·pha·ryn·ge·al (krye''ko·fa·rin'jee·ul, ·rin·jee'ul) *adj.* Of or pertaining to the cricoid cartilage and the pharynx.

cri·co·pha·ryn·ge·us (krye''ko·fa·rin'jee·us) *n.* The portion of the inferior constrictor muscle of the pharynx that arises from the cricoid cartilage.

cri·co·thy·re·ot·o·my (krye''ko·thigh·ree·ot'uh·mee) *n.* CRICOTHYROTOMY.

cri·co·thy·roid (krye''ko·thigh'roid) *adj. & n.* 1. Pertaining to the cricoid and thyroid cartilages. 2. The muscle, attached to the cricoid and thyroid cartilages, which tenses the vocal folds.

cricothyroid ligament. The sheet of fibroelastic connective tissue which is attached below to the upper margin of the cricoid cartilage. The central portion (the median cricothyroid ligament) of the upper margin is attached to the lower margin of the thyroid cartilage. The lateral portions of the upper margin of the connective-tissue sheet constitute the vocal ligaments. Syn. *elastic cone, cricovocal membrane.*

cricothyroid membrane. CRICOTHYROID LIGAMENT.

cri·co·thy·rot·o·my (krye''ko·thigh·rot'uh·mee) *n.* Incision of the larynx through the cricothyroid ligament.

cri·co·tra·che·al (krye''ko·tray'kee·ul) *adj.* Of or pertaining to the cricoid cartilage and the trachea.

cri·co·tra·che·ot·o·my (krye''ko·tray''kee·ot'uh·mee) *n.* Tracheotomy through the cricoid cartilage.

cri·du·chat syndrome (kree·due·shah') A syndrome of congenital defects, including a laryngeal anomaly which is associated with a cat-like cry in infants, hypertelorism, epicanthus, brachycephaly, moonface micrognathia, hypotonia, strabismus, and severe mental retardation. The somatic cells of affected individuals display a deletion of the short arm of one of the two number 5 chromosomes. Syn. *deletion-5 syndrome.*

Crig·ler-Naj·jar syndrome A recessively inherited defect in bilirubin conjugation by glucuronide associated with chronic icterus.

crim·i·nal abortion. Interruption of a pregnancy, or the attempt to do so, for reasons and under conditions not authorized by law; an illegal abortion.

criminally insane. *In law,* pertaining to an individual who is committed to a mental hospital by a court or courts after being found not guilty of a crime by reason of insanity.

criminal responsibility. *In forensic medicine,* the concept that a person is responsible for his crime if at the time of committing the act he knew what he was doing and knew it to be wrong.

-crine A suffix meaning *secretion* or *secreting* (as of a gland).

crino·gen·ic (krin″o·jen′ick) *adj.* Stimulating the production of secretions.

cri·sis (krye′sis) *n.,* pl. **cri·ses** (·seez) 1. A turning point for better or worse, as that of a disease or fever; especially, the sudden favorable termination of the acute symptoms of an infectious disease. 2. Paroxysmal disturbance of function accompanied with pain. 3. Paroxysmal intensification of symptoms. 4. The psychological events associated with a specific stage of life.

crisis intervention. *In psychiatry,* immediate brief treatment of a patient at a time of personal crisis by a therapist or a therapeutic team, utilizing medications, hospitalization, changes in environmental circumstances, referrals to community agencies, and other means.

cris·pa·tion (kris·pay′shun) *n.* 1. A puckering. 2. An annoying involuntary quivering of the muscles.

cris·ta (kris′tuh) *n.,* pl. & genit. sing. **cris·tae** (·tee) A crest or ridge. Adj. *cristal, cristate.*

cristae. 1. Plural and genitive singular of *crista.* 2. *In electron microscopy,* inward extensions of the inner membrane of the external double membrane system of mitochondria.

cristae cu·tis (kew′tis) [NA]. Ridges of the skin of the palm and sole, which are the basis for identification of fingerprints or toe prints.

crista gal·li (gal′eye) [NA]. The superior triangular process of the ethmoid bone, so called because it is shaped like a cock's comb.

crista ter·mi·na·lis atrii dex·tri (tur·mi·nay′lis ay′tree·eye decks′trye) [NA]. A crest on the wall of the right atrium derived from the cephalic part of the right valve of the sinus venosus; a point of attachment for the pectinate muscles of the right atrium.

crit, *n.* 1. In nuclear technology, the mass of a fissionable material which, under a given set of conditions, is critical. 2. HEMATOCRIT.

crit·i·cal (krit′i·kul) *adj.* 1. Pertaining to or characterized by a crisis. 2. Characterized by sharp discernment, severe assessment, or skillful judgement. 3. Of decisive importance as regards outcome; crucial. 4. Involving grave uncertainty or risk; perilous. 5. *In nuclear technology,* of or pertaining to the state of a fissionable material in which it is capable of sustaining, at constant level, a chain reaction.

critical illumination. Illumination in which the image of a small source of light is focused exactly at the object on the stage of the microscope.

critical ratio. A statistical term denoting the ratio of the difference between the mean of a series of observations and the true or hypothetical value to the standard deviation of the series.

CR lead. *In electrocardiography,* a precordial exploring electrode paired with an electrode on the right arm.

CRO Abbreviation for *cathode-ray oscillograph.*

croc·o·dile tears syndrome. A profuse, paroxysmal flow of tears observed in certain patients with peripheral facial paralysis, when they taste strongly flavored food.

Crohn's disease REGIONAL ENTERITIS.

Crohn's disease of the colon GRANULOMATOUS COLITIS.

Crooke's cells Beta cells of the adenohypophysis exhibiting Crooke's change.

Crooke's change Hyalinization and vacuolization of the cytoplasm of pituitary basophils; seen in Cushing's syndrome and other conditions.

crop, *n.* A dilatation of the esophagus of certain kinds of birds, in which relatively large quantities of food are stored, moistened, and released in small portions to the stomach.

cross·bite, cross bite, *n.* The abnormal occlusal relationship, in a facial or lingual version, of teeth in one arch to those in the opposite arch.

cross·breed·ing, *n.* Production of offspring from the mating of individuals of different breeds, varieties, or strains, or sometimes, different species. —**crossbreed,** *n. & v.*

crossed akinesia. Loss of motor activity on the side opposite that in which a lesion exists in the central nervous system.

crossed aphasia. Aphasia occurring in a clearly left-handed individual due to a lesion in the left cerebral hemisphere.

crossed cylinders. Two cylindrical lenses placed in apposition to each other with their axes at right angles; used by oculists to determine the strength and the axis of astigmatism.

crossed diplopia. Diplopia in which the false image of the right eye appears upon the left side, and that of the left eye upon the right side; a result of divergent strabismus.

crossed paralysis. Paralysis of the arm and leg on one side, associated with contralateral cranial nerve palsies due to a brainstem lesion involving cranial nerve nuclei and the ipsilateral pyramidal tract.

cross·fire treatment. A method of arranging beams in radiation therapy in such a manner that they overcross in the depth of the body at the site of the tumor, sparing the skin.

cross infection. Any infection which a patient contracts from another patient.

cross-link, *v.* To unite neighboring long-chain molecules by a chemical bond to form a complex molecule.

cross matching. A test to establish blood compatibility before transfusion by (a) mixing the prospective recipient's serum with the donor's cells (major cross match) or (b) mixing the donor's serum with the recipient's cells (minor cross match). If agglutination, or hemolysis, does not occur in either test when carried out by several acceptable techniques, the bloods are considered compatible, and the donor's blood may be used.

cross-over experiment. An experiment or clinical investigation in which subjects are divided randomly into at least as many groups as there are kinds of treatment to be given, and then the groups are interchanged until every subject has received each treatment. Thus it is possible to use each subject as his own control while compensating for any spontaneous time trends, and also to study how long effects persist after treatment is discontinued.

cross reaction. A reaction between an antibody and an antigen which is closely related to, but not identical with, the specific antigen.

cross section. 1. A slice of or a cut through an object made in a plane perpendicular to its longest axis. Syn. *transverse section.* 2. *In nuclear physics,* a measure, commonly expressed in barns, of the probability that a nuclear reaction will occur.

cross-striation. Lines running across the fibers of skeletal muscle in histologic preparations.

Cro·tal·i·dae (kro·tal'i·dee) *n. pl.* A family of venomous snakes, the pit vipers, differing from Viperidae (true vipers) in possessing a sensory pit situated between the eye and nostril. Found commonly in North and South America, southeastern Asia, and the East Indies.

crot·a·line (krot'uh·leen, ·lin) *adj. & n.* 1. Of or pertaining to the Crotalidae or, in particular, to the genus *Crotalus.* 2. A protein found in the venom of rattlesnakes. 3. A preparation of venom from the rattlesnakes *Crotalus horridus* and *C. adamanteus* which has been used subcutaneously for immunization against snake bites.

cro·tam·i·ton (kro·tam'i·ton) *n. N*-Ethyl-*o*-crotonotoluidide, $C_{13}H_{17}NO$, used as a scabicide and antipruritic.

crotch, *n.* The angle formed by the junction of the inner sides of the thighs and the trunk.

crotch·et (krotch'it) *n.* A hook used in extracting the fetus after craniotomy.

-crotic A combining form meaning *pulse, heartbeat.*

Cro·ton (kro'ton, ·tun) *n.* A genus of plants of the Euphorbiaceae. *Croton eluteria* yields cascarilla, and *C. tiglium* is the source of croton oil.

cro·ton·ism (kro'tun·iz·um) *n.* Poisoning by croton oil, characterized by hemorrhagic gastroenteritis.

croton oil. A fixed oil from the seed of *Croton tiglium;* a drastic purgative. Causes pustular eruptions when applied to the skin.

cro·tox·in (kro·tock'sin) *n.* A neurotoxin from the venom of the rattlesnake *Crotalus durissus terrificus.*

croup (kroop) *n.* Any condition of upper respiratory pathway obstruction, especially acute inflammation of the pharynx, larynx, and trachea of children, characterized by a hoarse, brassy, and stridulent cough and difficulties in breathing, and in some conditions (as in diphtheria), deposition of a localized membrane. —**croup·ous** (kroo'pus), **croupy** (kroo'pee) *adj.*

croup kettle. A kettle for the production of steam or medicated vapor, used for humidification.

crown, *n.* Corona; the top part of anything; any structure like a crown.

crown of a tooth. The part of the tooth covered with enamel.

CRT Cathode-ray tube.

cru·cial (kroo'shul) *adj.* 1. Resembling or pertaining to a cross. 2. Critical; decisive.

crucial incision. Two cuts at right angles, made deep into the tissues, usually to ensure free drainage.

cru·ci·ate (kroo'shee·ut, ·ate) *adj.* Resembling a cross; cross-shaped.

cru·ci·ble (kroo'si·bul) *n.* A vessel of clay or other refractory material used in melting or igniting substances that require a high degree of heat.

cru·ci·form (kroo'si·form) *adj.* Cruciate; shaped like a cross.

crude birth rate. The number of live births in a given year per 1,000 total population at midyear.

crude death rate. The number of deaths in a given year per 1,000 total population at midyear.

crup·per (krup'ur) *n.* 1. The buttocks of a horse. 2. The sacrococcygeal region in horses. 3. The base of the tail in mammals.

crura. Plural of *crus.*

cru·ral (kroo'rul) *adj.* 1. Pertaining to any of the crura of the body. 2. Pertaining to the lower leg. 3. Loosely, pertaining to the leg including the thigh.

crural hernia. FEMORAL HERNIA.

crural ring. FEMORAL RING.

cru·ro·scro·tal (kroo''ro·skro'tul) *adj.* Pertaining to the thighs and scrotum.

crus (krooce) *n.,* genit. **cru·ris** (kroo'ris), pl. **cru·ra** (kroo'ruh) 1. [NA] LEG (1). 2. Any of various parts of the body or of an organ suggestive of a leg. Adj. *crural.*

crus ce·re·bri (serr'e·brye) [NA]. CRUS OF THE CEREBRUM.

crush syndrome. A severe, often fatal condition that follows a severe crushing injury, particularly involving large muscle masses; characterized by extensive fluid and blood loss in the injured part, hypovolemic shock, hematuria, myoglobinuria, renal tubular necrosis, and renal failure. Syn. *compression syndrome, Bywaters' syndrome.*

crus of the cerebrum. Either of the two peduncles connecting the cerebrum with the pons.

crus of the fornix. Either one of the two bands of nerve fibers which pass from the hippocampus to the individual posterior portions of the fornix cerebri.

crus of the penis. The posterior part of either corpus cavernosum penis, attached to the pubic arch.

crus·ot·o·my (kroos·ot'uh·mee) *n.* PEDUNCULOTOMY.

crust, *n.* A barklike, hard covering; especially, a dried exudate on the skin.

crus·ta (krus'tuh) *n.,* pl. & genit. sing. **crus·tae** (·tee) CRUST.

crutch, n. A special staff used as a support in walking. The common form has a concave, padded crosspiece to fit the axilla, and a guiding and supporting grip for the hand.

Crutch·field tongs Hinged tongs whose points engage the skull; used to provide traction in the treatment of fracture dislocations of the cervical spine.

crutch paralysis or **palsy.** Weakness or paralysis of the muscles of the upper extremity, due to compression of the brachial plexus and especially of the radial nerve from pressure of the crutch head.

Cru·veil·hier-Baum·gar·ten syndrome or **cirrhosis** (krüᵉ·veh·ye′) Distention of the periumbilical veins, associated with a bruit and thrill, due to a large patent umbilical vein, occurring either as a developmental anomaly or as a response to portal hypertension.

crux (krucks) n., genit. **cru·cis** (kroo′sis), pl. **cru·ces** (-seez) A cross, or a crosslike structure.

cry-, cryo- A combining form meaning *cold, freezing.*

cry·al·ge·sia (krye′al·jee′zee·uh) n. Pain from the application of cold.

cry·anes·the·sia, cry·an·aes·the·sia (krye′an·es·theezh′uh, ·theez′ee·uh) n. 1. Loss of sensation or perception of cold by the skin. 2. Localized anesthesia of a part obtained by the application of cold.

cry·es·the·sia, cry·aes·the·sia (krye′es·theezh′uh, ·theez′ee·uh) n. 1. Temperature sense for cold. 2. Extreme sensitivity to cold.

crym-, crymo-, krymo- A combining form meaning *cold, frost.*

cry·mo·dyn·ia (krye′mo·din′ee·uh) n. CRYALGESIA; pain coming on in cold or damp weather.

cryo·bi·ol·o·gy (krye′o·bye·ol′uh·jee) n. The study of frozen or low-temperature life.

cryo·cau·tery (krye′o·kaw′tur·ee) n. The destruction of tissues by application of extreme cold which causes an obliterative thrombosis; used especially in removing moles.

cryo·ex·trac·tor (krye′o·eck·strack′tur) n. *In ophthalmology,* an instrument the tip of which can be cooled to extremely low temperatures by means of Freon, liquid carbon dioxide or nitrogen, or other agents; used in the extraction of cataracts.

cryo·glob·u·lin (krye′o·glob′yoo·lin) n. An abnormal protein which precipitates from plasma between 4° and 21°C (40 and 70°F).

cryo·glob·u·li·ne·mia, cryo·glob·u·li·nae·mia (krye′o·glob′yoo·li·nee′mee·uh) n. A disease state characterized by the presence of cryoglobulin in the blood, associated with malignant plasmacytoma (multiple myeloma) and certain other diseases.

cryo·hy·poph·y·sec·to·my (krye′o·high·pof′i·seck′tuh·mee) n. The partial or total destruction of the hypophysis by means of a freezing lesion.

cry·om·e·ter (krye·om′e·tur) n. An instrument for measuring low temperatures.

cryo·phake (krye′o·fake) n. A device for freezing the crystalline lens of the eye to aid in its removal during cataract surgery.

cryo·stat (krye′o·stat) n. 1. A device consisting of a freezing chamber containing a microtome,

so arranged as to allow operation from outside at normal temperature; used to make rapid sections of fresh tissue for microscopic study. 2. Any device for maintaining very low temperatures; as one that operates by compressing, regeneratively cooling, and then expanding helium gas until part of the gas becomes liquid; it can cool contents to −43°C (−45°F).

cryo·sur·gery (krye′o·sur′juh·ree) n. Surgery performed with aid of special instruments for local freezing of diseased tissues without significant harm to normal adjacent structures.

cryo·thal·a·mot·o·my (krye′o·thal·uh·mot′uh·mee) n. The stereotactical placement of a freezing lesion in the thalamus, primarily in the neurosurgical therapy of movement disorders, particularly parkinsonism, but sometimes to alleviate intractable pain.

cryo·tome (krye′o·tome) n. FREEZING MICROTOME.

crypt, n. 1. A small sac or follicle. 2. A glandular cavity.

crypt-, crypto-, krypto- A combining form meaning (a) *hidden, covered, occult;* (b) *latent;* (c) *crypt.*

cryp·ten·a·mine (krip·ten′uh·meen) n. A mixture of structurally unidentified alkaloids derived from an extract of *Veratrum viride;* used as an antihypertensive, in the form of the acetate or tannate salts.

cryp·ti·tis (krip·tye′tis) n. Inflammation of a crypt, or of crypts.

cryp·to·coc·co·sis (krip′to·kock·o′sis) n., pl. **cryp·tococco·ses** (-seez) A subacute or chronic infection caused by the yeast *Cryptococcus neoformans.* The infection may involve the lungs, bones, or skin, but has a predilection for the central nervous system, causing primarily meningitis. Syn. *torulosis.* European blastomycosis.

Cryp·to·coc·cus (krip′to·kock′us) n. A genus of true yeast whose species include the pathogen *Cryptococcus neoformans.*

Cryptococcus neo·for·mans (nee′o·for′manz). The causative organism of cryptococcosis.

cryp·to·gam (krip′to·gam) n. *In botany,* one of the Cryptogamia, a division of the vegetable kingdom comprising all plants without flowers or seeds, as the algae, fungi, mosses, and ferns. —**cryp·tog·a·mous** (krip·tog′uh·mus) adj.

cryp·to·gen·ic (krip′to·jen′ick) adj. Of unknown or obscure cause.

cryptogenic pyemia. A condition in which the primary suppuration occurs in a portion of the body where it is difficult to detect.

cryp·to·in·fec·tion (krip′to·in·feck′shun) n. A nonapparent, latent, or hidden infection.

cryp·to·lith (krip′to·lith) n. A concretion or calculus formed within a crypt, as in the tonsil.

cryp·to·men·or·rhea, cryp·to·men·or·rhoea (krip′′to·men′′o·ree′uh) n. A condition in which there is menstrual flow from the uterus, the external escape of which is prevented by an obstruction in the lower genital canal, usually an imperforate hymen.

cryp·to·mero·ra·chis·chi·sis, cryp·to·mer·or·rha·

chis·chi·sis (krip″to·merr″o·ra·kis′ki·sis) n. SPINA BIFIDA OCCULTA.

cryp·tom·ne·sia (krip″tom·nee′zhuh, ·zee·uh) n. The recall to mind of a forgotten episode which seems entirely new to the patient, and not a part of his experiences. Syn. *subconscious memory.*

cryp·toph·thal·mos (krip″tof·thal′mos) n. 1. Congenital union of the eyelids, usually over imperfect eyes. 2. An individual with this condition.

cryp·tor·chi·dec·to·my (krip″tor·kid·eck′tuh·mee) n. Removal of an undescended testis.

cryp·tor·chid·o·pexy (krip″tor·kid′o·peck·see, krip·tor′ki·do·) n. Fixation, within the scrotum, of an undescended testis.

cryp·tor·chism (krip·tor′kiz·um) n. A developmental defect in which the testes fail to descend, and remain within the abdomen or inguinal canal. —**cryptor·chid** (·kid) n. & adj.; **cryptor·chis** (·kis) n.

cryp·to·xan·thin (krip″to·zan′thin) n. Hydroxy-β-carotene, $C_{40}H_{56}O$, a carotenoid pigment widely distributed in natural sources; possesses vitamin A activity.

crys·tal (kris′tul) n. In chemistry, a substance that assumes a definite three-dimensional geometric form.

crys·tal·bu·min (kris″tal·bew′min) n. 1. Any crystallized albumin, such as bovine serum albumin. 2. A protein found in the crystalline lens.

crys·tal·line (kris′tuh·lin, ·line) adj. Like a crystal.

crystalline lens. The lens of the eye, a refractive organ of accommodation; a biconvex, transparent, elastic body lying in its capsule immediately behind the pupil of the eye, suspended from the ciliary body by the ciliary zonule.

crys·tal·li·za·tion (kris″tul·i·zay′shun) n. The process by which the molecules, atoms, or ions of a substance arrange themselves in geometric forms when passing from a gaseous or a liquid state to a solid state. —**crys·tal·lize** (kris′tul·ize) v.

crys·tal·loid (kris′tuh·loid) adj. Having a crystal-like nature, as distinguished from colloid.

crys·tal·lo·mag·net·ism (kris″tuh·lo·mag′ne·tiz·um) n. The property common to certain crystals of orienting themselves in a magnetic field.

crys·tal·lo·pho·bia (kris″tuh·lo·fo′bee·uh) n. An abnormal fear of glass or things made of glass.

Crystallose. A trademark for sodium saccharine.

crys·tal·lu·ria (kris″tuh·lew′ree·uh) n. The presence of crystals in the urine; usually a normal condition.

crystal violet. METHYLROSANILINE CHLORIDE.

Crysticillin. A trademark for procaine penicillin G.

Crystodigin. A trademark for digitoxin, a cardiotonic.

CS Abbreviation for *conditioned stimulus.*

CSF Abbreviation for *cerebrospinal fluid.*

C-substance. Among the hemolytic streptococci, antigenic group-specific complex polysaccharides of the cell wall which distinguish Group A, B, C, E, G, and probably others.

CT Abbreviation for *computed* or *computerized tomography.*

Cteno·ce·phal·i·des (ten″o·se·fal′i·deez, tee″no·) n. A genus of fleas which are cosmopolitan in distribution. The species *Ctenocephalides canis,* the dog flea, and *C. felis,* the cat flea, while they infest primarily dogs and cats, may attack man and other mammals. Members of this genus also serve as intermediate hosts of the dog tapeworm, *Dipylidium caninum.*

cten·oids (tee′noidz, ten′oidz) n.pl. In electroencephalography, 14- and 6-per-second positive spikes.

Cu Symbol for copper.

cu·beb (kew′beb) n. The dried, unripe, nearly full-grown fruit of *Piper cubeba,* cultivated in Java and the West Indies; contains a volatile oil. Has been used as a diuretic, urinary antiseptic, and expectorant.

cubic centimeter. A unit of volume represented by a cube one centimeter on edge; for all practical purposes it is equivalent in liquid measure to a milliliter. Abbreviated, c^3, cc.

cubital fossa. ANTECUBITAL FOSSA.

cu·bi·tus (kew′bi·tus) n., pl. & genit. sing. **cubi·ti** (·tye) 1. FOREARM. 2. [NA] ELBOW. 3. Obsol. ULNA. —**cubi·tal** (·tul) adj.

cubitus val·gus (val′gus). A decrease in the normal carrying angle of the arm.

cu·boid (kew′boid) adj. & n. 1. Resembling a cube. 2. The bone of the tarsus between the calcaneus and the fourth and fifth metatarsals.

cu·boi·deo·na·vic·u·lar (kew·boy″dee·o·na·vick′yoo·lur) adj. Pertaining to the cuboid and the navicular bones.

cu·boi·do·dig·i·tal (kew·boy″do·dij′i·tul) adj. Pertaining to the cuboid bone and the digits.

Cu·cu·mis (kew′kuh·mis) n. A genus of plants of the Cucurbitaceae that includes cucumbers and muskmelons, certain of which have been used medicinally.

Cu·cur·bi·ta (kew·kur′bi·tuh) n. A genus of plants of the Cucurbitaceae. Several species, such as *Cucurbita pepo,* the pumpkin, yield seeds that have been used as anthelmintics.

cuff, n. 1. Any bandlike structure that encircles a part. 2. A collection of cells, usually exudative, encircling a blood vessel, especially in the central nervous system.

cui·rass (kwee·ras′, kwee′ras) n. A close-fitting or immovable bandage or plate for the front of the chest.

cuirass respirator. An apparatus which, by means of an airtight chest piece of plastic and rubber, exerts intermittent negative pressure on the patient's thorax and thus aids breathing. Employed when the patient has some ability to breathe on his own.

cul-de-sac (kul′de·sack′) n. 1. A closed or blind pouch or sac. 2. RECTOUTERINE EXCAVATION.

cul·do·cen·te·sis (kul″do·sen·tee′sis) n., pl. **culdo·cente·ses** (·seez) Removal, by aspiration or incision, of intraperitoneal fluid material (transudate, exudate, or blood) through the vagina and the rectouterine excavation.

cul·do·plas·ty (kul′do·plas″tee) n. Plastic surgical repair of the rectouterine excavation.

cul·do·scope (kul′do·skope) n. An instrument for

the visualization of the female internal genitalia and pelvic tissues, entering through the vagina and a perforation into the rectouterine excavation. —**cul·dos·co·py** (kul·dos′kuh·pee) n.

cul·dot·o·my (kul″dot′uh·mee) n. *In surgery*, an incision through the rectouterine excavation.

Cu·lex (kew′lecks) n. A genus of mosquitoes which are vectors of disease.

Cu·lic·i·dae (kew·lis′i·dee) n.pl. A family of the Diptera comprising the mosquitoes.

cu·li·cide (kew′li·side) n. Any agent that destroys mosquitoes.

cu·lic·i·fuge (kew·lis′i·fewj) n. An agent to drive away mosquitoes.

Cullen's sign A sign for ruptured ectopic pregnancy in which a blue-red discoloration is seen about the umbilicus.

cul·men (kul′min) n., genit. **cul·mi·nis** (kul′mi·nis), pl. **cul·mi·na** (kul′mi·nuh) [NA]. The superior portion of the monticulus of the vermis of the cerebellum.

cul·ti·va·tion (kul″ti·vay′shun) n. Successive transferring of microorganisms to different media favorable to growth. —**cul·ti·vate** (kul′ti·vate) v.

cul·ture (kul′chur) n. & v. 1. The growth of microorganisms or tissue cells in artificial media. 2. A group of microorganisms or cells grown in an artificial medium. 3. *In cultural anthropology*, the total learned way of life of a society. 4. *In archeology*, the material evidence of a particular tradition or complex of traditions. 5. To grow or cultivate (microorganisms, cells) in an artificial medium.

culture medium. Any liquid, solid, or semisolid substance for the cultivation of microorganisms.

cu·mene (kew′meen) n. Isopropylbenzene, C_9H_{12}, a hydrocarbon occurring in pine tar, petroleum, and some volatile oils.

cumulative dose. *In radiology*, a total dose delivered in fractions over a period of time.

cu·mu·lus (kew′mew·lus) n., pl. & genit. sing. **cu·mu·li** (·lye) A heap or mound.

cune-, cuneo- A combining form meaning *cuneiform*.

cu·ne·ate (kew′nee·ate) adj. Wedge-shaped.

cuneate nucleus. The collection of nerve cells lying in the dorsal aspect of the medulla oblongata in which the fibers of the fasciculus cuneatus terminate and which give origin to part of the fibers of the medial lemniscus.

cu·ne·i·form (kew·nee′i·form, kew′nee·) adj. & n. 1. Wedge-shaped; cuneate. 2. Any of three tarsal bones. See Table of Bones in the Appendix. 3. TRIQUETRUM (1).

cuneiform cartilage. Either of two small, rod-shaped cartilages of the larynx, located in the aryepiglottic folds anterior to the corniculate cartilages. Syn. *Wrisberg's cartilages*.

cu·neo·cu·boid (kew″nee·o·kew′boid) adj. Pertaining to the cuneiform and cuboid bones.

cu·neo·na·vic·u·lar (kew″nee·o·na·vick′yoo·lur) adj. Pertaining to the cuneiform and the navicular bones.

cu·ne·us (kew′nee·us) n., pl. & genit. sing. **cu·nei** (·nee·eye) A wedge-shaped convolution on the medial aspect of the occipital lobe between the parieto-occipital and calcarine fissures.

cu·nic·u·lus (kew·nick′yoo·lus) n., pl. **cunicu·li** (·lye) A burrow made in the skin by an itch mite.

cun·ni·lin·gus (kun″i·lin′gus) n. The sexual practice in which the mouth and tongue are used to lick or stimulate the vulva.

cun·nus (kun′us) n., pl. & genit. sing. **cun·ni** (·eye) VULVA.

cup, v. To bleed by means of suction cups or cupping glasses.

cu·po·la (kew′po·luh) n. A dome-shaped structure.

cupped, adj. Having the upper surface depressed; applied to the coagulum of blood after phlebotomy.

cupped disk. Excavation of the optic disk, normally present in slight degree, but pathologic if excessive.

cup·ping, n. 1. A method of bloodletting by means of the application of cupping glasses to the surface of the body. 2. Formation of a cuplike depression.

cupping glass. A small bell-shaped glass capable of holding 3 to 4 ounces, in which the air is rarefied by heat or by exhaustion; the glass is applied to the skin, either with or without scarification of the latter.

cupr-, cupro-. A combining form meaning (a) *copper*; (b) *cupric*.

cu·prea bark (kew′pree·uh). The bark of certain species of *Remijia*, containing homoquinine and certain related alkaloids; once used as a substitute for cinchona bark.

cu·pre·ine (kew′pree·een, ·in) n. Hydroxycinchonine, $C_{19}H_{22}N_2O_2$, an alkaloid in cuprea bark.

cu·pric (kew′prik) adj. Pertaining to or containing copper in the bivalent state.

cu·prous (kew′prus) adj. Pertaining to or containing copper in the univalent state.

cu·pu·la (kew′pew·luh) n., pl. & genit. sing. **cupu·lae** (·lee). 1. A domelike structure. 2. A body of colorless substance on the crista ampullaris that coagulates and becomes visible upon applying fixing fluids.

cupular cecum. The blind sac which is the termination of the cochlear duct at the apex of the spiral lamina of the internal ear.

cu·rage (kewr′ij, kew·rahzh′) n. 1. Cleansing of the eye or of an ulcerated or carious surface. 2. Clearing the uterine cavity by means of the finger, as distinguished from the use of the curet.

cu·ra·re (kew·rahr′ee) n. A drug of uncertain and variable composition derived from several species of *Strychnos* and *Chondodendron* plants. Curare from *Chondodendron tomentosum* owes its characteristic action to the quaternary base *d*-tubocurarine, which paralyzes the skeletal muscles by a selective blocking of the neuromuscular junction and prevents response to nerve impulses and acetylcholine. Standardized preparations are used to control muscular spasms, particularly in the treatment of certain neurologic disorders; also to relax the skeletal muscles during anesthesia. In South America and elsewhere it is used as an arrow poison.

cu·ra·ri·mi·met·ic (kew·rahr″i·migh·met′ick) adj. Referring, or pertaining to, the action, similar to that of curare, of an agent that inhibits, at the neuromuscular junction, transmission of an impulse from a nerve to the skeletal muscle fibers that it innervates.

cu·ra·rine (kew·rah′reen, ·rin, kewr′uh·). n. 1. Any of several alkaloids obtained from curare species and identified by use of a preceding letter and a following numeral, as C-curarine I and C-curarine III, obtained from the calabash variety of curare. 2. Obsol. TUBO-CURARINE CHLORIDE.

cu·ra·ri·za·tion (kew′rahr·i·zay′shun) n. Administration of curare or one of its principles or derivatives to produce muscle relaxation or paralysis by blocking impulses at the myoneural junction. —**cu·ra·rize** (kew′ruh·rize) v.

cu·ra·tive (kew′ruh·tiv) adj. Having a healing tendency; pertaining to the cure of a disease.

cur·cu·ma (kur′kyoo·muh) n. The rhizome of Curcuma longa, of India, a plant of the Zingiberaceae, with properties similar to ginger; used as a condiment. It contains curcumin, and is occasionally employed as a yellow dye, to color ointments and other preparations.

cur·cu·min (kur′kyoo·min) n. Turmeric yellow, $C_{21}H_{20}O_6$, the coloring matter of curcuma. Used as an indicator; gives a brownish-red color with alkalies and a light yellow color with acids.

curd, n. The coagulum that separates from milk on the addition of rennin or acids.

cure, n. & v. 1. Recovery from an illness, or correction of a defect, as a result of therapeutic measures. 2. Colloq. A course of therapeutic measures. 3. Colloq. A remedy. 4. To restore (a patient) to health; to bring about recovery from (an illness); to correct (a defect). 5. To process (a material) from a plastic or raw state to a hard state or finish, usually by means of heat or by a chemical treatment, such as vulcanization or polymerization.

cu·ret, cu·rette (kew·ret′) n. & v. 1. An instrument, shaped like a spoon or scoop, for scraping away tissue. 2. To scape away tissue with such an instrument.

cu·ret·tage (kewr″e·tahzh′) n. In surgery, scraping of the interior of a cavity with a curet.

cu·rette·ment (kew·ret′munt) n. CURETTAGE.

cu·rie (kewr′ee, kew·ree′) n. 1. Formerly, the amount of radon in equilibrium with one gram of radium. 2. That quantity of any radioactive species (radioisotope) undergoing exactly 3.700×10^{10} disintegrations per second. Abbreviated, Ci.

cu·rie·gram (kewr′ee·gram, koor′ee·gram) n. A photographic print made by radium rays, similar to a radiograph.

cu·rie·ther·a·py (kew″ree·therr′uh·pee) n. Treatment with ionizing radiation from a radium source.

cu·rine (kewr′een, ·in) n. l-Bebeerine, $C_{36}H_{38}N_2O_6$, an alkaloid obtained from a kind of curare.

cu·ri·um (kew′ree·um) n. A metallic, artificially produced radioactive element, No. 96. Symbol, Cm.

Cur·ling's ulcer Acute peptic ulcer of the upper gastrointestinal tract, associated with skin burns.

cur·rant-jelly clot or **thrombus.** A red, gelatinous blood clot formed quickly after death, which contains all of the elements of blood.

cur·rent, n. 1. The flow of electricity (electrons) through a circuit; also, the rate of this flow. 2. The movement or flow of a liquid or gas, as of blood in vessels, or of air through the respiratory passages.

Cursch·mann's spirals (koorsh′mahⁿn) The spiral threads of mucin contained in the small pellets expectorated in asthmatic paroxysm.

cur·sive epilepsy. A form of psychomotor epilepsy manifested by uncontrollable forward running of the patient who appears oblivious to any obstacles in his course; the running phase may be followed by a generalized seizure.

cur·va·ture (kur′vuh·choor) n. A bending or curving; a curve.

curvature of the spine. Any of various kinds of persistent abnormal curvature of the vertebral column.

cus·co bark. The bark of Cinchona pelletierana (Rubiaceae), yielding several minor alkaloids of the quinoline group.

cush·ing·oid (koōsh′ing·oid) adj. 1. Having the appearance of a patient with Cushing's syndrome as the result of therapeutic administration of corticosteroid drugs. 2. Having the habitus of a patient with Cushing's syndrome, but without other features of that disorder.

Cushing's syndrome or **disease** 1. A clinical condition characterized by truncal and facial adiposity, hypertension, fatigability and weakness, polycythemia, amenorrhea or impotence, hirsutism, purplish striae, purpura-like ecchymoses, edema, glycosuria, osteoporosis, and increased susceptibility to infection, due to excess of the adrenocortical hormone cortisol from adrenal cortical tumor or hyperplasia, basophilic adenoma of the pituitary, certain tumors of nonendocrine origin, or administration of adrenal cortical hormones. 2. The symptoms of cerebellopontine angle tumors, usually acoustic neuromas, beginning with subjective noises, followed by hearing loss, ipsilateral paralysis of the abducens and facial nerves, vertigo, nystagmus, and later other cerebellar dysfunctions.

cush·ion (koōsh′un) n. In anatomy, an aggregate of adipose and fibrous tissue relieving pressure upon tissues lying beneath.

cusp, n. 1. A pointed or rounded eminence on or near the masticating surface of a tooth; designed to occlude in the sulcus of a tooth or between two teeth of the opposite dental arch. 2. One of the flaps or leaflets of a valve in the heart or a vessel. —**cus·pate** (kus′pate), **cuspated** (·id) adj.

cus·pid (kus′pid) adj. & n. 1. Unicuspid; having one cusp. 2. In the human dentition, CANINE TOOTH.

cus·pi·date (kus′pi·date) adj. 1. Pertaining to or having one or more cusps. 2. Pointed; coming to a point.

cu·ta·ne·ous (kew·tay′nee·us) adj. Pertaining to or involving the skin.

cutaneous anaphylaxis. An immunological response occurring 2 or 3 minutes after antigen is injected into the skin of a sensitive person; itching at the injected site is followed within a few minutes by a pale, elevated irregular wheal followed by a zone of erythema, with a complete return to normal appearance in 30 minutes.

cutaneous appendages. Organs and structures of ectodermal origin, attached to or embedded in the skin: the nails, hair, sebaceous glands, sweat glands, and mammary glands.

cutaneous diphtheria. Infection of the skin by *Corynebacterium diphtheriae*, usually manifested by an ulcer with a rolled edge, dirty base, and tending to bulla formation at the periphery; rarely associated with systemic manifestations.

cutaneous leishmaniasis. An infection characterized by localized cutaneous granulomas with a tendency to ulceration and chronicity; caused by *Leishmania tropica*, transmitted by the bite of the sandfly *Phlebotomus*.

cutaneous reaction. 1. Any change manifested in the outer layers of the skin, as in sunburn or the rash in measles. 2. The immediate reaction in the skin resulting from antigen-antibody union, such as follows the intracutaneous inoculation of foreign serum in a sensitized individual. 3. A delayed reaction at the site of introduction of the test material, such as tuberculin, based on the phenomenon of delayed hypersensitivity or specific cell mediated immunity. 4. Any reaction resulting from the directly injurious effect of inoculated material, such as diphtheria toxin in the Schick test.

cutaneous reflex. 1. Wrinkling or gooseflesh in response to irritation of the skin. 2. Any reflex, receptors for which are in the skin.

cut·down, *n.* An incision through skin, superficial fascia, or other tissues, permitting access to a cavity or vessel (usually a vein) for insertion of a cannula or other instrumentation.

cu·ti·cle (kew'ti·kul) *n.* 1. EPONYCHIUM. 2. EPIDERMIS. 3. Any fine covering. —**cu·tic·u·lar** (kew·tick'yoo·lur) *adj.*

cu·tig·er·al (kew·tij'ur·ul) *adj.* Made up of skin.

cu·tin (kew'tin) *n.* A waxlike substance found over most of the aerial parts of vascular plants. It serves to protect the underlying cells from too rapid loss of moisture.

cu·tis (kew'tis) *n.,* L. pl. **cu·tes** (·teez) SKIN.

cu·ti·sec·tor (kew'ti·seck"tur) *n.* An instrument for taking small sections of skin from the living subject. Syn. *biopsy punch.*

cutis hy·per·elas·ti·ca (high"pur·e·las'ti·kuh). EHLERS-DANLOS SYNDROME.

cutis mar·mo·ra·ta (mahr"mo·ray'tuh). Blue or purple mottling of the skin; seen in certain young persons as a constant phenomenon or upon exposure of the skin to cold air. Syn. *livedo reticularis, marble skin.*

cutis plate. DERMATOME; the lateral part of an embryonic somite.

cutis ve·ra (veer'uh, vehr'uh) DERMIS.

Cut·ler-Pow·er-Wil·der test A test of adrenal insufficiency (Addison's disease). A patient with adrenal insufficiency, given a diet with supplementary potassium and restricted sodium chloride, continues to excrete greater than normal amounts of sodium chloride in the urine.

cut·ting needle. A needle with a sharp edge, either curved or straight.

cu·vette, cu·vet (kew·vet') *n.* 1. The absorption cell for spectrophotometry. 2. A small transparent tube or vessel, used in colorimetric determinations.

CV Abbreviation for *cardiovascular.*

CVP Abbreviation for *central venous pressure.*

c wave. The positive pressure wave in the atrial and venous pulse produced by bulging of the atrioventricular valves at the onset of ventricular systole, and probably in the jugular venous pulse, by an impulse transmitted from the adjacent carotid artery.

cyan-, cyano- A combining form meaning (a) *dark blue;* (b) in chemistry, *the presence of the cyanogen group.*

cy·an·a·mide (sigh·an'uh·mide, ·mid) *n.* 1. Colorless deliquescent crystals, $H_2N.CN$. 2. CALCIUM CYANAMIDE.

cy·an·eph·i·dro·sis (sigh"an·ef"i·dro'sis) *n.* The excretion of sweat with a blue tint.

cy·an·he·mo·glo·bin, cy·an·hae·mo·glo·bin (sigh"an·hee'muh·glo"bin) *n.* A compound of hydrocyanic acid with hemoglobin formed in cases of poisoning with this acid. It gives the blood a bright red color.

cy·an·ic acid (sigh·an'ick). A poisonous liquid, HCNO, stable only at low temperatures.

cy·a·nide (sigh'uh·nide) *n.* 1. The univalent radical —CN. 2. Any compound containing this radical, as potassium cyanide, KCN.

cy·an·met·he·mo·glo·bin, cy·an·met·hae·mo·glo·bin (sigh"an·met·hee'muh·glo"bin) *n.* A relatively nontoxic compound formed by the combination of cyanide and methemoglobin.

cy·a·no·co·bal·a·min (sigh"uh·no·ko·bawl'uh·min, sigh·an") Antianemia vitamin B₁₂, $C_{63}H_{88}CoN_{14}O_{14}P$, a cobalt-containing substance usually produced by the growth of suitable microbial substances, or obtained from liver; dark-red crystals or powder sparingly soluble in water. Appears to be identical with the antianemia factor of liver.

cy·a·no·der·ma (sigh"uh·no·dur'muh) *n.* Blueness of the skin.

cy·a·no·gen (sigh·an'o·jen) *n.* 1. A colorless toxic gas, NCCN, having the odor of bitter almonds. 2. The radical —CN; cyanide (1).

cy·a·no·ge·net·ic (sigh"uh·no·je·net'ick) *adj.* Capable of producing hydrocyanic acid or a cyanide.

cy·a·no·pia (sigh"uh·no'pee·uh) *n.* A condition of the vision rendering all objects blue.

cy·a·nop·sia (sigh"uh·nop'see·uh) *n.* CYANOPIA.

cy·a·nosed (sigh'uh·noze'd) *adj.* Affected with cyanosis.

cy·a·no·sis (sigh"uh·no'sis) *n.,* pl. **cyano·ses** (·seez) A bluish-purple discoloration of the mucous membranes and skin, due to the presence of excessive amounts of reduced hemoglobin in capillaries, or less frequently to the presence of methemoglobin. —**cy·a·not·ic** (sigh"uh·not'ick) *adj.*

cyanotic congenital heart disease. Heart disease

present at birth, producing cyanosis by virtue of a significant right-to-left shunt.

cy·as·ma (sigh·az'muh) *n.*, *Obsol.* The peculiar pigmentation of the skin sometimes seen in pregnant women.

cy·ber·net·ics (sigh"bur·net'icks) *n.* The science dealing with communication and control in living and nonliving systems, including control by means of feedback mechanisms, i.e., servomechanisms. —**cybernet·ic** (·ick) *adj.*

cycl-, cyclo- A combining form meaning (a) *circle, circular, ring, cycle*; (b) *cyclic compound*; (c) *ciliary body*; (d) *fusion*.

Cyclaine. Trademark for hexylcaine, a local anesthetic used as the hydrochloride salt.

cy·cla·mate (sigh'kluh·mate, sick'luh·) *n.* A salt of cyclamic acid.

cy·clam·ic acid (sigh·klam'ick) Cyclohexanesulfamic acid, $C_6H_{11}NHSO_3H$, a nonnutritive sweetening agent; usually used in the form of the calcium or sodium salt.

Cyclamycin. A trademark for troleandomycin, an antibiotic substance.

cy·claz·o·cine (sigh·klaz'o·seen) *n.* 3-(Cyclopropylmethyl)-1,2,3,4,5,6-hexahydro-6,11-dimethyl-2,6-methano-3-benzazocin-8-ol, $C_{18}H_{25}NO$, an analgesic drug.

cy·cle, *n.* A regular series of changes which involve a return to the original state or condition, and repetition; a succession of events or symptoms, regularly recurring in an interval of time.

cy·clec·to·my (sigh·kleck'tuh·mee, sick·leck') *n.* Excision of part of the ciliary body.

cy·clic (sigh'klick, sick'lick) *adj.* 1. Having cycles or periods of exacerbation or change; intermittent. 2. Having a self-limited course, as certain diseases. 3. Of chemical compounds: having a closed-chain or ring structure of atoms.

cyclic adenosine monophosphate. Adenosine 3′,5′-monophosphate, a cyclic form of adenosine 5′-monophosphate, found in most animal cells and produced by the action of the enzyme adenyl cyclase on adenosine triphosphate. It mediates many of the actions of a great variety of hormones, performing the functions of the hormones at the intracellular level; it may also have an important role in brain function. A phosphodiesterase enzyme inactivates it by conversion to adenosine 5′-monophosphate. Abbreviated, cyclic AMP.

cyclic AMP. Abbreviation for *cyclic adenosine monophosphate.*

cyclic compound. *In chemistry,* an organic compound belonging to the closed-chain series.

cyclic fever. 1. A convulsive equivalent in which recurrent paroxysms of fever not associated with any specific cause are the most prominent symptom. 2. Any fever with a sequential pattern of appearance and disappearance.

cyclic headache. Any periodically occurring headache, as a vascular headache or headache associated with menstruation, or as a convulsive equivalent.

cyclic hemorrhage. 1. MENORRHAGIA. 2. Menstrual bleeding of ectopic endometrial implants, as in endometriosis.

cy·clit·ic (si·klit'ick) *adj.* 1. Pertaining to cyclitis. 2. Pertaining to the ciliary body.

cyclitic membrane. *In ophthalmology,* an inflammatory membrane forming along the plane of the anterior vitreous face anchored on each side at the pars plana.

cy·cli·tis (sigh·klye'tis, si·) *n.* Inflammation of the ciliary body, manifested by a zone of hyperemia in the scleritic coat surrounding the cornea. It may be serous, plastic, or suppurative.

cyclo-. See **cycl-.**

cy·clo·ceph·a·ly (sigh"klo·sef'uh·lee) *n.* A type of cyclopia in which there is more or less complete absence of the olfactory organs, and intimate union of rudimentary eyes, situated in a single orbit.

cy·clo·di·al·y·sis (sigh"klo·dye·al'i·sis) *n.*, pl. **cyclodialy·ses** (·seez) Detaching the ciliary body from the sclera in order to effect reduction of intraocular tension in certain cases of glaucoma, especially in aphakia.

cy·clo·di·a·ther·my (sigh"klo·dye'uh·thur·mee) *n.* Destruction, by diathermy, of the ciliary body.

Cyclogyl. Trademark for cyclopentolate, a cycloplegic and mydriatic drug used as the hydrochloride salt.

cy·cloid (sigh'kloid) *adj.* CYCLOTHYMIC.

Cyclopal. Trademark for 5-allyl-5-(2-cyclopenten-1-yl)barbituric acid, $C_{12}H_{14}N_2O_3$, a sedative and hypnotic of short duration of action.

cy·clo·pen·ta·mine (sigh"klo·pen'tuh·meen) *n.* N,α-Dimethylcyclopentaneëthylamine, $C_9H_{19}N$, a sympathomimetic amine used for systemic pressor and local vasoconstrictor effects; employed as the hydrochloride salt.

cy·clo·pen·to·late (sigh"klo·pen'to·late) *n.* 2-Dimethylaminoethyl 1-hydroxy-α-phenylcyclopentaneacetate, $C_{17}H_{25}NO_3$, a spasmolytic agent that produces cycloplegia and mydriasis and is used for these purposes in ophthalmology; employed as the hydrochloride salt.

cy·clo·pho·rase (sigh"klo·fo'race, ·raze). *n.* The group of mitochondria-associated enzymes that catalyze oxidations (as in the tricarboxylic acid cycle), oxidative phosphorylation, and certain reactions of synthesis.

cy·clo·pho·ria (sigh"klo·for'ee·uh) *n.* A tendency for the eyes to rotate around their vertical axes held in check by fusion.

cy·clo·phos·pha·mide (sigh"klo·fos'fuh·mide) *n.* N,N-Bis(2-chloroethyl)-N-3-(hydroxypropyl)phosphordiamidic acid cyclic ester, $C_7H_{15}Cl_2N_2O_2P$, a cyclic phosphamide of nitrogen mustard; used as an alkylating type of antineoplastic agent.

cy·clo·pia (sigh·klo'pee·uh) *n.* A large group of terata; characterized externally by fusion of the orbits and various degrees of fusion of the eyes; internally by severe defects of the facial skeleton and brain. A proboscis may or may not be present.

cy·clo·ple·gia (sigh"klo·plee'jee·uh) *n.* Paralysis of ciliary muscles of the eyes.

cy·clo·ple·gic (sigh"klo·plee'jick) *adj.* & *n.* 1. Causing temporary paralysis of the ciliary muscle. 2. Any agent that causes temporary paralysis of the ciliary muscle and the muscles of accommodation, such as atropine, homatropine, and other parasympatholytic compounds, used to facilitate ophthalmoscopic examination and refraction.

cy·clo·pro·pane (sigh″klo·pro′pane) *n.* Trimethylene, C_3H_6, a saturated cyclic hydrocarbon gas having an odor of petroleum benzin; a potent and explosive, but relatively nonirritating and nontoxic inhalation anesthetic which can be administered with a high concentration of oxygen.

cy·clops (sigh′klops) *n.*, pl. **cy·clo·pes** (sigh·klo′peez) An individual with a single eye or congenital fusion of the two eyes into one (synophthalmus).

Cyclops, *n.* A genus of minute crustaceans having a large, median eye; widely distributed throughout fresh and salt waters, but found most commonly in still water. Species have been found to be intermediate hosts of *Dracunculus medinesis, Diphyllobothrium latum, Drepanidotaenia lanceolata,* and *Gnathostoma spinigerum.*

cy·clo·ser·ine (sigh″klo·serr′een, ·seer′een) *n.* D-4-Amino-3-isoxazolidinone, $C_3H_6N_2O_2$, an antibiotic formed in cultures of several *Streptomyces* species. Used mainly in the treatment of tuberculosis and also in some cases of urinary tract infections.

cy·clo·thyme (sigh′klo·thime) *n.* An individual with a cyclothymic personality.

cy·clo·thy·mia (sigh″klo·thigh′mee·uh) *n.* A condition marked by alternating periods of elation and depression.

cy·clo·thy·mic (sigh″klo·thigh′mick) *adj. & n.* 1. Pertaining to or characterized by cyclothymia. 2. CYCLOTHYME.

cyclothymic personality. *In psychiatry,* a disposition marked by alternations of mood between elation and depression out of proportion to apparent external events and rather stimulated by internal factors; it may be hypomanic, depressed, or alternating.

cy·clo·tia (sigh·klo′shuh, ·shee·uh) *n.* Cyclopia associated with more or less complete absence of the lower jaw (agnathia) and approximation or fusion of the ears (synotia).

cy·clot·o·my (sigh·klot′uh·mee, si·) *n.* An operation for the relief of glaucoma, consisting of an incision through the ciliary body.

cy·clo·tron (sigh′klo·tron) *n.* A device for imparting high speeds to protons or deuterons by a combination of a constant powerful magnet and an alternating high-frequency charge. These high-speed particles can be directed to a target in order to produce neutrons, or they can be made to bombard various substances in order to make them artificially radioactive.

cyesio- A combining form meaning *pregnancy.*

cy·e·si·og·no·sis (sigh·ee″see·og·no′sis) *n.*, pl. **cyesiogno·ses** (·seez) Diagnosis of pregnancy.

cy·esi·ol·o·gy (sigh·ee″see·ol′uh·jee) *n.* The science of gestation in its medical aspects.

cy·e·sis (sigh·ee′sis) *n.*, pl. **cye·ses** (·seez) PREGNANCY.

Cyl. An abbreviation for (a) *cylinder;* (b) *cylindrical lens.*

cyl·in·der (sil′in·dur) *n.* 1. An elongated body of the same transverse diameter throughout and

circular on transverse section. 2. A cylindrical cast. 3. CYLINDRICAL LENS. Abbreviated, C., Cyl. —**cy·lin·dric** (si·lin′drick), **cylin·dri·cal** (·dri·kul) *adj.*

cylindr-, cylindro- A combining form meaning *cylinder, cylindrical.*

cylindrical bronchiectasis. Uniform dilatation of bronchi.

cylindrical-cell carcinoma. ADENOCARCINOMA.

cylindrical lens. A minus or plus lens, with a plane surface in one axis and a concave or convex surface in the axis at right angles to the first. Abbreviated, C., Cyl.

cyl·in·droid (sil′in·droid) *adj. & n.* 1. Resembling a cylinder or tube, i.e., resembling a cylinder with elliptic right sections. 2. One of the bodies sometimes seen on microscopical examination of urine, which resemble hyaline casts but differ by tapering to a slender tail; they have the same significance as casts.

cyl·in·dro·ma (sil′in·dro′muh) *n.*, pl. **cylindromas, cylindroma·ta** (·tuh) A tumor composed of groups of polygonal epithelial cells surrounded by bands of hyalinized stroma, forming cylinders of cells which give the tumor its name. In the skin, cylindromas are benign hamartomatous masses; in the respiratory tract and salivary glands, they are locally aggressive tumors which occasionally metastasize.

cyl·in·dru·ria (sil′in·droo′ree·uh) *n.* The presence of casts or cylindroids in the urine.

cym·bi·form (sim′bi·form) *adj. In biology,* boat-shaped.

cymbo- A combining form meaning *boat-shaped.*

cym·bo·ceph·a·ly (sim″bo·sef′uh·lee) *n.* SCAPHOCEPHALY. —**cymbo·ce·phal·ic** (·se·fal′ick), **cymbo·ceph·a·lous** (·sef′uh·lus) *adj.*

cy·mene (sigh′meen) *n.* 1-Methyl-4-isopropylbenzene, $C_{10}H_{14}$, a hydrocarbon that occurs in species of caraway, thyme, and other volatile oils. —**cy·mic** (·mick) *adj.*

cyn-, cyno- A combining form meaning *dog.*

cy·nan·thro·py (si·nan′thro·pee, sigh·) *n.* A psychotic disorder in which the patient believes himself to be a dog and imitates the actions of one.

cyn·o·dont (sin′o·dont, sigh′no·) *adj.* 1. Characterized by teeth with small pulp chambers. 2. One of a group of prehistoric reptiles having skulls and teeth relatively similar to those of mammals; considered possibly ancestral to mammals.

cyno·pho·bia (sin″o·fo′bee·uh, sigh′no·) *n.* 1. An abnormal fear of dogs. 2. A neurosis, usually hysterical in nature, reproducing the symptoms of rabies, sometimes precipitated by the bite of a dog.

cy·ot·ro·phy (sigh·ot′ruh·fee) *n.* Nutrition of the fetus.

cy·pri·do·pho·bia (sigh″pri·do·fo′bee·uh, si·prid′o·) *n.* An abnormal fear of acquiring a venereal disease or of coitus for that reason.

cyp·ri·pe·di·um (sip″ri·pee′dee·um) *n.* The dried rhizome and roots of lady's slipper, *Cypripedium pubescens,* containing a volatile oil, resins, and tannin. Has been used as an antispasmodic and stimulant tonic.

Cyredin. A trademark for cyanocobalamin.

cyrt-, cyrto- A combining form meaning *bent, curved.*

cyr·to·graph (sur'to·graf) *n.* An instrument used to measure and record the curves of the chest and head.

cyr·toid (sur'toid) *adj.* Resembling a hump or swelling.

cyr·tom·e·ter (sur·tom'e·tur) *n.* An instrument for measuring or delineating the curves of parts of the body. Used to demonstrate the dilation and deformation of the chest in certain diseases, or to measure the shape and size of the head. —**cyrtome·try** (·tree) *n.*

cyr·to·sis (sur·to'sis) *n.*, pl. **cyrto·ses** (·seez) KYPHOSIS.

cyst-, cysti-, cysto- A combining form meaning (a) *gallbladder;* (b) *urinary bladder;* (c) *pouch;* (d) *cyst.*

cyst, *n.* An enclosed space within a tissue or organ, lined by epithelium and usually filled with fluid or other material.

cyst·ad·e·no·car·ci·no·ma (sist·ad″·e·no·kahr·si·no'muh) *n.* An adenocarcinoma in which there is prominent cyst formation.

cyst·ad·e·no·fi·bro·ma (sist·ad″·e·no·figh·bro'muh) *n.* A fibroadenoma containing one or more cysts.

cyst·ad·e·no·ma (sist″·ad·e·no'muh) *n.* An adenoma containing one or more cysts.

cystadenoma pa·pil·lif·er·um (pap″·i·lif'ur·um). An adenoma containing cysts with papillae on the inner aspect of the cyst walls.

cyst·ad·e·no·sar·co·ma (sist·ad″·e·no·sahr·ko'muh) *n.* A cystic malignant mixed mesodermal tumor, including both glandular and supportive tissue elements.

cys·tal·gia (sis·tal'jee·uh) *n.* Pain in the urinary bladder.

Cystamin. A trademark for methenamine, a urinary antiseptic.

cys·ta·thi·o·nine (sis″·tuh·thigh'o·neen) *n.* A mixed thio ether, formed from homocysteine and serine as an intermediate in the conversion of methionine to cysteine.

cys·ta·thi·o·nin·uria (sis″·tuh·thigh″·o·nin·yoo'ree·uh) *n.* An inborn error of metabolism in which there is a deficiency of the cystathionine cleavage enzyme, resulting in large amounts of cystathionine in the urine and occasionally slight elevation in blood; manifested clinically by mental retardation, thrombocytopenia, acidosis, and sometimes acromegaly; probably transmitted as a homozygous recessive trait.

cyst·ec·ta·sia (sist·eck·tay'zhuh, ·zee·uh) *n.* Dilatation of the neck of the bladder.

cys·tec·to·my (sis·teck'tuh·mee) *n.* 1. Excision of the gallbladder, or part or all of the urinary bladder. 2. Removal of a cyst. 3. Removal of a piece of the anterior capsule of the lens for the extraction of a cataract.

cys·te·ine (sis'te·een, ·in, sis·tee'in) *n.* 2-Amino-3-mercaptopropanoic acid, $HSCH_2CH(NH_2)COOH$, obtained by reduction of cystine and important as a constituent of many proteins.

cys·tic (sis'tick) *adj.* 1. Pertaining to or resembling a cyst. 2. Of or pertaining to the urinary bladder or to the gallbladder.

cystic acne. Acne distinguished by the formation of cysts containing purulent or gelatinous material.

cystic calculus. A calculus in the urinary bladder or in the gallbladder.

cystic degeneration. Any form of degeneration with cyst formation.

cystic disease. 1. CYSTIC DISEASE OF THE BREAST. 2. CYSTIC FIBROSIS OF THE PANCREAS.

cystic disease of the breast. A condition affecting women, usually in their thirties or forties, characterized by the rapid development in the involuting breast of one or more fairly large cysts which can sometimes be transilluminated. At operation the cysts often show a thin blue dome and contain serous fluid. Syn. *chronic cystic mastitis, cystic mastopathy, fibrocystic disease.*

cystic duct or **canal.** The duct of the gallbladder.

cystic endometriosis. A focus of endometriosis which has undergone cavitation.

cys·ti·cer·coid (sis″·ti·sur'koid) *n.* A larval tapeworm that has a slightly developed bladder and a solid posterior; a stage in the life cycle of *Hymenolepis nana.*

cys·ti·cer·co·sis (sis″·ti·sur·ko'sis) *n.*, pl. **cysticerco·ses** (·seez) Infection of man with *Taenia solium* in the larval stages, resulting in invasion of striated muscle, brain, and many other tissues; manifested by fever, myalgia, and neurologic disturbances.

cys·ti·cer·cus (sis″·ti·sur'kus) *n.*, pl. **cysticer·ci** (·sigh) The larval tapeworm; develops in man after ingestion of the ova of *Taenia solium* or *T. saginata.*

Cysticercus, *n. Obsol.* A genus to which bladder worms were assigned before it was discovered that they were larval tapeworms. *Cysticercus cellulosae,* for example, is the larva of *Taenia solium* and *C. bovis* is that of *T. saginata.*

cystic fibrosis of the pancreas. A generalized heritable disease of unknown etiology, associated with dysfunction of exocrine and eccrine glands, including mucus-producing glands; observed chiefly in infants, children, and adolescents; manifested mainly by elevated sweat electrolyte concentration, absence of pancreatic enzymes with the clinical appearance of the celiac syndrome, and evidence of chronic lung disease; transmitted as a Mendelian recessive trait. Syn. *mucoviscidosis.*

cystic mastitis. CYSTIC DISEASE OF THE BREAST.

cystic mastopathy. CYSTIC DISEASE OF THE BREAST.

cys·tine (sis'teen, ·tin) *n.* Dicysteine, $(—S—CH_2CHNH_2COOH)_2$, an amino acid component of many proteins, especially keratin. It may be reduced to cysteine.

cys·ti·no·sis (sis″·ti·no'sis) *n.*, pl. **cystino·ses** (·seez). The form of the Fanconi syndrome in which cystinuria and storage of cystine crystals in the internal organs are prominent features.

cys·ti·nu·ria (sis″·ti·new'ree·uh) *n.* A congenital and hereditary anomaly of renal tubular function, in which there is impaired reabsorption of cystine, lysine, arginine, and ornithine, which may result clinically in the formation of urinary calculi composed of almost pure cystine but no other disability; transmitted as a recessive or incompletely recessive trait.

cys·ti·tis (sis·tye'tis) *n.*, pl. **cys·tit·i·des** (sis·tit'i·deez) Inflammation of the urinary bladder.

cystitis cys·ti·ca (sis'ti·kuh). Chronic inflammation of the urinary bladder characterized by the presence of minute translucent mucus-containing submucosal cysts.

cystitis em·phy·se·ma·to·sa (em''fi·sem·uh·to'suh, ·seem·uh·to'suh). Cystitis in which cystic spaces in the urinary bladder wall are filled with gas; this may result from bacterial fermentation of sugar in the urine, as in diabetes or after glucose infusion.

cystitis fol·lic·u·la·ris (fol·ick''yoo·lair'is). Cystitis in which there are lymphoid nodules or masses of lymphoid cells beneath the epithelium.

cystitis glan·du·la·ris (glan''dew·lair'is). A type of chronic cystitis in which there is metaplastic transformation of nests of transitional epithelium into columnar mucus-secreting epithelium.

cysto-. See *cyst-.*

cys·to·cele (sis'to·seel) *n.* Herniation of the urinary bladder into the vagina.

cys·to·en·tero·cele (sis''to·en'tur·o·seel) *n.* Herniation of the urinary bladder and intestine, usually into the vagina.

cys·to·gen·e·sis (sis''to·jen'e·sis) *n.*, pl. **cystogeneses** (·seez). The formation or genesis of cysts.

cys·to·gram (sis'to·gram) *n.* 1. A radiograph of the urinary bladder made after the injection of a contrast medium. 2. A radiograph for demonstration of cysts.

cys·tog·ra·phy (sis·tog'ruh·fee) *n.* Radiography of the urinary bladder after the injection of a contrast medium or contrast media. —**cys·to·graph·ic** (·graf'ick) *adj.*

cys·toid (sis'toid) *adj. & n.* 1. Having the form or appearance of a bladder or cyst. 2. Composed of a collection of cysts. 3. PSEUDOCYST.

cys·to·li·thec·to·my (sis''to·li·theck'tuh·mee) *n.* CYSTOLITHOTOMY.

cys·to·li·thi·a·sis (sis''to·li·thigh'uh·sis) *n.*, pl. **cys·tolithiases** (·seez) Calculi, or a calculus, in the urinary bladder.

cys·to·li·thot·o·my (sis''to·li·thot'uh·mee) *n.* Surgical removal of a calculus from the urinary bladder.

cys·to·ma (sis·to'muh) *n.*, pl. **cystomas, cystomata** (·tuh) A cystic mass, especially in or near the ovary; may be neoplastic or inflammatory, or due to retention.

cys·tom·e·ter (sis·tom'e·tur) *n.* An instrument used to determine pressure and capacity in the urinary bladder under standard conditions. —**cystome·try** (·tree) *n.*

cys·to·met·ro·gram (sis''to·met'ro·gram) *n.* Graphic demonstration of the pressure within the urinary bladder with gradual filling, as determined by cystometry.

cys·to·mor·phous (sis''to·mor'fus) *adj.* Having the structure of, or resembling, a cyst or a bladder.

cys·to·pexy (sis'to·peck''see) *n.* Surgical fixation

of the urinary bladder, or a portion of it, in a new location; vesicofixation.

cys·to·plas·ty (sis'to·plas''tee) *n.* A plastic operation upon the urinary bladder; used mainly to increase bladder capacity.

cys·to·pros·ta·tec·to·my (sis''to·pros''tuh·teck'tuh·mee) *n. In surgery,* excision of the urinary bladder and the prostate.

cys·to·py·eli·tis (sis''to·pye''e·lye'tis) *n.* Inflammation of the urinary bladder and the pelvis of the kidney.

cys·to·py·elo·ne·phri·tis (sis''to·pye''e·lo·nef·rye'tis) *n.* Inflammation of the urinary bladder, renal pelvis, and renal parenchyma.

cys·to·rec·to·cele (sis''to·reck'to·seel) *n.* Herniation of the urinary bladder and rectum into the vagina.

cys·tor·rha·phy (sis·tor'uh·fee) *n.* Suture of the urinary bladder.

cys·to·sar·co·ma (sis''to·sahr·ko'muh) *n.* Formerly, a fleshy mass containing cysts.

cystosarcoma phyl·lo·des (fi·lo'deez) [Gr. *phyllōdēs,* leafy]. A benign tumor of the mammary gland, which grows slowly but may attain great size, with nodular proliferation of connective tissue and lesser adenomatous proliferation.

cystosarcoma phyl·loi·des (fi·loy'deez). CYSTOSARCOMA PHYLLODES.

cys·to·scope (sis'tuh·skope) *n.* An instrument used in diagnosis and treatment of lesions of the urinary bladder, ureter, and kidney. It consists of an outer sheath bearing the lighting system, a well-fitted obturator, space for the visual system, and room for the passage of ureteral catheters and operative devices to be used under visual control. —**cys·to·scop·ic** (sis''to·skop'ick) *adj.*

cystoscopic lithotrite. A lithotrite which operates under visual control by means of a cystoscopic attachment.

cys·tos·co·py (sis·tos'kuh·pee) *n.* The procedure of using the cystoscope.

cys·to·sphinc·ter·om·e·try (sis''to·sfink''tur·om'e·tree) *n.* Simultaneous measurement of the pressure in the urinary bladder and in the urethra.

cys·tos·to·my (sis·tos'tuh·mee) *n. In surgery,* the formation of a fistulous opening in the urinary bladder wall.

cys·to·tome (sis'tuh·tome) *n.* 1. An instrument for incising the urinary bladder or gallbladder. 2. An instrument for incising the capsule of the lens.

cys·tot·o·my (sis·tot'uh·mee) *n.* 1. Incision into the urinary bladder or gallbladder. 2. Incision into the anterior capsule of the lens for the extraction of a cataract.

cys·to·ure·tero·cele (sis''to·yoo·ree'tur·o·seel) *n.* Herniation of the urinary bladder and one or both ureters into the vagina.

cys·to·ure·thri·tis (sis''to·yoo''re·thrigh'tis) *n.* Inflammation of the urinary bladder and the urethra.

cys·to·ure·thro·cele (sis''to·yoo·ree'thro·seel) *n.* Herniation of the urinary bladder and urethra into the vagina.

cys·to·ure·thro·gram (sis''to·yoo·ree'thro·gram) *n.* A radiograph of the urinary bladder and urethra, made after opacification of these structures.

cys·to·ure·throg·ra·phy (sis″to·yoo″re·throg′ruh·fee) *n.* Radiography of the urinary bladder and urethra. —**cystoure·thro·graph·ic** (·thro·graf′ick) *adj.*

cys·to·ure·thro·scope (sis″to·yoo·ree′thro·skope) *n.* An instrument for inspecting the urinary bladder and posterior urethra.

cyt-, cyto- A combining form meaning (a) *cell, cellular;* (b) *cytoplasm, cytoplasmic.*

cyt·ar·a·bine (sit′ār·uh·been) *n.* 1-Arabino-furanosylcytosine, $C_9H_{13}N_3O_5$, an inhibitor of deoxyribonucleic acid synthesis and of the proliferation of viruses containing this acid; used as the hydrochloride salt. Syn. *cytosine arabinoside, ara-C, arabinosyl cutosine.*

-cyte A combining form meaning *a cell.*

cyt·i·sine (sit′i·seen, ·sin) *n.* A poisonous alkaloid, $C_{11}H_{14}N_2O$, from *Laburnum anagyroides,* goldenchain laburnum, and from baptisia and other plants. It stimulates, then paralyzes, autonomic ganglions.

cyto-. See **cyt-**.

cy·to·ar·chi·tec·ton·ic (sigh″to·ahr″ki·teck·ton′ick) *adj.* Pertaining to the cellular arrangement of a region, tissue, or organ.

cy·to·ar·chi·tec·ture (sigh″to·ahr′ki·teck″chur) *n.* The cell pattern typical of a region, as of an area of the cerebral cortex.

cy·to·blast (sigh′to·blast) *n.* The nucleus of a cell.

cy·to·chem·ism (sigh″to·kem′iz·um) *n.* The reaction of the living cell to chemical agents.

cy·to·chem·is·try (sigh″to·kem′is·tree) *n.* The science dealing with the chemical constitution of cells and cell constituents, especially as demonstrated in histologic section by specific staining reactions.

cy·to·chrome (sigh′to·krome) *n.* One of several iron-protoporphyrin cellular pigments (cytochrome a_1, a_2, a_3, b_1, b_2, b_3, etc.) which function in cellular respiration (electron transport) by being alternately oxidized and reduced. Most cytochromes are bound to the protein-lipid complex of the mitochondria. Some 30 such compounds are now known.

cytochrome oxidase. An iron-porphyrin respiratory enzyme in mitochondria in which the prosthetic group undergoes reversible oxidation-reduction, accepting electrons which are transferred subsequently to oxygen. It is identical with indophenol oxidase.

cy·to·cide (sigh′to·side) *n.* An agent that is destructive to cells. —**cy·to·ci·dal** (sigh″to·sigh′dul) *adj.*

cy·tode (sigh′tode) *n.* The simplest form of cell, without nucleus or nucleolus.

cy·to·di·ag·no·sis (sigh″to·dye″ug·no′sis) *n.*, pl. **cytodiagno·ses** (·seez) The determination of the nature of an abnormal liquid by the study of the cells it contains.

cy·to·gen·e·sis (sigh″to·jen′e·sis) *n.*, pl. **cytogene·ses** (·seez) The genesis and differentiation of a cell. —**cy·to·ge·net·ic** (·je·net′ick) *adj.*

cy·to·ge·net·ics (sigh″to·je·net′icks) *n.* The hybrid science in which the methods of cytology are employed to study the chromosomes.

cy·toid (sigh′toid) *adj.* Resembling a cell.

cytoid bodies. Globular bodies located in the nerve fiber layer of the retina and which may represent terminal nerve fiber swellings. A collection of these cytoid bodies gives rise to the cotton-wool exudate.

cy·tol·o·gy (sigh·tol′uh·jee) *n.* 1. The subdivision of biology which deals with cells. 2. EXFOLIATIVE CYTOLOGY. —**cy·to·log·ic** (sigh″to·loj′ick), **cytolog·i·cal** (·i·kul) *adj.;* **cy·tol·o·gist** (sigh·tol′uh·jist) *n.*

cy·tol·y·sin (sigh·tol′i·sin, sigh″to·lye′sin) *n.* A specific protein or antibody of blood plasma which brings about the hemolysis of red cells (hemolysin), or the cytolysis of other tissue cells.

cy·tol·y·sis (sigh·tol′i·sis) *n.*, pl. **cytoly·ses** (·seez) The disintegration or dissolution of cells. —**cy·to·lyt·ic** (sigh″to·lit′ick) *adj.*

cy·to·ly·so·some (sigh″to·lye′so·sohm) *n.* An enlarged lysosome containing recognizable organelles such as mitochondria.

-cytoma A combining form meaning *a neoplasm made up of a* (specified) *kind of cell.*

cy·to·me·gal·ic (sigh″to·me·gal′ick) *adj.* Of, pertaining to, or characterizing the greatly enlarged cells, measuring 25 to 40 microns, with enlarged nuclei containing prominent inclusion bodies and sometimes also cytoplasmic inclusions; found in various tissues in cytomegalic inclusion disease.

cytomegalic inclusion disease. Infection with the cytomegaloviruses of man, monkeys, and other animals, characterized by a striking enlargement of epithelial cells of the salivary glands and other organs, and by prominent intranuclear inclusion bodies. In the neonatal period associated with hepatosplenomegaly, thrombocytopenic purpura, hepatitis, jaundice, microcephaly, and subsequent mental retardation; postnatally, may be asymptomatic or associated with pneumonitis and hepatitis. Abbreviated, CID. Syn. *salivary gland virus disease.*

cy·to·meg·a·lo·vi·rus (sigh″to·meg″uh·lo·vye′rus) *n.* A member of a group of DNA viruses closely related to the herpesviruses; the cause of cytomegalic inclusion disease.

Cytomel. Trademark for sodium liothyronine, a thyroid hormone.

cy·tom·e·ter (sigh·tom′e·tur) *n.* A device for counting cells, especially blood cells. —**cy·tom·e·try** (sigh·tom′e·tree) *n.;* **cy·to·met·ric** (sigh″to·met′rick) *adj.*

cy·to·mor·pho·sis (sigh″to·mor·fo′sis, ·mor′fuh·sis) *n.*, pl. **cytomopho·ses** (·seez) All the structural alterations which cells or successive generations of cells undergo from the earliest undifferentiated stage to their final destruction.

cy·to·my·co·sis (sigh″to·migh·ko′sis) *n.*, pl. **cyto·myco·ses** (·seez) 1. Fungal infection in which the organisms primarily grow within cells. 2. HISTOPLASMOSIS.

cy·to·patho·gen·ic (sigh″to·path″o·jen′ick) *adj.* Pertaining to the destruction of cells (in tissue culture) by a transmissible agent, such as a virus.

cy·to·pa·thol·o·gy (sigh″to·pa·thol′uh·jee) *n.* The branch of pathology concerned with alterations within cells, especially as demonstrated by techniques such as those of exfoliative cytology.

cy·top·a·thy (sigh·top'uth·ee) *n.* Disease of the living cell. —**cy·to·path·ic** (sigh''to·path'ick) *adj.*

cy·to·pemp·sis (sigh''to·pemp'sis) *n.* Transport of particulate matter or large molecules across an endothelial cell membrane by means of vesicles; of doubtful significance in vivo.

cy·to·pe·nia (sigh''to·pee'nee·uh) *n.* A cell count less than normal.

cy·toph·a·gy (sigh·tof'uh·jee) *n.* The engulfing of cells by other cells; PHAGOCYTOSIS. —**cytoph·a·gous** (·uh·gus) *adj.*

cy·to·phe·re·sis (sigh''to·fe·ree'sis) *n.* The removal of cells, especially leukocytes, from whole blood, with return of the remaining blood to the donor.

cy·to·phil (sigh'to·fil) *adj.* Having an affinity for cells; attracted by cells.

cy·to·phil·ic (sigh''to·fil'ick) *adj.* CYTOPHIL.

cy·to·plasm (sigh'to·plaz·um) *n.* The protoplasm of a cell other than that of the nucleus. —**cy·to·plas·mic** (sigh''to·plaz'mick) *adj.*

cy·to·poi·e·sis (sigh''to·poy·ee'sis) *n.* The formation and development of a cell.

cy·tos·co·py (sigh·tos'kuh·pee) *n.* CYTODIAGNOSIS. —**cy·to·scop·ic** (sigh''to·skop'ick) *adj.*

cy·to·sine (sigh'to·seen, ·sin) *n.* 4-Amino-2(1*H*)-pyrimidone, $C_4H_5N_3O$, a pyrimidine base important mainly as a component of ribonucleic and deoxyribonucleic acids.

cytosine ar·a·bi·no·side (ăr''uh·bin'o·side, a·rab'i·no·side). CYTARABINE.

cy·to·skel·e·ton (sigh''to·skel'e·tun) *n.* The structural framework of a cell, probably consisting of proteins.

cy·to·smear (sigh'to·smeer) *n.* A smear of some

cell-containing material, such as cervical scrapings, for the purpose of cytologic study.

cy·to·some (sigh''to·sohm) *n.* A cell body exclusive of the nucleus.

cy·to·stat·ic (sigh''to·stat'ick) *adj.* Preventing the multiplication and growth of cells.

cy·to·tax·is (sigh''to·tack'sis) *n.* The movement of cells toward or away from a stimulus. —**cyto·tac·tic** (·tack'tick) *adj.*

cy·to·tech·nol·o·gist (sigh''to·teck·nol'uh·jist) *n.* A person trained and skilled in the preparation and examination of exfoliated cells who conducts a preliminary study of such cells, referring abnormal smears to a specialized physician for final classification.

cy·toth·e·sis (sigh·toth'e·sis, sigh''to·thees'is) *n.* Cell repair.

cy·to·tox·in (sigh''to·tock'sin) *n.* 1. A serum, natural or immune, capable of injuring certain cells without lysis. 2. Any chemical agent which kills cells. —**cytotox·ic** (·sick) *adj.*

cy·to·tropho·blast (sigh''to·trof'o·blast) *n.* The innermost cellular layer of the trophoblast of embryonic placental mammals, which gives rise to the syntrophoblast layer which ultimately covers the placental villi. Syn. *Langhans' layer.*

cy·tot·ro·pism (sigh·tot'ruh·piz·um) *n.* 1. The tendency of cells to move toward or away from a stimulus. 2. The tendency of certain chemicals, viruses, and bacteria to be attracted to certain kinds of cells. —**cy·to·tro·pic** (sigh''to·tro'pick, ·trop'ick) *adj.*

Cytoxan. Trademark for cyclophosphamide, an alkylating type of antineoplastic agent.

cy·to·zyme (sigh'to·zime) *n.* A substance in various tissues, capable of activating thrombin, the fibrin ferment.

D

D Symbol for deuterium.

D., d. Abbreviation for (a) *da* (L., give); (b) day, days; (c) dead; (d) *density;* (e) *detur* (L., let it be given); (f) *dexter;* (g) died; (h) *diopter;* (i) *distal;* (j) *dorsal;* (k) *dose;* (l) duration.

D- *In chemistry,* a configurational descriptor placed before the stereoparent names of amino acids and carbohydrates. With amino acids it relates the configuration of the carbon bearing the amino acid group to serine and for carbohydrates the highest member asymmetric carbon atom to the reference compound, D-glyceraldehyde. Although the symbol D bears no relationship to the rotation of plane polarized light by the compound, the combined symbolic prefix DL always indicates an optically inactive form or a racemic mixture.

d- 1. *In chemistry,* a symbol formerly used for dextrorotatory, referring to the direction in which plane polarized light is rotated by a substance; this usage is superseded by the symbol (+). 2. *In chemistry,* a symbol formerly used to indicate the structural configuration of a particular asymmetric carbon atom in a compound, in the manner that the small capital letter D- is now used. 3. *In chemistry,* a chemical name followed by the symbol *d* indicates substitution of appropriate hydrogen atoms by deuterium and, if subscripted, also indicates the number of deuterium atoms inserted.

Da Cos·ta's syndrome NEUROCIRCULATORY ASTHENIA.

dacry-, dacryo- A combining form meaning (a) *tears;* (b) *lacrimal apparatus.*

dac·ry·ad·e·ni·tis (dack‴ree-ad″e-nigh′tis) *n.* DACRYOADENITIS.

dac·ry·ad·e·no·scir·rhus (dack‴ree-ad″e-no-skirr′us) *n.* An indurated tumor of the lacrimal gland.

dac·ry·ag·o·ga·tre·sia (dack‴ree-ag″o-ga-tree′zhuh, ‑zee‑uh, dack‴ree-uh-gog″uh‑) *n.* Obstruction of a lacrimal canaliculus.

dac·ry·a·gog·ic (dack‴ree-uh-goj′ick) *adj.* Pertaining to or having the character of a dacryagogue.

dac·ry·a·gogue (dack′ree-uh-gog) *n. & adj.* 1. An agent causing a flow of tears. 2. Causing a flow of tears; DACRYAGOGIC.

dacryo-. See *dacry-.*

dac·ry·o·ad·e·nal·gia (dack‴ree-o-ad″e-nal′jee-uh) *n.* Pain in a lacrimal gland.

dac·ry·o·ad·e·nec·to·my (dack‴ree-o-ad″e-neck′tuh-mee) *n.* Excision of a lacrimal gland.

dac·ry·o·ad·e·ni·tis (dack‴ree-o-ad″e-nigh′tis) *n.* Inflammation of a lacrimal gland.

dac·ry·o·ag·o·ga·tre·sia (dack‴ree-o-ag″o-ga-tree′zhuh) *n.* DACRYAGOGATRESIA.

dac·ry·o·blen·nor·rhea, dac·ry·o·blen·nor·rhoea (dack‴ree-o-blen″o-ree′uh) *n.* Chronic inflammation of and discharge of mucus from the lacrimal sac.

dac·ry·o·cele (dack′ree-o-seel) *n.* DACRYOCYSTOCELE.

dac·ry·o·cyst (dack′ree-o-sist) *n.* LACRIMAL SAC.

dac·ry·o·cys·tec·to·my (dack‴ree-o-sis-teck′tuh-mee) *n.* Excision of all or a part of the lacrimal sac.

dac·ry·o·cys·ti·tis (dack‴ree-o-sis-tye′tis) *n.* Inflammation of the lacrimal sac.

dac·ry·o·cys·to·blen·nor·rhea, dac·ry·o·cys·to·blen·nor·rhoea (dack‴ree-o-sis″to-blen-o-ree′uh) *n.* DACRYOCYSTITIS.

dac·ry·o·cys·to·cele (dack‴ree-o-sis′to-seel) *n.* Distention of a lacrimal sac.

dac·ry·o·cys·top·to·sis (dack‴ree-o-sis″top′to-sis) *n.* Prolapse or downward displacement of a lacrimal sac.

dac·ry·o·cys·to·rhi·nos·to·my (dack‴ree-o-sis″to-rye-nos′tuh-mee) *n.* An operation to restore drainage into the nose from the lacrimal sac when the nasolacrimal duct is obliterated or obstructed.

dac·ry·o·cys·tos·to·my (dack‴ree-o-sis-tos′tuh-mee) *n.* Incision into the lacrimal sac, particularly to promote drainage.

dac·ry·o·cys·tot·o·my (dack‴ree-o-sis-tot′uh-mee) *n.* Incision of the lacrimal sac.

dac·ry·o·lith (dack′ree-o-lith) *n.* A firm, laminated, stonelike structure that develops in the lacrimal sac with obstruction of the nasolacrimal duct.

dac·ry·o·li·thi·a·sis (dack"ree·o·li·thigh'uh·sis) *n.* The formation and presence of dacryoliths.

dac·ry·o·ma (dack"ree·o'muh) *n.*, pl. **dacryomas, dacryoma·ta** (·tuh) 1. A lacrimal tumor. 2. Obstruction of the lacrimal puncta, causing epiphora.

dac·ry·ops, dak·ry·ops (dack'ree·ops) *n.* 1. EPIPHORA. 2. A cyst of an excretory duct of a lacrimal gland.

dac·ry·or·rhea, dac·ry·or·rhoea (dack"ree·o·ree' uh) *n.* An excessive flow of tears.

dac·ry·o·so·le·ni·tis (dack"ree·o·so"le·nigh'tis) *n.* Inflammation of the lacrimal drainage system.

dac·ry·o·ste·no·sis (dack"ree·o·ste·no'sis) *n.* Stenosis or stricture of the lacrimal drainage system.

dac·ry·o·syr·inx (dack"ree·o·sirr'inks) *n.*, pl. **dac·ry·o·syr·in·ges** (·si·rin'jeez), **dacryosyrinxes** 1. LACRIMAL FISTULA. 2. A syringe for use in the lacrimal ducts.

Dactil. Trademark for piperidolate, an anticholinergic drug used as the hydrochloride salt.

dac·ti·no·my·cin (dack"ti·no·migh'sin) *n.* An actinomycin antibiotic, produced by *Streptomyces parvullus*, useful in the treatment of various tumors; also useful in the study of genetic transcription because it interferes with the synthesis of messenger RNA. Syn. *actinomycin D.*

dactyl-, dactylo- A combining form meaning *digit, finger, toe.*

dac·tyl (dack'til) *n. In zoology,* a digit; a finger or toe. —**dac·ty·lar** (·lur), **dac·ty·late** (·late) *adj.*

-dactylia A combining form designating *a condition or characteristic involving the digits.*

dac·ty·lif·er·ous (dack"ti·lif'uh·rus) *adj.* Having finger or fingerlike parts, organs, or appendages.

dac·ty·li·tis (dack"ti·lye'tis) *n.* Inflammation of a finger or a toe.

dac·ty·lo·gram (dack·til'o·gram, dack'ti·lo·) *n.* A fingerprint, generally used for purposes of identification and in genetic studies.

dac·ty·lol·y·sis (dack"ti·lol'i·sis) *n.* Loss or amputation of a digit.

dac·ty·lo·meg·a·ly (dack"ti·lo·meg'uh·lee) *n.* A condition in which one or more of the fingers or toes is abnormally large; MACRODACTYLY.

dac·ty·lo·sym·phy·sis (dack"ti·lo·sim'fi·sis) *n.* SYNDACTYLY.

Da·kin's solution A 0.4 to 0.5% solution of sodium hypochlorite, buffered with sodium bicarbonate; formerly used extensively as an antiseptic in the treatment of septic wounds.

Dall·dorf test A test for capillary fragility in which a suction cup is applied to the skin for a measured interval of time and the number of petechiae which result are counted. Syn. *suction test.*

dal·ton·ism (dawl'tun·iz·um, dal'tun·) *n.* COLOR BLINDNESS.

Dal·ton's law 1. The pressure of a mixture of gases equals the sum of the partial pressures of the constituent gases. 2. So long as no chemical change occurs, each gas in a mixture of gases is absorbed by a given volume of solvent in proportion not to the total pressure of the mixture but to the partial pressure of that gas.

dam, *n.* 1. A thin sheet of rubber used to isolate a tooth during dental operations. 2. A piece of dam used as a drain.

D and C Dilation of the cervix and curettage of the lining of the uterus; a diagnostic and therapeutic procedure in obstetrics and gynecology.

dan·der (dan'dur) *n.* Scales of animal skin, hair, or feathers; may act as an allergen.

dan·druff, *n.* Scales of greasy keratotic material shed from the scalp.

Dan·dy-Walk·er syndrome Distension of the fourth ventricle and hydrocephalus, generally attributed to congenital atresia or obstruction of the foramens of Luschka and Magendie.

dap·sone (dap'sone) *n.* 4,4'-Sulfonyldianiline or diaminodiphenylsulfone, $C_{12}H_{12}N_2O_2S$, a leprostatic drug and a suppressant for dermatitis herpetiformis; also used in prophylaxis of falciparum malaria.

Daraprim. Trademark for pyrimethamine, an antimalarial drug.

Darier's disease A genodermatosis transmitted as a dominant characteristic, consisting of keratotic papules which coalesce to form warty, crusted patches. Syn. *keratosis follicularis.*

dark adaptation. Adjustment of the iris and retina for vision in dim light or darkness.

dark-field microscopy or **illumination.** A system using a special condenser that transmits only light entering its periphery, so that particles in the object plane are obliquely illuminated and glow against a dark background. Submicroscopic particles and nearly transparent living organisms such as *Treponema* are thus visualized.

darm·brand (dahrm'brahnt) *n.* ENTERITIS NECROTICANS.

Dar·row's solution A solution of the electrolytes of plasma, containing added amounts of potassium, used in fluid therapy. It contains 122 mEq/liter sodium, 104 mEq/liter chloride, 35 mEq/liter potassium, and 53 mEq/liter lactate.

dar·tos (dahr'tos) *n.* The thin layer of smooth muscle in the deeper part of the corium and the subcutaneous tissue of the scrotum.

da·tu·rism (da·tew'riz·um, dat'yoo·riz·um) *n.* Poisoning by stramonium.

daugh·ter, *n.* 1. *In radiochemistry,* a radioactive or stable nuclide resulting from the disintegration of a radioactive nuclide, or parent. 2. (*Attributive use*) Resulting from cell division, as daughter nucleus, daughter chromosome.

daughter cell. A cell resulting from the division of a mother cell.

Da·vid·sohn differential test. A test for infectious mononucleosis in which is shown that the heterophil antibodies produced in infectious mononucleosis are not absorbed by guinea pig kidney whereas those produced in serum disease are readily absorbed.

Davidsohn presumptive test. A sheep cell agglutination test for the presence of heterophil agglutinin which is characteristically produced in the serum of patients with infectious mononucleosis.

Daw·son's encephalitis or **disease** SUBACUTE SCLEROSING PANENCEPHALITIS.

day blindness. Low visual acuity in good light; may be congenital, familial, or due to a lesion involving the cones of the fovea. Also considered to be a form of monochromatism or a frequently incomplete form of total color blindness. Syn. *hemeralopia.*

db Abbreviation for *decibel.*

D.C. 1. Doctor of Chiropractic. 2. Dental Corps.

D.D.S. Doctor of Dental Surgery.

DDT 1,1,1,-Trichloro-2,2-bis(*p*-chlorophenyl) ethane, an insecticide the medicinal grade of which is chlorophenothane.

de- A prefix meaning (a) *undoing, reversal;* (b) *removal, loss.*

de·ac·ti·vate (dee-ack'ti-vate) *v.* To become or render inactive. —**de·ac·ti·va·tion** (dee-ack''ti-vay'shun) *n.*

dead, *adj.* No longer living.

dead·ly night·shade. BELLADONNA.

dead space. A cavity left after the closure of a wound.

deaf, *adj.* Unable to hear because of a defect, disease, or dysfunction of the ear, the vestibulochlear nerve, or the brain. —**deaf·ness,** *n.*

deaf·ened. *adj.* Rendered deaf after having had normal hearing, especially after having learned to comprehend and produce speech. —**deaf·en,** *v.*

de·af·fer·en·ta·tion (dee-af''ur-en-tay'shun) *n.* The process of interrupting afferent nerve (sensory) fibers.

deaf-mute, *n.* A person who lacks the sense of hearing and the ability to speak.

deaf-mutism, *n.* The condition of being both deaf and mute.

de·am·i·dase (de-am'i-dace, -daze) *n.* An enzyme that catalyzes the hydrolysis of an amido compound. —**de·am·i·di·za·tion** (dee-am''i-di-zay'shun) *n.*

de·am·i·nate (dee-am'i-nate) *v.* To remove an amino (NH_2) group from an organic compound, particularly from an amino acid. —**de·am·i·na·tion** (dee-am''i-nay'shun) *n.*

deaminating enzyme. DEAMINIZING ENZYME.

deaminizing enzyme. An enzyme, such as guanase or adenase, that splits off —NH_2 groups; usually followed by a secondary oxidative reaction.

de·an·es·the·si·ant (dee-an''esth-ee'zhunt, -zee-unt) *n.* Any agent or means of arousing a patient from a state of anesthesia.

death, *n.* The cessation of life, beyond the possibility of resuscitation.

death certificate. A form, usually required by law, for recording the event of death, its time, place, cause, the name and age of the decedent, and other pertinent data.

death instinct. *In psychoanalytic theory,* the unconscious drive which leads the individual toward dissolution and death, and which coexists with the life instinct.

death rate. The proportion of deaths in a given year and area to the mid-year population of that area, usually expressed as the number of deaths per thousand of population.

death rattle. A gurgling sound heard in dying persons, due to the passage of air through fluid in the trachea.

de·bil·i·tant (de-bil'i-tunt) *adj. & n.* 1. Debilitating, weakening. 2. Any debilitating agent.

de·bil·i·tate (de-bil'i-tate) *v.* To weaken; to make feeble.

de·bil·i·ty (de-bil'i-tee) *n.* Weakness; lack of strength; ASTHENIA.

de·branch·er deficiency (de-branch'ur). LIMIT DEXTRINOSIS.

de·bride·ment (de-breed''mahn', de-breed'munt) *n.* Removal of foreign material and devitalized tissue from a wound, usually by sharp dissection, sometimes by means of enzymes or other chemical agents. —**de·bride** (de-breed', day-breed') *v.*

de·bris (de-bree', day-bree') *n.* 1. Foreign material or devitalized tissue. 2. *In dentistry,* soft foreign material loosely attached to the surface of a tooth, as the refuse from the drilling of a cavity.

debt, *n.* DEFICIT.

dec-, deca- A prefix meaning (a) *ten;* (b) *multiplied by ten.*

de·ca·dence (deck'uh-dunce, de-kay'dunce) *n.* Decay, decline, deterioration, as in aging process.

Decadron. A trademark for dexamethasone, an anti-inflammatory glucocorticoid.

deca·gram (deck'uh-gram) *n.* A metric measure of weight equal to 10 grams.

de·cal·ci·fi·ca·tion (de-kal''si-fi-kay'shun) *n.* Withdrawal or removal of the mineral salts of bone or other calcified substance. —**de·cal·ci·fy** (de-kal'si-fye) *v.*

deca·li·ter (deck'uh-lee''tur) *n.* A metric measure of volume equal to 10 liters.

de·cal·vant (de-kal'vunt) *adj.* Destroying or removing hair.

deca·me·ter (deck'uh-mee''tur) *n.* A metric measure of length equal to 10 meters.

de·can·cel·la·tion (dee-kan''se-lay'shun) *n.* The removal of cancellous bone either for use as bone chips in grafting operations or for correcting deformity.

dec·ane (deck'ane) *n.* Any of the isomeric hydrocarbons, $C_{10}H_{22}$, of the paraffin series.

deca·nor·mal (deck'uh-nor''mul) *adj.* Having 10 times the strength of the normal; said of solutions.

de·cant (dee-kant') *v.* To pour off a liquor or solution without disturbing the sediment. —**de·can·ta·tion** (dee-kan-tay'shun) *n.*

deca·pep·tide (deck''uh-pep'tide) *n.* A polypeptide composed of ten amino acids.

de·cap·i·tate (dee-kap'i-tate) *v.* To behead; to remove the head of a person, a fetus, an animal, or a bone. —**de·cap·i·ta·tion** (dee-kap''i-tay'shun) *n.*

Decapryn. Trademark for doxylamine, an antihistaminic drug used as the succinate salt.

de·cap·su·la·tion (dee-kap''sue-lay'shun) *n.* The removal of a capsule or enveloping membrane, as the capsule of a kidney.

de·car·box·yl·ase (dee''kahr-bock'sil·ace, -aze) *n.* An enzyme that removes carbon dioxide without oxidation from various carboxylic acids.

de·car·box·yl·ate (dee''kahr-bock'si·late) *v.* To

split off one or more molecules of carbon dioxide from organic acids, especially amino acids. —**decar·box·y·la·tion** (·bock''si·lay'shun) *n.*

de·ca·thec·tion (dee''ka·theck'shun) *n.* DECATHEXIS.

deca·vi·ta·min (deck''uh·vye'tuh·min) *n.* A U.S.P. formulation of vitamin A, vitamin D, ascorbic acid, calcium pantothenate, cyanocobalamin, folic acid, niacinamide, pyridoxine hydrochloride, riboflavin, thiamine, and a suitable form of alpha tocopherol. One capsule or tablet supplies the recommended daily requirement of the vitamins contained therein.

de·cay (de·kay') *n. & v.* 1. The progressive chemical decomposition of organic matter in the presence of atmospheric oxygen; due generally to aerobic bacteria and to fungi; rot. 2. A decline in health or strength. 3. SENILITY. 4. DENTAL CARIES. 5. *In physics,* the process or processes of nuclear disintegration by which an unstable, i.e., radioactive, atom is spontaneously converted to a stable one. 6. To undergo decay.

decay constant. The proportion of atoms of any radioactive substance that will disintegrate per unit of time. Radioactive disintegration (decay) is measured by the equation $N = N_0 e^{-kt}$, where N is the number of atoms unchanged at time t, N_0 is the number present initially, e is the base of natural logarithms, and k is the decay constant.

de·ce·dent (de·see'dunt) *n.* A deceased person.

decem- A combining form meaning *ten.*

de·cen·tered (dee·sen'turd) *adj.* Out of common center; said of a lens when the visual axis and the axis of the lens do not coincide. —**de·cen·tra·tion** (dee''sen·tray'shun) *n.*

decerebrate posture or **position.** The posture assumed by a patient in a state of decerebrate rigidity. The limbs are stiffly extended, the head retracted, and these postures become exaggerated in response to painful stimuli.

decerebrate rigidity. Markedly increased tone in the antigravity muscles resulting from interruption of the neuraxis at a point between the inferior and superior colliculi, with release of the facilitatory pathways of the reticular formation and the vestibulospinal tract.

de·cer·e·bra·tion (dee·serr''e·bray'shun) *n.* Experimental rendering of an animal's cerebrum and higher centers nonfunctional by interruption, usually transection, of the neuraxis at a point between the inferior and superior colliculi.

de·chlo·ri·da·tion (dee·klor''i·day'shun) *n.* Reduction of the quantity of chloride or salt present in tissues.

de·chlor·u·ra·tion (dee·klor''yoo·ray'shun, ·oo·ray'shun) *n.* Reduction of the amount of chlorides excreted in the urine.

Decholin. A trademark for dehydrocholic acid, a choleretic drug.

deci- A combining form meaning (a) *tenth;* (b) in the metric system, *a measure one-tenth as large as the unit.*

dec·i·bel (des'i·bel). *n.* One-tenth of a bel. Abbreviated, db.

de·cid·ua (de·sid'yoo·uh) *n.,* pl. **decid·u·ae** (·yoo·ee) The endometrium of pregnancy, which is cast off at parturition. —**decid·u·al** (·yoo·ul) *adj.*

decidua ba·sa·lis (ba·say'lis) [NA]. The part of the endometrium of pregnancy between the chorionic vesicle and the myometrium which forms the maternal part of the placenta.

decidua cap·su·la·ris (kap·sue·lair'is) [NA]. The part of the endometrium of pregnancy between the chorionic vesicle and the uterine lumen; the outer investing envelope of the fetus.

decidual cast. The entire decidua expelled from the uterus in a single piece, as with extrauterine gestation.

decidual endometritis. DECIDUITIS.

decidual fissure. One of the fissured spaces developing in the decidua basalis, parallel with the uterine wall, in the later months of pregnancy.

decidual membranes. The membranes formed by the superficial part of the endometrium during pregnancy.

decidual reaction. The reaction of tissues, especially the endometrium, to pregnancy; marked by the development of characteristic decidual cells from fibroblasts.

decidua mar·gi·na·lis (mahr''ji·nay'lis). The part of the endometrium of pregnancy at the junction of the decidua basalis, decidua parietalis, and decidua capsularis.

decidua men·stru·a·lis (men''stroo·ay'lis). The outer layer of the uterine mucosa which is shed during menstruation. Syn. *pseudodecidua.*

decidua pa·ri·e·ta·lis (pa·rye''e·tay'lis) [NA]. The endometrium of pregnancy exclusive of the region occupied by the embryo.

de·cid·u·ate (de·sid'yoo·ut) *adj.* 1. Having, or characterized by, a decidua. 2. Formed in part from a decidua.

de·cid·u·a·tion (de·sid''yoo·ay'shun) *n.* The act or process of dropping off or shedding.

de·cid·u·itis (de·sid''yoo·eye'tis) *n.* An acute inflammation of the decidua, frequently the result of attempts to induce abortion.

de·cid·u·o·ma (de·sid''yoo·o'muh) *n.* 1. Decidual tissue produced in the uterus by mechanical or other methods in the absence of an embryo. 2. An intrauterine tumor containing decidual remnants believed to arise from hyperplasia of a retained portion of the decidua.

de·cid·u·o·sis (de·sid''yoo·o'sis) *n.* A condition in which the decidual tissue develops in an ectopic site, such as the vagina or the cervix of the uterus.

de·cid·u·ous (de·sid'yoo·us) *adj.* Falling off or shed periodically or at a particular stage, as at maturity.

deciduous dentition. PRIMARY DENTITION.

deciduous teeth. The 20 teeth of the primary dentition; those which erupt first and are replaced by succedaneous permanent teeth; there are 8 incisors, 4 canines, and 8 molars. Syn. *primary teeth.*

deci·gram (des'i-gram) n. One-tenth of a gram. Abbreviated, dg.

deci·li·ter (des'i-lee"tur) n. One-tenth of a liter. Abbreviated, dl.

deci·me·ter (des'i-mee"tur) n. One-tenth of a meter. Abbreviated, dm.

deci·nor·mal (des'i-nor"mul) adj. Having one-tenth the strength of the normal.

de·cip·a·ra (de·sip'uh·ruh) n. A woman who has borne 10 children.

de·clive (de·klive') n. A lower or descending part.

Declomycin. Trademark for the antibiotic demeclocycline.

de·coc·tion (de·cock'shun) n. In pharmacy, a liquid dosage form obtained by boiling a medicinal vegetable substance in water.

de·col·la·tion (dee"kol·ay'shun) n. DECAPITATION.

de·col·or·ant (de·kul'ur·ant) adj. & n. 1. Employed or having the capacity to alter or remove color. 2. Any of a variety of decolorant chemical agents.

de·com·pen·sa·tion (dee·kom"pun·say'shun) n. Failure of compensation, as of the circulation or heart, or of the ego to stress. —**decompensate**, v., **decompensational**, adj.

de·com·po·si·tion (dee"kom·po·zi'shun, dee·kom") n. 1. The separation of the component principles of a body. 2. PUTREFACTION. —**decompose** (dee"kum·poze') v.

de·com·pres·sion (dee"kum·presh'un) n. The removal of compression or pressure; particularly, various techniques for reducing intracranial pressure, or for preventing decompression sickness in divers and caisson workers.

decompression chamber. 1. In aerospace medicine, an apparatus for the reduction of barometric pressure, used to study the biologic effects of high-altitude flying and to evaluate the endurance of flight personnel. 2. A compressed-air chamber for the gradual reduction of barometric pressure for deep-sea divers or caisson workers, designed to prevent or treat decompression sickness.

decompression sickness. A condition caused by the formation of nitrogen bubbles in the blood or body tissues due to an abrupt reduction in atmospheric pressure; occurring with rapid return from compressed-air chambers to normal atmospheric pressure or with rapid ascent either from depths in diving apparatus or to high altitudes in open airplanes; symptoms include severe pain in the joints and chest, itching of the skin, pulmonary edema, urticaria, paralysis, convulsions, and sometimes coma.

de·con·di·tion·ing (dee"kun·dish'un·ing) n. The breaking-up or extinction of a conditioned response. —**decondition**, v.

de·con·ges·tant (dee"kun·jes'tunt) n. & adj. 1. Any decongestive agent. 2. Any agent that reduces hyperemia. 3. DECONGESTIVE.

de·con·ges·tive (dee"kun·jes'tiv) adj. Relieving or reducing congestion.

de·con·tam·i·nate (dee"kun·tam'i·nate) v. To make an object or area safe for unprotected personnel by rendering chemical or biological agents harmless, or by removing or blanketing radiological agents. —**decon·tam·i·na·tion** (·tam"i·nay'shun) n.

de·cor·ti·cate (dee·kor'ti·kate) v. 1. To strip off the bark or husk of a plant. 2. To remove the cortex or external covering from any organ or structure; decapsulation. 3. Specifically, to remove part or all of the cerebral cortex. —**corti·cate** (·kate, ·kut) adj. **de·cor·ti·ca·tion** (dee·kor"ti·kay'shun) n.

decorticate posture or position. The posture assumed by a patient with a lesion at the level of the upper brainstem or above, i.e., whose cerebral cortex is essentially nonfunctioning, in which he lies rigidly motionless unless noxious stimuli are applied, with the arms tightly flexed and the fists clenched, and the legs and feet stiffly extended; the trunk may be opisthotonic.

dec·re·ment (deck're·munt) n. 1. Lessening or subtraction. 2. The amount of loss. 3. The stage in which the effects of a disease are decreasing. —**dec·re·men·tal** (deck"re·men'tul) adj.

de·cre·scen·do (dee"kre·shen'do) n. A gradual decrease in intensity or loudness; applied to cardiac murmurs.

de·cres·cent (de·kres'unt) adj. 1. Gradually becoming less; decreasing; waning. 2. INVOLUTIONAL; SENILE.

dec·ta·flur (deck'tuh·floor) n. 9-Octadecenylamine hydrofluoride, $C_{18}H_{37}N·HF$, a dental caries prophylactic.

de·cu·ba·tion (dee"kew·bay'shun) n. The period in the course of an infectious disease beginning with the disappearance of the symptoms and lasting until recovery and the absence of infectious organisms.

de·cu·bi·tus (de·kew'bi·tus) n., pl. **decubi·ti** (·tye) 1. The recumbent or horizontal posture. 2. DECUBITUS ULCER. —**decubi·tal** (·tul) adj.

decubitus ulcer. Ulceration of the skin and subcutaneous tissues, due to protein deficiency and prolonged unrelieved pressure on bony prominences; seen commonly in aged, cachectic, or paralytic bedridden persons. Syn. bedsore, pressure sore, pressure ulcer.

de·cus·sate (de·kus'ate) v. To intersect; to cross.

de·cus·sa·tion (dee"kuh·say'shun, deck"uh·) n. A chiasma or X-shaped crossing, especially of symmetrical parts, as of nerve fibers uniting unlike structures in the two sides of the brain or spinal cord.

de·dif·fer·en·ti·a·tion (dee"dif·ur·en"shee·ay'shun) n. The process of giving up or losing specific characters and reverting to a more generalized or primitive morphologic state. —**dediffer·en·ti·ate** (·en'shee·ate) v.

deep fascia. The fibrous tissue between muscles and forming the sheaths of muscles, or investing other deep, definitive structures, as nerves and blood vessels.

deep inguinal ring. The abdominal opening of the inguinal canal.

deep reflex. Any stretch or myotatic reflex of the phasic or jerk type.

deep sensation. Perception of pressure, tension,

and pain in the muscles, joints, tendons, and deep layers of the skin, as contrasted with sensations derived from the superficial layers of the skin.

deep tendon reflex. TENDON REFLEX.

deer fly. *Chrysops discalis*, a vector of tularemia; most common in western United States.

de·fat·ting (dee·fat'ing) *n.* 1. The removal of lipids from tissue by extraction with fat solvents. 2. The removal of adipose tissue by surgical means, especially from grafts of skin.

def·e·cate, def·ae·cate (def'e·kate) *v.* 1. To evacuate the bowels. 2. To purify or refine. —**def·e·ca·tion, def·ae·ca·tion** (def'e·kay'shun), *n.*

de·fect, *n.* 1. A lack, failure, or deficiency, as of a normal function. 2. Absence of a part or organ.

de·fec·tive, *adj. & n.* 1. Falling below an established standard of quality, composition, structure, or behavior. 2. A person lacking a physical or mental quality, especially the latter.

de·fem·i·ni·za·tion (de·fem''i·ni·zay'shun) *n.* 1. *In medicine,* the loss or diminution of female sex characteristics, usually as a result of ovarian dysfunction or removal. 2. *In psychiatry,* in cases of antipathic sexual instinct the psychic process in which there is a deep and permanent change of character in a woman, resulting in a giving up of feminine feelings, and the assumption of masculine qualities. —**de·fem·i·nize** (dee·fem'i·nize) *v.*

defense mechanism or reaction. Any psychic device for guarding oneself against blame, guilt, anxiety, and unpleasant or disagreeable memories or experiences, or for concealing unacceptable desires, feelings, and beliefs; an unconscious attempt at self-justification and the maintenance of self-esteem. Specific defense mechanisms are conversion, denial, dissociation, rationalization, repression, and sublimation.

def·er·ent (def'ur·unt) *adj.* 1. Carrying away or down; EFFERENT. 2. Pertaining to the ductus deferens.

def·er·en·tial (def''ur·en'shul) *adj.* Pertaining to the ductus deferens.

deferential artery. A small branch of the internal iliac artery, supplying the seminal vesicle, ductus deferens, and epididymis; the homologue in the male of the uterine artery.

def·er·en·tio·ves·i·cal (def''ur·en''shee·o·ves'i·kul) *adj.* Pertaining to both the ductus deferens and the urinary bladder.

def·er·en·ti·tis (def''ur·en·tye'tis) *n.* Inflammation of the ductus deferens.

de·fer·ves·cence (dee''fur·ves'unce, ·def'ur·) *n.* Disappearance of fever.

de·fer·ves·cent (dee''fur·ves'unt, def'ur·) *adj. & n.* 1. Of a fever; diminishing or disappearing. 2. Having the effect of allaying or reducing a fever. 3. A fever-reducing agent.

de·fi·bril·la·tion (dee·fib''ri·lay'shun, ·figh''bri·) *n.* 1. The arrest of fibrillation of the cardiac atria or ventricles. 2. Blunt dissection of tissue fibers along planes of cleavage. —**de·fi·bril·late** (dee·fib'ri·late, ·figh'bri·) *v.*

de·fi·bril·la·tor (dee·fib'ri·lay''tur, ·figh'bri·) *n.*

An apparatus for defibrillating the heart, by the application of electric current.

de·fi·bri·nate (dee·figh'bri·nate) *v.* To remove fibrin from blood or lymph. —**de·fi·bri·na·tion** (dee·figh''bri·nay'shun) *n.*

defibrination syndrome. DISSEMINATED INTRAVASCULAR COAGULATION.

de·fi·cien·cy, *n.* 1. The state or condition of lacking a substance, quality, or characteristic essential for completeness. 2. The amount or extent of lack of an essential substance, quality, or characteristic. 3. *In genetics,* the abnormal lack of a segment of a chromosome; DELETION.

de·fi·cient (de·fish'unt) *adj.* Lacking a substance, quality, or characteristic essential for completeness; below standard.

def·i·cit (def'i·sit) *n.* 1. A deficiency or lack. 2. An impairment in a particular function. 3. The amount by which something is short of a specified standard. Syn. *debt.*

def·i·ni·tion, *n.* 1. The quality of an image with respect to sharpness or clarity of outlines. 2. The quality of a lens with respect to sharpness or clarity of outlines in the images it forms.

de·fin·i·tive, *adj.* 1. Complete; fully developed. 2. Pertaining to the mature or fully developed stage of something. 3. Serving to define.

definitive host. A host in which the sexual stages of the parasite develop.

definitive treatment. Any treatment, including surgical and other generally accepted procedures, necessary to produce ultimate recovery of the patient.

de·fla·tion receptors. Vagal nerve fibers that are stimulated by deflation of the lung and reflexly induce inspiration.

de·flec·tion, *n.* A turning, or state of being turned, aside.

def·lo·ra·tion (def''lo·ray'shun) *n.* Natural loss of the external sexual characteristics which in women indicate virginity, usually typified by rupture of the hymen at the first sexual intercourse.

de·flo·res·cence (dee''flo·res'unce) *n.* Disappearance of the eruption of an exanthematous disease.

de·flu·vi·um (dee·floo'vee·um) *n.* DEFLUXIO.

de·flux·io (dee·fluck'see·o) *n.* 1. Loss, disappearance. 2. A flowing down.

de·for·mi·ty, *n.* 1. The state of being misshapen. 2. Marked deviation from the normal in size or shape of the body or of a part. —**deform,** *v.*

de·froth·i·cant (de·froth'ick·unt, ·froth') *n.* A chemical agent that reduces frothing.

de·fu·sion (dee·few'zhun) *n. In psychoanalysis,* the separation of the two primal, or life and death, instincts.

de·gan·gli·on·ate (dee·gang'glee·un·ate) *v.* To remove a ganglion or ganglia.

de·gen·er·a·cy (de·jen'ur·uh·see) *n.* 1. A state marked by the deterioration of the mind and body. 2. Sexual perversion as defined by existing social and legal codes; specifically, the committing of or the attempt to commit a sexual offense, such as rape, pederasty, or exhibitionism. 3. The existence in the genetic code of more than one codon for each amino acid.

de·gen·er·ate (de·jen'ur·ate) v. 1. To undergo the retrogressive changes of degeneration. 2. To deteriorate in physical, mental, or psychic characters.

de·gen·er·ate (de·jen'ur·ut) adj. & n. 1. Having undergone degeneration. 2. A person who has changed markedly for the worse in his moral, social, or biological, usually sexual, conduct, or who falls far short of the behavior expected of him in a particular society at a particular time; usually, an individual with markedly deviant sexual behavior.

de·gen·er·a·tion (de·jen'ur·ay'shun) n. 1. A retrogressive change in cells characterized by initial cytoplasmic deterioration, then nuclear death in some instances, all with little or no signs of a response to injury. 2. A retrogressive process including even the death of nerves, axons, or tracts of the central nervous system. 3. A sinking to a lower state; progressive deterioration of a physical, mental, or moral state. —**de·gen·er·a·tive** (de·jen'ur·uh·tiv) adj.

degenerative disease. Disease characterized by the progressive impairment of the function of an organ or organs and not attributable to some cause such as infection or a metabolic defect; for example, Alzheimer's disease or Parkinson's disease.

degenerative joint disease. A chronic joint disease characterized pathologically by degeneration of articular cartilage and hypertrophy of bone, clinically by pain on activity which subsides with rest; it occurs more commonly in older people, affecting the weight-bearing joints and the distal interphalangeal joints of the fingers; there are no systemic symptoms. Syn. degenerative arthritis, hypertrophic arthritis, osteoarthritis, senescent arthritis.

de·gen·i·tal·i·ty (dee·jen'i·tal'i·tee) n. In psychoanalysis, a condition wherein genital instincts are expressed through activities of a nongenital character. —**de·gen·i·tal·ize** (dee·jen'i·tul·ize) v.

de·germ (dee·jurm') v. To reduce the normal or abnormal bacterial flora of skin, mucosal surfaces, or open wounds by mechanical cleansing or antiseptic action. —**de·germ·a·tion** (dee''jur·may'shun) n.

de·glu·ti·tion (dee''gloo·tish'un, deg''loo·) n. The act of swallowing. —**de·glu·ti·tive** (de·gloo'ti·tiv), **deglu·ti·to·ry** (·to'ree) adj.

Degos' disease A combination of slowly evolving painless skin papules, that eventually develop an atrophic center, and multiple infarcts of the viscera, with angiitis common to both. Syn. malignant papulosis, papulosis atrophicans maligna.

deg·ra·da·tion (deg''ruh·day'shun) n. The conversion of one organic compound to another containing a smaller number of carbon atoms. —**de·grade** (de·grade') v.

de·gree, n. 1. A position in a graded series. 2. One of the units or intervals of a thermometric or other scale. 3. The unit for measuring arcs or angles. One degree is 1/360 of a circle. A right angle is 90° or one-quarter of a circle. 4. A rank or title conferred by a college or university in recognition of attainment. 5. In law, the relative amount of guilt. 6. One remove in the direct line of descent; one remove in the chain of relationship, as a cousin of fourth degree.

de·gus·ta·tion (dee''gus·tay'shun) n. The act of tasting.

de·his·cence (dee·his'unce) n. 1. The act of splitting open. 2. A defect in the boundary of a bony canal or cavity.

dehydr-, dehydro-. A combining form meaning (a) dehydrated; (b) dehydrogenated.

de·hy·drate (dee·high'drate) v. To remove water from (any source, including the body and its tissues). —**dehydrat·ed**, adj. **de·hy·dra·tion** (dee''high·dray'shun) n.

dehydrated alcohol. Ethyl alcohol containing not less than 99.5% by volume of C_2H_5OH. Syn. absolute alcohol.

de·hy·dro·ascor·bic acid (dee·high''dro·uh·skor'bick). The relatively inactive acid resulting from elimination of two hydrogen atoms from ascorbic acid when the latter is oxidized by air or other agents.

de·hy·dro·cho·late (dee·high''dro·ko'late) n. A salt of dehydrocholic acid.

7-de·hy·dro·cho·les·ter·ol (dee·high''dro·ko·les'tur·ole, ·ol) n. A provitamin of animal origin in the skin of man, in milk, and elsewhere, which upon irradiation with ultraviolet rays becomes vitamin D_3.

de·hy·dro·cho·lic acid (dee·high''dro·ko'lick, ·kol'ick). 3,7,12 -Triketocholanic acid, $C_{24}H_{34}O_5$, resulting when the three hydroxyl groups of cholic acid are oxidized to keto groups. Both the acid and its sodium salt are used for their hydrocholeretic and choleretic effects.

de·hy·dro·cor·ti·cos·ter·one (dee·high''dro·kor''ti·kos'tur·ohn) n. 11-Dehydrocorticosterone or 21-hydroxypregn-4-ene-3,11,20-trione, $C_{21}H_{28}O_4$, a steroid occurring in the adrenal cortex and possessing biologic activity similar to that of corticosterone.

de·hy·dro·gen·ase (dee·high''druh·je·nace, ·naze, dee''high·droj'e·) n. An enzyme that catalyzes the oxidation of a specific substrate by removal of hydrogen; a hydrogen acceptor may or may not be required.

de·hy·dro·gen·ate (dee·high''druh·je·nate, dee''high·droj'e·) v. To remove hydrogen from. —**de·hy·dro·gen·a·tion** (dee·high''druh·je·nay'shun) n.

de·hy·dro·iso·an·dros·ter·one (dee·high''dro·eye''so·an·dros'tur·ohn) n. Androst-5(6)-en-3-ol-17-one, $C_{19}H_{28}O_2$, an androgenic steroid found in the urine of men and women. Syn. dehydroepiandrosterone.

de·ion·ize (dee·eye'un·ize) v. To remove ionic constituents from (a liquid, especially water).

de·ion·iz·er (dee·eye'un·eye·zur) n. An apparatus, charged with suitable ion-exchanging and ion-removing substances, which effects removal of ionic constituents from liquids, notably from water.

dé·jà vu (deʸ·zhah vuᵉ') A feeling of familiarity; an illusionary or dream state in which experiences seem to have occurred before, as of a new scene or face that looks familiar; a symptom found in tumors or other lesions of the temporal lobe of the brain.

de·jec·ta (de·jeck'tuh) *n. pl.* EXCREMENT.

de·jec·tion (de·jeck'shun) *n.* 1. Depression, lowness of spirits. 2. The discharge of fecal matter; defecation. 3. Feces; excrement.

Dé·je·rine–Klump·ke's syndrome or **paralysis** (de"zh·reen' klump'keh) LOWER BRACHIAL PLEXUS PARALYSIS.

Déjerine–Rous·sy syndrome (roo·see') THALAMIC SYNDROME.

Déjerine's anterior bulbar syndrome Ipsilateral paralysis of the tongue, contralateral hemiplegia and occasionally contralateral loss of proprioceptive and tactile senses, due to occlusion of the anterior spinal artery.

Déjerine's cortical sensory syndrome Loss of proprioception, stereognosis, and other highly integrated sensory functions, but essentially normal appreciation of touch, pain, temperature, and vibration; seen in parietal lobe lesions.

Déjerine–Sot·tas disease or **neuropathy** HYPERTROPHIC INTERSTITIAL NEUROPATHY (1).

de·lac·ta·tion (dee"lack·tay'shun) *n.* 1. WEANING. 2. Cessation of lactation.

de·lam·i·na·tion (dee·lam"i·nay'shun) *n.* Separation or splitting into layers, as in the dividing of cells to form new layers.

delayed hypersensitivity. A specific state of sensitivity induced by infectious agents, chemicals, or foreign animal cells in which the onset of the reaction to the inducer is delayed, and which can be transferred passively by cells but not the serum of sensitive animals.

del·e·te·ri·ous (del"e·teer'ee·us) *adj.* Harmful, injurious.

de·le·tion (de·lee'shun) *n. In genetics,* the abnormal lack of a segment of a chromosome; DEFICIENCY (3).

de·lim·it, *v.* To fix limits or boundaries. **—de·lim·i·ta·tion,** *n.*

de·lin·quen·cy, *n.* 1. An offense or violation, especially when committed by a minor, as truancy, vandalism, stealing, or overt sex practices. The term implies a psychologic and therapeutic rather than a punitive attitude toward the offender. 2. The tendency to commit delinquencies; the committing of such offenses.

de·lin·quent, *adj. & n.* 1. Committing or constituting a delinquency. 2. A person who commits a delinquency.

de·lip·i·da·tion (dee·lip"i·day'shun) *n.* Removal of lipids by fat solvents from a tissue or microscopic sections.

del·i·quesce (del"i·kwes') *v.* To become liquid by absorption of water from the atmosphere. **—del·i·ques·cence** (·kwes'unce) *n.;* **deliques·cent** (·unt) *adj.*

de·lir·i·fa·cient (de·lirr"i·fay'shunt, ·shee·unt) *adj.* Producing or capable of producing delirium.

de·lir·i·um (de·lirr'ee·um) *n.,* pl. **delir·ia** (·ee·uh) A disordered mental state of acute onset and transient nature, characterized by confusion,

disorientation, disorders of perception (hallucinations and illusions), delusions, vigilance, and overactivity of psychomotor autonomic nervous system functions. Associated with febrile states, exogenous intoxications, withdrawal states, occasionally with trauma and other encephalopathies. **—deliri·ous** (·us) *adj.*

delirium tre·mens (tree'munz) A special and sometimes lethal form of delirium induced by the withdrawal of alcohol, following a prolonged period of alcoholic intoxication. Wakefulness, tremor, hallucinations, delusions, and signs of autonomic overactivity (fever, dilated pupils, sweating, tachycardia) are particularly prominent. An identical clinical state may follow withdrawal of barbiturates and other sedative-hypnotic drugs, and rarely may be associated with cerebral trauma and infections.

de·liv·ery, *n. In obstetrics,* the expulsion or extraction of a fetus and its membranes; parturition. **—deliver,** *v.*

del·le (del'eh) *n.,* pl. **del·len** (·un) 1. *In ophthalmology,* a small, saucerlike excavation at the margin of the cornea, occurring most often in processes that produce a localized break in the precorneal oily film layer of tears, which in turn causes the corneal dehydration and thinning. 2. *In hematology,* the central, discoid, usually more lightly colored portion of erythrocytes, as seen in a stained peripheral blood smear.

de·louse (dee·lowce', ·lowze') *v.* To free from lice; to destroy lice. **—delous·ing** (·ing) *n.*

del·ta (del'tuh) *n.* 1. The fourth of a series, or any particular member or subset of an arbitrarily ordered set; as in chemistry, the fourth carbon atom starting with the one adjacent to the characteristic functional group. Symbol, δ. 2. *In chemistry,* double bond. Symbol, Δ. 3. *In chemistry,* coefficient of diffusion. Symbol, Δ. 4. *In mathematics,* INCREMENT. Symbol, Δ.

delta cell. 1. A possible third type of cell in the islets of the pancreas. 2. A second type of beta cell of the adenohypophysis.

delta chain, δ chain. The heavy chain of the IgD immunoglobulin molecule.

delta rhythm. *In electroencephalography,* a succession of slow waves with a frequency of 4 or less per second. Predominate during deep sleep, but also seen in brain damage, especially that involving midline structures.

Deltasone. A trademark for prednisone, an anti-inflammatory adrenocortical steroid.

delta wave. See *delta rhythm.*

del·toid (del'toid) *adj. & n.* 1. Shaped like a Δ (capital delta). 2. DELTOID MUSCLE. 3. Pertaining to the deltoid muscle.

deltoid ligament. MEDIAL LIGAMENT.

deltoid muscle. The large, thick, delta-shaped muscle covering the shoulder joint.

del·to·pec·to·ral (del"to·peck'tuh·rul) *adj.* Pertaining to the deltoid and pectoral muscles.

Deltra. A trademark for prednisone, an anti-inflammatory adrenocortical steroid.

de·lu·sion (de·lew'zhun) *n.* A belief maintained in the face of incontrovertible evidence to the contrary, and not in line with the individual's level of knowledge and his cultural group. It results from unconscious needs and may therefore take on various forms.

dem-, demo- A combining form meaning *people, population.*

de·mar·ca·tion (dee″mahr·kay′shun) n. Separation; establishing of limits. —**de·mar·cate** (de·mahr′kate) v.

dem·e·clo·cy·cline (dem″e·klo·sigh′kleen) n. 7-Chloro-6-demethyltetracycline, $C_{21}H_{21}ClN_2O_8$, an antibiotic produced by a mutant strain of *Streptomyces aureofaciens;* used, as the hydrochloride salt, for the same purposes as other tetracycline antibiotics. Syn. *demethylchlortetracycline.*

de·ment·ed (de·men′tid) adj. Deprived of reason. —**dement,** n. & v.

de·men·tia (de·men′shuh) n., pl. **dementias, de·men·ti·ae** (·shee·ee) 1. Deterioration or loss of intellectual faculties, reasoning power, memory, and will due to organic brain disease; characterized by confusion, disorientation, apathy, and stupor of varying degrees. 2. Formerly, madness or insanity.

dementia par·a·lyt·i·ca (păr″uh·lit′i·kuh). GENERAL PARALYSIS.

dementia prae·cox or **pre·cox** (pree′kocks), pl. **dementiae prae·co·ces** (pree·ko′seez). Any of a group of psychotic disorders, beginning in adolescence or early adulthood, formerly thought to be a single entity, then categorized by Kraepelin as four, and now classified as simple, hebephrenic, paranoid, and catatonic types of schizophrenia.

Demerol. Trademark for meperidine, a narcotic analgesic used as the hydrochloride salt.

demi- A prefix signifying *half.*

demi·lune (dem′i·lewn) n. A crescent-shaped aggregation of serous cells capping mucous acini in mixed glands. Syn. *serous crescent.*

de·min·er·al·iza·tion (dee·min″ur·ul·i·zay′shun) n. Loss of mineral salts from the body, as from the bones. —**de·min·er·al·ize** (dee·min′ur·ul·ize) v.

demo-. See **dem-.**

dem·o·dec·tic (dem″o·deck′tick) adj. Of, pertaining to, or caused by mites of the genus *Demodex.*

Dem·o·dex (dem′o·decks, dee′mo·) n. A genus of parasitic mites.

de·mog·ra·phy (de·mog′ruh·fee) n. The science of populations; specifically, the statistical description of populations according to such characteristics of their members as age, sex, marital status, family structure, geographical distribution, and various other cultural, political, and socioeconomic factors, and of the determinants and consequences of population change. —**de·mo·graph·ic** (dem″uh·graf′ick, dee″muh·) adj.

de·mon·o·ma·nia (dee″mun·o·may′nee·uh) n. 1. A state in which one is oppressed by morbid dreams of demons. 2. The delusion of being possessed by evil spirits or a demon. —**demon·oma·niac** (·nee·ack) n.

de·mon·o·pho·bia (dee″mun·o·fo′bee·uh) n. Abnormal fear of devils and demons.

de·mul·cent (de·mul′sunt) adj. & n. 1. Soothing; allaying irritation of surfaces, especially mucous membranes. 2. A soothing substance, particularly a slippery, mucilaginous liquid.

de·my·e·lin·at·ed (dee·migh′uh·li·nay·tid) adj. Of a nerve or nerve tract: having had its myelin sheath removed or destroyed. —**demyelin·ate** (·nate) v., **demyelin·at·ing** (·nay·ting), **demyelin·at·ive** (·nay·tiv) adj.

de·my·e·lin·a·tion (dee·migh′e·li·nay′shun) n. Destruction of myelin; loss of myelin from nerve sheaths or nerve tracts.

de·my·e·lin·iza·tion (dee·migh″e·lin·i·zay′shun) n. DEMYELINATION.

de·na·tur·ant (dee·nay′chur·unt) n. 1. A substance added to another to make the latter unfit for certain uses, as when methyl alcohol is added to ethyl alcohol for the purpose of preventing beverage use of the ethyl alcohol. 2. *In nuclear science,* a nonfissionable isotope, which, when added to fissionable material, makes the latter unsuited for use in atomic weapons without considerable processing.

de·na·ture (dee·nay′chur) v. To modify, by physical or chemical action, the biological (secondary and tertiary) structure of an organic substance, especially a protein, in order to alter some properties of the substance, such as solubility. —**de·na·tur·a·tion** (de·nay″chur·ay′shun) n.

den·drite (den′drite) n. The process of a neuron which carries the nerve impulse to the cell body. It is usually branched, like a tree. Syn. *dendron.*

den·drit·ic (den·drit′ick) adj. 1. Branching in treelike or rootlike fashion; arborescent. 2. Pertaining to a dendrite.

dendritic keratitis. A superficial form of keratitis attributed to the virus of herpes simplex, also rarely seen with herpes zoster; characterized by a line of infiltration of the corneal tissue near the surface, developing later into an arborescent ulcer. Syn. *furrow keratitis, herpetic keratitis, keratitis arborescens.*

den·dro·phil·ia (den″dro·fil′ee·uh) n. *In psychiatry,* love of trees; a sexual attraction to trees which are symbolic for the phallus.

de·ner·vate (dee·nur′vate) v. To interfere with or cut off the nerve supply to a body part, or to remove a nerve; may occur by excision, drugs, or a disease process.

de·ner·va·tion (dee″nur·vay′shun) n. 1. The interruption of the nerve supply to a part by excision, drugs, or disease. 2. The cutting off of the nerve supply to the lower leg and foot to relieve certain types of lameness in a horse.

den·gue (deng′gay, ·ghee) n. An acute febrile, usually epidemic infectious disease caused by a group B togavirus and borne by the *Aëdes* mosquito; characterized by abrupt onset, diphasic course, prostration, muscle and joint pain, exanthems, lymphadenopathy, and leukopenia, with severe residual debility and weakness lasting for about a week.

de·ni·al, n. *In psychiatry,* the unconscious psychic mechanism or process whereby an observation is denied or refused recognition in order to avoid anxiety or pain; the simplest and commonest form of the ego defense mechanisms, and a part of many normal phenomena, as in the fantasies of children who deny the realities of their own lives to enjoy play.

den·i·da·tion (den"i·day'shun, dee"nigh·) n. Disintegration and ejection of the superficial part of the uterine mucosa.

den·i·grate (den'i·grate) v. 1. To render or become black. 2. To defame. —**den·i·gra·tion** (den"i·gray'shun, dee"nigh·) n.

de·ni·tri·fy (dee·nigh'tri·figh) v. To remove nitrogen.

de·ni·tro·gen·ate (dee·nigh'tro·je·nate, dee"nigh·troj'e·) v. To remove dissolved nitrogen from one's body by breathing nitrogen-free gas. —**de·ni·tro·gen·a·tion** (dee·nigh"tro·je·nay'shun, dee"nigh·troj'e·) n.

dens (denz) n., genit. **den·tis** (den'tis), pl. **den·tes** (·teez), genit. pl. **den·ti·um** (den'tee·um, ·shee·um) 1. TOOTH. 2. A toothlike process; specifically, the dens of the axis.

den·sim·e·ter (den·sim'e·tur) n. An instrument for determining density or specific gravity. —**den·si·met·ric** (den"si·met'rick) adj.

den·si·tom·e·ter (den"si·tom'e·tur) n. 1. An instrument utilizing the photoelectric principle for measuring the opacity of exposed and processed photographic film. 2. DENSIMETER.

den·si·ty n. 1. Closeness of any space distribution, as for example electron density, the number of electrons per unit volume, or population density, the number of inhabitants per unit area. 2. Any measure of the compactness of substances based on the ratio of weight or mass to volume. Abbreviated, d. 3. *In radiography and photography,* degree of opacity.

dens of the axis. The toothlike process on the body of the axis, going through the front part of the ring of the atlas. Syn. *odontoid process.*

dent-, denti-, dento- A combining form meaning *tooth, dental.*

den·tal (den'tul) adj. Pertaining to the teeth.

dental amalgam. An alloy of silver, tin, zinc, and copper with mercury, used as a tooth-filling material and in the making of dies.

dental calculus. A calcareous deposit on the teeth, consisting of organic and mineral matter; formerly divided into salivary calculus and serumal or sanguinary calculus. Syn. *tartar.*

dental caries. A localized, progressive, and molecular disintegration of the teeth believed to begin with the solution of tooth structure by lactic and pyruvic acids, which are the product of enzymic action of oral bacteria upon carbohydrates, followed by bacterial invasion of the dentinal tubules.

dental deposit. Mineralized or nonmineralized material adherent to the surface of a tooth.

dental floss. A string or thread used to clean interdental spaces and tooth surfaces, in the placement of rubber dam, and in the examination of proximal tooth surfaces.

dental hygienist. A person trained and licensed in the technique of removing calcareous deposits and stains from the teeth.

dental plaque. A thin, transparent film on the surfaces of a tooth made up of mucin and colloidal material secreted by the salivary glands. Depending on the predominant component, mucinous and bacterial plaques are recognized.

dental prophylaxis. The prevention of dental and oral diseases by preventive measures, such as fluoridation of water and, especially, the mechanical cleansing of the teeth.

dental prosthesis. An appliance to replace missing teeth, as a denture, crown, or bridgework.

dental pulp. The soft vascular tissue which fills the pulp chamber and the root canals of a tooth and is responsible for its vitality, consisting of connective tissue, blood vessels, and nerves with a superficial layer of cells, the odontoblasts, producing and maintaining dentin and supplying branching processes which occupy tubules in the dentin.

dental surgeon. DENTIST.

den·tate (den'tate) adj. 1. SERRATED; jagged. 2. Having a concavely scalloped edge or surface. 3. Pertaining to the dentate nucleus.

den·tat·ec·to·my (den"tait·eck'tuh·mee) n. The ablation of the dentate nucleus in the treatment of a movement disorder, particularly when due to erythroblastosis fetalis.

dentate gyrus. A narrow band of gray matter extending downward and forward above the gyrus parahippocampalis but separated from it by the hippocampal sulcus; anteriorly it is continued into the uncus.

dentate nucleus. An ovoid mass of nerve cells located in the center of each cerebellar hemisphere; the cells give rise to fibers which are found in the superior cerebellar peduncle.

den·ta·tion (den·tay'shun) n. 1. The quality or condition of being dentate. 2. A toothlike projection.

den·te·la·tion (den"te·lay'shun) n. The state of having tooth-like processes.

denti-. See *denti-.*

den·tia pre·cox (den'shuh pree'kocks) The presence of erupted teeth at birth, or shortly thereafter.

den·ti·cle (den'ti·kul) n. 1. A small tooth or projecting point. 2. A deposit of dentin-like or calcareous material within the pulp of the tooth, associated with degenerative or retrogressive changes of the pulp.

den·tic·u·late (den·tick'yoo·late) adj. Having minute dentations; furnished with small teeth or notches.

den·ti·fi·ca·tion (den"ti·fi·kay'shun) n. Formation of teeth.

den·ti·form (den'ti·form) adj. Tooth-shaped; ODONTOID (1).

den·ti·frice (den'ti·fris) n. A substance or preparation used to aid the mechanical cleaning of the teeth.

den·tig·er·ous (den·tij'ur·us) adj. Bearing, arising from, or containing teeth.

dentigerous cyst. A cyst originating in the enamel organ of a developing tooth.

den·tin (den'tin) n. The calcified tissue which forms the major part of a tooth. Dentin is related to bone but differs from it in the absence of included cells. It is covered by the enamel over the crown of the tooth, by the cementum over the roots, and itself surrounds the pulp chamber and root canals which contain the dental pulp. **—den·tin·al** (·ti·nul) *adj.*

dentinal tubules. Canals in the matrix of dentin occupied by odontoblastic processes.

den·ti·no·blas·to·ma (den"ti·no·blas·to'muh) *n.* A benign odontogenic tumor made up of poorly developed dentin.

den·ti·no·ce·men·tal (den"ti·no·se·men'tul) *adj.* Pertaining to the dentin and cementum of a tooth.

den·ti·no·enam·el (den"ti·no·e·nam'ul) *adj.* Pertaining to the dentin and the enamel of a tooth.

dentinogenesis im·per·fec·ta (im·pur·feck'tuh). A hereditary condition of the teeth characterized by a marked reduction in size or obliteration of the pulpal space and a rapid wearing away of the crowns; normal enamel which is weakly attached to the dentin and lost early; and ranging in color from opalescent to bluish to brown. Syn. *hereditary opalescent dentin, odontogenesis imperfecta.*

den·ti·noid (den'ti·noid) *n.* A calcified structure having some but not all of the characteristics of dentin.

den·ti·no·ma (den"ti·no'muh) *n.*, pl. **dentinomas, dentinoma·ta** (·tuh) A benign odontogenic tumor made up of dentin.

den·ti·nos·te·oid (den"ti·nos'tee·oid) *n.* A hard, calcified structure having some of the histologic appearance of both dentin and bone.

den·tip·a·rous (den·tip'uh·rus) *adj.* Producing or bearing teeth.

den·ti·phone (den'ti·fone) *n.* A device in which a vibrating disk is attached to or held in contact with the teeth, thus carrying vibration through the bony structures to the vestibulocochlear nerves; used in certain types of deafness.

den·tist (den'tist) *n.* One who practices dentistry.

den·tis·try (den'tis·tree) *n.* 1. The art and science of the prevention, diagnosis, and treatment of diseases of the teeth and adjacent tissues, and the restoration of missing dental and oral structures. 2. The practice of such art and science. 3. The dental profession collectively. 4. RESTORATION (3).

den·ti·tion (den·tish'un) *n.* 1. The teeth considered collectively and in place in the dental arch. 2. The character and arrangement of the teeth of an individual or species. 3. The eruption of the teeth.

dento-. See *dent-.*

den·to·al·ve·o·lar (den"to·al·vee'o·lur) *adj.* Pertaining to the alveolus of a tooth.

den·to·fa·cial (den"to·fay'shul) *adj.* Pertaining to the teeth and the face.

den·toid (den'toid) *adj.* Toothlike.

den·tu·lous (den'chuh·lus) *adj.* Having natural teeth.

den·ture (den'chur) *n.* The natural or artificial teeth of an individual, considered as a unit.

denture flange. The part of an artificial denture that extends from the cervical margins of the teeth to its border; the facial extension of an upper or lower denture and the lingual extension of a lower denture.

de·nu·cle·at·ed (dee·new'klee·ay"tid) *adj.* Deprived of a nucleus.

de·nude (de·newd') *v.* To deprive of covering; to strip, lay bare, as the root of a tooth. **—de·nu·da·tion** (dee"new·day'shun, den"yoo·) *n.*

de·ob·stru·ent (dee·ob'stroo·unt) *n.* Any agent or drug which removes an obstruction or obstructive material, as in the alimentary canal.

de·odor·ant (de·o'dur·unt) *n. & adj.* 1. A substance that removes or conceals offensive odors. 2. Having the action of a deodorant. **—deodor·ize** (·ize) *v.*

de·oral·i·ty (dee"o·ral'i·tee) *n. In psychoanalysis,* the shifting of instinctual activity away from gratification through oral expression.

de·os·si·fi·ca·tion (de·os"i·fi·kay'shun) *n.* 1. The absorption of bony material. 2. The deprivation of the bony character of any part.

deoxy-, desoxy-. A combining form designating (a) *loss of oxygen from a compound;* or specifically (b) *replacement of a hydroxyl group by a hydrogen atom.*

de·oxy·cho·lic acid (dee·ock"see·ko'lick, ·kol'ick). $3\alpha,12\alpha$-Dihydroxycholanic acid, $C_{24}H_{40}O_4$, one of the unconjugated bile acids; in bile it is largely conjugated with glycine or taurine. Used as a choleretic.

de·oxy·cor·ti·cos·ter·one (dee·ock"see·kor"ti·kos'tur·ohn) *n.* 4-Pregnene-3,20-dione-21-ol, $C_{21}H_{30}O_3$, an adrenocortical hormone. In man it causes an increase in retention of sodium ion and water, and an increase in excretion of potassium ion; it has no demonstrable effect on protein or carbohydrate metabolism. It is used, commonly as the acetate ester, in the management of adrenal insufficiency. Syn. *compound Q (Reichstein's), deoxycortone, deoxycostone.*

de·ox·y·gen·a·tion (dee·ock"si·je·nay'shun) *n.* The process of removing oxygen from a compound.

de·oxy·ri·bo·nu·cle·ase (dee·ock"see·rye"bo·new'klee·ace, ·aze) *n.* An enzyme, acting in the presence of magnesium ions, that causes depolymerization of deoxyribonucleic acids.

de·oxy·ri·bo·nu·cle·ic acid (dee·ock"see·rye"bo·new·klee'ick). Any of the high molecular weight polymers of deoxyribonucleotides, found principally in the chromosomes of the nucleus and varying in composition with the source, able to reproduce in the presence of the appropriate enzyme and substrates, and bearing coded genetic information. Abbreviated, DNA.

de·oxy·ri·bo·nu·cleo·pro·tein (dee·ock"see·rye"bo·new"klee·o·pro'tee·in, ·teen) *n.* Any nucleoprotein that yields a deoxyribonucleic acid as a hydrolysis product.

de·oxy·ri·bo·nu·cleo·tide (dee·ock"see·rye"bo·new"klee·o·tide) *n.* A nucleotide in which the sugar component is deoxyribose (2).

de·oxy·ri·bose (dee·ock"see·rye'bose, ·boze) *n.* 1. Any derivative of ribose in which an alcoholic hydroxyl group is replaced by hydrogen. 2. D-2-Deoxyribose, $CHOCH_2HCOH$-$HCOHCH_2OH$, the sugar component of deoxyribonucleic acid and deoxyribonucleo-tides.

de·par·af·fin·ize (dee-păr'uh·fin·ize) v. To remove the paraffin from something, as a tissue section.

de·pend, v. 1. To be contingent. 2. To rely, as for support or maintenance. 3. To hang, hang down.

de·pen·dence, n. 1. The quality or condition of being contingent upon, requiring the assistance of, being influenced by, or being subject or subservient to someone or something. 2. The causal relationship between two phenomena, as the degree to which one influences the other.

de·pen·den·cy, n. 1. DEPENDENCE (1). 2. The quality or condition of lacking independence, and particularly self-reliance, characterized by the need for mothering and the tendency to seek help in making decisions or in carrying out complex and demanding tasks. 3. The state of being dependent (3).

de·pen·dent, adj. 1. Determined or controlled by another factor. 2. Relying for support on another person. 3. Hanging down.

de·per·son·al·i·za·tion (dee-pur''sun·ul·i·zay' shun, -eye·zay'shun) n. 1. Loss of the sense of one's own reality or identity. 2. In psychopathology, a subjective feeling of estrangement or unreality within the personality, often manifested by symptoms of derealization and déjà vu. In mild form, the condition is common; in severe forms, it is a finding in various neuroses, depressive states, and beginning schizophrenias. It is considered to be a pathological defense mechanism.

de·pig·men·ta·tion (dee-pig''men·tay'shun) n. Loss of pigment, as from the skin.

dep·i·late (dep'i·late) v. To remove hair. —**de·pil·a·to·ry** (de·pil'uh·to·ree) adj. & n.

de·ple·tion (de·plee'shun) n. 1. The act of diminishing the quantity of fluid or stored materials in the body or in a part, especially by bleeding. 2. The condition of the system produced by the excessive loss of blood or other body constituents; reduction of strength; exhaustion. —**de·plete** (de·pleet') v.

de·po·lar·i·za·tion (dee·po''lur·i·zay'shun) n. The neutralization of polarity; the reduction of differentials of ion distributions across polarized semipermeable membranes, as in nerve or muscle cells in the conduction of impulses. —**de·po·lar·ize** (dee·po'lur·ize) v.

de·po·lym·er·ase (dee''po·lim'ur·ace, dee·pol'i·mur·ace) n. One of a group of enzymes which depolymerize high molecular weight plant and animal substances, as nucleic acids.

de·po·lym·er·i·za·tion (dee''po·lim''ur·i·zay'shun, dee·pol'i·mur·) n. The cleavage, by various means, of a polymer of high molecular weight into simpler units of the same composition. —**de·po·lym·er·ize** (dee''po·lim'ur·ize, dee·pol' i·mur·ize) v.

Depo-Medrol. A trademark for methylprednisolone acetate, a glucocorticoid.

Depo-Provera. A trademark for medroxyprogesterone acetate, a progestin.

de·pos·it, n. & v. 1. An accumulation of material that has settled, precipitated, or formed on surfaces or in hollow or permeable spaces. 2. To cause or allow to accumulate in such a way.

de·pot (dep'o, dee'po) n. In physiology, the site of accumulation, deposit, or storage of body products not immediately or actively involved in metabolic processes, such as a fat depot.

depot fat. Fat occurring in certain regions such as the abdominal wall or the buttocks, which are called fat depots.

de·pres·sant (de·pres'unt) n. & adj. 1. Any agent that diminishes functional activity. 2. Having the action of a depressant.

depressed fracture. A fracture of the skull in which the fractured part is depressed below the normal level.

de·pres·sion, n. 1. A hollow or fossa. 2. An inward displacement of a part. 3. A lowering or reduction of function. 4. In psychiatry, extreme sadness, melancholy, or dejection which, unlike grief, is unrealistic and out of proportion to any claimed cause; may be a symptom of any psychiatric disorder or the prime manifestation of a psychotic depressive reaction or of a neurosis. —**de·pressed, de·pres·sive,** adj.

depressive neurosis or **reaction.** A psychoneurotic disorder in which the anxiety due to an internal conflict is partially relieved by depression and self-depreciation, frequently precipitated by an identifiable event, such as the loss of a cherished person or object, and associated with guilt feelings. Syn. reactive depression.

depressive personality. In psychiatry, a type of personality in which there is a pattern of several kinds of character defenses, such as overseriousness, lowered spirits, increased vulnerability to letdown or disappointment, and excessive conscientiousness, dependability, compliance, subservience, and deliberateness; when sufficiently marked to cause interference with normal living or satisfactions, constitutes the depressive neurosis.

de·pres·sor (de·pres'ur) n. 1. A muscle, instrument, or apparatus that depresses or lowers. 2. DEPRESSOR NERVE.

depressor nerve. A nerve which, upon stimulation, lowers the blood pressure either in a local part or throughout the body.

dep·ri·va·tion (dep''ri·vay'shun) n. A condition of being in want of anything considered essential for physical or mental well-being; it may be due to a lack, denial, or loss of certain factors, powers, or stimuli. —**de·prive** (de·prive') v.

depth, n. 1. Distance from top to bottom, from front to back, or inward from a surface. 2. An inner or relatively inaccessible aspect of something.

depth perception. The ability to estimate depth or distance between points in the field of vision.

depth psychology. 1. The psychology of unconscious mental activity. 2. Any system of psychology in which the study of unconscious mental processes plays a major role, as in psychoanalysis.

de·pu·li·za·tion (dee·pew"li·zay'shun) n. The destruction or removal of fleas, as from infested animals or premises.

de Quer·vain's disease (duh·kehr·væn") 1. Subacute or stenosing fibrous tendovaginitis at the styloid process of the radius. 2. Chronic thyroiditis, a granulomatous inflammation of unknown etiology.

der-, dero- A combining form meaning *neck*.

de·range·ment (de·rainj'munt) n. 1. Disturbance of the regular arrangement or function of parts or a system. 2. Disorder of intellect; insanity.

de·re·al·iza·tion (de·ree"ul·i·zay'shun) n. *In psychiatry*, a subjective feeling that other people or objects are unreal, changed or changing, or strange in their particular characteristics and configuration; often accompanies depersonalization.

der·i·va·tion (derr"i·vay'shun) n. 1. The deflection of blood from one part of the body to another, as by counterirritation; formerly thought to relieve inflammatory hyperemia. 2. *In electrocardiography*, LEAD. 3. Synthesis of a chemical compound from another related to it. 4. The relationship of a substance to its source.

de·riv·a·tive (de·riv'uh·tiv) adj. & n. 1. Producing derivation. 2. Derived from another substance. 3. A derivative agent or substance.

derm-, derma-, dermo-. A combining form meaning (a) *dermis, dermal*; (b) *skin, cutaneous*.

der·ma·bra·sion (dur"muh·bray'zhun) n. The removal of skin in variable amounts or to variable depths by such mechanical means as revolving wire brushes or sandpaper, for the purpose of correcting scars.

Der·ma·cen·tor (dur"muh·sen'tur) n. A genus of ticks some species of which are vectors of disease.

Dermacentor an·der·so·ni (an·dur·so'nye). Medically, the most important North American species of tick, transmitting Rocky Mountain spotted fever and tularemia as well as producing tick paralysis. Syn. *wood tick*.

Dermacentor var·i·a·bi·lis (vār·ee·ay'bi·lis). A species of tick widely distributed in North America which has as its principal host the dog and sometimes man and other mammals; transmits Rocky Mountain spotted fever.

der·ma·fat (dur"muh·fat) n. The adipose tissue of the skin.

der·mal (dur'mul) adj. 1. Pertaining to the dermis. 2. CUTANEOUS.

der·ma·my·ia·sis (dur"muh·migh·eye'uh·sis) n., pl. **dermamyia·ses** (·seez) Dermal myiasis; any skin disease caused by fly larvae.

der·man·a·plas·ty (dur·man'a·plas"tee) n. SKIN GRAFTING.

dermat-, dermato- A combining form meaning *skin, cutaneous*.

der·ma·tal·gia (dur"muh·tal'jee·uh) n. Pain, burning, and other sensations of the skin, unaccompanied by any structural change.

der·ma·therm (dur'muh·thurm) n. An instrument made up of differential thermocouples, used to measure skin temperature. The apparatus consists of two sensitive thermopiles in parallel with a millivoltmeter, with one thermopile maintained at a constant known temperature and the other applied to the skin. The reading in degrees on the millivoltmeter added to or subtracted from the constant gives the skin temperature.

der·mat·ic (dur·mat'ick) adj. & n. 1. DERMAL; pertaining to the dermis. 2. CUTANEOUS. 3. A preparation for treating diseases of the skin.

der·ma·ti·tis (dur"muh·tye'tis) n., pl. **derma·tit·i·des** (·tit'i·deez) Inflammation of the skin.

dermatitis ex·fo·li·a·ti·va ne·o·na·to·rum (ecks·fo"lee·uh·tye'vuh nee·o·nay·to'rum). An acute dermatitis in infants, in which the epidermis is shed more or less freely in large or small scales; considered to be a consequence of staphylococcal impetigo. Syn. *Ritter's disease*.

dermatitis fac·ti·tia (fack·tish'ee·uh). An eruption induced by the patient; varies from simple erythema to gangrene. Syn. *dermatitis autofactitia*.

dermatitis her·pet·i·for·mis (hur·pet"i·for'mis, hur"pe·ti·). An inflammatory, recurring skin disease of a herpetic character, the various lesions showing a tendency to group. It is protean, appearing as erythema, vesicles, blebs, and pustules; associated with intense itching and burning. Syn. *Duhring's disease*.

dermatitis med·i·ca·men·to·sa (med"i·kuh·men·to'suh). A skin eruption due to the action of certain drugs.

dermatitis re·pens (ree'penz) A subacute peripherally spreading dermatitis due to *Staphylococcus aureus* (staphyloderma) usually following minor injuries, and commencing almost exclusively on the distal part of the upper extremity, marked by vesicles or pustules which dry and crust.

dermatitis se·bor·rhe·i·ca (seb·o·ree'i·kuh, see·bo·). SEBORRHEIC DERMATITIS.

dermatitis ve·ne·na·ta (ven·e·nay'tuh). CONTACT DERMATITIS.

Der·ma·to·bia (dur"muh·to'bee·uh) n. A genus of botflies whose larvae are obligatory sarcobionts, producing cutaneous myiasis in many animals.

der·ma·to·bi·a·sis (dur"muh·to·bye'uh·sis) n., pl. **dermatobia·ses** (·seez) Infection with *Dermatobia*.

der·ma·to·cha·la·sis (dur"muh·to·kuh·lay'sis) n. Diffuse relaxation and abnormal looseness of the skin. Syn. *cutis laxa*.

der·ma·to·cyst (dur"muh·to·sist") n. Any cyst of the skin.

der·ma·to·fi·bro·ma (dur"muh·to·figh·bro'muh) n. Firm, single, or multiple slowly growing nodules, red, yellow, or bluish-black, found most commonly on the extremities in adults. Histologically, the nodules are composed chiefly of fibroblasts.

der·ma·to·fi·bro·sar·co·ma (dur"muh·to·figh" bro·sahr·ko'muh) n. A fibrosarcoma arising in the skin.

dermatofibrosarcoma pro·tu·ber·ans (pro·tew' bur·anz). A tumor of dermal fibroblasts forming multinodular red protruding masses; it tends to recur but does not usually metastasize.

der·ma·to·glyph·ics (dur''muh·to·glif'icks) *n.* The skin-pattern lines and whorls of the fingertips, palms, and soles, systematically classified for identification purposes and used in medicine as ancillary findings in chromosomal abnormalities and in individuals with intrauterine exposure to viral infections, such as rubella, during the first trimester of pregnancy. These patterns are individually characteristic and never change.

der·ma·to·graph·ia (dur''muh·to·graf'ee·uh) *n.* DERMOGRAPHIA.

der·ma·tog·ra·phism (dur''muh·tog'ruh·fiz·um, ·to·graf'iz·um) *n.* DERMOGRAPHIA.

der·ma·to·het·er·o·plas·ty (dur''muh·to·het'ur·o·plas''tee) *n.* The grafting of heterogenous skin.

der·ma·tol·o·gist (dur''muh·tol'uh·jist) *n.* A skin specialist; a physician who makes a special study of diseases of the skin.

der·ma·tol·o·gy (dur''muh·tol'uh·jee) *n.* The medical specialty dealing with the skin, its structure, functions, diseases, and their treatment. —**derma·to·log·ic** (·to·loj'ick), **dermato·log·i·cal** (·i·kul) *adj.*

der·ma·tol·y·sis (dur''muh·tol'i·sis) *n.* Fibromas of the skin with masses of pendulous skin. Syn. *cutis laxa, cutis pendula.*

der·ma·tome (dur'muh·tome) *n.* 1. The areas of the skin supplied with sensory fibers from a single spinal nerve. 2. An instrument for cutting skin, as in grafting. 3. The lateral part of an embryonic somite; CUTIS PLATE. —**der·ma·tom·ic** (dur''muh·tom'ick) *adj.*

der·ma·to·meg·a·ly (dur''muh·to·meg'uh·lee) *n.* An excessive amount of skin, producing pendulous folds; may be congenital or acquired.

der·ma·to·my·co·sis (dur''muh·to·migh·ko'sis) *n.* Any fungous infection of the skin.

der·ma·to·my·o·ma (dur''muh·to·migh·o'muh) *n.* A leiomyoma located in the skin.

der·ma·to·my·o·si·tis (dur''muh·to·migh''o·sigh'tis) *n.* An inflammatory disorder involving skin and muscles, including the muscles of swallowing, often associated with visceral cancer in persons over 40 years old, or occurring as a manifestation of collagen disease.

dermatopathic lymphadenopathy. LIPOMELANOTIC RETICULOSIS.

der·ma·to·pa·thol·o·gy (dur''muh·to·pa·thol'uh·jee) *n.* A subspecialty of pathology concerning itself with diseases of the skin.

der·ma·to·path·o·pho·bia (dur''muh·to·path''o·fo'bee·uh) *n.* An abnormal fear of having a skin disease.

der·ma·top·a·thy (dur''muh·top'uth·ee) *n.* Any skin disease. —**derma·to·path·ic** (·to·path'ick) *adj.*

der·ma·to·phil·i·a·sis (dur''muh·to·fil·eye'uh·sis) *n.* Infection with the impregnated female flea, *Tunga penetrans*, which bores beneath the skin or nail, becomes distended with eggs, and appears as a pea-sized nodule.

der·ma·to·phyte (dur''muh·to·fite, dur·mat'o·) *n.* One of a group of keratinophilic fungi which invade the superficial keratinated areas of the body of man and animals, such as the skin,

hair, and nails. The dermatophytes include four genera: *Microsporum, Trichophyton, Epidermophyton,* and *Keratomyces.*

der·ma·to·phy·tid (dur''muh·to·figh'tid, ·tof'i·did) *n.* A skin eruption associated with a skin disease caused by a fungus; fungi are not found in the dermatophytids themselves.

der·ma·to·phy·to·sis (dur''muh·to·figh·to'sis) *n.* A skin eruption characterized by the formation of small vesicles on the hands and feet, especially between the toes, with cracking and scaling. There is sometimes secondary infection. The cause may be any one of the dermatophytes.

der·ma·to·plas·ty (dur''muh·to·plas''tee) *n.* A plastic operation on the skin whereby skin losses or defects are replaced by skin flaps or grafts.

der·ma·to·poly·neu·ri·tis (dur''muh·to·pol''ee·new·rye'tis) *n.* ACRODYNIA.

der·ma·tor·rha·gia (dur''muh·to·ray'jee·uh) *n.* Bleeding from the skin.

der·ma·tor·rhex·is (dur''muh·to·reck'sis) *n.* 1. Disruption of skin capillaries. 2. EHLERS-DANLOS SYNDROME.

der·ma·to·sis (dur''muh·to'sis) *n.,* pl. **dermato·ses** (·seez) Any disease of the skin.

der·ma·to·sto·ma·ti·tis (dur''muh·to·sto''muh·tye'tis) *n.* A severe form of erythema multiforme.

der·ma·to·thla·sia (dur''muh·to·thlay'zhuh, ·zee·uh) *n.* An abnormal state marked by an uncontrollable impulse to pinch or rub the skin.

der·ma·tro·phia (dur''muh·tro'fee·uh) *n.* Atrophy of the skin.

-dermia A combining form designating a *condition of the skin.*

der·mis (dur'mis) *n.* The layer of the skin below the epidermis, composed of collagen bundles, elastic fibers, and sparsely arranged fibroblasts, and bearing the appendages (as the hair apparatus, sebaceous glands, and sweat glands), the nerves, and the blood vessels. Syn. *corium [NA], cutis vera, true skin.*

dermo-. See *derm-.*

der·mo·blast (dur'mo·blast) *n.* The part of the mesoderm which develops into the dermis.

der·mo·epi·der·mal (dur''mo·ep''i·dur'mul) *adj.* Pertaining to both the superficial and the deeper layers of the skin; said of skin grafts.

dermoepidermal junction. The area of separation between the basal cell layer of the epidermis and the stratum papillare of the dermis.

der·mo·graph·ia (dur''mo·graf'ee·uh) *n.* A condition in which the skin is peculiarly susceptible to irritation; characterized by elevations or wheals with surrounding erythematous axon reflex flare, caused by tracing the fingernail or a blunt instrument over the skin. May or may not be accompanied by urticaria. Syn. *dermatographia, dermographism, autographism.* —**dermograph·ic** (·ick) *adj.*

der·mog·ra·phism (dur·mog'ruh·fiz·um) *n.* DERMOGRAPHIA.

der·moid (dur'moid) *adj. & n.* 1. Resembling skin. 2. DERMOID CYST.

dermoid cyst. A benign cystic teratoma with skin, skin appendages, and their products as the most prominent components, usually involving the ovary or the skin.

der·moid·ec·to·my (dur''moy·deck'tuh·mee) n. Excision of a dermoid cyst.

der·mo·la·bi·al (dur''mo·lay'bee·ul) adj. Having relation or pertaining to both the skin and the lips.

der·mo·li·po·ma (dur''mo·li·po'muh) n. A congenital increase in adipose tissue beneath the bulbar conjunctiva between the superior and external rectus muscles, appearing as a yellow mass.

der·mom·e·try (dur·mom'e·tree) n. The measurement of the resistance of the skin to the passage of an electric current; skin areas deprived of their autonomic innervation, where sweat glands are inactive, show increased resistance, and where sweat glands are active, resistance is low.

der·mo·ne·crot·ic (dur''mo·ne·krot'ick) adj. Causing necrosis of the skin.

der·mo·phle·bi·tis (dur''mo·fle·bye'tis) n. Inflammation of the cutaneous veins.

der·mo·ste·no·sis (dur''mo·ste·no'sis) n. A tightening of the skin, due to swelling or to disease.

der·mo·syn·o·vi·tis (dur''mo·sin''o·vye'tis) n. Inflammation of a subcutaneous bursa or tendon sheath and the adjacent skin.

des- A prefix designating (a) *reversing or undoing* (of an action); (b) *depriving, ridding of, or freeing from.*

Desacetyl-Lanatoside C. Trademark for deslanoside, a cardiotonic.

des·an·i·ma·nia (des·an''i·may'nee·uh) n. Any psychotic disorder with mental deficiency.

des·ce·me·ti·tis (des''e·me·tye'tis) n. KERATITIS PUNCTATA.

des·ce·met·o·cele (des''e·met'o·seel) n. A forward bulging of Descemet's membrane when the overlying cornea is destroyed.

Des·ce·met's membrane (des·meh', deh·se·meh') The posterior elastic lamina of the cornea which covers the posterior surface of the substantia propria; the thickened basement membrane of the corneal epithelium.

de·scen·dens (de·sen'denz) L. adj. DESCENDING.

descending aorta. That portion of the aorta between the distal end of the arch, in the thorax, and the bifurcation of the vessel into the iliac arteries in the abdomen.

descending colon. The portion of the colon that extends from the splenic flexure to the sigmoid colon.

descending tract. A collection of nerve fibers conducting impulses down the spinal cord. Syn. *efferent tract.*

de·scen·sus (de·sen'sus) n., pl. **descensus** Descent; fall, prolapse.

descensus ute·ri (yoo'tur·eye). PROLAPSE OF THE UTERUS.

de·scent (de·sent') n. 1. Movement or migration downward. 2. Derivation from an ancestor, especially in regard to evolutionary origin.

Descotone. A trademark for deoxycorticosterone acetate, an adrenocortical steroid.

Desenex. Trademark for a fungicidal ointment or powder that contains undecylenic acid and zinc undecylenate.

de·sen·si·tize (dee·sen'si·tize) v. 1. To render a person or experimental animal insensitive to an antigen or hapten by the appropriate administration of these agents. 2. *In psychiatry,* to alleviate or remove a mental complex, especially a phobia or an obsessive-compulsive neurosis, by repeated discussion of the stressful experience. —**de·sen·si·ti·za·tion** (dee·sen''si·ti·zay'shun) n.

de·ser·pi·dine (dee·sur'pi·deen) n. 11-Desmethoxyreserpine, $C_{32}H_{38}N_2O_8$, an alkaloid from *Rauwolfia canescens;* the pharmacologic actions are essentially the same as those of other active *Rauwolfia* alkaloids, including reserpine. Syn. *canescine.*

de·sex·u·al·iza·tion (dee·seck''shoo·ul·i·zay' shun, ·eye·zay'shun) n. 1. Depriving an individual of sexual powers; castration. 2. *In psychiatry,* the act of detaching or neutralizing sexual energy from an object or activity, or removing from an activity any apparent connection with the sexual drive, so that the energy released becomes available to the ego for its wishes and tasks.

des·ic·cant (des'ick·unt) adj. & n. 1. Drying; rendering dry. 2. A drying medicine or application.

des·ic·cate (des'i·kate) v. To deprive a substance of moisture. —**desic·cat·ed** (·kay'tid) adj., **des·ic·ca·tion** (des''i·kay'shun) n.

des·ic·ca·tor (des'i·kay'tur) n. A vessel containing some strongly hygroscopic substance, such as calcium chloride or sulfuric acid, used to absorb the moisture from any substance placed therein or to maintain it in a moisture-free state.

des·ic·cyte (des'ick·site) n. An erythrocyte with decreased water content, resulting from excessive membrane permeability to potassium as compared with sodium.

de·sid·er·ize (dee·sid'ur·ize) v. To deprive a pigment of its iron.

desm-, desmo- A combining form meaning (a) *bond, bound;* (b) *connective tissue;* (c) *ligament.*

des·mi·tis (dez·migh'tis, des·) n. Inflammation of a ligament.

des·mo·cyte (dez'mo·site, des') n. Any kind of supporting-tissue cell.

des·moid (dez'moid) adj. Like a ligament; fibrous.

desmoid tumor. A benign tumorlike lesion of subcutaneous tissues or of muscle, as of the rectus abdominis, probably a form of fibroma.

des·mo·lase (dez'mo·lace, ·laze) n. Any of a group of enzymes which catalyze rupture of atomic linkages that are not cleaved through hydrolysis, such as the bonds in the carbon chain of D-glucose.

des·mo·pla·sia (dez''mo·play'zhuh, ·zee·uh) n. 1. The formation and proliferation of connective tissue, especially fibrous connective tissue; frequently, prominent proliferation of connective tissue in the growth of tumors. 2. The formation of adhesions. —**desmo·plas·tic** (·plas'tick) adj.

des·mo·some (dez'mo·sohm, des') n. A very strong type of intercellular junction seen on intercellular bridges between epidermal and other epithelial cells and consisting of apposed dense plates (attachment plaques) separated by a narrow space filled with an extracellular substance which is presumed to act as a glue; in each half of the desmosome, delicate fibrils (tonofibrils) extend back from the plaque to the cytoplasm, perhaps to transmit mechanical tension away from the apposing cell membranes.

des·mot·o·my (dez·mot'uh·mee) *n.* Incision of a ligament.

desoxy-. See *deoxy-.*

des·oxy·cho·lic acid (des·ock"si·ko'lick, ·kol'ick). DEOXYCHOLIC ACID.

des·oxy·cor·ti·cos·ter·one (des·ock"see·kor"ti·kos'tur·ohn) *n.* DEOXYCORTICOSTERONE.

des·oxy·ri·bo·nu·cle·ic acid (des·ock"see·rye"bo·new·klee'ick). DEOXYRIBONUCLEIC ACID.

de·spe·ci·a·tion (dee·spee"shee·ay'shun) *n.* Change in properties characteristic of the species, as alteration of antigenic properties by digestion with taka-diastase. —**de·spe·ci·at·ed** (dee·spee'shee·ay·tid) *adj.*

des·qua·ma·tion (des"kwuh·may'shun) *n.* Shedding; a peeling and casting off of superficial epithelium, such as that of mucous membranes, renal tubules, or skin. —**des·qua·ma·tive** (de·skwam'uh·tiv, des"kwuh·may'tiv) *adj.;* **des·qua·mate** (des"kwuh·mate) *v.*

des·sert·spoon (de·zurt'spoon) *n.* A spoon of medium size, equal to approximately 2 fluidrachms or 8 ml.

destructive distillation. Decomposition of complex organic substances by heat and distillation of the products.

de·stru·do (de·stroo'do) *n. In psychiatry,* the basic energy associated with the death instinct; the counterpart of libido.

de·tach·ment of the retina. Separation of the neural portion of the retina from its pigment layer.

de·ter·gent (de·tur'junt) *adj. & n.* 1. Cleansing. 2. A cleansing agent or a preparation containing a cleansing agent, which may be useful for medical purposes and may also possess antibacterial activity. 3. A substance that enhances the cleansing action of water or other solvents.

de·te·ri·o·rate (de·teer'ee·uh·rate) *v.* To become impaired in functioning, quality, or condition from a previously better state; to grow worse; to degenerate. —**de·te·ri·o·ra·tion** (de·teer"ee·uh·ray'shun) *n.*

de·ter·mi·nant (de·tur'mi·nunt) *n.* 1. A fact, circumstance, influence, or factor that determines the nature of an entity or an event. 2. *In biology,* a hypothetical unit of the germ plasm which, according to Weismann's theory of heredity, determines the final fate of the cell or the part which receives it during development.

de·ter·mi·na·tion (de·tur"mi·nay'shun) *n.* 1. Tendency of the blood to collect in a part. 2. Fixation of the embryologic fate of a tissue or a part of an embryo by an evocator or other agent. 3. The performance of any measure-

ment, as of length, mass, or the quantitative composition of a substance.

de·ter·mi·nism (de·tur'mi·niz·um) *n.* The doctrine that no event, whether in the outer world or within a person, results from chance, but that each is the fixed result of antecedent conditions or forces, known or unknown, physical or emotional.

de To·ni-Fan·co·ni-Debré syndrome (de^y·toh"nee) FANCONI SYNDROME.

de·tor·sion (dee·tor'shun) *n.* The correction of a torsion, as the twisting of a spermatic cord or ureter.

de·tox·i·ca·tion (dee·tock"si·kay'shun) *n.* The process, usually consisting of a series of reactions, by which a toxic substance in the body is changed to a compound or compounds more easily excretable; the latter are not necessarily nontoxic. Syn. *detoxification.* —**de·tox·i·cant** (dee·tock'si·kunt) *n. & adj.;* **detoxi·cate** (·kate) *v.*

de·tox·i·fy (dee·tock'si·figh) *v.* To subject to detoxication. —**de·tox·i·fi·ca·tion** (dee·tock"si·fi·kay'shun) *n.*

de·tri·tion (de·trish'un) *n.* Wearing away by abrasion.

de·tri·tus (de·trye'tus) *n.,* pl. **detritus.** 1. Waste matter from disintegration. 2. Waste material adherent to a tooth, or disintegrated tooth substance.

de·trun·cate (dee·trung'kate) *v.* To decapitate, especially a fetus. —**de·trun·ca·tion** (dee"trung·kay'shun) *n.*

de·tru·sion (de·troo'zhun) *n.* An ejection or expulsion; thrusting down or out. —**de·trude** (de·trood') *v.*

de·tru·sor (de·troo'zur) *n.* Any muscle that detrudes or thrusts down or out.

de·tu·mes·cence (dee"tew·mes'unce) *n.* 1. Subsidence of any swelling. 2. Subsidence of the erectile sexual organs following orgasm.

deuter-, deutero- A combining form meaning (a) *second;* (b) *secondary.*

deu·ter·an·o·pia (dew"tur·uh·no'pee·uh) *n.* A form of color blindness in which only two of the three basic colors, blue and red, are perceived; green is seen inadequately and shades of red, green, and yellow are confused. Syn. *green blindness.* —**deuteran·op·ic** (·nop'ick, ·no'pick) *adj.*

deu·te·ri·um (dew·teer'ee·um) *n.* The isotope of hydrogen of atomic weight approximately 2.0. It constitutes approximately 1 part in 6000 of ordinary hydrogen. Symbol, ^2H, D. Syn. *heavy hydrogen.*

deu·ter·on (dew'tur·on) *n.* The nucleus of a deuterium atom.

deu·ter·op·a·thy (dew"tur·op'uth·ee) *n.* A disease occurring secondary to another disease. —**deu·tero·path·ic** (dew"tur·o·path'ick) *adj.*

de·vas·cu·lar·i·za·tion (de·vas"kew·lār·i·zay'shun) *n.* Removal of the blood supply to a given area by vascular destruction or obstruction.

de·vel·op·ment, *n.* 1. Change or growth with increase in complexity. 2. *In biology,* the series of events occurring in an organism during the change from the fertilized egg to the adult stage. —**de·vel·op·men·tal**, *adj.*

developmental age. Any index of development stated in age equivalent as determined by specified standardized measurements and observations; especially motor and mental tests, but also body measurements (height, weight), bone age (as measured by serial roentgenograms of the knee or wrist), or social or emotional development. Abbreviated, DA.

developmental alexia. Marked deficiency in learning to read, not based on obvious visual disturbance and out of line with the individual's mental age and accomplishment quotients in other subjects; may be familial and is seen more frequently in males.

developmental aphasia. A deficiency in learning to speak which is not commensurate with the individual's (child's) mental age or development and accomplishment quotients along other lines.

developmental crisis. *In psychiatry*, any brief, presumably transient period of stress in a child's life related to his attempts to complete successfully such psychosocial tasks as the establishment of trust, autonomy, initiative, and identity; internal forces predominate, as compared to a situational crisis.

developmental dyslexia. Greater than normal difficulties on the part of a school-age child in learning to read, or in reading ability and comprehension; may be hereditary or congenital.

developmental milestone. The achievement by an infant or young child of one of a series of sequentially acquired skills in the areas of motor and manipulative ability, general understanding and social behavior, language, and self-feeding, dressing, and toilet training, normally within a given time period.

developmental quotient. The score, obtained on the Gesell Developmental Schedules, derived by dividing the child's mental age (measured by the test) by his chronological age and multiplying by 100. Abbreviated DQ, D.Q.

de·vi·a·tion (dee"vee·ay'shun) *n.* 1. Variation from a given or accepted norm or standard. 2. Turning from a regular course, standard, or position; deflection. 3. *In ophthalmology*, the inability of the two eyes to focus upon an object at the same time; squint; strabismus. When the unaffected eye is fixed upon the object, the squinting eye is unable to fix and consequently deviates; this is known as primary deviation. When the squinting eye is the one fixed, there is a corresponding deviation of the unaffected eye, known as secondary deviation. The score, obtained on. —**de·vi·ate** (dee'vee·ate) *v.;* **de·vi·ate** (dee'vee·ut) *adj. & n.*

de·vi·tal·ize (dee·vye'tul·ize) *v.* To destroy vitality. —**de·vi·tal·i·za·tion** (dee·vye"tul·i·zay'shun) *n.*

dev·o·lu·tion (dev"o·lew'shun) *n.* The reverse of evolution; INVOLUTION. 2. CATABOLISM. 3. DEGENERATION.

dew·claw (dew'klaw) *n.* The vestigial first digit located on the medial surface of the feet of some animals, especially dogs and cattle.

dew·lap (dew'lap) *n.* A pendulous fold of skin extending downward from the neck of some animals.

dex·a·meth·a·sone (deck"suh·meth'uh·sone) *n.* 9α - Fluoro - 16α - methylprednisolone, $C_{22}H_{29}FO_5$, a potent anti-inflammatory adrenocortical steroid.

dex·am·phet·a·mine (decks"am·fet'uh·min, meen) *n.* DEXTROAMPHETAMINE.

dex·ter (decks'tur) *n.* Right; upon the right side. Abbreviated, d.

dextr-, dextro- A combining form meaning (a) *toward, of, or pertaining to the right;* (b) *dextrorotatory.*

dex·tral (decks'trul) *adj.* Pertaining to the right side; right-handed.

dex·tral·i·ty (decks·tral'i·tee) *n.* 1. The condition, common to most persons, in which, when there is a choice, the right side of the body is more efficient and hence used more than the left. 2. Specifically, RIGHT-HANDEDNESS.

dex·tral·i·za·tion (decks"trul·i·zay'shun) *n.* Development of the control of sensorimotor skill from a dominant area on the left side of the cerebral cortex in right-handed individuals.

dex·tran (decks'tran) *n.* A water-soluble, high molecular weight polymer of glucose produced by the action of *Leuconostoc mesenteroides* on sucrose. Purified forms are usually used to expand plasma volume and maintain blood pressure in emergency treatment of shock. Polymers of lower molecular weight may be useful in preventing intravascular thrombosis and in improving blood circulation in certain conditions. Often written with a number indicating average molecular weight in thousands, as dextran 40, dextran 70, dextran 75.

dex·trau·ral (decks·traw'rul) *adj.* 1. Right-eared; characterizing an individual who prefers to listen with the right ear, as with a telephone receiver, or who depends more on the right ear in binaural hearing. 2. Pertaining to the right ear.

dex·trin (decks'trin) *n.* A white or yellow amorphous powder, $(C_6H_{10}O_5)_n \cdot xH_2O$, produced by incomplete hydrolysis of starch; used as an emulsifying, protective, and thickening agent.

dex·tri·no·sis (deck"stri·no'sis) *n.* Accumulation within the body of abnormal polysaccharides.

dex·trin·u·ria (decks"tri·new'ree·uh) *n.* The presence of dextrin in the urine.

dextro-. See *dextr-.*

dex·tro·car·dia (decks"tro·kahr'dee·uh) *n.* The presence of the heart in the right hemithorax, with the cardiac apex directed to the right. —**dextrocar·di·al** (·dee·ul) *adj.*

dex·tro·car·dio·gram (decks"tro·kahr'dee·o·gram") *n.* 1. The component of the normal electrocardiogram or bicardiogram contributed by right ventricular forces. 2. The electrocardiographic complex derived from a unipolar lead facing the right ventricle.

dex·tro·con·dyl·ism (decks"tro·kon'dil·iz·um) *n.* Deviation of the mandibular condyles toward the right.

dex·troc·u·lar (deck·strock'yoo·lur) *adj.* RIGHT-

EYED. **—dex·troc·u·lar·i·ty** (deck·strock"yoo·lăr'i·tee) *n.*

dex·tro·duc·tion (deck"stro·duck'shun) *n.* Movement of the visual axis toward the right.

dex·tro·man·u·al (decks"tro·man'yoo·ul) *adj.* RIGHT-HANDED. **—dextro·man·u·al·i·ty** (·man"yoo·al'i·tee) *n.*

dex·tro·pe·dal (decks"tro·pee'dul, ·trop'e·dul) *adj.* RIGHT-FOOTED.

dex·tro·pho·bia (decks"tro·fo'bee·uh) *n.* Morbid fear of objects on the right side of the body.

dex·tro·po·si·tion (decks"tro·puh·zish'un) *n.* Displacement to the right.

dextroposition of the heart. Displacement of the heart toward the right or into the right half of the thorax.

dex·tro·ro·ta·to·ry (decks"tro·ro'tuh·tor"ee) *adj.* Rotating the rays of plane polarized light to the right.

dex·trose (decks'troce, ·troze) *n.* A dextrorotatory monosaccharide, $C_6H_{12}O_6 \cdot H_2O$, occurring as a white, crystalline powder; odorless and sweet, soluble in about one part of water, it is often prepared by the hydrolysis of starch. An important intermediate in carbohydrate metabolism. Used for nutritional purposes, for temporary increase of blood volume, as a diuretic, and for other purposes. Syn. *grape sugar, starch sugar, bread sugar, d-glucose.*

dex·tro·sin·is·tral (decks"tro·sin'is·trul) *adj.* Extending from right to left.

dex·tros·uria (decks"tro·sue'ree·uh) *n.* The presence of dextrose in the urine.

dex·tro·tor·sion (decks"tro·tor'shun) *n.* A twisting to the right.

dex·trous (decks'trus) *adj.* Skilled; expert.

dex·tro·ver·sion (deck"tro·vur'zhun) *n.* The act of turning to, or looking toward, the right.

DFP Abbreviation for *diisopropyl fluorophosphate.*

dg Abbreviation for *decigram.*

di-, dis- A prefix meaning *two, twice, double.*

dia-, di- A prefix meaning (a) *through, by way of, across, between;* (b) *apart, asunder.*

di·a·be·tes (dye"uh·bee'teez, ·bee'tis) *n.* 1. A disease characterized by the habitual discharge of an excessive quantity of urine and by excessive thirst. 2. Specifically, DIABETES MELLITUS.

diabetes in·si·pi·dus (in·sip'i·dus). A disorder resulting from a deficiency of antidiuretic hormone, characterized by the excretion of large volumes of dilute but otherwise normal urine, associated with compensatory polydipsia; relieved by replacement therapy with vasopressin.

diabetes mel·li·tus (mel·eye'tus) A chronic disorder of carbohydrate metabolism due to a disturbance of the normal insulin mechanism, characterized by hyperglycemia, glycosuria, and alterations of protein and fat metabolism, producing polyuria, polydipsia, weight loss, ketosis, acidosis, and coma; a hereditary predisposition is present in most if not all cases.

di·a·bet·ic (dye"uh·bet'ick) *adj. & n.* 1. Pertaining or relating to diabetes. 2. A person suffering from diabetes.

diabetic acidosis. The metabolic acidosis of uncontrolled diabetes mellitus, due to an excess

of ketone bodies; characterized by weakness, headache, thirst, air hunger, and coma.

diabetic diet. A diet used in the treatment of diabetes mellitus, containing calculated amounts of carbohydrate, protein, and fat, with restriction of free sugar.

diabetic gangrene. Moist or dry gangrene occurring in the course of diabetes mellitus, often as a consequence of slight injuries.

diabetic retinopathy. Retinal manifestations of diabetes mellitus characterized by capillary microaneurysms, small punctate hemorrhages, yellowish exudates, and neovascularization; saccular dilatations of the retinal veins may also occur and massive hemorrhages into the vitreous may result in blindness.

di·a·be·to·gen·ic (dye"uh·bee"to·jen'ick, ·bet'o·) *adj.* Causing diabetes.

di·a·be·to·pho·bia (dye"uh·bee"to·fo'bee·uh, ·bet'o·) *n.* Morbid fear of becoming a diabetic.

Diabinese. Trademark for chlorpropamide, an orally effective hypoglycemic agent.

di·a·bo·lep·sy (dye·ab'o·lep"see) *n.* Diabolical seizure or possession; delusion of supernatural possession. **—di·a·bo·lep·tic** (dye"uh·bo·lep'tick) *adj. & n.*

di·ac·e·te·mia, di·ac·e·tae·mia (dye"as"e·tee'mee·uh) *n.* The presence of diacetic acid (acetoacetic acid) in the blood.

di·ace·tic acid (dye"uh·see'tick, ·set'ick). ACETOACETIC ACID.

di·ac·e·tu·ria (dye·as"e·tew'ree·uh) *n.* The presence of diacetic acid (acetoacetic acid) in the urine.

di·a·cla·sis (dye"uh·klay'sis) *n.,* pl. **diacla·ses** (·seez) A fracture produced intentionally. **—di·a·clas·tic** (dye"uh·klas'tick) *adj.*

di·a·clast (dye'uh·klast) *n.* An instrument for breaking the fetal head.

di·a·crit·ic (dye"uh·krit'ick) *adj.* DIAGNOSTIC; distinctive.

dia·derm (dye'uh·durm) *n.* A two-layered blastoderm composed of ectoderm and entoderm.

di·ad·o·cho·ki·ne·sia, di·ad·o·ko·ki·ne·sia (dye·ad"uh·ko·ki·nee'zhuh, ·zee·uh) *n.* The normal power of performing alternating movements in rapid succession, such as flipping a hand back and forth.

di·ag·nos·able (dye"ug·no'zuh·bul, ·no'suh·bul) *adj.* Capable of being diagnosed.

di·ag·no·sis (dye"ug·no'sis) *n.,* pl. **diagno·ses** (·seez) 1. The art or the act of determining the nature of a patient's disease. 2. A conclusion reached in the identification of a patient's disease. **—diag·nose** (noce') *v.*

di·ag·nos·tic (dye"ug·nos'tick) *adj.* Pertaining to or serving as evidence in diagnosis; indicating the nature of a disease.

di·ag·nos·ti·cian (dye"ug·nos·tish'un) *n.* One skilled in making diagnoses.

di·ag·o·nal (dye·ag'uh·nul) *adj.* Pertaining to any plane or straight line that is not vertical, perpendicular, or horizontal.

di·al·y·sance (dye·al'i·sunce) *n.* A measure of the rate of exchange between blood and bath fluid used in connection with peritoneal dialysis or hemodialysis; it is the functional equivalent of physiologic renal clearance measurements, being expressed as the net exchange of a substance between blood and bath fluid, per minute.

di·al·y·sate (dye·al'i·sate) *n.* The portion of the liquid which passes through the membrane in dialysis, and contains the substances of greater diffusibility in solution.

di·al·y·sis (dye·al'i·sis) *n.*, pl. **dialy·ses** (·seez) Separation of substances from one another in solution by taking advantage of their differing diffusibility through porous membranes. —**di·a·lyt·ic** (dye·uh·lit'ick) *adj.*

di·al·y·zate (dye·al'i·zate) *n.* DIALYSATE.

di·a·lyz·er (dye·uh·lye·zur) *n.* 1. An apparatus for effecting dialysis. 2. The porous septum or diaphragm of such an apparatus.

di·am·e·ter (dye·am'e·tur) *n.* A straight line joining opposite points on the periphery of a body or figure and passing through its center. —**di·a·met·ric** (dye''uh·met'rick), **diametric·al** (·ul) *adj.*

diameter obli·qua pel·vis (o·blye'kwuh pel'vis) [NA]. Any oblique diameter of the pelvis, specifically the oblique diameter of the pelvic inlet.

diameter trans·ver·sa pel·vis (trans·vur'suh pel'vis) [NA]. Any transverse diameter of the pelvis, as the transverse diameter of the pelvic inlet or the transverse diameter of the pelvic outlet.

di·am·i·dine (dye·am'i·deen, ·din) *n.* Any compound consisting of two amidine groups, NH=C(NH₂)—, linked together by a hydrocarbon chain. Certain ones, of related chemical structure, have been found to possess, in varying degrees, trypanocidal and antibacterial activity.

di·a·min·uria (dye''uh·mi·new'ree·uh) *n.* The presence of diamine compounds in the urine.

Diamox. Trademark for acetazolamide, a carbonic anhydrase inhibitor used as an oral diuretic, in the treatment of hypercapnia, in chronic lung disease, in epilepsy, and in glaucoma.

di·am·tha·zole (dye·am'thuh·zole) *n.* 6-(β-Diethylaminoethoxy)-2-dimethylaminobenzothiazole, C₁₅H₂₃N₃OS, a topically applied antifungal agent.

Diaparene. A trademark for methylbenzethonium chloride, a quaternary ammonium salt used for bacteriostasis of urea-splitting organisms involved in ammonia dermatitis.

di·a·pe·de·sis (dye''uh·pe·dee'sis) *n.*, pl. **diapede·ses** (·seez) The passage of blood cells through the unruptured vessel walls into the tissues. —**diape·det·ic** (·det'ick) *adj.*

diaper rash. Maculopapular eruptions which tend to become confluent and may go on to excoriation, seen in the diaper area of infants, due to irritation from moisture, feces, the ammonia formed from decomposed urea, and often monilial infection.

di·aph·a·nom·e·ter (dye·af''uh·nom'e·tur) *n.* An instrument for measuring the transparency of gases, liquids, or solids.

di·aph·e·met·ric (dye·af''e·met'rick) *adj.* Pertaining to measurements of tactile sensibility.

di·aph·o·rase (dye·af'o·race) *n.* Mitochondrial flavoprotein enzymes which catalyze the reduction of dyes, such as methylene blue, by reduced pyridine nucleotides such as NADH.

di·a·pho·re·sis (dye''uh·fo·ree'sis) *n.*, pl. **diaphore·ses** (·seez) Perspiration, especially perceptible perspiration that is artificially induced.

di·a·pho·ret·ic (dye''uh·fo·ret'ick) *adj. & n.* 1. Causing an increase of perspiration. 2. A medicinal that induces diaphoresis.

di·a·phragm (dye'uh·fram) *n.* 1. *In anatomy,* a musculotendinous partition, especially that partition muscular at the circumference and tendinous at the center, which separates the thorax and abdomen and is the chief muscle of respiration and expulsion. 2. A thin septum such as is used in dialysis. 3. *In optics,* an aperture so placed as to control the amount of light passing through an optical system. 4. A device worn during copulation over the ostium uteri for preventing conception or infection; it is usually dome-shaped and of thin rubber or plastic material. 5. *In radiography,* a metal barrier plate with a central aperture designed to limit the beam of radiation to its smallest practical diameter.

dia·phrag·ma (dye·uh·frag'muh) *n.*, pl. **dia·phragma·ta** (·tuh) DIAPHRAGM.

diaphragma sel·lae (sel'ee) [NA]. DIAPHRAGM OF THE SELLA.

di·a·phrag·mat·ic (dye''uh·frag·mat'ick) *adj.* Of or pertaining to a diaphragm, especially in the anatomic sense.

diaphragmatic hernia. A hernia that passes through the diaphragm into the thoracic cavity; may be congenital, acquired, or traumatic, and may contain the stomach, small intestine, and colon; usually a false hernia.

diaphragmatic myocardial infarction. A myocardial infarction involving the diaphragmatic or inferior portion of the heart.

diaphragmatic respiration. Respiration effected primarily by movement of the diaphragm, changing the intrathoracic pressure.

diaphragmatic sign. The movement of the diaphragm during respiratory excursions, causing an altered contour of the chest wall. If the patient is observed by means of oblique illumination, a shadow is seen moving up or down the side of the chest. Syn. *Litten's sign.*

di·a·phrag·mato·cele (dye''uh·frag·mat'o·seel) *n.* A hernia through the diaphragm.

di·a·phrag·mi·tis (dye''uh·frag·migh'tis) *n.* Inflammation of the diaphragm.

diaphragm of the sella. The circular layer of dura mater which forms the roof of the hypophyseal fossa; its center is pierced by the stalk of the hypophysis.

di·aph·y·se·al (dye·af''i·see'ul, dye·uh·fiz'ee·ul) *adj.* Pertaining to or involving a diaphysis.

di·aph·y·sec·to·my (dye·af''i·seck'tuh·mee, dye''uh·fi-) *n.* Excision of a portion of the shaft of a long bone.

di·a·phys·i·al (dye''uh·fiz'ee·ul) *adj.* DIAPHYSEAL.

di·aph·y·sis (dye·af'i·sis) *n.*, pl. **diaphy·ses** (·seez) The shaft of a long bone.

di·ap·la·sis (dye·ap'luh·sis) *n.*, pl. **diapla·ses**

(·seez) Reduction of a dislocation or of a fracture.

di·a·poph·y·sis (dye″uh·pof′i·sis) *n.*, pl. **diapophyses** (·seez) The articular facet on the transverse process of a thoracic vertebra for articulation with the tubercle of the corresponding rib. Syn. *tubercular process.* —**di·a·po·phys·i·al** (dye″uh·po·fiz′ee·ul) *adj.*

di·ar·rhea, di·ar·rhoea (dye″uh·ree′uh) *n.* A common symptom of gastrointestinal disease; characterized by increased frequency and water content of the stools. —**diar·rhe·al** (·ree′ul), **diarrhe·al** (·ick) *adj.*

di·ar·rhe·o·gen·ic, di·ar·rhoe·o·gen·ic (dye″uh·ree″o·jen′ick) *adj.* Producing diarrhea.

di·ar·thric (dye·ahr′thrick) *adj.* Pertaining to two joints; DIARTICULAR.

di·ar·thro·di·al (dye″ahr·thro′dee·ul) *adj.* Pertaining to or exhibiting diarthrosis.

diarthrodial joint. SYNOVIAL JOINT.

di·ar·thro·sis (dye″ahr·thro′sis) *n.*, pl. **diarthro·ses** (·seez) 1. Freely movable articulation. 2. A freely movable joint; SYNOVIAL JOINT. Adj. *diarthrodial.*

di·ar·tic·u·lar (dye″ahr·tick′yoo·lur) *adj.* DIARTHRIC; pertaining to two different joints.

di·as·chi·sis (dye·as′ki·sis) *n.*, pl. **diaschi·ses** (·seez) An inhibition or loss of function in a region of the nervous system, due to a localized injury in another region with which it is connected by fiber tracts, such as loss of reflexes following a brain lesion comparable to spinal shock.

di·a·stal·sis (dye″uh·stal′sis, ·stahl′sis) *n.* The downward moving wave of contraction, occurring in the small intestine during digestion, in addition to peristalsis. —**diastal·tic** (·tick) *adj.*

di·a·stase (dye′uh·stace, ·staze) *n.* An enzyme preparation from malt that contains amylases and converts starch to dextrins and maltose by hydrolysis. Syn. *vegetable diastase.*

di·as·ta·sis (dye·as′tuh·sis) *n.*, pl. **diasta·ses** (·seez) 1. Any simple separation of parts normally joined together, as the separation of an epiphysis from the body of a bone without true fracture, or the dislocation of an amphiarthrosis. 2. The final phase of diastole, the phase of slow ventricular filling.

di·a·ste·ma (dye″uh·stee′muh) *n.*, pl. **diastema·ta** (·tuh) 1. A cleft or fissure, especially if congenital. 2. A space between teeth that are normally in approximal contact.

di·a·ste·ma·to·my·e·lia (dye″uh·stee″muh·to·migh·ee′lee·uh) *n.* A congenital, more or less complete doubling of the spinal cord associated with the formation of a bony or cartilaginous septum from the posterior wall of the vertebral canal, usually in spina bifida.

di·as·to·le (dye·as′tuh·lee) *n.* 1. The rhythmic period of relaxation and dilatation of a chamber of the heart during which it fills with blood. 2. Specifically, diastole of a cardiac ventricle. —**di·a·stol·ic** (dye″uh·tol′ick) *adj.*

diastolic blood pressure. Minimum arterial blood pressure during ventricular diastole.

diastolic murmur. A murmur occurring during ventricular diastole.

diastolic thrill. A vibratory sensation felt on precordial palpation during ventricular diastole.

di·a·ther·mic (dye″uh·thur′mick) *adj.* 1. Permitting passage of heat rays. 2. Of or pertaining to diathermy.

di·a·ther·mo·co·ag·u·la·tion (dye″uh·thur″mo·ko·ag″yoo·lay′shun) *n.* Coagulation secured by the use of a high-frequency electrosurgical knife.

dia·ther·mom·e·ter (dye″uh·thur·mom′e·tur) *n. In physics,* an instrument for measuring the heat-conducting capacity of substances.

di·a·ther·my (dye′uh·thur″mee) *n.* 1. The therapeutic use of an oscillating electric current of high frequency to produce local heat in the body tissues below the surface. 2. The electric current so used. 3. The machine producing the electric current. —**di·a·ther·mize** (dye″uh·thur′mize) *v.*

di·ath·e·sis (dye·ath′e·sis) *n.*, pl. **diathe·ses** (·seez) A condition or tendency of the body or a combination of attributes in one individual causing a susceptibility to some abnormality or disease. —**di·a·thet·ic** (dye″uh·thet′ick) *adj.*

di·a·tom (dye′uh·tom, ·tome) *n.* Any of the Diatomaceae, a small family of microscopic, unicellular algae having a cell wall of silica, the skeleton persisting after death of the organism.

di·a·to·ma·ceous (dye″uh·to·may′shus) *adj.* Consisting of diatoms or their siliceous remnants.

diatomaceous earth. A sedimentary rock composed of the empty shells of diatoms and other Protophyta; used as an absorbent, a filtration aid, and an insulating material. Syn. *purified kieselguhr, purified siliceous earth.*

di·atom·ic (dye″uh·tom′ick) *adj.* 1. Consisting of two atoms; commonly referring to a molecule. 2. Containing two replaceable univalent atoms or radicals.

dia·tri·zo·ic acid (dye″uh·tri·zo′ick, ·trye·zo′ick) 3,5-Diacetamido-2,4,6-triiodobenzoic acid, $C_{11}H_9I_3N_2O_4$, a roentgenographic contrast medium; used as the methylglucamine (meglumine) and sodium salts.

diaz-, diazo- A combining form signifying the presence (in an organic compound) *of two nitrogen atoms* as the —N≡N— or (RN≡N)⁺ group, where R is an organic radical.

di·az·e·pam (dye·az′e·pam) *n.* 7-Chloro-1,3-dihydro-1-methyl-5-phenyl-$2H$-1,4-benzodiazepin-2-one, $C_{16}H_{13}ClN_2O$, a tranquilizer.

di·a·zine (dye′uh·zeen) *n.* 1. A heterocyclic compound having the formula $C_4H_4N_2$, containing two nitrogen and four carbon atoms in the ring. Three isomers are possible, distinguished as 1,2-diazine (pyridazine), 1,3-diazine (pyrimidine), and 1,4-diazine (pyrazine). 2. Any derivative of any such compound.

di·a·zo·ni·um (dye″uh·zo′nee·um) *adj.* Pertaining to or characterizing a compound containing two nitrogen atoms in the form of the (RN≡N)⁺ group, where R is an organic radical, the compound being analogous to ammonium compounds in having saltlike properties.

diazo reaction. Any color test using Ehrlich's diazo reagent.

di·az·o·tize (dye·az'o·tize) v. To treat a primary aromatic amine with nitrous acid under conditions that produce a diazonium compound.

di·ba·sic (dye·bay'sick) adj. 1. Of a salt, containing two atoms of a monobasic element or radical. 2. Of an acid, having two replaceable hydrogen atoms.

Dibenamine. Trademark for N-(2-chloroethyl)-dibenzylamine, employed experimentally as a sympatholytic and adrenolytic agent, in the form of the hydrochloride salt.

di·bu·caine (dye·bew'kain) n. 2-n-Butoxy-N-(2-diethylaminoethyl) cinchoninamide, $C_{20}H_{29}N_3O_2$, a local anesthetic; used both as the base and the hydrochloride salt. Syn. cinchocaine.

Dibuline Sulfate. Trademark for dibutoline sulfate, a parasympatholytic drug.

di·bu·to·line sulfate (dye·bew'to·leen). Bis[(dibutylcarbamate) of ethyl (2-hydroxyethyl)dimethylammonium] sulfate, $C_{30}H_{66}N_4O_8S$, a parasympatholytic drug useful in the treatment of peptic ulcer and spastic disorders of the biliary and genitourinary tracts.

di·car·box·yl·ic acid (dye·kahr'bock·sil'ick). An organic compound with two —COOH groups.

di·ceph·a·lism (dye·sef'uh·liz·um) n. The condition of having two heads.

di·ceph·a·lous (dye·sef'uh·lus) adj. Having two heads.

di·chlor·a·mine (dye·klor'uh·meen) n. DICHLORAMINE-T.

di·chlo·ro·ace·tic acid (dye·klor'o·uh·see'tick). $CHCl_2COOH$. A colorless liquid at ordinary temperatures, crystallizing at lower temperatures; soluble in water. Has been used as an escharotic.

di·chlo·ro·phen·ar·sine hydrochloride (dye·klor'o·fen'ahr·seen, ·sin, ·fen·ahr'sin) 3-Amino-4-hydroxyphenyldichloroarsine hydrochloride, $C_6H_6AsCl_2NO.HCl$, formerly used as an antisyphilitic.

di·cho·ri·al (dye·kor'ee·ul) adj. DICHORIONIC.

di·cho·ri·on·ic (dye''ko·ree·on'ick) adj. Having two chorions.

di·chot·o·mize (dye·kot'uh·mize) v. To make a dichotomy; to divide a distribution, variable, or series into two parts according to a specified classification, as persons with or without a known disease or characteristic.

di·chot·o·my (dye·kot'uh·mee) n. 1. Division into two equal branches; BIFURCATION. 2. Division of a group into two classes on the basis of the presence or absence of a certain characteristic or characteristics. 3. The type of branching of plants in which there are repeated equal divisions of the stem.

di·chro·ic (dye·kro'ick) adj. Having or showing two colors; applied to doubly refracting crystals that show different colors when viewed from different directions, or to solutions that show different colors in varying degrees of concentration.

di·chro·mat (dye'kro·mat) n. A person affected with dichromatopsia.

di·chro·mate (dye'kro·mate) n. DICHROMAT.

di·chro·mat·ic (dye''kro·mat'ick) adj. 1. In biology, exhibiting two colors, regardless of sex or age. 2. In psychology, pertaining to that form of color blindness in which only two of the four fundamental colors can be seen, usually yellow and blue. 3. In hematology, pertaining to an immature nonnucleated erythrocyte.

di·chro·ma·top·sia (dye·kro''muh·top'see·uh) n. A condition in which an individual can perceive only two of the three basic hues (red, green, and blue).

di·chro·mic (dye·kro'mick) adj. 1. Marked by two colors. 2. Containing two atoms of chromium.

di·chro·mo·phil (dye·kro'mo·fil) adj. Characterizing a tissue or cell which takes both an acidic and a basic stain.

di·chro·moph·i·lism (dye''kro·mof'i·liz·um) n. The capacity for double staining.

Dick test A test for susceptibility or immunity to scarlet fever in which an intracutaneous inoculation of streptococcal erythrogenic toxin results in a red flush in susceptible individuals lacking the circulating antitoxin, and in no local reaction in individuals immune to scarlet fever.

di·cli·dot·o·my (dye''kli·dot'uh·mee) n. VALVOTOMY.

Dicodid. Trademark for hydrocodone (dihydrocodeinone), an antitussive drug used as the bitartrate salt.

di·co·phane (dye'ko·fane) n. A medicinal grade of DDT.

di·cou·ma·rin (dye·koo'muh·rin) n. DICUMAROL.

di·cou·ma·rol (dye·koo'muh·rol) n. DICUMAROL.

di·crot·ic (dye·krot'ick) adj. Pertaining to a secondary pressure wave on the descending limb of a main wave.

dicrotic notch. A notch on the descending limb of the normal arterial pulse tracing, corresponding to aortic valve closure.

dicrotic pulse. A double-beating arterial pulse, with the second beat occurring during ventricular diastole, due to accentuation of the dicrotic wave; occurs commonly with low diastolic blood pressure.

dicrotic wave. The positive wave following the dicrotic notch of the normal arterial pulse tracing, due to reflected waves from the periphery.

di·cro·tism (dye'kro·tiz·um) n. A condition of having a dicrotic pulse.

di·cu·ma·rol (dye·koo'muh·rol, ·kew') n. 3,3'-Methylene-bis(4-hydroxycoumarin), $C_{19}H_{12}O_6$, originally isolated from spoiled sweet clover, eating of which caused hemorrhagic disease in cattle; occurs as a white crystalline powder, practically insoluble in water; used as an anticoagulant. Syn. bishydroxycoumarin, dicoumarin, dicoumarol, melitoxin.

di·dac·tic (dye·dack'tick, di·dack'tick) adj. In medicine, pertaining to teaching by lectures and textbooks, as opposed to instruction by the clinical method.

di·dac·tyl·ism (dye·dack'til·izm) n. BIDACTYLY.

di·del·phia (dye·del'fee·uh) n. The condition of

having a double uterus. —**did·el·phic** (-fick) adj.

did·y·mi·tis (did''i·migh'tis) n. ORCHITIS.

did·y·mous (did'i·mus) adj. Growing in pairs; arranged in a pair, or in pairs.

¹die, v. To cease to live; to expire.

²die, n. An exact reproduction in metal, or other substance of suitable hardness, of a tooth, part, object, or cast; used in dentistry for forming an individual tooth restoration or dental appliance.

di·em·bry·o·ny (dye·em'bree·o·nee) n. The formation or production of two embryos from a single ovum; TWINNING.

di·en·ce·phal·ic (dye''en·se·fal'ick) adj. Of, pertaining to, or involving the diencephalon.

diencephalic syndrome. 1. A syndrome of early childhood, characterized by progressive emaciation in spite of high caloric intake, a euphoric appearance, and occasionally vertical nystagmus, tremor, and ataxia, due to a tumor in the diencephalon. **2.** CONVULSIVE EQUIVALENT.

di·en·ceph·a·lon (dye''en·sef'uh·lon) n. The part of the brain between the telencephalon and the mesencephalon, including the thalami and most of the third ventricle. Syn. *betweenbrain, interbrain.*

di·en·es·trol, di·en·oes·trol (dye''en·es'trol) n. 4,4'-(Diethylidineethylene)diphenol, $C_{18}H_{18}O_2$, a white, crystalline powder, practically insoluble in water; a nonsteroid estrogen.

Di·ent·amoe·ba (dye·en''tuh·mee'buh) n. A genus of parasitic protozoa having two nuclei.

Dientamoeba frag·i·lis (fraj'i·lis). A minute species of intestinal ameba found in the colon of man, lacking a cystic stage, and rarely associated with mild pathogenicity.

di·es·trum, di·oes·trum (dye·es'trum) n. DIESTRUS.

di·es·trus, di·oes·trus (dye·es'trus) n. The period of quiescence or sexual rest of a polyestrous animal; the longest stage of the estrous cycle in which there is a gradual reconstitution of the uterine mucosa or endometrium in preparation for the reception of a fertilized ovum. —**dies·trous, dioes·trous** (-trus) adj.

di·et, n. & v. **1.** Food and drink regularly consumed. **2.** Food prescribed, regulated, or restricted as to kind and amount, for therapeutic or other purposes. **3.** To take food according to a regimen. **4.** To cause to take food according to a regimen.

di·e·tary (dye'e·terr·ee) adj. & n. **1.** Of or pertaining to diet. **2.** A rule of diet. **3.** A treatise describing such a rule or rules. **4.** A fixed allowance of food.

di·e·tet·ic (dye''e·tet'ick) adj. Pertaining to diet or to dietetics.

di·e·tet·ics (dye''e·tet'icks) n. The science of the systematic regulation of the diet for hygienic or therapeutic purposes.

di·eth·a·zine (dye·eth'uh·zeen) n. 10-(-2-Diethylaminoethyl)phenothiazine, a drug possessing atropine-like actions and used in the treatment of parkinsonism.

di·eth·yl·ene glycol (dye·eth'il·een). β,β'-Dihydroxy-diethyl ether, $HOCH_2CH_2OCH_2$-CH_2OH, used in histology as a solvent for dyes and as a component of storage fixatives to prevent drying of tissues.

di·eth·yl·stil·bes·trol (dye·eth''il·stil·bes'trol) n. (E)α,α'-Diethyl-4,4'-stilbenediol, $C_{18}H_{20}O_2$, a white, crystalline powder, almost insoluble in water. A nonsteroid estrogen used as a substitute for the natural estrogenic hormones, more readily absorbed from the alimentary canal than most of the natural hormones and hence suitable for oral use. It is marketed under various trademarks. Abbreviated, DES. Syn. *stilbestrol.*

dietician. DIETITIAN.

di·e·ti·tian (dye''e·tish'un) n. A person trained in dietetics or the scientific management of the meals of individuals or groups; in institutions, one who arranges diet programs for purposes of adequate nutrition of the well and therapeutic nutrition of the sick.

Dietl's crisis (dee'tul) Recurrent attacks of radiating pain in the costovertebral angle, accompanied by nausea, vomiting, tachycardia, and hypotension, due to kinking or twisting of the ureter or renal vasculature; associated with ptosis of the kidney.

di·e·to·ther·a·py (dye''e·to·therr'uh·pee) n. The branch of dietetics that has to do with the use of food for therapeutic purposes.

dif·fer·en·tial (dif''ur·en'shul) adj. Pertaining to or creating a difference.

differential diagnosis. The distinguishing between diseases of similar character by comparing their signs and symptoms.

differential leukocyte count. The percentage of each variety of leukocyte, usually based on counting 100 leukocytes.

dif·fer·en·ti·ate (dif''ur·en'shee·ate) v. **1.** To distinguish or make different. **2.** To increase in complexity and organization during development; said of cells and tissues. —**differ·en·ti·a·tion** (-en''shee·ay'shun) n.

dif·frac·tion (di·frak'shun) n. The separation of light into component parts by means of prisms, parallel bars in a grating, or layers of atoms in a crystal, thus producing interference phenomena such as lines, bands, or spot patterns.

¹diffuse (di·fewce') adj. Scattered; not limited to one tissue or spot.

²diffuse (di·fewz') v. To spread, disperse.

diffuse goiter. Thyroid gland enlargement produced by the increased size of all the follicles, or by the increased number of follicles, without the nodule formation characteristic of nodular goiter.

diffuse hypergammaglobulinemia. The general increase in serum concentration of all or many different immunoglobulins, characterized electrophoretically by a diffuse broad band and clinically by hyperplasia of plasma cells throughout the reticuloendothelial system. Main causes include infection, hepatic disease, so-called collagen diseases, and advanced sarcoidosis.

diffuse lymphoma. A variety of malignant lymphoma, not seen in Hodgkin's disease, in which cellular proliferation is diffuse and without nodular structure; composed of well-differentiated lymphocytes, poorly differentiated lymphocytes, reticulum cells, or a mixture of the last two; prognosis is generally poorer than that of nodular lymphoma.

diffuse scleroderma. Scleroderma in which the cutaneous changes are accompanied by involvement of skeletal muscle and viscera.

dif·fus·ible (di·few′zi·bul) *adj.* Capable of being diffused. —**diffus·ibil·i·ty** (-few′′zi·bil′i·tee) *n.*

Diffusin. A trademark for lyophilized hyaluronidase.

di·gas·tric (dye·gas′trick) *adj.* 1. Of a muscle, having a fleshy part at each end and a tendinous portion in the middle. 2. Of or pertaining to the digastric muscle.

digastric fossa. 1. A depression on the inside of the mandible for the attachment of the anterior belly of the digastric muscle. 2. MASTOID NOTCH.

digastric muscle. A muscle of the neck having a posterior belly attached to the mastoid process and an anterior belly attached to the mandible with an intermediate tendon attached to the hyoid bone.

Di·ge·nea (dye·jee′nee·uh, dye′′je·nee′uh) *n. pl.* A subclass of the Trematoda, which in their life cycle exhibit alternation of generations and alternation of hosts. It includes all the species of flatworms parasitic in man, such as the liver flukes. —**di·ge·ne·ous** (dye·jee′nee·us) *adj.*

di·gen·e·sis (dye·jen′e·sis) *n.* ALTERNATION OF GENERATIONS.

di·ge·net·ic (dye′′je·net′ick) *adj.* 1. Characterized by or pertaining to alternation of generations. 2. Pertaining to the Digenea.

di·gen·ic (dye·jen′ick) *adj.* 1. Characterizing a genetic constitution of nondiploid organisms containing two different genes for any given locus. 2. Of hereditary characters, determined by two different genes.

Di George's syndrome THYMIC APLASIA.

di·ges·tant (di·jes′tunt, dye·) *adj. & n.* 1. Pertaining to or promoting digestion. 2. An agent that promotes digestion.

di·gest·er (di·jes′tur, dye·) *n.* An apparatus used to subject substances to the action of enzymes or of high temperature and pressure in order to decompose, soften, or cook them.

di·ges·tion (di·jes′chun, dye·jes′chun) *n.* 1. The act or process of converting food into assimilable form, principally through the action of various enzymes in the alimentary canal. 2. The softening of substances by moisture and heat. 3. The disintegration of materials by strong chemical agents. —**di·gest·ible** (di·jest′i·bul) *adj.;* **di·gest·ibil·i·ty** (di·jest′′i·bil′i·tee) *n.;* **di·gest** (dye·jest′, di·jest′) *v.*

di·ges·tive (di·jes′tiv) *adj.* Pertaining to digestion.

Digilanid. Trademark for a mixture of the cardioactive glycosides from the leaves of *Digitalis lanata* in the approximate proportion in which they occur in the crude drug. The respective glycosides are lanatosides A, B, and C.

dig·it (dij′it) *n.* 1. A finger or toe. 2. One of a set of elementary discrete symbols used for counting and calculating, such as the Arabic numerals (0–9).

dig·i·tal (dij′i·tul) *adj.* 1. Of or pertaining to the digits. 2. Executed or performed by a finger, as a maneuver or an examination. 3. Fingerlike. 4. Functioning, or manipulating data, in terms of digits or discrete units or pulses, as: digital clock, digital computer.

dig·i·tal·gia (dij′′i·tal′jee·uh) *n.* Pain in a digit.

digitalis, *n.* The dried leaf of *Digitalis purpurea,* the common foxglove, which is a powerful cardiac stimulant that increases contractility of heart muscle, but is frequently followed by a lengthened refractory period and diminished heart rate, and that also acts indirectly as a diuretic. Employed mainly in diseases of the heart where compensation is lost. A standardized preparation, powdered digitalis, should be employed medicinally.

dig·i·tal·i·za·tion (dij′′i·tal′i·zay′shun, ·dij′′i·tul·eye·zay′shun) *n.* Administration of a variety of digitalis preparations in a dosage schedule producing a therapeutic concentration of digitalis glycosides; maintenance dosage is continued subsequently. —**dig·i·tal·ize** (dij′i·tul·ize, dij′′i·tal′ize) *v.*

dig·i·tal·ose (dij′′i·tal′oce, ·tay′loce) *n.* 3-Methyl-D-fucose, $C_7H_{14}O_5$; one of the sugars obtained in the hydrolysis of certain digitalis glycosides.

digital pelvimetry. Measurement of the pelvis by means of the hand.

digital reflex. 1. Sudden flexion of the terminal phalanx of the thumb and of the second and third phalanges of some other finger, elicited by snapping the terminal phalanx or tapping the nail of the patient's middle or index finger, usually seen when the tendon reflexes are hyperactive, as in spastic hemiparesis. 2. Reflex finger flexion occurring upon tapping the palmar aspect of the terminal phalanges of the slightly flexed fingers.

digital tonometry. The estimation of intraocular pressure by the palpation of the eyeballs through the upper lids; pathologically high or low tension is readily perceived by the skilled examiner.

dig·i·tate (dij′i·tate) *adj.* Having digits or digitlike processes.

dig·i·ta·tion (dij′′i·tay′shun) *n.* A fingerlike process, or a succession of such processes, especially that of a muscle attachment.

dig·i·ti·form (dij′i·ti·form) *adj.* Finger-shaped.

dig·i·to·nin (dij′i·to′nin) *n.* A steroid glycoside, $C_{56}H_{92}O_{29}$, from digitalis, lacking in typical digitalis action and reputedly irritant.

dig·i·to·plan·tar (dij′′i·to·plan′tur, ·tahr) *adj.* Pertaining to the toes and the sole of the foot.

dig·i·tox·i·gen·in (dij′′i·tock′′si·jen′in) *n.* The steroid aglycone, $C_{23}H_{34}O_4$, formed by removal of three molecules of the sugar digitoxose from digitoxin; also obtained as the aglycone on hydrolysis of lanatoside A.

dig·i·tox·in (dij′′i·tock′sin) *n.* The principal active glycoside, $C_{41}H_{64}O_{13}$, of digitalis, introduced as Digitaline Nativelle; it occurs in crystals which are practically insoluble in water. The action is like that of digitalis. Syn. *digitoxoside.*

dig·i·tox·ose (dij′′i·tock′soce) *n.* 2-Deoxy-D-altromethylose, $C_6H_{12}O_4$, the sugar resulting when certain digitalis glycosides, notably digitoxin, gitoxin, and gitalin, are hydrolyzed.

di·gi·tus (dij'i-tus) *n.*, pl. & genit. sing. **digi·ti** (·tye), genit. pl. **digi·to·rum** (to'rum) A finger or toe; DIGIT.

di·glos·sia (dye-glos'ee-uh) *n.* A form of schistoglossia in which the lateral lingual swellings fail to fuse, producing a bifid tongue.

dig·ox·i·gen·in (dij·ock''si·jen'in) *n.* The steroid aglycone, $C_{23}H_{34}O_5$, of digoxin and of lanatoside C.

dig·ox·in (dij·ock'sin) *n.* A cardiotonic secondary glycoside, $C_{41}H_{64}O_{14}$, derived from lanatoside C, one of the glycosides of *Digitalis lanata*. On hydrolysis it yields the aglycone digoxigenin and three molecules of digitoxose. The actions and uses of digoxin are similar to those of digitalis.

di Gu·gliel·mo's syndrome or **disease** (dee·goo·lyel'mo)ERYTHREMIC MYELOSIS.

di·hy·drate (dye-high'drate) *n.* A compound containing two molecules of water.

di·hy·dro·co·en·zyme I (dye·high''dro·ko·en'zyme). A name given to the reduced form of diphosphopyridine nucleotide (coenzyme I), symbolized as DPNH, but now more often called the reduced form of nicotinamide-adenine dinucleotide and symbolized NADH.

dihydrocoenzyme II. A name given to the reduced form of triphosphopyridine nucleotide (coenzyme II), symbolized as TPNH, but now more often called the reduced form of nicotinamide-adenine dinucleotide phosphate and symbolized NADPH.

di·hy·dro·er·got·a·mine (dye·high''dro·ur·got'uh·meen, ·ur''goh·tam'een) *n.* A hydrogenated derivative, $C_{33}H_{37}N_5O_5$, of ergotamine, employed parenterally, as the methanesulfonate salt, in the treatment of migraine. It is less toxic than ergotamine and has no uterine effect.

di·hy·dro·strep·to·my·cin (dye·high''dro·strep''to·migh'sin) *n.* A hydrogenated derivative, $C_{21}H_{41}N_7O_{12}$, of streptomycin having the antibacterial action of, and used clinically like, streptomycin. It is available as the sulfate for intramuscular injection. Used in patients who cannot tolerate streptomycin, but is toxic to the eighth cranial nerve.

di·hy·dro·ta·chys·ter·ol (dye·high''dro·ta·kis'tuh·role, ·rol, ·tack''i·steer') *n.* A synthetic steroid, $C_{28}H_{46}O$, derived from ergosterol; possesses some of the biologic properties of vitamin D and of the parathyroid hormone. It produces hypercalcemia and increased urinary excretion of phosphorus. Used in treating hypoparathyroidism.

di·hy·dro·thee·lin (dye·high''dro·thee'lin) *n.* ESTRADIOL.

di·hy·droxy·ac·e·tone (dye''high·drock''see·as'e·tone) *n.* $CH_2OHCOCH_2OH$; a simple ketose derivable from glycerin or dextrose, important in metabolism of carbohydrates; also acts as a sunscreen and reacts with keratin in the stratum corneum to form a dark pigmentation which gives the appearance of a suntan.

di·hy·droxy·alu·mi·num ami·no·ac·e·tate (dye'' high·drock''see·uh·lew'mi·num a·mee''no·as'e·tate). A basic aluminum salt of aminoacetic acid, principally $NH_2CH_2COOAl(OH)_2$, a white powder, insoluble in water. It acts as a gastric antacid and is useful for control of hyperacidity in the management of peptic ulcer. It is available under various trade-marked names.

di·hy·droxy·es·trin (dye''high·drock''see·es'trin) *n.* ESTRADIOL.

di·hy·droxy·phen·yl·al·a·nine (dye''high·drock'' see·fen·il·al'uh·neen) *n.* 3-(3,4-Dihydroxyphenyl)-L-alanine, $C_9H_{11}NO_4$, an amino acid that can be formed by oxidation of tyrosine; it is converted by a series of biochemical transformations, utilizing the enzyme dopa oxidase, to black, pigments known as melanins, and is also the precursor of epinephrine and norepinephrine. Syn. *dopa.*

di·io·do·hy·droxy·quin (dye''eye·o''do·high·drock'see·kwin) *n.* 5,7-Diiodo-8-quinolinol, $C_9H_5I_2NO$, a light yellowish to tan microcrystalline powder, almost insoluble in water. It is used as an antiprotozoan agent in intestinal amebiasis and in the treatment of *Trichomonas hominis* infections.

di·iso·pro·pyl flu·o·ro·phos·phate (dye''eye·so·pro'pil floo''uh·ro·fos'fate). Diisopropyl phosphorofluoridate,

dik·ty·o·ma, dic·ty·o·ma (dick''tee·o'muh) *n.*, pl. **diktyomas, dictyomas, diktyoma·ta, dictyoma·ta** (·tuh) A tumor derived from the nonpigmented layer of the ciliary epithelium and structurally resembling the embryonic retina. Syn. *medulloepithelioma.*

di·lac·er·a·tion (dye·las''uh·ray'shun) *n.* 1. The act of tearing apart; being torn in pieces. 2. *In dentistry,* a partial alteration of the position of the formative organ during development, resulting in teeth with sharp angulation of the root and crown.

Dilantin. A trademark for phenytoin, an anticonvulsant in the treatment of epilepsy; the compound is also used as the sodium derivative.

di·lat·able (dye·lay'tuh·bul, di·) *adj.* Expandable.

dil·a·ta·tion (dil''uh·tay'shun, dye'') *n.* 1. The state of being stretched. 2. Enlargement, as of a hollow part or organ.

di·late (dye·late') *v.* To enlarge or expand. —**di·lat·ing** (dye·lay'ting) *adj.*

di·la·tor (dye·lay'tur, dye·lay'tur) *n.* 1. An instrument for stretching or enlarging a cavity or opening. 2. A dilating muscle.

Dilaudid. Trademark for hydromorphone (dihydromorphinone), a respiratory sedative and analgesic used as the hydrochloride salt.

dil·u·ent (dil'yoo·unt) *n.* An agent that dilutes the strength of a solution or mixture.

di·lute (di·lewt', dye·) *v. & adj.* 1. To make less concentrated, weaker, or thinner, as by addition of water to an aqueous solution. 2. Diluted.

di·lu·tion (di·lew'shun, dye·) *n.* 1. The process of diluting, as a solution with its solvent or a powder containing an active ingredient with an inactive diluent. 2. A diluted substance; the result of a diluting process. —**dilution·al** (·ul) adj.

dilution test. The administration of a water load to test the ability of the kidney to excrete a dilute urine; this ability is lost with renal failure.

di·men·hy·dri·nate (dye″men·high′dri·nate) n. 2-(Benzhydryloxy)-N,N-dimethylethylamine 8-chlorotheophyllinate, $C_{17}H_{21}NO.C_7H_7ClN_4O_2$, a white, crystalline powder, slightly soluble in water; an antihistaminic and antinauseant.

di·men·sion (di·men′shun, dye·) n. A measurable extent.

di·mer·cap·rol (dye″mur·cap′rol) n. 2,3-Dimercaptopropanol, $HSCH_2CHSHCH_2OH$, a colorless liquid with a mercaptan-like odor, soluble in water; an antidote for arsenic, gold, and mercury poisoning. Originally developed to counteract the effects of the chemical warfare agent lewisite. Syn. *British anti-lewisite.*

dimethyl-. A combining form indicating *the presence of two methyl groups.*

dimethyl sulfoxide. CH_3SOCH_3, a colorless liquid, practically odorless when pure, miscible with water. Rapidly absorbed through intact skin, it has local analgesic and anti-inflammatory activity; its use is disapproved. Abbreviated, DMSO.

di·meth·yl·tryp·ta·mine (dye·meth″il·trip′ta·meen, ·min) n. 3-[2-(Dimethylamino)ethyl]indole, $C_{12}H_{10}N_2$, a naturally occurring hallucinogenic agent extracted from the seeds of *Piptadenia peregrina.* Abbreviated, DMT.

di·meth·yl·xan·thine (dye·meth″il·zan′theen, ·thin) n. Either of two isomeric substances: (a) theobromine (3,7-dimethylxanthine); (b) theophylline (1,3-dimethylxanthine).

di·me·tria (dye·mee′tree·uh) n. UTERUS DUPLEX.

di·mor·phism (dye·mor′fiz·um) n. The property of existing in two distinct structural forms. —**dimor·phous** (·fus) adj.

dimp·ling, n. An abnormal skin depression from retraction occurring in subcutaneous carcinomas; most commonly seen in breast cancer.

di·ni·tro·phen·yl·hy·dra·zine (dye·nigh″tro·fen″il·high′druh·zeen, ·zin, dye·nigh″tro·fee″nil·) n. 2,4-Dinitrophenylhydrazine, C_6H_3·($NO_2)_2NHNH_2$, a red crystalline powder soluble in dilute acids; used in identification and analysis of aldehydes and ketones.

Di·oc·to·phy·ma (dye·ock″to·figh′muh) n. A genus of large nematodes of the superfamily Dioctophymoidea.

Dioctophyma re·na·le (re·nay′lee). A species of kidney worm which occasionally infects man, but principally a parasite of carnivorous and other animals.

di·o·done (dye′o·dohn) n. IODOPYRACET.

Diodoquin. A trademark for diiodohydroxyquin, an antiprotozoan drug.

Diodrast. Trademark for iodopyracet, a radiopaque medium.

di·oe·cious (dye·ee′shus) adj. Having separate sexes; used particularly for organisms belonging to larger groups in which hermaphroditism is also common.

Dionin. A trademark for ethylmorphine, a lym-

phagogue, analgesic, and antitussive; used as the hydrochloride salt.

di·op·ter, di·op·tre (dye·op′tur) n. A unit of measurement of the refractive power of an optic lens. It is the refractive power of a lens having a focal distance of one meter. Abbreviated, d. —**di·op·tral** (dye·op′trul) adj.

di·op·tom·e·ter (dye″op·tom′e·tur) n. An instrument for determining ocular refraction. —**dioptome** (·tree) n.

di·op·tric (dye·op′trick) adj. Pertaining to transmitted and refracted light.

di·op·trics (dye·op′tricks) n. The branch of optics that treats of the refraction of light, especially by the transparent medium of the eye, and by lenses.

di·or·tho·sis (dye″or·tho′sis) n., pl. **diortho·ses** (·seez) Surgical correction of a deformity or repair of an injury done to a limb, as diaplasis. —**dior·thot·ic** (·thot′ick) adj.

di·otic (dye·o′tick, ·ot′ick) adj. Pertaining to both ears; BINAURAL.

di·ovu·lar (dye·o′vyoo·lur) adj. BIOVULAR.

di·ox·ane (dye·ock′sane) n. 1,4-Diethylene dioxide, $C_4H_8O_2$, a colorless liquid miscible with water and many organic solvents. Employed as a solvent, and as a dehydrating agent in the process of paraffin embedding in histologic technique.

di·ox·ide (dye·ock′side, ·sid) n. A molecule containing two atoms of oxygen which was formed (or presumably formed) by oxidation of the basic molecule.

Di-Paralene. A trademark for chlorcyclizine, an antihistaminic drug used as the hydrochloride salt.

Diparcol. A trademark for diethazine, a drug used in parkinsonism; employed as the hydrochloride salt.

Dipaxin. Trademark for diphenadione, an orally effective anticoagulant drug.

di·pep·ti·dase (dye·pep′ti·dace, ·daze) n. An enzyme that splits dipeptides to amino acids.

di·pep·tide (dye·pep′tide) n. A chemical union of two molecules of amino acids obtained by condensation of the acids or by hydrolysis of proteins.

di·pet·a·lo·ne·mi·a·sis (dye·pet″uh·lo·ne·migh′uh·sis) n. Infection with *Dipetalonema perstans,* usually asymptomatic in man but sometimes causing cutaneous edema or elephantiasis.

di·phal·lus (dye·fal′us) n. 1. Partial or complete doubling of the penis or clitoris. 2. An individual with such a condition. —**diphal·lic** (·ick) adj.

di·pha·sic (dye·fay′zick) adj. Having two phases.

di·phem·a·nil methylsulfate (dye·fem′uh·nil). 4-Diphenylmethylene-1,1-dimethylpiperidinium methylsulfate, $C_{20}H_{24}N.CH_3SO_4$, a quaternary parasympatholytic agent used to inhibit gastric secretion and motility, relieve pylorospasm, and reduce sweating.

di·phen·a·di·one (dye·fen′duh·ohn) n. Diphenylacetylindandione, $C_{23}H_{16}O_3$, an orally effective anticoagulant.

di·phen·an (dye·fen′an) n. p-Benzylphenyl carbamate, $C_{14}H_{13}NO_2$, a white powder, almost insoluble in water; employed in the treatment of oxyuriasis.

di·phen·hy·dra·mine (dye″fen·high′druh·meen, ·min) *n.* 2-(Benzhydryloxy)-*N*,*N*-dimethylethylamine, $C_{17}H_{21}NO$, an antihistaminic drug; used as the hydrochloride salt.

di·phen·ox·yl·ate (dye″fen·ock′sil·ate) *n.* 1-(3-Cyano-3,3-diphenylpropyl)-4-phenylpiperidine-4-carboxylic acid ethyl ester, $C_{30}H_{32}N_2O_2$, an antidiarrheal drug; used as the hydrochloride salt.

di·phen·yl·amine (dye·fen″il·uh·meen′, ·am′een) *n.* $C_6H_5NHC_6H_5$. A reagent for nitrates, chlorates, and other oxidizing substances with which, in the presence of sulfuric acid, it gives a blue color.

di·phen·yl·hy·dan·to·in (dye·fen″il·high·dan′to·in, ·dan′toin, dye·fee″nil·) *n.* PHENYTOIN.

di·pho·nia (dye·fo′nee·uh) *n.* The production of two distinct tones during vocal utterance.

di·phos·pho·pyr·i·dine nucleotide (dye·fos″fo·pirr′i·deen, ·din). NICOTINAMIDE ADENINE DINUCLEOTIDE; NADIDE.

diph·the·ria (dif·theer′ee·uh) *n.* An acute infectious disease caused by *Corynebacterium diphtheriae*, characterized by local inflammation and the formation of a false membrane primarily in the pharyngeal area; absorption of toxin may affect the heart and peripheral nerves. —**diphtherial** (·ree·ul), **diph·ther·ic** (·therr′ick, ·theer′ick) *adj.*

diphtheria antitoxin. Any crude or purified serum containing antibodies that specifically neutralize diphtheria toxin.

diphtheria toxin. The crystallized protein purified from culture filtrates of *Corynebacterium diphtheriae* which has deleterious effects on the heart, peripheral nerves, and other tissues, as evidenced in the disease diphtheria.

diphtheria toxoid. A detoxified diphtheria toxin used to produce active immunity against diphtheria, having the advantage over toxinantitoxin of not producing sensitivity to serum.

diph·the·rit·ic (dif″the·rit′ick) *adj.* Pertaining to, caused by, or like diphtheria.

diph·the·roid (dif′the·roid) *adj. & n.* 1. Resembling diphtheria or the bacillus *Corynebacterium diphtheriae*. 2. Any of various unclassified bacteria morphologically resembling *Corynebacterium diphtheriae*. 3. PSEUDODIPHTHERIA.

di·phyl·lo·both·ri·a·sis (dye·fil″o·both·rye′uh·sis) *n.* Infection with *Diphyllobothrium latum*.

Di·phyl·lo·both·ri·um (dye·fil″o·both′ree·um) *n.* A genus of tapeworms.

Diphyllobothrium la·tum (lay′tum). The fish tapeworm, a large tapeworm found in the intestine. The head has two suckers or bothria. The adult worm ranges from 3 to 10 meters in length, and may have over 4,000 proglottids. The definitive hosts are man, dog, and cat. The first intermediate hosts are freshwater copepods, and the secondary intermediate hosts are various freshwater fishes. Infection in man may cause disorders of the nervous and digestive systems, malnutrition, and anemia.

di·phy·o·dont (dye·fee′o·dont″, dif′ee·o·) *adj.* Having two sets of teeth, as the deciduous teeth and the permanent teeth.

dipl-, diplo- A combining form meaning *twofold, double, twin.*

dip·la·cu·sis (dip″luh·kew′sis) *n.* The hearing of the same sound differently by one ear than by the other.

diplacusis bin·au·ra·lis (bin″aw·ray′lis). Perception of a single tone as having a higher fundamental pitch in one ear than in the other.

diplacusis uni·au·ra·lis (yoo″nee·aw·ray′lis). Hearing of two tones by one ear when only one tone is produced.

di·plas·mat·ic (dye″plaz·mat′ick) *adj.* Containing matter other than protoplasm, said of cells.

di·ple·gia (dye·plee′jee·uh) *n.* Paralysis of similar parts on the two sides of the body. —**diple·gic** (·jick) *adj.*

diplo-. See *dipl-.*

dip·lo·blas·tic (dip″lo·blas′tick) *adj.* Having two germ layers, ectoderm and entoderm.

dip·lo·car·di·ac (dip″lo·kahr′dee·ack) *adj.* Having a double heart, or one in which the two sides are more or less separate, as in birds and mammals.

dip·lo·coc·cus (dip″lo·kock′us) *n., pl.* **diplococ·ci** (·sigh) A micrococcus that occurs in groups of two, such as the pneumococcus.

Diplococcus, *n.* A genus of bacteria of the family Lactobacteriaceae of the tribe Streptococceae.

Diplococcus go·nor·rhoe·ae (gon″o·ree′ee). NEISSERIA GONORRHOEAE.

Diplococcus in·tra·cel·lu·la·ris men·in·git·i·dis (in·truh·sel·yoo·lair′is men·in·jit′i·dis) NEISSERIA MENINGITIDIS.

Diplococcus pneu·mo·ni·ae (new·mo′nee·ee). STREPTOCOCCUS PNEUMONIAE.

dip·loë (dip′lo·ee) *n.* The cancellous bone between the outer and inner tables of the bones of the skull. —**dip·lo·et·ic** (dip″lo·et′ick) *adj.*

dip·lo·gen·e·sis (dip″lo·jen′e·sis) *n.* Development of a double or twin monstrosity.

Dip·lo·go·nop·o·rus (dip″lo·go·nop′uh·rus) *n.* A genus of cestodes or tapeworms.

di·plo·ic (di·plo′ick) *adj.* Of or pertaining to the diploë.

dip·loid (dip′loid) *adj.* Having double the haploid or gametic number of chromosomes.

dip·lo·mate (dip′lo·mate) *n.* An individual who has received a diploma or certificate; specifically, one who is certified by an American specialty board as having satisfied all its requirements and passed its examinations, and as being qualified to practice that specialty.

dip·lo·mel·li·tu·ria (dip″lo·mel″i·tew′ree·uh) *n.* Coexistence or alternation of diabetic and nondiabetic glycosuria in the same individual.

dip·lo·neu·ral (dip″lo·new′rul) *adj.* Pertaining to a muscle supplied by two nerves from different sources.

di·plop·a·gus (di·plop′uh·gus) *n., pl.* **diplopa·gi** (·guy, ·jye) Equally developed conjoined twins.

di·plo·pia (di·plo′pee·uh) *n.* A disorder of sight in which one object is perceived as two. Syn. *double vision.*

di·plo·pi·om·e·ter (di·plo″pee·om′e·tur) *n.* An instrument for measuring the degree of diplopia.

dip·lo·scope (dip′lo·skope) *n.* An instrument for the investigation of binocular vision.

dip·lo·tene (dip′lo·teen) *n.* The stage in the first meiotic prophase in which the tetrads exhibit chiasmata.

di·pole (dye′pole) *n.* 1. A particle or object bearing opposite charges. 2. A pair of electric charges, positive and negative, situated near each other in a conducting medium.

dipole moment. The measure of the electric asymmetry of a molecule. It is equal to the product of the ionic charges and their spatial separation.

dip·ping, *n.* 1. Palpation of an abdominal organ, particularly the liver, by quick depression of the abdomen. 2. *In veterinary medicine,* the act of submerging an animal for the application of a dip.

di·pro·so·pia (dye″pro·so′pee·uh, dip″ro·) *n. In teratology,* duplication of the face.

di·pro·so·pus (dye·pro′so·pus, dye″pro·so′pus) *n.* An individual with doubling of the face.

dip·set·ic (dip·set′ick) *adj.* Causing or characterized by thirst.

dip·so·ma·nia (dip″so·may′nee·uh) *n.* Recurrent periodic compulsion to excessive drinking of alcoholic beverages. **—dipsoma·ni·ac** (·nee′ack) *n.*

dip·so·pho·bia (dip″so·fo′bee·uh) *n.* An abnormal fear of drinking, especially of alcoholic beverages.

dip·so·rex·ia (dip″so·reck′see·uh) *n.* The early stage of chronic alcoholism before the appearance of neurologic or systemic deficits.

dip·so·ther·a·py (dip″so·therr′uh·pee) *n.* Treatment of certain diseases by reducing the amount of fluid allowed the patient.

Dip·tera (dip′tur·uh) *n. pl.* An order of two-winged insects; includes mosquitoes, flies, midges.

dip·ter·ous (dip′tur·us) *adj. In biology,* having two wings or wing-like processes.

di·py·gus (di·pye′gus, dip′i·gus) *n.* A monster with more or less duplication of the pelvis, lower parts of the back, and inferior extremities.

dip·y·li·di·a·sis (dip″i·li·dye′uh·sis) *n.* Infection with *Dipylidium caninum,* the common tapeworm of dogs.

Di·py·lid·i·um (dye″pye·lid′ee·um) *n.* A genus of tapeworms.

Dipylidium ca·ni·num (ka·nigh′num). A species of tapeworm, 20 to 40 cm in length, of which the dog and cat are definitive hosts, and man is an occasional host; fleas and lice harbor the larval stage, thus acting as vectors.

direct Coombs test ANTIGLOBULIN TEST.

direct hernia. An inguinal hernia in which the sac does not leave the abdominal cavity through the abdominal inguinal ring but through a defect in the floor of the inguinal triangle, between the inferior epigastric artery and the outer edge of the rectus abdominis muscle.

direct laryngoscopy. Examination of the interior of the larynx by direct vision with the aid of a laryngoscope.

direct percussion. Percussion performed by striking the skin directly with the pads of one or two fingers without the interposition of a pleximeter.

Di·ro·fi·lar·ia (dye″ro·fi·lār′ee·uh, ·fi·lair′ee·uh) *n.* A genus of filarial worms. Members of the species *Dirofilaria immitis, D. magalhaesi,* and *D. repens* are parasites of dogs.

Dirofilaria im·mi·tis (i·migh′tis). The heartworm, an important filarial parasite of dogs and other Canidae, occurring primarily in tropical and subtropical regions, including the southern and southeastern coastal regions of the United States. The larvae are transmitted by the bite of mosquitoes and fleas, and the adult worms are found in the right ventricle and pulmonary artery of the canine host. Affected animals exhibit weakness, dyspnea, and cardiac hypertrophy, and may die from right heart failure or pulmonary embolism. Rare infections have been reported in man.

di·ro·fil·a·ri·a·sis (dye″ro·fil′uh·rye′uh·sis) *n.* Infection with worms of the genus *Dirofilaria.*

dir·rhi·nus, dir·rhy·nus (di·rye′nus) *n.* Partial or complete doubling of the nose; a mild degree of diprosopia.

dis-, di- A prefix meaning (a) *separation;* (b) *reversal;* (c) *apart from. Compare* di-, dis-.

dis·abil·i·ty, *n.* A persistent physical or mental defect, weakness, or handicap which prevents a person from engaging in ordinary activities or normal life, or from performing a specific job.

di·sac·cha·ri·dase (dye·sack′uh·ri·dace) *n.* An enzyme that causes hydrolysis of disaccharide, producing two monosaccharides.

di·sac·cha·ride (dye·sack′uh·ride, ·rid) *n.* A carbohydrate formed by the condensation of two monosaccharide molecules.

dis·ag·gre·ga·tion (dis·ag″re·gay′shun) *n.* 1. A state of perpetual distraction which prevents an individual from entertaining any idea other than the one which dominates or occupies his mind, as in the obsessive compulsive neurosis. 2. In hysteria, an inability to coordinate various new sensations and to connect them with visual impressions.

dis·ar·tic·u·la·tion (dis″ahr·tick″yoo·lay′shun) *n.* 1. Amputation at a joint. 2. Separation at a joint. **—disar·tic·u·late** (·tick′yoo·late) *v.*

dis·as·sim·i·la·tion (dis″uh·sim″i·lay′shun) *n.* CATABOLISM.

dis·as·sort·a·tive (dis″uh·sor′tuh·tiv) *adj.* Pertaining to selection on the basis of dissimilarity.

disc. DISK.

disc-, disco-. A combining form meaning *disk.*

¹dis·charge (dis·chahrj′) *v.* 1. To emit, unload. 2. To release, dismiss.

²dis·charge (dis·chahrj) *n.* 1. An emission, unloading, evacuation, or secretion. 2. That which is emitted. 3. *In electricity,* a setting free or escape of stored-up energy; the equalization of differences of potential between the poles of a condenser or other sources of electricity by connecting or nearly connecting them with a conductor. 4. The generation and transmission of impulses by a neuron.

dis·ci·form (dis'ki·form, dis'i·form) *adj.* Disk-shaped; DISCOID.

disciform keratitis. A localized, subacute, non-suppurative inflammation of the corneal stroma characterized by a discoid opacity, most commonly resulting from herpes simplex infection. Syn. *keratitis disciformis.*

dis·cis·sion (di·sish'un, ·sizh'un) *n.* 1. A tearing or being torn apart. 2. *In eye surgery*, an operation for soft cataract in which the capsule is lacerated a number of times to allow the lens substance to be absorbed.

dis·ci·tis, dis·ki·tis (disk·eye'tis) *n.* Inflammation of a disk, especially of an intervertebral or articular disk.

dis·coid (dis'koid) *adj. & n.* 1. Shaped like a disk. 2. Of or pertaining to a disk. 3. A dental carving instrument having a blade in the form of a disk.

discoid lupus erythematosus. CHRONIC DISCOID LUPUS ERYTHEMATOSUS.

dis·col·or·a·tion (dis·kul''ur·ay'shun) *n.* Change in color, as of a tissue, part, or fluid. —**dis·col·or** (dis·kul'ur) *v.*

dis·con·tin·u·ous phase. The particles, droplets, or bubbles of an insoluble or immiscible substance that are distributed through the dispersion medium in a colloidal system.

dis·cop·a·thy (dis·kop'uh·thee) *n.* Any disease process involving an intervertebral disk.

dis·co·pla·cen·ta (dis''ko·pluh·sen'tuh) *n.* DISCOID PLACENTA.

dis·cor·dance (dis·kor'dunce) *n.* A state of difference between twins with respect to a particular trait or disease.

dis·crete, *adj.* Not running together; separate.

dis·cus (dis'kus) *n.,* pl. & genit. sing. **dis·ci** (·kye, ·eye) DISK.

discus ar·ti·cu·la·ris (ahr·tick·yoo·lair'is) [NA]. ARTICULAR DISK.

dis·cu·tient (dis·kew'shee·unt) *adj. & n.* 1. Causing dispersion or disappearance, as of a swelling. 2. A discutient remedy.

dis·ease, *n.* 1. The failure of the adaptive mechanisms of an organism to counteract adequately the stimuli or stresses to which it is subject, resulting in a disturbance in function or structure of any part, organ, or system of the body. A response to injury; sickness or illness. 2. A specific entity which is the sum total of the numerous expressions of one or more pathological processes. The cause of a disease entity is represented by the cause of the basic pathological process in combination with important secondary causative factors.

disease potential. The sum of adverse health factors present in a population, which have a bearing upon the incidence of disease to be anticipated.

dis·en·gage·ment (dis''in·gaij'munt) *n.* 1. Emergence from a confined state; especially the emergence of the head of the fetus from the vagina during parturition. 2. The release from personal ties, obligations, occupation, or other constraints on one's life. —**disengage,** *v.*

dis·equi·lib·ri·um (dis·ee''kwi·lib'ree·um) *n.* Lack or loss of balance, as of bodily or mental balance, or as between the intellectual and moral faculties.

dis·gre·ga·tion (dis''gre·gay'shun) *n.* Dispersion; separation, as of molecules or cells. —**dis·gre·gate** (dis'gre·gate) *v.*

dis·im·pact (dis''im·pakt') *v.* To remove an impaction.

dis·in·fect (dis''in·fekt') *v.* To kill pathogenic agents by direct application of chemical or physical means, especially in the cleansing of inanimate objects. —**dis·in·fec·tion** (·feck'shun) *n.*

dis·in·fec·tant (dis''in·feck'tunt) *n. & adj.* 1. An agent that destroys or inhibits the microorganisms causing disease. 2. Used as or having the action of a disinfectant.

dis·in·fes·ta·tion (dis·in''fes·tay'shun) *n.* Extermination of insects, rodents, or animal parasites present on an individual or in his surroundings.

dis·in·ser·tion (dis''in·sur'shun) *n.* 1. Rupture of a tendon at its point of insertion into bone. 2. A circumferentially oriented tear in the extreme periphery of the retina where it terminates at the pars plana; common in juvenile retinal detachment and may occur following trauma. Syn. *retinodialysis.*

dis·in·te·grate (dis·in'te·grate) *v.* To break up or decompose. —**dis·in·te·gra·tion** (dis·in''te·gray'shun) *n.*

disintegration constant. DECAY CONSTANT.

Disipal. A trademark for orphenadrine, an antispasmodic and antitremor drug used as the hydrochloride salt.

dis·joint, *adj.* Disarticulate; separate, as bones from their natural relations.

dis·junc·tion (dis·junk'shun) *n.* 1. Moving apart, divergence. 2. Segregation of homologous chromosomes in first meiotic division or of products of chromosomal duplication in second meiotic division or in mitosis. —**disjunc·tive** (·tiv) *adj.*

disk, disc, *n.* A circular, platelike organ or structure.

dis·ko·gram, dis·co·gram (dis'ko·gram) *n.* A roentgenogram produced in radiographic examination of intervertebral disks employing the direct injection of radiopaque medium.

dis·lo·ca·tion (dis''lo·kay'shun) *n.* The displacement of one or more bones of a joint or of any organ from the original position. —**dis·lo·cate** (dis'lo·kate, dis·lo'kate) *v.*

dis·oc·clude (dis''uh·klude') *v.* To grind or level a tooth surface so that it will fail to touch the opposing tooth in the other jaw during mastication.

dis·or·der, *n.* A disturbance or derangement of regular or normal physical or mental health or function.

dis·ori·en·ta·tion (dis·or''ee·en·tay'shun) *n.* Loss of normal relationship to one's surroundings; particularly the ability to comprehend time, place, and people, such as occurs in organic brain syndromes.

dis·pa·rate (dis'pur·ut) *adj.* Not alike; unequal or unmated.

dis·par·i·ty (dis·păr'i·tee) *n*. Difference; inequality.

dis·pen·sa·ry (dis·pen'suh·ree) *n*. 1. A place where medicine or medical aid is given free or at low cost to ambulatory patients. 2. In a place of business, a medical office provided by the owner to serve sick or injured employees. 3. *In military medicine*, a medical treatment facility primarily intended to provide examination and treatment for ambulatory patients, to make necessary arrangements for the transfer of patients requiring bed care, and to provide first aid for emergency cases. 4. Any place where drugs or medications are dispensed.

dis·pen·sa·to·ry (dis·pen'suh·to''ree) *n*. A book containing a systematic discussion of medicinal agents, including origin, preparation, description, use, and mode of action.

dis·pense, *v*. To prepare and distribute (medicines).

di·sper·my (dye'spur·mee) *n*. Entrance of two spermatozoa into an ovum.

dispersed or **disperse phase.** DISCONTINUOUS PHASE.

dis·per·sion (dis·pur'zhun) *n*. 1. The act of scattering; any scattering of light, as that passed through ground glass. 2. A system consisting of an insoluble or immiscible substance dispersed throughout a continuous medium. —**dis·perse** (·purce') *v*. & *adj*.; **disper·sive** (·siv) *adj*.

dispersion medium. The homogeneous gas, liquid, or solid in which particles, droplets, or bubbles of an insoluble or immiscible substance are dispersed. Syn. *continuous medium*.

dis·place·ment, *n*. 1. Removal from the normal position; dislocation, luxation; dystopia. 2. *In pharmacy*, a process of percolation. 3. *In chemistry*, a change in which one element is replaced by another element. 4. *In psychiatry*, a defense mechanism in which an emotion is unconsciously transferred or displaced from its original object, as a person or situation that is disturbing to the ego, to a more acceptable, less disturbing substitute. —**dis·place,** *v*.

dis·po·si·tion, *n*. 1. PREDISPOSITION. 2. TEMPERAMENT.

dis·pro·por·tion, *n*. An abnormal size relationship between two elements.

dis·rup·tive, *adj*. Bursting; rending.

dis·sect (dis·sekt', dye·) *v*. 1. To divide or separate along natural lines of cleavage. 2. To cut or separate carefully and methodically, as in anatomical study or surgical operation.

dissecting aneurysm or **hematoma.** An aneurysm produced by blood forcing its way through a tear in the intima and between the layers of an arterial wall, usually that of the aorta.

dissecting microscope. A microscope with a long working distance, allowing adequate space for placement of large unmounted specimens in its stage so as to use magnification during dissection of the specimen.

dis·sec·tion (dis·seck'shun, dye·) *n*. 1. Division or separation along natural lines of cleavage.

2. The cutting of structures of the body for purposes of study or operative treatment.

dis·sec·tor (di·seck'tur) *n*. 1. One who makes a dissection. 2. A handbook or manual of anatomy and instructions for use in dissection.

dis·sem·i·nate (di·sem'i·nate) *v*. To scatter or disperse. —**dissemi·nat·ed** (·nay·tid) *adj*.

disseminated intravascular coagulation or **clotting.** A complex disorder of the clotting mechanisms, in which coagulation factors are consumed at an accelerated rate, with generalized fibrin deposition and thrombosis, hemorrhages, and further depletion of the coagulation factors. The process may be acute or chronic, and is usually triggered by the entry of large amounts of thromboplastic substances into the circulation, resulting from any of a wide variety of severe diseases and traumas. Abbreviated, DIC. Syn. *consumption coagulopathy, defibrination syndrome, diffuse intravascular coagulation*.

disseminated lipogranulomatosis. An inborn error of lipid metabolism, characterized by the diffuse development of granulomas in many tissues in infancy, resulting in feeding difficulties and hoarse cry due to laryngeal obstruction, periarticular changes suggestive of rheumatoid arthritis, and deposition of abnormal lipids in many other tissues, leading to motor and mental retardation and early death. Syn. *Farber's disease.*

disseminated lupus erythematosus. SYSTEMIC LUPUS ERYTHEMATOSUS.

disseminated sclerosis. MULTIPLE SCLEROSIS.

dis·sem·i·na·tion (di·sem''i·nay'shun) *n*. The scattering or dispersion of disease or disease germs.

dis·sim·u·la·tion (di·sim''yoo·lay'shun) *n*. The act of feigning, disguising, or malingering.

dis·so·ci·a·tion (di·so''see·ay'shun, ·shee·) *n*. 1. Separation; especially of a chemical compound into ions. 2. *In cardiology*, independent action of atria and ventricles; a form of heart block. 3. *In psychology*, the segregation from consciousness of certain components of mental processes, which then function independently as if they belonged to another person; the separation of ideas from their natural and appropriate affects or feelings. 4. *In bacteriology*, variations due to mutation in colony form and associated properties, including smooth, rough, mucoid, dwarf, gonidial, and L or pleuropneumonia-like colonial forms. —**dis·so·ci·ant** (·so'shee·unt) *adj*. & *n*.; **dis·so·ci·ate** (·so'shee·ate) *v*.; **dis·so·ci·a·tive** (·so'shee·uh·tiv) *adj*.

dissociation constant. The equilibrium constant pertaining to a reversible reaction in which a molecule breaks up into two or more products. Symbol, K.

dissociative reaction. DISSOCIATIVE TYPE OF HYSTERICAL NEUROSIS.

dissociative type of hysterical neurosis. The form of hysterical neurosis, leading to alterations in the person's identity or his state of consciousness, that may take the form of depersonalization, dissociation, multiple personality, amnesia, somnambulism, fugue, dream state, or of aimless running or freezing.

dis·so·lu·tion (dis″uh-lew′shun) *n.* 1. Separation of a body or compound into its parts. 2. Death; decomposition. 3. SOLUTION.

dis·solve, *v.* 1. To make a solution of. 2. To become a solution; to pass into solution. —**dis·sol·vent** (di-zol′vunt) *adj. & n.*

dist-, disto-. A combining form meaning *distal*.

dis·tad (dis′tad) *adv.* Toward the periphery; in a distal direction.

dis·tal (dis′tul) *adj.* 1. Farther or farthest from the point of origin along the course of any asymmetrical structure; nearest the end. 2. In any symmetrical structure, farther or farthest from the center or midline or median plane. 3. *In dentistry,* away from the sagittal plane along the curve of a dental arch.

dis·tance, *n.* The measure of space between two objects. —**dis·tant, dis·tan·tial** (dis-tan′shul) *adj.*

distant memory. REMOTE MEMORY.

dis·tem·per (dis-tem′pur) *n.* Any of several infectious, or sometimes contagious, diseases of animals, as: canine distemper, feline distemper (= FELINE PANLEUKOPENIA), equine distemper (= STRANGLES).

dis·ten·si·bil·i·ty (dis-ten″si-bil′i-tee) *n.* The property of being distensible.

dis·ten·si·ble (dis-ten′si-bul) *adj.* Capable of distention.

dis·ten·tion (dis-ten′shun) *n.* A state of dilatation.

dis·tich·ia (dis-tick′ee-uh) *n.* A congenital anomaly in which there is an accessory row of eyelashes at the inner lid border, which turn in and rub on the cornea. This row is additional to the two or three rows normally arising at the outer lid border; may be seen in Milroy's disease.

dis·ti·chi·a·sis (dis″ti-kigh′uh-sis) *n.* DISTICHIA.

dis·til·late (dis′ti-late) *n.* The condensate obtained by distillation.

dis·til·la·tion (dis″ti-lay′shun) *n.* Vaporization and subsequent condensation, used principally to separate liquids from nonvolatile substances. —**dis·till** (dis·til′) *v.*

disto-. See *dist-.*

dis·to·buc·cal (dis″to-buck′ul) *adj.* Pertaining to the distal and buccal surfaces of the premolar and molar teeth.

dis·to·buc·co·oc·clu·sal (dis″to-buck″o-uh-klew′zul) *adj.* Pertaining to the distal, buccal, and occlusal surfaces of a tooth.

dis·to·clu·sion (dis″to-klew′zhun) *n.* Malocclusion of the teeth in which those of the lower jaw are in distal relation to the upper teeth.

dis·to·in·ci·sal (dis″to-in-sigh′zul) *adj.* Pertaining to the distal and incisal surfaces of a tooth.

dis·to·la·bi·al (dis″to-lay′bee-ul) *adj.* Pertaining to the distal and labial surfaces of incisors and canines.

dis·to·lin·gual (dis″to-ling′gwul) *adj.* Pertaining to the distal and lingual surfaces of all teeth.

dis·to·lin·guo·oc·clu·sal (dis″to-ling″gwo-uh-klew′zul) *adj.* Pertaining to the distal, lingual, and occlusal surfaces of a tooth.

Di·sto·ma·ta (di-sto′muh-tuh) *n. pl.* A suborder of the Trematoda or flukes.

di·sto·mia (dye-sto′mee-uh) *n.* Congenital duplication of the mouth.

dis·to·mi·a·sis (dis″to-migh′uh-sis) *n.,* pl. **disto·mia·ses** (-seez) Infection with flukes or trematodes.

dis·to·mo·lar (dis″to-mo′lur) *n.* A supernumerary tooth distal to a third molar, hence in the position of a fourth molar.

dis·to·oc·clu·sal (dis″to-uh-klew′zul) *adj.* Pertaining to the distal and occlusal surfaces of premolar and molar teeth.

dis·tor·tion (dis-tor′shun) *n.* 1. A twisted or bent shape; deformity or malformation, acquired or congenital. 2. A writhing or twisting motion, as of the face. 3. *In optics,* a form of aberration in which objects viewed through certain lenses appear changed in shape but not broken in continuity. 4. *In psychiatry,* the adaptive alteration of an idea or memory to conform with the subject's wishes or prejudices.

dis·to·ver·sion (dis″to-vur′zhun) *n.* Tilting of a tooth so that the crown is directed distally.

distributing artery. Any of the arteries intermediate between the conducting arteries and arterioles, in which a well developed muscular coat of the arterial wall controls the size of the lumen and thereby also the volume of distributed blood.

dis·tri·bu·tion (dis″tri-bew′shun) *n. In anatomy,* the branching of a nerve or artery, and the arrangement of its branches within those parts that it supplies. —**dis·trib·u·tive** (dis-trib′yoo-tiv) *adj.*

dis·tri·chi·a·sis (dis″tri-kye′uh-sis) *n.* Two hairs growing from a single follicle.

di·sul·fide (dye-sul′fide, -fid) *n.* BISULFIDE.

di·sul·fi·ram (dye-sul′fi-ram) *n.* Bis(diethylthiocarbamoyl)disulfide, $C_{10}H_{20}N_2S_4$, an antioxidant that interferes with normal metabolic degradation of alcohol so that acetaldehyde is produced in high concentration; used in the treatment of alcoholism.

di·urese (dye″yoo-reece′) *v.* To effect diuresis in (someone).

di·ure·sis (dye″yoo-ree′sis) *n.,* pl. **diure·ses** (-seez) Increased excretion of urine.

di·uret·ic (dye″yoo-ret′ick) *adj. & n.* 1. Increasing the flow of urine. 2. Any diuretic agent.

Diuril. Trademark for chlorothiazide, an orally effective diuretic and antihypertensive drug.

di·ur·nal (dye-ur′nul) *adj.* Occurring in the daytime.

di·ur·nule (dye-urn′yool) *n.* A medicinal product that contains the full quantity of a drug to be administered in 24 hours.

di·va·ga·tion (dye″vuh-gay′shun) *n.* Rambling, incoherent speech and thought.

di·va·lent (dye-vay′lunt) *adj.* 1. BIVALENT. 2. Having the ability to exist in two valence states.

di·ver·gence (dye-vur′junce, di-) *n. In ophthalmology,* the abduction of both eyes simultaneously, or of one eye when the other is fixed. —**diver·gent** (-junt) *adj.*

divergent strabismus. EXOTROPIA.

diverticula. Plural of *diverticulum*.

diverticular disease. DIVERTICULITIS.

di·ver·tic·u·lec·to·my (dye″vur·tick″yoo·leck′

tuh·mee) *n. In surgery,* removal of a diverticulum.

di·ver·tic·u·li·tis (dye″vur·tick″yoo·lye′tis) *n.* Inflammation of a diverticulum; the clinical condition of inflammation of diverticula. Syn. *diverticular disease.*

di·ver·tic·u·lo·sis (dye″vur·tick″yoo·lo′sis) *n.* The presence of diverticula of the intestine, with or without clinical symptoms.

di·ver·tic·u·lum (dye″vur·tick′yoo·lum) *n., pl.* **diverticu·la** (·luh) An outpouching or sac arising from a hollow organ or structure; may be congenital or acquired. In the acquired form, it usually represents a herniation of the mucous membrane through the muscular wall of the organ.

diverticulum il·ei (il′ee·eye). A blind tube arising from the antimesenteric border of the terminal ileum at a variable distance from the ileocecal valve. It represents the persistent proximal end of the yolk stalk. Syn. *Meckel's diverticulum.*

di·vi·nyl ether (dye·vye′nil). VINYL ETHER.

di·vul·sion (dye·vul′shun, di·) *n.* A tearing apart. —**di·vulse** (dye·vulce′, di·) *v.*

di·vul·sor (dye·vul′sor, di·) *n.* An instrument for the forcible dilatation of a part or of stricture in any organ.

di·zy·got·ic (dye″zye·got′ick) *adj.* Developed from two fertilized ova at a single birth.

dizygotic twins. FRATERNAL TWINS.

diz·zi·ness, *n.* A sensation of disturbed relations to surrounding objects in space with feelings of rotation or whirling characteristic of vertigo as well as nonrotatory swaying, weakness, faintness, and unsteadiness characteristic of giddiness. —**diz·zy,** *adj.*

D.M.D. Doctor of Dental Medicine.

DMSO Abbreviation for *dimethyl sulfoxide.*

DMT Abbreviation for *dimethyltryptamine.*

DNA Abbreviation for *deoxyribonucleic acid,* any of the high molecular weight polymers of deoxyribonucleotides, found principally in the chromosomes of the nucleus and varying in composition with the source, able to reproduce in the presence of the appropriate enzyme and substrates, and bearing coded genetic information.

DNase Abbreviation for *deoxyribonuclease.*

DNA viruses. Viruses, such as adenoviruses, papovaviruses, herpesviruses, poxviruses, and most bacteriophages, in which the nucleic acid core consists of deoxyribonucleic acid.

D.O. Doctor of Osteopathy.

Do·bell's solution (do·bel′) Compound sodium borate solution, containing sodium borate, sodium bicarbonate, phenol, glycerin, and water; has been used as an antibacterial, mainly as a gargle and mouthwash.

Doca. A trademark for deoxycorticosterone (acetate), a salt-regulating adrenocortical hormone.

doc·tor, *n. & v.* 1. One licensed, usually after special study, and qualifying by examination, to practice medicine, dentistry, or veterinary medicine. 2. The recipient of an academic title signifying competence in a special branch of learning. 3. To treat as a physician; to practice medicine. 4. To tamper with or falsify.

doctrine of signatures. A theory that the medicinal uses of a plant can be determined from its fancied physical resemblance to normal or diseased organs (liverwort, lungwort, orchis).

dodec-, dodeca- A combining form meaning *twelve.*

Doeh·le bodies (dœh′le^h) Irregular peroxidase-negative clumps of ribonucleic acid, 1 to 2 microns in greatest dimension, occurring in the cytoplasm of granulocytes in persons with severe infections and in the May-Hegglin anomaly.

Dolantin. A trademark for meperidine, a narcotic analgesic used as the hydrochloride salt.

Dolene. A trademark for propoxyphene hydrochloride, an analgesic.

dolich-, dolicho- A combining form meaning (a) *long;* (b) *narrow.*

dol·i·cho·ceph·a·ly (dol″i·ko·sef′uh·lee) *n.* The condition in which the length-breadth index of the head is 75.9 or less, indicating that the head is much longer than it is broad. —**dolicho·ce·phal·ic** (·se·fal′ick), **dolicho·ceph·a·lous** (·sef′uh·lus) *adj.*

dol·i·cho·co·lon (dol″i·ko·ko′lun) *n.* An abnormally long colon.

dol·i·cho·de·rus (dol″i·ko·deer′us) *n.* A person having a disproportionately long neck.

dol·i·cho·fa·cial (dol″i·ko·fay′shul) *adj.* Having an unusually long face.

dol·i·cho·mor·phic (dol″i·ko·mor′fick) *adj.* Marked by a long or narrow form or build.

dol·i·cho·pel·lic (dol″i·ko·pel′ick) *adj.* Designating a pelvis the pelvic index of which is 95.0 or more.

dol·i·chor·rhine (dol′i·ko·rine, ·reen) *adj.* Having a long nose.

dol·i·cho·steno·me·lia (dol″i·ko·sten″o·mee′lee·uh) *n.* Abnormally long, thin extremities, as seen in Marfan's syndrome and in homocystinuria.

doll's-head phenomenon or **eye movements.** Involuntary turning of the eyes upward and downward on passive flexion and extension of the head, an action that has been likened to that of a mechanical doll's eyes. The presence of these movements indicates that the vestibulo-ocular connections are intact.

Dolophine. A trademark for methadone hydrochloride, a narcotic analgesic.

do·lor (do′lor) *n.,* pl. **do·lo·res** (do·lo′reez) Pain.

do·lo·rol·o·gy (do″luh·rol′uh·jee) *n.* The systematic study of the mechanisms and management of pain.

DOM 2,5-Dimethoxy-4-methylamphetamine, $C_{12}H_{20}NO_2$, a psychedelic agent, often abused and known colloquially as STP.

do·ma·to·pho·bia (do″muh·to·fo′bee·uh) *n.* Abnormal fear of being in a house; a variety of claustrophobia.

do·ma·zo·line (do″muh·zo′leen) *n.* 2-(3,6-Dimethoxy-2,4-dimethylbenzyl)-2-imidazoline, $C_{14}H_{20}N_2O_2$, an anticholinergic usually used as the fumarate salt.

dom·i·nance, *n.* 1. The state of being dominant. 2. *In biology,* the capacity of an allele of a gene for expression in the presence of a different allele which is not expressed. 3. *In psychiatry and psychology,* the disposition of one individual to play a prominent and controlling role in his relationship with another or other individuals.

dom·i·nant, *adj. & n.* 1. In any pattern or complex, the quality of being more important or prominent or of taking precedence. 2. DOMINANT CHARACTER.

dominant eye. The eye that is unconsciously and preferentially chosen to guide decision and action, as leading in reading and writing, or in sighting through a telescope.

dominant hemisphere. The cerebral hemisphere which controls certain motor activities, such as movements of speech; usually the left hemisphere in right-handed individuals. Syn. *categorical hemisphere.*

dom·i·na·tor, *n.* The receptive sense organ in light-adapted eyes representing the preponderant type, occurring in broad spectral response curves or absorption bands, having their maximum in the region of 5600 angstroms; it is regarded as responsible for the sensation of luminosity.

Do·nath-Land·stein·er test or **phenomenon** (do'nah^t) A test for paroxysmal hemoglobinuria based upon a thermolabile isohemolysin occurring in the blood of patients with paroxysmal hemoglobinuria. The cold hemolysin unites with the red cells at low temperatures and causes hemolysis after the cells are warmed to 37°C.

do·nee (do·nee') *n.* A patient who receives transfused blood or other tissues, as skin, bone, or cartilage, from a donor.

Don·nan equilibrium In a system in which a semipermeable membrane separates a solution of an electrolyte with diffusible ions, as sodium chloride, from one containing a salt NaR with a nondiffusible ion R^-, as proteinate, the product of the concentrations of diffusible ions on one side of the membrane is equal to the product of the concentrations of such ions on the other side of the membrane. Syn. *Gibbs-Donnan equilibrium.*

do·nor, *n.* A person who gives blood or other tissues and organs for use by another person.

donor area. An area, as of skin, from which a graft is taken.

Don·o·van bodies Chromatin masses at the ends of *Calymmatobacterium granulomatis* bacteria which give them the appearance of a closed safety pin.

Don·o·va·ni·a gran·u·lo·ma·tis (don-o-vay'nee-uh gran-yoo-lo'muh-tis) *CALYMMATOBACTERIUM GRANULOMATIS.*

do·pa (do'puh) *n.* DIHYDROXYPHENYLALANINE.

do·pa·man·tine (do''puh-man'teen) *n. N*-(3,4-Dihydroxyphenethyl)-1-adamantanecarboxamide, $C_{19}H_{25}NO_3$, an antiparkinsonian agent.

do·pa·mine (do'puh-meen) *n.* Hydroxytyramine, $C_8H_{11}NO_2$, the decarboxylation product of dopa; an intermediate in the biosynthesis of epinephrine and norepinephrine.

dopa oxidase. An enzyme of the skin that catalyzes the oxidation of dihydroxyphenylala-nine to melanin in the melanocytes of the epidermis, thus playing an important role in skin pigmentation.

dope, *n. & v.* 1. Any drug administered to stimulate or to stupefy, temporarily, or taken habitually. 2. To administer a narcotic, stimulant, or habit-forming drug.

dope addict. A person who has become psychologically and physiologically dependent on a narcotic or drug through habitual use.

Dopp·ler principle, phenomenon, or **effect** When a source of light or sound is moving rapidly, the wavelength appears to decrease as the object approaches the observer, or to increase as the object recedes; the pitch of sound becomes higher or lower.

do·ra·pho·bia (do''ruh-fo'bee-uh) *n.* Abnormal fear of touching the skin or fur of animals.

Doriden. Trademark for glutethimide, a hypnotic and sedative.

dor·mant (dor'munt) *adj.* Concealed; quiescent; inactive; potential.

do·ro·ma·nia (do''ro-may'nee-uh) *n.* An abnormal wish to give presents.

Dor·o·thy Reed cell REED-STERNBERG CELL.

dors-, dorsi-, dorso-. A combining form meaning (a) *of* or *on the back;* (b) *dorsal.*

Dorsacaine. Trademark for benoxinate, a surface anesthetic agent used as the hydrochloride salt.

dor·sad (dor'sad) *adv.* In a ventral-to-dorsal direction.

dor·sal (dor'sul) *adj.* 1. Pertaining to, situated at, or relatively near the back, that is, the "backbone side" of the trunk or the body as a whole; in human anatomy: POSTERIOR. 2. Pertaining to, situated at, or relatively near the back or dorsum of some part, such as a hand or foot. —**dorsal·ly** (·lee) *adv.*

dor·sal·gia (dor·sal'jee·uh) *n.* Pain in the back.

dorsal horn. The posterior column of gray matter in the spinal cord.

dor·sa·lis (dor·say'lis) *adj.* DORSAL.

dorsal motor nucleus of the vagus. The column of cells in the medulla oblongata in the floor of the fourth ventricle which gives origin to preganglionic parasympathetic fibers of the vagus nerve.

dorsal root ganglion. SPINAL GANGLION.

dor·si·flex·ion (dor''si·fleck'shun) *n.* Bending the foot toward the dorsum, or upper surface of the foot; opposed to plantar flexion. If used with reference to the toes, same as extension or straightening. —**dor·si·flex** (dor'si·flecks) *v.*

dor·si·flex·or (dor''si·fleck'sur) *n.* A muscle producing dorsiflexion.

dor·so·an·te·ri·or (dor''so·an·teer'ee·ur) *adj.* Characterizing the position of a fetus having its back toward the ventral aspect of the mother.

dor·so·ceph·a·lad (dor''so·sef'ul·ad) *adv.* Toward the dorsal aspect of the head.

dor·so·cu·boi·dal (dor''so·kew·boy'dul) *adj.* Pertaining to or situated on the dorsal aspect of the cuboid bone.

dor·so·lat·er·al (dor''so·lat'ur·ul) *adj.* Pertaining to or toward the back and the side.

dor·so·lum·bar (dor″so·lum′bur, ·bahr) adj. LUM-BODORSAL.

dor·so·me·di·al (dor″so·mee′dee·ul) adj. Pertaining to the back and toward the midline region of the back.

dor·so·me·di·an (dor″so·mee′dee·un) adj. Situated in or pertaining to the midline region of the back.

dor·so·pos·te·ri·or (dor″so·pos·teer′ee·ur) adj. Characterizing the position of a fetus having its back toward the dorsal aspect of the mother.

dor·so·ra·di·al (dor″so·ray′dee·ul) adj. Pertaining to or situated upon the dorsal aspect and radial border of the hand, finger, or forearm.

dor·so·sa·cral (dor″so·say′krul) adj. Pertaining to the dorsal and sacral regions.

dor·so·ul·nar (dor″so·ul′nur) adj. Pertaining to or situated upon the dorsal aspect and ulnar border of the arm, hand, or finger.

dor·so·ven·tral (dor″so·ven′trul) adj. Pertaining to the dorsal and ventral regions; extending in a direction from the dorsal surface toward the ventral.

dor·sum (dor′sum) n., genit. **dor·si** (dor′sigh), pl. **dor·sa** (·suh) 1. [NA] The back. 2. Any part analogous to the back, as the dorsum of the foot or hand.

dorsum sel·lae (sel′ee) [NA]. A quadrilateral plate of bone forming the posterior boundary of the sella turcica.

dos·age (do′sij) n. The proper amount of a medicine or other agent for a given patient or condition.

dose (doce) n. 1. A single prescribed, administered, or received portion or quantity of a therapeutic agent, as medicine or radiation. 2. In radiology, an administered quantity of radiation measured at a specific point, as: air dose, depth dose, exit dose, skin dose, and, especially, absorbed dose.

do·sim·e·ter (do·sim′e·tur) n. In radiology, an instrument for measuring exposure to x-rays or to radioactive emanations.

do·sim·e·try (do·sim′e·tree) n. 1. The accurate determination of medicinal doses. 2. The measurement of exposures or doses of x-rays, or of radioactive emanations. —**do·si·met·ric** (do″si·met′rick) adj.

double-blind experiment or **test.** An experiment or clinical investigation in which neither the subjects nor the investigator knows which kind of treatment is being given to each individual in order to obviate suggestion and bias of observation.

double knot. A knot in which the ends of the cord or suture are twisted twice around each other before tying. Syn. friction knot, surgeon's knot.

double pneumonia. Pneumonia involving both lungs.

double pupil. Polycoria in which there are two pupils. Syn. dicoria, diplocoria.

double refraction. The property of having more than one refractive index, according to the direction of the traversing light. It is possessed by all except isometric crystals, by transparent substances that have undergone internal strains (e.g., glass), and by substances that have different structures in different directions (e.g., fibers). Syn. birefringence.

douche (doosh) n. 1. A stream of water or air directed against the body or into a body cavity, commonly used on the body surface for its stimulating effect; may be hot, cold, or alternating. 2. In gynecology, lavage of the vagina; used for cleansing or for the application of heat or medication to the parts.

Down's syndrome A syndrome of congenital defects, especially mental retardation, typical facies responsible for the older descriptive term mongoloid idiocy, or mongolism, and cytogenetic abnormality consisting of trisomy 21 or its equivalent in the form of an unbalanced translocation.

dox·a·pram (dock′suh·pram) n. 1-Ethyl-4-(2-morpholinoethyl)-3,3-diphenyl-2-pyrrolidinone, $C_{24}H_{30}N_2O_2$, a respiratory and central stimulant; used as the hydrochloride salt.

dox·yl·a·mine (dock·sil′uh·meen) n. 2-[α-(2-Dimethylaminoethoxy)-α-methylbenzyl] pyridine, $C_{17}H_{22}N_2O$, an antihistaminic drug; used as the bisuccinate salt.

DPN Abbreviation for diphosphopyridine nucleotide, now called nicotinamide-adenine dinucleotide and abbreviated NAD.

drac·on·ti·a·sis (drack″on·tye′uh·sis) n. DRACUNCULIASIS.

dra·cun·cu·li·a·sis (dra·kunk″yoo·lye′uh·sis) n. Infection with the nematode Dracunculus medinensis; characterized by ulcers of the feet and legs produced by the gravid female worm; found in Africa, the Middle East, India, and Brazil. Syn. guinea worm infection.

dra·cun·cu·lo·sis (dra·kunk″yoo·lo′sis) n. DRACUNCULIASIS.

Dra·cun·cu·lus (dra·kunk′yoo·lus) n. A genus of threadworms belonging to the superfamily Dracunculoidea.

Dracunculus me·di·nen·sis (med·i·nen′sis). A species of filarial worm of which certain species of Cyclops are the intermediate hosts and man is a definitive host. Human infection is caused by drinking raw water containing infested Cyclops. Syn. guinea worm.

draft, draught (draft) n. 1. A current of air. 2. A quantity of liquid, usually medicine, taken at one swallow.

drain, n. & v. 1. A material, such as gauze, rubber tubing, rubber tissue, or twisted suture material, which affords a channel of exit for the discharge from a wound or cavity. 2. In surgery, to procure the discharge or evacuation of fluid from a cavity by operation, tapping, or otherwise.

drain·age, n. The method of draining; also, the fluid drained off.

dram, drachm (dram) n. 1. One-eighth of an apothecary ounce. Symbol, ℨ. 2. One-sixteenth of an avoirdupois ounce. Abbreviated, dr.

Dramamine. Trademark for dimenhydrinate, an antihistaminic and antinauseant drug.

dram·a·tism (dram′uh·tiz·um) n. Stilted and lofty speech or behavior, observed in some psychoses and neuroses.

dram·a·ti·za·tion, n. In psychoanalysis, the transformation of repressed desires into some symbolic form, usually into personifications.

drape, v. & n. 1. To cover a part with sterile sheets, so arranged as to leave exposed but protected the particular area to be examined or operated upon. 2. (plural) The sterile sheets or towels used to drape a part for examination or operation.

drap·e·to·ma·nia (drap''e·to·may'nee·uh) n. DROMOMANIA.

draw, v. & n. 1. To cause to soften and discharge; to cause to localize, said of a poultice. 2. The divergence of the walls of a dental cavity preparation that permits the seating and withdrawal of a wax pattern or an inlay.

draw-sheet, n. A narrow cloth sheet over a waterproof sheet, stretched across the center of the bed, which if soiled can be changed with minimal disturbance to the patient.

dream, n. & v. 1. An involuntary series of visual, auditory, or kinesthetic imagery, emotions, and thoughts occurring in the mind during sleep or a sleeplike state, which take the form of a sequence of events or of a story, have a feeling of reality, but totally lack a feeling of free will; believed by Freud to be a mental mechanism whereby impulses are conveyed from the unconscious to the conscious levels of mind. 2. To experience images and trains of thought during sleep, or as if asleep; to have a dream.

drench, n. 1. In veterinary medicine, the oral administration of a liquid medicinal agent to an animal. 2. The medicinal agent administered in that way.

drep·a·no·cyte (drep'uh·no·site, dre·pan'o·site) n. SICKLE CELL. —**drep·a·no·cyt·ic** (drep''uh·no·sit'ick) adj.

drepanocytic anemia. SICKLE CELL ANEMIA.

drep·a·no·cy·to·sis (drep''uh·no·sigh·to'sis, dre·pan''o·) n. The presence of sickle cells in blood.

dress·er, n. An attendant in British hospitals, usually a medical student, whose special duty is to dress and bandage wounds.

dress·ing, n. Material and medication applied to a wound or infection, and fastened in place to provide protection and to promote healing.

dressing combine. An incision or wound dressing consisting of an unwoven fabric cover which encloses absorbent material and a nonabsorbent layer of cotton or plastic to prevent fluid from passing through; designed to provide warmth and protection and absorb large quantities of fluid.

drib·ble, v. 1. To drool. 2. To void in drops, as urine from a distended or paralyzed bladder.

drill, n. A cutting instrument for excavating a tooth or bone by rotary motion.

Drinker respirator An iron lung, usually power driven, but also operated manually.

drip, n. & v. 1. The continuous slow introduction of fluid, usually containing nutrients or drugs. 2. To introduce fluid slowly.

drip treatment. The continuous infusion of fluid into the blood or a body cavity so slowly that the rate is measured in drops.

drive, n. 1. Instinct; basic urge; motivation. 2. In psychology and psychiatry, psychic phenomena such as the sexual or aggressive drives in contrast to the more purely biological and physical instincts. 3. In psychology, a hypothetical state of an organism necessary before a given stimulus will elicit a certain kind of response, as hunger must be present before the presence of food will elicit eating.

dromo·pho·bia (drom''o·fo'bee·uh) n. Morbid fear of walking or roaming about.

dromo·trop·ic (dro''mo·trop'ick, dromo''o·) adj. Affecting the speed and conduction of nerve fibers.

drool, v. 1. To let saliva flow out of the mouth, as seen normally in infants. 2. To secrete saliva profusely.

drop, n. 1. A minute mass of liquid which in falling or in hanging from a surface forms a spheroid. 2. Commonly, a volume of liquid equal to about 0.05 ml (approximately 1 minim). 3. A lozenge, as a cough drop. 4. In neurology, the falling of a part from paralysis, as a foot drop. 5. AKINETIC SEIZURE.

dro·per·i·dol (dro·perr'i·dol) n. 1-[1-[3-(p-Fluorobenzoyl)propyl]-1,2,3,6-tetrahydro-4-pyridyl]-2-benzimidazolinone, $C_{22}H_{22}FN_3O_2$, a tranquilizer and sedative.

drop·let, n. A minute particle of moisture, such as that expelled by talking, sneezing, or coughing, which may carry infectious microorganisms from one individual to another.

dropped beat. In second-degree heart block, an atrial deflection (P wave) not followed by a ventricular deflection (QRS complex).

dropped foot. A drop or plantar flexion of the foot, generally due to paralysis of the dorsiflexor muscles of the foot and toes.

drop·sy (drop'see) n. The abnormal accumulation of serous fluid in body tissues and cavities; ANASARCA. —**drop·si·cal** (·si·kul) adj.

Droptainer. A trademark for a plastic container which dispenses one drop of liquid when inverted and squeezed.

Dro·soph·i·la (dro·sof'i·luh) n. A genus of Diptera including common fruit flies.

Drosophila mel·a·no·gas·ter (mel'uh·no·gas''tur) The best known species of fruit fly because of its extensive use in genetic analysis.

Dr. P.H. Doctor of Public Health.

drug, n. & v. 1. Any substance other than food or water that is intended to be taken or administered (ingested, injected, applied, implanted, inhaled, etc.) for the purpose of altering, sustaining, or controlling the recipient's physical, mental, or emotional state. 2. In United States law, any article, other than a food or a device, that is intended for use in the diagnosis, cure, mitigation, treatment, or prevention of disease, or is intended to affect the structure or any function of the body of man or other animals, or is recognized in one or more of the official compendia which provide standards for the evaluation of such articles. 3. To administer a drug to; especially, to NARCOTIZE.

drug-fast, adj. Of microorganisms: resistant to antimicrobial drugs. —**drug-fast·ness,** n.

drug fever. Fever resulting from the administration of a drug.

drug·gist (drug'ist) n. A dealer in medicines.

drum, n. TYMPANIC MEMBRANE.

drunk·ard's arm paralysis. Paralysis due to compression of the radial nerve against the humerus during sleep, or when the arm is hung over the edge of a chair or bench during alcoholic stupor.

drunk·en·ness, n. INTOXICATION (2); especially as produced by drinking alcoholic liquor.

dru·sen (droo'zun) n. pl. 1. Colloid excrescences on the basal membrane. 2. Granules found in tissues in actinomycosis.

dry, adj. 1. Not wet; free from moisture or excess moisture; as dry heat sterilization, dry sponge. 2. Not accompanied by obvious bleeding; as dry operative wound. 3. Not accompanied by mucus or phlegm; as dry rales. 4. Marked by scantiness of effusions or secretions. 5. Dehydrated; as dry tissues.

dry gangrene. Local death of a part due to arterial obstruction without infection. Syn. mummification.

dry labor. Labor in which there is a deficiency of the liquor amnii, or in which there has been a premature rupture of the amniotic sac.

dry tap. A tap in which no fluid can be obtained.

Dryvax. A trademark for smallpox vaccine.

D. Sc., D. S. Doctor of Science.

D-state. REM SLEEP.

DTPA Tc 99m The diethylenetetraminepentaacetic acid chelate of technetium 99m, employed as a diagnostic agent for brain or kidney visualization and for vascular dynamic studies.

D.T.R. Abbreviation for deep tendon reflex.

du·al, adj. Consisting of two parts.

Du·bin-John·son syndrome A dominantly inherited defect in liver function in which icterus and hepatic pigmentation are associated with retention of conjugated bilirubin.

Du·bo·witz method A method, based on neurological function and maturity of skin, ears, genitalia, and other aspects of appearance, for estimating the gestational age of the newborn.

duck embryo vaccine. Vaccine prepared in duck embryos for use as active immunization following exposure to rabies.

duct, n. 1. A tube or channel, especially one for conveying the secretions of a gland. 2. Any enclosed channel conducting any fluid, as the cochlear duct. —**duc·tal** (duck'tul) adj.

duc·tile (duck'til, -tile) adj. Capable of being reshaped or drawn out without breaking.

duc·tion (duck'shun) n. The rotation of the eye around the horizontal axis or the vertical axis.

duc·tu·lar (duck'tew-lur) adj. Pertaining to a ductule.

duc·tule (duck'tewl) n. A small duct.

duc·tu·lus (duck'tew-lus) n., pl. **ductu·li** (-lye) [NA]. DUCTULE.

duc·tus (duck'tus) n., pl. & genit. sing. **ductus** (duck'tooss, duck'tus) DUCT.

ductus ar·te·ri·o·sus (ahr-teer''ee-o'sus) [NA]. The distal half of the left sixth aortic arch forming a fetal blood shunt between the left pulmonary artery and the aorta. Syn. Botallo's duct.

ductus cho·le·do·chus (ko-led'o-kus) [NA]. COMMON BILE DUCT.

ductus de·fe·rens (def'uh-renz), pl. **ductus de·fe·ren·tes** (def-e-ren'teez) [NA]. The portion of the excretory duct system of the testis which runs from the epididymal duct to the ejaculatory duct. Syn. deferent duct, vas deferens.

ductus epo·o·pho·ri lon·gi·tu·di·na·lis (ep''o-of'o-rye lon''ji·tew-di·nay'lis) [NA]. The vestigial remnant of the mesonephric duct.

ductus ve·no·sus (ve·no'sus) [NA]. A venous channel of the embryonic liver shunting blood from the left umbilical vein to the enlarging right sinus venosus of the heart. Syn. duct of Arantius.

du·ip·a·ra (dew·ip'uh·ruh) n. A woman who has given birth twice.

Duke test or **method** A test for bleeding time, performed by puncturing the lobe of the ear and determining the time which elapses until bleeding stops.

dul·cin (dul'sin) n. p-Phenetolcarbamide or 4-ethoxyphenylurea, $C_9H_{12}N_2O_2$, a crystalline substance, very sweet, that has been employed as a noncaloric sweetening agent but may be toxic on prolonged use.

dul·ci·tol (dul'si·tol) n. A sugar, $C_6H_{14}O_6$, found in a variety of plants.

Dulcolax. Trademark for bisacodyl, a laxative drug.

dull, adj. 1. Slow of perception; not clear of mind. 2. Not resonant on percussion; muffled. 3. Not bright in appearance. 4. Not sharp; blunt. —**dull·ness,** n.

dumb, adj. 1. MUTE. 2. Colloq. Stupid; lacking in intelligence. —**dumb·ness** n.

dumb·bell, n. 1. A weight consisting of two identical spheres connected by a short rod. 2. Something shaped like a dumbbell.

dum·my, n. 1. PONTIC. 2. British term for PLACEBO.

dump·ing, n. A sudden, rapid emptying.

dumping syndrome or **stomach.** Disagreeable or painful epigastric fullness, nausea, weakness, giddiness, sweating, palpitations, and diarrhea occurring after meals in patients who have had gastric surgery which interferes with the function of the pylorus.

duo- A combining form meaning two.

duoden-, duodeno-. A combining form meaning duodenum, duodenal.

du·o·de·nal (dew''o-dee'nul, dew-od'e-nul) adj. Of or pertaining to the duodenum.

duodenal bulb or **cap.** In radiology, the first part of the duodenum, immediately beyond the pylorus.

duodenal ulcer. A peptic ulcer situated in the duodenum.

du·o·de·nec·ta·sis (dew''o-de-neck'tuh-sis) n., pl. **duodenecta·ses** (-seez) Chronic dilatation of the duodenum.

du·o·de·nec·to·my (dew''o-de-neck'tuh-mee) n. Excision of part of the duodenum.

du·o·de·ni·tis (dew''o-de-nigh'tis) n. Inflammation of the duodenum.

du·o·de·no·chol·an·gi·tis (dew''o-dee''no-kol''an-jye'tis) n. Inflammation of the duodenum and the common bile duct.

du·o·de·no·chol·e·cys·tos·to·my (dew″o·dee″no·kol″e·sis·tos′tuh·mee) n. The formation of an anastomosis between the duodenum and gallbladder.

du·o·de·no·cho·led·o·chot·o·my (dew″o·dee″no·ko·led″o·kot′uh·mee) n. A modification of choledochotomy by incising the duodenum in order to approach the common duct.

du·o·de·no·col·ic (dew″o·dee″no·kol′ick, ·ko′lick) adj. Pertaining to the duodenum and the colon, as: duodenocolic fistula.

du·o·de·no·cys·tos·to·my (dew″o·dee″no·sis·tos′tuh·mee) n. DUODENOCHOLECYSTOSTOMY.

du·o·de·no·en·ter·os·to·my (dew″o·dee″no·en″tur·os′tuh·mee) n. In surgery, the formation of a passage between the duodenum and another part of the intestine.

du·o·de·nog·ra·phy (dew″o·de·nog′ruh·fee) n. Radiographic depiction of the duodenum using contrast material.

du·o·de·no·he·pat·ic (dew″o·dee″no·he·pat′ick) adj. Pertaining to the duodenum and the liver.

du·o·de·no·il·e·os·to·my (dew″o·dee″no·il″ee·os′tuh·mee) n. The formation of a passage between the duodenum and the ileum.

du·o·de·no·je·ju·nal (dew″o·dee″no·je·joo′nul) adj. Pertaining to the duodenum and the jejunum.

duodenojejunal flexure. The abrupt bend at the junction of the duodenum and jejunum.

du·o·de·no·je·ju·nos·to·my (dew″o·dee″no·jej″oo·nos′tuh·mee) n. In surgery, an anastomosis of the duodenum to the jejunum.

du·o·de·no·pan·cre·a·tec·to·my (dew″o·dee″no·pan″kree·uh·teck′tuh·mee) n. In surgery, excision of a portion of the duodenum together with the head of the pancreas.

du·o·de·no·plas·ty (dew″o·dee′no·plas″tee) n. A reparative operation upon some portion of the duodenum.

du·o·de·no·py·lo·rec·to·my (dew″o·dee″no·pye″lo·reck′tuh·mee) n. Resection of a portion of the duodenum and the pylorus.

du·o·de·nor·rha·phy (dew″o·de·nor′uh·fee) n. The suture and repair of the duodenum after incision, as for the closure of a ruptured duodenal ulcer.

du·o·de·nos·co·py (dew″o·de·nos′kuh·pee) n. Inspection and visual examination of the duodenum by instrumental means, as by a fiberoptic endoscope.

du·o·de·nos·to·my (dew″o·de·nos′tuh·mee) n. In surgery, the formation, temporarily, of a duodenal fistula.

du·o·de·not·o·my (dew″o·de·not′uh·mee) n. In surgery, incision of the duodenum.

du·o·de·num (dew·o·dee′num, dew·od′e·num) n., pl. **duode·na** (·nuh), **duodenums** The first part of the small intestine, beginning at the pylorus. It is 8 to 10 inches long and is the most fixed part of the small intestine; consists of superior, descending, and inferior portions, and contains the openings of the pancreatic duct or ducts and the common bile duct.

Duotal. A trademark for guaiacol carbonate, an expectorant.

du·plex (dew′plecks) adj. Having two parts.

du·pli·ca·tion, n. 1. The doubling of any structure which normally occurs singly. 2. In genetics, the occurrence of a segment of a chromosome in duplicate.

du·pli·ca·ture (dew′pli·kuh·chur, ·kay″chur) n. A fold, as a membrane folding upon itself.

du·plic·i·tas (dew·plis′i·tus, ·tahs) n. In teratology, an individual with duplication of either the cephalic or pelvic end, or both.

du·plic·i·ty (dew·plis′i·tee) n. In teratology, the condition of being double. Syn. duplexity.

Du·puy·tren's contracture (due͡·pwˈee·trænᵗ) A painless, chronic contracture of the hand, marked by thickening of the digital processes and of the palmar fascia and inability fully to extend the fingers, especially the third and fourth fingers. The disease is of uncertain etiology, and affects chiefly adult males.

du·ra (dew′ruh) n. DURA MATER.

Duracillin. A trademark for procaine penicillin G.

du·ral (dew′rul) adj. Pertaining to or involving the dura mater.

dural sheath. A strong fibrous membrane forming the external investment of the optic nerve.

dural sinus. SINUS OF THE DURA MATER.

du·ra ma·ter (dew′ruh may′tur, mah′tur) The fibrous membrane forming the outermost covering of the brain and spinal cord.

du·ra·plas·ty (dew′ruh·plas″tee) n. Repair of defects in the dura mater.

du·ro·ar·ach·ni·tis (dew″ro·ār″ack·nigh′tis) n. Inflammation of the dura mater and arachnoid membrane.

dust cell. ALVEOLAR MACROPHAGE; especially, one containing carbon or dust particles.

dust count. The number of particles of dust in a given atmosphere, usually expressed as the number of particles less than 10 microns in diameter per cubic foot of air when counted by the light field method. Used chiefly in evaluation of silicosis hazards in industry.

D.V.M. Doctor of Veterinary Medicine.

D.V.M.S. Doctor of Veterinary Medicine and Surgery.

D.V.S. 1. Doctor of Veterinary Science. 2. Doctor of Veterinary Surgery.

dwarf, n., adj., & v. 1. An abnormally small individual; especially, one whose bodily proportions are altered, as in achondroplasia. 2. Being an atypically small form or variety of something. 3. To prevent normal growth.

dwarf·ism, n. Abnormal underdevelopment of the body; the condition of being dwarfed.

dwarf tapeworm. HYMENOLEPIS NANA.

dwt Symbol for pennyweight.

Dx Symbol for diagnosis.

Dy Symbol for dysprosium.

dy·ad (dye′ad) n. 1. A pair or a couple. 2. One of the groups of paired chromosomes formed by the division of a tetrad during the first meiotic division. 3. In chemistry, a divalent element or radical.

Dyclone. Trademark for dyclonine, a topical anesthetic used as the hydrochloride salt.

dy·clo·nine (dye·klo′neen) n. 4′-Butoxy-3-piperidinopropiophenone, $C_{18}H_{27}NO_2$, a topical anesthetic; used as the hydrochloride salt.

dye test. A test for Toxoplasma antibodies

which, in the presence of a complement-like accessory factor, prevent the staining of *Toxoplasma* by alkaline methylene blue.

Dymelor. Trademark for acetohexamide, an oral hypoglycemic.

dynam-, dynamo- A combining form meaning *power, energy,* or *motion.*

dy·nam·ic (dye·nam'ick, di·nam'ick) *adj.* 1. Characterized by energy or great force. 2. Moving; changing; pertaining to motion or process.

dynamic ileus. SPASTIC ILEUS.

dy·nam·ics, *n.* The science that treats of matter in motion.

dy·na·mo, *n.* A machine for converting mechanical energy into electric energy by means of coils of insulated wire revolving through magnetic fields of force.

dy·na·mo·gen·e·sis (dye″nuh·mo·jen'e·sis) *n.* The generation of power, force, or energy.

dy·na·mo·graph (dye·nam'o·graf) *n.* An instrument designed to measure and graphically record muscular strength. —**dy·na·mog·ra·phy** (dye″nuh·mog'ruh·fee) *n.*

dy·na·mom·e·ter (dye″nuh·mom'e·tur) *n.* An instrument for measuring muscular strength, particularly of the hand.

dyne (dine) *n.* The amount of force which, when acting continuously on a mass of one gram for one second, will accelerate the mass one centimeter per second.

dys- A prefix meaning (a) *abnormal, diseased;* (b) *difficult, painful;* (c) *faulty, impaired;* (d) in biology, *unlike.*

dys·acou·sia, dys·acu·sia (dis″uh·koo'zhuh, ·zee·uh) *n.* 1. A condition in which pain or discomfort is caused by loud or even moderately loud noises. 2. The condition of being hard-of-hearing.

dys·ad·ap·ta·tion (dis·ad″ap·tay'shun) *n. In ophthalmology,* inability of the iris and retina to accommodate to variable intensities of light.

dys·an·ti·graph·ia (dis·an″tee·graf'ee·uh) *n.* A form of agraphia in which there is inability to copy writing or print.

dys·aphea (dis·ay'fee·uh, ·af'ee·uh) *n.* Disordered sense of touch.

dys·ar·te·ri·ot·o·ny (dis″ahr·teer″ee·ot'uh·nee) *n.* Abnormal blood pressure.

dys·ar·thria (dis·ahr'three·uh) *n.* Impairment of articulation caused by any disorder or lesion affecting the tongue or speech muscles. —**dys·ar·thric** (·thrick) *adj.*

dys·ar·thro·sis (dis″ahr·thro'sis) *n.,* pl. **disarthro·ses** (seez) 1. Deformity, dislocation, or disease of a joint. 2. PSEUDARTHROSIS. 3. DYSARTHRIA.

dys·au·to·no·mia (dis·aw″to·no'mee·uh) *n.* 1. Any dysfunction of the autonomic nervous system. 2. FAMILIAL DYSAUTONOMIA.

dys·bar·ism (dis·bar'iz·um) *n.* 1. Any disorder caused by excessive pressure differences between a tissue or part of the body and its surroundings. 2. Specifically, DECOMPRESSION SICKNESS.

dys·ba·sia (dis·bay'zhuh, ·zee·uh) *n.* Difficulty in walking; particularly when due to a nervous system disorder.

dys·bu·lia, dys·bou·lia (dis·boo'lee·uh) *n.* Impairment of will power.

dys·chei·ria, dys·chi·ria (dis·kigh'ree·uh) *n.* Inability to tell which side of the body is touched, though sensation of touch is not lost; partial allocheiria.

dys·che·zia (dis·kee'zee·uh) *n.* Painful or difficult defecation.

dys·chon·dro·pla·sia (dis·kon″dro·play'zhuh, ·zee·uh) *n.* ENCHONDROMATOSIS.

dys·chroia (dis·kroy'uh) *n.* Discoloration of the skin; a bad complexion.

dys·chro·nous (dis'kruh·nus) *adj.* Not agreeing as to time. —**dys·chro·na·tion** (dis″kro·nay'shun) *n.*

dys·co·ria (dis·ko'ree·uh) *n.* Abnormality of the form of the pupil.

dys·cra·sia (dis·kray'zhuh, ·zee·uh) *n.* 1. An abnormal state or disorder of the body. 2. Formerly, an abnormal mixture of the four humors of the body. —**dys·cra·sic** (·kray'zick), **dys·crat·ic** (krat'ick) *adj.*

dys·cri·nism (dis·krye'niz·um) *n.* DYSENDOCRINISM.

dys·di·ad·o·cho·ki·ne·sia, dys·di·ad·o·ko·ki·ne·sia (dis″dye·ad″o·ko·ki·nee'zhuh, ·zee·uh) *n.* Impairment of the power to perform alternating movements in rapid, smooth, and rhythmic succession, such as pronation and supination; a sign of cerebellar disease, but also seen in the so-called clumsy child with minimal brain damage.

dys·eco·ia (dis″e·koy'uh) *n.* DYSACOUSIA (2).

dys·eme·sia (dis″e·mee'zhuh, ·zee·uh) *n.* Painful vomiting; retching.

dys·emia, dys·ae·mia (dis·ee'mee·uh) *n.* Any disease of the blood.

dys·en·doc·rin·ism (dis″en·dock'rin·iz·um, dis·en″do·krin·iz·um) *n.* Any abnormality in the function of the endocrine glands. —**dys·en·do·crine** (dis·en'do·krin) *adj.*

dys·en·tery (dis'un·terr″ee) *n.* Inflammation of the intestine, particularly the colon, of varied causation, associated with abdominal pain, tenesmus, and diarrhea with blood and mucus. —**dys·en·ter·ic** (dis″un·terr'ick) *adj.*

dys·er·ga·sia (dis″ur·gay'zhuh, ·zee·uh) *n. In psychobiology,* a mental disturbance due to toxic factors which are capable of producing delirium, such as uremia or alcohol.

dys·es·the·sia, dys·aes·the·sia (dis″esth·ee'zhuh, ·zee·uh) *n.* 1. Impairment but not absence of the senses, especially of the sense of touch. 2. Painfulness or disagreeableness of any sensation not normally painful.

dys·flu·en·cy (dis·floo'un·see) *n.* Impairment of speech fluency, such as slow, halting delivery, difficulties in enunciation, or disordered rhythm, as seen in certain types of aphasia. —**dysflu·ent,** *adj.*

dys·func·tion (dis·funk'shun) *n.* Any abnormality or impairment of function, as of an organ.

dys·ga·lac·tia (dis″ga·lack'tee·uh, ·shee·uh) *n.* Loss or impairment of milk secretion.

dys·gam·ma·glob·u·li·ne·mia (dis″gam·muh·glob″yoo·li·nee'mee·uh) *n.* Any abnormality, quantitative or qualitative, of serum gamma globulins.

dys·gen·e·sis (dis·jen'e·sis) *n.*, pl. **dysgene·ses** (·seez) 1. Abnormal development of anything, usually of an organ or individual. 2. Impairment or loss of the ability to procreate.

dys·gen·ic (dis·jen'ick) *adj.* Detrimental to the hereditary constitution of a population.

dys·ger·mi·no·ma (dis·jur''mi·no'nuh) *n.* An ovarian tumor composed of large polygonal cells of germ-cell origin, resembling seminoma of the testis, but less malignant. Syn. *embryoma of the ovary.*

dys·geu·sia (dis·joo'zee·uh, ·see·uh) *n.* Abnormality, impairment, or perversion of the sense of taste.

dys·glan·du·lar (dis·glan'dew·lur) *adj.* Pertaining to any abnormality in the function of glands, particularly the glands of internal secretion.

dys·glob·u·li·ne·mia, dys·glob·u·li·nae·mia (dis·glob''yoo·li·nee'mee·uh) *n.* Any qualitative or quantitative abnormality of blood globulins.

dys·gnath·ic (dis·nath'ick, ·nay'thick) *adj.* Pertaining to jaws with improper development and in poor relation to each other.

dys·gno·sia (dis·no'zhuh, ·zee·uh) *n.* Disorder or distortion of intellectual function.

dys·graph·ia (dis·graf'ee·uh) *n.* Impairment of the power of writing as a result of a brain lesion.

dys·hi·dro·sis (dis·hi·dro'sis) *n.*, pl. **dishidro·ses** (·seez) 1. Any disturbance in sweat production or excretion. 2. CHEIROPOMPHOLYX. —**dyshidros·i·form** (·dros'i·form) *adj.*

dys·hor·ia (dis·hor'ee·uh) *n.* Any abnormality of vascular permeability. —**dyshor·ic** (·ick) *adj.*

dys·kar·y·o·sis (dis·kar''ee·o'sis) *n.* In *exfoliative cytology,* nuclear abnormalities, especially enlargement, hyperchromatism, irregularity in nuclear shape, and increased number of nuclei per cell without significant change in the cytoplasm or outline of the cell. —**dyskar·y·ot·ic** (·ee·ot'ick) *adj.*

dys·ker·a·to·sis (dis·kerr''uh·to'sis) *n.*, pl. **dysker·ato·ses** (·seez) 1. Imperfect keratinization of individual epidermal cells. 2. Keratinization of corneal epithelium. —**dyskera·tot·ic** (·tot'ick) *adj.*

dys·ki·ne·sia (dis''ki·nee'zhuh, ·zee·uh, dis''kigh'nee') *n.* 1. Any abnormal or disordered movement, particularly those seen in disorders affecting the extrapyramidal system as in parkinsonism or phenothiazine intoxication. 2. Impairment of the power of voluntary motion, resulting in partial movements. —**dyski·net·ic** (·net'ick) *adj.*

dys·la·lia (dis·lay'lee·uh, dis·lal'ee·uh) *n.* Impairment of the power of speaking, due to a defect of the organs of speech, especially the tongue.

dys·lex·ia (dis·leck'see·uh) *n.* Impairment of the ability to read, particularly in an individual who once knew how or is normally expected to know how to read. —**dys·lex·ic** (dis·leck'sick) *adj.* & *n.*

dys·lo·gia (dis·lo'jee·uh) *n.* 1. Difficulty in the expression of ideas by speech. 2. Impairment of reasoning or of the faculty to think logically.

dys·ma·se·sis (dis''ma·see'sis) *n.* Difficulty in chewing.

dys·me·lia (dis·mee'lee·uh) *n.* Congenital malformation or absence of a limb or limbs.

dys·men·or·rhea, dys·men·or·rhoea (dis·men''o·ree'uh) *n.* Difficult or painful menstruation.

dys·met·ria (dis·met'ree·uh) *n.* Inability to control accurately the range of movement in muscular acts, as observed in cerebellar lesions, with resultant overshooting of a mark; said particularly of hand movements.

dys·mim·ia (dis·mim'ee·uh) *n.* Impairment of the power to use signs and gestures as a means of expression; inability to imitate.

dys·mne·sia (dis·nee'zhuh, ·zee·uh) *n.* An impaired or defective memory.

dys·mor·phia (dis·mor'fee·uh) *n.* Deformity; abnormal shape.

dys·mor·phol·o·gy (dis''mor·fol'uh·jee) *n.* 1. Abnormal structure, especially as seen in congenital malformations. 2. The study and treatment of such abnormalities.

dys·mor·pho·pho·bia (dis·mor''fo·fo'bee·uh) *n.* Morbid fear of being deformed.

dys·my·e·lino·gen·ic (dis·migh''e·lin·o·jen'ick) *adj.* Characterizing or pertaining to any process that interferes with myelinization.

dys·odon·ti·a·sis (dis''o·don·tye'uh·sis, ·tee'uh·sis) *n.* Difficult or painful dentition.

dys·on·to·gen·e·sis (dis·on''to·jen'e·sis) *n.* Defective embryonic development of any tissue or organ. —**dys·on·to·ge·net·ic** (dis·on''to·je·net'ick) *adj.*

dys·orex·ia (dis''o·reck'see·uh) *n.* A disordered, diminished, or unnatural appetite.

dys·os·mia (dis·oz'mee·uh) *n.* Impairment of the sense of smell.

dys·os·to·sis (dis''os·to'sis) *n.*, pl. **dysosto·ses** (·seez) Defective formation of bone.

dys·para·thy·roid·ism (dis·păr''uh·thigh'roid·iz·um) *n.* Any disorder of parathyroid gland function.

dys·pa·reu·nia (dis''puh·roo'nee·uh) *n.* Painful or difficult sexual intercourse.

dys·pep·sia (dis·pep'see·uh, ·shuh) *n.* Disturbed digestion.

dys·pep·tic (dis·pep'tick) *adj.* Pertaining to or affected with dyspepsia.

dys·per·i·stal·sis (dis''perr·i·stal'sis, ·stahl'sis) *n.* Violent or abnormal peristalsis.

dys·pha·gia (dis·fay'jee·uh) *n.* Difficulty in swallowing, or inability to swallow.

dysphagia con·stric·ta (kun·strick'tuh) Difficulty in swallowing due to stenosis of the pharynx or esophagus.

dysphagia lu·so·ria (lew·so'ree·uh) Difficulty in swallowing due to compression of the esophagus by a persistent right aortic arch, a double aortic arch, or an anomalous right subclavian artery.

dys·phag·ic (dis·faj'ick) *adj.* Pertaining to or characterized by dysphagia.

dys·pha·sia (dis·fay'zhuh, ·zee·uh) *n.* Any aphasia which does not produce complete abolition of the facility to use language.

dys·phe·mia (dis·fee'mee·uh) *n.* STAMMERING.

dys·phoi·te·sis (dis''foy·tee'sis) *n.* Any learning disorder primarily neurophysiologic in character, and not due to mental retardation or to emotional and personality disturbances; often used in a specific sense, such as reading, calculation, graphic, or direction-sense dysphoitesis.

dys·pho·nia (dis·fo'nee·uh) *n.* An impairment of the voice.

dys·pho·ria (dis·fo'ree·uh) *n.* 1. The condition of not feeling well or of being ill at ease. 2. Morbid impatience and restlessness; anxiety; fidgetiness. 3. Physical discomfort. —**dys·phor·ic** (·for'ick) *adj.*

dys·pho·tia (dis·fo'shuh, ·shee·uh) *n.* MYOPIA.

dys·pi·tu·i·ta·rism (dis''pi·tew'i·tuh·riz·um) *n.* A condition due to abnormal function of the pituitary gland.

dys·pla·sia (dis·play'zhuh, ·zee·uh) *n.* 1. Abnormal development or growth, especially of cells. 2. The extent to which an individual presents different components (somatotypes) in different bodily regions, expressed quantitatively by regarding the body as made up of a specific number of regions and somatotyping each. They may be endomorphic, mesomorphic, or ectomorphic. Syn. *d component.*

dysplasia epi·phys·i·a·lis mul·ti·plex (ep''i·fiz·ee·ay'lis mul'ti·plecks). A rare congenital developmental disorder characterized by irregular ossification of several of the developing epiphyses, resulting in dwarfism, joint deformities, and short thick digits.

dys·plas·tic (dis·plas'tick) *adj.* Pertaining to or affected with dysplasia.

dys·pnea, dys·pnoea (disp·nee'uh, dis·nee'uh) *n.* Difficult or labored breathing. —**dys·pne·al** (·nee'ul), **dyspne·ic** (·ick) *adj.*

dys·po·ne·sis (dis''po·nee'sis) *n.* A physiopathologic state made up of errors in energy expenditure within the nervous system. —**dyspo·net·ic** (·net'ick) *adj.*

dys·prax·ia (dis·prack'see·uh) *n.* Disturbance in the ability to carry out skilled voluntary movements. —**dys·prac·tic** (dis·prack'tick) *adj.*

dys·pro·si·um (dis·pro'zee·um, ·see·um) *n.* Dy = 162.50. A rare-earth metal.

dys·pros·o·dy (dis·pros'uh·dee) *n.* Distortion or obliteration of the normal rhythm and melody of speech, as seen in certain types of aphasia.

dys·ra·phism (dis'ra·fiz·um) *n.* Defective raphe formation; defective fusion.

dys·rhyth·mia (dis·rith'mee·uh) *n.* Disordered rhythm, especially of brainwaves or of speech.

dys·so·cial (dis·so'shul) *adj. In psychiatry,* pertaining to behavior which is in manifest disregard of existing social codes and patterns, and often in conflict with them, but which is not due to a psychiatric disorder.

dys·som·nia (dis·som'nee·uh) *n.* Any disorder of sleep mechanisms.

dys·sper·ma·tism (dis·spur'muh·tiz·um) *n.* 1. Occurrence of pain or discomfort in discharge of seminal fluid. 2. Any disturbance in the formation of normal spermatozoa.

dys·sta·sia (dis·stay'see·uh, ·zee·uh) *n.* Difficulty in standing. —**dys·stat·ic** (·stat'ick) *adj.*

dys·syn·chro·nous (dis·sin'kruh·nus) *adj.* Characterized by a lack of synchronism; pertaining especially to children with the minimal brain dysfunction syndrome.

dys·syn·er·gia (dis''sin·ur'jee·uh) *n.* Faulty coordination of groups of organs or muscles normally acting in unison; particularly, the abnormal state of muscle antagonism in cerebellar disease.

dys·syn·er·gy (dis·sin'ur·jee) *n.* DYSSYNERGIA.

dys·tax·ia (dis·tack'see·uh) *n.* Complete or partial ataxia.

dys·the·sia (dis·theezh'uh, ·theez'ee·uh) *n.* Impatience; fretfulness; ill temper in the sick. —**dys·thet·ic** (·thet'ick) *adj.*

dys·thy·mia (dis·thigh'mee·uh, ·thim'ee·uh) *n.* 1. Any condition due to malfunction of the thymus during childhood. 2. *In psychiatry,* any despondent mood or depressive tendency, often associated with hypochondriasis. 3. Any abnormality of mentation.

dys·tith·ia (dis·tith'ee·uh) *n.* Difficulty of nursing or inability to nurse at the breast.

dys·to·cia (dis·to'shuh, ·see·uh) *n.* Difficult labor. —**dysto·cic** (·sick) *adj.*

dys·to·nia (dis·to'nee·uh) *n.* Disorder or lack of muscle tonicity. —**dys·ton·ic** (·ton'ick) *adj.*

dys·to·pia (dis·to'pee·uh) *n.* Displacement or malposition of any organ. —**dys·top·ic** (·top'ick) *adj.*

dys·tro·phia (dis·tro'fee·uh) *n.* DYSTROPHY.

dys·troph·ic (dis·trof'ick) *adj.* Pertaining to or characterized by dystrophy.

dys·tro·phy (dis'truh·fee) *n.* 1. Defective nutrition. 2. Defective or abnormal development; degeneration. 3. Specifically, MUSCULAR DYSTROPHY.

dys·uria (dis·yoo·ree'uh) *n.* Pain or burning on urination.

E

E. Abbreviation for (a) *eye*; (b) *emmetropia*; (c) *einstein*.

e Symbol for electron.

EAE Abbreviation for *experimental allergic encephalomyelitis*.

Ea·gle's media A variety of tissue culture media containing various vitamins, amino acids, inorganic salts and serous enrichments, and dextrose.

Eagle test 1. A complement-fixation test for syphilis. 2. A flocculation test for syphilis.

ear, *n.* The organ of hearing, consisting of the external ear, the middle ear, and the internal ear or labyrinth.

ear·ache, *n.* Pain in the ear; otalgia.

ear·drum, *n.* 1. TYMPANIC MEMBRANE. 2. MIDDLE EAR.

ear·lobe, *n.* The pendulous, fleshy lower portion of the auricle or external ear.

early syphilis. Primary, secondary, or latent acquired syphilitic infection of less than four years' duration.

ear·plug, *n.* A device made of rubber, cotton, or other pliable material, for insertion into the outer ear for protection against water or loud noises.

earth wax. CERESIN.

ear·wax, *n.* CERUMEN.

east·ern equine encephalitis. EASTERN EQUINE ENCEPHALITIS.

Ea·ton agent or **virus.** *MYCOPLASMA PNEUMONIAE.*

Eaton agent pneumonia. PRIMARY ATYPICAL PNEUMONIA (1).

Eber·thel·la (ee″bur·thel′uh, ay″bur′·) *n.* SALMONELLA.

Eb·ner's glands The serous glands opening into the trenches of the vallate papillae of the tongue.

ébran·le·ment (ay·brahn·luh·mahn′, F. eᵞ·brahⁿl·mahⁿ′) *n.* The removal of a polyp by twisting it until its pedicle ruptures.

Eb·stein's anomaly or **malformation** (ep′shtine) A symptomatic congenital anomaly of the tricuspid valve in which the septal and posterior leaflets are attached to the right ventricular wall, thus atrializing part of the right ventricle, producing a large right atrium and small ventricle, and sometimes causing obstruction to right ventricular outflow or filling; arrhythmias, cyanosis, and heart failure are common manifestations.

Ebstein's disease 1. ARMANNI-EBSTEIN LESION. 2. EBSTEIN'S ANOMALY.

ebur (ee′bur) *n.* A tissue similar to ivory in appearance or structure.

eb·ur·na·tion (ee″bur·nay′shun, eb″ur·) *n.* An increase in the density of tooth or bone following some pathologic change. —**eb·ur·nat·ed** (ee′bur·nay·tid, eb′ur·) *adj.*

EBV Abbreviation for *Epstein-Barr virus*.

EB virus. EPSTEIN-BARR VIRUS.

ec·bol·ic (eck·bol′ick) *adj. & n.* 1. Producing abortion or accelerating labor. 2. A drug that produces abortion or accelerates labor.

ec·cen·tric (eck·sen′trick) *adj. & n.* 1. Proceeding or situated away from the center or median line. 2. Deviating from the usual, normal, or generally expected behavior or reaction. 3. An individual whose behavioral patterns are generally unconventional or odd, but not necessarily symptomatic of a mental disorder. —**ec·centri·cal·ly** (·trick·lee) *adv.*

eccentric occlusion. The relation of the inclined planes of the teeth when the jaws are closed in any of the excursive movements of the mandible.

ec·cen·tro·cyte (eck·sen′tro·site) *n.* An erythrocyte with hemoglobin concentrated at the periphery.

ec·chon·dro·ma (eck″on·dro′muh) *n.* A nodular outgrowth from cartilage at the junction of cartilage and bone.

ec·chon·dro·sis (eck″on·dro′sis) *n.,* pl. **ecchondroses** (·seez) A cartilaginous outgrowth.

ec·chy·mo·sis (eck″i·mo′sis) *n.,* pl. **ecchymoses** (·seez) 1. Extravasation of blood into the subcutaneous tissues, discoloring the skin. 2. Any extravasation of blood into soft tissue. —**ec·chy·mot·ic** (·mot′ick) *adj.*

ec·crine (eck′rin, ·rine, ·reen) *adj.* 1. Of sweat

glands: MEROCRINE. 2. Of or pertaining to the eccrine glands or their secretion.

eccrine glands. The small sweat glands distributed all over the human body surface. Histologically, they are tubular coiled merocrine glands that secrete the clear aqueous sweat important for heat regulation and hydrating the skin and chemically different from apocrine sweat.

eccrine poroma. A benign skin tumor, usually on a sole and solitary, composed of bands of cuboidal cells suggesting origin from an eccrine sweat gland.

ec·cy·e·sis (eck″sigh·ee′sis) *n.,* pl. **eccye·ses** (·seez) EXTRAUTERINE GESTATION.

ec·dem·ic (eck·dem′ick) *adj.* Of diseases: brought into a region from without; not endemic or epidemic.

ec·dy·sis (eck′di·sis) *n.,* pl. **ecdy·ses** (·seez) Sloughing or casting off of the outer integument; molting, as of a crustacean, insect, or reptile.

ECG Abbreviation for *electrocardiogram.*

echid·nin (e·kid′nin) *n.* 1. Snake poison; the poison or venom of the viper and other similar snakes. 2. A nitrogenous and venomous principle found in poisonous secretion of various snakes.

Echid·noph·a·ga (eck″id·nof′uh·guh) *n.* A genus of fleas.

Echidnophaga gal·li·na·cea (gal″i·nay′see·uh). The species of flea which attacks chickens in many parts of the world; may also become a human pest.

echid·no·tox·in (e·kid″no·tock′sin) *n.* A principle of snake venom which produces a general reaction in the human body and has a powerful effect on the nervous system.

echin-, echino- A combining form meaning (a) spiny; (b) *echinoderm.*

echi·no·coc·co·sis (e·kigh″no·kock·o′sis) *n.* Infection of man with *Echinococcus granulosus* in its larval or hydatid stage. Most important site of infection is the liver, and secondly, the lungs.

Echi·no·coc·cus (eh·kigh″no·kock′us) *n.* A genus of tapeworms. —**echinoccus,** pl. **echinococ·ci** (·sigh), com. n.

echinococcus cyst. A cyst formed by growth of the larval form of *Echinococcus granulosus,* usually in the liver.

Echinococcus gran·u·lo·sus (gran·yoo·lo′sus). The species of tapeworm whose ova, when ingested by man or other intermediate hosts, develop into echinococcus cysts.

echi·no·derm (e·kigh′no·durm) *n.* One of the Echinodermata.

Echi·no·der·ma·ta (e·kigh″no·dur′muh·tuh) *n. pl.* A phylum of marine animals including starfish and sea urchins.

Echi·no·sto·ma (e·kigh″no·sto′muh, eck″i·nos′to·muh) *n.* A genus of flukes parasitic in man, but of little pathologic importance.

echi·no·sto·mi·a·sis (e·kigh″no·sto·migh′uh·sis, eck″i·no·) *n.,* pl. **echinostomia·ses** (·seez) Infection by flukes of the genus *Echinostoma* acquired by the ingestion of infected snails in the Far East, and causing diarrhea and abdominal pain.

echo·acou·sia (eck″o·a·koo′zhuh, ·zee·uh) *n.* A subjective disturbance of hearing in which there appears to be a repetition of a sound just heard.

echo·car·dio·gram (eck″o·kahr′dee·o·gram) *n.* A pictorial representation of the heart, using pulse-echo (ultrasound) techniques.

echo·en·ceph·a·lo·gram (eck″o·en·sef′uh·lo·gram) *n.* The pictorial representation of intracranial structures, obtained by echoencephalography.

echo·en·ceph·a·log·ra·phy (eck″o·en·sef″uh·log′ruh·fee) *n.* The study of intracranial structures and disease, employing pulse-echo techniques.

echo·gram (eck′o·gram) *n.* The pictorial display of anatomic structures, using pulse-echo techniques. Syn. *echosonogram, sonogram.*

echo·graph·ia (eck″o·graf′ee·uh) *n.* A form of aphasia in which the patient copies material presented to him without apparent comprehension.

echo·la·lia (eck″o·lay′lee·uh) *n.* The purposeless, often seemingly involuntary repetition of words spoken by another person; a disorder seen in certain psychotic states, as in the catatonic type of schizophrenia, in minimal brain dysfunction, and as the only form of speech in so-called isolation of the speech area. Syn. *echophrasia.* —**echo·lal·ic** (·lal′ick) *adj.*

echop·a·thy (eck·op′uth·ee) *n. In psychiatry,* a morbid condition marked by the automatic and purposeless repetition of a word or sound heard or of an act seen by the patient.

echoph·o·ny (eck·off′uh·nee) *n.* An echo of the vocal sound heard in auscultation of the chest.

echo·prax·ia (eck″o·prack′see·uh) *n.* Automatic imitation by the patient of another person's movements or mannerisms; seen in various psychoses, as in the catatonic type of schizophrenia.

echo·reno·gram (eck″o·ren′o·gram, ·ree′no·) *n.* The pictorial representation of the kidneys, using pulse-echo (ultrasound) techniques. Syn. *nephrosonogram.*

echo·vi·rus or **ECHO virus** A member of a large group of viruses of the picornavirus group which are small, contain RNA, and are ether-resistant. The cause of asymptomatic infection of man as well as a wide variety of syndromes, including aseptic meningitis, exanthems, and diarrhea.

Eck's fistula Anastomosis of the portal vein to the inferior vena cava, so that the portal blood bypasses the liver; performed in experimental animals.

eclamp·sia (e·klamp′see·uh) *n.* 1. A disease occurring in the latter half of pregnancy and sometimes in the puerperium, characterized by an acute elevation of blood pressure, proteinuria, edema, sodium retention, convulsions, and sometimes coma. 2. *Obsol.* Any of various conditions characterized by convulsions. —**eclamp·tic,** *adj.*

eclampsia nu·tans (new'tanz) *Obsol.* INFANTILE SPASM.

eclamp·sism (e·klamp'siz·um) *n.* The preeclamptic toxemia of pregnancy which may lead to convulsions and coma; includes the preconvulsive prodromes, nephritis, and vascular disease.

ec·lec·ti·cism (e·kleck'ti·siz·um) *n.* 1. The system of medicine involving the selection of doctrines or elements of various schools of therapeutics according to their utility and combining them into a set of practices. 2. A system of medicine depending primarily on indigenous plant remedies. —**ec·lec·tic** (·tick) *n. & adj.*

E. coli Abbreviation for *Escherichia coli.*

Ecolid Chloride. Trademark for chlorisondamine chloride, an antihypertensive drug.

ecol·o·gy (e·kol'uh·jee) *n.* The study of the environmental relations of organisms.

eco·ma·nia (ee''ko·may'nee·uh) *n.* A symptom complex characterized by a domineering, haughty, and irritable attitude toward members of one's own family, but an attitude of humility toward those in authority.

eco·sys·tem (ee''ko·sis''tum, eck''o·) *n.* A system comprised of the abiotic physicochemical environment and the biotic assemblage of plants, animals, and microbes in which an ecological kinship exists. A field, a forest, a pond, or an ocean may constitute such a system.

écra·seur (ay·kra·zur') *n.* A surgical instrument armed with a metal loop which can be tightened. Used in veterinary surgery, in castration of stallions, for example; infrequently in human surgery for the control of expected severe hemorrhage, as in excision of large pedicled tumors.

ECS Abbreviation for *electroconvulsive shock.*

ec·sta·sy (eck'stuh·see) *n.* 1. A trancelike state with mental and physical exaltation and often oblivion of environment. 2. *Obsol.* CATALEPSY. —**ec·stat·ic** (eck·stat'ick) *adj.*

ECT Abbreviation for *electroconvulsive therapy.*

ect-, ecto- A combining form meaning (a) *outside, outer;* (b) *out of place.*

ec·tad (eck'tad) *adv.* Outward.

ec·tal (eck'tul) *adj.* External; superficial.

ec·ta·sia (eck·tay'zhuh, ·zee·uh) *n.* Dilatation or distention, usually of a hollow structure. —**ec·tat·ic** (·tat'ick) *adj.*

ec·thy·ma (eck·thigh'muh) *n.* An inflammatory skin disease characterized by large, flat pustules that ulcerate and become crusted, and are surrounded by a distinct inflammatory areola. The lesions as a rule appear on the legs and thighs, and occur in crops which persist for an indefinite period.

ecto-. See *ect-.*

ec·to·car·dia (eck''to·kahr'dee·uh) *n.* An abnormal position of the heart. It may be outside the thoracic cavity (ectopia cordis) or misplaced within the thorax.

ec·to·cer·vix (eck''to·sur'vicks) *n.* The portio vaginalis of the uterine cervix; the portion of the cervix bearing stratified squamous epithelium.

ec·to·derm (eck'to·durm) *n.* The outermost of the three primary germ layers of the embryo.

From it arise the epidermis, epithelial lining of stomodeum and proctodeum, and the neural tube, with all derivatives of these. —**ec·to·der·mal** (eck''to·dur'mul) *adj.*

ectodermal dysplasia. Abnormal development or growth of tissues and structures arising from the ectoderm.

ec·to·der·mo·sis (eck''to·dur·mo'sis) *n.,* pl. **ecto·dermo·ses** (·seez) Any disease entity of the ectoderm.

ec·to·en·zyme (eck''to·en'zime, ·zim) *n.* 1. An enzyme so situated on the outer surface of a cell membrane that its active site is in contact with the exterior environment of the cell. 2. EXTRACELLULAR ENZYME.

ec·tog·e·nous (eck·toj'e·nus) *adj.* 1. Capable of growth outside the body of its host; applied to bacteria and other parasites. 2. Due to an external cause; not arising within the organism; exogenous.

ec·to·mere (eck'to·meer) *n.* A blastomere destined to take part in forming the ectoderm.

ec·to·meso·derm (eck''to·mez'o·durm, ·mes'o·durm) *n.* Mesoderm derived from the primary ectoderm of a bilaminar blastodisk or gastrula.

ec·to·morph (eck'to·morf) *n.* In the somatotype, an individual exhibiting relative predominance of ectomorphy.

ec·to·mor·phy (eck'to·mor''fee) *n.* Component III of the somatotype, representing relative predominance of linear and fragile body features; the skin or surface area, derived from ectoderm, is relatively great with respect to body mass. Ectomorphs appear to be more sensitive to their external environment. The counterpart on the behavioral level is cerebrotonia. —**ec·to·mor·phic** (eck''to·morf'ick) *adj.*

-ectomy A combining form meaning *surgical removal.*

ec·top·a·gus (eck·top'uh·gus) *n.,* pl. **ectopa·gi** (·guy, ·jye) An individual consisting of conjoined twins united laterally at the thorax. —**ectopagous,** *adj.*

ec·to·par·a·site (eck''to·pär'uh·site) *n.* A parasite that lives on the exterior of its host. —**ecto·par·a·sit·ic** (·pär·uh·sit'ick) *adj.*

ec·to·phyte (eck'to·fite) *n.* 1. An external parasitic plant growth. 2. *In dermatology,* a fungus that infects superficially.

ec·to·phyt·ic (eck''to·fit'ick) *adj.* 1. Of or pertaining to an ectophyte. 2. Characterizing a cutaneous tumor that enlarges outward.

ec·to·pia (eck·to'pee·uh) *n.* An abnormality of position of an organ or a part of the body; usually congenital.

ectopia cor·dis (kor'dis). A congenital anomaly in which the heart lies outside the thoracic cavity.

ectopia len·tis (len'tis). A subluxated lens, generally seen in Marfan's syndrome and homocystinuria.

ec·top·ic (eck·top'ick) *adj.* 1. Out of place, in an abnormal position. 2. Occurring at an abnormal time.

ectopic beat. PREMATURE BEAT.

ectopic gestation. EXTRAUTERINE GESTATION.

ectopic kidney. A congenital anomaly in which

the kidney is held in abnormal position on its own or on the opposite side, where fusion with the other kidney may occur.

ectopic pacemaker. An abnormal focus of impulse initiation in the heart, i.e., not in the sinoatrial node.

ectopic pregnancy. EXTRAUTERINE PREGNANCY.

ectopic testicle. A testis that has descended through the inguinal canal but does not reside in the scrotum.

ec·to·plasm (eck′to·plaz·um) *n.* The outer denser layer of cytoplasm of a cell or unicellular organism. —**ec·to·plas·mic** (eck″to·plaz′mick) *adj.*

ec·to·pot·o·my (eck″to·pot′uh·mee) *n.* Laparotomy for the removal of the contents of an extrauterine gestation sac.

ec·to·py (eck′to·pee) *n.* ECTOPIA.

ec·to·thrix (eck′to·thricks) *n.* A fungal parasite forming spores on the outside of hair shafts, as certain species of *Microsporum* and *Trichophyton.*

ectro- A combining form meaning *congenital absence.*

ec·tro·dac·tyl·ia (eck″tro·dack·til′ee·uh) *n.* Congenital absence of any of the fingers or toes or parts of them.

ec·trog·e·ny (eck·troj′e·nee) *n.* Loss or congenital absence of any part or organ. —**ec·tro·gen·ic** (eck″tro·jen′ick) *adj.*

ec·tro·me·lia (eck″tro·mee′lee·uh) *n.* Congenital absence or marked imperfection of one or more of the limbs.

ec·tro·pi·on (eck·tro′pee·on) *n.* Eversion of a part, especially of an eyelid. —**ectropi·on·ize** (·un·ize) *v.;* **ectropion·iza·tion** (·i·zay′shun) *n.*

ectropion iri·dis (eye′ri·dis). Eversion of a part of the iris.

ec·tro·syn·dac·ty·ly (eck″tro·sin·dack′ti·lee) *n.* A developmental defect in which some of the digits are missing while others are fused.

ec·trot·ic (eck·trot′ick) *adj.* 1. Tending to cut short; preventing the development of disease. 2. Abortive; abortifacient.

ec·tyl·urea (eck″til·yoo·ree′uh) *n.* 2-Ethyl-*cis*-crotonylurea, $C_7H_{12}N_2O_2$, a tranquilizing drug.

ec·ze·ma (eck′se·muh, eg·zee′muh) *n.* An acute or chronic, noncontagious, itching, inflammatory disease of the skin; usually characterized by irregular and varying combinations of edematous, vesicular, papular, pustular, scaling, thickened, or exudative lesions. The skin is reddened, the redness shading off into the surrounding unaffected parts. The cause is unknown. Eruptions of similar appearance due to such known causes as ingested drugs or local irritants are properly referred to as dermatitis medicamentosa, contact dermatitis, or dermatitis venenata.

eczema her·pet·i·cum (hur·pet′i·kum). A rare manifestation of primary herpes simplex infection occurring in patients with eczema or neurodermatitis, with grouped, varicella-like vesicles over large areas of the eczematous skin.

ec·ze·ma·ti·za·tion (eg·zem″uh·ti·zay′shun, eck·seem′) *n.* The formation or presence of eczema

or eczema-like lesions, as from continued physical or chemical irritation or from allergic or autoimmune reactions.

ec·ze·ma·toid (eck·sem′uh·toid, eck·seem′, eg·zem′, eg·zeem′) *adj.* Resembling eczema.

eczematoid reaction. A dermal and epidermal inflammatory response characterized by erythema, edema, vesiculation, and exudation in the acute stage, and in the chronic stage by erythema, edema, thickening (or lichenification) of the epidermis, and scaling.

ec·ze·ma·tous (eck·sem′uh·tus, eck·seem′, eg·zem′, ·zeem′) *adj.* Of or pertaining to eczema.

eczema vac·ci·na·tum (vack″si·nay′tum). The accidental inoculation of vaccinia virus on lesions of eczema, producing umbilicated vesicles and pustules on eczematous and normal skin, chiefly the former.

ede·ma, oe·de·ma (e·dee′muh) *n.,* pl. **edemas, edema·ta** (·tuh) Excessive accumulation of fluid in the tissue spaces, due to increased transudation of the fluid from the capillaries; dropsy. —**edem·a·tous** (e·dem′uh·tus, ·deem′) *adj.*

eden·tate (e·den′tate) *adj. & n.* 1. Without teeth. 2. Pertaining to the order of mammals Edentata. 3. A member of the Edentata.

eden·tia (e·den′shuh) *n.* ANODONTIA.

eden·tu·lous (e·den′chuh·lus) *adj.* Without teeth.

edes·tin (e·des′tin, ee′des·tin) *n.* A globulin type of simple protein; obtained from the seeds of hemp.

edet·ic acid (e·det′ick). (Ethylenedinitrilo)tetraacetic acid or ethylenediaminetetraacetic acid, $(HOOC·CH_2)_2NCH_2CH_2N·(CH_2COOH)_2$, salts of which, called edetates, are powerful chelating and sequestering agents that form water-soluble complexes with many cations, preventing these from exhibiting their characteristic properties.

ed·i·ble (ed′i·bul) *adj.* Fit to eat.

edis·yl·ate (e·dis′il·ate) *n.* Any salt or ester of 1,2-ethanedisulfonic acid, $(CH_2SO_3H)_2$; a 1,2-ethanedisulfonate.

ed·ro·phon·i·um chloride (ed″ro·fon′ee·um). Dimethylethyl(3-hydroxyphenyl)ammonium chloride, $C_{10}H_{16}ClNO$, a curare antagonist.

EDTA Abbreviation for *ethylenediaminetetraacetic acid* (= EDETIC ACID).

ed·u·ca·ble (ej′oo·kuh·bul) *adj.* 1. Capable of being educated. 2. Specifically, categorizing a mentally retarded individual who can, within limits, profit from educative efforts and become socially and economically self-maintaining or even independent as an adult.

ed·u·ca·tion·al age. The average achievement of a pupil or student in school subjects based on average performances for a given chronological age as measured by standard educational tests; achievement age for a person in school.

EEG Abbreviation for *electroencephalography, electroencephalogram,* or *electroencephalograph.*

ef·face·ment (e·face′munt) *n.* Loss of form or features; especially, the gradual flattening and obliteration of the uterine cervix during labor.

ef·fec·tor (e·feck′tur) *n.* A motor or secretory

nerve ending in an organ, gland, or muscle.

ef·fer·ent (ef'ur-unt) *adj.* Carrying or conducting away.

efferent duct. A duct that drains the secretion from an exocrine gland.

efferent ductules of the testis. The 8 to 15 coiled ducts that connect the rete testis with the duct of the epididymis and form the head of the epididymis; derived from paragenital mesonephric tubules.

efferent nerve. A nerve conducting impulses from the central nervous system to the periphery, as to a muscle.

ef·fer·ves·cence (ef''ur·ves'unce) *n.* 1. The escape of a gas from a liquid; a bubbling. 2. In infectious diseases, the period following the prodrome; the onset or invasion of the disease.

ef·fer·ves·cent (ef''ur·ves'unt) *adj.* Capable of producing effervescence.

ef·fleu·rage (ef''loo·rahzh', ef'lur·ahzh') *n.* The stroking movement used in massage.

ef·flo·res·cence (ef''lo·res'unce) *n.* 1. The spontaneous conversion of a crystalline substance into powder by a loss of its water of crystallization. 2. The eruption of an exanthematous disease.

ef·flu·ent (ef'lew·unt) *n.* 1. An outflow. 2. A fluid discharged from a basin or chamber for the treatment of sewage.

ef·flu·vi·um (e·floo'vee·um) *n.,* pl. **efflu·via** (·vee·uh) 1. An efflux, outflow. 2. An exhalation or emanation, especially when unpleasant or noxious.

ef·fort syndrome. NEUROCIRCULATORY ASTHENIA.

effort thrombosis. PAGET-SCHROETTER SYNDROME.

¹ef·fuse (e·fewce') *adj.* Of growth produced by bacteria on solid media: not projecting above the surface, in contrast with the raised type of growth.

²ef·fuse (e·fewz') *v.* Of a fluid: to pour or spread out, as into a body cavity or tissue. —**ef·fu·sion** (e·few'zhun) *n.*

eges·ta (e·jes'tuh) *n.pl.* Waste material discharged from the intestines or other excretory organs; excrement.

ego (ee'go) *n.* 1. *In psychology,* the self, regarded as a succession of mental states, or as the consciousness of the existence of the self as distinct from other selves. 2. *In psychoanalytic theory,* the part of the personality in conscious contact with reality, representing the sum of such mental mechanisms as perception, memory, and specific defense mechanisms, and serving to mediate between the demands of the instinctual drive (id), the superego, and reality.

ego·cen·tric (ee''go·sen'trick) *adj.* Self-centered. —**ego·cen·tric·i·ty** (·sen·tris'i·tee), **ego·cen·trism** (·sen'triz·um) *n.*

ego·ma·nia (ee''go·may'nee·uh) *n.* Pathological self-esteem.

egoph·o·ny (e·gof'uh·nee) *n.* A modification of bronchophony, in which the voice has a bleating character, like that of a goat; heard over areas of pleural effusion or lung consolidation.

ego-strength, *n.* The overall ability of a person to maintain himself and to make adjustments between his id, superego, and reality; the effectiveness with which the ego discharges its functions.

ego·tism (ee'guh·tiz·um, eg'uh·) *n.* A high degree of self-centeredness and conceit. —**ego·tist** (·tist) *n.;* **ego·tis·tic** (ee''guh·tis'tick, eg''uh·), **egotis·ti·cal** (·ti·kul) *adj.*

Eh·lers-Dan·los syndrome (eⁿlurss, dahⁿ·loce') An autosomal-dominantly inherited systemic connective tissue disorder manifested by skin fragility and hyperelasticity, easy bruising, atrophic scars and soft pseudotumors, subcutaneous ossifications, joint hyperextensibility with frequent luxation, bleeding tendency, and visceral anomalies. Syn. *cutis hyperelastica, dermatorrhexis.*

Ehrlich's diazo reagent A highly acid solution of sodium nitrite and sulfanilic acid used to detect and measure certain aromatic compounds.

ei·det·ic (eye·det'ick) *adj.* Pertaining to forms or images, especially those voluntarily reproducible.

eighth (VIIIth) cranial nerve. VESTIBULOCOCHLEAR NERVE.

eighth-nerve deafness. Deafness due to a lesion of the cochlear portion of the vestibulocochlear nerve.

eighth-nerve tumor. ACOUSTIC NEURILEMMOMA.

Ei·me·ria (eye·meer'ee·uh) *n.* A genus of protozoa of the order Coccidia which lives in the body fluids or tissues of vertebrates and invertebrates and has a life cycle characterized by alternation of generations; causes coccidiosis in cattle, sheep, rabbits, and chickens.

ein·stein (ine'stine) *n.* A unit of energy (6.06 × 10^{23} quanta) analogous to the faraday (6.06 × 10^{23} electrons); the amount of radiation absorbed by a system to activate one gram molecule of matter. Abbreviated, E.

Eisenmenger's complex or **tetralogy** A congenital cardiac anomaly, characterized by cyanosis, and consisting of a ventricular septal defect, dextroposition of the aorta, pulmonary artery dilatation, and right ventricular hypertrophy.

ejac·u·la·tion (e·jack'yoo·lay'shun) *n.* 1. A sudden expulsion. 2. Ejection of the semen during orgasm. —**ejac·u·late** (e·jack'yoo·late, ee·) *v.;* **ejac·u·la·to·ry** (e·jack'yoo·luh·to''ree) *adj.*

ejac·u·la·tio prae·cox (e·jack''yoo·lay'shee·o pree'kocks). PREMATURE EJACULATION.

ejaculatory duct. The terminal part of the ductus deferens after junction with the duct of a seminal vesicle, embedded in the prostate gland and opening into the urethra on the colliculus seminalis.

ejec·tion (e·jeck'shun) *n.* 1. The act of casting out, as of secretions, excretions, or excrementitious matter. 2. That which is cast out. —**eject** (e·jekt') *v.*

ejection phase. The phase of ventricular systole during which blood is pumped out of the heart.

eka- A combining form which, when prefixed to the name of a recognized chemical element, designates provisionally *a predicted but as yet undiscovered element which should adjoin the former in the same group of the periodic system.*

EKG An abbreviation for *electrocardiogram.*

elab·o·ra·tion (e·lab″uh·ray′shun) *n.* 1. *In physiology,* any anabolic process, such as the production or synthesis of complex substances from simpler precursors or the formation of secretory products in gland cells. 2. *In psychiatry,* an unconscious psychologic process of enlargement and embellishment of detail, especially of a symbol or representation in a dream; this process is also seen in certain psychoses.

Elap·i·dae (e·lap′i·dee) *n. pl.* A family of venomous snakes possessing short, erect, immovable front fangs; includes cobras, mambas, kraits, coral snakes, the death adder, and the tiger snake. **—el·a·pid** (el′uh·pid) *adj. & n.*

elast-, elasto-. A combining form meaning *elastic, elasticity.*

elas·tase (e·las′tace, ·taze) *n.* An enzyme that acts on elastin to render it soluble; has been isolated in crystalline form from pancreas.

elas·tic, *adj.* Capable of returning to the original form after being stretched or compressed. **—elas·tic·i·ty** (e·las″tis′i·tee) *n.*

elas·ti·ca (e·las′ti·kuh) *n.* The tunica intima of a blood vessel.

elastic bandage. A bandage of rubber or woven elastic material; used to exert continuous pressure on swollen extremities or joints, fractured ribs, the chest, or varicose veins.

elas·tin (e·las′tin) *n.* The protein base of yellow elastic tissue.

elas·to·fi·bro·ma (e·las″to·figh·bro′muh) *n.* A benign soft-tissue tumor, observed in elderly patients in the subscapular area, characterized by large bands of poorly cellular elastic and connective tissue, separated by fat lobules.

elas·to·ma (e·las·to′muh) *n.,* pl. **elastomas, elastoma·ta** (·tuh) A nevoid condition in which there is a localized thickening of the dermis due to increased elastin.

elas·to·sis (e·las″to′sis) *n.* 1. Retrogressive changes in elastic tissue. 2. Retrogressive changes in cutaneous connective tissue resulting in excessive amounts of material giving the usual staining reactions for elastin.

elastosis se·ni·lis (se·nigh′lis). Degeneration of the elastic connective tissue of the skin in old age.

Elavil. Trademark for amitriptyline, an antidepressant and mild tranquilizing drug used as the hydrochloride salt.

el·bow, *n.* The junction of the arm and forearm; the bend of the arm.

elective operation. An operation which is not urgent or mandatory, and which may be scheduled well in advance at a time of convenience.

Elec·tra complex The female analogue of the Oedipus complex.

electrical alternation An electrocardiographic pattern characterized by alternating amplitude or configuration of the QRS complex and/or the T wave, indicative of severe myocardial disease or abnormality of the innervation of the heart.

electrical axis. The single resultant vector of the electric activity of all myofibrils of the heart at any particular moment during the electric cycle of cardiac activity. Syn. *QRS axis.*

electric ophthalmia. Actinic keratoconjunctivitis following undue exposure to such bright lights as the electric arc used in welding and the arc lights used in motion-picture studios.

electric shock. The sudden violent effect of the passage of an electric current through the body.

electro-. A combining form meaning (a) *electric, electricity;* (b) *electron.*

elec·tro·an·es·the·sia, elec·tro·an·aes·the·sia (e·leck″tro·an″es·theezh′uh, ·theez′ee·uh) *n.* Local anesthesia induced by an electric current; electric anesthesia.

elec·tro·car·di·o·gram (e·leck″tro·kahr′dee·o·gram) *n.* A graphic record, made by an electrocardiograph, of the electrical forces that produce the contraction of the heart. A typical normal record shows P, Q, R, S, T, and U waves. Abbreviated, ECG, EKG.

elec·tro·car·di·o·graph (e·leck″tro·kahr′de·o·graf) *n.* An instrument that receives electrical impulses as they vary during the cardiac cycle and transforms them into a graphic record; an instrument for recording electrocardiograms. Abbreviated, ECG, EKG. **—elec·tro·car·di·o·graph·ic** (·kahr″dee·o·graf′ick) *adj.*

elec·tro·car·di·og·ra·phy (e·leck″tro·kahr″dee·og′ruh·fee) *n.* The specialty or science of recording and interpreting the electrical activity of the heart, i.e., electrocardiograms. Abbreviated, ECG, EKG.

elec·tro·cau·tery (e·leck″tro·kaw′tur·ee) *n.* Cauterization by means of a wire loop or needle heated by a direct galvanic current. Syn. *galvanocautery.*

elec·tro·chem·is·try (e·leck″tro·kem′is·tree) *n.* The science treating of chemical changes produced by electricity and of interconversion of electrical and chemical energy.

elec·tro·co·ag·u·la·tion (e·leck″tro·ko·ag″yoo·lay′shun) *n.* The destruction or hardening of tissues by coagulation induced by the passage of high-frequency currents; surgical diathermy.

elec·tro·con·trac·til·i·ty (e·leck″tro·kon″track·til′i·tee) *n.* The capacity of muscular tissue for contraction in response to electric stimulation.

elec·tro·con·vul·sive (e·leck″tro·kun·vul′siv) *adj.* Pertaining to a convulsive response to electrical stimulation.

electroconvulsive therapy or **treatment.** ELECTROSHOCK THERAPY. Abbreviated, ECT.

elec·tro·cor·ti·cal (e·leck″tro·kor′ti·kul) *adj.* Pertaining to the electrical activity of the cerebral cortex.

elec·tro·cor·ti·cog·ra·phy (e·leck″tro·kor·ti·kog′ruh·fee) *n.* The process of recording the electric activity of the brain by electrodes placed directly on the cerebral cortex, providing a much higher voltage, greater accuracy, and more exact localization than electroencephalography. —**electro·cor·ti·co·gram** (·kor'ti·ko·gram) n.

elec·tro·cu·tion (e·leck"truh·kew'shun) n. 1. Execution by electricity. 2. Loosely, any electric shock causing death. —**elec·tro·cute** (e·leck'truh·kewt) v.

elec·trode (e·leck'trode) n. 1. A surface of contact between a metallic and a nonmetallic conductor. 2. One of the terminals of metal, salts, or electrolytes through which electricity is applied to, or taken from, the body or an electric device or instrument.

elec·tro·des·ic·ca·tion (e·leck"tro·des"i·kay'shun) n. The diathermic destruction of small growths such as of the urinary bladder, skin, or cervix by means of a single terminal electrode with a small sparking distance.

elec·tro·di·al·y·sis (e·leck"tro·dye·al'i·sis) n. A method for rapidly removing electrolytes from colloids by dialysis of the colloidal sol while an electric current is being passed through it.

elec·tro·en·ceph·a·lo·gram (e·leck"tro·en·sef'uh·lo·gram) n. A graphic record of the minute changes in electric potential associated with the activity of the cerebral cortex, as detected by electrodes applied to the surface of the scalp. Abbreviated, EEG.

elec·tro·en·ceph·a·lo·graph (e·leck"tro·en·sef'ul·lo·graf) n. An instrument for recording the electric activity of the brain. Abbreviated, EEG. —**electro·en·ceph·a·lo·graph·ic** (·en·sef"uh·lo·graf'ick) adj.

elec·tro·en·ceph·a·log·ra·phy (e·leck"tro·en·sef"uh·log'ruh·fee) n. A method of recording graphically the electric activity of the brain, particularly the cerebral cortex, by means of electrodes attached to the scalp; used in the diagnosis of epilepsy, trauma, tumors, and degenerations of the brain, as well as in the study of the effect of drugs on the central nervous system and certain psychological and physiological phenomena. Abbreviated, EEG.

elec·tro·he·mos·ta·sis, elec·tro·hae·mos·ta·sis (e·leck"tro·hee·mos'tuh·sis) n. The arrest of hemorrhage by means of a high-frequency current, as in the reduction or prevention of bleeding in operations through use of an electrosurgical knife.

elec·tro·hys·ter·og·ra·phy (e·leck"tro·his"tur·og'ruh·fee) n. The recording of electric action potentials of the uterus.

elec·tro·ky·mog·ra·phy (e·leck"tro·kigh·mog'ruh·fee) n. The technique of recording the motions of an organ by means of an electrokymograph.

elec·trol·y·sis (e·leck"trol'i·sis) n. The decomposition of a chemical compound by a direct electric current. —**elec·tro·lyze** (e·leck'tro·lize) v.

elec·tro·lyte (e·leck'tro·lite) n. A substance which, in solution, is dissociated into ions and is capable of conducting an electric current, as the circulating ions of plasma and other body fluids. —**electro·lyt·ic** (e·leck"tro·lit'ick) adj.

elec·tro·mag·net (e·leck"tro·mag'nit) n. A core of soft iron surrounded by a coil of wire. A current passing through the wire will make the iron temporarily magnetic.

electromagnetic flowmeter. A flowmeter in which changes in the flow of blood are measured through impedance to electromagnetic lines of force introduced across a stream. It has the great advantage that an intact blood vessel can be used.

electromagnetic radiation. Radiation that is propagated through space or matter in the form of electromagnetic waves.

electromagnetic spectrum. The entire continuous range of electromagnetic waves from gamma rays of shortest wavelength to radio waves of longest wavelength.

electromagnetic waves. Any of a continuous spectrum of waves propagated by simultaneous oscillation of electric and magnetic fields perpendicularly to each other and both perpendicularly to the direction of propagation of the waves. Included in the spectrum, in order of increasing frequency (or decreasing wavelength) are the following types of waves: radio, microwave, infrared, visible light, ultraviolet, x-rays, and gamma rays.

elec·tro·mag·net·ism (e·leck"tro·mag'ne·tiz·um) n. 1. Magnetism produced by a current of electricity. 2. The science dealing with the relations between electricity and magnetism.

elec·tro·mas·sage (e·leck"tro·muh·sahzh') n. The transmission of an alternating electric current through body tissues accompanied by manual kneading.

electromotive force. The force that tends to alter the motion of electricity, measured in volts. Abbreviated, E, emf, EMF.

elec·tro·myo·gram (e·leck"tro·migh'o·gram) n. 1. A graphic record of the electric activity of a muscle either spontaneous or in response to artificial electric stimulation. 2. A record of eye movements during reading, obtained by measuring the potential difference between an electrode placed at the center of the forehead and one placed at the temple. Abbreviated, EMG.

elec·tro·my·og·ra·phy (e·leck"tro·migh·og'ruh·fee) n. Production and study of the electromyogram. Abbreviated, EMG. —**elec·tro·myo·graph·ic** (e·leck"tro·migh'o·graf'ick) adj.

elec·tron (e·leck'tron) n. Commonly the smallest particle of negative electricity, sometimes called negatron. The mass of an electron at rest is 9.109×10^{-28} gram or 1/1845 that of a hydrogen atom. Its electric charge is 4.77×10^{-10} electrostatic unit. Symbol, e.

elec·tro·nar·co·sis (e·leck"tro·nahr·ko'sis) n. Narcosis produced by the application of electric currents to the body for therapeutic purposes.

elec·tro·neg·a·tive (e·leck"tro·neg'uh·tiv) adj. Pertaining to or charged with negative electricity; tending to attract electrons.

elec·tro·neg·a·tiv·i·ty (e·leck"tro·neg"uh·tiv'i·tee) n. The power of an atom in a molecule to attract electrons to itself.

elec·tron·ic (e·leck"tron'ick) adj. 1. Of or pertaining to electrons. 2. Pertaining to the emission and transmission of electrons in a vacuum and in gases and semiconductors.

elec·tron microscope. A device for directing streams of electrons by means of electric and magnetic fields in a manner similar to the direction of visible light rays by means of glass lenses in an ordinary microscope. Since electrons carry waves of much smaller wavelengths than light waves, correspondingly greater magnifications are obtainable. The electron microscope will resolve detail 1,000 to 10,000 times finer than the optical microscope. Images can be studied on a fluorescent screen or recorded photographically.

elec·tro·pho·re·sis (e·leck″tro·fo·ree′sis) *n.* The migration of charged particles through the medium in which they are dispersed, when placed under the influence of an applied electric potential. Syn. *cataphoresis.* **—elec·tro·pho·ret·ic** (e·leck″tro·fo·ret′ick) *adj.*

elec·tro·pos·i·tive (e·leck″tro·poz′i·tiv) *adj.* Pertaining to or charged with positive electricity; tending to release electrons.

elec·tro·py·rex·ia (e·leck″tro·pye·reck′see·uh) *n.* The production of high body temperatures by means of an electric current; fever therapy.

elec·tro·ret·i·no·gram (e·leck″tro·ret′i·no·gram) *n.* A record of the electric variations of the retina upon stimulation by lights; made by placing one electrode over the cornea, the other over some indifferent region.

elec·tro·scis·sion (e·leck″tro·sizh′un, ·sish′un) *n.* Cutting of tissues by an electrocautery knife.

elec·tro·scope (e·leck″truh·skope) *n.* An instrument for detecting the presence of static electricity and its relative amount, and for determining whether it is positive or negative.

elec·tro·sec·tion (e·leck″tro·seck′shun) *n.* Tissue division by a knifelike electrode operated by a high-frequency machine.

elec·tro·shock (e·leck″tro·shock′) *n.* Shock produced by electricity.

electroshock therapy or treatment. The use of electric current to produce unconsciousness or convulsions in the treatment of psychotic, particularly depressive, disorders. Abbreviated, EST.

elec·tro·stat·ic (e·leck″tro·stat′ick) *adj.* Of or pertaining to static electricity.

electrostatic generator. An apparatus for producing up to several million volts of electrostatic energy by successive accumulation of small static charges on an insulated high-voltage metal collector.

elec·tro·sur·gery (e·leck″tro·sur′jur·ee) *n.* The use of electricity in surgery; surgical diathermy. **—electrosur·gi·cal** (·ji·kul) *adj.*

elec·tro·ther·a·peu·tics (e·leck″tro·therr·uh·pew′ticks) *n.* ELECTROTHERAPY.

elec·tro·ther·a·py (e·leck″tro·therr′uh·pee) *n.* The use of electricity to treat disease.

elec·tro·tome (e·leck″tro·tome) *n.* A surgical electrocautery device using low current, high voltage, and high frequency, which has a loop for engaging the part to be excised. No macroscopic coagulation of tissues is produced.

elec·trot·o·nus (e·leck″trot′o·nus, e·leck″tro·to′nus) *n.* The transient change of irritability in a nerve or a muscle during the passage of a current of electricity.

elec·tro·va·go·gram (e·leck″tro·vay′go·gram) *n.* A record of the electric changes occurring in the vagus nerve. Syn. *vagogram.*

el·e·ment, *n.* 1. Any one of the ultimate parts of which anything is composed, as the cellular elements of a tissue. 2. *In chemistry,* any one of the more than 100 ultimate chemical entities of which matter is believed to be composed. Each element is composed wholly of atoms of the same atomic number (having the same charge on their nuclei), although their atomic weights may differ due to differences in nuclear weight. For a list of elements see Table of Elements in the Appendix.

el·e·men·tal (el″e·men′tul) *adj.* 1. Of or pertaining to ultimate entities. 2. Not chemically combined; composed of a single element.

el·e·men·ta·ry (el″e·men′tuh·ree) *adj.* 1. Primary or first. 2. Rudimentary; introductory.

el·e·mi (el′e·mee) *n.* A resinous exudation frequently derived from *Canarium commune,* as well as from other plants of the Burseraceae. Its action is similar to that of the turpentines, and it has been used in plasters and ointments.

el·e·o·ma, el·ae·o·ma (el″ee·o′muh) *n.,* pl. **eleo·mas, eleoma·ta** (·tuh) A pathologic swelling caused by the injection of an oil into the tissues.

el·e·om·e·ter, el·ae·om·e·ter (el″ee·om′e·tur) *n.* An apparatus for ascertaining the specific gravity of oil.

el·e·op·tene, el·ae·op·tene (el″ee·op′teen) *n.* The permanent liquid portion of volatile oils.

el·e·phan·ti·a·sis (el″e·fan·tye′uh·sis) *n.,* pl. **elephantia·ses** (·seez) A chronic enlargement and thickening of the subcutaneous and cutaneous tissues as a result of lymphatic obstruction and lymphatic edema. In the form commonest in the tropics, the recurrent lymphangitis is caused by the filaria *Wuchereria bancrofti.* The legs and scrotum are most commonly affected. **—ele·phan·ti·ac** (·fan′tee·ack) *adj.* & *n.;* **ele·phan·ti·as·ic** (·fan·tee·az′ick) *adj.*

elephantiasis du·ra (dew′ruh). A variety of elephantiasis marked by density and sclerosis of the subcutaneous connective tissues.

elephantiasis fil·ar·i·en·sis (fi·lår″ee·en′sis). Elephantiasis due to infection with filaria, most commonly *Wuchereria bancrofti.*

elephantiasis neu·ro·ma·to·sa (new·ro″muh·to′suh). PACHYDERMATOCELE.

el·e·phan·toid (el″e·fan′toid, el′e·fun·toid″) *adj.* Pertaining to or resembling elephantiasis.

el·e·va·tor, *n.* An instrument for elevating or lifting a part, or for extracting the roots of teeth.

El·ford membrane. Graded collodion membrane filters employed for the determination of the relative size of different filtrable viruses.

elim·i·na·tion (e·lim″i·nay′shun) *n.* The process of expelling or casting out; especially, the expelling of the waste products of the body. **—elim·i·nate** (e·lim′i·nate) *v.*

elin·gua·tion (ee·ling·gway′shun) *n.* Surgical removal of the tongue.

eli·sion (e·lizh′un) *n.* The omission of one or

more sounds or syllables from words when speaking.

elix·ir (e·lik'sur) *n.* A sweetened, aromatic solution, usually hydroalcoholic, commonly containing soluble medicants, but sometimes not containing any medication; intended for use only as a flavor or vehicle, or both.

el·lip·sin (e·lip'sin) *n.* The protein constituents of the cell responsible for maintaining its form and structure.

el·lip·soid (e·lip'soid) *adj. & n.* 1. Ellipse-like or oval. 2. A solid figure of which all plane sections are ellipses, or of which some are ellipses and the rest circles. 3. The spindle-shaped sheathed arterial capillary (the second division of the penicillus) in the red pulp of the spleen, consisting of phagocytic cells and reticular fibers. Syn. *Schweigger-Seidel sheath.* —**el·lip·soi·dal** (e·lip'soy'dul) *adj.*

ellipsoid articulation. CONDYLAR JOINT.

el·lip·tic (e·lip'tick) *adj.* Shaped like an ellipse, or an elongated circle.

el·lip·to·cyte (e·lip'to·site) *n.* An elliptic erythrocyte.

el·lip·to·cy·to·sis (e·lip''to·sigh·to'sis) *n.* An autosomal dominant anomaly of erythrocytes characterized by an oval shape in 90% or more of peripheral blood erythrocytes, occasionally resulting in hemolysis but usually asymptomatic.

Ellis–van Cre·veld syndrome. CHONDROECTO-DERMAL DYSPLASIA.

elon·ga·tion factor. Any of the proteins required for the elongation of a growing polypeptide chain during the process of protein synthesis.

elope·ment (e·lope'munt) *n. In psychiatry,* the departure of a patient from a mental hospital without permission. —**elope,** *v.*

Elorine. Trademark for tricyclamol, an anticholinergic drug used as the methochloride salt.

Elsch·nig's pearls Nodules of proliferating ocular lens epithelium sometimes developing after trauma or cataract operations, and growing to visible size in the pupillary space.

el·u·ant, el·u·ent (el'yoo·unt) *n.* The solvent used in elution in chromatography.

el·u·ate (el'yoo·ate) *n.* The extract obtained from elution in chromatography; it represents a solution of the formerly adsorbed substance in the eluant.

elu·tion (e·lew'shun) *n.* 1. The process of extracting by means of a solvent the adsorbed substance from the solid adsorbing medium in chromatography. 2. The removal of antibody from the antigen to which it is attached. —**elute** (e·lewt') *v.*

elu·tri·a·tion (e·lew''tree·ay'shun) *n.* A process whereby the coarser particles of an insoluble powder are separated from the finer by mixing the substance with a liquid and decanting the upper layer after the heavier particles have settled. A form of water sifting.

elytr-, elytro- A combining form meaning *vagina, vaginal.*

ema·ci·a·tion (e·may''shee·ay'shun, e·may'see·) *n.* The process of losing flesh so as to become extremely lean, or the resultant state; a wasted

condition. —**ema·ci·ate** (e·may'shee·ate, e·may'see·ate) *v.*

em·a·na·tion (em''uh·nay'shun) *n.* 1. That which flows or is emitted from a substance; effluvium. 2. Gaseous, radioactive products formed by the loss of alpha particles from radium (radon), thorium X (thoron), and actinium X (actinon). —**em·a·nate** (em'uh·nate) *v.*

eman·sio (e·man'see·o, ·shee·o) *n.* A failing.

emansio men·si·um (men'see·um). Delay in the first appearance of the menses.

emas·cu·late (e·mas'kew·late) *v.* To castrate; to remove the testes, or the testes and penis. —**emas·cu·la·tion** (e·mas''kew·lay'shun) *n.*

em·balm (em·bahm') *v.* To treat a cadaver with antiseptic and preservative substances for burial or for dissection.

em·bar·rass·ment, *n.* Functional impairment; interference; difficulty.

Emb·den–Mey·er·hof scheme MEYERHOF PATHWAY.

em·bed (em·bed') *v. In histology,* to infiltrate a specimen with a substance, as paraffin or celloidin, to give support during the process of cutting it into sections for microscopical examination.

Em·be·lia (em·bee'lee·uh, em·beel'yuh) *n.* A genus of shrubs of the Myrsinaceae. The berries of *Embelia ribes,* an Asiatic species, have been used as an anthelmintic.

em·bo·lec·to·my (em''bo·leck'tuh·mee) *n.* Surgical removal of an embolus.

em·bo·le·mia, em·bo·lae·mia (em''bo·lee'mee·uh) *n.* The presence of emboli in the blood.

emboli. Plural of *embolus.*

em·bol·ic (em·bol'ick) *adj.* Pertaining to an embolus or an embolism.

em·bol·i·form (em·bol'i·form) *adj.* Shaped like or resembling an embolus.

em·bo·lism (em'bo·liz·um) *n.* The occlusion of a blood vessel by an embolus, causing various syndromes depending on the size of the vessel occluded, the part supplied, and the character of the embolus. —**em·bo·lize** (·lize) *v.*

em·bo·lo·la·lia (em''buh·lo·lay'lee·uh) *n.* 1. The insertion of meaningless words into speech, occurring in some aphasic and schizophrenic states. 2. A form of speech disorder, often seen in stutterers, in which short sounds or words are interpolated into the spoken sentence to cover hesitancy.

em·bo·lus (em'buh·lus) *n.,* pl. **embo·li** (·lye) A bit of matter foreign to the bloodstream, such as blood clot, air, tumor or other tissue cells, fat, cardiac vegetations, clumps of bacteria, or a foreign body (as a needle or bullet) which is carried by the bloodstream until it lodges in a blood vessel and obstructs it. —**embo·loid** (·loid) *adj.*

em·bo·ly (em'buh·lee) *n.* The process of invagination by which a two-layered gastrula develops from a blastula.

em·bra·sure (em·bray'zhur) *n.* The space formed by the sloping or curved proximal surfaces adjacent to the contact area of two teeth in the same arch; it may be facial, or buccal, or labial, lingual, gingival, incisal, or occlusal in accordance with the direction toward which it opens.

em·bro·ca·tion (em″bro·kay′shun) *n.* 1. The application, especially by rubbing, of a liquid to a part of the body. 2. The liquid so applied; liniment.

embry-, embryo-. A combining form meaning *embryo, fetus, embryonic, fetal.*

em·bry·ec·to·my (em″bree·eck′tuh·mee) *n.* The surgical removal of an extrauterine embryo.

em·bryo (em′bree·o) *n.* A young organism in the early stages of development; in human embryology, the product of conception from the moment of fertilization until about the end of the eighth week after fertilization.

em·bryo·car·dia (em″bree·o·kahr′dee·uh) *n.* A condition in which the heart sounds resemble those of a fetus, the first and second sounds being almost identical in intensity and duration.

em·bryo·ci·dal (em″bree·o·sigh′dul) *adj.* Capable of killing an embryo.

em·bryo·gen·e·sis (em″bree·o·jen′e·sis) *n.* EMBRYOGENY. —**embryo·ge·net·ic** (·je·net′ick) *adj.*

em·bry·og·e·ny (em″bree·oj′e·nee) *n.* The development of the embryo. —**embry·o·gen·ic** (·o·jen′ick), *adj.*

em·bry·oid (em′bree·oid) *adj.* Resembling an embryo.

em·bry·ol·o·gist (em″bree·ol′uh·jist) *n.* One skilled in embryology.

em·bry·ol·o·gy (em″bree·ol′uh·jee) *n.* The science dealing with the embryo and its development. —**embryo·o·log·ic** (·o·loj′ick), **embryolog·i·cal** (·i·kul) *adj.*

em·bry·o·ma (em″bree·o′muh) *n.,* pl. **embryo·mas, embryoma·ta** (·tuh) 1. MALIGNANT MIXED MESODERMAL TUMOR. 2. TERATOMA.

embryoma of the kidney. WILMS'S TUMOR.

embryoma of the ovary. DYSGERMINOMA.

em·bry·o·nal (em′bree·uh·nul) *adj.* EMBRYONIC.

em·bry·o·nate (em′bree·o·nate) *adj.* 1. Fecundated. 2. Containing an embryo.

em·bry·on·ic (em″bree·on′ick) *adj.* 1. Pertaining to an embryo. 2. Rudimentary; undifferentiated.

em·bry·op·a·thy (em″bree·op′uh·thee) *n.* Any type of embryonic or congenital defect resulting from faulty development, especially one caused by infection or toxicity from the mother or other damage in utero.

em·bry·ot·o·my (em″bree·ot′uh·mee) *n.* Any mutilation of the fetus in the uterus to aid in its removal when natural delivery is impossible.

em·bry·o·tox·ic·i·ty (em″bree·o·tock·sis′i·tee) *n.* The state of possessing qualities toxic to embryos.

em·bry·o·tox·on (em″bree·o·tocks′on) *n.* 1. A congenital opaque marginal ring in the cornea. 2. Specifically, ANTERIOR EMBRYOTOXON.

emer·gen·cy (e·mer′jen·see) *n.* 1. A suddenly developing pathologic condition in a patient, due to accident or disease, which requires urgent medical or surgical therapeutic attention. 2. A sudden threatening situation, as in warfare, disasters, or epidemics, which calls for immediate correction or defensive measures.

em·e·sis (em′e·sis) *n.,* pl. **eme·ses** (·seez) Vomiting; the act of vomiting.

emet-, emeto-. A combining form meaning (a) *emesis, vomiting;* (b) *emetic.*

em·e·ta·mine (em″e·tuh·meen′, e·met′uh·meen, ·min) *n.* An alkaloid, $C_{29}H_{36}N_2O_4$, occurring in small amounts in ipecac and obtainable from emetine by dehydrogenation.

emet·ic (e·met′ick) *adj. & n.* 1. Inducing emesis. 2. An agent that induces emesis.

em·e·tine (em′e·teen, ·tin) *n.* Cephaeline methyl ether, $C_{29}H_{40}N_2O_4$, the principal alkaloid of ipecac; a white powder, sparingly soluble in water; an emetic, diaphoretic, and expectorant, but used chiefly as an amebicide, in the form of emetine hydrochloride and emetine bismuth iodide.

em·e·to·ca·thar·sis (em″e·to·kuh·thahr′sis) *n.,* pl. **emetocathar·ses** (·seez) Vomiting and purgation at the same time, or produced by a common agent.

em·e·to·mor·phine (em″e·to·mor′feen, ·fin) *n.* APOMORPHINE.

emf, EMF An abbreviation for *electromotive force.*

EMG Abbreviation for *electromyography, electromyogram.*

-emia, -aemia A combining form designating *a* (specified) *condition of the blood or presence in the blood of a* (specified) *substance.*

emic·tion (e·mick′shun) *n.* URINATION.

em·i·gra·tion (em″i·gray′shun) *n.* The outward passage of wandering cells or leukocytes through the walls of a small blood vessel; DIAPEDESIS. —**em·i·grate** (em′i·grate) *v.*

em·i·nence (em′i·nunce) *n.* A projecting, prominent part of an organ, especially a bone.

em·i·nen·tia (em″i·nen′shee·uh) *n.* EMINENCE.

em·i·o·cy·to·sis (em″ee·o·sigh·to′sis) *n.* Fusion of intracellular granules with the cell membrane, followed by discharge of the granules into the surroundings; applied chiefly to insulin secretion by the islets of Langerhans. Syn. *reverse pinocytosis.*

em·is·sary (vein) (em′i·serr″ee) *n.* Any venous channel through the skull, connecting the venous sinuses with the diploic veins and veins of the scalp.

emis·sion (e·mish′un) *n.* 1. The action or process of emitting. 2. A seminal discharge or ejaculation.

em·men·a·gogue (e·men′uh·gog, e·mee′nuh·) *n.* An agent that stimulates the menstrual flow. —**emmen·a·gog·ic** (e·men″uh·goj′ick) *adj.*

em·men·ia (e·men′ee·uh, e·mee′nee·uh) *n.* MENSES.

em·men·i·op·a·thy (e·men″ee·op′uth·ee, e·mee″ nee·) *n.* Any menstrual disorder.

em·me·tro·pia (em″e·tro′pee·uh) *n.* Normal or perfect vision. The condition in which parallel rays are focused exactly on the retina without effort of accommodation. Abbreviated, E. —**em·me·trope** (em′e·trope) *n.;* **em·me·trop·ic** (em″e·trop′ick) *adj.*

em·o·din (em′o·din) *n.* 1,3,8-Trihydroxy-6-methylanthraquinone, $C_{15}H_{10}O_5$, a product of hydrolysis or oxidation of glycosidal compounds found in rhubarb, cascara, and other plants; it has also been synthesized. It is an irritant cathartic, acting mainly on the large intestine.

emol·lient (ee·mol'ee·unt, ·yunt) *adj.* & *n.* 1. Softening or soothing. 2. A substance used externally to soften the skin; or, internally, to soothe an irritated or inflamed surface.

emo·tion, *n.* 1. Affect, feeling, or sentiment. 2. Strong feeling, often of an agitated nature, accompanied frequently by physical and psychic reactions, as changes in heart action or gastrointestinal and vasomotor disturbances. —**emotion·al,** *adj.*

emotional deprivation. A lack of adequate and appropriate experience in interpersonal relationships or environmental stimulation or both, usually in the early formative years; may cause pseudoretardation.

emotionally disturbed. Characterized by inappropriate or disproportionate emotional responses to various life situations; emotionally unstable or labile; neurotic.

em·pa·thy (em'puth·ee) *n.* 1. The vicarious experience of another person's situation and psychological state, which may facilitate intuitive understanding of that person's feelings, thoughts, and actions. 2. Attribution of feelings or attitudes to a physical object or an animal.

em·phrac·tic (em·frack'tick) *n.* Any agent that obstructs the function of an organ, especially the excretory function of the skin.

em·phrax·is (em·frack'sis) *n.,* pl. **emphrax·es** (·eez) An obstruction, infarction, or congestion.

em·phy·se·ma (em'fi·see'muh) *n.* 1. An anatomic alteration of the lungs characterized by abnormal enlargement of the air spaces distal to the terminal respiratory bronchiole, often accompanied by destructive changes of the alveolar walls. 2. Abnormal presence of air or gas in the body tissues. —**emphy·se·ma·tous** (·sem'uh·tus, ·see'muh·tus) *adj.*

em·pir·ic (em·pirr'ick) *adj.* & *n.* 1. EMPIRICAL. 2. One who in practicing medicine relies solely on actual experience and experimentation.

em·pir·i·cal (em·pirr'i·kul) *adj.* Based on observation rather than on reasoning, assumption, or speculation.

em·pir·i·cism (em·pirr'i·siz·um) *n.* 1. Methodological preference for or tendency toward reliance on the directly observable rather than the theoretical, as, in psychology, partiality to behavioral data rather than unobservable mental entities and processes. 2. The philosophical view that all genuine knowledge is empirical.

em·pros·thot·o·nos, em·pros·thot·o·nus (em'pros·thot'uh·nus) *n.* A tetanic muscular spasm in which the head and feet are flexed forward, tensing the back in a curve with concavity forward.

em·py·e·ma (em'pye·ee'muh, em'pee·ee'muh) *n.,* pl. **empyema·ta** (·tuh), **empyemas** The presence of pus in a cavity, hollow organ, or body space. —**empy·em·a·tous** (·em'uh·tus), **empye·mic** (·mick) *adj.*

em·py·e·sis (em'pye·ee'sis) *n.,* pl. **empye·ses** (·seez) 1. A pustular eruption. 2. Any disease

characterized by phlegmonous vesicles filling with purulent fluid. 3. An accumulation of pus.

emul·si·fi·er (e·mul'si·figh"ur) *n.* An agent used to assist in the production of an emulsion.

emul·si·fy (e·mul'si·figh) *v.* To make into an emulsion. —**emul·si·fi·ca·tion** (e·mul"si·fi·kay' shun) *n.*

emul·sin (e·mul'sin) *n.* An enzyme, found in bitter almonds and other seeds, which selectively catalyzes hydrolysis of β-glucoside linkages; thus, it effects hydrolysis of amygdalin to benzaldehyde, hydrocyanic acid, and glucose. Syn. *amygdalase, glucosidase.*

emul·sion (e·mul'shun) *n.* A product consisting of minute globules of one liquid dispersed throughout the body of a second liquid. The portion that exists as globules is known as the internal, dispersed, or discontinuous phase; the other liquid is the external or continuous phase or the dispersion medium, for example, a suspension of silver halide salts in gelatin as a component of photographic and x-ray films.

emul·soid (e·mul'soid) *n.* A colloid system whose internal phase is liquid; a lyophilic colloid.

en-, em- A prefix meaning *in, inside, into.*

enam·el (e·nam'ul) *n.* The hard, calcified substance that covers the crown of a tooth.

enam·e·lo·blas·to·ma (e·nam"e·lo·blas·to'muh) *n.* AMELOBLASTOMA.

enam·e·lo·ma (e·nam"e·lo'muh) *n.* A benign dysontogenetic tumor composed of enamel-producing connective tissue. It commonly appears as a nodule attached to the root of a tooth, but may lie free in the periodontal ligament.

enam·e·lo·plas·ty (e·nam'e·lo·plas"tee) *n.* The act of grinding away a shallow developmental enamel fault or groove to create a smooth saucer-shaped surface which will be a self-cleansing or easily cleaned area; a prophylactic or preventive measure.

enamel organ. The epithelial ingrowth from the dental lamina which covers the dental papilla, furnishes a mold for the shape of a developing tooth, and forms the dental enamel.

en·an·them (e·nan'thum) *n.* An eruption on a mucous membrane, or within the body. —**en·an·them·a·tous** (en"an·them'uh·tus) *adj.*

en·an·the·ma (en"an·theem'uh) *n.,* pl. **enan·the·ma·ta** (·theem'uh·tuh, ·themm'uh·tuh). ENANTHEM.

en·an·tio·la·lia (en·an"tee·o·lay'lee·uh) *n.* Talking contrariwise; a disturbance in mental and speech function which prompts ideas and words opposite to those presented as a stimulus.

en·ar·thro·sis (en"ahr·thro'sis) *n.,* pl. **enarthro·ses** (·seez) A ball-and-socket joint, such as that of the hip. —**enarthro·di·al** (·dee·ul) *adj.*

en·can·this (en·kanth'is) *n.,* pl. **encan·thi·des** (·i·deez) A neoplasm in the inner canthus of the eye.

en·cap·su·la·tion (en·kap"sue·lay'shun) *n.* The process of surrounding a part with a capsule. —**en·cap·su·late** (en·kap'sue·late) *v.*

encephal-, encephalo-. A combining form meaning *encephalon, brain.*

en·ceph·al·at·ro·phy (en·sef''uh·lat'ruh·fee) *n.* Atrophy of the brain.

en·ce·phal·ic (en''se·fal'ick) *adj.* Pertaining to or involving the brain or encephalon.

en·ceph·a·li·tis (en·sef''uh·lye'tis) *n.,* pl. **encephali·ti·des** (·lit'i·deez) Inflammation of the brain. —**encepha·lit·ic** (·lit'ick) *adj.*

encephalitis le·thar·gi·ca (le·thahr'ji·kuh). Epidemic encephalitis reported in the first quarter of the 20th century, probably of viral etiology, characterized by lethargy, ophthalmoplegia, hyperkinesia, and at times residual neurologic disability, particularly parkinsonism with oculogyric crisis. Syn. *epidemic encephalitis, sleeping sickness, von Economo's disease.*

encephalo-. See *encephal-.*

en·ceph·a·lo·cele (en·sef'uh·lo·seel) *n.* Hernia of the brain through a congenital or traumatic opening in the cranium.

en·ceph·a·lo·dys·pla·sia (en·sef''uh·lo·dis·play'zhuh, ·zee·uh) *n.* Maldevelopment of the brain.

en·ceph·a·lo·fa·cial (en·sef''uh·lo·fay'shul) *adj.* Pertaining to the brain and face.

en·ceph·a·lo·gram (en·sef'uh·lo·gram) *n.* A roentgenogram of the brain made in encephalography.

en·ceph·a·log·ra·phy (en·sef''uh·log'ruh·fee) *n.* Radiography of the brain following removal of cerebrospinal fluid, by lumbar or cisternal puncture, and its replacement by air, other gas, or contrast material.

en·ceph·a·loid (en·sef'uh·loid) *adj.* 1. Resembling the brain or brain tissue. 2. Of soft, brainlike consistency.

en·ceph·a·lo·ma (en·sef''uh·lo'muh) *n.,* pl. **encephalomas, encephaloma·ta** (·tuh) 1. A tumor of the brain. 2. MEDULLARY CARCINOMA.

en·ceph·a·lo·ma·la·cia (en·sef''uh·lo·ma·lay'shuh, shee·uh) *n.* Softening of the brain due to infarction.

en·ceph·a·lo·men·in·gi·tis (en·sef''uh·lo·men''in·jye'tis) *n.* MENINGOENCEPHALITIS.

en·ceph·a·lo·me·nin·go·cele (en·sef''uh·lo·me·ning'go·seel) *n.* Hernia of the membranes and brain substance through an opening in the cranium.

en·ceph·a·lo·my·e·li·tis (en·sef''uh·lo·migh''e·lye'tis) *n.* Inflammation of the brain and spinal cord.

en·ceph·a·lo·my·e·lo·neu·rop·a·thy (en·sef''uh·lo·migh''e·lo·new·rop'uth·ee) *n.* Disease of the brain, spinal cord, and peripheral nervous system.

en·ceph·a·lo·my·e·lop·a·thy (en·sef''uh·lo·migh''e·lop'uth·ee) *n.* Any disease affecting both brain and spinal cord.

en·ceph·a·lo·myo·car·di·tis (en·sef''uh·lo·migh''o·kahr·dye'tis) *n.* An acute febrile illness, usually of infants and children, characterized by encephalitis and myocarditis; caused by a variety of viruses, including the encephalomyocarditis virus (named for this disease), and Columbia-SK, Mengo, and Coxsackie viruses.

en·ceph·a·lon (en·sef'uh·lon) *n.,* genit. **encepha·li** (lye), pl. **encepha·la** (·luh) The brain.

en·ceph·a·lop·a·thy (en·sef''uh·lop'uth·ee) *n.* Any disease of the brain.

en·ceph·a·lo·spi·nal (en·sef''uh·lo·spye'nul) *adj.* Pertaining to the brain and the spinal cord.

en·ceph·a·lo·tome (en·sef'uh·lo·tome) *n.* 1. An instrument for dissecting the brain. 2. A surgical instrument for incising the brain. 3. A surgical instrument for destroying the cranium of a fetus to facilitate delivery.

en·ceph·a·lot·o·my (en·sef''uh·lot'uh·mee) *n.* 1. Surgical incision of the brain. 2. Operative destruction of the fetal cranium to facilitate delivery. 3. Dissection of the brain.

en·ceph·a·lo·tri·gem·i·nal (en·sef''uh·lo·trye·jem'i·nul) *adj.* Pertaining to the brain and the trigeminal nerve.

en·chon·dral (en·kon'drul) *adj.* ENDOCHONDRAL.

en·chon·dro·ma (en''kon·dro'muh) *n.,* pl. **enchondroma·ta** (·tuh), **enchondromas** A benign tumor composed of dysplastic cartilage cells, occurring in the metaphysis of cylindric bones, especially of the hands and feet. —**enchondrom·a·tous** (·dro'muh·tus, ·drom'uh·tus) *adj.*

en·chon·dro·ma·to·sis (en·kon''dro·muh·to'sis, en''kon·dro'') *n.* A rare disorder principally involving tubular bones, especially those of the hands and feet, characterized by hamartomatous proliferation of cartilage in the metaphysis, indistinguishable in single lesions from enchondromas. Chondrosarcomas may appear in the involved areas in later life. Syn. *Ollier's disease.*

en·chon·dro·sis (en''kon·dro'sis) *n.* ENCHONDROMATOSIS.

en·clit·ic (en·klit'ick) *adj.* Presenting obliquely; not synclitic; designating the inclination of the pelvic planes to those of the fetal head.

en·cod·ing, *n.* The process whereby a message or code is transformed into signals or symbols in a communication system, or converted from one system of communication into another, as the translation of chemical into electrical data.

en·cop·re·sis (en''kop·ree'sis) *n.* Psychically caused incontinence of feces; soiling.

en·crust, in·crust (in·krust') *v.* To form a crust or hard coating on. —**encrust·ed, incrust·ed,** *adj.*

en·cys·ta·tion (en''sis·tay'shun) *n.* 1. Enclosure in a cyst or sac. 2. The process of forming a cyst. —**encyst** (en·sist') *v.*

en·cyst·ed (en·sis'tid) *adj.* Enclosed in a cyst or capsule.

encysted calculus. A calculus confined in a localized dilatation or diverticulum of the urinary bladder or gallbladder.

en·cyst·ment (en·sist'munt) *n.* ENCYSTATION.

end-, endo- A combining form meaning (a) *within;* (b) *inner, internal;* (c) *taking in, absorbing, requiring.*

End·amoe·ba (end''uh·mee'buh) *n.* ENTAMOEBA.

end·aor·ti·tis (end''ay·or·tye'tis) *n.* Inflammation of the intima of the aorta.

end·ar·te·ri·al (end''ahr·teer'ee·ul) *adj.* 1. Within an artery. 2. Pertaining to the intima of an artery.

end·ar·te·ri·tis (end''ahr·te·rye'tis) *n.* Inflammation of the inner coat or intima of an artery.

endarteritis de·for·mans (de-for'manz). Endarteritis obliterans with calcification.

endarteritis obli·te·rans (ob·lit'e·ranz). A degenerative arterial disease, chiefly of the small arteries of the extremities, in which muscular and fibrous hyperplasia of the media and intima lead to luminal stenosis and, sometimes, occlusion.

end artery. An artery without branches or anastomoses.

end·au·ral (end·aw'rul) *adj*. Pertaining to the inner surface or part of the external acoustic meatus.

end·brain, *n.* TELENCEPHALON.

en·dem·ic (en·dem'ick) *adj*. Peculiar to a certain region or people; said of a disease that occurs more or less constantly in any particular locality.

endemic cretinism. Cretinism due to maternal iodide deficiency occurring in regions where little iodide is naturally available in foods; now relatively uncommon as a result of the availability of iodinated salt and other foods.

endemic goiter. Goiter occurring commonly in mountainous or other geographic areas where the diet is deficient in iodine.

endemic typhus. MURINE TYPHUS.

end feet. Small terminal enlargements of nerve fibers which are in contact with the dendrites or cell bodies of other nerve cells; the synaptic endings of nerve fibers. Syn. *boutons terminaux, end bulbs.*

en·do·an·eu·rys·mor·rha·phy (en"do·an"yoo·riz·mor'uh·fee) *n.* An operation for aneurysm consisting of opening the sac, suturing the orifices of the communicating arteries, and folding and suturing the walls of the aneurysm, thus leaving a lumen of approximately normal size.

en·do·bron·chi·al (en"do·bronk'ee·ul) *adj*. 1. Within a bronchus. 2. Within the bronchial tree.

en·do·car·di·al (en"do·kahr'dee·ul) *adj*. 1. Pertaining to the endocardium. 2. Occurring or situated in the heart.

endocardial cushion. In the embryonic heart, either of two masses of embryonic connective tissue concerned with the development of the atrioventricular canals and valves.

endocardial fibroelastosis. Fibrous or fibroelastic thickening of the endocardium of unknown cause, but which may be congenital, hereditary, or secondary to other systemic or cardiac disease, usually associated with congestive heart failure and cardiac enlargement.

endocardial fibrosis. ENDOCARDIAL FIBROELASTOSIS.

endocardial sclerosis. ENDOCARDIAL FIBROELASTOSIS.

en·do·car·di·tis (en"do·kahr·dye'tis) *n.* Inflammation of the endocardium or lining membrane of the heart cavities and its valves. —**endocar·dit·ic** (·dit'ick) *adj*.

endocarditis len·ta (len'tuh) BACTERIAL ENDOCARDITIS.

en·do·car·di·um (en"do·kahr'dee·um) *n.,* pl. **en·docar·dia** (·dee·uh) The membrane lining the interior of the heart, consisting of endothelium and the subjacent connective tissue.

en·do·cel·lu·lar (en"do·sel'yoo·lur) *adj*. INTRACELLULAR.

en·do·cer·vi·cal (en"do·sur'vi·kul) *adj*. Pertaining to the inside of the uterine cervix.

endocervical canal. The portion of the uterine cavity situated in the cervix, extending from the isthmus to the ostium of the uterus. Syn. *canal of the cervix of the uterus.*

en·do·cer·vi·ci·tis (en"do·sur"vi·sigh'tis) *n.* Inflammation of the mucous membrane of the uterine cervix.

en·do·cer·vix (en"do·sur'vicks) *n.,* pl. **endocer·vi·ces** (·vi·seez) The glandular mucous membrane of the uterine cervix.

en·do·cho·le·doch·al (en"do·ko"le·dock'ul, ·ko·led'uh·kul) *adj*. Within the common bile duct.

en·do·chon·dral (en"do·kon'drul) *adj*. Situated within cartilage.

endochondral osteogenesis. A type of bone formation in which the osseous tissue produced largely replaces a preexisting mass of cartilage.

en·do·col·pi·tis (en"do·kol·pye'tis) *n.* MUCOUS VAGINITIS.

en·do·cra·ni·um (en"do·kray'nee·um) *n.,* pl. **en·docra·nia** (·nee·uh) The inner lining of the skull; DURA MATER. —**endocrani·al** (·ul) *adj*.

en·do·crine (en'do·krin, ·krine) *adj*. 1. Secreting directly into the bloodstream, as a ductless gland. 2. Of or pertaining to the endocrine glands or their secretions. —**en·do·crin·ic** (en"do·krin'ick) *adj*.

endocrine gland. Any gland that secretes hormonal substances directly into the bloodstream, as the hypophysis, the islets of the pancreas, the thyroid and parathyroid glands, the adrenal glands, the pineal body, the ovaries and testes.

endocrine obesity. Obesity due to dysfunction of the endocrine glands.

en·do·cri·nol·o·gy (en"do·kri·nol'uh·jee) *n.* The study of the endocrine glands and their function.

en·do·cri·nop·a·thy (en"do·kri·nop'uth·ee) *n.* A disorder resulting from abnormality in one or more of the endocrine glands or their secretions. —**endo·crino·path·ic** (·krin"o·path'ick) *adj*.

en·do·cyte (en'do·site) *n.* A cell inclusion of any type.

en·do·derm (en'do·durm) *n.* The innermost of the three primary germ layers, which forms the lining of the gut, from pharynx to rectum, and its derivatives. Syn. *entoderm.* —**en·do·der·mal** (en"do·dur'mul) *adj*.

en·do·der·mo·zo·o·no·sis (en"do·dur"muh·to·zo"uh·no'sis) *n.* A skin disease in which a parasite burrows deeply into and remains embedded within the skin, as certain ascarid and some oestrid larvae.

en·do·don·tics (en"do·don'ticks) *n.* The branch of dental practice that applies the science of endodontology. —**endodontic,** *adj*.

en·do·don·tist (en"do·don'tist) *n.* A dentist who specializes in endodontics.

en·do·don·tol·o·gy (en"do·don·tol'uh·jee) *n.* The

body of knowledge or science of disease of the dental pulp and associated processes; it deals with etiology, prevention, diagnosis, and treatment. Syn. *endodontia*.

en·do·en·ter·i·tis (en″do·en″tur·eye′tis) *n.* Inflammation of the mucous membrane lining the intestine.

en·do·en·zyme (en″do·en′zime, ·zim) *n.* An intracellular enzyme that is not excreted but is retained in the originating cell.

en·dog·a·my (en·dog′uh·mee) *n.* 1. Conjugation between gametes having the same chromatin ancestry. 2. *In anthropology*, marriage between members of the same tribe, community, or other social group, as established by law or custom. —**endoga·mous** (·mus) *adj.*

en·dog·e·nous (en·doj′e·nus) *adj.* 1. Produced within; due to internal causes; applied to the formation of cells or of spores within the parent cell. 2. Pertaining to the metabolism of the nitrogenous elements of tissues. 3. *In psychology*, pertaining to forms of mental disorders and deficiency based on hereditary or constitutional factors; originating within the body and directly affecting the nervous system.

en·dog·e·ny (en·doj′e·nee) *n. In biology*, growth from within; endogenous formation.

En·do·li·max (en″do·lye′macks) *n.* A genus of protozoans of the family Amoebidae, parasitic in man, but nonpathogenic.

Endolimax na·na (nay′nuh). An intestinal commensal ameba of man and other animals in which the nucleus contains a large karyosome; occurs as a trophozoite or as a cyst containing up to four nuclei.

en·do·lymph (en′do·limf) *n.* The fluid of the membranous labyrinth of the ear. —**en·do·lym·phat·ic** (en″do·lim·fat′ick), **endo·lym·phic** (·lim′fick) *adj.*

en·do·meso·derm (en″do·mes′o·durm, ·mez′o·) *n.* Mesoderm derived from the primary entoderm of a bilaminar blastodisk or gastrula.

en·do·me·tri·al (en″do·mee′tree·ul) *adj.* Pertaining to or consisting of endometrium.

en·do·me·tri·oid (en″do·mee′tree·oid) *adj.* Resembling endometrium.

en·do·me·tri·o·ma (en″do·mee″tree·o′muh) *n.*, pl. **endometriomas**, **endometrioma·ta** (·tuh) Endometriosis in which there is a discrete tumor mass.

en·do·me·tri·o·sis (en″do·mee″tree·o′sis) *n.*, pl. **endometrio·ses** (·seez) The presence of endometrial tissue in abnormal locations, including the uterine wall, ovaries, or extragenital sites. —**endometri·ot·ic** (·ot′ick) *adj.*

en·do·me·tri·um (en″do·mee′tree·um) *n.*, pl. **en·dome·tria** (·tree·uh) The mucous membrane lining the uterus.

en·dom·e·try (en·dom′e·tree) *n.* The measurement of the interior of an organ or cavity.

en·do·morph (en′do·morf) *n.* In the somatotype, an individual exhibiting relative predominance of endomorphy.

en·do·mor·phy (en′do·mor″fee) *n.* Component I of the somatotype, representing relative predominance of soft and round body features. In normal nutritional status, the abdominal viscera, whose functional elements are derived from entoderm, are prominent. Endomorphs tend to be fat. —**endomor·phic** (·fick) *adj.*

en·do·myo·car·di·tis (en″do·migh″o·kahr·dye′tis) *n.* Inflammation of the endocardium and myocardium.

en·do·mys·i·um (en″do·mis′ee·um, ·miz′ee·um) *n.*, pl. **endo·my·sia** (·ee·uh) The connective tissue between the fibers of a muscle bundle, or fasciculus. —**endomysi·al** (·ul) *adj.*

en·do·na·sal (en″do·nay′zul) *n.* Within the nasal cavity.

en·do·neu·ral (en″do·new′rul) *adj.* Pertaining to or situated in the interior of a nerve.

en·do·neu·ri·um (en″do·new′ree·um) *n.*, pl. **endo·neu·ria** (·ree·uh) The delicate connective tissue surrounding individual nerve fibers and forming intrafascicular partitions. —**endoneuri·al** (·ul) *adj.*

en·do·par·a·site (en″do·păr′uh·site) *n.* A parasite living within its host. —**endo·par·a·sit·ic** (·păr·uh·sit′ick) *adj.*

en·do·pha·ryn·ge·al (en″do·fa·rin′jee·ul) *adj.* Within the pharynx.

en·do·phle·bi·tis (en″do·fle·bye′tis) *n.* Inflammation of the intima of a vein.

en·doph·thal·mi·tis (en·dof″thal·migh′tis) *n.* Inflammation of the internal tissues of the eyeball.

en·do·plasm (en′do·plaz·um) *n.* The inner cytoplasm of a protozoon or of certain cells. —**en·do·plas·mic** (en″do·plaz′mick) *adj.*

endoplasmic reticulum. An intracytoplasmic membrane system as seen by electron microscopy.

end organ. The termination of a nerve fiber in muscle, skin, mucous membrane, or other structure.

end·or·phin (en·dor′fin) *n.* Any of a group of neurotransmitter peptides with morphine-like action, secreted by the central periaqueductal gray matter of the brain.

en·do·scope (en″duh·skope) *n.* An instrument used for the visual examination of the interior of a body cavity or viscus. —**endo·scop·ic** (·skop′ick) *adj.*; **en·dos·co·py** (·dos′kuh·pee) *n.*

en·dos·mo·sis (en″dos·mo′sis, en″doz·) *n.* The passage of a liquid through a porous septum or membrane into a cavity containing liquid of a different density. —**endosmo·sic** (·sick), **endos·mot·ic** (·mot′ick) *adj.*

en·do·sperm (en′do·spurm) *n. In biology*, the nutritional part of a seed, notable for its triploid state in normally diploid plants.

en·do·spore (en′do·spore) *n.* 1. A spore formed within the parent cell. 2. The inner coat of a spore. —**en·do·spor·u·late** (en″do·spor′yoo·late) *v.*

end·os·te·o·ma (en·dos″tee·o′muh) *n.* A tumor within a bone.

end·os·te·um (en·dos′tee·um) *n.*, pl. **endos·tea** (·tee·uh) The membranous layer of connective tissue lining the medullary cavity of a bone. —**endoste·al** (·ul) *adj.*

endotheli-, **endothelio-**. A combining form meaning *endothelium, endothelial*.

en·do·the·li·al (en''do-theel'ee-ul) *adj.* Pertaining to or involving endothelium.

endothelial cell. One of the thin, flat cells forming the lining (endothelium) of the heart and blood and lymph vessels.

endothelial leukocyte. HISTIOCYTE.

endothelial sarcoma. 1. HEMANGIOENDOTHELIOMA. 2. EWING'S SARCOMA.

en·do·the·lio·an·gi·i·tis (en''do-theel''ee-o-an''jee-eye'tis) *n.* An inflammatory process involving the endothelium of the blood vessels in many organs; used especially in reference to lupus erythematosus.

en·do·the·lio·cho·ri·al (en''do-theel''ee-o-ko'ree-ul) *adj.* Pertaining to maternal endothelium and chorionic ectoderm.

en·do·the·li·oid (en''do-theel'ee-oid) *adj.* Resembling endothelium.

en·do·the·li·o·ma (en''do-theel''ee-o'muh) *n.*, pl. **endotheliomas, endothelioma·ta** (·tuh) Any tumor arising from, or resembling, endothelium; usually a benign growth, but occasionally, a malignant tumor.

en·do·the·li·o·sis (en''do-theel''ee-o'sis) *n.* Overgrowth of endothelium from unknown cause.

en·do·the·li·um (en''do-theel''ee-um) *n.*, pl. **endo·the·lia** (ee-uh) 1. The simple squamous epithelium lining the heart, blood vessels, and lymph vessels; vascular endothelium. 2. *Obsol.* The mesodermally derived simple squamous epithelium lining any closed cavity in the body.

en·do·ther·mic (en''do-thur'mick) *adj.* 1. Pertaining to the absorption of heat. 2. Pertaining to diathermy.

en·do·ther·my (en'do-thur''mee) *n.* DIATHERMY.

en·do·thrix (en'do-thricks) *n.* A fungal parasite forming spores inside the hair shaft.

en·do·tox·i·co·sis (en''do-tock''si-ko'sis) *n.* Poisoning by an endotoxin.

en·do·tox·in (en''do-tock'sin) *n.* A substance containing lipopolysaccharide complexes found in the cell walls of microorganisms, principally gram-negative bacteria, associated with a wide variety of biological effects, such as fever, shock, transient leukopenia, and thrombocytopenia. Syn. *Boivin antigen.*

en·do·tra·che·al (en''do-tray'kee-ul) *adj.* Within the trachea.

endotracheal anesthesia. General anesthesia in which the anesthetic is administered by means of a tube which conducts the vapor directly into the trachea.

endotracheal tube. A large, specially constructed catheter which is passed through the glottis into the trachea to facilitate controlled, positive-pressure respiration, especially valuable in intrathoracic surgery, in operations on the head or neck, and in respiratory assistance.

en·do·vas·cu·li·tis (en''do-vas''kew-lye'tis) *n.* Inflammation of the intima of a blood vessel.

en·do·ven·tric·u·lar (en''do-ven-trick'yoo-lur) *adj.* Within a ventricle, as of the heart or brain.

end plate. 1. The structure in which motor nerves terminate in skeletal muscle, involved in the transmission of nerve impulses to mus-

cle. 2. The achromatic mass at the poles of the mitotic spindle of Protozoa.

end·pleas·ure, *n.* The pleasure accompanying sexual discharge or detumescence, brought about by a relief of the tension built up during the forepleasure.

end-point nystagmus. A physiologic, jerky type of nystagmus occurring on extreme lateral gaze after a short latency period, of small amplitude with the fast component in the direction of gaze, and generally exaggerated in fatigue states.

end-stage kidney. A scarred, shrunken kidney resulting from any of several chronic renal diseases, making an etiologic diagnosis difficult or impossible.

-ene. *In chemistry,* a suffix used in the naming of certain hydrocarbons; specifically, indicates *the presence of a double bond.*

en·e·ma (en'e-muh) *n.*, pl. **enemas, enem·a·ta** (e-nem'uh-tuh) A rectal infusion for therapeutic, diagnostic, or nutritive purposes.

en·er·get·ics (en''ur-jet'icks) *n.* The branch of physics dealing with energy and the laws and conditions governing its manifestations.

en·er·gy (en'ur-jee) *n.* The capacity for doing work. All forms of energy are mutually convertible one into the other. The quantity of work done in the process of transfer is a measure of energy. Therefore, work units are commonly used as energy units.

en·er·va·tion (en''ur-vay'shun) *n.* 1. Weakness, lassitude, neurasthenia; reduction of strength. 2. Removal of a nerve.

en·gage·ment, *n. In obstetrics,* the entrance of the presenting part of the fetus into the superior pelvic strait.

en·gorge·ment (en-gorj'munt) *n.* 1. HYPEREMIA. 2. The state of being completely filled, or overfilled, as a breast with milk. **—en·gorge,** *v.*

enol (ee'nol, ·nole) *n. In chemistry,* of or designating the form of a compound when it contains the $-C=C(OH)-$ group, as distinguished from that in which it contains the tautomeric $-CH_2CO-$ group, designated *keto*. The enol form is produced from the keto form by migration of a hydrogen atom from the carbon atom adjoining the carbonyl group of the keto form. **—eno·lize** (ee'no-lize) *v.*; **eno·li·za·tion** (ee''no-lye-zay'shun) *n.*

eno·lase (ee'no-lace, ·laze) *n.* The enzyme that converts 2-phosphoglyceric acid to phosphoenolpyruvic acid.

enol·py·ru·vic acid (ee''nol-pye-roo'vick) *n.* The enol form of pyruvic acid, $CH_2=C(OH)-COOH$; presumably formed in certain metabolic reactions involving pyruvic acid.

en·oph·thal·mos (en''off-thal'mus) *n.* Recession of the eyeball into the orbit.

en·o·si·ma·nia (en''o-si-may'nee-uh) *n.* 1. Extreme and irrational terror as a psychotic symptom. 2. The obsessional symptom of having perpetrated an unpardonable act or sin.

en·os·to·sis (en''os-to'sis) *n.*, pl. **enosto·ses** (·seez) A bony ingrowth within the medullary canal of a bone, or the cranium. Syn. *entostosis.*

Enovid. Trademark for a formulation of norethynodrel, a progestogen, and mestranol, an estrogen, used to inhibit ovulation and control fertility.

en·sheathed (en·sheethd′, en·sheetht′) *adj.* Enclosed, as within a sheath; invaginated; encysted.

en·si·form (en′si·form) *adj.* Shaped like a sword.

en·som·pha·lus (en·som′fuh·lus) *n.,* pl. **ensom·pha·li** (·lye) Conjoined twins (diplopagi) united by a band in the epigastric and lower sternal regions; Siamese twins. —**en·som·phal·ic** (en′som·fal′ick) *adj.*

en·stro·phe (en′stro·fee) *n.* Inversion, as of the margin of an eyelid.

ent-, ento- A combining form meaning (a) *within;* (b) *inner.*

en·tad (en′tad) *adv.* Inward; toward the center.

Ent·amoe·ba (en′tuh·mee′buh) *n.* A genus of protozoan parasites which includes species parasitic in man.

Entamoeba co·li (ko′lye). A nonpathogenic species of parasite inhabiting the intestinal tract.

Entamoeba his·to·lyt·i·ca (his·to·lit′i·kuh). The etiologic agent of amebiasis.

enter-, entero- A combining form meaning *intestine, intestinal.*

en·ter·ec·to·my (en″tur·eck′tuh·mee) *n.* Excision of a part of the intestine.

en·ter·ic (en·terr′ick) *adj.* Pertaining to the intestine.

enteric coating. A coating for pills or tablets or capsules, intended as a protection against solutions found in the stomach, but disintegrating or dissolving in the intestines.

enteric cyst. A congenital cyst formed from a duplicated segment of bowel.

enteric fever. 1. TYPHOID FEVER. 2. PARATYPHOID FEVER.

enteric plexus. The myenteric and submucous plexuses considered together.

en·ter·i·tis (en″tur·eye′tis) *n.,* pl. **enter·it·i·des** (·it′i·deez) Any inflammation of the intestinal tract, especially of the mucosa.

enteritis ne·crot·i·cans (ne·krot′i·kanz). A form of fulminant gangrenous inflammation of the small intestine, usually due to infection by *Clostridium perfringens.*

En·tero·bac·ter (en″tur·o·back′tur) *n.* A genus of the family Enterobacteriaceae, widely distributed in nature, composed of gram-negative motile or nonmotile rods which ferment glucose and lactose with the production of acid and gas. Reaction to the methyl red test is negative and to the Voges-Proskauer test, positive. —**enterobacter,** *com. n.*

Enterobacter aer·og·e·nes (air·oj′e·neez). A species of *Enterobacter* widely distributed in nature, found in soil, plants, water, milk, and intestinal canals of humans and animals; sometimes a secondary or opportunistic pathogen. Formerly called *Aerobacter aerogenes.*

En·tero·bac·te·ri·a·ce·ae (en″tur·o·back·teer″e·ay′see·ee) *n. pl.* A large family of gram-negative bacteria (rods), motile or nonmotile, attacking glucose with the production of acid or acid and gas, forming nitrites from nitrates, of complex antigenic composition with many cross-reactions, and including many animal

parasites and saprophytes. They do not possess cytochrome oxidase, and fail to liquefy sodium pectinate. Included are the following principal groups and genera: the *Klebsiella-Enterobacter-Serratia* group, *Salmonella, Shigella, Escherichia coli,* the Arizona group, *Citrobacter, Proteus,* and the Providence group.

en·ter·o·bi·a·sis (en″tur·o·bye′uh·sis) *n.* Infection of the intestinal tract with *Enterobius vermicularis,* characterized primarily by perianal pruritus. Syn. *oxyuriasis, pinworm infection.*

En·ter·o·bi·us (en″tur·o′bee·us) *n.* A genus of nematode parasites of man.

Enterobius ver·mic·u·la·ris (vur·mick·yoo·lair′is). The pinworm or seatworm; the etiologic agent of enterobiasis in man.

en·tero·cele (en′tur·o·seel) *n.* A hernia containing a loop of intestine.

en·tero·cen·te·sis (en″tur·o·sen·tee′sis) *n.,* pl. **en·terocente·ses** (·seez) Surgical puncture of the intestine.

en·tero·chro·maf·fin (en″tur·o·kro′muh·fin) *n.* An intestinal element having an affinity for chromium salts.

en·ter·oc·ly·sis (en″tur·ock′li·sis) *n.,* pl. **enterocly·ses** (·seez) Injection of a fluid preparation into the rectum or intestine for nutrient, medicinal, or cleansing purposes.

en·tero·coc·cus (en″tur·o·cock′us) *n.,* pl. **enterococ·ci** (·sigh) A streptococcus normally found in the intestinal tract of man and other species, but pathogenic when found elsewhere, as in urinary and respiratory tracts, and the cause of subacute bacterial endocarditis.

en·tero·col·ec·to·my (en″tur·o·ko·leck′tuh·mee, ·kol·eck′) *n.* Resection of parts of both small intestine and colon.

en·tero·col·ic (en″tur·o·ko′lick, ·kol′ick) *adj.* Pertaining to the small intestine and the colon.

en·tero·co·li·tis (en″tur·o·ko·lye′tis) *n.* Inflammation of small intestine and colon.

en·tero·co·los·to·my (en″tur·o·ko·los′tuh·mee) *n. In surgery,* the formation of a communication between the small intestine and colon; enterocolic anastomosis.

en·tero·cri·nin (en″tur·o·krin′in, ·krye′nin, en″tur·ock′rin·in) *n.* A hormonal extract from the intestinal mucosa which stimulates the glands of the small intestine.

en·tero·cyst (en′tur·o·sist) *n.* An intestinal cyst.

en·tero·cys·to·cele (en″tur·o·sis′tuh·seel) *n.* A hernia involving the urinary bladder and intestine.

en·tero·en·ter·os·to·my (en″tur·o·en″tur·os′tuh·mee) *n. In surgery,* the formation of a passage between two parts of the intestine.

en·tero·gas·trone (en″tur·o·gas′trone) *n.* A hormonal extract from the upper intestinal mucosa which inhibits gastric motility and secretion.

en·ter·og·e·nous (en″tur·oj′e·nus) *adj.* Originating in the intestine.

enterogenous cyanosis. 1. METHEMOGLOBINEMIA. 2. SULFHEMOGLOBINEMIA.

en·tero·graph (en′tur·o·graf″) *n.* An apparatus which records graphically the movements of the intestine.

en·tero·ki·nase (en″tur·o·kigh′nace, ·naze, ·kin′

ace, ·aze) n. An enzyme present in the succus entericus which converts inactive trypsinogen into active trypsin.

en·tero·lith (en'tur·o·lith) n. A concretion formed in the intestine.

en·ter·ol·y·sis (en''tur·ol'i·sis) n., pl. **enteroly·ses** (·seez) Removal of adhesions binding the intestine.

en·tero·meg·a·ly (en''tur·o·meg'uh·lee) n. Intestinal enlargement.

En·tero·mo·nas (en''tur·o·mo'nas, ·om'o·nas) n. A genus of the order of Polymastigida possessing four flagella, transmitted from one host to another in the encysted stage. *Enteromonas hominis* is commonly found in diarrheic stools of man.

en·tero·my·co·sis (en''tur·o·migh·ko'sis) n., pl. **enteromyco·ses** (·seez) Any intestinal fungus disease.

en·tero·my·ia·sis (en''tur·o·migh·eye'uh·sis) n., pl. **enteromyia·ses** (·seez) Disease due to the presence of the larvae of flies in the intestine.

en·tero·patho·gen·ic (en''tur·o·path·o·jen'ick) adj. Causing intestinal disease.

en·ter·op·a·thy (en''tur·op·uth·ee) n. Any disease of the intestine.

en·tero·plas·ty (en'tur·o·plas''tee) n. A plastic operation upon the intestine. —**en·tero·plas·tic** (en''tur·o·plas'tick) adj.

en·ter·or·rha·phy (en''tur·or'uh·fee) n. Suture of the intestine.

en·tero·scope (en'tur·o·skope) n. An endoscope for examining the inside of the intestine.

en·tero·ste·no·sis (en''tur·o·ste·no'sis) n., pl. **enterosteno·ses** (·seez) Stricture or narrowing of the intestinal lumen.

en·ter·os·to·my (en''tur·os'tuh·mee) n. 1. The formation of an artificial opening into the intestine through the abdominal wall. 2. An opening, temporary or permanent, in the small intestine for anastomosis or drainage. —**en·tero·sto·mal** (en''tur·o·sto'mul) adj.

en·tero·tome (en'tur·o·tome) n. An instrument for cutting open the intestine.

en·ter·ot·o·my (en''tur·ot'uh·mee) n. Incision of the intestine.

en·tero·tox·in (en''tur·o·tock'sin) n. A toxin that is specific for intestinal mucosa, such as the thermostable, trypsin-resistant toxin produced by some strains of *Staphylococcus aureus*, and which causes acute food poisoning.

en·tero·ves·i·cal (en''tur·o·ves'i·kul) adj. Pertaining to the intestine and the urinary bladder.

en·tero·vi·rus (en''tur·o·vye'rus) n. Any of a group of related viruses of human origin, including poliomyelitis, Coxsackie, and ECHO, which are members of the picornaviruses characterized by very small size and the RNA composition of the nucleic acid.

en·tero·zo·on (en''tur·o·zo'on) n., pl. **entero·zoa** (·zo'uh) An animal parasite of the intestine.

en·theo·ma·nia (enth''ee·o·may'nee·uh) n. A psychotic symptom in which the patient believes himself to be inspired or especially selected by God for his work.

en·the·sis (en'thuh·sis) n., pl. **enthe·ses** (·seez) The employment of metallic or other inorganic material to replace lost tissue.

ent·iris (ent·eye'ris) n. The uvea of the iris, forming its inner and pigmentary layer.

ento-. See *ent-*.

en·to·cone (en'to·kone) n. The posterior lingual cusp of a maxillary molar tooth.

en·to·derm (en'to·durm) n. The innermost of the three primary germ layers, which forms the lining of the gut, from pharynx to rectum, and its derivatives. Syn. *endoderm*. —**en·to·der·mal** (en''to·dur'mul) adj.

entom-, entomo- A combining form meaning *insect*.

en·to·mol·o·gist (en''tuh·mol'uh·jist) n. A specialist in that branch of zoology dealing with insects and other arthropods.

en·to·mol·o·gy (en''tuh·mol'uh·jee) n. The study of insects and other arthropods.

ent·op·tic (ent·op'tick) adj. Pertaining to the internal parts of the eye.

entoptic image. An image perceived by the retina of objects within the eye, as when one visualizes one's own vascular pattern on rubbing the illuminated bulb of a pocket flashlight against the lower lid while looking upward.

entoptic phenomena. Alterations in normal light perception resulting from intraoptic phenomena, as subjective perception of light resulting from mechanical compression of the eyeball.

ent·op·tos·co·py (ent''op·tos'kuh·pee) n. Examination of the interior of the eye, or of the shadows within the eye. —**entop·to·scop·ic** (·tuh·skop'ick) adj.

ent·otic (ent·ot'ick, ·ot'ick) adj. Pertaining to the internal ear.

en·to·zo·on (en''to·zo'on) n. An animal parasite living within another animal. —**entozo·al** (·ul) adj.

en·tro·pi·on (en·tro'pee·on) n. Inversion of the eyelid, so that the lashes rub against the globe of the eye. —**entropi·onize** (·un·ize) v.

en·tro·py (en'truh·pee) n. 1. The portion of the energy of a system, per degree of absolute temperature, that cannot be converted to work. All spontaneous changes—that is, those occurring in nature—are accompanied by an increase in the entropy of the system. 2. *In medicine*, diminished capacity for change such as occurs with aging.

enu·cle·ate (ee·new'klee·ate) v. To remove an organ or a tumor in its entirety, as an eye from its socket. —**enu·cle·a·tion** (ee·new''klee·ay' shun) n., **enuclea·tor** (·tur) n.

en·u·re·sis (en''yoo·ree'sis) n., pl. **enure·ses** (·seez) Urinary incontinence at an age when urethral sphincter control may normally be expected, usually a habit disturbance; bed-wetting. —**enu·ret·ic** (·ret'ick) adj. & n.

en·ven·om (en·ven'um) v. To inject or contaminate with venom, as from a poisonous insect or reptile. —**en·ven·om·a·tion** (en·ven''um·ay' shun) n.

en·vi·ron·ment, n. The external conditions which surround, act upon, and influence an organism or its parts.

en·zo·ot·ic (en''zo·ot'ick) adj. Pertaining to a disease afflicting animals in a limited district.

en·zyme (en'zime, ·zim) n. A catalytic substance, protein in nature, formed by living cells and having a specific action in promoting a chemical change. Enzymes are classified on the basis of types of reaction catalyzed as oxido-reductases, transferases, hydrolases, lyases, isomerases, and ligases. —**en·zy·mat·ic** (en·zi·mat'ick), **en·zy·mic** (en·zye'mick) adj.

en·zy·mol·y·sis (en''zye·mol'i·sis, en''zi·) n. A chemical change produced by enzymic action. —**en·zy·mo·lyt·ic** (en·zye''mo·lit'ick, en''zi·) adj.

en·zy·mo·pe·nia (en''zi·mo·pee'nee·uh) n. Deficiency or absence of an enzyme in the blood.

eon·ism (ee'on·iz·um) n. The adoption of feminine habits, manners, and costume by a male.

eo·sin, eo·sine (ee'uh·sin, eo'o·seen) n. A class of red acid dyes of the xanthene group, usually halogenated derivatives of fluorescein. They share the fluorescence of the parent substance to a greater or less extent. Usually eosin Y, $C_{20}H_6Br_4Na_2O_5$, the disodium salt of 2,4,5,7-tetrabromofluorescein, is meant, since it is the most used, but the class includes also ethyl and methyl eosin, eosin B, erythrosin, erythrosin B, phloxine, phloxine B, and rose Bengal. The eosins are variously used as histologic and clinical laboratory stains, and as dyes.

eo·sin·o·pe·nia (ee''o·sin''o·pee'nee·uh) n. A reduction below normal of the number of eosinophils per unit volume of peripheral blood. —**eosinope·nic** (·nick) adj.

eo·sin·o·phil (ee''o·sin'uh·fil) adj. & n. 1. Having an affinity for eosin or any acid stain. 2. EOSINOPHIL LEUKOCYTE. —**eo·sin·o·phil·ic** (ee''o·sin''uh·fil'ick) adj.

eo·sin·o·phil·ia (ee''o·sin''uh·fil'ee·uh) n. 1. An increase above normal in the number of eosinophils per unit volume of peripheral blood. 2. The occurrence of increased numbers of eosinophilic granulocytes in certain tissues and organs. 3. The assumption of a deeper shade of red by any cell or tissue in conventional hematoxylin- and eosin-stained material.

eosinophilic granuloma. A benign, chronic, localized, proliferative disorder of reticuloendothelial cells, accompanied by eosinophilic granulocytes and producing one or more bone lesions. Syn. *eosinophilic xanthomatous granuloma.*

eosinophilic pneumonitis. LOEFFLER'S SYNDROME.

eosinophil leukocyte. A leukocyte containing coarse round granules which stain pink to bright red (acid dye) with Wright's stain and usually having a bilobed nucleus.

ep-, epi- A prefix meaning (a) *upon, beside, among, above, anterior, over, on the outside;* (b) in chemistry, *relation of some kind to a (specified) compound.*

epac·tal (e·pack'tul) adj. & n. 1. INTERCALATED. 2. SUPERNUMERARY. 3. An epactal bone, as the interparietal bone, or one of the sutural or wormian bones.

ep·ar·te·ri·al (ep''ahr·teer'ee·ul) adj. Situated upon or above an artery.

eparterial bronchus. The first branch of the right primary bronchus, situated above the right pulmonary artery.

ep·ax·i·al (ep·ack'see·ul) adj. Situated above an axis.

ep·en·dy·ma (ep·en'di·muh) n. The nonnervous epithelial cells which abut on all cavities of the brain and spinal cord. —**ependy·mal** (·mul) adj.

ep·en·dy·mi·tis (ep·en''di·migh'tis) n. Inflammation of the ependyma.

ep·en·dy·mo·blas·to·ma (ep·en''di·mo·blas·to'muh) n. A poorly differentiated ependymoma.

ep·en·dy·mo·ma (ep·en''di·mo'muh) n., pl. **ependymomas, ependymoma·ta** (·tuh) A central nervous system tumor whose parenchyma consists of cells resembling, and derived from, the ependymal cells. Syn. *blastoma ependymale.*

ephe·bi·at·rics (e·fee''bee·at'ricks) n. The practice of adolescent medicine.

Ephed·ra (e·fed'rah, ef'e·druh) n. A genus of shrubs of the Gnetaceae, from some species of which is obtained the alkaloid ephedrine. Under the name *ma-huang,* species of *Ephedra* have been used in China for many years.

ephed·rine (e·fed'rin, ef'e·dreen, ·drin) n. *l-α-*(1-Methylaminoethyl)benzyl alcohol, $C_{10}H_{15}NO$, an alkaloid present in several *Ephedra* species and produced synthetically; white crystals, soluble in water. A sympathomimetic amine used in the form of the hydrochloride and sulfate salts for its action on the bronchi, blood pressure, blood vessels, and central nervous system.

ephe·lis (e·fee'lis) n., pl. **ephe·li·des** (·li·deez) FRECKLE.

ephem·er·al (e·fem'ur·ul) adj. Temporary; transient; applied to fevers that are of short duration.

Ephynal. A trademark for alpha tocopherol, a substance having vitamin E activity.

epi-. See *ep-.*

epi·ag·na·thus (ep''ee·ag'nuth·us, ·ag·nay'thus) n. An individual with a deficient upper jaw.

epi·an·dros·ter·one (ep''i·an·dros'tur·ohn) n. 3β-Hydroxy-17-androstanone, $C_{19}H_{30}O_2$, an androgenic ketosteroid of low activity present in normal human urine as a minor constituent. Syn. *isoandrosterone.*

epi·bleph·a·ron (ep''i·blef'uh·ron) n. A congenital fold of skin on the lower eyelid, causing lashes to turn inward.

epi·bul·bar (ep''ee·bul'bur) adj. Situated upon the globe of the eye.

epicanthic fold. EPICANTHUS.

epi·can·thus (ep''i·kanth'us) n. 1. A medial and downward fold of skin from the upper eyelid that hides the inner canthus and caruncle; a normal feature in some Asiatic races of man. Syn. *epicanthic fold.* 2. Any similar feature occurring as a congenital anomaly, as, for example, in Down's syndrome. —**epican·thic** (·ick), **epican·thal** (·ul) adj.

epi·car·dia (ep''i·kahr'dee·uh) n. 1. The lower end of the esophagus, between the diaphragm and the stomach. 2. Plural of *epicardium.*

epi·car·di·al (ep''i·kahr'dee·ul) adj. 1. Of or pertaining to the epicardium. 2. Of or pertaining to the epicardia.

epi·car·di·um (ep"i·kahr'dee·uh) n., pl. **epicar·dia** (·dee·uh) The visceral layer of serous pericardium.

epi·cho·ri·on (ep"i·ko'ree·on) n. DECIDUA CAPSULARIS.

epi·co·lic (ep"i·ko'lick, ·kol'ick) adj. Situated over the colon.

epicondylar fracture. A fracture involving an epicondyle of one of the long bones.

epi·con·dyle (ep"i·kon'dile, ep"ee·) n. An eminence on a bone upon its condyle. —**epicon·dy·lar** (·di·lur), **epi·con·dyl·i·an** (·kon·dil'ee·un), **epi·con·dyl·ic** (·kon·dil'ick) adj.

epi·con·dy·li·tis (ep"i·kon"di·lye'tis) n. 1. Inflammation of an epicondyle, or of tissues near an epicondyle. 2. Synovitis of the radiohumeral articulation. Syn. radiohumeral bursitis, tennis elbow.

epi·cra·ni·al (ep"i·kray'nee·ul) adj. Pertaining to or located on the epicranium.

epi·cra·ni·um (ep"i·kray'nee·um) n. The structures covering the cranium.

epi·cra·ni·us (ep"i·kray'nee·us) n. The muscle of the scalp, consisting of a frontal and an occipital portion with the galea aponeurotica between.

¹epi·cri·sis (ep'ee·krye'sis, ep"i·krye'sis) n. A secondary crisis in the course of a disease.

²epic·ri·sis (e·pick'ri·sis) n. A critical summary or analysis of the record of a case or of a scientific article.

epi·crit·ic (ep"i·krit'ick) adj. Characterized by or pertaining to fine sensory discriminations, especially of touch and temperature.

epi·cys·ti·tis (ep"i·sis·tye'tis) n. PERICYSTITIS (2).

epi·cys·tot·o·my (ep"i·sis·tot'uh·mee) n. Suprapubic incision of the urinary bladder.

epi·cyte (ep'i·site) n. 1. CELL WALL. 2. A cell of epithelial tissue.

ep·i·dem·ic (ep"i·dem'ick) adj. & n. 1. Of diseases, occurring or tending to occur in extensive outbreaks, or in unusually high incidence at certain times and places. 2. An extensive outbreak or period of unusually high incidence of a disease in a community or area. 3. Of or pertaining to epidemics.

epidemic cerebrospinal meningitis. Meningococcal meningitis of endemic and epidemic incidence.

epidemic diarrhea of the newborn. Contagious fulminating diarrhea with high mortality, seen in newborns in hospital nurseries, and caused by enteropathogenic strains of Escherichia coli, certain strains of Staphylococcus, other bacteria, and possibly viruses.

epidemic encephalitis. 1. ENCEPHALITIS LETHARGICA. 2. Loosely, any of various other encephalitides that occur epidemically, such as Japanese B encephalitis, eastern or western equine encephalomyelitis, Murray Valley encephalitis, St. Louis encephalitis, and others.

epidemic hemorrhagic fever. An acute febrile epidemic disease of northeast Asia, thought to be due to a virus transmitted by mites; characterized by widespread vascular damage, prostration, vomiting, proteinuria, hemorrhagic manifestations, shock, and renal failure. Syn. hemorrhagic fever, Far Eastern hemorrhagic fever, hemorrhagic nephrosonephritis.

epidemic keratoconjunctivitis. An infection caused by adenovirus types 6, 7, and 8, characterized by redness and chemosis of the conjunctiva, edema of periorbital tissues, preauricular lymphadenopathy, and mild constitutional symptoms. Superficial opacities of the cornea sometimes may result in persisting impairment of vision.

epidemic pleurodynia. An acute epidemic disease caused chiefly by Coxsackie B virus, characterized by severe paroxysmal pain in the lower thorax and upper abdomen increased by respiration, and associated with fever, headache, anorexia, and malaise. Syn. Bornholm disease.

epidemic typhus. An acute infectious louseborne disease caused by Rickettsia prowazekii, characterized by severe headache, high fever, skin rash, and vascular and neurologic disturbances. Syn. classic epidemic typhus, European typhus, louse-borne typhus.

ep·i·de·mi·ol·o·gist (ep"i·dee"mee·ol'uh·jist, ep"i·dem"ee·) n. One who has made a special study of epidemiology.

ep·i·de·mi·ol·o·gy (ep"i·dee"mee·ol'uh·jee, ep"i·dem"ee·) n. 1. The study of occurrence and distribution of disease; usually restricted to epidemic and endemic, but sometimes broadened to include all types of disease. 2. The sum of all factors controlling the presence or absence of a disease. —**epidemi·o·log·ic** (·o·loj'ick) adj.

epiderm-, epidermo-. A combining form meaning epidermis.

epi·der·mal (ep"i·dur'mul) adj. Of, pertaining to, or involving the epidermis. Syn. epidermic.

epidermal nevus. NEVUS VERRUCOSUS.

epi·der·ma·to·plas·ty (ep"i·dur'muh·to·plas"tee, ·dur·mat'o·) n. Skin grafting by transplanting small pieces to denuded areas.

epi·der·mi·dal·i·za·tion (ep"i·dur"mi·dul·i·zay'shun) n. The conversion of columnar into stratified squamous epithelium.

epi·der·mis (ep"i·dur'mis) n. The superficial portion of the skin, composed of a horny layer (stratum corneum) and a living, cellular part in layers named from outside inward: the stratum lucidum (when present), the stratum granulosum, the stratum spinosum, and the stratum germinativum.

epi·der·mi·za·tion (ep"i·dur"mi·zay'shun) n. 1. The formation of epidermis as a covering. 2. SKIN GRAFTING.

epi·der·mo·dys·pla·sia (ep"i·dur"mo·dis·play'zhuh, ·zee·uh) n. Abnormal development of the epidermis.

epidermodysplasia ver·ru·ci·for·mis (verr·oo"si·for'mis). A congenital defect in which verrucous lesions caused by a virus occur on the hands, feet, face, or neck.

epi·der·moid (ep"i·dur'moid) adj. & n. 1. Resembling epidermis. 2. Any tumor containing or resembling skin with its appendages.

epidermoid carcinoma. SQUAMOUS CELL CARCINOMA.

epi·der·moid·oma (ep"i·dur"moid·o'muh) *n.* An epidermal cyst involving the scalp, the bones of the calvaria, or the extradural space.

epi·der·mol·y·sis (ep"i·dur·mol'i·sis) *n.* The easy separation of various layers of skin, primarily of the epidermis from the dermis.

epidermolysis bul·lo·sa (buh·lo'suh, bŏŏl·o'suh). A genodermatosis characterized by the development of vesicles and bullae on slight, or even without, trauma.

epi·der·mo·ma (ep"i·dur·mo'muh) *n.* A skin mass of any sort, such as verruca vulgaris.

epi·der·moph·y·tid (ep"i·dur·mof'i·tid) *n.* A secondary allergic skin eruption thought to occur when the fungus *Epidermophyton floccosum,* or its products, is carried through the blood stream to sensitized areas of the skin.

Epi·der·moph·y·ton (ep"i·dur·mof'i·ton) *n.* A genus of fungi of the dermatophyte group; contains but one recognized species.

Epidermophyton floc·co·sum (flock·o'sum). The single species of this genus, found in infections of the skin and nails, and especially of the groin.

epi·der·mo·phy·to·sis (ep"i·dur"mo·figh·to'sis). Infection by *Epidermophyton floccosum.* It has been commonly used to include any fungus infection of the feet producing scaliness and vesicles with pruritus.

epi·der·mo·tro·pic (ep"i·dur"mo·tro'pick, ·trop' ick) *adj.* Having an affinity for epidermis.

epididym-, epididymo-. A combining form meaning *epididymis, epididymal.*

epi·did·y·mal (ep"i·did'i·mul) *adj.* Of or pertaining to the epididymis.

epididymal duct. The highly convoluted part of the duct of the testis which forms the main mass of the epididymis.

epi·did·y·mec·to·my (ep"i·did"i·meck'tuh·mee) *n.* Surgical removal of the epididymis.

epi·did·y·mis (ep"i·did'i·mis) *n.,* genit. **epi·di·dy·mi·dis** (ep"i·did·im'i·dis), pl. **epi·di·dy·mi·des** (·did'i·mi·deez, ·di·dim'i·deez) *n.* The portion of the seminal duct lying posterior to the testis and connected to it by the efferent ductules of the testis.

epi·did·y·mi·tis (ep"i·did"i·migh'tis) *n.* Inflammation of the epididymis.

epi·did·y·mo·or·chi·dec·to·my (ep"i·did"i·mo· or"ki·deck'tuh·mee) *n.* Surgical removal of a testis and epididymis.

epi·did·y·mo·or·chi·tis (ep"i·did"i·mo·or·kigh' tis) *n.* Inflammation of both the epididymis and testis.

epi·du·ral (ep"i·dew'rul) *adj.* Situated upon or over the dura mater.

epidural abscess. An abscess located outside the dura mater but within the cranium or spinal canal. Syn. *epidural pachymeningitis, extradural abscess, pachymeningitis externa.*

epidural hematoma. The localized accumulation of blood between the dura mater and the skull, usually as a result of rupture of the middle meningeal artery and skull fracture, characterized usually by a brief loss of consciousness, then a lucid interval, and later progressive neurologic involvement with depression of consciousness, hemiparesis, and

seizures due to compression of the brain by blood clot.

epidural space or **cavity.** The space between the spinal dura mater and the periosteum lining the canal.

epidural spinal hematoma or **hemorrhage.** Bleeding into the epidural space as a result of trauma, vascular abnormality, or bleeding tendency, as with anticoagulant therapy; manifested by signs and symptoms of rapidly progressive spinal cord compression.

epi·gas·tric (ep"i·gas'trick) *adj.* Of or pertaining to the epigastric region.

epigastric hernia. A hernia in the linea alba, between the umbilicus and the xiphoid process, generally found in young adult males; the contents of the sac are usually extraperitoneal fat, lipomas, and, only rarely, bowel.

epigastric region. The upper and middle part of the abdominal surface between the two hypochondriac regions. Syn. *epigastrium.*

epi·gas·tri·um, epi·gas·trae·um (ep"i·gas'tree· um) *n.,* pl. **epigas·tria** (·tree·uh) EPIGASTRIC REGION.

epi·gen·e·sis (ep"i·jen'e·sis) *n.* The theory that the fertilized egg gives rise to the organism by the progressive production of new parts, previously nonexistent as such in the egg's original structure. —**epi·ge·net·ic** (·je·net'ick) *adj.*

epi·glot·tic (ep"i·glot'ick) *adj.* Of or pertaining to the epiglottis; EPIGLOTTAL.

epi·glot·ti·dec·to·my (ep"i·glot"i·deck'tuh·mee) *n.* Excision of the epiglottis or a part of it.

epi·glot·tis (ep"i·glot'is) *n.* An elastic cartilage covered by mucous membrane, forming the superior part of the larynx which guards the glottis during swallowing.

epi·glot·ti·tis (ep"i·glot·eye'tis) *n.* Inflammation of the epiglottis, frequently caused by *Haemophilus influenzae.*

epilating forceps. Special forceps used for removing the hairs of the lashes, eyebrows, or other areas where hair is not desired.

ep·i·la·tion (ep"i·lay'shun) *n.* Removal of the hair roots, as by the use of forceps, chemical means, or roentgenotherapy. —**epi·late** (ep'i· late) *v.*

ep·i·lep·sia (ep"i·lep'see·uh) *n.* EPILEPSY.

ep·i·lep·sy (ep'i·lep'see) *n.* A disorder of the brain characterized by a recurring excessive neuronal discharge, manifested by transient episodes of motor, sensory, or psychic dysfunction, with or without unconsciousness or convulsive movements. The seizure is associated with marked changes in recorded electrical brain activity.

ep·i·lep·tic (ep"i·lep'tick) *adj.* & *n.* 1. Pertaining to or characterized by epilepsy. 2. An individual who suffers from epilepsy.

epileptic equivalent. CONVULSIVE EQUIVALENT.

ep·i·lep·ti·form (ep"i·lep'ti·form) *adj.* 1. Resembling epilepsy; specifically, resembling a generalized convulsion. 2. Having the electroencephalographic features characteristic of epilepsy, such as 3 per second spikes and waves, generalized paroxysmal activity, and spike or sharp wave discharges.

ep·i·lep·to·gen·ic (ep''i·lep''to·jen'ick) *adj.* Producing epilepsy.

epileptogenic focus. The exact location in the brain from which an epileptic discharge originates, sometimes identifiable by means of an electroencephalogram or electrocorticogram.

ep·i·lep·toid (ep''i·lep'toid) *adj.* Resembling epilepsy.

ep·i·loia (ep''i·loy'uh) *n.* TUBEROUS SCLEROSIS.

epi·mere (ep'i·meer) *n.* The dorsal portion of the trunk mesoderm of chordates, forming skeletal musculature and contributing to derma and axial skeleton.

epi·my·si·um (ep''i·miz'ee·um, ·mis'ee·um) *n.,* pl. **epimy·sia** (·ee·uh) The sheath of connective tissue surrounding a muscle. —**epimysi·al** (·ul) *adj.*

epi·neph·rine (ep''i·nef'rin, ·reen) *n. l-α-3,4-Di-hydroxyphenyl-β-methylaminoethanol,* $C_9H_{13}NO_3$, the chief catecholamine hormone of the adrenal medulla, occurring as colorless crystals that gradually darken on exposure to light and air; sparingly soluble in water. Increased levels cause a rise in blood glucose levels, elevation of blood pressure, acceleration of the heart, vasoconstriction in such organs as the skin and intestinal tract, but dilation of coronary and skeletal muscle vessels with increased alertness as a response to emergency. Obtained by extraction from the gland or prepared synthetically. In general, the effects of administration are those following stimulation of the sympathetic nervous system. The chief uses medically are as a vasoconstrictor to prolong the action of local anesthetics and as a source of symptomatic relief in allergic states. Its action is fleeting. Syn. *adrenaline.*

epi·neph·ri·ne·mia, epi·neph·ri·nae·mia (ep''i·nef''ri·nee'mee·uh) *n.* The presence of epinephrine in the blood.

epi·neu·ral (ep''ee·new'rul) *adj.* Attached to a neural arch.

epi·neu·ri·um (ep''i·new'ree·um) *n.* The connective-tissue sheath of a nerve trunk. —**epineuri·al** (·ul) *adj.*

epi·ot·ic (ep''ee·ot'ick, ·o'tick) *adj.* Situated above or on the cartilage of the ear.

ep·i·pas·tic (ep''i·pas'tick) *adj. & n.* 1. Having the qualities of a dusting powder. 2. A powder for use on the surface of the body, as talc.

epi·pa·tel·lar (ep''ee·puh·tel'ur) *adj.* Situated above the patella; SUPRAPATELLAR.

ep·i·phe·nom·e·non (ep''i·fe·nom'e·nun, ·non) *n.,* pl. **epiphenome·na** (·nuh) An unusual, accidental, or accessory event or process in the course of a disease, but not necessarily related to the disease.

epiph·o·ra (e·pif'o·ruh) *n.* A persistent overflow of tears, due to excessive secretion or to impeded outflow.

epi·phre·nal (ep''i·free'nul) *adj.* EPIPHRENIC.

epi·phren·ic (ep''i·fren'ick) *adj.* Originating or situated above the diaphragm.

epi·phy·lax·is (ep''i·fi·lack'sis) *n.,* pl. **epiphylax·es** (·seez) The reinforcing or increase of the natural defenses of the body, usually by specific therapy.

epi·phy·se·al (e·pif''i·see'ul, ep''i·fiz'ee·ul) *adj.* 1. Pertaining to or involving an epiphysis. 2. Of or pertaining to the pineal body (epiphysis cerebri).

epiphyseal line. 1. The area left at the site of the epiphyseal plate after fusion of an epiphysis with the diaphysis of a long bone. The site is commonly marked by a cribriform bony plate more or less easily demonstrable in sections. 2. *In radiology,* a strip of decreased density between the metaphysis and the ossified portion of the epiphysis.

epiphyseal plate. 1. The broad, articular surface with slightly elevated rim on each end of the centrum of a vertebra. Syn. *epiphyseal disk.* 2. The thin cartilage mass between an epiphysis and the shaft of a bone; the site of growth in length. It is obliterated by epiphyseal union.

ep·i·phys·e·op·a·thy (ep''i·fiz''ee·op'uth·ee) *n.* 1. Any disorder of an epiphysis of a bone. 2. Any disorder of the pineal body (epiphysis cerebri).

ep·i·phys·i·al (ep''i·fiz'ee·ul) *adj.* EPIPHYSEAL.

ep·i·phys·i·ol·y·sis, ep·i·phys·e·ol·y·sis (ep''i·fiz''ee·ol'i·sis) *n.,* pl. **epiphysioly·ses** (·seez) The separation of an epiphysis from the shaft of a bone.

epiph·y·sis (e·pif'i·sis) *n.,* pl. **epiphy·ses** (·seez) A portion of bone attached for a time to a bone by cartilage, but subsequently becoming consolidated with the principal bone.

epiphysis ce·re·bri (serr'e·brye). PINEAL BODY.

epiph·y·si·tis (e·pif''i·sigh'tis) *n.* Inflammation of an epiphysis.

epi·phyte (ep'i·fite) *n.* 1. A parasitic plant, such as a fungus, growing on the exterior of the body. 2. A plant growing upon another plant, but deriving the moisture required for its development from the air.

epi·pleu·ral (ep''i·ploor'ul) *adj.* 1. Pertaining to a pleurapophysis. 2. Located on the side of the thorax.

epiplo-. A combining form meaning *epiploon* or *omentum.*

epip·lo·cele (e·pip'lo·seel) *n.* A hernia containing omentum only.

ep·i·plo·ec·to·my (ep''i·plo·eck'tuh·mee) *n.* Excision of the greater omentum or part of it.

epip·lo·en·tero·cele (e·pip''lo·en'tur·o·seel) *n.* A hernia containing both omentum and intestine.

ep·i·plo·ic (ep''i·plo'ick) *adj.* Of or pertaining to the epiploon.

epiploic appendages. APPENDICES EPIPLOICAE.

epiploic foramen. An aperture of the peritoneal cavity situated between the liver and the stomach, bounded in front by the portal vein, hepatic artery, and common bile duct, behind by the inferior vena cava, below by the duodenum, and above by the liver. Formed by folds of the peritoneum, it establishes communication between the greater and lesser cavities of the peritoneum.

epip·lo·on (e·pip'lo·on) *n.,* pl. **epip·loa** (·lo·uh) OMENTUM; specifically, GREATER OMENTUM.

epip·lo·pexy (e·pip'lo·peck''see) *n.* Suturing the greater omentum to the anterior abdominal wall for the purpose of establishing a collateral venous circulation in cirrhosis of the liver.

epi·scle·ra (ep''i·skleer'uh) *n.* The loose connective tissue lying between the conjunctiva and the sclera.

epi·scle·ral (ep''i·skleer'ul) *adj.* 1. Situated on the outside of the sclerotic coat. 2. Pertaining to the episclera.

epi·scle·ri·tis (ep''i·skle·rye'tis) *n.* Inflammation of the episcleral tissue; can occur as a diffuse form in toxic, allergic, and infectious conditions or as a nodular episcleritis in diffuse connective-tissue diseases.

episio- A combining form meaning *vulva*.

epis·io·ely·tror·rha·phy (e·piz''ee·o·el''i·tror'uh·fee) *n.* Suturing a relaxed or lacerated perineum and narrowing the vagina.

epis·io·per·i·neo·plas·ty (e·piz''ee·o·perr''i·nee'o·plas''tee) *n.* Repair of the perineum and vestibule in the female.

epis·io·per·i·ne·or·rha·phy (e·piz''ee·o·perr''i·nee·or'ruh·fee) *n.* Surgical repair of lacerated vulva and perineum.

epis·io·plas·ty (e·piz'ee·o·plas''tee) *n.* A plastic operation upon the pubic region or the vulva.

epis·i·or·rha·phy (e·piz''ee·or'uh·fee, e·pee''see·, ep''i·sigh·) *n.* Surgical repair of lacerations about the vulva.

epis·i·ot·o·my (e·piz''ee·ot'uh·mee, e·pee''see·, ep''i·sigh·) *n.* Medial or lateral incision of the vulva during childbirth, to avoid undue laceration.

ep·i·sode, *n.* 1. An event having a distinct effect on a person's life, or on the course of a disease. 2. SEIZURE. 3. CEREBROVASCULAR ACCIDENT. —**ep·i·sod·ic** (·i·sod'ick) *adj.*

epi·spa·di·as (ep''i·spay'dee·us) *n.* A congenital defect of the anterior urethra in which the canal terminates on the dorsum of the penis and posterior to its normal opening or, rarely, above the clitoris. —**epispadi·ac** (·ack) *adj. & n.*; **epispadi·al** (·ul) *adj.*

ep·i·spas·tic (ep''i·spas'tick) *adj. & n.* 1. Causing blisters. 2. A blistering agent.

epi·spi·nal (ep''i·spye'nul) *adj.* 1. Upon the spinal column. 2. Upon the spinal cord. 3. Upon any spinelike structure.

epis·ta·sis (e·pis'tuh·sis) *n.*, pl. **epista·ses** (·seez) 1. A scum or film of substance floating on the surface of urine. 2. A checking or stoppage of a hemorrhage or other discharge. 3. The suppression of the effect of one gene by another, as in the suppression of genetically determined pigment variation in albinos. —**ep·i·stat·ic** (ep·i·stat'ick) *adj.*

ep·i·stax·is (ep''i·stack'sis) *n.* NOSEBLEED.

epi·ster·nal (ep''i·stur'nul) *adj.* 1. Situated on or above the sternum. 2. Of or pertaining to the episternum.

epi·ster·num (ep''i·stur'num) *n.* A dermal bone or pair of bones ventral to the sternum of certain fishes and reptiles.

ep·i·stro·phe·us (ep''i·stro'fee·us) *n.* AXIS (2); the second cervical vertebra.

epi·thal·a·mus (ep''i·thal'uh·mus) *n.*, pl. **epithalami** (·migh) The region of the diencephalon including the habenula, the pineal body, and the posterior commissure.

ep·i·tha·lax·ia (ep''i·tha·lack'see·uh) *n.* Shedding of epithelial cells, especially in the lining of the intestine.

epithelia. A plural of *epithelium*.

ep·i·the·li·al (ep''i·theel'ee·ul) *adj.* Pertaining to or involving epithelium.

ep·i·the·li·al·ize (ep·i·theel'ee·uh·lize) *v.* EPITHELIZE.

epithelial nevus. A nevoid proliferation, either present at birth or developing later in life, in which hyperplasia of epithelial cells occurs without the presence of melanocytes.

epithelial pearl. PEARL (1).

ep·i·the·li·i·tis (ep''i·theel''ee·eye'tis) *n.*, pl. **epitheliitis·es** (·iz), **epitheli·it·i·des** (·it'i·deez) Infiltration of an epithelial surface by inflammatory cells without ulceration or abscess formation.

ep·i·the·li·oid (ep''i·theel'ee·oid) *adj.* Resembling epithelium.

epithelioid cell. A cell evolved from macrophage and having abundant cytoplasm, which causes it to resemble an epithelial cell; found in granulomas such as those of tuberculosis. Syn. *alveolated cell.*

ep·i·the·li·o·ma (ep''i·theel''ee·o'muh) *n.*, pl. **epitheliomas, epithelioma·ta** (·tuh) A tumor derived from epithelium; usually a skin cancer, occasionally cancer of a mucous membrane. —**epithelioma·tous** (·tus) *adj.*

ep·i·the·li·tis (ep''i·thee·lye'tis) *n.* Inflammation and overgrowth of epithelium of a mucous membrane.

ep·i·the·li·um (ep''i·theel'ee·um) *n.*, pl. **epithe·lia** (·ee·uh) A tissue composed of contiguous cells with a minimum of intercellular substance. It forms the epidermis and lines hollow organs and all passages of the respiratory, digestive, and genitourinary systems. Epithelium is divided, according to the shape and arrangement of the cells, into columnar, cuboidal, and squamous; simple, pseudostratified, and stratified epithelium; according to function, into protective, sensory, and glandular or secreting.

ep·i·the·li·za·tion (ep''i·theel''i·zay'shun) *n.* The growth of epithelium over a raw surface.

ep·i·the·lize (ep''i·theel'ize) *v.* To cover or to become covered with epithelium. Syn. *epithelialize.*

ep·i·them (ep'i·them) *n.* Any local application, as a compress, fomentation, lotion, or poultice.

ep·i·to·nos (ep''i·to'nos) *n.* 1. The state of exhibiting abnormal tension or muscular tone, or of being overstretched from one point to another. 2. The state of being abnormally tense or overstrained. —**epi·ton·ic** (·ton'ick) *adj.*

ep·i·tope (ep'i·tope) *n.* Any structural component of an antigen molecule which is known to function as an antigenic determinant by allowing the attachment of certain antibody molecules.

ep·i·trich·i·um (ep''i·trick'ee·um) *n.* 1. PERIDERM. 2. The superficial layers of squamous cells overlying a hair shaft in its canal before it breaks through the epidermis. —**epitrichi·al** (·ul) adj.

epi·troch·lea (ep''i·trock'lee·uh) n. The medial epicondyle of the humerus.

epi·troch·le·ar (ep''i·trock'lee·ur) adj. 1. Of or pertaining to the epitrochlea. 2. Of or pertaining to a lymph node that lies above the trochlea of the elbow joint.

epi·tu·ber·cu·lo·sis (ep''i·tew·bur''kew·lo'sis) n., pl. **epituberculo·ses** (·seez) A prominent pulmonary shadow (lobar or lobular) seen in x-ray films in active juvenile tuberculosis, probably due to atelectasis secondary to bronchial obstruction; formerly thought to represent pneumonia or allergic reaction to tuberculosis.

epi·tym·pa·num (ep''i·tim'puh·num) n. The attic of the middle ear, or tympanic cavity. —**epi·tym·pan·ic** (·tim·pan'ick) adj.

epi·zo·on (ep''i·zo'on) n., pl. **epi·zoa** (·zo'uh) An animal parasite living upon the exterior of its host; ECTOZOON.

epi·zo·on·o·sis (ep''i·zo·on·o'sis) n., pl. **epizoono·ses** (·seez) A skin disease caused by an epizoon.

epi·zo·ot·ic (ep''i·zo·ot'ick) adj. & n. 1. Affecting many animals of one kind in any region simultaneously; widely diffused and rapidly spreading. 2. An extensive outbreak of an epizootic disease; a disease of animals which is widely prevalent in contiguous areas.

epizootic equine encephalomyelitis. EQUINE ENCEPHALOMYELITIS.

epizootic stomatitis. Foot-and-mouth disease in animals.

E point. The point of the apex cardiogram at the maximum outward deflection of the cardiac apex impulse, occurring at the onset of ventricular ejection.

Epon. Trademark for a synthetic embedding medium used in electron microscopy.

ep·o·nych·i·um (ep''o·nick'ee·um) n. 1. A horny condition of the epidermis from the second to the eighth month of fetal life, indicating the position of the future nail. 2. [NA] The horny layer (stratum corneum) of the nail fold attached to the nail plate at its margin, representing the remnant of the fetal eponychium.

ep·o·nym (ep'o·nim) n. A term formed or derived from the name of a person known or assumed to be the first, or one of the first, to discover or describe a disease, symptom complex, or theory. Eponyms often honor persons who are proponents of systems and procedures, methods, or surgical operations, even though these are not original with the person so honored. —**ep·o·nym·ic** (ep''o·nim'ick), **epon·y·mous** (e·pon'i·mus) adj.

ep·o·oph·o·ron (ep''o·off'uh·ron) n. A blind longitudinal duct (Gartner's) and 10 to 15 transverse ductules in the mesosalpinx near the ovary which represent remnants of the reproductive part of the mesonephros in the female; homologue of the head of the epididymis in the male. Syn. parovarium, Rosenmueller's organ. —**epoopho·ral** (·rul) adj.

Eprolin. A trademark for alpha tocopherol, a substance having vitamin E activity.

ep·si·lon (ep'si·lon, ·lun) n. A designation for the fifth in a series, or any particular member or subset of an arbitrarily ordered set in which other members or subjects are designated α (alpha), β (beta), γ (gamma), and δ (delta); or as a correlate of the letter E, e, in the Roman alphabet. Symbol, E, ε (or ε).

epsilon chain, ε chain. The heavy chain of the IgE immunoglobulin molecule.

Ep·som salt MAGNESIUM SULFATE.

Ep·stein-Barr virus. Herpes-like virus particles first noted in cultured human lymphoblasts from Burkitt's malignant lymphoma, and of uncertain significance as etiologic agents of such tumors. These viruses may be the cause of, or related to, infectious mononucleosis. Abbreviated, EBV.

epu·lis (e·pew'lis) n., pl. **epu·li·des** (·li·deez) Any benign solitary tumorlike lesion of the gingiva. —**epu·loid** (·po·loid) adj.

ep·u·lo·fi·bro·ma (ep''yoo·lo·figh·bro'muh) n. A fibroma of the gums.

ep·u·lo·sis (ep''yoo·lo'sis) n. Scarring.

Equanil. A trademark for meprobamate, a tranquilizer drug.

equa·tion (e·kway'zhun) n. A statement of equality between two parts, as mathematical expressions. —**equation·al** (·ul) adj.

equa·tor, ae·qua·tor (e·kway'tur) n. 1. Any imaginary circle that divides a body into two equal and symmetrical parts in the manner of the equator of a sphere. 2. Of a cell, the boundary of the plane in which division takes place. 3. (of the eye:) A line joining the four extremities of the transverse and the vertical axis of the eye. 4. (of the lens:) The margin of the crystalline lens. —**equa·to·ri·al** (ee''kwuh·to'ree·ul, ek''wuh·) adj.

equi-. A combining form meaning equal, equally.

equi·ax·i·al (ee''kwee·ack'see·ul) adj. Having equal axes.

equi·dom·i·nant (ee''kwi·dom'i·nunt, eck''wi·) adj. Having equal dominance.

eq·ui·len·in (eck''wi·len'in, ee''kwi·len'in) n. 3-Hydroxyestra-1,3,5(10),6,8-pentaen-17-one, $C_{18}H_{18}O_2$, an estrogenic steroid hormone, occuring in the urine of pregnant mares; structurally it differs from estrone in containing two additional double bonds.

equil·i·bra·tion (e·kwil''i·bray'shun, ee''kwi·li·) n. Development or maintenance of equilibrium. —**equil·i·brate** (e·kwil'i·brate) v.

equil·i·bra·to·ry (ee''kwi·lib'ruh·to·ree, e·kwil'i·bruh·to'ree) adj. Maintaining or designed to maintain equilibrium.

equi·lib·ri·um (ee''kwi·lib'ree·um) n., pl. **equilibri·ums, equilib·ria** (·ree·uh) 1. A state of balance; a condition in which opposing forces equalize one another so that no movement occurs. 2. A sense of being well balanced, whether pertaining to posture, or a condition of mind or feeling.

equilibrium constant. The constant pertaining to a reversible chemical reaction; the product of the concentrations or activities of the reaction products divided by the product of the concentrations or activities of the reactants, each concentration or activity term being raised to the power of the number of molecules (or ions) involved in the reaction, determined at the instant the rate of the forward and reverse reactions are equal. Symbol, K.

equi·mo·lec·u·lar (ee″kwi·mo·leck′yoo·lur) *adj.* 1. Containing or representing quantities of substances in the proportion of their molecular weights. 2. Containing or representing an equal number of molecules.

equine (ee′kwine, eck′wine) *adj.* Pertaining to, resembling, or derived from a horse.

equine encephalomyelitis or **encephalitis**. An epidemic viral disease of horses and mules, in which birds and reptiles are the main reservoirs and mosquitos the principal vectors of the virus; the disease mitted by mosquitoes; may be communicated to man, in whom it may result in severe illness with paralysis and a wide variety of other neurologic manifestations. Three causative viral strains are known: eastern, western, and Venezuelan.

equine infectious anemia. INFECTIOUS EQUINE ANEMIA.

equi·no·ca·vus (eck″wi·no·kay′vus, e·kwye′no·) *n.* TALIPES EQUINOCAVUS.

equi·no·val·gus (eck″wi·no·val′gus, e·kwye′no·) *n.* TALIPES EQUINOVALGUS.

equi·no·va·rus (eck″wi·no·vair′us, e·kwye′no·) *n.* TALIPES EQUINOVARUS.

equi·nus (e·kwye′nus) *n.* TALIPES EQUINUS.

equi·se·to·sis (eck″wi·se·to′sis, ee″kwi·) *n.* Poisoning of horses due to ingestion of plants of the genus *Equisetum*.

Equi·se·tum (eck″wi·see′tum, ee″kwi·) *n.* A genus of cryptogamous plants, some of which have a diuretic effect.

equiv·a·lent (e·kwiv′uh·lunt) *adj. & n.* 1. Having an equal value. 2. That which is equal in value, size, weight, or in any other respect, to something else. 3. *In chemistry,* the weight of a substance, usually in grams, which combines or otherwise reacts with a standard weight of a reference element or compound, as 8 weight units of oxygen; the weights of the substance and the reference element or compound are related to the respective atomic or molecular weights and the numerical proportions in which the atoms or molecules react.

Er Symbol for erbium.

era·sion (e·ray′zhun) *n.* 1. Surgical removal of tissue by scraping. 2. Excision of a joint; ARTHRECTOMY.

er·bi·um (ur′bee·um) *n.* Er = 167.26. A rare-earth metal.

Erb's palsy or **paralysis** UPPER BRACHIAL PLEXUS PARALYSIS.

erec·tile (e·reck′til) *adj.* Capable of erection.

erectile tissue. A spongelike arrangement of irregular vascular spaces as seen in the corpus cavernosum of the penis or clitoris.

erec·tion (e·reck′shun) *n.* The enlarged state of erectile tissue when engorged with blood, as of the penis or clitoris. —**erect** (e·rekt′) *adj. & v.*

erec·tor (e·reck′tur) *n.,* L. pl. **erec·to·res** (e·reck″-to′reez). A muscle that produces erection of a part.

erector spi·nae (spye′nee). A large, complex, deep muscle of the back, having three parts,

iliocostalis, longissimus, and spinalis, each with subdivisions.

er·e·mo·pho·bia (err″e·mo·fo′bee·uh) *n.* 1. An abnormal fear of being lonely. 2. An abnormal fear of large, desolate places; AGORAPHOBIA.

erep·sin (e·rep′sin) *n.* An enzyme mixture produced by the intestinal mucosa, consisting of various peptidases which split peptones and proteoses into simpler products; it has no effect on native proteins.

er·e·thism (err′e·thiz·um) *n.* 1. An abnormal increase of nervous irritability. 2. Quick response to stimulus. —**er·e·this·mic** (err′e·thiz′mick), **ere·this·tic** (·thiss′tick), **ere·thit·ic** (·thit′ick) *adj.*

erg-, ergo- A combining form meaning (a) *work;* (b) *activity.*

er·ga·sia (ur·gay′zhuh, ·zee·uh) *n.* 1. *In psychobiology,* the sum total of the functions and reactions of an individual; the actions or responses that spring from the whole organism or personality. 2. A tendency toward work.

er·ga·sio·ma·nia (ur·gay″see·o·may′nee·uh) *n.* An exaggerated or obsessive desire for work of any kind; seen in certain neuroses and psychoses.

er·gas·the·nia (ur″gas·theen′ee·uh) *n.* Weakness or debility due to overwork.

er·go·cal·cif·er·ol (ur″go·kal·sif′ur·ol) *n.* Vitamin D₂, prepared from ergosterol; CALCIFEROL.

er·go·cor·nine (ur″go·kor′neen, ·nin) *n.* A levorotatory alkaloid, $C_{31}H_{39}N_5O_5$, from ergot, isomeric with ergocorninine.

er·go·cor·ni·nine (ur″go·kor′ni·neen, ·nin) *n.* The dextrorotatory isomer of ergocornine, occurring in ergot; physiologically, it is relatively inactive.

er·go·cris·tine (ur″go·kris′teen, ·tin) *n.* A levorotatory alkaloid, $C_{35}H_{39}N_5O_5$, from ergot, isomeric with ergocristinine.

er·go·cris·ti·nine (ur″go·kris′ti·neen, ·nin) *n.* The dextrorotatory isomer of ergocristine, occurring in ergot; physiologically, it is relatively inactive.

er·go·graph (ur′go·graf) *n.* An instrument which, by means of a weight or spring against which a muscle can be contracted, records the extent of movement of that muscle or the amount of work it is capable of doing.

er·gom·e·ter (ur·gom′e·tur) *n.* An instrument that permits a calculation of the work performed (weight multiplied by shortening) by a muscle or muscles over a period of time.

er·go·met·ri·nine (ur″go·met′ri·neen, ·nin) *n.* The dextrorotatory, relatively inactive isomer of ergonovine. Syn. *ergobasinine.*

er·go·no·vine (ur″go·no′veen, ·vin) *n.* N-[α-(Hydroxymethyl)ethyl]-D-lysergamide, $C_{19}H_{23}N_3O_2$, an alkaloid obtained from ergot which causes sustained uterine contractions and is more prompt but less persistent in its action than other ergot alkaloids. Used in the form of its maleate and tartrate salts.

er·go·phore (ur′go·fore) *n.* The chemical group in a molecule, especially of a toxin or agglutinin, which is responsible for the specific activity of the molecule.

er·go·sine (ur′go·seen, ·sin) *n.* An alkaloid,

$C_{30}H_{37}N_5O_5$, of ergot, having physiologic activity similar to that of ergotoxine.

er·gos·ter·ol (ur·gos'tur·ol) *n.* Ergosta-5(6),7(8),22(23)-triene-3-ol, $C_{28}H_{44}O$, an unsaturated sterol found in ergot, yeast, and other fungi; it occurs as crystals, insoluble in water; it is provitamin D_2; on irradiation with ultraviolet light or activation with electrons, it may be converted to vitamin D_2 (ergocalciferol). Syn. *ergosterin.*

er·got (ur'got) *n.* The dried sclerotium of *Claviceps purpurea*, a fungus developed on rye plants. It contains at least five optically isomeric pairs of alkaloids; the levorotatory isomers are physiologically active, the dextrorotatory isomers nearly inactive. Originally ergot was used, and now certain of its alkaloids, for oxytocic action; the alkaloid ergotamine is also used for the treatment of migraine headache.

er·got·a·mine (ur·got'uh·meen, ·min) *n.* A levorotatory alkaloid, $C_{33}H_{35}N_5O_5$, from ergot; while it has oxytocic activity, its principal use, in the form of the tartrate salt, is to relieve pain in the symptomatic treatment of migraine.

er·got·i·nine (ur·got'i·neen, ·nin) *n.* A mixture, originally believed to be a chemical entity, of the ergot alkaloids ergocorninine, ergocristinine, and ergocryptinine; practically inert physiologically.

er·got·ism (ur'got·iz·um, ur'guh·tiz·um) *n.* Acute or chronic intoxication resulting from ingestion of grain infected with ergot fungus, *Claviceps purpurae*, or from the chronic use of drugs containing ergot; characterized by vomiting, colic, convulsions, paresthesias, psychotic behavior, and occasionally ischemic gangrene.

er·go·tox·ine (ur''go·tock'seen, ·sin) *n.* A crystalline alkaloidal substance, long believed to be a chemical entity, isolated from ergot and having pronounced physiologic activity, now known to be a mixture of ergocristine, ergocornine, and ergocryptine.

Ergotrate. A trademark for ergonovine, an oxytocic agent used as the maleate salt.

Erig·er·on (e·rij'ur·on) *n.* A genus of the Compositae, several species of which were formerly used, especially in the form of an oil, in treatment of urinary diseases, diarrhea, and dysentery. Syn. *fleabane.*

eris·o·phake (e·ris'o·fake) *n.* ERYSIPHAKE.

Eris·ta·lis (e·ris'tuh·lis) *n.* A genus of the Diptera of the Syrphidae; commonly called drone flies. The rat-tailed larvae of several species have been known to cause intestinal myiasis in man.

erog·e·nous (e·roj'e·nus) *adj.* EROTOGENIC.

eros (ee'ros, err'os) *n. In psychoanalysis,* all the instinctive tendencies that lead the organism toward self-preservation. Syn. *life instinct.*

ero·sion (e·ro'zhun) *n.* Superficial destruction of a surface area by inflammation or trauma. —**erode** (e·rode') *v.; ***ero·sive** (e·ro'siv) *adj.*

erosion of the cervix uteri. Congenital or acquired replacement of the squamous epithelium of the cervix by columnar cells of the endocervix due to inflammation.

erot·ic (e·rot'ick) *adj.* 1. Pertaining to the libido or sexual passion. 2. Moved by or arousing sexual desire.

erot·i·cism (e·rot'i·siz·um) *n.* EROTISM.

e·ro·tism (err'o·tiz·um) *n.* 1. Sexual excitement or desire. 2. *In psychoanalysis,* any manifestation of the sexual instinct and specifically, the erotic excitement derived from all mucous membranes and special sensory organs, such as anal erotism, oral erotism, or skin erotism.

ero·to·gen·ic (e·ro''to·jen'ick, err''o·to·, e·rot'o·) *adj.* Pertaining to, causing, or originating from sexual or libidinal feelings.

erotogenic zone. Any part of the body which, on being touched, causes sexual feelings or which most expresses libidinal impulses.

ero·to·ma·nia (e·ro''to·may'nee·uh, err''o·to·, e·rot'o·) *n.* 1. Exaggerated sexual passion, or exaggerated reaction to sexual stimulation. 2. A condition sometimes seen in schizophrenia (and elsewhere) in which one develops an unrealistic persistent infatuation for or sexual fixation upon a certain person, or a delusional belief that a certain person is in love with oneself. —**erotoma·ni·ac** (·nee·ack) *adj.*

er·o·top·a·thy (err''o·top'uth·ee) *n.* Any perversion of the sexual instinct. —**ero·to·path·ic** (·to·path'ick) *adj.; ***ero·to·path** (e·ro'to·path, e·rot'o·path) *n.*

ero·to·pho·bia (e·ro''to·fo'bee·uh, err''o·to·, e·rot'o·) *n.* An abnormal fear of love, especially of sexual feelings and their physical expression.

eruc·ta·tion (ee''ruck·tay'shun, err''uck·) *n.* BELCHING.

er·u·ga·tion (err·oo·gay'shun, err''yoo·) *n.* The procedure of removing wrinkles.

eru·ga·to·ry (e·roo'guh·to''ree, err·oo·guh·) *adj. & n.* 1. Pertaining to the removal of wrinkles. 2. A substance that removes wrinkles.

erup·tion (e·rup'shun) *n.* 1. The sudden appearance of lesions on the skin, especially in exanthematous diseases and sometimes as a result of a drug. 2. The appearance of a tooth through the gums.

erup·tive (e·rup'tiv) *adj.* Attended by or producing an eruption; characterized by sudden appearance or development.

er·y·sip·e·las (err''i·sip'e·lus) *n.* A form of acute streptococcal cellulitis involving the skin, with a well-demarcated, slightly raised red area having advancing borders, usually accompanied by constitutional symptoms. —**er·y·si·pel·a·tous** (err''i·si·pel'uh·tus) *adj.*

er·y·sip·e·loid (err''i·sip'e·loid) *n. & adj.* 1. An infection caused by *Erysipelothrix rhusiopathiae*, occurring on the hands of those who handle infected meat or fish and characterized by circumscribed, multiple red lesions with erythema present in some cases. 2. Resembling erysipelas.

Er·y·sip·e·lo·thrix (err''i·sip'e·lo·thricks) *n.* A genus of thin, gram-positive rod-shaped organisms, with a tendency to form long filaments, non-spore-forming and microaerophilic, and with pathogenicity for a wide range of animals, including man.

Erysipelothrix in·sid·i·o·sa (in·sid″ee·o′suh). *Obsol.* ERYSIPELOTHRIX RHUSIOPATHIAE.

Erysipelothrix rhu·si·o·path·i·ae (roo″see·o·path′ ee·ee). The causative organism of erysipelas, acute septicemia, and chronic arthritis of swine, and of erysipeloid in man.

erys·i·phake, eris·i·phake (e·ris′i·fake) *n.* A disk-shaped instrument with an opening on one side, capable of producing slight negative pressure and used in cataract extraction.

er·y·the·ma (err″i·thee′muh) *n.* A redness of the skin occurring in patches of variable size and shape. It can have a variety of causes, such as heat, certain drugs, ultraviolet rays, and ionizing radiation.

erythema ab ig·ne (ab ig′nee) An eruption of varying form and color, often with pigmentation; due to prolonged exposure to artificial heat; seen typically on the extremities of stokers or people who sit in front of fires.

erythema an·nu·la·re cen·trif·u·gum (an″yoo·lair′ee sen·trif′yoo·gum). A skin disease characterized by gyrate, annular red macules, with hard cordlike edges and peripheral enlargement.

erythema bul·lo·sum (buh·lo′sum, bŏŏl·o′sum). The bullous type of erythema multiforme.

erythema el·e·va·tum di·u·ti·num (el·e·vay′tum dye·oo′ti·num) A dermatosis characterized by firm, painless nodules, which, discrete at first, later coalesce to form flat, raised plaques or nodular tissues.

erythema in·du·ra·tum (in·dew·ray′tum). A chronic recurrent disorder characterized by deep-seated nodosities and subsequent ulcerations; usually involves the skin of the legs of younger women; occasionally tuberculous. Syn. *Bazin's disease.*

erythema in·fec·ti·o·sum (in·feck″shee·o′sum). A benign epidemic infectious disease of early childhood, probably viral in origin, characterized by a rose-red macular rash on the face which may spread to the limbs and the trunk. Syn. *acute infectious erythema, fifth disease, megalerythema.*

erythema mar·gi·na·tum (mahr″ji·nay′tum). A type of erythema multiforme in which an elevated, well-defined band remains as a sequela of an erythematous patch; seen in rheumatic fever.

erythema mul·ti·for·me (mul″ti·for′mee). An acute, inflammatory skin disease; characterized by red macules, papules, or tubercles; the lesions, varying in appearance, occur usually on neck, face, legs, and dorsal surfaces of hands, forearms, and feet; initial symptoms are often gastric distress and rheumatic pains. Ectodermosis erosiva pluriorificialis and Stevens-Johnson syndrome are clinical variants of erythema multiforme.

erythema no·do·sum (no·do′sum). An eruption, usually on the anterior surfaces of the legs below the knees, of pink to blue, tender nodules appearing in crops; more frequently seen in women; often associated with joint pains.

erythema so·la·re (so·lair′ee). SUNBURN.

er·y·the·ma·tous (err″i·theem′uh·tus, ·themm′ uh·tus) *adj.* Pertaining to or characterized by erythema.

erythr-, erythro- A combining form meaning (a) red; (b) *erythrocyte.*

er·y·thras·ma (err″i·thraz′muh) *n.* A skin disease seen in the axillas or the inguinal or pubic regions. It forms red or brown, sharply defined, slightly raised, desquamating patches which cause little or no inconvenience.

eryth·re·de·ma, eryth·roe·de·ma (e·rith″re·dee′ muh) *n.* ACRODYNIA.

erythremic myelosis or **disease.** A hemopoietic disease of uncertain nature, characterized by proliferation of atypical primitive red cells, often accompanied by anaplastic granulocytes, and often terminating in granulocytic leukemia. Syn. *DiGuglielmo's disease, erythroleukemia.*

eryth·ri·tol (e·rith′ri·tol) *n.* Butanetetrol, $C_4H_{10}O_4$, a polyhydric alcohol existing as several different optical isomers. The mesoisomer occurs in algae and fungi and is also obtained by synthesis; it is very soluble in water, and is about twice as sweet as sucrose.

erythritol tetranitrate. ERYTHRITYL TETRANITRATE.

eryth·ro·blast (e·rith′ro·blast) *n. In hematology,* generally a nucleated precursor of the erythrocyte in which cytoplasmic basophilia is retained. According to size and nuclear characteristics, these cells can be divided into early and late forms. —**eryth·ro·blas·tic** (e·rith″ro· blas′tick) *adj.*

eryth·ro·blas·te·mia, eryth·ro·blas·tae·mia (e·rith″ro·blas·tee′mee·uh) *n.* The abnormal presence of nucleated erythrocytes in the peripheral blood.

eryth·ro·blas·to·ma (e·rith″ro·blas·to′muh) *n.* A tumor of bone marrow composed of cells that resemble large erythroblasts; probably a variety of malignant plasmacytoma.

eryth·ro·blas·to·pe·nia (e·rith″ro·blas″to·pee′ nee·uh) *n.* A decrease in number of the erythroblasts in the bone marrow.

eryth·ro·blas·to·sis (e·rith″ro·blas·to′sis) *n.,* pl. **erythroblasto·ses** (·seez) 1. The presence of erythroblasts in the peripheral blood. 2. ERYTHROBLASTOSIS FETALIS. 3. A proliferative disorder of fowl hematopoiesis caused by a virus and characterized by atypical erythroblasts in the peripheral blood and tissues. —**erythroblas·tot·ic** (·tot′ick) *adj.*

erythroblastosis fe·ta·lis (fee·tay′lis). A hemolytic anemia of the fetus and newborn, occurring when the blood of the infant contains an antigen lacking in the mother's blood, stimulating maternal antibody formation against the infant's erythrocytes.

eryth·ro·chlo·ro·pia (e·rith″ro·klor·o′pee·uh) *n.* A form of subnormal color perception in which green and red are the only colors correctly distinguished.

Erythrocin. A trademark for the antibiotic substance erythromycin.

eryth·ro·cyte (e·rith′ro·site) *n.* The nonnucleated and agranular mature cell of vertebrate blood, whose oxygen-carrying pigment, hemoglobin, is responsible for the red color of fresh blood.

In man, the cells are generally disk-shaped and biconcave, normally 5 to 9 μm in diameter (mean 7.2 to 7.8) and 1 to 2 μm thick. They number around 5 million /mm³ in the adult, ranging somewhat higher in men and lower in women. Syn. *red blood cell, red cell.* For abnormal forms, see *elliptocyte, macrocyte, microcyte, poikilocyte, sickle cell, spherocyte, target cell.*

erythrocyte fragility test. A measure of the resistance of red blood cells to osmotic hemolysis in hypotonic salt solutions of graded dilutions.

erythrocyte sedimentation test. The settling rate of erythrocytes in a column of blood kept fluid by anticoagulants, as measured by any of several methods; it is related to content of various blood proteins, and may vary in health and disease.

eryth·ro·cy·the·mia, eryth·ro·cy·thae·mia (eh-rith″ro·sigh·theem′ee·uh) *n.* 1. ERYTHROCYTOSIS. 2. POLYCYTHEMIA VERA.

eryth·ro·cyt·ic (e·rith″ro·sit′ick) *adj.* Of or pertaining to erythrocytes.

erythrocytic series. In hemopoiesis, the cells at progressive stages of development from a primitive cell to the mature erythrocyte.

erythrocyto-. A combining form meaning *erythrocyte.*

eryth·ro·cy·tol·y·sis (e·rith″ro·sigh·tol′i·sis) *n.* Disruption of erythrocytes with discharge of their contents; HEMOLYSIS.

eryth·ro·cy·to·poi·e·sis (e·rith″ro·sigh″to·poy·ee′sis) *n.* ERYTHROCYTOPOIESIS. —**erythrocytopoi·et·ic** (·et·ick) *adj.*

eryth·ro·cy·tos·chi·sis (e·rith″ro·sigh·tos′ki·sis) *n.* The fragmentation or splitting up of erythrocytes, the parts retaining hemoglobin.

eryth·ro·cy·to·sis (e·rith″ro·sigh·to′sis) *n.,* pl. **erythrocyto·ses** (·seez) Elevation above normal of the numbers of peripheral blood erythrocytes accompanied by an increase in total red cell volume; usually secondary to hypoxia.

eryth·ro·der·ma (e·rith″ro·dur′muh) *n.* A dermatosis characterized by an abnormal redness of the skin; ERYTHEMA.

eryth·ro·dex·trin (e·rith″ro·decks′trin) *n.* A dextrin formed by the partial hydrolysis of starch with acid or amylase. It yields a red color with iodine.

eryth·ro·don·tia (e·rith″ro·don′chee·uh) *n.* Red discoloration of the teeth.

eryth·ro·gen·e·sis (e·rith″ro·jen′e·sis) *n.* The formation of erythrocytes; ERYTHROPOIESIS.

eryth·ro·gen·ic (e·rith″ro·jen′ick) *adj.* 1. Inducing a rash or redness of the skin. 2. ERYTHROPOIETIC. 3. Producing a color sensation of redness.

erythrogenic toxin. A toxin produced by certain hemolytic streptococci, which is responsible for the rash of scarlet fever. Syn. *Dick toxin.*

er·y·throid (err′i·throid) *adj.* Reddish; of a red color; used of cells of the erythrocytic series.

eryth·ro·ker·a·to·der·mia (e·rith″ro·kerr″uh·to·dur′mee·uh) *n.* Papulosquamous erythematous plaques on the skin.

eryth·ro·leu·ke·mia (e·rith″ro·lew·kee′mee·uh) *n.* ERYTHREMIC MYELOSIS.

eryth·ro·leu·ko·sis (e·rith″ro·lew·ko′sis) *n.,* pl. **erythroleuko·ses** (·seez) ERYTHROBLASTOSIS (3).

er·y·throl·y·sis (err″i·throl′i·sis) *n.,* pl. **erythroly·ses** (·seez) ERYTHROCYTOLYSIS.

eryth·ro·me·lal·gia (e·rith″ro·me·lal′jee·uh) *n.* A cutaneous vasodilatation of the feet or, more rarely, of the hands; characterized by redness, mottling, changes in skin temperature, and neuralgic pains. Syn. *acromelalgia, Mitchell's disease.*

eryth·ro·my·cin (e·rith″ro·migh′sin) *n.* An antibiotic substance, $C_{37}H_{67}NO_{13}$, isolated from cultures of the red-pigment-producing organism *Streptomyces erythreus.* Erythromycin is effective orally against many gram-positive and some gram-negative pathogens. It is used in the form of various salts and esters, as the estolate (propionate lauryl sulfate), ethylcarbonate, ethyl succinate, gluceptate (glucoheptonate), lactobionate, and stearate.

eryth·ro·neo·cy·to·sis (e·rith″ro·nee″o·sigh·to′sis) *n.* The presence of regenerative forms of erythrocytes in the circulating blood.

eryth·ro·pe·nia (e·rith″ro·pee′nee·uh, err″i·thro>) *n.* Deficiency in the number of erythrocytes.

eryth·ro·phago·cy·to·sis (e·rith″ro·fag″o·sigh·to′sis) *n.* The ingestion of an erythrocyte by a phagocytic cell, such as a blood monocyte or a tissue macrophage.

eryth·ro·pho·bia (e·rith″ro·fo′bee·uh) *n.* 1. An abnormal fear of red colors; may be associated with a fear of blood. 2. Fear of blushing.

eryth·ro·pla·sia of Queyrat (e·rith″ro·play′zhuh, ·zee·uh). QUEYRAT'S ERYTHROPLASIA.

eryth·ro·poi·e·sis (e·rith″ro·poy·ee′sis) *n.,* pl. **erythropoie·ses** (·seez) The formation and development of erythrocytes. —**erythropoi·et·ic** (·et′ick) *adj.*

erythropoietic porphyria. A rare inborn error of porphyrin metabolism, probably transmitted as a recessive trait, appearing in infancy or early childhood; characterized clinically by photosensitivity with development of blisters, pigmentation and hypertrichosis of the skin exposed to light, redness of the teeth at the gingival margins, splenomegaly, hemolytic anemia, and chemically by the presence of uroporphyrin I and coproporphyrin I in bone marrow, erythrocytes, and urine, and absence of porphobilinogen. Syn. *congenital porphyria, photosensitive porphyria.*

erythropoietic protoporphyria. A congenital and probably inherited form of erythropoietic porphyria in which exposure to sunlight results in intense pruritus, erythema, and edema of the uncovered areas of the body, usually subsiding within one day, and marked increase in the concentration of a free form of protoporphyrin in circulating erythrocytes and its excretion in stools.

eryth·ro·poi·e·tin (e·rith″ro·poy′e·tin) *n.* A humoral substance concerned in the regulation of erythrocyte production, found in a variety of animals including man, and characterized as a glycoprotein migrating in blood plasma with alpha-2 globulins.

er·y·throp·sia (err″i·throp′see·uh) *n.* An abnormality of vision in which all objects appear red. Syn. *red vision.*

er·y·thro·sis (err"i·thro'sis) *n.*, pl. **erythro·ses** (-seez) 1. Overproliferation of erythrocytopoietic tissue as found in polycythemia. 2. The unusual red skin color of individuals with polycythemia.

eryth·ro·sta·sis (e·rith"ro·stay'sis) *n.* The processes to which erythrocytes are subjected when denied free access to fresh plasma, resulting from stasis of the blood.

er·y·thru·ria (err"i·throo'ree·uh) *n.* Passage of red urine.

Es·bach's method (ess·bahk') A method for detecting protein in urine in which picric acid is added to urine to precipitate protein which settles to the bottom of a graduated tube.

Esbach's reagent A picric acid–citric acid–water solution used for quantitative protein testing of urine.

es·cape *n.* 1. *In medicine,* leakage or outflow, as of nervous impulses; release from control. 2. *In psychiatry,* the departure of a patient confined to the maximum security unit of a mental hospital without permission. **—es·cap·ee** (es·kay·pee') *n.*

escape mechanism. *In psychiatry,* a mode of adjustment to difficult or unpleasant situations by utilizing a means easier or pleasanter than that required for a permanent solution of the difficulty, often resulting in an evasion of responsibility.

-escent A suffix meaning (a) *becoming;* (b) *-like, somewhat.*

es·char (es'kahr, es'kur) *n.* A dry slough, especially that produced by heat or a corrosive or caustic substance.

es·cha·rot·ic (es"kuh·rot'ick) *adj. & n.* 1. Caustic; producing a slough. 2. A substance that produces an eschar; a caustic or corrosive. **—es·cha·ro·sis** (·ro'sis) *n.*

Esch·e·rich·ia (esh"e·rick'ee·uh) *n.* A genus of non-spore-forming gram-negative bacteria, widely distributed in nature, belonging to the family Enterobacteriaceae.

Escherichia co·li (ko'lye). A group of normal bacterial inhabitants of the intestine of man and all vertebrates. Toxic strains may cause enteritis, peritonitis, and infections of the urinary tract. Abbreviated, *E. coli.* Syn. *colon bacillus.*

es·cu·lin, aes·cu·lin (es'kew·lin) *n.* 6,7-Dihydrocoumarin 6-glucoside, $C_{15}H_{16}O_9$, a constituent of the leaves and bark of the horse chestnut, *Aesculus hippocastanum.* Being fluorescent, it absorbs ultraviolet rays and has been used as a sunburn protective.

es·cutch·eon (e·skutch'un) *n.* The pattern of pubic hair growth, which differs in men and women.

es·er·ine (es'ur·een, ·in, ez') *n.* PHYSOSTIGMINE.

-esis A suffix meaning (a) *action;* (b) *process.*

Esmarch's operation A method of amputation at the hip joint.

esophag-, esophago-, oesophag-, oesophago-. A combining form meaning *esophagus, esophageal.*

esoph·a·gal·gia, oe·soph·a·gal·gia (e·sof"uh·gal'jee·uh) *n.* Pain in the esophagus.

esoph·a·ge·al, oe·soph·a·ge·al (e·sof"uh·jee'ul, ee"so·faj'ee·ul) *adj.* Of or pertaining to the esophagus.

esophageal diverticulum. 1. A herniation through the posterior pharyngeal wall, pulsion in type, presenting most frequently on the left side of the neck. 2. A traction diverticulum of small size and no clinical significance, usually noted only at autopsy.

esophageal fistula. An abnormal tract of congenital origin, communicating between the esophagus and some portion of the skin through an external opening, or between esophagus and some viscus or organ through an internal opening. A similar fistula may result from trauma or disease.

esophageal hiatus. The opening in the diaphragm for the esophagus.

esophageal lead. *In electrocardiography,* an exploring electrode placed in the esophagus adjacent to the heart and paired with an indifferent electrode; used to study atrial waves or posterior myocardial infarction.

esophageal speech *or* **voice.** Speech produced after laryngectomy by swallowing air into the esophagus and expelling it with an eructation past the pharyngeal opening to produce a sound that is then modulated by the lips, tongue, and palate.

esophageal varices. Dilated anastomosing veins of the esophageal plexus, resulting from persistent portal hypertension.

esoph·a·gec·to·my, oe·soph·a·gec·to·my (e·sof" uh·jeck'tuh·mee) *n.* Surgical resection of part of the esophagus.

esoph·a·gi·tis, oe·soph·a·gi·tis (e·sof"uh·jye'tis) *n.* Inflammation of the esophagus.

esoph·a·go·bron·chi·al, oe·soph·a·go·bron·chi·al (e·sof"uh·go·brong'kee·ul) *adj.* Pertaining to the esophagus and a bronchus or the bronchi.

esoph·a·go·cele, oe·soph·a·go·cele (e·sof"uh·go·seel) *n.* 1. An esophageal hernia. 2. An acquired hernia of the inner coats of the esophagus through the tunica muscularis. 3. Abnormal distention of the esophagus.

esoph·a·go·du·o·de·nos·to·my, oe·soph·a·go·du·o·de·nos·to·my (e·sof"uh·go·dew"o·de·nos' tuh·mee) *n. In surgery,* an anastomosis between the esophagus and the jejunum.

esoph·a·go·en·ter·os·to·my, oe·soph·a·go·en·ter·os·to·my (e·sof"uh·go·en"tur·os'tuh·mee) *n. In surgery,* anastomosis of the cardiac end of the esophagus to the intestine, following total gastrectomy.

esoph·a·go·gas·trec·to·my, oe·soph·a·go·gas·trec·to·my (e·sof"uh·go·gas·treck'tuh·mee) *n.* Excision of parts of the stomach and esophagus.

esoph·a·go·gas·tric, oe·soph·a·go·gas·tric (e·sof"uh·go·gas'trick) *adj.* Pertaining to the esophagus and the stomach.

esophagogastric sphincter. CARDIAC SPHINCTER.

esoph·a·go·gas·tro·du·o·de·no·scope (e·sof"uh·go·gas"tro·dew"o·dee'no·skope) *n.* An instrument for examining the interior of the esophagus, stomach, and duodenum.

esoph·a·go·gas·tro·plas·ty, oe·soph·a·go·gas·tro·plas·ty (e·sof''uh·go·gas'tro·plas''tee) *n. In surgery,* repair of the stomach and esophagus.

esoph·a·go·gas·tros·to·my, oe·soph·a·go·gas·tros·to·my (e·sof''uh·go·gas·tros'tuh·mee) *n. In surgery,* establishment of an anastomosis between the esophagus and the stomach; may be performed by the abdominal route or by transpleural operation.

esoph·a·go·gram, oe·soph·a·go·gram (e·sof'uh·go·gram) *n.* A radiographic image of the esophagus.

esoph·a·go·hi·a·tal, oe·soph·a·go·hi·a·tal (e·sof'uh·go·high·ay'tul) *adj.* Pertaining to the esophagus and the opening in the diaphragm through which that organ passes.

esoph·a·go·je·ju·nos·to·my, oe·soph·a·go·je·ju·nos·to·my (e·sof''uh·go·je·joo''nos'tuh·mee) *n. In surgery,* an anastomosis between the esophagus and the jejunum.

esoph·a·gop·a·thy, oe·soph·a·gop·a·thy (e·sof'uh·gop''uhth·ee) *n.* Any disease of the esophagus.

esoph·a·go·pha·ryn·geal (e·sof''uh·go·fa·rin'jee·ul) *adj.* Pertaining to the esophagus and pharynx.

esoph·a·go·plas·ty, oe·soph·a·go·plas·ty (e·sof'uh·go·plas''tee) *n.* Plastic surgery of the esophagus.

esoph·a·go·scope, oe·soph·a·go·scope (e·sof'uh·go·skope'') *n.* An endoscopic instrument for examination of the interior of the esophagus. —**esoph·a·go·co·py** (e·sof''uh·gos'kuh·pee) *n.*

esoph·a·go·spasm, oe·soph·a·go·spasm (e·sof'uh·go·spaz·um) *n.* Spasmodic contraction of the esophagus.

esoph·a·go·ste·no·sis, oe·soph·a·go·ste·no·sis (e·sof''uh·go·ste·no'sis) *n.* Constriction of the lumen of the esophagus.

esoph·a·gos·to·ma, oe·soph·a·gos·to·ma (e·sof'uh·gos'tuh·muh) *n.* An abnormal aperture or passage into the esophagus.

esoph·a·gos·to·my, oe·soph·a·gos·to·my (e·sof'uh·gos'tuh·mee) *n.* The formation of an artificial opening in the esophagus.

esoph·a·got·o·my, oe·soph·a·got·o·my (e·sof'uh·got'uh·mee) *n.* Opening of the esophagus by an incision.

esoph·a·gus, oe·soph·a·gus (e·sof'uh·gus) *n.,* pl. *& genit. sing.* **esopha·gi** (·guy, ·jye) The musculomembranous canal, about nine inches in length, extending from the pharynx to the stomach; the gullet.

eso·pho·ria (es''o·fo'ree·uh, ee''so·) *n.* A form of heterophoria in which the visual lines tend inward.

eso·tro·pia (es''o·tro'pee·uh) *n.* Convergent strabismus, occurring when one eye fixes upon an object and the other deviates inward.

es·pun·dia (es·pun'dee·uh, Sp. es·pōōn'dya) *n.* A form of American mucocutaneous leishmaniasis caused by *Leishmania brasiliensis,* characterized by erosions of the mucosal surfaces of the nose and mouth and respiratory obstruction, accompanied by fever, anemia, and weight loss, often leading to death, but treatable in the early stages with pentavalent antimonials.

ESR Abbreviation for *erythrocyte sedimentation rate.*

es·sence, *n.* 1. That which gives to anything its character or peculiar quality. 2. A solution of an essential oil in alcohol.

es·sen·tial, *adj.* 1. Pertaining to the essence of a substance. 2. Of a disease or condition, idiopathic; occurring without a known cause. 3. Necessary in the life of an organism but not producible by it, as an essential amino acid or an essential fatty acid, which cannot be synthesized in the body and must be obtained from the diet.

essential amino acid. An amino acid which must be supplied in the diet because of the inability of an organism to synthesize it; the essential amino acids in humans and other animals are histidine, isoleucine, leucine, lysine, methionine, phenylalanine, threonine, tryptophan, valine, and, on some criteria, arginine.

essential fatty acid. Any of the polyunsaturated fatty acids that are required in the diet of mammals; probably needed as precursors of the prostaglandins.

essential hypertension. A familial and possibly a genetic form of elevation of blood pressure of unknown origin, which may result in anatomic and physiologic abnormalities of the heart, blood vessels, kidneys, and nervous system. Syn. *primary hypertension.*

essential oil. VOLATILE OIL.

EST Abbreviation for *electroshock therapy.*

es·ter (es'tur) *n.* A compound formed from an alcohol and an acid by elimination of water, as ethyl acetate, $CH_3COOC_2H_5$.

es·ter·ase (es'tur·ace, ·aze) *n.* Any enzyme that catalyzes the hydrolysis of an ester into an alcohol and an acid.

es·the·sia, aes·the·sia (es·theezh'uh, ·theez'ee·uh) *n.* Capacity for perception, feeling, or sensation.

-esthesia A combining form designating *a condition involving sensation or sense perception.*

esthesio-, aesthesio- A combining form meaning *sense, sensory, sensation.*

es·the·si·om·e·ter, aes·the·si·om·e·ter (es·theez''ee·om'e·tur) *n.* A two-pronged instrument for measuring tactile sensibility by finding the least distance between two pressure points on the skin which can be perceived as distinct.

es·the·sio·neu·ro·blas·to·ma, aes·the·sio·neu·ro·blas·to·ma (es·theez''ee·o·new''ro·blas·to'muh) *n. Obsol.* A neuroblastoma arising in the olfactory apparatus.

es·the·sio·phys·i·ol·o·gy, aes·the·sio·phys·i·ol·o·gy (es·theez''ee·o·fiz''ee·ol'uh·jee) *n.* The physiology of sensation and the sense organs.

es·thi·om·e·ne (es''thee·om'e·nee) *n.* The chronic ulcerative lesion of the vulva in lymphogranuloma venereum.

es·ti·va·tion, aes·ti·va·tion (es''ti·vay'shun) *n.* 1. The adaptation of certain animals to the conditions of summer, or the taking on of certain modifications, which enables them to survive a hot dry summer. 2. The dormant condition of an organism during the summer.

es·ti·vo·au·tum·nal, aes·ti·vo·au·tum·nal (es''ti·

vo·aw·tum′nul) *adj.* Pertaining to the summer and fall seasons.

es·tra·di·ol, oes·tra·di·ol (es·truh-dye′ol) *n.* Estra-1,3,5(10)-triene-3,17-diol, $C_{18}H_{24}O_2$, an estrogenic hormone secreted by the ovary and by the placenta. Two isomers exist: the active isomer 17β-estradiol (once designated α-estradiol) and the inactive isomer 17α-estradiol (once designated β-estradiol). The former is used as an estrogen, commonly as one of its esters: the benzoate, cyclopentylpropionate, dipropionate, undecylate, or valerate. Syn. *dihydrotheelin.*

es·tri·ol, oes·tri·ol (es′tree-ole, ·ol, es·trye′ol) *n.* An estrogenic hormone, estra-1,3,5(10)-triene-3,16,17-triol, $C_{18}H_{24}O_3$, which comprises about 90 percent of the estrogen excreted in maternal urine during pregnancy. Since its synthesis then is regulated by enzymes of the placenta and the fetal adrenal gland, the amounts excreted serve as a measure of placental and fetal status, a decline suggesting abnormal function.

es·tro·gen, oes·tro·gen (es′tro·jin) *n.* Any substance possessing the biologic activity of estrus-producing hormones, either occurring naturally or prepared synthetically. —**es·tro·gen·ic, oes·tro·gen·ic** (es′tro·jen′ick) *adj.*

es·tro·gen·iza·tion, oes·tro·gen·iza·tion (es′tro·jin·i·zay′shun) *n.* The administration of estrogenic substances.

es·trone, oes·trone (es′trone) *n.* 3-Hydroxyestra-1,3,5(10)-trien-17-one, $C_{18}H_{22}O_2$, an estrogenic hormone present in the ovary, adrenal glands, placenta, and urine. Syn. *theelin, folliculin.*

estrous cycle. The periodically recurring series of changes in uterus, ovaries, and accessory sexual structures associated with estrus and diestrus in lower mammals.

es·trus, oes·trus (es′trus) *n.* 1. Sexual desire in the lower animals; the mating period of animals, especially of the female. 2. The whole sequence of changes in the uterine mucosa of mammals, corresponding to the various phases of ovarian activity. —**estrous, oestrous, es·tru·al, oes·tru·al** (es′troo-ul) *adj.*

eth·a·cry·nic acid (eth″uh·krye′nick, ·krin′ick). [2,3-Dichloro-4-(2-methylenebutyryl)phenoxyacetic acid, $C_{13}H_{12}Cl_2O_4$, a diuretic drug.

eth·ane (eth′ane) *n.* A saturated, gaseous hydrocarbon, C_2H_6, a constituent of natural gas. Syn. *methylmethane.*

eth·a·nol (eth′uh·nol) *n.* ETHYL ALCOHOL.

eth·a·nol·amine (eth″uh·nol′uh·meen) *n.* 2-Aminoethanol, $HOCH_2CH_2NH_2$, a colorless liquid, miscible with water. In animals it may be formed by reduction of glycine or decarboxylation of serine; when methylated by methionine it forms choline. It is the basic component of certain cephalins. Syn. *cholamine, monoethanolamine.*

eth·chlor·vy·nol (eth″klor·vye′nol) *n.* 1-Chloro-3-ethyl-1-penten-4-yn-3-ol, C_7H_9ClO, a sedative-hypnotic with short duration of action.

ether, ae·ther (ee′thur) *n.* 1. An all-pervading and permeating medium, formerly believed to exist and to transmit light and similar energy. 2. A compound of the general formula ROR,

formed hypothetically from H_2O by the substitution of two hydrocarbon radicals for the H. 3. Ethyl ether, $(C_2H_5)_2O$; a thin, colorless, volatile, and highly inflammable liquid. The ether of the U.S.P. contains 96 to 98% by weight of $(C_2H_5)_2O$, the remainder consisting of alcohol and water. Its chief use is as an anesthetic. Syn. *ethyl oxide, sulfuric ether, diethyl ether, diethyl oxide.* —**ethe·re·al, ae·the·re·al** (ee·theer′ee·ul) *adj.*

eth·ics (eth′icks) *n.* A system of moral principles.

eth·i·nam·ate (eth″i·nam′ate) *n.* 1-Ethynylcyclohexyl carbamate, $C_9H_{13}NO_2$, a central depressant drug of short duration of action; used as a hypnotic.

ethinyl estradiol. 17-Ethynylestradiol, $C_{20}H_{24}O_2$, an orally effective estrogen.

eth·is·ter·one (e·thiss′tur·ohn) *n.* 17α-Ethynyltestosterone or anhydrohydroxyprogesterone, $C_{21}H_{28}O_2$, a synthetic progestational steroid.

ethmo-. A combining form meaning *ethmoid.* *ethmoidal.*

eth·mo·fron·tal (eth″mo·frun′tul) *adj.* Pertaining to the ethmoid and frontal bones.

eth·moid (eth′moid) *n. & adj.* 1. ETHMOID BONE. 2. Pertaining to the ethmoid bone or related structures. —**eth·moi·dal** (eth·moy′dul) *adj.*

ethmoidal or **ethmoid air cells.** ETHMOIDAL CELLS.

ethmoidal cells. The small air spaces, lined with mucous membrane and separated by thin bony partitions, which honeycomb the lateral portions of the ethmoid bone, forming the two ethmoid labyrinths, with the anterior cells and middle cells communicating with the middle nasal meatus and the posterior cells with the superior nasal meatus.

ethmoid bone. A delicate bone in the anterior portion of the base of the skull, forming the medial wall of each orbit and part of the lateral wall of each nasal cavity.

eth·moid·ec·to·my (eth″moy·deck′tuh·mee) *n.* Removal of the ethmoid sinuses or part of the ethmoid bone.

eth·moid·itis (eth″moy·dye′tis) *n.* Inflammation of the ethmoid bone or of the ethmoid sinuses.

eth·moid·ot·o·my (eth″moy·dot′uh·mee) *n.* Incision of an ethmoid sinus.

ethmoid sinus. Either of the paranasal sinuses in the ethmoid bone, each occupying one of the two lateral portions of the bone and consisting of several small air-filled spaces, the ethmoidal cells.

eth·mo·lac·ri·mal (eth″mo·lack′ri·mul) *adj.* Pertaining to the ethmoid and lacrimal bones.

eth·mo·max·il·lary (eth″mo·mack′si·lerr″ee) *adj.* Pertaining to the ethmoid and the maxillary bone.

eth·mo·na·sal (eth″mo·nay′zul) *adj.* Pertaining to the ethmoid and the nasal bones.

eth·mo·sphe·noid (eth″mo·sfee′noid) *adj.* Pertaining to the ethmoid and the sphenoid bones.

eth·mo·tur·bi·nal (eth″mo·tur′bi·nul) *adj.* Pertaining to the turbinal portions of the ethmoid bone, forming what are known as the superior and middle turbinates.

eth·nic (eth′nick) *adj.* Pertaining to races and peoples, and to their traits and customs.

eth·nol·o·gy (eth·nol'uh·jee) *n.* The anthropological study of peoples and societies. **—eth·no·log·ic** (eth''nuh·loj'ick), **ethnolog·i·cal** (·i·kul) *adj.*

ethol·o·gy (e·thol'uh·jee) *n.* 1. *In psychology and zoology*, the study of innate behavior patterns; particularly, the study of animal behavior. 2. The empirical study of human character. 3. The study of social behavior, as manners and mores. 4. The study of ethics.

etho·pro·pa·zine (eth''o·pro'puh·zeen) *n.* 10-(2-Diethylaminopropyl)phenothiazine, $C_{19}H_{24}N_2S$, used for the treatment of parkinsonism; administered as the hydrochloride salt. Syn. *profenamine.*

eth·o·to·in (eth''o·to'in, eth·o'toin) *n.* 3-Ethyl-5-phenylhydantoin, $C_{11}H_{12}N_2O_2$, an anticonvulsant used in the management of generalized epilepsy.

eth·oxy (eth·ock'see) *n.* The univalent radical $C_2H_5O—$.

eth·ox·zol·a·mide (eth''ocks·zo'luh·mide) *n.* 6-Ethoxy-2-benzothiazolesulfonamide, $C_9H_{10}N_2O_3S_2$, a diuretic chemically related to acetazolamide but about twice as active.

eth·yl (eth'il) *n.* The univalent radical $C_2H_5—$.

ethyl acetate. A colorless, pleasantly odorous liquid, $CH_3COOC_2H_5$, used chiefly as a solvent and in artificial fruit essences. Syn. *acetic ether.*

ethyl alcohol. C_2H_5OH, a colorless, volatile liquid which, as the basis of alcoholic beverages, acts as a central nervous system depressant valued for its euphoric effect but which in immoderate or prolonged use leads to acute or chronic alcoholism. It is used as a pharmaceutical solvent and in medicine as a sedative, for its calorific value in the debilitated, and for its cutaneous vasodilative effect. On the skin, it is antiseptic and astringent. Syn. *ethanol.*

ethyl aminobenzoate. Ethyl *p*-aminobenzoate, $H_2NC_6H_4COOC_2H_5$, a white crystalline powder, slightly soluble in water; a local anesthetic. Syn. *benzocaine.*

ethyl biscoumacetate. 3,3'-Carboxymethylene bis(4-hydroxycoumarin) ethyl ester, $C_{22}H_{16}O_8$, a white, crystalline powder practically insoluble in water; an anticoagulant.

ethyl bromide. A rapid and transient anesthetic, C_2H_5Br, more dangerous than ethyl chloride.

ethyl carbamate. URETHAN (1).

ethyl chloride. A colorless, mobile, very volatile liquid, CH_3CH_2Cl. It acts as a local anesthetic of short duration through the superficial freezing produced by rapid vaporization from the skin. Occasionally used by inhalation as a rapid and fleeting general anesthetic, comparable to nitrous oxide but somewhat more dangerous.

eth·yl·ene (eth'i·leen) *n.* A colorless gas, $CH_2=CH_2$, used as an inhalation anesthetic. Syn. *ethene, olefiant gas.*

eth·yl·ene·di·amine (eth''i·leen·dye'uh·meen, ·min) *n.* 1,2-Diaminoethane, $H_2NCH_2·CH_2NH_2$, a colorless strongly alkaline liquid of ammoniacal odor; used as a solvent and to increase the solubility of certain medicinal substances.

eth·yl·ene·di·amine·tet·ra·ace·tic acid (eth''il·een·dye''uh·meen·tet''ruh·uh·see'tick). EDETIC ACID.

ethylene glycol. 1,2-Ethanediol, $HOCH_2·CH_2OH$, a slightly viscous liquid, miscible with water. It has many industrial uses, and is used as a solvent and humectant.

ethylene oxide. $(CH_2)_2O$. A colorless gas used as a fumigant, insecticide, and sterilizing agent.

ethylene series. A group of hydrocarbons of the general formula, C_nH_{2n}, having one double bond. Syn. *ethene series, alkene series.*

eth·yl·hy·dro·cu·pre·ine (eth''il·high''dro·kew'pree·een, ·in) *n.* A synthetic derivative, $C_{21}H_{28}N_2O_2$, of cupreine; it is also chemically related to quinine. Has been used internally, as the base, in the treatment of pneumonia and locally, as the hydrochloride, in the treatment of pneumococcal infections of the eye.

eth·yl·mor·phine (eth''il·mor'feen, ·fin) *n.* An ethyl ether of morphine; $C_{19}H_{23}NO_3$. The hydrochloride is used topically as a lymphagogue in inflammatory disease of the eye, in rhinitis, and in otitis media, and internally as a narcotic analgesic and antitussive.

etio-, aetio- A combining form meaning (a) *cause;* (b) *formed by chemical degradation of a compound.*

etio·cho·lan·o·lone (ee''tee·o·ko·lan'o·lone) *n.* Etiocholane-3(α)-ol-17-one, $C_{19}H_{30}O_2$, an isomer of androsterone found in urine.

etiocholanolone fever. Recurrent fever, abdominal pain, arthralgia, and leukocytosis, associated with the presence of unconjugated etiocholanolone in the plasma and elevated urinary etiocholanolone levels. It may be associated with a variety of underlying disease states, including a condition resembling the adrenogenital syndrome, familial Mediterranean fever, and such conditions as malignant lymphoma.

eti·o·la·tion (ee''tee·o·lay'shun) *n.* Pallor caused by the exclusion of light.

eti·ol·o·gy, ae·ti·ol·o·gy (ee''tee·ol'uh·jee) *n.* 1. The science or study of the causes of disease, both direct and predisposing, and the mode of their operation. 2. PATHOGENESIS. **—eti·o·log·ic** (·o·loj'ick) *adj.*

etio·patho·gen·e·sis, aetio·patho·gen·e·sis (ee''tee·o·path''o·jen'e·sis) *n.* The cause and course of development of a disease or lesion.

eu- A combining form meaning (a) *good, well, easily;* (b) *normal, true, typical;* (c) *improved derivative of a substance.*

Eu·bac·te·ri·a·les (yoo''back·teer''ee·ay'leez) *n. pl.* An order of bacteria, class Schizomycetes, including forms least differentiated and least specialized; the true bacteria.

eu·ca·lyp·tol (yoo''kuh·lip'tol) *n.* Cineol, $C_{10}H_{18}O$, the chief constituent of the volatile oils of eucalyptus and cajeput; a mild local irritant; used in bronchitis and coryza, and formerly as a vermifuge and antimalarial.

eu·ca·lyp·tus (yoo''kuh·lip'tus) *n.* The leaf of *Eucalyptus globulus,* used medicinally.

euc·at·ro·pine (yook·at'ro·peen, ·pin) *n.* 4-Hydroxy-1,2,2,6-tetramethylpiperidine mandelate, $C_{17}H_{25}NO_3$, used as the hydrochloride salt as a mydriatic.

eu·chlor·hy·dria (yoo″klor·high′dree·uh) *n.* The presence of a normal amount of hydrochloric acid in the gastric juice.

eu·chro·ma·tin (yoo·kro′muh·tin) *n.* 1. The part of the chromatin which in interphase is dispersed and not readily stainable, and is thought to be genetically and metabolically active. 2. The substance of the autosomes (euchromosomes) in contrast to the substance of heterochromosomes. —**eu·chro·mat·ic** (yoo″kro·mat′ick) *adj.*

eu·chro·ma·top·sia (yoo·kro″muh·top′see·uh) *n.* Ability to recognize colors correctly; normal color vision.

eu·co·dal (yoo′ko·dal) *n.* A trade name for oxycodone hydrochloride, a narcotic analgesic.

Eucupin. Trademark for euprocin, a local anesthetic used as the dihydrochloride salt.

eu·es·the·sia, eu·aes·the·sia (yoo″es·theez′ee·uh) *n.* The sense of well-being; vigor and normal condition of the senses.

Eu·ge·nia (yoo·jeen′yuh) *n.* A genus of trees and shrubs of the Myrtaceae, mostly tropical. The species *Eugenia caryophyllata* yields cloves.

eu·gen·ic (yoo·jen′ick) *adj.* 1. Of or pertaining to eugenics. 2. Beneficial to the hereditary constitution of a population.

eu·gen·ics (yoo·jen′icks) *n.* The applied science concerned with improving the genetic constitution of populations, and specifically, of human populations. Positive eugenics involves selection for desirable types; negative eugenics involves selection against undesirable types.

eu·ge·nol (yoo′je·nol) *n.* 4-Allyl-2-methoxyphenol, $C_{10}H_{12}O_2$, a colorless or pale yellow liquid having a clove odor and spicy, pungent taste; obtained from clove oil and other sources. Used in dentistry as a local anesthetic and disinfectant in root canals; in ointments, as an anesthetic and antiseptic.

eu·glob·u·lin (yoo·glob′yoo·lin) *n.* True globulin. A globulin fraction soluble in distilled water and dilute salt solutions.

eu·gnath·ic (yoo·nath′ick, ·nay′thick) *adj.* Pertaining to jaws that are well developed and in proper relation to each other.

eu·gon·ic (yoo·gon′ick) *adj.* Growing luxuriantly; used to describe bacterial cultures.

eu·kary·ote, eu·cary·ote (yoo·kăr′ee·ote) *n.* An organism with a true nucleus, in contrast to bacteria and viruses. —**eu·kary·otic** (yoo″kăr″ee·ot′ick) *adj.*

eu·ker·a·tin (yoo·kerr′uh·tin) *n.* One of the two main groups of keratins. Eukeratins are insoluble in water, dilute alkali, and acids; are not digested by common proteolytic enzymes; and contain histidine, lysine, and arginine in the ratio of approximately 1:4:12.

eu·ki·ne·sia (yoo″ki·nee′shuh, ·zee·uh) *n.* Normal power of movement.

Eu·my·ce·tes (yoo″migh·see′teez) *n. pl.* A class of thallophytes containing all the true fungi.

eu·nuch (yoo′nuck) *n.* A man who has undergone complete loss of testicular function from castration, inflammation, or mechanical in-

jury. If this occurs before puberty, it is associated with failure of development of secondary sex characters and typical changes in skeletal maturation, with increased height and span and disproportionate length of the lower extremities to trunk. —**eunuch·ism** (·iz·um) *n.*

eu·nuch·oid (yoo′nuh·koid) *adj.* Characteristic of, or manifesting, eunuchoidism.

eu·nuch·oid·ism (yoo′nuh·koy·diz·um) *n.* Deficiency or absence of testicular secretion causing deficient sexual development with persistence of prepuberal characteristics.

eu·on·y·mus (yoo·on′i·mus) *n.* The dried bark of *Euonymus atropurpureus;* formerly used as a cathartic.

Eu·pa·to·ri·um (yoo″puh·to′ree·um) *n.* A genus of composite-flowered plants. The leaves and flowering tops of *Eupatorium perfoliatum,* the thoroughwort or boneset, have been used commonly as a bitter tonic, diaphoretic, and feeble emetic.

eu·pho·nia (yoo·fo′nee·uh) *n.* A normal, harmonious sound of the voice.

Eu·phor·bia (yoo·for′bee·yuh) *n.* A genus of plants of the Euphorbiaceae. *Euphorbia corollata* and *E. ipecacuanhae,* the American species, were formerly employed in medicine because of their emetic and cathartic properties. *E. pilulifera* of South America and Australia is used in asthma and bronchitis. *E. resinifera* of Africa produces euphorbium.

eu·phor·bi·um (yoo·for′bee·um) *n.* The dried resinous latex obtained from *Euphorbia resinifera.* It is strongly purgative and vesicant; sometimes employed in veterinary medicine.

eu·pho·ria (yoo·fo′ree·uh) *n.* 1. Elation. 2. *In psychiatry,* an exaggerated sense of physical and emotional well-being, especially when not in keeping with real events; may be of psychogenic origin or due to neurologic or toxic disorders, or as a result of drugs. —**eu·phor·ic** (yoo·for′ick) *adj.*

Euphthalmine. Trademark for eucatropine, a mydriatic used as the hydrochloride salt.

eu·ploid (yoo′ploid) *n. In biology,* having an exact multiple of the basic haploid number of chromosomes. —**eu·ploidy** (yoo′ploy·dee) *n.*

eup·nea, eup·noea (yoop·nee′uh) *n.* Normal or easy respiration.

eu·prax·ia (yoo·prack′see·uh) *n.* Normal and controlled performance of coordinated movements.

Eurax. Trademark for crotamiton, a scabicide and antipruritic.

Euresol. Trademark for resorcinol monoacetate, a drug used in the treatment of certain skin diseases.

Eu·ro·pe·an blastomycosis. CRYPTOCOCCOSIS.

eu·ro·pi·um (yoo·ro′pee·um) *n.* Eu = 151.96. A rare-earth metal found in cerium minerals.

eury- A combining form meaning *broad, wide.*

eu·ry·ce·phal·ic (yoo″ree·se·fal′ick) *adj.* 1. Having or characterizing a head that is unusually broad. 2. Sometimes, designating a brachycephalic head with a cephalic index of 81 to 85.4.

eu·ryg·na·thism (yoo·rig′nuh·thiz·um, yoo″ree·nath′iz·um) *n.* A condition in which the jaws are unusually broad. —**eu·ryg·nath·ic** (yoo''rig-nath'ick, yoo''ree·), **eu·ryg·na·thous** (yoo-rig'nuth·us) *adj.*

eu·sta·chian (yoo-stay'kee·un, ·stay'shun) *adj.* 1. Described by or named for Bartolomeo Eustachio, Italian anatomist, 1520–1574. 2. Pertaining to the auditory (eustachian) tube.

eustachian catheter. A small catheter with a bend at the leading end, used to relieve obstruction of the auditory tube.

eustachian salpingitis. Inflammation of the auditory tube.

eustachian tube. AUDITORY TUBE.

eu·sys·to·le (yoo-sis'tuh·lee) *n.* Normal systole.

eu·tec·tic (yoo-teck'tick) *adj. In physical chemistry,* of, pertaining to, or designating the specific mixture of two or more substances which has the lowest melting point of any mixture of the substances.

eu·tha·na·sia (yoo''thuh·nay'zhuh, ·zee·uh) *n.* The intentional bringing about of an easy and painless death to a person suffering from an incurable or painful disease.

eu·then·ics (yoo·thenn'icks) *n.* The science of rendering the environment optimal for the particular phenotype, as by the administration of specific diets or drugs. —**euthenic,** *adj.*

eu·thy·roid (yoo·thigh'roid) *adj.* Characterized by or pertaining to normal thyroid function. —**euthyroid·ism,** *n.*

eu·to·cia (yoo·to'shee·uh, ·see·uh) *n.* Natural or easy childbirth; normal labor.

Eu·trom·bic·u·la (yoo''trom·bick'yoo·luh) *n.* The genus of mites of the Trombiculidae to which chiggers belong.

Eutrombicula al·fred·du·ge·si (al''fred·dew·jee'-sigh). The mite species that causes a common type of dermatitis; widely distributed in North and South America; a chigger.

evac·u·ant (e·vack'yoo·unt) *adj. & n.* 1. Causing evacuation; purgative. 2. Medicine which empties an organ, especially the bowels; a purgative.

evac·u·ate (e·vack'yoo·ate) *v.* To empty or remove.

evac·u·a·tion (e·vack''yoo·ay'shun) *n.* 1. The voiding of any matter either by the natural passages of the body or by an artificial opening; specifically, defecation. 2. *In military medicine,* the withdrawal of sick and wounded personnel, or material, or both, as from a battle area.

evac·u·a·tor (e·vack'yoo·a''tur) *n.* An instrument for the removal of fluid or particles from the urinary bladder or intestine.

evag·i·na·tion (e·vaj''i·nay'shun) *n.* 1. The turning inside out of an organ or part. 2. The protrusion of an organ or part by eversion of its inner surface or from its covering. Syn. *outpouching.* —**evag·i·nate** (e·vaj'i·nate) *v.*

ev·a·nes·cent (ev''uh·nes'unt) *adj.* Unstable; tending to vanish quickly.

Ev·ans blue Tetrasodium salt of 4,4'-bis[7-(1-amino-8-hydroxy-2,4-disulfo)naphthylazo]-3,3'-bitolyl, $C_{34}H_{24}N_6Na_4O_{14}S_4$, a diazo dye, occurring as a bluish-green or brown iridescent powder, very soluble in water; it is used as an intravenous diagnostic agent for colorimetric determination of blood volume, cardiac output, and residual blood volume in the heart; when injected into the bloodstream it combines with plasma albumin and leaves the circulation slowly. Syn. *T 1824.*

Evans blue method A dye-dilution method using Evans blue (T 1824) for the determination of blood volume, cardiac output, and residual blood volume in the heart.

even·tra·tion (ee''ven·tray'shun) *n.* Protrusion of the abdominal viscera through the abdominal wall, as in ventral hernia.

eventration of the diaphragm. A condition where there is defective muscular action of the diaphragm, the left leaf being abnormally high, not moving through the normal excursion.

ever·sion (e·vur'zhun) *n.* A turning outward. —**evert** (e·vurt') *v.*

eversion of the eyelid. 1. A method of folding the lid upon itself for the purpose of exposing the conjunctival surface or sulcus. 2. ECTROPION.

ev·i·dence, *n. In legal medicine,* any type of proof or material, as testimony of witnesses, records, or x-ray films, presented at a trial for the purpose of convincing the court or jury as to the truth and accuracy of an alleged fact.

evil eye. The ability to cause misfortune, disease, or death indirectly, or by a glance, believed in many parts of the world to be possessed by certain individuals. The delusion of being a victim of or threatened by the evil eye is frequent among individuals with the paranoid type of schizophrenia.

Evipal. Trademark for hexobarbital, a sedative and hypnotic of short duration of action.

ev·i·ra·tion (ev''i·ray'shun) *n.* 1. Castration; emasculation. 2. Loss of potency. 3. A psychic process in which there is a deep and permanent assumption of feminine qualities, with corresponding loss of manly virtues.

evis·cer·a·tion (e·vis''ur·ay'shun) *n.* 1. Removal of the abdominal or thoracic viscera. 2. Protrusion of viscera postoperatively through a disrupted abdominal incision. 3. Removal of the contents of an organ, such as the eyeball.

evo·lu·tion, *n.* 1. A gradual, usually developmental or directional change in kind or type. 2. *In biology,* specifically, phylogenetic evolution, which is believed to result mainly from natural selection of variants produced by genetic mutations (some few of which are not deleterious and may allow adaptation to new conditions or environments); especially, the totality of those changes whereby the more complex life forms have generally developed from simpler forms. —**evolution·ary,** *adj.*

evul·sion (e·vul'shun) *n.* AVULSION.

Ew·ing's sarcoma or **tumor** (yoo'ing) A malignant tumor of bone whose parenchyma consists of cells resembling endothelial or reticulum cells.

¹**ex-, e-, ef-** A prefix meaning (a) *out, away, off;* (b) *without, -less.*

²**ex-.** See *exo-.*

ex·ac·er·ba·tion (eg·zas''ur·bay'shun, eck·sas''-

ur·) *n.* Increase in the manifestations or severity of a disease or symptom. —**ex·ac·er·bate** (eg·zas′ur·bait) *v.*

ex·al·ta·tion (eg″zawl·tay′shun) *n.* A mental state characterized by self-satisfaction, ecstatic joy, abnormal cheerfulness, optimism, or delusions of grandeur.

ex·am·i·na·tion (eg·zam″i·nay′shun) *n.* 1. Investigation or inspection for the purpose of diagnosis. 2. A formal test of the proficiency or competence of an individual in a given area of learning or training, as for a licensure or certification. —**ex·am·ine** (eg·zam′in) *v.*

ex·am·in·ee (eg·zam″i·nee′) *n.* A patient undergoing examination or any person taking an examination.

ex·an·them (eck·san′thum, eg·zan′thum) *n.* 1. An eruption upon the skin. 2. Any eruptive fever or disease. —**exan·them·a·tous** (·themm′uh·tus), **exan·the·ma·ic** (·thi·mat′ick) *adj.*

ex·an·the·ma (eck″san·theem′uh) *n.*, pl. **exan·them·a·ta** (·tuh), **exanthemas.** EXANTHEM.

ex·ca·va·tion (eks″kuh·vay′shun) *n.* 1. A hollow or cavity, especially one with sharply defined edges. 2. The act or process of making hollow. 3. Removal of carious material from a tooth.

excavation of the optic disk. The depression or cupping in the center of the optic disk.

ex·ca·va·tor (eks″kuh·vay″tur) *n.* 1. An instrument like a gouge or scoop used to scrape away tissue. 2. A dental instrument for removing decayed matter from a tooth cavity.

exchange transfusion. The replacement of most or all of the recipient's blood in small amounts at a time by blood from a donor, a technique used particularly in cases of erythroblastosis fetalis, in certain types of poisoning such as salicylism, and occasionally in liver failure. Syn. *replacement transfusion.*

ex·cip·i·ent (eck·sip′ee·unt) *n.* Any substance combined with an active drug to make of the latter an agreeable or convenient dosage form.

ex·ci·sion (eck·sizh′un) *n.* 1. The cutting out of a part. 2. Removal of a foreign body, growth, or devitalized or infected tissue from a part, organ, or wound. —**ex·cise** (eck·size′) *v.*

ex·cit·abil·i·ty (eck·sight″uh·bil′i·tee) *n.* Readiness of response to a stimulus; IRRITABILITY. —**ex·cit·able** (eck·sight′uh·bul) *adj.*

ex·ci·tant (eck·sigh′tunt, eck′si·tunt) *adj. & n.* 1. Stimulating the activity of an organ. 2. An agent that stimulates the activity of an organ.

ex·ci·ta·tion (eck″sigh·tay′shun) *n.* 1. Stimulation or irritation of an organ or tissue. 2. *In physics and chemistry,* the addition of energy to a system, thereby transferring it from its ground state to an excited state. Excitation of a nucleus, atom, or molecule can result from absorption of photons or from inelastic collisions with various atomic or nuclear particles. —**ex·cit·ing** (eck·sigh′ting) *adj.;* **ex·cite** (eck·sight′) *v.*

excitation wave. The progressive wavelike activation of successive muscle fibers in the excitatory process.

ex·cit·ato·ry (eck·sight′uh·to″ree) *adj.* 1. Tending to stimulate or excite. 2. Tending to facilitate or catalyze.

ex·clu·sion (ecks·kloo′zhun) *n.* 1. The process of extruding or shutting out. 2. *In surgery,* an operation by which part of an organ is disconnected from the rest, but not excised.

ex·coch·le·a·tion (ecks·kock″lee·ay′shun) *n.* Removal by scraping.

ex·co·ri·a·tion (ecks·ko″ree·ay′shun) *n.* Abrasion of a portion of the skin or other epithelial surface. —**ex·co·ri·ate** (ecks·ko′ree·ate) *v.*

ex·cre·ment (ecks′kre·munt) *n.* An excreted substance; specifically, feces. —**ex·cre·men·ti·tious** (ecks″kre·men·tish′us) *adj.*

ex·cres·cence (ecks·kres′unce) *n.* Abnormal outgrowth upon the body.

ex·cre·ta (eck·skree′tuh) *n. pl.* The waste material cast out or separated from an organism.

ex·cre·tion (ecks·skree′shun) *n.* 1. The expulsion of waste-containing substances from cells, tissues, organ systems, or the whole body. 2. EXCRETA. —**ex·cre·to·ry** (eck′skre·tor″ee) *adj. & n.;* **ex·crete** (ecks·skreet′) *v.*

excretion threshold. The critical concentration of a substance in the blood, above which the substance is excreted by the kidneys.

excretory urography. The radiographic visualization of the urinary tract, including the renal parenchyma and renal collecting system, ureters, urinary bladder, and sometimes the urethra, following intravenous injection of a contrast medium.

ex·cur·sion (eck·skur′zhun) *n.* 1. A wandering from the usual course. 2. The extent of movement, as of the eyes from a central position, or of the chest during respiration. —**ex·cur·sive** (eck·skur′siv) *adj.*

ex·cy·clo·pho·ria (eck·sigh″klo·fo′ree·uh) *n.* A form of cyclophoria in which the eyes rotate outward.

ex·cy·clo·tro·pia (eck·sigh″klo·tro′pee·uh) *n.* Cyclotropia outward.

ex·cys·ta·tion (ecks″sis·tay′shun) *n.* The escape from a cyst by the bursting of the surrounding envelope; a stage in the life of an intestinal parasite which occurs after the parasite has been swallowed by the host.

ex·en·ter·a·tion (eck·sen″tur·ay′shun) *n.* EVISCERATION (1, 3). —**ex·en·ter·ate** (eck·sen′tur·ate) *v.*

ex·er·cise (eck′sur·size) *n.* Muscular exertion for the purpose of preservation or restoration of health, or development of physical prowess or athletic skill.

exercise tolerance test. Any of several standardized exercise tests in which the development of chest pain and electrocardiographic abnormalities are interpreted as indicating myocardial ischemia, supporting the diagnosis of angina pectoris.

ex·fe·ta·tion (ecks″fe·tay′shun) *n.* Ectopic or extrauterine fetation.

ex·fo·li·a·tion (ecks·fo″lee·ay′shun) *n.* 1. The separation of bone or other tissue in thin layers; a superficial sequestrum. 2. A peeling and shedding of the horny layer of the skin, a normal process that may be exaggerated after an inflammation or as part of a skin disease.

—ex·fo·li·ate (ecks·fo'lee·ate) *v.;* **ex·fo·li·a·tive** (ecks·fo'lee·uh·tiv) *adj.*

exfoliative cytology. The study of desquamated cells.

exfoliative dermatitis. Any dermatitis in which there is extensive involvement of the skin with denudation of large areas, involving hair loss.

exfoliative erythroderma. A dermatosis having a scarlatiniform eruption lasting from 6 to 8 weeks, with free desquamation. Syn. *pityriasis rubra.*

ex·ha·la·tion (ecks"ha·lay'shun) *n.* 1. The giving off or sending forth in the form of vapor; expiration. 2. That which is given forth as vapor; emanation. **—ex·hale** (ecks·hail', ecks') *v.*

ex·haus·tion (eg·zaws'chun) *n.* 1. The act of using up or consuming all possibilities or resources. 2. Loss of physical and mental power from fatigue, protracted disease, psychogenic causes, or excessive heat or cold. 3. The pharmaceutical process of dissolving out one or more of the constituents of a crude drug by percolation or maceration.

ex·hi·bi·tion (eck"si·bish'un) *n.* The administration of a remedy. **—ex·hib·it** (eg·zib'it) *v. & n.*

ex·hi·bi·tion·ism (eck"si·bish'un·iz·um) *n.* 1. A sexual perversion in which pleasure is obtained by exposing the genitalia. 2. *In psychoanalysis,* gratification of early sexual impulses in young children by physical activity, such as dancing. **—exhibition·ist** (·ist) *n.*

ex·hil·a·rant (eg·zil'uh·runt) *adj. & n.* 1. Exhilarating; causing a rise in spirits. 2. An agent that enlivens or elates. **—ex·hil·a·rate** (eg·zil' uh·rate) *v.;* **ex·hil·a·ra·tion** (eg·zil"uh·ray'shun) *n.*

ex·hu·ma·tion (ecks"hew·may'shun) *n.* Removal from the ground after burial; disinterment. **—ex·hume** (·hewm') *v.*

ex·is·ten·tial (eg"zis·ten'shul) *adj.* 1. Pertaining to or grounded in existence; readily perceived, experienced, or implied from actuality as opposed to ideal or metaphysical. 2. Specifically, pertaining to human existence.

ex·i·tus (eck'si·tus) *n.* 1. Exit; outlet. 2. Death.

exo-, ex- A combining form meaning (a) *outside;* (b) *outer layer;* (c) *out of.*

exo·bi·ol·o·gy (eck"so·bye·ol'uh·jee) *n.* The science that is concerned with life forms occurring outside the earth and its atmosphere.

exo·car·di·ac (eck"so·kahr'dee·ack) *adj.* Originating, occurring, or situated outside the heart.

exo·car·di·al (eck"so·kahr'dee·ul) *adj.* EXOCARDIAC.

exo·cer·vix (eck"so·sur'vicks) *n.* ECTOCERVIX.

exo·crine (eck'so·krin, ·krine) *adj.* Secreting externally; of or pertaining to glands that deliver their secretion to an epithelial surface, either directly or by ducts.

ex·odon·tia (eck"so·don'chee·uh) *n.* The art and science of the extraction of teeth.

ex·odon·tist (eck"so·don'tist) *n.* Formerly, one who specialized in tooth extraction.

exo·eryth·ro·cyt·ic (eck"so·e·rith"ro·sit'ick) *adj.* Outside of erythrocytes; said of the development of some of the malaria plasmodia in the

cells of the lymphatic system of birds, and of human malarial parasites in parenchymal cells of the liver.

ex·og·a·my (ecks·og'uh·mee) *n.* 1. Union of gametes of different ancestry; outbreeding; cross-fertilization. 2. *In anthropology,* marriage between members of different clans, communities, or other social groups, as established by law or custom. **—exoga·mous** (·mus) *adj.*

exo·gen·ic (eck"so·jen'ick) *adj.* EXOGENOUS.

ex·og·e·nous (eck·soj'e·nus) *adj.* 1. Due to an external cause; not arising within the organism. 2. *In physiology,* pertaining to those factors in the metabolism of nitrogenous substances obtained from food. 3. Growing by addition to the outer surfaces.

exo·pho·ria (eck"so·fo'ree·uh) *n.* A type of heterophoria in which the visual lines tend outward.

ex·oph·thal·mic (eck"sof·thal'mick) *adj.* Characterized by or pertaining to exophthalmos.

exophthalmic goiter. Hyperthyroidism with exophthalmos.

exophthalmic ophthalmoplegia. Extraocular muscle weakness causing strabismus usually accompanied by diplopia, seen with exophthalmos.

ex·oph·thal·mos, ex·oph·thal·mus (eck"sof·thal' mus) *n.* Abnormal prominence or protrusion of the eyeball.

exo·phyt·ic (eck"so·fit'ick) *adj.* ECTOPHYTIC.

exo·skel·e·ton (eck"so·skel'e·tun) *n.* 1. The usually chitinous external skeleton of invertebrates. 2. The bony or horny supporting structures in the skin of many vertebrates, such as fish scales or the carapace of a turtle.

ex·os·mo·sis (eck"sos·mo'sis, eck"soz·) *n.* Passage of a liquid outward through a porous membrane. **—exos·mot·ic** (·mot'ick) *adj.*

ex·os·to·sis (eck"sos·to'sis) *n.,* pl. **exosto·ses** (·seez) A benign cartilage-capped protuberance from the surface of long bones but also seen on flat bones; due to chronic irritation as from infection, trauma, or osteoarthritis. **—exos·tot·ic** (·tot'ick), **ex·os·tosed** (eck·sos' toze'd, eg·zos') *adj.*

exostosis car·ti·la·gin·ea (kahr"ti·la·jin'ee·uh). A limited or abortive form of multiple hereditary exostosis in which a benign protruding bony lesion capped by growing cartilage appears usually by the end of the second decade of life.

exo·ther·mic (eck"so·thur'mick) *adj.* Pertaining to the giving out of energy, especially heat energy.

exo·tox·in (eck"so·tock'sin) *n.* A toxin which is excreted by a living microorganism and which can afterward be obtained in bacteria-free filtrates without death or disintegration of the microorganisms. **—exotox·ic** (·sick) *adj.*

exo·tro·pia (eck"so·tro'pee·uh) *n.* Divergent strabismus, occurring when one eye fixes upon an object and the other deviates outward.

exo·tro·pic (eck"so·tro'pick, ·trop'ick) *adj.* 1. Turning outward. 2. Pertaining to exotropia.

ex·pan·sile (eck·span'sil, ·sile) *adj.* Prone to or capable of expansion.

ex·pan·sive, *adj.* 1. Comprehensive; extensive. 2. *In psychiatry,* characterized by megalomania, euphoria, talkativeness, overgenerosity, grandiosity. **—expansive·ness,** *n.*

ex·pect·ant, *adj.* 1. In expectation or anticipation of an outcome, as expectant mother. 2. Characterized by expectations, but also uncertainty as to result, as expectant treatment.

ex·pec·ta·tion of life. 1. *In biometry,* the average number of years lived by a group of individuals after reaching a given age, as determined by the mortality experience of a specific time and geographic area. 2. Commonly, the probable number of years of survival for an individual of a given age.

ex·pec·to·rant (eck·speck'to·runt) *adj. & n.* 1. Promoting expectoration. 2. A medicinal that promotes or modifies expectoration.

ex·pec·to·ra·tion (eck·speck''tuh·ray'shun) *n.* 1. Ejection of material from the mouth. 2. The fluid or semifluid matter from the lungs and air passages expelled by coughing and spitting; sputum.

ex·pel, *v.* To drive or force out, as the fetus, by means of muscular contractions.

ex·pe·ri·en·tial (eck·speer''ee·en'shul) *adj.* Pertaining to or derived from experience.

ex·per·i·ment, *n.* 1. A trial or test. 2. A procedure undertaken to discover some unknown principle or effect, to test a hypothesis, or to illustrate a known principle or fact. **—ex·per·i·men·tal,** *adj.;* **ex·per·i·men·ta·tion,** *n.*

experimental allergic encephalomyelitis. A demyelinating encephalomyelitis arising from hypersensitivity to neural tissues, induced in experimental animals by injection of brain, spinal cord, or peripheral nerve tissue and important as a laboratory model of acute disseminated encephalomyelitis and similar diseases. Abbreviated, EAE.

ex·pert testimony or **evidence.** The testimony given before a court of law by an expert witness.

expert witness. An individual skilled in a profession, science, art, or occupation, who testifies before a court or jury to facts within his own sphere of competence, or who gives an opinion on assumed facts.

ex·pi·ra·tion (eck''spi·ray'shun) *n.* The act of breathing forth or expelling air from the lungs; exhalation. **—ex·pi·ra·to·ry** (eck·spye'ruh·tor·ee) *adj.*

expiratory reserve volume. The maximal volume of air that can be expired after involuntary exhalation, as from the end expiratory level. Abbreviated, ERV.

ex·pire (eck·spire') *v.* 1. To breathe out; exhale. 2. To die.

¹**ex·plant** (ecks·plant') *v.* To remove (living tissue) from an organism for tissue culture. **—ex·plan·ta·tion** (ecks''plan·tay'shun) *n.*

²**ex·plant** (ecks'plant) *n.* Tissue that has been explanted for tissue culture.

ex·plode, *v.* 1. To burst violently and noisily because of sudden release of energy. 2. To cause to burst violently. 3. To discredit and reject, as a theory. 4. To break out suddenly, as an epidemic. **—ex·plo·sive,** *adj.;* **ex·plo·sion,** *n.*

ex·plo·ra·tion, *n.* The act of exploring for diagnostic purposes, through investigation of a part hidden from sight, by means of operation, by touch, by artificial light, or by instruments. **—ex·plor·a·to·ry,** *adj.*

exploratory operation. An operation performed for the purpose of diagnosis, often an abdominal operation.

ex·plor·er, *n.* A probe; an instrument for use in exploration.

exploring electrode. *In electrocardiography,* an electrode designed to determine the potential at single points, paired with an indifferent electrode which registers near-zero potential.

explosive decompression. *In aerospace medicine,* a reduction of barometric pressure which is so rapid as to cause expansion of the involved gases in an explosive manner.

explosive speech. CEREBELLAR SPEECH.

ex·po·sure, *n.* 1. The act of exposing or laying open. 2. Subjection to some condition or influence that may affect detrimentally, as excessive heat, cold, radiation, or infectious agents. 3. *In radiology,* the dose delivered.

exposure of person. *In legal medicine,* the public display of sexual organs before persons of the opposite sex for gratification or erotic purposes. Syn. *indecent exposure.*

ex·press, *v.* 1. To press or squeeze out. 2. To show, bring out, manifest, as thoughts or feelings.

ex·pres·sion, *n.* 1. The act of pressing or squeezing out. 2. The means or the results of expressing something.

ex·san·gui·nate (eck·sang'gwi·nate) *v.* To drain of blood. **—exsangui·nat·ed** (·nay·tid) *adj.;* **ex·san·gui·na·tion** (eck·sang''gwi·nay'shun) *n.*

exsanguinate, *adj.* EXSANGUINE.

ex·san·guine (eck·sang'gwin) *adj.* Bloodless; anemic. **—ex·san·guin·i·ty** (eck''sang·gwin'i·tee) *n.*

ex·sic·cant (eck·sick'unt) *adj. & n.* Drying or absorbing moisture. 2. DUSTING POWDER.

ex·sic·ca·tion (eck''si·kay'shun) *n.* The act of drying; especially, depriving a crystalline body of its water of crystallization. **—ex·sic·cate** (eck'si·kate) *v.;* **ex·sic·ca·tive** (eck·sick'uh·tiv) *adj.*

ex·stro·phy (eck'stro·fee) *n.* Eversion; the turning inside out of a part.

exstrophy of the bladder. A rare congenital malformation due to failure of the cloaca to close anteriorly, in which the lower anterior part of the abdominal wall, the anterior wall of the urinary bladder, and usually the symphysis pubis are wanting, and the posterior wall of the bladder presents through the opening; associated with epispadias.

ex·suf·fla·tion (eck''suf·lay'shun) *n.* Forcible expiration; forcible expulsion of air from the lungs by a mechanical apparatus.

ex·ten·sion, *n.* 1. A straightening out, especially the muscular movement by which a flexed part is made straight. 2. Traction upon a fractured or dislocated limb. 3. *In psychiatry,* a mental mechanism operating outside and beyond conscious awareness in which an emotional process comes to include areas associated by physical or psychologic contiguity or by continuity, as for example the progression of a phobia to include related objects and areas. 4. Growth (of a neoplasm) into adjacent structures.

ex·ten·sor (eck·sten'sur) *n.* A muscle which extends or stretches a limb or part.

extensor di·gi·to·rum (dij''i·to'rum). The extensor of the fingers. See Table of Muscles in the Appendix.

extensor hallucis lon·gus (long'gus). The long extensor of the great toe. See Table of Muscles in the Appendix.

ex·te·ri·or·iza·tion (ecks·teer''ee·ur·i·zay'shun) *n.* 1. *In psychiatry,* the turning of one's interests outward. 2. *In surgery,* an operation that brings an internal organ or part to the surface or exterior of the body, and fixes it in that position.

ex·ter·nal (ecks·tur'nul) *adj.* 1. Exterior; acting from without. 2. *In anatomy,* on or near the outside of the body; away from the center or middle line of the body. 3. Not essential; superficial. **—exter·nad** (·nad) *adv.*

external acoustic meatus. The passage in the external ear from the auricle or pinna to the tympanic membrane.

external anal sphincter. Bundles of striate muscle fibers surrounding the anus.

external auditory meatus or canal. EXTERNAL ACOUSTIC MEATUS.

external ballottement. *In obstetrics,* the rebound of the fetal head against the examiner's hand, felt on pressure of the abdominal wall.

external carotid artery. An artery which originates at the common carotid and has superior thyroid, ascending pharyngeal, lingual, facial, sternocleidomastoid (occasionally), occipital, posterior auricular, superficial temporal, and maxillary branches. It distributes blood to the anterior portion of the neck, face, scalp, side of the head, ear, and dura mater.

external carotid plexus. A network of sympathetic nerve fibers surrounding the external carotid artery, formed by the external carotid nerves and providing fibers which form networks along the branches of the artery.

external conjugate diameter. The distance from the depression above the spine of the first sacral vertebra to the middle of the upper border of the symphysis pubis. Syn. *Baudeloque's diameter.*

external ear. The part of the ear that is external to the tympanic membrane, consisting of the external acoustic meatus and the pinna.

external genitalia. In the male, the penis and testes; in the female, the vulva, vagina, and clitoris.

external hemorrhoid or pile. A hemorrhoid protruding below the anal sphincter.

ex·ter·nal·ize (ecks·tur'nul·ize) *v.* 1. *In psychology,* to transform an idea or impression which is on the percipient's mind into an external phantasm. 2. To refer to some outside source,

as the voices heard by the subject of hallucinations.

external limiting membrane. 1. In the eye, the thin layer between the outer nuclear layer of the retina and that of the rods and cones; not actually a membrane but a series of junctional complexes between Müller's fibers and the rods and cones. 2. *In embryology,* the membrane investing the outer surface of the neural tube.

external os. OSTIUM UTERI.

external respiration. The interchange of gases between the atmosphere and the air in the lungs and between the air in the lungs and pulmonary capillaries.

external spermatic fascia. The outer covering of the spermatic cord and testis, continuous with the aponeurosis of the external oblique muscle at the subcutaneous inguinal ring.

external strabismus. EXOTROPIA.

external version. ABDOMINAL VERSION.

ex·tero·cep·tive (eck''stur·o·sep'tiv) *adj.* Activated by or pertaining to stimuli impinging on an organism from outside.

ex·tero·cep·tor (eck''stur·o·sep'tur) *n.* An end organ, in or near the skin or a mucous membrane, which receives stimuli from the external world.

ex·tinc·tion (eck·stink'shun) *n.* 1. The act of putting out or extinguishing; destruction. 2. *In neurophysiology,* the disappearance of excitability of a nerve, synapse, or nervous tissue to a previously adequate stimulus. 3. *In clinical neurology,* the failure to recognize one of two simultaneously presented stimuli. 4. *In psychology,* the disappearance of a conditioned reflex when excited repeatedly without reinforcement.

ex·tir·pa·tion (eck''stur·pay'shun) *n.* Complete removal of a part or surgical destruction of a part.

Exton's reagent Either of two slightly different watery solutions of sulfosalicylic acid and sodium sulfate; used in a qualitative and a quantitative urine protein test.

Exton's test A test for urine protein in which equal volumes of clear urine and Exton's qualitative reagent are mixed in a test tube. Cloudiness appearing upon heating indicates protein.

ex·tor·sion (ecks·tor'shun) *n.* 1. Outward rotation of a part. 2. *In ophthalmology,* a turning outward of the vertical meridians.

extra- A prefix meaning (a) *outside of;* (b) *beyond the scope of.*

ex·tra·ar·tic·u·lar (ecks''truh·ahr·tick'yoo·lur) *adj.* Outside a joint.

ex·tra·buc·cal (ecks''truh·buck'ul) *adj.* Outside the mouth. Syn. *extraoral.*

ex·tra·bul·bar (ecks''truh·bul'bur) *adj.* Exterior to a bulb; specifically, exterior to the medulla oblongata.

ex·tra·cap·su·lar (ecks''truh·kap'sue·lur) *adj.* Outside a capsule; outside the capsular ligament of a joint.

extracapsular ankylosis. Ankylosis due to rigidity of the parts external to the joint, as interference resulting from bony block, adhesions of tendons and tendon sheaths, contractures due to muscles, scars, or thickening of skin in scleroderma, or from heterotopic periarticular bone formation following injury or operation. Syn. *false ankylosis, spurious ankylosis.*

ex·tra·car·di·ac (eck″struh·kahr′dee·ack) *adj.* Outside the heart.

ex·tra·car·di·al (eck″struh·kahr′dee·ul) *adj.* EXTRACARDIAC.

ex·tra·car·pal (ecks″truh·kahr′pul) *adj.* Exterior to the wrist bones.

ex·tra·cel·lu·lar (ecks″truh·sel′yoo·lur) *adj.* External to the cells of an organism.

extracellular enzyme. An enzyme which retains its activity when removed from the cell in which it is formed, or which normally exerts its activity at a site removed from the place of formation. Syn. *lyoenzyme.*

ex·tra·cer·e·bral (ecks″truh·serr′e·brul) *adj.* Outside the brain, but within the cranial cavity.

ex·tra·cor·po·re·al (ecks″truh·kor·po′ree·ul) *adj.* Outside the body.

ex·tra·cor·pus·cu·lar (ecks″truh·kor·pus′kew·lur) *adj.* Outside a corpuscle; especially, outside a blood cell.

ex·tra·cra·ni·al (ecks″truh·kray′nee·ul) *adj.* Outside the cranial cavity.

ex·tract (eck′strakt) *n.* 1. A pharmaceutical preparation obtained by dissolving the active constituents of a drug with a suitable solvent, evaporating the solvent, and adjusting to prescribed standards, often so that one part of the extract represents four to six parts of the drug. Abbreviated, ext. 2. A preparation, usually in a concentrated form, obtained by treating plant or animal tissue with a solvent to remove desired odoriferous, flavorful, or nutritive components of the tissue.

ex·trac·tion (eck·strack′shun) *n.* 1. The act of drawing out. 2. The process of making an extract. 3. The surgical removal of a tooth. —**ex·tract** (eck·strakt′) *v.*

ex·trac·tor (eck·strack′tur) *n.* 1. An instrument or forceps for extracting bullets, sequestra, or foreign bodies. 2. *In dentistry,* an instrument for extracting the root of a tooth.

ex·tra·cyst·ic (ecks″truh·sist′ick) *adj.* Outside a cyst, the urinary bladder, or the gallbladder.

ex·tra·du·ral (ecks″truh·dew′rul) *adj.* EPIDURAL.

extradural abscess. EPIDURAL ABSCESS.

ex·tra·em·bry·on·ic (ecks″truh·em″bree·on′ick) *adj.* Situated outside, or not forming a part of, the embryo.

extraembryonic mesoderm. The earliest mesoderm of the embryo, derived from the trophoblast, that forms a part of the amnion, chorion and yolk sac, and the body stalk.

ex·tra·gen·i·tal (ecks″truh·jen′i·tul) *adj.* Situated outside of, or unrelated to, the genitals.

extragenital syphilis. Syphilis in which the primary lesion is situated elsewhere than on the genital organs.

ex·tra·gin·gi·val (ecks″truh·jin′ji·vul) *adj.* Situated outside or above the gingiva.

ex·tra·he·pat·ic (ecks″truh·he·pat′ick) *adj.* Outside, or not connected with, the liver; especially, referring to disease affecting the liver, in which the primary lesion is external to the organ, as an extrahepatic biliary obstruction.

ex·tra·mam·ma·ry (eck″struh·mam′uh·ree) *adj.* Outside the mammary gland; usually referring to a condition associated with the breast but occurring in another location.

ex·tra·med·ul·lary (ecks″truh·med′yoo·lerr″ee) *adj.* 1. Situated or occurring outside the spinal cord or brainstem. 2. Situated or occurring outside the bone marrow.

extramedullary hemopoiesis. Formation of blood outside the bone marrow.

ex·tra·mu·ral (ecks″truh·mew′rul) *adj.* Outside the wall of an organ.

ex·tra·oc·u·lar (eck″struh·ock′yoo·lur) *adj.* Extrinsic to the eyeball.

ex·tra·os·se·ous (ecks″struh·os′ee·us) *adj.* Outside a bone or bones.

ex·tra·pel·vic (ecks″truh·pel′vick) *adj.* Situated or occurring outside the pelvis.

ex·tra·peri·to·ne·al (ecks″truh·perr″i·tuh·nee′ul) *adj.* External to the peritoneal cavity.

ex·tra·pla·cen·tal (ecks″truh·pluh·sen′tul) *adj.* Not connected with the placenta.

ex·tra·pleu·ral (ecks″truh·ploo′rul) *adj.* Outside the pleura or the pleural cavity, or both.

ex·trap·o·late (ecks·trap′uh·late) *v.* 1. *In statistics,* to estimate a quantity which depends on one or more variables not known by projecting, extending, or expanding such data as are known. 2. To interpret or explain any phenomenon, whether physical or mental, of which the causative factors are secondary or circumstantial. —**ex·trap·o·la·tion** (ecks·trap″uh·lay′shun) *n.*

ex·tra·pros·tat·ic (ecks″truh·pros·tat′ick) *adj.* Outside or away from the prostate.

ex·tra·psy·chic (ecks″truh·sigh′kick) *adj.* Occurring outside the mind or psyche.

ex·tra·pul·mo·nary (ecks″truh·pul′muh·nerr″ee) *adj.* Outside of or independent of the lungs.

ex·tra·py·ram·i·dal (ecks″truh·pi·ram′i·dul) *adj.* 1. Outside the pyramidal tracts, applied to other descending motor pathways. 2. Pertaining to or involving the extrapyramidal system.

extrapyramidal disorder or syndrome. Any manifestation or complex of symptoms due to a disorder or disease of the extrapyramidal system; manifestations include tremors, muscular rigidity, and dyskinesias, as in hepatolenticular degeneration, Parkinson's disease, or phenothiazine intoxication.

extrapyramidal system. A widespread and complicated system of descending fiber tracts arising in the cortex and subcortical motor centers; in the widest sense it includes all nonpyramidal motor tracts; in the usual clinical sense it includes the striatopallidonigral and cerebellar motor systems.

ex·tra·re·nal (ecks″truh·ree′nul) *adj.* Outside of or not involving a kidney or kidneys.

extrarenal uremia. PRERENAL UREMIA.

ex·tra·sen·so·ry (eck″struh·sen′suh·ree) *adj.* 1. Of or pertaining to phenomena outside the realm normally perceived through the senses; not sensory. 2. Of or pertaining to certain capacities of perception unexplainable in relation to the senses.

extrasensory perception. Direct awareness

without the use of the senses; telepathy; clairvoyance; precognition. Abbreviated, ESP.

ex·tra·sphinc·ter·ic (ecks″truh·sfink·terr′ick) *adj.* Outside a sphincter.

extraspinal plexus. A large venous plexus extending the length of the vertebral column and lying between it and the multifidus muscle.

ex·tra·sys·to·le (ecks″truh·sis′tuh·lee) *n.* PREMATURE BEAT.

ex·tra·tu·bal (ecks″truh·tew′bul) *adj.* Outside a tube, as the uterine tube.

ex·tra·uter·ine (ecks″truh·yoo′tur·in, ·ine) *adj.* Outside the uterus.

extrauterine pregnancy or **gestation.** Development of the fertilized ovum outside the uterine cavity.

ex·tra·vag·i·nal (ecks″truh·vaj′i·nul, ·va·jye′nul) *adj.* Outside the vagina or any sheath.

ex·trav·a·sa·tion (ecks·trav″uh·say′shun) *n.* 1. The passing of a body fluid out of its proper place, as blood into surrounding tissues after rupture of a vessel. 2. Material so discharged. —**ex·trav·a·sate** (ecks·trav′uh·sate) *v. & n.*

ex·tra·vas·cu·lar (ecks″truh·vas′kew·lur) *adj.* Outside a vessel.

ex·tra·ver·sion (ecks″truh·vur′zhun) *n.* EXTROVERSION.

ex·trem·i·ty, *n.* 1. The distal, or terminal, end of any part. 2. An upper or lower limb.

ex·trin·sic (eck·strin′zick, ·sick) *adj.* Originating outside.

extrinsic asthma. Asthma caused by inhalants, foods, or drugs.

extrinsic factor. VITAMIN B₁₂.

extrinsic muscle. A muscle which has its origin outside, and its insertion into, an organ, as a rectus muscle of the eye.

extro-. A prefix meaning (a) *outside*; (b) *outward.*

ex·tro·phia (eck·stro′fee·uh) *n.* EXSTROPHY.

ex·tro·phy (ecks′tro·fee) *n.* 1. Malformation of an organ. 2. EXSTROPHY.

ex·tro·ver·sion (ecks″tro·vur′zhun) *n.* 1. A turning outward. 2. *In psychoanalytic theory,* the turning of the libido outward, as to a love object. 3. *In psychiatry,* a turning to things and persons outside oneself rather than to one's own thoughts and feelings. 4. Unusual widening of the dental arch.

ex·tro·vert (ecks′tro·vurt) *v. & n.* 1. To turn one's interests to external things rather than to oneself. 2. A person whose interests center in the outside world rather than in subjective activity.

ex·tru·sion (eck·stroo′zhun) *n.* 1. A forcing out; expulsion. 2. *In dentistry,* movement of a tooth beyond the occlusal plane. —**ex·trude** (eck·strood′) *v.*

exuberant granulation. An excess of granulation tissue in the base of an ulcer or in a healing wound. Syn. *fungous granulation, proud flesh.*

ex·u·date (ecks′yoo·date) *n.* 1. A material, with a high content of protein and cells, that has passed through the walls of vessels into adjacent tissues or spaces, especially in inflammation. 2. Any exuded substance.

ex·u·da·tion (ecks″yoo·day′shun) *n.* The passage of various constituents of the blood through the walls of vessels into adjacent tissues or spaces, especially in inflammation. —**ex·u·da·tive** (ecks·yoo′duh·tiv, ecks″yoo·day″tiv) *adj.;* **ex·ude** (eck·sue′d′) *v.*

ex·u·vi·a·tion (eg·zew″vee·ay′shun) *n.* The shedding of the primary teeth, or of epidermal structures.

ex vi·vo (ecks vee′vo) Outside the living organism; characterizing an operation or other procedure performed on a living organ or tissue that has been removed from the body.

ex vivo surgery. BENCH SURGERY.

eye, *n.* The organ of vision which occupies the anterior part of the orbit and which is nearly spherical. It is composed of three concentric coats: the sclera and cornea; the choroid, ciliary body, and iris; and the retina. Abbreviated, E.

eye·ball, *n.* The globe of the eye.

eye·brow, *n.* 1. The arch above the eye. 2. The hair covering the eye.

eye·cup, *n.* 1. OPTIC VESICLE. 2. A small cup that fits over the eye; used for bathing the conjunctiva.

eye dominance. The almost universal condition in which one eye is unconsciously relied on and used more than the other. Syn. *ocular dominance.*

eye ground. The fundus of the eye; the internal aspect of the eye as seen through an ophthalmoscope.

eye·lash, *n.* One of the stiff hairs growing on the margin of the eyelid.

eye·lid, *n.* One of the two protective coverings of the eyeball; a curtain of movable skin lined with conjunctiva, having the tarsus, glands, and cilia in the distal part, muscle in the proximal part.

eye·piece, *n.* The lens or combination of lenses of an optical instrument, as a microscope or telescope, nearest the eye.

eyepiece micrometer. A micrometer to be used with the eyepiece of a microscope.

eye·strain, *n.* ASTHENOPIA.

eye·tooth, *n.* A canine tooth of the upper jaw.

eye·wash, *n.* A medicated solution for the eye; a collyrium.

eye worm. *LOA LOA.*

F

F Symbol for fluorine.

F Abbreviation for (a) *Fahrenheit*; (b) *fellow*; (c) *field of vision*; (d) *formula.*

F₁ Symbol for first filial generation, offspring of a given mating.

F₂ Symbol for second filial generation, grandchildren of a given mating.

fa·bel·la (fa-bel′uh) *n.*, pl. **fabel·lae** (·ee) A sesamoid fibrocartilage or small bone occasionally developed in the lateral head of the gastrocnemius muscle.

Fab fragment. The antigen-binding fraction of an immunoglobulin molecule.

fab·ri·ca·tion (fab″ri·kay′shun) *n.* CONFABULATION.

Fa·bry's disease (fah′bree) ANGIOKERATOMA CORPORIS DIFFUSUM UNIVERSALE.

fab·u·la·tion (fab″yoo·lay′shun) *n.* CONFABULATION.

F.A.C.D. Fellow of the American College of Dentists.

face, *n.* The anterior part of the head including forehead and jaws, but not the ears.

face-bow, *n.* A device used to record the spatial relationship between the jaws and the temporomandibular joints and to aid in mounting the dental casts to an articulator.

face-lift, *n.* RHYTIDOPLASTY.

face presentation. The fetal presentation of the face at the cervix, where the chin is used as the point of reference.

fac·et (fas′it) *n.* 1. A small plane surface, especially on a bone or a hard body. 2. A worn spot on a surface, as of a tooth.

facet syndrome. A form of traumatic arthritis involving the articular facets of the spinal column, usually in the lumbar region; manifested by sudden onset, with low back pain relieved in certain postures and exaggerated in others, the pain being described as of the locking type.

fac·ial (fay′shul) *adj.* 1. Of, pertaining to, or involving the face. 2. BUCCAL. 3. LABIAL.

facial canal. A channel in the temporal bone for the passage of the facial nerve.

facial nerve. The seventh cranial nerve, which is attached to the brainstem at the inferior border of the pons and innervates the stapedius, stylohyoid, posterior belly of the digastric, and the muscles of facial expression. It also has parasympathetic and sensory components, running by way of the nervus intermedius.

facial neuralgia. TRIGEMINAL NEURALGIA.

facial palsy or **paralysis.** Partial or total weakness of the muscles of the face. There are two types: the central, or supranuclear, type; and the peripheral, nuclear, or infranuclear, type.

-facient A combining form meaning (a) *making;* (b) *causing.*

fa·ci·es (fay′shee-eez) *n.*, genit. **fa·ci·ei** (fay″shee-ee′eye), pl. **facies** 1. The appearance of the face. 2. A surface. 3. [NA] FACE.

facies ab·do·min·a·lis (ab·dom″i·nay′lis). The pinched, dehydrated facial mien of a person with severe abdominal disease, such as peritonitis. Syn. *face gripée.*

facies hip·po·crat·i·ca (hip-o-krat′i·kuh). An appearance of the face indicative of the rapid approach of death: the nose is pinched, the temples are hollow, the eyes sunken, the ears leaden and cold, the lips relaxed, the skin livid.

facies le·on·ti·na (lee-on-tye′nuh). The "lionlike" face seen in some patients with leprosy.

fa·cil·i·ta·tion (fa·sil″i·tay′shun) *n.* 1. Increased ease in carrying out an action or function. 2. Enhanced or reinforced reflex or other neural activity by impulses arising other than from a reflex center. 3. An increase in excitatory postsynaptic potential by a slight added quantity of neurotransmitter which enables excitation of the postsynaptic cell.

fa·cil·i·ty (fa·sil′i·tee) *n.* 1. Anything that makes it possible for some particular function to be performed, or which serves toward some specific end. 2. Ease in performance, as the facility to run; freedom from some impediment. 3. Any specific structure, building, establishment, or installation, or part thereof, designed to promote some particular end or purpose, as a hospital or a center for learning or recreation.

fac·ing, *n.* A veneer of porcelain or resin cemented or processed to an artificial tooth crown or pontic to achieve a greater esthetic effect.

facio-. A combining form meaning *face, facial.*

fa·cio·ple·gic (fay″shee·o·plee′jick) *adj.* Pertaining to weakness or paralysis of the facial muscles.

facioplegic migraine. Transient paralysis of facial muscles sometimes accompanying migraine.

fa·cio·scap·u·lo·hu·mer·al (fay″shee·o·skap″yoo-lo·hew′mur·ul) *adj.* Pertaining to the muscles involving the face, scapula, and humerus.

F.A.C.O.G. Fellow of the American College of Obstetricians and Gynecologists.

F.A.C.P. Fellow of the American College of Physicians.

F.A.C.S. Fellow of the American College of Surgeons.

fac·ti·tious (fack·tish′us) *adj.* Pertaining to a state or substance brought about or produced by means other than natural.

fac·tor, *n.* 1. A circumstance, fact, or influence which tends to produce a result; a constituent or component. 2. *In biology,* GENE. 3. An essential or desirable element in diet. 4. A substance promoting or functioning in a particular physiologic process, as a coagulation factor.

factor I. FIBRINOGEN.

factor II. PROTHROMBIN.

factor III. *Obsol.* THROMBOPLASTIN.

factor IV. Calcium when it participates in the coagulation of blood.

factor V. A labile procoagulant in normal plasma but deficient in the blood of patients with parahemophilia; essential for rapid conversion of prothrombin to thrombin. It is suggested that during clotting this factor is transformed from an inactive precursor into an active accelerator of prothrombin conversion. Syn. *proaccelerin.*

factor VI. A hypothetical substance believed to be derived from factor V during coagulation.

factor VII. A stable procoagulant in normal plasma but deficient in the blood of patients with a hereditary bleeding disorder; formed in the liver by action of vitamin K. Syn. *proconvertin.*

factor VIII. A procoagulant present in normal plasma but deficient in the blood of patients with hemophilia A.

factor IX. A procoagulant in normal plasma but deficient in the blood of patients with hemophilia B. Syn. *Christmas factor.*

factor X. A procoagulant present in normal plasma but deficient in the blood of patients with a hereditary bleeding disorder. May be closely related to prothrombin since both are formed in the liver by action of vitamin K. Syn. *Stuart-Prower factor.*

factor XI. A procoagulant present in normal plasma but deficient in the blood of patients with a hereditary bleeding disorder.

factor XII. A factor necessary for rapid coagulation in vitro, but apparently not required for hemostasis, present in the normal plasma but deficient in the blood of patients with a hereditary bleeding disorder. Syn. *Hageman factor.*

factor XIII. A factor present in normal plasma which, in the presence of calcium, causes the formation of a highly insoluble fibrin clot resistant to urea and weak acid. Syn. *fibrinase, fibrin stabilizing factor.*

fac·ul·ta·tive (fack′ul·tay″tiv) *adj.* 1. Voluntary; optional; having the power to do or not to do a thing. 2. *In biology,* capable of existing under differing conditions, as a microorganism that can grow aerobically or anaerobically.

facultative aerobe. An organism which is normally or usually anaerobic but which, under certain circumstances, may grow aerobically.

facultative anaerobe. An organism which usually grows aerobically, but which can also grow in the absence of molecular oxygen.

facultative hyperopia. Manifest hyperopia that can be concealed by accommodation.

fac·ul·ty (fack′ul·tee) *n.* 1. A function, power, or capability inherent in a living organism, often in the sense of exceptional development of the function, power, or capability. 2. The teaching staff of an educational institution or one of its divisions. 3. An area of learning or teaching in an institution of higher education.

fag·o·py·rism (fag″o·pye′riz·um) *n.* Photosensitization of the skin and mucous membranes, accompanied by convulsions; produced in white and piebald animals by feeding with the flowers or seed husks of the buckwheat plant (*Fagopyrum sagittatum*) or clovers and grasses containing flavin or carotin and xanthophyll.

Fahr. An abbreviation for *Fahrenheit.*

Fahr·en·heit (făr′un·hite, ferr′) *adj.* Pertaining to or designating the Fahrenheit temperature scale in which the interval between the freezing point of water (32°) and its boiling point (212°) is divided into 180 degrees. Abbreviated F, Fahr.

fail·ure, *n. In medicine,* profound inability of an organ to carry out its physiologic functions or the demands upon it, usually resulting in severe impairment of the individual's health.

faint, *adj., n. & v.* 1. Weak or lacking strength or consciousness. 2. Barely perceptible. 3. A sudden, transient loss of consciousness; swoon; syncope. 4. To swoon; lose strength and/or consciousness suddenly.

faint·ness, *n.* A sudden lack of strength with a sensation of impending faint.

fal·ci·form (fal′si·form) *adj.* Having the shape of a sickle.

falciform ligament of the liver. The ventral mesentery of the liver. Its peripheral attachment extends from the diaphragm to the umbilicus and contains the round ligament of the liver.

fal·cip·a·rum malaria (fal·sip′ur·um, fawl·). A form of malaria caused by *Plasmodium falciparum* characterized by paroxysms of fever occurring at irregular intervals and often by the localization of the organism in a specific organ, causing capillary blockage in the brain, lungs, intestinal mucosa, spleen, and kidney. Syn. *estivo-autumnal malaria, malignant tertian malaria, subtertian malaria.*

falling sickness. EPILEPSY.

fal·lo·pi·an (fa·lo'pee·un) *adj.* Pertaining to or designating anatomic structures associated with Gabriele Fallopio (Fallopius), Italian anatomist, 1523–1562.

fallopian tube. UTERINE TUBE.

false aneurysm. 1. An aneurysm due to a rupture of all the coats of an artery, the effused blood being retained by the surrounding tissues. 2. A swelling in the course of an artery, usually caused by a hematoma, which mimics the appearance of an aneurysm, but does not involve the wall of the artery.

false hernia. A hernia that has no sac covering the hernial contents.

false hypertrophy. An increase in size of an organ due to an increase in amount of tissue not associated with functional activity, such as connective tissue.

false labor. Painful uterine contractions which simulate labor but are not associated with progressive dilation or effacement of the cervix or descent of the presenting part.

false membrane. A fibrinous layer formed on a mucous membrane or cutaneous surface and extending downward for a variable depth. It is the result of coagulation necrosis, generally seen in croup and diphtheria. Syn. *pseudomembrane.*

false pelvis. The part of the pelvis above the iliopectineal line.

false-positive reaction. An erroneous or deceptive positive reaction, such as a positive serological test for syphilis in the presence of infectious mononucleosis, leprosy, or malaria.

false pregnancy. PSEUDOCYESIS.

false proteinuria. Proteinuria from sources other than the usual pathologic states (such as bleeding into the lower urinary tract) associated with this condition. Syn. *accidental proteinuria, false albuminuria.*

false ribs. The five lower ribs on each side not attached to the sternum directly.

fal·si·fi·ca·tion, *n.* The act of distorting or altering a fact or object. —**fal·si·fy,** *v.*

falx (falks, fawlks) *n.,* genit. **fal·cis** (fal'sis), pl. **fal·ces** (fal'seez) A sickle-shaped structure.

falx ce·re·bel·li (serr·e·bel'eye) [NA]. A sickle-like process of dura mater between the lobes of the cerebellum.

falx ce·re·bri (serr'e·brye) [NA]. The process of the dura mater separating the hemispheres of the cerebrum.

fa·mil·ial (fa·mil'ee·ul, ·mil'yul) *adj.* Occurring among or pertaining to the members of a family, as a familial disease.

familial benign pemphigus. A dominantly inherited vesicular and bullous dermatitis localized to the sides of the neck, the axillary spaces, and other flexor surfaces. It is possibly a variant of Darier's disease. Syn. *Hailey-Hailey disease.*

familial disease. Any disorder occurring in several members of the same family; sometimes restricted to mean several members of the same generation.

familial dysautonomia. A hereditary disease, transmitted as an autosomal recessive trait, most common in Jewish children, characterized from infancy by feeding difficulties, absence of overflow tears, indifference to pain, absent or hypoactive deep tendon reflexes, absent corneal reflexes, absence of fungiform papillae on tongue, postural hypotension, emotional lability, abnormal intradermal histidine response, and frequently abnormal temperature control with excessive sweating, abnormal esophageal motility, abnormal pupillary response to methacholine, and excess urinary homovanillic acid, as well as other evidence of autonomic nervous system dysfunctions.

familial fat-induced hyperlipemia. Familial hyperlipoproteinemia, type I, due to a defect in removal of chylomicrons and other lipoproteins rich in triglycerides, probably as a result of a genetically determined low lipoprotein lipase activity; characterized by an excess of chylomicrons in serum with an ordinary diet and their disappearance with a fat-free diet. Clinically there may be paroxysms of abdominal pain, hepatosplenomegaly, pancreatitis, and xanthomas of various tissues. Syn. *familial lipoprotein lipase deficiency.*

familial hemolytic anemia. HEREDITARY SPHEROCYTOSIS.

familial hyperbetalipoproteinemia. The most common form of familial hyperlipoproteinemia, type IIA, characterized by an increase in total serum cholesterol and phospholipids and normal glycerides with an ordinary diet; associated with the formation of xanthelasmas, tendon and tuberous xanthomas, frequently early atheromatosis, and generally a positive family history.

familial hyperbetalipoproteinemia and hyperprebetalipoproteinemia. Familial hyperlipoproteinemia, type III, similar to familial hyperbetalipoproteinemia, but with an increase in total serum cholesterol accompanied by an increase in glycerides which is endogenous and induced by carbohydrates. The plasma very-low-density lipoproteins have unusual electrophoretic mobility, extending from the β to the α_2 zone on paper electrophoresis. Generally, there is an abnormal glucose tolerance curve, as well as tuberous and planar xanthomas, and early ischemic heart disease. Peripheral arteriosclerosis obliterans is often present. Syn. *familial broad-beta hyperlipoproteinemia.*

familial hyperchylomicronemia with hyperprebetalipoproteinemia. Familial hyperlipoproteinemia, type V, characterized by the increase in total serum chylomicrons and prebetalipoproteins which appears to be a combination of fat- and carbohydrate-induced hyperlipemia. There is usually associated moderate diabetes mellitus or other metabolic disorder. Bouts of abdominal pain, eruptive xanthomas of various tissues, and other clinical features similar to those seen in familial fat-induced hyperlipemia may occur.

familial hyperlipoproteinemia. One of several inherited disorders of lipoprotein metabolism, separated on clinical and chemical basis thus far into six types.

familial hyperprebetalipoproteinemia. Familial hyperlipoproteinemia, type IV, clinically similar to types II and III, characterized by elevated levels of plasma very-low-density lipoproteins, which migrate into the pre-beta region on electrophoresis. Plasma triglyceride levels are elevated with normal diet but there is little or no elevation of total cholesterol. Abdominal pain similar to that seen in other hypertriglyceridemic states is seen clinically.

familial hypophosphatemia. An inborn error of metabolism in which hypophosphatemia is the most consistent and often the only anomaly, and where there are various degrees of vitamin D–refractory rickets or osteomalacia, diminished tubular reabsorption of calcium, and at times unusual histologic changes in bone; transmitted as a sex-linked dominant trait.

familial Mediterranean fever. An inherited disorder occurring mainly in people of Sephardic Jewish, Armenian, and Arabic ancestry, of unknown etiology characterized by recurrent episodes of fever, abdominal and chest pain, arthralgia, and rash, terminating in some cases in chronic renal failure due to amyloidosis. Abbreviated, FMF. Syn. *familial recurring polyserositis, periodic disease, periodic peritonitis.*

familial neurovisceral lipidosis. G$_{M1}$ GANGLIOSIDOSIS. Deficiency of beta-galactosidase; characterized by peculiar facies, radiologically characteristic bone deformities, visceral enlargement, and vacuolated renal glomerular epithelial cells. Foamy histiocytes and swollen ganglion cells have been observed in most cases, increased gangliosides in liver, spleen, and brain in one. Clinically, there is progressive coarsening of facies, repeated infections, and failure of brain maturation.

familial periodic paralysis. PERIODIC PARALYSIS.

familial polyposis. An autosomal dominant disease characterized by the appearance before age 30 to 40 of multiple discrete adenomas of the colon; in Type I malignant transformation is common; in Type II (Peutz-Jeghers syndrome) mucocutaneous pigmentation occurs, but malignant transformation is rare; and in Type III (Gardner syndrome) there are sebaceous and inclusion cysts, osteomata of the face, jaw, and calvarium; and the polyps are predisposed to malignancy.

familial tremor. A variety of postural or action tremor, inherited as a dominant trait, which begins in childhood and grows more marked with age and which may be limited to the hands and arms, but often involves the head.

fam·i·ly, *n.* 1. A group of closely related persons; parents and children; those descended from a common ancestor. 2. *In biology,* a classification group higher than a genus; the principal division of an order.

fa·nat·i·cism (fa-nat'i-siz-um) *n.* Perversion and excess of the religious sentiment; unreasoning zeal in regard to any subject. Sometimes a manifestation of mental disease.

Fanconi syndrome A heritable recessive or sometimes acquired disorder of renal tubular function seen most commonly in children, in which there is rickets or osteomalacia resistant to vitamin D in usual doses, as well as renal glycosuria, generalized aminoaciduria, and hyperphosphaturia in spite of normal or decreased plasma levels of these constituents, and, usually, chronic acidosis and hypokalemia, and sometimes marked growth retardation. (The names of de Toni and Debré are often linked to designate this form of the syndrome.) In many childhood cases, cystinosis, characterized by an excess of cystine in the urine and the deposition of cystine crystals in internal organs and the eyes, is a prominent feature. (The names of Abderhalden, Kaufmann, and Lignac are often associated with this form.)

fang, *n.* A sharp or pointed tooth; especially, the tooth of a wild beast or serpent.

fan·go (fang'go) *n.* Clay from the hot springs of Battaglio, Italy; used as a local application.

fan·go·ther·a·py (fang''go-therr'uh-pee) *n.* Treatment with fango or other mud; used in arthritis or gout.

fan·ning, *n. In neurology,* the spreading apart of the fingers or toes like the ribs of an open fan; seen as a normal or abnormal reflex sign, as in the Babinski sign.

fan·ta·sy, *n.* 1. Imagination; the ability to form mental pictures of scenes, occurrences, or objects not actually present; fanciful or dreamlike image making. 2. An image or series of images which may be an expression of unconscious conflicts or a gratification of unconscious wishes.

far·ad (far'ad) *n.* The unit of electric capacitance; the capacitance of a capacitor that is charged to a potential of 1 volt by 1 coulomb of electricity.

far·a·day (far'uh-day) *n.* The quantity of electricity which will liberate one gram equivalent of an element, specifically 107.88 g of silver, on electrolysis. It equals $96{,}494 \pm 10$ international coulombs.

fa·rad·ic (fa-rad'ick) *adj.* Pertaining to induced rapidly alternating currents of electricity.

faradic contractility. Ability of muscle to contract in response to a rapidly alternating current.

far·a·dism (far'uh-diz-um) *n.* The application of a rapidly alternating current of electricity; FARADIZATION.

far·a·di·za·tion (far''uh-di-zay'shun) *n.* The therapeutic application of induced rapidly alternating current to a diseased part; FARADISM. **—far·a·dize** (far'uh-dize) *v.*

far·a·do·con·trac·til·i·ty (far''uh-do-kon''track-til'i-tee) *n.* Contractility in response to faradic stimulus.

far·a·do·mus·cu·lar (far''uh-do-mus'kew-lur) *adj.* Pertaining to the reaction of a muscle when a faradic current is applied.

far·a·do·ther·a·py (făr"uh·do·therr'uh·pee) *n.* Therapeutic use of faradism; FARADIZATION.

Far·ber's disease DISSEMINATED LIPOGRANULOMATOSIS.

far·cy (fahr'see) *n.* The cutaneous form of glanders, characterized by skin ulcers and thickening of superficial lymphatics.

fardel-bound, *n. & adj.* 1. A condition of cattle or sheep in which the omasum becomes static and the food dry and impacted. 2. Affected with this condition.

farm·er's lung. An acute or chronic inflammatory reaction in the lungs caused by hypersensitivity to thermophilic actinomycetes in moldy hay or grain, characterized by dyspnea, fever, cough, cyanosis, and patchy infiltrates in the lung; may also be caused by other organic dusts.

farmer's skin. SAILOR'S SKIN.

far point. The most distant point at which an eye can see distinctly when accommodation is completely relaxed.

far sight. HYPEROPIA.

far·sight·ed·ness, *n.* HYPEROPIA.

fas·cia (fash'uh, ·ee·uh) *n.*, L. pl. & genit. sing. **fasci·ae** (·shee·ee) 1. The areolar tissue layers under the skin (superficial fascia). 2. The fibrous tissue between muscles and forming the sheaths of muscles, or investing other deep, definitive structures, as nerves and blood vessels (deep fascia). Adj. *fascial.*

fas·cial (fas'ee·ul) *adj.* Pertaining to or involving a fascia.

fascia la·ta (lay'tuh) [NA]. The deep fascia surrounding the muscles of the thigh.

fascial graft. A strip of fascia lata or aponeurosis; used either for the repair of a defect in muscle or fascia, or for suturing.

fascial plane. Any plane in the body which is oriented along a layer of fascia. It usually represents a cleavage plane, and is used for exposure in surgery; it may limit or direct the spread of infection.

fas·ci·cle (fas'i·kul) *n.* FASCICULUS.

fas·cic·u·lar (fa·sick'yoo·lur) *adj.* Of or pertaining to a fasciculus or to fasciculi.

fascicular degeneration. Degeneration, usually with necrosis, in fasciculi of muscle supplied by diseased or interrupted motor neurons.

fas·cic·u·lat·ed (fa·sick'yoo·lay'tid) *adj.* United into bundles or fasciculi.

fas·cic·u·la·tion (fa·sick"yoo·lay'shun) *n.* 1. An incoordinate contraction of skeletal muscle in which groups of muscle fibers innervated by the same neuron contract together. 2. The formation of fasciculi.

fas·cic·u·li·tis (fa·sick"yoo·lye'tis) *n.* Inflammation of a small bundle of muscle or nerve fibers, usually the latter.

fas·cic·u·lus (fa·sick'yoo·lus) *n.*, pl. & genit. sing. **fascicu·li** (·lye) 1. *In histology,* a bundle of nerve, muscle, or tendon fibers separated by connective tissue; as that of muscle fibers, by perimysium. 2. *In neurology,* a bundle or tract of nerve fibers presumably having common connections and functions.

fas·ci·ec·to·my (fash"ee·eck'tuh·mee, fas"ee·) *n. In surgery,* excision of fascia; specifically, excision of strips from the lateral part of the fascia lata (iliotibial tract) for use in plastic surgery.

fas·ci·i·tis (fas"ee·eye'tis, fash") *n.* 1. Inflammation of fascia. 2. A benign proliferative disorder of fascia of unknown cause, often producing nodules.

fas·ci·num (fas'i·num) *n.* 1. Literally, a spell, a bewitching; specifically, a spell cast by the evil eye. 2. The belief that certain individuals can cause injury by casting an evil eye upon a person, frequently expressed by patients suffering from the paranoid type of schizophrenia. 3. Any amulet or charm worn to protect against the evil eye, as, in Roman times, a tiny image of a penis hung around the necks of children as a protection against the evil eye and other forms of witchcraft.

fascio-. A combining form meaning *fascia, fascial.*

fas·ci·od·e·sis (fash"ee·od'e·sis, fas"ee·) *n.*, pl. **fasciode·ses** (·seez) The operation of suturing a fascia to another fascia, to a tendon, or to a skeletal attachment.

Fas·ci·o·la (fa·sigh'o·luh) *n.* A genus of trematodes; hermaphroditic flukes.

Fasciola he·pat·i·ca (he·pat'i·kuh). A species of liver fluke worldwide in distribution, especially in sheep-raising areas, which lives in the biliary passages of the host, producing fascioliasis. Occurs in many mammals, including sheep, goats, camels, elephants, rabbits, monkeys, and man.

fas·ci·o·li·a·sis (fas"ee·o·lye'uh·sis, fa·sigh"o·) *n.*, pl. **fasciolia·ses** (·seez) Infection with liver flukes, especially *Fasciola hepatica,* occurring in sheep and other herbivorous animals; man has served as an accidental host. The liver is usually the site of infection.

fas·ci·o·lop·si·a·sis (fas"ee·o·lop·sigh'uh·sis, fa·sigh"o·) *n.* An intestinal infection of man and hogs by *Fasciolopsis buski,* characterized by diarrhea, abdominal pain, anasarca, and eosinophilia. Generally acquired by the ingestion of water plants, such as the water chestnut, contaminated by infected snails.

Fas·ci·o·lop·sis (fas"ee·o·lop'sis, fa·sigh'o·) *n.* A genus of flukes parasitic in both man and hogs.

Fasciolopsis bus·ki (bus'kye). The largest intestinal fluke of man; endemic only in the Orient; the causative organism of fasciolopsiasis.

fas·cio·plas·ty (fash"ee·o·plas'tee) *n.* Plastic surgery upon fascia.

fas·ci·or·rha·phy (fash"ee·or'uh·fee) *n.* Suture of cut or lacerated fascia.

fas·ci·ot·o·my (fash"ee·ot'uh·mee) *n.* Incision of a fascia.

fas·ci·tis (fas·eye'tis, fash·eye'tis) *n.* FASCIITIS.

¹fast, *adj.* 1. Fixed, usually permanently; unable to leave, as a place or thing; immobile. 2. Resistant to change or destructive action.

²fast, *v. & n.* 1. To abstain from eating. 2. To restrict one's diet. 3. To deny food to someone. 4. Abstention from food.

-fast. A combining form meaning (a) *securely attached, narrowly confined,* as in bedfast; (b) *resistant to a* (specified) *dye, chemical agent, or microorganism,* as in acid-fast.

fas·tid·i·ous (fas·tid'ee·us) *adj.* Having exacting nutritional and other requirements for growth, said of microorganisms.

fas·tig·i·al (fas·tij'ee·ul) *adj.* Of or pertaining to the fastigium.

fas·tig·io·bul·bar (fas·tij''ee·o·bul'bur) *adj.* Pertaining to the fastigium and the medulla oblongata.

fas·tig·i·um (fas·tij'ee·um) *n.* 1. [BNA] The most rostral part of the roof of the fourth ventricle at the junction of the superior medullary velum of each side with the tela choroidea of the fourth ventricle. 2. The acme of a disease or fever.

fa·tal, *adj.* 1. Causing death; deadly; disastrous. 2. Of or pertaining to whatever is destined or decreed. —**fatal·ly** (·ee) *adv.*

fa·tal·i·ty (fay·tal'i·tee) *n.* 1. Death resulting from a disease, ingestion of a poisonous substance, or a disaster; a fatal outcome. 2. A victim of a fatal outcome.

fat·i·ga·ble (fat'i·guh·bul) *adj.* Susceptible to fatigue; easily tired. —**fat·i·ga·bil·i·ty** (fat''i·guh·bil'i·tee) *n.*

fa·tigue (fa·teeg') *n. & v.* 1. Exhaustion of strength; weariness from exertion. 2. Condition of cells or organs in which, through overactivity, the power or capacity to respond to stimulation is diminished or lost. 3. To tire; make or become exhausted.

fat-induced familial hypertriglyceridemia. A deficiency of lipoprotein lipase, transmitted as an autosomal recessive, resulting in chylomicron accumulation due to defective clearing of dietary fat; manifested clinically by xanthomas, hepatosplenomegaly, attacks of abdominal pain, and lipemia retinalis.

fat infiltration. 1. Deposit of neutral fats in tissues or cells as the result of transport. 2. FATTY INFILTRATION.

fat necrosis. Necrosis in adipose tissue, commonly accompanied by the production of soaps from the hydrolyzed fat, and seen in association with pancreatitis and in injuries to adipose tissue (traumatic fat necrosis).

fat pad. *In anatomy,* any mass of fatty tissue.

fat-soluble, *adj.* Soluble in fats or fat solvents; specifically used with a letter to designate certain vitamins, as fat-soluble A.

fatty acid. An acid derived from the series of open-chain hydrocarbons, usually obtained from the saponification of fats.

fatty cirrhosis. Early Laennec's cirrhosis with prominent fatty metamorphosis of liver cells.

fatty degeneration. Fatty metamorphosis, fatty infiltration, or both together.

fatty heart. 1. Fatty degeneration of the cardiac muscle fibers. 2. An increase in the quantity of subpericardial and intramyocardial adipose tissue.

fatty infiltration. Excessive accumulation of fat cells in the interstitial tissue of an organ.

fatty liver. A liver which is the seat of fatty change, as fat infiltration.

fau·ces (faw'seez) *n.pl.* genit. pl. **fau·ci·um** (faw'see·um) The space surrounded by the soft palate, palatoglossal and palatopharyngeal arches, and base of the tongue. —**fau·cial** (faw'shul) *adj.*

fau·na (faw'nuh) *n.,* pl. **faunas, fau·nae** (·nee) The entire animal life peculiar to any area or period.

fa·ve·o·late (fa·vee'uh·late) *adj.* Honeycombed; alveolate.

fa·vism (fay'viz·um) *n.* An acute hemolytic anemia, usually in those of Mediterranean area descent, occurring when a person with glucose 6-phosphate dehydrogenase deficiency of erythrocytes eats the beans of *Vicia faba* and inhales its pollen, presumed to be an antigen-antibody interaction with the red blood cells.

fa·vus (fay'vus) *n.* A fungal infection of the scalp, usually caused by *Trichophyton schoenleini,* characterized by round, yellow cup-shaped crusts (scutula, favus cups) having a peculiar mousy odor, which may form honeycomb-like masses; other body areas may occasionally be affected. Syn. *tinea favosa.*

F.C.A.P. Fellow of the College of American Pathologists.

F.C.C.P. Fellow of the American College of Chest Physicians.

Fc fragment. The crystallizable fraction of immunoglobulin heavy chains.

FDA Abbreviation for *Food and Drug Administration.*

Fe Symbol for iron.

fear, *n.* An emotion marked by dread, apprehension, or alarm, sometimes with the visceral manifestations accompanying anxiety.

fear reaction. A neurosis, particularly one developed in combat, in which anxiety is manifested by the conscious fear of a particular object or event.

fea·ture, *n.* Any single part or lineament of a structure, as of the face.

febri- A combining form meaning *fever.*

feb·ri·fa·cient (feb''ri·fay'shunt) *adj.* Producing fever.

feb·ri·fuge (feb'ri·fewj) *n. & adj.* 1. A substance that mitigates or reduces fever; an antipyretic. 2. Tending to reduce fever.

febrile convulsion. A generalized (sometimes focal) convulsive seizure accompanying fever, usually in children; febrile seizures in infants with a familial history of epilepsy or with prenatal and birth difficulties often presage recurrent seizures in later life.

febrile pulse. A pulse that is full, rapid, and often exhibiting dicrotism; common in fever.

feb·ri·pho·bia (feb''ri·fo'bee·uh) *n.* PYREXIOPHOBIA.

fe·cal, fae·cal (fee'kul) *adj.* Pertaining to or containing feces.

fecal abscess. An abscess containing feces and communicating with the lumen of the intestine.

fecal fistula. An opening from an intestine through the abdominal wall to the skin, with discharge of intestinal contents; usually applied to openings from the ileum and colon.

fe·ca·lith (fee'kuh·lith) *n.* A concretion formed from intermingled fecal material and calcium salts; coprolith.

fe·cal·oid (fee'kuh·loid) *adj.* Resembling feces.

fe·ces, fae·ces (fee'seez) *n.pl.* The excretions of the bowels; the excretions from the intestine of unabsorbed food, indigestible matter, intestinal secretions, and bacteria. —**fe·cal, fae·cal** (·kul) *adj.*

fe·co·lith (fee'ko·lith) *n.* FECALITH.

fec·u·la (feck'yoo·luh) *n.,* pl. **fec·u·lae** (·lee) 1. The starchy part of a seed. 2. The sediment subsiding from an infusion.

fec·u·lent, fae·cu·lent (feck'yoo·lunt, fee'kew·) *adj.* 1. Having sediment. 2. Excrementitious.

fe·cun·da·tion (fee"kun·day'shun) *n.* The act of fertilizing; fertilization. —**fe·cun·date** (fee'kun·date, feck'un·) *v.*

fe·cun·di·ty (fe·kun'di·tee) *n.* The innate potential reproductive capacity of the individual organism, as denoted by its ability to produce offspring. —**fe·cund** (fee'kund) *adj.*

fee·ble·mind·ed (-mind'ed) *adj.* Mentally deficient or retarded. —**feeblemindedness,** *n.*

feed·back, *n.* 1. The return to the input, as of a electric, endocrine, or other system, of a part of its output, which frequently leads to an adjustment in this system. 2. The partial redistribution of the effects or products of a given process to its source so as to modify it.

feeling tone. *In psychiatry,* the affective aspect, as the pleasingness or unpleasingness of a person, object, or act.

fee splitting. The practice of dividing fees paid for professional services without informing the patient, as between consultants and referring physicians.

Feh·ling's reagent or **solution** (fey'ling) A reagent prepared by mixing an aqueous solution of copper sulfate with an aqueous solution of Rochelle salt and either potassium or sodium hydroxide; used to test for glucose and other reducing substances in urine.

Fehling's test A test for reducing substances in urine in which an equal amount of Fehling's reagent and urine are boiled. In the presence of reducing substances, chiefly glucose, a green, yellow, or red precipitate forms, the color depending on the amount of glucose present.

feld·sher (feld'shur) *n.* In the Soviet Union and other countries, a trained medical worker without the full training or status of a qualified physician, who delivers initial medical care and performs other tasks according to qualifications under the supervision of a physician or medical team; a physician's assistant.

fe·line (fee'line) *adj. & n.* 1. Pertaining to or derived from cats (genus *Felis*) or the family (Felidae) which includes cats, tigers, lions, leopards. 2. Catlike. 3. A member of the family Felidae.

feline distemper. FELINE PANLEUKOPENIA.

feline enteritis. FELINE PANLEUKOPENIA.

feline infectious anemia. An anemia of cats caused by the rickettsial agent *Hemobartonella felis* and characterized by anorexia, depression, fever, and hemolytic anemia.

feline infectious peritonitis. An invariably fatal disease of domestic cats, suspected to be caused by a virus and characterized by fever, severe depression, anorexia, weight loss, and ascites.

feline leukemia virus. A virus which is widespread in the cat population and known to cause myeloproliferative disorders and lymphosarcoma; probably also responsible for a variety of disease problems related to immunosuppression; horizontal transmission of the virus from cat to cat is possible.

feline panleukopenia. A highly contagious usually fatal virus disease of cats, wild Felidae and mink, characterized by severe leukopenia of the granulocytic series, enteritis, and fever. Syn. *feline distemper, infectious feline enteritis.*

fel·la·tio (fe·lay'shee·o) *n.* Sexual stimulation of the penis by oral contact.

¹**fel·on** (fel'un) *n.* An infection in the closed space of the terminal phalanx of a finger.

²**felon.** *n.* A person who has committed a felony.

fe·lo·ni·ous (fe·lo'nee·us) *adj.* Pertaining to or constituting a felony.

fel·o·ny (fel'uh·nee) *n.* A grave crime; usually one declared such by statute because of the attendant severe punishment.

felt·work, *n.* A tissue composed of closely interwoven fibers.

Fel·ty's syndrome Adult rheumatoid arthritis, with splenomegaly resulting in granulocytopenia due to hypersplenism.

fe·male (fee'male) *adj. & n.* 1. Belonging or pertaining to the sex that produces the ovum. Symbol, ♀. 2. Designating that part of a double-limbed instrument that receives the complementary element. 3. A female organism or individual.

female pseudohermaphroditism. A condition simulating hermaphroditism in which the external sexual characteristics are in part or wholly of male aspect, but internal female genitalia are present. Syn. *gynandry.*

fem·i·nine (fem'i·nin) *adj.* Having the appearance or qualities of a woman; female.

fem·i·nism (fem'i·niz·um) *n.* The presence in a male of secondary characteristics of the female sex. —**fem·i·ni·za·tion** (fem"i·ni·zay'shun) *n.;* **fem·i·nize** (fem'i·nize) *v.*

femora. Plural of *femur.*

fem·o·ral (fem'uh·rul) *adj.* Of or pertaining to the femur or to the thigh.

femoral canal. The medial compartment of the femoral sheath behind the inguinal ligament.

femoral hernia. A hernia involving the femoral canal; found most often in women, it is usually small and painless, often remaining unnoticed. The neck lies beneath the inguinal ligament and lateral to the tubercle of the pubic bone. Syn. *crural hernia.*

femoral ring. The abdominal opening of the femoral canal.

femoral triangle. A triangle formed laterally by the medial margin of the sartorius, medially by the lateral margin of the adductor longus, and superiorly by the inguinal ligament. Syn. *Scarpa's triangle.*

femoro-. A combining form meaning *femur, femoral.*

fem·o·ro·pop·lit·e·al (fem"uh·ro·pop·lit'ee·ul) *adj.* 1. Pertaining to the femur and the popliteal space. 2. Pertaining to the femoral and popliteal arteries.

fem·o·ro·tib·i·al (fem"uh-ro-tib'ee-ul) *adj.* Pertaining to the femur and the tibia.

fe·mur (fee'mur) *n.,* genit. **fe·mo·ris** (fem'o-ris), pl. **femurs, fe·mo·ra** (fem'o-ruh) The long bone of the thigh; thighbone. Adj. *femoral.*

fen·clo·nine (fen-klo'neen) *n.* DL-3-(*p*-Chlorophenyl)alanine, C₉H₁₀ClNO₂, an inhibitor of serotonin biosynthesis.

fe·nes·tra (fe-nes'truh) *n.,* pl. & genit. sing. **fenestrae** (·tree) 1. A small opening. 2. *In anatomy,* an aperture of the medial wall of the middle ear. 3. An opening in a bandage or plaster splint for examination or drainage. 4. The open space in the blade of a forceps. **—fenestral** (·trul) *adj.*

fenestra coch·le·ae (kock'lee-ee) [NA]. COCHLEAR WINDOW (= ROUND WINDOW).

fen·es·tra·tion (fen"e-stray'shun) *n.* 1. The creation of an opening or openings; perforation. 2. The presence of fenestrae in a structure. 3. An operation to create a permanently mobile window in the lateral semicircular canal; used in cases of deafness caused by stapedial impediment of sound waves. Syn. *Lempert's operation.* 4. *In dentistry,* an isolated area in which a root is denuded of bone and the root surface is covered only by periosteum and the overlying gingiva; usually occurring in the facial alveolar plate in the anterior region, rarely on the lingual surface. **—fen·es·trat·ed** (fen'e-stray-tid) *adj.*

fenestra ves·ti·bu·li (ves-tib'yoo-lye) [NA]. VESTIBULAR WINDOW (= OVAL WINDOW).

fen·nel (fen'ul) *n.* The dried, ripe fruit of cultivated varieties of *Foeniculum vulgare;* contains a volatile oil. It is used as a carminative.

fennel oil. The volatile oil from the fruit of *Foeniculum vulgare,* containing anethol; a carminative and flavoring oil.

Feosol. A trademark for certain preparations of ferrous sulfate.

fe·ral (ferr'ul, feer'ul) *adj.* 1. Characteristic of or suggestive of an animal, particularly a ferocious one, in its natural state; wild. 2. Living in or being in a natural state; not domesticated, socialized, or humanized, as a child reared in isolation with few human contacts.

fer-de-lance (fair" duh lahnce') *n.* A large, venomous pit viper of Central and South America; the *Bothrops atrox.*

fer·ment (fur'ment) *n.* A catalytic agent produced by, and associated with, a living organism (organized ferment), as distinguished from an enzyme which may be separated from the living organism (unorganized ferment).

fer·men·ta·tion (fur"men·tay'shun) *n.* The decomposition of complex molecules under the influence of ferments or enzymes. **—fer·men·ta·tive** (fur·men'tuh-tiv) *adj.*

fern·ing, *n.* The formation of a crystallized fern pattern in dried mucus from the uterine cervix before ovulation, resulting from estrogen stimulation. Pregnancy and progestational changes prevent ferning; in pregnancy ferning indicates the presence of amniotic fluid in the

vagina following premature rupture of membranes. Syn. *arborization.*

fern test. See *ferning.*

-ferous, -iferous A combining form meaning *bearing, producing.*

fer·rat·ed (ferr'ay-tid) *adj.* Combined with iron; containing iron.

ferri-. A combining form meaning *ferric, containing iron as a trivalent element.*

fer·ric (ferr'ick) *adj.* 1. Pertaining to or of the nature of iron. 2. Containing iron as a trivalent element.

ferric chloride. FeCl₃ + water. Has been used as an astringent and styptic.

ferric sulfate. Fe₂(SO₄)₃; a salt occurring as a grayish-white powder, very hygroscopic, slowly soluble in water, and forming an acid solution. It is largely used industrially.

fer·ri·cy·a·nide (ferr"eye-sigh'uh-nide, ferr"i·) *n.* A salt containing the trivalent [Fe (CN)₆] anion.

fer·ri·heme (ferr'eye-heem, ferr'i·) *n.* Heme in which the ferrous iron normally present is in the ferric (oxidized) state; the resulting higher valence imparts a positive charge which in alkaline solution attracts a hydroxyl ion, forming hematin, and in hydrochloric acid solution attracts a chloride ion, forming hemin.

fer·ri·he·mo·glo·bin, fer·ri·hae·mo·glo·bin (ferr"i-hee'muh-glo"bin, ferr"eye·) *n.* Methemoglobin, characterized by containing iron in the ferric state.

fer·ri·tin (ferr'i-tin) *n.* An iron-protein complex occurring in tissues, probably being a storage form of iron. It is in many characteristics similar to hemosiderin.

ferro-. A combining form meaning (a) *ferrous;* (b) *containing metallic iron.*

fer·ro·he·mo·glo·bin, fer·ro·hae·mo·glo·bin (ferr"o-hee'muh-glo"bin) *n.* Hemoglobin in which the iron is in the normal ferrous state.

fer·ro·ther·a·py (ferr"o-therr'uh-pee) *n.* Treatment of disease by the use of iron and iron compounds or chalybeates.

fer·rous (ferr'us) *adj.* Containing iron in divalent form.

ferrous chloride. FeCl₂.4H₂O; pale-green, deliquescent crystals or crystalline powder, soluble in acidulated water; used largely industrially.

ferrous gluconate. Fe(C₆H₁₁O₇)₂.2H₂O. A yellowish-gray or pale, greenish-yellow powder; soluble in water. A hematinic better tolerated than other iron salts.

ferrous iodide. FeI₂.4H₂O, occurring as almost black, very deliquescent masses, rapidly decomposing in air with liberation of iodine. It has been used in chronic tuberculosis. Ferrous iodide syrup, containing about 5% of FeI₂ by weight, has been used as a hematinic.

ferrous sulfate. FeSO₄.7H₂O. Pale bluish-green crystals or granules. A widely used and effective hematinic, used also as a deodorant. Syn. *copperas, green vitriol.*

fer·ru·gi·na·tion (fe-roo"ji-nay'shun) *n.* Depositions of iron in tissues.

fer·ru·gi·nous (fe-roo'ji-nus) *adj.* 1. Of, containing, or pertaining to iron. 2. Having the color of iron rust.

fer·tile (fur′til) adj. 1. Prolific; fruitful. 2. Of an organism: able to reproduce. 3. Of a gamete: able to bring about or undergo fertilization. 4. Of an ovum: fertilized. —**fer·til·i·ty** (fur·til′i·tee) n.

fertility clinic. A clinic to diagnose the causes of infertility in human beings and to assist reproductive ability. Syn. sterility clinic.

fertility factor. A factor which imparts to host bacteria the ability to donate genetic material by conjugation to bacteria lacking it, thereby permitting genetic recombination in the recipient. The factor may be transmitted independently to recipient cells and may under certain conditions become associated with its host deoxyribonucleic acid; this ability to exist in two states qualifies the factor as an episome. Syn. F factor, sex factor.

fer·til·iza·tion (fur′ti·li·zay′shun) n. The act of making fruitful; impregnation; union of male and female gametes. —**fer·til·ize** (fur′til·ize) v.

Fer·u·la (ferr′yoo·luh, ferr′oo·luh) n. A genus of the family Umbelliferae whose genera and species yield asafetida, galbanum, and sumbul.

fes·ter, v. 1. To suppurate superficially; to generate pus. 2. To become inflamed and suppurate.

festinating gait. The gait of patients with Parkinson's syndrome, marked by rigidity, shuffling, and festination.

fes·ti·na·tion (fes′ti·nay′shun) n. An involuntary increase or hastening in gait, seen in Parkinson's syndrome, both paralysis agitans and postencephalitic parkinsonism. —**fes·ti·nate** (fes′ti·nate) v. & adj.

fes·toon (fes·toon′) n. & v. 1. The scalloped appearance that is the natural arrangement of the marginal gingiva. 2. To recreate or reshape the gingival margin to its ideal physiologic contour. 3. To shape the base material in a dental prosthesis to simulate the form of the natural gingiva.

fe·tal, foe·tal (fee′tul) adj. Pertaining to, involving, or characteristic of a fetus.

fetal adenoma. A follicular adenoma of the thyroid made up of numerous small follicles of a primitive or fetal type, containing little or no colloid.

fetal age. The age of a fetus computed from the time of conception to any point in time prior to birth.

fetal alcohol syndrome. A syndrome of various defects, principally small size for gestational age, microcephaly, and retardation, observed in offspring of mothers with excessive alcohol intake during pregnancy.

fetal appendages. The placenta, amnion, chorion, and umbilical cord.

fetal asphyxia. Asphyxia of the fetus while in the uterus caused by interference with its blood supply, as by cord compression or premature placental separation.

fetal circulation. The circulation of the fetus, including the circulation through the placenta and the umbilical cord.

fetal cortex. ANDROGENIC ZONE.

fetal heart sounds. The sounds produced by the beating of the fetal heart, best heard near the umbilicus of the mother.

fetal hemoglobin. The dominant type of hemoglobin in the fetus, small amounts being produced throughout life; it differs in many chemical properties from adult hemoglobin. Syn. hemoglobin F.

fe·tal·ism (fee′tul·iz·um) n. The presence or persistence of certain prenatal conditions in the body after birth.

fetal membranes. The chorion, amnion, and allantois.

fetal rest. A portion of embryonic tissue, or cells, which remain in the mature tissue or organ.

fetal souffle. FUNICULAR SOUFFLE.

fe·ta·tion (fee·tay′shun) n. 1. The formation of the fetus. 2. PREGNANCY.

fe·ti·cide, foe·ti·cide (fee′ti·side) n. The killing of the fetus in the uterus.

fet·id, foet·id (fet′id, fee′tid) adj. Having a foul odor.

fet·ish, fet·ich (fet′ish, fee′tish) n. 1. Any inanimate object thought to have magical power or to bring supernatural aid. 2. In psychiatry, a personalized inanimate object, love object, or any maneuver or body part which, through association, arouses erotic feelings. —**fetish·ism** (·iz·um) n.; **fetish·ist** (·ist) n.

fet·lock, n. The region of a horse's leg that extends from the lower extremity of the metacarpal or metatarsal bone to the pastern joint.

fe·to·am·ni·ot·ic (fee′to·am·nee·ot′ick) adj. Pertaining to the fetus and the amnion.

fe·to·glob·u·lin, foe·to·glob·u·lin (fee′to·glob′yoo·lin) n. FETOPROTEIN.

fe·to·gram (fee′to·gram) n. A radiographic depiction of a fetus, including skin outline and bowel.

fe·tog·ra·phy (fee·tog′ruh·fee) n. A method of demonstrating fetal features by injecting the amniotic sac with contrast media designed to show the skin and the intestinal tract.

fe·tol·o·gy (fee·tol′uh·jee) n. The study, science, and treatment of the fetus. —**fetolo·gist,** n.

fe·tom·e·try (fee·tom′e·tree) n. The measurement of the fetus, especially of its cranial diameters.

fe·tor, foe·tor (fee′tur, ·tor) n. Stench.

fetor ex ore (ecks o′ree) Bad breath; halitosis.

fetor he·pat·i·cus (he·pat′i·kus). A peculiar musty or sweetish odor of the breath occurring in the terminal stage of hepatocellular liver disease.

fe·tu·in (fee′tew·in) n. A fetoprotein found in fetal calf serum.

fe·tus, foe·tus (fee′tus) n., pl. **fetuses, foetuses** The unborn offspring of viviparous mammals in the later stages of development; in human beings, from about the beginning of the ninth week after fertilization.

fetus cy·lin·dri·cus (si·lin′dri·kus). A malformed fetus with little indication of head and extremities, roughly cylindrical in form.

fetus pa·py·ra·ce·us (pap·i·ray′shee·us). A dead twin fetus which has been compressed by the growth of its living twin.

Feul·gen reaction (foil'g'n) A reaction specific for aldehydes based on formation of a purple-colored compound when aldehydes react with fuchsin-sulfuric acid. Deoxyribonucleic acid, but not ribonucleic acid, gives this reaction after the removal of its purine bases by acid hydrolysis.

fe·ver (fee'vur) *n.* 1. Elevation of the body temperature above the normal; in human beings, above an average value of 37°C (98.6°F) orally. Syn. *pyrexia.* 2. A disease whose distinctive feature is elevation of body temperature. —**fe·ver·ish** (·ish) *adj.*

fever blister. HERPES FACIALIS.

F factor. FERTILITY FACTOR.

F.F.P.S. Fellow of the Faculty of Physicians and Surgeons (Glasgow).

FFT Abbreviation for (a) *flicker fusion test;* (b) *flicker fusion threshold.*

fiant. Plural of *fiat.*

fi·at (figh'at) *v.,* pl. **fi·ant** (·ant, ·unt) Let there be made; used in the writing of prescriptions. Abbreviated, ft.

fi·ber, fi·bre (figh'bur) *n.* A filamentary or thread-like structure. —**fi·brous** (·brus) *adj.*

fi·ber·op·tic (figh''bur·op'tick) *adj.* Pertaining to or characterizing fine glass or plastic fibers with optical refraction properties such that light can be conveyed along them and reflected around corners; used especially for illumination in endoscopy. —**fiberoptics,** *n.*

fi·ber·scope (figh'bur·skope) *n.* An instrument that has a flexible shaft of light-conducting fibers and a source of illumination and that is used for viewing certain internal tissues.

fibr-, fibro-. A combining form meaning *fiber, fibrous.*

fibre. FIBER.

fi·bri·form (figh'bri·form) *adj.* Shaped like a fiber.

fi·bril (figh'bril, fib'ril) *n.* A component filament of a fiber, as of a muscle or of a nerve. —**fi·bril·lar** (·bri·lur), **fibril·lary** (·lăr·ee) *adj.*

fi·bril·late (figh'bri·late, fib'ri·) *v.* 1. To undergo fibrillation. 2. To cause to undergo fibrillation.

fi·bril·la·tion (figh''bri·lay'shun, fib''ri·) *n.* 1. A noncoordinated twitching involving individual muscle fibers that have been separated from their nerve supply. 2. Very rapid irregular noncoordinated contractions of the heart.

fi·bril·lo·gen·e·sis (figh·bril''o·jen'e·sis, figh''bri·lo·) *n.* The formation and development of fibrils.

fibril sheath. A sheath formed by connective-tissue fibrils and surrounding individual nerve fibers.

fi·brin (figh'brin) *n.* The fibrous insoluble protein formed by the interaction of thrombin and fibrinogen.

fibrin-, fibrino-. A combining form meaning *fibrin, fibrinous.*

fibrin film. A pliable, elastic, translucent film of fibrin, prepared from human blood plasma; used in neurosurgery and for the repair of dural defects and in the prevention of meningocerebral adhesions.

fibrin foam. A spongy material made from human fibrin which, when soaked in human thrombin, is a useful hemostatic agent in neurosurgery, in wounds of parenchymatous organs, and in cases of jaundice and hemophilia. It causes little tissue reaction and is absorbable.

fi·brin·o·cel·lu·lar (figh''bri·no·sel'yoo·lur) *adj.* Containing both fibrin and cells; usually refers to an exudate.

fi·brin·o·gen (figh·brin'o·jen) *n.* A protein, which may be bactericidal, of the globulin class present in blood plasma and serous transudations and increasing in quantity during the acute phase of an inflammatory reaction or trauma. The soluble precursor of fibrin. Syn. *factor I.* —**fi·brin·o·gen·ic** (figh''brin·o·jen'ick), **fi·bri·nog·e·nous** (figh''bri·noj'e·nus) *adj.*

fi·brin·o·geno·pe·nia (figh·brin''o·jen''o·pee'nee·uh) *n.* A decrease in the fibrinogen content of the blood plasma.

fi·bri·no·hem·or·rhag·ic (figh''bri·no·hem''o·raj'ick) *adj.* Containing fibrin and blood; usually describes an exudate.

fi·brin·oid (figh'brin·oid) *adj. & n.* 1. Having the appearance and the staining properties of fibrin. 2. A homogeneous, refractile, oxyphilic substance occurring in degenerating connective tissue, in term placentas, in rheumatoid nodules, in Aschoff bodies, and in pulmonary alveoli in some prolonged pneumonitides.

fibrinoid degeneration. A form of degeneration in which the tissue involved is converted to a homogeneous or granular acellular mass with bright acidophilic staining reaction resembling that of fibrin.

fi·bri·nol·y·sin (figh''bri·nol'i·sin) *n.* Any enzyme that digests fibrin; a less specific term than plasmin.

fi·bri·nol·y·sis (figh''bri·nol'i·sis) *n.* The digestion or degradation of fibrin; may be applied to the proteolysis of fibrin by plasmin, but applies also to other mechanisms. —**fi·bri·no·lyt·ic** (·no·lit'ick) *adj.*

fi·brin·ous (figh'bri·nus) *adj.* Of, containing, or resembling fibrin.

fibrinous exudate. An exudate in which fibrin is a prominent constituent.

fibrinous inflammation. Inflammation in which the noncellular portion of the exudate is composed largely of fibrin.

fi·bro·ad·e·no·ma (figh''bro·ad·e·no'muh) *n.* A benign tumor containing both fibrous and glandular elements.

fi·bro·ad·i·pose (figh''bro·ad'i·poce) *adj.* Both fibrous and fatty.

fi·bro·am·e·lo·blas·to·ma (figh''bro·am''e·lo·blas·to'muh) *n.* An ameloblastoma with an especially abundant fibrous stroma.

fi·bro·an·gio·li·po·ma (figh''bro·an''jee·o·li·po'muh) *n.* A benign tumor whose parenchyma contains fibrous, vascular, and adipose tissue components.

fi·bro·an·gi·o·ma (figh''bro·an''jee·o'muh) *n.* A benign tumor composed of blood or lymph vessels, with abundant connective tissue.

fi·bro·are·o·lar (figh''bro·a·ree'o·lur) *adj.* Both fibrous and areolar.

fi·bro·blast (figh'bro·blast) *n.* A large stellate cell (spindle-shaped in edge view) in which the nucleus is large, oval, and pale-staining with one or two nucleoli. Fibroblasts are common in developing or repairing tissues where they are concerned in protein and collagen synthesis.

fi·bro·blas·tic (figh″bro·blas′tick) *adj.* 1. Pertaining to fibroblasts. 2. FIBROPLASTIC.

fibroblastic meningioma. A meningioma in which the meningioma cells are highly elongated, resembling fibroblasts, and form interlacing bundles.

fi·bro·blas·to·ma (figh″bro·blas·to′muh) *n.* A tumor whose parenchyma consists of fibroblasts, as fibromas and fibrosarcomas.

fi·bro·bron·chi·tis (figh″bro·brong·kye′tis) *n.* Bronchitis with expectoration of fibrinous casts.

fi·bro·cal·cif·ic (figh″bro·kal·sif′ick) *adj.* Consisting of fibrous and calcific elements, the fibrous element being primary.

fi·bro·car·ci·no·ma (figh″bro·kahr·si·no′muh) *n.* A carcinoma with fibrous elements.

fi·bro·car·ti·lage (figh″bro·kahr′ti·lij) *n.* Dense, white, fibrous connective tissue in which the cells have formed small masses of cartilage between the fibers. **—fibro·car·ti·lag·i·nous** (·kahr″ti·laj′i·nus) *adj.*

fi·bro·ca·se·ous (figh″bro·kay′see·us) *adj.* Containing both fibrous and caseous elements, said of certain forms of pulmonary tuberculosis.

fi·bro·cav·i·tary (figh″bro·kav′i·terr·ee) *adj.* Having both fibrosis and cavity formation; said of certain forms of pulmonary tuberculosis.

fi·bro·cel·lu·lar (figh″bro·sel′yoo·lur) *adj.* Both fibrous and cellular.

fi·bro·ce·men·to·ma (figh″bro·see″men·to′muh) *n.* A type of cementoma in which the fibrous component overshadows the cementum component.

fi·bro·chon·dro·ma (figh″bro·kon·dro′muh) *n.* A benign tumor containing both fibrous and cartilaginous elements.

fi·bro·chon·dro·os·te·o·ma (figh″bro·kon·dro·os·tee·o′muh) *n.* A type of osteochondroma with a prominent fibrous element.

fi·bro·col·lag·e·nous (figh″bro·kol·aj′e·nus) *adj.* Pertaining to fibrous tissue in which there is a great deal of collagen and relatively few cells.

fi·bro·cys·tic (figh″bro·sis′tick) *adj.* Having both fibrous and cystic aspects; usually applied to the development of cysts in a gland which is the seat of chronic retrogressive or inflammatory changes accompanied by fibrosis.

fibrocystic disease. CYSTIC DISEASE OF THE BREAST.

fibrocystic disease of the pancreas. CYSTIC FIBROSIS OF THE PANCREAS.

fi·bro·cys·to·ma (figh″bro·sis·to′muh) *n.* A benign tumor containing both fibrous and cystic elements.

fi·bro·cyte (figh′bro·site) *n.* A connective-tissue cell present in fully differentiated or mature tissue in which the cytoplasm is less abundant and less basophilic than that of a fibroblast. Fibrocytes are relatively immobile; however,

they regain proliferative capacity following tissue injury.

fi·bro·dys·pla·sia (figh″bro·dis·play′zhuh, ·zee·uh) *n.* FIBROUS DYSPLASIA.

fi·bro·elas·tic (figh″bro·e·las′tick) *adj.* Having interlacing collagenous fibers interspersed by more or less strongly developed networks of elastic fibers; applied to connective tissue.

fi·bro·elas·to·sis (figh″bro·e·las·to′sis) *n.* 1. Proliferation of fibrous and elastic tissues. 2. ENDOCARDIAL FIBROELASTOSIS.

fi·bro·en·chon·dro·ma (figh″bro·en″kon·dro′muh) *n.* An enchondroma containing fibrous elements.

fi·bro·en·do·the·li·o·ma (figh″bro·en″do·theel·ee·o′muh) *n.* A tumor containing fibrous and endothelium-like structures, as a synovioma.

fi·bro·fat·ty (figh″bro·fat′ee) *adj.* Both fibrous and fatty.

fi·brog·lia (figh·brog′lee·uh, fi·) *n.* The ground substance of connective tissue.

fi·bro·he·mo·tho·rax, fi·bro·hae·mo·tho·rax (figh″bro·hee″mo·tho′racks) *n.* The presence of blood and fibrin in the pleural space.

fi·broid (figh′broid) *adj.* 1. Composed largely of fibrous tissue. 2. LEIOMYOMA UTERI. 3. Any fibrous tumor.

fi·broid·ec·to·my (figh″broy·deck′tuh·mee) *n.* Removal of a uterine fibroid; MYOMECTOMY.

fibroid tumor. 1. FIBROMA. 2. LEIOMYOMA UTERI.

fi·bro·leio·my·o·ma (figh″bro·lye″o·migh·o′muh) *n.* A leiomyoma containing a fibrous component.

fi·bro·li·po·ma (figh″bro·li·po′muh) *n.* A lipoma with a considerable amount of fibrous tissue. **—fibroli·po·ma·tous** (·pom″uh·tus, ·po′muh·tus) *adj.*

fi·bro·lipo·sar·co·ma (figh″bro·lip″o·sahr·ko′muh) *n.* A malignant tumor with both fibrosarcomatous and liposarcomatous elements.

fi·brol·y·sis (figh·brol′i·sis) *n.,* pl. **fibroly·ses** (·seez) Resolution of abnormal fibrous tissue, as in a scar.

fi·bro·ma (figh·bro′muh) *n.,* pl. **fibromas, fibroma·ta** (·tuh) A benign tumor composed principally of fibrous connective tissue.

fibroma du·rum (dew′rum). 1. A hard fibroma, firm because of large quantities of collagenous material in comparison with the number of cells. 2. DERMATOFIBROMA.

fibroma mol·le (mol′ee). A soft fibroma, containing many cellular components, as compared with collagenous fibers.

fibroma pen·du·lum (pen′juh·lum, pend′yoo·lum). A benign, pendulous fibrous tumor attached to the skin by a narrow neck.

fibromata. A plural of *fibroma.*

fi·bro·ma·to·gen·ic (figh″bro″muh·to·jen′ick) *adj.* Pertaining to any process or agent that promotes fibrous connective-tissue formation or fibroma.

fi·bro·ma·toid (figh·bro′muh·toid) *adj.* Resembling a fibroma.

fi·bro·ma·to·sis (figh·bro″muh·to′sis) *n.,* pl. **fibromato·ses** (·seez) 1. The occurrence of multiple fibromas. 2. Localized proliferation of fibroblasts without apparent cause.

fibromatosis gin·gi·vae (jin·jye′vee). A generalized form of gingival hyperplasia of unknown etiology, but having a strong familial or hereditary background. Syn. *diffuse fibromatosis, familial fibromatosis, hereditary gingival fibromatosis.*

fi·bro·ma·tous (figh·bro'muh·tus, ·brom'uh·tus) *adj.* Of or pertaining to a fibroma.

fi·bro·mus·cu·lar (figh"bro·mus'kew·lur) *adj.* Made up of connective tissue and muscle.

fi·bro·my·o·ma (figh"bro·migh·o'muh) *n.* A benign tumor, usually of smooth muscle, with a prominent fibrous stroma; commonly a LEIO-MYOMA UTERI.

fi·bro·my·o·mec·to·my (figh"bro·migh"o·meck' tuh·mee) *n.* Excision of a fibromyoma.

fi·bro·my·o·si·tis (figh"bro·migh"o·sigh'tis) *n.* 1. FIBROSITIS. 2. FIBROUS MYOSITIS.

fi·bro·myxo·li·po·ma (figh"bro·mick"so·li·po' muh) *n.* A benign mixed mesodermal tumor of hamartomatous nature, containing fibrous, myxoid, and fatty components.

fi·bro·myx·o·ma (figh"bro·mick·so'muh) *n.* A benign mixed mesodermal tumor of hamartomatous nature, composed of fibrous and myxoid elements.

fi·bro·myxo·sar·co·ma (figh"bro·mick"so·sahr· ko'muh) *n.* A malignant mixed mesodermal tumor with fibrosarcomatous and myxosarcomatous components.

fi·bro·os·teo·chon·dro·ma (figh"bro·os"tee·o· kon·dro'muh) *n.* An osteochondroma with a prominent fibrous element.

fi·bro·os·te·o·ma (figh"bro·os·tee·o'muh) *n.* An osteoma with a prominent fibrous component.

fi·bro·os·teo·sar·co·ma (figh"bro·os"tee·o·sahr· ko'muh) *n.* An osteosarcoma with a significant fibrosarcomatous element.

fi·bro·pap·il·lo·ma (figh"bro·pap"i·lo'muh) *n.* FIBROADENOMA.

fi·bro·pla·sia (figh"bro·play'zhuh, ·zee·uh) *n.* The growth of fibrous connective tissue, as in the second phase of wound healing. —**fibro·plas·tic** (·plas'tick) *adj.*

fi·bro·plate (figh'bro·plate) *n.* A disk of interarticular fibrocartilage.

fi·bro·psam·mo·ma (figh"bro·sa·mo'muh) *n.* A benign tumor, chiefly fibrous, containing psammoma bodies.

fi·bro·pu·ru·lent (figh"bro·pewr'yoo·lunt, ·pewr' uh·lunt) *adj.* Pertaining to purulent exudate with a prominent fibrinous element.

fi·bro·sar·co·ma (figh"bro·sahr·ko'muh) *n.* A malignant tumor whose parenchyma is composed of anaplastic fibrocytes. —**fibrosarcoma·tous** (·tus) *adj.*

fibrosarcoma phyl·lo·des (fi·lo'deez). CYSTOSARCOMA PHYLLODES.

fi·brose (figh'broce) *adj. & v.* 1. FIBROUS. 2. To form fibrous tissue.

fi·bro·se·rous (figh"bro·seer'us) *adj.* Having both fibrous and serous elements.

fi·bros·ing (figh'bro·sing) *adj.* 1. Undergoing fibrosis. 2. Having the property of stimulating fibrous tissue production.

fi·bro·sis (figh·bro'sis) *n.,* pl. **fibro·ses** (·seez) An increment in fibrous connective tissue. —**fi·brot·ic** (figh·brot'ick) *adj.*

fi·bro·si·tis (figh"bro·sigh'tis) *n.* A clinical disease entity characterized by pain, stiffness, and tenderness associated with muscle sheaths and fascial layers. Syn. *muscular rheumatism.* —**fibro·sit·ic** (·sit'ick) *adj.*

fi·bro·tho·rax (figh"bro·tho'racks) *n.* Complete adhesion between the visceral and parietal layers of the pleura of a hemithorax, together with fibrosis of the joined surfaces.

fi·brous (figh'brus) *adj.* Containing fibers; similar to fibers.

fibrous adhesion. Firm attachment of adjacent serous membranes by bands or masses of fibrous connective tissue.

fibrous ankylosis. Ankylosis due to fibrosis in the joint capsule or fibrous adhesions between the joint surfaces.

fibrous connective tissue. The densest connective tissue of the body, including tendons, ligaments, and fibrous membranes. Collagenous fibers form the main constituent and are arranged in parallel bundles between which are rows of connective-tissue cells.

fibrous dysplasia. 1. Fibrous hyperplasia and osseous metaplasia in one bone (monostotic) or several bones (polyostotic); the latter form is often accompanied by segmental café-au-lait spots with ragged edges and, usually in girls, with precocious puberty (Albright's syndrome). 2. A form of mammary dysplasia characterized by abnormal amounts of fibrous tissue in relation to glandular tissue.

fibrous investment. General term describing an outer sheath of connective tissue found about various organs outside the proper capsule of the organ.

fibrous myositis. Chronic myositis with formation of fibrous tissue.

fi·bro·vas·cu·lar (figh"bro·vas'kew·lur) *adj.* Having both fibrous and vascular components.

fi·bro·xan·tho·ma (figh"bro·zan·tho'muh) *n.* A xanthoma with a prominent fibrous stroma. —**fibroxanthoma·tous** (·tus) *adj.*

fib·u·la (fib'yoo·luh) *n.,* L. pl. & genit. sing. **fibu·lae** (·lee) The slender bone at the outer part of the leg, articulating above with the tibia and below with the talus and tibia. —**fibu·lar** (·lur) *adj.*

fibular artery. PERONEAL ARTERY.

fib·u·lo·cal·ca·ne·al (fib"yoo·lo·kal·kay'nee·ul) *adj.* Pertaining to or connecting the fibula and the calcaneus.

fib·u·lo·tib·i·a·lis (fib"yoo·lo·tib·ee·ay'lis) *adj.* Pertaining to the fibula and the tibia.

F.I.C.D. Fellow of the International College of Dentists.

fi·cin (figh'sin) *n.* A proteolytic enzyme from the sap of the fig-tree. It is an active *Ascaris* and *Trichuris* vermicide.

Fick principle, method, or **equation** A method for determining cardiac output based on the principle that the uptake or release of oxygen by an organ is the product of the organ blood flow and the arteriovenous oxygen concentration difference; cardiac output = (oxygen consumption)/(arteriovenous oxygen difference) × 100.

F.I.C.S. Fellow of the International College of Surgeons.

Fiedler's myocarditis An acute interstitial myocarditis of unknown etiology, with a predominant mononuclear cell infiltrate and varying muscle necrosis.

field, *n.* 1. A space or area of varying size or boundaries. 2. A concept of development in which the whole and the parts of a structure or organism are dynamically interrelated, reacting to each other and to the environment. 3. A region of the embryo that is the anlage of some organ or part. 4. The area within which objects can be seen through a microscope at one time. 5. *In surgery,* the area exposed to the surgeon's vision. 6. A specialty or special branch of knowledge, as the field of neurology. 7. In diagnostic radiology, the projected image of an anatomic organ or region, as lung field. 8. In therapeutic radiology, the area directly encompassed by an external therapy beam; port.

field of fixation. *In optics,* the region bounded by the utmost limits of distinct or central vision, which the eye has under its direct control throughout its excursions when the head is not moved.

field of vision. The space visible to an individual when the eye is fixed steadily on an object in the direct line of vision. Abbreviated, F.

fifth (Vth) cranial nerve. TRIGEMINAL NERVE.

fifth disease. ERYTHEMA INFECTIOSUM.

fight-or-flight reaction. 1. *In physiology,* according to W. B. Cannon, the response of the sympathetic nervous system and the adrenal medulla to stress, which results in adjustments in blood flow and metabolism adapted to the preservation of the organism in an emergency situation. 2. *In psychiatry,* the manner in which a person responds to stress. In the "fight" reaction he strives for adjustment; if he fails he may adopt a neurosis as a compromise. In the "flight" reaction, the patient may take refuge in a psychosis, permitting him to fancy a situation in which he can control the problem or ignore its reality.

fig·ure, *n.* 1. The visible form of anything; the outline of an organ or part. 2. A group of impressions derived from a single sense and perceived as a whole or one unit set apart from adjacent impressions. 3. A person who represents the essential aspects of a certain role; in particular, a father or mother figure.

figure-ground, *n. In psychology,* a general property of perception or awareness, according to which the perceived is divided into two or more parts, each endowed with a different shape or other attribute, but all influencing each other; the most distinct part being the figure and the least formed one, the ground. Inability to separate figure from ground is seen in certain organic brain syndromes.

figure-of-eight bandage. A bandage in which the successive turns cross like the figure eight.

fila. Plural of *filum.*

fi·la·ceous (fi-lay'shus) *adj.* Consisting of threads or threadlike fibers or parts.

fil·a·ment (fil'uh-munt) *n.* A small, threadlike structure. —**fil·a·men·tous** (fil''uh·men'tus), **fil·a·men·ta·ry** (fil''uh·men'tuh·ree) *adj.*

fil·a·men·ta·tion (fil''uh·men·tay'shun) *n.* THREAD REACTION.

fila ol·fac·to·ria (ol·fack·to'ree·uh). The component fasciculi of the olfactory nerve before and during their passage through the cribriform plate of the ethmoid bone.

fi·lar (figh'lur) *adj.* Filamentous; having or being threadlike structures.

fi·lar·ia (fi·lār'ee·uh) *n.,* pl. **filar·i·ae** (·ee·ee) A worm of the superfamily Filarioidea: long filiform nematodes, the adults of which may live in the circulatory or lymphatic systems, the connective tissues, or serous cavities of a vertebrate host. The larval forms, or microfilariae, are commonly found in the circulating blood or lymph spaces from which they are ingested by some form of bloodsucking arthropod. After a series of metamorphoses in the body of the arthropod, the larvae migrate to the proboscis as infestive forms. —**filari·al** (·ul) *adj.*

filarial fever. A recurrent fever occurring irregularly at intervals of months or years in most forms of filariasis. Syn. *elephantoid fever.*

fil·a·ri·a·sis (fil''uh·rye'uh·sis) *n.,* pl. **filaria·ses** (·seez) An infection with filariae, with or without the production of manifest disease.

fi·lar·i·cide (fi·lār'i·side) *n.* A drug that destroys filariae. —**fi·lar·i·ci·dal** (fi·lār''i·sigh'dul) *adj.*

fi·lar·i·form (fi·lār'i·form) *adj.* In the form of, or resembling, filariae.

fil·ial (fil'ee·ul) *adj.* 1. Pertaining to an offspring. 2. *In genetics,* indicating the sequence of an offspring from the original parents, the first being designated F_1, the second F_2, and so forth.

filial regression. The tendency for the mean phenotypic value of offspring to deviate less from a population mean than do parents who demonstrate large deviations.

fili·form (fil'i·form, figh'li·) *adj.* Threadlike.

filiform catheter. A catheter the leading end of which is molded into an extremely slender or thread-shaped form in order to facilitate passage of the larger, following portion through a constricted or irregular passage. Syn. *whip catheter.*

filiform papilla. Any one of the papillae occurring on the dorsum and margins of the oral part of the tongue, consisting of an elevation of connective tissue covered by a layer of epithelium, giving the tongue a velvety appearance.

fil·let (fil'it) *n.* 1. A loop for the purpose of making traction on the fetus. 2. LEMNISCUS.

fill·ing, *n.* A dental restoration; may be applied to a restoration of a temporary nature or for treatment.

fil·mat·ed gauze (fil'may·tid). A folded absorbent gauze with a thin layer of cotton or rayon evenly distributed over every layer giving ample dressing volume, rapid absorption and extreme softness.

film badge. A device containing photographic film, worn by personnel exposed to radiation to record dosage received.

film-coated tablet. A compressed tablet covered with a thin film of a water-soluble substance.

fil·ter, n. & v. 1. An apparatus that separates one or more components of a mixture from the others. 2. A special part of a high-frequency circuit which suppresses or admits certain frequencies of electric waves. 3. *In acoustics.* a device that suppresses certain frequencies of sound waves. 4. *In photography.* a colored glass or gelatin plate used in front of the photographic lens to alter the relative intensity of different wavelengths in the light beam. 5. To separate one or more components of a mixture from the others.

fil·ter·able (fil'tur·uh·bul) *adj.* FILTRABLE.

filtering operation. A surgical procedure performed for various types of glaucoma to form a new route of egress for the aqueous humor.

fil·tra·ble (fil'truh·bul) *adj.* Able to pass through a filter; usually applied to living agents of disease smaller than the common pathogenic bacteria.

filtrable virus. VIRUS.

fil·trate (fil'trate) *n.* The liquid that has passed through a filter.

fil·tra·tion (fil·tray'shun) *n.* The operation of straining through a filter.

filtration angle. The angle marking the periphery of the anterior chamber of the eye, formed by the attached margin of the iris and the junction of the sclera and cornea and functioning as a drainage route for aqueous humor. Syn. *anterior chamber angle, iridocorneal angle.*

fil·trum (fil'trum) *n.*, pl. **fil·tra** (-truh) A filter or strainer.

fi·lum (figh'lum) *n.*, pl. **fi·la** (-luh) Any threadlike or filamentous structure.

filum ter·mi·na·le (tur·mi·nay'lee) [NA]. The atrophic slender inferior end of the spinal cord, the caudal part of which is mostly pia mater.

fim·bria (fim'bree·uh) *n.*, pl. **fim·bri·ae** (-bree·ee) 1. A fringe. 2. The fringelike process of the outer extremity of the uterine tube. 3. A flattened band of white fibers along the medial margin of the hippocampus, continuous with the crus of the fornix. —**fim·bri·al** (fim'bree·ul) *adj.*

fimbria hip·po·cam·pi (hip·o·kam'pye) [NA]. FIMBRIA (3).

fim·bri·ate (fim'bree·ate) *adj.* Fringed with slender processes that are larger than filaments; possessing pili; said of bacterial cells and of the ostium of the uterine tube.

fim·bri·at·ed (fim'bree·ay''tid) *adj.* FIMBRIATE.

fim·bri·ec·to·my (fim''bree·eck'tuh·mee) *n.* Surgical resection of the fimbriated portion of the uterine tube.

fim·brio·den·tate (fim''bree·o·den'tate) *adj.* Pertaining to the fimbria (3) and to the dentate gyrus.

fine, *adj.* Involving movement through a narrow range. Said of tremors and other involuntary oscillatory movement of skeletal muscle.

fine structure. Ultramicroscopic structure.

fin·ger, *n.* A digit of the hand.

finger agnosia. Inability to recognize, name, and select individual fingers when looking at the hands; frequently a component of the Gerstmann syndrome.

finger anomia. A form of aphasia in which the patient has lost the ability to name his fingers though still able to recognize them.

finger cot. A covering of rubber or other material to protect the finger or to prevent infection.

finger-finger test. A cerebellar function test in which the patient is asked to bring the tips of his index fingers together from a position in which the arms are outstretched, or to place his index finger on the examiner's index finger with eyes open. Normally this is carried out smoothly and accurately.

finger-nose test. A cerebellar function test in which the patient is asked to put the tip of the index finger of each hand on the tip of the nose in rapid succession with eyes open. Abnormalities in the rate, range, and force of movement and an ataxic tremor betray the presence of cerebellar disease.

fin·ger·print, *n.* 1. An impression of the cutaneous ridges of a finger tip. May be a direct pressure print or a rolled print, the latter recording the entire flexor and lateral aspects of the phalanx. 2. Hydrolization of polypeptides into a pattern on a two-dimensional chromatogram. —**fingerprint·ing** (-ing) *n.*

fin·ger·stall (fing'gur·stawl) *n.* FINGER COT.

finger-thumb reflex. Apposition and adduction of the thumb, associated with flexion at the metacarpophalangeal joint on firm passive flexion of the third to the fifth finger at the proximal joints. Syn. *Mayer's reflex.*

fire·damp, *n.* An explosive mixture of methane and air.

first aid. Emergency treatment given to a casualty before regular medical or surgical care can be administered by trained individuals. —**first-aid**, *adj.*; **first-aider**, *n.*

first-aid kit. A pouch, bag, or box containing sterilized dressings, antiseptics and simple medications, bandages, an emergency airway, and simple instruments; for use in first aid.

first-degree burn. A mild burn, characterized by pain and reddening of the skin.

first-degree heart block. An atrioventricular block producing prolongation of the PR interval, but not completely blocking the conduction of any sinus beats to the ventricle.

first heart sound. The heart sound complex related primarily to closure of the atrioventricular valves and rapid ejection of blood from the ventricles. Symbol, S_1 or SI.

first-set, *adj.* Pertaining to a graft of a genetic constitution to which the recipient has had no previous exposure.

Fish·berg's test. A concentration test for kidney function in which urinary specific gravity is determined 12 hours after fluid deprivation.

fishskin disease. ICHTHYOSIS.

fish tapeworm. DIPHYLLOBOTHRIUM LATUM.

fis·sion (fish'un) *n.* 1. Any splitting or cleaving. 2. *In biology.* asexual reproduction by the division of the body into two or more parts, each of which grows into a complete organism. It is the common method of reproduction among the bacteria and protozoa. 3. *In nuclear physics.* the splitting of an atomic nucleus, by bombardment with elementary particles, with release of energy. —**fission,** v.; **fission·able,** *adj.*

fis·su·la (fish'oo·luh, fis'yoo·luh) *n.,* pl. & genit. sing. **fissu·lae** (·lee) A small fissure.

fis·su·ra (fi·shoo'ruh, fi·syoo'ruh) *n.,* pl. & genit. sing. **fissu·rae** (·ree) FISSURE.

fis·su·ral (fish'yoo·rul) *adj.* Of or pertaining to a fissure.

fis·sure (fish'ur) *n.* 1. Any groove or cleft normally occurring in a part or organ such as the skull, liver, or spinal cord. 2. A crack in skin or an ulcer in mucous membrane. 3. A lineal developmental fault in the surface of a tooth caused by imperfect union of the enamel of adjoining dental lobes. —**fis·sured** (fish'urd) *adj.;* **fis·su·ra·tion** (fish″uh·ray'shun) *n.*

fissured tongue. A condition of the tongue in which there are deep furrows in the mucous membrane.

fissure in ano (in ay'no) ANAL FISSURE.

fissure of Rolando CENTRAL SULCUS (1).

fis·tu·la (fis'tew·luh) *n.,* pl. **fistulas, fistu·lae** (·lee) An abnormal congenital or acquired communication between two surfaces or between a viscus or other hollow structure and the exterior. —**fistu·lar** (·lur) **fistu·late** (·late), **fistu·lous** (·lus) *adj.*

fistula in ano (in ay'no) ANAL FISTULA.

fis·tu·la·tion (fis'tew·lay'shun) *n.* FISTULIZATION.

fis·tu·lec·to·my (fis″tew·leck'tuh·mee) *n. In surgery,* excision of a fistula.

fis·tu·li·za·tion (fis″tew·li·zay'shun) *n.* The development or formation of a fistula or the surgical creation of a fistula.

fis·tu·lize (fis'tew·lize) *v.* To cause the formation of a fistula.

fis·tu·lo·en·ter·os·to·my (fis″tew·lo·en·tur·os'tuh·mee) *n. In surgery,* the establishment of an anastomosis between a biliary fistula and the duodenum.

fis·tu·lo·gram (fis'tew·lo·gram) *n.* A radiographic depiction of a fistulous tract using contrast material.

fis·tu·lot·o·my (fis″tew·lot'uh·mee) *n.* Incision of a fistula.

fit, *n.* Any sudden paroxysm of a disease, especially a seizure.

five-glass test. Collection of a urine sample in five containers, sequentially, to aid in localization of disease.

fix, *v.* 1. To render firm, stable, permanent; to fasten. 2. *In histology,* to treat tissue so that it hardens with preservation of the elements in the same relation and form as in life. 3. *In ophthalmology,* to turn the eye so that the image in the field of vision falls on the foveola or other point of fixation. 4. *In genetics,* to establish permanently some character of plants or animals by selective inbreeding.

fix·ate (fick'sate) *v.* 1. To become fixed. 2. To render fixed or stable.

fix·a·tion (fick·say'shun) *n.* 1. The act of fixing, establishing firmly, or making permanent. 2. *In surgery,* the immobilization of a part, as of a floating kidney by operative means or of a fractured bone by the use of a metal nail.

3. The intent focusing of the eyes upon an object. 4. *In psychology,* the strengthening of a learned tendency or habit formation; especially, the establishment of a strong or excessive attachment for a person, object, or way of doing something. 5. *In psychiatry,* the arrest of personality development or of psychosexual maturation at a certain stage. 6. *In microscopy,* the process of preservation of tissue elements in form, position, and reactivity by means of chemical or physical hardening or coagulating agents.

fixation muscle. A muscle that holds a part from moving to allow more accurate control of a distal part, as a muscle that holds the wrist steady to allow more precise control of finger movement.

fixation point. The point of sharpest vision in the retina; the point where the visual axis meets the retina.

fix·a·tive (fick'suh·tiv) *n.* 1. *In microscopy,* any substance used to fasten a section on a slide. 2. Any substance used to preserve tissues for microscopic study.

fixed, *adj.* 1. *In clinical medicine,* characterizing a persistent, nongrowing lesion, or one recurring frequently at the same site. 2. *In dermatology,* characterizing a drug eruption that recurs in the same site over and over again upon reexhibition of the causative drug.

fixed cell. A reticular cell attached to the reticular fibers in reticuloendothelium.

fixed idea. 1. A delusional idea which the patient refuses to relinquish even after its disproof. 2. Any compulsive drive or obsessive idea.

fixed macrophage. A scavenger cell with the capacity to ingest particulate matter, as found in loose connective tissue fixed to reticular fibers, or lining the sinuses in the liver, spleen, bone marrow, or lymph nodes.

fixed rabies virus. A rabies virus that is injected into rabbits and passed from one animal to another until it acquires a shorter and more constant incubation period than the naturally occurring virus; used in the Pasteur-type vaccines.

fl. Abbreviation for *fluid.*

flac·cid (flack'sid) *adj.* Soft; flabby; relaxed. —**flac·cid·i·ty** (flack·sid'i·tee) *n.*

flaccid paralysis. Paralysis of the bladder due to interruption of peripheral motor or sensory innervation of detrusor muscles.

Flack's node SINOATRIAL NODE.

flagella. Plural of *flagellum.*

flag·el·lant (flaj'e·lunt) *n.* A person practicing flagellation.

flag·el·lant·ism (flaj'e·lun·tiz·um) *n.* The masochistic or sadistic need for flagellation.

fla·gel·lar (fla·jel'ur) *adj.* Pertaining to a flagellum.

¹**flag·el·late** (flaj'e·late) *v.* To practice or indulge in flagellation.

²**flag·el·late** (flaj'e·lut, ·late) *n.* A protozoon with slender, whiplike processes.

flag·el·la·tion (flaj″e·lay'shun) *n.* 1. Flogging or beating, especially as a means of producing erotic or religiously oriented stimulation or gratification. 2. Massage by strokes or blows. 3. By extension, stabbing or cutting with a knife. 4. Having flagella; the pattern of flagella.

flag·el·lo·ma·nia (flaj″e·lo·may′nee·uh) n. Erotic excitement from flagellation.

fla·gel·lum (fla·jel′um) n., pl. **flagel·la** (·luh) A whiplike process consisting of an axial filament enclosed in thin cytoplasmic sheath; the organ of locomotion of sperm cells, and of certain bacteria and protozoa.

Flagyl. Trademark for metronidazole, a systemic trichomonacide.

flail, adj. Abnormally mobile or active; lacking normal control; flaccid.

flail chest. A condition in which there are multiple rib fractures, with or without fracture of the sternum, allowing the occurrence of paradoxic motion of the chest wall and the attendant physiologic disturbances; "stove-in chest."

flail joint. A condition of excessive mobility often following resection of a joint or paralysis.

flame photometer. An instrument for the quantitative determination of sodium, potassium, and sometimes other elements, especially in biological fluids. A sample when sprayed into a flame emits light which is resolved into its spectrum; a photoelectric cell measures the intensity of light of the wavelength corresponding to the particular element for which the analysis is made.

flam·ma·ble (flam′uh·bul) adj. INFLAMMABLE.

flange (flanj) n. DENTURE FLANGE.

flank, n. The fleshy or muscular part of an animal or a man between the ribs and the hip.

flap, n. A partially detached portion of skin or other tissue, either accidentally formed, or created by a surgeon to be used as a graft to fill a defect or to improve contour. Flaps that are composed of special tissue, such as mucous membrane, conjunctiva, dura, wall of intestinal tract, omentum, or muscle are named after the tissue contained, as muscle flap. They may also be named according to the special purpose for which they are used, as a rhinoplastic flap for repair of the nose.

flash·eye, n. ELECTRIC OPHTHALMIA.

flask, n. 1. A glass, plastic, or metal vessel having a narrow neck. 2. A sectional metal case in which a sectional mold is made of plaster of paris or artificial stone for the processing of artificial dentures or other resinous dental restorations.

flat, adj. 1. Lying in one plane. 2. Having a smooth or even surface. 3. Of a percussion note or a voice sound, lacking in resonance. —**flat·ness,** n.

flat film. A plain radiograph of the abdomen made with the patient in the supine position.

flat·foot, n. A depression of the plantar arch of varying degree, which may be congenital or acquired; PES PLANUS.

flat·u·lence (flatch′oo·lunce) n. The presence or sensation of excessive gas in the stomach and intestinal tract. —**flatu·lent** (·lunt) adj.

fla·tus (flay′tus) n. 1. Gas, especially gas or air in the gastrointestinal tract. 2. Air or gas expelled via any body orifice.

flat·worm, n. Any worm of the phylum Platyhelminthes.

fla·ve·do (fla·vee′do) n. Yellowness or sallowness, usually referring to the skin.

fla·vin (flay′vin, flav′in) n. 1. One of a group of yellow pigments, derived from isoalloxazine, isolated from various plant and animal sources. 2. QUERCITRIN.

Fla·vo·bac·te·ri·um (flay″vo·back·teer′ee·um) n. A genus of the Achromobacteriaceae consisting of gram-negative rod-shaped bacteria characteristically producing yellow-orange, red, or yellow-brown pigments on media. Commonly proteolytic, they occur widely in water and soil, and are rarely pathogenic.

fla·vone (flay′vone, flav′ohn) n. 1. 2-Phenyl-1,4-benzopyrone, $C_{15}H_{10}O_2$. 2. One of the yellow vegetable dye derivatives of flavone (1).

fla·vo·noid (flay′vuh·noid, flav′uh·) n. 1. A substance derived from flavone (1), or one of its derivatives. 2. Any of the flavone derivatives, including citrin, hesperetin, hesperidin, rutin, quercetin, and quercitrin, which may reduce capillary fragility in certain cases. 3. Pertaining to or like a flavonoid.

fla·vo·nol (flay′vo·nol, flav′·) n. 1. 3-Hydroxyflavone, $C_{15}H_{10}O_3$. 2. One of a group of vegetable dyes, including the anthocyanins, derived from flavonol (1).

fla·vo·none (flay′vuh·nohn, flav′uh·) n. 2,3-Dihydroflavone, $C_{15}H_{12}O_2$, derivatives of which include hesperetin and citrin.

fla·vo·pro·tein (flay″vo·pro′teen, ·tee·in, flav″o·) n. One of a group of conjugated proteins of the chromoprotein type which constitute the yellow enzymes. The prosthetic group in the known enzymes of this type is either a phosphoric acid ester of riboflavin or the latter combined with adenylic acid.

Flaxedil Triethiodide. Trademark for gallamine triethiodide, a curarimimetic drug employed as a skeletal muscle relaxant.

flaxseed oil. LINSEED OIL.

flea, n. Any bloodsucking, laterally compressed, wingless insect of the order Siphonaptera. Fleas are of medical importance as hosts and transmitters of disease, and their bites produce a form of dermatitis.

flea-borne typhus. MURINE TYPHUS.

flesh, n. The soft tissues of the body, especially the muscles. —**fleshy** (flesh′ee) adj.

flesh fly. One of the Sarcophagidae.

fleshy mole. 1. A blood mole that has become more solid and has assumed a fleshy appearance. 2. The more or less amorphous remains of a dead fetus in the uterine cavity.

flex, v. To bend.

flex·i·ble, adj. Capable of being bent, without breaking; pliable. —**flex·i·bil·i·ty** (fleck″si·bil′i·tee) n.

flex·im·e·ter (fleck·sim′e·tur) n. An instrument for measuring the amount of flexion possible in a joint.

flex·ion (fleck′shun) n. 1. The bending of a joint, or of parts having joints. 2. The condition of being bent.

Flexner's bacillus *Shigella flexneri.* See *Shigella.*
flex·or (fleck'sur, ·sor) *n.* A muscle that bends or flexes a limb or a part.
flexor retinaculum. A thickening of deep fascia overlying tendons of flexor muscles.
flex·u·ous (fleck'shoo-us, flecks'yoo-us) *adj.* Curving in an undulating manner.
flex·u·ra (fleck·shoor'uh, ·syoor'uh) *n.*, pl. & genit. sing. **flexu·rae** (·ree) FLEXURE.
flex·ure (fleck'shur) *n.* A bend or fold. —**flexur·al** (·ul) *adj.*
flick·er *n.* A sensation of fluctuating vision, caused by a light of such slow intermittence that the visual impressions produced do not fuse.
flicker fusion test. An application of the flicker fusion threshold in a test for fatigue and for tolerance to hypoxia; formerly used in the evaluation of hypertension and angina pectoris.
flicker fusion threshold. The minimal frequency of standard flashes of light that will be seen as steady illumination.
flight of ideas. The rapid skipping from one idea to another, even before the last one is thought through, the ideas bearing only a superficial relation to one another and often associated by chance; seen in the manic phase of manic depressive illness or in schizophrenia.
float·ers *n.* Floating specks in the field of vision, due to opacities in the media of the eye. Syn. *muscae volitantes, mouches volantes.*
float·ing *adj.* 1. Free or partly free from firm attachment, as a floating rib. 2. Abnormally movable, as a floating kidney. 3. Buoyed up freely, as in a fluid.
floating kidney. A kidney that is displaced from its bed, becoming more freely movable, sometimes causing symptoms, as by kinking the ureter. Syn. *wandering kidney, ren mobilis.*
floating rib. One of the last two ribs which have the anterior end free.
floc·cu·lar (flock'yoo-lur) *adj.* 1. Of or pertaining to the flocculus. 2. Tuftlike.
floccular lobule. One of the paired, small lobules on the inferior surface of the cerebellar hemisphere forming part of the flocculonodular lobe.
floc·cu·la·tion (flock''yoo-lay'shun) *n.* The coagulation or coalescence of finely divided or colloidal particles into larger particles which precipitate. —**floc·cu·late** (flock'yoo-late) *v. & n.*
flocculation test. A test in which the antibody reacts directly with the soluble antigen to produce flocculent, as in toxin-antitoxin reactions.
floc·cu·lent (flock'yoo-lunt) *adj. & n.* 1. Flaky, downy, or woolly, said of such particles in a liquid medium. 2. Causing flocculation. 3. A substance which causes flocculation.
floc·cu·lo·nod·u·lar (flock''yoo·lo·nod'yoo·lur) *adj.* Pertaining to the flocculus and nodulus of the cerebellum.
flocculonodular lobe. The part of the cerebellum consisting of the nodule of the vermis and the paired lateral flocculi.

floc·cu·lus (flock'yoo-lus) *n.*, pl. **floccu·li** (·lye) FLOCCULAR LOBULE.
floor, *n.* The lower inside surface of a hollow organ or open space.
floppy-infant syndrome. The constellation in infancy of marked deficiency in tone and muscular activity, and usually also delay in motor development; may be due to any of several systemic, neurologic, muscular, and connective-tissue disorders. Syn. *infantile hypotonia.*
flo·ra (flo'ruh) *n.*, pl. **floras, flo·rae** (·ree) 1. The entire plant life of any geographic area or geologic period. 2. The entire bacterial and fungal life normally inhabiting an area of the body, as: intestinal flora, vaginal flora.
flor·an·ty·rone (flor·an'ti·rone) *n.* γ-Oxo-γ-(8-fluoranthene)butyric acid, $C_{20}H_{14}O_3$, a hydrocholeretic drug.
flo·res (flor'eez) *n.pl.* 1. The flowers or blossoms of a plant. 2. A flocculent or pulverulent form of certain substances after sublimation.
flor·id (flor'id) *adj.* 1. Bright red. 2. Fully developed; manifesting a completely developed clinical syndrome.
flo·ta·tion, *n.* The process of separating the valuable constituents (minerals) of ores from the valueless gangue by agitation with water, a small proportion of an oil, and a foaming agent, the mineral rising with the foam and the gangue sinking.
flotation method. A technique employed for separating ova and larvae from stool specimens. The stool is put into a salt solution where it sinks while the ova and larvae, due to their lower specific gravity, rise to the surface.
flow, *v. & n.* 1. To move freely like liquid or particulate matter. 2. A quantity that flows within a set amount of time, as liquid through an organ. 3. To menstruate. 4. MENSTRUATION.
flowers of sulfur. A form of sulfur that has been refined by sublimation; sublimed sulfur.
flow·me·ter, *n.* 1. A physical device for measuring the rate of flow of a gas or liquid. 2. An apparatus for measuring flow characteristics of various substances.
fluc·tu·ance (fluck'tew·uns) *n.* The quality of fluctuation.
fluc·tu·a·tion (fluck''choo·ay'shun) *n.* 1. The wavelike motion produced by palpation or percussion of a body cavity when it contains fluid. 2. In an organism, a slight structural variation that is not inherited. 3. A recurrent, and often cyclic, alteration. 4. A variation about a fixed value or quantity.
flu·dro·cor·ti·sone acetate (floo''dro·kor'ti·sone). 9α-Fluoro-17-hydroxycorticosterone-21-acetate, $C_{23}H_{31}FO_6$, a fluorine derivative of hydrocortisone acetate with potent anti-inflammatory action.
flu·id, *adj. & n.* 1. Of substances: in a state in which the molecules move freely upon one another; flowing. 2. A fluid substance, such as any liquid secretion of the body. Abbreviated, fl.
fluid balance. A state of dynamic equilibrium in the body between the outgo and intake of water. Optimum water content is maintained by homeostatic physiologic mechanisms.

flu·id·ex·tract (floo″id·eck′strakt) *n.* A hydroalcoholic solution of vegetable principles usually so made that each milliliter contains the therapeutic constituents of 1 g of the standardized drug which it represents. Maceration and percolation with suitable solvent are employed as the means of obtaining solution of the desired constituents.

fluid level. In *radiology,* the interface between gas and liquid or aqueous liquid and liquid fat shown on radiographs as a line when the x-ray beam parallels the interface; seen on films made with the patient in the erect or decubitus positions and using a horizontal x-ray beam.

flu·id·ounce (floo″id·æownce′) *n.* A liquid measure; 8 fluidrams. Equivalent to approximately 29.57 ml. Symbol, f℥.

flu·i·dram, flu·i·drachm (floo′i·dram″) *n.* A liquid measure equal to one-eighth fluidounce, roughly equivalent to one teaspoonful. 60 minims = 1 fluidram. Symbol, f℈.

fluke, *n.* A trematode worm of the order Digenia.

fluo-, fluor-, fluori-, fluoro-. A combining form meaning (a) *fluorine;* (b) *fluorescence, fluorescent.*

flu·o·cin·o·lone acet·o·nide (floo″o·sin′uh·lohn a·set′o·nide). 6α,9α-Difluoro-16α-hydroxyprednisolone-16,17-acetonide, $C_{24}H_{30}F_2O_6$, an anti-inflammatory glucocorticoid.

flu·or·chrome (floo′ur·krome) *n.* A dye that fluoresces when irradiated with ultraviolet radiation.

flu·o·res·ce·in (floo·uh·res′ee·in) *n.* A fluorescent dye, the simplest of the fluorine dyes and the mother substance of eosin, commonly used intravenously to determine the state and adequacy of circulation in the retina, optic nerve head, and to a lesser degree, the choroid and iris and to detect corneal and conjunctival epithelial lesions. Peak excitation occurs with light at a wavelength between 485 and 500 millimicrons, and peak emission occurs between 520 and 530 millimicrons. From 50 to 84 percent of the dye is bound to albumin in the blood.

fluorescein funduscopy and angiography. Observation, and usually photography, of the vascular pattern of the fundus of the eye by special techniques following the injection into a peripheral vein of fluorescein; used in the diagnosis of vascular and neoplastic lesions of the eye and changes of the optic disk.

flu·o·res·cence (floo″uh·res′unce) *n.* A property possessed by certain substances of radiating, when illuminated, a light of a different, usually greater, wavelength. —**fluores·cent,** *adj.;* **flu·o·resce** (floo″uh·res′) *v.*

fluorescence microscope. A microscope equipped with a source of ultraviolet radiation for detection or examination of fluorescent specimens.

fluorescent stain method. 1. A staining method using a fluorescent dye, such as the method for demonstrating *Mycobacterium tuberculosis* in smears using auramine O, and a fluorescence microscope. 2. Fluorescein labeling of antibodies for identifying and localizing the antigens.

fluorescent treponemal-antibody absorption test. A serologic test for syphilis utilizing *Treponema pallidum* and fluorescein-tagged antibodies, more sensitive than and as specific as the *T. pallidum* immobilization test.

flu·o·ri·date (floo′ur·i·date) *v.* To add a fluoride compound to drinking water in such concentration that the incidence rate of caries will be diminished.

flu·o·ri·da·tion (floo″ur·i·day′shun) *n.* The addition of a fluoride to water, especially to the water supply of a community, as an aid in control of dental caries.

flu·o·ride (floo′ur·ide, ·id) *n.* A salt of hydrofluoric acid.

flu·o·ri·dize (floo′ur·i·dize) *v.* To use a fluoride, especially as a therapeutic measure for the prevention of dental caries. —**flu·o·ri·di·za·tion** (floo″ur·i·di·zay′shun) *n.*

flu·o·rine (floo′ur·een, ·in) *n.* F = 18.9984. A gaseous element belonging to the halogen group. Certain of its salts, the fluorides, have been used in the treatment of goiter and in rheumatism. Fluorides have been shown to prevent dental caries, but in excessive amounts in drinking water they may cause mottling of tooth enamel.

flu·o·rite (floo′ur·ite) *n.* Native calcium fluoride, CaF_2; used as a source of fluorine, as a flux, and in the manufacture of certain lenses.

flu·o·rog·ra·phy (floo″ur·og′ruh·fee) *n.* A combination of fluoroscopy and photography whereby a photograph of small size is made of the fluoroscopic image; used for making large numbers of chest examinations for tuberculosis surveys. —**fluo·ro·graph·ic** (·o·graf′ick) *adj.*

flu·o·ro·pho·tom·e·try (floo″ur·o·fo·tom′e·tree) *n.* The quantitative assay of fluorescent substances in solution. The exciting radiation is concentrated upon the substance under investigation, and the intensity of fluorescence is compared, either visually or photoelectrically, against the fluorescence of a standard solution. —**fluoropho·to·met′ric** (·to·met′rick) *adj.*

flu·o·ro·scope (floo′ur·uh·skope) *n.* An instrument used for examining the form and motion of the internal structures of the body by means of roentgen rays. It consists of a fluorescent screen composed of fluorescent crystals and excited by x-rays. —**flu·o·ro·scop·ic** (floo″ur·uh·skop′ick) *adj.*

flu·o·ros·co·py (floo″ur·os′kuh·pee) *n.* Examination of internal body structures by means of a fluoroscope.

flu·o·ro·sis (floo″ur·o′sis) *n.,* pl. **fluoro·ses** (·seez) 1. Poisoning by absorption of toxic amounts of fluorine. 2. A condition of generalized increased density of the skeleton, resulting from prolonged ingestion of fluorides. In endemic areas, this may lead to rigidity of the spinal column, increased bone fragility, and other symptoms referable to bone and joint changes.

flu·o·ro·ura·cil (floo″ur·o·yoo′ruh·sil) *n.* 5-Fluorouracil, $C_4H_3FN_2O_2$, an antineoplastic agent believed to function as an antimetabolite. Abbreviated, 5-FU.

Fluothane. Trademark for halothane, a general anesthetic.

flu·oxy·mes·ter·one (floo″ock-see-mes′tur-ohn) *n.* 9α-Fluoro-11β-hydroxy-17α-methyltestosterone, $C_{20}H_{29}FO_3$, an anabolic and androgenic steroid.

flur·az·e·pam (floo·raz′e-pam, ·ray′ze·) *n.* 7-Chloro-1-[2-(diethylamino)ethyl]-5-(o-fluorophenyl)-1,3-dihydro-2H-1,4-benzodiazepin-2-one, $C_{21}H_{23}ClFN_3O$, a hypnotic agent; used as the dihydrochloride salt.

Flury strain. A strain of rabies virus, used in the prophylactic immunization of dogs, that has been modified by prolonged cultivation in chick embryos.

flush, *n. & v.* 1. A sudden suffusion and reddening caused by cutaneous vasodilation, as of the face and neck; a blush. 2. A subjective transitory sensation of extreme heat; a hot flush. 3. A more or less persistent reddening of the face, as seen with fever, hyperthyroidism, certain drugs, or in emotional states. 4. To blush; to become suffused, as the cheeks, due to vasodilation of small arteries and arterioles. 5. To cleanse a wound or cavity by a rapid flow of water.

flut·ter, *n.* Quick, irregular motion; agitation; tremulousness.

flux, *n.* 1. An excessive flow of any of the excretions of the body, especially the feces. 2. The rate of flow or transfer of a liquid, particles, or energy across a unit area. 3. *In chemistry,* material added to minerals or metals to promote fusion.

fly, *n.* Any of numerous insects of the order Diptera, especially those that are relatively large or thick-bodied. In compound names, also applied to certain non-dipteran flying insects, as caddis fly, ichneumon fly.

foam, *n.* A heterogeneous mixture of a gaseous phase, or finely divided gas bubbles, suspended in a liquid. —**foamy** (fo′mee) *adj.*

foam cell. A cell containing lipids in small vacuoles, as seen in leprosy and xanthoma, often a histiocyte but may be some other cell, for example smooth muscle.

fo·cal, *adj.* 1. Of, pertaining to, or possessing a focus. 2. Limited to one area or part of an organ or of the body; localized.

focal embolic glomerulonephritis. The renal lesion seen in subacute bacterial endocarditis, of unknown cause, although allergic mechanisms, rather than embolization are thought responsible; the glomerular tufts are damaged and the kidney appears "flea-bitten." Infarcts may be present. Glomeruli show a lesion characteristic of focal glomerulonephritis. Deposits of IgG, IgM, and C3 within glomeruli have been described. Renal failure is uncommon.

focal epilepsy. Recurrent focal seizures.

focal infection. Infection in a limited area, such as the tonsils, teeth, sinuses, or prostate, to which remote clinical effects have been attributed, often erroneously.

focal length. For a thin lens, the image distance

of a point object on the lens axis at an infinite distance from the lens.

focal motor seizure. A focal seizure manifested by tonic or clonic movements in one part of the body, as in a hand, arm, face, or leg; may spread (Jacksonian march) to involve the rest of the body.

focal seizure. An epileptic manifestation of a restricted nature, usually without loss of consciousness, due to irritation of a localized area of the brain, often associated with organic lesions such as scar, inflammation, or tumor. May be manifested by the single motor, sensory, or sensorimotor component (Jacksonian convulsion), or may be psychomotor in type; the seizure may also spread to other regions of the brain and develop into a generalized convulsion with loss of consciousness.

focal status. Continuous focal seizures lasting in the order of an hour or more.

fo·cus (fo′kus) *n.,* pl. **focuses, fo·ci** (·sigh) 1. The principal seat of a disease. 2. The point at which rays of any radiant energy, such as light, heat, or sound converge. 3. Adjustment or the position of adjustment for clear, distinct vision. 4. *In cardiology,* the site or locus of a pacemaker.

fog·ging, *n.* 1. In repression treatment of esophoria, the reduction of vision to about 20/80 by combining prisms (varying with the muscular imbalance), bases in, with a convex sphere; the patient reads with these glasses for a half hour at night before retiring. 2. A method of refracting the eye by using a convex lens sufficiently strong to cause the eye to become artificially myopic and fog the vision. Astigmatism is then corrected by means of minus cylinders, after which the fog is removed by gradually reducing the convex lens. Generally used in adults or when cycloplegia might precipitate glaucoma. 3. The darkening of a radiograph due to any factor other than the intended radiation, caused by light, processing, or stray or scattered radiation.

fo·go sel·va·gem (fo′goo sel·vah′zhem, Pg. ·zheyⁿ) A severe endemic bullous disease found in certain lowland areas of Brazil, believed to be an attenuated tropical form of pemphigus foliaceus.

foil, *n.* A thin sheet of metal used in dentistry for restoration.

Foix syndrome Unilateral paralysis of all muscles innervated by the third, fourth and sixth cranial nerves and sensory defect in the distribution of the ophthalmic division of the fifth nerve; indicative of a lesion in the cavernous sinus and the region of the superior orbital fissure. Syn. *Tolosa-Hunt syndrome.*

fo·la·cin (fo′luh-sin) *n.* FOLIC ACID.

fo·late (fo′late) *n.* A salt of folic acid.

fold, *n.* A plication or doubling, as of various parts of the body.

Fo·ley catheter A balloon-tipped rubber catheter used in the urinary bladder.

folia. Plural of *folium.*

fo·li·a·ceous (fo″lee·ay′shus) *adj.* Leaflike.

fo·li·ate (fo′li·ate) *adj.* Shaped like a leaf.

fo·lic acid (fo′lick). Pteroylglutamic acid, or N-

{*p*-{[(2-amino-4-hydroxy-6-pteridinyl)methyl] amino} benzoyl} glutamic acid, $C_{19}H_{19}N_7O_6$, a substance occurring in green leaves, liver, and yeast, and also produced synthetically. It is essential for growth of *Lactobacillus casei.* It is effective in the treatment of various megaloblastic anemias and gastrointestinal malabsorption states. In pernicious anemia, it should be used only as an adjunct to treatment with cyanocobalamin or liver injection as it does not prevent or improve the spinal cord lesions.

fo·lie (foʰ·lee′) *n.* A mental disorder or psychosis; insanity.

folie à deux (aʰ dœh′) A type of communicated delusion involving two persons, one of whom suffers from an essential psychosis, and whose control of and influence over the other person is so potent that the latter will simulate or accept elements of the psychosis without question.

folie du doute (duᵉ doot′) A symptom of anxiety, as seen in anxiety neurosis or obsessive-compulsive neurosis, in which a person checks and rechecks an act, such as locking a door, doubting its having been properly done before, so that he may be unable to proceed beyond the act in question, or even to be able to make a simple decision.

Folin and Wu's method 1. A method for protein-free blood filtrate in which blood is laked and the proteins removed by precipitation with tungstic acid. 2. A method for nonprotein nitrogen in which the nitrogen in the blood filtrate is estimated by the Kjeldahl method; the ammonia formed is determined colorimetrically after direct nesslerization. 3. A method for reducing substances in blood in which the blood filtrate is heated with a copper solution and phosphomolybdic acid is added to form a blue color which is compared with a standard. 4. A method for total acidity in which 25 ml of a mixed 24-hour urine is titrated with O.1N sodium hydroxide using phenolphthalein for an indicator.

fo·lin·ic acid (fo·lin′ick). 1. Any of a group of factors occurring in liver extracts and also obtained from pteroylglutamic acid by synthesis; essential for growth of *Leuconostoc citrovorum.* 2. 5-Formyl-5,6,7,8-tetrahydrofolic acid, $C_{20}H_{23}N_7O_7$, the form in which folic acid exists and is active in tissues. It is identical with leucovorin and closely related, if not identical, to citrovorum factor. In the form of calcium leucovorin, it is used to counteract the toxic effects of folic acid antagonists and also in the treatment of megaloblastic anemias.

fo·li·um (fo′lee·um) *n.*, pl. **fo·lia** (·lee·uh) Any lamina or leaflet of gray matter, forming a part of the arbor vitae of the cerebellum.

fol·li·cle (fol′i·kul) *n.* 1. A lymph nodule. 2. A small secretory cavity or sac, as an acinus or alveolus. —**fol·lic·u·lar** (fol·ick′yoo·lur) *adj.*

follicle-stimulating hormone. An adenohypophyseal hormone which stimulates follicular growth in the ovary and spermatogenesis in the testis. Abbreviated, FSH.

follicular cell. One of the epithelial cells of the ovarian follicle exclusive of the ovum.

follicular conjunctivitis. Conjunctivitis characterized by discrete lymphoid follicles in the superficial conjunctival stroma, which often suggest a viral or chlamydial etiology.

follicular cyst. 1. A cyst due to retention of secretion in a follicular space, as in the ovary. 2. DENTIGEROUS CYST.

follicular hyperkeratosis. That form of hyperkeratosis occurring about the openings of the hair follicles.

follicular lymphoma. NODULAR LYMPHOMA.

follicular tonsillitis. A form of tonsillitis in which the crypts are involved and their contents project as white or yellow spots from the surface of the tonsil.

folliculi. Plural of *folliculus.*

fol·lic·u·li·tis (fol·ick″yoo·lye′tis) *n.* Inflammation of a follicle or group of follicles, usually hair follicles.

folliculitis de·cal·vans (de·kal′vanz). An inflammatory condition of hair follicles of the scalp that results in baldness.

fol·lic·u·loid (fol·ick′yoo·loid) *adj.* Resembling a follicle.

fol·lic·u·lo·ma (fol·ick″yoo·lo′muh) *n.*, pl. **folliculomas, folliculoma·ta** (·tuh) A granulosa cell tumor of the ovary.

fol·lic·u·lo·sis (fol·ick″yoo·lo′sis) *n.* An excess of lymph follicles caused by a disease process.

fol·li·cu·lus (fol·ick′yoo·lus) *n.*, pl. **follicu·li** (·lye) [NA]. FOLLICLE.

Follutein. Trademark for a preparation of chorionic gonadotropin obtained from the urine of pregnant women.

fo·men·ta·tion (fo″men·tay′shun) *n.* 1. The application of heat and moisture to a part to relieve pain or reduce inflammation. 2. The substance applied to a part to convey heat or moisture; a poultice.

fo·mes (fo′meez, fom′eez) *n.*, pl. **fomi·tes** (fom′i·teez, fo′mi·) FOMITE.

fo·mite (fo′mite) *n.* Any inanimate object which may be contaminated with infectious organisms and thus serve to transmit disease.

fon·ta·nel, fon·ta·nelle (fon″tuh·nel′) *n.* A membranous space between the cranial bones in fetal life and infancy.

fontanel sign. Constant bulging and tenseness of the anterior fontanel in infants observed in meningitis and other conditions where intracranial pressure is increased.

fon·ti·cu·lus (fon·tick′yoo·lus) *n.*, pl. **fonticu·li** (·lye) 1. JUGULAR NOTCH OF THE STERNUM. 2. A small artificial ulcer or issue. 3. [NA] FONTANEL.

food, *n.* Any organic substance which, when ingested or taken into the body of an organism through some alternate means and assimilated, may be used either to supply energy or to build tissue; classified in three groups: proteins, carbohydrates, and fats, all of which may occur in animal or vegetable substance.

Food and Drug Administration. An agency of the United States federal government responsible for ensuring that food, drugs, and cosmetics sold in the United States are safe, fulfill their stated functions, and are correctly labeled and packaged. Abbreviated, FDA.

food poisoning. 1. A type of poisoning due to food contaminated by bacterial toxins or by certain living bacteria, particularly those of the *Salmonella* group. 2. The symptoms due to foods naturally poisonous, such as certain fungi, or foods that contain allergens or toxic chemical residues.

foot, *n.* 1. The terminal extremity of the leg. Skeletally, it consists of the tarsus, metatarsus, and phalanges. 2. A measure of length equal to 12 inches, or 30.479 cm. Abbreviated, ft.

foot-and-mouth disease. A highly infectious and acute febrile viral disease producing a vesicular eruption of the mucous membranes of the nose and mouth and of the skin near the interdigital space of cloven-hoofed animals. It is contagious among domestic animals and is occasionally transmitted to man. Syn. *aphthous fever, epidemic stomatitis, epizootic stomatitis.*

foot-candle, *n.* The illumination received at a surface one foot from a standard source of one candela.

foot drop, foot-drop. DROPPED FOOT.

foot·ling presentation. Presentation of the fetus with the feet foremost.

foot plate. The flat part of the stapes.

foot-pound, *n.* The work performed when a constant force of one pound is exerted on a body which moves a distance of one foot in the same direction as the force.

foot-print, *n.* An ink impression of the sole of the foot; used for identification of infants and in the study of dermatoglyphics.

foot process. One of the cytoplasmic processes by which the visceral epithelial cells of a glomerular capsule of the kidney attach to the glomerular basement membrane.

fo·ra·men (fo-ray′mun) *n.,* genit. **fo·ra·mi·nis** (fo-ram′i·nis, fo-ray′mi·nis), pl. **forami·na, fora·mens** A perforation or opening, especially in a bone.

foramen ce·cum (see′kum). A blind foramen, specifically: 1. (of the frontal bone:) A small pit or channel located between the frontal crest and the crista galli. When it is a channel it may transmit an emissary vein. 2. (of the medulla oblongata:) a small pit at the rostral termination of the anterior median fissure of the medulla oblongata. 3. (of the tongue:) a small pit located in the posterior termination of the median raphe of the tongue; the site of the thyroglossal duct.

foramen eth·moi·da·le an·te·ri·us (eth-moy·day′lee an·teer′ee·us) [NA]. ANTERIOR ETHMOID FORAMEN.

foramen in·ter·ven·tri·cu·la·re (in″tur·ven·trick′yoo·lair′ee) [NA]. INTERVENTRICULAR FORAMEN.

foramen ju·gu·la·re (jug·yoo·lair′ee) [NA]. JUGULAR FORAMEN.

foramen la·ce·rum (las′e·rum) [NA]. An irregular aperture in the cranium between the apex of the petrous portion of the temporal bone and the body and great wing of the sphenoid, and the basilar process of the occipital bone.

The internal carotid artery with its venous and sympathetic plexuses ascends through the upper end of the foramen.

foramen mag·num (mag′num) [NA]. A large oval aperture centrally placed in the lower and anterior part of the occipital bone; it gives passage to the spinal cord and its membranes and venous plexuses, the spinal accessory nerves, and the vertebral arteries.

foramen man·di·bu·lae (man·dib′yoo·lee) [NA]. MANDIBULAR FORAMEN.

foramen mas·toi·de·um (mas·toy′dee·um) [NA]. MASTOID FORAMEN.

foramen of Lusch·ka (loosh′kah) LATERAL APERTURE OF THE FOURTH VENTRICLE.

foramen of Ma·gen·die (ma·zhahⁿ·dee′) MEDIAN APERTURE OF THE FOURTH VENTRICLE.

foramen of Mon·ro INTERVENTRICULAR FORAMEN.

foramen of Wins·low EPIPLOIC FORAMEN.

foramen op·ti·cum (op′ti·kum) [BNA]. CANALIS OPTICUS.

foramen ova·le (o·vay′lee). 1. FORAMEN OVALE OF THE HEART. 2. FORAMEN OVALE OF THE SPHENOID.

foramen ovale of the heart. A fetal opening between the two atria of the heart, situated at the lower posterior portion of the septum secundum. Through this opening, blood is shunted from the right atrium to the left atrium.

foramen ovale of the sphenoid. An oval opening near the posterior margin of the great wing of the sphenoid, giving passage to the mandibular branch of the trigeminal nerve, the accessory meningeal artery, and occasionally the lesser petrosal nerve.

foramen pa·la·ti·num ma·jus (pal·uh·tye′num may′jus) [NA]. GREATER PALATINE FORAMEN.

foramen pri·mum (prye′mum). The temporary interatrial opening bounded by the growing margins of the septum primum and the endocardial cushions.

foramen ro·tun·dum (ro·tun′dum) [NA]. A round opening in the great wing of the sphenoid bone of the maxillary division of the trigeminal nerve.

foramen se·cun·dum (se·kun′dum). The secondary opening in the septum primum due to thinning and perforation of its cranial portion.

foramen spi·no·sum (spye·no′sum) [NA]. A passage in the great wing of the sphenoid bone, near its posterior angle, giving passage to the middle meningeal artery and spinosal nerve.

foramen ver·te·bra·le (vur·te·bray′lee) [NA]. VERTEBRAL FORAMEN.

foramina. Plural of *foramen.*

fo·ram·i·nal (fo·ram′i·nul) *adj.* Of or pertaining to a foramen.

foraminal hernia. A false hernia of a loop of bowel through the epiploic foramen.

fo·ram·i·not·o·my (fo·ram″i·not′uh·mee) *n.* Surgical removal of a portion of an intervertebral foramen.

force, *n. & v.* 1. That which initiates, changes, or arrests motion or results in acceleration of movement of a body. 2. To cause to change or move against resistance.

forced feeding or **alimentation.** 1. The administration of food to a resistant individual, especially feeding through a nasogastric or gastric tube. 2. The administration of food in excess of the amount required by the patient's appetite.

forced movement. 1. PASSIVE MOVEMENT. 2. Involuntary movement as a result of injury or exogenous stimulation of the motor centers or the conducting pathways of the nervous system.

forced respiration. Respiration induced by blowing air into the lungs by means of a pump or respirator, or in some other way, as in physiologic experiments or during artificial respiration.

for·ceps (for'seps) n. 1. A surgical instrument with two opposing blades or limbs; controlled by handles or by direct pressure on the blades. Used to grasp, compress, and hold tissue, a part of the body, needles, or other surgical material. 2. Fiber bundles in the brain resembling forceps.

Forch·heimer's sign A maculopapular, rose-red eruption on the soft palate, seen in early rubella before the skin rash appears.

for·ci·pres·sure (for'si·presh'ur) n. Pressure exerted on a blood vessel by means of a forceps, to prevent hemorrhage.

fore-. Combining form meaning (a) *before, preceding;* (b) *in front, anterior;* (c) *the front* (as of a part of structure).

fore·arm, n. The part of the upper extremity between the wrist and the elbow.

fore·brain, n. PROSENCEPHALON.

fore·con·scious, n. & adj. 1. The portion of the unconscious containing mental experiences that are not in the focus of immediate attention, but which may be recalled to consciousness. 2. Capable of being recalled into the conscious mind, although not in the realm of consciousness.

fore·fin·ger, n. INDEX FINGER.

fore·foot, n. 1. The anterior part of the foot; from a clinical standpoint, the portion of the foot that includes the toes and the metatarsal, cuneiform, and cuboid bones. 2. Of a quadruped: the foot of the foreleg.

fore·gut, n. The cephalic part of the embryonic digestive tube that develops into pharynx, esophagus, stomach, part of the small intestine, liver, pancreas, and respiratory ducts.

fore·head, n. The part of the face above the eyes.

for·eign, adj. 1. Derived from other than self, as in tissue transplantation or antigens. 2. Not belonging in the location where found.

foreign body. A substance occurring in any organ or tissue where it is not normally found, especially a substance of extrinsic origin.

foreign-body giant cell. A large cell derived from macrophages, with multiple nuclei and abundant cytoplasm which may contain foreign material; found in granulomatous inflammation in response to foreign bodies.

foreign-body reaction. An inflammation around a foreign body in a tissue or organ. Syn. *perialienitis, perixenitis.*

foreign protein. A protein that differs from the proteins of the animal or person into whom it is introduced.

fore-milk, n. 1. The milk first withdrawn at each milking. 2. COLOSTRUM.

fo·ren·sic (fo·ren'sik) adj. 1. Pertaining or belonging to a court of law. 2. Pertaining to use in legal proceedings or in public discussions.

forensic psychiatry. The branch of psychiatry concerned with the legal aspects of mental disorders.

fore·play, n. The fondling of erotogenic zones which usually precedes sexual intercourse and may lead to orgasm; contrectation.

fore·pleas·ure, n. The erotic pleasure, both physical and emotional, accompanied by a rise in tension, which precedes the culmination of the sexual act, or end pleasure.

fore·skin, n. PREPUCE.

fore·wa·ters, n. HYDRORRHEA GRAVIDARUM.

-form, -iform. A combining form meaning *having the form of, -shaped, resembling.*

form·al·de·hyde (for·mal'de·hide) n. Formic aldehyde or methanal, HCHO, a colorless gas obtained by the oxidation of methyl alcohol. It is a powerful disinfectant, generally used in aqueous solution; employed also as a reagent.

formaldehyde solution. An aqueous solution containing not less than 37% by weight of formaldehyde. It is a powerful antiseptic. By means of oxidizing agents or heat, it may be converted into a gas, a procedure that has been used for disinfection of rooms and dwellings previously exposed to contagion.

for·ma·lin. 1. FORMALDEHYDE SOLUTION. 2. A 4% aqueous solution of formaldehyde; the most common histologic fixative.

form·am·ide (form·am'ide, ·am'id, for'muh·mide") n. 1. HCONH₂, the amide of formic acid. 2. A compound containing the HCONH — radical.

for·mate (for'mate) n. A salt of formic acid.

for·ma·tion (for·may'shun) n. 1. The process of developing shape or structure. 2. That which is formed; a structure or arrangement.

for·ma·tive (for'muh·tiv) adj. 1. Pertaining to the process of development, as of tissue or of the embryo. 2. Forming, producing, creating.

form·a·zan (form'uh·zan) n. A generic name for a deeply colored pigment obtained by reducing 2,3,5-triphenyltetrazolium chloride or certain other related tetrazolium salts by highly labile enzyme systems. The reaction is utilized in testing the ability of seeds to germinate and the function of granulocytes.

forme fruste (form froost, F. frue⁵t) An incomplete, abortive, or atypical form or manifestation of a syndrome or disease.

for·mic (for'mick) adj. 1. Of or pertaining to ants. 2. Pertaining to or derived from formic acid.

formic acid. 1. The anhydrous liquid HCOOH; a strong reducing agent, dangerously caustic to the skin. Syn. *methanoic acid.* 2. An aqueous solution containing about 25% HCOOH; it is counterirritant and astringent.

for·mi·cant (for'mi·kunt) adj. Producing a tactile sensation like the crawling of small insects.

for·mi·ca·tion (for"mi·kay'shun) n. An abnormal sensation as of insects crawling in or upon the skin; a common symptom in diseases of the spinal cord and the peripheral nerves; a form of paresthesia; may be a hallucination.

for·mim·i·no·glu·tam·ic acid (for·mim″i·no·gloo·tam′ick). Glutamic acid in which an amino hydrogen is replaced by a formimino (—CH =NH) group. An intermediate in the metabolic conversion of histidine to glutamic acid, it is also involved in the metabolism of tetrahydrofolic acid.

for·mim·i·no·glu·tam·ic·ac·i·du·ria (for·mim″i·no·gloo·tam″ick·as″i·dew′ree·uh) n. An inborn error of amino acid metabolism of which there are two types: type A characterized biochemically by a deficiency of formiminotransferase and increased formiminoglutamic acid excretion in urine after a histidine load, and clinically by physical and mental retardation, obesity, and hypersegmentation of polymorphonuclear cells; and type B characterized biochemically by increased formiminoglutamic acid excretion both before and after histidine load, and probably a defect in folic acid transport, and clinically by mental retardation, ataxia, convulsions, and megaloblastic anemia.

for·mu·la (for′mew·luh) n., pl. **formulas, formulae** (·lee) 1. A prescribed method. 2. The representation of a chemical compound by symbols. 3. A recipe or prescription. Abbreviated, F.

for·mu·lary (for′mew·lerr″ee) n. A collection of formulas for making medicinal preparations.

Formvar. A trademark for plastic film used to coat grids to support tissue sections for examination in electron microscopy.

for·myl (for′mil) n. HCO—, the radical of formic acid.

for·ni·cal (for′ni·kul) adj. Of or pertaining to a fornix.

for·ni·cate (for′ni·kut, ·kate) adj. Arched or vaulted.

for·ni·ca·tion (for″ni·kay′shun) n. Legally, coitus between unmarried persons. —**for·ni·cate** (for′ni·kate) v.

for·nix (for′nicks) n., genit. **for·ni·cis** (for′ni·sis), pl. **for·ni·ces** (·seez) An arched body or surface; a concavity or cul-de-sac.

fornix ce·re·bri (serr′e·brye) [NA]. An arched fiber tract lying under the corpus callosum; anteriorly it divides into two columns, projecting mainly to the mamillary bodies; posteriorly it divides into two crura, projecting mainly to the hippocampus on each side.

fornix of the conjunctiva. The cul-de-sac at the line where the bulbar conjunctiva is reflected upon the lid.

fornix of the vagina. The vault of the vagina; the upper part of the vagina which surrounds the cervix of the uterus. May be divided into anterior, posterior, and lateral in relation to the cervix.

Forss·man antigens (fors′mahn) A widely distributed group of heterophil antigens that are thermostable and carbohydrate lipoprotein complex in structure; found in sheep red blood cells, in the tissue of many animals, in bacteria, and in plant cells, but absent in some

species, as the rabbit; and detectable by the induction of antibodies reacting with sheep red blood cells by antigens from genetically unrelated species.

for·ward failure. Left heart failure in which symptoms result predominantly from low cardiac output; there is weakness and fatigue.

Fo·shay's test A delayed skin test for the diagnosis of tularemia made by the intradermal injection of a killed suspension of *Francisella tularensis*. A local erythema is considered a positive reaction.

fossa ace·ta·bu·li (as·e·tab′yoo·lye) [NA]. ACETABULAR FOSSA.

fossa axil·la·ris (ack·si·lair′is) [NA]. Axillary fossa; AXILLA.

fossa cra·nii anterior (kray′nee·eye) [NA]. ANTERIOR CRANIAL FOSSA.

fossa cranii me·dia (mee′dee·uh) [NA]. MIDDLE CRANIAL FOSSA.

fossa cranii posterior [NA]. POSTERIOR CRANIAL FOSSA.

fossa di·gas·tri·ca (dye·gas′tri·kuh) [NA]. DIGASTRIC FOSSA (1).

fossa is·chio·rec·ta·lis (is″kee·o·reck·tay′lis) [NA]. ISCHIORECTAL FOSSA.

fossa la·te·ra·lis ce·re·bri (lat·e·ray′lis serr′e·brye) [NA]. A depression on the lateral aspect of the cerebral hemisphere of the fetus; in the adult brain a portion remains as the lateral sulcus.

fossa na·vi·cu·la·ris ure·thrae (na·vick″yoo·lair′is yoo·ree′three) [NA]. NAVICULAR FOSSA (2).

fossa ova·lis (o·vay′lis). 1. An oval depression in the interatrial septum; its floor is derived from the embryonic septum primum, and its rim (limbus) from the septum secundum. 2. An opening in the fascia lata of the thigh which gives passage to the great saphenous vein.

fos·sette (fos·et′) n. 1. A dimple; a small depression. 2. A small, deep ulcer of the cornea.

fossil wax. CERESIN.

fos·su·la (fos′yoo·luh) n., pl. **fossu·lae** (·lee) A small fossa.

Fos·ter Ken·ne·dy syndrome Unilateral blindness and optic atrophy, contralateral papilledema, and sometimes anosmia, usually due to a frontal lobe or sphenoid crest tumor or abscess on the side of the atrophy.

Fou·chet's reagent (foo·sheh′) A solution of trichloracetic acid and ferric chloride, used in urine bilirubin testing.

foun·der, n. & v. 1. An acute gastroenteritis in cattle, horses, and sheep caused by the overeating of foods with a high caloric content. 2. Lameness in horses, especially that caused by laminitis. 3. To be afflicted with such lameness.

found·ling, n. An infant found after being abandoned by its parents.

four·chette, four·chet (foor·shet′) n. 1. A fold of skin just inside the posterior commissure of the vulva. 2. A fork used in dividing the frenulum of the tongue.

fourth disease. EXANTHEM SUBITUM.

fourth heart sound. The heart sound following atrial contraction, immediately preceding the first heart sound, to which it may sometimes contribute. Symbol, S_4, or SIV. Syn. *presystolic extra sound.*

fourth venereal disease. LYMPHOGRANULOMA VENEREUM.

fourth ventricle. The cavity that overlies the pons and medulla and extends from the central canal of the upper cervical spinal cord to the aqueduct of the midbrain. Its roof is the cerebellum and the superior and inferior medullary vela and its floor is the rhomboid fossa.

fo·vea (fo'vee·uh) *n.*, pl. **fo·ve·ae** (·vee·ee) 1. A small pit or depression. 2. *In ophthalmology.* FOVEA CENTRALIS.

fovea cen·tra·lis (sen·tray'lis) [NA]. The small depression, measuring approximately 1.85 mm in diameter with a floor of 0.4 mm in the center of the macula lutea of the retina. Its center is 4.0 mm temporal and 0.8 mm inferior to the center of the optic disk.

fo·ve·al (fo'vee·ul) *adj.* 1. Pertaining to a fovea, especially the fovea centralis. 2. Like a fovea; pitted.

foveal reflex. FOVEOLAR REFLEX.

fo·ve·o·la (fo·vee'o·luh) *n.*, pl. **foveo·lae** (·lee), **foveolas** 1. A small fovea or depression. 2. The basal part of the fovea centralis of the retina, containing closely packed, elongated cones.

fo·ve·o·lar (fo·vee'uh·lur) *adj.* Of or pertaining to a foveola.

foveolar reflex. The bright reflection of light seen with the ophthalmoscope when it is directed upon the fovea. Syn. *foveal reflex.*

Fowl·er's position A semireclining or sitting position in bed, formerly used in the treatment of peritonitis.

Fowler's solution Potassium arsenite solution, containing the equivalent of 1% of As_2O_3; formerly frequently employed as a dosage form of arsenic and more recently employed as an antileukemic drug.

fowl plague or **pest.** An acute septicemic disease of chickens, turkeys, and other avian species caused by one of the highly pathogenic myxoviruses of the avian influenza group and characterized by edema of the head, hemorrhage, and focal necrosis of various organs.

fowl pox. AVIAN POX in chickens and turkeys.

fowl typhoid. An infectious disease of domesticated birds, caused by *Salmonella gallinarum.*

fox·glove, *n.* DIGITALIS.

frac·tion·al (frack'shun·ul) *adj.* 1. Pertaining to a fraction. 2. *In chemistry,* divided successively; applied to any one of the several processes for separating a mixture into its constituents through differences in solubility, boiling point, or other characteristic.

frac·tion·a·tion (frack"shun·ay'shun) *n.* 1. *In chemistry,* the separation of a mixture into its constituents, as in fractional distillation. 2. *In microbiology,* the process of obtaining a pure culture by successive culturing of small portions of a colony. Syn. *fractional cultivation.* 3. *In physiology,* the phenomenon whereby maximal stimulation of a given efferent nerve innervating a limb does not evoke as powerful a muscular contraction as direct stimulation of the muscles themselves. Thus the fractiona-

tion phenomenon occurs within the motor neuron pool of the spinal cord. —**frac·tion·ate** (frack'shun·ate) *v. & adj.*

frac·ture (frack'chur) *n. & v.* 1. A break in a bone, cartilage, tooth, or solid organ, such as the spleen, usually caused by trauma.

fracture dislocation. A dislocation accompanied by a fracture.

fragilitas os·si·um (os'ee·um). OSTEOGENESIS IMPERFECTA.

fra·gil·i·ty (fra·jil'i·tee) *n.* The quality of being easily broken or destroyed. —**frag·ile** (fraj'il) *adj.*

fragility test. 1. A test of osmotic fragility of erythrocytes. 2. A test of integrity of blood capillaries.

frag·men·ta·tion (frag"men·tay'shun) *n.* 1. Division into small portions. 2. AMITOSIS.

fram·be·sia, fram·boe·sia (fram·bee'zhuh, ·zee·uh) *n.* YAWS.

Fran·ci·sel·la (fran"si·sel'uh) *n.* The genus of pleomorphic, nutritionally fastidious, cytotropic gram-negative rods, belonging to the family Brucellaceae, of which the type species is *Francisella tularensis.*

Francisella tu·la·ren·sis (too"luh·ren'sis). The causative organism of tularemia in wild mammals, birds, and insects, transmissible to man. Formerly designated *Pasteurella tularensis.*

fran·ci·um (fran'see·um) *n.* Fr = 223. Element number 87.

fran·gu·la (frang'gew·luh) *n.* The bark of *Rhamnus frangula,* or glossy buckthorn. The fresh bark is strongly irritant and causes violent catharsis; when dried it is laxative.

fran·gu·lin (frang'gew·lin) *n.* 4,5,7-Trihydroxy-2-methylanthraquinone-L-rhamnoside, $C_{21}H_{20}O_9$, a glycoside occurring in *Rhamnus* species. On hydrolysis it yields emodin and L-rhamnose.

frank breech presentation. A breech presentation of the fetus with the buttocks alone presenting at the cervix with the hips flexed and the knees extended along the body so that the feet are near the head.

frank·in·cense (frank'in·sense) *n.* An aromatic gum resin.

Frank-Star·ling law of the heart (fra^nk) The force developed by cardiac contraction is proportional to the length of the myocardial fibers in diastole.

fra·ter·nal (fra·tur'nul) *adj.* 1. Of or pertaining to brothers or siblings. 2. Of twins, not identical.

fraternal twins. Twins resulting from the simultaneous fertilization of two ova. They may be of the same or opposite sex, have a different genetic constitution, and each has a separate chorion. Syn. *biovular twins, dizygotic twins.*

frat·ri·cide (frat'ri·side) *n.* 1. Murder of one's own sibling. 2. One who murders one's own sibling.

F.R.C.P. Fellow of the Royal College of Physicians.

F.R.C.P.E. Fellow of the Royal College of Physicians of Edinburgh.

F.R.C.P.I. Fellow of the Royal College of Physicians of Ireland.

F.R.C.S. Fellow of the Royal College of Surgeons.

F.R.C.S.E. Fellow of the Royal College of Surgeons of Edinburgh.

F.R.C.S.I. Fellow of the Royal College of Surgeons of Ireland.

freak, *n.* 1. *In medicine,* any organism that varies markedly, especially in its physical aspects, from the organisms of its kind or species; a mutation; a monster. 2. Any odd, startling, or unexpected phenomenon, idea, or event.

freck·le, *n.* A pigmented macule resulting from focal increase of melanin, usually associated with exposure to sunlight, commonly on the face. Syn. *ephelis.*

Fre·det-Ram·stedt operation (fruh·deh′, rahm′ shtet) PYLOROMYOTOMY.

free association. Spontaneous consciously unrestricted association of ideas or mental images, used to gain an understanding of the organization of the content of the mind in psychoanalysis.

free-floating anxiety. *In psychiatry,* severe, generalized, persistent anxiety which often precedes panic.

free graft. A graft of any type of tissue which is cut free and transplanted to another area.

free macrophage. An actively ameboid macrophage found in the normal connective tissues and in areas of inflammation.

free-mar·tin (free′mahr′tin) *n.* An intersexual, usually sterile female calf twinborn with a male; produced by masculinization by sex hormones of the male twin when the placental circulations are partially fused.

free radical. A nonionic compound, highly reactive and of relatively short life, in which the central element is linked to an abnormal number of atoms or groups of atoms, and characterized by the presence of at least one unpaired electron.

freezing microtome. A microtome used for cutting frozen tissue, sometimes equipped with a cooling device for the knife or a cold chamber to encase the microtome.

Frei test An intracutaneous test for immunologic changes resulting from infection with the virus of lymphogranuloma venereum, performed by injecting material processed from bubo pus or from infected mouse brain or chick embryo.

frem·i·tus (frem′i·tus) *n.* A palpable vibration or thrill.

fre·nec·to·my (fre·neck′tuh·mee) *n. In surgery,* removal of a frenum.

fre·not·o·my (fre·not′uh·mee) *n.* The cutting of any frenum, particularly of the frenulum of the tongue for tongue-tie.

Frenquel. Trademark for azocyclonol, a drug used as the hydrochloride salt for control of psychotic symptoms.

fren·u·lum, frae·nu·lum (fren′yoo·lum, freen′) *n.,* pl. **frenu·la, fraenu·la** (·luh) A small frenum; any small fold of mucous membrane or tissue that restrains a structure or part.

frenulum cli·to·ri·dis (kli·tor′i·dis) [NA]. FRENULUM OF THE CLITORIS.

frenulum la·bii in·fe·ri·o·ris (lay′bee·eye in·feer·ee·o′ris) [NA]. A fold of mucous membrane on the inside of the median portion of the lower lip attached to the gingiva.

frenulum lin·guae (ling′gwee) [NA]. FRENULUM OF THE TONGUE.

frenulum of the clitoris. Either of two folds of skin coming from the labia minora and being united under the glans of the clitoris.

frenulum of the prepuce. The fold on the lower surface of the glans penis connecting it with the prepuce.

frenulum of the tongue. The vertical fold of mucous membrane under the tongue.

fre·num, frae·num (free′num) *n.,* pl. **frenums, fraenums, fre·na, frae·na** (·nuh) A fold of integument or mucous membrane that checks or limits the movements of any organ.

fren·zy, *n.* 1. Violent temporary mental derangement; the manic phase of manic-depressive illness. 2. Delirious excitement.

Freon. Trademark for a group of halogenated hydrocarbons containing one or more fluorine atoms; widely used as refrigerants and propellants for the dispersion of insecticidal mists.

fre·quen·cy, *n.* 1. The rate of occurrence of a periodic or cyclic process. 2. *In biometry,* the ratio of the number of observations falling within a classification group to the total number of observations made.

frequency distribution. *In biometry,* a statistical table showing the frequency, or number, of observations (as test scores, ages) falling in each of certain classification groups or intervals (as 10–19, 20–29).

Freud·i·an (froy′dee·un) *adj. & n.* 1. Pertaining to Freud, his psychoanalytic theories and methods. 2. A person, often a psychiatrist, who adheres to the basic tenets of Freud's theories and methods.

Freud·i·an·ism (froy′dee·un·iz·um) *n.* The psychoanalytic theories and psychotherapeutic methods developed by Freud and his followers.

Freund's adjuvant (froind) An immunological adjuvant consisting of an emulsion of water in oil, and described as incomplete or complete depending on whether it is mixed with antigen only or with antigen and a killed microorganism (usually *Mycobacterium tuberculosis*).

F.R.F.P.S. Fellow of the Royal Faculty of Physicians and Surgeons.

F.R.F.P.S.G. Fellow of the Royal Faculty of Physicians and Surgeons of Glasgow.

fri·a·ble (frye′uh·bul) *adj.* Easily broken or crumbled.

fric·tion (frick′shun) *n.* 1. The act of rubbing, as the rubbing of the body for stimulation of the skin. 2. The resistance offered to motion between two contacting bodies. —**friction·al** (·ul) *adj.*

friction fremitus. The vibrations produced by the rubbing together of two dry and often inflamed surfaces.

friction rub, murmur, or **sound.** The sounds heard on auscultation produced by the rubbing of two dry or roughened surfaces, such as inflamed serous surfaces, upon each other.

Fried·län·der cells (freet′len·dur) The large clear

connective-tissue cells of the uterine decidua.

Friedländer pneumonia Pneumonia caused by *Klebsiella pneumoniae.*

Friedländer's bacillus KLEBSIELLA PNEUMONIAE.

Fried·man test A pregnancy test in which a female rabbit is given an intravenous injection of urine from the patient. Formation of corpora hemorrhagica and corpora lutea in the ovaries indicates a positive test.

Fried·reich's ataxia (freed'rye*^k*h) A hereditary spinocerebellar degenerative disease beginning in childhood and characterized by ataxia, diminished or absent deep tendon reflexes, Babinski signs, dysarthria, nystagmus, scoliosis, and clubfoot. There is degeneration of lateral and posterior columns of the spinal cord and to a variable extent in the cerebellum and medulla.

fri·gid·i·ty (fri-jid'i-tee) *n.* Lack of libido or interest in sex, usually of psychic origin.

Froeh·lich's syndrome (frœh'lik*h*) ADIPOSOGENITAL DYSTROPHY.

frog, *n.* 1. Any of various tailless, smooth-skinned, web-footed amphibians, primarily of the family Ranidae. 2. An elastic, horny pad, in the middle of the sole of a horse's hoof; it is triangular in shape and serves to separate the two bars.

frog face. A facial deformity due to growth of polyps or other tumors in the nasal cavities. A temporary condition of this kind may be due to orbital cellulitis or facial erysipelas.

frog position or **posture.** An attitude frequently assumed by premature infants and infants with various central nervous system diseases, especially those resulting in flaccid paralysis, in which the lower extremities are kept flexed and externally rotated at the hips and flexed at the knees.

frog test. A pregnancy test in which urine containing chorionic gonadotropin is injected into the dorsal lymph sac of the male leopard frog (*Rana pipiens*). If spermatozoa are demonstrable in the frog's urine within 3 hours after injection, the test is positive.

Froin's syndrome A sign of spinal subarachnoid block in which the cerebrospinal fluid below the lesion shows xanthochromia, few or no cells, hyperglobulinemia, and spontaneous clotting.

frôle·ment (frole"mahn') *n.* 1. A succession of slow, brushing movements in massage, done with the palmar surfaces of the hand. 2. A rustling sound sometimes heard on auscultation in pericardial disease.

fron·tal (frun'tul) *adj.* 1. In humans, pertaining to the anterior part or aspect of an organ or body. 2. Pertaining to the forehead.

frontal bone. A large cranial bone including the squama-frontalis, the superciliary arches, the glabella, and part of the roofs of the orbital and nasal cavities.

frontal gyrectomy. Surgical excision of a block of cortex, bilaterally, from the frontal lobes of the brain, formerly used as a treatment for certain mental illnesses.

fron·ta·lis (frun-tah'lis, fron-tay'lis) *n.* The frontal portion of the epicranius.

frontal lobe. The part of the cerebral hemisphere in front of the central sulcus and above the lateral cerebral sulcus.

frontal plane. 1. Any plane parallel with the long axis of the body and perpendicular to the sagittal plane, dividing the body of bipeds into front and back parts. 2. The plane of the limb leads in electrocardiography. 3. The plane defined by combining the Y, or vertical, lead with the X, or horizontal, lead in vectorcardiography.

frontal region. The area or surface of the forehead.

frontal sinus. The paranasal sinus situated in the frontal bone.

frontal suture. A suture which at birth joins the two frontal bones from the vertex to the root of the nose, but which afterward becomes obliterated.

fronto-. A combining form meaning (a) *frontal;* (b) *forehead.*

fron·to·eth·moid (frun"to-eth'moid) *adj.* Pertaining to the frontal and ethmoid bones.

fron·to·lac·ri·mal (frun"to-lack'ri-mul) *adj.* Of or pertaining to the frontal bone and lacrimal bones.

fron·to·ma·lar (frun"to-may'lur) *adj.* Pertaining to the frontal and zygomatic bones.

fron·to·max·il·lary (frun"to-mack'si-lerr"ee) *adj.* Pertaining to the frontal bone and the maxilla.

fron·to·men·tal (frun"to-men'tul) *adj.* 1. Running from the top of the forehead to the point of the chin. 2. Pertaining to the forehead and chin.

fron·to·na·sal (frun"to-nay'zul) *adj.* Pertaining to the frontal and nasal bones.

fron·to·oc·cip·i·tal (frun"to-ock-sip'i-tul) *adj.* OCCIPITOFRONTAL.

fron·to·pa·ri·e·tal (frun"to-pa-rye'e-tul) *adj.* PARIETOFRONTAL.

fron·to·pon·tine (frun"to-pon'tine, -teen) *adj.* Pertaining to the frontal lobe of the cerebrum and the pons.

fron·to·pon·to·cer·e·bel·lar (frun"to-pon"to-serr"e-bel'ur) *adj.* Pertaining to the frontal lobe, the pons, and the cerebellum.

fron·to·sphe·noid (frun"to-sfee'noid) *adj.* Pertaining to the frontal and sphenoid bones.

fron·to·tem·po·ral (frun"to-tem'pur-ul) *adj.* Pertaining to the frontal and temporal bones.

fron·to·zy·go·mat·ic (frun"to-zye-go-mat'ick) *adj.* Pertaining to the frontal and zygomatic bones.

frost·bite, *n.* Injury to skin and subcutaneous tissues, and in severe cases to deeper structures also, from exposure to extreme cold; blood vessel damage and cessation of local circulation lead to edema, vesiculation, and tissue necrosis.

frot·tage (frot-ahzh') *n.* 1. Massage, rubbing. 2. A form of masturbation in which orgasm is induced by rubbing against someone, especially in a crowd.

frot·teur (frot-ur') *n.* One who practices frottage to achieve sexual gratification.

frozen section. 1. A histologic section cut from frozen tissues or organs to permit rapid microscopic study. 2. In the teaching of gross anatomy, one of a series of divisions of the body or part which has been frozen before being sectioned.

frozen shoulder. A chronic tenosynovitis of unknown cause, associated with increased vascularity, degeneration, and fibrosis of collagen fibers in and about the shoulder joint, and characterized by pain and limitation of motion.

F.R.S. Fellow of the Royal Society.

F.R.S.E. Fellow of the Royal Society of Edinburgh.

fruc·to·fu·ra·nose (fruck″to-few′ruh-noce) n. A fructose with a 2, 5-butylene oxide or furanose ring.

fruc·to·fu·ran·o·side (fruck″to-few-ran′o-side) n. A glycoside of fructofuranose.

fruc·to·ki·nase (fruck″to-kigh′nace, -naze) n. An enzyme catalyzing transfer of phosphate from a donor to fructose, forming fructose 1-phosphate.

fruc·to·py·ra·nose (fruck″to-pye′ruh-noce) n. A fructose with a 2, 6-pyranose ring.

fruc·tose (fruck′toce, frook′toce) n. L. A monosaccharide, $C_6H_{12}O_6$, occurring as such in many fruits and obtainable also by hydrolysis of sucrose and inulin; a white, crystalline powder, freely soluble in water, at least as sweet as sucrose; used for parenteral alimentation. Syn. *fruit sugar, levulose.*

fructose intolerance. A hereditary disease characterized by vomiting, sweating, and aversion to fructose-containing foods.

fruc·to·side (fruck′to-side) n. A glycoside that yields fructose on hydrolysis.

fruc·tos·uria (fruck″to-syoo′ree-uh) n. The presence of fructose in the urine. Syn. *levulosuria.*

fru·giv·o·rous (froo-jiv′uh-rus) adj. Fruit-eating.

fruit, n. The developed ovary of a plant, including the succulent, fleshy parts gathered about it.

fruit sugar. FRUCTOSE.

fru·men·tum (froo-men′tum) n. Wheat or other grain.

frus·tra·tion (frus-tray′shun) n. 1. The condition that results when an impulse to act or the completion of an act is blocked or thwarted, preventing the satisfaction of attainment. 2. The blocking or thwarting of an impulse, purpose, or action. —**frus·trate** (frus′trate) v.

Frutabs. A trademark for fructose.

FSH Abbreviation for *follicle-stimulating hormone.*

ft Abbreviation for (a) in pharmacy, *fiat* or *fiant;* let there be made; (b) *foot.*

ft-lb Abbreviation for *foot-pound.*

5-FU FLUOROURACIL.

Fuadin. Trademark for stibophen, an organic antimonial employed in the treatment of granuloma inguinale and of schistosomiasis.

Fuchs' dystrophy (fooks) A familial degenerative condition of the eye, beginning in late middle life and affecting more women than men, progressing from cornea guttata to edema of the epithelium with clouding of the corneal stroma and impaired corneal sensitivity to subepithelial connective-tissue formation and often complicated by glaucoma or infection.

fuch·sin (fook′sin, fyook′sin) n. A red dyestuff which can be prepared in two forms, acid fuchsin and basic fuchsin.

fuchsin bodies. Inclusion bodies of keratohyalin, sometimes seen in the cytoplasm of epithelial tumor cells.

fuch·sin·o·phil (fyook·sin′o·fil, fook·) adj. Stainable with fuchsin.

fu·cose (few′koce) n. 6-Deoxygalactose, $C_6H_{12}O_5$, an aldose terminating in a methyl group at the number 6 carbon atom, existing in D- and L- forms. D-Fucose is obtained by hydrolysis of convolvulin, jalapin, and other glycosides; L-fucose is a component of certain glycoproteins and occurs also in some seaweeds. Syn. D-*galactomethylose.*

fu·co·si·do·sis (few″ko-si-do′sis) n. A familial neurovisceral degenerative disease, due to the absence of the enzyme alpha-fucosidase, characterized by normal early development followed by progressive neurologic deterioration, cardiomegaly with myocarditis, thick skin, hyperhidrosis, and early death, with accumulation of fucose-containing sphingolipids and glycoprotein fragments in all tissues and of abnormal carbohydrates especially in brain and liver; inherited as an autosomal recessive trait.

-fuge A combining form meaning *that which causes to flee, or drives away.*

fu·gi·tive (few′ji-tiv) adj. Wandering or transient; inconstant, as a pain.

fugue (fewg) n. A dissociative reaction in hysterical neurosis characterized by amnesia of considerable duration and frequently flight from familiar surroundings. During the fugue, the patient appears to act in a conscious way and retains his mental faculties, but after recovery has no remembrance of the state.

fulgurant pains. LIGHTNING PAINS.

ful·gu·rate (ful′gew-rate) v. 1. To produce fulguration. 2. To wax and wane with lightning-like speed.

ful·gu·rat·ing (ful′gew-ray″ting) adj. Lightning-like; used to describe sudden, lancinating, excruciating pain.

ful·gu·ra·tion (ful″gew-ray′shun) n. Destruction of tissue, usually malignant tumors, by means of electric sparks.

fu·lig·i·nous (few-lij′i-nus) adj. Smokelike; very dark; soot-colored.

fuller's asthma. A pneumoconiosis due to the inhalation of lint and dust in the manufacture of wool cloth.

fuller's earth. A clay related to kaolin, and used similarly, as an adsorbent and protective.

full-thickness graft. A skin graft including all layers of the skin. Syn. *Krause-Wolfe graft.*

ful·mi·nant (ful′mi-nunt) n. Sudden, severe, intense, and rapid in course.

ful·mi·nat·ing (ful′mi-nay″ting) adj. FULMINANT.

Fulvicin-U/F. A trademark for griseofulvin, an orally effective fungistatic antibiotic.

fu·ma·rate (few′muh-rate, few-mar′ate) n. A salt or ester of fumaric acid.

Fu·mar·i·a·ce·ae (few-mâr″ee-ay′see-ee) n.pl. A family of plants including the genera *Adlumia, Corydalis, Dicentra,* and *Fumaria;* by some authorities this family is ranked as a subfamily (Fumaroidae) of the Papaveraceae. Many alkaloids are found among the plants of the Fumariaceae.

fu·mar·ic acid (few·măr'ick). *trans*-Ethylenedicarboxylic acid, HOOCCH=CHCOOH, the *trans*-isomer of maleic acid. It occurs in *Fumaria officinalis* and in mammalian tissues as an intermediate in the metabolism of carbohydrate.

fu·mig·a·cin (few·mig'uh·sin) *n*. HELVOLIC ACID.

fu·mi·gate (few'mi·gate) *v*. To expose to the fumes of a vaporized disinfectant. —**fumi·gant** (·gunt) *n*.: **fu·mi·ga·tion** (few''mi·gay'shun) *n*.

fum·ing (few'ming) *adj*. Emitting smoke or vapor, as fuming nitric acid or fuming sulfuric acid.

func·tio (funk'shee·o) *n*. FUNCTION.

func·tion (funk'shun) *n*. 1. The normal or special action of a part. 2. The chemical character, relationships, and properties of a substance contributed by a particular, atom, group of atoms, or type of bond in the substance. 3. A factor related to or dependent upon other factors.

func·tion·al (funk'shun·ul) *adj*. 1. Of or pertaining to a specific function, process, or activity. 2. Pertaining to the physiology or working of a part or system, but not its structure. 3. Useful; able to carry out appropriate tasks though structurally not intact. 4. Pertaining to a condition or illness in which the normal activities are disturbed or cannot be carried out, though there is no apparent organic explanation.

functional disease. A disease in which no definite organic cause or no demonstrable pathologic lesion can be discovered.

functional dysmenorrhea. Dysmenorrhea without anatomic or pathologic explanation.

functional impotence. Impotence due to a psychologic disturbance, usually depression.

functional lesion. An alteration of function or functional capacity without demonstrable morphologic alteration.

functional menorrhagia. Excessive menstruation due to no demonstrable anatomic or pathologic lesion; usually assumed to be due to endocrine dysfunction. Syn. *primary menorrhagia*.

functional murmur. INNOCENT MURMUR.

fun·dal (fun'dal) *adj*. FUNDIC.

fun·da·ment, *n*. 1. The foundation or base. 2. The buttocks.

fun·da·men·tal, *adj*. 1. Basic; underlying. 2. Of essential nature, property, or quality. 3. Elementary.

fun·dec·to·my (fun·deck'tuh·mee) *n*. FUNDUSECTOMY.

fundi. Plural of *fundus*.

fun·dic (fun'dick) *adj*. Pertaining to or involving a fundus.

fun·di·form (fun'di·form) *adj*. Shaped like a sling, or loop.

fun·do·plasty (fun'do·plas''tee) *n*. Plastic repair of the fundus of an organ.

fun·do·pli·ca·tion (fun''do·pli·kay'shun) *n*. Plication of the gastric fundus around the esophagus.

fun·dos·co·py (fun·dos'kuh·pee) *n*. Examination of the interior of the eye with the use of an ophthalmoscope or slit lamp (biomicroscope) and contact lens; OPHTHALMOSCOPY. —**fun·do·scop·ic** (fun''duh·skop'ick) *adj*.

fun·dus (fun'dus) *n*., pl. **fun·di** (·dye) The part farthest removed from the opening (exit) of the organ.

fun·du·scope (fun'duh·skope) *n*. OPHTHALMO-SCOPE.

fun·dus·co·py (fun·dus'kuh·pee) *n*. FUNDOSCOPY. —**fun·du·scop·ic** (fun''duh·skop'ick) *adj*.

fun·du·sec·to·my (fun''duh·seck'tuh·mee) *n*. 1. Surgical removal of the fundus of an organ, as of the uterus. 2. Surgical removal of a wedge-shaped portion of the fundus of the stomach, used in the treatment of postoperative jejunal ulcer.

fundus ocu·li (ock'yoo·lye). The posterior portion of the interior of the eye.

fundus of the gallbladder. The wide, anterior end of the gallbladder.

fundus of the uterus. The part of the uterus most remote from the cervix.

fundus ute·ri (yoo'tur·eye) [NA]. FUNDUS OF THE UTERUS.

fundus ven·tri·cu·li (ven·trick'yoo·lye) [NA]. The large, rounded cul-de-sac cephalad to the cardia of the stomach, when that organ is dilated. Syn. *fornix of the stomach*.

fundus ve·si·cae fel·le·ae (ve·sigh'kee fel'ee·ee, ve·sigh'see) [NA]. FUNDUS OF THE GALLBLADDER.

fun·gal (fun'gul) *adj*. Of or pertaining to fungi.

fun·gate (fung'gate) *v*. & *adj*. 1. To grow upward from a surface in a fashion resembling a fungus, as certain tumors. 2. Grown into a funguslike form. —**fungat·ing** (·ing) *adj*.

fungating carcinoma. A centrally necrotic carcinoma growing in a sessile polypoid fashion from a surface or into a lumen, giving a resemblance to a fungus.

fun·ge·mia, fun·gae·mia (fun·jee'mee·uh) *n*. The presence of fungi in the blood.

fungi. Plural of *fungus*.

fun·gi·cide (fun'ji·side) *n*. An agent that destroys fungi. —**fun·gi·ci·dal** (fun''ji·sigh'dul) *adj*.

fun·gi·form (fun'ji·form) *adj*. Having the form of a mushroom.

fungiform papilla. One of the low, broad papillae scattered over the dorsum and margins of the tongue.

Fungi Im·per·fec·ti (im''pur·feck'tye). Fungi which lack a known sexual phase of reproduction in their life history.

fun·gi·sta·sis (fun''ji·stay'sis) *n*. The inhibition of fungus growth by a chemical or physical agent; to be distinguished from fungicidal action, which involves the killing of fungi. —**fungi·stat·ic** (·stat'ick) *adj*.

fun·goid (fung'goid) *adj*. Resembling a fungus.

fun·gous (fung'gus) *adj*. 1. Of or pertaining to fungi; FUNGAL. 2. Caused by or infected with a fungus. 3. Funguslike; FUNGOID.

fun·gus (fung'gus) *n*., pl. **fun·gi** (fun'jye), **funguses** 1. A low form of plant life, a division of the Thallophytes without chlorophyll. The chief classes of fungi are the Phycomycetes, Ascomycetes, Basidiomycetes, and Fungi Imperfecti. Most of the pathogenic fungi belong to the last group. 2. A spongy morbid excrescence.

fu·nic (few'nick) *adj.* Pertaining to the umbilical cord.

fu·ni·cle (few'ni·kul) *n.* A slender cord, a funiculus.

funic souffle. FUNICULAR SOUFFLE.

fu·nic·u·lar (few·nick'yoo·lur) *adj.* Of or pertaining to a funiculus.

funicular hernia. A variety of congenital, indirect hernia confined to the spermatic cord.

funicular process. The portion of the tunica vaginalis that surrounds the spermatic cord.

funicular souffle. A blowing murmur usually synchronous with the fetal heartbeat, heard over the pregnant uterus; thought to originate in the umbilical cord.

funiculi. Plural of *funiculus*.

fu·nic·u·li·tis (few·nick''yoo·lye'tis) *n.* 1. Inflammation of a funiculus, specifically of the spermatic cord. 2. Inflammation of a spinal nerve root within the vertebral canal.

fu·nic·u·lus (few·nick'yoo·lus) *n.*, pl. **funic·u·li** (·lye) 1. One of the three main divisions of white matter, which are named with reference to the gray matter of the cord as dorsal, lateral, and ventral. 2. *Obsol.* FASCICULUS. 3. *Obsol.* The umbilical or spermatic cord.

funiculus se·pa·rans (sep'uh·ranz) A white ridge of thickened ependyma, separating the ala cinerea from the area postrema.

fu·nis (few'nis) *n.* A cord, particularly the umbilical cord.

fun·nel, *n.* A wide-mouthed conical vessel ending in an open tube; for filling bottles or other containers, and as a support for filter papers.

funnel chest *or* **breast.** A deformity of the sternum, costal cartilages, and anterior portions of the ribs, producing a depression of the lower portion of the chest; usually associated with development of kyphoscoliosis.

funnel pelvis. A deformity in which the usual external measurements are normal while the outlet is contracted, the transverse diameter of the latter being 8 cm or less.

funny bone. The region at the back of the medial condyle of the humerus, crossed superficially by the ulnar nerve. Compression of the nerve at this point induces a painful tingling sensation to the cutaneous area supplied by the ulnar nerve.

F.U.O. Fever of undetermined or unknown origin.

fur, *n.* 1. A coating of epithelial debris, as on the tongue. 2. The hairy coat of some animals. —**furred,** *adj.*

Furacin. Trademark for nitrofurazone, a local antibacterial agent.

Furadantin. Trademark for nitrofurantoin, an antibacterial agent for oral administration in the treatment of bacterial infections of the urinary tract.

fu·ran (few'ran) *n.* CH=CH—CH=CH. A constituent of wood tars; a colorless liquid, insoluble in water.

fu·rane (few'rane) *n.* FURAN.

fu·ra·nose (few'ruh·noce) *n.* A sugar having a ring structure resembling that of furan.

fur·cu·la (fur'kew·luh) *n.*, pl. **furcu·lae** (·lee) 1. A crescentic median elevation of the floor of the embryonic pharynx, at the level of the third and fourth visceral arches; differentiates into the epiglottis and aryepiglottic folds. Syn. *hypobranchial eminence.* 2. A forked process, especially the joined clavicles of a bird; wishbone.

fur·fur (fur'fur) *n.* Dandruff; a branny desquamation of the epidermis. —**fur·fu·ra·ceous** (fur''fur·ay'shus, fur''few'ray'shus) *adj.*

fur·fu·ral (fewr'fuh·ral, fur'few-) *n.* 2-Furaldehyde, $C_5H_4O_2$, a liquid used as a solvent and reagent, and as an insecticide and fungicide.

fur·fu·ryl (fewr'fuh·ril, fur'few-) *n.* The monovalent radical C_5H_5O— derived from furfuryl alcohol.

fu·ri·bund (few'ri·bund) *adj.* Raging; maniacal.

furious rabies. The commoner form of rabies, in which the cerebral involvement is prominent.

fu·ror (few'ror) *n.* 1. Madness. 2. The manic phase of manic depressive illness; maniacal attack.

fur·o·sem·ide (fewr''o·sem'id, ·ide) *n.* 4-Chloro-*N*-furfuryl-5-sulfamoylanthranilic acid, $C_{12}H_{11}ClN_2O_5S$, a diuretic drug.

furred tongue. The tongue the papillae of which are coated.

fur·row (fur'o) *n.* A groove.

fu·run·cle (few'rung·kul) *n.* A localized infection, usually staphylococcal, of skin and subcutaneous tissue, which usually originates in or about a hair follicle and develops into a solitary abscess that drains externally through a single suppurating tract; a boil. —**fu·run·cu·lar** (few·runk'yoo·lur) *adj.*

fu·run·cu·lo·sis (few·run·ku''yoo·lo'sis) *n.*, pl. **furun·culo·ses** (·seez) A condition in which multiple furuncles form or in which outbreaks of furuncles rapidly succeed one another.

Fu·sar·i·um (few·zar'ee·um) *n.* A genus of fungi, including species that may act as allergens and that are pathogenic for plants. Produces verticillate conidiophores, which give rise to sickle-shaped, multiseptate conidia. The spores are airborne.

fus·cin (fus'in, few'sin) *n.* The melanin pigment of the eye.

fused kidney. Connection of the inferior poles of the two kidneys anterior to the aorta by an isthmus of renal parenchyma. The most common anomaly is the horseshoe kidney and the sigmoid kidney. Fusion is also seen in the cake kidney.

fu·sel oil (few'zul) A by-product, formed from protein materials, in the production of ethyl alcohol by fermentation; it consists chiefly of isoamyl alcohol with varying quantities of other alcohols.

fusi-, fuso- A combining form meaning (a) *spindle;* (b) *fusiform.*

fu·si·ble (few'zi·bul) *adj.* Capable of being melted.

fu·si·form (few'zi·form, few'si·) *adj.* Spindle-shaped.

fusiform aneurysm. A spindle-shaped dilatation of an artery.

fusiform bacillus. A bacterium of spindle-shaped or cigar-shaped morphology, belonging to the genus *Fusobacterium.*

fusiform bougie. A bougie with a spindle-shaped shaft.

Fu·si·for·mis (few'zi·for'mis, few'si·) *n.* FUSOBACTERIUM.

fu·si·mo·tor (few'zi·mo'tur) *adj. In neurophysiology,* pertaining to the motor or efferent innervation of the intrafusal muscle fibers, derived from the gamma efferent neurons of the anterior gray matter of the spinal cord.

fusion frequency. The lowest frequency at which flashes of light produce on the retina the impression of a steady light rather than a flicker.

Fu·so·bac·te·ri·um (few'zo·back·teer'ee·um) *n.* A genus of strictly anaerobic or microaerophilic bacteria, consisting of gram-negative rods which are slender, of various length, and often fusiform in shape. They form part of the indigenous flora of man, are found in the mouth, intestinal and genital tracts; in association with spirochetes; and in necrotizing lesions. —**fusobacterium,** pl. **fusobacte·ria,** *com. n.*

fu·so·cel·lu·lar (few'zo·sel'yoo·lur) *adj.* Consisting of spindle-shaped cells.

fu·so·spi·ro·che·tal, fu·so·spi·ro·chae·tal (few'zo·spye''ro·kee'tul) *adj.* Pertaining to the association of fusiform bacteria and spirochetes.

fusospirochetal bronchitis. An infection of the respiratory tract characterized by foul sputum containing anaerobes including fusiform rods and spirilla, probably representing lung abscess or bronchiectasis rather than bronchitis.

fusospirochetal gangrene. Foul, gangrenous lesions of the oropharynx, genitalia, respiratory tract, and other tissues; characterized by the presence of a mixed, largely anaerobic microbial flora, generally including fusobacteria and spirochetes.

fu·so·spi·ro·che·to·sis, fu·so·spi·ro·chae·to·sis (few'zo·spye''ro·kee·to'sis) *n.* Infection with *Fusobacterium fusiforme* and spirochetes, associated with Vincent's infection, lung abscess, vulvovaginitis, or balanitis.

f waves. FIBRILLATION WAVES.

F waves. FLUTTER WAVES.

G, Ĝ, g, ĝ *In electrocardiography,* a symbol for the ventricular gradient, usually as projected on the frontal plane of the body.

G, g 1. Symbol for gravitation constant or Newtonian constant, a constant in Newton's law of gravitation which gives the attraction f between two particles m_1 and m_2 at a distance r as $f = G(m_1 m_2)/r^2$. G is a constant whose value depends on the units in which f, m_1, m_2, and r are expressed. If f is given in dynes, m_1 and m_2 in grams, and r in centimeters, then G is 6.673×10^{-8} dyne cm^2/g^2. 2. A unit of force of acceleration, equal to that exerted on a body by gravity at the earth's surface, allowing the expression of force of acceleration as a multiple of earth's gravitation.

g Abbreviation for *gram.*

gad·fly, *n.* Any of various flies of the Tabanidae.

Gaffkya te·trag·e·na (te-traj′e-nuh). A species of micrococci forming tetrads, found in the mucous membranes of the respiratory tract and occasionally pathogenic in man. Syn. *Micrococcus tetragenus.*

gag, *n. & v.* 1. An instrument placed between the jaws to prevent closure of the mouth. 2. To insert a gag. 3. To retch or heave.

gage. GAUGE.

gag reflex. Contraction of the constrictor muscles of the pharynx in response to stimulation of the posterior pharyngeal wall or neighboring structures.

Gais·böck's disease or **syndrome** (gice′bœck) Polycythemia vera and hypertension without splenomegaly. Syn. *polycythemia hypertonica.*

gait, *n.* Manner of walking.

galact-, galacto- A combining form meaning (a) *milk;* (b) *milky fluid.*

ga·lac·ta·cra·sia (ga·lack′′tuh·kray′zhuh, ·zee·uh) *n.* Deficiency of or abnormality in mother's milk.

ga·lac·ta·gogue (ga·lack′tuh·gog) *n.* An agent that induces or increases the secretion of milk.

ga·lac·tan (ga·lack′tan) *n.* Any polysaccharide composed of galactose units; on hydrolysis it yields galactose. Syn. *galactosan.*

ga·lac·tase (ga·lack′tace, ·taze) *n.* A soluble proteolytic enzyme present normally in milk.

gal·ac·te·mia, gal·ac·tae·mia (gal′′ack·tee′mee·uh) *n.* A milky state or appearance of the blood.

ga·lact·hi·dro·sis (ga·lakt′′hi·dro′sis) *n.* Sweating of a milklike fluid.

ga·lac·tic (ga·lack′tick) *adj.* Pertaining to or promoting the flow of milk.

gal·ac·tis·chia (gal′′ack·tis′kee·uh) *n.* Suppression of the secretion of milk; GALACTOSCHESIS.

ga·lac·to·cele (ga·lack′to·seel) *n.* 1. A retention cyst caused by obstruction of one or more of the mammary ducts. 2. A hydrocele with milky contents.

ga·lac·to·gram (ga·lack′to·gram) *n.* A radiograph of the mammary ductal system.

gal·ac·tog·ra·phy (gal′′ack·tog′ruh·fee) *n.* Radiographic depiction of the mammary ductal system.

ga·lac·toid (ga·lack′toid) *adj.* Resembling milk.

gal·ac·to·ma (gal′′ack·to′muh) *n.,* pl. **galactomas, galactoma·ta** (·tuh) GALACTOCELE (1).

gal·ac·tom·e·ter (gal′′ack·tom′e·tur) *n.* 1. A graduated glass funnel for determining the fat in milk. 2. An instrument for determining the specific gravity of milk.

gal·ac·ton·ic acid (gal′′ack·ton′ick). Pentahydroxyhexoic acid, $C_6H_{12}O_7$, a monobasic acid derived from galactose.

gal·ac·toph·a·gous (gal′′ack·tof′uh·gus) *adj.* Subsisting on milk.

ga·lac·to·phore (ga·lack′to·fore) *n.* A lactiferous duct. —**gal·ac·toph·o·rous** (gal′′ack·tof′uh·rus) *adj.*

gal·ac·toph·o·ri·tis (gal′′ack·tof′′uh·rye′tis) *n.* Inflammation of a lactiferous duct.

gal·ac·toph·y·gous (gal′′ack·tof′i·gus) *adj.* Arresting the secretion of milk.

ga·lac·to·py·ra (ga·lack′to·pye′ruh) *n.* MILK FEVER. —**galacto·py·ret·ic** (·pye·ret′ick) *adj.*

ga·lac·tor·rhea, ga·lac·tor·rhoea (ga·lack′′to·ree′uh) *n.* Excessive or spontaneous flow of milk.

ga·lac·tos·a·mine (ga·lack′′to′suh·meen, ·toce·am′een) *n.* Galactose containing an amine group in 2-position, hence 2-amino-D-galactose. Syn. *chondrosamine.*

ga·lac·to·san (ga·lack'to·san) *n.* GALACTAN.

gal·ac·tos·che·sis (gal''ack·tos'ke·sis) *n.* Retention or suppression of milk secretion.

ga·lac·tose (ga·lack'toce, ·toze) *n.* A D-aldohexose, $C_6H_{12}O_6$, obtained by hydrolysis of lactose, occurring also as a component of cerebrosides and of many oligosaccharides and polysaccharides; it exists in α- and β- forms. On oxidation it yields mucic acid. L-Galactose occurs in small amounts in certain polysaccharides, as the mucilage of agar and flaxseed.

galactose diabetes. GALACTOSEMIA.

ga·lac·tos·emia, ga·lac·tos·ae·mia (ga·lack''to·see'mee·uh) *n.* An inborn error of metabolism due to absence of galactose 1-phosphate uridyl transferase resulting in inability to convert galactose into glucose; manifested by failure to thrive in infancy, jaundice, involvement of liver and spleen, cataract formation, and mental retardation.

galactose tolerance test. A test of the glycogenic function of the liver, performed by administering 40 g of galactose to a fasting individual. The elimination of more than 3 g of galactose over a 5-hour period indicates hepatic dysfunction.

ga·lac·to·sid·ase (ga·lack''to·sigh'dace, ·daze) *n.* Any enzyme that catalyzes the hydrolysis of a galactoside. Two varieties are known, α- and β-, which act on α- and β- forms, respectively, of galactosides.

ga·lac·to·side (ga·lack'to·side) *n.* A glycoside which, on hydrolysis, yields the sugar galactose and an aglycone.

ga·lac·to·sis (gal''ack·to'sis) *n.* The secretion of milk by the mammary glands.

gal·ac·tos·ta·sis (gal''ack·tos'tuh·sis) *n.* 1. Suppression of milk secretion. 2. An abnormal collection of milk in a breast.

ga·lac·tos·uria (ga·lack''to·sue'ree·uh) *n.* Passage of urine containing galactose.

ga·lac·to·ther·a·py (ga·lack''to·therr'uh·pee) *n.* 1. Treatment by a milk diet; particularly treatment of newborn infants by feeding breast milk. 2. The treatment of disease in nursing infants by the administration of drugs to the mother which are subsequently secreted in the milk. 3. Hypodermic injection of sterile milk as a form of protein therapy.

ga·lac·to·tox·in (ga·lack''to·tock'sin) *n.* A poisonous substance formed in milk by growth of microorganisms.

ga·lac·to·tox·ism (ga·lack''to·tock'siz·um) *n.* Poisoning resulting from ingestion of contaminated or spoiled milk.

gal·ac·tot·ro·phy (gal''ack·tot'ruh·fee) *n.* Nourishing with milk only.

ga·lac·to·zy·mase (ga·lack''to·zye'mace, ·maze) *n.* An enzyme found in milk that is capable of hydrolyzing starch.

gal·ac·tu·ria (gal''ack·tew'ree·uh) *n.* Milkiness of the urine; CHYLURIA.

gal·ba·num (gal'buh·num) *n.* A gum resin of *Ferula galbaniflua;* formerly used as a stimulant and expectorant and externally in plasters.

ga·lea (gay'lee·uh, gal'ee·uh) *n.,* pl. **galeas, ga·le·ae** (·lee·ee) 1. Any structure resembling a helmet. 2. A form of head bandage.

galea apo·neu·ro·ti·ca (ap''o·new·rot'i·kuh) [NA]. The aponeurotic portion of the occipitofrontal muscle. NA alt. *aponeurosis epicranialis.*

gal·e·an·thro·py (gal''ee·an'thruh·pee, gay'lee·) *n.* A form of zoanthropy in which the patient believes himself to be transformed into a cat.

ga·le·na (ga·lee'nuh) *n.* Native lead sulfide, PbS.

ga·len·ic (ga·len'ick, ·lee'nick) *adj.* Pertaining to, or consistent with, the system of medicine and teachings of Galen.

ga·len·i·cal (ga·len'i·kul) *adj. & n.* 1. GALENIC. 2. Any medicine prepared from plants, according to standard formulas, as contrasted with chemical entities.

gal·eo·phil·ia (gal''ee·o·fil'ee·uh) *n.* Excessive love of cats.

gal·eo·pho·bia (gal''ee·o·fo'bee·uh) *n.* An abnormal fear of cats.

gal·e·ro·pia (gal''e·ro'pee·uh) *n.* An abnormally clear and light appearance of objects due to some defect in the visual apparatus.

gall (gawl) *n.* BILE.

gal·la·mine tri·eth·io·dide (gal'uh·meen trye''eth·eye·o·dide). 1,2,3-Tris(2-triethylammonium ethoxy)benzene triiodide, $C_{30}H_{60}I_3N_3O_3$, a curarimimetic drug employed as a skeletal muscle relaxant.

gall·blad·der (gawl'blad·ur) *n.* A hollow, pear-shaped, musculomembranous organ, situated on the undersurface of the right lobe of the liver, for the storage and concentration of bile and the secretion of mucus.

gal·lic acid (gal'ick) 3,4,5-Trihydroxybenzoic acid, $C_7H_6O_5$, formerly used internally as an astringent; esters of the acid are used as antioxidants.

gal·lon, *n.* A standard unit of volume equivalent in the United States to 3785.3 ml or to 231 cubic inches; 4 quarts. Syn. *congius.*

galloping consumption. *Colloq.* A rapidly fatal form of pulmonary tuberculosis. Syn. *florid phthisis.*

gallop rhythm. A three-sound sequence resulting from the intensification of the normal third or fourth heart sounds, occurring usually, but not invariably, with a rapid ventricular rate.

gallop sound. A third or fourth heart sound.

gall·stone, *n.* A concretion formed in the gallbladder or the biliary ducts, composed, in varying amounts, of cholesterol, bilirubin, and other elements found in bile.

gal·van·ic (gal·van'ick) *adj.* Of, pertaining to, or caused by galvanism.

galvanic skin response. The electrical reactions of the skin to any stimulus as detected by a sensitive galvanometer; most often used experimentally to measure the resistance of the skin to the passage of a weak electric current.

gal·va·nism (gal'vuh·niz·um) *n.* Primary direct current electricity produced by chemical action, as opposed to that produced by heat, friction, or induction.

gal·va·nize (gal'vuh·nize) *v.* To apply or stimulate with galvanic current. **—gal·va·ni·za·tion** (gal"vuh·ni·zay'shun) *n.*

galvano-. A combining form meaning *galvanic* or *direct current* of electricity.

gal·vano·cau·tery (gal"vuh·no·kaw'tur·ee) *n.* ELECTROCAUTERY.

gal·vano·con·trac·til·i·ty (gal"vuh·no·kon"track'til·i·tee) *n.* The property of being contractile under stimulation by a galvanic current.

gal·va·nom·e·ter (gal"vuh·nom'e·tur) *n.* An instrument for measuring or detecting the presence of relatively small electric currents.

gal·vano·mus·cu·lar (gal"vuh·no·mus'kew·lur) *adj.* Denoting a reaction produced by the application of a galvanic current to a muscle.

gal·vano·sur·gery (gal"vuh·no·sur'jur·ee) *n.* The surgical use of direct or galvanic current.

gal·vano·ther·a·py (gal"vuh·no·therr'uh·pee) *n.* Treatment of disease with direct or galvanic currents.

gal·vano·ther·my (gal'vuh·no·thur"mee, gal·van'o·) *n.* The production of heat by direct or galvanic currents.

gal·va·not·o·nus (gal"vuh·not'o·nus) *n.* 1. ELECTROTONUS. 2. The continued tetanus of a muscle between the make and break contraction of direct or galvanic current. **—gal·vano·ton·ic** (gal"vuh·no·ton'ick) *adj.*

gal·va·not·ro·pis·um (gal"vuh·not'ro·piz·um) *n.* The turning movements of a living organism under the influence of direct current.

gam-, gamo- A combining form meaning (a) *marriage;* (b) in biology, *sexual union;* (c) in botany, *union* or *fusion of parts.*

Gambian trypanosomiasis. Infection of man with *Trypanosoma brucei gambiense,* acquired by the bite of the tsetse fly, occurring widely throughout central Africa, and characterized by parasitemia, lymphadenitis, and central nervous system lesions causing a chronic, lethal meningoencephalitis. Syn. *mid-African sleeping sickness.*

gam·boge (gam·boje') *n.* The gum resin obtained from *Garcinia hanburyi;* a drastic, hydragogue cathartic.

gam·ete (gam'eet, ga·meet') *n.* A male or female reproductive cell capable of entering into union with another in the process of fertilization or of conjugation. In higher animals, these sex cells are the egg and sperm; in higher plants, the male gamete is part of the pollen grain, while the ovum is contained in the ovule. In lower forms, the gametes are frequently similar in appearance. **—ga·met·ic** (ga·met'ick) *adj.*

ga·me·to·cyte (ga·mee'to·site, gam'e·to·site) *n.* A cell which by division produces gametes; a spermatocyte or oocyte.

gam·e·to·gen·e·sis (gam"e·to·jen'e·sis) *n.* The origin and formation of gametes. **—gameto·gen·ic** (·ick) *adj.*

gam·e·tog·o·ny (gam"e·tog'uh·nee) *n.* A process of reproduction leading to the formation of gametocytes and gametes in the sexual phase of the life cycle in certain protozoa.

gam·ma (gam'uh) *n.* 1. The third of a series, or any particular member or subset of an arbitrarily ordered set. For many terms so desig-

nated, see under the specific noun. Symbol, γ. 2. *In photography,* the contrast of a negative or print, usually controlled by developing time, and expressed as a relationship between the density of the negative and the time of exposure. 3. One-millionth of a gram; MICROGRAM.

gamma-A globulin. The immunoglobulin which comprises about 10 percent of the antibodies of human serum, where it occurs as a monomer with a sedimentation constant of 7 Svedberg units, and which constitutes the principal immunoglobulin in such secretions as parotid saliva, tears, colostrum, and gastrointestinal fluid, where it occurs as a dimer possessing an added peptide (the secretory piece) and having a sedimentation constant of 11 Svedberg units. Symbol, IgA, γA.

gamma angle. *In ophthalmology,* the angle formed by the line of fixation and the optic axis.

gamma chain, γ chain. The heavy chain of the IgG immunoglobulin molecule.

gam·ma·cism (gam'uh·siz·um) *n.* Guttural stammering; difficulty in pronouncing velar consonants, especially hard g and k.

gamma-D globulin. An immunoglobulin found in small amounts in normal human serum and on fetal and umbilical cord lymphocytes, having a light chain similar to that of other immunoglobulins, but possessing a heavy chain of unique properties. Symbol, IgD, γD.

gamma-E globulin. The immunoglobulin associated with reaginic antibodies. Symbol, IgE, γE.

gamma-G globulin. The immunoglobulin comprising about 80% of the serum antibodies of the adult, readily transported across the human placenta, having a sedimentation constant of 6.7 Svedberg units and an estimated molecular weight of 145,000. Symbol, IgG, γG.

gamma globulin, γ-globulin. 1. A broad designation for immunoglobulins of differing molecular weights and for certain proteins related to them by chemical structure, many of which have known antibody activity. 2. Sterile concentrated solutions of globulins obtained from pooled human blood of placental or venous origin, containing protective antibodies, and used clinically in viral hepatitis, measles, German measles, or hypogammaglobulinemia. Syn. *immune serum globulin.* 3. Originally, the fraction of serum proteins migrating most slowly toward the anode upon separation by electrophoresis.

gamma-M globulin. The immunoglobulin comprising 5 to 10% of the total serum antibodies, and including heterophile and Wassermann antibodies, cold agglutinins, isohemagglutinins, and antibodies to the endotoxins of gram-negative bacteria; characterized by a sedimentation constant of 19 Svedberg units and a molecular weight of about 900,000. Symbol, IgM, γM. Syn. *macroglobin.*

gamma ray. Electromagnetic radiation of high energy and short wavelength emitted by the nucleus of a radioactive atom when it has excess energy.

gamma rhythm. *In electroencephalography,* very fast waves whose functional significance is unknown; 40 to 50 per second are recorded from the anterior head regions.

gamma roentgen. A unit of radium dosage such that the same amount of ionization in air is produced as by one roentgen unit of gamma rays. Syn. *gamma-ray roentgen.*

gam·mop·a·thy (ga·mop'uth·ee) *n.* A condition in which disturbance of immunoglobulin synthesis is presumed to play a primary role; reflected in significant changes of the immunoglobulin profile in the serum of the host.

Gamna-Gandy bodies (gahn·dee') Brown nodules noted in the spleen in chronic passive hyperemia, composed of calcium salts and hemosiderin encrusting fibrous connective and reticular tissues.

gamo-. See *gam-.*

gamo·ma·nia (gam''o·may'nee·uh) *n.* Excessive desire for marriage.

gamo·pho·bia (gam''o·fo'bee·uh) *n.* An abnormal fear of marriage.

gangli-, ganglio-. A combining form meaning *ganglion.*

ganglia. A plural of *ganglion.*

gan·gli·at·ed (gang'glee·ay''tid) *adj.* Supplied with ganglia; GANGLIONATED.

gan·gli·ec·to·my (gang''glee·eck'tuh·mee) *n.* GANGLIONECTOMY.

gan·gli·form (gang'gli·form) *adj.* Formed like or resembling a ganglion.

gan·gli·itis (gang''glee·eye'tis) *n.* GANGLIONITIS.

gan·glio·gli·o·ma (gang''glee·o·glye·o'muh) *n.* A tumor of the central nervous system composed of nerve cells in various stages of differentiation and glial elements.

gan·gli·o·ma (gang''glee·o'muh) *n.,* pl. **ganglio·mas, ganglioma·ta** (·tuh) GANGLIOGLIOMA.

gan·gli·on (gang'glee·un) *n.,* pl. **gan·glia** (·glee·uh), **ganglions** 1. A group of nerve cell bodies, usually located outside the brain and spinal cord, as the dorsal root ganglion of a spinal nerve. 2. A cystic, tumorlike, localized lesion in or about a tendon sheath or joint capsule, especially of the hands, wrists, and feet, but also occasionally within other connective tissues. It is composed of stellate cells in a matrix of mucoid hyaluronic acid and reticular fibers. Syn. *cystic tumor of a tendon sheath, cyst of a joint capsule, cyst of a semilunar cartilage, weeping sinew.*

gan·gli·on·ec·to·my (gang''glee·un·eck'tuh·mee) *n.* Excision of a ganglion.

gan·glio·neu·ro·blas·to·ma (gang''glee·o·new''ro·blas·to'muh) *n.* A tumor sharing features of ganglioneuroma and neuroblastoma that contains incompletely differentiated nerve cells, ranging from embryonal to anaplastic, and that may metastasize.

gan·glio·neu·ro·ma (gang''glee·o·new·ro'muh) *n.* A tumor composed predominantly of mature ganglion cells, often lying in groups within abundant interlacing reticulin fibers and Schwann cells, and commonly showing cystic degeneration and microscopic calcification. There is considerable histological variation, even within the same tumor, depending on the

degree of neoplastic evolution and the tumor site, with those located in the cerebral hemispheres and brainstem very different from those in the cerebellum and those along the sympathetic ganglia and adrenal medulla. Transitional forms with neuroblastomas, hamartomatous variants, and metastases may occur. Syn. *gangliocytoma.*

ganglionic block. Blockade by local anesthetic of an autonomic or central nervous system ganglion.

ganglionic layer of the retina. The layer of the retina which contains the bipolar cells.

gan·gli·on·itis (gang''glee·un·eye'tis) *n.* Inflammation of a ganglion.

ganglion nodosum tumor. A tumor of the inferior ganglion of the vagus nerve, histologically indistinguishable from a carotid-body tumor.

ganglion of the cervix uteri. A ganglion of the craniosacral autonomic system, located at the cervix of the uterus. Syn. *Frankenhafuser's ganglion.*

gan·gli·o·side (gang'glee·o·side) *n.* One of a group of glycosphingolipids found in neuronal surface membranes and spleen. They contain an *N*-acyl fatty acid derivative of sphingosine linked to a carbohydrate (galactose or glucose). They also contain *N*-acetylglucosamine or *N*-acetylgalactosamine, and *N*-acetylneuraminic acid.

gan·gli·o·si·do·sis (gang''glee·o·si·do'sis, ·sigh·do'sis) *n.,* pl. **gangliosido·ses** (·seez) 1. Any disorder of the biosynthesis or breakdown of ganglioside, including (a) the generalized or G_{M1} gangliosidosis, (b) the G_{M2} gangliosidoses, and (c) G_{M3} gangliosidosis. 2. *Especially,* a disorder of the breakdown of ganglioside; that is, any of the G_{M1} or G_{M2} gangliosidoses.

gan·go·sa (gang·go'suh) *n.* Destructive lesions of the nose and hard palate, sometimes more extensive, considered to be a tertiary stage of yaws. Syn. *rhinopharyngitis mutilans.*

gan·grene (gang'green, gang·green') *n.* 1. Necrosis of a part; due to failure of the blood supply, to disease, or to direct injury. 2. The putrefactive changes in dead tissue. —**gan·gre·nous** (·gre·nus) *adj.*

gangrene of the appendix. Necrosis of the vermiform appendix in appendicitis, with sloughing of the organ.

gangrene of the lung. A diffuse, putrefactive necrosis of the lung or of a lobe; due to anaerobic or other bacteria; usually a termination of lung abscess in a patient with low resistance.

gangrenous blepharitis. Carbuncle of the eyelids.

gangrenous cystitis. An acute, severe, diffuse inflammation of the urinary bladder involving principally the mucosa and submucosa, due principally to severe infection, x-ray therapy, injection of chemicals, or impaired blood supply and characterized by gross suppuration, necrosis, and gangrene of the involved tissues.

gangrenous inflammation. Severe inflammation complicated by secondary infection with putrefactive bacteria.

gan·ja, gan·jah (gan'juh, ·zhuh) *n.* The tops,

stems, leaves, and twigs of the female hemp plant as used in India for mixing into cakes and for smoking; a form of cannabis more potent than marijuana.

gan·o·blast (gan'o·blast) *n.* AMELOBLAST.

Gantrisin. Trademark for sulfisoxazole, an antibacterial sulfonamide of high solubility in body fluids.

gapes, *n.* A disease of young fowl caused by the presence of gapeworms in the trachea.

gape·worm (gaip'wurm) *n.* SYNGAMUS TRACHEALIS.

Gard·ner's syndrome An autosomal dominant trait manifested in childhood by multiple osteomas, fibrous and fatty tumors of the skin and the mesentery, epidermoid inclusion cysts of the skin, and the development of intestinal polyps predisposed to malignancy; other tumors, such as carcinoma of the thyroid, may occur.

gar·get (gahr'ghit) *n.* A progressive inflammation of the udder, usually of cattle.

gar·gle, *v.* & *n.* 1. To rinse the oropharynx. 2. A solution for rinsing the oropharynx.

gar·goyl·ism (gahr'goil·iz·um) *n.* MUCOPOLYSACCHARIDOSIS.

gar·lic, *n.* The fresh bulb of *Allium sativum*, containing allyl sulfides; has been used medicinally. —**gar·licky,** *adj.*

Gar·ré's osteomyelitis or **disease** (ga·rey') Chronic sclerosing osteomyelitis with little suppuration, characterized by small areas of necrosis.

gar·rot·ing (ga·ro'ting, ga·rot'ing) *n. In legal medicine,* forcible compression of a victim's neck from behind with intent to rob or kill.

Gart·ner's cyst A benign cyst arising in the anterolateral vaginal walls from incompletely obliterated remnants of Gartner's duct.

Gartner's duct The ductus epoophori longitudinalis. It may persist in the mesosalpinx near the ovary or in the lateral wall of the vagina.

gas, *n.* & *v.* 1. The vaporous or airlike state of matter. A fluid that distributes itself uniformly throughout any space in which it is placed, regardless of its quantity. 2. Any combustible gas used as a source of light or heat. 3. To drench an area with poisonous gas. 4. To execute or attempt to execute a person by means of toxic gas. —**gas·e·ous** (gas'ee·us, gash'us) *adj.*

gas gangrene. A form of gangrene occurring in massive wounds, where there is crushing and devitalization of tissue and contamination with dirt. The specific organisms found are anaerobes, including *Clostridium perfringens, C. novyi, C. septicum,* and *C. histolyticum;* nonspecific aerobic pyogens are commonly present also. The condition is characterized by high fever, an offensive, thin, purulent discharge from the wound, and the presence of gas bubbles in the tissues.

gas gangrene bacillus. CLOSTRIDIUM PERFRINGENS, type A.

gas myelography. Radiographic examination of the spinal cord after injecting gas into the subarachnoid spaces.

gas·om·e·ter (gas·om'e·tur) *n.* A device for holding and measuring gas. —**gas·o·met·ric** (gas''o·met'rick) *adj.*

gas·se·ri·an ganglion (ga·seer'ee·un) TRIGEMINAL GANGLION.

gas·ter (gas'tur) *n.* STOMACH. NA alt. *ventriculus.*

Gas·ter·oph·i·lus (gas''tur·off'i·lus) *n.* A genus of botflies. The larvae are parasites of horses and occasionally infest the cutaneous and subcutaneous tissues in man.

Gasterophilus in·tes·ti·na·lis (in·tes''ti·nay'lis). A species of horse botfly that lays its eggs on the hairs of the foreparts of the horse, with the larvae excavating tunnels under the mucosa of the mouth, and ultimately migrating to the stomach. Human infection similar to the larva migrans caused by *Ancylostoma braziliense* occurs.

gastr-, gastro-. A combining form meaning (a) *stomach, gastric;* (b) *belly, abdominal.*

gas·tral·gia (gas·tral'jee·uh) *n.* Pain in the stomach.

gas·tral·go·ke·no·sis (gas·tral''go·ke·no'sis) *n.* Paroxysmal pain due to emptiness of the stomach; relieved by taking food.

gas·tra·tro·phia (gas''tra·tro'fee·uh) *n.* Atrophy of the stomach.

gas·trec·ta·sis (gas·treck'tuh·sis) *n.,* pl. **gastrectases** (·seez) Dilatation of the stomach.

gas·trec·to·my (gas·treck'tuh·mee) *n.* Excision of the whole or a part of the stomach.

gas·tric (gas'trick) *adj.* Of or pertaining to the stomach.

gastric antrum. PYLORIC ANTRUM.

gastric canal. A longitudinal groove of the mucous membrane of the stomach near the lesser curvature.

gastric fever. BRUCELLOSIS.

gastric juice. The secretion of the glands of the stomach; a clear, colorless liquid having an acid pH and a specific gravity of about 1.006 and containing about 0.5% of solid matter; contains hydrochloric acid, pepsin, mucin, and, in infants, rennin.

gastric motility. The movements of the stomach walls, including antral peristalsis and fundic contraction in the smooth muscle walls of the stomach.

gastric plexus. Any of the nerve plexuses associated with the stomach. The anterior gastric plexus lies along the anterior surface of the lesser curvature of the stomach; its fibers are derived mainly from the left vagus, a few from the right vagus, and some sympathetic fibers. The posterior gastric plexus lies along the posterior surface of the lesser curvature; its fibers are derived mainly from the right vagus. The inferior gastric plexus accompanies the left gastroepiploic artery; its fibers are derived from the splenic plexus. The superior gastric plexus accompanies the left gastric artery, and receives fibers from the celiac plexus.

gastric prolapse. Protrusion of gastric mucosa through the pylorus or a surgical stoma.

gas·tric·sin (gas·trick'sin) *n.* One of the two principal gastric proteases, the other being pepsin.

gastric ulcer. An ulcer affecting the wall of the stomach.

gas·trin (gas'trin) *n.* A polypeptide hormone,

secreted by the mucosa of the gastric antrum in response to eating or alkalinization of the stomach; it causes gastric secretion of pepsin and hydrochloric acid and promotes growth of the gastrointestinal mucosa.

gas·tri·tis (gas·trye'tis) n., pl. **gas·trit·i·des** (gas·trit'i·deez) Inflammation of the stomach. —**gas·trit·ic** (gas·trit'ick) adj.

gas·tro·anas·to·mo·sis (gas''tro·uh·nas''tuh·mo'sis) n. GASTROGASTROSTOMY.

gas·tro·cam·era (gas''tro·kam'e·ruh) n. A tiny camera with attached light designed to be introduced through the esophagus into the stomach to obtain pictures from within the lumen.

gas·tro·cele (gas'tro·seel) n. A hernia of the stomach.

gas·tro·cne·mi·us (gas''tro·nee'mee·us, -·k'nee'mee·us) n., pl. **gastrocne·mii** (-·mee·eye) A muscle on the posterior aspect of the leg, arising by two heads from the posterior surfaces of the lateral and medial condyles of the femur, and inserted with the soleus muscle into the calcaneal tendon, and through this into the back of the calcaneus.

gas·tro·col·ic (gas''tro·kol'ick, -·ko'lick) adj. Pertaining to the stomach and the colon.

gastrocolic reflex or **response.** Motility of the colon induced by the entrance of food into the stomach.

gas·tro·col·pot·o·my (gas''tro·kol·pot'uh·mee) n. Cesarean section in which the opening is made through the linea alba and continued into the upper part of the vagina.

gas·tro·dis·ci·a·sis (gas''tro·dis·kigh'uh·sis, -·di·sigh'uh·sis) n. Infection of the cecum by *Gastrodiscoides hominis*, causing inflammation and producing diarrhea.

Gastrodiscoides hom·i·nis (hom'i·nis). A species of small intestinal fluke which has as its natural host the hog; man serves as an accidental host, the fluke attaching to the cecum and ascending colon; the cause of gastrodisciasis.

gas·tro·du·o·de·nal (gas''tro·dew''o·dee'nul, dew·od'e·nul) adj. Pertaining to the stomach and the duodenum.

gas·tro·du·o·de·ni·tis (gas''tro·dew''o·de·nigh'tis, -dew·od''e·nigh'tis) n. Inflammation of the stomach and duodenum.

gas·tro·du·o·de·nos·to·my (gas''tro·dew''o·de·nos'tuh·mee) n. Establishment of an anastomosis between the stomach and duodenum.

gas·tro·en·ter·ic (gas''tro·en·terr'ick) adj. Pertaining to the stomach and the intestines; GASTROINTESTINAL.

gas·tro·en·ter·i·tis (gas''tro·en·tur·eye'tis) n. Inflammation of the mucosa of the stomach and intestines. —**gastroenter·it·ic** (-·it'ick) adj.

gas·tro·en·tero·anas·to·mo·sis (gas''tro·en''tur·o·uh·nas''tuh·mo'sis) n. Anastomosis between the intestine and the stomach.

gas·tro·en·ter·ol·o·gist (gas''tro·en·tur·ol'uh·jist) n. A physician specializing in gastroenterology.

gas·tro·en·ter·ol·o·gy (gas''tro·en''tur·ol'uh·jee) n. The study of the stomach and intestine and their diseases.

gas·tro·en·ter·op·a·thy (gas''tro·en''tur·op'uh·thee) n. Any disease of the stomach and intestines.

gas·tro·en·ter·op·to·sis (gas''tro·en''tur·op·to'sis) n. Sagging or prolapse of the stomach and intestines.

gas·tro·en·ter·os·to·my (gas''tro·en·tur·os'tuh·mee) n. The formation of a communication between the stomach and the small intestine, usually the jejunum.

gas·tro·ep·i·plo·ic (gas''tro·ep'i·plo'ick) adj. Pertaining to the stomach and greater omentum.

gas·tro·esoph·a·ge·al, gas·tro·oe·soph·a·ge·al (gas''tro·e·sof''uh·jee'ul) adj. Pertaining to or involving the stomach and esophagus.

gas·tro·esoph·a·gi·tis (gas''tro·e·sof''uh·jye'tis) n. Inflammation of the stomach and the esophagus.

gas·tro·esoph·a·go·plas·ty, gas·tro·oe·soph·a·go·plas·ty (gas''tro·e·sof''uh·go·plas''tee) n. Plastic surgical repair of the stomach and esophagus.

gas·tro·gas·tros·to·my (gas''tro·gas·tros'tuh·mee) n. *In surgery,* anastomosis of one portion of the stomach with another, as the surgical formation of a communication between the two pouches of an hourglass stomach.

gas·tro·ga·vage (gas''tro·ga·vahzh') n. Artificial feeding through an opening in the stomach wall.

gas·tro·gen·ic (gas''tro·jen'ick) adj. Originating in the stomach.

gas·tro·graph (gas'tro·graf) n. An apparatus for recording the peristaltic movements of the stomach.

gas·tro·he·pat·ic (gas''tro·he·pat'ick) adj. Pertaining to the stomach and liver.

gas·tro·hy·per·ton·ic (gas''tro·high''pur·ton'ick) adj. Pertaining to or characterized by morbid or excessive tonicity or irritability of the stomach.

gastroileac reflex. Altered, usually increased, motility of the ileum resulting from the presence of food in the stomach.

gas·tro·in·tes·ti·nal (gas''tro·in·tes'ti·nul) adj. Pertaining to the stomach and intestine.

gastrointestinal tract. ALIMENTARY CANAL.

gas·tro·je·ju·nal (gas''tro·je·joo'nul) adj. Pertaining to the stomach and the jejunum.

gas·tro·je·ju·ni·tis (gas''tro·jee''joo·nigh'tis, -·jej'oo·) n. Inflammation of both the stomach and jejunum, sometimes occurring after gastrojejunostomy.

gas·tro·je·ju·nos·to·my (gas''tro·jee''joo·nos'tuh·mee) n. *In surgery,* anastomosis of the jejunum to the anterior or posterior wall of the stomach.

gas·tro·la·vage (gas''tro·la·vahzh') n. The washing out of the stomach; gastric lavage.

gas·tro·li·e·nal (gas''tro·lye'e·nul) adj. GASTROSPLENIC.

gas·tro·lith (gas'tro·lith) n. A calcareous formation in the stomach.

gas·tro·li·thi·a·sis (gas''tro·li·thigh'uh·sis) n. The formation or presence of gastroliths.

gas·trol·o·gy (gas·trol'uh·jee) n. The science of the stomach, its functions and diseases.

gas·trol·y·sis (gas·trol'i·sis) n., pl. **gastroly·ses**

(·seez) The breaking up of adhesions between the stomach and adjacent organs.

gas·tro·ma·la·cia (gas''tro·ma·lay''shee·uh, ·see· uh) *n.* An abnormal softening of the walls of the stomach.

gas·tro·meg·a·ly (gas''tro·meg''uh·lee) *n.* Abnormal enlargement of the stomach.

gas·trom·e·lus (gas·trom'e·lus) *n.,* pl. **gastrome·li** (·lye) An individual with an accessory limb attached to the abdomen.

gas·tro·mes·en·ter·ic (gas''tro·mes''in·terr'ick) *adj.* Pertaining to the stomach and the mesentery.

gas·tro·my·co·sis (gas''tro·migh·ko'sis) *n.,* pl. **gastromyco·ses** (·seez) Gastric disease due to fungi.

gas·tro·my·ot·o·my (gas''tro·migh·ot'uh·mee) *n.* Incision of the circular muscle fibers of the stomach.

gas·tro·pan·cre·at·ic (gas''tro·pan''kree·at'ick) *adj.* Pertaining to the stomach and the pancreas.

gas·trop·a·thy (gas·trop'uth·ee) *n.* Any disease or disorder of the stomach.

gas·tro·pexy (gas'tro·peck''see) *n.* The fixation of a prolapsed stomach in its normal position by suturing it to the abdominal wall or other structure.

gas·tro·phren·ic (gas''tro·fren'ick) *adj.* Pertaining to the stomach and diaphragm.

gas·tro·plas·ty (gas'tro·plas''tee) *n.* Plastic operation on the stomach.

gas·tro·pli·ca·tion (gas''tro·pli·kay'shun) *n.* An operation for relief of chronic dilatation of the stomach, consisting of suturing a large horizontal fold in the stomach wall; plication of the stomach wall for redundancy due to chronic dilatation.

gas·trop·to·sis (gas''trop·to'sis) *n.* Prolapse or downward displacement of the stomach.

gas·tro·py·lo·rec·to·my (gas''tro·pye''lo·reck'tuh·mee) *n.* Excision of the pyloric portion of the stomach.

gas·tror·rha·gia (gas''tro·ray'jee·uh) *n.* Hemorrhage from the stomach.

gas·tror·rha·phy (gas·tror'uh·fee) *n.* 1. Repair of a stomach wound. 2. GASTROPLICATION.

gas·tror·rhea, gas·tror·rhoea (gas''tro·ree'uh) *n.* Excessive secretion of gastric mucus or of gastric juice.

gas·tro·sal·i·vary reflex (gas''tro·sal'i·verr·ee). Salivation following the introduction of food into the stomach.

gas·tros·chi·sis (gas·tros'ki·sis) *n.* A congenital malformation in which the abdomen remains open to the exterior.

gas·tro·scope (gas'truh·skope) *n.* A fiberoptic endoscope for examining the interior of the stomach. —**gas·tros·co·py** (gas·tros'kuh·pee) *n.*

gas·tro·spasm (gas'tro·spaz·um) *n.* Spasm or contraction of the stomach wall.

gas·tro·splen·ic (gas''tro·splen'ick) *adj.* Pertaining to the stomach and the spleen.

gas·tro·stax·is (gas''tro·stack'sis) *n.* The oozing of blood from the mucous membrane of the stomach.

gas·tros·to·my (gas·tros'tuh·mee) *n.* The establishing of a fistulous opening into the stomach,

with an external opening in the skin; usually for artificial feeding.

gas·trot·o·my (gas·trot'uh·mee) *n.* Incision into the stomach.

gas·tro·tox·in (gas''tro·tock'sin) *n.* A cytotoxin which has a specific action on the cells lining the stomach. —**gastrotox·ic** (·sick) *adj.*

gas·tro·tym·pa·ni·tes (gas''tro·tim''puh·nigh'teez) *n.* Gaseous distention of the stomach.

gas·tru·la (gas'troo·luh) *n.,* pl. **gastrulas, gastru·lae** (·lee) An embryo at that stage of its development when it consists of two cellular layers, the primary ectoderm and entoderm, and a primitive gut or archenteron opening externally through the blastopore. The simplest type is derived by the invagination of the spherical blastula, but this is greatly modified in the various animal groups. —**gas·tru·la·tion** (gas''troo·lay'shun) *n.*

Gatch bed A jointed bed frame that permits a patient to be placed in a sitting or semireclining position.

Gau·cher lipid (go·shey') KERASIN.

Gaucher's cells Altered macrophages found in Gaucher's disease, 20 to 80 microns in diameter, with single small spherical nuclei and abundant striated cytoplasm containing the characteristic cerebrosides of the disease.

Gaucher's disease A rare chronic familial deficiency of a glucocerebroside-cleaving enzyme resulting in abnormal storage of cerebrosides in reticuloendothelial cells and characterized by splenomegaly, hepatomegaly, skin pigmentation, pingueculae of the scleras, and bone lesions. Syn. *cerebroside lipidosis, familial splenic anemia.*

gauge (gaje) *n.* An instrument for measuring the dimensions or extent of a structure, or for testing the status of a process or phenomenon.

gaunt·let (gawnt'lit) *n.* A bandage that covers the hand and fingers like a glove.

gauntlet flap. A pedicle flap that is raised and applied to a movable part, as from the abdominal wall to a hand.

gauss (gowss) *n.* A unit of magnetic induction, equal to one line of flux per square centimeter.

gauze (gawz) *n.* A thin, open-meshed absorbent cloth of varying degrees of fineness, used in surgical operations and for surgical dressings. When sterilized it is called aseptic gauze.

gauze sponge. A flat folded piece of gauze of varying size, used by a surgical assistant to absorb blood from the wound during an operation.

ga·vage (ga·vahzh') *n.* The administration of nourishment through a stomach tube.

Gee-Her·ter disease INFANTILE CELIAC DISEASE.

ge·gen·hal·ten (gay'gun·hahl''tun) *n.* PARATONIA.

Geiger-Mül·ler counter (mue'l·ur) An instrument for the detection of individual ionizing particles; entry of a charged particle into the apparatus produces ionization and a momentary flow of current which is relayed to a counting device.

Geiger-Müller tube A tube which, when the proper voltage is imposed, will produce an electric pulse each time an ionizing particle penetrates its walls.

gel (jel) *n.* A colloidal system comprising a solid and a liquid phase which exists as a solid or semisolid mass.

ge·las·mus (je·laz'mus) *n.* Insane or hysterical spasmodic laughter.

gelastic epilepsy. A form of epilepsy characterized by laughing.

gel·a·tin (jel'uh·tin) *n.* The product obtained by partial hydrolysis of collagen, occurring in sheets, flakes, shreds, or as a coarse or fine powder, insoluble in cold water but soluble in hot water; used in many pharmaceutical preparations, in formulations for histochemical examinations, as an ingredient of bacteriologic culture mediums, as a food, as a plasma extender, and as an absorbable film or sponge in operative procedures.

ge·lat·i·nase (je·lat'i·nace, ·naze) *n.* An enzyme, found in some yeasts and molds, that hydrolyzes and liquefies gelatin.

ge·lat·i·nize (je·lat'i·nize) *v.* To convert into a jellylike mass.

ge·lat·i·nous (je·lat'i·nus) *adj.* 1. Resembling gelatin; jelly-like. 2. Of or pertaining to gelatin.

gelatinous ascites or **peritonitis.** PSEUDOMYXOMA PERITONEI.

gelatinous carcinoma. MUCINOUS CARCINOMA.

ge·la·tion (je·lay'shun) *n.* 1. The change of a colloid from a sol to a gel. 2. Freezing.

gel·a·tose (jel'uh·toce) *n.* An intermediate product in the hydrolysis of gelatin.

geld (gheld) *v.* To castrate, as a horse; EMASCULATE.

geld·ing (ghel'ding) *n.* A castrated male horse.

gel electrophoresis. Electrophoresis employing a gel as the supporting medium.

gel filtration chromatography. A type of column chromatography which separates molecules on the basis of size, the substances of higher molecular weight passing through the column first. Syn. *molecular exclusion chromatography, molecular sieve chromatography.*

Gelfoam. Trademark for an absorbable gelatin sponge material used as a local hemostatic.

gel·ose (jel'oce, je·loce') *n.* The gelatinizing principle of agar, being the calcium salt of a complex carbohydrate substance composed of galactose units.

gel·o·to·lep·sy (jel'uh·to·lep''see) *n.* A sudden loss of muscle tone (cataplexy) induced by uproarious laughter.

¹gem·i·nate (jem'i·nit, ·nate) *adj.* In pairs, coupled.

²gem·i·nate (jem'i·nate) *v.* 1. To double. 2. To become doubled.

gem·i·na·tion (jem''i·nay'shun) *n.* An anomaly that represents the attempt of a tooth germ to divide by invagination; it usually presents a tooth having two completely or incompletely separated crowns and a common root or roots and pulp chamber.

ge·mis·to·cyte (je·mis'to·site) *n.* A large, round type of astrocyte with pale, acidophilic, homogeneous cytoplasm and eccentrically displaced nucleus, observed in certain neuropathologic conditions. —**ge·mis·to·cyt·ic** (je·mis''to·sit'ick) *adj.*

gem·ma (jem'uh) *n.*, pl. **gem·mae** (·ee) An asexual budlike body, either unicellular or multicellular.

gem·ma·tion (jem·ay'shun) *n.* BUDDING.

gem·mule (jem'yool) *n.* 1. A small bud or gemma. 2. The short thorny processes of the dendrites of pyramidal nerve cells.

Gemonil. Trademark for metharbital, a barbituric acid derivative useful in treating epilepsy.

-gen, -gene A combining form meaning (a) *substance or organism that produces or generates;* (b) *thing produced or generated.*

gen-, geno-. A combining form meaning (a) *gene, genetic;* (b) *genital, sexual;* (c) *generating;* (d) *race, kind.*

ge·na (jee'nuh) *n.*, pl. **ge·nae** (·nee) CHEEK. —**ge·nal** (·nul) *adj.*

gender identity. The sum of those aspects of personal appearance and behavior culturally attributed to masculinity or femininity. While usually based on the external genitalia and body physique, parental attitudes and expectations as well as those of society determine what is masculine and what is feminine, and may cause conflicts.

gender role. The image or behavior a person presents to society whereby that person is categorized as a boy or man, or girl or woman. While gender identity and gender role are usually congruent, the former represents what society or the parents expect, and the latter, what an individual delivers; the two may be in conflict.

gene (jeen) *n.* A hereditary factor; the unit of transmission of hereditary characteristics, capable of self-reproduction, which usually occupies a definite locus on a chromosome, although some genes are nonchromosomal. Genes in general are constituted of DNA, although in some viruses they are RNA.

-gene. See *-gen.*

gene frequency. The relative frequency, usually expressed as a decimal, with which an allele of a gene occurs among all the alleles at a given locus in a population.

gene pool. The totality of reproductively available genes in a breeding population, characterized by the alleles that are present and their relative frequency.

genera. Plural of *genus.*

gen·er·al, *adj.* 1. Common to a class. 2. Distributed through many parts, diffuse. —**general·ly,** *adv.*

general adaptation syndrome. According to Hans Selye, the sum of all nonspecific systemic reactions of the body which ensue upon long-continued exposure to systemic stress. It is divided into three stages: (a) alarm reaction (shock and countershock), (b) stage of resistance, and (c) stage of exhaustion.

general anesthesia. Loss of sensation with loss of consciousness, produced by administration of anesthetic drugs.

gen·er·al·iza·tion (jen''rul·i·zay'shun) *n.* 1. The act or process of generalizing; the making of a general assumption or statement on the basis of one or only a few specifics. 2. *In psychiatry,* a mental mechanism operating outside and beyond conscious awareness by which an emotional process extends to include additional areas, as a fear of bridges may progress to a fear of tall buildings, mountains, or any high place.

gen·er·al·ize (jen'ur·ul·ize, jen'rul·) *v.* 1. To make general. 2. To become diffused or widespread.

generalized seizure. An epileptic seizure characterized by sudden loss of consciousness, tonic convulsion, cyanosis, and dilated pupils, followed by a clonic spasm of all voluntary muscles, with the eyes rotated upward, the head extended, frothing at the mouth, and, frequently, incontinence of urine. After the convulsion subsides, the patient is confused and frequently falls into a deep sleep. Syn. *grand mal seizure, major motor seizure.*

generalized Shwartzman phenomenon. SHWARTZMAN PHENOMENON (2).

general paralysis or **paresis.** A chronic progressive form of central nervous system syphilis occurring 15 to 20 years after the initial infection, taking the form of a meningoencephalitis and resulting in physical and mental dissolution. Syn. *paretic neurosyphilis, syphilitic meningoencephalitis, dementia paralytica.*

gen·er·a·tion (jen''ur·ay'shun) *n.* 1. Production; REPRODUCTION, procreation. 2. The aggregate of individuals descended in the same number of life cycles from a common ancestor or from ancestors that are in some respect equivalent; also, any aggregate of contemporaneous individuals. 3. An aggregate of cells or individuals in the same stage of development from a precursor. 4. The period spanning one life cycle of an organism, from the conception (or birth) of an individual to the conception (or birth) of his offspring.

generative organs. The gonads and secondary sexual organs that are functional in reproduction.

gen·er·a·tor, *n.* 1. A machine that transforms mechanical power into electric power. 2. *In radiology,* a machine that supplies the roentgen-ray tube with the electric energy necessary for the production of roentgen rays. 3. *In chemistry,* an apparatus for the formation of vapor or gas from a liquid or solid by heat or chemical action.

ge·ner·ic (je·nerr'ick) *adj.* 1. Of or pertaining to a genus. 2. Not specific. 3. Nonproprietary, as of a drug not registered or protected by a trademark.

ge·nes·ic (je·nes'ick, je·nee'zick) *adj.* Of or pertaining to generation or the genital organs.

gen·e·sis (jen'e·sis) *n.,* pl. **gen·e·ses** (·seez) 1. The origin or generation of anything. 2. The developmental evolution of a specific thing or type.

-genesis A combining form meaning (a) *origination;* (b) *development;* (c) *evolution* of a thing or type.

ge·net·ic (je·net'ick) *adj.* 1. Pertaining to or having reference to origin, mode of production, or development. 2. Pertaining to genetics. 3. Produced by genes.

genetic code. The code of the molecules of heredity; the nucleotide "dictionary" that permits the translation of specific gene DNA and messenger RNA molecules into proteins of specific amino acid sequence. The code is triplet and degenerate; each amino acid found in proteins is coded for by more than one triplet. The code is evidently universal for all species.

ge·net·i·cist (je·net'i·sist) *n.* A specialist in genetics.

genetic load. The accumulated deleterious mutant genes in a population, including those maintained by mutation and selection.

ge·net·ics (je·net'icks) *n.* The branch of biology that deals with the phenomena of heredity and variation. It seeks to understand the causes of the resemblances and differences between parents and progeny, and, by extension, between all organisms related to one another by descent.

Ge·ne·va convention. An agreement signed by the European powers in Geneva, Switzerland, in 1864, guaranteeing humane treatment of the wounded and those caring for them in time of war. Later revisions were accepted by the majority of nations.

geni-, genio- A combining form meaning *chin.*

ge·ni·al (jee'nee·ul) *adj.* Of or pertaining to the chin. Syn. *mental.*

-genic A combining form meaning (a) *producing, forming;* (b) *produced by, formed from;* (c) *of* or *pertaining to a gene.*

ge·nic·u·lar (je·nick'yoo·lur) *adj.* Of or pertaining to the knee joint.

ge·nic·u·late (je·nick'yoo·lut) *adj.* Abruptly bent.

geniculate body. See *medial geniculate body, lateral geniculate body.*

ge·nic·u·lo·cal·ca·rine (je·nick''yoo·lo·kal'kuh·reen) *adj.* Pertaining to the lateral geniculate body and the calcarine sulcus.

ge·nic·u·lo·tem·po·ral (je·nick''yoo·lo·temp'ur·ul) *adj.* Pertaining to the medial geniculate body and the temporal cortex.

ge·nic·u·lum (je·nick'yoo·lum) *n.,* pl. **genic·u·la** (·luh) A small, kneelike structure; a sharp bend in any small organ.

genio-. See *geni-.*

ge·nio·glos·sus (jee''nee·o·glos'us) *n.,* pl. **genioglos·si** (sigh) An extrinsic muscle of the tongue, arising from the superior mental spine of the mandible.

ge·nio·hy·oid (jee''nee·o·high'oid) *n.* A muscle arising from the inferior mental spine of the mandible and inserted into the body of the hyoid.

ge·nio·plas·ty (jee''nee·o·plas''tee, je·nigh'o·) *n.* Plastic operation on the chin.

gen·i·tal (jen'i·tul) *adj.* Of or pertaining to the organs of generation or to reproduction.

genital herpes. HERPES PROGENITALIS.

gen·i·ta·lia (jen''i·tay'lee·uh) *n. pl.* The organs of generation, comprising in the male the two testes or seminal glands, their excretory ducts, the prostate, the penis, and the urethra, and in the female the vulva, the vagina, the ovaries, the uterine tubes, and the uterus.

genital ridge. A medial ridge or fold on the ventromedial surface of the mesonephros in the embryo produced by growth of the peritoneum; the primordium of the gonads and their ligaments.

genito-. A combining form meaning *genital*.

gen·i·to·cru·ral (jen″i·to·kroo′ul) *adj.* Pertaining to the genitalia and the lower limb.

gen·i·to·fem·o·ral (jen″i·to·fem′uh·rul) *adj.* Pertaining to the genitalia and the thigh; GENITO-CRURAL.

gen·i·to·u·ri·nary (jen″i·to·yoor′i·nerr″ee) *adj.* Pertaining to the genitalia and the urinary organs or functions.

genitourinary tract. UROGENITAL SYSTEM.

gen·i·to·ves·i·cal (jen″i·to·ves′i·kul) *adj.* Pertaining to the genitalia and the urinary bladder.

ge·nius (jee′nee·us, jeen′yus) *n.* 1. Distinctive character or inherent nature. 2. Unusual creative ability; mental superiority. 3. An individual with unusual creative ability or mental superiority.

geno·cide (jen′uh·side) *n.* The systematic extermination of an entire human group.

geno·der·ma·to·sis (jen″o·dur″muh·to′sis) *n.* Any hereditary skin disease, as ichthyosis, pachyonychia congenita, or epidermolysis bullosa.

ge·nome, ge·nom (jee′nome) *n.* A complete set of the hereditary factors, such as is contained in a haploid set of chromosomes.

geno·pho·bia (jen″o·fo′bee·uh) *n.* An abnormal fear of sex.

ge·no·type (jee′no·tipe, jen′o·) *n.* 1. The hereditary constitution of an organism resulting from its particular combination of genes. 2. A class of individuals having the same genetic constitution. —**ge·no·typ·ic** (jee″no·tip′ick, jen″o·), **genotyp·i·cal** (·i·kul) *adj.*

–genous A combining form meaning (a) *producing*; (b) *produced by, arising in.*

gen·ta·mi·cin (jen″tuh·migh′sin) *n.* A mixture of two isomeric antibiotics, gentamicin C_1 and gentamicin C_2, produced by the fungi *Micromonospora purpurea* and *M. echinospora.* It is active against many gram-negative pathogens, especially *Pseudomonas aeruginosa,* and also against many gram-positive bacteria; used medicinally, as the sulfate salt, by parenteral injection.

gen·tian (jen′shun) *n.* 1. The common name for species of *Gentiana.* 2. The dried rhizome and roots of *Gentiana lutea,* containing a number of glycosides; has been used as a bitter tonic.

gentian violet. A form of methylrosaniline chloride.

gen·tis·ic acid (jen·tis′ick). 2,5-Dihydroxybenzoic acid, $C_7H_6O_4$; occurs in gentian and in urine after ingestion of salicylates.

Gentran. A trademark for dextran, a plasma-expanding and blood-pressure-maintaining glucose polymer.

ge·nu (jen′yoo) *n.,* genit. **ge·nus** (jen′ooss), pl. **ge·nua** (jen′yoo·uh) 1. [NA] KNEE. 2. Any of various angular or curved structures suggestive of a bent knee. 3. (of the corpus callosum:) The sharp curve of the anterior portion of the corpus callosum. 4. (of the internal capsule:) The portion of the internal capsule which, in

cross section, appears bent at an angle; it occurs where the capsule approaches the cavity of the lateral ventricle. 5. (of the facial nerve:) Either of the sharp curves in the facial nerve. —**ge·nu·al** (jen′yoo·ul) *adj.*

genu·cu·bi·tal (jen″yoo·kew′bi·tul) *adj.* Pertaining to or supported by the knees and elbows.

genu·fa·cial (jen″yoo·fay′shul) *adj.* Pertaining to or resting on the knees and face.

genu·pec·to·ral (jen″yoo·peck′tur·ul) *adj.* Pertaining to or resting on the knees and the chest.

genu re·cur·va·tum (ree″kur·vay′tum, reck″ur·). The backward curvature of the knee joint.

genu val·gum (val′gum). Inward or medial curving of the knee. Syn. *knock-knee.*

-geny A combining form meaning *genesis* or *generation.*

geny-, genyo- A combining form meaning the *under jaw.*

geny·chei·lo·plas·ty (jen″i·kigh′lo·plas″tee) *n.* Plastic operation on both cheek and lip.

geny·plas·ty (jen′i·plas″tee) *n.* Plastic operation on the lower jaw.

geo·graph·ic (jee″uh·graf′ick) *adj.* 1. Pertaining to or characteristic of features and regions of the earth. 2. Resembling land masses on a map.

geo·med·i·cine (jee″o·med′i·sin) *n.* The study of the effects of climate and other environmental conditions on health and disease.

geometric mean. The antilogarithm of the arithmetic mean of the logarithms of a series of observations; the *n*th root of the product of *n* observations.

geometric-optic agnosia. A form of agnosia in which a person can recognize objects, but has lost appreciation of direction or dimension, or both.

geo·pha·gia (jee·o·fay′jee·uh) *n.* GEOPHAGY.

ge·oph·a·gism (jee·off′uh·jizm) *n.* GEOPHAGY.

ge·oph·a·gy (jee·off′uh·jee) *n.* The practice of eating earth or clay. —**geopha·gous** (·gus) *adj.;* **geopha·gist** (·jist) *n.*

ge·ot·ri·cho·sis (jee·ot″ri·ko′sis) *n.,* pl. **geotricho·ses** (·seez) An infection possibly caused by one or more species of the fungus *Geotrichum.* Lesions may occur in the mouth, intestinal tract, bronchi, and lungs.

ge·ot·ro·pism (jee·ot′ruh·piz·um) *n. In biology,* the gravitational factor which in plants causes roots to grow downward toward the earth and shoots to grow up, and in some animals causes the climbing, swimming, or right-side-up orientation.

ge·phy·ro·pho·bia (je·figh″ro·fo′bee·uh, jef″i·ro·) *n.* An abnormal fear of crossing a bridge.

ger-, gera-, gero- A combining form meaning *old age.*

ge·ra·ni·ol (je·ray′nee·ol) *n.* 3,7-Dimethyl-2,6-octadien-1-ol, $C_{10}H_{18}O$, a terpene alcohol constituent of many volatile oils.

ge·rat·ic (je·rat′ick) *adj.* Of or pertaining to old age; GERONTIC.

ger·a·tol·o·gy (jerr″uh·tol′uh·jee) *n.* The scientific study of senescence and its related phenomena; GERONTOLOGY.

ger·i·at·ric (jerr″ee·at′rick) *adj.* Of or pertaining to geriatrics or to the process of aging.

ger·i·a·tri·cian (jerr''ee·uh·trish'un) n. A physician who specializes in the treatment of the diseases of aging.

ger·i·at·rics (jerr''ee·at'ricks) n. The branch of medical science that is concerned with aging and its diseases.

ger·i·a·trist (jerr''ee·uh·trist) n. GERIATRICIAN.

gerio- A combining form meaning *old* or *aged*.

ger·io·psy·cho·sis (jerr''ee·o·sigh·ko'sis) n., pl. **geriopsycho·ses** (·seez) SENILE DEMENTIA.

germ, n. 1. A small bit of protoplasm capable of developing into a new individual, especially an egg, spore, or seed; any of the early stages in the development of an organism. 2. Any microorganism.

Ger·man measles. RUBELLA.

ger·mi·cide (jur'mi·side) n. An agent that destroys germs. —**germi·ci·dal** (jur''mi·sigh'dul) adj.

ger·mi·nal (jur'mi·nul) adj. 1. Of, pertaining to, or within a germ or seed. 2. Pertaining to the early developmental stages of an embryo or organism.

germinal center. The actively proliferating region of a lymphatic nodule in which lymphocytes are being formed; the site of the high-level antibody formation characteristic of a secondary immune response. Syn. *germ center.*

germinal disk. 1. The protoplasm area in the eggs of reptiles, birds, and lower animals which becomes the blastoderm, in the center of which arises the definitive embryo. 2. In placental mammals, the inner cell mass which becomes the embryonic disk while the rest of the blastocyst becomes amnion, yolk sac, and trophoblast.

germinal epithelium. A region of the dorsal coelomic epithelium, lying between the dorsal mesentery and the mesonephros, becoming the covering epithelium of the gonad when it arises from the genital ridge; once falsely believed to give rise to the germ cells. Syn. *germ epithelium.*

germinal inclusion cyst. A cyst located near the surface of an ovary, arising from inclusions of germinal epithelium.

ger·mi·na·tion (jur''mi·nay'shun) n. The beginning of growth of a spore or seed. —**germi·nate** (jur'mi·nate) v.

ger·mi·na·tive (jur'mi·nuh·tiv, ·nay''tiv) adj. Having the power to begin growth or to develop.

ger·mi·no·ma (jur''mi·no'muh) n. A tumor whose parenchyma is composed of germ cells; usually a malignant teratoma, a seminoma, or a dysgerminoma.

germ plasm. The material basis of inheritance; it is located in the chromosomes.

germ theory. The theory that contagious and infectious diseases are caused by microorganisms.

ge·roc·o·my (je·rock'o·mee) n. The medical and hygienic care of old people. —**ger·o·com·i·cal** (jerr''o·kom'i·kul) adj.

gero·der·ma (jerr''o·dur'muh) n. The skin of old age, showing atrophy, loss of fat, and loss of elasticity.

ger·o·don·tia (jerr''o·don'chee·uh) n. Dentistry for the aged.

gero·ma·ras·mus (jerr''o·ma·raz'mus) n. Emaciation characteristic of extreme old age.

gero·mor·phism (jerr''o·mor'fiz·um) n. The condition of appearing prematurely aged.

geront–, geronto– A combining form meaning *old age.*

ge·ron·tic (je·ron'tick) adj. Pertaining to old age; GERATIC. —**geron·tism** (·tiz·um) n.

ger·on·tol·o·gy (jerr''on·tol'uh·jee) n. Scientific study of the phenomena and problems of aging; GERATOLOGY.

ge·ron·to·phil·ia (je·ron''to·fil'ee·uh) n. Love for and understanding of old people.

ge·ron·to·pho·bia (je·ron''to·fo'bee·uh) n. Unusual fear or dislike of old people or old age.

ge·ron·to·ther·a·py (je·ron''to·therr'uh·pee) n. 1. Treatment of the aging process. 2. Therapeutic management of aged persons.

Gerota's fascia RENAL FASCIA.

Gerst·mann's syndrome A disorder of cerebral function due to a lesion in the angular gyrus of the dominant cerebral hemisphere and the adjoining area of the middle occipital gyri, consisting of right-left disorientation, finger agnosia, agraphia and acalculia.

Ge·sell developmental schedule (guh·zel') A test of the mental growth of the preschool child which includes motor development, adaptive behavior, language development, and personal-social behavior.

ge·stalt (guh·shtahlt') n. The configuration of separate units, both experiential and behavioral, into a pattern or shape which itself seems to function as a unit.

gestalt psychology. A system or theory of psychology that emphasizes the wholeness and organized structure of every experience, maintaining that psychologic processes and behavior cannot be described adequately by analyzing the elements of experience alone, but rather by their integration into one perceptual configuration, and emphasizing sudden learning by insight rather than by trial and error or association.

ges·ta·tion (jes·tay'shun) n. PREGNANCY. —**ges·tate** (jes'tate) v.; **ges·ta·tion·al** (jes·tay'shun·ul) adj.

gestational age. The age of a conceptus computed from the first day of the last menstrual period to any point in time thereafter, but usually not calculated beyond the first few months of life after birth.

gestational psychosis. Any serious mental disorder in association with pregnancy or the postpartum period.

gestation period. The period of pregnancy. The average length of human gestation is taken as 10 lunar months (280 days) from the onset of the last menstrual period with a variation between 250 and 310 days.

ges·to·sis (jes·to'sis) n., pl. **gesto·ses** (·seez) Any toxemic manifestation in pregnancy.

geu·ma·pho·bia (gew''muh·fo'bee·uh) n. A morbid fear of tastes.

-geusia A combining form meaning *condition of the taste sense.*

GFR Glomerular filtration rate.

ghat·ti gum (gat'ee). The gummy exudate from

stems of *Anogeissus latifolia*, a tree of India and Ceylon. It forms a viscous mucilage, and is sometimes used in place of acacia.

Ghon complex (gohn) The combination of a focus of subpleural tuberculosis (Ghon tubercle) with associated hilar and mediastinal lymph node tuberculosis, usually in children. Syn. *primary complex, Kufss-Ghon focus.*

Ghon primary focus or **lesion.** GHON TUBERCLE.

Ghon tubercle The primary lesion of pulmonary tuberculosis, appearing as a radiographic shadow in the lung.

ghost cells or **corpuscles.** 1. The still visible stromata of hemolyzed erythrocytes. Syn. *phantom cells.* 2. *In exfoliative cytology,* the cells of squamous lung cancer in which the nuclei are compressed or destroyed by large amounts of intracytoplasmic keratin.

GI Abbreviation for *gastrointestinal.*

gi·ant cell. 1. Any large cell. 2. A multinucleate large cell.

giant-cell arteritis. 1. An arterial inflammatory disease characterized by multinucleated cells (giant cells), affecting the carotid artery branches, particularly the temporal artery, in elderly people, accompanied by fever, headache, and a variety of neurologic disturbances, including blindness. Syn. *cranial arteritis, temporal arteritis.* 2. POLYARTERITIS NODOSA. 3. AORTIC ARCH SYNDROME.

giant-cell tumor. 1. A distinctive tumor of bone, thought to arise from nonosteogenic connective tissue or marrow, composed of a richly vascularized reticulum of stromal cells interspersed with multinuclear giant cells. It generally appears after the second decade of life near the end of long limb bones, and it causes thinning of the compact bone. Syn. *central giant-cell tumor, osteoclastoma, myeloid sarcoma, myeloplaxic tumor, chronic hemorrhagic osteomyelitis.* 2. EPULIS. 3. CHONDROBLASTOMA. 4. NONOSSIFYING FIBROMA. 5. XANTHOMATOUS GIANT-CELL TUMOR OF TENDON SHEATH.

giant colon. MEGACOLON.

giant follicular lymphoblastoma. NODULAR LYMPHOMA.

giant follicular lymphoma. NODULAR LYMPHOMA.

giant intracanalicular fibroadenomyxoma. CYSTOSARCOMA PHYLLODES.

Gi·ar·dia (jee·ahr'dee·uh) *n.* A genus of flagellated protozoan parasites.

Giardia lam·blia (lam'blee·uh). A species of parasites found in the small intestine of man. It is not a tissue invader but is the cause of giardiasis.

gi·ar·di·a·sis (jee″ahr·dye'uh·sis) *n.,* pl. **giardiases** (·seez) The presence of the *Giardia lamblia* in the small intestine of man, usually without symptoms, but occasionally producing diarrhea and abdominal discomfort. Syn. *lambliasis.*

gib·bos·i·ty (gi·bos'i·tee) *n.* KYPHOSIS.

gib·bous (gib'us) *adj.* KYPHOTIC; swollen, convex, or protuberant, especially on one side.

gib·bus (gib'us) *n.* A hump; usually the dorsal convexity seen in tuberculosis of the spine (Pott's disease) or fracture.

gid, *n.* A chronic brain disease of sheep, less frequently of cattle; characterized by forced movements of circling, rolling. Caused by the larval form of the dog tapeworm *Multiceps multiceps.*

gid·di·ness, *n.* An unpleasant sensation of disturbed relation to surrounding objects in space, differing from vertigo in that there is no experience of the external world, or of the patient, being in motion. —**gid·dy,** *adj.*

Giem·sa's stain (gyem'zah) A stain for hemopoietic tissue and hemoprotozoa consisting of a stock glycerol methanol solution of eosinates of Azure B and methylene blue with some excess of the basic dyes.

gi·gan·tism (jye·gan'tiz·um) *n.* In man, excessive growth, with a height greater than 78 to 80 inches.

Gigli's saw A flexible wire saw with detachable handles at either end. Adapted to cranial and other bone operations.

Gilbert's syndrome or **disease** An asymptomatic disorder associated with a hereditary (autosomal dominant) glucuronyl transferase deficiency, a compensated hemolytic process, or a nonhemolytic overproduction of bilirubin; characterized by mild fluctuating indirect hyperbilirubinemia and usually with an impaired hepatic uptake or transport of bilirubin, or both.

Gil·christ's disease NORTH AMERICAN BLASTOMYCOSIS.

¹gill (jil) *n.* One-fourth of a pint.

²gill (gil) *n.* A respiratory organ of water-breathing animals.

Gilles de la Tou·rette disease or **syndrome** (zheel″duh·la·too·ret') A severe form of habit spasm, beginning in late childhood and adolescence and characterized by multiple tics associated with echolalia, obscene utterances, and other compulsive acts.

gin·ger, *n.* The dried rhizome of *Zingiber officinale,* formerly used as a carminative and flavoring agent.

ginger paralysis. TRIORTHOCRESYL PHOSPHATE NEUROPATHY.

gin·gi·va (jin'ji·vuh, jin·jye'vuh) *n.,* pl. & genit. sing. **gingi·vae** (·vee) The mucous membrane and underlying soft tissue that covers the alveolar process and surrounds a tooth. —**gin·gi·val** (·vul) *adj.;* **gingival·ly** (·ee) *adv.*

gingival margin. 1. The more or less rounded crest of the gingival tissue. 2. The margin of a dental cavity or restoration nearest the apex.

gingival pocket. An abnormally deep gingival sulcus due to inflammatory gingival enlargement, gingival hyperplasia, or incomplete eruption of a tooth; it does not involve the gingival attachment.

gingival septum. The mucous membrane projecting into the interproximal space between two teeth.

gingival sulcus. The space between the free gingiva and the surface of a tooth.

gin·gi·vec·to·my (jin″ji·veck'tuh·mee) *n.* Excision of a portion of the gingiva.

gin·gi·vi·tis (jin″ji·vye'tis) *n.* Inflammation of the gingiva.

gin·gi·vo·buc·cal (jin″ji·vo·buck′ul) adj. Pertaining to the gingivae and the mucous membranes of the lips or cheeks.

gin·gi·vo·glos·sal (jin″ji·vo·glos′ul) adj. Pertaining to the gums and the tongue.

gin·gi·vo·plas·ty (jin′ji·vo·plas″tee) n. The surgical recontouring or reshaping of the gingiva for the achievement of physiologic form.

gin·gi·vo·sis (jin″ji·vo′sis) n. CHRONIC DESQUAMATIVE GINGIVITIS.

gin·gi·vo·sto·ma·ti·tis (jin″ji·vo·sto″muh·tye′tis) n. An inflammation of the gingiva and oral mucosa.

gin·gly·mus (jing′gli·mus, ging′) n., pl. **gingly·mi** (-migh) HINGE ARTICULATION. —**gingly·moid** (-moid) adj.

gir·dle, n. 1. A band designed to go around the body. 2. A structure resembling a circular belt or band.

girdle anesthesia. A zone of anesthesia encircling the body.

girdle pain. A painful sensation as of a cord tied about the waist, symptomatic of disease of the nerve roots.

git·a·lin (jit′uh·lin, ji·tay′lin, ji·tal′in) n. 1. A crystalline glycoside, $C_{35}H_{56}O_{12}$, from digitalis leaves. 2. An amorphous mixture of digitalis glycosides.

Git·lin's syndrome PRIMARY LYMPHOPENIC IMMUNOLOGIC DEFICIENCY.

git·o·gen·in (jit″o·jen′in, ji·toj′e·nin) n. The steroid aglycone of gitonin.

git·o·nin (jit′o·nin, ji·to′nin) n. A saponin from *Digitalis purpurea.* On acid hydrolysis it yields the steroid aglycone gitogenin, galactose, and L-xylose.

gi·tox·i·gen·in (ji·tock″si·jen′in, ji·tock′si·ji·nin) n. The steroid aglycone, $C_{23}H_{34}O_5$, of gitoxin and of lanatoside B.

gi·tox·in (ji·tock′sin) n. One of the partially hydrolyzed glycosides, $C_{41}H_{64}O_{14}$, obtained from both *Digitalis purpurea* and *D. lanata;* on complete hydrolysis it yields the steroid aglycone gitoxigenin and three molecules of the sugar digitoxose.

git·ter cell (git′ur) COMPOUND GRANULE CELL.

giz·zard (giz′urd) n. The muscular portion of the upper digestive system of some birds. Syn. *ventriculus.*

gla·bel·la (gla·bel′uh) n., pl. **glabel·lae** (-ee) 1. The bony prominence on the frontal bone joining the supraorbital ridges. 2. *In craniometry,* a point found in the sagittal plane of the bony prominence joining the supraorbital ridges, usually the most anteriorly projecting portion of this region. —**glabel·lar** (-ur) adj.

gla·brous (glay′brus) adj. Smooth; devoid of hairs.

glacial acetic acid. A colorless liquid containing not less than 99.4% CH_3COOH; formerly used as a caustic for removing warts and corns.

glad·i·ol·ic acid (glad″ee·ol′ick). An antibiotic substance, $C_{11}H_{10}O_5$, isolated from cultures of *Penicillium gladioli;* it is active against some bacteria and has marked fungistatic properties.

glairy (glair′ee) adj. 1. Slimy; VISCOUS; MUCOID. 2. Resembling the white of an egg.

gland, n. 1. A cell, tissue, or organ that elaborates and discharges a substance that is used elsewhere in the body (secretion), or is eliminated (excretion). 2. GLANS. 3. *Obsol.* LYMPH NODE. Adj. *glandular.*

glan·ders (glan′durz) n. A highly contagious acute or chronic disease of horses, mules, and asses, caused by *Pseudomonas mallei* and communicable to dogs, goats, sheep, and man, but not to bovines; characterized by fever, inflammation of mucous membranes (especially of the nose); enlargement and hardening of the regional lymph nodes, formation of nodules which have a tendency to coalesce and then to degenerate to form deep ulcers. In man, the disease runs an acute febrile or a chronic course with granulomas and abscesses in the skin, lungs and elsewhere. Syn. *equinia.*

glan·du·la (glan′dew·luh) n., pl. **glandu·lae** (-lee) GLAND (1).

glan·du·lar (glan′dew·lur) adj. 1. Of or pertaining to a gland or glands. 2. Of or pertaining to the glans of the penis or of the clitoris; BALANIC.

glandular cheilitis. A chronic inflammation of the lower lip; characterized by swelling of the labial mucous glands and their ducts. Syn. *cheilitis glandularis, cheilitis glandularis apostematosa, myxadenitis labialis, Puente's disease.*

glandular epithelium. An epithelium in which the cells are predominantly secretory in function.

glandular fever. INFECTIOUS MONONUCLEOSIS.

glandular tuberculosis. *Obsol.* Tuberculosis affecting the lymph nodes, especially the cervical, bronchial, and mesenteric.

glans (glanz) n., pl. **glan·des** (glan′deez) The conical body that forms the distal end of the clitoris or of the penis.

glans cli·to·ri·dis (kli·tor′i·dis) [NA]. The erectile body at the distal end of the clitoris.

glans pe·nis (pee′nis) [NA]. The erectile body at the distal end of the penis, an expansion of the corpus spongiosum.

Glanzmann's disease THROMBOASTHENIA.

glass·blow·er's cataract. HEAT-RAY CATARACT.

glassblower's disease. Infection of the parotid gland.

glass test. A gross test for localizing infection of the urinary tract, in which the urine is voided in sequential fractions into two or more glass containers.

glassy, adj. 1. Having the appearance of glass; VITREOUS; HYALINE. 2. Expressionless; dull; lifeless (as applied to the appearance of the eyes).

Glau·ber's salt (glaw′bur) SODIUM SULFATE.

glau·co·ma (glaw·ko′muh, glaw·ko′muh) n. An eye disease, the complete clinical picture of which is characterized by increased intraocular pressure, excavation and degeneration of the optic nerve head, and typical nerve fiber bundle defects which produce characteristic defects in the visual field. May be primary, secondary, or congenital.

glau·co·ma·to·cy·clit·ic (glaw·ko″muh·to·si·klit′ick) adj. Pertaining to the combination of increased intraocular tension and inflammation of the ciliary body.

glaucomatocyclitic crisis. A discrete, self-limited form of secondary open-angle glaucoma, usually unilateral and recurrent, characterized by inflammatory signs and usually with no synechias. Inflammation may be confined to the trabecular meshwork.

glau·co·ma·tous (glaw·ko′muh·tus, ·kom′uh·tus) adj. Pertaining to or affected with glaucoma.

glaucomatous cup. A depression in the optic disk seen in cases of glaucoma.

gleet, n. The slight mucopurulent discharge that characterizes the chronic stage of gonorrheal urethritis. —**gleety,** adj.

gleno·hu·mer·al (glen″o·hew′mur·ul, glee″no·) adj. Pertaining to the glenoid cavity and the humerus.

gle·noid (glee′noid, glen′oid) adj. Having a shallow cavity; resembling a shallow cavity or socket.

glenoid cavity. The articular surface on the scapula for articulation with the head of the humerus.

gli-, glio- A combining form meaning (a) gluey, gelatinous; (b) glia, glial, neuroglia.

glia (glye′uh, glee′uh) n. NEUROGLIA.

-glia. A combining form meaning neuroglia of a specified kind or size.

gli·a·din (glye′uh·din) n. A protein derived from gluten of wheat, rye, oats, and other grains.

gli·al (glye′ul, glee′ul) adj. Of or pertaining to neuroglia.

glid·ing joint. A synovial joint that allows only gliding movements; formed by the apposition of plane surfaces, or one slightly convex, the other slightly concave.

gliding movement. The simplest movement that can take place in a joint, one surface gliding or moving over another, without any angular or rotatory movement.

glio·blas·to·ma (glye″o·blas·to′muh, glee″) n. GLIOBLASTOMA MULTIFORME.

glioblastoma mul·ti·for·me (mul″ti·for′mee). A central nervous system tumor whose parenchyma is composed of embryonal astrocytes presenting a pleomorphic appearance, accompanied by necrosis, hemorrhages, and reaction and involvement of connective tissue.

gli·o·ma (glye·o′muh, glee·) n., pl. **gliomas, gli·oma·ta** (·tuh) A tumor composed of cells and fibers representative of the special supporting tissue of the central nervous system, and derived from neuroglial cells or their antecedents; occurs principally in the central nervous system. —**gli·om·a·tous** (·om′uh·tus, ·o′muh·tus) adj.

gli·o·ma·to·sis (glye″o·muh·to′sis, glee·o″) n., pl. **gliomato·ses** (·seez) 1. Multiple hamartomatous nodules of glial cells in the cerebrum. 2. Multifocal gliomas.

gli·o·sis (glye·o′sis, glee·) n., pl. **glio·ses** (·seez) Proliferation of neuroglia in the brain or spinal cord, as a replacement process or a reaction to low-grade inflammation; may be diffuse or focal.

glob·al (glo′bul) adj. 1. Spherical; shaped like a sphere. 2. Total; comprehensive. 3. Of or pertaining to the eyeball.

global aphasia. Loss of both expression and perception of language and communicative skills.

globe, n. 1. A sphere or ball. 2. The earth or the world. 3. In ophthalmology, the eyeball.

globi. 1. Plural of globus. 2. Rounded masses of lepra bacilli, as seen in tissue sections.

glo·bid·i·o·sis (glo·bid″ee·o′sis) n., pl. **globidio·ses** (·seez). BESNOITIOSIS.

glo·bin (glo′bin) n. One of a class of proteins, histone in nature, obtained from the hemoglobins of various animal species; soluble in water, acids, and alkalies and coagulable by heat.

globin zinc insulin. A preparation of insulin modified by the addition of globin (derived from the hemoglobin of beef blood) and zinc chloride; it has intermediate duration of action.

glo·boid (glo′boid) adj. Shaped somewhat like a globe; SPHEROID.

globoid leukodystrophy. A heredodegenerative disease transmitted as an autosomal recessive trait, affecting the nervous system of infants with onset in the first months of life and a rapidly progressive course characterized by fretfulness, blindness, dementia, and rigidity. There is a generalized deficit of myelin, more marked in the central than in the peripheral nervous system. Syn. Krabbe's disease.

glo·bose (glo′boce) adj. GLOBULAR.

globu·lar (glob′yoo·lur) adj. 1. Shaped like a ball or globule. 2. Made up of globules.

globular process. One of the inferior, bilateral bulbous expansions of the median nasal process that fuse in the midline to form the philtrum of the upper lip and adjacent premaxilla.

glob·ule (glob′yool) n. A small spherical droplet of fluid or semifluid material.

glob·u·li·cide (glob′yoo·li·side) n. & adj. 1. An agent that destroys blood cells. 2. Destructive to blood cells. —**glob·u·li·ci·dal** (glob″yoo·li·sigh′dul) adj.

glob·u·lin (glob′yoo·lin) n. Any of a group of animal and plant proteins, including alpha, beta, and gamma globulins, characterized by solubility in dilute salt solutions and differentiated from albumins by lesser solubility, more alkaline isoelectric points, greater molecular weight, faster sedimentation rates, and slower electrophoretic mobilities.

α-**globulin.** ALPHA GLOBULIN.

β-**globulin.** BETA GLOBULIN.

γ-**globulin.** GAMMA GLOBULIN.

glob·u·lin·uria (glob″yoo·li·new′ree·uh) n. The presence of globulins in the urine.

glob·u·lo·max·il·lary (glob″yoo·lo·mack′si·lerr·ee) adj. Pertaining to the globular and maxillary processes.

globulomaxillary cyst. A cystic embryonal inclusion in the alveolar process between upper lateral incisor and canine teeth, at the site of fusion of the globular and maxillary processes of the upper jaw.

glo·bus (glo′bus) n., pl. **glo·bi** (·bye) A ball or globe.

globus hys·ter·i·cus (hi·sterr′i·kus). The choking sensation, or so-called lump in the throat, occurring in hysteria.

globus pal·li·dus (pal′i·dus) [NA]. The inner and lighter part of the lenticular nucleus of the corpus striatum.

glo·man·gi·o·ma (glo″man·jee·o′muh) *n.* GLOMUS TUMOR.

glom·er·ate (glom′ur·ut, ·ate) *adj.* Rolled together like a ball of thread.

glomerul-, glomerulo-. A combining form meaning *glomerulus, glomerular.*

glo·mer·u·lar (glom·err′yoo·lur) *adj.* Pertaining to, produced by, or involving a glomerulus.

glomerular capsule. The sac surrounding the glomerulus of the kidney; the first part of the uriniferous tubule. Syn. *Bowman's capsule.*

glomeruli. Plural of *glomerulus.*

glo·mer·u·li·tis (glo·merr″yoo·lye′tis) *n.* Inflammation of renal glomeruli, one or more than one.

glo·mer·u·lo·ne·phri·tis (glom·err″yoo·lo·ne·frye′tis) *n.* An acute, subacute, or chronic, usually bilateral, diffuse nonsuppurative inflammatory kidney disease primarily affecting the glomeruli; characterized by proteinuria, cylindruria, hematuria, and often edema, hypertension, and nitrogen retention.

glo·mer·u·lo·scle·ro·sis (glom·err″yoo·lo·skle·ro′sis) *n.* Fibrosis of the renal glomeruli.

glo·mer·u·lus (glom·err′yoo·lus) *n.,* pl. **glo·mer·u·li** (·lye) 1. A small rounded mass. 2. [NA]. The tuft of capillary loops projecting into the lumen of a renal corpuscle.

glo·mus (glo′mus) *n.,* pl. **glom·er·a** (glom′ur·uh) 1. A small mass of tissue composed of a tuft of small arterioles connected with veins and having an abundant nerve supply. 2. A prominent portion of the choroid plexus of the lateral ventricle located at the beginning of the inferior horn. —**glo·mic** (·mick) *adj.*

glomus bodies. Arteriovenous anastomoses that have a special arrangement of muscle and nerve tissue; usually present in the cutis and subcutis of fingers and toes.

glomus coc·cy·ge·um (kock·sij′ee·um) [BNA]. CORPUS COCCYGEUM.

glomus ju·gu·la·re (jug·yoo·lair′ee). Any of a number of tiny masses of epithelioid tissue similar in structure to that of the carotid body, usually situated in the adventitia of the superior bulb of the internal jugular vein.

glomus jugulare tumor. A tumor histologically resembling a carotid body tumor, arising mainly in the dome of the jugular bulb but also in many other sites in and around the temporal bone. The clinical syndrome consists of slowly progressive deafness, facial palsy, dysphagia, and unilateral atrophy of the tongue, combined with a vascular polyp in the external auditory meatus.

glomus tumor. A tumor derived from an arteriovenous plexus of the skin, especially of the digits; usually small, blue, painful, and benign.

gloss-, glosso-. A combining form meaning (a) *tongue;* (b) *language.*

glos·sa (glos′uh) *n.,* pl. & genit. sing. **glos·sae** (·ee) TONGUE. —**glos·sal** (·ul) *adj.*

-glossa A combining form meaning *tongue.*

glos·sal·gia (glos·al′jee·uh) *n.* Pain in the tongue.

glos·sec·to·my (glos·eck′tuh·mee) *n.* Excision of the tongue.

-glossia A combining form meaning *condition of the tongue.*

Glos·si·na (glos·eye′nuh) *n.* A genus of bloodsucking flies, known as tsetse flies; confined to tropical and subtropical Africa. The species *Glossina fusca, G. palpalis,* and *G. morsitans* transmit the trypanosomes of sleeping sickness in man and of nagana and the souma disease of horses, cattle, and sheep.

glos·si·tis (glos·eye′tis) *n.* Inflammation of the tongue. —**glos·sit·ic** (glos·it′ick) *adj.*

glos·so·dyn·ia (glos″o·din′ee·uh) *n.* Pain in the tongue.

glos·so·epi·glot·tic (glos″o·ep·i·glot′ick) *adj.* Pertaining to the tongue and epiglottis.

glos·so·hy·al (glos″o·high′ul) *adj.* Pertaining to the tongue and the hyoid bone.

glos·so·kin·es·thet·ic, glos·so·kin·aes·thet·ic (glos″o·kin″es·thet′ick) *adj.* Pertaining to the sensations produced by the motions of the tongue in speech.

glos·so·la·bi·al (glos″o·lay′bee·ul) *adj.* Relating to the tongue and lips.

glos·so·la·bio·la·ryn·ge·al (glos″o·lay″bee·o·la·rin′jee·ul) *adj.* Pertaining to the tongue, lips, and larynx.

glos·so·la·lia (glos″o·lay′lee·uh) *n.* Gibberish, jargon; speech simulating an unknown foreign language.

glos·so·pal·a·tine (glos″o·pal′uh·tine, ·tin) *adj.* PALATOGLOSSAL.

glos·so·pal·a·to·la·bi·al (glos″o·pal″uh·to·lay′bee·ul) *adj.* Pertaining to the tongue, palate, and lips.

glos·so·pha·ryn·ge·al (glos″o·fa·rin′jee·ul) *adj.* Pertaining to tongue and pharynx.

glossopharyngeal nerve. The ninth cranial nerve with motor, sensory (special and visceral), and parasympathetic components. Motor fibers pass from the nucleus ambiguus to the stylopharyngeus and muscles of the soft palate and pharynx; sensory fibers supply the posterior third of the tongue and taste buds there, the pharynx, middle ear and mastoid air cells; parasympathetic fibers pass from the inferior salivatory nucleus via the otic ganglion to the parotid gland.

glos·so·pha·ryn·geo·la·bi·al (glos″o·fa·rin″jee·o·lay′bee·ul) *adj.* Pertaining to the tongue, pharynx, and lips.

glos·so·pha·ryn·ge·us (glos″o·fa·rin′jee·us) *n.* PARS GLOSSOPHARYNGEA MUSCULI CONSTRICTORIS PHARYNGIS SUPERIORIS.

glos·so·plas·ty (glos″o·plas′tee) *n.* Plastic surgery of the tongue.

glos·sop·to·sis (glos″op·to′sis) *n.* Downward displacement or a dropping backward of the tongue, usually secondary to underdevelopment of the mandible as in the Robin syndrome.

glos·sor·rha·phy (glos·or′uh·fee) *n.* Surgical suturing of the tongue.

glos·sot·o·my (glos·ot′uh·mee) *n.* 1. The dissection of the tongue. 2. An incision of the tongue.

glot·tal (glot'ul) *adj.* Of or pertaining to the glottis.

glot·tic (glot'ick) *adj.* GLOTTAL.

glot·tis (glot'is) *n.,* genit. **glot·ti·dis** (·i·dis), L. pl. **glot·ti·des** (·i·deez) The two vocal folds and the space (rima glottidis) between them.

glove-and-stocking anesthesia or **hypalgesia.** Distal, symmetrical loss or diminution of sensation in the hands and feet corresponding more or less to the area covered by gloves and stockings; may accompany inflammatory or degenerative diseases affecting peripheral nerves. Absolute loss of all sensations in such a distribution, unaccompanied by objective neurologic findings, is usually a hysterical phenomenon.

gluc-, gluco-. A combining form meaning *glucose.*

glu·ca·gon, glu·ca·gone (gloo'kuh·gon) *n.* A polypeptide hormone composed of 29 amino acid residues, secreted by the alpha cells of the islets of Langerhans. Its primary effect is to elevate blood glucose concentration through an adenyl cyclase-dependent mobilization of hepatic glycogen. Its other effects include inhibition of fatty acid synthesis and stimulation of ketone body production. Syn. *hyperglycemic factor, hyperglycemic-glycogenolytic factor, glycogenolytic hormone.*

glu·case (gloo'kace) *n.* Obsol. An enzyme that converts starch into glucose.

glu·cide (gloo'side) *n.* A group term for carbohydrates and glycosides. —**glu·cid·ic** (gloo·sid'ick) *adj.*

glu·co·cor·ti·coid (gloo"ko·kor'ti·koid) *n.* 1. An adrenal cortex hormone, such as cortisol, that affects the metabolism of glucose. 2. Any related natural or synthetic substance that functions similarly.

glu·co·ki·nase (gloo"ko·kigh'nace, ·naze, ·kin'ace, ·aze) *n.* An enzyme, present in liver, which in the course of glycogenesis catalyzes phosphorylation of D-glucose, by adenosine triphosphate, to glucose 6-phosphate.

glu·co·neo·gen·e·sis (gloo"ko·nee"o·jen'e·sis) *n.* The formation of glucose by the liver from noncarbohydrate sources.

glu·con·ic acid (gloo·kon'ick). D-Gluconic acid, $C_6H_{12}O_7$, resulting from oxidation of dextrose and other sugars. Several of its salts, notably calcium gluconate and ferrous gluconate, are used medicinally.

glu·co·no·ki·nase (gloo"kuh·no·kigh'nace, ·naze, ·kin'ace) *n.* An enzyme, present in microorganisms, in muscle, and in liver, which catalyzes phosphorylation of D-gluconic acid, by adenosine triphosphate, to 6-phospho-D-gluconic acid.

glu·co·no·lac·tone (gloo"kuh·no·lack'tone) *n.* A ring form of D-gluconic acid.

glu·co·py·ra·nose (gloo"ko·pye'ruh·noce) *n.* A cyclic form of glucose having a pyranose structure in which carbon atoms 1 and 5 are bridged by an oxygen atom.

glu·co·sa·mine (gloo"ko·suh·meen', ·sam'in) *n.* An amino sugar, $C_6H_{13}NO_5$, derived from D-glucose; it is a structural component of chitin, chondroitin, and heparin, and occurs also in mucus, fungi, and lichens. Syn. *2-aminoglucose, chitosamine, glycosamine.*

glu·co·san (gloo'ko·san) *n.* A polysaccharide that yields glucose on hydrolysis.

glu·cose (gloo'koce, ·koze) *n.* 1. The crystalline monosaccharide dextrose, $C_6H_{12}O_6$, sometimes called dextro-glucose, but properly designated D-glucose. 2. A product obtained by the incomplete hydrolysis of starch, consisting chiefly of dextrose (D-glucose), dextrins, maltose, and water; being liquid, it is more correctly designated liquid glucose; employed for its food value, local dehydrating effect, and diuretic action, and in various pharmaceutical and industrial manufacturing operations.

D-glucose. DEXTROSE.

glucose 6-phosphatase. An enzyme, found in liver but not in muscle, which catalyzes the hydrolysis of glucose 6-phosphate to free glucose and inorganic phosphate; important in the conversion of glycogen to glucose and in the process of gluconeogenesis.

glucose 6-phosphate. Glucose 6-phosphoric acid, $C_6H_{13}O_9P$, an ester intermediate formed in the biochemical interactions of glucose. Syn. *Robison ester.*

glucose tolerance test. Evaluation of the ability of the body to metabolize glucose by administration of a standard dose of glucose to a fasting individual and measurement of blood and urine glucose at regular intervals thereafter.

glu·co·si·dase (gloo·ko'si·dace, ·daze) *n.* 1. An enzyme that catalyzes the hydrolysis of glucosides. 2. EMULSIN.

glu·co·side (gloo'ko·side) *n.* 1. Any member of a series of compounds, usually of plant origin, that may be hydrolyzed into dextrose (D-glucose) and another principle; the latter is often referred to as an aglycone. 2. Any substance, commonly a plant principle, which on hydrolysis yields a sugar and another principle.

glu·co·sin (gloo'ko·sin) *n.* Any one of a series of bases obtained by the action of ammonia on dextrose.

glu·cos·uria (gloo"ko·syoo'ree·uh) *n.* Glucose in the urine.

glu·cu·ron·ic acid (gloo"kew·ron'ick). D-Glucuronic acid, $C_6H_{10}O_7$, the acid resulting from oxidation of the CH_2OH group of D-glucose to COOH; a component of many polysaccharides, and certain vegetable gums. It is a conjugating compound in the metabolism and excretion of many medicinal substances, forming glucuronides. Syn. *glycuronic acid.*

glu·cu·ron·i·dase (gloo"kew·ron'i·dace, ·daze) *n.* An enzyme that catalyzes hydrolysis of glucuronides. Syn. *glycuronidase.*

glu·cu·ro·nide (gloo·kew'ro·nide) *n.* A compound resulting from the interaction, commonly referred to as conjugation, of glucuronic acid with a phenol, an alcohol, or an acid containing a carboxyl group. In man, many of these substances are excreted in the form of glucuronides. Syn. *conjugated glucuronate, glycuronide.*

glu·ta·mate (gloo'tuh-mate) n. A salt of glutamic acid.

glu·tam·ic acid (gloo-tam'ick) 2-Aminopentane-dioic acid or α-aminoglutaric acid, $C_5H_9NO_4$, an amino acid obtained on hydrolysis of various proteins. The sodium salt of the naturally occurring L- form of glutamic acid is used for symptomatic treatment of encephalopathies associated with diseases of the liver and for various other therapeutic purposes; it imparts a meat flavor to foods. Syn. *glutaminic acid.*

glu·tam·ic·ac·i·de·mia, glu·tam·ic·ac·i·dae·mia (glew·tam·ick·as''i-dee'mee·uh) n. An inborn error of metabolism in which there is an increased amount of glutamic acid in plasma and a slight generalized increase in total urinary amino nitrogen; characterized clinically by sparse, coarse unpigmented hair, mental retardation, failure to thrive, and various congenital malformations.

glutamic-oxaloacetic transaminase. An enzyme that catalyzes transfer of the amino group of glutamic acid to oxaloacetic acid, forming α-ketoglutaric acid and aspartic acid. Measurement of the levels of this enzyme in serum is of importance in the diagnosis of liver disease and myocardial infarction. Abbreviated, GOT. Syn. *glutamic-aspartic transaminase, aspartate aminotransferase, l-aspartate:2-oxoglutarate aminotransferase.*

glutamic-pyruvic transaminase. An enzyme that catalyzes transfer of the amino group of glutamic acid to pyruvic acid, forming α-ketoglutaric acid and L-alanine. Measurement of the levels of this enzyme in serum is of importance in the diagnosis of hepatocellular injury. Abbreviated, GPT. Syn. *glutamic-alanine transaminase, alanine aminotransferase, l-alanine:2-oxoglutarate aminotransferase.*

glu·tam·i·nase (gloo-tam'i·nace, ·naze) n. The enzyme that catalyzes the conversion of glutamine to glutamic acid and ammonia.

glu·ta·mine (gloo'tuh-meen, ·min) n. The monamide of glutamic acid, $C_5H_{10}N_2O_3$, found in many plant and animal tissues.

glutamine synthetase. An enzyme catalyzing the formation of glutamine from glutamic acid and ammonia, using ATP as a source of energy.

glu·ta·ral (gloo'tuh-ral) n. $C_5H_8O_2$, an effective agent against bacteria and spores; employed for cold sterilization of surgical instruments.

glu·tar·al·de·hyde (gloo''tuh-ral'de·hide) n. GLUTARAL.

glu·tar·ic acid (gloo·tăr'ick, ·tahr'ick). Pentane-dioic acid or 1,3-propanedicarboxylic acid, $C_5H_8O_4$, a constituent of beets and crude wool; formed from lysine by liver homogenates of certain animals.

glu·ta·thi·one (gloo''tuh·thigh'ohn) n. The tripeptide γ-L-glutamyl-L-cysteinylglycine, $C_{10}H_{17}N_3O_6S$, widely distributed in plant and animal tissues. It is important in tissue oxidations, acting through the sulfhydryl group (—SH) with the formation of disulfide (—S—S—) in oxidation and reduction. Syn. *GSH.*

glu·te·al (gloo·tee'ul, gloo'tee·ul) adj. Pertaining to the buttocks.

gluteal fold. The crease between the buttock and thigh.

glu·ten (gloo'tin) n. A mixture of gliadin and glutelin types of proteins found in the seeds of cereals; imparts cohesiveness to dough.

gluten bread. Bread made from wheat flour from which all the starch has been removed; used as a substitute for ordinary bread in diabetes.

gluten sensitivity. Hypersensitivity to the gliadin fraction of gluten, leading to infantile celiac disease and some cases of sprue.

glu·teo·fas·cial (gloo'tee·o·fash'ee·ul) adj. Pertaining to the gluteus maximus and the deep fascia of the thigh.

glu·teo·fem·o·ral (gloo''tee·o·fem'o·rul) adj. Pertaining to the gluteal muscles and the femur.

glu·teo·tro·chan·ter·ic (gloo''tee·o·tro''kan·terr'ick) adj. Pertaining to the gluteal muscles and the greater trochanter of the femur.

glu·teth·i·mide (gloo·teth'i·mide) n. 2-Ethyl-2-phenylglutarimide, $C_{13}H_{15}NO_2$, a central nervous system depressant used as a short-acting sedative and hypnotic.

glu·te·us, glu·tae·us (gloo·tee'us, gloo·tee'us) n. & adj., pl. & genit. sing. **glu·tei, glu·taei** (gloo·tee'eye, gloo'tee·eye) Being or pertaining to any of the three large muscles of the buttock.

gluteus max·i·mus (mack'si·mus). The largest and most superficial gluteal muscle.

glu·tin (gloo'tin) n. 1. A protein obtained from gelatin. 2. VEGETABLE CASEIN.

glu·ti·nous (gloo'ti·nus) adj. VISCID; gluelike.

glut·tony (glut'un·ee) n. Excessive indulgence in eating.

glyc-, glyco- A combining form meaning (a) *sweet;* (b) *sugar;* or sometimes specifically (c) *glucose;* (d) *glycerin;* (e) *glycine.*

gly·case (glye'kase, ·kaze) n. MALTASE.

gly·ce·mia, gly·cae·mia (glye·see'mee·uh) n. 1. The presence of glucose in the blood. 2. HYPERGLYCEMIA.

glyc·er·al·de·hyde (glis''ur·al'de·hide) n. The simplest aldose exhibiting optical activity, formed by mild oxidation of glycerin. It exists as D-glyceraldehyde, as L-glyceraldehyde, or as a racemic mixture of the two (DL-glyceraldehyde). The D- and L- forms are the configurational reference standards for carbohydrates. Glyceraldehyde and phosphoric acid derivatives of it are intermediates in certain biochemical reactions of carbohydrates. Syn. *glyceric aldehyde.*

glyc·er·ide (glis'ur·ide, ·id) n. Any ester of glycerin and an organic acid radical. Fats are glycerides of certain long-chain organic acids.

glyc·er·in, glyc·er·ine (glis'ur·in) n. 1. Trihydroxypropane, $C_3H_5(OH)_3$, a clear, colorless, syrupy liquid of sweet taste, miscible with water. Obtained by hydrolysis of fats, and also by synthesis, it is the manufactured form of the natural substance glycerol. Used as a vehicle, emollient, and, rectally, as a laxative, particularly in the form of suppositories. 2. British term for GLYCERITE.

glyc·er·ite (glis'ur·ite) n. A solution of one or more medicinal substances in glycerin.

glyc·ero·gel·a·tin (glis''ur·o·jel'uh·tin) n. One of a class of pharmaceutical preparations composed of glycerin, gelatin, water, and one or more medicinal substances; they are soft solids, melting at body temperature, and can be applied to the skin or molded as suppositories.

glyc·er·ol (glis'ur·ole, ·ol) n. Trihydroxypropane, $C_3H_5(OH)_3$, an important intermediate component in carbohydrate and lipid metabolism.

glyc·ero·phos·pha·tase (glis''ur·o·fos'fuh·tace, ·taze) n. An enzyme, found in pancreatic juice, and generally in cells, capable of liberating phosphoric acid from glycerophosphoric acid and certain of its derivatives.

glyc·er·yl (glis'ur·il) n. The trivalent radical, $C_3H_5\equiv$, combined with fatty acids in fats and in animal and vegetable oils.

glyceryl trinitrate. NITROGLYCERIN.

gly·cine (glye'seen, ·sin) n. Aminoethanoic acid, NH_2CH_2COOH, a nonessential amino acid. It is a constituent of many proteins from which it may be obtained by hydrolysis. It has been used for treatment of muscular dystrophy and myasthenia gravis. Syn. *aminoacetic acid.*

gly·ci·nu·ria (glye''si·new'ree·uh) n. A defect in renal tubular reabsorption, associated with many disorders resulting in the presence of large amounts of glycine in the urine.

glyco-. See glyc-.

gly·co·bi·ar·sol (glye''ko·bye·ahr'sol) n. Bismuthyl N-glycoloylarsanilate, $C_8H_9AsBiNO_6$, an amebicide employed only for treatment of intestinal amebiasis.

gly·co·cho·late (glye''ko·ko'late, ·kol'ate) n. Any salt of glycocholic acid.

gly·co·cho·lic acid (glye''ko·kol'ick, ·ko'lick). An acid, $C_{26}H_{43}NO_6$, obtained by the conjugation of cholic acid with glycine; found in bile.

gly·co·gen (glye'kuh·jin) n. A polysaccharide, $(C_6H_{10}O_5)_n$, in liver cells, all tissues in the embryo, testes, muscles, leukocytes, fresh pus cells, cartilage, and other tissues. It is formed from carbohydrates and is stored in the liver, where it is converted, as the system requires, into sugar (glucose). Syn. *animal starch.*

gly·co·ge·nase (glye'ko·je·nace, glye·koj'e·nace) n. An enzyme found in the liver, which hydrolyzes glycogen to maltose and dextrin.

gly·co·gen·e·sis (glye''ko·jen'e·sis) n. The process of formation of glycogen in the animal body. —**glyco·ge·net·ic** (·je·net'ick), **gly·cog·e·nous** (glye·koj'e·nus) adj.

gly·co·gen·ic (glye''ko·jen'ick) adj. Pertaining to glycogen or to glycogenesis.

gly·co·gen·ol·y·sis (glye''ko·je·nol'i·sis) n., pl. **glycogenol·y·ses** (·seez) The liberation of glucose from glycogen in the liver or other tissues. —**gly·co·gen·o·lyt·ic** (·jen''uh·lit'ick) adj.

gly·co·gen·o·sis (glye''ko·je·no'sis) n., pl. **glycogeno·ses** (·seez) One of several inborn errors in the metabolism of glycogen, classified on the basis of the enzyme deficiency and clinical findings by the Coris as: type I, von Gierke's disease; type II, Pompe's disease; type III, limit dextrinosis; type IV, amylopectinosis; type V, McArdle's disease; type VI, Hers' disease.

glycogen storage disease. 1. GLYCOGENOSIS. 2. VON GIERKE'S DISEASE.

gly·col (glye'kol) n. 1. Any dihydric aliphatic alcohol. 2. ETHYLENE GLYCOL.

gly·col·ic acid (glye·kol'ick). Hydroxyacetic acid, $CH_2OHCOOH$, a possible intermediate in protein metabolism.

glycolic aciduria. OXALOSIS, type I.

gly·co·lip·id, gly·co·lip·ide (glye''ko·lip'id) n. Any cerebroside or similar lipid.

gly·col·y·sis (glye·kol'i·sis) n., pl. **glycoly·ses** (·seez) The process of conversion of carbohydrate, in tissues, to pyruvic acid or lactic acid, with release of energy. Commonly it is considered to begin with hydrolysis of glycogen to glucose (glycogenolysis), which subsequently undergoes a series of chemical changes. —**gly·co·lyt·ic** (glye''ko·lit'ick) adj.

gly·co·me·tab·o·lism (glye''ko·me·tab'uh·liz·um) n. The metabolism of sugar in the body. —**gly·co·met·a·bol·ic** (·met''uh·bol'ick) adj.

gly·co·pe·nia (glye''ko·pee'nee·uh) n. HYPOGLYCEMIA.

gly·co·pro·tein (glye''ko·pro'teen, ·pro'tee·in) n. One of a group of conjugated proteins which upon decomposition yield a protein and a carbohydrate, or derivatives of the same.

gly·co·pty·a·lism (glye''ko·tye'uh·liz·um) n. Excretion of glucose in the saliva.

gly·cor·rha·chia (glye''ko·ray'kee·uh, ·rack'ee·uh) n. 1. Glucose in the cerebrospinal fluid. 2. HYPERGLYCORRHACHIA.

gly·cor·rhea, gly·cor·rhoea (glye''ko·ree'uh) n. Discharge of sugar-containing fluid from the body.

gly·co·si·al·ia (gly''ko·sigh·al'ee·uh, ·ay'lee·uh) n. The presence of glucose in the saliva.

gly·co·side (glye'ko·side) n. Any natural or synthetic compound that yields on hydrolysis a sugar and another substance designated as an aglycone. In order to indicate the specific sugar which is formed, a more descriptive term such as glucoside or galactoside may be used. Many glycosides are therapeutically valuable. —**gly·co·si·dal** (glye''ko·sigh'dul), **gly·co·sid·ic** (·sid'ick) adj.

gly·co·sphin·go·lip·id (glye''ko·sfing''go·lip'id) n. A sphingolipid containing galactose or glucose.

gly·cos·uria (glye''ko·syoor'ee·uh) n. The presence of sugar in the urine. —**glycos·uric** (·syoor'ick) adj.

gly·cu·ro·nu·ria (glye''kew·ro·new'ree·uh) n. The presence of glucuronic acid in the urine.

gly·cyl (glye'sil) n. The univalent radical $H_2NCH_2CO—$, of the amino acid glycine.

glyc·yr·rhi·za (glis''i·rye'zuh) n. The dried rhizome and roots of several varieties of *Glycyrrhiza glabra*. Glycyrrhiza extract is used as a flavor. Glycyrrhiza fluid extract is used as a vehicle. Compound opium and glycyrrhiza mixture, called brown mixture, is an expectorant. Glycyrrhiza elixir is used as a vehicle for disguising the taste of bitter substances. Syn. *licorice.*

glyc·yr·rhi·zic acid (glis''i·rye'zick). A crystalline glycoside, $C_{42}H_{62}O_{16}$, salts of which occur in glycyrrhiza; on hydrolysis it yields two molecules of glucuronic acid and one molecule of glycyrrhetinic acid. It appears to have certain of the physiologic actions of deoxycorticosterone.

gly·ox·a·lase (glye·ock'suh·lace, ·laze) *n.* An enzyme present in various body tissues which catalyzes the conversion of methylglyoxal into lactic acid.

gly·ox·al·ic acid (glye''ock·sal'ick). GLYOXYLIC ACID.

Gm, gm A former abbreviation for *gram.*

G$_{M1}$ gangliosidosis. Any disorder of the breakdown of the ganglioside G$_{M1}$. G$_{M1}$ gangliosidoses are due to deficiency of the enzyme ganglioside G$_{M1}$ β-galactosidase, and have been recognized in both infantile (type 1) and juvenile (type 2) forms. The clinical picture in both includes bony deformities and mental and motor deterioration progressing to decerebrate rigidity and death; pathological findings include neuronal lipidosis, visceral histiocytosis, and renal glomerular cytoplasmic ballooning.

G$_{M2}$ gangliosidosis. Any disorder of the breakdown of the ganglioside G$_{M2}$. G$_{M2}$ gangliosidoses are due to deficiency of one or both of two enzymes, hexosaminidase A and B. Two infantile forms (type 1, or Tay-Sachs disease, and type 2, or Sandhoff's disease) and a juvenile form (type 3) are recognized.

gnat, *n.* Any of various small pestiferous dipteran insects such as black flies, biting midges, sand flies, or (in British usage) mosquitos.

gnath-, gnatho- A combining form meaning *jaw* or *jaws.*

gnath·ic (nath'ick, nay'thick) *adj.* Pertaining to a jaw, or the jaws.

gnatho·dy·na·mom·e·ter (nath''o·dye''nuh·mom'e·tur) *n.* An instrument for recording the force of the bite by measuring the pressure exerted on two rubber pads. Syn. *occlusometer.*

gnatho·plas·ty (nay'tho·plas''tee, nath''o·) *n.* Plastic surgery of the cheek or jaw.

gna·thos·chi·sis (na·thos'ki·sis) *n.* Cleft alveolar process, or jaw.

Gna·thos·to·ma (na·thos'to·muh) *n.* A genus of nematode worms of the family Gnathostomatidae.

gna·thos·to·mi·a·sis (na·thos''to·mye'uh·sis) *n.* Infection with *Gnathostoma spinigerum* larvae; deep burrows, boils, and abscesses in the skin are caused by this parasite.

gno·sis (no'sis) *n.*, pl. **gno·ses** (·seez) The faculty of knowing in contradistinction to the function of feeling, in respect to any external stimulus.

gnos·tic (nos'tick) *adj.* Pertaining to discriminative or epicritic sensations in contradistinction to vital or protopathic sensations.

gno·to·bi·ot·ics (no''to·bye·ot'icks) *n.* The science of raising germ-free animals into which a defined microflora is introduced. —**gnotobiot·ic** (·ick), *adj.*; **gnoto·bi·ote** (·bye'ote) *n.*

Goa powder (go'uh) ARAROBA.

goat·pox, *n.* A cutaneous viral disease of goats in Europe, North Africa, and the Middle East, characterized by vesicular skin lesions.

gob·let cell. One of the unicellular mucous glands found in the epithelium of certain mucous membranes, such as those of the respiratory passages and the intestine.

goi·ter, goi·tre (goy'tur) *n.* Enlargement of the thyroid gland; characterized as aberrant when the gland is supernumerary or ectopic.

goiter heart. A condition characterized by atrial fibrillation, cardiac enlargement, and congestive cardiac failure; due to hyperthyroidism. Syn. *thyroid heart, thyrotoxic heart.*

goi·tro·gen·ic (goy''tro·jen'ick) *adj.* Producing goiter; such as iodine-deficient diets or, experimentally, diets of cabbage and other *Brassica* plants, or administration of sulfonamides or drugs of the thiourea group. —**goi·tro·gen** (goy'tro·gen) *n.*

goi·trous (goy'trus) *adj.* Pertaining to or afflicted with goiter.

gold, *n.* Au = 196.967. A yellow metallic element, easily malleable and ductile. Gold salts are used principally for treatment of rheumatoid arthritis.

gold Au 198. The radioactive isotope of gold of mass number 198, with a half-life of 2.70 days, used in colloidal solution, by injection, principally for irradiation of closed serous cavities in palliative treatment of ascites and pleural effusion associated with metastatic malignancies.

Goldblatt kidney A kidney to which blood flow is reduced by various experimental procedures in animals or by vascular disease in man. Such kidneys may be associated with hypertension, attributed either to release of vasoconstrictor substances by the kidney or to failure of the ischemic kidney to oppose the action of endogenous vasoconstrictor substances.

gold·en·rod, *n.* The common name for several species of the genus *Solidago* of the Compositae.

gold sodium thiomalate. [(1,2-Dicarboxyethyl)·thio] gold disodium salt, C$_4$H$_3$AuNa$_2$O$_4$S·H$_2$O, a white to yellowish-white powder, very soluble in water, used in the treatment of rheumatoid arthritis.

gold sodium thiosulfate. Na$_3$Au(S$_2$O$_3$)$_2$·2H$_2$O, sodium aurothiosulfate, occurring in white crystals, freely soluble in water; used for treatment of rheumatoid arthritis.

Gol·gi apparatus (gohl'jee) An organelle, present in the centrosome of virtually all cells but prominent in secretory cells, which encloses secretory material in membrane and may also add a carbohydrate moiety thereto; can be visualized by light microscopy as a branched or reticular apparatus associated with vesicles; by electron microscopy it commonly appears as an array of parallel crescentic membranes about 60Å in thickness, but also frequently as flattened sacs or vesicles and vacuoles of diverse size.

Golgi cells Nerve cells of two types: type I, those with long axons; and type II, those with short axons that branch repeatedly and terminate near the cell body.

Golgi complex. GOLGI APPARATUS.

gom·phi·a·sis (gom·fye'uh·sis) *n.* Obsol. Looseness of the teeth in their sockets; PERIODONTO-SIS.

gom·pho·sis (gom-fo'sis) *n.*, pl. **gompho·ses** (·seez) A form of synarthrosis, as a tooth in its alveolus.

gon-, gono- A combining form meaning (a) *sexual, generative*; (b) *seed, semen*; (c) *genitalia.*

gon·a·cra·tia (gon''uh-kray'shuh) *n.* SPERMATOR-RHEA.

go·nad (go'nad) *n.* 1. A gland or organ producing gametes; a general term for ovary or testis. 2. The embryonic sex gland before morphologic identification as ovary or testis is possible. Syn. *indifferent gonad.* —**go·nad·al** (go-nad' ul) *adj.*

gonadal dysgenesis, aplasia, or **hypoplasia.** A chromosomal disorder resulting in failure of the development of the gonads, characterized clinically by various combinations of short stature, webbed neck, deformities of the chest, spine, and extremities, particularly cubitus valgus; abnormalities of skin, face, ears, eyes, and palate; cardiac anomalies; lymphedema of the hands and feet; sexual infantilism; and elevated excretion of urinary gonadotropin. Usually there is a 45,X chromosome complement or sometimes mosaicism. Syn. *Bonnevie-Ullrich syndrome. Turner's syndrome. XO syndrome.*

go·nad·ec·to·my (go''nad.eck'tuh.mee) *n.* In surgery, removal of a gonad.

go·na·do·blas·to·ma (go·nad''o·blas·to'muh, gon''uh.do·) *n.* A complex ovarian neoplasm containing primitive sex cords, germ cells, and mesenchyme; occasionally associated with defeminization.

go·nad·o·cen·tric (go·nad''o·sen'trick, gon''uh.do·) *adj.* Relating to a focusing of the libido upon the genitalia; a phase of psychosexual development normally occurring in puberty.

go·nad·o·rel·in (go·nad''o·rel'in) *n.* A polypeptide, $C_{55}H_{75}N_{17}O_{13}$, obtained from sheep or swine, used as the acetate or hydrochloride; a gonad-stimulating principle.

go·na·do·ther·a·py (go·nad''o·therr'uh.pee, gon''uh.do·) *n.* Treatment with gonadal extracts or hormones.

go·na·do·tro·phin (go·nad''o·tro'fin, gon''uh.do·) *n.* GONADOTROPIN.

gonadotropic hormone. Any gonad-stimulating hormone.

go·na·do·tro·pin (go·nad''o·tro'pin, gon''uh.do·) *n.* A gonad-stimulating hormone, the principal sources of which are the adenohypophysis of various animal species, the urine of pregnant women (chorionic gonadotropin), and the serum of pregnant mares (serum gonadotropin). —**gonado·trop·ic** (·trop'ick, ·tro'pick) *adj.*

gona·duct, gono·duct (gon'uh·dukt) *n.* The duct of a gonad; oviduct or sperm duct.

go·nag·ra (go·nag'ruh, go·nay'gruh) *n.* Gout of the knee joint.

go·nal·gia (go·nal'jee·uh) *n.* Pain in the knee joint.

gon·an·gi·ec·to·my (gon''an·jee·eck'tuh·mee) *n.* Excision of part of the ductus deferens; VASEC-TOMY.

gon·ar·thri·tis (gon''ahr·thrye'tis) *n.* Inflammation of the knee joint.

gon·ar·throt·o·my (gon''ahr·throt'uh·mee) *n.* Incision into the knee joint.

go·nato·cele (go·nat'o·seel) *n.* A swelling or tumor of the knee.

gon·e·cyst (gon'e·sist) *n.* SEMINAL VESICLE. —**gon·e·cys·tic** (gon''e·sis'tick) *adj.*

gon·e·cys·ti·tis (gon''e·sis·tye'tis) *n.* Inflammation of the seminal vesicles.

gon·e·cys·to·lith (gon''e·sis'to·lith) *n. Obsol.* A concretion or calculus in a seminal vesicle.

gon·e·cys·to·py·o·sis (gon''e·sis''to·pye·o'sis) *n. Obsol.* Suppuration of a seminal vesicle.

gon·gy·lo·ne·mi·a·sis (gon''ji·lo·ne·migh'uh·sis) *n.* Infection with filarial nematodes of the genus *Gongylonema.*

goni-, gonio- A combining form meaning (a) *corner, angle*; (b) *gonion.*

go·ni·al (go'nee·ul) *adj.* Of or pertaining to the gonion.

gon·ic (gon'ick) *adj.* Pertaining to semen or to generation.

go·nio·chei·los·chi·sis (go''nee·o·kigh·los'ki·sis) *n.* TRANSVERSE FACIAL CLEFT.

go·ni·om·e·ter (go''nee·om'e·tur) *n.* An instrument for measuring angles, as the angle of the mandible.

go·ni·on (go'nee·on) *n.*, pl. **go·nia** In craniometry, the tip of the angle of the mandible.

go·nio·punc·ture (go'nee·o·punk''chur) *n.* A filtering operation for congenital glaucoma achieved by puncturing the filtration angle with a goniotomy knife and extending it through the sclera.

go·nio·scope (go'nee·o·skope) *n.* A special optical instrument for studying in detail the angle of the anterior chamber of the eye. —**go·ni·os·co·py** (go''nee·os'kuh·pee) *n.*

go·ni·ot·o·my (go''nee·ot'uh·mee) *n.* An operation for congenital glaucoma in which a segment of the angle is swept with a goniotomy knife in order to cut through mesodermal remnants, allow the iris to fall back, and enable the drainage angle to function.

go·ni·tis (go·nigh'tis) *n.* Inflammation of the knee joint.

gono·coc·cal (gon''uh·kock'ul) *adj.* Of, pertaining to, or caused by gonococci.

gonococcal salpingitis. Salpingitis due to infection with gonococci.

gonococcal urethritis. Urethritis due to infection with gonococci.

gonococcal vaginitis. Vaginitis due to infection with gonococci.

gono·coc·ce·mia, gono·coc·cae·mia (gon''o·cock·see'mee·uh) *n.* The presence of gonococci in the blood.

gonococci. Plural of *gonococcus.*

gono·coc·cus (gon''uh·kock'us) *n.*, pl. **gonococ·ci** (·sigh) The common name for *Neisseria gonorrhoeae,* the organism causing gonorrhea.

gon·or·rhea, gon·or·rhoea (gon''uh·ree'uh) *n.* A venereal disease caused by *Neisseria gonorrhoeae,* characterized by mucopurulent inflammation of the mucosa of the genital tract; may produce septicemia with involvement of synovial tissues and serosal surfaces, causing arthritis, endocarditis, or meningitis. —**gonor·rhe·al, gonorrhoe·al** (·ul) *adj.*

gonorrheal ophthalmia or **conjunctivitis.** An acute and severe form of purulent conjunctivitis, caused by infection by the *Neisseria gonorrhoeae.*

gony·camp·sis (gon″ee·kamp′sis) *n.* Deformity of knee due to abnormal bending or curving.

gony·on·cus (gon″ee·onk′us) *n.* A tumor or swelling of the knee.

Good·ell's sign (gŏŏ·del′) Softening of the cervix of the uterus, considered to be evidence of pregnancy.

Goodpasture's syndrome Rapidly progressive glomerulonephritis associated with pulmonary hemorrhage and hemosiderosis; basement membrane antibodies are present in the blood serum and are linearly deposited along the glomerular basement membrane.

gor·get (gor′jit) *n.* A channeled instrument similar to a grooved director, formerly used in lithotomy.

GOT Abbreviation for *glutamic-oxaloacetic transaminase.*

gouge (gæwj) *n.* A transversely curved chisel for cutting or removing bone or other hard structures.

goun·dou (goon′doo) *n.* An exostosis of the face; probably a sequela of yaws, involving the nasal and adjacent bones to produce a projecting tumorlike mass. Syn. *anakhre, henpue.*

gout (gæwt) *n.* 1. Primary gout, an inborn error of uric acid metabolism characterized by hyperuricemia and recurrent attacks of acute arthritis, most often of the great toe, and eventually by tophaceous deposits of urates. 2. Secondary gout, the gouty symptom complex which may be acquired as a complication of polycythemia vera and other myeloproliferative disorders, as well as of diuretic therapy. 3. *In veterinary medicine,* a condition usually found in adult hens characterized by the presence of pathologic accumulations of urates in the viscera or joints. —**gouty,** *adj.*

Gowers' solution A dilution fluid used in the erythrocyte count, made up of sodium sulfate and glacial acetic acid dissolved in distilled water.

GPT Abbreviation for *glutamic-pyruvic transaminase.*

gr Abbreviation for *grain* (3).

graaf·i·an follicle (graf′ee·un) A mature ovarian follicle.

grac·ile (gras′il) *adj.* Long and slender.

grac·i·lis (gras′i·lis) *L. adj.* Gracile; long and slender.

gracilis muscle. A long and slender muscle on the medial aspect of the thigh.

gracilis nucleus. A nucleus in the dorsal aspect of the medulla oblongata in which fibers of the fasciculus gracilis terminate and which gives origin to part of the fibers of the medial lemniscus. Syn. *nucleus of Goll.*

Gra·de·ni·go's sign or **syndrome** (grahᵇdehᵇnee′go) Intense pain in the temporoparietal region, with paralysis of the lateral rectus muscle of the eye associated with otitis media and mastoiditis; indicative of extradural abscess or

mass involving the apex of the petrous part of the temporal bone.

gra·di·ent (gray′dee·unt) *n.* 1. The rate of change in a variable magnitude, such as electrical potential, pressure, or concentration, or the curve that represents it. 2. *In biology,* a system of relations within the organism, or a part of it, which involves progressively increasing or decreasing differences in respect to rate of growth, rate of metabolism, or of any other structural or functional property of the cells.

grad·u·ate (graj′oo·ut) *n.* A vessel, usually of glass or plastic, marked with lines at different levels; used for measuring liquids.

grad·u·at·ed (graj′oo·ay·tid) *adj.* Divided into units by a series of lines, as on a barometer, a graduate, or a thermometer.

graft, *n. & v.* 1. A portion of tissue, such as skin, periosteum, bone, fascia, or sometimes an entire organ, used to replace a defect in the body. 2. To replace a defect in the body with a portion of suitable tissue.

graft-versus-host reaction. The reaction of transferred immunologically competent allogenic cells against host antigens which may take place when immunologically immature or otherwise immunologically deficient animals or humans are the recipients. In animals, the reaction may include runting, failure to thrive, lymph node atrophy, splenomegaly, hepatomegaly, anemia, and death. In humans, the syndrome includes a diffuse rash, diarrhea, hepatosplenomegaly, and sometimes death.

Gra·ham-Cole test CHOLECYSTOGRAPHY.

Graham Steell murmur The murmur of pulmonary insufficiency, associated with pulmonary hypertension of any cause, but often due to mitral stenosis.

grain, *n.* 1. The seed or seedlike fruit of the cereal grasses. 2. A minute portion or particle, as of sand, or of starch. 3. A unit of weight of the troy, the avoirdupois, and the apothecaries' systems of weights. Abbreviated, gr.

grain alcohol. Alcohol (especially ethyl alcohol) prepared by fermentation of grain.

grain itch. An eruption due to *Pediculoides ventricosus,* acquired by contact with grain or straw, which harbors the parasite. Syn. *prairie itch.*

-gram A combining form designating a *drawing, writing,* or *record.*

gram, gramme, *n.* The basic unit of mass, and of weight, in the metric system, and one of the fundamental units of physical measurement; corresponds almost exactly to the weight of a milliliter, or cubic centimeter, of water at the temperature of maximum density. Abbreviated, g, Gm, gm.

gram·i·ci·din (gram″i·sigh′din) *n.* One of the components of tyrothricin, an antibacterial substance produced by the growth of *Bacillus brevis;* used topically for treatment of localized bacterial infections of the skin.

gram-meter, gramme-metre, *n.* A unit of work, equal to the energy used in raising one gram to a height of one meter.

gram molecule. The weight of any substance, in

grams, equivalent to its molecular weight. Syn. *gram mole.*

gram-negative, *adj.* In Gram's stain, pertaining to microorganisms that do not retain gentian or crystal violet when decolorized by alcohol or acetone-ether, being stained only by the counterstain; they appear pink.

gram-positive, *adj.* In Gram's stain, pertaining to microorganisms that retain the gentian or crystal violet stain; they appear blue.

Gram's stain (grahᵐ) Bacteria are stained with solutions of crystal violet and iodine, followed by exposure to alcohol and then to a counterstain. If the blue color is retained, the organisms are called gram-positive; if it is removed, the organisms appear pink and are called gram-negative.

gran·di·ose (gran'dee·oce) *adj. In psychiatry,* characterized by a feeling of being important, wealthy, or influential, when there is no true basis for such feeling.

grand mal seizure (grahn mahl, grahⁿ mahl) GENERALIZED SEIZURE.

gran·u·lar (gran'yoo·lur) *adj.* Composed of, containing, or having the appearance of, granules.

granular cell myoblastoma. A tumor, usually benign, composed of large cells with granular cytoplasm; the nature of the cells is unknown. The tongue and skin are common sites, though it may occur in many other places.

granular conjunctivitis. TRACHOMA.

granular corneal dystrophy. Bilateral corneal opacities, occurring in the first decade of life and slowly progressive, consisting of discrete stromal lesions in the axial area. The intervening stroma and peripheral cornea are clear and vision is usually unaffected. Inherited as an autosomal dominant trait.

granular layer. 1. GRANULAR LAYER OF THE CEREBELLUM. 2. GRANULAR LAYER OF THE EPIDERMIS.

granular layer of the cerebellum. The innermost of the three layers of the cerebellar cortex, lying deep to the molecular and Purkinje-cell layers; it contains a large number of granule cells.

granular layer of the epidermis. The layer of cells containing keratohyalin granules in the epidermis.

granular leukocyte. A leukocyte containing granules in its cytoplasm.

granulated lids. 1. Chronic blepharitis. 2. TRACHOMA.

gran·u·la·tion (gran"yoo·lay'shun) *n.* 1. The tiny red granules that are grossly visible in a wound during healing, as in the base of an ulcer; made up of loops of newly formed capillaries and fibroblasts. 2. The process of forming granulation tissue in or around a focus of inflammation. 3. The formation of granules. —**gran·u·lat·ed** (gran'yoo·lay·tid) *adj.*

granulation tissues. Newly formed capillaries filled with granulocytes, mixed with proliferating fibrocytes, the spaces between them containing an inflammatory exudate, representing a stage in repair of damage associated with inflammation.

gran·ule (gran'yool) *n.* 1. A minute particle or

mass. 2. A small, intracellular particle, usually staining selectively. 3. A small pill.

granule cell. One of the small nerve cells of the cerebellar and cerebral cortex.

gran·u·lo·cyte (gran'yoo·lo·site) *n.* A mature granular leukocyte; especially, a polymorphonuclear leukocyte, which may be eosinophilic, basophilic, or neutrophilic. —**gran·u·lo·cyt·ic** (gran''yoo·lo·sit'ick) *adj.*

granulocytic leukemia. Leukemia in which the predominant cell types belong to the granulocytic series.

granulocytic sarcoma. A focal tumorous proliferation of granulocytes, with or without the blood findings of granulocytic leukemia; the sectioned surfaces of the mass are often green. Syn. *chloroma.*

granulocytic series. The cells concerned in the development of the granular leukocytes (basophil, eosinophil, or neutrophil) from the primitive myeloblasts to the adult segmented cells. Syn. *myeloid series, myelocytic series, leukocytic series.*

gran·u·lo·cy·to·pe·nia (gran''yoo·lo·sigh''to·pee'nee·uh) *n.* A deficiency of granular leukocytes in the blood.

gran·u·lo·cy·to·poi·e·sis (gran''yoo·lo·sigh''to·poy·ee'sis) *n.* The process of development of the granular leukocytes, occurring normally in the bone marrow. —**granulocytopoi·et·ic** (·et'ick) *adj.*

gran·u·lo·ma (gran''yoo·lo'muh) *n.,* pl. **granulomas, granuloma·ta** (·tuh) 1. The aggregation and proliferation of macrophages to form small nodules or granules. 2. A swelling composed of granulation tissue. Adj. *granulomatous.*

granuloma an·nu·la·re (an·yoo·lair'ee). A chronic, self-limiting disease of the skin, usually on the extremities; characterized by reddish nodules, arranged in a circle.

granuloma fa·ci·a·le (fay''shee·ay'lee). An idiopathic, asymptomatic skin disorder, usually limited to the face, and characterized by soft, purple-red, slowly enlarging patches which usually show marked eosinophilic infiltration microscopically.

granuloma fis·su·ra·tum (fis''yoo·ray'tum). A discoid mucous membrane inflammatory mass indented by a deep fissure and located in the groove between the lip and the jaw.

granuloma in·gui·na·le (ing·gwi·nay'lee). A chronic, often serpiginous, destructive ulceration of the external genitalia due to a gram-negative rod, *Calymmatobacterium granulomatis,* and exhibiting encapsulated forms (Donovan bodies) in infected tissue.

granuloma py·o·ge·ni·cum (pye''o·jen'i·kum). A hemangioma with superimposed inflammation, affecting the skin or other epithelial surfaces.

granulomata. A plural of *granuloma.*

gran·u·lo·ma·to·sis (gran''yoo·lo''muh·to'sis) *n.* A disease characterized by multiple granulomas.

granulomatosis in·fan·ti·sep·ti·ca (in·fan''ti·sep'ti·kuh). Fetal infection with *Listeria monocytogenes.*

gran·u·lom·a·tous (gran″yoo·lom′uh·tus, ·lo′ muh·tus) adj. 1. Of or pertaining to granulomas. 2. Composed of or characteristic of granulomas or granulation tissue.

granulomatous colitis. An inflammatory disease of the colon, differing from ulcerative colitis by being patchy in distribution and being characterized pathologically by granulomas.

granulomatous cystitis. Cystitis in which the urinary bladder has been affected by a granulomatous reaction, commonly tuberculosis.

granulomatous inflammation. Inflammation characterized by proliferation of macrophages, usually forming nodules of various sizes.

gran·u·lo·mere (gran′yoo·lo·meer) n. The mottled purple central portion of a platelet as seen in a peripheral blood film stained with a Romanovsky-type stain.

gran·u·lo·pe·nia (gran″yoo·lo·pee′nee·uh) n. GRANULOCYTOPENIA.

gran·u·lo·pex·is (gran″yoo·lo·peck′sis) n. Removal of particulate matter by the cells of the reticuloendothelial system; PHAGOCYTOSIS. —**granulo·pec·tic** (·peck′tick) adj.

gran·u·lo·poi·e·sis (gran″yoo·lo·poy·ee′sis) n. GRANULOCYTOPOIESIS. —**granulopoi·et·ic** (·et′ick) adj.

gran·u·lo·sa (gran″yoo·lo′suh) adj. Pertaining to the layer of epithelial cells lining the ovarian follicle.

granulosa cell. One of the epithelial cells lining the ovarian follicle and constituting the granulosa membrane.

granulosa cell tumor. An ovarian neoplasm composed of cells resembling those lining the primordial follicle, associated with clinical signs of feminization.

granulosa membrane. The layer of small polyhedral cells within the theca of the graafian follicle.

gran·u·lo·sis (gran″yoo·lo′sis) n., pl. **granulo·ses** (·seez) The development of a collection of granules or granulomas.

granulosis ru·bra na·si (roo′bruh nay′zigh). An uncommon condition of unknown cause characterized by an eruption of small, red papules and diffuse redness on the nose, cheeks, and chin and by persistent hyperhidrosis; seen in children with delicate constitutions and tending to disappear at puberty.

graph, n. A representation of statistical data by means of points, lines, surfaces, or solids, their positions being determined by a system of coordinates. —**graph·ic** (·ick) adj.

-graph A combining form meaning something written or recorded.

graph·an·es·the·sia, graph·an·aes·the·sia (graf″ an·es·theezh′uh) n. Loss of ability to recognize letters or numbers traced on the skin; in the presence of intact peripheral sensation, a contralateral cortical lesion is implied.

graph·es·the·sia, graph·aes·the·sia (graf″es·theezh′uh, ·theez·ee·uh) n. The sense or sensation of recognizing a symbol, such as a number, figure, or letter, traced on the skin.

-graphia A combining form designating (a) writing characteristic of a (specified) psychologic disorder; (b) a condition characterized by (a specified kind of) markings or tracings.

graph·ite (graf′ite) n. Plumbago, or black lead; an impure allotropic form of carbon.

grapho-. See graph-.

gra·phol·o·gy (gra·fol′uh·jee) n. The study of the handwriting; may be used for personal identification, for the analysis of specific psychologic or neurologic states at the time of writing, or for personality analysis.

grapho·ma·nia (graf″o·may′nee·uh) n. An excessive impulse to write; frequently observed in the paranoid personality and in paranoia. —**graphoma·ni·ac** (·nee·ack) n.

grapho·mo·tor (graf″o·mo′tur) n. Pertaining to or affecting the movements of writing.

grapho·pho·bia (graf″o·fo′bee·uh) n. An abnormal fear of writing.

graph·or·rhea, graph·or·rhoea (graf″o·ree′uh) n. In psychiatry, an uncontrollable desire to write, in which pages are covered with usually unconnected and meaningless words; an intermittent condition, most often seen in manic patients.

grasp reflex. A grasping motion of the fingers or toes, induced by tactile and then proprioceptive stimulation of the palm of the hand or the sole of the foot, seen in frontal lobe disease. A grasp reflex is normal in young infants.

grat·tage (gra·tahzh′) n. A method, sometimes used in treatment of trachoma, in which a hard brush, as a toothbrush, is used to scrub the conjunctival surface of the eyelid in order to remove the granulations.

grave, adj. Extremely serious; threatening to life; indicating a poor prognosis or fatal outcome.

grav·el (grav′ul) n. 1. A granular, sandlike material forming the substance of renal or vesical calculi. 2. Informal. Small calculi.

Graves' disease A disease of unknown cause, tending to be familial and most commonly affecting women, characterized typically by hyperthyroidism (with diffuse goiter and exophthalmos) and circumscribed myxedema. Syn. Basedow's disease.

grav·id (grav′id) adj. Pregnant; of the uterus, containing a fetus; also, pertaining to other than human females when carrying young or eggs. —**gra·vid·i·ty** (grav′id′i·tee) n.

grav·i·da (grav′i·duh) n., pl. **gravidas, gravi·dae** (·dee) A pregnant woman.

gra·vid·ic (gra·vid′ick) adj. Taking place during pregnancy.

grav·i·do·car·di·ac (grav″i·do·kahr′dee·ack) adj. Obsol. Pertaining to cardiac disorders associated with pregnancy.

gra·vim·e·ter (gra·vim′e·tur) n. An instrument used in determining the specific gravity of a substance, especially a hydrometer, aerometer, or urinometer. —**grav·i·met·ric** (grav′i·met′rick) adj.; **grav·im·e·try** (gra·vim′e·tree) n.

grav·i·ta·tion (grav′i·tay′shun) n. The force by which bodies are drawn together. —**gravitation·al** (·ul) adj.; **grav·i·tate** (grav′i·tate) v.

grav·i·ty (grav′i·tee) n. 1. Seriousness. 2. The effect of the attraction of the earth upon matter.

Gra·witz's tumor (grah'vits) RENAL CELL CARCINOMA.

gray hepatization. The gross appearance of the lungs in lobar pneumonia just prior to resolution.

gray substance or **matter.** The part of the central nervous system composed of nerve cell bodies, their dendrites, and the proximal and terminal unmyelinated portions of axons.

grease (greece) *n.* GREASE HEEL.

grease heel. An infection of the fetlock joint of a horse; characterized by cracking of the skin and an oily exudate.

greater omentum. A fold of peritoneum attached to the greater curvature of the stomach above and, after dipping down over the intestine, returning to fuse with the transverse mesocolon. Between the ascending and descending folds is the variable cavity of the greater omentum.

greater palatine foramen. The lower opening of the greater palatine canal; it is formed on the medial side by a notch in the horizontal part of the palatine bone and on the lateral side by the adjacent part of the maxilla. Syn. *major palatine foramen.*

greater splanchnic nerve. A nerve that arises from the fifth to ninth or tenth thoracic ganglions and supplies visceral nerve plexuses in the thorax and to the celiac plexus.

greater trochanter. A process situated on the outer side of the upper extremity of the femur.

greater tubercle of the humerus. A prominence on the upper lateral end of the shaft of the humerus into which are inserted the supraspinatus, infraspinatus, and teres minor muscles.

green diarrhea. Infantile diarrhea, characterized by the passage of green stools.

green-stick fracture. An incomplete fracture of a long bone, seen in children; the bone is bent but splintered only on the convex side.

green sweat. Sweat having a bluish or greenish color, seen mainly in copper workers.

grenz rays (grents) Electromagnetic radiations of about two angstroms, used in x-ray therapy of the skin because of their limited power of penetration.

grief, *n.* The appropriate, self-limited emotional response to an external and consciously recognized loss.

grief reaction. *In psychiatry,* an overintense and prolonged reaction to a loss, particularly the death of someone close.

grip. Grippe (= INFLUENZA).

gripe, *n.* A spasmodic intestinal or abdominal pain. —**grip·ing,** *adj.*

grippe, *n.* INFLUENZA.

Grit·ti-Stokes amputation (greet'tee) A supracondylar osteoplastic operation in which the patella is retained in the flap and is attached to the cut end of the femur.

groin, *n.* The depression between the abdomen and thigh.

groove, *n.* An elongated depression. —**grooved,** *adj.*

gross (groce) *adj.* 1. Large enough to be seen without magnification. 2. Pertaining to or describing general aspects or distinctions; not concerned with minute details. 3. Growing or spreading excessively.

gross pathology. 1. The description of grossly visible changes in the tissues and organs of the body resulting from disease. 2. Grossly visible pathologic changes.

ground itch. Local irritation of the skin resulting from the entrance of the larvae of any variety of *Ancylostoma* into the skin.

ground substance. The fluid, semifluid, or solid material, in the connective tissues, cartilage, and bone, which fills in part or all of the space between the cells and fibers. Syn. *matrix, interstitial substance.*

group medicine. 1. The practice of medicine by a number of physicians working in systematic association, with joint use of equipment and technical personnel, and with centralized administrative and financial organization. Its objectives are increased professional efficiency, improved medical care of the patient, and increased economic efficiency. 2. The practice of medicine carried on under a legal agreement in a community, by a body of registered physicians and surgeons, for the purpose of caring for a group of persons who have subscribed to such service by the payment of a definite sum for a specified time, which entitles each subscriber to medical care and hospitalization under definite rules and regulations.

group psychotherapy. *In psychiatry,* the therapy given to a group of patients by a professional therapist, and based on the effect of the group upon the individual and his interaction with the group.

group-specific substances. Substances derived from a source other than blood which reduce the amount of naturally occurring anti-A or anti-B agglutinins in bloods of the appropriate ABO blood groups. Syn. *Witebsky's substances.*

growth factor. 1. GROWTH HORMONE. 2. Any substance, either genetic or extrinsic, which affects growth.

growth hormone. An adenohypophyseal hormone that promotes growth and also has direct influence on the metabolism of carbohydrates, fats, and proteins. Syn. *somatotropin.*

grume, *n.* A clot, as of blood; a thick and viscid fluid. —**gru·mose** (groo'moce), **gru·mous** (·mus) *adj.*

gry·po·sis (grye·po'sis, gri·) *n.* Abnormal curvature, especially of the nails.

gt. Abbreviation for *gutta,* drop.

gtt. Abbreviation for *guttae,* drops.

GU Abbreviation for *genitourinary.*

guai·ac (gwye'ack) *n.* The resin of the wood of *Guajacum officinale* or of *G. sanctum,* formerly used in treatment of syphilis, chronic rheumatism, and gout; now used in testing for occult blood.

guai·a·col (gwye'uh·kol) *n.* o-Methoxyphenol, $C_7H_8O_2$, a constituent of guaiac and wood creosote, also prepared synthetically; has been used internally as an expectorant, and externally as an antiseptic and anesthetic.

guaiac test. A test for blood in which an acetic acid or alcoholic solution of guaiac resin and hydrogen peroxide is mixed with the unknown. The development of a blue color is a positive test.

gua·nase (gwah'nace, ·naze) n. A deaminizing enzyme, widely distributed in animal tissues, that catalyzes conversion of guanine into xanthine, with release of ammonia.

guan·eth·i·dine (gwahn·eth'i·deen) n. {2-[Hexahydro-1(2H)-azocinyl]ethyl}guanidine, $C_{10}H_{22}N_4$, a potent hypotensive drug used as the sulfate salt.

gua·ni·dine (gwah'ni·deen, ·din, gwan'i·) n. Aminomethanamidine, $NH=C(NH_2)_2$, a normal product of protein metabolism found in the urine. The hydrochloride has been used for the treatment of myasthenia gravis. Syn. *carbamidine, iminourea.*

gua·nine (gwah'neen, ·nin, gwan'een, ·in) n. 2-Aminohypoxanthine, $C_5H_5N_5O$, a purine base important mainly as a component of ribonucleic and deoxyribonucleic acids; occurs also in guano.

gua·no·sine (gwah'no·seen, ·sin) n. Guanine riboside, $C_{10}H_{13}N_5O_5$, a nucleoside composed of one molecule each of guanine and D-ribose. One of the four main riboside components of ribonucleic acid. Syn. *vernine.*

gua·ra·na (gwah''rah·nah', gwah·rah'nuh) n. A dried paste prepared from the seeds of *Paullinia cupana,* a Brazilian tree; contains caffeine. Used as an astringent and stimulant.

guard, n. An appliance placed on a knife to prevent too deep an incision.

Guar·nie·ri bodies (gwar·nyeh'ree) Eosinophilic cytoplasmic inclusion bodies found in the epidermal cells of patients with smallpox or vaccinia.

gu·ber·nac·u·lum (gew''bur·nack'yoo·lum) n., pl. **gubernacu·la** (·luh) A guiding structure. **—gubernacu·lar** (·lur) adj.

gubernaculum tes·tis (tes'tis) [NA]. A fibrous cord extending from the fetal testis to the scrotal swellings; it occupies the potential inguinal canal and guides the testis in its descent.

Guil·lain-Bar·ré disease or **syndrome** (ghee·læⁿ', ba·reyʸ') An acute, more or less symmetrical lower motor neuron paralysis of unknown cause, with areflexia and variable sensory involvement. Proximal as well as distal muscles of the limbs are involved, and, in advanced cases, trunk and cranial muscles as well, with progression to respiratory failure and death within several days. The protein level of the spinal fluid rises after several days, usually without an increase in cells. Syn. *acute idiopathic polyneuritis, acute inflammatory polyradiculoneuropathy, Landry-Guillain-Barrea syndrome.*

guil·lo·tine amputation (gil'uh·teen, gee'o·teen) n. CIRCULAR AMPUTATION.

guinea worm infection. DRACUNCULIASIS.

gul·let, n. ESOPHAGUS.

¹gum, n. GINGIVA.

²gum, n. A concrete vegetable juice exuded from many plants, insoluble in alcohol or ether, but swelling or dissolving in water into a viscid mass. Gums consist of glycosidal hexoseuronic acids, partly or wholly combined with calcium, potassium, or magnesium.

gum arabic. ACACIA.

gum·boil, n. The aspect of a periodontal abscess that has extended through the periodontal tissues and involved the gingiva.

gum ghatti. GHATTI GUM.

gum·ma (gum'uh) n., pl. **gummas, gumma·ta** (·tuh) A mass of rubberlike necrotic tissue found in any of various organs and tissues in tertiary syphilis. **—gumma·tous** (·tus) adj.

Gum·precht's shadows (goōm'preᵏht) A degenerated nucleus and its contained nucleolus from the abnormal cells of chronic lymphocytic leukemia, where they are commonly seen in peripheral blood films.

gun·cot·ton, n. PYROXYLIN.

gun·ja, gun·jah (gun'juh) n. GANJA.

gur·ney, guer·ney (gur'nee) n. A stretcher with wheels for transporting a recumbent patient.

gus·ta·tion (gus·tay'shun) n. The sense of taste; the act of tasting.

gus·ta·to·ry (gus'tuh·to''ree) adj. Pertaining to or involving the sense of taste.

gustatory fit or **seizure.** A form of psychomotor or temporal lobe seizure announced by an aura of peculiar taste; frequently followed by disturbance of consciousness and automatisms, such as smacking movements of the tongue and lips; usually indicative of an irritation of the inframtemporal cortex.

gustatory hyperhidrosis. The phenomenon of sweating over facial areas, particularly about the mouth and nose, accompanied by flushing of the involved areas, upon smelling or ingestion of spicy or acid foods, or some foods such as chocolate. May be caused even by the thought of these foods, and is found to varying degrees in most people.

gut, n. 1. INTESTINE. 2. The embryonic digestive tube, consisting of foregut, midgut, and hindgut. 3. Catgut or other suturing material.

Guthrie test A screening test for the detection of phenylketonuria in which the inhibition of growth of a strain of *Bacillus subtilis* by a phenylalanine analogue is reversed by L-phenylalanine, as found in elevated concentration in the plasma of patients with phenylketonuria. Syn. *Guthrie inhibition assay test.*

gut·ta (gut'uh) n., pl. **gut·tae** (·ee) A drop. Abbreviated, gt.

guttae. Plural of *gutta.* Abbreviated, gtt.

gut·ta-per·cha (gut'uh pur'chuh) n. The latex of various trees of the family Sapotaceae; essentially a polymerized hydrocarbon of the general formula $(C_5H_8)_n$ with other resinous substances. Used to make splints, as a wound dressing, or as an insulator.

gut·tate (gut'ate) adj. *In biology,* spotted as if by

drops of something colored; resembling a drop.

gut·ta·tim (guh·tay'tim) *adv.* Drop by drop.

gut·ter, *n. & v.* 1. A shallow groove. 2. To form a shallow groove; specifically, SAUCERIZE.

gut·ti·form (gut'i·form) *adj.* Drop-shaped.

gut·tur·al (gut'ur·ul) *adj.* 1. Pertaining to the throat. 2. Throaty, as certain voice sounds. 3. *Erron.* Of consonant sounds: VELAR; or loosely: velar, uvular, pharyngeal, or laryngeal.

guttural pouch. One of a pair of mucomembranous sacs which are ventral diverticula of the auditory tube in Equidae, located between the base of the cranium and the atlas dorsally and the pharynx ventrally.

gut·tur·oph·o·ny (gut''ur·off'uh·nee) *n.* A form of dysphonia characterized by a throaty quality of the voice sounds.

gut·turo·tet·a·ny (gut''ur·o·tet'uh·nee) *n.* A stammering with difficulties in pronouncing "guttural" sounds due to spasm of the laryngeal muscles.

gym·no·pho·bia (jim''no·fo'bee·uh) *n.* An abnormal fear of nudity.

gyn-, gyno- A combining form meaning (a) *woman, female;* (b) *female reproductive organ.*

gyn·an·der (ji·nan'dur) *n.* PSEUDOHERMAPHRODITE.

gyn·an·dria (ji·nan'dree·uh) *n.* 1. FEMALE PSEUDOHERMAPHRODITISM. 2. A condition involving secondary characteristics of the opposite sex.

gyn·an·drism (ji·nan'driz·um) *n.* 1. FEMALE PSEUDOHERMAPHRODITISM. 2. A condition involving secondary characteristics of the opposite sex.

gyn·an·dro·blas·to·ma (ji·nan''dro·blas·to'muh) *n.* An ovarian tumor, histologically characterized by elements resembling arrhenoblastoma and granulosa cell tumor, associated with hyperestrogenism and masculinization.

gyn·an·dro·mor·phism (ji·nan''dro·mor'fiz·um) *n.* An abnormality in which the individual contains both genetically male and genetically female tissue.

gyn·an·dro·mor·phy (ji·nan'dro·mor''fee) *n.* 1. GYNANDROMORPHISM. 2. In the somatotype, the degree or prominence of feminine characteristics in a male physique, or vice versa, expressed numerically as the g-component.

gyn·an·dry (ji·nan'dree) *n.* FEMALE PSEUDOHERMAPHRODITISM. —**gynan·droid** (·droid) *adj. & n.*

gyn·atre·sia (jin''uh·tree'zhuh, ·zee·uh) *n.* 1. An imperforate condition of the vagina or of other areas of the female genital system. 2. Occlusion of any portion of the female genital system.

-gyne A combining form meaning *woman* or *female.*

gy·ne·cic, gy·nae·cic (ji·nee'sick) *adj.* Pertaining to women or the female sex.

gy·ne·co·gen·ic (jin''e·ko·jen'ick, guy''ne·ko·) *adj.* Causing or producing female characteristics.

gy·ne·cog·ra·phy, gy·nae·cog·ra·phy (jin''e·kog'ruh·fee, guy''ne·) *n.* A roentgenologic method of visualization of the female pelvic organs by means of the injection of air or carbon dioxide intraperitoneally.

gy·ne·coid, gy·nae·coid (jin'e·koid, guy'ne·) *adj.* 1. Pertaining to or like a woman. 2. Specifically, of a pelvis: having a shape typical of that of the female, with a round or nearly round inlet.

gy·ne·col·o·gist, gy·nae·col·o·gist (jin''e·kol'uh·jist, guy''ne·, guy''ne·) *n.* A physician who practices gynecology.

gy·ne·col·o·gy, gy·nae·col·o·gy (jin''e·kol'uh·jee, guy''ne·, jye''ne·) *n.* The science of the diseases of women, especially those affecting the sexual organs. —**gyne·co·log·ic, gynae·co·log·ic** (·ko·loj'ick), **gynecolog·i·cal, gynaecolog·i·cal** (·i·kul) *adj.*

gy·ne·co·ma·nia, gy·nae·co·ma·nia (jin''e·ko·may'nee·uh, guy''ne·) *n.* SATYRIASIS.

gy·ne·co·mas·tia, gy·nae·co·mas·tia (jin''e·ko·mas'tee·uh, guy''ne·) *n.* Mammary glandular hyperplasia in the male.

gy·ne·cop·a·thy, gy·nae·cop·a·thy (jin''e·kop'uth·ee, guy''ne·, jye''ne·) *n.* Any disease of, or peculiar to, women.

gy·ne·co·pho·bia (jin''e·ko·fo'bee·uh, guy''ne·, jye''ne·) *n.* GYNEPHOBIA.

gy·ne·phor·ic (jin''e·for'ick, guy''ne·) *adj.* Pertaining to inheritance sex-linked to the X chromosome.

Gynergen. A trademark for ergotamine used as the tartrate salt principally to relieve migraine pain.

gy·ni·a·tri·cian (jin''ee·uh·trish'un, jye·, guy·) *n.* A physician who specializes in gyniatrics.

gy·ni·at·rics (jin''ee·at'ricks, jye''nee·, guy''nee·) *n.* Treatment of the diseases of women.

gyno-. See *gyn-.*

gy·no·plas·ty (jin'o·plas·tee, jye'no·, guy'no·) *n.* Plastic surgery of the female genitalia. —**gy·no·plas·tic** (jin''o·plas'tick, guy''no·) *adj.*

gyp·sum (jip'sum) *n.* Native calcium sulfate, $CaSO_4.2H_2O$. Deprived of the major portion of its water of crystallization, it constitutes plaster of paris.

gy·ral (jye'rul) *adj.* Of, pertaining to, or involving a gyrus.

gy·rate (jye'rate) *adj.* Coiled; in rings; convoluted.

gy·ra·tion (jye·ray'shun) *n.* 1. A turning in a circle. 2. *Obsol.* The arrangement of gyri in the cerebral hemisphere.

gy·rec·to·my (jye·reck'tuh·mee) *n.* Excision of any gyrus of the brain.

gyri. Plural and genitive singular of *gyrus.*

gy·rose (jye'roce) *adj.* Marked with curved or undulating lines.

gy·ro·spasm (jye'ro·spaz·um) *n.* SPASMUS NUTANS.

gy·rus (jye'rus) *n.*, pl. & genit. sing. **gy·ri** (·rye) A convolution on the surface of the cerebral hemisphere.

gyrus cin·gu·li (sing'gew·lye) [NA]. CINGULATE GYRUS.

gyrus ol·fac·to·ri·us (ol·fack·to'ree·us). Either of

the small gyri on the undersurface of the frontal lobe; there is a medial and a lateral one.

gyrus pa·ra·hip·po·cam·pa·lis (păr″uh·hip·o·kam·pay′lis) [NA]. PARAHIPPOCAMPAL GYRUS.

gyrus pa·ra·ter·mi·na·lis (păr″uh·tur·mi·nay′lis) [NA]. A convolution at the rostrum of the corpus callosum limited anteriorly by the paraolfactory sulcus.

gyrus rec·tus (reck′tus) [NA]. A narrow strip of cortex medial to the olfactory sulcus on the inferior surface of the frontal lobe and continuous with the superior frontal gyrus on the medial surface. Syn. *straight gyrus.*

H

H Symbol for hydrogen.

H, H *In electrocardiography*, symbol for the longitudinal anatomic axis of the heart as projected on the frontal plane. —**habe·nar** (·nur) *adj.*

¹H Symbol for protium.

²H Symbol for deuterium.

³H Symbol for tritium.

H⁺ Symbol for hydrogen ion.

h Abbreviation for (a) height; (b) *hora,* hour; (c) hundred.

h Symbol for Planck's constant.

ha·be·na (ha·bee'nuh) *n.* 1. FRENUM. 2. A bandage. —**habe·nar** (·nur) *adj.*

ha·ben·u·la (ha·ben'yoo·luh) *n.,* pl. & genit. sing. **habenu·lae** (·lee), genit. pl. **ha·be·nu·la·rum** (ha·ben''yoo·lair'um) 1. The stalk of the pineal body, attaching it to the thalamus. 2. A ribbonlike structure. —**habenu·lar** (·lur) *adj.*

ha·ben·u·lo·pe·dun·cu·lar (ha·ben''yoo·lo·pe·dunk'yoo·lur) *adj.* Pertaining to the habenular and the interpeduncular nuclei.

hab·it, *n.* 1. A behavior pattern fixed by repetition. 2. HABITUS. —**ha·bit·u·al,** *adj.*

hab·i·tat (hab'i·tat) *n.* The natural place or environment of an organism.

ha·bit·u·a·tion, *n.* 1. The gradual adaptation to environment, accompanied by the feeling of certainty that a particular situation will produce a particular response. 2. The gradual increase in efficiency by the elimination of unnecessary motions as a result of repeated reaction to a given stimulus. 3. A condition of tolerance to the effects of a drug or a poison, acquired by its continued use; marked by a craving for the drug when it is withdrawn. 4. Drug addiction, especially a mild form in which withdrawal does not result in severe abstinence symptoms.

hab·i·tus (hab'i·tus) *n.* The general appearance of the body, especially as associated with a disease or a predisposition thereto.

Hab·ro·ne·ma (hab''ro·nee'muh) *n.* A genus of nematodes parasitic in the stomach of horses and mules, and whose larvae may produce dermatitis and conjunctival infection in horses and also in man.

hab·ro·ne·mi·a·sis (hab''ro·ne·migh'uh·sis) *n.,* pl. **habronemia·ses** (·seez) Infection of horses by nematodes of the genus *Habronema.*

hab·ro·ne·mic (hab''ro·nee'mick) *adj.* Pertaining to or caused by nematodes of the genus *Habronema.*

habronemic ophthalmomyiasis. A granulomatous disease of the eyelids of the horse, caused by any of three species of the nematode *Habronema.*

hack·ing, *adj. & n.* 1. Harsh, racking, as hacking cough. 2. A form of massage consisting of a succession of chopping strokes with the edge of the extended fingers or the whole hand, or with firm patting strokes with the extended finger and the whole hand. Syn. *hachement.*

ha·de·pho·bia (hay''de·fo'bee·uh) *n.* A morbid fear of hell.

Hae·ma·phy·sa·lis (hee''muh·figh'suh·lis, hem'' uh·) *n.* A genus of ticks which includes the dog tick and the rabbit tick.

Haemaphysalis lep·o·ris pa·lus·tris (lep'o·ris pa·lus'tris). A species of ticks limited to rabbits as hosts, and known to be a natural reservoir of Rocky Mountain spotted fever rickettsia.

Hae·ma·to·si·phon (hee''muh·to·sigh'fon, hem'' uh·to·) *n.* A genus of bugs of the family Cimicidae. *Haematosiphon inodora,* a poultry chinch of Central and North America, attacks man as well as fowl.

Haem·a·to·ther·ma (hem''uh·to·thur'muh, hee'' muh·to·) *n.pl.* The warm-blooded vertebrates; birds and mammals.

Hae·mon·chus (hee·mong'kus) *n.* A genus of nematode worms infecting sheep and cattle.

Haemonchus con·tor·tus (kon·tor'tus). A species of nematode worm parasitic to sheep and other herbivores throughout the world; occasionally infects man.

Haemophilus ae·gyp·ti·us (e·jip'shee·us). A causative agent of catarrhal conjunctivitis. Syn. *Koch-Weeks bacillus.*

For words beginning HAEM... not found here, see HEM... .

Haemophilus du·creyi (dew·kray'eye). A species of small, gram-negative bacilli tending to grow in short chains; the cause of chancroid.

Haemophilus in·flu·en·zae (in''flew·en'zee). A causative agent of serious pyogenic infection, especially in children, including meningitis, epiglottitis, bacteremia, pneumonia, arthritis, otitis media, and sinusitis.

Haemophilus pertussis. BORDETELLA PERTUSSIS.

Hae·mo·spo·rid·ia (hee''mo·spo·rid'ee·uh, hem''o·) *n.pl.* An order of sporozoa that live for a part of their life cycle within the red blood cells of their hosts. —**haemosporidia,** *com. n. pl.,* sing. **haemosporid·i·um; haemosporid·i·an,** *adj. & n.*

Haenel's variant Progressive muscular atrophy affecting only the upper extremities.

Haff disease (hahff) A disease characterized by muscular weakness, pain in the limbs, and myoglobinuria; caused by ingestion of fish poisoned by industrial wastes from cellulose factories.

Hageman factor FACTOR XII. Abbreviated, HF.

hair, *n.* 1. A keratinized filament growing from the skin of mammals; a modified epidermal structure consisting of a shaft, which is the hair itself, exclusive of its sheaths and papilla, and a root. 2. Collectively, the hairs covering the skin.

hair bulb. The part of the hair apparatus from which the hair shaft develops.

hair cell. An epithelial cell with delicate, hair-like processes, as that of the spiral organ of Corti, which responds to the stimuli of sound waves, and those of the crista ampullaris, macula utriculi, and macula sacculi, which are concerned with equilibrium.

hair follicle. An epithelial ingrowth of the dermis that surrounds a hair.

hair matrix tumor. PILOMATRICOMA.

hairy nevus or **mole.** A pigmented nevus covered with downy or stiff hairs.

hal-, halo- A combining form meaning (a) *salt;* (b) *halogen.*

ha·la·tion (hay·lay'shun) *n.* Blurring of the visual image under a powerful direct light coming from a direction different from the line of vision.

hal·a·zone (hal'uh·zone) *n.* p-Dichlorosulfamoylbenzoic acid, $C_7H_5Cl_2NO_4S$, a disinfectant for drinking water.

half-life, *n.* 1. The time required for half of any amount of a substance or property to disappear from a mathematically or physically defined space. 2. *In radiology,* the time in which half of any given amount of a radioactive substance will have undergone transmutation; a constant for any given radioactive isotope. Symbol, $t\frac{1}{2}$. 3. *In pharmacology,* the time required for half the amount of a radioactive or nonradioactive substance or drug introduced into an organism to undergo radioactive decay or to be metabolized or excreted.

hal·i·but-liver oil. The vitamin A-rich fixed oil from the livers of *Hippoglossus hippoglossus;* has been used for prophylaxis and treatment of vitamin A-deficiency states.

hal·ide (hal'ide, hay'lide) *n.* A binary salt in which a halogen serves as anion.

hal·i·ste·re·sis (hal''i·ste·ree'sis) *n.,* pl. **halisteresses** (·seez) The loss of lime salts from previously well-calcified bone. —**halisteret·ic** (·ret'ick) *adj.*

hal·i·to·sis (hal''i·to'sis) *n.,* pl. **halito·ses** (·seez) The state of having offensive breath. Syn. *bromopnea, fetor ex ore.*

hal·i·tus (hal'i·tus) *n.* An exhalation or vapor, as that expired from the lung.

Hal·ler·vor·den-Spatz disease or **syndrome** (ha^{b}l'ur·for''dun, shpa^{b}ts) An inherited (autosomal recessive) disease beginning in late childhood or early adolescence and characterized clinically by a slowly progressive pyramidal and extrapyramidal motor syndrome and dementia. There is intense brown pigmentation of the globus pallidus, substantia nigra, and red nucleus. Microscopically, in these parts, there is a loss of neurons and medullated fibers, swollen axon fragments, and deposits of iron mixed with calcium. Syn. *progressive pallidal degeneration syndrome.*

hal·lu·ci·na·tion (ha·lew'si·nay'shun) *n.* A sensory experience of an object not actually existing in the external world or an alteration in perception, which may be in the auditory, visual, tactile (haptic), olfactory, or gustatory fields or any combination; usually occurring in psychosis, in response to certain drugs and toxic substances, following withdrawal of alcohol and barbiturates, and with diseases of and trauma to the brain, particularly in the temporal lobes and diencephalon and in febrile conditions. Syn. *phantasm, socordia, waking dream.* —**hal·lu·ci·nate** (ha·lew'si·nate) *v.;* **hal·lu·ci·na·tive** (ha·lew'si·nuh·tiv), **hallucina·to·ry** (·to''ree) *adj.*

hal·lu·cino·gen (ha·lew'sin·o·jen, hal''yoo·sin'o·jen) *n.* A drug or substance that produces hallucinations.

hal·lu·ci·no·gen·ic (ha·lew''si·no·jen'ick, hal''yoo·sin''o·jen'ick) *adj.* 1. Pertaining to hallucinogens. 2. Pertaining to any stimuli, such as rapidly revolving and changing colored lights, which create the impression of experiencing a hallucination.

hal·lu·ci·no·sis (ha·lew''si·no'sis) *n.,* pl. **hallucino·ses** (·seez) *In psychiatry,* the condition of experiencing persistent hallucinations, especially while fully conscious.

hal·lux (hal'ucks) *n.,* genit. **hal·lu·cis** (hal'yoo·sis), pl. **hallu·ces** (·seez) GREAT TOE. NA alt. *digitus I.*

hallux flex·us (fleck'sus). A condition allied to and perhaps identical with hammertoe, or flexion of the first phalanx of the great toe. The second phalanx is usually extended upon the first, and there is more or less rigidity of the metatarsophalangeal joint.

hallux rig·i·dus (rij'i·dus). A condition in which there is restriction in the range of motion in the first metatarsophalangeal joint; it is frequently secondary to degenerative joint disease.

hallux val·gus (val'gus). A deformity of the great toe, in which the head of the first metatarsal deviates away from the second metatarsal and the phalanges are deviated toward the second toe, causing undue prominence of the metatarsophalangeal joint.

hallux va·rus (vair'us). A deformity of the great toe, in which the head of the first metatarsal deviates toward the second metatarsal and the phalanges are deviated away from the second toe.

ha·lo (hay'lo) *n.* 1. *In cytology,* a clear area surrounding the nucleus under certain abnormal conditions, especially in cervical cell smears. 2. A luminous circle seen around lights resulting from edema of the cornea or lens; a symptom of glaucoma. 3. The imprint made on the vitreous humor by the ciliary body of the eye. 4. A ring observed ophthalmoscopically around the macula lutea.

halo-. See *hal-.*

halo·gen (hal'o·jin) *n.* Any one of the nonmetallic elements chlorine, iodine, bromine, and fluorine.

hal·o·gen·ate (hal'o·je·nate) *v.* To combine or treat with a halogen. —**halogen·at·ed** (·nay·tid) *adj.*

hal·oid (hal'oid, hay'loid) *adj.* Resembling or derived from a halogen.

halo nevus. A pigmented nevus surrounded by a depigmented zone, usually occurring as a part of self-involution of the nevus.

halo symptom. The colored circles seen around lights in glaucoma.

Halotestin. A trademark for fluoxymesterone, an anabolic and androgenic steroid.

hal·o·thane (hal'o·thane) *n.* 2-Bromo-2-chloro-1,1,1-trifluoroethane, $C_2HBrClF_3$, a colorless, nonflammable liquid; employed as a general anesthetic, by inhalation.

Halsted's forceps 1. A delicate, sharp-pointed hemostat. Syn. *mosquito forceps.* 2. A standard-sized artery forceps with relatively narrow jaws designed to catch blood vessels with precision and with minimal crushing of tissues.

ham, *n.* 1. The posterior portion of the thigh above the popliteal space and below the buttock. 2. POPLITEAL SPACE. 3. The buttock, hip, and thigh.

ha·mar·tia (ha·mahr'shee·uh) *n.* A nodular or localized defect of embryonal development; cells and structures natural to the part are not in normal orderly arrangement, giving rise to a hamartoma.

ha·mar·to·blas·to·ma (ha·mahr''to·blas·to'muh) *n.* A neoplasm arising from a hamartoma.

ham·ar·to·ma (ham''ahr·to'muh) *n.,* pl. **hamartomas, hamartoma·ta** (·tuh) A developmental anomaly resulting in the formation of a mass composed of tissues normally present in the locality of the mass, but of improper proportion and distribution with dominance of one type of tissue. —**hamar·tom·a·tous** (·tom'uh·tus, ·to'muh·tus) *adj.*

ha·mar·to·pho·bia (ha·mahr''to·fo'bee·uh, ham'' ur·to·) *n.* A morbid fear of error or sin.

ha·mate (hay'mate) *adj. & n.* 1. Hook-shaped. 2. HAMATUM.

Ham·man-Rich syndrome Progressive idiopath-

ic diffuse interstitial pulmonary fibrosis, with progressive hypoxia, dyspnea, and right ventricular failure.

ham·mer, *n.* 1. *In anatomy,* MALLEUS. 2. An instrument for striking.

hammer finger. A flexion deformity of the distal interphalangeal joint of a finger due to avulsion or disruption of the extensor tendon.

ham·mer·toe, *n.* A condition of the toe, usually the second, in which the proximal phalanx is extremely extended while the two distal phalanges are flexed.

ham·ster, *n.* A short-tailed rodent with large cheek pouches, belonging to the family Cricetidae. Found in Europe, western Asia, and Africa. It is susceptible to a variety of microorganisms, and is used for laboratory purposes.

ham·string, *n.* 1. One of the tendons bounding the ham on the outer and inner side. 2. To cripple by cutting the hamstring tendons.

hamstring muscles. The biceps femoris, semitendinosus, and semimembranosus collectively.

ham·u·lus (ham'yoo·lus) *n.* A hook-shaped process, as of the hamatum, of the medial plate of the pterygoid process of the sphenoid bone, and of the osseous cochlea at the cupula (hamulus laminae spiralis). —**hamu·lar** (·lur), **hamu·late** (·late) *adj.*

hand, *n.* The organ of prehension, the part of the upper limb at the end of the forearm, composed of the carpus, metacarpus, and phalanges.

hand·ed·ness, *n.* 1. The favoring of either the right or the left hand for intricate, complex acts, according to cerebral dominance. 2. CHIRALITY.

hand·i·cap, *n.* 1. A condition that imposes difficulties on functioning and achievement. 2. A mental or physical disability.

hand·piece, *n.* A device used in connection with the dental engine for engaging such instruments as burs and mandrels during operative procedures; held in the hand of the operator.

Hand-Schül·ler-Chris·tian disease or **syndrome** A syndrome of childhood, of unknown cause, insidious in onset and progressive, characterized by exophthalmos, diabetes insipidus, and softened or punched-out areas in the bones, particularly in the femurs and those of the skull, shoulder, and pelvic girdle, and with foci of reticuloendothelial proliferation which may be found in every part of the body.

hang·nail, *n.* A partly detached piece of skin of the nail fold, friction against which has caused inflammation.

hang·over, *n.* The disagreeable aftereffects following use of alcohol or of certain drugs, such as barbiturates, in large or excessive doses.

Ha·not's cirrhosis or **disease** (a^h·no') BILIARY CIRRHOSIS.

Han·sen's bacillus MYCOBACTERIUM LEPRAE.

Hansen's disease LEPROSY.

Hapamine. Trademark for a histamine-protein complex used subcutaneously for histamine desensitization.

haph·al·ge·sia (haf''al·jee'zee·uh) *n.* A sensation

of pain experienced upon the mere touching of an object.

haph·e·pho·bia (haf″e·fo′bee·uh) *n.* A morbid fear of being touched or having to touch objects. Syn. *haptephobia.*

hapl-, haplo- A combining form meaning (a) *single;* (b) *simple.*

hap·lo·dont (hap′lo·dont) *adj.* In biology, having or pertaining to molar teeth having simple or single crowns.

ha·plo·pia (ha·plo′pee·uh) *n.* Single vision.

hap·lo·scope (hap′lo·skope) *n.* An instrument for measuring the visual axes.

hap·ten (hap′ten) *n.* A low-molecular-weight substance which reacts with a specific antibody but which by itself is unable to elicit the formation of that antibody. It is antigenic (immunogenic) if coupled to an antigenic carrier. —**hap·ten·ic** (hap·ten′ick) *adj.*

hap·tic (hap′tick) *adj.* Pertaining to the sense of touch; tactile.

hap·tics (hap′ticks) *n.* The branch of psychology dealing with the sense of touch.

hap·to·dys·pho·ria (hap″to·dis·fo′ree·uh) *n.* The disagreeable sensation sometimes aroused by touching certain objects, such as nylon or fine sandpaper.

hap·to·glo·bin (hap′to·glo″bin) *n.* A hemoglobin-binding $α_2$-globulin of serum, which occurs in at least three different antigenic types.

hard·ness, *n.* In radiology, a quality of roentgen rays; increased hardness is associated with increased penetrating power, greater energy, and shorter wavelength.

hard pad. A disease of dogs, probably associated with the canine distemper virus; often characterized by encephalitis and hardening of the foot pads.

hard palate. The anterior part of the palate which is formed by the palatal processes of the maxillary bones and the palatine bones with their covering mucous membranes.

hard·ware disease. Traumatic results of the ingestion of hardware or other metal objects in cattle.

hare·lip, *n.* A congenital cleft, or clefts, in the upper lip, resulting from a failure of the union of the maxillary and median nasal processes which may be bilateral and sometimes involves the maxilla and palate. Syn. *cheiloschisis.*

har·paxo·pho·bia (hahr″pack·so·fo′bee·uh) *n.* An abnormal fear of robbers.

Har·ri·son Narcotic Act The federal law regulating the possession, sale, purchase, and prescription of habit-forming drugs.

Harrison spot test. A test for bilirubin in urine in which urine and barium chloride are mixed and dried on filter paper, and a drop of Fouchet's reagent is added. A green color indicates the presence of bilirubin, which is oxidized to biliverdin.

Hart·man·nel·la (hahrt′mun·el″uh) *n.* A genus of nonparasitic, free-living amebas, commonly found in soil and water. Some varieties are pathogenic for the central nervous system of mammals. This organism was formerly incriminated in human meningoencephalitis on the basis of the morphological appearance of the trophozoites, but on culture these cases have proved to be due to an ameboflagellate, *Naegleria fowleri.*

Hart·nup disease A hereditary metabolic disorder in which there is defective intestinal absorption and renal tubular reabsorption of monoamino-monocarboxylic acids, with indicanuria resulting from the bacterial conversion to indole of tryptophan reaching the colon in large amounts; usually manifested by short stature, and clinically by a pellagra-like dermatitis on exposure to sunlight, episodic and reversible ataxia, nystagmus and sometimes pyramidal tract signs, transient psychiatric disorders, and often mild mental retardation; thought to be transmitted as a homozygous autosomal recessive trait. Syn. *H disease.*

harvest mite. EUTROMBICULA ALFREDDUGESI.

Ha·shi·mo·to's disease STRUMA LYMPHOMATOSA.

hash·ish, hash·eesh (hash′eesh, ha·sheesh′) *n.* The pure resinous exudate of the female hemp plant, *Cannabis sativa,* prepared as a tincture and formerly used in medicine, or prepared as a hardened resin and smoked or eaten as an intoxicant and mild hallucinogen.

Hassall's body or **corpuscle** THYMIC CORPUSCLE.

haunch, *n.* The part of the body which includes the hip and the buttock of one side.

haus·tra·tion (haw·stray′shun) *n.* 1. HAUSTRUM. 2. The formation of a haustrum.

haus·trum (haw′strum) *n.,* pl. **haus·tra** (·truh) One of the pouches or sacculations of the colon. —**haus·tral** (·trul) *adj.*

Ha·ver·hill fever An acute infection due to *Streptobacillus moniliformis,* usually acquired by rat bite, and characterized by acute onset, intermittent fever, erythematous rash, and polyarthritis. Syn. *erythema arthriticum epidemicum, streptobacillary fever.*

ha·ver·sian (ha·vur′zhun, ha·) *adj.* Described by or associated with Clopton Havers, English anatomist, 1650–1702.

haversian canal. Any one of the canals penetrating the compact substance of bone in a longitudinal direction and anastomosing with one another by transverse or oblique branches. They contain blood vessels and connective tissue.

haversian system. The concentric layers of bone about a haversian canal; concentric lamellar system.

Hayem's solution A solution of mercuric chloride, anhydrous sodium sulfate, and sodium chloride in water; used as a diluent for erythrocyte counting.

hay fever. A seasonal form of allergic rhinitis characterized by sneezing, rhinorrhea, itching of the eyes, and lacrimation; attributed to pollen antigens in the air.

Hb 1. An abbreviation for *hemoglobin.* 2. A symbol for reduced hemoglobin.

HBD Abbreviation for *α-hydroxybutyric dehydrogenase.*

HCG Human chorionic gonadotropin.

h. d. Abbreviation for *hora decubitus,* at the hour of going to bed.

He Symbol for helium.

head, *n.* 1. The uppermost part of the body, containing the brain, organs of sight, smell, taste, hearing, and part of the organs of speech. 2. The top, beginning, or most prominent part of anything.

head-ache, *n.* Pain in the head. Syn. *cephalalgia.*

head louse. The louse *Pediculus humanus capitis,* a vector of disease and the cause of pediculosis capitis.

Head's areas or **zones** The segments of skin exhibiting reflex hyperesthesia and hyperalgesia due to disease of the viscera.

heal-er, *n.* 1. One who effects cures. 2. A Christian Science practitioner. 3. A person without formal medical education who claims to cure by some form of suggestion.

heal-ing, *n.* The process or act of getting well or of making whole; the restoration of diseased parts; curing. **—heal,** *v.*

healing by first intention. The primary union of a wound when the incised skin edges are approximated and so held and union takes place without the process of granulation.

healing by second intention. The process of wound closure where the edges remain separated; the wound becomes closed after granulation tissue has filled the cavity to the skin level so that epithelium can grow over the unhealed area.

health, *n.* 1. The state of dynamic equilibrium between the organism and its environment which maintains the structural and functional integrity of the organism within the normal limits for the particular form of life (race, genus, species) and the particular phase of its life cycle. 2. The state of being sound in body and mind; well-being. **—health-ful, healthy** *adj.*

health physics. The study and practice of various methods of protection from the undesirable effects of ionizing radiation.

hearing aid. An instrument that amplifies the intensity of sound waves, used by persons with impaired hearing.

hearing loss. Impairment of ability to hear, sometimes only within certain frequency ranges.

heart, *n.* A hollow muscular organ in the thorax which functions as a pump to maintain the circulation of the blood.

heart-beat, *n.* The throb or pulsation of the heart with each ventricular systole.

heart block. Any partial or complete interruption in the transmission of the activation process from the sinoatrial node to the ventricular myocardium; especially, ATRIOVENTRICULAR BLOCK.

heart-burn, *n.* A burning sensation over the precordium or beneath the sternum, usually from the esophagus; gastric pyrosis.

heart failure. 1. The condition in which the heart is no longer able to pump an adequate supply of blood in relation to venous return and to meet the metabolic needs of body tissues. 2. CONGESTIVE HEART FAILURE. 3. CIRCULATORY FAILURE.

heart rate. The number of ventricular contractions per minute.

heart sounds. The sounds produced by normal hemodynamic events heard on auscultation over the heart; the first and second heart sounds are related to closure of the atrioventricular and semilunar valves, respectively, as well as to ventricular systole; the third and fourth are softer, often inaudible, and are related to the early rapid (passive) phase of ventricular filling, and the late (presystolic) active phase produced by atrial contraction, respectively.

heart-wa-ter disease. A tick-borne disease of ruminants seen in South Africa; due to *Cowdria ruminantium* and characterized by serous exudate in the pericardium.

heart-worm, *n.* DIROFILARIA IMMITIS.

heat, *n.* 1. A form of kinetic energy communicable from one body to another by conduction, convection, or radiation; it is that form of molecular motion which is appreciated by a special thermal sense. 2. The periodic sexual excitement in animals.

heat and acid test. A test for protein in urine in which urine is boiled in a test tube for 1 or 2 minutes and then 3 to 5 drops of 5% acetic acid are added. A white precipitate indicates protein.

heat capacity. The amount of heat necessary to raise the temperature of a body from 15° to 16°C.

heat exhaustion, collapse, or **prostration.** A heat-exposure syndrome characterized by weakness, vertigo, headache, nausea, and peripheral vascular collapse, usually precipitated by physical exertion in a hot environment.

heat rash. MILIARIA.

heat-ray cataract. A slowly progressing posterior cortical lens opacity due to prolonged exposure to high temperatures, sometimes seen in persons engaged in the glassblowing or iron-puddling industries.

heat-regulating centers. Centers in the hypothalamus for the control of heat production and heat elimination and for regulating the relation of these.

heat-stroke, *n.* A heat-exposure syndrome characterized by hyperpyrexia and prostration due to diminution or cessation of sweating, occurring most commonly in persons with underlying disease.

heaves, *n.* 1. Chronic diffuse alveolar emphysema of the horse, characterized by difficult and laborious respiration. Syn. *broken wind.* 2. Retching or vomiting.

heavy, *adj.* 1. Of substances: high in density or specific gravity. 2. Of elements: high in atomic weight. 3. Of isotopes: higher in atomic weight than the most common or stable isotope.

heavy chain. Any of the polypeptide subunits (molecular weight 50,000 to 70,000) of immunoglobulin molecules which determine the distinctive properties of each immunoglobulin class and which are classified, depending on the immunoglobulin molecule in which they occur, as alpha chains (IgA), gamma chains (IgG), delta chains (IgD), epsilon chains (IgE), or mu chains (IgM).

heavy hydrogen. DEUTERIUM.

he·be·phre·nia (hee''be·free'nee·uh) *n.* HEBE-PHRENIC TYPE OF SCHIZOPHRENIA. —**hebe-phren·ic** (·fren'ick) *adj.*

hebephrenic type of schizophrenia. A form of schizophrenia marked by disorganized thinking, mannerisms, and regressive behavior caricaturing that seen in some adolescents, such as silliness, unpredictable giggling, and posturing; delusions and hallucinations, if present, are not well organized and are transient. Syn. *pubescent insanity.*

Heberden's arthritis Degenerative joint disease of the terminal joints of the fingers, producing enlargement (Heberden's nodes) and flexion deformities. Most common in older women; prominent hereditary pattern.

Heberden's node Nodose deformity of the fingers in degenerative joint disease. Syn. *Heberden-Rosenbach node.*

he·bet·ic (he·bet'ick) *adj.* Relating to, or occurring at, puberty or adolescence.

heb·e·tude (heb'e·tewd) *n.* Dullness of the special senses and intellect. —**heb·e·tu·di·nous** (heb''e·tew'di·nus) *adj.*

hect-, hecto- A combining form meaning *one hundred.*

hec·tic (heck'tick) *adj.* 1. Of a fever: recurring daily and tending to rise in the afternoon, as in tuberculosis or septicemia. 2. Consumptive; tuberculous.

hecto-. See *hect-.*

hec·to·gram (heck'to·gram) *n.* One hundred grams, or 1,543.2349 grains. Abbreviated, hg.

hec·to·li·ter (heck'to·lee''tur) *n.* One hundred liters; equal to 22 imperial or 26.4 United States gallons. Abbreviated, hl.

hec·to·me·ter (heck'to·mee''tur) *n.* One hundred meters, or 328 feet 1 inch. Abbreviated, hm.

he·do·nia (he·do'nee·uh) *n.* Abnormal cheerfulness; AMENOMANIA (2).

he·don·ism (hee'dun·iz·um) *n.* 1. The philosophy in which the attainment of pleasure and happiness is the supreme good. 2. *In psychology and psychiatry,* the doctrine that every act is motivated by the desire for pleasure or the aversion from pain and unpleasantness.

he·do·no·pho·bia (hee''duh·no·fo'bee·uh) *n.* An abnormal fear of pleasure.

heel, *n.* The hinder part of the human foot below the ankle.

heel cord. CALCANEAL TENDON.

heel-to-knee-to-toe test. A test for nonequilibratory coordination in which the patient is asked to place the heel of one foot on the opposite knee, then push the heel along the shin to the big toe. Normally, this is done smoothly and accurately.

He·gar's sign (hey'gar) Softening of the isthmic portion of the uterus which occurs at about six weeks of gestation in pregnancy.

he·gem·o·ny (he·jem'uh·nee) *n.* Leadership, domination; as the supremacy of one function over a number of others.

Heim·lich maneuver The abrupt application of upward pressure to the upper abdomen, used as a technique for explusion of a choking object from the windpipe.

Heinz bodies Refractile areas in red cells, probably representing denatured globin or methemoglobin; seen in hemolytic anemia due to toxic agents.

helc-, helco- A combining form meaning *ulcer.*

hel·coid (hel'koid) *adj.* Resembling an ulcer; ulcerative.

heli-, helio- A combining form meaning (a) *the sun;* (b) *sunlight.*

helic-, helico-. A combining form meaning (a) *helix, helical;* (b) *spiral;* (c) *snail.*

hel·i·cal (hel'i·kul) *adj.* 1. Pertaining to a helix. 2. Having the form of a helix.

hel·i·cine (hel'i·seen, ·sine, ·sin) *adj.* 1. Spiral, coiled. 2. Pertaining to a helix.

hel·i·cis (hel'i·sis) *n.* A vestigial muscle associated with the helix of the external ear; a helicis major and helicis minor have been described.

helico-. See *helic-.*

hel·i·coid (hel'i·koid) *adj.* Spiral; coiled like a snail shell.

hel·i·co·tre·ma (hel''i·ko·tree'muh) *n.* The opening connecting the scalae tympani and vestibuli of the spiral canal of the perilymphatic space of the cochlea.

he·li·en·ceph·a·li·tis (hee''lee·en·sef''uh·lye'tis) *n.* HEATSTROKE.

he·lio·phobe (hee'lee·o·fobe) *n.* One who is abnormally sensitive to the effects of the sun's rays, or afraid of them.

he·lio·pho·bia (hee''lee·o·fo'bee·uh) *n.* An abnormal fear of exposure to the sun's rays.

he·lio·tax·is (hee''lee·o·tack'sis) *n.* A form of taxis in which there is attraction toward (positive heliotaxis) or repulsion from (negative heliotaxis) the sun or sunlight.

he·lio·ther·a·py (hee''lee·o·therr'uh·pee) *n.* SOLAR THERAPY.

he·li·um (hee'lee·um) *n.* He = 4.0026. A chemically inert, colorless, odorless, nonflammable, gaseous element, occurring in certain natural gases and in small amount in the atmosphere; next to the lightest element known. A mixture with oxygen, being less dense than ordinary air, is useful in various types of dyspnea and in cases involving respiratory obstruction.

he·lix (hee'licks) *n.,* genit. **he·li·cis** (hee'li·sis, hel'i·), L. pl. **hel·i·ces** (hel'i·seez, hee'li·) 1. [NA] The rounded convex margin of the pinna of the ear. 2. An object or other entity spiral in form, as a coil of wire, the native structure of deoxyribonucleic acid, or a three-dimensional curve with one or more turns about an axis.

hel·le·bore (hel'e·bore) *n.* A plant of the genus *Helleborus,* particularly *Helleborus niger,* black hellebore, which has been used as a purgative.

hel·minth (hel'minth) *n.* Originally any parasitic worm; now includes those worm-like animals, either parasitic or free-living, of the phyla Platyhelminthes and Nemathelminthes as well as members of the phylum Annelida.

hel·min·tha·gogue (hel·min'thuh·gog) *n.* ANTHELMINTIC.

hel·min·them·e·sis (hel''min·them'e·sis) *n.* The vomiting of worms.

hel·min·thi·a·sis (hel''min·thigh'uh·sis) *n.,* pl. **hel-**

minthia·ses (·seez) A disease caused by parasitic worms in the body.

hel·min·thic (hel·min'thick) adj. Pertaining to or caused by a worm.

hel·min·tho·ma (hel''min·tho'muh) n., pl. **helminthomas, helminthoma·ta** (·tuh) A mass caused by the presence of a parasitic worm.

hel·min·tho·pho·bia (hel·min''tho·fo'bee·uh) n. An abnormal fear of worms or of becoming infected with worms.

helo- A combining form meaning (a) horny, studded; (b) corn, callosity.

he·lo·ma (he·lo'muh) n., pl. **helomas, heloma·ta** (·tuh) CALLOSITY.

he·lot·o·my (he·lot'uh·mee) n. The cutting of a corn; surgery upon a corn.

hel·vol·ic acid (hel·vol'ick) n. An antibiotic substance, $C_{33}H_{44}O_8$, produced by Aspergillus fumigatus; identical with fumigacin.

hem-, hema-, hemo-, haem-, haema-, haemo- A combining form meaning blood, of or pertaining to blood.

he·mag·glu·ti·na·tion, hae·mag·glu·ti·na·tion (hee''muh·gloo''ti·nay'shun, hem'·uh·) n. The clumping of red blood cells, as by specific antibodies or by hemagglutinating viruses.

hem·ag·glu·ti·nin, haem·ag·glu·ti·nin (hee''muh·gloo'ti·nin, hem'·uh·) n. 1. An antibody which agglutinates red blood cells. 2. The protein antigen of some viruses, such as the myxoviruses, thought to be the enzyme neuraminidase which reacts with the neuraminic acid of red blood cells to lead to agglutination. 3. Any agent which agglutinates red blood cells.

he·mal, hae·mal (hee'mul) adj. 1. Pertaining to the blood or the vascular system. 2. Pertaining to the part of the body containing the heart and major blood vessels.

hemal node or **gland.** A node of lymphatic tissue, situated in the course of blood vessels, and containing large numbers of erythrocytes; frequently found in ruminants.

he·man·gi·ec·ta·sis, hae·man·gi·ec·ta·sis (he·man''jee·eck'tuh·sis) n., pl. **hemangiecta·ses, haemangiecta·ses** (·seez) Dilatation of blood vessels. —**hemangi·ec·tat·ic, haemangi·ec·tat·ic** (·eck·tat'ick) adj.

he·man·gi·o·am·e·lo·blas·to·ma, hae·man·gio·am·e·lo·blas·to·ma (he·man''jee·o·am''e·lo·blas·to'muh) n. An ameloblastoma with a prominent vascular stroma.

he·man·gio·blas·to·ma, hae·man·gio·blas·to·ma (he·man''jee·o·blas·to'muh) n. A variety of hemangioma whose vascular spaces are lined by prominent endothelial cells, found especially in the cerebellum.

he·man·gio·blas·to·ma·to·sis, hae·man·gio·blas·to·ma·to·sis (he·man''jee·o·blas''to·muh·to'sis) n. Widespread occurrence of hemangioblastomas.

he·man·gi·o·en·do·the·li·o·ma, hae·man·gi·o·en·do·the·li·o·ma (he·man''jee·o·en''do·theel·ee·o'muh) n. 1. A highly cellular benign hemangioma seen in children. Syn. benign hemangioendothelioma. 2. A malignant tumor composed of anaplastic endothelial cells forming vascular spaces in some instances. Syn. angiosarcoma, malignant hemangioendothelioma.

he·man·gio·en·do·the·lio·sar·co·ma, hae·man·gio·en·do·the·lio·sar·co·ma (he·man''jee·o·en''do·theel''ee·o·sahr·ko'muh) n. HEMANGIOENDOTHELIOMA (2).

he·man·gio·li·po·ma, hae·man·gio·li·po·ma (he·man''jee·o·li·po'muh) n. A hamartomatous mass having hemangiomatous and lipomatous elements.

he·man·gi·o·ma, hae·man·gi·o·ma (he·man''jee·o'muh) n. An angioma made up of blood vessels. —**hemangioma·tous, haemangioma·tous** (·tus) adj.

he·man·gi·o·ma·to·sis, hae·man·gi·o·ma·to·sis (he·man''jee·o·muh·to'sis) n., pl. **hemangiomato·ses, haemangiomato·ses** (·seez) The occurrence of multiple hemangiomas.

he·man·gio·myo·li·po·ma, hae·man·gio·myo·li·po·ma (he·man''jee·o·migh''o·li·po'muh) n. A hamartomatous mass containing hemangiomatous, muscular, and lipomatous elements.

he·man·gio·peri·cy·to·ma, hae·man·gio·peri·cy·to·ma (he·man''jee·o·perr''i·sigh·to'muh) n. A tumor composed of endothelium-lined tubes or cords of cells, surrounded by spherical cells with supporting reticulin network; the parenchymal cells are presumed to be related to pericytes.

he·man·gio·sar·co·ma, hae·man·gio·sar·co·ma (he·man''jee·o·sahr·ko'muh) n. HEMANGIOENDOTHELIOMA (2).

hem·ar·thro·sis, haem·ar·thro·sis (hee''mahr·thro'sis, hem''ahr·) n., pl. **hemarthro·ses, haemarthro·ses** (·seez) Extravasation of blood into a joint.

hemat-, hemato-, haemat-, haemato- A combining form meaning blood, of or pertaining to the blood.

he·ma·tem·e·sis, hae·ma·tem·e·sis (hee''muh·tem'e·sis, hem'·uh·) n. The vomiting of blood.

he·mat·hi·dro·sis, hae·mat·hi·dro·sis (hee''mat·hi·dro'sis, hem''at·) n. The appearance of blood or blood products in sweat gland secretions.

he·mat·ic, hae·mat·ic (hee·mat'ick) adj. Pertaining to, full of, or having the color of, blood.

he·ma·tin, hae·ma·tin (hee'muh·tin, hem'uh·tin) n. Ferriheme hydroxide, $C_{34}H_{32}N_4O_4 \cdot FeOH$, formed from hemin by treatment with alkali; contains iron in the ferric state.

he·ma·ti·ne·mia, hae·ma·ti·nae·mia (hem''uh·ti·nee'mee·uh, hee''muh·) n. The presence of heme in the blood.

he·ma·tin·ic, hae·ma·tin·ic (hee''muh·tin'ick, hem''uh·tin'ick) n. & adj. 1. An agent that tends to increase the hemoglobin content of the blood. 2. Pertaining to or containing hematin. 3. Pertaining to or acting like a hematinic.

hemato-. See hemat-.

he·ma·to·bil·ia (hee''muh·to·bil'ee·uh, hem''uh·) n. A condition in which there is blood in the bile ducts. Syn. hemobilia.

he·ma·to·blast, hae·ma·to·blast (hee'muh·to·blast, hem'uh·, hee·mat'o·) n. An immature form of hematopoietic cell.

he·ma·to·cele, hae·ma·to·cele (hee'muh·to·seel, hem'uh·, he·mat'o·) n. The extravasation and collection of blood in a part, especially in the cavity of the tunica vaginalis testis.

he·ma·to·che·zia, hae·ma·to·che·zia (hee''muh·to·kee'zee·uh, hem''uh·) n. HEMOCHEZIA.

he·ma·to·chy·lo·cele, hae·ma·to·chy·lo·cele (hee''muh·to·kigh'lo·seel, hem''uh·to·) n. The extravasation and collection of chyle and blood in a part, especially in the tunica vaginalis testis, complicating filariasis.

he·ma·to·chy·lu·ria, hae·ma·to·chy·lu·ria (hee''muh·to·kigh·lew'ree·uh, hem''uh·to·) n. The presence of blood and chyle in the urine.

he·ma·to·col·pos, hae·ma·to·col·pos (hee''muh·to·kol'pus, hem''uh·to·) n. A retained collection of blood within the vagina, resulting from an imperforate hymen or other obstruction.

he·ma·to·crit, hae·ma·to·crit (he·mat'o·krit, hee'muh·to·krit) n. 1. Hematocrit reading. 2. A small centrifuge used to separate blood cells in clinical analysis. 3. The centrifuge tube in which the blood cells are separated.

hematocrit reading. The percentage of the whole blood volume occupied by the red cells after centrifugation.

he·ma·to·cyst, hae·ma·to·cyst (he·mat'o·sist, hee'muh·to·) n. A cyst containing blood.

he·ma·to·cy·tol·y·sis, hae·ma·to·cy·tol·y·sis (hee''muh·to·sigh·tol'i·sis, hem''uh·to·) n. HEMOLYSIS.

he·ma·to·en·ce·phal·ic, hae·ma·to·en·ce·phal·ic (hee''muh·to·en''se·fal'ick, hem''uh·to·) adj. Pertaining to the blood and the brain.

he·ma·tog·e·nous, hae·ma·tog·e·nous (hee''muh·toj'e·nus, hem''uh·) adj. 1. Pertaining to the production of blood or its constituents. 2. Disseminated via the circulation or transported by the bloodstream. 3. Derived from the blood.

he·ma·toi·din, hae·ma·toi·din (hee''muh·toy'din) n. A golden yellow, orange, or reddish-brown amorphous or crystalline iron-negative pigment found free or sometimes in macrophages in areas of hemorrhagic infarction.

he·ma·tol·o·gist, hae·ma·tol·o·gist (hee''muh·tol'uh·jist, hem''uh·) n. A person who specializes in the study of blood.

he·ma·tol·o·gy, hae·ma·tol·o·gy (hee''muh·tol'uh·jee, hem''uh·) n. The science of the blood, its nature, functions, and diseases. —**hema·to·log·ic, haema·to·log·ic** (·to·loj'ick) adj.

he·ma·to·lymph·uria, hae·ma·to·lymph·uria (hee''muh·to·lim·few'ree·uh, hem''uh·to·) n. The discharge of urine containing lymph and blood.

he·ma·to·lymph·an·gi·o·ma, hae·ma·to·lymph·an·gi·o·ma (hee''muh·to·lim·fan''jee·o'muh, hem''uh·to·) n. A benign tumor composed of blood vessels and lymph vessels.

he·ma·to·lyt·o·poi·et·ic, hae·ma·to·lyt·o·poi·et·ic (hee''muh·to·lit''o·poy·et'ick, hem''uh·to·) adj. HEMOLYTOPOIETIC.

he·ma·to·ma, hae·ma·to·ma (hee''muh·to'muh, hem''uh·) n., pl. **hematomas, hematoma·ta** (·tuh) A circumscribed extravascular collection of blood, usually clotted, which forms a mass.

he·ma·to·me·tra, hae·ma·to·me·tra (hee''muh·

to·mee'truh, hem''uh·to·) n. An accumulation of blood or menstrual fluid in the uterus.

he·ma·to·mole, hae·ma·to·mole (hee''muh·to·mole) n. BREUS'S MOLE.

he·ma·to·my·e·lia, hae·ma·to·my·e·lia (hee''muh·to·migh·ee''lee·uh, hem''uh·to·) n. Hemorrhage into the spinal cord.

he·ma·to·my·e·li·tis, hae·ma·to·my·e·li·tis (hee''muh·to·migh''e·lye'tis, hem''uh·to·) n. An acute myelitis together with an effusion of blood into the spinal cord.

he·ma·ton·ic, hae·ma·ton·ic (hee''muh·ton'ick, hem''uh·) n. HEMATINIC.

he·ma·toph·a·gous, hae·ma·toph·a·gous (hee''muh·tof'uh·gus, hem''uh·) adj. Bloodsucking, subsisting on blood.

he·ma·to·poi·e·sis, hae·ma·to·poi·e·sis (hee''muh·to·poy·ee'sis, he·mat''o·, hem''uh·to·) n. The formation and maturation of blood cells and their derivatives. Syn. *hemopoiesis*.

he·ma·to·poi·et·ic, hae·ma·to·poi·et·ic (hee''muh·to·poy·et'ick, he·mat''o·, hem''uh·to·) adj. Blood-forming; of or pertaining to hematopoiesis. Syn. *hemopoietic*.

he·ma·to·por·phy·rin, hae·ma·to·por·phy·rin (hee''muh·to·por'fi·rin, hem''uh·to·) n. HEMOPORPHYRIN.

he·ma·to·por·phy·rin·uria, hae·ma·to·por·phy·rin·uria (hee''muh·to·por''fi·ri·new'ree·uh, hem''uh·to·) n. The presence of hemoporphyrin in the urine.

he·ma·tor·rha·chis, hae·ma·tor·rha·chis (hee''muh·to·ray'kis, hee''muh·tor'uh·kis) n. Hemorrhage into the spinal canal.

he·ma·tor·rhea, hae·ma·tor·rhoea (hee''muh·to·ree'uh, hem''uh·to·, he·mat'o·) n. Copious or profuse hemorrhage.

he·ma·to·sal·pinx, hae·ma·to·sal·pinx (hee''muh·to·sal'pinks, hem''uh·to·) n. A collection of blood in a uterine tube.

he·ma·to·scope, hae·ma·to·scope (hee''muh·to·skope, hem''uh·to·, he·mat'o·) n. An instrument used in the spectroscopic or optical examination of the blood.

he·ma·tose, hae·ma·tose (hee'muh·toce) adj. Full of blood; bloody.

he·ma·to·sis, hae·ma·to·sis (hee''muh·to'sis, hem''uh·) n. Obsol. 1. HEMATOPOIESIS. 2. Oxygenation of the blood, especially in the lungs.

he·ma·to·sper·ma·to·cele, hae·ma·to·sper·ma·to·cele (hee''muh·to·spur'muh·to·seel, ·spur·mat'o·seel, hem''uh·to·) n. A spermatocele containing blood.

he·ma·to·sper·mia, hae·ma·to·sper·mia (hee''muh·to·spur'mee·uh, hem''uh·to·) n. The discharge of bloody semen. Syn. *hemospermia*.

he·ma·to·tox·ic, hae·ma·to·tox·ic (hee''muh·to·tock'sick, hem''uh·to·) adj. Poisonous to the hematopoietic tissues. —**hemato·tox·ic·i·ty** (·tock·sis'i·tee) n.

he·ma·to·tox·i·co·sis, hae·ma·to·tox·i·co·sis (hee''muh·to·tock''si·ko'sis, hem''uh·to·) n. A state of toxic damage to the hematopoietic system.

he·ma·tox·y·lin, hae·ma·tox·y·lin (hee''muh·tock'si·lin, hem''uh·) n. 1. A colorless crystalline compound, $C_{16}H_{14}O_6$, occurring in hematoxylon. Upon oxidation, it is converted to hematein which forms deeply colored lakes with various metals. Used as a stain in microscopy. 2. ALUM HEMATOXYLIN.

he·ma·tox·y·lino·phil·ic, hae·ma·tox·y·lino·phil·ic (hee″muh·tock″so·lin·o·fil′ick) *adj.* Having an affinity for hematoxylin.

he·ma·tox·y·lon, hae·ma·tox·y·lon (hee″muh·tock′si·lon, hem′uh·) *n.* The heartwood of *Haematoxylon campechianum;* contains tannic acid and hematoxylin. Has been used as a mild astringent. Syn. *logwood.*

he·ma·to·zo·on, hae·ma·to·zo·on (hee″muh·to·zo′on, hem″uh·to·) *n.,* pl. **hemato·zoa, haemato·zoa** (·zo′uh) Any animal parasite living in the blood. **—hematozo·al, haematozo·al** (·ul), **hematozo·ic, haematozo·ic** (·ick) *adj.*

he·ma·tu·ria, hae·ma·tu·ria (hee″muh·tew′ree·uh, hem′uh·) *n.* The discharge of urine containing blood.

heme, haem (heem) *n.* $C_{34}H_{32}N_4O_4Fe$; the ferrous complex of protoporphyrin 9, constituting the prosthetic component of hemoglobin. Syn. *ferroheme, reduced heme, ferroprotoporphyrin 9.*

hem·er·a·lo·pia (hem″ur·uh·lo′pee·uh) *n.* 1. DAY BLINDNESS. 2. *Erron.* NIGHT BLINDNESS.

hemi- A prefix meaning (a) *half, partial;* (b) in biology and medicine, either *the right or the left half of the body;* (c) in chemistry, *a combining ratio of one-half.*

hemi·achro·ma·top·sia (hem″ee·a·kro″muh·top′see·uh) *n.* A loss of color vision in corresponding halves of each visual field due to a lesion of one occipital lobe.

hemi·agen·e·sis (hem″ee·a·jen′e·sis) *n.* Failure of development of one half or one side of a part, usually one consisting of two nearly symmetrical halves, as the cerebellum.

hemi·ageu·sia (hem″ee·a·gew′zee·uh, ·a·joo′see·uh) *n.* Loss of the sense of taste on one side of the tongue.

hemi·al·bu·mose (hem″ee·al′bew·moce) *n.* A product of the digestion of certain kinds of proteins. It is a normal constituent of bone marrow, and is found also in the urine of patients with osteomalacia. Syn. *propeptone, pseudopeptone.*

hemi·al·bu·mo·su·ria (hem″ee·al″bew·mo·sue′ree·uh) *n.* The presence of hemialbumose in the urine. Syn. *propeptonuria.*

hemi·an·a·cu·sia (hem″ee·an″uh·kew′zhuh, ·zee·uh) *n.* Deafness in one ear.

hemi·an·al·ge·sia (hem″ee·an″uh·jee′zee·uh) *n.* Insensibility to pain on one side of the body.

hemi·an·en·ceph·a·ly (hem″ee·an″en·sef′uh·lee) *n.* Anencephaly on one side only.

hemi·an·es·the·sia, hemi·an·aes·the·sia (hem″ee·an″es·theez′uh, ·theez′ee·uh) *n.* Loss of sensation on one side of the body; unilateral anesthesia.

hemi·an·o·pia (hem″ee·an·o′pee·uh) *n.* HEMIANOPSIA. **—hemiano·pic** (·pick) *adj. & n.*

hemi·an·op·sia (hem″ee·an·op′see·uh) *n.* Blindness in one half of the visual field; may be bilateral or unilateral.

hemi·atax·ia (hem″ee·uh·tack′see·uh) *n.* Ataxia affecting one side of the body.

hemi·ath·e·to·sis (hem″ee·ath″e·to′sis) *n.,* pl. **hemiatheto·ses** (·seez) Athetosis of one side of the body.

hemi·at·ro·phy (hem″ee·at′ruh·fee) *n.* Atrophy confined to one side of an organ or region of the body.

hemi·azy·gos, hemi·azy·gous (hem″ee·az′i·gus, uh·zye′gus) *adj.* Partially paired.

hemi·bal·lis·mus (hem″ee·ba·liz′mus) *n.* Sudden, violent, flinging movements involving particularly the proximal portions of the extremities of one side of the body; caused by a destructive lesion of the contralateral subthalamic nucleus or its neighboring structures or pathways; HEMICHOREA.

he·mic, hae·mic (hee′mick) *adj.* Pertaining to or developed by the blood.

hemi·car·dia (hem″ee·kahr′dee·uh) *n.* The presence of only a lateral half of the usual four-chambered heart.

hemi·ce·phal·ic (hem″ee·se·fal′ick) *adj.* Pertaining to or involving one side of the head.

hemicephalic vasodilation. CLUSTER HEADACHE.

hemi·ceph·a·ly (hem″ee·sef′uh·lee) *n.* HEMIANENCEPHALY; anencephaly on one side only.

hemi·cho·rea (hem″ee·ko·ree′uh) *n.* Chorea in which the involuntary movements are largely confined to one side of the body.

hemic murmur. A cardiac or vascular murmur, usually systolic, heard with anemia or other high cardiac output state; due to increased velocity of blood flow.

hemi·co·lec·to·my (hem″ee·ko·leck′tuh·mee) *n.* Excision of one side of the colon.

hemi·con·vul·sion (hem″ee·kun·vul′shun) *n.* A form of epilepsy characterized by tonic-clonic movements of one side of the body.

hemi·cra·nia (hem″i·kray′nee·uh) *n.* 1. MIGRAINE. 2. Pain or headache on one side of the head only.

hemi·cra·ni·o·sis (hem″i·kray″nee·o′sis) *n.* Enlargement of one half of the cranium or face.

hemi·cys·tec·to·my (hem″ee·sis·teck′tuh·mee) *n.* Removal of half of the urinary bladder.

hemi·de·cor·ti·ca·tion (hem″ee·dee·kor″ti·kay′shun) *n.* Removal of the cortex from one cerebral hemisphere.

hemi·di·a·phragm (hem″ee·dye′uh·fram) *n.* 1. A lateral half of the diaphragm. 2. A diaphragm in which the muscle development is deficient on one side.

hemi·dys·es·the·sia, hemi·dys·aes·the·sia (hem″ee·dis″es·theezh′uh, ·theez′ee·uh) *n.* Impairment of the cutaneous senses, especially of touch, and paresthesias on one side of the body.

hemi·fa·cial (hem″ee·fay′shul) *adj.* Pertaining to one side of the face.

hemi·glos·sec·to·my (hem″ee·glos·eck′tuh·mee) *n.* Removal of one side of the tongue.

hemi·glos·so·ple·gia (hem″ee·glos″o·plee′jee·uh) *n.* Unilateral paralysis of the tongue with relatively minor disturbances of motility; the tongue deviates toward the palsied side upon protrusion.

hemi·gna·thia (hem″i·nay′thee·uh, ·nath′ee·uh) *n.* Partial or complete absence of the lower jaw on one side. —**hemi·gnath·us** (·nath'us, nayth'us) *n.*

hemi·hyp·al·ge·sia (hem''ee·high''pal·jee'zee·uh) *n.* Decreased sensitivity to pain on one side of the body.

hemi·hy·per·es·the·sia, hemi·hy·per·aes·the·sia (hem''ee·high''pur·es·theezh'uh, ·theez'ee·uh) *n.* Increased sensitivity to tactile stimulation on one side of the body.

hemi·hy·per·hi·dro·sis (hem''ee·high''pur·hi·dro'sis) *n.* Excessive sweating on one side of the body.

hemi·hy·per·to·nia (hem''ee·high''pur·to'nee·uh) *n.* Increased muscular tone confined to one side of the body.

hemi·hy·per·tro·phy (hem''ee·high·pur'truh·fee) *n.* Hypertrophy of one side of the body or unilateral hypertrophy of one or more bodily regions (e.g., the head, an arm).

hemi·hyp·es·the·sia, hemi·hyp·aes·the·sia (hem''ee·high''pes·theezh'uh, theez'ee·uh) *n.* Decreased cutaneous sensitivity in one side of the body.

hemi·hy·po·to·nia (hem''ee·high''po·to'nee·uh) *n.* Decreased muscular tone of one side of the body.

hemi·lab·y·rin·thec·to·my (hem''ee·lab''i·rin·theck'tuh·mee) *n.* Removal of one or more of the membranous semicircular canals while leaving the ampullated ends and the saccule.

hemi·lam·i·nec·to·my (hem''ee·lam''i·neck'tuh·mee) *n.* Laminectomy in which laminae of only one side are removed.

hemi·lar·yn·gec·to·my (hem''ee·lãr''in·jeck'tuh·mee) *n.* Extirpation of one side of the larynx.

hemi·lar·ynx (hem''ee·lãr'inks) *n.* Half of the larynx.

hemi·man·dib·u·lec·to·my (hem''ee·man''dib·yoo·leck'tuh·mee) *n.* The surgical removal of one side of the mandible.

hemi·man·di·bu·lo·glos·sec·to·my (hem''ee·man·dib''yoo·lo·glos·eck'tuh·mee) *n.* Surgical removal of half of the mandible and of the tongue.

hemi·max·il·lec·to·my (hem''ee·mack''si·leck'tuh·mee) *n.* Excision of half of the maxilla.

hemi·me·lia (hem''i·mee'lee·uh) *n.* Congenital absence of all or part of the distal portion of an extremity.

hemi·me·lus (hem''i·mee'lus) *n.,* pl. **hemime·li** (·lye) An individual with incomplete or stunted arms or legs.

he·min, hae·min (hee'min) *n.* $C_{34}H_{32}N_4O_4 \cdot FeCl$; the chloride of ferriprotoporphyrin, containing iron in the ferric state.

hemi·ne·phrec·to·my (hem''ee·ne·freck'tuh·mee) *n.* Removal of part of a kidney; partial nephrectomy.

hemi·o·pia (hem''ee·o'pee·uh) *n.* HEMIANOPSIA. —**hemi·op·ic** (·op'ick, ·o'pick) *adj.*

hemi·pal·at·ec·to·my (hem''ee·pal''uh·teck'tuh·mee) *n.* Excision of half of the palate.

hemi·pal·a·to·la·ryn·go·ple·gia (hem''ee·pal''uh·to·la·ring''go·plee'jee·uh) *n.* Paralysis of the muscles of the soft palate and larynx on one side.

hemi·pa·ral·y·sis (hem''ee·pa·ral'i·sis) *n.* HEMIPLEGIA.

hemi·pa·re·sis (hem''ee·pa·ree'sis) *n.,* pl. **hemi·pare·ses** (·seez) Muscle weakness of one side of the body. —**hemipa·ret·ic** (·ret'ick) *adj.*

hemi·par·kin·son·ism (hem''ee·pahr'kin·sun·iz·um) *n.* Disease of the extrapyramidal system of the brain, manifested by tremor and rigidity of the extremities confined to or predominantly on one side.

hemi·pel·vec·to·my (hem''ee·pel·veck'tuh·mee) *n.* The surgical removal of an entire posterior extremity including the hipbone.

hemi·pel·vis (hem''ee·pel'vis) *n.* Half of a pelvis.

hemi·ple·gia (hem''i·plee'jee·uh) *n.* Paralysis of one side of the body. —**hemiple·gic** (·jick) *adj.*

He·mip·tera (he·mip'te·ruh) *n.pl.* 1. An order of insects; the true bugs. 2. Formerly the suborder Heteroptera of the order Hemiptera which also included the suborder Homoptera.

hemi·ra·chis·chi·sis (hem''ee·ra·kis'ki·sis) *n.* SPINA BIFIDA OCCULTA.

hemi·sec·tion (hem''ee·seck'shun) *n.* 1. The act of division into two lateral halves; bisection. 2. The division of the crown and separation of the roots of a tooth for the removal of the diseased or affected part to accomplish endodontic therapy. —**hemi·sect** (·sekt') *v.*

hemi·sep·tum (hem''i·sep'tum) *n.* The remaining portion of an interdental septum after the mesial or distal portion has been destroyed in periodontal disease.

hemi·so·mus (hem''i·so'mus) *n.* An individual with one side of the body imperfectly developed.

hemi·spasm (hem''ee·spaz·um) *n.* A spasm affecting only one side of the body or part of the body, as in facial hemispasm.

hemi·sphere (hem''i·sfeer) *n. In neuroanatomy,* one half of the cerebrum or of the cerebellum. —**hemi·spher·ic** (hem''i·sfeer'ick, ·sferr'ick) *adj.*

hemi·spher·ec·to·my (hem''i·sfeer·eck'tuh·mee) *n.* Surgical excision of one cerebral hemisphere.

hemi·sys·to·le (hem''ee·sis'tuh·lee) *n.* Contraction of the ventricle after every second atrial contraction so that for each two beats of the atrium only one pulse beat is felt.

hemi·tho·rax (hem''ee·tho'racks) *n.* One side of the thorax.

hemi·thy·roid·ec·to·my (hem''ee·thigh''roy·deck'tuh·mee) *n.* Removal of one lateral lobe of the thyroid gland.

hemi·ver·te·bra (hem''ee·vur'te·bruh) *n.* A congenital anomaly of the spine in which one half of a vertebra fails to develop.

hemi·zy·gote (hem''ee·zye'gote) *n.* An individual with only one of a given pair of genes, as in the case of the sex-linked genes in the human male; or with only one of each of all the pairs of genes, as the male bee. —**hemizy·gous** (·gus) *adj.*

Hem·me·ler's thrombopathy. A familial anomaly characterized by poor granulation of megakaryocytes, large platelets, normal platelet count, and a bleeding tendency.

hemo-, haemo-. See *hem-.*

he·mo·bil·ia (hee''mo·bil'ee·uh) *n.* HEMATOBILIA.

he·mo·bil·i·ru·bin, hae·mo·bil·i·ru·bin (hee''mo·bil·i·roo'bin) *n.* 1. Bilirubin as it occurs normally in serum before passing through the hepatic cells. 2. A form of bilirubin present normally in blood serum, which is increased in amount in hemolytic jaundice. It gives a negative direct van den Bergh's test.

he·mo·che·zia, hae·mo·che·zia (hee"mo·kee'zee·uh) *n.* The passage of blood, especially bright red blood, in the feces. Sometimes used to distinguish this type of blood from the dark blood characteristic of melena.

he·mo·cho·ri·al, hae·mo·cho·ri·al (hee"mo·kor'ee·ul) *adj.* Pertaining to maternal blood and chorionic ectoderm (trophoblast), especially in their intimate contact in the hemochorial placenta.

hemochorial placenta. A type of placenta in which the chorionic ectoderm is in direct contact with maternal blood; found in insectivores, bats, and anthropoids.

he·mo·chro·ma·to·sis, hae·mo·chro·ma·to·sis (hee"mo·kro"muh·to'sis) *n.* A chronic disease characterized pathologically by excessive deposits of iron in the body and clinically by hepatomegaly with cirrhosis, skin pigmentation, diabetes mellitus, and frequently cardiac failure; it may be idiopathic, erythropoietic, dietary, or due to blood transfusion. The idiopathic form is heritable, but the mechanism of its inheritance has not been elucidated. Syn. *bronze diabetes.* —**hemochromatot'ic, haemochromatot'ic** (·tot'ick) *adj.*

he·mo·chro·mo·gen, hae·mo·chro·mo·gen (hee"mo·kro'muh·jen) *n.* The class of substances formed by the union of heme with a nitrogen-containing substance, as a protein or base.

he·mo·co·ag·u·la·tion, hae·mo·co·ag·u·la·tion (hee"mo·ko·ag"yoo·lay'shun) *n.* Blood coagulation.

he·mo·con·cen·tra·tion, hae·mo·con·cen·tra·tion (hee"mo·kon"sin·tray'shun) *n.* An increase in the concentration of blood cells resulting from the loss of plasma or water from the bloodstream without a concomitant loss of formed elements, as in extensive burns; ANHYDREMIA.

he·mo·co·nia, hae·mo·co·nia (hee"mo·ko'nee·uh) *n.pl.* Round or dumbbell-shaped refractile, colorless particles found in blood plasma.

he·mo·cyte, hae·mo·cyte (hee'mo·site) *n.* BLOOD CELL.

he·mo·cy·to·blast, hae·mo·cy·to·blast (hee"mo·sigh'to·blast) *n.* The cell considered by some to be the primitive stem cell, giving rise to all blood cells. —**hemo·cy·to·blas'tic, haemo·cy·to·blas·tic** (·sigh'to·blas'tick) *adj.*

he·mo·cy·tom·e·ter, hae·mo·cy·tom·e·ter (hee"mo·sigh·tom'e·tur) *n.* An instrument for counting the number of blood cells. —**hemocytome·try, haemocytome·try** (·tree) *n.*

he·mo·cy·to·zo·on, hae·mo·cy·to·zo·on (hee"mo·sigh"to·zo'on) *n.,* pl. **hemocyto·zoa, haemocyto·zoa** (·zo'uh) A protozoan parasite inhabiting the red blood cells.

he·mo·di·ag·no·sis, hae·mo·di·ag·no·sis (hee"mo·dye·ug·no'sis) *n.,* pl. **hemodiagno·ses, haemodiagno·ses** (·seez) Diagnosis by examination of the blood.

he·mo·di·al·y·sis, hae·mo·di·al·y·sis (hee"mo·dye·al'i·sis) *n.* The process of exposing blood

to a semipermeable membrane, thereby removing from it or adding to it diffusible materials, rate and direction being a function of the concentration gradient across that membrane.

he·mo·di·lu·tion, hae·mo·di·lu·tion (hee"mo·di·lew'shun) *n.* A condition of the blood in which the ratio of blood cells to plasma is reduced.

he·mo·dy·nam·ics, hae·mo·dy·nam·ics (hee"mo·dye·nam'icks) *n.* The study of the interrelationship of blood pressure, blood flow, vascular volumes, physical properties of the blood, heart rate, and ventricular function. —**hemodynamic,** *adj.*

he·mo·dy·na·mom·e·ter, hae·mo·dy·na·mom·e·ter (hee"mo·dye"nuh·mom'e·tur) *n.* An instrument for measuring the pressure of the blood within the arteries. —**hemodynamome·try** (·tree) *adj.*

he·mo·flag·el·late, hae·mo·flag·el·late (hee"mo·flaj'e·late) *n.* Any protozoan flagellate living in the blood of its host.

he·mo·fus·cin, hae·mo·fus·cin (hee"mo·fus'in) *n.* An insoluble lipid pigment found in liver cells.

hemogenic-hemolytic balance. The balance in the body between the production of normal erythrocytes and their destruction, which maintains the count and the hemoglobin at the optimum level by physiologic processes.

he·mo·glo·bin, hae·mo·glo·bin (hee'muh·glo"bin) *n.* The respiratory pigment of erythrocytes, having the reversible property of taking up oxygen (oxyhemoglobin, HbO_2) or of releasing it (reduced hemoglobin, Hb), depending primarily on the oxygen tension of the medium surrounding it. At tensions of 100 mmHg or more, hemoglobin is fully saturated with oxygen; at 50 mmHg, oxygen is progressively more rapidly dissociated. Other factors affecting dissociation of oxyhemoglobin are temperature, electrolytes, and carbon dioxide tension (Bohr effect). Human hemoglobin consists of four heme molecules (iron-protoporphyrin) linked to the protein globin, which is composed of complexly folded polypeptide chains. Globin may vary in its essential properties, resulting in definite normal and genetically determined abnormal types, which may be differentiated on biochemical, pathophysiological, and genetic bases; it may differ in the fetus and in the adult, and also in different animal species. The average molecular weight of hemoglobin is about 67,000. Hemoglobin combines with carbon monoxide to form the stable compound carboxyhemoglobin. Oxidation of the ferrous iron of hemoglobin to the ferric state produces methemoglobin. Abbreviated, Hb.

hemoglobin A. The type of hemoglobin found in normal adults, which moves as a single component in an electrophoretic field, is rapidly denatured by highly alkaline solutions, and contains two titratable sulfhydryl groups per molecule. It forms orthorhombic crystals. Specific hemoglobin A antibodies have been obtained.

hemoglobin C. A slow-moving abnormal hemoglobin associated with intraerythrocytic crystal formation, target cells, and chronic hemolytic anemia; it may occur together with sickle-cell hemoglobin.

hemoglobin C disease. A disease largely of blacks, characterized by anemia, splenomegaly, target erythrocytes, intraerythrocytic hemoglobin crystals, and presence of hemoglobin C.

hemoglobin E. An abnormal hemoglobin found in Southeast Asia, migrating slightly faster than hemoglobin C; in the homozygous form it causes a mild hemolytic anemia with normochromic target cells.

he·mo·glo·bi·ne·mia, hae·mo·glo·bi·nae·mia (hee″muh·glo″bi·nee′mee·uh) n. The presence in the blood plasma of hemoglobin.

hemoglobin F. FETAL HEMOGLOBIN.

hemoglobin H. An abnormal hemoglobin migrating more rapidly than normal hemoglobin on electrophoresis, and usually associated with thalassemia.

hemoglobin M. An abnormal hemoglobin associated with hereditary methemoglobinemia, which can be differentiated from normal hemoglobin in its electrophoretic mobility by the starch-block method.

he·mo·glo·bi·nom·e·ter, hae·mo·glo·bi·nom·e·ter (hee″muh·glo″bi·nom′e·tur) n. An instrument for determining the hemoglobin concentration of the blood. —**hemoglobinome·try, haemoglobinome·try** (·tree) n.; **hemoglobi·no·met·ric, haemoglobi·no·met·ric** (·no·met′rick) adj.

he·mo·glo·bin·op·a·thy (hee″muh·glo·bi·nop′uh·thee) n. Any disease caused by abnormal hemoglobin.

hemoglobin S. SICKLE CELL HEMOGLOBIN.

he·mo·glo·bin·uria, hae·mo·glo·bin·uria (hee″muh·glo″bi·new′ree·uh) n. The presence of hemoglobin in the urine. —**hemoglobin·uric, haemoglobin·uric** (·new′rick) adj.

hemoglobinuric nephrosis. ACUTE TUBULAR NECROSIS.

he·mo·gram, hae·mo·gram (hee′mo·gram) n. 1. The number of erythrocytes and leukocytes per cubic millimeter of blood plus the differential leukocyte count and hemoglobin level in grams per 100 ml blood. 2. The differential leukocyte count.

he·mo·his·tio·blast, hae·mo·his·tio·blast (hee″mo·his′tee·o·blast) n. The hypothetical reticuloendothelial cell from which all the cells of the blood are eventually differentiated; a stem cell.

he·mo·hy·dro·sal·pinx, hae·mo·hy·dro·sal·pinx (hee″mo·high″dro·sal′pinks) n. A state in which blood and watery fluid distend a uterine tube.

he·mo·lith, hae·mo·lith (hee′mo·lith) n. A stone or concretion within the lumen of a blood vessel, or incorporated in the wall of a blood vessel.

he·mol·y·sate (he·mol′i·sate) n. The product obtained when blood or a material containing blood undergoes hemolysis.

he·mol·y·sin, hae·mol·y·sin (he·mol′i·sin, hee″mo·lye′sin) n. A substance that frees hemoglobin from the red cells.

he·mol·y·sis, hae·mol·y·sis (he·mol′i·sis) n., pl. **hemoly·ses, haemoly·ses** (·seez) The destruction of red blood cells and the resultant escape of hemoglobin. —**he·mo·lyt·ic, hae·mo·lyt·ic** (hee″mo·lit′ick, hem″o·) adj.

α-hemolytic. ALPHA-HEMOLYTIC.

β-hemolytic. BETA-HEMOLYTIC.

hemolytic anemia. Anemia resulting from excessive destruction of erythrocytes.

hemolytic jaundice. 1. Jaundice due to excessive red blood cell destruction. 2. HEREDITARY SPHEROCYTOSIS.

hemolytic streptococci. A group of β-hemolytic streptococci, especially varieties of *Streptococcus pyogenes*, that produce complete hemolysis on blood agar. It includes Lancefield groups A, B, C, E, F, G, H, K, L, M, O. Occasionally strains not producing complete hemolysis elaborate C-substance identical with the above Lancefield groups, and are therefore classified in this group. Group A and less commonly groups C and G are pathogenic for man. Group A is subdivided into 40 or more types on the basis of a type-specific protein (M-substance) produced by matt colonies; especially, types 12 and 4 are thought to be associated with acute glomerulonephritis. Members of this group also cause scarlet fever, erysipelas, sore throat, and other infections.

hemolytic-uremic syndrome. An acute illness of unknown cause, principally of infants and sometimes of older children and adults, that may follow a nonspecific respiratory infection; characterized clinically by bloody diarrhea, hemolytic anemia with abnormally shaped erythrocytes, thrombocytopenia, and azotemia, and pathologically by findings similar to those seen in the Shwartzman phenomenon, as well as by fibrin deposits, endothelial proliferation, and hyalin necrosis of the walls of blood vessels.

he·mo·lyto·poi·et·ic, hae·mo·lyto·poi·et·ic (hee″mo·lit″o·poy·et′ick, hem″o·) adj. Pertaining to the processes of blood destruction and blood formation.

he·mo·lyze, hae·mo·lyze (hee′mo·lize, hem′o·) v. To produce hemolysis. —**he·mo·ly·za·tion, hae·mo·ly·za·tion** (hee″mo·li·zay′shun, hem″o·) n.

he·mo·ma·nom·e·ter, hae·mo·ma·nom·e·ter (hee″mo·ma·nom′e·tur) n. A manometer for determining blood pressure.

he·mo·me·di·as·ti·num, hae·mo·me·di·as·ti·num (hee″mo·mee″dee·uh·stye′num) n. The presence of blood in the mediastinal space.

he·mo·me·tra, hae·mo·me·tra (hee″mo·mee′truh) n. HEMATOMETRA.

he·mo·pa·thol·o·gy, hae·mo·pa·thol·o·gy (hee″mo·pa·thol′uh·jee) n. The science of the diseases of the blood.

he·mo·peri·car·di·um, hae·mo·peri·car·di·um (hee″mo·perr″i·kahr′dee·um) n. The presence of blood or bloody effusion in the pericardial sac.

he·mo·peri·to·ne·um, hae·mo·peri·to·ne·um (hee″mo·perr″i·tuh·nee′um) n. An effusion of blood into the peritoneal cavity.

he·mo·pex·in, hae·mo·pex·in (hee·mo·peck′sin)

n. A heme-binding protein in human plasma that may be a regulator of heme and drug metabolism, and a distributor of heme. Measurement of its levels in serum and amniotic fluid may aid in assessing the severity of porphyria and certain hemolytic conditions.

he·mo·phage, hae·mo·phage (hee'mo-faij) *n.* A phagocytic cell that destroys red blood cells. —**he·mo·phag·ic, hae·mo·phag·ic** (hee''mo-faj'ick, hem''o·). **he·moph·a·gous, hae·moph·a·gous** (he-mof'uh-gus) *adj.*

he·mo·pha·gia, hae·mo·pha·gia (hee''mo·fay'jee·uh, hem''o·) *n.* 1. Ingestion of blood as a therapeutic agent. 2. Feeding on the blood of another organism. 3. Phagocytosis of the red blood cells.

he·mo·phil, hae·mo·phil (hee'mo·fil) *adj.* Characterizing an organism that grows preferably on blood media.

he·mo·phil·ia, hae·mo·phil·ia (hee''mo·fil'ee·uh) *n.* 1. An X-linked recessive hereditary bleeding disorder caused by factor VIII or factor IX deficiency and characterized clinically by hemarthrosis, hematomas, ecchymoses, gastrointestinal and genitourinary bleeding, and excessive traumatic bleeding. 2. Broadly, any of various other hereditary procoagulant deficiencies clinically similar to hemophilia A or B.

hemophilia A. Hemophilia resulting from deficiency of factor VIII; the typical and most common hemophilia.

hemophilia B. CHRISTMAS DISEASE; hemophilia resulting from deficiency of factor IX.

he·mo·phil·i·ac, hae·mo·phil·i·ac (hee''mo·fil'ee·ack) *n.* An individual who is affected with hemophilia.

he·mo·phil·ic, hae·mo·phil·ic (hee''mo·fil'ick, hem''o·) *adj.* 1. *In biology,* pertaining to bacteria growing well in culture media containing hemoglobin. 2. Pertaining to hemophilia or to a hemophiliac.

hemophilic arthritis. Arthritis that is the result of repeated bleeding into the joints in a hemophilic patient.

he·mo·phil·i·oid, hae·mo·phil·i·oid (hee''mo·fil'ee-oid) *adj.* Designating any coagulation disorder that resembles hemophilia, but that is the result of a genetic defect different from that in hemophilia.

Hemophilus. HAEMOPHILUS.

he·mo·pho·bia, hae·mo·pho·bia (hee''mo·fo'bee·uh) *n.* An abnormal fear of the sight of blood or of bleeding.

he·moph·thal·mia, hae·moph·thal·mia (hee''mof·thal'mee·uh) *n.* Hemorrhage into the vitreous.

he·mo·plas·tic, hae·mo·plas·tic (hee''mo·plas'tick) *adj.* Blood-forming.

he·mo·pneu·mo·tho·rax, hae·mo·pneu·mo·tho·rax (hee''mo·new''mo·thor'acks) *n.* A collection of blood and air within the pleural cavity.

he·mo·poi·e·sis, hae·mo·poi·e·sis (hee''mo·poy·ee'sis, hem''o·), **hemopoie·ses, haemopoie·ses** (·seez) HEMATOPOIESIS. —**hemo·poi·et·ic, haemo·poi·et·ic** (·poy·et'ick) *adj.*

he·mo·por·phy·rin, hae·mo·por·phy·rin (hee''mo·por'fi·rin) *n.* Iron-free heme, $C_{34}H_{38}N_4O_6$;

a porphyrin obtained in vitro by treating hemoglobin with sulfuric acid. It is closely related to the naturally occurring porphyrins.

he·mop·ty·sis, hae·mop·ty·sis (hee·mop'ti·sis) *n.* The spitting of blood or blood-stained sputum from the lungs, trachea, or bronchi.

hem·or·rhage, haem·or·rhage (hem'uh·rij) *n.* An escape of blood from the vessels, either by diapedesis through intact capillary walls or by flow through ruptured walls; bleeding. —**hem·or·rhag·ic, haem·or·rhag·ic** (hem''uh·raj'ick) *adj.*

hemorrhagic diathesis. An abnormal bleeding tendency as in hemophilia, purpura, scurvy, or vitamin K deficiency.

hemorrhagic disease of the newborn. A bleeding tendency occurring in the neonatal period as a result of vitamin K deficiency.

hemorrhagic measles. A grave variety of measles with a hemorrhagic eruption and severe constitutional symptoms. Syn. *black measles.*

hemorrhagic septicemia. SHIPPING FEVER.

he·mor·rhe·ol·o·gy (hee''mo·ree·ol'uh·jee, hem''o·) *n.* A branch of medical science which seeks to ascertain physical laws obeyed by circulating blood.

hem·or·rhoid, haem·or·rhoid (hem'uh·roid) *n.* A varix in the lower rectal or anal wall; a pile.

hem·or·rhoi·dal, haem·or·rhoi·dal (hem''uh·roy'dul) *adj.* 1. Pertaining to or affected with hemorrhoids. 2. Of or pertaining to blood vessels or nerves of the anus.

hemorrhoidal ring. A circular swelling of the wall of the anal canal at the level of the external sphincter muscle; it contains the rectal venous plexus. When enlarged, it forms hemorrhoids.

hem·or·rhoid·ec·to·my, haem·or·rhoid·ec·to·my (hem''o·roy·deck'tuh·mee) *n.* Surgical removal of hemorrhoids.

he·mo·sal·pinx, hae·mo·sal·pinx (hee''mo·sal'pinks) *n.* HEMATOSALPINX.

he·mo·sid·er·in, hae·mo·sid·er·in (hee''mo·sid'ur·in) *n.* An iron-containing glycoprotein pigment found in liver and in most tissues, representing colloidal iron in the form of granules much larger than ferritin molecules. It is insoluble in water and differs from ferritin in electrophoretic mobility. Pathologic accumulations are known to occur in a number of disease states.

he·mo·sid·er·ino·pe·nia, hae·mo·sid·er·ino·pe·nia (hee''mo·sid''ur·in·o·pee'nee·uh) *n.* HEMOSIDEROPENIA.

he·mo·sid·er·in·uria, hae·mo·sid·er·in·uria (hee''mo·sid''ur·i·new'ree·uh) *n.* The presence of hemosiderin in the urine.

he·mo·sid·er·o·pe·nia, hae·mo·sid·er·o·pe·nia (hee''mo·sid''ur·o·pee'nee·uh) *n.* Hemosiderin deficiency in the bone marrow and other storage sites.

he·mo·sid·er·o·sis, hae·mo·sid·er·o·sis (hee''mo·sid''ur·o'sis) *n.,* pl. **hemosider·ses, haemosidero·ses** (·seez) Deposition of hemosiderin in body tissues without tissue damage, reflecting an increase in body iron stores.

he·mo·sta·sis, hae·mo·sta·sis (hee''mo·stay'sis hee·mos'tuh·sis) *n.,* pl. **hemosta·ses, haemosta·ses** (·seez) 1. The arrest of a flow of blood or hemorrhage either physiologically via vaso-constriction and clotting or by surgical intervention. 2. The stopping or slowing of the circulation through a vessel or area of the body.

he·mo·stat, hae·mo·stat (hee′mo·stat) *n.* An agent or instrument that arrests the flow of blood.

he·mo·stat·ic, hae·mo·stat·ic (hee″mo·stat′ick) *n.* An agent that arrests hemorrhage. Syn. *hemostyptic.*

he·mo·ther·a·py, hae·mo·ther·a·py (hee″mo·therr′uh·pee) *n.* The treatment of disease by means of blood or blood derivatives.

he·mo·tho·rax, hae·mo·tho·rax (hee″mo·tho′racks) *n.* An accumulation of blood in the pleural cavity. Syn. *hemopleura.*

he·mo·tox·ic·i·ty, hae·mo·tox·ic·i·ty (hee″mo·tock·sis′i·tee) *n.* The property of being injurious to blood or blood-forming organs.

he·mo·tox·in, hae·mo·tox·in (hee″mo·tock′sin) *n.* A cytotoxin capable of destroying red blood cells. **—hemotox·ic, haemotox·ic** (·sick) *adj.*

he·mot·ro·phe, hae·mot·ro·phe (hee′mo·trofe, ·trof, he·mot′ro·fee) *n.* All the nutritive substances supplied to the embryo from the maternal bloodstream in viviparous animals having a deciduate placenta. **—he·mo·troph·ic, hae·mo·troph·ic** (hee″mo·trof′ick) *adj.*

he·mo·tym·pa·num, hae·mo·tym·pa·num (hee″mo·tim′puh·num) *n.* The presence of blood in the tympanic cavity.

he·mo·zo·in, hae·mo·zo·in (hee″mo·zo′in) *n.* A dark-brown or red-brown pigment, seen within plasmodia; formed from the disintegrated hemoglobin.

Hen·der·son-Has·sel·balch equation An equation expressing the pH of a buffer solution as a function of the concentrations of weak acid (or weak base) and salt components of the buffer. For a weak acid-salt buffer system, the equation is pH = pK_a + log (salt/acid), where pK_a is the negative logarithm of the ionization constant of the acid.

He·noch-Schön·lein purpura (he′y′nokh, shoehn′line) Purpura having features of both Henoch's purpura and Schönlein's purpura, such as abdominal pain, gastrointestinal bleeding, joint pain, and nephritis.

Henoch's purpura A type of allergic, nonthrombocytopenic purpura associated with attacks of gastrointestinal pain and bleeding and with erythematous or urticarial exanthema.

hen·ry (hen′ree) *n.,* pl. **hen·rys, hen·ries** (·reez) The unit of electric inductance; the inductance in a circuit such that an electromotive force of 1 volt is induced in the circuit by variation of an inducing current at the rate of 1 ampere per second. Abbreviated, h.

he·par (hee′pahr) *n.* 1. [NA] LIVER. 2. *Obsol.* A substance having the color of liver, generally a compound of sulfur, as hepar sulfuris.

hep·a·rin (hep′uh·rin) *n.* An acid mucopolysaccharide acting as an antithrombin, antithromboplastin, and antiplatelet factor to prolong the clotting time of whole blood; it occurs in a variety of tissues, most abundantly in the liver. Employed parenterally as an anticoagu-

lant, in the form of the sodium salt. **—heparin·ize** (·ize) *v.;* **heparin·oid** (·oid) *adj.*

hep·a·ri·ne·mia, hep·a·ri·nae·mia (hep″uh·ri·nee′mee·uh) *n.* The presence of heparin in the circulating blood.

hep·a·ri·tin sulfate (hep′uh·ri·tin). A sulfate ester of an acetylated heparin.

hepar lo·ba·tum (lo·bay′tum). The nodular lobulated liver of syphilitic cirrhosis; gummatous pseudolobation.

hepat-, hepato- A combining form meaning *liver, hepatic.*

hep·a·tal·gia (hep″uh·tal′jee·uh) *n.* Pain in the liver. **—hepatal·gic** (·jick) *adj.*

hep·a·tec·to·my (hep″uh·teck′tuh·mee) *n.* Excision of the liver or of a part of it.

he·pat·ic (he·pat′ick) *adj.* Of, pertaining to, or involving the liver.

hepatic artery. One of the three branches of the celiac trunk. The common hepatic artery (arteria hepatica communis) gives off the right gastric and gastroduodenal arteries and continues as the proper hepatic artery (arteria hepatica propria) to the liver.

hepatic coma. 1. A state of unconsciousness seen in patients severely ill with liver disease. 2. The precomatose state of hepatic encephalopathy.

hepatic duct. The common hepatic duct or any of its branches.

hepatic encephalopathy. Disturbance of central nervous function involving the changes in consciousness, mentation, behavior, and neurologic status occurring in advanced liver disease.

hepatic flexure. An abrupt bend where the ascending colon becomes the transverse colon.

he·pat·i·co·du·o·de·nos·to·my (he·pat″i·ko·dew″o·de·nos′tuh·mee) *n.* Establishment of an anastomosis between the hepatic duct and the duodenum.

he·pat·i·co·en·ter·os·to·my (he·pat″i·ko·en″tur·os′tuh·mee) *n.* Establishment of an anastomosis between the hepatic duct and the intestine.

he·pat·i·co·gas·tros·to·my (he·pat″i·ko·gas·tros′tuh·mee) *n.* Establishment of an anastomosis between the hepatic duct and the stomach.

he·pat·i·co·je·ju·nos·to·my (he·pat″i·ko·jej″oo·nos′tuh·mee) *n.* Surgical connection of the hepatic duct and the jejunum.

he·pat·i·co·li·thot·o·my (he·pat″i·ko·li·thot′uh·mee) *n.* Removal of a biliary calculus from the liver or any of its ducts.

he·pat·i·co·pan·cre·at·ic (he·pat″i·ko·pan″kree·at′ick) *adj.* Pertaining to the liver and the pancreas.

hepaticopancreatic ampulla. The dilation of the common bile duct and pancreatic duct where they join the duodenum.

he·pat·i·cos·to·my (he·pat″i·kos′tuh·mee) *n.* The formation of a fistula in the hepatic duct for the purpose of drainage.

he·pat·i·cot·o·my (he·pat″i·kot′uh·mee) *n.* Incision into the hepatic duct.

hep·a·ti·tis (hep″uh·tye′tis) *n.,* pl. **hepa·tit·i·des** (·tit′i·deez) Inflammation of the liver.

hepatitis A. INFECTIOUS HEPATITIS.

hepatitis–associated antigen. An antigen associated with a spherical lipid-containing particle 200 to 250 Å in diameter and virus-like in appearance, found in the blood of most individuals with serum hepatitis. Abbreviated, HAA. Syn. *Australia antigen.*

hepatitis B. SERUM HEPATITIS.

hepatitis virus A. The virus of infectious hepatitis.

hepatitis virus B. The virus of serum hepatitis.

hep·a·ti·za·tion (hep"uh·ti·zay'shun) *n.* The conversion of tissue, as of the lungs during the exudative stage of pneumonia, into a liverlike substance. **—hep·a·tized** (hep'uh·tize'd) *adj.*

hep·a·to·can·a·lic·u·lar (hep"uh·to·kan"uh·lick' yoo·lur) *adj.* Pertaining to the intrahepatic bile duct tributaries, especially the very small ones.

hep·a·to·cel·lu·lar (hep"uh·to·sel'yoo·lur) *adj.* Of or pertaining to the liver cells.

hepatocellular jaundice. Jaundice due to destruction or functional impairment of the liver cells.

hep·a·to·chol·an·gio·du·o·de·nos·to·my (hep" uh·to·ko·lan"jee·o·dew"o·de·nos'tuh·mee) *n.* Establishment of a communication between the hepatic duct and the duodenum.

hep·a·to·chol·an·gio·gas·tros·to·my (hep"uh·to· ko·lan"jee·o·gas·tros'tuh·mee) *n.* Establishment of an anastomosis between the hepatic duct and the stomach.

hep·a·to·chol·an·gio·je·ju·nos·to·my (hep"uh·to· ko·lan"jee·o·jej·oo·nos'tuh·mee) *n.* Establishment of a communication between the hepatic duct and the jejunum.

hep·a·to·co·lic (hep"uh·to·ko'lick, ·kol'ick) *adj.* Pertaining to the liver and the colon.

hep·a·to·cys·tic (hep"uh·to·sist'ick) *adj.* Pertaining to the liver and the gallbladder.

hep·a·to·du·o·de·nal (hep"uh·to·dew"o·dee'nul, ·dew·od'e·nul) *adj.* Pertaining to the liver and the duodenum.

hep·a·to·gen·ic (hep"uh·to·jen'ick) *adj.* HEPATOGENOUS.

hep·a·tog·e·nous (hep"uh·toj'e·nus) *adj.* Produced by or originating in the liver.

hep·a·to·gram (hep'uh·to·gram) *n.* 1. A graphic record of the liver pulse. 2. A radiograph of the liver, usually a phase of hepatic angiography.

hep·a·to·je·ju·nal (hep"uh·to·je·joo'nul) *adj.* Pertaining to the liver and jejunum.

hep·a·to·len·tic·u·lar (hep"uh·to·len·tick'yoo·lur) *adj.* Pertaining to the liver and the lentiform nucleus.

hepatolenticular degeneration. A recessive autosomal disorder associated with abnormalities of copper metabolism, characterized by decreased serum ceruloplasmin and copper values and increased urinary copper excretion. Untreated patients develop tissue copper deposits associated with hepatic cirrhosis, deep marginal pigmentation of the cornea (Kayser-Fleischer rings), and extensive degenerative changes in the central nervous system, particularly the basal ganglions. Syn. *Wilson's disease.*

hep·a·to·li·enal (hep"uh·to·lye·ee'nul, ·lye'e·nul) *adj.* Pertaining to the liver and the spleen.

hep·a·to·li·en·og·ra·phy (hep"uh·to·lye"e·nog' ruh·fee) *n.* Radiographic examination of the liver and the spleen.

hep·a·to·lith (hep'uh·to·lith) *n.* A calculus in the biliary passages of the liver.

hep·a·to·li·thi·a·sis (hep"uh·to·li·thigh'uh·sis) *n.* The presence or formation of calculi in the biliary passages of the liver.

hep·a·tol·o·gy (hep"uh·tol'uh·jee) *n.* The medical study and treatment of the liver. **—hepatolo·gist,** *n.*

hep·a·to·ma (hep"uh·to'muh) *n.*, *pl.* **hepatomas,** **hepatoma·ta** (·tuh) 1. A malignant tumor whose parenchymal cells resemble those of the liver. 2. Any tumor of the liver.

hep·a·to·meg·a·ly (hep"uh·to·meg'uh·lee) *n.* Enlargement of the liver.

hep·a·to·pan·cre·at·ic (hep"uh·to·pan"kree·at' ick) *adj.* HEPATICOPANCREATIC.

hep·a·to·pexy (hep"uh·to·peck"see) *n.* Surgical fixation of a movable, or ptosed, liver; usually by utilizing additional supportive power of the round and the falciform ligaments.

hep·a·top·to·sis (hep"uh·top·to'sis, hep"uh·to·to' sis) *n.* Abnormally low position of the liver in the abdomen.

hep·a·to·re·nal (hep"uh·to·ree'nul) *adj.* Pertaining to both the liver and the kidney.

hepatorenal syndrome. 1. Hyperpyrexia, oliguria, azotemia, and coma; the renal failure once thought to be of toxic origin, related to hepatic decompensation, now is generally agreed to be concomitant hepatic and renal failure, due to infection, dehydration, hemorrhage, or shock. Syn. *Heyd's syndrome.* 2. Renal failure occurring in any severe chronic hepatic disease, probably related to change in renal blood flow.

hep·a·tor·rha·phy (hep"uh·tor'uh·fee) *n.* Suturing of the liver following an injury or an operation.

hep·a·tor·rhex·is (hep"uh·to·reck'sis) *n.*, *pl.* **hepatorrhex·es** (·seez) Rupture of the liver.

hep·a·tos·co·py (hep"uh·tos'kuh·pee) *n.* Inspection of the liver, as by laparotomy or peritoneoscopy.

hep·a·to·sis (hep"uh·to'sis) *n.*, *pl.* **hepato·ses** (·seez) Any noninflammatory disorder of the liver.

hep·a·to·sple·no·meg·a·ly (hep"uh·to·splee"no· meg'uh·lee) *n.* Enlargement of the liver and spleen.

hep·a·tot·o·my (hep"uh·tot'uh·mee) *n.* Incision into the liver.

hep·a·to·tox·in (hep"uh·to·tock'sin) *n.* 1. A substance that produces injury or death of parenchymal liver cells. 2. A poisonous or deleterious product elaborated in the liver. **—hepatotox·ic** (·sick) *adj.*

hept-, hepta- A combining form meaning *seven, seventh.*

herb, *n.* 1. A plant without a woody stem. 2. A plant used for medicinal purposes or for its odor or flavor.

herb·al, *adj. & n.* 1. Of or pertaining to herbs. 2. A book on the medicinal virtues of herbs.

herd instinct. The fundamental psychic urge to identify oneself with a group and to function in the same manner as the group; group feeling. Syn. *gregariousness.*

he·red·i·tary (he·red'i·terr-ee) *adj.* 1. Of or pertaining to heredity. 2. Of or pertaining to inheritance; inborn; inherited.

hereditary anhidrotic ectodermal dysplasia. One of a very large group of primarily cutaneous congenital abnormalities, marked chiefly by deficient or absent sweat-gland function (anhidrosis), deficient development of the teeth (hypodontia) or their absence (anodontia), and by congenital alopecia. Transmitted in a mild form as a dominant trait, and in a severe form as an X-linked recessive trait. Syn. *Siemen's syndrome.*

hereditary cerebellar ataxia. 1. FRIEDREICH'S ATAXIA. 2. MARIE'S ATAXIA.

hereditary cerebral sclerosis. MARIE'S ATAXIA.

hereditary chorea. HUNTINGTON'S CHOREA.

hereditary deforming chondrodysplasia. MULTIPLE HEREDITARY EXOSTOSES.

hereditary disease. A disorder transmitted from parent to offspring through the genes; may be dominant or recessive, sex-linked or autosomal.

hereditary hemorrhagic telangiectasia. A hereditary disease characterized by multiple telangiectases and a tendency to habitual hemorrhages, most commonly epistaxis. Syn. *Osler-Rendu-Weber disease.*

hereditary multiple polyposis. Any of various hereditary polypoid conditions of the gastrointestinal tract, such as Peutz-Jeghers syndrome and familial polyposis.

hereditary nephritis. ALPORT'S SYNDROME.

hereditary progressive ar·thro·oph·thal·mop·a·thy (ahr''thro-off''thal·mop'uth·ee). A dominantly inherited disease, manifesting abnormal epiphyseal development, degenerative joint changes beginning in childhood, progressive myopia with retinal detachment and blindness, and sensorineural loss.

hereditary spherocytosis. A chronic dominantly inherited disorder characterized by spherocytosis, increased osmotic fragility of the red corpuscles, splenomegaly, and a variable degree of hemolytic anemia. Syn. *chronic acholuric jaundice, chronic familial jaundice, congenital hemolytic anemia, hemolytic splenomegaly, spherocytic anemia.*

he·red·i·ty (he·red'i-tee) *n.* The inborn capacity of the organism to develop ancestral characteristics; it is dependent upon the constitution and organization of the cell or cells that form the starting point of the new individual. In biparental reproduction, this starting point is the fertilized egg.

heredo- A combining form meaning *hereditary.*

her·e·do·de·gen·er·a·tion (herr''e·do·de·jen''uh·ray'shun) *n.* A degenerative process or state which results from a hereditary defect. **—her·edode·gen·er·a·tive** (·jen'ur·uh-tiv) *adj.*

her·e·do·fa·mil·i·al (herr''e·do·fa·mil'ee·ul) *adj.* Characterizing a disease or condition that occurs in more than one member of a family and is suspected of being inherited.

her·e·do·mac·u·lar (herr''e·do·mack'yoo·lur) *adj.* Of hereditary diseases, involving the macular part of the retina.

He·ring-Breu·er reflex (he'y·ring, broy'ur) The neural mechanism that controls respiration automatically by impulses transmitted via the pulmonary fibers of the vagus nerves.

her·i·ta·bil·i·ty, *n.* The ratio of the variance due to genetic effects to the total variance, used as an index of the extent to which the phenotype is genetically determined and responsive to selection.

her·i·ta·ble, *adj.* Able to be inherited.

her·i·tage, *n.* In *genetics,* the sum total of the genes of characteristics transmitted from parents to their children.

her·maph·ro·dite (hur·maf'ro·dite) *n.* An individual showing hermaphroditism. **—hermaph·ro·dit·ic** (hur·maf''ro·dit'ick) *adj.*

her·maph·ro·dit·ism (hur·maf'ro·dye·tiz·um) *n.* A condition characterized by the coexistence in an individual of ovarian and testicular tissue.

her·met·ic (hur·met'ick) *adj.* Protected from exposure to air; airtight. **—hermet·i·cal·ly** (·ick·uh·lee) *adv.*

her·nia (hur'nee·uh) *n.,* pl. **hernias, her·ni·ae** (·nee·ee) The abnormal protrusion of an organ or a part through the containing wall of its cavity, usually the abdominal cavity, beyond its normal confines. Syn. *rupture.* **—her·nial** (·nee·ul) *adj.*

hernial sac. The pouch or protrusion of peritoneum containing a herniated organ or part, formed gradually by pressure against a defect in the containing wall or present at birth.

her·ni·ate (hur'nee·ate) *v.* To form a hernia. **—herni·at·ed** (·ay·ted) *adj.;* **her·ni·a·tion** (hur''nee·ay'shun) *n.*

herniated disk. An intervertebral disk in which the nucleus pulposus has protruded through the surrounding fibrocartilage, occurring most frequently in the lower lumbar region, less commonly in the cervical region. Mild to severe symptoms may result from pressure on spinal nerves. Syn. *ruptured intervertebral disk, slipped disk.*

hernio-. A combining form meaning *hernia.*

her·ni·og·ra·phy (hur''nee·og'ruh·fee) *n.* The radiographic depiction of a hernia aided by injection of contrast medium into the sac.

her·nio·plas·ty (hur'nee·o·plas''tee) *n.* Plastic operation for the radical cure of hernia.

her·ni·or·rha·phy (hur''nee·or'uh·fee) *n.* Any operation which includes suturing for the repair of hernia.

her·ni·ot·o·my (hur''nee·ot'uh·mee) *n.* 1. An operation for the relief of irreducible hernia, by cutting through the neck of the sac. 2. HERNIOPLASTY.

her·o·in (herr'o·in) *n.* Diacetylmorphine, $C_{21}H_{23}NO_5$, a morphine derivative, a white, crystalline, odorless powder, formerly used as an analgesic, a sedative, and to relieve coughs, but since 1956 banned from use or manufacture because of its addictive properties.

her·o·in·ism (herr'o·in·iz·um) *n.* Addiction to heroin.

her·pan·gi·na (hur''pan·jye'nuh, hur·pan'ji·nuh)

n. A mild disease caused by any of various Coxsackie group A viruses and characterized by fever, anorexia, dysphagia, and grayish-white papules or vesicles surrounded by a red areola on the pharynx, uvula, palate, and tonsils, or tongue.

her·pes (hur'peez) *n.* HERPES SIMPLEX.

herpes fa·ci·a·lis (fay-shee-ay'lis). A type of herpes simplex occurring on the face, usually about the lips. May also occur in the mouth and pharynx. Syn. *cold sore, herpes febrilis.*

herpes ges·ta·ti·o·nis (jes-tay"shee-o'nis). A vesicular or bullous skin eruption occurring during pregnancy; probably related to erythema multiforme.

herpes iris (eye'ris). A form of erythema multiforme, characterized by vesicles growing in a ring. It is usually seen on the backs of the hands and feet.

herpes la·bi·a·lis (lay"bee-ay'lis). Herpes facialis on the lip.

herpes pro·gen·i·ta·lis (pro-jen"i-tay'lis). Vesicles on the genitalia caused by herpes simplex virus, type 2. Syn. *herpes praeputialis, herpes genitalis.*

herpes sim·plex (sim'plecks). A viral disorder, characterized by groups of vesicles on an erythematous base. Commonly recurrent, and at times seen in the same place.

herpes simplex virus. A herpesvirus that causes a variety of human diseases notable for their persistence in a latent state and tendency to recur at irregular intervals. The virus usually enters the body through breaks in mucous membranes or skin. Of the two principal strains, type 1 usually causes oral, ocular, cutaneous, and encephalitic infections and type 2, genital (and various congenital) infections. Syn. *Herpesvirus hominis.*

herpes ton·su·rans (ton'sue·ranz, ton'sue·ranz). TINEA CAPITIS.

Her·pes·vi·rus (hur"peez-vye'rus) *n.* A group of ether-sensitive, large DNA viruses that form eosinophilic intranuclear inclusion bodies, and include among others the viruses of herpes simplex, varicella, herpes zoster, pseudorabies, infectious bovine rhinotracheitis, and equine abortion. —**herpesvirus,** *com. n.*

Herpesvirus sim·i·ae (sim'ee-ee). A virus that causes a usually mild disease similar to herpes simplex in Old World monkeys, but which may cause fatal myelitis or encephalomyelitis in man. Syn. *B virus.*

herpes zos·ter (zos'tur). An acute viral infectious disease of man, characterized by unilateral segmental inflammation of the posterior root ganglia and roots (and sometimes of anterior roots and posterior horn), or sensory ganglia of cranial nerves and by a painful vesicular eruption of the skin or mucous membranes in the peripheral distribution of the individual nerve or nerves. Syn. *shingles.*

her·pet·ic (hur-pet'ick) *adj.* Of or pertaining to herpes.

herpetic encephalitis. An acute encephalitis, frequently lethal, which occurs sporadically throughout the year in all age groups and throughout the world, usually caused by type

1 herpes simplex virus. Type 2 virus causes acute encephalitis rarely and only in the neonate, in relation to maternal genital herpetic infection.

herpetic fever. A herpetic eruption on the face associated with chills, fever, and sore throat.

her·pet·i·form (hur-pet'i-form) *adj.* Resembling herpes; having groups of vesicles.

Hers' disease Glycogenosis caused by a deficiency of the enzyme liver phosphorylase, with abnormal storage of glycogen in liver, and clinically similar to von Gierke's disease with marked hepatomegaly and varying degrees of hypoglycemia and its manifestations. Syn. *type VI of Cori.*

het·a·flur (het'uh-flure) *n.* Hexadecylamine hydrofluoride, $C_{16}H_{35}N\cdot HF$, a dental caries prophylactic.

heter-, hetero- A combining form meaning (a) *other, another;* (b) *different, unlike;* (c) *various, diverse;* (d) *irregular, abnormal.*

het·er·es·the·sia, het·er·aes·the·sia (het"ur·es·theez'ee·uh) *n.* Variations in the degree of response to a cutaneous stimulus from one point to another on the body.

hetero-. See *heter-.*

het·er·o·ag·glu·ti·nin (het"ur·o·uh·gloo'ti·nin) *n.* An agglutinin in normal blood having the property of agglutinating foreign cells, including the blood corpuscles of other species of animals.

het·er·o·blas·tic (het"ur·o·blas'tick) *adj.* Arising from tissue of a different kind.

het·er·o·cel·lu·lar (het"ur·o·sel'yoo·lur) *adj.* Formed of cells of different kinds.

het·er·o·chro·ma·tin (het"ur·o·kro'muh·tin) *n.* 1. BASICHROMATIN. 2. Originally, the substance of heterochromosomes (allosomes), as of the Y chromosome. —**hetero·chro·mat·ic** (·kro·mat'ick) *adj.*

het·er·o·chro·mia (iri·dis) (het"ur·o·kro'mee·uh eye'ri·dis) *n.* A condition in which the two irises are of different colors, or a portion of an iris is a different color from the remainder. Syn. *anisochromia, chromheterotropia.* —**heterochro·mous** (·mus), **heterochro·mic** (·mick) *adj.*

het·er·o·cy·clic (het"ur·o·sigh'click, ·sick'lick) *adj. In chemistry,* pertaining to compounds of the closed-chain or ring type in which the ring atoms are of two or more dissimilar elements.

Heterodera ra·di·ci·o·la (rad"i·sick'o·luh). A species of minute nematodes parasitic on the roots and stems of many edible plants. The ova are sometimes found in human feces and may be mistaken for hookworm eggs.

het·er·o·dont (het'ur·o·dont) *adj. In biology,* having teeth of more than one shape, as does man.

het·er·o·er·o·tism (het"ur·o·err'o·tiz·um) *n.* The direction of the sexual desire toward another person or toward any object other than oneself. —**hetero·erot·ic** (·e·rot'ick) *adj.*

het·er·o·ge·ne·ous (het"ur·o·jee'nee·us) *adj.* 1. Differing in kind or nature; composed of different substances or constituents. 2. Not uniform in composition or structure. —**het·ero·ge·ne·i·ty** (·je·nee'i·tee) *n.*

het·er·og·e·nous (het"ur·oj'e·nus) *adj.* 1. Of, relating to, or derived from a different species. 2. Not originating within the same body.

het·ero·graft (het″ur·o·graft) *n.* A graft of tissue obtained from an animal of one species and transferred to the body of another animal of a different species. Syn. *xenograft.*

het·ero·hyp·no·sis (het″ur·o·hip·no′sis) *n.* Hypnosis induced by another.

het·ero·in·tox·i·ca·tion (het″ur·o·in·tock″si·kay′shun) *n.* Intoxication by a poison not produced within the body.

het·ero·la·lia (het″ur·o·lay′lee·uh) *n.* 1. The unconscious saying of one thing when something else is intended. 2. A form of motor aphasia in which the patient habitually says one thing but means something else. 3. ECHOLALIA; the echoing of someone else's words.

het·ero·lat·er·al (het″ur·o·lat′ur·ul) *adj.* Pertaining to or situated on the opposite side.

het·er·ol·o·gous (het″ur·ol′uh·gus) *adj.* 1. Characterized by heterology. 2. Derived from an organism of a different species.

het·er·ol·o·gy (het″ur·ol′uh·jee) *n.* Deviation from the normal in structure, organization, or time or manner of formation.

het·ero·me·tro·pia (het″ur·o·me·tro′pee·uh) *n.* The condition in which the refraction in the two eyes is dissimilar.

het·ero·mor·phic (het″ur·o·mor′fick) *adj.* 1. Differing in size or form as compared with the normal. 2. *In chemistry,* crystallizing in different forms. 3. *In zoology,* having different forms at different stages of the life history. 4. *In cytology,* unlike in form or size; applied to either chromosome of a synaptic pair of unlike chromosomes, as an X and a Y chromosome. **—heteromor·phism** (·fiz″um) *n.*

het·ero·mor·phous (het″ur·o·mor′fus) *adj.* 1. Differing from the normal in form. 2. Of varied or irregular form.

het·er·on·y·mous (het″ur·on′i·mus) *adj. In optics,* pertaining to crossed images of an object seen double.

het·ero·os·teo·plas·ty (het″ur·o·os′tee·o·plas″tee) *n.* The grafting, by operation, of bone taken from an animal.

het·er·op·a·thy (het″ur·op′uth·ee) *n.* 1. The condition of being abnormally sensitive to stimuli; hypersensitivity. 2. ALLOPATHY. **—het·ero·path·ic** (het″ur·o·path′ick) *adj.*

het·ero·phil (het′ur·o·fil) *adj.* Of or pertaining to antigens occurring in apparently unrelated animals and microorganisms that are closely related immunologically so that antibodies produced against one antigen cross-react with the others.

heterophil antibody. An antibody that is produced in response to a heterophil antigen, as exemplified in the Paul-Bunnell test for infectious mononucleosis.

het·ero·pho·nia (het″ur·o·fo′nee·uh) *n.* Abnormal quality or change of voice.

het·ero·pho·ria (het″ur·o·fo′ree·uh) *n.* Any tendency of the eyes to turn away from the position correct for binocular vision; latent squint or deviation.

Het·er·oph·y·es (het″ur·off′e·eez) *n.* A genus of trematode worms, found in Egypt and the Far East, which produces heterophyidiasis in humans.

Heterophyes heterophyes. A trematode species that has as definitive hosts man, cats, dogs, foxes, hogs, and other fish-eating animals; as first intermediate hosts, the snails; and as second intermediate hosts, mullet fish.

het·er·o·phy·id·i·a·sis (het″ur·o·figh″id·eye′uh·sis) *n.* Infection by any fluke of the family Heterophyidae, of which the species *Heterophyes heterophyes* and *Metagonimus yokogawai* are the most important and most common in humans. The flukes inhabit the small intestine but may also pass into the muscles of the heart through the lymphatics.

het·ero·pla·sia (het″ur·o·play′zhuh, ·zee·uh) *n.* 1. The presence of a tissue in an abnormal location. 2. A process whereby tissues are displaced to or developed in locations foreign to their normal habitats. **—hetero·plas·tic** (·plas′tick) *adj.*

het·ero·plas·ty (het′ur·o·plas″tee) *n.* The operation of grafting parts taken from another species. **—het·ero·plas·tic** (het″ur·o·plas′tick) *adj.*

het·er·op·sia (het″ur·op′see·uh) *n.* Inequality of vision in the two eyes.

het·ero·sex·u·al·i·ty (het″ur·o·seck″shoo·al′i·tee) *n.* Sexual orientation toward the opposite sex.

het·ero·sug·ges·tion (het″ur·o·sug·jes′chun) *n.* Suggestion originating from a source outside the individual's mind; suggestion by another.

het·ero·tax·is (het″ur·o·tack′sis) *n.,* pl. **heterotax·es** (·seez) Anomalous position or transposition of organs.

het·ero·to·nia (het″ur·o·to′nee·uh) *n.* Variability in tension or tone.

het·ero·to·pia (het″ur·o·to′pee·uh) *n.* Displacement or deviation from natural position, as of an organ or a part.

het·ero·top·ic (het″ur·o·top′ick) *adj.* 1. Occurring in an abnormal location, as intestinal epithelial cells occurring in the gastric epithelium. 2. Of or pertaining to a graft transplanted to an abnormal anatomic location in the host, as bone of the donor to muscle of the recipient.

het·ero·tox·in (het″ur·o·tock′sin) *n.* A toxin introduced into, but formed outside of, the body.

het·ero·trans·plan·ta·tion (het″ur·o·trans·plan·tay′shun) *n.* Transplantation of a tissue or part from one species to another. **—hetero·transplant** (·trans′plant) *n.*

het·ero·troph (het′ur·o·trof, ·trofe) *n.* Any of those bacteria, including all those pathogenic for man, which require for growth a source of carbon more complex than carbon dioxide. Wide variation exists in respect to utilizable organic carbon sources and requirements for accessory growth factors.

het·ero·tro·pia (het″ur·o·tro′pee·uh) *n.* STRABISMUS.

het·ero·zy·go·sis (het″ur·o·zye·go′sis) *n.* In the genotype, the presence of one or many pairs of genes in the heterozygous phase, which results from crossbreeding.

het·ero·zy·gote (het″ur·o·zye′gote) *n.* A heterozygous individual.

het·ero·zy·gous (het″ur·o·zye′gus) *adj.* Having

the two members of one or more pairs of genes dissimilar. **—heter·o·zy·gos·i·ty** (·zye-gos'i-tee) *n.*

HEW Department of Health, Education and Welfare, a United States federal agency.

hex·a·canth (heck'suh-kanth) *n.* A six-hooked larva of a tapeworm.

hexa·chlo·ro·phene (heck''suh-klor'uh-feen) *n.* 2,2'-Methylenebis(3,4,6-trichlorophenol), $C_{13}H_6Cl_6O_2$, a germicide active in the presence of soap. Syn. *compound G-11.*

hexa·chro·mic (heck''suh-kro'mick) *adj.* Capable of distinguishing only six of the seven spectrum colors, indigo not being distinguished.

hex·ad (heck'sad) *n.* An element which has a valence of six.

hexa·dac·ty·lism (heck''suh-dack'ti-liz-um) *n.* The state of having six fingers or toes.

hexa·di·meth·rine bromide (heck''suh-dye-meth'reen) Poly[(1,5-dimethyl)-1,5-diazaundecamethylene dimethobromide], $(C_{13}H_{30}Br_2N_2)_x$, a heparin-neutralizing agent.

hexa·hy·dric (heck''suh-high'drick) *adj.* Containing six atoms of replaceable hydrogen.

hex·ane (heck'sane) *n.* Any one of the isomeric liquid hydrocarbons, C_6H_{14}, of the paraffin series.

hexa·va·lent (heck''suh-vay'lunt) *adj.* Having a valence of six.

hexo·ki·nase (heck''so-kigh'nace, ·naze) *n.* An enzyme that catalyzes the transfer of phosphate from adenosine triphosphate to glucose or fructose, forming glucose 6-phosphate or fructose 6-phosphate and adenosine diphosphate.

hex·one base (heck'sohn). One of the diaminomonocarboxylic acids (arginine, lysine, and histidine) each containing six carbon atoms, basic in reaction.

hex·os·a·mine (heck''so-suh-meen', heck-so'suh-meen'') *n.* A primary amine derivative of a hexose resulting from replacement of hydroxyl in the latter by an amine group. Glucosamine is an important hexosamine.

hex·o·san (heck'so-san) *n.* Any complex carbohydrate yielding a hexose on hydrolysis. Cellulose, starch, and glycogen are important hexosans.

hex·ose (heck'soce) *n.* Any monosaccharide that contains six carbon atoms in the molecule.

hex·u·ron·ic acid (heck''syoo-ron'ick) *n.* 1. An acid formed by oxidation of the primary alcohol group of a hexose sugar, as glucuronic acid from glucose. 2. *Obsol.* ASCORBIC ACID.

hex·yl·caine (heck'sil-kane) *n.* 1-Cyclohexylamino-2-propyl benzoate, $C_{16}H_{23}NO_2$, a local anesthetic suitable for infiltration, spinal anesthesia, surface anesthesia, and nerve block; used as the hydrochloride salt, primarily for surface anesthesia.

hex·yl·res·or·cin·ol (heck''sil-re-zor'sin-ole, -ol) *n.* 4-Hexylresorcinol, $C_{12}H_{18}O_2$; an anthelmintic active against intestinal roundworms and trematodes and also employed as an antiseptic and germicide.

Hg Symbol for mercury.

hgb An abbreviation for *hemoglobin.*

hi·a·tus (high-ay'tus) *n.* A space or opening. **—hi·a·tal** (·tul) *adj.*

hiatus hernia. A form of hernia through the esophageal hiatus; usually a small, intermittent hernia of a part of the stomach.

hi·ber·na·tion (high''bur-nay'shun) *n.* The dormant condition of certain animals in the winter, characterized by twilight sleep, muscle relaxation, a fall in metabolic rate, and, hence, lowered body temperature. **—hi·ber·nate** (high'bur-nate) *v.*

hi·ber·no·ma (high''bur-no'muh) *n.* A benign tumor composed of adipose tissue cells with a high lipochrome content, giving it the appearance of the brown fat organs of hibernating animals.

hic·cough (hick'up, ·off) *n.* HICCUP.

hic·cup (hick'up) *n.* A sudden contraction of the diaphragm causing inspiration, followed by a sudden closure of the glottis.

hidr-, hidro- A combining form meaning *sweat, perspiration.*

hi·drad·e·ni·tis, hy·drad·e·ni·tis (hi-drad''e-nigh'tis, high-) *n.* Inflammation of the sweat glands.

hidradenitis sup·pu·ra·ti·va (sup''yoo-ruh-tye'vuh). Suppurative inflammation of apocrine glands, usually of the axillae. A characteristic condition marked by abscesses, sinus formation, and great chronicity.

hi·drad·e·no·car·ci·no·ma (hi-drad''e-no-kahr''si-no'muh, high-) *n.* SWEAT GLAND CARCINOMA.

hi·drad·e·no·ma, hy·drad·e·no·ma (hi-drad''e-no'muh, high-) *n.* 1. Any benign sweat-gland tumor. 2. HIDRADENOMA PAPILLIFERUM. 3. SYRINGOMA. 4. CYLINDROMA.

hidradenoma pap·il·lif·e·rum (pap''il-lif'e-rum). A benign sweat-gland tumor whose parenchymal cells are arranged into papillary processes extending into a cystic space, usually occurring on the vulva or perineum.

hidro-. See hidr-.

hid·ro·cyst·ad·e·no·ma (hid''ro-sist''ad-e-no'muh, high''dro-) *n.* HIDROCYSTOMA.

hid·ro·cys·to·ma (hid''ro-sis-to'muh, high''dro-) *n., pl.* **hidrocystomas, hidrocystoma·ta** (·tuh) A retention cyst of a sweat gland.

hid·ro·poi·e·sis (hid''ro-poy-ee'sis, high''dro-) *n.* The formation and secretion of sweat. **—hidro·poi·et·ic** (·et'ick) *adj.*

hid·ror·rhea, hid·ror·rhoea (hid''ro-ree'uh, high'dro-) *n.* Excessive flow of sweat.

hi·dro·sis (hi-dro'sis, high-) *n., pl.* **hidro·ses** (·seez) 1. The formation and excretion of sweat. 2. Abnormally profuse sweating. **—hi·drose** (high'droce) *adj.*

hi·drot·ic (hi-drot'ick, high-) *adj. & n.* 1. Diaphoretic or sudorific. 2. A medicine that causes sweating.

hidrotic, *n.* A medicine that causes sweating.

hi·ero·pho·bia (high''ur-o-fo'bee-uh) *n.* Morbid fear of religious objects or rituals, clergymen, or places of religious worship.

high-altitude pulmonary edema. Pulmonary edema occurring in certain predisposed individuals after a rapid change from low to high altitude, usually over 3,000 m.

high forceps. An obstetric forceps applied to the fetal head which has descended into the pelvic canal, when its greatest diameter is still above the superior strait.

high hyperopia. Manifest hyperopia, especially the absolute form.

high myopia. A degree of myopia greater than 6.5 diopters.

high-performance liquid chromatography. A separation process similar to gas chromatography in which the mobile phase is a liquid.

hi·lar (high'lur) *adj.* Pertaining to or located near a hilus.

hilar dance. Increased amplitude of pulsation of the pulmonary arteries on fluoroscopic examination.

hi·lum (high'lum) *n.*, pl. **hi·la** (·luh) 1. *In botany,* the scar on a seed marking its point of attachment. 2. *In anatomy,* HILUS.

hi·lus (high'lus) *n.*, pl. & genit. sing. **hi·li** (·lye) A pit, recess, or opening in an organ, usually for the entrance and exit of vessels or ducts.

hilus-cell tumor. ADRENOCORTICOID ADENOMA OF THE OVARY.

hind·brain, *n.* RHOMBENCEPHALON.

hind·gut, *n.* The caudal part of the embryonic digestive tube formed by the development of the tail fold.

hinge articulation or **joint.** A synovial joint in which a convex cylindrical surface is grooved at right angles to the axis of the cylinder, or trochlea, and meets a concave cylindrical surface that is ridged to fit the trochlea in such a manner as to permit motion in only one plane.

Hin·ton test A macroscopic flocculation test for syphilis.

hip·bone, *n.* The irregular bone forming one side and the anterior wall of the pelvic cavity, and composed of the ilium, ischium, and pubis. Syn. *innominate bone.*

Hip·pel-Lin·dau disease Angiomatosis of the retina (von Hippel's disease) associated with cerebellar angioma (Lindau's disease) and angioma of other viscera.

hip·po·cam·pal (hip″o·kam′pul) *adj.* Of or pertaining to the hippocampus.

hippocampal sulcus. A fissure situated between the parahippocampal gyrus and the fimbria hippocampi.

hip·po·cam·pus (hip″o·kam′pus) *n.*, pl. & genit. sing. **hippocam·pi** (·pye) A curved elevation consisting largely of gray matter, in the floor of the inferior horn of the lateral ventricle.

hip·pu·ric acid (hi·pew′rick) Benzoylaminoacetic acid, $C_9H_9NO_3$, an acid found in high concentration in the urine of herbivorous animals and to a lesser extent in the urine of man; it is a metabolic product of benzoic acid. Syn. *urobenzoic acid.*

hip·pus (hip′us) *n.* Spasmodic pupillary movement, independent of the action of light.

hir·cis·mus (hur·siz′mus, hear·sis′mus) *n.* The peculiar odor of axillary apocrine secretion.

Hirsch·sprung's disease A congenital, often familial disorder manifested by inability to defecate due to absence of ganglion cells in the submucosal or myenteric plexuses in a given segment of the colon or proximal rectum, which is unable to relax to permit passage of the stool. The normal colon proximal to the

aganglionic segment is narrow, with dilatation above. Treatment is surgical, and if untreated, the disease results in growth retardation.

hir·sute (hur′sewt) *adj.* Shaggy; hairy.

hir·su·ti·es (hur·sue′shee·eez) *n.* Excessive growth of hair; HYPERTRICHOSIS.

hir·sut·ism (hur′sewt·iz·um) *n.* A condition characterized by growth of hair in unusual places and in unusual amounts.

hiru·din (hirr′yoo·din) *n.* The active principle of a secretion derived from the buccal glands of leeches. It prevents the coagulation of blood.

Hir·u·din·ea (hirr″yoo·din′nee·uh) *n.pl.* A class of predatory or parasitic annelids; the leeches.

hir·u·di·ni·a·sis (hirr″yoo·di·nigh′uh·sis) *n.*, pl. **huridinia·ses** (·seez) Infestation by leeches.

his·tam·i·nase (his·tam′i·nace, ·naze, his″tuh·mi·naze′) *n.* An enzyme, obtainable from extracts of kidney and intestinal mucosa, capable of inactivating histamine and other diamines; has been used in the treatment of anaphylactic shock, asthma, hay fever, serum sickness, and other allergic conditions which may be due to, or accompanied by, liberation of histamine in the body. Syn. *diamine oxidase.*

his·ta·mine (his′tuh·meen, ·min) *n.* 4-(2-Aminoethyl)imidazole, $C_5H_9N_3$, an amine occurring as a decomposition product of histidine and prepared synthetically from that substance. It stimulates visceral muscles, dilates capillaries, and stimulates salivary, pancreatic, and gastric secretions. Used as the hydrochloride or phosphate salt as a diagnostic agent in testing gastric secretion. **—his·ta·min·ic** (his″tuh·min′ick) *adj.*

histamine test. 1. The subcutaneous injection of histamine stimulating the gastric secretion of hydrochloric acid. 2. The precipitation of an attack of cephalalgia (vasomotor headache) by the injection of histamine done for purposes of diagnosis. 3. The intradermal injections of histamine at various points along a limb, resulting normally in the appearance within 5 minutes of a wheal with an erythematous areola. Absence of these phenomena indicates insufficient pressure in skin vessels, arterial spasm, or nonfunctioning sensory nerves of the skin.

his·ta·nox·ia (his″tuh·nock′see·uh) *n.* Decreased tissue oxygenation due to diminution of the blood supply.

Histaspan. A trademark for chlorpheniramine maleate, an antihistaminic.

his·ti·dase (his″ti·dace, ·daze) *n.* An enzyme, found in the liver of higher animals, acting on L-histidine, but not on D-histidine or other imidazole compounds, to open the imidazole ring with formation of urocanic acid.

his·ti·dine (his′ti·deen, ·din) *n.* β-Imidazole-α-alanine, $C_6H_9N_3O_2$, an amino acid resulting from hydrolysis of many proteins. By elimination of a molecule of carbon dioxide, it is converted to histamine. The hydrochloride has been used for the treatment of peptic ulcers.

his·ti·di·ne·mia, his·ti·di·nae·mia (his″ti·di·nee′mee·uh) *n.* A rare hereditary (probably autosomal recessive) metabolic disorder in which there is a deficiency of histidase (L-hystidine ammonia lysase) with a high blood level of histidine and often alanine, increased urinary excretion of imidazolepyruvate, imidazole-acetate, and imidazolelactate, as well as absence of urocanic acid in sweat and urine after an oral histidine load; manifested clinically by speech disorders and often mild mental retardation, as well as lowered growth rates and heightened susceptibility to infection.

his·tio·cyte (his'tee-o-site) *n.* A fixed macrophage of the loose connective tissue, usually one which has not ingested material and which, in common with other cells belonging to the reticuloendothelial system, stores electively certain dyes such as trypan blue or lithium carmine. —**his·tio·cyt·ic** (his''tee-o-sit'ick) *adj.*

his·tio·cy·to·ma (his''tee-o-sigh-to'muh) *n.*, pl. **histiocytomas, histiocytoma·ta** (-tuh) 1. A benign tumor composed of histiocytes. 2. DERMATOFIBROMA.

his·tio·cy·to·sis (his''tee-o-sigh-to'sis) *n.*, pl. **histiocyto·ses** (-seez) An excessive number of histiocytes, usually generalized.

histiocytosis X. Any of a group of proliferative disorders of the reticuloendothelial system of unknown cause, characterized by local or general proliferation of histiocytes which often show phagocytosis. Among the subtypes are Letterer-Siwe disease, Hand-Schüller-Christian disease, and eosinophilic granuloma of bone. Syn. *reticuloendotheliosis.*

his·tio·troph·ic (his''tee-o-trof'ick) *adj.* Having a protective or anabolic influence on the energy of cells, as the histiotrophic functions of the autonomic nervous system.

his·to·chem·is·try (his''to-kem'is-tree) *n.* 1. The chemistry of the tissues of the body. 2. The study of microscopic localization and analysis of substances in cells and tissues. —**histochem·i·cal** (-i·kul) *adj.*

his·to·com·pat·i·bil·i·ty (his''to·kum·pat''i·bil'i·tee) *n.* Sufficient compatibility between different tissues for a graft to be accepted and remain functional without rejection. —**histo·com·pat·i·ble** (-pat'i·bul) *adj.*

his·to·flu·o·res·cence (his''to·floo''uh·res'unce) *n.* Fluorescence of the tissues during x-ray treatment, produced by the prior administration of fluorescing drugs.

his·to·gram (his'to·gram) *n.* A type of chart used in descriptive statistics to show the frequency distribution of a set of data.

his·toid (his''toid) *adj.* 1. Resembling tissue. 2. Composed of only one kind of tissue.

his·to·in·com·pat·i·bil·i·ty (his''to·in''kum·pat·i·bil'i·tee) *n.* Lack of histocompatibility; incompatibility of tissues. —**histoincom·pat·i·ble** (-pat'i·bul) *adj.*

his·to·log·ic (his''tuh·loj'ick) *adj.* 1. Of or pertaining to tissues. 2. Of or pertaining to histology. —**histolog·i·cal** (-i·kul) *adj.*; **histologi·cal·ly** (-kuh·lee) *adv.*

his·tol·o·gy (his·tol'uh·jee) *n.* The branch of biology that deals with the minute structure of tissues, including the study of cells and of organs. —**histolo·gist,** *n.*

his·tol·y·sis (his·tol'i·sis) *n.* Disintegration and dissolution of organic tissue. —**his·to·lyt·ic** (his''to·lit'ick) *adj.*

his·to·meta·plas·tic (his''to·met''uh·plas'tick) *adj.* Causing the transformation of one tissue into another type.

his·tom·o·ni·a·sis (his·tom''o·nigh'uh·sis, his''to·mo·) *n.* A disease of the ceca and liver of poultry, and wild gallinaceous birds caused by the protozoan *Histomonas meleagridis.* Syn. *blackhead enterohepatitis.*

his·to·mor·phol·o·gy (his''to·mor·fol'uh·jee) *n.* The morphology of the tissues of the body; histology.

his·to·my·co·sis (his''to·migh·ko'sis) *n.* Fungal infection of the deep tissues, as opposed to surface growth.

his·tone (his'tone) *n.* Any one of a group of strongly basic proteins found in cell nuclei, such as thymus histone; soluble in water but insoluble in, or precipitated by, ammonium hydroxide, and coagulable by heat.

his·to·nu·ria (his''to·new'ree·uh) *n.* The presence of histone in the urine.

his·to·pa·thol·o·gy (his''to·puh·thol'uh·jee) *n.* The study of microscopically visible changes in diseased tissue. —**histo·patho·log·ic** (·path''uh·loj'ick) *adj.*

his·to·phys·i·ol·o·gy (his''to·fiz''ee·ol'uh·jee) *n.* The science of tissue functions.

His·to·plas·ma (his''to·plaz'muh) *n.* A genus of parasitic fungi.

Histoplasma cap·su·la·tum (kap·sue·lay'tum). The species of parasitic fungi that is the causative agent of histoplasmosis.

his·to·plas·min (his''to·plaz'min) *n.* A standardized liquid concentrate of soluble growth factors developed by the fungus *Histoplasma capsulatum*; used as a dermal reactivity indicator in the diagnosis of histoplasmosis.

his·to·plas·mo·ma (his''to·plaz·mo'muh) *n.* A tumorlike swelling produced by an inflammatory reaction to *Histoplasma capsulatum.*

his·to·plas·mo·sis (his''to·plaz·mo'sis) *n.*, pl. **histoplasmo·ses** (-seez) A reticuloendothelial cell infection with the fungus *Histoplasma capsulatum,* varying from a mild respiratory infection to severe disseminated disease, usually characterized by fever, anemia, hepatomegaly, splenomegaly, leukopenia, pulmonary lesions, gastrointestinal ulcerations, and suprarenal necrosis. Syn. *cytomycosis, Darling's histoplasmosis.*

his·to·ra·di·og·ra·phy (his''to·ray·dee·og'ruh·fee) *n.* MICRORADIOGRAPHY.

his·to·ry (his'tur·ee) *n.* MEDICAL HISTORY.

his·tot·o·my (his·tot'uh·mee) *n.* 1. The dissection of tissues. 2. The cutting of thin sections of tissues; microtomy.

his·to·tox·ic (his''to·tock'sick) *adj.* Deleterious or poisonous to the tissues, wholly or in part.

his·tri·on·ic (his''tree·on'ick) *adj.* 1. Characterized by exaggerated, dramatic gestures, attitudes, speech, and facial expressions, as are used by some actors. 2. Pertaining to the muscles producing facial expression.

hives, *n.pl.* URTICARIA.

HLA The complex of antigens controlled by the

major histocompatibility complex of gene loci for leukocyte antigens in man. Also written *HL-A.*

hoarse, *adj.* 1. Of the voice: harsh, grating. 2. Having a harsh, discordant voice, caused by an abnormal condition of the larynx or throat. —**hoarse·ness,** *n.*

hoary, *adj.* Gray or white with age; said of the hair. —**hoar·i·ness,** *n.*

hob·ble, *v. & n.* 1. To have an uneven gait; to limp. 2. *In veterinary medicine,* a bond or shackle used to confine the foot of an animal. 3. Anything that restrains motion.

hob·nail liver. The liver as seen in Laennec's cirrhosis, in which masses of regenerated liver cells among weblike fibrous septa form a nodular or "hobnail" surface.

hock, *n.* The joint on the hind leg of a quadruped between the knee and the fetlock, corresponding to the ankle joint in man.

Hodg·kin's disease or **lymphoreticuloma** A malignant lymphoma composed of anaplastic reticuloendothelial cells of a distinctive type (Reed-Sternberg cells) and varying numbers of stromal cells including fibrocytes, lymphocytes, and eosinophils, with or without foci of necrosis.

ho·do·pho·bia (ho″do·fo′bee·uh) *n.* An abnormal fear of travel.

hoe, *n.* 1. A scraping instrument used in operations for cleft palate. 2. A type of instrument used in the preparation of a dental cavity for restoration. 3. A periodontal instrument with a single blade, usually at a right angle to the shank, used for removing deposits of calculus from the tooth surface.

Hof·bau·er cell A large, sometimes binucleate, apparently phagocytic cell found in chorionic villi.

Hoffmann's syndrome Muscle enlargement, weakness, and fatigue, accompanied by slow, clumsy movements, associated with myxedema in adults.

hog cholera. An epizootic infectious disease of swine caused by a filtrable virus. *Salmonella choleraesuis* is a common secondary invader. The disease is characterized by fever, diarrhea, emaciation, patchy redness of the skin with inflammation and ulceration of the intestines. Syn. *swine fever.*

hol-, holo- A combining form meaning (a) *complete, entire;* (b) *homogeneous, like.*

hol·an·dric (hol·an′drick, ho·lan′) *adj.* Pertaining to genes carried by the Y chromosomes; inherited only through the paternal line. —**hol·an·dry** (hol′an·dree) *n.*

hol·er·ga·sia (hol″ur·gay′zhuh, ·zee·uh, ho″lur·) *n.* A mental disorder, or major psychosis, that disrupts the entire structure of the personality, such as schizophrenia.

ho·lism (ho′liz·um) *n.* A concept in modern biological and psychological thinking which states that for complex systems such as a cell, an organism, or a personality the whole is greater than the sum of its parts from a functional point of view. Syn. *organicism.* —**ho·lis·tic** (ho·lis′tick) *adj.*

Hol·lan·der test A test for the presence of intact vagus nerves based on the rise in gastric acidity after the production of hypoglycemia by giving insulin.

ho·lo·di·as·tol·ic (hol″o·dye″as·tol′ick, ho″lo·) *adj.* Lasting throughout diastole, especially as the murmurs of major aortic or pulmonic valve insufficiency or the diastolic portion of a continuous murmur.

ho·lo·en·zyme (hol″o·en′zyme, ho″lo·) *n.* A complete enzyme formed from the purely protein part, or apoenzyme, combined with the coenzyme.

ho·lo·gas·tros·chi·sis (hol″o·gas·tros′ki·sis, ho″lo·) *n.* A congenital fissure involving the entire length of the abdominal wall, exposing the abdominal organs.

ho·lo·gram (hol′o·gram, ho′lo·) *n.* The record of the diffraction pattern of the image of an object obtained by holography.

ho·log·ra·phy (ho·log′ruh·fee) *n.* A lensless type of photography in which monochromatic light, as from a laser, is split into two beams, one of which enters the lensless camera directly, while the other enters after passing through a transparent image of the object; the two beams combine to form a diffraction pattern of the image which is recorded on film, this record being the hologram. To reconstruct the image, a beam of laser light is transmitted through the hologram to generate a second diffraction pattern, a component of which reproduces the original image on a screen.

ho·lo·gyn·ic (hol″o·jin′ick, ·jye′nick, ho″lo·) *adj.* Pertaining to genes transmitted only in the female line from mother to daughter generation after generation, as in the case of attached X chromosomes.

ho·lo·ra·chis·chi·sis (hol″o·ra·kis′ki·sis, ho″lo·) *n.* The type of spina bifida in which the entire spinal canal is open.

ho·lo·sys·tol·ic (hol″o·sis·tol′ick, ho″lo·) *adj.* Lasting throughout systole, as the murmurs of major mitral or tricuspid valve insufficiency or ventricular septal defect.

hom-, homo- A combining form meaning (a) *common, like, same;* (b) in chemistry and biology, *homologous.*

Ho·mans' sign Pain in the calf and popliteal area on passive dorsiflexion of the foot, indicating deep venous thrombosis of calf. Syn. *dorsiflexion sign.*

hom·at·ro·pine (ho·mat′ro·peen, ·pin) *n.* An alkaloid, $C_{16}H_{21}NO_3$, prepared from atropine and mandelic acid. It causes dilatation of the pupil and paralysis of accommodation, as does atropine, but its effects pass off more quickly, usually in two or three days. Variously used, in the form of its hydrobromide, hydrochloride, or methylbromide salt, as a parasympatholytic drug.

homeo-, homoeo-, homoio- A combining form meaning *like, similar.*

ho·meo·ki·ne·sis (ho″mee·o·ki·nee′sis) *n.,* pl. **ho·meokine·ses** (·seez) A mitosis in which equal amounts of chromatin go to each daughter nucleus.

ho·meo·path·ic, ho·moeo·path·ic (ho″mee·o·

path'ick) *adj.* Of or pertaining to homeopathy, and to its practice and principles.

ho·me·op·a·thy, ho·moe·op·a·thy (ho''mee·op'uth·ee) *n.* A system of medicine expounded by Samuel Hahnemann based on the simile phenomenon (*similia similibus curantur*). Cure of disease is effected by minute doses of drugs which produce the same signs and symptoms in a healthy person as are present in the disease for which they are administered. Syn. *Hahnemannism.* —**ho·meo·path, ho·moeo·path** (ho'mee·o·path) **ho·me·op·a·thist, ho·moe·op·a·thist** (ho''mee·op'uh·thist) *n.*

ho·meo·sta·sis (ho''mee·os'tuh·sis, ho''mee·o·stay'sis) *n.,* pl. **homeosta·ses** (·seez) The maintenance of steady states in the organism by coordinated physiologic processes or feedback mechanisms. Thus all organ systems are integrated by automatic adjustments to keep within narrow limits disturbances excited by, or directly resulting from, changes in the organism or in the surroundings of the organism. —**ho·meo·stat·ic** (ho''mee·o·stat'ick) *adj.*

ho·meo·therm (ho'mee·o·thurm) *n.* A homeothermic organism.

ho·meo·ther·mic (ho''mee·o·thur'mick) *adj.* Of an organism: able to regulate physiologically the rate of heat production and heat loss so as to maintain itself at constant temperature independently of the environmental temperature; WARM-BLOODED. —**ho·meo·ther·my** (ho'mee·o·thur''mee) *n.*

home·sick·ness, *n.* An urgent desire to return to one's home, which may be accompanied by a morbid sluggishness of the functions of the various organs of the body, and may develop into depression and morbid anxiety.

Ho·mo (ho'mo) *n.* The hominid genus that includes *Homo sapiens,* modern man, together with extinct species known from fossil remains such as *H. erectus* (formerly assigned to another genus, *Pithecanthropus*) and *H. neanderthalensis* (regarded by some as *H. sapiens neanderthalensis,* conspecific with modern man).

homo-. See **hom-.**

ho·mo·cy·clic (ho''mo·sigh'click, ·sick'lick) *adj. In chemistry,* pertaining to compounds of the closed-chain or ring type in which all the ring atoms are of the same element, usually carbon.

ho·mo·cys·ti·nu·ria (ho''mo·sis·ti·new'ree·uh) *n.* A recessively inherited disorder clinically resembling Marfan's syndrome; manifested by subluxated lenses regularly developing after the age of 10, frequently thromboembolic phenomena, and usually mental retardation. Homocystine is excreted in the urine as a result of absence of cystathionine synthetase activity.

ho·mo·erot·i·cism (ho''mo·e·rot'i·siz·um) *n.* HOMOEROTISM.

ho·mo·er·o·tism (ho''mo·err'o·tiz·um) *n.* 1. The direction of the libido toward a member of the same sex; HOMOSEXUALITY. 2. Specifically, homosexual orientation in which the erotic feeling is well sublimated, not requiring genital expression. —**homo·erot·ic** (·e·rot'ick) *adj. & n.*

ho·mo·ga·met·ic (ho''mo·ga·met'ick) *adj.* Producing one kind of germ cell in regard to the sex chromosomes. The female, being XX in constitution, is the homogametic sex.

ho·mog·e·nate (ho·moj'e·nate) *n.* The substance produced by homogenization.

ho·mo·ge·ne·ous (ho''mo·jee'nee·us, hom''o·) *adj.* Having the same nature or qualities; of uniform character in all parts. —**homo·ge·nei·ty** (·je·nee'i·tee) *n.*

ho·mo·ge·net·ic (ho''mo·je·net'ick) *adj.* HOMOGENOUS.

ho·mo·gen·i·tal·i·ty (ho''mo·jen''i·tal'i·tee) *n.* Homoerotism in which the sexual impulses are given genital expression; HOMOSEXUALITY (1). —**ho·mo·gen·i·tal** (·jen'i·tul) *adj.*

ho·mog·e·ni·za·tion (ho·moj''e·ni·zay'shun) *n.* 1. The process of becoming homogeneous. 2. The production of a uniform dispersion, suspension, or emulsion from two or more normally immiscible substances. —**ho·mog·e·nize** (huh·moj'e·nize) *v.*

ho·mog·e·nous (ho·moj'e·nus) *adj.* 1. Of or derived from an individual of a closely related or similar strain of the same species. 2. Of two or more individuals, genetically or otherwise identical in certain characteristics.

ho·mo·gen·tis·ic acid (ho''mo·jen·tiz'ick, ·jen·tis'ick, hom''o·) 2,5-Dihydroxyphenylacetic acid, $C_8H_8O_4$, found in urine in alkaptonuria; it is an intermediate in the oxidation of tyrosine and phenylalanine.

ho·mo·graft (ho'mo·graft) *n.* A tissue graft taken from a genetically nonidentical donor of the same species as the recipient. Syn. *allograft, homologous graft.*

homograft rejection. The immunologic process by which an animal causes the destruction or sloughing of tissue transplanted to it from an animal of the same species.

ho·mo·lat·er·al (ho''mo·lat'ur·ul) *adj.* IPSILATERAL.

ho·mol·o·gous (ho·mol'uh·gus) *adj.* 1. Corresponding in structure, either directly or as referred to a fundamental type. 2. Derived from a different organism of the same species. 3. *In chemistry,* being of the same type or series; differing by a multiple, such as CH_2, or by an arithmetic ratio in certain constituents.

homologous chromosomes. Chromosomes that have like gene loci in the same sequence; in man there are 23 pairs of homologous chromosomes; one member of each pair is derived from the mother and one from the father.

homologous serum hepatitis or **jaundice.** SERUM HEPATITIS.

ho·mon·y·mous (ho·mon'i·mus) *adj.* 1. Having the same name; of words, having the same form. 2. *In ophthalmology,* pertaining to the same sides of the field of vision. —**homony·my** (·mee) *n.*

homonymous hemianopsia. Loss of vision affecting the inner half of one and the outer half of the other visual field; generally caused by lesions involving the optic radiations posterior to the optic chiasm; the more congruous the defect, the closer the lesion to the occipital cortex.

ho·mo·plas·ty (ho'mo·plas"tee) *n.* Surgery using grafts from another individual of the same species. **—ho·mo·plas·tic** (ho''mo·plas'tick) *adj.*

Homo sa·pi·ens (say'pee·unz, sap'ee·enz) The human species; the species of *Homo* that includes all extant races of man.

ho·mo·sex·u·al·i·ty (ho''mo·seck''shoo·al'i·tee) *n.* 1. The practice of sexual relations with members of one's own sex. 2. The disposition to be sexually attracted to, or to fall in love with, members of one's own sex. 3. *Colloq.* Male homosexuality. **—homo·sex·u·al** (·seck'shoo·ul) *adj. & n.*

homosexual panic. An acute undifferentiated syndrome that comes as the climax of prolonged tension from unconscious homosexual conflicts or sometimes bisexual tendencies. The attack is characterized by a high degree of fear, paranoid ideas, great excitement, and a tendency toward disorganization. It may mark the onset of schizophrenia.

ho·mo·tope (hom'o·tope, ho'mo·) *n.* Any member of a particular group of elements in the periodic table, thus, sodium is a homotope of lithium, potassium, rubidium, cesium, and francium.

ho·mo·type (ho'mo·tipe, hom'o·) *n.* A part corresponding to a part on the lateral half of the body. **—ho·mo·typ·ic** (ho·mo·tip'ick) *adj.*

ho·mo·typ·i·cal (ho·mo·tip'i·kul) *adj.* Pertaining to a common structure.

ho·mo·zy·gous (ho''mo·zye'gus) *adj.* Having both members of a given pair of genes alike. **—homo·zy·gos·i·ty** (·zye·gos'i·tee) *n.*

Hong Kong influenza An acute respiratory illness which first appeared in a moderate pandemic in 1968; due to certain strains of influenza A virus.

hook, *n. & v.* 1. An elongate structure with a bend or curve at one end which serves to exert traction or to perform functions based on traction. 2. To exert traction in the manner of a hook; a function of the hand with fingers flexed but without participation of the opposed thumb.

hook·worm, *n.* Any nematode belonging to the superfamily Strongyloidea, particularly the species *Ancylostoma duodenale* and *Necator americanus.*

ho·ra (ho'ruh) *n.* Hour; at the hour. Abbreviated, h.

hora de·cu·bi·tus (de·kew'bi·tus) At bedtime. Abbreviated, h. d.

hora som·ni (som'nigh) At bedtime. Abbreviated, h. s.

hor·de·o·lum (hor·dee'o·lum) *n.,* pl. **hordeo·la** (·luh) A suppurative infection of the tarsal glands or the ciliary glands of the eyelid; a sty.

hor·i·zon·tal, *adj.* In a plane parallel to the ground or a base line.

hor·me·pho·bia (hor''me·fo'bee·uh) *n.* Morbid fear of shock.

hor·mone (hor'mone) *n.* A specific chemical product of an organ or of certain cells of an organ, transported by the blood or other body fluids, and having a specific regulatory effect upon cells remote from its origin. **—hor·mo·**

nal (hor·mo'nul), **hor·mon·ic** (hor·mon'ick) *adj.*

hor·mo·no·poi·e·sis (hor·mo''no·poy·ee'sis) *n.* The production of hormones. **—hormonopoi·et·ic** (·et'ick) *adj.*

horn, *n.* 1. A substance composed chiefly of keratin. 2. CORNU. **—horny,** *adj.*

Horner's syndrome Unilateral ptosis, miosis, enophthalmos, diminished sweating on the same side of the face and neck, and redness of the conjunctiva due to interruption of the sympathetic nerve fibers on the affected side.

ho·rop·ter (ho·rop'tur) *n.* The sum of all the points seen singly by the two retinas while the fixation point remains stationary. **—ho·rop·ter·ic** (hor''op·terr'ick) *adj.*

horse·fly, *n.* A large fly of the family Tabanidae.

horse·pox, *n.* A virus disease of horses characterized by fever, mucopurulent discharge, and pox lesions on the mouth, vulva, leg, and occasionally over the entire body.

horse serum. Serum obtained from the blood of horses. Some therapeutically useful serums are obtained from horses immunized against a specific organism or its toxin.

horse·shoe, *n.* 1. A metal bow for the attachment of Steinmann pins and threaded (Kirschner) wires. 2. Something shaped like a horseshoe.

horseshoe kidney. Greater or lesser degree of congenital fusion of the two kidneys, usually at the lower poles.

Hor·ton's headache or **syndrome** CLUSTER HEADACHE.

hos·pice (hos'pis) *n.* 1. A shelter or lodging for paupers, destitute travelers, or abandoned children, usually maintained by a charitable institution. 2. An institution for the care and comfort of the terminally ill.

hos·pi·tal, *n.* A medical treatment facility intended, staffed, and equipped to provide diagnostic and therapeutic service in general medicine and surgery or in some circumscribed field or fields of restorative medical care, together with bed care, nursing, and dietetic service to patients requiring such care and treatment.

hos·pi·tal·i·za·tion, *n.* Placement of patients in a hospital for diagnostic study or treatment.

host, *n.* 1. An organism on or in which another organism, known as a parasite, lives and from which the parasite obtains nourishment during all or part of its existence. 2. *In teratology,* a relatively normal fetus to which a less complete fetus or fetal part is attached. 3. The recipient of a transplanted organ or tissue. 4. The tissue invaded by a tumor.

hos·tile, *adj.* Marked by hostility.

hos·til·i·ty, *n.* Antagonism, animosity, anger, or resistance toward an individual or group.

hot, *adj. Slang.* Highly radioactive.

hot atom. An atom that has high internal energy or high kinetic energy as a result of a nuclear process, such as neutron capture or beta decay.

hot flush. A vasomotor symptom of menopause; sudden vasodilatation and sensation of heat involving the upper portion of the body, often accompanied by sweating. Syn. *menopausal flush.*

hourglass contraction. A contraction of an organ, as the stomach or uterus, at the middle.

hourglass stomach. A stomach divided more or less completely into two compartments by an equatorial constriction, usually resulting from chronic gastric ulcer. Syn. *bilocular stomach, ectasia ventricula paradoxa.*

house-fly, *n.* A fly of the genus *Musca.*

house physician. A physician employed by, and constantly available at, a particular place, as an intern at a hospital or a physician at a hotel.

house staff. The group of physicians and surgeons employed by a hospital, and receiving postgraduate training there; those having the status of intern or resident.

house surgeon. A surgeon employed by a hospital and constantly available.

Houssay phenomenon Occasional abrupt amelioration of preexisting diabetes mellitus, with sudden lowering of insulin requirement, after pituitary destruction.

Houston's valves TRANSVERSE RECTAL FOLDS.

How-ell-Jol-ly bodies Dot-shaped basophilic inclusions of nuclear material occurring in the peripheral blood erythrocytes of splenectomized persons.

h.s. Abbreviation for *hora somni,* bedtime.

H-substance, *n.* A substance similar to, if not identical with, histamine; believed to play a prominent role in the response of local blood vessels to tissue damage.

Hub-bard tank A large, specially designed tank in which a patient may be immersed for various therapeutic underwater exercises.

Huh-ner's test An examination of seminal fluid obtained from the vaginal fornix and cervical canal after a specified interval following coitus; used in fertility studies to evaluate spermatozoal survival and activity in the lower female genital tract.

hum, *n.* A low murmuring sound.

hu-man, *adj. & n.* 1. Belonging or pertaining to the species *Homo sapiens.* 2. A human being; a member of the species *Homo sapiens.*

human immune serum. A sterile serum obtained from the blood of a healthy person who has survived an attack of a disease, administered during the incubation period to prevent or modify the expected attack of a specific disease; immune sera exist for measles, varicella, vaccinia, diphtheria, etc.

hu-mec-tant (hew-meck'tunt) *adj. & n.* 1. Moistening. 2. A substance used to retain moisture.

hu-mer-al (hew'mur-ul) *adj.* Of or pertaining to the humerus.

hu-mero-ra-di-al (hew''mur-o-ray'dee-ul) *adj.* Pertaining to the humerus and the radius; applied to the joint between these two bones and to the ligaments joining them.

hu-mer-us (hew'mur-us) *n.,* pl. & genit. sing. **hu-meri** (-mur-eye) The bone of the upper arm, or brachium.

hu-mid-i-fi-ca-tion (hew-mid''i-fi-kay'shun) *n.* The process of moistening or humidifying air; specifically, in respiration, by moisture from mucous membranes.

hu-mid-i-ty, *n.* The state or quality of being moist; moisture; dampness. —**hu-mid** (hew'mid) *adj.*

hu-mor, hu-mour, *n.* 1. Any fluid or semifluid part of the body. 2. *In old physiology,* one of the four cardinal body fluids of Galen: the choleric, the melancholic, the phlegmatic, and the sanguine, said to determine a person's health and temperament. 3. Disposition, temperament. —**humor-al** (-ul) *adj.*

humoral antibody. Any antibody found in solution in lymph, plasma, or another fluid part of the body, as contrasted with antibody bound to the surface of a cell.

humoral immunity. Immunity which is maintained by antibody molecules secreted by B lymphocytes and plasma cells and circulating freely throughout the plasma, lymph, and other body fluids, as distinguished from cell-mediated immunity, which is maintained by T lymphocytes; seen in immune response to bacterial infections and reinfection by virus.

hump-back, *n.* KYPHOSIS.

hunch-back, *n.* 1. A person with kyphosis. 2. KYPHOSIS.

hun-ger, *n.* A sensation of longing for food.

hunger contractions. Movements of the stomach formerly thought to be associated with hunger.

Hun-ner's ulcer A chronic ulcer of the urinary bladder, of unknown etiology, found frequently near the vertex and in association with interstitial cystitis. Syn. *elusive ulcer.*

Hun-te-ri-an chancre (hun-teer'ee-un) A syphilitic chancre.

Hun-ter's canal ADDUCTOR CANAL.

Hunter's glossitis Glossitis associated with pernicious anemia, characterized by atrophy of the papillae and by redness, burning, and pain. Syn. *atrophic glossitis.*

Hunter's syndrome Mucopolysaccharidosis II, transmitted as an X-linked recessive, characterized chemically by excessive dermatan sulfate and heparitin sulfate in tissues and urine, and clinically by an appearance similar to that seen in the more common Hurler's syndrome, but a milder course. Mental deterioration progresses more slowly, lumbar gibbus does not occur, and clouding of the cornea of clinically evident degree does not appear.

Hunt-ing-ton's chorea or **disease** A dominantly heritable disorder of the central nervous system characterized by the onset, usually in adult life, of progressive choreoathetosis, emotional disturbances, and dementia.

Hur-ler's syndrome (hoor'lur) Mucopolysaccharidosis I, transmitted as an autosomal recessive, characterized chemically by excessive dermatan sulfate and heparitin sulfate in tissues and urine, and clinically by a rather grotesque appearance due to a disproportionately large head and coarse facies with flat nose and thick lips, skeletal changes including shortness of stature, gibbus, chest deformities, marked limitation in extensibility of joints, spadelike hands, enlarged tongue and hepatosplenomegaly, skin and cardiac changes, and early progressive clouding of the cornea, mental deficit, and often deafness.

Hürth·le-cell adenoma (huᵉrt′leʰ) A thyroid adenoma whose parenchyma is composed of Hürthle cells.

Hürthle cells 1. Thyroid follicular epithelial cells that are enlarged and have acidophilic cytoplasm, seen especially in adenomas. 2. Sometimes, cells of similar appearance in the parathyroid.

Hutchinson-Gil·ford syndrome or **disease** A disorder of unknown cause appearing in early childhood, characterized by cessation of growth, senile-like changes, large skull, "birdlike" features with crowding of teeth, atrophic skin, and loss of subcutaneous fat in the face, chest, and extremities, often with severe mental defects, high levels of serum lipoproteins and consequent atherosclerosis and its complications. Syn. *progeria of children.*

hutch·in·so·ni·an (hutch′in·so′nee·un) *adj.* Described by or associated with Jonathan Hutchinson, English surgeon, 1828–1913.

Hutchinson's freckle LENTIGO MALIGNA.

Hutchinson's teeth Deformity of permanent incisor teeth associated with congenital syphilis. The crown of such a tooth is wider in the cervical portion than at the incisal edge; the incisal edge has a characteristic crescent-shaped notch.

Hutchinson's triad Interstitial keratitis, eighth-nerve deafness, and notched permanent teeth signifying congenital syphilis.

hyal-, hyalo- A combining form meaning (a) *glass;* (b) *glassy, transparent;* (c) *vitreous, hyaloid;* (d) *hyaline.*

hy·a·line, hy·a·lin (high′uh·lin) *n. & adj.* 1. A clear, structureless, homogeneous, glassy material occurring normally in matrix of cartilage, vitreous body, colloid of thyroid gland, mucin, glycogen, Wharton's jelly; occurs pathologically in degenerations of connective tissue, epithelial cells, and in the form of mucinous and colloid degenerations and glycogen infiltration. 2. Consisting of or pertaining to hyaline.

hyaline thrombus. A thrombus found in the smaller blood vessel as a glossy fibrinous mass.

hy·a·li·tis (high′uh·lye′tis) *n.* Inflammation of the vitreous body, or of the hyaloid membrane of the vitreous body.

hy·a·lo·cap·su·li·tis (high′uh·lo·kap′sue·lye′tis) *n.* Hyalinization of a capsule, usually of the liver or spleen.

hy·a·loid (high′uh·loid) *adj.* 1. Transparent; glasslike. 2. Pertaining to the vitreous body.

hyaloid membrane. The dense layer of fibrils surrounding the vitreous body.

hy·a·lo·mere (high′uh·lo·meer) *n.* The clear part of a blood platelet after staining with stains of the Romanovsky type.

hy·a·lo·nyx·is (high′uh·lo·nick′sis) *n.* Puncture of the vitreous body of the eye.

hy·a·lo·pho·bia (high′uh·lo·foe′bee·uh) *n.* A morbid fear of glass.

hy·a·lo·plasm (high′uh·lo·plaz·um) *n.* The fluid portion of the protoplasm. Syn. *enchylema, interfilar mass, paraplasm, paramitome.*

hy·al·uron·ic acid (high″uh·lew·ron′ick). A viscous mucopolysaccharide occurring in connective tissues and in bacterial capsules.

hy·a·lu·ron·i·dase (high″uh·lew·ron′i·dace, -daze) *n.* An enzyme occurring in pathogenic bacteria, snake venoms, and sperm capable of catalyzing depolymerization and hydrolysis of hyaluronic acid in protective polysaccharide barriers, promoting penetration of cells and tissues by an agent in contact with them; it is a spreading factor. Hyaluronidase is used to promote diffusion and absorption of various injected medicaments.

hy·brid, *n. & adj.* 1. The offspring of parents belonging to different species, varieties, or genotypes. 2. Being or pertaining to a hybrid. —**hybrid·ism** (-iz·um), **hy·brid·i·ty** (high·brid′i·tee) *n.*

hy·brid·iza·tion (high″brid·i·zay′shun) *n.* 1. CROSSBREEDING. 2. *In chemistry,* a distribution of electrons in different types of orbitals in an atom to give equivalent orbitals and bonds. 3. The pairing of single complementary strands of deoxyribonucleic acid and ribonucleic acid to form a double-stranded molecule.

hy·dan·to·in (high·dan′to·in, high″dan·to′in) *n.* 2,4-($3H,5H$)-Imidazoledione or glycolylurea, $C_3H_4N_2O_2$, a crystalline substance derived from allantoin and related to urea.

hy·dat·id (high·dat′id) *n.* 1. A cyst formed in tissues due to growth of the larval stage of *Echinococcus granulosus* (dog tapeworm). 2. A cystic remnant of an embryonal structure. —**hydat·ic** (-ick), **hy·da·tid·i·form** (high″duh·tid′i·form) *adj.*

hydatidiform mole. Transformation of all or part of the placenta into grapelike cysts, characterized by poorly vascularized and edematous villi and trophoblastic proliferation. Syn. *hydatid mole.*

hydatid of Morgagni APPENDIX TESTIS.

hydr-, hydro- A combining form meaning (a) *water;* (b) *presence of hydrogen or the addition of hydrogen to a compound;* (c) *a disease characterized by an accumulation of water or other fluid in a bodily part.*

hy·drac·id (high·dras′id) *n.* An acid containing no oxygen.

hy·dra·gogue, hy·dra·gog (high″druh·gog) *adj. & n.* 1. Causing the discharge of watery fluid, especially from the bowel. 2. A purgative that causes copious watery discharges.

hy·dral·a·zine (high·dral′uh·zeen) *n.* 1-Hydrazinophthalazine, $C_8H_8N_4$, an antihypertensive drug; used as the hydrochloride salt.

hy·dram·ni·os (high·dram′nee·os) *n.* POLYHYDRAMNIOS.

hy·dran·en·ceph·a·ly (high″dran·en·sef′uh·lee) *n.* A developmental disorder of the nervous system due to a failure of evagination of the greater part of the cerebral hemispheres, resulting in large fluid-filled cavities in communication with the third ventricle. The disorder is characterized clinically by postnatal enlargement and transillumination of the head, retention of brainstem reflexes, and a failure of development of cerebral functions.

hy·drar·gyr·ia (high″drahr·jirr′ee·uh, ·jye′ree·uh) n. Chronic mercurial poisoning.

hy·drar·gy·rum (high·drahr′ji·rum) n. MERCURY.

hy·drar·thro·sis (high″drahr·thro′sis) n., pl. **hy·drar·thro·ses** (·seez) An accumulation of fluid in a joint.

hy·drase (high′drace, ·draze) n. An enzyme that catalyzes removal or addition of water to a substrate without hydrolyzing it.

hy·drate (high′drate) n. 1. A compound containing water in chemical combination; water of crystallization. 2. Obsol. HYDROXIDE. —**hydrat·ed** (·id) adj.

hy·dra·tion n. 1. Absorption of, or combination with, water. 2. In histologic procedures, successively transferring a specimen from an anhydrous reagent or solvent through mixtures of solvent with an increasing proportion of water and finally to water alone. 3. Fluid replacement.

hy·drau·lics (high·draw′licks) n. The science that deals with the mechanical properties of liquids. —**hydrau·lic** (·lick) adj.

hy·dra·zine (high′druh·zeen, ·zin) n. 1. H_2NNH_2. Diamine; a colorless liquid, soluble in water, having a strong alkaline reaction. The sulfate is used as a reducing agent. 2. One of a class of bodies derived from hydrazine by replacing one or more hydrogen atoms by a radical.

hy·dre·lat·ic (high″dre·lat′ick) adj. Pertaining to the secretory effect of nerves or hormones upon glands, causing them to discharge the watery part of their secretion.

hy·dre·mia, hy·drae·mia (high·dree′mee·uh) n. An excessive amount of water in the blood; disproportionate increase in plasma volume as compared with red blood cell volume. —**hydre·mic, hydrae·mic** (·mick) adj.

hy·dren·ceph·a·lo·cele (high″dren·sef′uh·lo·seel) n. Protrusion through a defect in the cranium of a sac and brain substance in which a cystic cavity contains fluid.

hy·dren·ceph·a·lo·me·nin·go·cele (high″dren·sef″uh·lo·me·ning′go·seel) n. A hernia through a cranial defect of meninges and brain substance, fluid filling the space between these.

hy·dride (high′dride) n. A compound containing hydrogen united to a more positive element or to a radical.

hy·dri·on (high·drye′on, high′dree·on) n. Hydrogen in the ionized form.

hydro-. See hydr-.

hy·droa (high·dro′uh) n. Any skin disease characterized by vesicles or bullae.

hydroa vac·ci·ni·for·me (vack·sin″i·for′mee) n. A dermatosis consisting of delicate blisters that appear on exposed skin during the summer and that heal by scarring. Erythropoietic protoporphyria is the underlying condition.

hy·dro·bro·mate (high″dro·bro′mate) n. A hydrobromic acid salt; a hydrobromide.

hydrobromic acid. 1. Hydrogen bromide, HBr; a heavy, colorless gas with a pungent irritating odor. 2. An aqueous solution of hydrogen bromide.

hy·dro·bro·mide (high″dro·bro′mide) n. A bromide formed by interaction of an organic nitrogenous base with hydrobromic acid.

hy·dro·cal·y·co·sis, hy·dro·cal·i·co·sis (high″dro·kal″i·ko′sis, ·kay″li·ko′sis) n. CALICEAL DIVERTICULUM.

hy·dro·ca·lyx, hy·dro·ca·lix (high″dro·kay′licks) n. Cystic dilatation of a renal calix, usually solitary.

hy·dro·car·bon (high″dro·kahr′bun) n. Any compound composed only of hydrogen and carbon.

hy·dro·cele (high′dro·seel) n. An accumulation of clear, slightly viscid fluid in the processus vaginalis or sac of the tunica vaginalis of the testis. In communicating hydrocele, a patent processus vaginalis permits peritoneal fluid to distend the tunica vaginalis in the upright position. In hydrocele of the cord, there is loculation of fluid along the incompletely involuted processus vaginalis.

hy·dro·ce·lec·to·my (high″dro·se·leck′tuh·mee) n. Surgical removal of part of the tunica vaginalis or drainage of the tunica vaginalis.

hy·dro·ce·phal·ic (high″dro·se·fal′ick) adj. Of or pertaining to hydrocephalus.

hy·dro·ceph·a·lus (high″dro·sef′uh·lus) n. 1. Distention of the cerebral ventricles with cerebrospinal fluid due to obstruction of the flow of spinal fluid within the ventricular system or in the subarachnoid space, preventing its absorption. 2. An individual with hydrocephalus.

hy·dro·ceph·a·ly (high″dro·sef′uh·lee) n. HYDROCEPHALUS(1).

hy·dro·chlo·ride (high″druh·klor′ide) n. A chloride formed by interaction of an organic nitrogenous base with hydrochloric acid.

hy·dro·chlo·ro·thi·a·zide (high″druh·klor″o·thigh″uh·zide) n. 6-Chloro-3,4-dihydro-2H-1,2,4-benzothiadiazine-7-sulfonamide 1,1-dioxide, $C_7H_8ClN_3O_4S_2$, an orally effective diuretic and antihypertensive drug.

hy·dro·chol·e·re·sis (high″dro·kol″ur·ee′sis, ·ko′lur·ee′sis) n. Choleresis characterized by an increase of water output, or of a bile relatively low in specific gravity, viscosity, and content of total solids. —**hydrochol·er·et·ic** (·et′ick) adj.

hy·dro·co·done (high″dro·ko′dohn) n. Dihydrocodeinone, $C_{18}H_{21}NO_3$, a compound isomeric with codeine and prepared from it by catalytic rearrangement. Used mainly as an antitussive, as the bitartrate salt.

hy·dro·col·loid (high″dro·kol′oid) n. A type of dental impression material derived from marine kelp. It is introduced into the mouth as a viscous sol which sets into an elastic, insoluble gel.

hy·dro·col·pos (high″dro·kol′pos) n. A vaginal retention cyst containing a watery fluid.

hy·dro·cor·ti·sone (high″dro·kor′ti·sone) n. 11β,17,21-Trihydroxypregn-4-ene-3,20-dione or 17-hydroxycorticosterone, $C_{21}H_{30}O_5$, an adrenocortical steroid occurring naturally and prepared synthetically; its metabolic and therapeutic effects are qualitatively similar to those of cortisone, but it is considerably more active. Used therapeutically in the form of free hydrocortisone, hydrocortisone acetate, hydrocortisone cypionate, and hydrocortisone sodium succinate. Syn. *Kendall's compound F. Reichstein's substance M.*

hy·dro·cy·an·ic acid (high″dro·sigh·an′ick, ·see· an′ick). Hydrogen cyanide, HCN, a liquid boiling at 26°C; used as a fumigant to rid vessels, buildings, or orchards of vermin. It is a powerful, rapidly acting blood and nerve poison. Syn. *prussic acid.*

hy·dro·cyte (high′dro·site) n. An erythrocyte containing excess water, resulting from excessive membrane permeability to sodium as compared with potassium.

hy·dro·dip·so·ma·nia (high″dro·dip″so·may′nee· uh) n. Periodic attacks of uncontrollable thirst; psychogenic thirst.

hy·dro·elec·tric bath (high″dro·e·leck′trick). A process of immersing the body, or parts of it, in water through which faradic, galvanic, or sinusoidal currents are running.

hy·dro·gel (high′dro·jel) n. A colloidal gel in which water is the dispersion medium.

hy·dro·gen (high′druh·jin) n. H = 1.0080. A univalent, flammable, gaseous element; the lightest element known. It occurs in water and in practically all organic compounds. It is used in various syntheses, as a reducing agent, for the hydrogenation of vegetable oils to form solid products, and in many other industrial applications. Three isotopes of hydrogen (namely, protium, deuterium, and tritium, having atomic masses of approximately one, two, and three, respectively) have been discovered.

hydrogen acceptor. A substance that, on reduction, accepts hydrogen atoms from another substance (hydrogen donor).

hydrogen donor. A chemical compound capable of transferring hydrogen atoms to another substance (hydrogen acceptor), thereby reducing the latter and oxidizing the donor.

hydrogen ion. The positively charged nucleus of the hydrogen atom, a proton. Acids are characterized by their ability to liberate hydrogen ions when in aqueous solution. Symbol, H^+.

hydrogen peroxide. H_2O_2, a colorless, caustic liquid, highly explosive in contact with oxidizable material. A 3% solution is used as an antiseptic and germicide.

hydrogen sulfide. H_2S. A colorless, highly toxic gas of unpleasant odor.

hy·dro·glos·sa (high″dro·glos′uh) n. RANULA.

hy·dro·gym·nas·tics (high″dro·jim·nas′ticks) n. Active exercises performed in water; the buoyancy thus obtained enables weakened muscles to move the limbs more easily.

hy·dro·he·ma·to·ne·phro·sis, hy·dro·hae·ma·to· ne·phro·sis (high″dro·hee″muh·to·ne·fro′sis, ·hem″uh·to·) n. The presence of blood and urine in a dilated renal pelvis.

hy·dro·he·ma·to·sal·pinx, hy·dro·hae·ma·to·sal· pinx (high″dro·hee″muh·to·sal′pincks) n. HE· MOHYDROSALPINX.

hy·dro·ki·net·ics (high″dro·ki·net′icks) n. The science of the motion of liquids. —**hydrokinet· ic**, *adj.*

An instrument used in estimating the percentage of water in milk.

hy·dro·lase (high′dro·lace, ·laze) n. An enzyme catalyzing hydrolysis.

hy·drol·y·sate (high·drol′i·sate) n. The product of hydrolysis.

hy·drol·y·sis (high·drol′i·sis) n. Any reaction with water, frequently of the type $AB + HOH \rightarrow AOH + HB$, the latter being the reverse reaction of neutralization. —**hy·dro·lyt·ic** (high″dro·lit′ick) *adj.*; **hy·dro·lyze** (high′dro· lize) v.

hy·dro·lyte (high′dro·lite) n. The substance undergoing hydrolysis.

hy·dro·ma·nia (high″dro·may′nee·uh) n. 1. Abnormal thirst, especially for water. 2. A severe depressive neurosis with a morbid desire for suicide by drowning.

hy·dro·mas·sage (high″dro·ma·sahzh′) n. Massage by means of moving water.

hy·dro·me·nin·go·cele (high″dro·me·ning′go· seel) n. A meningocele with prominent distention by cerebrospinal fluid.

hy·drom·e·ter (high·drom′e·tur) n. An instrument for determining the specific gravity of liquids. —**hy·dro·met·ric** (high·dro·met′rick) *adj.*; **hy·drom·e·try** (high·drom′e·tree) n.

hy·dro·me·tra (high″dro·mee′truh) n. Accumulation of watery fluid in the uterus.

hy·dro·me·tro·col·pos (high″dro·mee″tro·kol′ pos) n. Accumulation of watery fluid in the uterus and vagina.

hy·dro·mi·cro·ceph·a·ly (high″dro·migh″kro·sef′ uh·lee) n. Microcephaly with increased cerebrospinal fluid.

hy·dro·mor·phone (high″dro·mor′fone) n. Dihydromorphinone, $C_{17}H_{19}NO_3$, prepared by hydrogenation of morphine; a respiratory sedative and analgesic considerably more powerful than morphine. Used as the hydrochloride salt.

hy·dro·my·e·lia (high″dro·migh·ee′lee·uh) n. A dilatation of the central canal of the spinal cord.

hy·dro·my·e·lo·cele (high″dro·migh′e·lo·seel″) n. HYDROMYELIA.

hy·dro·ne·phro·sis (high″dro·ne·fro′sis) n. Dilation of the pelvis and calyces of the kidney secondary to urinary tract obstruction; eventually kidney parenchymal atrophy results. —**hydrone·phrot·ic** (·frot′ick) *adj.*

hy·dro·ni·um (high·dro′nee·um) n. The solvated hydrogen ion, $H^+(H_2O)$ or H_3O^+, considered to be present in aqueous solutions of all acids.

hy·drop·a·thy (high·drop′uth·ee) n. The system of internal and external use of water in attempting to cure disease. —**hy·dro·path·ic** (high″dro·path′ick) *adj.*

hy·dro·pel·vis (high″dro·pel′vis) n. Distention of the renal pelvis by urine, with little or no calyceal distention; PELVIECTASIS.

hy·dro·peri·car·di·tis (high″dro·perr″i·kahr·dye′ tis) n. Pericarditis accompanied by serous effusion into the pericardial cavity.

hy·dro·peri·car·di·um (high″dro·perr″i·kahr′dee· um) n. A collection of a serous effusion in the pericardial cavity.

Hy·droph·i·dae (high·drof′i·dee) n.pl. A family of

poisonous snakes, the sea snakes, which because of certain modifications are adapted to life in the sea. These snakes occur most abundantly in the waters of northern Australia and southern Asia; although their venom is the most toxic known, bites are relatively rare.

hy·dro·phil (high'dro·fil) n. & adj. 1. A substance, usually in the colloidal state, which is capable of combining with, or attracting, water. 2. Capable of combining with, or attracting, water.
—**hy·dro·phil·ic** (high''dro·fil'ick) adj.

hydrophilic colloid. A colloid that has a strong affinity for water and forms stable dispersions in water by virtue of this property.

hy·droph·i·lism (high·drof'i·liz·um) n. The property of colloids, cells, and tissues of attracting and holding water.

hy·dro·phobe (high'dro·fobe) n. 1. A substance, usually in the colloidal state, which lacks affinity for water. 2. A person who has a fear of water.

hy·dro·pho·bia (high''dro·fo'bee·uh) n. 1. Spasticity and paralysis of the muscles of deglutition, with consequent aversion to liquids, as a manifestation of rabies. 2. RABIES. 3. Morbid fear of water.

hy·dro·pho·bo·pho·bia (high''druh·fo''bo·fo'bee·uh) n. An intense dread of hydrophobia, sometimes producing a state simulating true hydrophobia.

hy·dro·phone (high'druh·fone) n. An instrument used in auscultatory percussion, the sound being conveyed to the ear through a liquid column.

hy·droph·thal·mos (high'drof·thal'mus) n. CONGENITAL GLAUCOMA.

hy·drop·ic (high·drop'ick) adj. Characterized by swelling or retention of fluid; specifically, characterized by or pertaining to hydrops.

hy·dro·pneu·ma·to·sis (high''dro·new''muh·to'sis) n. A collection of liquid and gas within the tissues.

hy·dro·pneu·mo·peri·car·di·um (high''dro·new''mo·perr·i·kahr'dee·um) n. A collection of fluid and gas in the pericardial sac.

hy·dro·pneu·mo·peri·to·ne·um (high''dro·new''mo·perr·i·tuh·nee'um) n. A collection of fluid and gas within the peritoneal cavity.

hy·dro·pneu·mo·tho·rax (high''dro·new''mo·tho'racks) n. The presence of fluid and gas in the pleural cavity.

hy·drops (high'drops) n. The accumulation of fluid in body tissues or cavities; dropsy.

hydrops fe·ta·lis (fee·tay'lis). A severe form of erythroblastosis fetalis characterized by marked anasarca; the fetus is usually dead at delivery.

hydrops of the labyrinth. A condition of the labyrinth caused by increased endolymphatic pressure producing tinnitus, hearing loss, and vertigo.

hy·dro·pyo·ne·phro·sis (high''dro·pye''o·ne·fro'sis) n. Dilatation of the pelvis of the kidney with urine and pus, usually caused by bacterial infection complicating an obstruction of the urinary tract.

hy·dror·rhea, hy·dror·rhoea (high''dro·ree'uh) n. A copious flow of a watery fluid.

hydrorrhea grav·i·da·rum (grav·i·dair'rum). A chronic discharge from the vagina, prior to parturition, of watery fluid resembling amniotic fluid, but with no evidence of ruptured membranes. It may be formed by the decidua.

hy·dro·sal·pinx (high''dro·sal'pinks) n. A distention of a uterine tube with fluid.

hy·dro·sol·u·ble (high''dro·sol'yoo·bul) adj. Soluble in water.

hy·dro·sper·ma·to·cyst (high''dro·spur'muh·to·sist, ·spur·mat'o·) n. A hydrocele whose fluid contains spermatozoa.

hy·dro·spi·rom·e·ter (high''dro·spye·rom'e·tur) n. A spirometer in which air pressure is indicated by the rise and fall of a column of water.

hy·dro·stat·ic (high''dro·stat'ick) adj. 1. Functioning by means of a liquid in equilibrium. 2. Pertaining to hydrostatics.

hydrostatic pressure. A pressure created in a fluid system.

hy·dro·stat·ics (high''dro·stat'icks) n. The branch of hydraulics that treats of the properties and characteristics of liquids in a state of equilibrium.

hy·dro·sy·rin·go·my·e·lia (high''dro·si·ring''go·migh·ee'lee·uh) n. Dilatation of the central canal of the spinal cord by cerebrospinal fluid, accompanied by degeneration and the formation of cavities.

hy·dro·tax·is (high''dro·tack'sis) n. The response of organisms to the stimulus of moisture.

hy·dro·ther·a·peu·tics (high''dro·therr·uh·pew'ticks) n. The branch of therapeutics that deals with the curative use of water.

hy·dro·ther·a·py (high''dro·therr'uh·pee) n. The treatment of disease by the external use of water.

hy·dro·ther·mal (high''dro·thur'mul) adj. Of or pertaining to warm water; said of springs.

hy·dro·tho·rax (high''dro·tho'racks) n. A collection of fluid in the pleural cavity. —**hydro·rac·ic** (·tho·ras'ick) adj.

hidrotic. HIDROTIC.

hy·dro·tis (high·dro'tis) n. Watery effusion into the external ear, the middle ear, or the inner ear, seldom in combination.

hy·drot·ro·py (high·drot'ruh·pee) n. The power that certain substances have of making water-insoluble substances dissolve in water without any apparent chemical alteration of the dissolved substances, as the solubilizing action of bile salts on fatty acids.

hy·dro·tym·pa·num (high''dro·tim'puh·num) n. Effusion of fluid into the cavity of the middle ear.

hy·dro·ure·ter (high''dro·yoo·ree'tur, ·yoor'e·tur) n. Abnormal distention of the ureter with urine, usually due to partial obstruction.

hy·dro·ure·tero·ne·phro·sis (high''dro·yoo·ree''tur·o·ne·fro'sis) n. Abnormal unilateral or bilateral distention and dilatation of both kidney and ureter with urine or other watery fluid, from obstructed outflow.

hy·dro·ure·ter·o·sis (high''dro·yoo·ree''tur·o'sis) n. HYDROURETER.

hy·drous (high'drus) adj. Containing water.

hydrous wool fat. LANOLIN.

hy·drox·ide (high·drock'side, ·sid) n. Any compound formed by the union of a metal, or of an inorganic or organic radical, with one or more hydroxyl (OH) groups.

hydroxy-. A combining form indicating *the hydroxyl group —OH.*

β-hy·droxy·bu·tyr·ic acid (high·drock″see·bew·tirr′ick). 3-Hydroxybutanoic acid, $C_4H_8O_3$, an intermediate acid formed in fat metabolism. It is a member of a group of compounds called acetone bodies or ketone bodies. In ketosis, increased amounts of these compounds appear in blood and urine.

α-hydroxybutyric dehydrogenase. Any of a group of isoenzymes of lactic dehydrogenase, largely the isoenzyme chiefly found in cardiac muscle; determination of serum levels is sometimes used in the diagnosis of myocardial infarction.

hy·droxy·chlo·ro·quine (high·drock″see·klo′ro·kween) *n.* 7-Chloro-4-{4-[ethyl(2-hydroxyethyl)amino]-1-methylbutylamino}-quinoline, $C_{18}H_{26}ClN_3O$, used as the sulfate salt for the treatment of malaria, lupus erythematosus, and rheumatoid arthritis.

17-hy·droxy·cor·ti·cos·ter·one (high·drock″see·kor″ti·kos′tur·ohn) *n.* HYDROCORTISONE.

17-hydroxy-11-dehydrocorticosterone, *n.* CORTISONE.

5-hy·droxy·in·dole·ace·tic acid (high·drock″see·in″dole·a·see′tick). $C_{10}H_9NO_3$. A metabolite of serotonin present in cerebrospinal fluid and in small amounts in normal urine, and markedly increased in some cases of carcinoid syndrome.

hy·drox·yl (high·drock′sil) *n.* The univalent radical —OH, the combination of which with a basic element or radical forms a hydroxide.

hy·drox·yl·amine (high·drock″sil·uh·meen′) *n.* A basic substance, NH_2OH, known only in solution in water or in combination with acids. The hydrochloride salt is used as a reagent.

hy·drox·yl·ase (high·drock′si·lace, ·laze) *n.* Any enzyme that results in the formation or introduction of a hydroxyl group in a substrate.

hy·drox·yl·ation (high·drock″si·lay′shun) *n.* Introduction or formation, by various chemical procedures, of one or more hydroxyl radicals in a compound. **—hy·drox·yl·at·ed** (high·drock′si·lay·tid) *adj.*

hy·droxy·ly·sine (high·drock″see·lye′seen) *n.* The amino acid 2,6-diamino-3-hydroxycaproic acid, $C_6H_{14}N_2O_3$.

hy·droxy·pro·line (high·drock″see·pro′leen, ·lin) *n.* 4-Hydroxy-2-pyrrolidinecarboxylic acid, $C_5H_9NO_3$, a naturally occurring amino acid.

hy·droxy·pro·lin·emia, hy·droxy·pro·lin·ae·mia (high·drock″see·pro·lin·ee′mee·uh) *n.* An inborn error of metabolism in which there is a deficiency of hydroxyproline oxidase with increased blood levels of hydroxyproline; mental retardation is the main clinical manifestation.

hy·droxy·quin·o·line (high·drock″see·kwin′o·leen, ·lin) *n.* 8-Hydroxyquinoline, C_9H_7NO, used as an analytical reagent for metals and for arginine. The base and certain of its salts, especially the citrate and sulfate, have been used as fungicides, antiseptics, and deodorants. Syn. *oxyquinoline.*

hy·droxy·urea (high·drock″see·yoo·ree′uh) *n.* Hydroxycarbamide, $H_2NCONHOH$, an antineoplastic agent.

hy·droxy·zine (high·drock′si·zeen) *n.* 1-(p-Chlorobenzhydryl)-4-[2-(2-hydroxyethoxy)-ethyl]piperazine, $C_{21}H_{27}ClN_2O_2$, a tranquilizer also possessing antiemetic and antihistaminic effects; used as the hydrochloride or pamoate salt.

hy·dru·ria (high·droo′ree·uh) *n.* The passage of large amounts of urine of low specific gravity, as in diabetes insipidus; polyuria. **—hydru·ric** (·rick) *adj.*

Hy·ge·ia (high·jee′uh) *n.* In Greek mythology, the goddess of health; daughter of Asklepios.

hy·giene (high′jeen) *n.* The science that treats of the laws of health and the methods of their observation. **—hy·gien·ic** (high·jee·en′ick) *adj.*

hy·gien·ist (high′jeen·ist, high·jen′ist) *n.* 1. One trained in the science of health. 2. A dental hygienist.

hygr-, hygro- A combining form meaning *moist, moisture, humidity.*

hy·gre·che·ma (high″gre·kee′muh) *n.* The sound produced by a liquid in a body tissue or cavity as heard by auscultation.

hy·gro·ble·phar·ic (high″gro·ble·făr′ick) *adj.* Serving to moisten the eyelid.

hy·gro·ma (high·gro′muh) *n., pl.* **hygromas, hy·groma·ta** (·tuh) A cystic cavity derived from distended lymphatics and filled with lymph; a congenital malformation, most often seen in young children. Syn. *cavernous lymphangioma, cystic hygroma.* **—hy·grom·a·tous** (high·grom′uh·tus) *adj.*

hygroma cys·ti·cum col·li (sis′ti·kum kol′eye). A hygroma in the neck.

hy·grom·e·ter (high·grom′e·tur) *n.* An instrument for determining quantitatively the amount of moisture in the air. **—hygrome·try** (·tree) *n.*

hy·gro·pho·bia (high″gro·fo′bee·uh) *n.* Morbid fear of liquids or of moisture.

hy·gro·scope (high′gro·skope) *n.* An instrument for indicating the humidity of the atmosphere. **—hy·gros·co·py** (high·gros′kuh·pee) *n.*

hy·gro·scop·ic (high″gro·skop′ick) *adj.* 1. Pertaining to a hygroscope. 2. Sensitive to moisture; readily absorbing moisture.

hyl-, hylo- A combining form meaning (a) *wood;* (b) *material, substance, matter.*

hy·lo·pho·bia (high″lo·fo′bee·uh) *n.* Morbid fear of forests.

hy·lo·trop·ic (high″lo·trop′ick) *adj.* Characterizing a substance capable of changing its form without changing its composition, as a solid that can be melted or distilled.

hy·men (high′mun) *n.* A membranous partition partially, or in some cases wholly, blocking the orifice of the vagina. It may be of several forms, such as circular, or crescentic; it may be multiple, entirely lacking, or imperforate. **—hymen·al** (·ul) *adj.*

hymen-, hymeno-. A combining form meaning (a) *hymen;* (b) *membrane.*

hymenal caruncles. The small irregular nodules which are the remains of the hymen.

hy·men·ec·to·my (high''me·neck'tuh·mee) n. Excision of the hymen.

hy·me·no·le·pi·a·sis (high''me·no·le·pye'uh·sis) n., pl. **hymenolepia·ses** (·seez) Infection of the intestines by tapeworms of the genus *Hymenolepis*, usually producing only mild abdominal distress.

Hy·me·nol·e·pis (high''me·nol'e·pis) n. A genus of tapeworms; any dwarf tapeworm.

Hymenolepis na·na (nay'nuh). A species of tapeworm, cosmopolitan in distribution, which infects man; the smallest of the dwarf tapeworms.

hy·men·or·rha·phy (high''me·nor'uh·fee) n. 1. Suture of the hymen to occlude the vagina. 2. Suture of any membrane.

hy·meno·tome (high·men'uh·tohm) n. A surgical instrument used for cutting membranes.

hy·men·ot·o·my (high''me·not'uh·mee) n. 1. Surgical incision of the hymen. 2. Dissection or anatomy of membranes.

hyo·epi·glot·tic (high''o·ep·i·glot'ick) adj. Relating to the hyoid bone and the epiglottis.

hyo·glos·sal (high''o·glos'ul) adj. 1. Pertaining to the hyoglossus. 2. Extending from the hyoid bone to the tongue.

hyo·glos·sus (high''o·glos'us) n., pl. **hyoglos·si** (·sigh) An extrinsic muscle of the tongue arising from the hyoid bone.

hy·oid (high'oid) n. & adj. 1. A bone between the root of the tongue and the larynx, supporting the tongue and giving attachment to several muscles. 2. Of or pertaining to the hyoid.

hyoid arch. The second visceral arch.

hyo·man·dib·u·lar (high''o·man·dib'yoo·lur) adj. & n. 1. Pertaining to the hyoid and mandibular arches of the embryo or to the groove and pouch between them. 2. The upper cartilaginous or osseous element of the hyoid arch in fishes.

hy·o·scine (high'o·seen, ·sin) n. SCOPOLAMINE.

hyo·scy·a·mine (high''o·sigh'uh·meen, ·min) n. An alkaloid, $C_{17}H_{23}NO_3$, occurring in many of the Solanaceae, notably belladonna, hyoscyamus, and stramonium. It is the levorotatory component of racemic atropine, the pharmacologic activity of the latter being due largely to hyoscyamine. Used as the hydrobromide and sulfate salts.

hyo·scy·a·mus (high''o·sigh'uh·mus) n. Henbane. The dried leaf, with or without flowering tops, of *Hyoscyamus niger*; contains the alkaloids hyoscyamine and scopolamine. Its therapeutic effects are similar to those of belladonna but it is variable in its action. An extract and tincture were popular dosage forms.

hyo·ver·te·brot·o·my (high''o·vur''te·brot'uh·mee) n. *In veterinary medicine*, the operation of incising the guttural pouch. Syn. *hypospondylotomy.*

hyp-, hypo- A prefix meaning (a) *deficiency, lack;* (b) *below, beneath;* (c) (of acids and salts) *having the least number of atoms of oxygen* (as in a series of compounds of the same elements).

hyp·acu·sia (hip''a·kew'zhuh, ·zee·uh, high''pa·) n. Impairment of hearing. Syn. *hypoacusia.*

hyp·al·ge·sia (hip''al·jee'zee·uh, high''pal·) n. Diminished sensitivity to pain. —**hypalge·sic** (·zick) adj.

hyp·am·ni·on (hip·am'nee·on, high·pam') n. A small amount of amniotic fluid; OLIGOHYDRAMNIOS.

hyp·an·i·sog·na·thism (hi·pan''i·sog'nuth·iz·um, high·pan''i·) n. The condition of having the upper teeth broader than the lower, with a lack of correspondence between the jaws. —**hypanisogna·thous** (·us) adj.

Hypaque. Trademark for sodium diatrizoate, a roentgenographic contrast medium for excretory urography and angiography.

hyp·ar·te·ri·al (high''pahr·teer'ee·ul, hip''ahr·) adj. Situated beneath an artery; specifically applied to branches of the stem bronchi.

hyparterial bronchus. Any one of the first collateral branches of the stem bronchi except the eparterial bronchus.

hyp·as·the·nia (high''pas·theen'ee·uh, hip''as·) n. Slight loss of strength.

hyp·ax·i·al (high·pack'see·ul, hip·ack') adj. Situated beneath the vertebral column; ventral.

hy·pen·gyo·pho·bia (high·pen''jee·o·fo'bee·uh) n. Morbid fear of responsibility.

hyper- A prefix meaning (a) *excessive, excessively;* (b) *above normal;* (c) in anatomy and zoology, *situated above.*

hy·per·ab·duc·tion (high''pur·ab·duck'shun) n. Excessive abduction of a limb or part. Syn. *superabduction.*

hy·per·acid·i·ty (high''pur·a·sid'i·tee) n. Excessive acidity.

hyperactive child syndrome. MINIMAL BRAIN DYSFUNCTION SYNDROME.

hy·per·ac·tiv·i·ty (high''pur·ack·tiv'i·tee) n. Excessive or abnormal activity. —**hy·per·ac·tive** (high''pur·ack'tiv) adj.

hy·per·acu·i·ty (high''pur·uh·kew'i·tee) n. Unusual sensory acuity or sharpness, especially of vision.

hy·per·acu·sia (high''pur·a·kew'zhuh, ·zee·uh) n. Abnormal acuteness of the sense of hearing; painful sensitivity to sounds, as in cases of Bell's palsy, with involvement of the nerve to the stapedius.

hy·per·acu·sis (high''pur·a·kew'sis) n. HYPERACUSIA.

hy·per·ad·e·no·sis (high''pur·ad''e·no'sis) n. Enlargement of the lymph nodes.

hy·per·adre·nal·ism (high''pur·uh·dree'nul·iz·um) n. A condition due either to hyperfunction of the adrenal cortex or prolonged or excessive treatment with adrenal cortical hormones, resulting in several clinical syndromes reflecting excessive glucocorticoid, mineralocorticoid, estrogen, or androgen secretion. Syn. *hyperadrenocorticism.*

hy·per·adre·no·cor·ti·cism (high''pur·a·dree''no·kor'ti·siz·um) n. HYPERADRENALISM.

hy·per·aer·a·tion (high''pur·ay·ur·ay'shun) n. HYPERVENTILATION (1).

hy·per·af·fec·tiv·i·ty (high''pur·a·feck·tiv'i·tee) n. A pathologic increase in reaction to normal or mild sensory stimuli.

hy·per·al·do·ste·ron·ism (high″pur·al″do·sterr′o·niz·um, al″do·ste·ro′niz·um) *n*. The clinical syndrome of muscle weakness, polyuria, hypertension, hypokalemia, and alkalosis associated with hypersecretion of the mineralocorticoid aldosterone by the adrenal cortex; described as primary hyperaldosteronism when due to adrenal hyperplasia or tumor and as secondary hyperaldosteronism when due to stimuli external to the adrenal gland.

hy·per·al·ge·sia (high″pur·al·jee′zee·uh) *n*. Excessive sensitivity to pain. —**hyperalge·sic** (·zick) *adj*.

hy·per·al·i·men·ta·tion (high″pur·al″i·men·tay′shun) *n*. 1. Overfeeding; superalimentation. 2. Prolonged maintenance of full nutritional requirements by intravenous infusion of carbohydrate, fat, amino acids, electrolytes, and vitamins.

hy·per·al·i·men·to·sis (high″pur·al″i·men·to′sis) *n*. Any disease due to excessive eating.

hy·per·am·i·no·ac·id·uria (high″pur·am′in·o·as″i·dew′ree·uh, high″pur·a·mee″no·) *n*. Abnormally high urinary excretion of amino acids.

hy·per·am·mo·ne·mia, hy·per·am·mo·nae·mia (high″pur·am″o·nee′mee·uh) *n*. 1. An elevation of ammonia in blood; characteristic of a number of metabolic diseases and hepatic encephalopathy. 2. A rare inborn error of metabolism divided into types I and II according to the location of the metabolic block in the urea cycle. Type I is carbamylphosphate synthetase deficiency. Type II is ornithine carbamyl transferase deficiency. Both are accompanied by elevation of ammonia in blood and cerebrospinal fluid; manifested clinically, especially after a meal rich in proteins, by vomiting, agitation and then lethargy, and later by ataxia, slurred speech, ptosis, and mental retardation. Pneumoencephalography may reveal cortical atrophy.

hy·per·an·a·ki·ne·sia (high″pur·an″uh·ki·nee′zhuh, zee·uh, ·an″uh·kigh·nee′·) *n*. Excessive activity of a part; hyperkinesia.

hy·per·aphia (high″pur·ay′fee·uh, ·af′ee·uh) *n*. An abnormally acute sense of touch. —**hyperaph·ic** (·af′ick) *adj*.

hy·per·az·o·te·mia, hy·per·az·o·tae·mia (high″pur·az″o·tee·mee·uh) *n*. AZOTEMIA.

hy·per·bar·ic (high″pur·băr′ick) *adj*. 1. Of greater weight, density, or pressure. 2. Of an anesthetic solution: having a specific gravity greater than that of the cerebrospinal fluid.

hyperbaric oxygen treatment. The administration of oxygen, under greater than atmospheric pressure, usually by placing the patient within a room or chamber especially designed for this purpose.

hy·per·bar·ism (high″pur·băr′iz·um) *n*. A condition resulting from an excess of the ambient gas pressure over that within the body tissues, fluids, and cavities.

hy·per·beta·al·a·ni·ne·mia, hy·per·beta·al·a·ni·nae·mia (high″pur·bay″tuh·al″uh·neen·ee′mee·uh) *n*. An inborn error of metabolism in which there appears to be a deficiency of beta-alanyl-alpha-ketoglutaric amino transferase, resulting in elevated levels of beta-alanine and gamma-aminobutyric acid in blood and cerebrospinal fluid, and increased excretion of beta-aminoisobutyric acid, gamma-aminobutyric acid, and taurine in the urine; manifested clinically by excessive somnolence and seizures.

hy·per·beta·lipo·pro·tein·emia (high″pur·bay″tuh·lip″o·pro·tee·nee′mee·uh) *n*. Abnormally high concentration of low-density lipoproteins in the plasma.

hy·per·bil·i·ru·bi·ne·mia, hy·per·bil·i·ru·bi·nae·mia (high″pur·bil″i·roo″bi·nee·mee·uh) *n*. 1. Excessive amount of bilirubin in the blood. 2. A severe and prolonged physiologic jaundice, sometimes seen in a premature newborn.

hy·per·bu·lia (high″pur·bew′lee·uh) *n*. Exaggerated willfulness.

hy·per·cal·ce·mia, hy·per·cal·cae·mia (high″pur·kal·see′mee·uh) *n*. Excessive quantity of calcium in the blood. Syn. *calcemia*.

hy·per·cal·ci·nu·ria (high″pur·kal·si·new′ree·uh) *n*. An abnormally high level of calcium in the urine.

hy·per·cal·ci·uria (high″pur·kal·si·yoo′ree·uh) *n*. HYPERCALCINURIA.

hy·per·cap·nia (high″pur·kap′nee·uh) *n*. Excessive amount of carbon dioxide in the blood.

hy·per·ca·thar·sis (high″pur·ka·thahr′sis) *n*. Excessive purgation of the bowels. —**hyperca·thar·tic** (·tick) *adj*.

hy·per·ca·thex·is (high″pur·ka·theck′sis) *n*. Excessive concentration of the psychic energy upon a particular focus.

hy·per·ce·men·to·sis (high″pur·see″men·to′sis, ·sem″en·to′sis) *n*., *pl*. **hypercemento·ses** (·seez) Excessive formation of cementum on the root of a tooth.

hy·per·ce·nes·the·sia, hy·per·coe·naes·the·sia (high″pur·see″nes·theezh′uh, ·theez′ee·uh, ·sen′es·) *n*. EUPHORIA (2).

hy·per·chlo·re·mia, hy·per·chlo·rae·mia (high″pur·klo·ree′mee·uh) *n*. An increase in the chloride content of the blood. —**hyperchlo·re·mic, hyperchlo·rae·mic** (·ree′mick) *adj*.

hyperchloremic acidosis. A metabolic acidosis characterized by low blood pH, low blood carbon dioxide, and elevated blood chloride; most commonly seen with renal disease.

hy·per·chlor·hy·dria (high″pur·klor·high′dree·uh) *n*. Excessive secretion of hydrochloric acid in the stomach.

hy·per·cho·les·ter·emia, hy·per·cho·les·ter·ae·mia (high″pur·ko·les″ter·ee′mee·uh) *n*. HYPERCHOLESTEROLEMIA.

hy·per·cho·les·ter·ol·emia, hy·per·cho·les·ter·ol·aemia (high″pur·ko·les″tur·o·lee′mee·uh) *n*. An excess of cholesterol in the blood. —**hypercholesterole·mic** (·mick) *adj*.

hy·per·cho·lia (high″pur·ko′lee·uh) *n*. Excessive secretion of bile.

hy·per·chro·mat·ic (high″pur·kro·mat′ick) *adj*. Pertaining to a cell or a portion of a cell which stains more intensely than is normal. —**hyperchro·ma·sia** (·may′zhuh, ·zee·uh) *n*.

hy·per·chro·ma·tism (high″pur·kro′muh·tiz·um) *n*. 1. Excessive formation of the pigment of the skin. 2. A condition in which cells or parts of cells stain more intensely than is normal.

hy·per·chro·ma·to·sis (high"pur·kro"muh·to'sis) *n.* Excessive pigmentation, as of the skin.

hy·per·chro·mia (high"pur·kro'mee·uh) *n.* HYPERCHROMATISM.

hy·per·chro·mic (high"pur·kro'mick) *adj.* Pertaining to or describing the microscopic appearance of cells of the erythropoietic series, in which dense staining is due not to increased concentration of hemoglobin, but to increased thickness of the cells.

hyperchromic anemia. 1. Anemia in which the erythrocytes are more deeply colored than usual as a result of increased thickness. 2. Anemia associated with a lack of vitamin B_{12} and related substances. 3. Megaloblastic anemia associated with pregnancy.

hy·per·chy·lia (high"pur·kigh'lee·uh) *n.* Excess secretion or formation of chyle.

hy·per·chy·lo·mi·cro·ne·mia, hy·per·chy·lo·mi·cro·nae·mia (high"pur·kigh"lo·migh"kro·nee'mee·uh) *n.* FAT-INDUCED FAMILIAL HYPERTRIGLYCERIDEMIA.

hy·per·co·ag·u·la·bil·i·ty (high"pur·ko·ag"yoo·luh·bil'i·tee) *n.* A condition in which the blood coagulates more readily than normally.

hy·per·cor·ti·cism (high"pur·kor'ti·siz·um) *n.* HYPERADRENALISM.

hy·per·cor·ti·sol·ism (high"pur·kor'ti·so·liz·um) *n.* Excessive production of hydrocortisone (cortisol) by the adrenal cortex, as in Cushing's syndrome.

hy·per·cry·al·ge·sia (high"pur·krye"al·jee'zee·uh) *n.* Abnormal sensitivity to cold.

hy·per·cu·pri·uria (high"pur·koo"pri·yoo'ree·uh) *n.* Excessive urinary excretion of copper.

hy·per·cy·a·not·ic (high"pur·sigh"uh·not'ick) *adj.* Characterized by an extreme degree of cyanosis.

hy·per·di·crot·ic (high"pur·dye·krot'ick) *adj.* Pertaining to the dicrotic wave of the peripheral pulse which is increased in amplitude, so that it may be detected by palpation. —**hyperdicrotism** (·dye'kro·tiz·um) *n.*

hy·per·dis·ten·tion (high"pur·dis·ten'shun) *n.* Forcible or extreme distention.

hy·per·dy·na·mia (high"pur·dye·nay'mee·uh, ·di·nay'mee·uh, ·dye·nam'ee·uh) *n.* Excessive strength or exaggeration of function, as of nerves or muscles. —**hyperdynamic** (·nam'ick) *adj.*

hyperdynamic ileus. SPASTIC ILEUS.

hy·per·em·e·sis (high"pur·em'e·sis) *n.* Excessive vomiting. —**hyperemetic** (·e·met'ick) *adj.*

hyperemesis gra·vi·da·rum (grav·i·dair'rum). PERNICIOUS VOMITING in pregnancy.

hyperemesis lac·ten·ti·um (lack·ten'tee·um, ·chee·um). Vomiting of nurslings.

hy·per·emia, hy·per·ae·mia (high"pur·ee'mee·uh) *n.* Increased blood in a part, resulting in distention of the blood vessels. Hyperemia may be active, when due to dilatation of blood vessels, or passive, when the drainage is hindered. —**hyperemic, hyper·ae·mic** (ee'mick) *adj.*

hy·per·er·gy (high"pur·ur·jee) *n.* An altered state of reactivity, in which the response is more marked than usual; hypersensitivity. It is one form of allergy or pathergy.

hy·per·eso·pho·ria (high"pur·es"o·fo'ree·uh) *n.* A form of heterophoria in which the visual axis tends to deviate upward and inward.

hy·per·es·the·sia, hy·per·aes·the·sia (high"pur·es·theezh'uh, ·theez'ee·uh) *n.* Increased sensitivity (usually cutaneous) to tactile, painful, thermal, and other stimuli. —**hyperes·thet·ic, hyperaes·thet·ic** (·thet'ick) *adj.*

hy·per·es·trin·ism, hy·per·oes·trin·ism (high"pur·es'trin·iz·um) *n.* Excessive or prolonged secretion, or both, of the female estrogenic hormones.

hy·per·es·tro·gen·ism, hy·per·oes·tro·gen·ism (high"pur·es'tro·je·niz·um) *n.* HYPERESTRINISM.

hy·per·ex·cit·abil·i·ty (high"pur·eck·sight"uh·bil'i·tee) *n.* 1. Excessive excitability. 2. A lowered threshold to excitation.

hy·per·ex·ten·sion (high"pur·ick·sten'shun) *n.* Overextension of a limb or part for the correction of deformity or for the retention of fractured bones in proper position and alignment.

hy·per·fer·re·mia, hy·per·fer·rae·mia (high"pur·ferr·ee'mee·uh) *n.* Excessive amounts of iron in the blood plasma. —**hyperferre·mic** (·mick) *adj.*

hy·per·fi·bri·nol·y·sis (high"pur·fye"bri·nol'i·sis) *n.* Markedly increased fibrinolysis.

hy·per·flex·ion (high"pur·fleck'shun) *n.* Overflexion of a limb or part of the body.

hy·per·func·tion (high"pur·funk'shun) *n.* Excessive function; excessive activity.

hy·per·gam·ma·glob·u·li·ne·mia, hy·per·gam·ma·glob·u·li·nae·mia (high"pur·gam"uh·glob"yoo·lin·ee'mee·uh) *n.* The increased concentration of immunoglobulins in the blood seen in a wide variety of clinical disorders.

hy·per·geu·sia (high"pur·gew'see·uh, ·joo'see·uh) *n.* Abnormal acuteness of the sense of taste.

hy·per·glob·u·li·ne·mia, hy·per·glob·u·li·nae·mia (high"pur·glob"yoo·lin·ee'mee·uh) *n.* Increased amount of globulin in the blood plasma or serum.

hy·per·gly·ce·mia, hy·per·gly·cae·mia (high"pur·glye·see'mee·uh) *n.* Excess of sugar in the blood. —**hyperglyce·mic, hyperglycae·mic** (·mick) *adj.*

hy·per·gly·cor·rha·chia (high"pur·glye"ko·ray'kee·uh, ·rack'ee·uh) *n.* An excess of glucose in the cerebrospinal fluid; usually secondary to an elevated concentration of glucose in the blood.

hy·per·gly·cos·uria (high"pur·glye"ko·sue'ree·uh) *n.* The presence of excessive amounts of sugar in the urine.

hy·per·go·nad·ism (high"pur·go'nad·iz·um, ·gon'uh·diz·um) *n.* Excessive internal secretion of the sexual glands (testes or ovaries).

hy·per·go·nia (high"pur·go'nee·uh) *n.* Increase in size of the gonial angle.

hy·per·he·do·nia (high"pur·he·do'nee·uh) *n.* 1. An excessive feeling of pleasure in any sensation or the gratification of a desire. 2. Erethism relating to the sexual organs.

hy·per·he·mo·lyt·ic, hy·per·hae·mo·lyt·ic (high"pur·hee"mo·lit'ick) *adj.* Of, pertaining to, or caused by excessive hemolysis.

hy·per·hi·dro·sis (high″pur·hi·dro′sis, ·high·dro′ sis) *n.* Excessive sweating; may be localized or generalized, chronic or acute; the sweat often accumulates in visible drops on the skin. Syn. *ephidrosis, polyhidrosis, sudatoria.*

hy·per·his·ta·mi·ne·mia, hy·per·his·ta·mi·nae· mia (high″pur·his″tuh·min·ee′mee·uh) *n.* An increase of histamine in the blood.

hy·per·hor·mo·nal (high″pur·hor·mo′nul) *adj.* Containing, or due to, excess of a hormone.

hy·per·in·su·lin·ism (high″pur·in′sue·lin·iz·um) *n.* The presence of high circulating blood levels of endogenous insulin, seen in a variety of conditions, such as obesity and insulin-producing tumors, and in newborns of diabetic mothers. Symptoms may or may not be present.

hy·per·in·vo·lu·tion (high″pur·in·vuh·lew′shun) *n.* A rapid shrinking to less than normal size of an organ that has been enlarged, as of the uterus after delivery.

hy·per·ir·ri·ta·bil·i·ty (high″pur·irr″i·tuh·bil′i· tee) *n.* The pathologically excessive reaction of an individual, organ, or part to a given stimulus.

hy·per·ka·le·mia (high″pur·ka·lee′mee·uh) *n.* An elevation above normal of potassium in the blood. **—hyperkale·mic** (·mick) *adj.*

hy·per·ker·a·tin·iza·tion (high″pur·kerr″uh·tin·i· zay′shun) *n.* Excessive production of keratin.

hy·per·ker·a·to·sis (high″pur·kerr″uh·to′sis) *n.,* pl. **hyperkerato·ses** (·seez) Hypertrophy of the horny layer of the skin, usually associated with hypertrophy of the granular and prickle-cell layers.

hy·per·ker·a·tot·ic (high″pur·kerr″uh·tot′ick) *adj.* Of, pertaining to, or characterized by hyperkeratosis.

hy·per·ke·to·nu·ria (high″pur·kee″to·new′ree· uh) *n.* The presence of an excess of ketone in the urine.

hy·per·ki·ne·mia, hy·per·ki·nae·mia (high″pur· ki·nee′mee·uh) *n.* A condition marked by an abnormally increased cardiac output at rest and lying supine.

hy·per·ki·ne·sia (high″pur·ki·nee′zhuh, ·zee·uh, ·kigh·nee′) *n.* Excessive movement; excessive muscular activity. **—hyperki·net·ic** (·net′ick) *adj.*

hy·per·ki·ne·sis (high″pur·ki·nee′sis) *n.* HYPERKINESIA.

hyperkinetic heart syndrome. A syndrome of unknown cause in young adults, characterized by an increased cardiac output at rest, increased rate of ventricular ejection, and in some patients, the development of heart failure.

hy·per·lac·ta·tion (high″pur·lack·tay′shun) *n.* Excessive or prolonged secretion of milk.

hy·per·leu·ko·cy·to·sis (high″pur·lew″ko·sigh·to′ sis) *n.* An excessive increase in leukocytes per unit volume of blood.

hy·per·lip·ac·i·de·mia (high″pur·lip·as″i·dee′ mee·uh) *n.* Excessive blood levels of fatty acids.

hy·per·li·pe·mia, hy·per·li·pae·mia (high″pur·li· pee′mee·uh) *n.* An excess of lipemic sub-stances in the blood. **—hyperlipe·mic, hyperli· pae·mic** (·mick) *adj.*

hy·per·lip·id·emia, hy·per·lip·id·ae·mia (high″ pur·lip′i·dee′mee·uh) *n.* HYPERLIPEMIA.

hy·per·lipo·pro·tein·emia, hy·per·lipo·pro·tein· ae·mia (high″pur·lip″o·pro·tee·nee′mee·uh) *n.* An excess of lipoproteins in the blood.

hy·per·li·thu·ria (high″pur·lith·yoo′ree·uh) *n.* An excess of uric (lithic) acid in the urine.

hy·per·lo·gia (high″pur·lo′jee·uh) *n.* Excessive or manic loquacity.

hy·per·ly·si·ne·mia, hy·per·ly·si·nae·mia (high″ pur·lye″si·nee′mee·uh) *n.* A hereditary metabolic disorder of unknown cause, in which there is an abnormally high blood level of lysine and excessive urinary excretion of ornithine, gamma-aminobutyric acid and ethanolamine, and delayed conversion of injected lysine to carbon dioxide; the disorder is manifested clinically by physical and mental retardation, lax ligaments and hypotonia, seizures in early life, and impaired sexual development.

hy·per·mag·ne·se·mia (high″pur·mag″ne·see′mee·uh) *n.* Abnormally high serum magnesium levels.

hy·per·ma·nia (high″pur·may′nee·uh) *n.* An advanced manic type of manic-depressive illness. **—hyper·man·ic** (·man′ick) *adj.*

hy·per·mas·tia (high″pur·mas′tee·uh) *n.* Overgrowth of the mammary gland.

hy·per·ma·ture (high″pur·muh·tewr′) *adj.* Overmature; overripe.

hy·per·men·or·rhea, hy·per·men·or·rhoea (high″ pur·men″o·ree′uh) *n.* MENORRHAGIA.

hy·per·me·tab·o·lism (high″pur·me·tab′uh·liz· um) *n.* Any state in which there is an abnormal increase in metabolic rate. **—hyper·met·a· bol·ic** (·met″uh·bol′ick) *adj.*

hy·per·me·tro·pia (high″pur·me·tro′pee·uh) *n.* HYPEROPIA. **—hyper·met·rope** (·met′rope) *n.* **—hyperme·tro·pic** (·trop′ick, ·tro′pick) *adj.*

hy·per·mi·cro·so·ma (high″pur·migh″kro·so′ muh) *n.* Extreme dwarfism.

hy·per·mim·ia (high″pur·mim′ee·uh) *n.* Excessive emotional expression or mimetic movement.

hy·per·min·er·alo·cor·ti·coid·ism (hy″pur·min′ ur·uh·lo·kor′ti·koid·iz·um) *n.* A pathologic state resulting from the excessive production of adrenal cortical steroids affecting mineral metabolism.

hy·perm·ne·sia (high″purm·nee′zhuh, ·zee·uh) *n.* Unusual ability of memory.

hy·per·mo·til·i·ty (high″pur·mo·til′i·tee) *n.* Increased motility, as of the stomach or intestines.

hy·per·na·tre·mia, hy·per·na·trae·mia (high″ pur·na·tree′mee·uh) *n.* Abnormally high sodium level in the blood. **—hypernatre·mic** (·mick) *adj.*

hy·per·neph·roid (high″pur·nef′roid) *adj.* Resembling the adrenal gland.

hy·per·ne·phro·ma (high″pur·ne·fro′muh) *n.,* pl. **hypernephromas, hypernephroma·ta** (·tuh) 1. Originally, a variety of tumor of the kidney supposed to be derived from embryonal inclusions of adrenocortical tissue in the kidney. 2. RENAL CELL CARCINOMA.

hy·per·on·to·morph (high"pur·on'to·morf) *n.* A person of a long, thin body type.

hy·per·ope (high'pur·ope) *n.* A person with hyperopia.

hy·per·opia (high"pur·o'pee·uh) *n.* A refractive error in which, with suspended accommodation, the focus of parallel rays of light falls behind the retina; due to an abnormally short anteroposterior diameter of the eye or to subnormal refractive power. Abbreviated, H. Syn. *hypermetropia, farsightedness.*

hy·per·os·mia (high"pur·oz'mee·uh, ·os'mee·uh) *n.* An abnormally acute sense of smell.

hy·per·os·mo·lar (high"pur·oz'mo'lur) *n.* Of solutions: having an osmotic pressure greater than that of normal plasma.

hy·per·os·te·og·e·ny (high"pur·os"tee·og'e·nee) *n.* Excessive development of bone.

hy·per·os·to·sis (·seez) Exostosis or hypertrophy of bone tissue. —**hyperos·tot·ic** (·tot'ick) *adj.*

hyperostosis fron·ta·lis in·ter·na (fron·tay'lis in·tur'nuh). An idiopathic condition occurring almost exclusively in women, in which new bone is formed in a symmetrical pattern on the inner aspect of the frontal bone; usually of no clinical significance but historically associated with the Stewart-Morel-Morgagni syndrome.

hy·per·ox·al·uria (high"pur·ock"suh·lew'ree·uh) *n.* The excessive excretion of oxalates in the urine.

hy·per·ox·emia, hy·per·ox·ae·mia (high"pur·ock·see'mee·uh) *n.* Extreme acidity of the blood.

hy·per·ox·ia (high"pur·ock'see·uh) *n.* An excessive amount of oxygen.

hy·per·ox·y·gen·a·tion (high"pur·ock"si·je·nay'shun) *n.* An excessive amount of oxygen in the body.

hy·per·para·thy·roid·ism (high"pur·păr"uh·thigh'roy·diz·um) *n.* A state produced by an increased functioning of the parathyroid glands.

hy·per·path·ia (high"pur·path'ee·uh) *n.* 1. An exaggerated or excessive perception of or response to any painful stimulus. 2. A condition in which all tactile, painful, and thermal stimuli have a severely painful and unpleasant quality, usually associated with an elevated threshold to these stimuli.

hy·per·peri·stal·sis (high"pur·perr"i·stal'sis, ·stahl'sis) *n.* An increase in the occurrence, rate, or depth of peristaltic waves.

hy·per·pex·ia (high"pur·peck'see·uh) *n.* The binding of an excessive amount of a substance by a tissue.

hy·per·pha·gia (high·pur·fay'jee·uh) *n.* BULIMIA.

hy·per·pha·lan·gism (high"pur·fuh·lan'jiz·um) *n.* The presence of supernumerary phalanges.

hy·per·phen·yl·al·a·nin·emia, hy·per·phen·yl·al·a·nin·ae·mia (high"per·fen"il·al"uh·ni·nee'mee·uh) *n.* The presence of abnormally high blood levels of phenylalanine, which may or may not be associated with elevated tyrosine levels, observed in premature and also in full-term newborn infants and associated with the heterozygous state of phenylketonuria, maternal phenylketonuria, or transient deficiency of phenylalanine hydroxylase or *p*-hydroxyphenylpyruvic acid oxidase.

hy·per·pho·ne·sis (high"pur·fo·nee'sis) *n.* Increased intensity of the percussion note or of the voice sound on auscultation.

hy·per·pho·nia (high"pur·fo'nee·uh) *n.* Excessive utterance of vocal sounds, especially in stuttering.

hy·per·pho·ria (high"pur·fo'ree·uh) *n.* A condition of latent strabismus or intermittent hypertropia in which the visual axis of one eye tends to deviate upward as compared with that of the other.

hy·per·phos·pha·te·mia, hy·per·phos·pha·tae·mia (high"pur·fos·fay·tee'mee·uh, ·fos·fuh·tee'mee·uh) *n.* Increased levels of inorganic phosphate in serum.

hy·per·phos·pha·tu·ria (high"pur·fos"fay·tew'ree·uh, ·fos·fuh·tew') *n.* An excess of phosphates in the urine.

hy·per·pi·e·sia (high"pur·pye·ee'zhuh, ·zee·uh) *n.* Abnormally high blood pressure; especially, essential hypertension. —**hyperpi·et·ic** (·et'ick) *adj.*

hy·per·pig·men·ta·tion (high"pur·pig"men·tay'shun) *n.* Excessive or increased pigmentation.

hy·per·pi·tu·i·ta·rism (high"pur·pi·tew'i·tuh·riz·um) *n.* 1. Increased growth-hormone secretion from the anterior lobe of the hypophysis with resultant gigantism or acromegaly. 2. Increased secretion of any anterior pituitary trophic hormone, particularly ACTH, producing Cushing's syndrome.

hy·per·pla·sia (high"pur·play'zhuh, ·zee·uh) *n.* Excessive formation of tissue; an increase in the size of a tissue or organ owing to an increase in the number of cells. —**hyper·plas·tic** (·plas'tick) *adj.*

hy·per·pnea, hy·per·pnoea (high"pur·nee'uh, ·pnee'uh) *n.* Increase in depth and rate of respiration.

hy·per·po·ro·sis (high"pur·po·ro'sis) *n.* An excessive formation of callus in the reunion of fractured bones.

hy·per·po·tas·se·mia, hy·per·po·tas·sae·mia (high"pur·po·ta·see'mee·uh) *n.* HYPERKALEMIA.

hy·per·pra·gia (high"pur·pray'jee·uh) *n.* An excess of thinking and feeling, commonly observed in the manic type of the manic-depressive illness. —**hyper·prag·ic** (·praj'ick) *adj.*

hy·per·prax·ia (high"pur·prack'see·uh) *n.* Restlessness of movement; HYPERACTIVITY.

hy·per·cho·re·sis (high"pur·pro"ko·ree'sis) *n.* Excessive motor function of the gastrointestinal tract.

hy·per·pro·lin·emia, hy·per·pro·lin·ae·mia (high"pur·pro"li·nee'mee·uh) *n.* A hereditary metabolic disorder in which there is an abnormally high blood level of proline, and mental retardation clinically. In type I of this disorder, there is a deficiency of proline oxidase, increased urinary excretion of hydroxyproline and glycine, and an association with renal disease. In type II, there is a deficiency of Δ^1-

pyrroline-5-carboxylate dehydrogenase, excessive urinary excretion of Δ^1-pyrroline-5-carboxylate, as well as proline, hydroxyproline, and glycine; clinically there are seizures and mental retardation.

hy·per·pro·sex·ia (high″pur·pro·seck′see·uh) *n.* Marked attention to one subject, as to one idea or symptom.

hy·per·pro·tein·emia, hy·per·pro·tein·ae·mia (high″pur·pro″tee·in·ee′mee·uh) *n.* Abnormally high blood protein level.

hy·per·psy·cho·sis (high″pur·sigh·ko′sis) *n.* Exaggerated mental activity.

hy·per·py·rex·ia (high″pur·pie·reck′see·uh) *n.* Excessively high fever. —**hyperpy·ret·ic** (·ret′ick) *adj.*

hy·per·re·flex·ia (high″pur·re·fleck′see·uh) *n.* A condition in which reflexes are increased above normal, due to a variety of causes. —**hyperreflex·ic** (·sick) *adj.*

hy·per·res·o·nance (high″pur·rez′uh·nunce) *n.* Exaggeration of normal resonance on percussion; heard chiefly in pulmonary emphysema and pneumothorax.

hy·per·ru·gos·i·ty (high″pur·roo·gos′i·tee) *n.* An excessive number of folds or excessively prominent folds.

hy·per·sal·i·va·tion (high″pur·sal′i·vay′shun) *n.* Abnormally increased secretion of saliva.

hy·per·se·cre·tion (high″pur·se·kree′shun) *n.* Excessive secretion. —**hypersecre·to·ry** (·tuh·ree′) *adj.*

hy·per·seg·men·ta·tion (high″pur·seg·men·tay′shun) *n.* Division into more than the usual number of segments or lobes.

hy·per·sen·si·tiv·i·ty (high″pur·sen″si·tiv′i·tee) *n.* The state of being abnormally sensitive or susceptible, as to the action of allergens.

hy·per·sen·si·ti·za·tion (high″pur·sen″si·ti·zay′shun) *n.* The process of producing hypersensitivity.

hy·per·se·ro·to·nin·emia, hy·per·se·ro·to·nin·ae·mia (high″pur·serr″o·to″ni·nee′mee·uh, ·seer′o·) *n.* 1. Excessive amounts of circulating serotonin. 2. A rare inborn error of metabolism of unknown cause in which abnormally high blood levels of serotonin are associated over a long period of time with episodes of flushing, rage attacks, ataxia, seizures, intermittent hypertension, and other manifestations of disturbances of the autonomic and central nervous systems.

hy·per·som·nia (high″pur·som′nee·uh) *n.* Excessive sleepiness.

hy·per·splen·ism (high″pur·splen′iz·um, ·spleen′iz·um) *n.* A pattern of reaction in which the peripheral blood lacks one or more formed elements whose precursors in the bone marrow are present in normal or increased numbers; removal of the spleen leads, at least temporarily, to return toward normal levels. The reaction may accompany any recognized splenic disease, or may occur idiopathically. Syn. *dyssplenism.*

hy·per·sthe·nia (high″pur·sthee′nee·uh) *n.* A condition of exalted strength or tone of the body. —**hyper·sthen·ic** (·sthen′ick) *adj.*

hy·per·tel·or·ism (high″pur·tel′ur·iz·um) *n.* Excessive width between two organs or parts.

hy·per·ten·sin·o·gen (high″pur·ten·sin′uh·jen) *n.* ANGIOTENSINOGEN. —**hyperten·sin·o·gen·ic** (·sin·o·jen′ick) *adj.*

hy·per·ten·sion (high″pur·ten′shun) *n.* 1. Excessive tension or pressure, especially that exerted by bodily fluids such as blood or aqueous humor. 2. Specifically, high blood pressure. See *essential hypertension, malignant hypertension, portal hypertension.*

hy·per·ten·sive (high″pur·ten′siv) *adj. & n.* 1. Pertaining to, characterized by, or causing hypertension. 2. A person affected with hypertension.

hypertensive retinopathy. A vascular retinopathy associated with arteriolar sclerosis; characterized by cotton-wool exudates, linear hemmorrhages, and AV nicking.

hy·per·ten·sor (high″pur·ten′sur, ·sor) *n.* A substance capable of raising blood pressure.

hy·per·the·co·sis (high″pur·thee·ko′sis) *n.* Hyperplasia of the ovarian theca interna, with increased luteinization of the cells.

hy·per·the·lia (high″pur·theel′ee·uh) *n.* The presence of supernumerary nipples.

hy·per·therm·al·ge·sia (high″pur·thur″mal·jee′zee·uh, ·see·uh) *n.* Abnormal sensitivity to heat.

hy·per·ther·mia (high″pur·thur′mee·uh) *n.* 1. HYPERPYREXIA. 2. The treatment of disease by the induction of fever, as by inoculation with malaria, by injection of foreign proteins, or by physical means.

hy·per·thy·mia (high″pur·thigh′mee·uh) *n.* 1. Excessive sensibility or oversensitiveness. 2. Vehement cruelty or foolhardiness as a symptom of mental disorder. 3. Pathologically labile or unstable emotionality.

hy·per·thy·ro·tro·pin·ism (high″pur·thigh″ro·tro′pin·iz·um, ·thigh·rot′ro·pin·iz·um) *n.* Excessive secretion of thyrotropic hormone by the adenohypophysis.

hy·per·to·nia (high″pur·to′nee·uh) *n.* Abnormally great muscular tonicity or contractility.

hy·per·ton·ic (high″pur·ton′ick) *adj.* 1. Excessive or above normal in tone or tension. 2. Having an osmotic pressure greater than that of physiologic salt solution or of any other solution taken as a standard. —**hyper·to·nic·i·ty** (·to·nis′i·tee) *n.*

hy·per·to·nus (high″pur·to′nus) *n.* HYPERTONIA.

hy·per·tri·cho·sis (high″pur·tri·ko′sis) *n.* Excessive growth of normal hair; superfluous hair; abnormal hairiness. —**hypertri·chot·ic** (·kot′ick) *adj.*

hy·per·tri·glyc·er·id·emia, hy·per·tri·glyc·er·id·ae·mia (high″pur·trye·glis″ur·i·dee′mee·uh) *n.* An excessively high level of serum triglycerides.

hy·per·tro·phic (high″pur·trof′ick) *adj.* Pertaining to or characterized by hypertrophy.

hypertrophic arthritis. DEGENERATIVE JOINT DISEASE.

hypertrophic gastritis. A chronic form of gastritis with increased thickness of mucosa, exaggerated granulation, and larger, more numerous rugae.

hypertrophic interstitial neuropathy or **radiculo-**

neu·ropathy. 1. A rare genetically determined syndrome of undetermined etiology, characterized by onset between 10 to 40 years of age, a slowly progressive motor and sensory radiculoneuropathy with palpable thickening of nerve trunks, weakness, atrophy, kyphoscoliosis, impaired coordination, nystagmus, and other neurologic deficits. Microscopically, the nerves show a nonspecific "onion-bulb" formation, which may be the result of successive demyelination and regeneration. Syn. *Dejerine-Sottas disease.* 2. Any condition which may result in thickening of the nerves with the "onion-bulb" microscopic appearance mentioned above.

hypertrophic pulmonary osteoarthropathy. The clubbing of the fingers and toes associated with enlargement of the ends of the long bones, encountered in chronic pulmonary disease. Syn. *osteopulmonary arthropathy, pseudoacromegaly.*

hy·per·tro·phy (high-pur'truh-fee) *n.* An increase in size of an organ, independent of natural growth, due to enlargement of its constituent cells; usually with an accompanying increase in functional capacity.

hy·per·tro·pia (high"pur-tro'pee-uh) *n.* Vertical strabismus in which the visual axis of one eye deviates upward. **—hypertro·pic,** *adj.*

hy·per·uri·ce·mia, hy·per·uri·cae·mia (high"pur-yoo"ri-see'mee-uh) *n.* Abnormally high level of uric acid in the blood.

hy·per·vas·cu·lar (high"pur-vas'kew-lur) *adj.* Excessively vascular.

hy·per·ven·ti·la·tion (high"pur-ven"ti-lay'shun) *n.* 1. Abnormally rapid, deep breathing. 2. Overbreathing, usually due to anxiety, producing hypocapnia and symptoms of dizziness, paresthesia, and carpopedal spasm caused by the respiratory alkalosis that develops.

hy·per·vis·cos·i·ty (high"pur-vis-kos'i-tee) *n.* Abnormally high viscosity. **—hyper·vis·cous** (·vis'kus) *adj.*

hy·per·vi·ta·min·osis (high"pur-vye"tuh-min-o'sis) *n.,* pl. **hypervitamin·oses** (·o'seez) A condition due to administration of excessive amounts of a vitamin, as: hypervitaminosis A, hypervitaminosis D.

hy·per·vo·le·mia, hy·per·vo·lae·mia (high"pur-vo·lee'mee-uh) *n.* A total circulating blood volume greater than normal. **—hypervole·mic, hypervolae·mic** (·mick) *adj.*

hyp·es·the·sia, hyp·aes·the·sia (hip"es-thee'zhuh, -theez'ee-uh, high"pes·) *n.* Impairment of sensation; lessened tactile sensibility. **—hypesthe·sic, hypaesthe·sic** (·zick), **hypes·thet·ic, hypaes·thet·ic** (·thet'ick) *adj.*

hy·pha (high'fuh) *n.,* pl. **hy·phae** (·fee) A filament that develops from the germ tube of a fungus. The septate hyphae are those divided into a chain of cells by cross walls forming at regular intervals. Those without cross walls, the nonseptate hyphae, are described as being coenocytic. **—hy·phal** (·ful) *adj.*

hyp·he·do·nia (hip"he·do'nee-uh, hype"he·do'nee-uh) *n.* Abnormal diminution of pleasure.

hy·phe·ma, hy·phae·ma (high-fee'muh) *n.* Blood in the anterior chamber of the eye.

hy·phe·mia, hy·phae·mia (high-fee'mee-uh) *n.* 1. HYPHEMA. 2. OLIGEMIA.

hyp·hi·dro·sis (hip"hi-dro'sis, hipe"hi·) *n.* Deficiency of perspiration.

hyp·i·no·sis (hip"i·no'sis) *n.* A deficiency of fibrin factors in the blood.

hypn-, hypno- A combining form meaning (a) *sleep;* (b) *hypnotism, hypnosis.*

hyp·na·gog·ic (hip"nuh-goj'ick) *adj.* 1. Pertaining to the inception or the induction of sleep. 2. Occurring at the inception or induction of sleep, before stage 1 is reached.

hyp·na·gogue (hip'nuh-gog) *n.* A hypnotic drug.

hyp·nal·gia (hip-nal'jee-uh) *n.* Pain occurring during sleep.

hyp·nic (hip'nick) *adj. & n.* 1. Pertaining to or inducing sleep; hypnotic. 2. An agent that induces sleep.

hyp·no·anal·y·sis (hip"no·uh-nal'i·sis) *n.,* pl. **hypnoanal·ses** (·seez) A form of psychotherapy combining psychoanalytic techniques with hypnosis.

hyp·no·ge·net·ic (hip"no·je·net'ick) *adj.* HYPNOGENIC.

hyp·no·gen·ic (hip"no·jen'ick) *adj.* 1. Producing or inducing sleep. 2. Inducing hypnosis. **—hypnogen·e·sis** (·e·sis) *n.*

hyp·no·lep·sy (hip'no-lep"see) *n.* NARCOLEPSY.

hyp·nol·o·gy (hip·nol'uh-jee) *n.* 1. The science dealing with sleep 2. The scientific study of hypnosis.

hyp·no·nar·co·sis (hip"no-nahr·ko'sis) *n.* 1. Deep sleep induced through hypnosis. 2. Combined hypnosis and narcosis.

hyp·no·pho·bia (hip"no·fo'bee-uh) *n.* Morbid dread of sleep or of falling asleep. **—hypnopho·bic** (·bick) *adj.*

hyp·no·phre·no·sis (hip"no·fre·no'sis) *n.,* pl. **hyp·nophreno·ses** (·seez) Any sleep disorder.

hyp·no·pom·pic (hip"no-pom'pick) *adj.* Pertaining to or occurring during the process of awakening.

hyp·no·sis (hip·no'sis) *n.,* pl. **hypno·ses** (·seez) A state of altered consciousness, sleep, or trance; induced artificially in a subject by means of verbal suggestion by the hypnotist or by the subject's concentration upon some object; characterized by extreme responsiveness to suggestions made by the hypnotist. The degree of the hypnotic state may vary from mild increased suggestibility to that comparable to surgical anesthesia.

hyp·no·ther·a·py (hip"no·therr'uh-pee) *n.* 1. The treatment of disease by means of hypnotism. 2. The induction of sleep for therapeutic purposes.

hyp·not·ic (hip-not'ick) *adj. & n.* 1. Inducing sleep. 2. Pertaining to hypnosis or to hypnotism. 3. A drug that causes sleep. 4. A person who is susceptible to hypnotism; one who is hypnotized.

hypnotic somnambulism. A condition of hypnosis in which the subject is possessed of his or her senses and often has the appearance of one awake, though his or her consciousness is under the control of the hypnotizer.

hyp·no·tism (hip'nuh·tiz·um) *n.* The practice and principles of inducing hypnosis. —**hypno·tist** (·tist) *n.*

hyp·no·tize (hip'nuh·tize) *v.* 1. To bring into a state of hypnosis. 2. To influence another person, usually by suggestion or strong personal attributes. —**hyp·no·ti·za·tion** (hip'nuh·ti·zay'shun) *n.*

¹hypo, *n.* Short for *hypodermic* syringe or medication.

²hypo, *n.* SODIUM THIOSULFATE.

hy·po·acid·i·ty (high''po·a·sid'i·tee) *n.* Deficiency in acid constituents.

hy·po·ac·tiv·i·ty (high''po·ack·tiv'i·tee) *n.* Diminished activity.

hy·po·adre·nal·ism (high''po·uh·dree'nul·iz·um) *n.* 1. Abnormally diminished adrenal gland function; adrenal insufficiency. 2. HYPOADRENOCORTICISM. —**hypoadrenal,** *adj.*

hy·po·adre·no·cor·ti·cism (high''po·uh·dree'no·kor'ti·siz·um) *n.* Diminished activity of the adrenal cortex.

hy·po·ag·na·thus (high''po·ag'nuth·us) *n.* An individual with no lower jaw.

hy·po·al·bu·min·emia, hy·po·al·bu·min·ae·mia (high''po·al·bew''min·ee·mee·uh) *n.* Abnormally low blood content of albumin.

hy·po·al·do·ste·ro·nism (high''po·al·do·sterr'o·niz·um) *n.* Deficient production or secretion of aldosterone.

hy·po·al·i·men·ta·tion (high''po·al'i·men·tay'shun) *n.* The state produced by insufficient or inadequate food intake.

hy·po·az·o·tu·ria (high''po·az''o·tew'ree·uh) *n.* A diminished amount of nitrogenous substances in the urine.

hy·po·bar·ic (high''po·bār'ick) *adj.* 1. Of less weight or pressure. 2. Pertaining to an anesthetic solution of specific gravity lower than the cerebrospinal fluid.

hy·po·bar·ism (high''po·bār'iz·um) *n.* A condition resulting from an excess of gas pressure within the body fluids, tissues, or cavities over the ambient gas pressure.

hy·po·ba·rop·a·thy (high''po·ba·rop'uth·ee) *n.* ALTITUDE SICKNESS.

hy·po·bil·i·ru·bi·ne·mia, hy·po·bil·i·ru·bi·nae·mia (high''po·bil''i·roo''bi·nee'mee·uh) *n.* A reduction below normal of bilirubin in the blood.

hy·po·bu·lia (high''po·bew'lee·uh) *n.* Deficiency of will power.

hy·po·cal·ce·mia, hy·po·cal·cae·mia (high''po·kal·see'mee·uh) *n.* A condition in which there is a diminished amount of calcium in the blood. —**hypocalce·mic** (·mick) *adj.*

hy·po·cal·ci·fi·ca·tion (high''po·kal''si·fi·kay'shun) *n.* Reduction of the normal amount of mineral salts in calcified tissues, as bone, dentin, or dental enamel. —**hypo·cal·cif·ic** (·kal·sif'ick) *adj.;* **hypo·cal·ci·fy** (·kal'si·figh) *v.*

hy·po·cal·ci·uria (high''po·kal''see·yoo'ree·uh) *n.* Decreased urinary calcium excretion.

hy·po·cap·nia (high''po·kap'nee·uh) *n.* Subnormal concentration of carbon dioxide in the blood. Syn. *acapnia.*

hy·po·ca·thex·is (high''po·ka·theck'sis) *n.* A lack

of concentration of the psychic energy upon a particular object, as a parent or spouse.

hy·po·cel·lu·lar (high''po·sel'yoo·lur) *adj.* Characterized by an abnormally low number or density of cells. —**hypo·cel·lu·lar·i·ty** (·sel''yoo·lār'i·tee) *n.*

hy·po·ce·ru·lo·plas·min·emia, hy·po·ce·ru·lo·plas·min·ae·mia (high''po·se·roo''lo·plaz''min·ee'mee·uh) *n.* Decreased amounts of ceruloplasmin in the blood plasma.

hy·po·chlo·re·mia, hy·po·chlo·rae·mia (high''po·klor·ee'mee·uh) *n.* Reduction in the amount of blood chlorides.

hy·po·chlor·hy·dria (high''po·klor·high'dree·uh, ·klor·hid'ree·uh) *n.* Diminished hydrochloric acid secretion by the stomach.

hy·po·chlo·ri·za·tion (high''po·klo''ri·zay'shun) *n.* Reduction in the dietary intake of sodium chloride.

hy·po·chlor·uria (high''po·klor·yoo'ree·uh) *n.* A diminution in the amount of chlorides excreted in the urine.

hy·po·cho·les·ter·emia, hy·po·cho·les·ter·ae·mia (high''po·ko·les''tur·ee'mee·uh) *n.* HYPOCHOLESTEROLEMIA. —**hypocholester·emic, hypocho·lester·ae·mic** (·ee'mick) *adj.*

hy·po·cho·les·ter·ol·emia, hy·po·cho·les·ter·ol·ae·mia (high''po·ko·les''tur·ol·ee'mee·uh) *n.* An abnormally low level of serum cholesterol.

hy·po·chon·dria (high''po·kon'dree·uh) *n.* 1. HYPOCHONDRIASIS. 2. Plural of *hypochondrium.*

hy·po·chon·dri·ac (high''po·kon'dree·ack) *adj. & n.* 1. Pertaining to the hypochondriac region. 2. Affected with or caused by hypochondriasis. 3. A person who is affected with hypochondriasis.

hy·po·chon·dri·a·cal (high''po·kon·drye'uh·kul) *adj.* Of, pertaining to, or characterized by hypochondriasis.

hypochondriac region. The right or the left upper lateral region of the abdomen below the lower ribs. Syn. *hypochondrium.*

hypochondrial reflex. Sudden inspiration produced by sudden pressure below the costal border.

hy·po·chon·dri·a·sis (high''po·kon·drye'uh·sis) *n.*, *pl.* **hypochondria·ses** (·seez) A chronic condition in which one is morbidly concerned with one's own physical or mental health, and believes himself or herself to be suffering from a grave, usually bodily, disease often focused upon one organ, without demonstrable organic findings; this condition is traceable to some longstanding intrapsychic conflict.

hy·po·chon·dri·um (high''po·kon'dree·um) *n.*, *pl.* **hypochon·dria** (·dree·uh) HYPOCHONDRIAC REGION.

hy·po·chon·dro·pla·sia (high''po·kon''dro·play'zhuh, ·zee·uh) *n.* A type of chondrodystrophy with radiologic changes similar to, but less pronounced than, achondroplasia.

hy·po·chro·ma·sia (high''po·kro·may'zee·uh, ·zhuh) *n.* HYPOCHROMIA.

hy·po·chro·mat·ic (high''po·kro·mat'ick) *adj.* HYPOCHROMIC.

hy·po·chro·ma·tism (high''po·kro'muh·tiz·um) *n.* HYPOCHROMIA.

hy·po·chro·mia (high''po·kro'mee·uh) *n.* 1. A

lack of color. 2. A lack of complete saturation of the erythrocytic stroma with hemoglobin, as judged by pallor of the unstained or stained erythrocytes when examined microscopically. —**hypochro·mic** (·mick) *adj.*

hypochromic microcytic anemia. Anemia characterized by erythrocytes of decreased size and decreased hemoglobin content such as iron-deficiency anemia.

hy·po·com·ple·men·te·mia (high″po·kom″ple·men·tee′mee·uh) *n.* Abnormally low blood levels of one or more complement components, most frequently secondary to fixation or activation of complement by antigen-antibody reactions, but sometimes the result of decreased production or excessive loss of complement. —**hypocomplemente·mic** (·mick) *adj.*

hy·po·cone (high′po·kone) *n.* The distolingual cusp of an upper molar tooth.

hy·po·con·id (high″po·kon′id) *n.* The distobuccal cusp of a lower molar tooth.

hy·po·con·ule (high″po·kon′yool) *n.* The fifth, or distal, cusp of an upper molar tooth.

hy·po·con·u·lid (high″po·kon′yoo·lid) *n.* The fifth or distal cusp of a lower molar tooth.

hy·po·cu·pre·mia, hy·po·cu·prae·mia (high″po·kew·pree′mee·uh) *n.* An abnormally low amount of copper in the blood plasma.

hy·po·cy·clo·sis (high″po·sigh·klo′sis) *n.*, pl. **hy·pocyclo·ses** (·seez) *In ophthalmology,* deficient accommodation.

hy·po·der·mic (high″po·dur′mick) *adj. & n.* 1. Pertaining to the region beneath the skin. 2. Placed or introduced beneath the skin. 3. A substance, as a medicine or drug, introduced or injected beneath the skin. 4. A syringe used for a hypodermic injection.

hy·po·der·mis (high″po·dur′mis) *n.* 1. The outermost layer of cells of invertebrates, which corresponds to the epidermis. It secretes the cuticular exoskeleton of arthropods, annelids, mollusks, and other forms. 2. In human anatomy, SUBCUTANEOUS TISSUE.

hy·po·der·moc·ly·sis (high″po·dur·mock′li·sis) *n.*, pl. **hypodermocly·ses** (·seez) The therapeutic introduction into the subcutaneous tissues of large quantities of fluids.

hy·po·don·tia (high″po·don′chee·uh) *n.* Partial anodontia.

hy·po·eso·pho·ria (high″po·es″o·fo′ree·uh) *n.* A type of heterophoria in which the visual lines tend downward and inward.

hy·po·es·the·sia, hy·po·aes·the·sia (high″po·es·theezh′uh, ·theez·ee·uh) *n.* HYPESTHESIA.

hy·po·es·trin·ism, hy·po·oes·trin·ism (high″po·es′trin·iz·um) *n.* The state of deficient production of estrogen by the ovaries.

hy·po·exo·pho·ria (high″po·eck″so·fo′ree·uh) *n.* A type of heterophoria in which the visual lines tend downward and outward.

hy·po·fer·re·mia, hy·po·fer·rae·mia (high″po·ferr·ee′mee·uh) *n.* Diminished or abnormally low iron level in the blood.

hy·po·fi·brin·o·gen·emia, hy·po·fi·brin·o·gen·ae·mia (high″po·figh″bri·no·je·nee′mee·uh) *n.* A decrease in plasma fibrinogen level.

hy·po·func·tion (high″po·funk′shun) *n.* Diminished function. —**hypofunction·al** (·ul) *adj.*

hy·po·ga·lac·tia (high″po·ga·lack′shee·uh) *n.* Decreased milk secretion.

hy·po·gam·ma·glob·u·lin·emia, hy·po·gam·ma·glob·u·lin·ae·mia (high″po·gam″uh·glob″yoo·li·nee′mee·uh) *n.* A decrease in plasma gamma globulin.

hy·po·gan·gli·on·o·sis (high″po·gang″glee·uh·no′sis) *n.* A reduction in the number of ganglia, especially of the ganglia of the myenteric plexus.

hy·po·gas·tric (high″po·gas′trick) *adj.* Of or pertaining to the hypogastrium or pubic region.

hy·po·gas·tri·um (high″po·gas′tree·um) *n.*, pl. **hypogas·tria** (·tree·uh) PUBIC REGION.

hy·po·gen·e·sis (high″po·jen′e·sis) *n.* Underdevelopment.

hy·po·gen·i·tal·ism (high″po·jen′i·tul·iz·um) *n.* Underdevelopment of the genital system.

hy·po·geu·sia (high″po·gew′see·uh, ·joo′see·uh) *n.* Diminution in the sense of taste.

hy·po·glos·sal (high″po·glos′ul) *adj.* Situated under the tongue.

hypoglossal nerve. The twelfth cranial nerve; a motor nerve, attached to the medulla oblongata, which innervates the intrinsic and extrinsic muscles of the tongue.

hy·po·glos·si·tis (high″po·glos·eye′tis) *n.* Inflammation of the tissue under the tongue.

hy·po·glot·tis (high″po·glot′is) *n.* The underpart of the tongue.

hy·po·gly·ce·mia, hy·po·gly·cae·mia (high″po·glye·see′mee·uh) *n.* 1. A reduction below normal in blood glucose. 2. The clinical state associated with decrease of blood glucose below a critical level for the individual, characterized by hunger, nervousness, profuse sweating, faintness, and sometimes convulsions.

hy·po·gly·ce·mic, hy·po·gly·cae·mic (high″po·glye·see′mick) *adj.* 1. Of or pertaining to hypoglycemia. 2. Lowering the concentration of glucose in the blood.

hy·po·gly·cin (high″po·glye′sin) *n.* A toxin (L-α-amino-β-methylenecyclopropanepropionic acid) found in the unripe fruit of the akee, associated with Jamaican vomiting sickness; it produces marked hypoglycemia by interfering with oxidation of long-chain fatty acids and gluconeogenesis.

hy·po·gly·cor·rha·chia (high″po·glye″ko·ray′kee·uh) *n.* Abnormally low concentration of glucose in the cerebrospinal fluid; usually values below 40 mg per 100 ml or less than two-thirds of the blood sugar value.

hy·po·gnath·us (high″po·nath′us) *n. In teratology,* an individual having a parasite attached to the lower jaw.

hy·po·go·nad·ism (high″po·go′nad·iz·um, ·gon″uh·diz·um) *n.* Diminished internal secretion of the testes or ovaries which may be due to a primary defect or secondary to insufficient stimulation by the adenohypophysis.

hy·po·hi·dro·sis (high″po·hi·dro′sis) *n.* Deficient perspiration.

hy·po·in·su·lin·ism (high″po·in′sue·lin·iz·um) *n.*

Diminished secretion of insulin by the pancreas.

hy·po·io·dism (high″po·eye′uh·diz·um) *n.* Iodine deficiency.

hy·po·ka·le·mia, hy·po·ka·lae·mia (high″po·ka·lee′mee·uh) *n.* A deficiency of potassium in the blood. —**hypokale·mic, hypokalae·mic** (·mick) *adj.*

hy·po·ki·ne·sia (high″po·ki·nee′zhuh, ·zee·uh, ·kigh·nee′) *n.* Abnormally decreased muscular movement. —**hypoki·net·ic** (·net′ick) *adj.*

hy·po·ki·ne·sis (high″po·ki·nee′sis, ·kigh·nee′) *n.* HYPOKINESIA.

hy·po·lem·mal (high″po·lem′ul) *adj.* Lying under a sheath, as the motor end plates under the sarcolemma or sheath of a muscle fiber.

hy·po·ley·dig·ism (high″po·lye′dig·iz·um) *n.* Retarded sexual development, or loss of some male sexual characteristics, as a result of a decrease or absence in the function of the interstitial (Leydig) cells of the testes.

hy·po·lo·gia (high″po·lo′jee·uh) *n.* Poverty of speech as a symptom of cerebral disease.

hy·po·mag·ne·se·mia, hy·po·mag·ne·sae·mia (high″po·mag′ne·see′mee·uh) *n.* An abnormally low level of magnesium in the blood.

hy·po·ma·nia (high″po·may′nee·uh) *n.* A common, mild form of the manic type of manic depressive illness, in which the person generally exhibits rapid fluctuations between elation and irritation, great energy, impatience, euphoria, and occasionally bouts of depression; in an otherwise normal person, this state of stimulation may be very productive. —**hypo·man·ic** (man′ick) *adj.*

hy·po·mas·tia (high″po·mas′tee·uh) *n.* Abnormal smallness of the mammary glands.

hy·po·ma·ture (high″po·muh·tewr′) *adj.* IMMATURE.

hy·po·mel·a·no·sis (high″po·mel′′uh·no′sis) *n.* Decrease in melanin pigmentation. —**hypo·mela·not·ic** (·not′ick) *adj.*

hy·po·men·or·rhea, hy·po·men·or·rhoea (high″po·men′o·ree′uh) *n.* A small amount of menstrual flow over a shortened duration at the regular period.

hy·po·me·tab·o·lism (high″po·me·tab′uh·liz·um) *n.* Metabolism below the normal rate.

hy·po·me·tro·pia (high″po·me·tro′pee·uh) *n.* MYOPIA.

hy·po·mi·cro·so·ma (high″po·migh′kro·so′muh) *n.* The lowest stature that is not dwarfism.

hy·po·mne·sia (high″pom·nee′zhuh, ·zee·uh) *n.* Poor or defective memory.

hy·po·mo·til·i·ty (high″po·mo·til′i·tee) *n.* 1. Decreased movement or motility, especially of the gastrointestinal tract. 2. HYPOKINESIA.

hy·po·na·tre·mia, hy·po·na·trae·mia (high″po·na·tree′mee·uh) *n.* Abnormally low blood sodium level. —**hyponatre·mic** (·mick) *adj.*

hy·po·ovar·i·an·ism (high″po·o·vâr′ee·un·iz·um, ·o·vair′) *n.* Decrease in ovarian endocrine activity.

hy·po·para·thy·roid·ism (high″po·pâr′′uh·thigh′roy·diz·um) *n.* The functional state resulting from insufficiency of parathyroid hormone, characterized by hypocalcemia, hyperphosphatemia, and increased neuromuscular ex-

citability, sometimes progressing to seizures or tetany. —**hypoparathyroid,** *adj.*

hy·po·per·fu·sion (high″po·pur·few′zhun) *n.* A reduction of blood flow through a part.

hy·po·per·me·abil·i·ty (high″po·pur′′mee·uh·bil′i·tee) *n.* A state in which membranes have reduced permeability for electrolytes, and other solutes, or colloids.

hy·po·pha·lan·gism (high″po·fuh·lan′jiz·um) *n.* Congenital absence of one or more phalanges in a finger or toe.

hy·po·phar·yn·gi·tis (high″po·fâr′′in·jye′tis) *n.* Inflammation of the laryngopharynx.

hy·po·phar·ynx (high″po·fâr′inks) *n.* LARYNGOPHARYNX.

hy·po·pho·ria (high″po·fo′ree·uh) *n.* A tendency of the visual axis of one eye to deviate below that of the other.

hy·po·phos·pha·ta·sia (high″po·fos′fuh·tay′zee·uh) *n.* 1. A deficiency of alkaline phosphatase, as in rickets. 2. An inborn error of metabolism, probably due to an autosomal recessive trait, characterized by a deficiency of tissue alkaline phosphatase; manifested by skeletal abnormalities resembling rickets or osteomalacia, defective development of teeth, and the presence of phosphoethanolamine (ethanolamine phosphate) in the urine.

hy·po·phos·pha·te·mia, hy·po·phos·pha·tae·mia (high″po·fos′fuh·tee′mee·uh, ·fos′′fay·) *n.* Abnormally low concentration of phosphates in the blood serum.

hy·po·phos·pha·tu·ria (high″po·fos′fuh·tew′ree·uh, ·fos′′fay·) *n.* Reduced urinary phosphate excretion.

hy·po·phre·nia (high″po·free′nee·uh) *n.* MENTAL RETARDATION. —**hypo·phren·ic** (·fren′ick) *adj.*

hy·poph·y·se·al (high·pof′′i·see′ul, high″po·fiz′ee·ul) *adj.* Of or pertaining to the hypophysis.

hypophyseal-duct tumor. Any of the tumors derived from epithelial remnants of the involuted pouch of Rathke. Usually suprasellar, they include the craniopharyngioma and teratoma, which originate in the residual stalk, and cystic neoplasms, which originate from the residual cleft. More frequent in children than in adults.

hy·poph·y·sec·to·my (high·pof′′i·seck′tuh·mee) *n.* Surgical removal of the hypophysis or pituitary gland. —**hypophysecto·mize** (·mize) *v.*

hy·poph·y·seo·por·tal (high″po·fiz′ee·o·por′tul, high″po·fiz′ee·o·) *adj.* Related to the hypophysis and its portal type of circulation.

hy·po·phys·io·priv·ic, hy·po·phys·io·priv·ic (high″po·fiz′ee·o·priv′ick) *adj.* Lacking in hypophyseal hormones.

hy·poph·y·sis (high·pof′i·sis) *n.*, genit. **hy·po·phys·e·os** (high″po·fiz′ee·os), pl. **hypophy·ses** (·seez) A small, rounded, bilobate endocrine gland, averaging about 0.5 g in weight, which lies in the sella turcica of the sphenoid bone, is attached by a stalk, the infundibulum, to the floor of the third ventricle of the brain at the hypothalamus, and consists of an anterior lobe, the adenohypophysis, which produces and secretes various important hormones, including several which regulate other endocrine glands, and a less important posterior lobe, the neurohypophysis, which holds and secretes antidiuretic hormone and oxytocin produced in the hypothalamus. Syn. *pituitary gland.* NA alt. *glandula pituitaria.*

hypophysis cer·e·bri (serr'e·brye). HYPOPHYSIS.

hy·po·pi·e·sia (high″po·pye·ee′zhuh, ·zee·uh) *n.* Subnormal arterial blood pressure resulting from an organic or specific cause.

hy·po·pi·tu·i·ta·rism (high″po·pi·tew′i·tuh·riz·um) *n.* The clinical condition resulting from hypofunction of the anterior pituitary gland with secondary atrophy of the gonads, thyroid gland, and/or adrenal cortex; due to tumor or metastasis of neoplastic disease or to postpartum necrosis of the hypophysis. Syn. *adult hypopituitarism, pituitary insufficiency.*

hy·po·pla·sia (high″po·play′zhuh, ·zee·uh) *n.* Underdevelopment of a tissue or organ, usually associated with a decreased number of cells.

hy·po·plas·tic (high″po·plas′tick) *adj.* Pertaining to or characterized by hypoplasia.

hypoplastic anemia. PRIMARY REFRACTORY ANEMIA.

hypoplastic dwarf. An individual with usual proportions of bodily parts, but markedly smaller than normal.

hypoplastic left-heart syndrome. Aortic atresia, or severe aortic stenosis, aortic arch atresia, or mitral atresia with hypoplasia of the left ventricle; there is severe cyanosis and heart failure.

hy·po·pnea (high″po·nee′uh) *n.* Diminution of breathing; abnormally slow or shallow breathing.

hy·po·po·tas·se·mia, hy·po·po·tas·sae·mia (high″po·po·ta·see′mee·uh) *n.* HYPOKALEMIA.

hy·po·prax·ia (high″po·prack′see·uh) *n.* 1. Deficient activity; inactivity. 2. Listlessness.

hy·po·pro·sex·ia (high″po·pro·seck′see·uh) *n.* Inadequate attention or inability to pay attention.

hy·po·pro·tein·emia, hy·po·pro·tein·ae·mia (high″po·pro″tee·in·ee′mee·uh) *n.* Abnormally low concentration of protein in the blood.

hy·po·pro·throm·bin·emia, hy·po·pro·throm·bin·ae·mia (high″po·pro·throm″bin·ee′mee·uh) *n.* Deficient supply of prothrombin in the blood.

hy·po·psel·a·phe·sia (high″po·sel″uh·fee′zee·uh, ·zhuh) *n. Obsol.* Diminution of sensitivity to tactile impressions.

hy·po·psy·cho·sis (high″po·sigh·ko′sis) *n.* Diminution or blunting of thought.

hy·po·py·on (high·po′pee·on, high′i·po′) *n.* A collection of pus in the anterior chamber of the eye.

hy·po·re·ac·tive (high″po·ree·ack′tiv) *adj.* Characterized by decreased responsiveness to stimuli.

hy·po·re·flex·ia (high″po·re·fleck′see·uh) *n.* Reflexes below normal. —**hyporeflex·ic** (·sick) *adj.*

hy·po·scle·ral (high″po·skleer′ul, ·sklerr′ul) *adj.* Beneath the sclera.

hy·po·se·cre·tion (high″po·se·kree′shun) *n.* Diminished secretion.

hy·po·sen·si·tiv·i·ty (high″po·sen″si·tiv′i·tee) *n.* A state of diminished sensitivity, especially

to appropriate external stimuli. —**hypo·sen·si·tive** (·sen′si·tiv) *adj.;* **hyposensitive·ness** (·nis) *n.*

hy·pos·mia (high·poz′mee·uh, hi·poz′) *n.* Diminution of the sense of smell.

hy·po·spa·di·as (high″po·spay′dee·us) *n.* 1. A congenital anomaly of the penis and urethra in which the urethra opens upon the ventral surface of the penis or in the perineum. 2. A congenital malformation in which the urethra opens into the vagina.

hy·po·sper·ma·to·gen·e·sis (high″po·spur″muh·to·jen′e·sis, ·spur·mat″o·) *n.* A decreased production of male germ cells, caused by such factors as diseased testes or hypoleydigism.

hy·po·spon·dy·lot·o·my (high″po·spon″di·lot′uh·mee) *n.* HYOVERTEBROTOMY.

Hypospray. Trademark for a device for administering jet injections.

hy·pos·ta·sis (high·pos′tuh·sis, hi·) *n.,* pl. **hyposta·ses** (·seez) 1. A deposit that forms at the bottom of a liquid; a sediment. 2. The formation of a sediment, especially the settling of blood in dependent parts of the body.

hy·po·stat·ic (high″po·stat′ick) *adj.* 1. Due to, or of the nature of, hypostasis. 2. *In genetics,* subject to being suppressed, as a gene whose effect is suppressed by another gene that affects the same part of the organism.

hypostatic pneumonia. Pneumonia in dependent parts of lungs which are hyperemic, seen in patients who remain in one position for long periods of time.

hy·po·sthe·nia (high″po·sthee′nee·uh) *n.* ASTHENIA. —**hyposthe·ni·ant** (·nee·unt), **hypo·sthen·ic** (·sthen′ick) *adj.*

hy·pos·the·nu·ria (high·pos″thi·new′ree·uh) *n.* The constant secretion of urine of low specific gravity.

hy·po·syn·er·gia (high″po·sin·ur′jee·uh) *n.* DYSSYNERGIA.

hy·po·tax·ia (high″po·tacks′ee·uh) *n.* A condition of emotional rapport existing in the beginning of hypnosis between the subject and the hypnotizer.

hy·po·tax·is (high″po·tack′sis) *n.* Light hypnotic sleep.

hy·po·tel·or·ism (high″po·tel·ur′iz·um) *n.* Decrease in distance between two organs or parts.

hy·po·ten·sion (high″po·ten′shun) *n.* 1. Diminished or abnormally low tension. 2. Specifically, low blood pressure.

hy·po·ten·sive (high″po·ten′siv) *adj.* 1. Pertaining to or characterized by hypotension. 2. Serving to reduce tension or to lower blood pressure.

hy·po·ten·sor (high″po·ten′sur) *n.* Any substance capable of lowering blood pressure. It implies a persistent effect, as opposed to the fleeting effect of a depressor.

hy·po·tha·lam·ic (high″po·thuh·lam′ick) *adj.* Pertaining to or involving the hypothalamus.

hypothalamic inhibitory factors. Hormonelike substances released from the hypothalamus which inhibit the release of specific hormones from the anterior pituitary gland.

hypothalamic obesity. Obesity resulting from a

disturbance of function of the appetite-regulating centers of the hypothalamus.

hypothalamic releasing factors. Hormones secreted by the hypothalamus which travel via nerve fibers to the anterior pituitary where they cause selective release of specific pituitary hormones.

hy·po·thal·a·mus (high"po·thal'uh·mus) *n.* The region of the diencephalon forming the floor of the third ventricle, including neighboring, associated nuclei. It is divided into three regions: (a) The anterior region, or pars supraoptica, which is superior to the optic chiasma, and includes the supraoptic and paraventricular nuclei and a less differentiated nucleus that merges with the preoptic area (the anterior hypothalamic nucleus). (b) The middle region, the pars tuberalis or tuber cinereum, including the lateral hypothalamic and tuberal nuclei, lateral to a sagittal plane passing through the anterior column of the fornix, and the dorsomedial, ventromedial, and posterior hypothalamic nuclei, medial to the above plane. (c) The caudal region, pars mamillaris or mamillary bodies, including medial, lateral, and intercalated mamillary nuclei and premamillary and supramamillary nuclei.

hy·po·the·nar (high"po·theen'ur, high·poth'e·nahr) *adj.* Designating or pertaining to the fleshy prominence on the ulnar side of the palm of the hand.

hy·po·therm·es·the·sia, hy·po·therm·aes·the·sia (high"po·thur"mes·theezh'uh) *n.* Decreased temperature sensibility.

hy·po·ther·mia (high"po·thur'mee·uh) *n.* 1. Subnormal temperature of the body. 2. The artificial reduction of body temperature to below normal to slow physiologic processes for operative or therapeutic purposes. —**hypothermal** (·mul), **hypother·mic** (·mick) *adj.*

hy·poth·e·sis (high·poth'e·sis) *n.*, pl. **hypothe·ses** (·seez) A supposition or conjecture put forth to account for known facts.

hy·po·thy·mia (high"po·thigh'mee·uh) *n.* 1. Despondency; depression of spirits. 2. A diminution in the intensity of emotions.

hy·po·thy·roid (high"po·thigh'roid) *adj.* Characterized or caused by, or pertaining to, hypothyroidism.

hy·po·thy·roid·ism (high"po·thigh'roid·iz·um) *n.* The functional state resulting from insufficiency of thyroid hormones; the clinical manifestations depend upon the stage of development of the patient and the degree of insufficiency.

hy·po·to·nia (high"po·to'nee·uh) *n.* Decrease of normal tonicity or tension; especially diminution of intraocular pressure or of muscle tone.

hy·po·ton·ic (high"po·ton'ick) *adj.* 1. Below the normal strength or tension. 2. Characterizing or pertaining to a solution whose osmotic pressure is less than that of sodium chloride solution, or any other solution taken as standard. —**hypo·to·nic·i·ty** (·to·nis'i·tee) *n.*

hypotonic diplegia. A form of spastic diplegia (2), characterized by atonicity of the muscles of the extremities with retention of postural reflexes, preservation of tendon reflexes, and mental backwardness.

hypotonic solution. A solution that produces a change in the tone of a tissue immersed in it through passage of water from the solution into the tissue. With reference to erythrocytes, a hypotonic solution of sodium chloride is one that contains less than 0.9 g of sodium chloride in each 100 ml.

hy·po·tri·chi·a·sis (high"po·tri·kigh'uh·sis) *n.* HYPOTRICHOSIS.

hy·po·tri·cho·sis (high"po·tri·ko'sis) *n.* A condition in which there is less than normal hair.

hy·po·tro·pia (high"po·tro'pee·uh) *n.* A form of strabismus in which one eye looks downward.

hy·po·tym·pa·num (high"po·tim'puh·num) *n.* The part of the tympanum lying below the level of the tympanic membrane. —**hypo·tym·pan·ic** (tim·pan'ick) *adj.*

hy·po·veg·e·ta·tive (high"po·vej'e·tay"tiv) *adj.* Characterizing or pertaining to a human biotype in which purely somatic systems dominate over the visceral or nutritional organs.

hy·po·ven·ti·la·tion (high"po·ven·ti·lay'shun) *n.* 1. Reduced respiratory effort. 2. Reduced alveolar ventilation.

hy·po·vi·ta·min·osis (high"po·vye"tuh·min·o'sis) *n.*, pl. **hypovitamin·oses** (·o'seez) A condition due to deficiency of one or more vitamins in the diet.

hy·po·vo·le·mia, hy·po·vo·lae·mia (high"po·vo·le'mee·uh) *n.* Low, or decreased, blood volume. —**hypovole·mic, hypovolae·mic** (·mick) *adj.*

hypovolemic shock. Shock caused by a reduced circulating blood volume which may be due to loss of blood or plasma as in burns, the crush syndrome, perforating wounds, or other trauma. Syn. *wound shock.*

hy·po·xan·thine (high"po·zan'theen, ·thin) *n.* 6-Oxypurine or 6-ketopurine, $C_5H_4N_4O$, an intermediate product resulting when adenine, an amino purine formed by hydrolysis of nucleic acid, is transformed into uric acid and allantoin.

hyp·ox·emia, hy·pox·ae·mia (high"pock·see'mee·uh) *n.* HYPOXIA. —**hypoxe·mic, hypoxae·mic** (·mick) *adj.*

hyp·ox·ia (high·pock'see·uh, hi·pock') *n.* Oxygen want or deficiency; any state wherein a physiologically inadequate amount of oxygen is available to, or utilized by, tissue without respect to cause or degree. —**hypox·ic** (·sick) *adj.*

hypoxic hypoxia. Reduction in availability of oxygen to tissue due to a decrease in the partial pressure of oxygen in the arterial blood, as in low oxygen tension in inspired air, interference with gas exchange in the lungs, and arteriovenous shunts.

hyp·sar·rhyth·mia, hyp·sa·rhyth·mia (hip"sa·rith'mee·uh) *n.* An electroencephalographic abnormality consisting of continuous multifocal spikes and slow waves of large amplitude; characteristic of, but not specific for, infantile spasms.

hyp·so·pho·bia (hip"so·fo'bee·uh) *n.* Morbid dread of being at a great height.

hys·ter·al·gia (his″tur·al′jee·uh) *n.* Neuralgic pain in the uterus. —**hysteral·gic** (·jick) *adj.*

hys·ter·ec·to·my (his″tur·eck′tuh·mee) *n.* Total or partial surgical removal of the uterus.

hys·te·ria (his·teer′ee·uh, ·terr′) *n.* 1. *In psychiatry,* a neurosis resulting from repression of emotional conflicts from the conscious; characterized by immature, impulsive, dependent, and attention-seeking behavior, and conversion and dissociation symptoms. Usually through a process of suggestion or autosuggestion, the symptoms may take any form and involve any mental or bodily function under voluntary control. 2. *Loosely,* any excessive emotional response.

hysteric, *n. & adj.* 1. An individual in a state of hysteria. 2. An overemotional individual. 3. HYSTERICAL.

hys·ter·i·cal (his·terr′i·kul) *adj.* Pertaining to or characterized by hysteria.

hysterical amblyopia or blindness. A unilateral or bilateral functional loss of vision involving great variations in the extent of the visual fields; seen in hysteria.

hysterical dysbasia. The apparent difficulty in gait seen in hysterical individuals, often characterized by marked swaying, zigzag steps, superfluous movements, and faked falling by which the person dramatizes the disability.

hysterical neurosis. A form of neurosis in which there is an involuntary disturbance or loss of psychogenic origin of motor, sensory, or mental function. Characteristically, the symptoms begin and end suddenly in situations which are emotionally charged and which are symbolic of underlying, usually repressed conflicts; frequently the symptoms can be modified by suggestion. It can be classified as conversion type or dissociative type.

hysterical personality. An individual whose behavior is characterized by excitability, instability under, and overreaction to, minor stress; self-dramatization; attention-seeking; and often seductiveness. Such individuals tend to be immature, undependable in their judgment, self-centered, vain, and dependent on others.

hys·ter·ics (his·terr′icks) *n.* 1. A hysterical attack. 2. Extreme emotional display, as a fit of laughing, crying, or anger.

hys·ter·i·form (his·terr′i·form) *adj.* Resembling hysteria.

hys·tero·cele (his′tur·o·seel) *n.* A hernia containing all or part of the uterus.

hys·tero·clei·sis (his″tur·o·klye′sis) *n.* The closure of the uterus by suturing the edges of the os.

hys·tero·cys·tic (his″tur·o·sis′tick) *adj.* Pertaining to the uterus and the urinary bladder.

hys·tero·cys·to·pexy (his″tur·o·sis′to·peck″see) *n.* Suturing of the uterus to the bladder and abdominal wall.

hys·ter·o·dyn·ia (his″tur·o·din′ee·uh) *n.* Pain in the uterus.

hys·tero·ep·i·lep·sy (his″tur′uh·o·ep′i·lep·see) *n.* Hysteria in which seizures usually occur only in the presence of others; they are frequently triggered by some emotional situation, are imitative of true epileptic phenomena including disorganized violent muscular movements, and are abruptly terminated without the confusion and lethargy which frequently occur in true epilepsy.

hys·tero·fren·ic (his″tur·o·fren′ick) *adj.* Capable of arresting an attack of hysteria, as pressure on a certain point or part of the body.

hys·tero·gen·ic (his″tur·o·jen′ick) *adj.* Producing hysterical phenomena or symptoms.

hys·tero·gram (his′tur·o·gram) *n.* A roentgenogram obtained after the injection of the uterine cavity with contrast material.

hys·ter·og·ra·phy (his″tur·og′ruh·fee) *n.* Roentgenologic examination of the uterus after the introduction of a contrast medium.

hys·ter·ol·y·sis (his″tur·ol′i·sis) *n.*, pl. **hysteroly·ses** (·seez) Severing the attachments or adhesions of the uterus.

hys·tero·ma·nia (his″tur·o·may′nee·uh) *n.* 1. Psychomotor overactivity seen in hysteria. 2. NYMPHOMANIA.

hys·ter·om·e·ter (his″tur·om′e·tur) *n.* An instrument for measuring the length of the intrauterine cavity. —**hysterome·try** (·tree) *n.*

hys·tero·my·o·ma (his″tur·o·migh·o′muh) *n.* A uterine leiomyoma.

hys·tero·my·o·mec·to·my (his″tur·o·migh″o·meck′tuh·mee) *n. In surgery,* removal of a fibroid tumor of the uterus.

hys·tero·my·ot·o·my (his″tur·o·migh·ot′uh·mee) *n.* Incision into the uterus for removal of a solid tumor.

hys·tero·oo·pho·rec·to·my (his″tur·o·o″uh·fo·reck′tuh·mee) *n. In surgery,* removal of the uterus and ovaries.

hys·ter·op·a·thy (his″tur·op′uth·ee) *n.* Any disease or disorder of the uterus. —**hystero·path·ic** (his″tur·o·path′ick) *adj.*

hys·tero·pexy (his′tur·o·peck″see) *n.* Fixation of the uterus by a surgical operation to correct displacement.

hys·tero·phil·ia (his″tur·o·fil′ee·uh) *n.* A tendency to develop symptoms of the conversion type of hysterical neurosis.

hys·tero·plas·ty (his′tur·o·plas″tee) *n.* A plastic operation on the uterus.

hys·ter·op·to·sis (his″tur·op·to′sis) *n.* Falling or inversion of the uterus.

hys·ter·or·rha·phy (his″tur·or′uh·fee) *n.* The closure of a uterine incision or rent by suture.

hys·ter·or·rhex·is (his″tur·o·reck′sis) *n.*, pl. **hys·terorrhex·es** (·seez) Rupture of the uterus.

hys·tero·sal·pin·gec·to·my (his″tur·o·sal″pin·jeck′tuh·mee) *n.* Excision of the uterus and oviducts.

hys·tero·sal·pin·gog·ra·phy (his″tur·o·sal″ping·gog′ruh·fee) *n.* Radiographic examination of the uterus and oviducts after injection of a radiopaque substance into their cavities.

hys·tero·sal·pin·go·oo·pho·rec·to·my (his″tur·o·sal·ping″go·o″uh·fo·reck′tuh·mee) *n.* Excision of the uterus, oviducts, and ovaries.

hys·tero·sal·pin·go·oo·the·cec·to·my (his″tur·o·sal·ping″go·o″o·thi·seck′tuh·mee) *n. Obsol.* HYSTEROSALPINGO-OOPHORECTOMY.

hys·tero·sal·pin·gos·to·my (his″tur·o·sal″ping·gos′tuh·mee) *n.* The establishment of an anastomosis between an oviduct and the uterus.

hys·tero·scope (his′tur·o·skope) *n.* A uterine speculum with a reflector. —**hys·ter·os·co·py** (his″tur·os′kuh·pee) *n.*

hys·tero·tome (his′tur·o·tome) *n.* An instrument for incising the uterus.

hys·ter·ot·o·my (his″tur·ot′uh·mee) *n.* 1. Incision of the uterus. 2. CESAREAN SECTION.

hys·tero·trach·e·lec·to·my (his″tur·o·tray″ke·leck′tuh·mee, ·track″e·leck′) *n.* Amputation of the cervix of the uterus.

hys·tero·trach·e·lo·plas·ty (his″tur·o·tray′ke·lo·plas″tee, ·track′e·lo·) *n.* Plastic surgery on the cervix of the uterus.

hys·tero·trach·e·lor·rha·phy (his″tur·o·tray″ke·lor′uh·fee, ·track″e·lor′) *n.* A plastic operation for the restoration of a lacerated cervix of the uterus.

hys·tero·trach·e·lot·o·my (his″tur·o·tray″ke·lot′uh·mee, ·track″e·lot′) *n.* Surgical incision of the cervix of the uterus.

hys·tero·trau·ma·tism (his″tur·o·traw′muh·tiz·um, ·traw′) *n.* Hysterical symptoms arising in association with a severe injury.

hys·trix (his′tricks) *n.* NEVUS VERRUCOSUS.

H zone. The region of low density bisecting the A disk of a striated myofibril, occupied by myosin filaments only. Syn. *Hensen's disk.*

I

I Symbol for iodine.

131I Symbol for the radioactive isotope of iodine of atomic weight 131. Formerly written I^{131}.

i- *In chemistry,* symbol for is-, iso-.

-ia A suffix indicating a *condition, especially an abnormal or pathologic condition.*

-iasis A suffix indicating a *diseased condition caused by or resembling.*

iatro- A combining form signifying a *relation to medicine or to physicians.*

iat·ro·chem·is·try (eye·at''ro·kem'is·tree) *n.* 1. The application of chemistry to therapeutics; the treatment of disease by chemical means. 2. A seventeenth century theory that physiology and disease and its treatment are explicable on a chemical basis.

iat·ro·gen·ic (eye·at''ro·jen'ick) *adj.* Induced by a physician or by medical treatment; of or pertaining to the effects of a physician's words, actions, or treatments upon the patient. —**iat·ro·gen·e·sis** (·jen'e·sis) *n.*

-ic 1. A general adjective-forming suffix meaning *of or pertaining to.* 2. *In chemistry,* a suffix designating the higher of two valencies assumed by an element and, incidentally, in many cases, a larger amount of oxygen.

ice, *n.* Water in its solid state, which at 1 atmosphere it assumes at a temperature of 0°C, or 32°F.

iced spleen. A spleen with a clear, translucent, pearl-gray or pale-blue hyalinized capsule. Syn. *sugar-coated spleen, zuckerguss spleen.*

ich·no·gram (ick'no·gram) *n. In legal medicine,* the record of a footprint.

ichor (eye'kor, eye'kur) *n.* A thin discharge from an ulcer or wound. —**ichor·ous** (·us), **ichor·oid** (·oid) *adj.*

ichor·rhea, ichor·rhoea (eye''ko·ree'uh) *n.* A copious flow of ichor.

ichor·rhe·mia, ichor·rhae·mia (eye''ko·ree'mee·uh) *n.* 1. PYEMIA. 2. SEPTICEMIA.

ich·tham·mol (ick'thuh·mole, ·mol) *n.* A reddish-brown to brownish-black, viscid fluid of characteristic odor; obtained by the destructive distillation of certain bituminous schists, followed by sulfonation of the distillate and neu-tralization with ammonia. It is used as a weak antiseptic and stimulant in skin diseases, usually in ointment form; it has been occasionally used internally as an expectorant.

ichthy-, ichthyo- A combining form meaning *fish.*

ich·thy·ism (ikth'ee·iz·um) *n.* Poisoning from eating fish containing toxic substances, as of bacterial origin.

ich·thy·oid (ikth'ee·oid) *adj.* Resembling or shaped like a fish.

ich·thyo·pho·bia (ikth''ee·o·fo'bee·uh) *n.* 1. A morbid fear of fish. 2. An intense dislike for the taste or smell of fish. —**ichthyopho·bic** (·bick) *adj.*

ich·thy·o·si·form (ikth''ee·o·si'form) *adj.* Resembling ichthyosis.

ich·thy·o·sis (ikth''ee·o'sis) *n.,* pl. **ichthyo·ses** (·seez) A genodermatosis characterized by a dry harsh skin with adherent scales, most severe on the extensor surfaces of the extremities. —**ichthy·ot·ic** (·ot'ick) *adj.*

ichthyosis con·gen·i·ta (kon·jen'i·tuh). A severe, probably familial form of ichthyosis present at birth; the fetus may be stillborn or live a few days. The skin and mucous membranes are markedly cracked and thickened, producing a bizarre checked appearance. Syn. *harlequin fetus.*

ichthyosis fol·lic·u·la·ris (fol·ick'yoo·lair'is). The genodermatosis with moderate ichthyosis and associated baldness, absence of eyebrows and eyelashes, thickened lens, and conjunctivitis.

ichthyosis sim·plex (sim'plecks). The common form of ichthyosis developing in early life; characterized by large, finely corrugated, papery scales with deficient secretions of the sebaceous glands and sometimes of the sweat glands.

ich·thyo·tox·ism (ikth''ee·o·tock'siz·um) *n.* ICHTHYISM.

icon (eye'kon) *n.* An image or model. —**icon·ic** (eye·kon'ick) *adj.*

icon-, icono- A combining form meaning *image.*

icon·o·lag·ny (eye·kon''o·lag'nee, eye·kon'o·lag')

nee) *n.* Sexual stimulation induced by the sight of statues or pictures.

icono·ma·nia (eye·kon"o·may'nee·uh) *n.* A morbid interest in images.

ic·tal (ick'tul) *adj.* Pertaining to or caused by ictus.

icter-, ictero-. A combining form meaning *icterus, jaundice.*

ic·ter·ic (ick·terr'ick) *adj.* Pertaining to or characterized by jaundice.

ic·tero·gen·ic (ick"tur·o·jen'ick) *adj.* Causing jaundice.

ic·tero·hem·or·rhag·ic fever (ick"tur·o·hem·o·raj'ick) WEIL'S DISEASE.

ic·ter·oid (ick'tur·oid) *adj.* Resembling the color of, or having the nature of, jaundice.

ic·ter·us (ick'tur·us) *n.* JAUNDICE.

icterus grav·is (grav'is). ACUTE YELLOW ATROPHY.

icterus gravis neonatorum. ERYTHROBLASTOSIS FETALIS.

icterus index. A measurement of the yellow color of blood serum when compared with standard solutions of potassium dichromate; roughly correlated with serum bilirubin levels.

icterus index test. A colorimetric test for jaundice in which blood serum is compared with a standard solution of sodium dichromate.

icterus neonatorum. JAUNDICE OF THE NEWBORN.

ic·tus (ick'tus) *n.* 1. An acute attack, or stroke, as a cerebrovascular accident. 2. Specifically, an epileptic attack, usually a generalized or psychomotor seizure.

ICU Abbreviation for *intensive care unit.*

id, *n. In psychoanalysis,* an unconscious part of the personality consisting of those wishes and needs which are the mental representations of the sexual and aggressive instinctual drives as well as of wishes resulting from perceptions and memories of the earlier gratification of basic physiologic needs.

-idae. *In biology,* a suffix indicating a taxonomic *family.*

idea, *n.* 1. A mental impression or thought; a belief or object existing in the mind or thought. 2. *In psychology,* an experience or thought not directly due to an external sensory stimulation.

ide·al·iza·tion, *n.* 1. Seeing or conceiving a person, situation, or object as ideal, perfect, or far better than it is, with an exaggeration of the virtues and an overlooking of faults. 2. *In psychiatry,* a defense mechanism in which there is a gross overestimation of another person or a situation. 3. *In psychoanalysis,* a sexual overevaluation of the love object.

ideas of influence. *In psychiatry,* a clinical manifestation of certain psychoses in which one may believe that one's thoughts are read, that one's limbs move involuntarily, or that one is under the control of someone else or some external force or influence.

ideas of reference. *In psychopathology,* the symptom complex in which, through the mechanism of projection, every casual remark or incident is believed directed at the individual with hostile intent; observed in various paranoid states, the paranoid type of schizophrenia, and in manic-depressive illness.

ide·a·tion (eye"dee·ay'shun) *n.* The formation of a mental conception; the mental action by which, or in accord with which, an idea is formed. **—ideation·al** (·ul) *adj.*

ideational apraxia. One of the now largely abandoned divisions of the apractic syndromes, including those syndromes thought to be due to affection of a presumed ideation area rather than of motor association cortex or of fibers connecting the ideation area with it.

idée fixe (ee·day feeks) FIXED IDEA.

identical twins. Twins developed from a single ovum, always of the same sex, the same genetic constitution, and ordinarily the same chorion. Syn. *monozygotic twins.*

iden·ti·fi·ca·tion, *n.* 1. Verification of identity. 2. Establishment of a specimen's classification or composition. 3. *In psychiatry,* a defense mechanism whereby one unconsciously patterns one's self, on the basis of love or aggression, after the characteristics of another. Identification normally plays a major role in the development of the personality and especially of the superego, but when used to excess, may disturb the development of an integrated and independent ego.

iden·ti·ty, *n.* 1. Exact sameness; selfsameness. 2. *In psychiatry,* the sense of unity and of continuity of one's own self in the face of changing experiences. Syn. *ego-identity.*

ileal bladder. ILEAL CONDUIT.

ileal conduit. A segment of ileum which is surgically prepared to receive both ureters and to serve as a substitute bladder.

identity crisis. The critical period in emotional maturation and personality development, occurring usually during adolescence, which involves the reworking and abandonment of childhood identifications and the integration of new personal and social identifications.

ideo-. A combining form meaning (a) *idea;* (b) *pertaining to the mind.*

ideo·ge·net·ic (id"ee·o·je·net'ick, eye"dee·o·) *adj.* 1. Pertaining to mental activity in which primary sense impressions are employed in place of completed ideas that are ready for expression. 2. Produced within the mind, as the assumption that judgment or a sense of responsibility is a primary mental activity and not due to experience.

ideo·glan·du·lar (id"ee·o·glan'dew·lur, eye"dee·o·) *adj.* Pertaining to glandular activity as evoked by a mental concept, as salivating at the thought of a good meal.

ideo·ki·net·ic (id"ee·o·ki·net'ick, eye"dee·o·) *adj.* IDEOMOTOR.

ide·ol·o·gy (id"ee·ol'uh·jee, eye"dee·) *n.* 1. The science of ideas and of intellectual operations. 2. A program of ideas or world view.

ideo·mo·tor (id"ee·o·mo'tur) *adj.* 1. Pertaining to involuntary movement resulting from or accompanying some mental activity, as moving the lips while reading. 2. Pertaining to both ideation and motor activity.

ideomotor apraxia. One of the now largely abandoned divisions of the apractic syndromes, including those syndromes thought to be due to disconnection of a presumed ideation area in the supramarginal gyrus of the dominant hemisphere from association cortex, either by interruption of long association fibers within the dominant hemisphere (causing an apraxia of both sides of the body) or by disconnection of the motor areas of the two hemispheres by a callosal lesion (causing an apraxia on the non-dominant side only).

ideo·mus·cu·lar (id″ee·o·mus′kew·lur) *adj.* IDEOMOTOR.

ideo·pho·bia (id″ee·o·fo′bee·uh, eye″dee·o·) *n.* A morbid fear of ideas.

ideo·vas·cu·lar (id″ee·o·vas′kew·lur, eye″dee·o·) *adj.* Designating a vascular change resulting from a mental or emotional activity, as blushing in response to an embarrassing memory.

idio- A combining form meaning (a) *one's own;* (b) *separate, distinct;* (c) *self-produced.*

id·io·chro·mo·some (id″ee·o·kro′muh·sohm) *n.* SEX CHROMOSOME.

id·i·oc·to·nia (id″ee·ock·to′nee·uh) *n.* SUICIDE.

id·i·o·cy (id′ee·uh·see) *n.* The lowest grade of mental deficiency, in which the subject's mental age is under 3 years, or if a child, the intelligence quotient is under 20. Custodial or complete protective care is usually required.

id·i·og·a·mist (id″ee·og′uh·mist) *n.* A man capable of coitus only with his marital partner or with certain women, but impotent with women in general.

id·io·glos·sia (id″ee·o·glos′ee·uh) *n.* Any form of speech invented by an individual and unique, usually incomprehensible to others; in a very young child, a transition stage toward normal speech which may be understood by parents and associates; in one in whom normal speech development may be expected, it represents a neuropathological process, such as congenital auditory aphasia or auditory imperception. —**idio·glot·tic** (·glot′ick) *adj.*

id·io·gram (id′ee·o·gram) *n.* Schematic representation of the karyotype.

id·io·hyp·no·tism (id″ee·o·hip′nuh·tiz·um) *n.* The practice of self-hypnosis.

id·i·o·lo·gism (id″ee·ol′uh·jiz·um) *n.* A form of utterance peculiar to and constantly employed by a particular person, and incomprehensible to all others, as seen in certain psychoses.

id·io·mus·cu·lar (id″ee·o·mus′kew·lur) *adj.* Characterizing phenomena occurring in a muscle which are independent of outside stimuli.

id·io·path·ic (id″ee·o·path′ick) *adj.* 1. Primary, spontaneous; not resulting from another disease. 2. Of a pathological condition: having an unknown or obscure cause.

idiopathic anemia. Anemia of unknown origin.

idiopathic epilepsy. Recurrent seizures of unknown cause.

idiopathic eunuchoidism. A type of eunuchoidism without enlargement of the mammary glands, in which the testes are similar in histologic appearance to those of a prepubertal male. There is a normal to low level of urinary 17-ketosteroids.

idiopathic hypertrophic subaortic stenosis. A cardiomyopathy characterized by left ventricular hypertrophy, particularly marked hypertrophy of the interventricular septum. During systole, left ventricular ejection is obstructed. Abbreviated, IHSS.

idiopathic megacolon. Hypertrophy and dilatation of the colon resulting in moderate constipation; sometimes due to a congenital anomaly of the colon, but usually due to psychogenic causes and faulty bowel habits.

idiopathic parkinsonism. PARKINSON'S DISEASE.

idiopathic thrombocytopenic purpura. Thrombocytopenic purpura of unknown cause but suspected to be immunogenic in character. Abbreviated, ITP.

id·i·op·a·thy (id″ee·op′uth·ee) *n.* 1. A primary disease; one not a result of any other disease, but of spontaneous origin. 2. Disease for which no cause is known. *Adj.* **idiopathic.**

id·io·psy·chol·o·gy (id″ee·o·sigh·kol′uh·jee) *n.* The psychological study by a person of his own mental acts and dynamics.

id·io·syn·cra·sy (id″ee·o·sing′kruh·see) *n.* 1. Any special or peculiar characteristic or temperament by which a person differs from other persons. 2. A peculiarity of constitution that makes an individual react differently from most persons to drugs, diet, treatments, or other situations. —**idio·syn·crat·ic** (·sing·krat′ick) *adj.*

id·i·ot, *n.* A person afflicted with idiocy.

idi·ot sa·vant (ee·dee·o′ sa·vahn′) An individual with general mental retardation as measured by the intelligence quotient, but capable of performing some isolated mental feat, such as calculating or puzzle-solving.

id·io·ven·tric·u·lar (id″ee·o·ven·trick′yoo·lur) *adj.* Pertaining to the cardiac ventricles alone, and not involving the atria.

idox·uri·dine (eye″docks·yoor′i·deen) *n.* 2′-Deoxy-5-iodouridine, $C_9H_{11}IN_2O_5$, a topical antiviral agent used for the treatment of dendritic keratitis. Abbreviated, IDU.

id reaction Papulovesicular exanthematic eruptions that appear suddenly after exacerbation of foci of some superficial fungous infections, particularly on the hands from tinea pedis and on the trunk from tinea cruris.

IgA A symbol for gamma-A globulin.

IgD A symbol for gamma-D globulin.

IgE A symbol for gamma-E globulin.

IgG A symbol for gamma-G globulin.

IgM A symbol for gamma-M globulin.

ig·ni·punc·ture (ig′ni·punk″chur) *n.* Puncture with metal needles heated to either red or white heat.

ig·ni·tion, *n.* The process of heating solids until all volatile matter has been driven off. When performed in the presence of air, oxidizable matter such as carbon is burned.

IHSA Radioactive iodine-tagged human serum albumin.

IH virus. HEPATITIS VIRUS A.

ile-, ileo-. A combining form meaning *ileum, ileal.*

il·e·ac (il′ee·ack) *adj.* ILEAL.

il·e·al (il′ee·ul) *adj.* Pertaining to, or involving the ileum.

ileal bladder. ILEAL CONDUIT.

ileal conduit. A segment of ileum which is surgically prepared to receive both ureters and to serve as a substitute bladder.

il·e·ec·to·my (il″ee-eck'tuh·mee) *n.* Excision of the ileum.

il·e·itis (il″ee-eye'tis) *n.*, pl. **il·e·it·i·des** (il″ee-it'i-deez) Inflammation of the ileum. **—il·e·it·ic** (·it'ick) *adj.*

il·eo·ce·cal, il·eo·cae·cal (il″ee-o·see'kul) *adj.* Pertaining to or involving the ileum and the cecum.

ileocecal valve. The valve at the junction of the terminal ileum and the cecum which consists of a superior and inferior lip and partially prevents reflux from the cecum into the ileum.

il·eo·ce·cos·to·my, il·eo·cae·cos·to·my (il″ee-o·see·kos'tuh·mee) *n.* The formation of an anastomosis between the cecum and the ileum.

il·eo·co·lic (il″ee-o·ko'lick) *adj.* Pertaining conjointly to the ileum and the colon.

il·eo·co·li·tis (il″ee-o·ko·lye'tis) *n.* Inflammation of the ileum and the colon.

il·eo·co·lon·ic (il″ee-o·ko·lon'ick) *adj.* ILEOCOLIC.

il·eo·co·los·to·my (il″ee-o·ko·los'tuh·mee) *n.* The establishment of an anastomosis between the ileum and the colon.

il·eo·cu·ta·ne·ous (il″ee-o·kew·tay'nee·us) *adj.* Pertaining to the ileum and the skin, usually to a fistulous connection between the two.

il·eo·cys·to·plas·ty (il″ee-o·sis'to·plas″tee) *n.* An operation in which a segment of ileum is sutured to the urinary bladder, to increase bladder capacity.

il·eo·il·e·al (il″ee-o·il'ee·ul) *adj.* Pertaining to two different portions of the ileum, usually to a communication or other connection between two parts of the ileum.

il·eo·il·e·os·to·my (il″ee-o·il·ee·os'tuh·mee) *n.* The establishment of an anastomosis between two different parts of the ileum.

il·eo·proc·tos·to·my (il″ee-o·prock·tos'tuh·mee) *n.* The surgical formation of a connection between the ileum and the rectum.

il·e·or·rha·phy (il″ee-or'uh·fee) *n.* Suture of the ileum.

il·eo·sig·moid·os·to·my (il″ee-o·sig″moid·os'tuh·mee) *n.* The surgical formation of an anastomosis between the ileum and the sigmoid colon.

il·e·os·to·my (il″ee-os'tuh·mee) *n.* The surgical formation of a fistula or artificial anus through the abdominal wall into the ileum.

il·e·ot·o·my (il″ee-ot'uh·mee) *n.* Surgical incision of the ileum.

il·eo·trans·verse (il″ee-o·trans·vurce′) *adj.* Pertaining to the ileum and transverse colon.

il·eo·trans·ver·sos·to·my (il″ee-o·trans·vur·sos'tuh·mee) *n. In surgery,* the formation of a connection between the ileum and the transverse colon.

il·eo·typh·li·tis (il″ee-o·tif·lye'tis) *n.* Inflammation of the cecum and the ileum.

il·eo·ves·i·cal (il″ee-o·ves'i·kul) *adj.* Pertaining to the ileum and the urinary bladder.

Iletin. A trademark for insulin.

il·e·um (il'ee·um) *n.*, genit. **ilei** (il'ee·eye), pl. **il·e·a** (·ee·uh) The lower portion of the small intestine, extending from the jejunum to the large intestine.

il·e·us (il'ee·us) *n.* Acute intestinal obstruction characterized by diminished or absent intestinal peristalsis, distention, obstipation, abdominal pain, and vomiting.

ili-, ilio-. A combining form meaning *ilium, iliac.*

ilia. Plural of *ilium.*

il·i·ac (il'ee·ack) *adj.* Pertaining to the ilium.

iliac crest. The thickened and expanded upper border of the ilium.

iliac fossa. A wide depression on the internal surface of the ilium.

ili·a·cus (i·lye'uh·kus) *n.* The portion of the iliopsoas muscle arising from the iliac fossa and sacrum.

ilio-. See *ili-.*

il·io·coc·cyg·e·al (il″ee-o·cock·sij'ee·ul) *adj.* Pertaining to the ilium and the coccyx.

il·io·fem·o·ral (il″ee-o·fem'o·rul) *adj.* Pertaining to the ilium and the femur.

il·io·hy·po·gas·tric (il″ee-o·high″po·gas'trick) *adj.* Pertaining to the ilium and the pubic (hypogastric) region.

il·io·in·gui·nal (il″ee-o·ing'gwi·nul) *adj.* Pertaining to the ilium and the groin.

il·io·lum·bar (il″ee-o·lum'bur) *adj.* Pertaining to the ilium and the lumbar vertebrae, or to the iliac and lumbar regions.

il·io·pec·tin·e·al (il″ee-o·peck·tin'ee·ul) *adj.* Pertaining jointly to the ilium and the pecten of the pubic bone.

iliopectineal line. The bony ridge marking the brim of the true pelvis, the pecten of the pubic bone, plus its lateral extension to the iliopubic eminence.

il·io·pso·as (il″ee-o·so'us, il″ee-op'so·us) *n.* The combined iliacus and psoas muscles.

il·io·pu·bic (il″ee-o·pew'bick) *adj.* Pertaining to the ilium and the pubis.

iliopubic eminence. A ridge on the hipbone marking the site of union of ilium and pubis.

il·io·tib·i·al (il″ee-o·tib'ee·ul) *adj.* Pertaining to the ilium and the tibia.

iliotibial tract or **band.** A thickened portion of fascia lata extending from the lateral condyle of the tibia to the iliac crest.

il·i·um (il'ee·um) *n.*, genit. **ilii** (il'ee·eye), pl. **il·ia** (·ee·uh) 1. The flank. 2. The superior broad portion of the hipbone.

ill, *adj. & n.* 1. Not healthy; sick; indisposed. 2. An ailment, illness, disease, or misfortune.

il·laq·ue·ate (i·lack'wee·ate) *v.* To correct an ingrowing eyelash by drawing it with a loop through an opening in the lid. **—il·laq·ue·a·tion** (i·lack″wee·ay'shun) *n.*

il·le·git·i·mate, *adj.* 1. Not in accordance with statutory law. 2. Not recognized by statutory law as a lawful offspring; bastard. **—illegiti·ma·cy,** *n.*

ill·ness, *n.* 1. The state of being ill or sick. 2. A malady; sickness; disease; disorder.

il·lu·mi·na·tion, *n.* 1. The lighting up or illuminating, as of a surface or cavity in the examination of a patient or of an object under microscopical examination. 2. The quantity of light thrown upon an object. **—il·lu·mi·nate,** *v.*

il·lu·mi·nism (i·lew'mi·niz·um) *n.* The mental

state in which one imagines that one receives messages from or converses with supernatural beings.

il·lu·sion, *n.* A false interpretation of a real sensation; a perception that misinterprets the object perceived. —**illusion·al, illu·so·ry,** *adj.*

Ilotycin. A trademark for the antibiotic substance erythromycin.

I.M., i.m. Abbreviation for *intramuscular.*

im-. See *in-.*

ima (eye'muh) *L. adj.* Lowest.

im·age, *n.* 1. A more or less accurate representation of an object. 2. The picture of an object formed by a lens; a collection of foci, each corresponding to a point in the object. 3. A mental picture of an object in the absence of viewing or directly perceiving that object. 4. IMAGO (2).

imag·i·nary, *adj.* Produced by the picture-making power of the mind; fictitious; often used in relation to pain or other sensations or ailments for which no objective cause can be demonstrated.

imag·i·na·tion, *n.* The picture-making power of the mind. The faculty by which one creates new ideas or mental pictures by means of separate data derived from experience, ideally revivified, extended, and combined in new forms.

im·ag·ing, *n.* Production of an image; usually refers to the production of a photographable image by a radionuclide concentrated in an organ or other part of the body.

ima·go (i·may'go) *n.*, pl. **imagoes, imag·i·nes** (i·maj'i·neez) 1. The adult, sexually mature stage of an insect. 2. *In analytic psychology,* an unconscious mental picture, usually idealized, of a parent or loved person important in the early development of an individual and carried into adulthood.

im·bal·ance, *n.* 1. Lack of balance. 2. Lack of muscular balance, especially between the muscles of the eyes. 3. Absence of biological equilibrium, as between the number of males and females in a population. 4. Lack of physiologic balance between parts or functions of the body.

im·be·cile (im'bi·sil) *n.* A person afflicted with imbecility.

im·be·cil·i·ty (im''be·sil'i·tee) *n.* An intermediate grade of mental deficiency, in which the subject's mental age is between 3 and 7 years with an intelligence quotient between 20 and 45.

im·bi·bi·tion, *n.* The absorption of liquid by a solid or a gel. —**imbibe,** *v.*

im·bri·ca·tion (im''bri·kay'shun) *n. In surgery,* the closing of wounds or the covering of deficiencies with tissue arranged in layers overlapping one another. —**im·bri·cate** (im'bri·kate) *v.*; **im·bri·cat·ed** (·kay·tid) *adj.*

Imferon. Trademark for iron-dextran complex, a preparation for parenteral treatment of iron-deficiency anemias.

imid-, imido-. A combining form meaning *imide.*

im·id·az·ole (im''id·az'ole, ·ay'zole, im'id·uh·zole'') *n.* 1,3-Diaza-2,4-cyclopentadiene, $C_3H_4N_2$, a compound, readily synthesized, which is of interest because of the importance

of a number of its derivatives, such as histamine, histidine, privine. Syn. *glyoxaline.*

im·id·az·o·line (im''id·az'o·leen) *n.* Any of three dihydro derivatives of imidazole, or compounds derived from the former.

im·ide (im'ide) *n.* Any compound containing the radical NH= united to a divalent acid radical.

imin-, imino-. A combining form designating *the bivalent group NH= when attached to or in nonacid radicals.*

im·i·no acid (im'i·no). An organic acid that contains the bivalent imino group (=NH). Imino acids are in some instances intermediaries in the metabolism of amino acids.

im·i·tate, *v.* To copy an act, a manner of behavior, or a characteristic of another.

im·i·ta·tive, *adj.* Having some of the qualities of or imitating an original model, pattern, or process.

im·ma·ture, *adj.* Not yet adult or fully developed; unripe. —**imma·tur·i·ty,** *n.*

im·me·di·ate, *adj.* Direct; without the intervention of anything.

immediate auscultation. The direct application of the examiner's ear to the patient's skin overlying the area to be auscultated in order to listen to the heart and lungs without a stethoscope.

immediate hypersensitivity. Hypersensitivity in which reaction commences within seconds or minutes of exposure to antigens; always associated with prior presence of serum antibodies, generally of the IgE class.

immediate percussion. DIRECT PERCUSSION.

im·med·i·ca·ble (i·med'i·kuh·bul) *adj.* Characterizing that which does not yield to medicine or treatment; incurable.

im·mer·sion, *n.* The plunging of a body or an object into a liquid so that it is completely covered by the liquid. —**im·merse,** *v.*

immersion foot. Skin, peripheral vessel, nerve, and muscle damage of the foot due to prolonged exposure to low but not freezing temperatures, combined with dampness or actual immersion in water.

immersion lens. A microscope objective lens designed for use with a liquid (usually oil) filling the space between it and the cover glass over the specimen.

immersion oil. An oil, such as cedar, used as a medium of contact between the objective of a microscope and the object being examined.

im·mis·ci·ble (i·mis'i·bul) *adj.* Not capable of being mixed.

im·mo·bi·lize, *v.* To render motionless or to fix in place, as by splints or surgery. —**im·mo·bi·li·za·tion,** *n.*

im·mune, *adj.* 1. Safe from attack; protected against a disease by an innate or an acquired immunity. 2. Pertaining to or conferring immunity.

immune-adherence phenomenon. An immunologically specific in vitro reaction involving microorganisms sensitized with antibody, phagocytic cells, and complement resulting in enhanced phagocytosis. Syn. *adhesion phenomenon.*

immune body. ANTIBODY.

immune complex. A complex of antigen and antibody molucules bound together, either circulating in the blood or forming a precipitate; often associated with such pathologic lesions as glomerulonephritis, vasculitis, and arthritis.

immune reaction or **response.** Any reaction involving demonstrated specific antibody response to antigen, or the specifically altered reactivity of host cells following antigenic stimulation.

immune serum. The serum of an immunized animal or person, which carries specific antibodies for the organism or antigen introduced.

im·mu·ni·ty (i·mew'ni·tee) n. The condition of a living organism whereby it resists and overcomes infection or disease.

im·mu·ni·za·tion (im''yoo·ni·zay'shun) n. The act or process of rendering immune.

im·mu·nize (im'yoo·nize) v. To render immune.

immuno-. A combining form meaning immune, immunity.

im·mu·no·blast (im'yoo·no·blast'') n. An immature cell of the plasmacytic series, actively synthesizing antibodies. —**im·mu·no·blas·tic** (im''yoo·no·blas'tick) adj.

im·mu·no·chem·is·try (im''yoo·no·kem'is·tree) n. The branch of science that deals with the chemical changes and phenomena of immunity; specifically, the chemistry of antigens, antibodies, and their reactions.

im·mu·no·con·glu·ti·nin (im''yoo·no·kon·gloo'ti·nin) n. A gamma-M antibody to altered complement, measured by reacting the serum with sensitized erythrocytes coated with complement.

im·mu·no·de·fi·cien·cy (im''yoo·no·de·fish'un·see) n. Any deficiency of immune reaction, involving humoral immunity or cell-mediated immunity only, or both, as in severe combined immunodeficiency.

im·mu·no·dif·fu·sion (im''yoo·no·di·few'zhun) n. Any of a number of techniques favoring the formation of immune precipitates by the diffusion of antigens and antibodies in gels.

im·mu·no·elec·tro·pho·re·sis (im''yoo·no·e·leck''tro·fo·ree'sis) n. The technique of first separating antigens according to their migration in an electric field in a supporting medium, such as agar, and then demonstrating their presence by means of precipitation zones with antibody. —**immunoelectrophoret·ic** (·ret'ick) adj.

im·mu·no·flu·o·res·cence (im''yoo·no·floo''ur·es'unce) n. Fluorescence as the result of, or identifying, an immune response.

im·mu·no·gen (im'yoo·no·jen) n. Any substance capable of stimulating an immune response.

im·mu·no·ge·net·ics (im''yoo·no·je·net'icks) n. The discipline encompassing the study of immunoglobulins, including genetic markers and histocompatibility antigens.

im·mu·no·gen·ic (im''yoo·no·jen'ick) adj. 1. Producing immunity. 2. Pertaining to an immunogen.

im·mu·no·ge·nic·i·ty (im''yoo·no·je·nis'i·tee) n. The capacity to produce an immune response; the state or quality of being an immunogen.

im·mu·no·glob·u·lin (im''yoo·no·glob'yoo·lin) n. Any one of the proteins of animal origin having known antibody activity, or a protein related by chemical structure and hence antigenic specificity; may be found in plasma, urine, spinal fluid, and other body tissues and fluids, and includes such proteins as myeloma and Bence Jones protein. Abbreviated, Ig.

immunoglobulin chain. Any of the major groups of polypeptide chains found in immunoglobulin molecules.

immunoglobulin fragments. Portions of the molecule of immunoglobulins obtained by cleavage of the peptide bonds by proteolytic enzymes, and further subdivided into such fractions as Fab and Fc fragments.

im·mu·no·gran·u·lom·a·tous disease (im''yoo·no·gran''yoo·lom'uh·tus, ·lo'muh·tus). A disease in which an aberration in immune mechanisms is thought to be associated with the development of granulomas in various organs, as in sarcoidosis.

im·mu·no·he·ma·tol·o·gy, im·mu·no·hae·ma·tol·o·gy (im''yoo·no·hee''muh·tol'uh·jee) n. The branch of immunology and hematology concerned with immunologic aspects of normal and diseased blood; includes studies of antigen-antibody systems of the formed blood elements, hemolytic anemias, and other autoimmune phenomena.

im·mu·no·log·ic (im''yoo·no·loj'ick) adj. Pertaining to immunology.

immunologic tolerance. 1. A condition, natural or induced, in which a graft will be accepted without the occurrence of homograft rejection. 2. A state of specific unresponsiveness to an antigen or antigens in adult life as a consequence of exposure to the antigen in utero or in the neonatal period, administration of modified antigen, administration of specific blocking antibody, or administration of antigen with immunosuppressive agents.

im·mu·nol·o·gist (im''yoo·nol'uh·jist) n. A specialist in immunology.

im·mu·nol·o·gy (im''yoo·nol'uh·jee) n. The science dealing with specific mechanisms, including antigen-antibody and cell-mediated reactions, by which living tissues react to foreign or autologous biological material that may result in enhanced resistance or immunity or, as in allergy, in heightened reactivity that may be damaging to the host.

im·mu·no·pa·thol·o·gy (im''yoo·no·pa·thol'uh·jee) n. 1. The study of diseases and other changes caused by immunologic reactions in the host. 2. The changes caused by immunologic reactions.

im·mu·nop·a·thy (im''yoo·nop'uth·ee) n. Any disorder of the immune system of the body.

im·mu·no·pho·re·sis (im''yoo·no·fo·ree'sis) n. IMMUNOELECTROPHORESIS.

im·mu·no·re·ac·tant (im''yoo·no·ree·ack'tunt) n. Any of the substances involved in immunologically mediated reactions, including immunoglobulins, complement components, and specific antigens.

im·mu·no·sup·pres·sant (im''yoo·no·suh·press'unt) n. & adj. IMMUNOSUPPRESSIVE.

im·mu·no·sup·pres·sion (im''yoo·no·suh·presh'

un) *n.* Suppression of immune responses produced primarily by any of a variety of immunosuppressive agents or secondarily during any of a number of diseases.

im·mu·no·sup·pres·sive (im″yoo·no·suh·pres′iv) *adj. & n.* 1. Capable of suppressing an immune response. 2. An agent, such as a chemical, a drug, or x-rays, for suppressing immunologic reactions, as in autoimmune diseases or for enhancing successful foreign tissue grafts.

im·mu·no·ther·a·py (im″yoo·no·therr′uh·pee) *n.* 1. SEROTHERAPY. 2. Therapy utilizing immunosuppressives. 3. Therapy using vaccines or allergenic extracts.

im·mu·no·trans·fu·sion (im″yoo·no·trans·few′zhun) *n.* Transfusion with the blood or plasma of a donor previously rendered immune to a specific infection.

im·pac·tion, *n.* 1. The state of being lodged and retained in a part or strait. 2. Confinement of a tooth in the jaw so that its eruption is prevented. 3. A condition in which one fragment of a fractured bone is driven into another and is fixed in that position. 4. A large accumulation of inspissated feces in the rectum or colon, difficult to move. **—im·pact·ed,** *adj.*

im·pal·pa·ble, *adj.* Not capable of being felt; imperceptible to the touch.

im·par (im′pahr) *adj.* Without a fellow; AZYGOUS.

im·ped·ance (im·peed′unce) *n.* The apparent resistance of a circuit to the flow of an alternating electric current. Symbol, Z.

im·per·a·tive, *adj.* Peremptory, absolute; compulsory; binding.

im·per·cep·tion, *n.* Defective or absent perception.

im·per·fo·rate (im·pur′fuh·rit, ·rate) *adj.* Without the normal opening. **—im·per·fo·ra·tion** (im·pur″fuh·ray′shun) *n.*

imperforate anus. Congenital closure of the anal opening, usually by a membranous septum.

im·per·me·able, *adj.* Not permitting passage through a substance.

im·per·vi·ous, *adj.* Not permitting a passage; impermeable.

im·pe·tig·i·ni·za·tion (im″pe·tij″i·ni·zay′shun) *n.* Lesions of impetigo occurring on a previous skin lesion.

im·pe·ti·go (im″pe·tye′go, ·tee′go) *n.* An acute, inflammatory skin disease caused by streptococci or staphylococci, and characterized by subcorneal vesicles and bullae which rupture and develop distinct yellow crusts. **—impe·tig·i·nous** (·tij′i·nus) *adj.*

impetigo cir·ci·na·ta (sur″si·nay′tuh). A form of impetigo characterized by a circle or a semicircle of small vesicles or pustules; there are usually many such circles.

impetigo fol·lic·u·la·ris (fol·ick″yoo·lair′is). A form of staphylococcal infection of hair follicles characterized by vesicles at the pilosebaceous orifice, which form yellowish crusts. Syn. *Bockhart's impetigo, impetigo circumpilaris.*

impetigo her·pet·i·for·mis (hur·pet″i·for′mis). A variant form of psoriasis resembling pustular psoriasis, but occurring in hypocalcemic pa-

tients following parathyroidectomy or during pregnancy, and not associated with pre-existing psoriasis.

¹im·plant (im·plant′) *v.* To embed, set in.

²im·plant (im′plant) *n.* 1. A small tube or needle which contains radioactive material, placed in a tissue or tumor to deliver therapeutic doses of radiation. 2. A tissue graft placed in depth.

im·plan·ta·tion, *n.* 1. The act of implanting, as the transplantation of a tissue, tooth, duct, or organ from one place in the body to another, or from the body of one person to that of another, implying the placement of the tissue in depth, as distinguished from the placement of a surface graft. Tissue implants are sometimes used as guides or ladders for the restoration of damaged nerve trunks and tendons. 2. The placement within the body tissues of a substance, such as tantalum, vitallium, or wire filigree, for restoration by mechanical means; as, for example, the closure of a bone defect or the repair of a ventral hernia. 3. The embedding of the embryo into, or on, the endometrium.

im·pon·der·a·ble, *adj.* Incapable of being weighed, evaluated, or measured.

im·po·tence (im′puh·tunce) *n.* 1. Inability in the male to perform the sexual act, most frequently for psychologic reasons. 2. By extension, lack of sexual vigor or of power generally. **—impo·tent** (·tunt) *adj.*

im·preg·nate (im·preg′nate) *v.* 1. To inseminate and fertilize; make pregnant. 2. To saturate or mix with another substance. **—im·preg·na·tion** (im″preg·nay′shun) *n.*

im·pres·sio (im·pres′ee·o) *n.,* pl. **im·pres·si·o·nes** (im·pres″ee·o′neez) IMPRESSION (1).

im·pres·sion, *n.* 1. A mark produced upon a surface by pressure. 2. A mold or imprint of a bodily part or parts from which a positive likeness or cast is made, usually from material, as plaster of Paris, wax compounds, or hydrocolloids. 3. The effect or sensation, usually the initial one, produced by a person, situation, or other phenomenon upon an individual's mind or feelings.

im·print·ing, *n.* A particular mode of learning in animals occurring at critical periods in early development, characterized by patterning on adult models, rapid acquisition, and relative resistance to forgetting or extinction. Observed chiefly in animal behavior; the extent to which it applies to human behavior has not been determined. **—imprint,** *v.*

im·pu·ber·al (im·pew′bur·ul) *adj.* 1. Destitute of hair on the pubes. 2. Not of adult age; immature.

im·pulse, *n.* 1. A push or communicated force. 2. A mechanical or electrical force or action generally of brief duration. 3. *In neurophysiology,* NERVE IMPULSE. 4. A sudden mental urge to an action.

im·pul·sion, *n.* 1. The act of driving or urging onward, either mentally or physically. 2. The sudden and spontaneous drive to perform a usually forbidden or illegal act. **—impul·sive,** *adj.*

im·put·abil·i·ty (im·pew″tuh·bil′i·tee) *n. In legal*

medicine, the degree of mental soundness which makes a person responsible for his own acts.

Imuran. Trademark for azathioprine, a drug used in treating leukemia, as a suppressive agent in diseases produced by altered immune mechanisms, in the induction of immune tolerance, and in the prevention of rejection of allografts.

¹in-, im- A prefix meaning *not, non-, un-.*

²in-, im- A prefix meaning *in, into, on, onto, toward.*

in·ac·ti·vate, *v.* To render inactive, as by heating fresh serum to destroy its complement.

in·ac·tive, *adj.* 1. Of a substance: exhibiting no activity of a given sort, as optical, chemical, or biological. 2. Of a disease: exhibiting no activity or progress; in remission. —**inactiv·i·ty,** *n.*

in·ad·e·qua·cy, *n.* Insufficiency of function or capacity. —**inade·quate,** *adj.*

in·a·ni·tion (in″a·nish′un) *n.* A pathologic state of the body due to the lack of food and water; starvation.

in·ar·tic·u·late (in″ahr·tick′yoo·lut) *adj.* Not articulate.

in ar·tic·u·lo mor·tis (in ahr·tick′yoo·lo mor′tis) At the moment of death; in the act of dying.

in·as·sim·i·la·ble (in″a·sim′i·luh·bul) *adj.* Incapable of being assimilated.

in·born, *adj.* Of a constitutional characteristic: inherited or implanted during intrauterine life; innate; congenital.

in·bred, *adj.* Derived from closely related parents.

in·breed·ing, *n.* Any system of mating which gives a smaller number of ancestors than the maximum possible, the closest inbreeding being self-fertilization, as in plants, or brother-by-sister mating in animals.

in·cap·a·ri·na (in·kap″uh·rye′nuh, ·ree·nuh) *n.* A cereal food mixture with added yeast and vitamin A supplied to increase protein intake to combat kwashiorkor in Central America.

in·car·cer·ate (in·kahr′sur·ate) *v.* To imprison, confine, or enclose. —**incarcer·at·ed** (·ay·tid) *adj.*

incarcerated hernia. An irreducible hernia, frequently due to adhesions, particularly of the omentum, to the sac. If bowel is present in the hernia, it may become obstructed.

in·car·cer·a·tion (in·kahr″sur·ay′shun) *n.* The abnormal imprisonment of a part, as in some forms of hernia.

in·car·nant (in·kahr′nunt) *adj. & n.* 1. Flesh-forming; promoting granulation. 2. An agent that promotes granulation.

in·cest (in′sest) *n.* Sexual intercourse between persons of such close genetic relationship that their marriage is prohibited by law.

inch, *n.* The twelfth part of a foot; 2.54 cm.

in·ci·dence, *n.* 1. The act or manner of falling upon; the way in which one body strikes another. 2. The rate of occurrence, as of a disease.

incidence rate. The number of new cases of a disease or injury that occur per population at risk in a particular geographic area within a

defined time interval such as a year; usually expressed as the number of new cases of a disease or injury per 1,000 or 100,000 population.

in·ci·dent, *adj.* 1. Falling upon, as an incident ray. 2. External. 3. Likely to occur. —**in·ci·den·tal** (in″si·dent′ul) *adj.*

in·cin·er·ate, *v.* To heat an organic substance until all the organic matter is driven off and only ash remains; to cremate. —**in·cin·er·a·tion,** *n.;* **in·cin·er·a·tor,** *n.*

in·cip·i·ent, *adj.* Initial, commencing; coming into being, as a disease. —**incipi·ence, incipi·en·cy,** *n.*

in·ci·sal (in·sigh′zul) *adj.* Of or pertaining to the cutting edge of incisor and canine teeth.

in·cise (in·size′) *v.* To cut into a body tissue or organ with a knife or scalpel.

in·ci·sion (in·sizh′un) *n.* 1. A cut or wound of the body tissue, as an abdominal incision or a vertical or oblique incision. 2. The act of cutting. —**incision·al** (·ul) *adj.*

in·ci·sive (in·sigh′siv, ·ziv) *adj.* 1. Cutting; penetrating. 2. Pertaining to the incisor teeth.

incisive bone. The intermaxillary bone which bears the upper incisor teeth. Fused with the maxilla in man; a separate bone in most mammals.

in·ci·so·la·bi·al (in·sigh″zo·lay′bee·ul) *adj.* Pertaining to the incisal and labial surfaces of an anterior tooth.

in·ci·so·lin·gual (in·sigh″zo·ling′gwul) *adj.* Pertaining to the incisal and lingual surfaces of an anterior tooth.

in·ci·so·prox·i·mal (in·sigh″zo·prock′si·mul) *adj.* Pertaining to the incisal and proximal surfaces of an anterior tooth.

in·ci·sor (in·sigh′zur) *n.* A cutting tooth; in the human dentition, one of the four front teeth of either jaw.

in·ci·sure (in·sigh′zhur) *n.* A notch, fissure, or groove.

incisure of the cerebellum. One of the notches separating the cerebellar hemispheres.

in·cli·na·tion (in″kli·nay′shun) *n.* 1. A propensity; a leaning. 2. The deviation of the long axis of a tooth from the vertical. 3. A slope. —**in·cline** (in·kline′) *v.;* **in·cline** (in′kline) *n.*

in·cli·nom·e·ter (in″kli·nom′e·tur) *n.* A device for determining the diameter of the eye from the horizontal and vertical lines.

inclusion body. A minute foreign particle found in cells under special conditions; especially in cells infected by any of various viruses.

inclusion body encephalitis. Encephalitis characterized pathologically by large intranuclear inclusion bodies in astrocytes, oligodendrocytes, and nerve cells; classified as acute (HERPETIC ENCEPHALITIS) and subacute (SUBACUTE SCLEROSING PANENCEPHALITIS).

inclusion conjunctivitis. An acute purulent conjunctivitis, caused by *Chlamidia trachomatis,* and having a different clinical appearance in the neonate than in the adult. In the neonate the organism is transmitted from the mother's genital tract during birth, and the condition is characterized by swelling and redness of the lids, purulent discharge, and chemosis, involving both eyes. In the adult the condition is less severe and often acquired in swimming pools or venereally; it is characterized by a less purulent discharge, but by larger papillae and preauricular adenopathy, frequently involving one eye only. Confirmed clinically in both instances by finding of epithelial-cell inclusion bodies in conjunctival scrapings.

inclusion cyst. A cyst due to embryonal or traumatic implantation of epithelium into another structure, as an epidermal inclusion cyst.

in·co·ag·u·la·ble (in″ko·ag′yoo·luh·bul) *adj.* Incapable of coagulating or curdling.

in·com·pat·i·ble (in″kum·pat′i·bul) *adj.* Incapable of being used or put together because of resulting chemical change or of antagonistic qualities, as two drugs or two types of blood. —**incom·pat·i·bil·i·ty** (·pat″i·bil′i·tee) *n.*

in·com·pe·tence (in·kom′pe·tunce) *n.* 1. Insufficiency; inadequacy in performing natural functions. 2. *In legal medicine,* incapacity; want of legal fitness, as the incompetence of a drunken man to drive a car. —**incompe·tent** (·tunt) *adj.*

incomplete (inguinal) hernia. An inguinal hernia in which the sac has not passed through the subcutaneous inguinal ring.

in·con·gru·i·ty (in″kong·groo′i·tee) *n.* Absence of agreement, correspondence, or needful harmony.

in·con·stant (in·kon′stunt) *adj.* Not always present.

in·con·ti·nence (in·kon′ti·nunce) *n.* Inability to control the natural evacuations, as the feces or the urine; specifically, involuntary evacuation due to organic causes.

in·co·or·di·na·tion (in″ko·or″di·nay′shun) *n.* Inability to bring into common, harmonious movement or action, as inability to produce voluntary muscular movements in proper order or sequence. —**inco·or·di·nate** (·or′di·nut) *adj.*

in·co·sta·pe·di·al (ing″ko·stay·pee′dee·ul) *adj.* INCUDOSTAPEDIAL.

in·cre·ment (in′kre·munt) *n.* The amount of increase or growth in a given period of time. —**in·cre·men·tal** (in″kre·men′tal) *adj.*

incremental lines of Ret·zi·us (ret′see·ōōs) Brownish bands that represent the successive apposition of layers of enamel matrix; seen in ground sections of dental enamel.

in·crust, en·crust (in·krust′) *v.* To form a crust or hard coating on.

in·crus·ta·tion (in″krus·tay′shun) *n.* The formation of a crust or hard coating, as from an exudate; scab, scale.

in·cu·ba·tion (ing″kew·bay′shun) *n.* 1. The act or process of hatching or developing, as eggs or bacteria. 2. The phase of an infectious disease from the time of infection to the appearance of symptoms. 3. The process of culturing bacteria for qualitative or quantitative growth studies, as in microbiologic assays. 4. The process of maintaining mixtures of substances in suspension or solution at definite temperatures for varying periods of time for the study of enzyme action or other chemical reactions. 5. In ancient Greek medicine, sleep within the

precincts of the temples of healing gods, for the purpose of curing disease. —**in·cu·bate** (ing′kew·bate) *v.*

in·cu·ba·tor (ing′kew·bay″tur) *n.* 1. A small chamber with controlled oxygen, temperature, and humidity for newborns requiring special care. 2. A laboratory cabinet with controlled temperature for the cultivation of bacteria or for facilitating biologic tests. 3. A device for the artificial hatching of eggs.

in·cu·bus (ing′kew·bus) *n.,* pl. **incu·bi** (·bye), **incu·buses** 1. A demon supposed to have sexual intercourse with sleeping men or women or to enter their bodies and thus direct and influence their behavior. 2. A stifling or suffocating dream; NIGHTMARE.

in·cu·dec·to·my (ing″kew·deck′tuh·mee) *n.* Surgical removal of the incus.

in·cu·do·mal·le·al (in″kew·do·mal′ee·ul, ·ing″) *adj.* Pertaining to the incus and the malleus, as the ligaments joining these two bones.

in·cu·do·sta·pe·di·al (in″kew·do·stay·pee′dee·ul, ·ing″) *adj.* Pertaining to the incus and the stapes, as the ligaments joining these two bones.

in·cur·able (in·kewr′uh·bul) *adj. & n.* 1. Not capable of being cured. 2. A person suffering from an incurable disease.

in·cur·va·tion (in·kur·vay′shun) *n.* A state or condition of being turned inward. —**incur·vate** (in′kur·vate) *v. & adj.*

in·cus (ing′kus) *n.,* genit. **in·cu·dis** (ing·kew′dis), pl. **in·cu·des** (ing·kew′deez) The middle one of the chain of ossicles in the middle ear, so termed from its resemblance to an anvil. —**in·cu·dal** (ing′kew·dul, ing·kew′dul) *adj.*

in·cy·clo·pho·ria (in″sigh″klo·fo′ree·uh) *n.* Cyclophoria in which the eyes rotate inward.

in·da·ga·tion (in″duh·gay′shun) *n.* 1. Close investigation or examination. 2. Digital examination.

in·de·cent (in·dee′sunt) *adj.* Characterizing any act or material that is lewd or obscene, or specifically designed to arouse the kind of sexual interest that is outside the accepted mores of the community.

in·de·ci·sion (in″de·sizh′un) *n.* 1. A state characterized by inability to make up one's mind; want of firmness or of will. 2. Abnormal irresolution, usually a symptom of anxiety and depression.

indentation tonometry. A method of determining the intraocular pressure by measuring the depth of the impression produced upon the ocular wall by a given force represented by a plunger which has a small bearing area.

in·dex (in′decks) *n.,* genit. **in·di·cis** (in′di·sis), pl. **in·di·ces** (in′di·seez) 1. [NA]. INDEX FINGER. NA alt. *digitus II.* 2. The ratio, or the formula expressing the ratio, of one dimension of a thing to another dimension.

index case. A case of a disease or abnormality whose identification leads to the investigation and identification of further cases in other members of the same family; PROBAND; PROPOSITUS.

index finger. The second digit of the hand, next to the thumb. Syn. *forefinger.*

Indian hemp. See *cannabis*.

in·di·can (in'di·kan) *n.* 1. Indoxyl glucoside, $C_{14}H_{17}NO_6.3H_2O$, occurring in indigo plants; upon hydrolysis and subsequent oxidation, it is converted to indigotin, the chief constituent of indigo. 2. Indoxyl sulfuric acid or, more commonly, its potassium salt, $C_8H_6NSO_4K$, a substance occurring in urine and formed from indole.

in·di·can·uria (in''di·kuh·new'ree·uh) *n.* The presence of an excess of indican in the urine.

in·di·ca·tion, *n.* Any symptom, sign, or occurrence in a disease which points out its cause, diagnosis, course of treatment, or prognosis.

in·di·ca·tor, *n.* In chemistry, a substance used to show by a color or other change when a reaction has taken place or a chemical affinity has been satisfied.

indices. Plural of *index*.

in·dif·fer·ent (in·dif'runt) *adj.* Neutral; undifferentiated or nonspecialized, as indifferent cells.

indifferent electrode. INDIRECT LEAD.

in·dig·e·nous (in·dij'e·nus) *adj.* 1. Native; originating or belonging to a certain locality or country. 2. INBORN.

in·di·ges·tion (in''di·jesh'chun) *n.* 1. Imperfect or disturbed digestion. Failure to digest.

in·dig·i·ta·tion (in·dij''i·tay'shun) *n.* 1. INTUSSUSCEPTION. 2. Interlocking of fibers, as between muscle and tendons.

in·di·go (in'di·go) *n.* A blue pigment formed by the hydrolysis and oxidation of the indican contained in various species of the shrub *Indigofera* (*Indigofera tinctoria, I. anil, I. argentea*); the chief constituent of indigo is indigotin, but varying amounts of such dyes as indigo brown, indigo red, and indigo yellow are also present.

indigo carmine test. A test of kidney function. Indigo carmine should appear in the urine 5 to 7 minutes after intramuscular or intravenous injection if the kidneys are functioning normally.

in·di·go·uria (in''di·go·yoo'ree·uh) *n.* The presence of indigo in the urine, due to a decomposition of indican.

indirect hernia. An inguinal form of hernia that follows the spermatic cord into the scrotum or, in the female, the round ligament into the labium majus. The hernial sac leaves the abdomen through the deep inguinal ring, traverses the inguinal canal, and passes through the superficial inguinal ring. Syn. *lateral hernia, oblique hernia*.

indirect laryngoscopy. Examination of the interior of the larynx by means of a laryngeal mirror.

indirect lead. An electrical connection in which all electrodes or the exploring electrodes are not in direct contact with, but are distant from, the current source, such as the heart, brain, muscle, or spinal cord; body tissues or fluids serving as a conducting medium.

indirect percussion. Percussion effected by placing a pleximeter against the skin surface to receive the tap. Syn. *mediate percussion*.

in·dis·po·si·tion (in·dis''po·zish'un) *n.* The state of being slightly ill or somewhat unwell. —**in·dis·posed** (in''dis·spoze'd') *adj.*

in·di·um (in'dee·um) *n.* In = 114.82. A rare metal that is very soft, resembles lead in its properties, and is used in many alloys.

in·di·vid·u·al·iza·tion (in''di·vij''oo·ul·i·zay'shun) *n.* 1. The process whereby an organism becomes an individual, distinct and independent from others in the same category. 2. The process by which an observer recognizes an organism, in particular a person, as an individual with distinctive qualities. 3. The adaptation of any method, such as a therapeutic or educational process, to the needs of a particular person. —**indi·vid·u·al·ize** (·vij'oo·ul·ize) *v.*

in·di·vid·u·a·tion (in''di·vij''oo·ay'shun) *n.* The process whereby a part of a whole becomes progressively more independent and distinct. 2. INDIVIDUALIZATION.

Indocin. Trademark for indomethacin, a drug with anti-inflammatory, antipyretic, and analgesic activities used in the management of arthritic disorders.

in·dole (in'dole) *n.* 2,3-Benzopyrrole, C_8H_7N, a substance formed from tryptophan during intestinal putrefaction. It is responsible, in part, for the odor of feces. In intestinal obstruction it is converted to indican, which is eliminated in the urine.

in·dole·ace·tic acid (in''dole·a·see'tick). Indole-3-acetic acid, $C_{10}H_9NO_2$, a bacterial decomposition product of tryptophan, found in the urine and feces. It promotes and accelerates rooting of plant clippings.

in·do·lent (in'duh·lunt) *adj.* 1. Painless. 2. Sluggish; of tumors: slow in developing; of ulcers: slow in healing.

in·do·lu·ria (in''do·lew'ree·uh) *n.* The excretion of indole in the urine.

in·do·meth·a·cin (in''do·meth'uh·sin) *n.* 1-(*p*-Chlorobenzoyl)-5-methoxy-2-methylindole-3-acetic acid, $C_{19}H_{16}ClNO_4$, a drug with anti-inflammatory, antipyretic, and analgesic activities used in the management of arthritic disorders.

in·do·phe·nol (in''do·fee'nole, ·nol) *n.* Any of a series of dyes, derived from quinone imine, used as electron acceptors in biological oxidation studies.

indophenol oxidase. The oxidizing enzyme, present in animal and plant tissues, that catalyzes formation of indophenol blue from dimethyl-*p*-phenylenediamine and α-naphthol when these are injected into tissue; it is identical with cytochrome oxidase.

in·dor·a·min (in·dor'uh·min) *n.* N-[1-(2-Indol-3-ylethyl)-4-piperidyl]benzamide, $C_{22}H_{25}N_3O$, an antihypertensive.

in·duce, *v.* To bring on, produce, as by application of a stimulus.

induced abortion. Intentional premature termination of pregnancy by medicinal or mechanical means. Syn. *artificial abortion*.

induced labor. Labor brought on by artificial means.

in·duc·ible enzyme (in·dew'si·bul). An enzyme normally present in extremely minute quantities within a cell but whose concentration increases dramatically in the presence of substrate molecules.

in·duc·tion, *n.* 1. The act of bringing on or causing. 2. The bringing about of an electric or magnetic state in a body by the proximity (without actual contact) of an electrified or magnetized body. 3. The period from first administration of the anesthetic until consciousness is lost and the patient is stabilized in the desired surgical plane of anesthesia. 4. *In embryology*, the specific morphogenetic effect brought about by the action of one tissue upon another, acting through organizers or evocators. 5. The process whereby a lysogenic bacterium is caused to produce infective bacteriophage. 6. The process of initiating or increasing cellular production of an inducible enzyme. —**in·duct**, *v.;* —**in·duc·tor**, *n.*

in·duc·to·py·rex·ia (in-duck″to-pye-reck′see-uh) *n.* ELECTROPYREXIA.

in·duc·to·ther·my (in-duck′to-thur″mee) *n.* The application of energy to tissue through the agency of a high-frequency magnetic field; usually applied to local parts, but may be used to produce general artificial fever.

in·du·ra·tion (in″dew-ray′shun) *n.* 1. The hardening of a tissue or part, resulting from hyperemia, inflammation, or infiltration by neoplasm. 2. A hardened area of tissue. —**in·du·rate** (in′dew-rate) *v.;* —**in·du·ra·tive** (in′dew-ray″tiv) *adj.*

in·du·si·um (in-dew′zee-um) *n.,* pl. **indu·sia** (·zee-uh) A membranous covering.

indusium gri·se·um (gris′e-um) [NA]. A thin layer of gray matter in contact with the upper surface of the corpus callosum and continuous laterally with the gyrus fasciolaris and the dentate gyrus. Syn. *supracallosal gyrus.*

in·dus·tri·al (in-dus′tree-ul) *adj.* 1. Of or pertaining to industry. 2. Caused by certain types of work or by processes used in industry.

in·dwell·ing (in′dwel·ing) *adj.* Of a catheter or similar tube: left within an organ, duct or vessel for a time to provide drainage, prevent obstruction, or maintain a passage for administration of food or drugs.

-ine. A suffix designating (a) a *basic nitrogenous compound*, as morphine or purine; (b) a *halogen*, as bromine.

in·e·bri·ant (in-ee′bree-unt) *adj. & n.* 1. Inebriating; causing inebriation. 2. An agent that causes inebriation; an intoxicant.

in·e·bri·ate (in-ee′bree-ate) *v.* To make drunk; to intoxicate. —**in·e·bri·a·tion** (in-ee″bree-ay′shun) *n.*

in·ef·fi·ca·cious (in″ef-i-kay′shus) *adj.* Failing to produce the desired effect. —**in·ef·fi·ca·cy** (in-ef′i-kuh·see) *n.*

in·e·las·tic (in″e-las′tick) *adj.* Not elastic.

in·ert (in-urt′) *adj.* Lacking in physical activity, in chemical reactivity, or in an expected biologic or pharmacologic effect.

in·er·tia, *n.* 1. Dynamic opposition to acceleration, common to all forms of matter, including electrons and quanta. 2. Lack of activity; sluggishness.

in·ev·i·ta·ble abortion. An abortion that has advanced to a stage where termination of the pregnancy no longer can be prevented.

in ex·tre·mis (in ecks·tree′mis) At the end; at the last; at the point of death.

in·fant, *n.* A baby; often more specifically, a child 12 months old or less or, by some criteria, two years old or less. —**in·fan·cy,** *n.*

in·fan·ti·cide (in·fan′ti·side) *n.* 1. The murder of an infant. 2. The murderer of an infant.

in·fan·tile (in′fun·tile, ·til) *adj.* 1. Pertaining to or occurring during infancy or early childhood. 2. Like or characteristic of an infant.

infantile amaurotic familial idiocy. Either or both of the infantile forms of G_{M2} gangliosidosis: TAY-SACHS DISEASE and SANDHOFF'S DISEASE.

infantile autism. AUTISM (2).

infantile celiac disease. A form of the celiac syndrome of infants and young children, associated with an intolerance to the gliadin fraction of gluten found in wheat, oats, and rye. The patient presents marked abdominal distention, characteristic bulky, greasy, and foul-smelling stools, malnutrition, and growth retardation.

infantile cortical hyperostosis. A self-limited painful swelling of the soft parts of the lower jaw, associated with irritability and fever and characterized by periosteal proliferation of the mandible, occurring in the first 3 months of life. The clavicles, scapulae, and long bones are sometimes affected. Syn. *Caffey's disease.*

infantile diarrhea. An acute form of diarrhea in infants, frequently during the summer, caused by bacterial and viral infection of the intestinal tract or other body systems. The pathogens cannot always be identified, and there may be predisposing factors, such as allergic or nutritional ones.

infantile hypothyroidism. Hypothyroidism in infancy or early childhood, frequently congenital but may be acquired. Of the congenital types, cretinism is the most severe, but milder forms, often diagnosed later, exist. The acquired forms may be the result of pituitary dysfunction, ingestion of medications containing iodides or cobalt, deficiency of iodides, surgical excision of the thyroid, or lymphocytic thyroiditis or various chronic infections.

infantile sexuality. *In psychoanalysis*, the infant's or young child's capacity for, and pleasure derived from, experiences that are essentially sexual in nature, which may include excitation of erotogenic zones, as well as the sexual coloring of the child's relation to close and significant persons, especially the parents.

infantile spasm. A type of seizure seen in infants and young children, characterized by a sudden, brief, massive myoclonic jerk. The commonest form is the flexion spasm, salaam or jack-knife seizure in which the arms are flung forward and out and the legs flex at the hips, resembling the Moro reflex, or there may be simply a sudden nodding of the head or extension of the legs at the hips. Frequently there is an associated cry. The spasms tend to occur on waking or going to sleep and to run in series, and to be accompanied by hypsar-rhythmia and mental regression.

infantile spinal muscular atrophy. The commonest and most rapidly progressive heredo-familial form of progressive spinal muscular atrophy, becoming clinically manifest in the prenatal period or in the three months after birth and characterized by general hypotonia and atrophy of skeletal muscle, with death occurring in infancy or childhood. Syn. *Werdnig-Hoffmann atrophy.*

infantile uterus. A uterus normally formed, but arrested in development.

in·fan·ti·lism (in·fan'ti·liz·um, in'fun·ti·liz·um) *n.* 1. The persistence of infantile or childish physical, sexual, or mental characteristics into adolescent and adult life. 2. Specifically such a condition due to a malfunctioning organ or to a disease state, as in Down's syndrome. 3. In *psychiatry,* a behavioral pattern characteristic of the state of infancy prolonged into childhood or adult life, such as temper tantrums.

infant mortality rate. The number of deaths reported among infants under 1 year of age in a calendar year per 1,000 live births reported in the same year and place.

in·farct (in'fahrkt, in·fahrkt') *n.* A localized or circumscribed area of ischemic tissue necrosis due to inadequate blood flow.

in·farc·tec·to·my (in·fahrk·teck'tuh·mee) *n.* Removal by surgery of an infarct.

in·farc·tion (in·fahrk'shun) *n.* 1. The process leading to the formation or development of an infarct. 2. INFARCT.

in·fect, *v.* 1. To contaminate with a disease or a pathogenic organism. 2. To invade a body or organ, as by disease-producing pathogens; to cause an infection.

in·fec·tion, *n.* 1. The invasion of a host by organisms such as bacteria, fungi, viruses, protozoa, helminths, or insects, with or without manifest disease. 2. The pathologic state caused in the host by such organisms.

in·fec·tious (in·feck'shus) *adj.* Caused by infection.

infectious abortion. An infectious disease in animals which causes premature termination of gestation. The specific organisms are *Brucella abortus* for cattle, *Salmonella abortivoequina* for horses, and *Salmonella abortusovis* for sheep.

infectious arthritis. An acute or chronic inflammatory disease of a joint caused by invasion of the articular tissue by microorganisms. Infection is usually hematogenous in origin.

infectious disease. A disease due to invasion of the body by pathogenic organisms, which subsequently grow and multiply.

infectious equine anemia. A virus disease of solipeds (horse, mule, ass), characterized by fever, progressive anemia, edema, and emaciation. Syn. *swamp fever of horses.*

infectious hepatitis. An acute infectious inflammatory disease of the liver, often epidemic, due to hepatitis A virus, characterized in many cases by fever, hepatomegaly, and jaundice. There is oral transmission of the virus, and the incubation period varies from 2 to 6 weeks. Syn. *hepatitis A, short-incubation hepatitis.*

infectious lymphocytosis. A self-limited contagious and infectious disease, chiefly of children, with or without such systematic manifestations as fever and diarrhea, and characterized by a marked increase in small lymphocytes in the peripheral blood.

infectious mononucleosis. A usually benign, probably infectious disorder, now associated with the Epstein-Barr virus, characterized by irregular fever, sore throat, lymphadenopathy, splenomegaly, lymphocytosis with abnormal lymphocytes, and the development of an abnormally high serum concentration of a specific type of heterophil antibodies against sheep erythrocytes. Syn. *glandular fever, kissing disease, lymphocytic angina, monocytic angina, Pfeiffer's disease.*

infectious oral papillomatosis of dogs. A viral disease of young dogs, characterized by the formation of multiple pedunculated growths on the oral mucosa. The growths disappear spontaneously and leave the animal with a high degree of immunity.

in·fec·tive (in·feck'tiv) *adj.* 1. Capable of producing infection. 2. INFECTIOUS.

in·fe·cun·di·ty (in''fe·kun'di·tee) *n.* Sterility; barrenness.

in·fe·ri·ad (in·feer'ee·ad) *adv.* In anatomy, downward; in a superior-to-inferior direction.

in·fe·ri·or (in·feer'ee·ur) *adj.* In anatomy (with reference to the human or animal body as poised for its usual manner of locomotion): lower; nearer the ground or surface of locomotion. —**inferior·ly,** *adv.*

inferior articular process. One of a pair of processes projecting downward from a vertebral arch and articulating with a superior articular process of the vertebra next below.

inferior colliculus. One of the posterior pair of rounded eminences arising from the dorsal portion of the mesencephalon. It contains centers for reflexes in response to sound. Syn. *inferior quadrigeminal body.*

inferior dental canal. MANDIBULAR CANAL.

inferior frontal gyrus. The most inferior of the three frontal convolutions, situated in relation to the horizontal and ascending branches of the lateral sulcus.

inferior ganglion. 1. (of the glossopharyngeal nerve:) The lower sensory ganglion on the glossopharyngeal nerve located in the lower part of the jugular foramen. 2. (of the vagus nerve:) The lower sensory ganglion on the vagus nerve located below the jugular foramen and anterior to the upper part of the internal jugular vein.

in·fe·ri·or·i·ty complex. Repressed unconscious fears and feelings of physical or social inadequacy or both, which may result in excessive anxiety, and inability to function, or actual failure; or because of overcompensation, the individual may exhibit excessive ambition and develop skills, often in the area of the real or imagined handicaps.

inferior nasal concha. The scroll-like bone covered with mucous membrane situated in the lower part of the lateral nasal wall.

inferior olive. OLIVARY NUCLEUS.

inferior orbital fissure. A fissure of the orbit which gives passage to the infraorbital blood vessels, and ascending branches through the pterygopalatine ganglion.

inferior salivatory nucleus. An ill-defined nucleus anterior to the ambiguous nucleus which sends preganglionic autonomic fibers to the otic ganglion via the lesser petrosal nerve. Concerned in the regulation of secretion of the parotid gland.

in·fe·ro·lat·er·al (in″fur·o·lat′ur·ul) *adj.* Located below and to one side.

in·fe·ro·me·di·al (in″fur·o·mee′dee·ul) *adj.* Located below and in the middle.

in·fe·ro·pa·ri·etal (in″fur·o·pa·rye′e·tul) *adj.* Pertaining to the inferior portion of the parietal bone or parietal lobe of the brain.

in·fe·ro·pos·te·ri·or (in″fur·o·pos·teer′ee·ur) *adj.* Located below and behind.

in·fer·til·i·ty (in″fur·til′i·tee) *n.* Involuntary reduction in reproductive ability. —**in·fer·tile** (in·fur′til) *adj.*

in·fest, *v.* To live on or within the skin of the host, as in the case of certain insects and other arthropods in relation to their hosts.

in·fes·ta·tion, *n.* The state or condition of being infested. Often used as a synonym for infection in reference to animal parasites but, more properly, restricted to the presence of animal parasites, such as arthropods, on the surface of the host or in his environment.

in·fib·u·la·tion (in·fib″yoo·lay′shun) *n.* The act of clasping or fastening a ring, clasp, or frame to the genital organs to prevent copulation.

in·fil·trate (in·fil′trate, in′fil·) *v. & n.* 1. To pass into tissue spaces or cells, as fluids, cells, or other substances. 2. The material that has infiltrated.

in·fil·tra·tion, *n.* 1. A process by which cells, fluid, or other substances pass into tissue spaces or into cells. The various substances may be natural to the part or cell, but in excess; or they may be foreign to the part or cell. 2. The material taking part in the process.

in·firm, *adj.* In poor health; feeble.

in·fir·ma·ry, *n.* 1. A medical facility serving a live-in institution providing beds and treatment primarily on a short-term or nonintensive basis. 2. A hospital.

in·fir·mi·ty, *n.* 1. Poor health; feebleness. 2. An illness or disability.

in·flamed, *adj.* Exhibiting or in a state of inflammation.

in·flam·ma·ble, *adj.* Tending to ignite and burn readily.

in·flam·ma·tion, *n.* The reaction of the tissues to injury, characterized clinically by heat, swelling, redness, pain, and loss of function; pathologically, by vasoconstriction followed by vasodilatation, stasis, hyperemia, accumulation of leukocytes, exudation of fluid, and deposition of fibrin; and according to some authorities, the processes of repair, the production of new capillaries and fibroblasts,

organization, and cicatrization. —**in·flam·ma·to·ry,** *adj.;* **in·flame,** *v.*

inflammatory carcinoma. A fast-spreading carcinoma which may clinically resemble a benign inflammatory process, usually of the breast.

inflammatory polyps. A structure of polypoid configuration resulting from inflammation rather than epithelial proliferation.

in·fla·tion, *n.* Distention with air or fluid; or the process of filling with air or fluid to produce distention. —**in·flate,** *v.*

in·flu·en·za (in″floo·en′zuh) *n.* genit. sing. **influenzae** (-zee) An acute respiratory infection of specific viral etiology, usually epidemic, characterized by sudden onset of headache, myalgia, fever, and prostration. Three major antigenic types of the causative organism exist: the influenza A, B, and C viruses. Syn. **flu** *(colloq.).* —**influen·zal** (-zul) *adj.*

in·fold, *v.* To enclose within folds.

in·formed consent. Consent, preferably in writing, obtained from a patient regarding the use of specific therapy, especially in case of operative intervention, radiation, new or unusual use of drugs, or other unconventional treatment, or participation in a research project, or to allow use of medical or other records for research purposes, after the proposed procedure and risks involved have been explained fully in nontechnical terms. If the patient is a minor, or is incapable of understanding or communicating, such consent may be obtained from a close adult relative or legal guardian.

infra- A prefix meaning (a) *below, beneath, inferior;* (b) *within.*

in·fra·al·ve·o·lar (in″fruh·al·vee′uh·lur) *adj.* Below an alveolus, especially of a tooth.

in·fra·au·ric·u·lar (in″fruh·aw·rick′yoo·lur) *adj.* Below the external ear.

in·fra·ax·il·lary (in″fruh·ack′si·lerr·ee) *adj.* Situated below the axilla.

in·fra·car·di·ac (in″fruh·kahr′dee·ack) *adj.* Situated below or beneath the heart.

infracardiac bursa. The cephalic end of the embryonic mesenteric recess lying in the mesentery between the esophagus and right lung bud, or a small cyst in the right pulmonary ligament derived from it.

in·fra·cla·vic·u·lar (in″fruh·kla·vick′yoo·lur) *adj.* Below the clavicle.

in·fra·cli·noid (in″fruh·klye′noid) *adj.* Below one or more of the clinoid processes of the sphenoid bone.

in·fra·clu·sion (in″fruh·kloo′zhun) *n.* INFRAOCCLUSION.

in·fra·con·dyl·ism (in″fruh·kon′di·liz·um) *n.* Downward deviation of the mandibular condyles.

in·frac·tion (in·frack′shun) *n.* Incomplete fracture of a bone.

in·fra·den·ta·le (in″fruh·den·tay′lee) *n.* The highest anterior point on the gums between the central incisors of the mandible.

in·fra·di·an (in·fray′dee·un) *adj.* Recurring in or manifesting cycles less frequent than once a day.

in·fra·di·a·phrag·mat·ic (in″fruh-dye″uh-frag-mat′ick) *adj.* Situated below the diaphragm.

in·fra·ge·noid (in″fruh-glee′noid, -glen′oid) *adj.* Located below the glenoid cavity of the scapula.

in·fra·glot·tic (in″fruh-glot′ick) *adj.* Below the glottis.

in·fra·hy·oid (in″fruh-high′oid) *adj.* Situated below the hyoid bone.

in·fra·mam·ma·ry (in″fruh-mam′uh-ree) *adj.* Below a breast.

in·fra·nu·cle·ar (in″fruh-new′klee-ur) *adj.* In the nervous system, peripheral to a nucleus; below or away from the nucleus of a nerve.

in·fra·oc·clu·sion (in″fruh-o-klew′zhun) *adj.* Failure of one or more teeth to reach the plane of occlusion.

in·fra·or·bit·al (in″fruh-or′bi-tul) *adj.* Beneath or below the floor of the orbit.

in·fra·pa·tel·lar (in″fruh-puh-tel′ur) *adj.* Below the patella.

in·fra·red (in″fruh-red′) *adj. & n.* 1. Beyond the red end of the spectrum of visible light; pertaining specifically to the thermal region of the electromagnetic spectrum with wavelengths longer than those of the red end of the visible spectrum and shorter than those of microwaves. 2. Radiation or waves in the infrared region of the electromagnetic spectrum.

in·fra·scap·u·lar (in″fruh-skap′yoo-lur) *adj.* Below the scapula.

in·fra·spi·na·tus (in″fruh-spye-nay′tus) *n.* A muscle arising from the infraspinous fossa of the scapula and inserted into the greater tubercle of the humerus.

in·fra·spi·nous (in″fruh-spye′nus) *adj.* Below the spine of the scapula.

in·fra·ster·nal (in″fruh-stur′nul) *adj.* Below the sternum.

in·fra·tem·po·ral (in″fruh-tem′puh-rul) *adj.* Situated below the temporal fossa.

in·fra·ten·to·ri·al (in″fruh-ten-to′ree-ul) *adj.* Below the tentorium.

in·fra·troch·le·ar (in″fruh-trock′lee-ur) *adj.* Below a trochlea.

in·fra·um·bil·i·cal (in″fruh-um-bil′i-kul) *adj.* Below the navel; caudal to a transverse plane at the umbilicus.

in·fra·va·gi·nal (in″fruh-vaj′i-nul, -va-jye′nul) *adj.* Below the vagina.

in·fra·ver·sion (in″fruh-vur′zhun) *n.* 1. Downward turning of an eye. 2. INFRAOCCLUSION.

in·fra·ves·i·cal (in″fruh-ves′i-kul) *adj.* Below the urinary bladder.

in·fra·zy·go·mat·ic (in″fruh-zye-go-mat′ick) *adj.* Below the cheekbone.

in·fric·tion (in-frick′shun) *n.* The rubbing of a body surface with an ointment or liniment.

in·fun·dib·u·lar (in″fun-dib′yoo-lur) *adj.* 1. Resembling a funnel. 2. Pertaining to an infundibulum.

in·fun·dib·u·li·form (in″fun-dib′yoo-li-form) *adj.* Funnel-shaped.

in·fun·dib·u·lo·ma (in″fun-dib-yoo-lo′muh) *n.* A glioma, characteristically a pilocytic astrocytoma, involving the infundibulum (2).

in·fun·dib·u·lum (in″fun-dib′yoo-lum) *n.*, genit. **infundibu·li** (-lye), pl. **infundibu·la** (-luh) 1. A

funnel-shaped passage or part. 2. (of the hypophysis:) The stalk by which the neurohypophysis is attached to the tuber cinereum of the hypothalamus; consists of the medial eminence and infundibular stem. 3. (of the uterine tube:) The wide, funnel-shaped portion of the uterine tube at its fimbriated end. 4. (of the frontal sinus:) NASOFRONTAL DUCT. 5. [NA alt.] CONUS ARTERIOSUS.

in·fu·sion (in-few′zhun) *n.* 1. The process of extracting the active principles of a substance by means of water, but without boiling. 2. The product of such a process. 3. The slow injection of a solution into a vein or into subcutaneous or other tissue of the body, from which it is absorbed into the bloodstream.

infusion reaction. An acute febrile response to the infusion of pyrogenic agents present as contaminants in parenteral fluids.

In·fu·so·ria (in″few-sor′ee-uh, -zor′ee-uh) *n.pl.* 1. CILIATA. 2. Originally, a group including diverse kinds of microorganisms, principally protozoans. —**infuso·ri·al** (-ee-ul) *adj.*; **infuso·ri·an** (-ee-un) *n. & adj.*

in·ges·ta (in-jes′tuh) *n.pl.* Substances taken into the body, especially foods.

in·ges·tion (in-jes′chun) *n.* 1. The act of taking substances, especially food, into the body. 2. The process by which a cell takes up nutrients or foreign matter, such as bacilli or smaller cells. —**ingest,** *v.*; **inges·tive,** *adj.*

in·gra·ves·cent (in″gruh-ves′unt) *adj.* Increasing in severity.

in·gre·di·ent, *n.* Any substance that enters into the formation of a compound or mixture.

in·grown, *adj.* Of a hair or nail, grown inward so that the normally free end is embedded in or under the skin. —**in·grow·ing,** *adj.*; **in·growth,** *n.*

inguin-, inguino- A combining form meaning *groin, inguinal.*

in·gui·nal (ing′gwi-nul) *adj.* Pertaining to or in the vicinity of the groin.

inguinal canal. A canal about 4 cm long, running obliquely downward and medially from the deep to the superficial inguinal ring; the channel through which an inguinal hernia descends; it gives passage to the ilioinguinal nerve and to the spermatic cord in the male and to the round ligament of the uterus in the female.

inguinal hernia. A hernia through the inguinal canal. This variety constitutes more than four-fifths of all hernias.

inguinal ligament. The lower portion of the aponeurosis of the external oblique muscle extending from the anterior superior spine of the ilium to the tubercle of the pubis and the pectineal line. Syn. *Poupart's ligament.*

inguinal reflex. In the female, contraction of muscle fibers above the inguinal ligament, induced by stimulation of the skin over the upper and inner aspect of the thigh; comparable to the cremasteric reflex in the male.

inguinal region. The right or left lower abdominal region, on either side of the pubic region. The right inguinal region includes the abdominal surface covering the cecum and the vermiform appendix, the ureter, and the spermatic vessels. The left inguinal region includes the abdominal surface covering the sigmoid flexure of the colon, the ureter, and the spermatic vessels. Syn. *iliac region*.

inguinal triangle. An area bounded laterally by the inferior epigastric artery, medially by the rectus abdominis, and inferiorly by the medial half of the inguinal ligament.

inguino-. See *inguin-*.

in·gui·no·cru·ral (ing″gwi·no·kroo'rul) *adj*. Pertaining to the groin and the thigh.

in·gui·no·dyn·ia (ing″gwi·no·din'ee·uh) *n*. Pain in the groin.

in·gui·no·la·bi·al (ing″gwi·no·lay'bee·ul) *adj*. Pertaining to the groin and the labium.

in·gui·no·scro·tal (ing″gwi·no·skro'tul) *adj*. Relating to the groin and the scrotum.

INH Abbreviation for *isonicotinic acid hydrazide (isoniazid)*.

in·hal·ant (in·hay'lunt) *n. & adj*. 1. That which is inhaled, either from the atmosphere or as a medicine. 2. Occurring as, or used as, an inhalant.

in·ha·la·tion (in″huh·lay'shun) *n*. 1. The process of inhaling. 2. A medicinal substance to be inhaled; an inhalant.

in·ha·la·tor (in'huh·lay″tur, in″huh·lay'tur) *n*. A device for facilitating the inhalation of a gas or spray, as for providing oxygen or oxygen-carbon dioxide mixtures for respiration in resuscitation.

in·hale, *v*. To breathe in, as air or vapor; inspire.

in·hal·er (in·hail'ur) *n*. 1. A device containing a solid medication through which air is drawn into the air passages. 2. An atomizer. 3. An apparatus used to filter or condition air, etc., for inhalation, to protect the lungs against the entry of damp or cold air, dust, smoke, or gases.

inherent filter. The intrinsic filtration of a roentgen-ray tube, consisting of tube wall plus any oil layer or plastic layer in the mounting covering the aperture.

in·her·it, *v*. To derive from an ancestor.

in·her·i·tance, *n*. 1. The acquisition of characteristics by transmission of germ plasm from ancestor to descendant. 2. The sum total of characteristics dependent upon the constitution of the fertilized ovum; also, the total set of genes in the fertilized ovum.

in·hib·in (in·hib'in) *n*. 1. A postulated testicular hormone inhibiting the gonadotropic secretion of the adenohypophysis. 2. Generic name for various antibacterial substances occurring in normal saliva, urine, and other body fluids. 3. An antibiotic substance present in honey.

in·hi·bi·tion, *n*. 1. The act of checking or restraining the action of an organ, cell, or chemical, as the process of rusting, or the action of an enzyme. 2. *In psychiatry*, an unconscious restraining of or interference with an instinctual drive, leading to restricted patterns of behavior. —**in·hib·i·to·ry** (in·hib'i·to·ree) *adj*.; **in·hib·it**, *v*.

in·hib·i·tor, *n*. 1. A substance that checks or stops a chemical action. 2. A neuron whose stimulation stops, or suppresses, the activity of the part it innervates, or of a neuron on which it synapses. 3. Any substance or structure that prevents, slows, or stops a process.

in·i·on (in'ee·on) *n. In craniometry*, the external protuberance of the occipital bone.

ini·ti·a·tor, *n*. Any substance capable of starting a reaction as peroxide in the polymerization of acrylic resins.

in·ject, *v*. To introduce into, as a fluid into the skin, subcutaneous tissue, muscle, blood vessels, spinal canal, or any body cavity.

in·ject·able (in·jeck'tuh·bul) *adj. & n*. 1. Suitable for injection into the body. 2. Any drug preparation intended for injection.

in·jec·tion, *n*. 1. The act of injecting. 2. The substance injected. 3. A state of hyperemia.

in·ju·ry, *n*. 1. Any stress upon an organism that disrupts its structure or function, or both, and results in a pathologic process. 2. The resultant hurt, wound, or damage.

in·lay, *n*. A dental restoration that is formed outside the tooth cavity and subsequently secured in place with a cementing medium; usually made of metal or porcelain.

in·let, *n*. The entrance to a cavity.

inlet of the pelvis. The space within the brim of the pelvis; the superior pelvic strait.

in·ly·ing, *adj*. INDWELLING.

in·nate, *adj*. Dependent upon the genetic constitution; inherent; natural to the organism.

inner ear. INTERNAL EAR.

in·ner·va·tion, *n*. 1. The distribution of nerves to a part. 2. The amount of nerve stimulation received by a part. —**innervation·al**, *adj*.

in·no·cent, *adj*. Benign; not malignant; not apparently harmful.

innocent murmur. A murmur, systolic in time, occurring in the absence of any cardiac abnormality. Syn. *functional murmur, inorganic murmur, physiologic murmur*.

in·noc·u·ous, *adj*. Not injurious; harmless.

in·nom·i·nate (i·nom'i·nut) *adj. & n*. 1. Unnamed, nameless; a designation traditionally applied to certain anatomical structures. 2. The innominate bone (= HIPBONE).

innominate artery. BRACHIOCEPHALIC TRUNK.

innominate bone. HIPBONE.

in·nox·ious (i·nock'shus, in·nock'shus) *adj*. Innocuous; not harmful.

ino-, in- A combining form meaning (a) *fiber, fibrous;* (b) *muscle fiber, muscle*.

ino·chon·dri·tis (in″o·kon·drye'tis) *n*. Inflammation of fibrocartilage.

in·oc·u·la·ble (in·ock'yoo·luh·bul) *adj*. 1. Capable of transmission by inoculation. 2. Susceptible to inoculation for a disease. —**in·oc·u·la·bil·i·ty** (in·ock″yoo·luh·bil'i·tee) *n*.

in·oc·u·late (in·ock'yoo·late) *v*. 1. To introduce a small amount of a pathogenic substance such as bacteria, viruses, spores, antibodies, or antigens into (an organism), as for therapeutic, prophylactic, or experimental purposes. 2. *In bacteriology*, to plant microorganisms in or on (a culture medium). —**in·oc·u·la·tion** (in·ock″yoo·lay'shun) *n*.

in·oc·u·la·tor (in·ock'yoo·lay″tur) *n*. One who or

that which inoculates; an instrument used in inoculation.

in·oc·u·lum (in·ock'yoo·lum) *n.*, pl. **inocu·la** (·luh) A substance containing bacteria, spores, viruses, or other material for use in inoculation.

in·op·er·a·ble (in·op'ur·uh·bul) *adj.* Not to be operated upon; of or pertaining to a condition in which the prognosis is unfavorable if an operation is undertaken.

in·or·gan·ic (in''or·gan'ick) *adj.* Not organic.

inorganic murmur. INNOCENT MURMUR.

in·os·cu·late (in·os'kew·late) *v.* To unite by small openings, as in anastomosis.

in·os·cu·la·tion (in·os''kew·lay'shun) *n.* The joining of blood vessels by direct communication.

in·o·se·mia, in·o·sae·mia (in''o·see'mee·uh) *n.* 1. An excess of fibrin in the blood. 2. The presence of inositol in the blood.

ino·si·tol (i·no'si·tole, ·tol) *n.* Hexahydroxycyclohexane, $C_6H_6(OH)_6$, a sugarlike alcohol widely distributed in plants and animals. It is a growth factor for animals and microorganisms.

in·o·si·tu·ria (in''o·si·tew'ree·uh) *n.* The presence of inositol in the urine.

ino·trop·ic (in''o·trop'ick) *adj.* Modifying the force of muscular contractions.

in·pa·tient, *n.* A person admitted to a hospital who receives lodging and food as well as treatment.

in·put, *n.* 1. Energy or matter entering a structure or system of structures. 2. A stimulus or contribution; may be emotional or physical.

in·quest, *n. In legal medicine,* a judicial inquiry, as a coroner's inquest, for the purpose of determining the cause of death of one who has died by violence or in some unknown way.

in·qui·si·tion, *n.* An inquiry, especially one into the sanity or mental incompetence of a person.

in·sa·lu·bri·ty (in''sa·lew'bri·tee) *adj.* Unwholesomeness or unhealthfulness, as of air or climate.

in·san·i·tary, *adj.* Not sanitary; not in a proper condition to preserve health.

in·san·i·ty, *n.* 1. Loosely, any mental disorder or derangement. 2. *In legal medicine,* a mental disorder of such severity that the individual (a) is unable to manage his or her own affairs and fulfill social duties, (b) cannot distinguish "right from wrong," or (c) is dangerous to him- or herself or to others. —**in·sane,** *adj.*

in·scrip·tion, *n.* 1. The body or main part of a prescription that specifies the ingredients and amounts to be used. 2. *In anatomy,* INTERSECTIO.

in·sect, *n.* A member of the class Insecta of the phylum Arthropoda. In the adult, the body is segmented and is divided into head, thorax, and abdomen; there are three pairs of legs and a single pair of antennae. Usually there are one pair or two pairs of wings, but sometimes none.

in·sec·ti·cide (in·seck'ti·side) *n.* A substance that is used to kill insects. —**in·sec·ti·ci·dal** (in·seck''ti·sigh'dul) *adj.*

in·sec·ti·fuge (in·seck'ti·fewj) *n.* A substance that is used to repel insects.

in·se·cu·ri·ty, *n.* The state, feeling, or quality of being uncertain or unsafe; an attitude of apprehensiveness, as in respect to one's social status, circumstances, or safety.

in·sem·i·na·tion (in·sem''i·nay'shun) *n.* The introduction of semen into the female genital tract.

in·sen·si·ble, *adj.* 1. Incapable of sensation or feeling; unconscious. 2. Incapable of being perceived or recognized by the senses. —**in·sen·si·bil·i·ty** (in·sen''si·bil'i·tee) *n.*

in·ser·tion, *n. In anatomy,* the attachment of a muscle that is relatively more movable during contraction of that muscle.

in·sid·i·ous, *adj.* Coming on gradually or almost imperceptibly, as a disease whose onset is gradual or inappreciable.

in·sight, *n.* 1. Self-understanding; a person's ability to understand the origin, nature, mechanisms, and meaning of his behavior, feelings, and attitudes. 2. Superficially, the ability of a mentally disturbed person to recognize that he is ill.

in si·tu (in sigh'too, sigh'tew) In a given or natural position; undisturbed.

in·so·la·tion (in''so·lay'shun) *n.* 1. Exposure to the rays of the sun. 2. Treatment of disease by such exposure. 3. HEATSTROKE.

in·sol·u·ble (in·sol'yoo·bul) *adj.* Not soluble; incapable of dissolving in a liquid. —**in·sol·u·bil·i·ty** (in·sol''yoo·bil'i·tee) *n.*

in·som·ni·a (in·som'nee·uh) *n.* Sleeplessness; disturbed sleep; prolonged inability to sleep.

in·som·ni·ac (in·som'nee·ack) *n.* A person who is susceptible to insomnia.

in·spec·tion, *n. In medicine,* the examination of the body or any part of it by the eye.

in·sper·sion (in·spur'zhun) *n.* Sprinkling.

in·spi·ra·tion, *n.* The drawing in of the breath; inhalation. —**in·spire,** *v.*

in·spi·ra·to·ry (in·spye'ruh·to·ree) *adj.* Pertaining to the act of inspiration.

in·spis·sate (in·spis'ate, in'spi·sate) *v.* To make thick by evaporation or by absorption of fluid. —**inpissat·ed,** *adj.;* **in·spis·sa·tion** (in''spi·say'shun) *n.*

in·sta·bil·i·ty, *n.* 1. Lack of stability; insecurity of support or balance. 2. Lack of fixed purpose; inconstancy in opinions or beliefs.

in·stance, *n. In psychoanalysis,* the dominance or perseverance of one level of mental function in comparison to others.

in·step, *n.* The arch on the medial side of the foot.

in·stil·la·tion (in''sti·lay'shun) *n.* The introduction of a liquid into a cavity drop by drop.

in·stinct, *n.* 1. A precise, inherited pattern of unlearned behavior in which there is an invariable association of a particular series of responses with specific stimuli; an unconditioned complex reflex. 2. *In psychiatry,* a primary tendency or inborn drive, as toward life, sexual reproduction, and death.

in·stinc·tive, *adj.* Prompted or determined by instinct; of the nature of instinct.

in·stinc·tu·al (in·stink'choo·ul, ·tew·ul) *adj.* 1. INSTINCTIVE. 2. *In psychiatry,* pertaining to a psychic process or behavior which is a function of, or motivated by, the id, and which is more or less emotional, impulsive, and unreasoned.

in·stru·ment, *n.* A mechanical tool or implement; a mechanical device having a specific function. —**in·stru·men·tal,** *adj.*

in·stru·men·ta·tion (in″stroo·men·tay′shun) *n.* The use of instruments in treating a patient.

in·suf·fi·cien·cy (in″suh·fish′un·see) *n.* The state of being inadequate; incapacity to perform a normal function. —**insuffi·cient** (·unt) *adj.*

in·suf·fla·tion (in″suh·flay′shun) *n.* The act of blowing into, as blowing a gas, powder, or vapor into one of the cavities of the body.

in·suf·fla·tor (in′suh·flay″tur) *n.* An instrument used in insufflation.

in·su·la (in′sue·luh) *n.*, pl. & genit. sing. **insu·lae** (·lee) The portion of the cortex overlying the corpus striatum; it lies hidden from view in the adult brain at the bottom of the lateral fissure.

in·su·lar (in′sue·lur) *adj.* Pertaining to or characterized by islands or islets.

in·su·lin (in′suh·lin, ·sue·) *n.* The hypoglycemic hormone secreted by the beta cells of the islets of the pancreas; a protein with a molecular weight of about 6000. It participates, together with other biochemical entities, in regulating carbohydrate and fat metabolism. The principal effect of insulin may be to facilitate conversion of extracellular glucose to intracellular glucose 6-phosphate. Deficiency of insulin causes diabetes mellitus, for the treatment of which one or more forms of insulin may be used; these differ in speed and duration of action, mainly because of difference in solubility. Globin zinc insulin, which is insulin modified by addition of globin and zinc, has longer duration of action than regular insulin. Protamine zinc insulin, prepared by adding protamine and zinc to insulin, is a long-acting insulin. Isophane insulin contains crystals of insulin, protamine, and zinc, in such proportion (the isophane ratio) as to produce an intermediate-acting preparation. By using insulin modified by the addition of zinc, it is possible to prepare amorphous or crystalline forms of insulin, which differ in particle size and hence in solubility and duration of action; long-acting, intermediate-acting, and rapid-acting forms are available.

in·su·lin·ase (in′suh·li·nace, ·naze) *n.* An enzyme, present in liver, capable of inactivating insulin.

insulin atrophy. Atrophy of the subcutaneous, chiefly fatty tissues about the site of injection of insulin.

in·su·lin·emia, in·su·lin·ae·mia (in″sue·li·nee′mee·uh) *n.* The presence of insulin in the circulating blood.

in·su·li·no·ma (in″sue·li·no′muh) *n.* An islet-cell tumor that produces insulin.

insulin shock. Hypoglycemia with coma as a result of overdosage of insulin in diabetes or in the treatment of psychoses.

in·su·li·tis (in″sue·lye′tis) *n.* Inflammation of the islets of the pancreas.

in·su·lo·ma (in″sue′lo·muh) *n.* 1. ISLET-CELL TUMOR. 2. Specifically, INSULINOMA.

in·sult, *n.* Trauma or other harmful stress to tissues or organs.

in·sus·cep·ti·bil·i·ty, *n.* Lack of susceptibility.

in·take, *n. In medicine,* the total amount of fluid and other substances entering the body by ingestion or parenterally.

in·te·gra·tion, *n.* 1. The process of unifying different elements into a single whole. 2. The combination of bodily activities to cooperate in the welfare of the whole organism. 3. *In neurology,* the impingement of impulses from various centers upon one final, common pathway, resulting in an adaptive response. 4. The useful and harmonious incorporation and organization of old and new information and experiences into the personality, including the amalgamation of functions at different levels of psychosexual development.

in·teg·u·ment (in·teg′yoo·munt) *n.* A covering, especially the skin. —**in·teg·u·men·ta·ry** (in·teg″yoo·men′tuh·ree) *adj.*

in·tel·lect, *n.* The mind, the understanding, the reasoning or thinking power. —**in·tel·lec·tu·al,** *adj.*

in·tel·lec·tu·al·iza·tion, *n.* 1. Analysis of an emotional or social problem in rational, intellectual terms to the exclusion or neglect of feelings or practical considerations. 2. *In psychiatry,* a defense mechanism utilizing reasoning against consciously facing an unconscious conflict and the stress and affect connected with it.

in·tel·li·gence, *n.* 1. The understanding, intellect, or mind. 2. The ability to perceive qualities and attributes of the objective world, and to employ purposively a means toward the attainment of an end. 3. The general capacity of an organism endowed with a cerebrum to meet a novel situation by improvising a novel adaptive response, that is, to solve a problem and to engage in abstract thought. 4. Mental astuteness, insight, sagacity.

intelligence quotient. A numerical rating used to designate a person's intelligence; a ratio of an individual's performance on some standardized mental test as compared to the normal or average for age and even social situation. The most common such ratio is arrived at by dividing the mental age by the chronologic age (up to 16 years) and multiplying by 10. The most common scale employed in the United States is the Stanford-Binet test. The three grades of mental deficiency are marked by intelligence quotients of 69 or lower. Above 69 the classification is as follows: dull normal, 70 to 90; normal 90 to 110; superior, 110 to 125; very superior, 125 to 140; and genius, 140 and above. Abbreviated, I.Q.

intelligence test. Any task or series of problems presented to an individual to carry out or solve with a view toward determining the level of ability to think, conceive, or reason. Such tests seek to measure innate capacity rather than achievement resulting from formal education and are standardized by finding the average level of performance of individuals who by other, independent criteria are judged to have a certain degree of intelligence. Among the most widely used tests are the Cattell infant intelligence scale, the Stanford-Binet test, and the Wechsler-Bellevue intelligence scale.

in·tem·per·ance, n. Lack of moderation; immoderate indulgence, especially in alcoholic beverages. —**intemper·ate,** adj. & n.

in·tense, adj. 1. Extreme in degree; showing to a high degree the characteristic attribute. 2. Feeling deeply.

in·ten·si·fi·ca·tion, n. 1. An increase in intensity, concentration, or strength of any kind. 2. The condition occurring in cutaneous sensory disturbances in which certain sensations are abnormally vivid. 3. In radiology, the enhancement of the radiographic image produced on film by the use of intensifying screens or in fluoroscopy by means of an electron multiplier tube. —**in·ten·si·fy,** v.

in·ten·si·ty, n. 1. The state or condition of being intense. 2. Amount or degree of strength or power. 3. In radiology, the amount of energy per unit time passing through a unit area perpendicular to the line of propagation.

in·ten·sive, adj. Characterized by intensity; occurring or administered in high concentration.

intensive care. 1. The services, such as continuous close medical and nursing attention and the use of complex equipment, offered in a hospital for care of certain critically ill patients, with a view to restoring, when possible, normal life processes. 2. Informal. INTENSIVE CARE UNIT.

intensive care unit. An area within a hospital facility for patients whose health conditions require close medical attention, constant nursing care, and the use of complex medical equipment. Abbreviated, ICU.

in·ten·tion, n. 1. Aim, purpose. 2. A process or manner of healing.

intention tremor. A jerky, four-to-six-per-second tremor, which is absent when the limbs are inactive, but becomes more prominent as action continues and fine adjustment of the movement is demanded; indicative of disease of the cerebellum or its connections. Syn. ataxic tremor.

inter- A prefix meaning (a) between, among; (b) mutual, reciprocal.

in·ter·ac·i·nar (in″tur·as′i·nur) adj. Situated between acini.

in·ter·al·ve·o·lar (in″tur·al·vee′uh·lur) adj. Between alveoli.

in·ter·an·nu·lar (in″tur·an′yoo·lur) adj. 1. Between two cardiac valve rings. 2. Between nodes of Ranvier.

in·ter·ar·tic·u·lar (in″tur·ahr·tick′yoo·lur) adj. Situated between articulating surfaces.

in·ter·ar·y·te·noid (in″tur·ar′i·tee′noid) adj. Between arytenoid cartilages or muscles.

in·ter·atri·al (in″tur·ay′tree·ul) adj. Between the atria of the heart.

interatrial septum. The septum between the right and left atria of the heart. Syn. atrial septum.

in·ter·ax·o·nal (in″tur·ack′suh·nul) adj. Occurring between nerve fibers.

in·ter·brain, n. DIENCEPHALON.

in·ter·ca·lary (in·tur′kuh·lerr″ee) adj. Situated between; intercalated.

in·ter·ca·lat·ed (in·tur′kuh·lay″tid) adj. Placed or inserted between.

intercalated disk. Transverse thickening, representing an intercellular junction, occurring at the abutting surface of cardiac muscle cells.

in·ter·can·a·lic·u·lar (in″tur·kan″uh·lick′yoo·lur) adj. Situated between canaliculi, particularly of the small ducts of the breasts.

in·ter·cap·il·lary (in″tur·kap′i·lerr·ee) adj. Between capillaries.

intercapillary glomerulosclerosis. A nodular eosinophilic hyalin deposit at the periphery of the renal glomerular tufts in diabetic patients, usually associated with the clinical syndrome of hypertension, proteinuria, and edema.

in·ter·car·pal (in″tur·kahr′pul) adj. Between carpal bones.

in·ter·cav·ern·ous (in″tur·kav′ur·nus) adj. Situated between the two cavernous sinuses.

in·ter·cel·lu·lar (in″tur·sel′yoo·lur) adj. Between cells.

intercellular bridge. An attachment structure formed by the protrusion of apposing cell membrane processes from adjacent epidermal and other stratified squamous epithelial cells; once thought to constitute a continuous cytoplasmic connection between cells, but now known to include a narrow space separating the apposing processes.

in·ter·chon·dral (in″tur·kon′drul) adj. Between cartilages.

in·ter·cil·i·um (in″tur·sil′ee·um) n. The space between the eyebrows.

in·ter·cla·vic·u·lar (in″tur·kla·vick′yoo·lur) adj. Between the clavicles.

in·ter·col·um·nar (in″tur·kuh·lum′nur) adj. Between pillars or columns.

in·ter·con·dy·lar (in″tur·kon′di·lur) adj. Between condyles.

in·ter·con·dy·loid (in″tur·kon′di·loid) adj. INTERCONDYLAR.

in·ter·cor·o·nary (in″tur·kor′uh·nerr·ee) adj. Among or between coronary arteries.

in·ter·cos·tal (in″tur·kos′tul) adj. Between the ribs.

in·ter·cos·to·bra·chi·al (in″tur·kos″to·bray′kee·ul) adj. Associated with an intercostal space and the arm.

in·ter·coup·lur (in″tur·kup′lur) n. An apparatus used during the administration of an inflammable anesthetic to equalize the electric potential among anesthetist, patient, operating table, and anesthetic machine; designed to prevent explosions or fires due to static electricity.

in·ter·course, n. 1. Personal communication or interaction. 2. Specifically, sexual intercourse; coitus.

in·ter·cri·co·thy·rot·o·my (in″tur·krye″ko·thigh·rot′uh·mee) n. A cut into the larynx by transverse section of the cricothyroid ligament.

in·ter·cru·ral (in″tur·kroo′rul) adj. Situated between the crura, particularly of the superficial inguinal ring.

in·ter·cu·ne·i·form (in″tur·kew·nee′i·form) *adj.* Between cuneiform bones.

in·ter·cur·rent (in″tur·kur′unt) *adj.* Partially concurrent; occurring during the course of another condition.

intercurrent disease. COMPLICATING DISEASE.

in·ter·cus·pa·tion (in″tur·kus·pay′shun) *n.* The fitting together of the occlusal surfaces of the maxillary and mandibular teeth in jaw closure.

in·ter·cusp·ing (in″tur·kus′ping) *n.* INTERCUSPATION.

in·ter·den·tal (in″tur·den′tul) *adj.* Located or placed between teeth in the same arch.

in·ter·den·ti·um (in″tur·den′shee·um) *n.* The space between any two approximating teeth.

in·ter·dic·tion, *n. In legal medicine,* a judicial or voluntary restraint placed upon a person suffering from, or suspected of suffering from, a mental disorder, preventing that person from managing his or her own affairs or the affairs of others.

in·ter·dig·i·tal (in″tur·dij′i·tul) *adj.* Between digits.

in·ter·dig·i·ta·tion (in″tur·dij″i·tay′shun) *n.* 1. The locking or dovetailing of similar parts, as the fingers of one hand with those of the other; or of the ends of the obliquus abdominis externus muscle with those of the serratus anterior. 2. In closure of the jaws, the fitting of the cusps of the teeth of one arch fairly into the occluding sulci of the other arch. —**inter·dig·i·tate** (·dij′i·tate) *v.*

in·ter·duc·tal (in″tur·duck′tul) *adj.* Between ducts.

in·ter·face, *n.* A surface which forms the boundary between two phases or systems. —**in·ter·fa·cial,** *adj.*

in·ter·fas·cic·u·lar (in″tur·fa·sick′yoo·lur) *adj.* Between fasciculi or fascicles.

in·ter·fere, *v.* In horses, to strike one hoof against the shoe of one hoof against the opposite leg or fetlock.

in·ter·fer·ence, *n.* 1. *In physics,* the mutual action of two beams of light, or of two series of sound vibrations, or, in general, of two series of any types of waves when they coincide or cross. 2. The mutual extinction of two excitation waves that meet in any portion of the heart.

in·ter·fer·om·e·ter (in″tur·fe·rom′e·tur) *n.* An apparatus for the production and demonstration of interference fringes between two or more wave trains of light from the same area. It is chiefly used to compare wavelengths with a standard wavelength, by means of interference fringes.

in·ter·fer·on (in″tur·feer′on) *n.* A protein, formed by animal cells in the presence of a virus, or other inducing agent, that prevents viral reproduction and that is capable of inducing in fresh cells of the same animal species resistance to a variety of viruses.

in·ter·fi·bril·lar (in″tur·figh′bri·lur, ·fib′ri·lur) *adj.* Situated between the fibrils of tissues, as interfibrillar substances.

in·ter·fol·lic·u·lar (in″tur·fol·ick′yoo·lur) *adj.* Between follicles.

in·ter·fur·ca (in″tur·fur′kuh) *n.,* pl. **interfur·cae** (·kee, ·see) The region between, and at the base of, three or more normally divided tooth roots.

in·ter·gem·mal (in″tur·jem′ul) *adj.* Situated between the taste buds, or other buds.

in·ter·glu·te·al (in″tur·gloo·tee′ul) *adj.* Between the buttocks.

in·ter·go·ni·al (in″tur·go′nee·ul) *adj.* Between the two gonia (angles of the lower jaw).

in·ter·he·mal cartilages (in″tur·hee′mul). Nodules of cartilage which aid in the formation of the hemal arch of a vertebra.

in·ter·hemi·sphe·ric (in″tur·hem·is·ferr′ick, ·feer′ick) *adj.* Situated between the cerebral hemispheres.

in·ter·ic·tal (in″tur·ick′tul) *adj.* Between seizures or paroxysms.

in·te·ri·or (in·teer′ee·ur) *adj.* Situated within, with reference to a cavity, part, or organ.

in·ter·ja·cent (in″tur·jay′sunt) *adj.* Being, falling, or lying between or among others.

in·ter·la·bi·al (in″tur·lay′bee·ul) *adj.* Between the lips, or between the labia pudendi.

in·ter·la·mel·lar (in″tur·la·mel′ur) *adj.* Between lamellas.

in·ter·lam·i·nar (in″tur·lam′i·nur) *adj.* Situated between laminas.

in·ter·lig·a·men·tous (in″tur·lig″uh·men′tus) *adj.* Between ligaments.

in·ter·lo·bar (in″tur·lo′bur) *adj.* Situated or occurring between lobes of an organ or structure.

in·ter·lob·u·lar (in″tur·lob′yoo·lur) *adj.* Between lobules.

in·ter·mam·ma·ry (in″tur·mam′uh·ree) *adj.* Between breasts.

in·ter·mar·riage, *n.* 1. Marriage of blood relations. 2. Marriage between persons of different ethnic groups.

in·ter·max·il·lary (in″tur·mack′si·lerr″ee) *adj. & n.* 1. Between the maxillary bones. 2. INCISIVE BONE.

in·ter·me·di·ary, *adj. & n.* Intermediate; mediating, mediator.

in·ter·me·di·ate, *n.* 1. A biological substance or type necessary in the change of one form into another. 2. A chemical substance formed as part of a necessary step between one organic compound and another, as an amino acid or dye intermediate.

intermediate disk. In a muscle fiber, the thin, dark, doubly refractive disk in the middle of the isotropic disk. Not confined to a single myofibril, it passes through the entire diameter of a striated muscle fiber. Syn. *Krause's membrane, Z disk.*

intermediate host. A host in which the parasite passes its larval or asexual stage.

intermediate lobe of the hypophysis. PARS INTERMEDIA (1).

in·ter·me·din (in″tur·mee′din) *n.* A hypophyseal substance influencing pigmentation and found in greatest concentration in the intermediate portion of the hypophysis in certain animal species. A similar or identical principle active in man is now called melanocyte-stimulating hormone (MSH).

in·ter·me·dio·lat·er·al (in"tur-mee"dee-o-lat'ur-ul) *adj.* Both lateral and intermediate.

in·ter·me·dio·me·di·al (in"tur-mee"dee-o-mee'dee-ul) *adj.* Both intermediate and medial.

in·ter·me·di·us (in"tur-mee'dee-us) *adj. & n.* 1. Intermediate, middle. 2. NERVUS INTERMEDIUS.

in·ter·mem·bra·nous (in"tur-mem'bruh-nus) *adj.* Lying between membranes.

in·ter·me·nin·ge·al (in"tur-me-nin'jee-ul) *adj.* Between the dura mater and the arachnoid, or between the arachnoid and the pia mater, as intermeningeal hemorrhage.

in·ter·men·stru·al (in"tur-men'stroo-ul) *adj.* Between menstrual periods.

in·ter·ment (in-tur'munt) *n.* The burial of a body.

in·ter·meta·tar·sal (in"tur-met-uh-tahr'sul) *adj.* Between metatarsal bones.

in·ter·mi·tot·ic (in"tur-migh-tot'ick) *adj.* Pertaining to the interphase stage of mitosis.

in·ter·mit·tent (in"tur-mit'ent) *adj.* Occurring at intervals; not continuous; recurring periodically.

intermittent claudication. Cramplike pains and weakness in the legs, particularly the calves; induced by walking and relieved by rest; associated with atherosclerosis and perhaps with vascular spasm. Syn. *angina cruris, dysbasia intermittens angiosclerotica.*

intermittent fever. 1. MALARIA. 2. Any febrile state interrupted by periods of normal temperature.

intermittent pulse. A pulse in which one or more beats are absent or dropped.

in·ter·mu·ral (in"tur-mew'rul) *adj.* Situated between the walls of an organ.

in·ter·mus·cu·lar (in"tur-mus'kew-lur) *adj.* Situated between muscles.

in·tern, in·terne, *n.* A resident physician in a hospital, usually in the first year of service following graduation from medical school.

in·ter·nal, *adj.* Situated within or on the inside. —**in·ter·nad** (-nad) *adv.*

internal acoustic meatus. A passage in the petrous portion of the temporal bone which gives passage to the facial and eighth cranial nerves and internal labyrinthine or internal auditory vessels.

internal anal sphincter. A thickening of the inner circular (smooth) muscle layer of the anal canal.

internal arcuate fibers. Arching fibers within the substance of the medulla oblongata.

internal auditory meatus or **canal.** INTERNAL ACOUSTIC MEATUS.

internal capsule. A layer of nerve fibers on the outer side of the thalamus and caudate nucleus, which it separates from the lenticular nucleus; it is continuous with the cerebral peduncle and the corona radiata and consists of fibers to and from the cerebral cortex.

internal carotid plexus. A network of sympathetic fibers from the internal carotid nerve, surrounding the internal carotid artery and supplying fibers to its branches as well as to the abducens nerve, the pterygopalatine gan-

glion, the tympanic plexus, and the cerebral arteries.

internal derangement of the knee. A condition of abnormal joint mobility with painful symptoms, usually due to injury to a semilunar cartilage or cruciate ligament.

internal ear. The labyrinth, containing the essential organs of hearing and equilibrium, the sensory receptors of the vestibulocochlear nerve. The osseous labyrinth, consisting of the vestibule, the osseous semicircular canals, and the cochlea, houses the membranous labyrinth, which consists of the membranous semicircular canals, the cochlear duct, the utricle, saccule, and associated structures.

internal elastic coat. The internal elastic membrane of an artery.

internal genitalia. In the female, the uterus, uterine tubes, and ovaries; in the male, the prostate, ductus deferentes, and seminal vesicles.

internal hemorrhage. Bleeding that is concealed by escape into a cavity, as the intestine, peritoneal cavity, or within the cranium.

internal hemorrhoids. Hemorrhoids within the anal orifice or sphincter.

in·ter·nal·iza·tion (in-tur"nul-i-zay'shun) *n. In psychiatry,* an unconscious process by which the attributes, attitudes, or standards of the parents and cultural environment are taken within oneself.

internal medicine. The branch of medicine which deals with the diagnosis and medical therapy of diseases of the internal organ systems; the nonsurgical management of disease.

internal os. OS UTERI INTERNUM.

internal spermatic fascia. The inner covering of the spermatic cord and testis, continuous with the transversalis fascia at the deep inguinal ring.

in·ter·nar·i·al (in"tur-năr'ee-ul, -nair'ee-ul) *adj.* Situated between the nostrils.

internasal suture. The union between the nasal bones.

in·ter·na·tal (in"tur-nay'tul) *adj.* Situated between the nates, or buttocks.

international unit. The amount of a substance, commonly a vitamin, hormone, enzyme, or antibiotic, that produces a specified biological effect and is internationally accepted as a measure of the activity or potency of the substance. Such units are usually used only when the substance is not sufficiently pure to express its activity or potency in units of weight or volume. Abbreviated, I.U.

in·ter·neu·ron (in"tur-new'ron) *n.* Any neuron that is intermediary in position in a chain of neurons. Syn. *internuncial neuron, intercalated neuron.*

in·ter·neu·ro·nal (in"tur-new'ruh-nul) *adj.* Between neurons.

in·ter·nist (in-tur'nist) *n.* A physician who specializes in internal medicine.

in·ter·no·dal (in"tur-no'dul) *adj.* Between nodes.

in·ter·node (in'tur-node) *n.* The space between two nodes of a nerve fiber, as the internode between the nodes of Ranvier. Syn. *internodal segment.*

in·ter·nun·ci·al (in″tur·nun′see·ul, ·shul) *adj.* Serving as a connecting or announcing medium.

in·ter·oc·clu·sal (in″tur·uh·kloo′zul) *adj.* Situated between the occlusal surfaces of teeth in opposite arches.

interocclusal record. A record of the positional relationship of the teeth of opposite arches made of a plastic material, such as wax, plaster of Paris, or zinc oxide and eugenol paste.

in·tero·cep·tive (in″tur·o·sep′tiv) *adj.* Pertaining to an interoceptor.

in·tero·cep·tor (in″tur·o·sep′tur) *n.* Any sensory receptor situated in the viscera and responding to such stimuli as digestion, excretion, and blood pressure. Syn. *visceroceptor.*

in·tero·fec·tive (in″tur·o·feck′tiv) *adj.* Bringing about internal changes; referring specifically to the nerves of the autonomic nervous system. —**interofection** (·shun).

in·tero·ges·tate (in″tur·o·jes′tate) *adj. & n.* 1. Forming in the uterus. 2. During gestation. 3. An intrauterine fetus.

in·ter·ol·i·vary (in″tur·ol′i·verr·ee) *adj.* Between the olivary nuclei.

in·ter·os·se·ous (in″tur·os′ee·us) *adj.* Between bones.

in·ter·pal·a·tine (in″tur·pal′uh·tine) *adj.* Between the palatine bones.

in·ter·pal·pe·bral (in″tur·pal′pe·brul) *adj.* Between the palpebrae, or eyelids.

in·ter·pa·ri·etal (in″tur·pa·rye′e·tul) *adj.* 1. Between walls or layers. 2. Between the parietal bones. 3. Between the parietal lobules.

in·ter·pe·dun·cu·lar (in″tur·pe·dunk′yoo·lur) *adj.* Situated between the cerebral peduncles.

interpeduncular nucleus. A nucleus of the brainstem located between the cerebral peduncles, in which terminate the fibers of the habenulopeduncular tract.

in·ter·pha·lan·ge·al (in″tur·fuh·lan′jee·ul) *adj.* Between the phalanges of the fingers or toes.

in·ter·pleu·ral (in″tur·ploo′rul) *adj.* Between two layers of pleura, particularly of the visceral and parietal pleurae.

in·ter·po·si·tion (in″tur·puh·zish′un) *n.* The act of placing in between or in an intermediate position. —**interpose** (·poze′) *v.*

in·ter·pre·ta·tion, *n.* In psychiatry, the process by which the therapist communicates to the patient understanding or insight into some particular aspect of his or her problems or behavior on a deep level.

in·ter·prox·i·mal (in″tur·prock′si·mul) *adj.* Between two adjacent teeth.

interproximal space. The V-shaped space between the proximal surfaces of the teeth and the alveolar septum which is normally occupied by gingival tissue.

in·ter·pu·pil·lary (in″tur·pew′pi·lerr·ee) *adj.* Between the pupils.

interrupted respiration. Respiration in which either inspiration or expiration is not continuous but is divided into two or more sounds. Syn. *jerky respiration, cogwheel respiration.*

interrupted suture. A type of suture in which each stitch is tied and cut individually.

in·ter·scap·u·lar (in″tur·skap′yoo·lur) *adj.* Situated between the scapulae.

in·ter·sec·tio (in″tur·seck′shee·o) *n.,* pl. **inter·sec·ti·o·nes** (·seck″shee·o′neez) A cross line marking the site of union of two structures; intersection.

in·ter·seg·men·tal (in″tur·seg·men′tul) *adj.* Situated between or involving segments.

in·ter·sep·to·val·vu·lar (in·tur·sep″to·val′vew·lur) *adj.* Situated between a septum and a valve.

in·ter·sex (in′tur·secks) *n.* An individual whose constitution is intermediate between male and female, and who may be a true or a pseudohermaphrodite. —**in·ter·sex·u·al** (in″tur·seck′shoo·ul) *adj.;* **inter·sex·u·al·i·ty** (in″tur·seck″shoo·al′i·tee) *n.*

in·ter·sig·moid (in″tur·sig′moid) *adj.* Between portions of the sigmoid colon.

intersigmoid fossa. INTERSIGMOID RECESS.

intersigmoid recess. A peritoneal diverticulum occasionally found at the apex of the attachment of the sigmoid mesocolon.

in·ter·space, *n.* An interval between the ribs or the fibers or lobules of a tissue or organ.

in·ter·spi·nal (in″tur·spye′nul) *adj.* Situated between or connecting spinous processes; interspinous.

in·ter·spi·nous (in″tur·spye′nus) *adj.* Situated between or connecting spines or spinous processes.

in·ter·sti·ces (in·tur·sti′siz) *n.,* sing. **inter·stice** (·stis) Spaces or intervals.

in·ter·sti·tial (in″tur·stish′ul) *adj.* 1. Situated between parts; occupying the interspaces or interstices of a part. 2. Pertaining to the finest connective tissue of organs.

interstitial cell. A cell that lies between the germ cells or germinal tubules of a gonad, poorly represented in the adult human ovary. In the testis they are the Leydig cells.

interstitial-cell stimulating hormone. LUTEINIZING HORMONE. Abbreviated, ICSH.

interstitial-cell tumor. A usually benign tumor of the testis composed of interstitial cells (Leydig cells), which may be associated with hypersecretion of male sex hormones. Syn. *interstitioma, Leydig-cell tumor.*

interstitial cystitis. Chronic cystitis of unknown etiology with painful inflammation principally in the subepithelial connective tissue, extending in variable degree into the deeper tissues. Ulcers frequently accompany the process and are known as Hunner's ulcer or elusive ulcer.

interstitial irradiation therapy. Therapy of tumors with various types of implants or seeds containing radioactive material.

interstitial keratitis. An inflammatory process that involves the corneal stroma, characteristically seen in congenital syphilis.

interstitial myocarditis. 1. Inflammation of the myocardium characterized primarily by cellular infiltration of the interstitial tissues. 2. FIEDLER'S MYOCARDITIS.

interstitial nephritis. 1. Inflammation primarily localized in the renal interstitium and involving the tubules. It may be seen as an acute form in drug-induced reactions, a chronic form in congenital renal diseases, and an accompanying lesion in many cases of chronic glomerulonephritis. It is characterized by various degrees of mononuclear cell infiltrates, tubular atrophy and dilatation, and interstitial fibrosis and edema. 2. PYELONEPHRITIS.

interstitial pneumonia. Inflammation particularly of the stroma of the lungs including the peribronchial tissues and the septa between alveoli, often viral or rickettsial in origin.

interstitial pregnancy. Gestation in the uterine part of a uterine tube. Syn. *intramural pregnancy.*

interstitial salpingitis. Salpingitis marked by excessive formation of connective tissue in response to an inflammatory stimulus.

interstitial tissue. The intercellular connective tissue.

in·ter·sti·ti·o·ma (in″tur·stish·ee·o′muh) *n.* INTERSTITIAL-CELL TUMOR.

in·ter·sti·ti·um (in″tur·stish′ee·um) *n.* The interstitial tissue; intercellular connective tissue.

in·ter·tho·ra·ci·co·scap·u·lar (in″tur·tho·ras″i·ko·skap′yoo·lur) *adj.* Between the thorax and the scapula.

in·ter·tra·gic (in″tur·tray′jick) *adj.* Situated between the tragus and the antitragus.

in·ter·trans·verse (in″tur·tranz·vurce′) *adj.* Connecting the transverse processes of contiguous vertebrae.

in·ter·tri·go (in″tur·trye′go) *n.* An erythematous eruption of the skin produced by friction of adjacent parts. —**inter·trig·i·nous** (·trij′i·nus) *adj.*

in·ter·tro·chan·ter·ic (in″tur·tro″kan·terr′ick) *adj.* Between the trochanters.

in·ter·tu·ber·al (in″tur·tew′bur·ul) *adj.* Between tubers or tuberosities; specifically, between the ischial tuberosities.

in·ter·tu·ber·cu·lar (in″tur·tew·bur′kew·lur) *adj.* Situated between tubercles.

in·ter·tu·bu·lar (in″tur·tew′bew·lur) *adj.* Between tubes or tubules.

in·ter·ure·ter·ic (in″ter·yoo″re·terr′ick) *adj.* Situated between the ureters.

in·ter·vag·i·nal (in″tur·vaj′i·nul) *adj.* Situated between sheaths.

in·ter·val, *n.* 1. The time intervening between two points of time. 2. The lapse of time between two recurrences of the same phenomenon. 3. The space between any two things or parts of the same thing.

in·ter·vas·cu·lar (in″tur·vas′kew·lur) *adj.* Situated between vessels.

in·ter·ven·tric·u·lar (in″tur·ven·trick′yoo·lur) *adj.* Situated between or connecting ventricles.

interventricular foramen. Either one of the two foramina that connect the third ventricle with each lateral ventricle. Syn. *foramen of Monro.*

interventricular septum. The wall between the ventricles of the heart, largely muscular, partly membranaceous.

in·ter·ver·te·bral (in″tur·vur′te·brul) *adj.* Between vertebrae.

intervertebral disks. The masses of fibrocartilage between adjacent surfaces of most of the vertebrae.

intervertebral foramen. The aperture formed by the notches opposite to each other in the laminas of the adjacent vertebrae; a passage for the spinal nerves and vessels.

in·ter·vil·lous (in″tur·vil′us) *adj.* Between villi.

intervillous thrombosis. Coagulation of blood in the intervillous spaces of the placenta, usually seen near the end of pregnancy. Syn. *placentosis.*

in·tes·ti·nal (in·tes′ti·nul) *adj.* Of or pertaining to the intestine.

intestinal angina. ABDOMINAL ANGINA.

intestinal capillariasis. A chronic wasting disease caused by the nematode worm *Capillaria philippinensis*, characterized clinically by abdominal pain, muscle wasting, and edema, often leading to death within several months; observed in epidemics in the Philippines since 1966.

in·tes·tine (in·tes′tin) *n.* The part of the digestive tube extending from the pylorus to the anus. It consists of the small and large intestine. The small intestine extends from the pylorus to the junction with the large intestine at the cecum. Three divisions are described: the duodenum, the jejunum, and the ileum. The large intestine consists of the cecum (with the vermiform appendix), the colon, the rectum, and the anal canal.

in·tes·ti·num (in″tes·tye′num) *n.,* genit. **intesti·ni** (nye), pl. **intesti·na** (·nuh) INTESTINE.

in·ti·ma (in′ti·muh) *n.* TUNICA INTIMA; the innermost of the three coats of a blood vessel. —**inti·mal** (·mul) *adj.*

in·ti·mate, *adj.* 1. Pertaining to something which is innermost or of an essential character, as something which is reflective of the deepest part of oneself or someone very close to oneself. 2. Pertaining to highly personal matters, especially to emotions and drives, marriage, coitus. 3. Pertaining to detailed knowledge of a person or subject matter, as from a close and long association.

in·ti·mec·to·my (in″ti·meck′tuh·mee) *n.* Surgical removal of a portion of the intima of an artery, especially to relieve obstruction of blood flow.

in·toe·ing, *adj. & n.* Walking pigeon-toed.

in·tol·er·ance, *n.* 1. Lack of capacity to endure, as intolerance of light or pain. 2. Sensitivity, as to a drug.

in·tor·sion, in·tor·tion (in·tor′shun) *n.* 1. Inward rotation of a part. 2. *In ophthalmology,* an inward rotation of the vertical meridan, so that the superior point of the cornea turns nasally.

in·tort (in·tort′) *v.* To tilt the vertical meridian of the eye inward.

in·tox·i·cant (in·tock′si·kunt) *n. & adj.* 1. An agent capable of producing intoxication. 2. Producing intoxication.

in·tox·i·ca·tion (in·tock″si·kay′shun) *n.* 1. Poisoning, or the pathological state produced by a drug, a serum, alcohol, or any toxic substance. 2. The state of being intoxicated, especially the acute condition produced by overindulgence in alcohol; drunkenness. 3. A state of mental excitement or emotional frenzy.

intra- A prefix meaning *within, inside, inward, into.*

in·tra·ab·dom·i·nal (in″truh·ab·dom′i·nul) *adj.* Within the cavity of the abdomen.

in·tra·ac·i·nar (in″truh·as′i·nur) *adj.* Situated or occurring within an acinus.

in·tra·al·ve·o·lar (in″truh·al·vee′uh·lur) *adj.* Within an alveolus.

in·tra·am·ni·ot·ic (in″truh·am″nee·ot′ick) *adj.* Within or into the amniotic sac.

in·tra·ar·te·ri·al (in″truh·ahr·teer′ee·ul) *adj.* Within or directly into an artery.

in·tra·ar·tic·u·lar (in″truh·ahr·tick′yoo·lur) *adj.* Within a joint.

in·tra·atri·al (in″truh·ay′tree·ul) *adj.* Within an atrium, usually of the heart.

in·tra·bron·chi·al (in″truh·bronk′ee·ul) *adj.* Within a bronchus; for use within or by way of a bronchus, as an intrabronchial catheter.

in·tra·bron·chi·o·lar (in″truh·brong·kigh′o·lur, brong·kee·o′lur) *adj.* Within a bronchiole.

in·tra·cal·i·ce·al, in·tra·cal·y·ce·al (in″truh·kal′i·see·ul) *adj.* Within a calix.

in·tra·can·a·lic·u·lar (in″truh·kan″uh·lick′yoo·lur) *adj.* Located within a canaliculus.

intracanalicular fibroadenoma. A benign breast tumor with proliferation of connective tissue causing distortion of the glands and ducts in the tumor.

in·tra·cap·su·lar (in″truh·kap′sue·lur) *adj.* Within the fibrous capsule of a joint.

in·tra·car·di·ac (in″truh·kahr′dee·ack) *adj.* Within the heart.

in·tra·cav·ern·ous (in″truh·kav′ur·nus) *adj.* Within a cavernous sinus.

intracavernous aneurysm. A nonfistulous aneurysm of the internal carotid artery within the cavernous sinus. Syn. *subclinoid aneurysm.*

in·tra·cav·i·tary (in″truh·kav′i·terr·ee) *adj.* Within a cavity.

in·tra·cel·lu·lar (in″truh·sel′yoo·lur) *adj.* Within a cell.

in·tra·cer·e·bel·lar (in″truh·serr″e·bel′ur) *adj.* Within the cerebellum.

in·tra·cer·e·bral (in″truh·serr′e·brul, ·se·ree′brul) *adj.* Within or into the cerebrum.

in·tra·cis·ter·nal (in″truh·sis·tur′nul) *adj.* In a cistern, usually the cisterna magna.

in·tra·cor·ne·al (in″truh·kor′nee·ul) *adj.* 1. Within the cornea of the eye. 2. Within the horny layer of the skin.

in·tra·cor·pus·cu·lar (in″truh·kor·pus′kew·lur) *adj.* Within a corpuscle, usually an erythrocyte.

in·tra·cra·ni·al (in″truh·kray′nee·ul) *adj.* Within the cranium, as intracranial pressure or calcifications.

in·trac·ta·ble (in·track′tuh·bul) *adj.* Not easily managed.

in·tra·cu·ta·ne·ous (in″truh·kew·tay′nee·us) *adj.* Within the skin.

in·tra·cu·tic·u·lar (in″truh·kew·tick′yoo·lur) *adj.* Within the epidermis.

in·tra·cys·tic (in″truh·sis′tick) *adj.* Situated or occurring within a cyst or bladder.

in·tra·cy·to·plas·mic (in″truh·sigh″to·plaz′mick) *adj.* Within or surrounded by cytoplasm.

in·tra·der·mal (in″truh·dur′mul) *adj.* Within the dermis.

intradermal nevus. A skin lesion containing melanocytes located chiefly or entirely in the dermis, with little or no dermoepidermal junctional proliferation.

in·tra·duc·tal (in″truh·duck′tul) *adj.* Within a duct.

in·tra·du·ral (in″truh·dew′rul) *adj.* Within the dura mater.

in·tra·epi·der·mal (in″truh·ep·i·dur′mul) *adj.* Within the epidermis.

in·tra·epi·the·li·al (in″truh·ep·i·theel′ee·ul) *adj.* Within the epithelial layer.

in·tra·eryth·ro·cyt·ic (in″truh·e·rith″ro·sit′ick) *adj.* Within erythrocytes.

in·tra·esoph·a·ge·al (in″truh·e·sof″uh·jee′ul) *adj.* Within the esophagus.

in·tra·gen·ic (in″truh·jen′ick, ·jee′nick) *adj.* Within a gene.

in·tra·glu·te·al (in″truh·gloo·tee′ul, ·gloo′tee·ul) *adj.* Within a buttock.

in·tra·group (in″truh·groop′) *adj.* Within a group.

in·tra·he·pat·ic (in″truh·he·pat′ick) *adj.* Within the liver.

in·tra·le·sion·al (in″truh·lee′zhun·ul) *adj.* Within a lesion, either by natural occurrence or introduction.

in·tra·lig·a·men·ta·ry (in″truh·lig·uh·men′tuh·ree) *adj.* INTRALIGAMENTOUS.

in·tra·lig·a·men·tous (in″truh·lig·uh·men′tus) *adj.* 1. Within the broad ligament of the uterus. 2. Within a ligament.

in·tra·lo·bar (in″truh·lo′bar) *adj.* Within a lobe.

in·tra·lob·u·lar (in″truh·lob′yoo·lur) *adj.* Within a lobule.

in·tra·lu·mi·nal (in″truh·lew′mi·nul) *adj.* Within the lumen of a hollow or tubelike structure.

in·tra·mam·ma·ry (in″truh·mam′uh·ree) *adj.* Within breast tissue.

in·tra·med·ul·lary (in″truh·med′yoo·lerr·ee) *adj.* 1. Within the substance of the spinal cord or medulla oblongata. 2. Within the substance of the bone marrow, as an intramedullary nail. 3. Within the substance of the adrenal medulla.

intramedullary nail. A metal rod or nail inserted into the medullary canal of a tubular bone to provide internal immobilization of fractures. It is long enough to pass across the fracture site to obtain fixation of both fragments of the bone.

in·tra·mem·bra·nous (in″truh·mem′bruh·nus) *adj.* Developed or taking place within a membrane.

intramembranous bone formation. The formation of bone by or within a connective tissue without involvement of a cartilage stage.

in·tra·men·stru·al (in″truh·men′stroo·ul) *adj.* Occurring during a menstrual period.

in·tra·mu·co·sal (in″truh·mew·ko′sul, ·zul) *adj.* Within a mucous membrane.

in·tra·mu·ral (in″truh·mew′rul) *adj.* Within the substance of the walls of an organ, as intramural fibroid of the uterus.

intramural pregnancy. INTERSTITIAL PREGNANCY.

in·tra·mus·cu·lar (in″truh·mus′kew·lur) *adj.* Within or into the substance of a muscle.

in·tra·myo·car·di·al (in″truh·migh·o·kahr′dee·u) *adj.* Within the myocardium.

in·tra·myo·me·tri·al (in"truh·migh"o·mee'tree-ul) *adj.* Within the muscular part of the uterine wall.

in·tra·na·sal (in"truh·nay'zul) *adj.* Within the cavity of the nose.

in·tra·neu·ral (in"truh·new'rul) *adj.* Within a nerve.

in·tra·nu·cle·ar (in"truh·new'klee·ur) *adj.* Within a nucleus.

in·tra·oc·u·lar (in"truh·ock'yoo·lur) *adj.* Within the globe of the eye.

intraocular pressure or **tension.** The pressure within the eyeball, which in the normal population usually ranges between 14 and 20 mm of mercury; aqueous humor dynamics are mainly responsible for maintaining the intraocular pressure.

in·tra·op·er·a·tive (in"truh·op'ur·uh·tiv) *adj.* During the time of a surgical operation.

in·tra·op·tic (in"truh·op'tick) *adj.* Within the eye.

in·tra·oral (in"truh·o'rul) *adj.* Within the mouth.

in·tra·or·bit·al (in"truh·or'bi·tul) *adj.* Within an orbit.

in·tra·pan·cre·at·ic (in"truh·pan"kree·at'ick) *adj.* Within the pancreas.

in·tra·pa·ren·chy·mal (in"truh·pa·renk'i·mul) *adj.* Within the parenchyma of an organ.

in·tra·pa·ri·e·tal (in"truh·pa·rye'e·tul) *adj.* 1. Within the wall of an organ. 2. Within the parietal region of the cerebrum. 3. Within the body wall.

in·tra·par·tum (in"truh·pahr'tum) *adj.* Occurring during parturition.

in·tra·pel·vic (in"truh·pel'vick) *adj.* Within the pelvic cavity.

in·tra·peri·car·di·al (in"truh·perr·i·kahr'dee·ul) *adj.* Within the pericardial sac.

in·tra·peri·to·ne·al (in"truh·perr·i·tuh·nee'ul) *adj.* Within the peritoneum, or peritoneal cavity.

in·tra·pha·lan·ge·al (in"truh·fuh·lan'jee·ul) *adj.* Within a phalanx or phalanges.

in·tra·pleu·ral (in"truh·ploo'rul) *adj.* Within the pleura or pleural cavity.

in·tra·psy·chic (in"truh·sigh'kick) *adj.* Pertaining to that which takes place within the mind or psyche.

in·tra·pul·mo·nary (in"truh·pool'muh·nerr·ee) *adj.* Within the parenchyma of a lung.

in·tra·re·nal (in"truh·ree'nul) *adj.* Within a kidney or kidneys.

in·tra·scap·u·lar (in"truh·skap'yoo·lur) *adj.* Within the scapula.

in·tra·scro·tal (in"truh·skro'tul) *adj.* Within the scrotal sac.

in·tra·seg·men·tal (in"truh·seg·men'tul) *adj.* Within a segment.

in·tra·sel·lar (in"truh·sel'ur) *adj.* Within the sella turcica.

in·tra·spi·nal (in"truh·spye'nul) *adj.* Within the spinal canal.

in·tra·spi·nous (in"truh·spye'nus) *adj.* Within a spinous process, usually of a vertebra.

in·tra·splen·ic (in"truh·splen'ick, splee'nick) *adj.* Within the spleen.

in·tra·stro·mal (in"truh·stro'mul) *adj.* Within the stroma of an organ, part, or tissue.

in·tra·sy·no·vi·al (in"truh·si·no'vee·ul) *adj.* 1. Within a synovial cavity. 2. Within a synovial membrane.

in·tra·the·cal (in"truh·theek'ul) *adj.* In the subarachnoid space.

in·tra·tho·rac·ic (in"truh·tho·ras'ick) *adj.* Within the thoracic cavity.

in·tra·ton·sil·lar (in"truh·ton'si·lur) *adj.* Within a tonsil.

in·tra·tra·che·al (in"truh·tray'kee·ul) *adj.* Within the trachea.

in·tra·tro·chan·ter·ic (in"truh·tro'kan·terr'ick) *adj.* Within a trochanter.

in·tra·tu·bal (in"truh·tew'bul) *adj.* Within a tube; specifically, within a uterine tube.

in·tra·tu·bu·lar (in"truh·tew'bew·lur) *adj.* Within a tubule.

in·tra·um·bil·i·cal (in"truh·um·bil'i·kul) *adj.* Within the umbilicus.

in·tra·ure·ter·al (in"truh·yoo·ree'tur·ul) *adj.* Within a ureter.

in·tra·ure·thral (in"truh·yoo·ree'thrul) *adj.* Within the urethra.

in·tra·uter·ine (in"truh·yoo'tur·in, ·ine) *adj.* Within the uterus.

intrauterine contraceptive device. Any mechanical device placed in the uterine cavity to prevent implantation or growth of the embryo. Abbreviated, IUD.

in·tra·vag·i·nal (in"truh·vaj'i·nul) *adj.* 1. Within the female vagina. 2. Within a tendon sheath.

in·tra·vas·cu·lar (in"truh·vas'kew·lur) *adj.* Within the blood vessels.

in·tra·ve·nous (in"truh·vee'nus) *adj.* Within, or into, the veins.

intravenous pyelogram. A pyelogram in which the contrast material is given intravenously and excreted by the kidneys to permit their radiographic visualization; an intravenous urogram.

in·tra·ven·tric·u·lar (in"truh·ven·trick'yoo·lur) *adj.* Located, or occurring, within a ventricle.

in·tra·ver·te·bral (in"truh·vur'te·brul) *adj.* Within a vertebra.

in·tra·ves·i·cal (in"truh·ves'i·kul) *adj.* Within the urinary bladder.

in·tra·vi·tal (in"truh·vye'tul) *adj.* Occurring during life; pertaining to the tissues or cells of living organisms.

intravital stain. A dye, introduced by injection into the body of man or animal, which stains certain tissues or cells selectively; the stain must be minimally toxic so as not to kill cells. Syn. *vital stain.*

in·trin·sic (in·trin'sick) *adj.* Inherent; situated within; peculiar to a part; originating from or due to causes or factors within a body, organ, or part.

intrinsic asthma. Asthma caused by factors such as bronchial or other infection of the respiratory tract or by unknown factors.

intrinsic factor. A substance, produced by the stomach, which combines with the extrinsic factor (vitamin B_{12}) in food to yield an antianemic principle; lack of the intrinsic factor is believed to be a cause of pernicious anemia. Syn. *intrinsic factor of Castle.*

intrinsic thromboplastin. Any of several lipid-rich clot accelerators present in blood, primarily in blood platelets.

in·tro- A prefix meaning *inward, into.*

in·tro·ces·sion (in″tro·sesh′un) *n.* A depression, as of a surface.

in·tro·flex·ion (in″tro·fleck′shun) *n.* A bending in; inward flexion.

in·troi·tus (in·tro′i·tus) *n.,* pl. **introitus** An aperture or entrance, particularly the entrance to the vagina. —**introi·tal** (·tul) *adj.*

in·tro·jec·tion (in″tro·jeck′shun) *n. In psychiatry* and *psychoanalysis,* the symbolic absorption into and toward oneself of concepts and feelings generated toward another person or object; an unconscious process which may serve as a defense against conscious recognition of overwhelming or intolerable impulses. Its effect in mental disorders is to motivate irrational behavior toward oneself, such as self-neglect or suicide arising from aggression stimulated by others, then introjected.

in·tro·mis·sion (in″tro·mish′un) *n.* Insertion, the act of putting in, the introduction of one body into another, as of the penis into the vagina.

in·tro·mit·tent (in″tro·mit′unt) *adj.* Conveying or allowing to pass into or within, as into a cavity; refers usually to the penis, which carries the semen into the vagina.

Intropin. A trademark for dopamine.

in·tro·spec·tion (in″tro·speck′shun) *n.* The act of looking inward, as into one's own mind and feelings.

in·tro·ver·sion (in″tro·vur′zhun) *n.* 1. A turning within, as a sinking within itself of the uterus. 2. *In psychiatry,* the preoccupation with oneself, with concomitant reduction of interest in the outside world.

[1]in·tro·vert (in″tro′vurt′) *v.* To turn one's interests to oneself rather than to external things.

[2]in·tro·vert (in′tro·vurt) *n.* A person whose interests are directed inwardly upon himself and not toward the outside world.

in·tu·ba·tion (in″tew·bay′shun) *n.* The introduction of a tube into a hollow organ to keep it open, especially into the trachea to ensure the passage of air.

intubation tube. A tube for insertion through the larynx into the trachea to maintain an airway, primarily used in anesthesia or cardiopulmonary resuscitation.

in·tu·i·tion, *n.* 1. Knowledge of something attained without conscious reasoning. 2. A sudden understanding or insight. —**intuition·al,** *adj.*

in·tu·mes·cence (in″tew·mes′unce) *n.* 1. A swelling of any kind, as an increase of the volume of any organ or part of the body. 2. The process of becoming swollen. 3. *Obsol. In neuroanatomy,* the cervical and lumbar enlargements. —**intumes·cent** (·unt) *adj.*

intumescent cataract. A cataract presenting a swollen appearance from breakdown of lens protein with an increase in osmotic pressure, resulting in imbibition of water.

in·tus·sus·cep·tion (in″tuh·suh·sep′shun) *n.* The receiving of one part within another; especially, the invagination, slipping, or passage of one part of the intestine into another, occurring usually in young children. Acute intussusception is characterized by paroxysmal pain, vomiting, the presence of a sausage-shaped tumor in the lower abdomen, and the passage of blood and mucus per rectum.

in·tus·sus·cep·tum (in″tuh·suh·sep′tum) *n.* In intussusception, the invaginated portion of intestine.

in·tus·sus·cip·i·ens (in″tuh·suh·sip′ee·enz) *n.* In intussusception, the segment of the intestine receiving the other segment.

in·u·lin (in′yoo·lin) *n.* A polysaccharide, $(C_6H_{10}O_5)_n$, in Jerusalem artichoke and certain other plants, made up of polymerized fructofuranose units, and yielding fructose on hydrolysis; used to measure glomerular filtration rate (inulin clearance).

in·unc·tion (in·unk′shun) *n.* 1. The act of rubbing an oily or fatty substance into the skin. 2. The substance thus used.

in ute·ro (in yoo′te·ro) Within the uterus; not yet born.

in vac·uo (in vack′yoo·o) In a vacuum; in a space from which most of the air has been exhausted.

in·vade, *v.* To enter or penetrate into an area or sphere of which one is not naturally a part, usually with resultant injury to that part, as a virus invades a cell, or cancer invades healthy tissue. —**in·vad·er,** *n.*

in·vag·i·na·tion (in·vaj′i·nay′shun) *n.* 1. The act of ensheathing or becoming ensheathed. 2. The process of burrowing or infolding to form a hollow space within a previously solid structure, as the invagination of the nasal mucosa within a bone of the skull to form a paranasal sinus. 3. INTUSSUSCEPTION. 4. *In embryology,* the infolding of a part of the wall of the blastula to form a gastrula. —**in·vag·i·nate** (in·vaj′i·nate) *v.*

[1]in·va·lid (in′vuh·lid) *n.* A person with a long-term, usually acquired, disability or illness which seriously limits self-sufficiency, as one confined to bed or wheelchair. —**invalid·ism** (·iz·um) *n.*

[2]in·val·id (in·val′id) *adj.* Not valid; unsound.

invariably lethal dose. The dose of an injurious agent (drug, virus, radiation) given to a population of animals or man, such that 100 percent die within a given time period. Symbol, LD 100.

in·va·sion, *n.* 1. One period in the course of disease, especially an infectious disease, during which the pathogen multiplies and is distributed preceding prodromal signs and symptoms. 2. The process whereby bacteria or other microorganisms enter the body.

in·va·sive (in·vay′siv) *adj.* 1. Tending to invade healthy cells or tissues; said of microorganisms or tumors. 2. Characterized by instrumental penetration of the viscera or nonsuperficial tissues of the body; said especially of diagnostic or therapeutic techniques such as biopsy, catheterization. —**invasive·ness** (·nis) *n.*

in·verse, *adj.* Inverted, reversed; reciprocal; opposite.

in·ver·sion (in·vur′zhun) *n.* 1. Reversal in order

form, or structure; specifically, a change in configuration or orientation resulting in a structure that is inside out, upside down, backward, or opposite with respect to a prior or more usual one, as: *in chemistry*, the alteration of configuration about a chiral center to produce the enantiomorphic isomer, or, *in genetics*, the reattachment of a detached chromosome segment in its original place but reversed end for end, so that the order of its genetic material with respect to the rest of the chromosome is the opposite of what it was. 2. A turning inward. 3. HOMOSEXUALITY.

¹in·vert (in·vurt′) v. 1. To turn inside out, outside in, upside down; to reverse in position or relationship, especially from one that is natural to one less usual. 2. To turn inward.

²in·vert (in′vurt) adj. & n. 1. INVERTED. 2. A homosexual.

invert sugar. A mixture of equal parts of glucose and levulose obtained by hydrolysis of sucrose, the sign of optical rotation having been inverted from (+) for sucrose, to (−) for the mixture.

in·vest, v. To envelop, enclose, cover.

in·vest·ment, n. A sheath; a covering.

in·vet·er·ate (in·vet′ur·ut) adj. Long established, chronic, resisting treatment.

in·vi·ril·i·ty (in″vi·ril′i·tee) n. IMPOTENCE.

in vi·tro (in vee′tro) In glass; referring to a process or reaction carried out in a culture dish or test tube.

in vi·vo (in vee′vo) In the living organism.

in·vo·lu·crum (in″vo·lew′krum) n., pl. involu·cra (·kruh) 1. The covering of a part. 2. New bone laid down by periosteum around a sequestrum in osteomyelitis.

in·vol·un·tary, adj. 1. Performed or acting independently of the will, as involuntary contractions of visceral muscles. 2. Resulting from an irresistible impulse or accident, rather than from a conscious or purposeful act.

involuntary movements. Unintentional bodily movements; applied particularly to movements that characterize extrapyramidal disorders, such as athetosis, chorea, and ballism.

involuntary nervous system. AUTONOMIC NERVOUS SYSTEM.

in·vo·lute (in′vo·lewt) adj. In biology, rolled up, as the edges of certain leaves in the bud.

in·vo·lu·tion (in″vo·lew′shun) n. 1. A turning or rolling inward. 2. The retrogressive change to their normal condition that certain organs undergo after fulfilling their functional purposes, as the uterus after pregnancy. 3. The period of regression or the process of decline or decay that occurs in all organ systems of the body after middle life. —involution·al (·ul) adj.

involutional depression. INVOLUTIONAL MELANCHOLIA.

involutional melancholia. A sometimes prolonged severe mental disorder occurring in late middle life, usually characterized by depression and sometimes by paranoid ideas; manifested by excessive worry, narrow mental interests, lack of adaptability, severe insomnia, guilt, anxiety, agitation, delusional and nihilistic ideas, and somatic concerns.

involutional psychosis. INVOLUTIONAL MELANCHOLIA.

involution of the uterus. The return of the uterus to its usual mass and physiologic state after childbirth.

iod-, iodo-. A combining form meaning (a) *iodine*; (b) *violet*.

Iodamoeba bütsch·lii (bootch′lee·eye). A species of small, sluggish ameba that is nonpathogenic but is parasitic in the large intestine of man.

io·dide (eye′uh·dide) n. Any binary compound, such as a salt or ester, containing iodine having a negative valence of 1.

io·dip·a·mide (eye″o·dip′uh·mide) n. 3,3′-(Adipoyldiimino)-bis[2,4,6-triiodobenzoic acid], $C_{20}H_{14}I_6N_2O_6$, a roentgenographic contrast medium; used as the methylglucamine (meglumine) and sodium salts.

io·dism (eye′uh·diz·um) n. A condition arising from the excessive or prolonged use of iodine or iodine compounds; marked by frontal headache, coryza, ptyalism, and various skin eruptions, especially acne.

iodized oil. An iodine addition product of vegetable oils, containing 38 to 42% of organically combined iodine. Used for the therapeutic effect of iodine and as an x-ray contrast medium.

io·do·al·phi·on·ic acid (eye·o″do·al′fee·on·ick). 3-(4-Hydroxy-3,5-diiodophenyl)-2-phenylpropionic acid, $C_{15}H_{12}I_2O_3$, used orally as a contrast medium in cholecystography.

io·do·chlor·hy·droxy·quin (eye·o″do·klor″high·drock′see·kwin) n. 5-Chloro-7-iodo-8-quinolinol, C_9H_5ClINO, a brownish-yellow powder; formerly used for treatment of amebiasis, trichomonas vaginitis, and coccogenic infections of the skin; now used mainly for treatment of dermatitides.

io·do·form (eye·o′duh·form, eye·od′uh·) n. Triiodomethane, CHI_3, a yellow, crystalline powder, used locally as an antiseptic and anesthetic.

io·do·phil·ia (eye·o″duh·fil′ee·uh, eye·od″o·) n. A pronounced affinity for iodine; applied to the protoplasm of leukocytes in purulent conditions.

io·do·phor (eye·o′duh·fore, eye·od′o·fore) n. A type of antiseptic in which iodine is combined with a detergent, a solubilizing agent, or other carrier in relatively stable form, which produces its effect by slow release of the iodine when in contact with tissues or bacteria.

io·dop·sin (eye″o·dop′sin) n. The visual pigment found in the cones, consisting of retinene₁ combined with photopsin.

io·do·pyr·a·cet (eye·o″do·pirr′uh·set) n. Diethanolamine 3,5-diiodo-4-pyridone-N-acetate, $C_{11}H_{16}I_2N_2O_5$, a radiopaque medium for urography, pyelography, and angiocardiography. Syn. *diodone*.

ion (eye′on) n. An atom or group of atoms which, by a suitable application of energy (for example, by collision with alpha or beta particles or gamma rays, or by dissociation of a molecule), has lost or gained one or more orbital electrons and has thereby become capable of conducting electricity.

ion exchange. The reversible exchange of ions in a solution with ions present in an ion exchanger.

ion-exchange chromatography. Separation of charged molecules by differential evolution from a column containing ion-exchange resin.

ion-exchange resin. A synthetic polymer containing fixed ionizable groups capable of exchanging ions of opposite charge in a solution in contact with the polymer.

ion·ic (eye-on'ick) *adj.* Pertaining to, characterized by, or existing as ions.

ionic strength. A measure of the intensity of the electric field in a solution; half the sum of the activity of each ion in solution, multiplied by the square of its ionic charge.

ion·iza·tion (eye''un·i·zay'shun) *n.* The production of ions. **—ion·ize** (eye'un·ize) *v.;* **ion·iz·ing** (-eye·zing) *adj.*

ionizing event. Any occurrence of a process in which an ion or group of ions is produced, as by passage of alpha or beta particles or gamma rays through a gas.

ionizing radiation. Radiation which directly or indirectly produces ionization.

ion·o·sphere (eye·on'uh·sfeer) *n.* The part of the earth's atmosphere which is sufficiently ionized by solar ultraviolet radiation for the concentration of free electrons to affect the propagation of radio waves; extends upward an indefinite distance from the upper boundary of the stratosphere at roughly 70 or 80 kilometers from the earth's surface.

ionto- A combining form meaning *ion, ionic.*

ion·to·pho·re·sis (eye·on''to·fo·ree'sis) *n.,* pl. **ion·tophore·ses** (-seez) 1. ELECTROPHORESIS. 2. *In medicine,* a method of introducing therapeutic particles into the skin or other tissues by means of an electric current.

io·phen·dyl·ate (eye''o·fen'di·late) *n.* A mixture of isomers of ethyl iodophenylundecanoate, $C_{19}H_{29}IO_2$, a radiopaque medium for myelography, cisternography, and sialography.

io·pho·bia (eye''o·fo'bee·uh) *n.* A morbid fear of poison or being poisoned.

ip·e·cac (ip'e·kack) *n.* The dried rhizome and roots of *Cephaëlis ipecacuanha,* known as Rio or Brazilian ipecac, or of *C. acuminata,* known as Cartagena, Nicaragua, or Panama ipecac. It contains emetine, cephaeline, and other alkaloids. Used, in various dosage forms, as an emetic and nauseating expectorant.

ipro·ni·a·zid (eye''pro·nigh'uh·zid) *n.* Isonicotinic acid 2-isopropylhydrazide, $C_9H_{13}N_3O$, formerly used as an antituberculosis drug and psychic energizer.

ip·sa·tion (ip·say'shun) *n.* MASTURBATION.

ip·si·lat·er·al (ip''si·lat'ur·ul) *adj.* Situated on the same side, as for example paralytic (or similar) symptoms which occur on the same side as the lesion causing them.

IQ, I.Q. Abbreviation for *intelligence quotient.*

iras·ci·bil·i·ty (i·ras''i·bil'i·tee) *n.* The quality of being choleric, irritable, or of hasty temper;

frequently a symptom in some mental disorders.

irid-, irido- A combining form meaning *iris.*

iri·dal (eye'ri·dul, irr'i·dul) *adj.* Pertaining to the iris.

iri·dal·gia (eye''ri·dal'jee·uh, irr''i·) *n.* Pain referable to the iris.

irid·avul·sion (eye''ri·duh·vul'shun, irr''i·) *n.* Surgical avulsion of the iris; iridoavulsion.

iri·dec·tome (eye''ri·deck'tome, irr''i·) *n.* A cutting instrument used in iridectomy.

iri·dec·to·mize (eye''ri·deck'tuh·mize, irr''i·) *v.* To excise a part of the iris; to perform iridectomy.

iri·dec·to·my (eye''ri·deck'tuh·mee, irr''i·) *n.* The cutting out of part of the iris.

iri·dec·tro·pi·um (eye''ri·deck·tro'pee·um, irr''i·) *n.* Eversion of a part of the iris; ECTROPION IRIDIS.

iri·de·mia, iri·dae·mia (eye''ri·dee'mee·uh, irr''i·) *n.* Hemorrhage of the iris.

iri·den·clei·sis (eye''ri·den·klye'sis, irr·i·) *n.,* pl. **iridenclei·ses** (·seez) An operation, as for glaucoma, in which, in addition to inclusion of iris in the wound, a piece of limbus may be excised to permit better drainage of aqueous humor under the conjunctiva.

iri·den·tro·pi·um (eye''ri·den·tro'pee·um, irr''i·) *n.* Inversion of a part of the iris.

irides. Plural of iris.

ir·i·des·cence (irr''i·des'unce) *n.* A rainbow-like display of intermingling and changing colors, as in mother-of-pearl. **—irides·cent** (·unt) *adj.*

irid·i·al (eye·rid'ee·ul, i·rid') *adj.* IRIDAL.

irid·ic (eye·rid'ick, i·rid'ick) *adj.* Pertaining to the iris.

irid·i·um (i·rid'ee·um, eye·rid'ee·um) *n.* Ir = 192.2. An element of the platinum family; alloyed in small proportion with platinum, it confers rigidity upon the latter.

iri·di·za·tion (eye''ri·di·zay'shun) *n.* The appearance of an iridescent halo, seen by persons affected with glaucoma.

iri·do·avul·sion (eye''ri·do·a·vul'shun, irr''i·) *n.* Avulsion of the iris.

iri·do·cap·su·li·tis (eye''ri·do·kap·sue·lye'tis, irr''i·) *n.* Inflammation involving the iris and the capsule of the lens.

iri·do·cap·su·lot·o·my (eye''ri·do·kap''sue·lot'uh·mee, irr''i·) *n.* An incision through the iris and adherent secondary membrane to create a pupillary opening.

iri·do·cele (i·rid'o·seel, eye·rid'o·, irr''i·do·) *n.* Protrusion of part of the iris through a wound or ulcer.

iri·do·cho·roid·itis (eye''ri·do·ko''roy·dye'tis, irr''i·) *n.* Inflammation of both the iris and the choroid of the eye.

iri·do·col·o·bo·ma (eye''ri·do·kol''uh·bo'muh, irr''i·) *n.* A coloboma of the iris.

iri·do·cy·clec·to·my (eye''ri·do·si·kleck'tuh·mee, irr''i·) *n.* En bloc excision of the iris and of the ciliary body.

iri·do·cy·cli·tis (eye''ri·do·sigh·klye'tis, irr''i·) *n.* Inflammation of the iris and the ciliary body; IRITIS.

iri·do·cy·clo·cho·roid·itis (eye''ri·do·sigh''klo·ko''roy·dye'tis, irr''i·) *n.* Combined inflammation of the iris, the ciliary body, and the choroid; uveitis.

iri·do·cys·tec·to·my (eye"ri·do·sis·teck'tuh·mee, irr'i·) n. An operation for making a new pupil; the edge of the iris and the capsule are drawn out through an incision in the cornea and cut off.

iri·do·di·al·y·sis (eye"ri·do·dye·al'i·sis, irr'i·) n. A separation of the base of the iris from its normal insertion.

iri·do·di·la·tor (eye"ri·do·dye·lay'tur, irr'i·do·) n. Anything which dilates the iris.

iri·do·do·ne·sis (eye"ri·do·do·nee'sis, irr'i·) n., pl. **irido·done·ses** (·seez) Quivering movements of the iris with motion of the eye, seen in aphakia or as a sign of subluxation of the lens; HIPPUS.

iri·do·ki·ne·sia (eye"ri·do·kigh·nee'zee·uh, irr'i·) n. Any movement of the iris, normal or otherwise, as in contracting and dilating the pupil.

iri·do·ma·la·cia (eye"ri·do·ma·lay'shuh, ·see·uh, irr'i·) n. Pathologic softening of the iris.

iri·do·pa·re·sis (eye"ri·do·pa·ree'sis, ·pâr'e·sis, irr'i·) n. A slight or partial paralysis of the smooth muscle of the iris.

iri·dop·a·thy (eye"ri·dop'uth·ee, irr'i·) n. 1. Any disease of the iris. 2. A degenerative disease of the iris generally localized to the pigment epithelium. Consists of vacuoles forming in the pigment epithelium and can occur in diabetes and in some systemic mucopolysaccharidoses.

iri·do·ple·gia (eye"ri·do·plee'jee·uh, irr'i·) n. Paralysis of the sphincter pupillae of the iris.

iri·dop·to·sis (eye"ri·dop·to'sis, eye"ri·) n., pl. **iri·dopto·ses** (·seez) Prolapse of the iris.

iri·do·pu·pil·lary (eye"ri·do·pew'pi·lerr·ee, irr'i·) adj. Pertaining to the iris and the pupil.

iri·dor·rhex·is, iri·dor·rhex·is (eye"ri·do·reck'sis, irr'i·) n., pl. **iridorhex·es, iridorrhex·es** (·seez) 1. Rupture of the iris. 2. The tearing away of the iris from its attachment.

iri·do·scle·rot·o·my (eye"ri·do·skle·rot'uh·mee, irr'i·) n. Puncture of the sclera with division of the iris.

iri·dot·a·sis (eye"ri·dot'uh·sis, irr'i·) n., pl. **iri·dota·ses** (·seez) Stretching the iris, as in glaucoma; in place of iridotomy. The stretched iris is left in the wound, under the conjunctiva.

iri·do·tome (eye"ti·duh·tome, irr'i·) n. An instrument for incising the iris.

iri·dot·o·my (eye"ri·dot'uh·mee, irr'i·) n. A small incision into the iris.

iris (eye'ris) n., genit. **iri·dis** (eye'ri·dis), L. pl. **iri·des** (eye'ri·deez) The anterior portion of the uvea of the eye, suspended in the aqueous humor from the ciliary body. Its posterior surface rests on the lens; hence it separates the anterior and posterior chambers. It is perforated by the adjustable pupil. It consists of loose stroma with radial vessels and melanocytes, a layer of smooth muscle (sphincter and dilator of the pupil), and pigmented epithelium. The two smooth muscles control the size of the pupil; one, circularly arranged in the pupillary border, forms the sphincter pupillae; the other, radially arranged, is the dilator pupillae. The color is governed by the number of melanocytes in the stroma.

iris bom·bé (bom·bay') A condition in which the iris bulges forward at the periphery due to an accumulation of the intraocular fluid in the posterior chamber; due to seclusion of the pupil.

Irish moss. See *Chondrus crispus.*

iri·tis (eye·rye'tis, irr·eye'tis) n. 1. Inflammation of the iris. 2. Inflammation of the iris and the ciliary body; IRIDOCYCLITIS. —**irit·ic** (eye·rit'ick) adj.

iri·to·ec·to·my (eye"ri·to·eck'tuh·mee, irr'i·to·) n. The removal of a portion of the iris for occlusion of the pupil.

iron, n. Fe = 55.847. A silver-white or gray, hard, ductile, malleable metal. Iron forms two classes of salts: ferrous, in which it has a valence of 2; and ferric, in which it has a valence of 3. In medicine, iron is used in the form of one of its salts in the treatment of certain anemias, especially of the hypochromic type.

iron-deficiency anemia. Hypochromic microcytic anemia due to excessive loss, deficient intake, or poor absorption of iron.

iron-dextran complex. A colloidal solution of ferric hydroxide in complex with partially hydrolyzed dextran of low molecular weight; used parenterally for treatment of iron-deficiency anemias.

iron lung. A metal tank respirator which encloses the body up to the neck; alternating negative and positive pressure within the respirator produces expansion and contraction of the patient's chest, inducing artificial breathing. Syn. *artificial lung, Drinker respirator.*

ir·ra·di·ate (i·ray'dee·ate) v. To treat with radiation, either roentgen rays or radiation from radioactive isotopes; to expose to radiation.

ir·ra·di·a·tion (i·ray"dee·ay'shun) n. Exposure to radiation such as infrared, ultraviolet, roentgen rays, gamma rays.

irradiation cataract. A slowly developing cataract, beginning peripherally and progressing centrally in the posterior cortex, occurring 6 months to 2 years after prolonged or intense exposure to radium or roentgen rays. Syn. *cyclotron cataract, radiation cataract.*

ir·ra·tio·nal, adj. 1. Contrary to reason or logical thinking. 2. Of a personality type, tending to rely on the affective, intuitive features, rather than on reason and logic.

ir·re·duc·ible (irr"e·dew'si·bul) adj. Not reducible; not capable of being replaced in a normal position.

ir·reg·u·lar·i·ty, n. In medicine, a deviation from a rhythmic activity or regular interval.

ir·re·me·di·a·ble, adj. Not capable of correction.

ir·re·sus·ci·ta·ble (irr"e·sus'si·tuh·bul) adj. Not capable of being resuscitated or revived.

ir·re·vers·i·ble, adj. Not capable of being reversed; characterizing a state or process from which recovery is impossible. —**irre·ver·si·bil·i·ty,** n.

ir·ri·ga·tion n. The act of washing out by a stream of water, as irrigation of the urinary bladder or a wound.

ir·ri·ga·tor (irr'i·gay"tur) n. An apparatus, or

device, for accomplishing the irrigation or washing of a part, surface, or cavity.

ir·ri·ta·bil·i·ty, n. 1. A condition or quality of being excitable; the ability to respond to a stimulus. 2. A condition of abnormal excitability of an organism, organ, or part, when it reacts excessively to a slight stimulation.

ir·ri·ta·ble, adj. 1. Capable of reacting to appropriate stimuli. 2. Easily excited; susceptible to irritation. 3. Likely to become disturbed, or otherwise mentally distraught.

irritable colon. Any of a variety of disturbances of colonic function, with accompanying emotional tension, which participate in the general bodily adaptation to nonspecific stress. Syn. *adaptive colitis, mucous colitis, spastic colon, unstable colon.*

irritable heart. NEUROCIRCULATORY ASTHENIA.

ir·ri·tant, adj. & n. 1. Causing or giving rise to irritation. 2. An agent that induces irritation.

ir·ri·ta·tion, n. 1. A condition of excitement or irritability. 2. The act of irritating or stimulating. 3. The stimulus necessary to elicit a response.

ir·ru·ma·tion (irr″oo·may′shun) n. FELLATIO.

is-, iso- A combining form indicating (a) *equality, similarity, uniformity;* (b) in biology, *for or from different individuals of the same species;* (c) in chemistry, *a compound isomeric with another, or a compound with a straight chain of carbon atoms containing a functional group at one end and an isopropyl group at the opposite end.* Symbol, *i-.*

isch-, ischo- A combining form meaning *suppression, checking, stoppage,* or *deficiency.*

isch·e·mia, isch·ae·mia (is·kee′mee·uh) n. Local diminution in the blood supply, due to obstruction of inflow of arterial blood or to vasoconstriction; localized tissue anemia. —**isch·e·mic, isch·ae·mic** (is·kee′mick) adj.

ischemic contracture. Shortening of muscle, often with fibrosis, due to interference with the blood supply.

ischemic necrosis. Death of tissue due to lack of blood flow.

is·che·sis (is·kee′sis, is′ki·sis) n. Retention of a discharge or secretion.

ischi-, ischio-. A combining form meaning *ischium, ischial.*

ischia. Plural of *ischium.*

is·chi·ad·ic (is″kee·ad′ick) adj. ISCHIAL; SCIATIC.

is·chi·al (is′kee·ul) adj. Of or pertaining to the ischium.

is·chi·al·gia (is″kee·al′jee·uh) n. Obsol. SCIATICA. —**ischial·gic** (·jick) adj.

ischial spine. SPINE OF THE ISCHIUM.

ischial tuber or **tuberosity.** A protuberance on the posterior portion of the superior ramus of the ischium, upon which the body rests in sitting.

is·chi·dro·sis (is″ki·dro′sis) n. Suppression of the secretion of sweat. —**ischi·drot·ic** (·drot′ick) adj.

is·chi·ec·to·my (is″kee·eck′tuh·mee) n. Resection of the ischium.

is·chio·bul·bo·sus (is″kee·o·bul′bo′sus) n. A variable part of the bulbospongiosus muscle.

is·chio·cap·su·lar (is″kee·o·kap′sue·lur) adj. Pertaining to the ischium and the fibrous capsule of the hip, as in ischiocapsular ligament of the hip joint.

is·chio·ca·ver·no·sus (is″kee·o·kav″ur·no′sus) n. A muscle arising from the ischium, encircling each crus of the penis or clitoris.

is·chio·coc·cyg·e·al (is″kee·o·cock·sij′ee·ul) adj. Pertaining to the ischium and the coccyx.

is·chio·my·e·li·tis (is″kee·o·migh″e·lye′tis) n. Lumbar myelitis.

is·chi·op·a·gus (is″kee·op′uh·gus) n. Conjoined twins united by their sacral or ischial regions.

is·chio·pu·bic (is″kee·o·pew′bick) adj. Pertaining to the ischial and pubic bones.

is·chio·rec·tal (is″kee·o·reck′tul) adj. Pertaining to both the ischium and the rectum.

ischiorectal fossa. The region on either side of the rectum, bounded laterally by the obturator internus muscle, medially by the levator ani and coccygeus muscles, and posteriorly by the gluteus maximus muscle.

is·chi·um (is′kee·um) n., genit. **is·chii** (is′kee·eye), pl. **is·chia** (·kee·uh) The inferior part of the hipbone; the bone upon which the body rests in sitting.

isch·no·pho·nia (isk″no·fo′nee·uh) n. STAMMERING.

is·cho·ga·lac·tic (is″ko·guh·lack′tick) adj. & n. 1. Suppressing the secretion of milk. 2. An agent that suppresses the secretion of milk.

is·cho·gy·ria (is″ko·jye′ree·uh) n. Obsol. A jagged appearance of the cerebral convolutions, produced by atrophy.

is·cho·me·nia (is″ko·mee′nee·uh) n. Suppression of the menstrual flow.

isch·uria (is·kew′ree·uh) n. Retention or suppression of the urine. —**isch·uret·ic** (is″kew·ret′ick) adj.

is·ei·ko·nia (eye″sigh·ko′nee·uh) n. The condition in which the images are of equal size in the two eyes. Syn. *isoiconia.*

is·land, n. 1. An isolated structure; particularly, a group of cells differentiated from the surrounding tissue by staining or arrangement. 2. INSULA.

island of Lang·er·hans (lahng′ur·hah′nss) ISLET OF THE PANCREAS.

is·let, n. A small island.

islet-cell tumor. A benign tumor arising from cells of the islets of the pancreas, clinically classified as functioning, producing insulin or other polypeptide hormones, or as nonfunctioning. Syn. *Langerhansian adenoma, insuloma.*

islet of Lang·er·hans (lahng′ur·hah′nss) ISLET OF THE PANCREAS.

islet of the pancreas. One of the small irregular islands of cell cords, found in the pancreas; it has no connection with the functioning duct system, and is delimited from the acini by a reticular membrane. It is of an endocrine nature, as indicated by its great vascularity and consists mainly of alpha and beta cells the former secreting a hormone believed to be glucagon, and the latter secreting insulin. The islets also secrete a growth-hormone-release inhibiting factor, somatostatin. Syn. *island of Langerhans.*

-ism A suffix indicating (a) *a condition or disease resulting from or involving*, as embolism, alcoholism; (b) *a doctrine or practice*, as Freudianism, hypnotism; (c) *-ismus*.

-ismus A suffix meaning *spasm, contraction, displacement*.

iso·ag·glu·ti·nin (eye″so·uh·gloo′ti·nin) *n.* An agglutinin which acts upon the cells of members of the same species.

iso·ag·glu·ti·no·gen (eye″so·a·gloo′ti·no·jen, ·ag″ lew·tin′o·jen) *n.* An antigen which distinguishes the cells of some individuals from those of other individuals of the same species.

iso·an·ti·body (eye″so·an′ti·bod″ee) *n.* An antibody in certain members of a species against cells or cell constituents of certain other members of the same species.

iso·an·ti·gen (eye″so·an′ti·jin) *n.* An antigen found in an animal, capable of stimulating the production of a specific antibody in some other animal of the same species but not in itself.

iso·bar (eye′so·bahr) *n.* 1. Any one of two or more atoms which have the same atomic mass but different atomic numbers. 2. A line drawn through points having equal barometric or manometric pressure. —**iso·bar·ic** (eye″so·băr′ick) *adj.*

iso·car·box·a·zid (eye″so·kahr·bock′suh·zid) *n.* 1-Benzyl-2-(5-methyl-3-isoxazolylcarbonyl)-hydrazine, $C_{12}H_{13}N_3O_2$, a monoamine oxidase inhibitor used in treating mental depression and angina pectoris.

iso·cel·lu·lar (eye″so·sel′yoo·lur) *adj.* Composed of cells of the same size or character.

iso·cho·les·ter·ol (eye″so·ko·les′tur·ol) *n.* A substance isolated from wool fat; originally considered to be a sterol but now believed to consist of several complex terpene alcohols.

iso·chro·mat·ic (eye″so·kro·mat′ick) *adj.* Having the same color throughout.

iso·chro·ma·to·phil (eye″so·kro′muh·to·fil, ·kro·mat′o·) *adj.* Of cells and tissues: equally stainable by the same dye.

isoch·ro·nal (eye·sock′ruh·nul, eye″so·kro′nul) *adj.* Occurring at or occupying equal intervals of time. —**isochro·nism** (·niz″um) *n.*

iso·com·ple·ment (eye″so·kom′ple·munt) *n.* A complement from an individual of the same species.

iso·co·ria (eye″so·ko·ree·uh) *n.* Equality in diameter of the two pupils.

iso·cor·tex (eye″so·kor′tecks) *n.* The parts of the cerebral cortex exhibiting the six characteristic layers or strata, each layer having certain predominant cells and histologic features common to all isocortical areas; NEOCORTEX. Syn. *homogenetic cortex.*

iso·cy·tol·y·sin (eye″so·sigh·tol′i·sin, ·sigh″to·lye′sin) *n.* A cytolysin capable of acting against the cells of other animals of the same species.

iso·dac·tyl·ism (eye″so·dack′ti·liz·um) *n.* The condition of having fingers or toes of equal length. —**isodacty·lous** (·lus) *adj.*

iso·dose (eye″so·doce) *adj.* Pertaining to surfaces that receive equal radiation intensities.

iso·dy·nam·ic (eye″so·dye·nam′ick, ·di·nam′ick) *adj.* Having or generating equal amounts of force, or energy, as isodynamic foods. —**isody·nam·ia** (·nam′ee·uh) *n.*

iso·e·lec·tric (eye″so·e·leck′trick) *adj.* Having the same electric properties throughout.

isoelectric level or **line.** *In electrocardiography,* the zero position of the string, needle, pen, or heated stylus of a galvanometer when no current from the heart is flowing through it. The base line of the electrocardiogram, from which all deflections are measured.

isoelectric point. The pH at which the concentration of an amphoteric electrolyte in cation form equals that in anion form; the pH at which the net electric charge on the electrolyte is zero.

iso·en·zyme (eye″so·en′zime) *n.* Any of the electrophoretically distinct forms of an enzyme having the same function. Syn. *isozyme.*

iso·flur·ane (eye″so·floo′rane) *n.* 1-Chloro-2,2,2-trifluoroethyl difluoromethyl ether, $C_3H_2ClF_5O$, an inhalation anesthetic.

iso·flu·ro·phate (eye″so·floo′ro·fate) *n.* Diisopropyl phosphorofluoridate, $[(CH_3)_2CHO]_2PFO$, a colorless, oily liquid. It is a powerful inhibitor of cholinesterase, produces marked and prolonged miosis, and is used topically in the treatment of a variety of ophthalmic afflictions.

iso·gen·e·sis (eye″so·jen′e·sis) *n.* Identity of origin of development.

iso·gen·ic (eye″so·jen′ick) *adj.* Having the same genotype.

iso·graft (eye′so·graft) *n.* A graft between a genetically identical donor and recipient; transplantation of tissues between identical twins.

iso·haem·ag·glu·ti·nin, iso·haem·ag·glu·ti·nin (eye″so·hee″muh·gloo′ti·nin, eye″so·hem′ uh·) *n.* An agglutinin in the serum of an individual which agglutinates the red blood cells of another individual of the same species.

iso·he·mol·y·sin, iso·hae·mol·y·sin (eye″so·he·mol′i·sin) *n.* A hemolysin produced by injecting red blood cells into an animal of the same species. An isohemolysin will destroy the red blood cells of any animal of the same species except the immunized individual. Syn. *isolysin.* —**iso·he·mo·lyt·ic, iso·hae·mo·lyt·ic** (eye″so·hee″mo·lit′ick, ·hem″o·) *adj.*

iso·ico·nia, iso·iko·nia (eye″so·eye·ko′nee·uh) *n.* ISEIKONIA. —**iso·icon·ic** (·eye·kon′ick) *adj.*

iso·im·mune (eye″so·i·mewn′) *adj.* Pertaining to or characterized by isoimmunization.

isoimmune hemolytic disease of the newborn. ERYTHROBLASTOSIS FETALIS.

iso·im·mu·ni·za·tion (eye″so·im″yoo·ni·zay′ shun) *n.* Immunization of a species of animal with antigens of the same species; for example, the development of anti-Rh serum may be produced by transfusing Rh-positive blood into an Rh-negative individual or by an Rh-negative woman being pregnant with an Rh-positive fetus.

iso·lat·er·al (eye″so·lat′ur·ul) *adj.* 1. IPSILATERAL. 2. Equilateral.

iso·la·tion, *n. In medicine,* the separation of a patient from the rest of the community or from other patients because of a communicable disease or for other reasons. **2.** *In psychoanalysis*, the dissociation of an idea or memory from its emotional content or the feelings attached to it, or from other facts related to it, so as to render it a matter of indifference; a common defense mechanism against anxiety. **3.** *In microbiology*, the derivation of a pure culture of an organism. **4.** *In chemistry*, the purification or separation of a substance or compound. **5.** *In physiology and experimental medicine*, the separation of cells, a body part, organ, tissue, or system from the organism for the purpose of studying its functions. —**isolate,** *v.*

Isolette. Trade name for a self-contained incubator permitting isolation and manipulations of an infant, usually a premature or neonate requiring special care.

iso·leu·cine (eye″so·lew′seen, ·sin) *n.* α-Amino-β-methylvaleric acid, $C_2H_5CH(CH_3)CH(NH_2)COOH$; an essential amino acid.

isol·o·gous (eye·sol′uh·gus) *adj.* ISOGENIC.

iso·logue, iso·log (eye′so·log) *n.* One of a series of compounds of similar structure, but having different atoms of the same valency and usually of the same periodic group.

iso·mer (eye′suh·mur) *n.* **1.** One of two or more compounds having the same molecular formula but differing in the relative positions of the atoms within the molecule. **2.** *In nuclear science*, one of two or more nuclides with the same numbers of neutrons and protons in the nucleus, but different energy.

isom·er·ase (eye·som′ur·ace, ·aze) *n.* An enzyme that catalyzes an intramolecular rearrangement with the formation of an isomeric compound, such as the interconversion of aldose and ketose sugars.

iso·mer·ic (eye″so·merr′ick) *adj.* **1.** Pertaining to isomerism. **2.** Existing as an isomer of another substance.

isom·er·ism (eye·som′ur·iz·um) *n.* The relationship between two isomers. The phenomenon wherein two or more compounds possess the same molecular formula but differ in the relative position of the atoms within the molecule and may have different properties.

iso·me·thep·tene (eye″so·me·thep′teen) *n.* N,1,5-Trimethyl-4-hexenylamine, $C_9H_{19}N$, an antispasmodic and vasoconstrictor drug used as the hydrochloride or mucate salt.

iso·met·ric (eye″so·met′rick) *adj.* **1.** Having equal measurements in several dimensions. **2.** Characterized by maintenance of equal distance, area, or volume.

isometric exercise. Muscular exercise in which contraction, and bodily movement ordinarily produced thereby, is counteracted in equal force by opposing muscles, in the same individual.

iso·me·tro·pia (eye″so·me·tro′pee·uh) *n.* Equality of kind and degree in the refraction of the two eyes.

iso·morph (eye′so·morf) *n.* **1.** *In chemistry*, one of two or more substances of different composition which have the same crystalline form. **2.** *In chemistry*, one of a group of elements

whose compounds with the same other atoms or radicals have the same crystalline form. **3.** *In biology*, an animal or plant having superficial similarity to another which is phylogenetically different.

iso·mor·phic (eye″so·mor′fick) *adj.* **1.** Identical or similar in form or structure. **2.** *In genetics*, descriptive of genotypes of polysomic or polyploid organisms which, although containing the same number of linked genes in different combinations on homologous chromosomes, yet are similar in the series of gametes which they can produce. **3.** *In chemistry*, pertaining to similar crystalline forms. —**isomor·phism** (·fiz·um) *n.*

iso·mor·phous (eye″so·mor′fus) *adj.* ISOMORPHIC.

isomorphous provocative reaction. The appearance of cutaneous lesions at sites of trauma, originally observed in psoriasis, now applied equally to diseases such as lichen planus, atopic dermatitis, necrobiosis lipoidica. Syn. *isomorphous irritation effect, Koebner's phenomenon.*

iso·ni·a·zid (eye″so·nigh′uh·zid) *n.* Isonicotinic acid hydrazide, $C_6H_7N_3O$, a tuberculostatic drug.

iso·nic·o·tin·ic acid hydrazide (eye″so·nick·o·tin′ick). ISONIAZID.

iso·os·mot·ic (eye″so·oz·mot′ick) *adj.* Characterizing or pertaining to a solution which has the same osmotic pressure as that of any reference physiological fluid, particularly that enclosed in red blood cells. An isoosmotic solution is also isotonic only when the tissue concerned, by virtue of its lack of permeability to the solutes present or to any interaction with them, maintains its normal state or tone. Syn. *isosmotic.*

isop·a·thy (eye·sop′uth·ee) *n.* The treatment of a disease by the administration of the causative agent or of its products, as the treatment of smallpox by the administration of variolous matter. Syn. *isotherapy.* —**iso·path·ic** (eye″so·path′ick) *adj.*

iso·phane insulin (eye′so·fane). A preparation of protamine and insulin, commonly zinc-insulin, in which the two substances are present in their combining proportion (isophane ratio); has intermediate duration of action. NPH insulin is an isophane insulin.

iso·pho·ria (eye″so·fo·ree·uh) *n.* A condition in which the eyes lie in the same horizontal plane, the tension of the vertical muscles being equal in both eyes, and the visual lines lying in the same plane.

iso·pia (eye·so′pee·uh) *n.* Equal acuteness of vision in the two eyes.

iso·pre·cip·i·tin (eye″so·pre·sip′i·tin) *n.* A precipitin which is active only against the serum of animals of the same species as that from which it is derived.

iso·pro·pa·nol (eye″so·pro′puh·nole, ·nol) *n.* ISOPROPYL ALCOHOL.

iso·pro·pyl (eye″so·pro′pil) *n.* The univalent hydrocarbon radical $(CH_3)_2CH—$.

isopropyl alcohol. 2-Propanol, $CH_3CH(OH)CH_3$, a homologue of ethyl alcohol; used as a solvent and rubefacient. Syn. *isopropanol.*

iso·pro·ter·e·nol (eye''so·pro·teer'e·nole, ·terr'e·nole) *n.* 3,4-Dihydroxy-α-[(isopropylamino)-methyl]benzyl alcohol, $C_{11}H_{17}NO_3$, a sympathomimetic amine; used principally as a bronchodilator as the hydrochloride and sulfate salts. Syn. *isopropylarterenol.*

isop·ters (eye·sop'turz) *n.pl.* The curves of relative visual acuity of the retina, at different distances from the macula, for form and for color.

iso·scope (eye'so·skope) *n.* An instrument consisting of two sets of parallel vertical wires, one of which can be superimposed on the other; it is designed to show that the vertical lines of separation of the retina do not correspond exactly to the vertical meridians.

iso·sex·u·al (eye''so·seck'shoo·ul) *adj.* Characteristic of or pertaining to the same sex, as: isosexual precocity, precocious sexual development appropriate to the sex of the individual undergoing it.

isosmotic solution. A solution which has the same osmotic pressure as that of a selected reference solution; commonly accepted as synonymous with isotonic solution, but the two are identical only when there is no diffusion of solute across the membrane of a tissue immersed in the solution. Syn. *isoosmotic solution.*

Isos·po·ra (eye·sos'puh·ruh) *n.* A genus of coccidia.

iso·spo·ro·sis (eye''so·spo·ro'sis) *n.* Human infection by members of the genus *Isospora.*

isos·the·nu·ria (eye''sos·thi·new'ree·uh) *n.* Inability of the kidneys to produce either a concentrated or dilute urine.

iso·tel (eye'so·tel) *n.* A food factor capable of replacing another in a given diet for a specified species; thus, for the human species, carotene is isotelic with vitamin A; for the cat, it is not, since the cat is incapable of converting carotene into vitamin A. —**iso·tel·ic** (eye''so·tel'ick) *adj.*

iso·therm (eye'so·thurm) *n.* A graph or curve representing the dependence of one quantity upon another at constant temperature, such as the dependence of gas pressure upon volume.

iso·ther·mal (eye''so·thur'mul) *adj.* Of equal or uniform temperature; without change in temperature.

iso·ton·ic (eye''so·ton'ick) *adj.* Pertaining to a solution in which cells or a tissue, especially erythrocytes, maintain the normal state without undergoing lysis or crenation. 2. *In physiology,* having uniform tension under pressure.

iso·tope (eye'suh·tope) *n.* An element which has the same atomic number as another but a different atomic weight. Many elements have been shown to consist of several isotopes, the apparent atomic weight of the element actually representing an average of the atomic weights of the isotopes. —**iso·top·ic** (·top'ick) *adj.*

iso·tro·pic (eye''so·tro'pick, trop'ick) *adj.* 1. Having the same values of a property (as refractive index, tensile strength, elasticity, electrical or heat conductivity, or rate of solution) in different directions, especially in crystal. 2. Having the same shape and appearance from whatever point observed. 3. *In biology,* having equal growth tendency in all directions. 4. In an ovum, lacking a predetermined axis or axes.

isovaleric acidemia. Elevated serum isovaleric acid content associated with recurrent episodes of coma, acidosis, and malodorous sweat.

iso·vol·u·met·ric (eye''so·vol''yoo·met'rick) *adj.* Isometric in volume.

is·sue, *n.* 1. Offspring. 2. A bloody or purulent discharge from a wound or cavity.

isth·mec·to·my (is·meck'tuh·mee, isth·) *n.* Excision of an isthmus; specifically, excision of the isthmus of the thyroid gland in goiter.

isthmic nodular salpingitis. Follicular inflammation of the small constricted portion (isthmus) of the oviduct, with formation of small nodules of muscular and connective tissue. Syn. *endosalpingiosis.*

isth·mus (is'mus, isth'mus) *n.* The neck or constricted part of an organ. —**isth·mic** (·mick) *adj.*

isthmus of the fauces. The passage between the oral cavity and the oral pharynx.

isthmus of the thyroid gland. The narrow transverse part connecting the lobes of the thyroid gland.

Isuprel. A trademark for isoproterenol, a sympathomimetic amine used principally as a bronchodilator in the form of the hydrochloride salt.

isu·ria (eye·sue'ree·uh, i·sue'ree·uh) *n.* Excretion of equal amounts of urine in equal periods of time.

Italian juice root. GLYCYRRHIZA.

itch, *n.* 1. An irritating sensation in the skin. 2. Any of various skin diseases accompanied by itching, particularly scabies.

itch mite. *SARCOPTES SCABIEI.*

¹-ite A suffix designating (a) *a mineral or rock;* (b) *a division of the body or of a part.*

²-ite. A suffix designating *the salt or ester from an acid with the termination -ous.*

iter (eye'tur, it'ur) *n.* A passageway.

it·er·a·tion (it''ur·ay'shun) *n.* Repetition.

-itis A suffix meaning *inflammation of a* (specified) *part.*

Ito cells (ee'to) Lipid-containing cells of mesenchymal origin found in human liver in certain diseases.

-itol. A suffix designating *a polyhydroxy alcohol, usually related to a sugar.*

Ito-Reen·stier·na test or **reaction.** An allergic skin test of aid in the diagnosis or exclusion of chancroid, performed by the intradermal injection of a vaccine of killed *Haemophilus ducreyi.*

ITP Abbreviation for *idiopathic thrombocytopenic purpura.*

IUD Abbreviation for *intrauterine contraceptive device.*

Ive·mark syndrome (ee've·mark'') A syndrome of unknown etiology, characterized by visceral symmetry, absence, rudimentary development, or situs inversus of the spleen, and complex cardiac malformations leading to early death. Syn. *asplenia syndrome*.

ivory bones. Very dense bones, as seen in osteopetroses, osteoblastic metastases, etc.

IVP Abbreviation for *intravenous pyelogram*.

Ivy method or **test.** A test for bleeding time, in which a small puncture wound is made in a relatively avascular part of the forearm and the time which elapses until bleeding stops is recorded.

Ix·o·des (ick·so'deez) *n.* A genus of parasitic ticks, some species of which cause tick paralysis and are important vectors of diseases of cattle, sheep, and dogs, as well as transmitters of encephalomyelitis and tularemia to man.

ix·od·ic (ick·sod'ick, ·so'dick) *adj.* Caused by or pertaining to ticks.

Ix·od·i·dae (ick·sod'i·dee) *n.pl.* A family of hard-bodied ticks, which includes the genera *Boöphilus, Amblyomma, Dermacentor, Haemaphysalis, Hyalomma, Ixodes,* and *Rhipicephalus,* all of some pathologic significance to man.

J Symbol for joule.

j Used as a Roman numeral (in prescriptions) as the equivalent of i for one, usually at the end of a number, as j, ij, iij, vj, vij.

jaag·siek·te (yahk'seek''te) *n.* A contagious disease of sheep, sometimes of goats and guinea pigs, resembling the more benign and diffuse forms of bronchiolar carcinoma in man.

Jac·coud's arthritis (zhah⸳koo') Progressive periarticular fibrosis with later pain or loss of mobility developing after severe recurrent rheumatic fever arthritis.

jack bean. The seed of *Canavalia*, from which urease is prepared for use in the estimation of urea.

jack·et, *n.* 1. *In medicine*, a supporting, therapeutic, or restraining apparatus covering the upper part or trunk of the body. 2. JACKET CROWN.

jacket crown. An artificial crown of a tooth consisting of a covering of porcelain or resin.

jackknife position. A position in which the patient reclines on his back with the shoulders elevated, the legs flexed on the thighs, and the thighs at right angles to the abdomen; a position for urethral instrumentation.

jack·screw, *n.* A threaded screw in a socket, used in various types of appliances to exert orthodontic forces or to position the parts of a fracture.

Jack·son-Bab·cock operation An operation for radical removal of an esophageal diverticulum.

Jack·so·nian convulsion or **seizure** (jack·so'nee·un) A focal seizure originating in one part of the motor or sensorimotor cortex, and manifested usually by spasmodic contractions or paroxysmal paresthesias of part of the fingers, toes, and face, whence it spreads to involve one side of the body with retention of consciousness (Jacksonian march); or it may become generalized with loss of consciousness.

Jacksonian epilepsy Epilepsy characterized by recurrent focal seizures.

Jacksonian march A focal motor or sensorimotor seizure of the fingers, toes, or face, spreading to involve the rest of the body.

Ja·cod's syndrome or **triad** (zhah⸳ko') Unilateral optic atrophy with blindness, total ophthalmoplegia, and trigeminal neuralgia involving the distribution of the ophthalmic branch, due to tumors or aneurysms in the petrosphenoid space.

jac·ti·ta·tion (jack''ti·tay'shun) *n.* A tossing about, great restlessness; seen with acute illness, high fever, and great exhaustion.

jac·u·lif·er·ous (jack''yoo·lif'ur·us) *adj.* Prickly, bearing spines.

Jadassohn's nevus NEVUS SEBACEUS.

Jadassohn-Tièche nevus (tyesh) BLUE NEVUS.

Jaf·fé-Lich·ten·stein disease or **syndrome** The monostotic form of fibrous dysplasia.

jail fever. EPIDEMIC TYPHUS.

jake palsy or **paralysis.** TRIORTHOCRESYL PHOSPHATE NEUROPATHY. Polyneuropathy and myelopathy from triorthocresylphosphate poisoning.

Jakob-Creutzfeldt disease or **syndrome.** CREUTZFELDT-JAKOB DISEASE.

jal·ap (jal'up) *n.* The tuberous root of *Exogonium purga*, a plant of the Convolvulaceae. Its active principle is a resin that contains a glycoside, convolvulin. Jalap is an active hydragogue cathartic.

Jamaican neuropathy. STRACHAN'S SYNDROME.

ja·mais vu (zha·meh' vue') A psychic phenomenon in which the patient has the sensation of never having seen or being an utter stranger to surroundings which are normally thoroughly familiar to him; observed particularly in lesions of the temporal lobe and in temporal lobe epilepsy.

jam·bul (jam'bul) *n. Eugenia jambolana*, the bark and seeds of which have been variously used in medicine.

Jane·way lesions Small painless hemorrhagic macular lesions on the palms of the hand and soles of the feet in bacterial endocarditis.

Janeway nodes or **spots** JANEWAY LESIONS.

jan·i·ceps (jan'i·seps) *n.* CEPHALOTHORACOPAGUS DISYMMETROS.

Jan·ský's classification or **groups** (yahn'skee) An early system of classification of the ABO blood groups in which O,A,B, and AB were designated groups I,II,III, and IV, respectively.

Japanese B encephalitis. An arbovirus encephalitis, epidemic in Japan, most commonly producing subclinical infection; symptomatic disease is characterized by fever, cortical, cerebellar, motor, and sensory deficits, and coma.

jar·gon (jahr'gun) n. The production, as a manifestation of aphasia, of linguistic segments whose combinations cannot be recognized as vocabulary items of a language; gibberish.

jargon aphasia. Aphasia characterized by the occurrence of jargon; usually central aphasia.

Ja·risch-Herx·hei·mer reaction (yah'rish, hehrks'high-mur) An acute systemic reaction following initial dose of a therapeutic agent, characterized by fever, chill, malaise, headache, and myalgia, with exacerbations of the clinical signs of the infection being treated, most commonly seen in the treatment of syphilis; thought to be due to rapid release of large amounts of the antigen.

jaun·dice (jawn'dis) n. Yellowness of the skin, mucous membranes, and secretions; due to hyperbilirubinemia. Syn. *icterus.*

jaundice of the newborn. Yellowness of skin and hyperbilirubinemia observed in infants during the first few days after birth. The causes are various and range from physiologic jaundice, which has no aftereffects, through that of erythroblastosis fetalis and septic jaundice, to the severe jaundice due to absence of the bile ducts.

jaw, n. Either of the two structures that constitute the framework of the mouth; skeletally, the upper jaw is formed by the maxillae, and the lower jaw by the mandible.

jaw·bone, n. One of the bones of the jaw; especially, the mandible.

jaw jerk. Contraction of the muscles of mastication and elevation of the mandible, elicited by striking the relaxed and dependent jaw with a percussion hammer, the mouth being open. Absent in nuclear and peripheral lesions of the trigeminal nerve, and exaggerated with supranuclear lesions, when jaw clonus may be elicited.

jejun-, jejuno-. A combining form meaning *jejunum.*

je·ju·nal (je·joo'nul) adj. Of or pertaining to the jejunum.

je·ju·nec·to·my (jej''oo·neck'tuh·mee) n. Excision of part or all of the jejunum.

je·ju·ni·tis (jej''oo·nigh'tis) n. Inflammation of the jejunum.

je·ju·no·ce·cos·to·my, je·ju·no·cae·cos·to·my (je·joo''no·se·kos'tuh·mee, jej''oo·no·) n. In surgery, formation of an anastomosis between the jejunum and the cecum.

je·ju·no·co·los·to·my (je·joo''no·ko·los'tuh·mee, jej''oo·no·) n. In surgery, the formation of an anastomosis between the jejunum and the colon.

je·ju·no·gas·tric (je·joo''no·gas'trick, jej''oo·no·) adj. GASTROJEJUNAL.

je·ju·no·il·e·i·tis (je·joo''no·il''ee·eye'tis, jej''oo·no·) n. Inflammation of the jejunum and the ileum.

je·ju·no·il·e·os·to·my (je·joo''no·il·ee·os'tuh·mee, jej''oo·no·) n. In surgery, the formation of an anastomosis between the jejunum and the ileum.

je·ju·no·il·e·um (jej''oo·no·il·ee·eum, je·joo''no·) n. The part of the small intestine extending from the duodenum to the cecum.

je·ju·no·je·ju·nos·to·my (je·joo''no·jej''oo·nos'tuh·mee) n. Formation of an anastomosis between two parts of the jejunum.

je·ju·nor·rha·phy (jej''oo·nor'uh·fee) n. Suture of the jejunum.

je·ju·nos·to·my (jej''oo·nos'tuh·mee) n. The making of an artificial opening (jejunal fistula) through the abdominal wall into the jejunum.

je·ju·not·o·my (jej''oo·not'uh·mee) n. Incision into the jejunum.

je·ju·num (je·joo'num) n., pl. **jeju·na** (·nuh) The portion of the small intestine extending between the duodenum and the ileum. It is usually considered to be about the proximal two-fifths of the combined jejunum and ileum.

Jel·li·nek's sign (yel'i·neck) Increased pigmentation of the lids and area around the eyes in hyperthyroidism.

jel·ly, n. A semisolid colloidal system of a liquid suspended in a solid, as water in gelatin.

Jen·dras·sik's maneuver (yen'drah·sick) A method used in neurologic examination to facilitate testing of a peripheral reflex, particularly the knee jerk, wherein the patient is asked to interlink his hands and pull them apart at time of testing.

jerk, n. 1. A sudden, spasmodic movement. 2. A muscle stretch reflex, as jaw jerk, knee jerk. —**jerky,** adj.

jerky pulse. A pulse in which the artery is suddenly and markedly distended, as in aortic regurgitation.

Je·su·its' balsam. COMPOUND BENZOIN TINCTURE.

Jesuits' bark. CINCHONA.

jet injection. A technique for administering injections intracutaneously and subcutaneously; the fluid is ejected with high velocity through an orifice 75 to 80 µm in diameter and penetrates the unbroken skin without pain.

jig·ger, n. TUNGA PENETRANS.

Jim·son weed STRAMONIUM.

jock itch. TINEA CRURIS.

jock·strap, n. A scrotal supporter.

Joh·ne's bacillus (yo'nuh) MYCOBACTERIUM PARATUBERCULOSIS.

Johne's disease A chronic granulomatous enteritis of cattle, sheep, and deer, caused by *Mycobacterium paratuberculosis* and characterized by intermittent diarrhea and progressive emaciation without fever. Gross thickening of the mucosa of the small intestine and enlargement of the mesenteric lymph nodes without ulceration may occur. Syn. *paratuberculosis.*

joint, n. Any junction of two or more bones or skeletal parts, including the fibrous joints (syndesmoses, sutures, and gomphoses), cartilaginous joints (synchondroses and symphyses), and synovial joints (the movable joints). Syn. *articulation*. For synovial joints listed by name, see Table of Synovial Joints and Ligaments in the Appendix.

joint capsule. The fibrous sheet enclosing a synovial joint. Syn. *capsular ligament*.

joint cavity. The closed space in a synovial joint, formed by the synovial membrane and containing synovial fluid; the cavity enclosed by the synovial sac.

joint-ill, *n.* A pyosepticemia of newborn animals resulting from an infection of the navel, characteristically accompanied by a suppurative arthritis.

joint mouse. A small loose body within a synovial joint, frequently calcified, derived from synovial membrane, organized fibrin fragments of articular cartilage, or arthritic osteophytes. Syn. *joint body*.

Jones criteria A listing of findings of major and minor importance for making the diagnosis of acute rheumatic fever.

Jo·seph's syndrome (zhoh'zef') A hereditary defect in renal tubular reabsorption resulting in exceedingly high urinary excretion of proline, hydroxyproline, and glycine; manifested clinically by generalized seizures beginning in early life, terminal status epilepticus, and elevated cerebrospinal fluid protein. Syn. *familial hyperprolinemia*.

joule (jool) *n.* 1. The absolute joule: an mks unit of work or energy equivalent to 10^7 ergs. 2. The international joule: a unit equivalent to the work done when a current of 1 international ampere is passed for 1 second through a conductor having a resistance of 1 international ohm; an international joule = 1.00019 absolute joules. Symbol, J.

J point. The junction point of the QRS complex and the S-T segment of the electrocardiogram.

J stomach. A long, longitudinally oriented stomach.

Ju·det prosthesis (zhu^e.deh') A femoral head prosthesis consisting of an acrylic head component attached to an acrylic or metalic stem.

juga. Plural of *jugum*.

ju·gal (joo'gul) *adj.* 1. Connecting or uniting, as by a yoke. 2. Pertaining to the zygoma.

jug·u·lar (jug'yoo-lur) *adj. & n.* 1. Pertaining to the neck above the clavicle. 2. Any of the jugular veins. See Table of Veins in the Appendix.

jugular foramen. The space formed by the jugular notches of the occipital and temporal bones, divided into two portions, the posterior portion giving passage to an internal jugular vein and the anterior portion giving passage to the ninth, tenth, and eleventh cranial nerves and the inferior petrosal sinus.

jugular foramen syndrome. Paralysis of the ipsilateral glossopharyngeal, vagus, and spinal accessory nerves; caused by a lesion involving the jugular foramen, usually a basilar skull fracture.

jugular notch of the sternum. The depression on

the upper surface of the manubrium between the two clavicles.

jugular pulse. Pulsation of the jugular veins.

jugular vein. Any of several major veins of the neck. See *anterior jugular*, *external jugular*, and *internal jugular* in Table of Veins in the Appendix.

ju·gum (joo'gum) *n.*, pl. **ju·ga** (·guh) A yoke or bridge.

juice, *n.* 1. The liquid contained in vegetable or animal tissues. 2. Any of the secretions of the body.

Jukes. A fictitious name given to the descendants of certain sisters in a study of the occurrence among them of crime, immorality, pauperism, and disease in relation to heredity.

ju·men·tous (joo-men'tus) *adj.* Similar to that of a horse; applied to the odor of urine.

jumping disease or **spasm.** JUMPING FRENCHMEN OF MAINE.

jumping Frenchmen of Maine. A bizarre paroxysmal disorder of unknown cause characterized by episodes of a single, violent jump evoked by sound, touch, or a sudden movement, and accompanied by echolalia; usually the disorder begins in childhood, is lifelong, familial, and observed only in males of French-Canadian descent.

junc·tion (junk'shun) *n.* The point or line of union of two parts; juncture. interface. —**junc·tion·al** (·ul) *adj.*

junctional rhythm. A regular cardiac rhythm with the dominant pacemaker located in the atrioventricular junctional tissues. The rate is usually between 40 and 70 per minute. The P wave of the electrocardiogram is usually abnormal and may precede, follow, or be hidden in the QRS complex. Syn. *nodal rhythm*.

junction nevus. A benign skin lesion containing nevus cells at the junction of the epidermis and dermis, but not in the dermis.

junc·tu·ra (junk-tew'ruh) *n.*, pl. & genit. sing. **junctu·rae** (·ree) A joint or junction.

Jung·i·an (yoong'ee-un) *adj.* Pertaining to Jung, his psychoanalytic theories and methods.

Jungian psychology ANALYTIC PSYCHOLOGY.

jun·gle yellow fever. A form of yellow fever endemic in South and Central America and Africa; occurs in or near forested areas where the disease is present in monkeys and is transmitted by *Haemagogus* and some *Aëdes* mosquitoes. Syn. *sylvan yellow fever*.

ju·ry, *n.* A body of adult persons chosen according to law to attend a judicial tribunal and sworn to determine upon the evidence to be placed before them the true verdict concerning a matter being tried or inquired into.

jury mast. An iron rod fixed in a plaster jacket; used to support the head in disease or fracture of the cervical spine.

jus·to major (jus'to) Greater than normal, larger in all dimensions than normal, applied to a pelvis.

justo minor Abnormally small in all dimensions, applied to a pelvis.

ju·ve·nile (joo've-nil, ·nile) *adj.* 1. Pertaining to or characteristic of youth or childhood. 2. Young; immature.

juvenile acanthosis. A variety of acanthosis nigricans.

juvenile amaurotic familial idiocy. SPIELMEYER-VOGT DISEASE.

juvenile cell. METAMYELOCYTE.

juvenile macular degeneration. The most common familial form of macular degeneration, with onset between ages 8 to 20, characterized by slowly progressive loss of foveal reflex, granular appearance of the macula, and eventually pigmentary or atrophic macular changes; resulting in loss of central vision and markedly decreased visual acuity, but with no mental or neurologic dysfunctions. Inherited as either a dominant or recessive trait. Syn. *Stargardt's disease.*

juvenile melanoma. A type of benign compound nevus, principally occurring in young people, whose histologic appearance superficially resembles that of malignant melanoma.

juvenile-onset diabetes. Diabetes mellitus which develops early in life, presenting much more severe symptoms than the more common maturity-onset diabetes.

juvenile rheumatoid arthritis. Rheumatoid arthritis beginning before puberty, often ushered in by symptoms such as fever, erythematous rash, and weight loss, which often precede the onset of arthritis, and with lymphadenopathy, hepatosplenomegaly, and pericarditis.

juvenile spinal muscular atrophy. A hereditary, slowly progressive degenerative disorder of the anterior horn cells of the spinal cord, with onset in the first or second decade of life, usually affecting the larger proximal muscles first, especially of the pelvic girdle, and those of the arms and the distal muscles later. Commonly inherited as an autosomal recessive. Syn. *Kugelberg-Welander syndrome.*

juvenile xanthogranuloma. A benign self-limited disorder of unknown cause, often familial and found at birth or early childhood, characterized clinically by yellowish-brown or red nodules on the extensor surfaces of the extremities as well as on the face, scalp, and trunk, and histologically by the presence of many histiocytes, foam cells, and Touton giant cells. The lesions disappear gradually. Lack of bone and other systemic involvement differentiates the disorder from Hand-Schüller-Christian disease, Letterer-Siwe disease, and eosinophilic granuloma. Syn. *nevoxantho-endothelioma, juvenile histiocytoma, juvenile xanthoma.*

juvenile xanthoma. JUVENILE XANTHOGRANU-LOMA.

juxta- A combining form meaning *near, next to.*

jux·ta·ar·tic·u·lar (jucks″tuh·ahr·tick′yoo·lur) *adj.* Near a joint.

juxta-articular node or **nodule.** 1. A nodule adjacent to a joint. 2. A very hard, well-outlined tumefaction about a joint, frequently multiple, usually found about the elbows; most often seen in patients with syphilis, yaws, or pinta. Syn. *Jeanselme's nodule, Steiner's tumor.*

jux·ta·cor·ti·cal (jucks″tuh·kor′ti·kul) *adj.* Near the cortex.

jux·ta·glo·mer·u·lar (jucks″tuh·glom·err′yoo·lur) *adj.* Next to a glomerulus.

juxtaglomerular apparatus. A cuff of epithelioid cells in the muscularis of an afferent arteriole near its entrance into the renal glomerulus and in contact with the distal convoluted tubules; it is concerned with renin production and sodium metabolism.

jux·ta·pap·il·lary (jucks″tuh·pap′i·lerr·ee) *adj.* Situated near the optic disk.

juxtapapillary choroiditis. Choroiditis adjacent to the optic disk, resulting in a visual field defect; may be confused in the active stage with optic neuritis. Syn. *Jensen's chorioretinitis.*

jux·ta·po·si·tion (juck″stuh·po·zish′un) *n.* Situation adjacent to another; close relationship; apposition. —**juxta·pose** (·poze′) *v.*

jux·ta·py·lo·ric (jucks″tuh·pye·lor′ick, ·pi·lor′ick) *adj.* Near the pylorus.

K Symbol for potassium.

K_a Symbol for the dissociation constant of an acid.

K_b Symbol for the dissociation constant of a base.

K_m Symbol for Michaelis constant.

Kader's operation A gastrostomy with a fold which acts like a valve when the tube is removed.

Kaf·fir pox (kaf´ur). A mild form of smallpox; VARIOLA MINOR.

Kahn test A precipitin test for syphilis.

kai·no·pho·bia (kigh´´no·fo´bee·uh). A morbid fear of anything new. **—kai·no·phobe** (kigh´no·fobe) *n.*

kak·or·rhaph·io·pho·bia (kack´´o·raf´´ee·o·fo´bee·uh) *n.* Morbid fear of failure.

ka·la azar, kala-azar (kah´lah ah·zahr´, ah´zahr, kal´´uh ay´zur, az´ur) Visceral leishmaniasis due to the protozoan *Leishmania donovani,* transmitted by sandflies of the genus *Phlebotomus.* It is characterized by irregular fever of long duration, chronicity, enlargement of the spleen and liver, emaciation, anemia, leukopenia, and hyperglobulinemia.

ka·le·mia (ka·lee´mee·uh) *n.* HYPERKALEMIA.

kal·io·pe·nia (kal´´ee·o·pee´nee·uh) *n.* Low potassium concentration in the blood; HYPOKALEMIA. **—kaliope·nic** (·nick) *adj.*

ka·li·um (kay´lee·um) *n.* POTASSIUM.

kal·li·din (kal´i·din) *n.* Either or both of two polypeptide plasma kinins released from the plasma alpha globulin kallidinogen (bradykininogen) by a kallikrein. The individual kallidins are identified as kallidin-9 (identical with bradykinin), which contains nine amino acid residues, and kallidin-10, which contains an additional amino acid residue. Kallidins cause vasodilatation, increase capillary permeability, produce edema, and contract or relax a variety of extravascular smooth muscles.

kal·li·din·o·gen (kal´´i·din´o·jen) *n.* An alpha globulin present in blood plasma which serves as the precursor for the kallidins and the substrate for the kallikreins. Kallidinogen appears to be identical with bradykininogen.

Kal·li·kak (kal´i·kack) *n.* A fictitious name given to the descendants of a Revolutionary War soldier in a study of the occurrence among them of feeblemindedness and of immorality and the bearing of heredity on intelligence, personality, and behavior.

kal·li·kre·in (kal´´i·kree´in) *n.* A proteolytic enzyme present in pancreatic juice, blood plasma, urine, saliva, and other body fluids that releases a kallidin from the plasma alpha globulin kallidinogen (bradykininogen). Kallikrein from blood plasma releases only kallidin-9, but kallikrein from urine releases kallidin-9 and kallidin-10.

Kall·mann's syndrome. An inherited form of hypogonadotropic hypogonadism associated with infertility and anosmia.

ka·ma·la (kuh·may´luh, kam´uh·luh) *n.* The glands and hairs from the capsules of *Mallotus philippinensis* (kamala tree); has been used as a purgative and anthelmintic.

kan·a·my·cin (kan´´uh·migh´sin) *n.* An antibiotic substance, $C_{18}H_{36}N_4O_{11}$, derived from strains of *Streptomyces kanamyceticus;* used as the sulfate salt. Absorbed rapidly from intramuscular sites but only slightly from the gastrointestinal tract. It is active against many bacteria.

Ka·na·vel's operation (ka·nay´vul) An operation in which full-thickness skin grafts, with all fat removed, are used for the relief of Dupuytren's contracture.

kan·ga·roo tendon. A tendon obtained from the tail of the kangaroo; used for surgical ligatures and sutures.

"kan·gri basket" cancer. (kang´gree, kung´gree). A nonmetastasizing squamous cell carcinoma of the abdominal skin occurring in Kashmir and Tibet where people warm the belly by means of a wicker-covered clay pot (kangri) of hot coals.

Kan·ner's syndrome AUTISM (2).

Kantrex. Trademark for the antibiotic kanamycin.

ka·o·lin (kay´o·lin) *n.* A native, hydrated alumi num silicate, powdered and freed from gritty particles by elutriation. Used externally as a protective and absorbent; internally it is sometimes used as an adsorbent.

ka·o·li·no·sis (kay"o·li·no'sis) *n.* A pneumoconiosis due to the inhalation of kaolin dust.

Ka·po·si's disease (kah'po·zee) 1. XERODERMA PIGMENTOSUM. 2. MULTIPLE IDIOPATHIC HEMORRHAGIC SARCOMA. 3. ECZEMA HERPETICUM.

Kaposi's sarcoma or **syndrome** MULTIPLE IDIOPATHIC HEMORRHAGIC SARCOMA.

Kaposi's varicelliform eruption ECZEMA HERPETICUM.

kappa chain, κ chain. See *light chain.*

ka·ra·ya gum (ka·rah'yuh, kär'ay·uh). An exudate from trees of the *Sterculia* or *Cochlospermum* species; with water, it swells to form a bulky mass. Karaya gum is sometimes employed as a mechanical laxative. Syn. *sterculia gum.*

Kar·ta·ge·ner's syndrome or **triad** (kar·tah'ge·nur) A hereditary symptom complex consisting of transposition of the viscera, maldevelopment of the sinuses leading to sinusitis, and bronchiectasis.

kary-, karyo- *In biology,* a combining form meaning *nucleus, nuclear.*

karyo·chrome (kär'e·o·krome) *n.* KARYOCHROME CELL.

karyochrome cell. *Obsol.* 1. A nerve cell which has a high nucleocytoplasmic ratio. 2. A nerve cell in which the nucleus stains intensely.

kary·oc·la·sis (kär"ee·ock'luh·sis) *n.* KARYORRHEXIS. **—karyo·clas·tic** (kär"ee·o·klas'tick) *adj.*

karyo·gram (kär'ee·o·gram) *n.* KARYOTYPE (2).

karyo·ki·ne·sis (kär"ee·o·ki·nee'sis, ·kigh·nee'sis) *n.* Mitosis, especially the nuclear transformations. Syn. *karyomitosis.* **—karyoki·net·ic** (·net'ick) *adj.*

kary·ol·y·sis (kär"ee·ol'i·sis) *n.* The dissolution of the nucleus of the cell. **—karyo·lit·ic** (kär"ee·o·lit'ick) *adj.*

karyo·meg·a·ly (kär"ee·o·meg'uh·lee) *n. In exfoliative cytology,* slight but uniform nuclear enlargement in superficial and intermediate squamous cells of the uterine cervical epithelium.

karyo·mere (kär'ee·o·meer) *n.* A segment of a chromosome.

kar·y·on (kär'ee·on) *n.* The nucleus of a cell.

karyo·phage (kär'ee·o·faje, ·fahzh) *n.* A cell capable of phagocytizing the nucleus of an infected cell.

karyo·plasm (kär'ee·o·plaz·um) *n.* NUCLEOPLASM. **—karyo·plas·mic** (kär"ee·o·plaz'mick) *adj.*

kary·or·rhex·is (kär"ee·o·reck'sis) *n.,* pl. **karyor·rhex·es** (·seez) Fragmentation or splitting up of a nucleus into a number of pieces which become scattered in the cytoplasm. **—karyor·rhec·tic** (·reck'tick) *adj.*

karyo·some (kär'ee·o·sohm) *n.* 1. An aggregated mass of chromatin in the nucleus, confused with the nucleolus. 2. A large, deeply staining body in the nucleus of many Protista, associated with the chromosomes or other structures.

·aryo·type (kär'ee·o·tipe) *n.* 1. The total of char-

acteristics, including number, form, and size, of chromosomes and their grouping in a cell nucleus; it is characteristic of an individual, race, species, genus, or larger grouping. 2. The arrangement of chromosome photomicrographs according to a standard classification.

Kas·a·bach-Mer·ritt syndrome Giant capillary hemangioma, thrombocytopenia, and purpura, occurring principally in childhood; HEMANGIOMA-THROMBOCYTOPENIA SYNDROME.

Ka·shin-Beck disease (kah'shin) A chronic degenerative generalized osteoarthrosis occurring chiefly in children in Siberia, northern China, and northern Korea; believed to be a form of mycotoxicosis due to ingestion of cereals infected with the fungus *Fusarium sporotrichiella.* Syn. *Urov disease.*

Kast's syndrome (kahᵇst) Multiple cavernous hemangiomas associated with chondromas or enchondromatosis. Some patients show pigmentary skin changes. It is thought to be a variant of Maffucci's syndrome.

kata-. See *cata-.*

kata·did·y·mus (kat"uh·did'i·mus) *n.* Duplication of the superior pole, as in diprosopia or dicephalism. Has been incorrectly used for inferior duplicity. Syn. *superior duplicity.*

kata·ther·mom·e·ter, cata·ther·mom·e·ter (kat"uh·thur·mom'e·tur) *n.* An alcohol thermometer, with a dry bulb and a wet bulb, that measures how quickly air is cooling, thus permitting an estimate of evaporation of moisture from the body.

Ka·ta·ya·ma (kat"uh·yah'muh, kah"tuh·) *n.* A genus of amphibious snails, usually included in the genus *Oncomelania.*

Katayama formosana. ONCOMELANIA FORMOSANA.

Katayama nosophora. ONCOMELANIA NOSOPHORA.

kath·i·so·pho·bia (kath"i·so·fo'bee·uh) *n.* Morbid fear of or anxiety about sitting down; AKATHISIA (2).

Katz-Wach·tel sign High-voltage QRS complexes in the midprecordial leads of the electrocardiogram; a sign of ventricular septal defect.

ka·va (kah'vuh, kav'uh) *n.* 1. An intoxicating beverage prepared in the Hawaiian Islands from the root of *Piper methysticum.* 2. The root of *Piper methysticum,* containing a resin, kawine, and other constituents; formerly used for treatment of genitourinary tract inflammation.

Kayexalate. Trademark for sodium polystyrene sulfonate, an ion-exchange resin used for the treatment of hyperkalemia.

Kayser-Fleischer ring A ring of golden-brown or brownish green pigmentation in the periphery of the cornea due to the deposition of copper in the area of Descemet's membrane and deep corneal stroma; diagnostic of hepatolenticular degeneration. It may be visible only on slit-lamp examination.

kcal Abbreviation for *kilocalorie.*

Keflex. A trademark for cephalexin, an antibacterial agent.

Keflin. Trademark for cephalothin, a bactericidal antibiotic drug.

Keith's node SINOATRIAL NODE.

ke·lis (kee'lis) n. 1. Localized scleroderma. 2. KELOID.

Kell blood group system A family of antigens, first described in 1946, found in erythrocytes designated as K,k, Kp^a, Kp^b, and Ku. Antibodies to the K antigen, which occurs in about 10 percent of the population of England, have been associated with hemolytic transfusion reactions and with hemolytic disease.

Kelly forceps A curved surgical clamp which can be used either as a hemostat for large vessels or to grasp bundles of vascular tissues prior to dividing them.

Kelly plication. Surgical plication of the bladder neck and urethra for stress incontinence of urine.

ke·loid, che·loid (kee'loid) n. A fibrous hyperplasia usually at the site of a scar, elevated, rounded, firm, and with ill-defined borders. There is predilection for the upper trunk and face, and the condition is observed especially in young female adults and in blacks. —**ke·loid·al** (kee·loy'dul) adj.

keloid acne. Follicular infection, resembling acne in papular and pustular form, and resulting in hypertrophic or keloidal scarring. The nape of the neck is the commonest site of such process; blacks are frequently affected. Syn. folliculitis keloidalis, dermatitis papillaris capillitii.

keloid sycosis. Sycosis in which keloidal change occurs in the cicatrices resulting from the follicular inflammation.

ke·lo·ma (kee'lo'muh) n. KELOID.

kelp, n. 1. A common name for a group of large brown algae growing in the cool ocean waters. 2. Burnt seaweed from which potassium salts and iodine formerly were prepared.

kel·vin, n. A commercial unit of electricity; 1,000 watt-hours.

Kelvin scale An absolute scale of temperature which has its zero at −273°C.

Kemp·ner rice diet A rigid diet of rice, fruit, and sugar, providing about 7 mEq per day of sodium and averaging about 2000 calories per day; used in the treatment of hypertension.

ken-, keno- A combining form meaning empty.

Kenacort. A trademark for the adrenocortical steroid triamcinolone and its diacetate ester.

Kenalog. A trademark for triamcinolone acetonide.

Kendall's compound A DEHYDROCORTICOSTERONE.

Kendall's compound B CORTICOSTERONE.

Kendall's compound C COMPOUND C.

Kendall's compound D COMPOUND D.

Kendall's compound E CORTISONE.

Kendall's compound F HYDROCORTISONE.

Ken·ny treatment Treatment of weak or paralyzed muscles in poliomyelitis with hot moist packs, followed by passive and then active exercises with muscle reeducation.

keno·pho·bia (ken''o.fo'bee·uh) n. A morbid fear of large, empty spaces.

keno·tox·in (ken''o·tock'sin) n. A hypothetical poisonous substance developed in the tissues during their activity which has been said to be responsible for their fatigue and for sleep.

kephir, kephyr. KEFIR.

ker·a·phyl·lo·cele (kerr''uh·fil'o·seel) n. A horny tumor on the inner side of the wall of a horse's hoof.

ker·a·phyl·lous (kerr''uh·fil'us, ker·af'i·lus) adj. In veterinary medicine, composed of horny layers.

ker·a·sin (kerr'uh·sin) n. A cerebroside separated from the brain; contains sphingosine, galactose, and fatty acid.

kerat-, kerato- A combining form meaning (a) horn, horny; (b) cornea, corneal.

ker·a·tal·gia (kerr''uh·tal'jee·uh) n. Pain in the cornea.

ker·a·tec·ta·sia (kerr''uh·teck·tay'zhuh) n. Thinning with protrusion of the cornea as seen following ulceration or with keratoconus.

ker·a·tec·to·my (kerr''uh·teck'tuh·mee) n. Surgical excision of a part of the cornea, usually for removal of a localized opacity or for diagnostic purposes.

ke·rat·ic (ke·rat'ick) adj. Pertaining to the cornea.

keratic precipitates. Clumps of inflammatory cells deposited upon the endothelial surface of the cornea, occurring with intraocular inflammations such as uveitis. Round-cell precipitates are generally the result of an acute, nongranulomatous infection, while the larger "mutton-fat" precipitates of epithelioid cells indicate a chronic, granulomatous process.

ker·a·tin (kerr'uh·tin) n. Any of a group of albuminoids or scleroproteins characteristic of horny tissues, hair, nails, feathers, insoluble in protein solvents, and having a high content of sulfur. Two main groups are distinguished: eukeratins, which are not digested by common proteolytic enzymes, and pseudokeratins, which are partly digested. Both contain various amino acids; cystine and arginine generally predominate.

ker·a·tin·iza·tion (kerr''uh·tin·i·zay'shun) n. 1. Development of a horny quality in a tissue. 2. The process whereby keratin is formed. 3. The coating of pills with keratin. —**ker·a·tin·ize** (kerr''uh·tin·ize) v.; **keratin·ized** (·ize'd) adj.

ke·rat·i·no·cyte (ke·rat'i·no·site) n. An epidermal cell that synthesizes keratin.

ke·rat·i·no·phil·ic (ke·rat''i·no·fil'ick) adj. Having an affinity for horny or keratinized tissue, as certain fungi.

ke·rat·i·nous (ke·rat'i·nus) adj. 1. Of or pertaining to keratin. 2. HORNY.

keratinous degeneration. The appearance of keratin granules in the cytoplasm of a cell which does not ordinarily undergo keratinization.

ker·a·ti·tis (kerr''uh·tye'tis) n., pl. **kera·tit·i·des** (·tit'i·deez) Inflammation of the cornea. —**kera·tit·ic** (·tit'ick) adj.

keratitis bul·lo·sa (bool·o'suh). The formation of large or small blebs upon the cornea in cases of iridocyclitis, glaucoma, interstitial keratitis, or Fuch's dystrophy. Syn. bullous keratitis.

keratitis dis·ci·for·mis (dis''i·for'mis, dis''ki·). DISCIFORM KERATITIS.

keratitis hypopyon. Keratitis with accumulation of neutrophils, gravitating inferiorly, in the anterior chamber; seen most commonly with pneumococcal and aspergillus infections.

keratitis pa·ren·chy·ma·to·sa (pa·renk''i·muh·to'suh). INTERSTITIAL KERATITIS.

keratitis punc·ta·ta (punk'tay'tuh). The presence of leukocytes on the back of Descemet's membrane. Not a primary inflammation of Descemet's membrane, since the cells derive from the ciliary body as a result of its inflammation. Syn. *descemetitis*.

keratitis ro·sa·cea (ro·zay'see·uh, ·shee·uh). The occurrence of small, sterile infiltrates at the periphery of the cornea, which are approached but not invaded by small blood vessels. They are most frequently seen unaccompanied by acne rosacea, but are most severe in this connection.

ker·a·to·ac·an·tho·ma (kerr''uh·to·ack''an'tho·muh) *n.* A firm skin nodule with a center of keratotic material, occurring on the hairy parts of the body, especially the exposed sites, developing and regressing over a period usually less than six months; it has a histologic resemblance to squamous cell cancer of the skin, and is usually solitary.

ker·a·to·cele (kerr'uh·to·seel) *n.* A hernia of Descemet's membrane through the cornea; DESCEMETOCELE.

ker·a·to·cen·te·sis (kerr''uh·to·sen·tee'sis) *n.*, pl. **keratocente·ses** (·seez) Corneal puncture.

ker·a·to·chro·ma·to·sis (kerr''uh·to·kro·muh·to'sis) *n.* Discoloration of the cornea.

ker·a·to·con·junc·ti·vi·tis (kerr''uh·to·kun·junk·ti·vye'tis) *n.* Simultaneous inflammation of the cornea and the conjunctiva.

keratoconjunctivitis sic·ca (sick'uh). Keratinization of the cornea and conjunctiva resulting from dryness.

ker·a·to·co·nus (kerr''uh·to·ko'nus) *n.* Conical axial ectasia of the cornea. The anterior form is an acquired lesion for adults, may be associated with an allergic diathesis, and is also a component of Down's syndrome; posterior keratoconus is a congenital lesion considered to be the mildest form of Peter's anomaly.

ker·a·to·der·ma (kerr''uh·to·dur'muh) *n.* A horny condition of the skin, especially of the palms and soles.

keratoderma blen·nor·rhag·i·cum (blen''o·raj'i·kum). KERATOSIS BLENNORRHAGICA.

keratoderma cli·mac·ter·i·cum (klye''mack·terr'i·kum). A circumscribed hyperkeratosis of the palms and soles occurring in women during the menopause, and accompanied chiefly by obesity and hypertension. Syn. *Haxthausen's disease*.

ker·a·to·der·ma·to·cele (kerr''uh·to·dur·mat'o·seel, ·dur'muh·to·) *n.* KERATOCELE.

ker·a·to·gen·e·sis (kerr''uh·to·jen'e·sis) *n.* Development of horny growths.

ker·a·to·glo·bus (kerr''uh·to·glo'bus) *n.* A globular protrusion of the cornea due to thinning of the entire cornea. May be congenital or acquired as with arrested congenital or juvenile glaucoma.

ker·a·to·hel·co·sis (kerr''uh·to·hel·ko'sis) *n.* Ulceration of the cornea.

ker·a·to·he·mia, ker·a·to·hae·mia (kerr''uh·to·hee'mee·uh) *n.* The presence of blood or its breakdown products in or staining the cornea.

ker·a·to·hy·a·lin (kerr''uh·to·high'uh·lin) *n.* The substance of the granules in the stratum granulosum of keratinized stratified squamous epithelium; an early phase in the formation of keratin. —**keratohya·line** (·lin, ·leen) *adj.*

ker·a·toid (kerr'uh·toid) *adj.* Hornlike.

ker·a·to·iri·tis (kerr''uh·to·eye·rye'tis, ·i·rye'tis) *n.* Combined inflammation of the cornea and the iris, as seen especially in herpetic keratouveitis.

ker·a·to·leu·ko·ma (kerr''uh·to·lew·ko'muh) *n.* A leukoma or whitish opacity of the cornea.

ker·a·tol·y·sis (kerr''uh·tol'i·sis) *n.* 1. Exfoliation of the epidermis. 2. A congenital anomaly in which the skin is shed periodically.

keratolysis neonatorum. DERMATITIS EXFOLIATIVA NEONATORUM.

ker·a·to·lyt·ic (kerr''uh·to·lit'ick) *adj. & n.* 1. Characterized by or pertaining to keratolysis. 2. An agent which causes exfoliation of the epidermis to a greater degree than that which occurs normally.

ke·ra·to·ma (kerr''uh·to'muh) *n.* CALLOSITY.

ker·a·to·ma·la·cia (kerr''uh·to·ma·lay'shee·uh) *n.* Degeneration of the cornea characterized by keratinization of the epithelium, eventually leading to ulceration and perforation of the cornea; seen in vitamin A deficiency.

ker·a·tome (kerr'uh·tome) *n.* A knife with a trowel-like blade, for incising the cornea.

ker·a·to·meg·a·ly (kerr''uh·to·meg'uh·lee) *n.* MEGALOCORNEA.

ker·a·tom·e·ter (kerr''uh·tom'e·tur) *n.* An instrument for measuring the curves of the cornea. —**keratome·try** (·tree) *n.*

ker·a·to·my·co·sis (kerr''uh·to·migh·ko'sis) *n.* A fungus disease of the cornea.

ker·a·top·a·thy (kerr''uh·top'uth·ee) *n.* A degenerative process of the cornea.

ker·a·to·plas·ty (kerr''uh·to·plas''tee) *n.* A plastic operation upon the cornea, especially the transplantation of a portion of cornea; may be full thickness or partial. —**ker·a·to·plas·tic** (kerr''uh·to·plas'tick) *adj.*

ker·a·tor·rhex·is (kerr''uh·to·reck'sis) *n.*, pl. **kera·torrhex·es** (·seez) Rupture of the cornea, due to ulceration or trauma.

ker·a·to·scle·ri·tis (kerr''uh·to·skle·rye'tis) *n.* Inflammation of the cornea and the sclera.

ker·a·to·scope (kerr''uh·to·skope) *n.* An instrument for examining the cornea and testing the symmetry of its meridians of curvature. Syn. *Placido's disk.*

ker·a·tos·co·py (kerr''uh·tos'kuh·pee) *n.* Examination of the cornea with the keratoscope.

ker·a·tose (kerr''uh·toce) *adj.* Horny.

ker·a·to·sis (kerr''uh·to'sis) *n.* 1. Any disease of the skin characterized by an overgrowth of the cornified epithelium. 2. ACTINIC KERATOSIS.

keratosis blen·nor·rhag·i·ca (blen''o·raj'i·kuh). A disease characterized by rupial, pustular, and crusted lesions, usually on the palms and soles. Found in association with gonococcal arthritis or with Reiter's disease. Syn. *keratoderma blennorrhagicum.*

keratosis fol·lic·u·la·ris (fol·ick″yoo·lair′is). DA-RIER'S DISEASE.

keratosis nigricans. ACANTHOSIS NIGRICANS.

keratosis pal·ma·ris et plan·ta·ris (pal·mair′is et plan·tair′is). A marked, congenital thickening of the volar surfaces of the hands and feet, frequently complicated by painful fissures; occurs as a dominant hereditary trait.

keratosis pi·la·ris (pi·lair′is). A chronic disorder of the skin marked by hard, conical elevations in the pilosebaceous orifices on the arms and thighs.

keratosis punc·ta·ta (punk·tay′tuh). Keratosis of the palms and soles, characterized by numerous minute, crateriform pits set in patches of thickening of the stratum corneum. Syn. *keratoderma punctatum.*

keratosis seb·or·rhe·i·ca (seb″o·ree′i·kuh). SEB-ORRHEIC KERATOSIS.

keratosis se·ni·lis (se·nigh′lis). ACTINIC KERATO-SIS.

ker·a·to·sul·fate (kerr″uh·to·sul′fate) *n.* A sulfated mucopolysaccharide in which the uronic acid component is replaced by D-galactose.

ker·a·to·sul·fa·tu·ria (kerr″uh·to·sul″fuh·tew′ree·uh, ·sul″fay·) *n.* MORQUIO'S SYNDROME.

ker·a·tot·ic (ker·uh·tot′ick) *adj.* Pertaining to or affected with keratosis.

keratotic nevus. NEVUS VERRUCOSUS.

ker·a·tot·o·my (kerr″uh·tot′uh·mee) *n.* Incision of the cornea.

ke·rau·no·pho·bia (ke·raw″no·fo′bee·uh) *n.* Abnormal excessive fear of lightning and thunderstorms.

kerion cel·si (sel′sigh) A type of dermatophytosis of the scalp or beard, with deep, boggy infiltration.

Ker·ley lines Thickened interlobular septa visible radiographically usually in the region of the costophrenic angles (Kerley B lines) but also in the upper and middle portion of the lungs as longer lines or extending peripherally from the hilum (Kerley A lines). The thickening is due to edema and lymphatic distention in chronic pulmonary venous hypertension, but may be due to cellular infiltrate or fibrous tissue in other conditions.

ker·nic·ter·us (kair·nick′tur·us, kur·) *n.* Bilirubin pigmentation of gray matter of the central nervous system, especially basal ganglions, accompanied by degeneration of nerve cells; occurring as complication of erythroblastosis fetalis and other causes of severe hyperbilirubinemia of the newborn, and accompanied and followed by a variety of severe neurological deficits or death. Syn. *nuclear icterus.*

Ker·nig's sign (kʸerr′nʸik) In meningeal irritation, with the patient supine and the thigh flexed at the hip, an attempt to completely extend the leg at the knee causes pain and spasm of the hamstring muscles.

ker·o·sene oil (kerr′uh·seen). A liquid mixture of hydrocarbons distilled from petroleum. Syn. *coal oil.*

ket-, keto-. *In chemistry,* a combining form designating the presence of the ketone group.

ke·ta·mine (kee′tuh·meen) *n.* 2-(o-Chlorophenyl)-2-(methylamino) cyclohexanone, $C_{13}H_{16}ClNO$, an anesthetic given intravenously or intramuscularly as the hydrochloride salt; may produce vivid and sometimes unpleasant dreams.

ke·tene (kee′teen) *n.* Ethenone, $H_2C{=}CO$, a colorless gas that forms acetic acid on hydrolysis; used to effect acetylization of free amino and hydroxyl groups.

ke·to (kee′to) *adj.* Characterizing the tautomeric and usually most stable form of certain ketones, which exhibit keto-enol tautomerism.

ke·to acid (kee′to). Any compound containing both a ketone (—CO—) and a carboxyl (—COOH) group.

ke·to·ac·i·do·sis (kee″to·as″i·do′sis) *n.* Acidosis accompanied by an increase in the blood of such ketone bodies as β-hydroxybutyric and acetoacetic acids.

ke·to·ac·i·du·ria (kee″to·as·i·dew′ree·uh) *n.* The excretion, especially the excessive excretion, in the urine of organic molecules which have both a ketone and an acid group.

ke·to·cho·lan·ic acid (kee″to·ko·lan′ick). Cholic acid in which one or more of the secondary alcohol groups have been oxidized to ketone groups.

Keto-Diastix. A trademark for a reagent strip containing sodium nitroprusside used to test for glucose and ketones in urine.

ke·to·gen·e·sis (kee″to·jen′e·sis) *n.* The production of ketone bodies.

ke·to·gen·ic (kee″to·jen′ick) *adj.* Producing ketone bodies.

ketogenic diet. A diet in which an excessive proportion of the allotted calories is derived from fats, which are reduced to ketones; used in the therapy of epilepsy, especially in children with myoclonic and akinetic seizures and absence attacks refractory to conventional anticonvulsant drugs.

ketogenic hormone. Originally, the factor in crude extract of the anterior hypophysis which stimulated the rate of fatty acid metabolism. The metabolic actions which the term designates are now known to be induced by adrenocorticotropin and the growth hormone. Syn. *fat-metabolizing hormone.*

ke·to·glu·tar·ic acid (kee″to·gloo·tar′ick, ·tahr′ick). A dibasic keto acid, $HOOC(CH_2)_2CO{-}COOH$, an intermediate product in the metabolism of carbohydrates and proteins.

ke·to·hep·tose (kee″to·hep′toce) *n.* A general term for monosaccharides consisting of a seven-carbon chain and containing a ketone group.

ke·to·hex·ose (kee″to·heck′soce) *n.* A general term for monosaccharides consisting of a six-carbon chain and containing a ketone group.

ke·tol (kee′tole, ·tol) *n.* Any compound containing both a ketone (—CO—) group and an alcohol (—OH) group.

ke·tol·y·sis (kee·tol′i·sis) *n.* The dissolution of ketone bodies. —**ke·to·lyt·ic** (kee″to·lit′ic) *adj.*

ke·tone (kee′tone) *n.* An organic compound derived by oxidation from a secondary alcohol; it contains the characterizing group —CO—.

ketone acid. KETO ACID.

ketone body. A group name for any of the compounds, β-hydroxybutyric acid, acetoacetic acid, or acetone, which simultaneously increase in blood and urine in diabetic acidosis, starvation, pregnancy, after ether anesthesia, and in other conditions.

ke·to·ne·mia, ke·to·nae·mia (kee''to·nee'mee·uh) *n.* The presence of increased concentrations of ketone bodies in the blood.

ke·to·nu·ria (kee''to·new'ree·uh) *n.* The presence of ketone bodies in the urine.

ke·tose (kee'toce) *n.* A carbohydrate containing the ketone group.

ke·to·sis (kee·to'sis) *n.,* pl. **keto·ses** (·seez) 1. A condition in which ketones are present in the body in excessive amount. 2. The acidosis of diabetes mellitus. —**ke·tot·ic** (kee·tot'ick) *adj.*

ke·to·ste·roid (kee''to·sterr'oid, ·steer'oid, ke·tos'te·roid) *n.* One of a group of neutral steroids possessing ketone substitution, which produces a characteristic red color with *m*-dinitrobenzene in alkaline solution. The ketosteroids are principally metabolites of adrenal cortical and gonadal steroids. Syn. *17-ketosteroid.*

17-ketosteroid. KETOSTEROID.

key·way (kee'way) *n.* The receptacle attachment of a precision prosthodontic partial denture.

kg Abbreviation for *kilogram.*

khel·lin (kel'in) *n.* 2-Methyl-5,8-dimethoxyfuranochromone, $C_{14}H_{12}O_5$, a constituent of the umbelliferous plant *Ammi visnaga,* the fruits of which have been used in Egypt as an antispasmodic in renal colic and ureteral spasm. Khellin has been used as a coronary vasodilator and bronchodilator. Syn. *kellin, chellin, visammin.*

Kidd blood group system. The erythrocyte antigens defined by reactions to anti-Jk^a antibodies originally found in the mother (Mrs. Kidd) of an erythroblastotic infant, and to anti-Jk^b.

kid·ney, *n.* One of the pair of glandular organs of the urinary system which, by filtration and excretory activity of its component units, the nephrons, elaborates the urine. Comb. form *nephr-, ren-.*

kidney basin. A kidney-shaped basin; emesis basin.

kidney stone. A concretion in the kidney. Syn. *renal calculus.*

kidney worm. *DIOCTOPHYMA RENALE.*

kidney worm infection. Infection of the dog, mink, and occasionally of man by *Dioctophyma renale.*

Kien·böck's atrophy (keen'bœck) Acute atrophy of bone seen in inflammatory conditions of the extremities.

Kienböck's disease Osteochondrosis of the lunate bone.

kie·sel·guhr (kee'zul·goor'') *n.* DIATOMACEOUS EARTH.

Kies·sel·bach's area or **triangle** (kee'sul·baʰkh) An area of the anterior of the nasal septum which may be the site of epistaxis or of perforation.

kilo- A prefix meaning *thousand.*

kil·o·cal·o·rie, kilo·cal·o·ry (kil'o·kal''o·ree) *n.* Any one of several heat units that represent the quantity of heat required to raise the temperature of one kilogram of water 1 degree centigrade but that differ slightly from each other in the specific 1-degree interval of temperature selected. Kilocalorie units are used in metabolic studies, when they are also called large calories or Calories.

kilo·gram (kil'uh·gram) *n.* One thousand grams, or about 2.2 pounds avoirdupois. Abbreviated, kg.

kilo·gram-me·ter, kilo·gram-me·tre (kil'uh·gram mee'tur) *n.* A unit of energy; the amount of energy required to raise one kilogram one meter; approximately 7.233 foot-pounds.

kilo·joule (kil'o·jool'') *n.* A unit of heat, equivalent to 239.1 small calories.

kilo·li·ter, kilo·li·tre (kil'o·lee''tur) *n.* One thousand liters, or 35.31 cubic feet. Abbreviated, kl.

ki·lo·me·ter, ki·lo·me·tre (ki·lom'e·tur, kil'uh·mee''tur) *n.* One thousand meters, or 1093.6 yards. Abbreviated, km.

kilo·nem (kil'o·nem) *n.* A nutritional unit representing 1000 nems, equivalent to approximately 667 calories.

kilo·volt (kil'o·vohlt) *n.* A unit of electric power equal to 1000 volts. Abbreviated, kv.

kilo·watt (kil'uh·wot) *n.* A unit of electric power; one thousand watts. Abbreviated, kw.

Kim·mel·stiel-Wil·son syndrome Hypertension, proteinuria, edema, and renal failure in association with diabetic glomerulosclerosis.

kin-, kine-, kino- A combining form meaning *action, motion.*

ki·nase (kigh'nace, kin'ace, kin'aze) *n.* An enzyme that catalyzes the transfer of phosphate from adenosine triphosphate to an acceptor.

kin·dred, *n.* 1. A more or less broad and cohesive kinship group such as an extended family or a clan. 2. Any aggregate of relatives, such as might be studied for genetic purposes, that is broader than an immediate family of parents and offspring.

ki·ne·mat·ic (kin·e·mat'ick, kigh''ne·) *adj.* 1. Of or pertaining to motion. 2. Of or pertaining to kinematics.

kinematic amputation. An amputation in which a muscular stump is left so as to allow for movement of an artificial limb; KINEPLASTY.

ki·ne·mat·ics (kin''e·mat'icks, kigh''ne·) *n.* The science of motion.

ki·ne·mato·graph (kin''e·mat'o·graf, kigh''ne·) *n.* A device for making and demonstrating a continuous record or pictures of a moving body such as a motion picture camera.

kineplastic amputation. KINEPLASTY.

kin·e·plas·ty (kin'e·plas''tee) *n.* An amputation in which tendons are arranged in the stump to permit their use in moving parts of the prosthetic appliance. Types of kineplastic amputations include the club, the loop, the tendon tunnel, and the muscle tunnel. —**kin·e·plas·tic** (kin''e·plas'tick) *adj.*

ki·ne·ra·dio·ther·a·py (kin″e·ray″dee·o·therr′uh·pee) *n.* X-ray therapy whereby the tube is moved in relation to the patient, or the patient in relation to the stationary tube. The object is the attainment of larger depth doses with sparing of the skin.

kin·e·scope (kin′e·skope) *n.* An instrument for testing the refraction of the eye; consists of a moving disk with a slit of variable width, through which the patient observes a fixed object.

kinesi-, kinesio-. A combining form meaning *kinesis, movement.*

ki·ne·sia (ki·nee′zhuh, ·see·uh, kigh·nee′) *n.* Motion sickness or other disorder caused by motion. Syn. *kinetosis.*

-kinesia A combining form meaning *a condition involving movements.*

ki·ne·si·at·rics (ki·nee″see·at′ricks) *n.* The treatment of disease by systematic active or passive movements. Syn. *kinesitherapy, kinesiotherapy.*

ki·ne·si·es·the·si·om·e·ter, ki·ne·si·aes·the·si·om·e·ter (ki·nee″see·es·theez″ee·om′e·tur) *n.* 1. An instrument for testing the proprioceptive sense; kinesthesiometer. 2. Specifically: an instrument employed to measure the perception of changes in the angles of joints.

ki·ne·si·gen·ic (ki·nee″si·jen′ick) *adj.* Brought on or triggered by movements.

ki·ne·sim·e·ter (kin″e·sim′e·tur, kigh″ne·) *n.* An instrument for determining quantitatively the motions of a part.

ki·ne·si·ol·o·gy (ki·nee″see·ol′uh·jee) *n.* The science of the anatomy, physiology, and mechanics of purposeful muscle movement in man.

ki·ne·si·om·e·ter (ki·nee″see·om′e·tur) *n.* KINESIMETER.

ki·ne·sis (ki·nee′sis, kigh·nee′sis) *n.,* pl. **kine·ses** (·seez) The general term for physical movement, including that induced by stimulation, as by light.

ki·ne·so·pho·bia (ki·nee″so·fo′bee·uh) *n.* Morbid fear of motion.

kin·es·the·sia, kin·aes·the·sia (kin″es·theezh′uh, ·theez′ee·uh) *n.* The proprioceptive sense; the sense of perception of movement, weight, resistance, and position. —**kines·thet·ic** (·thet′ick) *adj.*

kin·es·the·si·om·e·ter, kin·aes·the·si·om·e·ter (kin″es·theez″ee·om′e·tur) *n.* An instrument for measuring the degree of proprioceptive sense.

kinet-, kineto-. A combining form meaning *motion, movement, kinesis, kinetic.*

ki·net·ic (ki·net′ick, kigh·net′ick) *adj.* Pertaining to motion; producing motion.

kinetic apraxia. APRAXIA.

kinetic ataxia. MOTOR ATAXIA.

kinetic energy. The part of the total energy of a body in motion which is caused by its motion.

kinetic reflex. Any reflex that results in movement.

ki·net·ics (ki·net′icks, kigh·) *n.* 1. The science of the effects of forces on the motions of matter. 2. *In chemistry,* the study of the rates of reaction of systems; often referred to as reaction kinetics.

kinetic tremor. ACTION TREMOR.

ki·ne·tism (ki·nee′tiz·um, kin′e·) *n.* The ability to initiate or perform independent movement such as muscular activity.

ki·neto·car·dio·gram (ki·net″o·kahr′dee·o·gram) *n.* The record of the pulsations and vibrations over the anterior chest, used in the diagnosis of cardiac disease. —**kineto·car·di·og·ra·phy** (·kahr·dee·og′ruh·fee) *n.*

kin·e·to·sis (kin″e·to′sis) *n.,* pl. **kineto·ses** (·seez) Motion sickness or any other disorder caused by motion. Syn. *kinesia.*

king's evil. SCROFULA.

ki·nin (kin′in, kigh′nin) *n.* Any of a group of polypeptides, as bradykinin, that are hypotensive, contract most isolated smooth muscle preparations, increase capillary permeability, and have certain other pharmacologic properties in common. Certain other polypeptides that are hypertensive, such as angiotensins, may also be included in the group.

kink, *n.* ANGULATION.

kinky hair disease. A sex-linked recessive disorder of unknown cause, with onset in early infancy, characterized clinically by light, kinky hair, developmental failure, death in early childhood, and focal cerebral and cerebellar degeneration. Syn. *Menkes' syndrome.*

ki·no (kee′no, kigh′no) *n.* The dried juice obtained from the trunk of *Pterocarpus marsupium;* a powerful astringent that has been used in the treatment of diarrhea.

Kirch·ner's diverticulum (kirr^{kh}′nur) A small diverticulum of the lower portion of the auditory tube.

Kirsch·ner's traction (kirrsh′nur) A form of skeletal traction used in the treatment of bone fractures. Kirschner's wires, passed through holes drilled in the bones, and attached to stirrups, are used to apply the traction.

Kirschner's wires Metallic wires, usually 9 inches in length, either threaded or smooth, usually supplied in three diameters of .035, .045, and .062 inches, used for the application of percutaneous skeletal traction or internal fixation of small fractures.

kiss·ing bug. 1. ASSASSIN BUG. 2. Specifically, REDUVIUS PERSONATUS.

kissing disease. INFECTIOUS MONONUCLEOSIS.

kissing ulcer. An ulcer that appears to be due to transmission from one apposing part to another, or due to pressure of apposing parts.

Kjel·dahl method (kel′dahl) A method to determine the amount of nitrogen in an organic compound by interaction with sulfuric acid to produce ammonium ion which is converted to ammonia by alkali and distilled into standard acid.

kl Abbreviation for *kiloliter.*

Kleb·si·el·la (kleb″zee·el′uh) *n.* A genus of bacteria of the family Enterobacteriaceae; frequently associated with infections of the respiratory tract and pathologic conditions of other parts of the body.

Klebsiella ozae·nae (o·zee′nee). A gram-negative encapsulated rod found in association with ozena and atrophic rhinitis.

Klebsiella pneu·mo·ni·ae (new·mo′nee·ee). A species of short, plump, heavily capsulated, nonmotile, and gram-negative bacteria, responsible for severe pneumonitis in man. Syn. *Bacillus mucosus capsulatus, Friedländer's bacillus, pneumobacillus.*

Klebsiella rhi·no·scle·ro·ma·tis (rye″no-skle-ro′ muh-tis). Encapsulated gram-negative rod recovered from nasal granulomas of patients with rhinoscleroma. Syn. *Frisch's bacillus.*

Klebs-Loeffler bacillus CORYNEBACTERIUM DIPH-THERIAE.

Klei·ne-Le·vin syndrome (klye′neh, le·vin′) Periodic attacks of excessive sleepiness and food intake (bulimia) frequently associated with mild mental confusion, irritability, and amnesia for portions of the attacks; of unknown cause.

klept-, klepto- A combining form meaning *stealing, theft.*

klep·to·lag·nia (klep″to·lag′nee·uh) *n.* Sexual gratification induced by theft.

klep·to·ma·nia (klep″to·may′nee·uh) *n.* A morbid desire to steal; obsessive stealing; a mental disorder in which the objects stolen are usually of symbolic value only, being petty and useless items.

klep·to·pho·bia (klep″to·fo′bee·uh) *n.* 1. A morbid fear of thieves or of suffering theft. 2. A morbid dread of becoming a kleptomaniac.

Klinefelter's syndrome The clinical syndrome of hypogonadism including gynecomastia, eunuchoidism, elevated urinary gonadotropins, and decreased testicular size associated with hyalinization of the tubules. The sex chromosome constitution of somatic cells is abnormal in that a Y chromosome is associated with more than one X chromosome.

Kline test A flocculation test for syphilis.

Klip·pel-Feil syndrome or **deformity** (klee·pel′, fel) Congenital fusion of the bodies of two or more cervical vertebrae; the spines are small, deficient, or bifid; atlanto-occipital fusion is common. As a result the neck is short and wide with markedly limited movements. Platybasia and its associated neurologic deficits may occur.

Klippel-Tré·nau·nay-We·ber syndrome (trey·no· neh′, wee′bur) Cutaneous hemangioma of an extremity, often extending to the trunk, followed as the child grows by hypertrophy of the involved limb and, if a leg, by varicose veins. Mild mental retardation is frequently present.

Klump·ke's paralysis or **palsy** (klump′kee) LOW-ER BRACHIAL PLEXUS PARALYSIS.

km Abbreviation for *kilometer.*

knee, *n.* 1. The part of the leg containing the articulation of the femur, tibia, and patella. 2. The knee joint. 3. An analogous part or joint in the leg of certain animals, as for example the carpus of ungulates.

knee-chest position. A position assumed by a patient resting on the knees and chest as an exercise after childbirth, or for the purposes of examination and treatment.

knee jerk. PATELLAR REFLEX.

knee-sprung, *adj.* Of a horse: having bucked knees, anterior deviation of the carpus resulting in constant partial flexion.

knife, *n.* A cutting instrument of varying shape, size, and design, used in surgery and in dissecting; a scalpel.

knit·ting, *n.* A lay term to indicate the process of union in a fractured bone.

knob, *n.* 1. A rounded prominence or protuberance. 2. An end foot.

knock-knee, *n.* GENU VALGUM.

knock-out drops. Chloral hydrate solution; so called because of the rapid action of small doses of the compound, sometimes given in food or drink to render a victim helpless.

knuck·le, *n.* 1. An articulation of the phalanges with the metacarpal bones or with each other. 2. The distal convex ends of the metacarpals.

knuck·ling, *n.* A condition in which the hoof of a horse is turned under; due to excessive flexion of the fetlock joint.

Ko·belt's cyst A small cystic remnant of the mesonephric duct in the vicinity of the ovary and broad ligament.

Kocher forceps A strong surgical clamp having serrated jaws and sharp interlocking teeth at the tip.

Kocher's sign A sign of hyperthyroidism in which, as the patient looks up, the eyelid retracts faster than the eyeball is raised, thus exposing the sclera above the cornea. Syn. *globe lag.*

Koch phenomenon (koʻh) The altered reactivity of guinea pigs, previously infected with tubercle bacilli, to reinoculation with living or killed tubercle bacilli, or with tuberculin, characterized by an acceleration and intensification of the reaction at the local site. Serves as the basis of the general concept of delayed hypersensitivity.

Koch's law or **postulate** The four conditions that are required to establish an organism as the causative agent of a disease are: (a) the microorganism must be present in every case of the disease; (b) it must be capable of cultivation in pure culture; (c) it must, when inoculated in pure culture, produce the disease in susceptible animals; (d) it must be recovered and again grown in pure culture. Syn. *law of specificity of bacteria.*

Koch-Weeks bacillus HAEMOPHILUS AEGYPTICUS.

Koch-Weeks conjunctivitis Catarrhal conjunctivitis due to infection by *Haemophilus aegyptius.*

Koeb·ner's phenomenon (kœb′nur) ISOMOR-PHOUS PROVOCATIVE REACTION.

Köh·ler's disease (kœh′lur) 1. Osteochondrosis of the navicular bone; a variety of aseptic necrosis of bone. Syn. *Kofhler's tarsal scaphoiditis.* 2. Osteochondrosis of the second metatarsal head. Syn. *Freiberg's disease.*

Köhler's method of illumination A method of microscopical illumination in which an image of the source is focused in the lower focal plane of the microscope condenser, and the condenser, in turn, focuses an image of the lamp lens in the object field.

koi·lo·cy·to·sis (koy″lo·sigh·to′sis) *n.* The hollow appearance of a cell due to large perinuclear vacuoles, as seen in certain desquamated cells of the uterine cervix. —**koilocy·tot·ic** (·tot′ick) *adj.*

koilocytotic atypia. A pattern of nuclear abnormalities of the stratified squamous epithelium of the uterine cervix, associated with vacuolization and ballooning of the upper layer of cells.

koil·onych·ia (koy″lo·nick′ee·uh) *n.* A spoon-shaped deformity of the nails; may be familial, or associated with other diseases, such as iron-deficiency anemia and lichen planus. Syn. *spoon nail.*

koi·lo·ster·nia (koy″lo·stur′nee·uh) *n.* FUNNEL CHEST.

koi·not·ro·py (koy·not′ruh·pee) *n. In psychobiology,* the state of being socialized; the condition of being identified with the common interest of the people. —**koi·no·trop·ic** (koy″no·trop′ick) *adj.*

ko·la (ko′luh) *n.* The dried cotyledon of *Cola nitida* or of other species of *Cola* (cola nut); the chief constituent is caffeine, with traces of theobromine also present. The effect of kola is the same as that of other sources of caffeine, as coffee and tea.

Kol·mer's test 1. A complement-fixation test for syphilis. 2. A complement-fixation test for bacterial, spirochetal, viral, protozoal, or metazoal diseases.

Kon·do·le·on's operation An operation for elephantiasis, in which extensive strips of skin, subcutaneous tissue, and scarred fascia are excised.

koni·, konio·. See *coni-.*

Kö·nig's disease (kœh′nikh) OSTEOCHONDRITIS DISSECANS.

ko·nio·cor·tex (ko″nee·o·kor′tecks) *n.* Granular cortex characteristic of sensory areas.

Kop·lik's spots or **sign** The characteristic oral enanthem of measles, at the end of the prodromal stage, consisting of tiny gray-white areas on a bright red base, grouped around the orifice of the parotid duct opposite the premolar teeth.

kop·o·pho·bia (kop″o·fo′bee·uh) *n.* Morbid fear of fatigue or exhaustion.

Ko·rot·kov's method (kor′ut·kuf) The auscultatory method for determining the blood pressure, by applying a stethoscope to the brachial artery below the pressure cuff of a sphygmomanometer.

Korotkov sounds The sounds heard with the stethoscope during the auscultatory determination of the blood pressure.

Kor·sa·koff's syndrome, psychosis, or **neurosis** (kor′suh·kuf) An amnestic-confabulatory syndrome characterized by confusion, retrograde and anteograde amnesia, confabulation, and apathy seen most often in chronic alcoholism and other causes of vitamin B deficiency as well as in other diseases that involve the diencephalon or hippocampal formations bilaterally.

Kr Symbol for krypton.

Krab·be's disease GLOBOID LEUKODYSTROPHY.

Krae·pe·lin-Mo·rel disease (kreh′pe·leen, moh.rel′) DEMENTIA PRAECOX.

Kraepelin's classification An extensive systematic, descriptive classification of mental disorders, which employed the term dementia praecox for schizophrenia and divided it into the simple, hebephrenic, catatonic, and paranoid types.

kra·tom·e·ter (kra·tom′e·tur) *n.* A device consisting of prisms, used for correcting nystagmus or in orthoptic exercises.

krau·ro·sis (kraw·ro′sis) *n.* A progressive, sclerosing, shriveling process of the skin.

kraurosis of the vulva. A disease of elderly women, characterized by pruritus, atrophy, and dryness of the external genitalia. Stenosis of the vaginal orifice and carcinoma may develop.

Krebs cycle CITRIC ACID CYCLE.

Krebs-Hen·se·leit cycle (hen′ze·lite) UREA CYCLE.

kreo·tox·in (kree″o·tock′sin) *n.* A meat poison that is formed by bacteria.

Kretsch·mer type The type of physique associated with certain psychic or temperamental traits a person possesses, such as the pyknic, asthenic, athletic, or dysplastic type.

Krukenberg's tumor Bilateral primary ovarian carcinoma, as originally described, but most widely used to denote metastatic ovarian carcinoma, usually of gastric origin.

kry·mo·ther·a·py (krye″mo·therr′uh·pee) *n.* CRYOTHERAPY.

kryp·ton (krip′ton) *n.* Kr = 83.80; a colorless, inert gaseous element which occurs in the atmosphere.

KUB (kay yoo bee) A plain film of the abdomen, including the areas of the kidneys, ureters, and the bladder.

Ku·gel·berg-We·lan·der syndrome (ku″gᵉl·bærʸ, veʸ′laʰn·dur) JUVENILE SPINAL MUSCULAR ATROPHY.

Kulchitsky. See *Kultschitzsky.*

Kun·kel test A test for gamma globulin in which the turbidity resulting on addition of zinc sulfate solution is compared with suitable standards.

Kupf·fer cells (kööp′fur) Fixed macrophages lining the hepatic sinusoids.

ku·ru (koo′roo) *n.* A subacute degenerative disease of the central nervous system unique to certain groups, especially the Fore tribe of New Guinea, but now disappearing, characterized clinically by cerebellar ataxia, trembling, spasticity and progressive dementia, due to a transmissible agent once acquired by ritual cannibalism.

Kus·ko·kwim disease Arthrogryposis occurring in the Yupik Eskimos of southwestern Alaska.

Kuss·maul-Mai·er disease (kōōs′mɑwl, migh′ur) POLYARTERITIS NODOSA.

Kussmaul's respiration, breathing, or **sign** AIR HUNGER.

kv Abbreviation for *kilovolt.*

Kveim antigen Emulsified material from a lymph node proved to be sarcoid, which, on injection into an individual with sarcoidosis, usually results in the formation of sarcoid tubercles. Used in the Kveim test.

Kveim test A test for the diagnosis of sarcoidosis, in which intradermal administration of

Kveim antigen results in the appearance of noncaseating granulomas at the site of injection 4 to 8 weeks later. Syn. *Nickerson-Kveim test.*

kwa·shi·or·kor (kwah″shee·or′kor) *n.* A disease of infants and young children, mainly in the tropics and subtropics, occurring soon after weaning, due primarily to deficient quality and quantity of dietary protein; characterized by edema, skin and hair changes, impaired growth, fatty liver, severe apathy, and weakness.

Kya·sa·nur forest disease. One of the Russian tick-borne encephalitides.

ky·mo·gram (kigh′mo·gram) *n.* The record made on a kymograph.

ky·mo·graph (kigh′mo·graf) *n.* An instrument for recording physiologic cycles or actions in a patient, an experimental animal, or in an isolated muscle or heart; consists of a clock- or motor-driven cylinder, covered with paper on which the record is made. Time intervals can be recorded simultaneously with the phenomena. —**ky·mo·graph·ic** (kigh″mo·graf′ick) *adj.*

ky·mog·ra·phy (kigh·mog′ruh·fee) *n.* Any method or technique for recording motions or contractions in an organ, usually by means of a kymograph or electrokymograph.

kyn·uren·ic acid (kin″yoo·ree′nick, ·ren′ick, kigh″new·). γ-Hydroxy-β-quinolinecarboxylic acid, $C_{10}H_7NO_3$, a product of the metabolism of tryptophan occurring in the urine of mammals.

kyn·uren·ine (kigh·new′ri·neen, kin″yoo·ree′nin) *n.* An intermediate product, $C_{10}H_{12}N_2O_3$, of tryptophan metabolism isolated from the urine of mammals.

kyphorachitic pelvis. A deformity of the pelvis associated with rickets in which changes are slight because the effect of kyphosis tends to counterbalance that of rickets.

ky·pho·ra·chi·tis (kigh″fo·ra·kigh′tis) *n.* Rachitic deformity of the thorax and spine, resulting in an anteroposterior hump. The pelvis is sometimes involved. —**kyphora·chit·ic** (·kit′ick) *adj.*

ky·phos (kye′fos) *n.* The convex part (the hump) of the deformed back in kyphoscoliosis.

kyphoscoliorachitic pelvis. A deformity of the pelvis resembling the kyphorachitic type because the kyphotic and rachitic effects counterbalance each other. However, a considerable degree of oblique deformity of the superior strait is usually present.

ky·pho·sco·lio·ra·chi·tis (kigh″fo·sko″lee·o·ra·kigh′tis) *n.* A combined kyphosis and scoliosis due to rickets. The pelvis and thorax may be involved in the deformity. —**kyphoscoliora·chit·ic** (·kit′ick) *adj.*

ky·pho·sco·li·o·sis (kigh″fo·sko″lee·o′sis) *n.* Lateral curvature of the spine with vertebral rotation, associated with an anteroposterior hump in the spinal column. —**kyphoscoli·ot·ic** (·ot′ick) *adj.*

kyphoscoliotic heart disease. Cardiorespiratory disease or failure due to functional abnormalities imposed by kyphoscoliosis.

kyphoscoliotic pelvis. A deformity of the pelvis varying in character with the predominance of the kyphosis or scoliosis of the vertebral column.

ky·pho·sis (kigh·fo′sis) *n.,* pl. **kypho·ses** (·seez) Angular curvature of the spine, the convexity of the curve being posterior, usually situated in the thoracic region, and involving few or many vertebrae; the result of such diseases as tuberculosis, osteochondritis or ankylosing spondylitis of the spine, or an improper posture habit. Syn. *humpback, hunchback.* —**ky·phot·ic** (kigh·fot′ick) *adj.*

kyphotic pelvis. A pelvis characterized by increase of the conjugata vera, but decrease of the transverse diameter of the outlet, through approximation of the ischial spines and tuberosities. Associated with kyphosis of the vertebral column.

L

l. Abbreviation for (a) *left*; (b) *left eye*; (c) *libra*; (d) *lethal*; (e) *liter*.

L+ Symbol for limes death.

L0 Symbol for limes zero.

l- 1. *In chemistry,* a symbol formerly employed for levorotatory, referring to the direction in which the plane of polarized light is rotated by a substance; this usage is superseded by the symbol (−). 2. *In chemistry,* a symbol formerly used to indicate the structural configuration of a particular asymmetric carbon atom in a compound, in the manner that the small capital letter L- is now used.

La Symbol for lanthanum.

-labe A combining form designating *something that takes, removes, takes up, or absorbs.*

la·bel, *v.* To convert a small portion of the atoms of a specific element in a compound or system to a radioactive isotope, or to add a radioactive isotope or an isotope of unusual mass of the element for the purpose of tracing the element through one or more chemical reactions. Syn. *tag.* **—la·beled, la·belled,** *adj.*

labia. Plural of *labium.*

la·bi·al (lay'bee·ul) *adj.* Pertaining to a lip or labium.

labial hernia. Complete, indirect inguinal hernia into the labium majus.

la·bi·al·ism (lay'bee·ul·iz·um) *n.* 1. The tendency to substitute labial sounds, as *b, p, m,* or *w,* for other speech sounds. 2. The addition of a labial or labiodental quality to any speech sound. 3. The tendency to confuse one labial consonant with any other.

labial occlusion. A situation in which the alignment of a tooth is external to the line of occlusion.

labia ma·jo·ra (ma·jo'ruh). Plural of *labium majus.*

labia mi·no·ra (mi·no'ruh). Plural of *labium minus.*

labia oris (o'ris) [NA]. The lips of the mouth, including the upper lip and the lower lip.

labia pu·den·di (pew·den'dye). The lips of the vulva, including the labia majora and the labia minora.

la·bile (lay'bil, ·bile) *adj.* 1. Unstable, particularly when applied to moods. 2. Readily changed as by heat, oxidation, or other processes, particularly when applied to chemical substances, microorganisms, antibodies, and so on. 3. Moving from place to place. 4. Fluctuating widely.

la·bil·i·ty (lay·bil'i·tee) *n.* The quality of being labile. Specifically: 1. *In neurology and psychiatry,* very rapid fluctuations in intensity and modality of emotions, without apparent adequate cause and with inadequate control of their expression, seen most dramatically in the affective reactions or in pseudobulbar palsy. 2. *In chemistry,* readily susceptible to change, such as a rearrangement or cleavage of an organic molecule.

labio- A combining form meaning *lip, labial.*

la·bio·al·ve·o·lar (lay''bee·o·al·vee'uh·lur) *adj.* Pertaining to the lip and to the alveolar process of maxilla or mandible.

la·bio·cer·vi·cal (lay''bee·o·sur'vi·kul) *adj.* 1. Pertaining to a lip and a neck. 2. Pertaining to the labial surface of the neck of a tooth.

la·bio·den·tal (lay''bee·o·den'tul) *adj.* Pertaining to the lips and the teeth.

la·bio·gin·gi·val (lay''bee·o·jin'ji·vul, ·jin·jye'vul) *adj.* Pertaining to the lips and gums.

la·bio·glos·so·la·ryn·ge·al (lay''bee·o·glos''o·la·rin'jee·ul) *adj.* Pertaining conjointly to the lips, tongue, and larynx.

la·bio·glos·so·pha·ryn·ge·al (lay''bee·o·glos''o·fa·rin'jee·ul) *adj.* Pertaining to the lips, tongue, and pharynx.

la·bio·men·tal (lay''bee·o·men'tul) *adj.* Pertaining to the lip and chin.

la·bio·pal·a·tine (lay''bee·o·pal'uh·tine, ·tin) *adj.* Pertaining to the lip and palate.

la·bio·plas·ty (lay·bee·o·plas'tee) *n.* CHEILOPLASTY.

la·bi·um (lay'bee·um) *n.,* genit. **la·bii** (·bee·eye), pl. **la·bia** (·bee·uh) 1. A lip. 2. *In invertebrate zoology,* the lower lip, as opposed to the labrum, the upper lip.

labium lep·o·ri·num (lep·o·rye'num) HARELIP.

labium ma·jus (may'jus). One of two folds (labia

majora) of the female external genital organs, arising just below the mons pubis, and surrounding the vulval entrance or rima pudendi. Syn. *major lip.*

labium mi·nus (migh'nus). One of the two folds (labia minora) at the inner surfaces of the labia majora. Syn. *minor lip.*

labium vo·ca·le (vo·kay'lee) [BNA]. VOCAL LIP.

la·bor, la·bour, *n.* The series of processes, especially the coordinated, periodic uterine contractions, whereby the fetus is expelled in parturition.

lab·o·ra·to·ry, *n.* 1. A place for experimental work in any branch of science. 2. In the 17th and 18th century, a place where medicines were prepared.

labor pains. The pains associated with parturition due to uterine contractions.

la·brum (lay'brum, lab'rum) *n.* 1. A liplike structure. 2. *In invertebrate zoology,* the upper lip, as opposed to the labium, the lower lip.

Labstix. A trademark for reagent strips employed to test urine for pH, proteins, glucose, ketones, or blood.

lab·y·rinth (lab'i·rinth) *n.* 1. An intricate system of connecting passageways; maze. 2. The system of intercommunicating canals and cavities that makes up the inner ear. —**lab·y·rin·thine** (lab''i·rin'theen) *adj.*

lab·y·rin·thec·to·my (lab''i·rin·theck'tuh·mee) *n.* The complete removal of the membranous labyrinth of the inner ear.

labyrinthine nystagmus. Nystagmus occurring when the labyrinths are stimulated or diseased.

labyrinthine reflex. A reflex initiated by stimulation of the vestibular apparatus of the inner ear.

labyrinthine test. Any test to check the function of the vestibular nerve and labyrinth.

lab·y·rin·thi·tis (lab''i·rin·thigh'tis) *n.* Inflammation of the labyrinth of the inner ear. Syn. *otitis interna.*

lab·y·rin·thot·o·my (lab''i·rin·thot'uh·mee) *n.* Incision into the labyrinth, specifically, into that of the inner ear.

la·by·rin·thus (lab''i·rinth'us) *n.,* pl. & genit. sing. **labyrin·thi** (·eye) LABYRINTH.

lac (lack) *n.,* pl. **lac·ta** (·tuh) MILK (1).

lac·er·ate (las'ur·ate) *v.* To wound by tearing. —**lacer·at·ed** (·ay·tid) *adj.*

lacerated foramen. FORAMEN LACERUM.

lac·er·a·tion (las''ur·ay'shun) *n.* 1. A tear, or a wound made by tearing. 2. The act of tearing or lacerating.

la·cin·i·ate (la·sin'ee·ate) *adj.* Jagged, fringed; cut into narrow flaps.

lac·ri·ma (lack'ri·muh) *n.,* pl. **lacri·mae** (·mee) Tear.

lac·ri·mal (lack'ri·mul) *adj. & n.* 1. Pertaining to tears, or to the organs secreting and conveying tears. 2. LACRIMAL BONE.

lacrimal apparatus. The mechanism for secreting tears and draining them into the nasal cavity, consisting of the lacrimal gland, lake, puncta, canaliculi, sac, and the nasolacrimal duct.

lacrimal canaliculus. A small tube lined with

stratified squamous epithelium which runs vertically a short distance from the punctum of each eyelid and then turns horizontally in the lacrimal part of the lid margin to the lacrimal sac.

lacrimal caruncle. A small, rounded elevation covered by modified skin lying in the lacrimal lake at each medial palpebral commissure.

lacrimal duct. LACRIMAL CANALICULUS.

lacrimal fistula. A fistula communicating with a lacrimal canaliculus.

lacrimal gland. The compound tubuloalveolar gland secreting the tears, situated in the orbit in a depression of the frontal bone.

lacrimal lake. The space at the inner canthus of the eye, near the lacrimal punctum, in which there is some pooling of tear fluid.

lacrimal punctum. The orifice of either lacrimal canaliculus at the inner canthus of the eye.

lacrimal sac. The dilated upper portion of the nasolacrimal duct.

lac·ri·ma·tion (lack''ri·may'shun) *n.* 1. Normal secretion of tears. 2. Excessive secretion, as in weeping.

lac·ri·ma·tor (lack'ri·may''tur) *n.* Any substance, as a tear gas, which irritates the conjunctiva and causes secretion of the tears.

lac·ri·ma·to·ry (lack''ri·muh·to'ree) *adj.* Pertaining to or causing lacrimation.

lac·ri·mo·na·sal (lack''ri·mo·nay'zul) *adj.* Pertaining to the lacrimal apparatus and the nose.

lac·ri·mot·o·my (lack''ri·mot'uh·mee) *n.* Incision of the nasolacrimal duct.

lac·tac·i·de·mia, lac·tac·i·dae·mia (lack·tas''i·dee'mee·uh) *n.* The presence of lactic acid in the blood.

lac·tac·i·du·ria (lack·tas''i·dew'ree·uh) *n.* The presence of lactic acid in the urine.

lac·ta·gogue (lack'tuh·gog) *n.* GALACTAGOGUE.

lac·tal·bu·min (lack''tal·bew'min) *n.* A simple protein contained in milk which resembles serum albumin and is of high nutritional quality.

lac·tase (lack'tace, ·taze) *n.* A soluble enzyme found in the animal body which hydrolyzes lactose to dextrose and galactose.

lactase deficiency syndrome. Diarrhea induced by ingestion of a lactose-containing food such as milk, secondary to a congenital or acquired deficiency of the disaccharide-splitting enzyme lactase in the intestinal mucosa.

¹**lac·tate** (lack'tate) *n.* A salt or ester of lactic acid. —**lac·tat·ed** (·tay·tid) *adj.*

²**lactate,** *v.* To secrete milk.

lactate dehydrogenase. LACTIC ACID DEHYDROGENASE.

lactated Ringer's injection A sterile solution of 0.6 g sodium chloride, 0.03 g potassium chloride, 0.02 g calcium chloride, and 0.31 g sodium lactate in sufficient water for injection to make 100 ml. Used intravenously as a systemic alkalizer, and as a fluid and electrolyte replenisher. Syn. *Hartmann's solution, Ringer lactate solution.*

lac·ta·tion (lack·tay'shun) *n.* 1. The period during which the child is nourished from the breast. 2. The formation or secretion of milk. —**lactation·al** (·ul) *adj.*

lac·te·al (lack'tee·ul) *adj. & n.* 1. Pertaining to milk. 2. Milky. 3. Any of the lymphatics of the small intestine that take up the chyle.

lac·tes·cence (lack·tes'unce) *n.* Milkiness; often applied to the chyle.

lac·tic (lack'tick) *adj.* Pertaining to milk or its derivatives.

lactic acid. 2-Hydroxypropanoic acid or α-hydroxypropionic acid, existing in three forms: (a) D(−)-lactic acid, $CH_3HCOHCOOH$, levorotatory, biochemically produced from methylglyoxal under certain conditions; (b) L(+)-lactic acid, $CH_3HOCHCOOH$, dextrorotatory, the product of anaerobic glycolysis in muscle, hence called sarcolactic acid; (c) DL-lactic acid, a racemic mixture of (a) and (b), produced by the action of bacteria on sour milk and other foods, and prepared synthetically by fermentation. The last occurs as a colorless, syrupy liquid, miscible with water. It is used as an ingredient of infant-feeding formulas, and has been variously used for medicinal purposes.

lactic acid dehydrogenase. A polymeric enzyme in mammalian tissues that exists in different forms and that catalyzes dehydrogenation of L(+)-lactic acid to pyruvic acid. Measurement of the levels of this enzyme in serum is useful in the diagnosis of myocardial infarction. Abbreviated, LAD.

lactic dehydrogenase. LACTIC ACID DEHYDROGENASE.

lac·tif·er·ous (lack·tif'ur·us) *adj.* Conveying or secreting milk. Syn. *lactigerous.*

lactiferous ducts. The excretory ducts of the mammary gland, opening on the nipple. Syn. *milk ducts.*

lac·ti·fuge (lack'ti·fewj) *n. & adj.* 1. A drug or agent that lessens the secretion of milk. 2. Having the action of a lactifuge.

lac·tim (lack'tim) *n.* An organic compound, containing a —NCOH— group in ring form, produced by the elimination of a molecule of water from certain amino acids. It is the enol form of its isomer, lactam.

Lac·to·ba·cil·lus (lack"to·ba·sil'us) *n.* A genus of bacteria that are capable of producing lactic acid from carbohydrates and carbohydrate-like compounds, and which are able to withstand a degree of acidity usually destructive to nonsporulating bacteria. —**lactobacillus,** pl. **lactobacilli** (·eye), *com. n.*

Lactobacillus ac·i·doph·i·lus (as"i·dof'i·lus). A gram-positive rod-shaped microorganism found in milk, feces, saliva, and carious teeth, nonpathogenic and unusually resistant to acid. Formerly called *Bacillus acidophilus, B. gastrophilus, Lactobacillus gastrophilus.*

Lactobacillus bul·gar·i·cus (bul·gār'i·kus). A species of bacteria isolated from Bulgarian fermented milk.

Lactobacillus ca·sei factor (kay'see·eye). FOLIC ACID.

lactobacillus count. A count of the number of *Lactobacillus acidophilus* in a sample of saliva; used in testing for dental caries activity.

lac·to·cele (lack'to·seel) *n.* GALACTOCELE.

lac·to·fla·vin (lack"to·flay'vin, ·flav'in) *n.* RIBOFLAVIN.

lac·to·gen (lack'to·jen) *n.* Any agent or substance that stimulates the secretion of milk.

lac·to·gen·ic (lack"to·jen'ick) *adj.* Activating or stimulating the mammary glands.

lactogenic hormone. PROLACTIN.

lac·to·glob·u·lin (lack"to·glob'yoo·lin) *n.* One of the proteins of milk.

lac·tom·e·ter (lack·tom'e·tur) *n.* An instrument for determining the specific gravity of milk.

lac·tone (lack'tone) *n.* An anhydro-ring compound produced by elimination of water from a molecule of an oxyacid.

lac·ton·ic acid (lack·ton'ick). GALACTONIC ACID.

lac·to·pro·te·in (lack"to·pro'tee·in, ·pro'teen) *n.* A protein of milk.

lac·tose (lack'toce) *n.* 4-(β-D-Galactopyranosido)-D-glucopyranose or 4-D-glucopyranosyl-β-D-galactopyranoside, $C_{12}H_{22}O_{11}$, a disaccharide representing D-glucose and D-galactose joined by a 1,4-glycosidic bond; on hydrolysis it is converted to these sugars. Two forms are known, alpha-lactose and beta-lactose; milk of mammals contains an equilibrium mixture of the two. Lactose is commonly the alpha form; crystallization at higher temperatures yields the beta form, which is more soluble in water. Both are used as nutrients and occasionally as diuretic agents; in pharmacy both are widely used as diluents and tablet excipients. Syn. *lactin, milk sugar.*

lac·tos·uria (lack"to·sue'ree·uh) *n.* The presence of lactose in the urine.

lac·to·veg·e·tar·i·an (lack"to·vej"e·terr'ee·un) *adj. & n.* 1. Subsisting on or pertaining to a diet of milk and vegetables. 2. One who lives on a diet of milk and vegetables.

lac·to·vo·veg·e·tar·i·an (lack·to"vo·vej"e·terr'ee·un) *n.* A person who lives on a diet of milk, eggs, and vegetables.

la·cu·na (la·kew'nuh) *n.*, pl. **lacunas, lacu·nae** (·nee) 1. A little depression or space. 2. The space in the matrix occupied by a cartilage cell or by the body of a bone cell. 3. Gap; lapse; something missing.

lacunar abscess. An abscess involving a lacuna, usually of the urethra.

lacunar amnesia. Amnesia characterized by gaps or hiatuses in recall of a given stretch of time; spotty memory loss.

LAD Abbreviation for *lactic acid dehydrogenase.*

La·en·nec's cirrhosis (la·eh·neck') Replacement of normal liver structure by abnormal lobules of liver cells, often hyperplastic, delimited by bands of fibrous tissue, giving the gross appearance of a finely nodular surface; alcoholism and malnutrition are chronically associated factors. Syn. *atrophic cirrhosis, diffuse nodular cirrhosis.*

La·e·trile (lay'e·tril) *n.* A British trademark for *l*-mandelnitrile-β-glucuronic acid, $C_{14}H_{15}HO_7$, a product obtained by hydrolysis of amygdalin and oxidation of the resulting glycoside. It has been proposed as a valuable agent in the treatment of cancer, but, to date, this has not been confirmed by scientific studies.

La·fo·ra bodies (lah·fo'rah) Basophilic, cytoplasmic bodies composed of an unusual polyglucosan and found in the dentate, brainstem, and thalamic neurons in progressive familial myoclonic epilepsy.

Lafora's disease PROGRESSIVE FAMILIAL MYOCLONIC EPILEPSY.

lag, *n.* 1. The time between the application of a stimulus and resulting response; LATENT PERIOD. 2. LAG PHASE.

la·ge·ni·form (la·jee′ni·form, la·jen′i·) *adj.* Flask-shaped.

lag·neia (lag·nigh′uh) *n.* EROTOMANIA.

lagophthalmic keratitis. Keratitis due to the failure of the eyelids to close completely; a form of exposure keratitis.

lag·oph·thal·mos (lag″off·thal′mus) *n.* A condition in which the eyelids do not entirely close. —**lagophthal·mic** (·mick) *adj.*

lag phase or **period.** The early period of slow growth of bacteria when first inoculated in a culture medium.

La·grange's operation (la·grahⁿzh′) A combination of iridectomy and sclerectomy for relief of glaucoma.

la grippe (lah greep) INFLUENZA.

¹lake, *n.* A small, fluid-filled hollow or cavity.

²lake, *n.* A pigment prepared by precipitating a vegetable or animal coloring matter or synthetic dye with a metallic compound.

³lake, *v.* To hemolyze.

laky (lay′kee) *adj.* Purplish red; said of blood serum which has a transparent red color after hemolysis.

-lalia A combining form designating a *condition involving speech.*

lal·io·pho·bia (lal″ee·o·fo′bee·uh) *n.* Morbid fear of talking or of stuttering.

lal·la·tion (lal·ay′shun) *n.* 1. Any unintelligible stammering of speech, particularly that in which difficult consonants are avoided so that the speech sounds like the prattling of a baby. 2. Pronunciation of *l* sounds in place of *r* sounds.

lal·og·no·sis (lal″og·no′sis) *n.* Recognition of words.

la·lop·a·thy (la·lop′uth·ee) *n.* Any disorder of speech or disturbance of language.

lalo·pho·mi·a·trist (lal″o·fo·migh′uh·trist) *n.* SPEECH PATHOLOGIST.

lalo·ple·gia (lal″o·plee′jee·uh) *n.* Inability to speak, due to paralysis of the muscles concerned in speech, except those of the tongue.

La·marck·ism (la·mahrk′iz·um) *n.* The theory that organic evolution takes place through the inheritance of modifications caused by the environment, and by the effects of use and disuse of organs.

lamb·da·cism (lam′duh·siz·um) *n.* 1. Difficulty in uttering the sound of the letter *l.* 2. Too frequent use of the *l* sound, or its substitution for the *r* sound.

lamb·doid (lam′doid) *adj.* Resembling the Greek letter lambda (Λ, λ).

lambdoid suture. The union between the two superior borders of the occipital bone with the parietal bones.

lam·bert (lam′burt) *n.* A photometric unit for describing the brightness of light reflected

from a surface. One lambert is the equivalent of one lumen per square centimeter.

Lam·blia (lam′blee·uh) *n.* GIARDIA.

lam·bli·a·sis (lam·blye′uh·sis) *n.* GIARDIASIS.

Lambl's excrescences. Fine, hairlike proliferations of fibrous connective tissue in the region of the nodules of the aortic valves.

lame, *adj.* Having a weakness or partial loss of function of a leg, so that the gait is abnormal, whether due to acute disease, shortening, atrophy of muscle, pain, or to any other disturbance of the member. —**lame·ness,** *n.*

la·mel·la (la·mel′uh) *n.,* pl. **lamellas, lamel·lae** (·ee) 1. A thin scale or plate. 2. Specifically: a thin layer of bone deposited during one period of osteogenic activity. 3. *In ophthalmology,* a medicated disk, usually prepared with gelatin, intended to be inserted under the eyelid.

la·mel·lar (la·mel′ur) *adj.* Resembling a thin plate; composed of lamellas or thin plates.

lamellar cataract. ZONULAR CATARACT.

lames fo·li·a·cées (lam fo·lee·a·say′) Fibrous tissue in a concentric arrangement, resembling Meissner corpuscles found in the intradermal type of nevus pigmentosus.

lam·i·na (lam′i·nuh) *n.,* pl. **laminas, lami·nae** (·nee) A thin plate or layer.

lamina du·ra (dew′ruh). 1. DURA MATER. 2. The bone lining a dental alveolus which appears more radiopaque than the surrounding spongy bone; ALVEOLAR BONE (2).

lam·i·na·gram (lam′i·nuh·gram) *n.* TOMOGRAM.

lam·i·nag·ra·phy (lam″i·nag′ruh·fee) *n.* SECTIONAL RADIOGRAPHY.

lamina propria mu·co·sae (mew·ko′see) [NA]. The connective tissue of a mucous membrane. Syn. *tunica propria mucosae.*

lam·i·nar (lam′i·nur) *adj.* Of or pertaining to a lamina.

lam·i·nate (lam′i·nut, ·nate) *adj.* Consisting of layers or laminae; laminated.

lam·i·na·tion (lam″i·nay′shun) *n.* 1. Arrangement in plates or layers. 2. An operation in embryotomy consisting in cutting the skull in slices.

lam·i·nec·to·my (lam″i·neck′tuh·mee) *n.* Surgical removal of one or more laminas of the vertebrae, often including the spinous processes of the vertebrae.

lam·i·ni·tis (lam″i·nigh′tis) *n.* An inflammatory disease of the laminae of a horse's hoof which may follow a variety of stressful events including acute gastroenteritis, parturition, overdosing with strong purgatives, temperature extremes, septicemic infections, and trauma.

lam·i·nog·ra·phy (lam″i·nog′ruh·fee) *n.* SECTIONAL RADIOGRAPHY. —**lam·i·no·gram** (lam′i·no·gram) *n.*

lam·i·not·o·my (lam″i·not′uh·mee) *n.* Division of a lamina of a vertebra.

lam·pas (lam′pus) *n. In veterinary medicine,* hyperemia of the mucous membrane of the hard palate just posterior to the incisor teeth in horses.

lamp·black, *n.* A fine black substance, almost pure carbon, made by burning oils, tars, fats, or resins in an atmosphere deficient in oxygen. The similar product (sometimes called lamp-black), obtained by allowing a gas flame to impinge on a cold surface, is more properly designated gas black or carbon black.

lam·proph·o·ny (lam·prof´uh·nee) n. Clearness of voice. —**lam·pro·phon·ic** (lam´´pro·fon´ick) adj.

la·nat·o·side (la·nat´o·side) n. A natural glycoside from the leaves of *Digitalis lanata*; three such glycosides have been isolated and are designated lanatoside A, lanatoside B, and lanatoside C, formerly called digilanid A, digilanid B, and digilanid C, respectively. The aglycones are, respectively, digitoxigenin, gitoxigenin, and digoxigenin. All three lanatosides yield, on hydrolysis with acid, one molecule of D-glucose, three molecules of digitoxose, and one molecule of acetic acid. They are cardioactive.

lance, v. To cut or open, as with a lancet or bistoury.

Lancefield groups An antigenic classification of streptococci.

lan·cet (lan´sit) n. A small, pointed, double-edged surgical knife; rarely used nowadays.

lan·ci·nat·ing (lan´si·nay·ting) adj. Tearing; shooting, sharply cutting, as lancinating pain. —**lanci·nate** (·nate) v.

land·marks, n.pl. Superficial marks, as eminences, lines, and depressions, that serve as guides to, or indications of, deeper parts.

Landolt's broken C test A test for visual acuity wherein the subject is to determine in which segment the gap in the ring (or letter C) lies, a factor which is determined by the size of the image of the gap on the retina.

Landry-Guillain-Barré disease or **syndrome.** GUILLAIN-BARRÉ DISEASE.

Lan·dry's ascending paralysis (lahn·dree´) GUILLAIN-BARRÉ DISEASE.

Land·stei·ner classification Designation of the major blood groups as O, A, B, and AB.

Lang·er·hans cell (lahng´ur·hahnss) A star-shaped structure of the mammalian epidermis and dermis, revealed by gold impregnation and containing nonmelanized disklike organelles.

Langhans' giant cell A multinucleated giant cell with peripheral, radially arranged nuclei found in certain granulomatous lesions, as tuberculosis, leprosy, and tularemia.

Langhans' layer CYTOTROPHOBLAST.

lan·o·lin (lan´uh·lin) n. Wool fat containing about 30% water; used as an ointment base. Syn. *hydrous wool fat.*

la·nos·ter·ol (la·nos´tur·ol) n. 8,24-Lanostadien-3-ol, $C_{30}H_{50}O$, an unsaturated sterol in wool fat.

Lanoxin. Trademark for the cardioactive glycoside digoxin.

Lan·sing virus. Poliomyelitis virus type 2; a strain of virus that can infect human beings. It was adapted to the cotton rat and white mouse in 1937, and is useful in vaccines and in serologic studies of poliomyelitis.

lan·tha·nic (lan´thuh·nick, lan·than´ick) adj. Pertaining to patients who are medically diagnosed as having a particular disease but have a symptom or complaint that is not attributable to that disease.

lan·tha·num (lan´thuh·num) n. La = 138.9055. A rare metallic element.

la·nu·go (la·new´go) n. 1. [NA] The downlike hair that covers the fetus from about the fifth month of gestation. 2. VELLUS. —**lanu·gi·nous** (·ji·nus) adj.

lan·u·lous (lan´yoo·lus) adj. Covered with short, fine hair.

la·pac·tic (la·pack´tick) n. 1. An evacuant. 2. Any purgative substance.

lap·a·ror·rha·phy (lap´´uh·ror´uh·fee) n. Suture of the abdominal wall.

lap·a·ro·scope (lap´uh·ro·skope) n. PERITONEOSCOPE.

lap·a·ros·co·py (lap´´uh·ros´kuh·pee) n. PERITONEOSCOPY.

lap·a·rot·o·my (lap´´uh·rot´uh·mee) n. 1. An incision through the abdominal wall; CELIOTOMY. 2. The operation of cutting into the abdominal cavity through the loin or flank.

lap·a·ro·trach·e·lot·o·my (lap´´uh·ro·tray´´ke·lot´ uh·mee, ·track´´e·lot´uh·mee) n. A low cervical cesarean section in which the uterine incision is made in the lower uterine segment following entry into the peritoneal cavity.

la·pis (lap´is, lay´pis) n. A stone; an alchemic term applied to any nonvolatile substance.

lap·pa (lap´uh) n. The root of the common burdock, *Arctium lappa*, or of *A. minus*; has been used as an aperient, diuretic, and alterative.

lap·sus (lap´sus) n. 1. *In psychiatry*, a slip thought to reveal an unconscious desire. 2. PTOSIS.

lapsus lin·guae (ling´gwee). Slip of the tongue, considered by psychoanalysts to reveal an unconscious desire.

lard, n. The purified internal fat of the abdomen of the domestic hog. Has been used in pharmacy as an ingredient of ointment and cerate bases.

lar·da·ceous (lahr·day´shus) adj. 1. Resembling lard. 2. Containing diffuse amyloid deposits.

Largactil. A trademark for chlorpromazine, a tranquilizer used as the hydrochloride salt.

large alveolar cell. GREAT ALVEOLAR CELL.

large calorie. KILOCALORIE.

large intestine. The distal portion of the intestine, extending from the ileum to the anus, and consisting of the cecum, the colon, and the rectum.

lark·spur, n. The dried ripe seed of *Delphinium ajacis*; preparations of the seed have been used as a pediculicide.

Larodopa. A trademark for levodopa, an anticholinergic.

lar·va (lahr´vuh) n., pl. **lar·vae** (·vee) An immature and independent developmental stage in the life cycle of various animals which reach the adult form by undergoing metamorphosis.

lar·val (lahr´vul) adj. 1. Pertaining to or in the condition of a larva. 2. LARVATE.

larval seizures. *In electroencephalography,* subliminal seizures which produce no clinical symptoms but which are recognized by abnormal brain-wave discharges.

larva mi·grans (migh´granz). Invasion of the epidermis by various larvae, characterized by bizarre red irregular lines which are broad at one end and fade at the other, produced by burrowing larvae, most commonly in the United States by those of *Ancylostoma braziliense.* Syn. *creeping eruption.*

lar·vate (lahr'vate) *adj.* Concealed; masked; applied to diseases and conditions that are hidden or atypical.

lar·vi·cide (lahr'vi·side) *n.* Any agent destroying insect larvae.

laryng-, laryngo-. A combining form meaning *larynx, laryngeal.*

lar·yn·gal·gia (lăr''in·gal'jee·uh) *n.* Pain or neuralgia of the larynx.

lar·yn·ge·al (la·rin'jee·ul, ·jul, lăr''in·jee'ul) *adj.* Of or pertaining to the larynx.

laryngeal crisis. An acute laryngeal spasm, sometimes occurring in tabes dorsalis.

laryngeal mirror. 1. A small circular mirror affixed to a long handle, used in laryngoscopy. 2. A similar instrument used by dentists in the examination of the teeth.

laryngeal prominence. The tubercle of the thyroid cartilage and the bulging in the midline of the neck caused by it. Syn. *Adam's apple, laryngeal protuberance.*

laryngeal reflex. A cough resulting from irritation of the larynx.

laryngeal speech. Speech produced by means of an artificial larynx following laryngectomy; less commonly employed than esophageal speech.

laryngeal stridor. Stridor due to laryngeal obstruction.

laryngeal ventricle. The portion of the cavity of the larynx between the vestibular and the vocal folds.

lar·yn·gec·to·my (lăr''in·jeck'tuh·mee) *n.* Extirpation or partial excision of the larynx.

lar·yn·gis·mus (lăr''in·jiz'mus) *n.,* pl. **laryngis·mi** (·migh). A spasm of the larynx. —**laryngis·mal** (·mul) *adj.*

laryngismus stri·du·lus (strye'dew·lus, strid'yoo·lus). 1. SPASMODIC CROUP. 2. The laryngeal spasm sometimes seen in hypocalcemic states.

lar·yn·gi·tis (lăr''in·jye'tis) *n.,* pl. **laryn·git·i·des** (·jit'i·deez) Inflammation of the larynx. It may be acute or chronic, catarrhal, suppurative, croupous (diphtheritic), tuberculous, or syphilitic. —**laryn·git·ic** (·jit'ick) *adj.*

laryngo-. See *larynge-.*

la·ryn·go·cele (la·ring'go·seel) *n.* An aerocele connected with the larynx.

la·ryn·go·cen·te·sis (la·ring''go·sen·tee'sis) *n.* Puncture of the larynx.

la·ryn·go·fis·sure (la·ring''go·fish'ur) *n.* 1. Surgical division of the larynx for the removal of tumors or foreign bodies. 2. The aperture made in the operation of laryngofissure.

la·ryn·go·gram (la·ring'go·gram) *n.* A representation of the larynx, usually radiographic, after the introduction of contrast material.

la·ryn·go·graph (la·ring'go·graf) *n.* An instrument for recording laryngeal movements. —**laryn·gog·ra·phy** (la''rin·gog'ruh·fee) *n.*

lar·yn·gol·o·gist (lăr''ing·gol'uh·jist) *n.* A person who specializes in laryngology.

lar·yn·gol·o·gy (lăr''ing·gol'uh·jee) *n.* The science of the anatomy, physiology, and diseases of the larynx. —**laryn·go·log·ic** (·go·loj'ick) *adj.*

la·ryn·go·pa·ral·y·sis (la·ring''go·puh·ral'i·sis) *n.* Paralysis of the laryngeal muscles.

lar·yn·gop·a·thy (lăr''ing·gop'uh·thee) *n.* Any disease of the larynx.

la·ryn·go·pha·ryn·ge·al (la·ring''go·fa·rin'jee·ul) *adj.* Pertaining conjointly to the larynx and pharynx.

la·ryn·go·phar·yn·gec·to·my (la·ring''go·făr''in·jeck'tuh·mee) *n.* Surgical removal of the larynx and a portion of the pharynx.

la·ryn·go·phar·yn·gi·tis (la·ring''go·făr''in·jye'tis) *n.* 1. Inflammation of the laryngopharynx. 2. Inflammation of the larynx and the pharynx.

la·ryn·go·phar·ynx (la·ring''go·făr'inks) *n.* The inferior portion of the pharynx. It extends from the level of the greater cornua of the hyoid bone to that of the inferior border of the cricoid cartilage. Syn. *hypopharynx, laryngeal pharynx.*

lar·yn·goph·o·ny (lăr''ing·gof'uh·nee) *n.* The sound of the voice observed in auscultation of the larynx.

la·ryn·go·plas·ty (la·ring'go·plas''tee) *n.* Plastic reparative operation upon the larynx.

la·ryn·go·ple·gia (la·ring''go·plee'jee·uh) *n.* Paralysis of the laryngeal muscles.

la·ryn·gop·to·sis (la·ring''go·to'sis) *n.* Mobility and falling of the larynx; sometimes occurs in old age.

lar·yn·gor·rha·phy (lăr''ing·gor'uh·fee) *n.* Suture of the larynx.

la·ryn·gor·rhea, la·ryn·gor·rhoea (la·ring''go·ree'uh) *n.* Excessive secretion of mucus from the larynx, especially when it is used in phonation.

la·ryn·go·scope (la·ring'go·skope) *n.* A tubular instrument, combining a light system and a telescopic system, used in the visualization of the interior larynx and adaptable for diagnostic, therapeutic, and surgical procedures. —**la·ryn·go·scop·ic** (la·ring''go·skop'ick) *adj.*

lar·yn·gos·co·py (lăr''ing·gos'kuh·pee) *n.* Examination of the interior of the larynx directly with a laryngoscope or indirectly with a laryngeal mirror or telescope.

la·ryn·go·spasm (la·ring'go·spaz·um) *n.* Spasmodic closure of the glottis; LARYNGISMUS STRIDULUS.

lar·yn·gos·ta·sis (lăr''ing·gos'tuh·sis) *n.* CROUP.

la·ryn·go·ste·no·sis (la·ring''go·ste·no'sis) *n.* Contraction or stricture of the larynx.

lar·yn·gos·to·my (lăr''ing·gos'tuh·mee) *n.* The establishing of a permanent opening into the larynx through the neck.

lar·yn·got·o·my (lăr''ing·got'uh·mee) *n.* The operation of incising the larynx.

la·ryn·go·tra·che·al (la·ring''go·tray'kee·ul) *adj.* Pertaining conjointly to the larynx and the trachea.

la·ryn·go·tra·che·i·tis (la·ring''go·tray''kee·eye'tis) *n.* Inflammation of the larynx and the trachea.

la·ryn·go·tra·cheo·bron·chi·tis (la·ring''go·tray''kee·o·brong·kigh'tis) *n.* Acute inflammation of the mucosa of the larynx, trachea, and bronchi.

la·ryn·go·tra·che·ot·o·my (la·ring"go·tray"kee·ot'uh·mee) *n.* Incision of the larynx and trachea.

la·ryn·go·xe·ro·sis (la·ring"go·ze·ro'sis) *n.* Dryness of the larynx or throat.

lar·ynx (lăr'inks) *n.*, genit. **la·rin·gis** (la·rin'jis), pl. **larynxes, la·ryn·ges** (la·rin'jeez) The organ of the voice, situated between the trachea and the base of the tongue. It consists of a series of cartilages: the thyroid, the cricoid, and the epiglottis, and three pairs of cartilages: the arytenoid, corniculate, and cuneiform, all of which are lined by mucous membrane and are moved by the muscles of the larynx. The mucous membrane is, on each side, thrown into two transverse folds that constitute the vocal bands or folds, the upper being the false, the lower the true, vocal folds.

Lasègue's sign A sign elicited in patients with low back pain and sciatica. With the patient supine, the entire lower extremity is raised gently keeping the knee in full extension. The sign becomes positive at whatever angle of elevation pain or muscle spasm is produced, resulting in limitation of movement.

la·ser (lay'zur) *n.* An operating assembly for utilizing the property of certain molecules to emit essentially monochromatic radiation when stimulated with radiation of optical frequencies (near ultraviolet, visible, and infrared). The emitted radiation may be produced as a directional beam of great power, which has been used as a surgical tool, and in research. Syn. *optical maser.*

lash, *n.* 1. EYELASH. 2. FLAGELLUM.

Lasix. Trademark for furosemide, a diuretic drug.

Lassa virus. A highly infectious, virulent, and pathogenic arenavirus, antigenically related to the virus of lymphocytic choriomeningitis and to some South American hemorrhagic fevers. Believed to be spherical, with a lipid envelope and having ribonucleic acid as its genetic material.

Las·sar's paste A paste containing zinc oxide, starch, and salicylic acid, dispersed in white petrolatum, used in dermatologic practice.

las·si·tude ('as'i·tewd) *n.* A state of exhaustion or weakness; debility.

late infantile amaurotic familial idiocy. BIELSCHOWSKY-JANSKÝ DISEASE.

late juvenile amaurotic familial idiocy. KUFS' DISEASE.

la·ten·cy (lay'tun·see) *n.* 1. The state or quality of being latent. 2. *In psychoanalytic theory,* the phase between the oedipal period and adolescence, lasting approximately 5 to 7 years, and characterized by an apparent cessation in psychosexual development. 3. LATENT PERIOD (1, 2).

la·tent (lay'tunt) *adj.* Not manifest; dormant; potential.

latent content. *In psychiatry,* the hidden unconscious meaning of thoughts or actions, especially in dreams and fantasies, where such meaning appears in condensed, disguised, and symbolic form.

latent gout. Hyperuricemia without gouty symptoms.

latent heat. The quantity of heat necessary to convert a body into another state without changing its temperature.

latent homosexuality. *In psychiatry,* an erotic desire for a member of the same sex, present in the unconscious but not felt or expressed overtly.

latent hyperopia. The part of the total hyperopia which cannot be overcome by the accommodation, or the difference between the manifest and the total hyperopia, detected only after using a cycloplegic. Symbol, Hl.

la·ten·ti·a·tion (la·ten"shee·ay'shun) *n.* The chemical modification of an active drug to form a new compound or precursor, which upon enzymatic or other action in vivo will liberate or form the parent compound, for the purpose of delaying the action or prolonging the effect of the parent drug or avoiding any local reaction or unpleasant taste it may produce.

latent neurosyphilis. ASYMPTOMATIC NEUROSYPHILIS.

latent period. 1. Any stage of an infectious disease in which there are no clinical signs or symptoms of the infection. 2. *In physiology,* the period of time which elapses between the introduction of a stimulus and the response to it. Syn. *inertia time.* 3. *In radiology,* the elapsed time between the exposure to radiation and the appearance of morphologic or physiologic effects.

latent schizophrenia. A form of mental disorder in which there are definite symptoms of schizophrenia, but because of the absence of a history of a psychotic schizophrenic episode, the disorder is regarded as incipient, prepsychotic, pseudoneurotic, pseudopsychopathic, or borderline.

latent syphilis. Absence of clinical manifestations in syphilis as after spontaneous healing of primary and secondary lesions; the existence of the disease is recognized only by serologic tests.

lat·er·ad (lat'ur·ad) *adv.* Toward the lateral aspect.

lat·er·al (lat'ur·ul) *adj.* 1. At, belonging to, or pertaining to the side; situated on either side of the median vertical plane. 2. External, as opposed to medial (internal), away from the midline of the body.

lateral aperture of the fourth ventricle. The aperture at the tip of each of the lateral recesses of the fourth ventricle, through which cerebrospinal fluid passes into the subarachnoid space. Syn. *foramen of Luschka.*

lateral arcuate ligament. A thick band of fascia extending from the tip of the transverse process of the second lumbar vertebra to the twelfth rib.

lateral cerebral sulcus. A deep fissure of the brain, beginning on the outer side of the anterior perforated space, and extending outward to the lateral surface of the hemisphere. It has two branches, a short vertical and a long horizontal, the latter separating the temporal from the frontal and parietal lobes.

lateral corticospinal tract. The fibers of the corticospinal tract that run in the dorsolateral zone of the spinal cord. Most of these fibers originate in the contralateral motor cortex and decussate in the medulla; a smaller number originate in the ipsilateral motor cortex.

lateral decubitus. 1. A position employed in radiography, with the patient lying on his side on a table and the x-ray beam directed through the patient parallel to the tabletop and perpendicular to the x-ray film. Described as left lateral decubitus when patient's left side is down, and as right lateral decubitus when patient's right side is down. 2. A position also used in lumbar puncture.

lateral fistula of the neck. A congenital fistula opening lateral to the midline, anywhere from the mandible to the sternum, and communicating with the pharynx, a cyst, a fetal rest, or a duct; due to faulty closure of pharyngeal pouches or the thymopharyngeal duct, or to other developmental defects.

lateral geniculate body. A flattened area in the posterolateral surface of the thalamus containing nerve cells which receive impulses from the retinas and relay them to the occipital cortex via the geniculocalcarine tracts.

lateral hermaphroditism. The form of human hermaphroditism in which there is an ovary on one side and a testis on the other. Syn. *alternating hermaphroditism.*

lateral hypothalamic nucleus. A group of cells located in the lateral part of the middle region of the hypothalamus.

lat·er·al·i·ty (lat″ur·al′i·tee) *n.* Functional predominance of one side of an anatomically bilateral structure, such as greater proficiency in the use of one side of the body or language-related dominance of one cerebral hemisphere.

lat·er·al·iza·tion (lat″ur·ul·i·zay′shun) *n.* Localization on one side of the body, as in one of the cerebral hemispheres. **—lat·er·al·ize** (lat′ur·ul·ize) *v.*

lateral malleolus. The distal end of the fibula. Syn. *external malleolus.*

lateral meniscus. The articular disk in the knee joint between the lateral condyles of the tibia and femur; a crescentic, nearly circular fibrocartilaginous disk attached to the margin of the lateral condyle of the tibia, resting on and serving to deepen the tibia's lateral articular surface. Syn. *external semilunar cartilage.*

lateral nystagmus. Horizontal nystagmus that appears on right or left lateral gaze.

lateral rectus. An extrinsic muscle of the eye. See *rectus lateralis bulbi* in Table of Muscles in the Appendix.

lateral region of the abdomen. The right or left abdominal region on either side of the umbilical region.

lateral sclerosis. See *amyotrophic lateral sclerosis, primary lateral sclerosis.*

lateral sinus. The sinus of the dura mater running from the internal occipital protuberance, following for part of its course the attached margin of the tentorium cerebelli, then over the jugular process of the occipital bone to reach the jugular foramen. Syn. *transverse sinus.*

lateral spinothalamic tract. A tract of nerve fibers which arise from cells of the posterior horn of spinal gray matter, cross in the anterior white commissure, ascend in the lateral funiculus, and terminate in the posterior nuclei of the thalamus; it conducts mainly pain and temperature impulses.

lateral ventricle. The cavity of either cerebral hemisphere communicating with the third ventricle through the interventricular foramen, and consisting of a triangular central cavity or body and three smaller cavities or cornua.

lateral vestibular nucleus. One of four vestibular nuclei, consisting of large cells at the caudal border of the pons between the inferior cerebellar peduncle and the spinal tract of the trigeminal nerve. Syn. *Deiter's nucleus.*

late rickets. OSTEOMALACIA.

lat·er·i·ver·sion (lat″ur·i·vur′zhun) *n.* LATEROVERSION.

lat·ero·ab·dom·i·nal (lat″ur·o·ab·dom′i·nul) *adj.* Pertaining to either lateral portion of the abdomen.

lateroabdominal position. SIM'S POSITION.

lat·ero·duc·tion (lat″ur·o·duck′shun) *n.* Lateral movement, as of the eye.

lat·ero·flex·ion (lat″ur·o·fleck′shun) *n.* Lateral flexion, as the alteration in position of the uterus in which the uterine axis is bent upon itself to one side.

lat·ero·mar·gin·al (lat″ur·o·mahr′ji·nul) *adj.* Situated on the lateral edge.

lat·ero·pul·sion (lat″ur·o·pul′shun) *n.* An involuntary tendency to move to one side in forward locomotion.

lat·ero·tor·sion (lat″ur·o·tor′shun) *n.* A twisting to one side.

lat·ero·ver·sion (lat″ur·o·vur′zhun) *n.* Lateral version, as the alteration in position of the uterus in which the entire uterine axis is displaced to one side.

late syphilis. Stages of infection occurring after secondary syphilis, and including asymptomatic and symptomatic neurosyphilis, cardiovascular syphilis, and gumma.

la·tex (lay′teks) *n.,* pl. **lat·i·ces** (lat′i·seez), **la·texes** The milky juice of certain plants and trees. Rubber and gutta-percha are commercial products of latex.

lath·y·rism (lath′i·riz·um) *n.* 1. An affection attributed to the ingestion of the peas or meal from varieties of the chickpea, chiefly *Lathyrus sativus* and toxins derived from the common vetch, *Vicia sativa,* characterized by spastic paraplegia with tremor, hyperreflexia, and Babinski responses, but normal sensation. 2. A disease produced by feeding experimental animals extracts of *Lathyrus odoratus* seeds, or more commonly, beta-aminopropionitrile; it is characterized in rats by gross bony deformity of the limb epiphyses and vertebrae, hind limb paresis, aortic medial hemorrhage and, in some cases, hernias.

la·tis·si·mus (la·tis′i·mus) *adj.* Widest.

la·trine (la·treen′) *n.* A water closet or other place for urination or defecation, especially any of a number of types used in military installations, permanent or temporary.

Lat·ro·dec·tus (lat′ro·deck′tus) *n.* A genus of spiders of the family Theridiidae, of which the females are sedentary in webs, have globose abdomens, and a bite poisonous to man. Excepting the more northerly parts of Europe, Asia, and North America, species are found in most parts of the inhabited world, including almost all of the contiguous United States. The most dangerous species is *Latrodectus mactans*, the black widow.

LATS Abbreviation for *long-acting thyroid stimulator.*

lat·tice (lat′is) *n.* 1. A network or framework, as of fibers or filaments; a reticulum. 2. *In physics*, the structural pattern of ions or molecules in a crystal.

lattice corneal dystrophy. A type of primary localized amyloidosis inherited as an autosomal dominant trait, clinically manifest as progressive corneal opacities which include a filamentous branching network rarely associated with systemic amyloidosis.

la·tus (lay′tus, lat′us) *n.* FLANK.

laud·able (law′duh·bul) *adj.* Healthy; formerly used to describe thick, copious pus thought to indicate an improved condition of a wound.

lau·dan·o·sine (law·dan′o·seen, ·sin) *n. l-N-*Methyltetrahydropapaverine, $C_{21}H_{27}NO_4$, an alkaloid from opium.

lau·da·num (law′duh·num) *n.* A tincture of opium.

laughing gas. NITROUS OXIDE.

laugh·ter, *n.* A succession of rhythmic, spasmodic expirations with open glottis and vibration of the vocal folds normally expressing mirth, but also a response to tickling, or a manifestation of pseudobulbar palsy or rarely of epilepsy.

Laurence–Moon–Biedl syndrome A heredodegenerative disease probably due to recessive mutations of two genes in the same chromosome, and more frequent in males; characterized by girdle-type obesity, hypogenitalism, mental retardation, polydactyly, skull deformations, pigmentary retinal degeneration, and generally a shortened life-span.

lau·ric acid (law′rik). Dodecanoic acid, $CH_3(CH_2)_{10}COOH$, a fatty acid from the glycerides of laurel oil, coconut oil, and other fats.

lau·ryl (law′ril) *n.* The univalent radical $C_{12}H_{25}$ — present in lauric acid.

la·vage (lah·vahzh, la′vij) *n.* The irrigation or washing out of an organ, such as the stomach, bowel, urinary bladder, or paranasal sinus.

lav·en·der, *n.* The flowers of *Lavandula officinalis;* formerly used as an aromatic stimulant.

law, *n.* 1. Statement of a relation or sequence of phenomena invariable under the same conditions. 2. A rule of conduct prescribed by authority.

law of filial regression. Children whose parents deviate from the average of the population likewise deviate from the average in the same direction as the parents, but regress by about one-third of the parental deviation toward the mean. For example, children whose parents are 3 inches above the average stature are themselves on the average about 2 inches above the mean stature of the population. Syn. *Galton's law of filial regression.*

law of inverse squares. For point sources of radiant energy, the intensity of the radiation at any point varies inversely as the square of the distance from the point source.

law of mass action. The speed of a chemical reaction is proportional to the active masses of the reacting substances. Syn. *Guldberg-Waage law.*

law of multiple proportions. If more than one compound is formed by two elements, the weight of one of the elements remains constant, that of the other element varies as a multiple of the lowest amount of that element in the series of compounds.

law of reciprocal proportions. Two elements, which unite with each other, will unite singly with a third element in proportions which are the same as, or multiples of, the proportions in which they unite with each other.

law of refreshment. The rate of recovery of muscle from fatigue is proportional to its blood supply.

law of the intestines. A stimulus applied to a given point in the intestinal wall initiates a band of constriction on the proximal side and relaxation on the distal side of the stimulated point.

law of universal affect. *In psychology*, the premise that every idea, thought, or object, no matter how apparently minor or neutral, possesses a distinct quantum of affect.

lax·a·tion (lack·say′shun) *n.* DEFECATION.

lax·a·tive (lack′suh·tiv) *adj. & n.* 1. Relieving constipation; causing evacuation of the bowels. 2. An agent employed for its laxative properties; a cathartic of the least potent category.

lax·i·ty (lack′si·tee) *n.* 1. Absence or loss of tone, tension, or firmness. 2. Lack of strictness or precision. —**lax,** *adj.*

lay·er, *n.* A deposited material of uniform or nearly uniform thickness, spread over a comparatively considerable area; cover. Syn. *stratum.*

layer of Langhans CYTOTROPHOBLAST.

lay·ette (lay·et′) *n.* A full outfit of garments and bedding for a newborn child.

laz·ar (laz′ur) *n.* A patient with leprosy, or any person having a repulsive disease.

laz·a·ret·to (laz′uh·ret′o) *n.* 1. A public hospital for the care of persons suffering from contagious diseases, especially lepers; a pesthouse. 2. A building or vessel used for quarantine.

laz·a·rine leprosy (laz′uh·rine, ·reen) A form of lepromatous leprosy marked by continuous ulceration and resultant scarring.

lb. Abbreviation for *libra,* pound.

LBBB. Left bundle branch block.

L.C.L. bodies Clusters of minute spherical or coccoid elementary inclusion bodies found within reticuloendothelial cells and in body fluids of birds and humans infected with psittacosis (ornithosis).

LD Abbreviation for (a) *lethal dose*; (b) *light difference*.

LD 50, LD$_{50}$ Symbol for median lethal dose.

LD 100, LD$_{100}$ Symbol for invariably lethal dose.

L.D.A. Abbreviation for *left dorsoanterior* position of the fetus.

L.D.P. Abbreviation for *left dorsoposterior* position of the fetus.

L.E. Abbreviation for *lupus erythematosus*.

leach, *v.* To wash or extract the soluble constituents from insoluble material.

¹lead (leed) *n.* 1. A pair of terminals or electrodes or electrode arrays situated within or upon the body, each connected either directly or through resistors to a recording instrument for the purpose of measuring the difference in electrical potential between them. 2. The electrocardiogram or other recording obtained from a pair of electrodes.

²lead (led) *n.* Pb = 207.2. A soft, bluish-gray, malleable metal, occurring in nature chiefly as the sulfide, PbS, known as galena. Its soluble salts are violent irritant poisons, formerly used as local astringents. Insoluble lead salts at one time were used as protectives, but because of the danger of absorption, the therapeutic use of lead compounds has been discontinued.

lead acetate. $(CH_3COO)_2Pb.3H_2O$. Occurs as white crystals. Has been used as a local astringent. Syn. *sugar of lead*.

lead anemia. Anemia resulting from lead poisoning.

lead arsenate. Approximately $PbHAsO_4$; a dense, white powder, insoluble in water, used as a constituent of insecticides.

lead arsenite. Approximately $Pb(AsO_2)_2$; a white powder, insoluble in water, used as a constituent of insecticides.

Lead·bet·ter's maneuver or **procedure** A method of reduction in fracture of the femoral neck.

lead encephalopathy. A form of lead poisoning, occurring mainly in children, characterized by swelling of the brain, herniation of the temporal lobes and cerebellum, multiple ischemic foci, and perivascular deposition of proteinaceous material and mononuclear inflammatory cells. The clinical syndrome consists of vomiting, seizures, stupor, and coma.

lead equivalent. The thickness of lead which absorbs a specific radiation which is the same amount as the material in question.

lead·er, *n. Obsol.* 1. A sinew or tendon. 2. An inflamed lymphatic channel.

lead line. The blue line at the dental margin of the gums in chronic lead poisoning.

lead monoxide. PbO; a yellowish or reddish powder, almost insoluble in water. Has been used as an ingredient of external applications for relieving inflammation. Syn. *litharge, yellow lead oxide*.

lead-pencil stools. Fecal discharges of very small caliber.

lead poisoning. Poisoning caused by prolonged ingestion or absorption of lead or lead-containing materials, manifested by colic, encephalopathy, polyneuropathy, and hemolytic anemia.

lead polyneuropathy. A distal symmetrical polyneuropathy, affecting mainly the wrists and hands, seen principally in adults with chronic lead poisoning; characterized by weakness, paresthesias, pain, and less often by sensory loss.

lead tetraethyl. $Pb(C_2H_5)_4$, a colorless, flammable liquid; used as an antiknock ingredient in motor fuels. Acute or chronic poisoning may result from its inhalation.

learning disorder, disturbance, or **defect.** Any specific defect in the ability of a child to learn one of the basic academic disciplines, or a general defect in learning to read or write, or in learning mathematics. It is often complicated by behavior disturbances.

leather bottle stomach. LINITIS PLASTICA.

Le·ber's disease or **optic atrophy** (le'ber) A hereditary form of optic atrophy, characterized by loss of central vision with usually relatively well-preserved peripheral vision, occurring in young males; usually acute in onset, often preceded by transient optic neuritis, and commonly reaching its maximum within a few weeks, it rarely progresses to total blindness; it is transmitted as a sex-linked recessive through the female.

L.E. cell. Abbreviation for *lupus erythematosus cell*.

L.E. cell test. Any procedure that provides optimum conditions for the formation and detection of lupus erythematosus cells.

lec·i·thal (les'i·thul) *adj.* Having a yolk; used especially in combination, as alecithal and telolecithal.

lec·i·thin (les'i·thin) *n.* A phospholipid in which phosphatidic acid is esterified to choline. Syn. *phosphatidyl choline*. **—leci·thoid** (·thoid) *adj.*

lec·i·thi·nase (les'i·thi·nace, ·naze) *n.* An enzyme that catalyzes the hydrolysis of a lecithin to its constituents.

lec·i·tho·pro·te·in (les"i·tho·pro'tee·in, ·teen) *n.* A compound of lecithin with a protein molecule.

lec·tin (leck'tin) *n.* A substance occurring in seeds and other parts of certain plants which displays specific antibody-like activity toward animal cells or their components, as in specific agglutination of mammalian erythrocytes.

Led·der·hose's disease (led'ur·ho'zeʰ) Dupuytren's contracture involving the plantar aponeurosis.

leech, *n.* Any parasitic annelid of the class Hirudinea; some leeches have been detrimental, and some have aided medically. Infestation by leeches (hirudiniasis) may be either internal or external.

Lee-White method. A test-tube method for estimating the coagulation time of whole blood.

L.E. factor. A substance occurring in the blood and other body fluids of patients with systemic lupus erythematosus and, occasionally, in other diseases. Syn. *lupus erythematosus factor, L.E. plasma factor, L.E. serum factor.*

left axis deviation or **shift.** Leftward deviation of the mean frontal plane axis of the QRS complex of the electrocardiogram less than O°; usually beyond −15 or −30° for the adult.

left-eyed, *adj.* Tending to use the left eye in preference to the right, as in looking through a monocular telescope.

left-footed, *adj.* Tending to use the left foot in preference to the right, as in hopping or kicking.

left-handed, *adj.* Having the left hand stronger or more expert than the right, or using the left hand in preference to the right.

left heart. The part of the heart which pumps blood to the systemic and coronary vessels; the left atrium and left ventricle.

left lateral. A position assumed by a patient for x-ray examination, with his left side closest to the film and the x-ray beam perpendicular to the film.

left posterior oblique. A position assumed by a patient for x-ray examination, with the posterior aspect of his left side closest to the film so that x-ray beam passes diagonally through his body.

left-to-right shunt. A cardiac defect characterized by the return of oxygenated blood from the left side of the heart directly to the right side of the heart or pulmonary artery, without passage through the systemic circulation.

leg, *n.* 1. *In human anatomy,* the lower extremity between the knee and the foot. 2. Popularly, the lower extremity including the thigh, but usually excluding the foot.

le·gal medicine. The branch of medicine, involving any and all of its disciplines, employed by the legal authorities for the solution of legal problems. Syn. *forensic medicine.*

Legal's test An alkaline urine distillate containing acetone produces a red color in the presence of sodium nitroferricyanide.

Legg-Calvé-Perthes disease or **syndrome** OSTEOCHONDRITIS DEFORMANS JUVENILIS.

Legg-Perthes disease OSTEOCHONDRITIS DEFORMANS JUVENILIS.

Le·gion·naires' bacillus (lee′juh·nairz′). A small gram-negative bacillus, the causative organism of Legionnaires' disease.

Legionnaires' disease. An acute lobar pneumonia often producing renal, intestinal, neurologic, and hepatic symptoms, due to the Legionnaires' bacillus; first recognized in an outbreak at a convention of the American Legion in July 1976.

leio-, lio- A combining form signifying *smooth.*

leio·der·ma·tous (lye′′o·dur′muh·tus) *adj.* Smooth-skinned.

leio·der·mia, lio·der·mia (lye′′o·dur′mee·uh) *n.* A condition of abnormal smoothness and glossiness of the skin.

leio·myo·fi·bro·ma (lye′′o·migh′′o·figh·bro′muh) *n.* A benign tumor composed of smooth muscle cells and fibrocytes.

leio·my·o·ma (lye′′o·migh·o′muh) *n.*, *pl.* **leio·myomas, leiomyoma·ta** (·tuh) A benign tumor whose parenchyma is composed of smooth muscle cells; occurs most often in the uterus.

leiomyoma ute·ri (yoo′tur·eye). A leiomyoma of the uterus. Syn. *fibroid tumor, uterine fibroid.*

leio·myo·sar·co·ma (lye′′o·migh′′o·sahr·ko′muh) *n.* A malignant tumor whose parenchyma is composed of anaplastic smooth muscle cells. Syn. *malignant leiomyosarcoma, metastasizing leiomyosarcoma.*

lei·ot·ri·chous (lye·ot′ri·kus) *adj.* Having smooth or straight hair.

Leish·man-Don·o·van bodies (leesh′mun). Small, oval protozoa lacking flagellum and undulating membrane, occurring in the vertebrate host intracellularly in macrophages of areas such as the skin, liver, spleen, and common to leishmanial infections such as kala azar, oriental sore, and mucocutaneous leishmaniasis.

Leish·man·ia (leesh·man′ee·uh, ·may′nee·uh) *n.* A genus of the Trypanosomatidae whose species are morphologically similar but differ in serologic reactions; transmitted to man by the bite of species of *Phlebotomus.* They have a single flagellum when in the invertebrate host, but assume the leishmania (nonflagellated) form in the vertebrate host. **—leishma·ni·al** (·nee·ul) *adj.*

Leishmania don·o·va·ni (don′′o·vay′nigh, ·van′ eye). A species of protozoan flagellate which is the etiologic agent of kala azar, the visceral form of leishmaniasis.

leish·man·i·a·sis (leesh′′muh·nigh′uh·sis) *n.*, *pl.* **leishmania·ses** (·seez) A variety of visceral and tegumentary infections caused by protozoan parasites of the genus *Leishmania.* Several species of biting flies of the genus *Phlebotomus* are responsible for transmission. In India, man constitutes the main reservoir, but in the Mediterranean region infected dogs are the reservoirs for the infantile form of the disease.

le·ma (lee′muh) *n.* A collection of dried secretion of the tarsal glands at the inner canthus of the eye.

Lem·bert's suture (lahⁿ·behr′) An interrupted suture used to approximate serous surfaces of the intestine.

-lemma A combining form meaning *a sheath or envelope.*

lemmo- A combining form meaning *neurilemma.*

lem·mo·blas·to·ma (lem′′o·blas·to′muh) *n.* NEURILEMMOMA.

lem·nis·cus (lem·nis′kus) *n.*, *pl.* **lemnis·ci** (·kigh, ·igh) A secondary sensory pathway of the central nervous system, which usually decussates and terminates in the thalamus. **—lemin·is·cal** (·kul) *adj.*

lem·on, *n.* The fruit of *Citrus limon.*

lemon oil. The volatile oil obtained from the fresh peel of the fruit of *Citrus limon;* characteristic odor is due chiefly to citral, an aldehyde. Used as a flavor.

le·mo·pa·ral·y·sis (lee′′mo·pa·ral′i·sis) *n.* Paralysis of the esophagus.

le·mo·ste·no·sis (lee′′mo·ste·no′sis) *n.* Constriction or narrowing of the pharynx or esophagus.

Len·drum's inclusion-body stain A hematoxylin-phloxine stain which colors certain inclusion bodies red.

len·i·ceps (len'i-seps) *n.* Obstetric forceps with short handles.

Len·nox-Gas·taut syndrome (gahs·to') The occurrence, in infants and young children, of akinetic seizures, succeeded by tonic seizures and mental retardation, and associated with slow spike-and-wave complexes in the electroencephalogram.

lens (lenz) *n.*, genit. sing. **len·tis** (len'tis). L. pl. **len·tes** (·teez) 1. A piece of glass or crystal for the refraction of rays of light. 2. [NA] CRYSTALLINE LENS.

lens·om·e·ter (len·zom'e·tur) *n.* An instrument for determining the optical centers and refractive power of spheres and lenses, to locate the axes of cylindrical lenses, and to measure the power and locate the direction of prisms. Syn. *phacometer.*

lent-, lenti- A combining form meaning *lens, lenticular.*

len·te insulin (len'tee). One of a series of protein-free injectable preparations of insulin, with adjustable duration of action, obtained by mixing proper proportions of crystalline, long-acting zinc insulin with amorphous, short-acting zinc insulin, the mixture being suspended in an acetate-buffered medium of pH 7.3. A mixture of approximately 7 parts of the crystalline form and 3 parts of the amorphous variety is known as insulin zinc suspension.

len·ti·co·nus (len''ti·ko'nus) *n.* A rare, usually congenital, anomaly of the lens; marked by a conical prominence upon its anterior or, more rarely, upon its posterior surface; may be seen in Alport's syndrome.

len·tic·u·lar (len·tick'yoo·lur) *adj.* 1. Pertaining to or resembling a lens. 2. Pertaining to the crystalline lens. 3. Pertaining to the lentiform nucleus of the brain.

lenticular astigmatism. Astigmatism due to defective curvature or refractive surface of the lens of an eye.

lenticular nucleus. The globus pallidus and putamen together. Syn. *lentiform nucleus.*

len·tic·u·lo·stri·ate (len·tick''yoo·lo·stry'ate) *adj.* Pertaining to the lenticular nucleus of the corpus striatum, as lenticulostriate arteries.

len·tic·u·lo·tha·lam·ic (len·tick''yoo·lo·tha·lam'ick) *adj.* Extending from the lentiform nucleus to the thalamus.

len·ti·form (len'ti·form) *adj.* Lens-shaped or lentil-shaped.

lentiform nucleus. The globus pallidus and putamen together. Syn. *lenticular nucleus.*

len·ti·glo·bus (len''ti·glo'bus) *n.* A spherical bulging of the lens of the eye, as in intumescent cataract.

len·ti·go (len·tye'go) *n.*, pl. **len·tig·i·nes** (len·tij'i·neez) A smooth, dark brown spot on the skin, usually of an exposed part, of a person of middle years or older. Histologically there is elongation of rete ridges with increased numbers of melanocytes.

lentigo ma·lig·na (muh·lig'nuh). A slowly growing variety of junction nevus characteristically occurring on the face of people over age 50, which may evolve into an invasive malignant melanoma. Syn. *Hutchinson's freckle, malignant freckle, melanosis circumscripta preblastomatosa of Dubreuilh, melanotic freckle, senile freckle.*

le·on·ti·a·sis (lee''on·tye'uh·sis) *n.*, pl. **leontia·ses** (·seez) A "lionlike" appearance of the face, seen in lepromatous leprosy.

leontiasis os·sea (os'ee·uh). An overgrowth of the bones of the face and cranium as the result of which the features acquire a "lionlike" appearance.

Leon virus. POLIOMYELITIS VIRUS, type 3.

lep·er (lep'ur) *n.* One affected with leprosy.

lepid-, lepido- A combining form meaning *a scale, scaly.*

Lep·i·dop·te·ra (lep''i·dop'te·ruh) *n.pl.* An order of insects distinguished by featherlike scales and spirally coiled suctorial apparatus. The order includes butterflies, moths, and skippers. The larvae of certain species cause caterpillar dermatitis.

L.E. plasma factor. L.E. FACTOR.

lep·o·thrix (lep'o·thricks) *n.* A skin disorder in which masses of reddish, black, and yellow fungous material are found in nodular or diffuse distribution about the axillary or genital hair; usually seen in those who sweat freely. Syn. *trichomycosis nodosa.*

lepr-, lepro-. A combining form meaning *leprous, leprosy.*

lep·ra (lep'ruh) *n.* LEPROSY.

lepra cell. A large mononuclear cell associated with lepromatous lesions, which often contains the acid-fast organisms of leprosy.

lepra reaction. Exacerbation of the inflammatory process in lepromatous leprosy, either spontaneous or provoked by treatment.

lep·re·chaun·ism (lep're·kawn'iz·um) *n.* A congenital disorder, presumably autosomal recessive, in which the infant is small and cachectic, with a small hirsute face but nearly normal-sized ears, eyes, and nasal tip, giving it a gnome-like appearance; there is also premature ovarian follicular maturation, enlargement of the nipples and external genitalia, and various visceral abnormalities. Syn. *Donahue's syndrome.*

lep·rid (lep'rid) *n.* 1. Any skin lesion of leprosy. 2. A type of skin lesion seen in tuberculoid leprosy.

lep·rol·o·gist (lep·rol'uh·jist) *n.* An individual who specializes in the study and treatment of leprosy.

lep·rol·o·gy (lep·rol'uh·jee) *n.* The study of leprosy. —**lep·ro·log·ic** (lep''ro·loj'ick) *adj.*

lep·ro·ma (lep·ro'muh) *n.*, pl. **lepromas, leproma·ta** (·tuh) The cutaneous nodular lesion of leprosy. —**lep·rom·a·tous** (lep·rom'uh·tus) *adj.*

lepromatous leprosy. One of the two principal forms of leprosy, characterized by the presence of large numbers of *Mycobacterium leprae* in the lesions, a negative lepromin reaction, and diffuse skin lesions which may be macular or nodular, with later involvement of peripheral nerve trunks. In advanced cases, destructive lesions of the nose, mouth, throat, and larynx and deformities of the extremities are common.

lep·ro·min (lep'ro-min) *n.* An emulsion prepared from ground and sterilized tissue containing the leprosy bacillus (*Mycobacterium leprae*); used for intradermal skin tests in leprosy but of little diagnostic utility although of prognostic significance.

lepromin test. The intradermal injection of lepromin as a skin test, useful in the classification and prognosis of leprosy, generally positive in the tuberculoid and negative in the lepromatous form.

lep·ro·pho·bia (lep''ro-fo'bee-uh) *n.* Morbid dread of leprosy.

lep·ro·sar·i·um (lep''ro-sãr'ee-um) *n., pl.* **leprosariums, leprosar·ia** (-ee-uh). An institution for the treatment of persons affected with leprosy.

lep·ro·stat·ic (lep''ro-stat'ick) *adj.* Having an action inhibiting the growth of *Mycobacterium leprae*, the organism causing leprosy.

lep·ro·sy (lep'ruh-see) *n.* An infectious disease of low communicability, due to invasion of nerves by acid-fast *Mycobacterium leprae*; followed by progressive local invasion of tissues or hematogenous spread to skin, ciliary bodies, testes, lymph nodes, and nerves.

lep·rous (lep'rus) *adj.* 1. Pertaining to, or characteristic of leprosy. 2. Affected with leprosy.

lept-, lepto- A combining form meaning (a) *thin, narrow, fine;* (b) *small;* (c) *slight, mild.*

lep·to·ceph·a·lus (lep''to-sef'uh-lus) *n., pl.* **leptocephali** (-lye) An individual with an abnormally small head from premature union of the frontal and sphenoid bones.

lep·to·chro·mat·ic (lep''to-kro-mat'ick) *adj.* Having chromatin of a thin-stranded or fine appearance.

lep·to·cyte (lep'to-site) *n.* An abnormally thin erythrocyte, often characterized also by other abnormalities of shape.

lep·to·cy·to·sis (lep''to-sigh'to'sis) *n.* A preponderance of leptocytes in the blood.

lep·to·dac·ty·lous (lep''to-dack'ti-lus) *adj.* Characterized by slenderness of the fingers or toes, or both.

lep·to·don·tous (lep''to-don'tus) *adj.* Having thin or slender teeth.

lep·to·me·nin·ges (lep''to-me-nin'jeez) *n.pl.* The arachnoid and the pia mater considered together.

lep·to·men·in·gi·tis (lep''to-men''in-jye'tis) *n.* Inflammation of the pia mater and arachnoid of the brain or the spinal cord or both.

lep·to·me·ninx (lep''to-mee'ninks) *n., pl.* **lepto·me·nin·ges** (-me-nin'jeez) PIA-ARACHNOID.

lep·to·pel·lic (lep''to-pel'ick) *adj.* Having a very narrow pelvis.

lep·to·pho·nia (lep''to-fo'nee-uh) *n.* Delicacy, gentleness, or weakness of the voice. —**lepto·phon·ic** (-fon'ick) *adj.*

lep·to·pro·so·pia (lep''to-pro·so'pee-uh) *n.* Narrowness of the face. —**leptopro·sop·ic** (-sop'ick, -'sop'ick) *adj.*

Lep·to·spi·ra (lep''to-spye'ruh) *n.* A genus of spirochetes able to survive in water; characterized by sharply twisted filaments with one

or both extremities hooked or recurved. These organisms are not predominantly blood parasites, but are also found in other tissues. —**leptospira,** pl. **leptospiras, lep·to·spi·rae** (lep''to-spye'ree) *com. n.*

Leptospira au·tum·na·lis (aw-tum-nay'lis). The causative agent of pretibial fever.

Leptospira ca·nic·o·la (ka-nick'o-luh) The etiologic agent of Stuttgart disease in dogs and of canicola fever in man.

Leptospira grip·po·ty·pho·sa (grip-o-ty-fo'suh). One of the etiological agents of leptospirosis.

Leptospira ic·tero·hae·mor·rha·gi·ae (ick''tur-o-hem-o-ray'jee-ee). A species of spirochete which produces leptospirosis in man, in common with other species such as *Leptospira canicola, L. grippotyphosa.*

lep·to·spi·ro·sis (lep''to-spye-ro'sis) *n., pl.* **lepto·spiro·ses** (-seez) A systemic infection with spirochetal microorganisms of the genus *Leptospira,* usually a short self-limited febrile illness, but at times producing distinctive clinical syndromes of aseptic meningitis, hemorrhagic jaundice, or glomerulonephritis. Syn. *Landouzy's disease.*

leptospirosis ic·te·ro·he·mor·rhag·i·ca (ick''tur-o-hem-o-raj''i-kuh). WEIL'S DISEASE.

Lep·to·thrix (lep'to-thricks) *n.* A genus of unbranched filamentous organisms of the Chlamydobacteriaceae.

lep·to·tri·chal (lep''to-trye'kul, -trick'ul) *adj.* Pertaining to or caused by organisms of the genus *Leptothrix.*

lep·to·tri·cho·sis (lep''to-tri-ko'sis) *n., pl.* **leptotri·cho·ses** (-seez) Any disease caused by a species of *Leptothrix.*

le·re·sis (le-ree'sis) *n.* Garrulousness; senile loquacity.

Le·riche's operation (le-reesh') A periarterial sympathectomy for relief of vasomotor disturbances.

Leriche syndrome Thrombotic obliteration or occlusion of the aortic bifurcation producing intermittent claudication of the low back, buttocks, thighs, or calves; symmetrical atrophy and pallor of the legs; impotence; and weakness or absence of the femoral pulses.

les·bi·an (lez'bee-un) *adj. & n.* 1. Pertaining to or practicing female homosexuality. 2. One who practices female homosexuality.

les·bi·an·ism (lez'bee-un-iz-um) *n.* Female homosexuality. Syn. *sapphism.*

Lesch-Ny·han disease or syndrome. A disease of male children characterized by hyperuricemia, deficiency of hypoxanthine-guanine phosphoribosyltransferase, mental retardation, spasticity, tremor, choreoathetosis, and self-mutilating biting; transmitted as an X-linked recessive.

L. E. serum factor. L. E. FACTOR.

le·sion (lee'zhun) *n.* An alteration, structural or functional, due to disease; most commonly applied to morphological alterations.

lesser curvature of the stomach. The right border of the stomach, to which the lesser omentum is attached.

lesser omentum. A fold of peritoneum passing from the lesser curvature of the stomach to the transverse fissure of the liver. On the right its edge is free and encloses all the structures issuing from or entering the transverse fissure of the liver: portal vein, hepatic artery, bile duct, nerves, and lymphatics. Behind the free edge is the epiploic foramen. Syn. *gastrohepatic omentum.*

lesser pelvis. TRUE PELVIS.

lesser peritoneal cavity. OMENTAL BURSA.

lesser sac. OMENTAL BURSA.

lesser trochanter. A process situated on the inner side of the upper extremity of the femur below the neck.

L. E. test. 1. L. E. CELL TEST. 2. Any test for systemic lupus erythematosus.

le·thal (lee'thul) *adj.* Deadly; pertaining to or producing death. Abbreviated, l.

lethal dose. A dose sufficient to kill. Abbreviated, LD.

lethal gene. An allele that causes the death of the gamete or the zygote before development is completed, or at least before the organism reaches sexual maturity.

lethal mutation. A mutation causing death of the organism during any stage of its development prior to reproduction.

lethargic encephalitis. ENCEPHALITIS LETHARGICA.

leth·ar·gy (leth'ur·jee) *n.* Drowsiness or stupor; mental torpor. —**le·thar·gic** (le·thahr'jick) *adj.*

Let·ter·er-Si·we disease (let'ur·ur, see'vuh) A usually fatal disease of infancy and childhood, of unknown cause, characterized by hyperplasia of the reticuloendothelial system without lipid storage. Manifestations include enlargement of spleen, liver, and lymph nodes, histiocytic infiltration of the lungs, perivascular white matter of brain and meninges, osseous defects particularly in the skull, and involvement of the bone marrow resulting in secondary anemia. Cutaneous eruptions and purpura are frequently observed. Syn. *nonlipid reticuloendotheliosis, nonlipid histiocytosis.*

leu·cine (lew'seen, ·sin) *n.* $CH_3CH\cdot(CH_3)CH_2CH(NH_2)COOH$. The α-amino-isocaproic acid, an amino acid obtainable by the hydrolysis of milk and other protein-containing substances, and found in various tissues of the human body. It is essential to the growth of man. —**leu·cic** (lew'sick) *adj.*

leucine aminopeptidase. An enzyme acting on peptides which have a terminal free α-amino group, causing the sequential liberation of free amino acids from the peptide. The enzyme acts most rapidly on terminal leucine residues, and is useful in determining the structure of proteins. Marked increase in the serum level of the enzyme has been observed in pancreatic carcinoma but also in certain other diseases.

leucine intolerance or **sensitivity.** A condition of hypoglycemia primarily in infants caused by the ingestion of proteins rich in leucine. Thought to be genetic in origin, the condition appears to be caused by stimulation of insulin secretion.

Leu·co·nos·toc (lew"ko·nos'tock) *n.* A genus of saprophytic bacteria of the family Lactobacteriaceae. Species of this genus are found in milk, fermenting vegetables, and slimy sugar solutions. Used in the manufacture of dextrans.

leu·co·sin (lew'ko·sin) *n.* A simple protein of the albumin type found in wheat and other cereals.

leu·co·vor·in (lew"ko·vor'in, lew·kov'uh·rin) *n.* Folinic acid (2); used as the calcium salt to counteract the toxic effects of folic acid antagonists and for treatment of megaloblastic anemias.

leuk-, leuc-, leuko-, leuco- A combining form meaning (a) *white, colorless, weakly colored;* (b) *leukocyte, leukocytic.*

leu·ke·mia, leu·kae·mia (lew·kee'mee·uh) *n.* Any disease of the hemolytopoietic system characterized by uncontrolled proliferation of the leukocytes. Anaplastic leukocytes usually are present in the blood, often in large numbers, and characteristically involve various organs. Leukemias are classified on the basis of rapidity of course (acute, subacute, or chronic), the cell count, the cell type, and the degree of differentiation. Syn. *leukosis, leukocythemia.*

leu·ke·mic (lew·kee'mick) *adj.* 1. Of or pertaining to leukemia. 2. Characterized by an increase in leukocytes.

leu·ke·mid (lew·kee'mid) *n.* A cutaneous lesion which accompanies leukemia; sometimes restricted to those which do not contain leukemic cells.

leu·ke·moid, leu·kae·moid (lew·kee'moid) *adj.* Similar to leukemia, but due to other conditions; usually refers to the presence of immature cells in the blood in conditions other than leukemia.

Leukeran. Trademark for chlorambucil, an antineoplastic drug.

leu·ker·gy (lew'kur·jee) *n.* The tendency of leukocytes in the bloodstream of subjects with various inflammatory states to aggregate in groups of cytologically similar cells.

leu·ko·blast, leu·co·blast (lew'ko·blast) *n.* A general term for the parent cell of the leukocytes.

leu·ko·blas·to·sis, leu·co·blas·to·sis (lew"ko·blas·to'sis) *n.* Excessive proliferation of immature leukocytes.

leu·ko·ci·din, leu·co·ci·din (lew·ko·sigh'din, lew·ko'si·din) *n.* A toxic substance capable of killing and destroying neutrophil leukocytes.

leu·ko·cyte, leu·co·cyte (lew'ko·site) *n.* 1. One of the colorless, more or less ameboid cells of the blood, having a nucleus and cytoplasm. Those found in normal blood are usually divided according to their staining reaction into granular leukocytes, including neutrophils, eosinophils, and basophils, and nongranular leukocytes, including lymphocytes and monocytes. The kinds found in abnormal blood are myeloblasts, promyelocytes, neutrophilic myelocytes, eosinophilic myelocytes, basophilic myelocytes, lymphoblasts, and plasma cells. Syn. *white blood cell, white corpuscle.* 2 Specifically, NEUTROPHIL LEUKOCYTE.

leukocyte antigens. Transplantation antigens found on leukocytes, used for clinical pur poses because easily detectable and roughly representative of the antigenic content of body tissue.

leu·ko·cyt·ic (lew"ko·sit'ick) *adj.* Of or pertaining to leukocytes.

leu·co·cy·to·ma, leu·co·cy·to·ma (lew"ko·sigh'to'muh) *n.* A tumor composed of leukocytes.

leu·ko·cy·to·pe·ni·a, leu·co·cy·to·pe·ni·a (lew"ko·sigh"to·pee'nee·uh) *n.* LEUKOPENIA.

leu·ko·cy·to·poi·e·sis, leu·co·cy·to·poi·e·sis (lew" ko·sigh"to·poy·ee'sis) *n.*, pl. **leukocytopoie·ses, leucocytopoie·ses** (·seez) The formation of leukocytes. Syn. *leukopoiesis.* —**leukocytopoi·et·ic, leucocytopoi·et·ic** (·et'ick) *adj.*

leu·ko·cy·to·sis, leu·co·cy·to·sis (lew"ko·sigh·to'sis) *n.*, pl. **leukocyto·ses, leucocyto·ses** (·seez) An increase in the leukocyte count above the upper limits of normal. —**leukocy·tot·ic, leuco·cy·tot·ic** (·tot'ick) *adj.*

leu·ko·der·ma (lew"ko·dur'muh) *n.* Loss of skin melanin secondary to a cause which is known or reasonably certain. —**leukoder·mic** (·mick) *adj.*

leukoderma ac·qui·si·tum cen·trif·u·gum (ak"wi·sigh'tum sen·trif'yoo·gum). HALO NEVUS.

leukoderma pso·ri·at·i·cum (so"ree·at'i·kum). Areas of skin hypopigmentation following psoriatic inflammation.

leu·ko·dys·tro·phy, leu·co·dys·tro·phy (lew"ko·dis'truh·fee) *n.* Any disorder characterized by progressive degeneration of the cerebral white matter, or by defective building up of myelin, and most often due to an inborn error of metabolism.

leu·ko·en·ceph·a·li·tis, leu·co·en·ceph·a·li·tis (lew"ko·en·sef"uh·lye'tis) *n.* Any inflammatory disease affecting chiefly the cerebral white matter; may be acute, subacute, or chronic.

leu·ko·en·ceph·a·lop·a·thy, leu·co·en·ceph·a·lop·a·thy (lew"ko·en·sef"uh·lop'uth·ee) *n.* Any pathologic condition involving chiefly the white matter; may be inflammatory (leukoencephalitis) or degenerative (leukodystrophy).

leu·ko·eryth·ro·blas·tic anemia (lew"ko·e·rith'ro·blas'tick) Anemia accompanied by immature erythrocytes and leukocytes in the peripheral blood.

leu·ko·eryth·ro·blas·to·sis, leu·co·eryth·ro·blas·to·sis (lew"ko·e·rith"ro·blas·to'sis) *n.* Immature erythrocytes and leukocytes simultaneously present in the peripheral blood.

leu·ko·ker·a·to·sis, leu·co·ker·a·to·sis (lew"ko·kerr·uh·to'sis) *n.* LEUKOPLAKIA.

leu·ko·lym·pho·sar·co·ma, leu·co·lym·pho·sar·co·ma (lew"ko·lim"fo·sahr·ko'muh) *n.* LEUKOSARCOMA (1).

leu·ko·ma, leu·co·ma (lew"ko·muh) *n.*, pl. **leuko·mas, leucomas, leukoma·ta, leucoma·ta** (·tuh) 1. A dense opacity of the cornea as a result of an ulcer, wound, or inflammation, which presents an appearance of ground glass. 2. LEUKOPLAKIA BUCCALIS. 3. LEUKOSARCOMA. —**leukoma·tous, leucoma·tous** (·kom'uh·tus), **leukoma·toid, leucoma·toid** (·toid) *adj.*

leuk·onych·ia, leuc·onych·ia (lew"ko·nick'ee·uh) *n.* Whitish discoloration of the nails.

—**leuk·ony·chit·ic, leuc·ony·chit·ic** (·ni·kit'ick) *adj.*

leukonychia stri·a·ta (strye·ay'tuh). Horizontal streaks of whiteness of the nails.

leu·kop·a·thy, leu·cop·a·thy (lew·kop'uth·ee) *n.* 1. Any deficiency of coloring matter. 2. ALBINISM.

leu·ko·pe·de·sis, leu·co·pe·de·sis (lew"ko·pe·dee'sis) *n.* Diapedesis of leukocytes through the walls of blood vessels, especially the capillaries.

leu·ko·pe·ni·a, leu·co·pe·ni·a (lew"ko·pee'nee·uh) *n.* A decrease below the normal number of leukocytes in the peripheral blood. Syn. *leukocytopenia.* —**leukope·nic, leucope·nic** (·nick) *adj.*

leu·ko·phe·re·sis (lew"ko·fe·ree'sis) *n.* LEUKAPHERESIS.

leu·ko·pla·ki·a, leu·co·pla·ki·a (lew"ko·play'kee·uh) *n.* Abnormal thickening and whitening of the epithelium of a mucous membrane; it is considered to be precancerous in some cases. —**leukopla·ki·al** (·kee·ul) *adj.*

leukoplakia buc·ca·lis (buh·kay'lis). Leukoplakia characterized by pearly-white or bluish-white patches on the surface of the tongue or the mucous membrane of the cheeks.

leukoplakia oris (o'ris). LEUKOPLAKIA BUCCALIS.

leukoplakia vul·vae (vul'vee). Irregular white patches on the mucosa of the vulva. There is thickening of the epithelium, and the papillae may be hypertrophied. Carcinoma may develop.

leu·ko·poi·e·sis, leu·co·poi·e·sis (lew"ko·poy·ee'sis) *n.*, pl. **leukopoie·ses, leucopoie·ses** (·seez) LEUKOCYTOPOIESIS.

leu·ko·pro·te·ase, leu·co·pro·te·ase (lew"ko·pro'tee·ace, ·aze) *n.* An enzyme in leukocytes which splits protein. In inflammation, it causes liquefaction of necrotic tissue.

leu·kop·sin, leu·cop·sin (lew·kop'sin) *n.* Visual white, produced by reaction of light on rhodopsin (visual purple) derived from vitamin A.

leu·kor·rhea, leu·cor·rhoea (lew"ko·ree'uh) *n.* A whitish, mucopurulent discharge from the female genital canal. —**leukor·rhe·al, leucor·rhe·al** (·ree'ul) *adj.*

leu·ko·sar·co·ma, leu·co·sar·co·ma (lew"ko·sahr·ko'muh) *n.* 1. Lymphosarcoma accompanied by involvement of the peripheral blood with anaplastic lymphoid cells. Syn. *leukolymphosarcoma, sarcoleukemia.* 2. LYMPHOCYTIC LEUKEMIA.

leu·ko·sar·co·ma·to·sis, leu·co·sar·co·ma·to·sis (lew"ko·sahr·ko"muh·to'sis) *n.* A generalized form of leukosarcoma.

leu·ko·sis, leu·co·sis (lew·ko'sis) *n.*, pl. **leuko·ses, leuco·ses** (·seez) An excess of white blood cells.

leu·ko·tome, leu·co·tome (lew"ko·tome) *n.* An instrument for dividing nerve fibers of the white matter of the brain in lobotomy.

leu·kot·o·my, leu·cot·o·my (lew·kot'uh·mee) *n.* LOBOTOMY.

leu·ko·tox·ic, leu·co·tox·ic (lew"ko·tock'sick) *adj.* Destructive to leukocytes.

leu·ko·tox·in, leu·co·tox·in (lew"ko·tock'sin) *n.* A cytotoxin obtained from lymph nodes.

leu·ko·trich·ia (lew"ko·trick'ee·uh) n. Whiteness of the hair; CANITIES. —**leu·kot·ri·chous** (lew·kot'ri·kus) adj.

leu·ko·uro·bil·in, leu·co·uro·bil·in (lew"ko·yoor" o·bil'in, ·bye'lin) n. A colorless decomposition product of bilirubin.

leu·ro·cris·tine (lew"ro·kris'teen) n. VINCRISTINE.

lev·ar·ter·e·nol (lev"ahr·teer'e·nole, ·ahr·terr'e·nole) n. l-α-(Aminomethyl)-3,4-dihydroxybenzyl alcohol, $C_8H_{11}NO_3$, the levo isomer of the pressor amine l-arterenol (l-norepinephrine); used as a vasopressor in the form of the bitartrate salt.

le·va·tor (le·vay'tur) n., pl. **le·va·to·res** (lev"uh·to' reez) 1. Any of various muscles that raise or elevate. 2. An instrument used for raising a depressed portion of the skull.

levator ani (ay'nigh). The chief muscle of the pelvic diaphragm.

levator pal·pe·brae su·pe·ri·o·ris (pal·pee'bree sue·peer·ee·o'ris). The muscle that raises the upper eyelid.

levator sign. In paralysis of the facial nerve, when the patient is asked to look down and then close his eyes slowly, the upper lid on the paralyzed side moves upward slightly, being elevated by the levator palpebrae superioris whose action is no longer opposed by the orbicularis. Syn. Cestan's sign.

levator ve·li pa·la·ti·ni (vee'lye pal·uh·tye'nigh). The muscle that raises the soft palate.

le·ver (lee'vur, lev'ur) n. A vectis or one-armed tractor, used in obstetrics.

Lé·vi-Lo·rain disease or **dwarfism** (ley·vee', loh· ra$e^{n\prime}$) PITUITARY DWARFISM.

Le·vin tube A nasal gastroduodenal catheter, used in connection with gastric and intestinal operations.

lev·i·ta·tion (lev"i·tay'shun) n. 1. The subjective sense of rising into the air or being aloft without support, as in dreams or certain mental disorders. 2. The illusion of the suspension of a body in air; performed by modern magicians.

le·vo·car·dia (lee"vo·kahr'dee·uh) n. 1. Normal position of the heart in the left hemithorax. 2. A form of congenital heart disease associated with situs inversus, in which the heart paradoxically remains in the left chest, usually with intrinsic anomalies of its own.

le·vo·car·dio·gram (lee"vo·kahr'dee·o·gram) n. 1. That component of the normal electrocardiogram contributed by left ventricular forces. 2. The electrocardiographic complex derived from a unipolar lead facing the left ventricle.

le·vo·con·dy·lism (lee"vo·kon'di·liz·um) n. Deviation of the mandibular condyles toward the left.

le·vo·cy·clo·ver·sion (lee"vo·sigh"klo·vur'zhun, ·sick"lo·) n. Counterclockwise torsional movement of both eyes to the left.

le·vo·do·pa (lee"vo·do'puh) n. (−)-3-(3,4-Dihydroxyphenyl)-l-alanine, $C_9H_{11}NO_4$, an antiparkinson drug.

le·vo·duc·tion (lee"vo·duck'shun) n. Movement to the left, said especially of an eye.

le·vo·gy·rous (lee"vo·jye'rus) adj. LEVOROTATORY.

Levophed. Trademark for levarterenol, a pressor amine used as the bitartrate salt.

le·vo·pho·bia (lee"vo·fo'bee·uh) n. Morbid fear of objects on the left side of the body.

le·vo·ro·ta·tion (lee"vo·ro·tay'shun) n. Rotation toward the left, especially of the plane of polarization of light.

le·vo·ro·ta·to·ry (lee"vo·ro'tuh·to"ree, lev"o·) adj. Rotating the plane of polarized light from right to left (counterclockwise).

le·vo·thy·rox·ine (lee"vo·thigh·rock'seen, ·sin) n. l-3-[4-(4-Hydroxy-3,5-diiodophenoxy)-3,5-diiodophenyl]alanine, or l-3,3',5,5'-tetraiodothyronine, $C_{15}H_{11}I_4NO_4$, the active isomer of thyroxine occurring in the thyroid gland.

le·vo·ver·sion (lee"vo·vur'zhun) n. A turning to the left.

lev·u·lose (lev'yoo·loce) n. FRUCTOSE.

lev·u·lo·su·ria (lev"yoo·lo·sue'ree·uh) n. Presence of levulose in the urine.

Lew·is blood group system. First recognized in a Mrs. Lewis in 1946, an antigen occurring in some 22% of the population, designated Le^a and detected by anti-Le^a antibodies. Le^b and Le^c antigens and antibodies have since been recognized. The system is unique in being primarily composed of soluble antigens of serum and body fluids like saliva, with secondary adsorption by erythrocytes, in that Le^a positive individuals are nonsecretors of blood group substances A,B, and H, and in that the frequency of Le^a positives is highest in infancy up to the age of 5 years.

lew·is·ite (lew'is·ite) n. Chlorovinyldichloroarsine, ClCH=CHAsCl$_2$, an oily substance having vesicant, lacrimatory, and lung irritant effects; it was developed for use as a chemical warfare agent.

Lewy body. A concentric hyaline cytoplasmic inclusion, especially numerous in pigmented neurons of the substantia nigra and locus ceruleus, characteristic of idiopathic Parkinson's disease.

-lexia A combining form meaning (a) impairment of reading; (b) impairment of word recognition.

Leydig cell (lye'dik^h) One of the interstitial cells of the testis; it produces the male sex hormone.

Leydig-cell tumor. INTERSTITIAL-CELL TUMOR.

L.F.A. Abbreviation for left frontoanterior position of the fetus.

L.F.P. Abbreviation for left frontoposterior position of the fetus.

LH Abbreviation for luteinizing hormone.

Lher·mitte's sign (lehr·meet') Flexion of the neck is accompanied by the sensation of an electric shock shooting into the extremities in multiple sclerosis and other diseases involving the cervical spinal cord.

LHRF Abbreviation for luteinizing hormone releasing factor.

Li Symbol for lithium.

li·bid·i·nal (li·bid'i·nul) adj. Of or pertaining to the libido.

li·bi·do (li·bee'do, li·bye'do) n. 1. Sexual desire. 2. In psychoanalysis, psychic energy or drive usually associated with the sexual instinct that is, for pleasure and the seeking out of a love object. —**li·bid·i·nous** (li-bid'i·nus) adj.

Lib·man-Sacks endocarditis, syndrome, or **disease** Verrucous endocarditis complicating systemic lupus erythematosus.

li·bra (lye'bruh, lee'bruh) n., pl. **li·brae** (·bree) A pound; a weight of 12 troy ounces. Abbreviated, l. Symbol, ℔.

Librium. Trademark for chlordiazepoxide, a tranquilizer used as the hydrochloride salt.

lice. Plural of louse.

li·cense, n. An official permit or authority conferring on the recipient the right and privilege of practicing his profession.

li·cen·ti·ate (lye·sen'shee·ut, ·ate) n. 1. One who practices a profession by the authority of a license. 2. Specifically, in some countries, a licensed medical practitioner who has no medical degree and whose professional training is less than those who do have such a degree.

li·chen (lye'kin) n. 1. A plant consisting of a symbiotically associated alga and fungus, usually growing as an incrustation on dry rock or wood. 2. Any of various lesions of the skin which consist of solid papules with exaggerated skin markings.

lichen chron·i·cus sim·plex (kron'i·kus sim'plecks). The chronic stage of neurodermatitis characterized by lichenification of lesions in various regions. Syn. neurodermatitis circumscripta.

lichen cor·ne·us hy·per·troph·i·cus (kor'nee·us high'pur·trof'i·kus). Thickening and induration of the skin, found in lichen chronicus simplex and the plaque type of lichen planus. Syn. lichenificatio gigantea.

li·chen·i·fi·ca·tion (lye·ken'i·fi·kay'shun) n. The process whereby the skin becomes leathery and hardened; often the result of chronic pruritis and the irritation produced by scratching or rubbing eruptions.

lichen myx·e·de·ma·to·sus (mick''se·dee''muh·to'sus). A widespread eruption of asymptomatic nodules resulting from focal mucinosis of the upper dermis. Syn. papular mucinosis.

lichen nit·i·dus (nit'i·dus). A chronic, inflammatory skin disease characterized by groups of tiny papules which are asymptomatic; found frequently in the genital region and the flexor region of a joint.

li·chen·oid (lye'ke·noid) adj. Resembling lichen.

lichenoid amyloidosis. A primary amyloidosis involving only the skin, usually of the legs, characterized by small subepidermal amyloid deposits producing papules resembling those of lichen planus; they are conical or flat, discrete, brown-red, and may coalesce to form plaques.

lichen pla·nus (play'nus). A subacute or chronic idiopathic skin disease characterized by small, flat violaceous papules, often combining to form plaques; it is often pruritic and chiefly affects the flexor surfaces of the wrist, the legs, penis, and buccal mucosa.

lichen scrof·u·lo·sus (skrof''yoo·lo'sus). TUBERCULOSIS LICHENOIDES.

lichen stri·a·tus (strye·ay'tus). A rare, sudden,

self-limited disorder of the skin, occurring mostly in children, appearing as long strips of small lichenoid papules, usually on the extremities.

lick, n. A term used in the jargon of sports medicine to denote a dazed state following a blow to the head.

lic·o·rice, liq·uo·rice (lick'ur·is) n. GLYCYRRHIZA.

lid, n. EYELID.

lid lag. Lagging of the upper lid behind the eyeball when the patient looks downward, seen in thyrotoxic exophthalmos (von Graefe's sign) and other myopathies.

lid·o·caine (lid'o·kane) n. 2-(Diethylamino)-2',6'-acetoxylidide, $C_{14}H_{22}N_2O$, a local anesthetic; usually used as the hydrochloride salt. Syn. lignocaine. (Brit.)

Lie·ber·mann-Bur·chard reaction or **test** (lee'bur·mahn) A test for cholesterol, in which a solution of cholesterol in acetic anhydride, when treated with concentrated sulfuric acid, develops a color display going from red to purple to green.

lie detector. An instrument such as a polygraph used to record graphically changes in pulse rate, respiration, blood pressure, and perspiration in a person confronted by questions pertaining to past behavior; sudden marked changes are assumed to be indicative of a repressed sense of guilt or fear of detection when answering a question untruthfully.

li·en (lye'en) n., genit. **li·e·nis** (lye·ee'nis) SPLEEN. —**li·e·nal** (lye·ee'nul, lye'e·nul) adj.

lien-, lieno- A combining form meaning spleen, splenic.

li·en·cu·lus (lye·eng'kew·lus) n., pl. **liencu·li** (·lye) ACCESSORY SPLEEN.

li·en·i·tis (lye''e·nigh'tis) n. SPLENITIS.

li·e·no·cele (lye·ee'no·seel, lye''e·no·) n. Hernia of the spleen.

li·en·og·ra·phy (lye''e·nog'ruh·fee) n. Radiography of the spleen.

li·e·no·ma·la·cia (lye·ee''no·ma·lay'shee·uh, lye''e·no·) n. Abnormal softening of the spleen.

li·e·no·re·nal (lye·ee''no·ree'nul, lye''e·no·) adj. Pertaining to the spleen and the kidneys; SPLENORENAL.

lienteric diarrhea. Diarrhea with stools containing undigested food.

li·en·un·cu·lus (lye''un·ung'kew·lus) n., pl. **lienun·cu·li** (·lye) ACCESSORY SPLEEN.

Liep·mann's apraxia (leep'mahⁿn) APRAXIA.

life, n. The sum of properties by which an organism grows, reproduces, maintains its structure, and adapts itself to its environment; the quality by which an organism differs from inorganic or dead organic bodies.

life cycle. 1. The characteristic sequence of changes beginning with any given stage in the life of a particular kind of organism and ending with the first recurrence of that stage in its descendants. 2. The sequence of biologically significant periods in the lifetime of an individual.

lig·a·ment (lig'uh·munt) n. 1. A band of flexible, tough, dense white fibrous connective tissue connecting the articular ends of the bones, and sometimes enveloping them in a capsule.

Syn. *ligamentum.* 2. Certain folds and processes of the peritoneum.

ligament of Cooper 1. Any of the suspensory ligaments of the breast. See *suspensory ligament.* 2. A band of fibrous connective tissue overlying the pecten of the pubis.

ligament of Treitz The suspensory ligament of the duodenum. See *suspensory ligament.*

ligament of Zinn The fibrous ring from which arise the four rectus muscles of the eye and which is attached to the dural sheath of the optic nerve and to the upper and medial margins of the optic canal; it bridges the superior orbital fissure.

lig·a·men·to·pexy (lig″uh·men′to·peck″see) *n.* Suspension of the uterus by shortening or fixation of the round ligaments.

lig·a·men·tous (lig″uh·men′tus) *adj.* Of or pertaining to a ligament or ligaments.

ligamentous ankylosis. FIBROUS ANKYLOSIS.

lig·a·men·tum (lig″uh·men′tum) *n.,* pl. **ligamen·ta** (·tuh) LIGAMENT.

ligamentum carpi ra·di·a·tum (ray·dee·ay′tum) [NA]. RADIATE CARPAL LIGAMENT.

ligamentum vo·ca·le (vo·kay′lee) [NA]. VOCAL LIGAMENT.

lig·and (lig′and, lye′gand) *n.* 1. *In biochemistry,* a molecule which is bound by a protein surface. 2. *In inorganic chemistry,* any ion or molecule that by donating one or more pairs of electrons to a central metal ion is coordinated with it to form a complex ion or molecule, as in the compound $[CoCl(NH_3)_5] Cl_2$, in which Cl and NH_3 in the bracketed portion are ligands coordinated with Co.

li·gase (lye′gace, ·gaze, lig′ace) *n.* Any enzyme that catalyzes the joining of two molecules and that involves also the participation of a nucleoside triphosphate, such as adenosine triphosphate, which is converted to nucleoside diphosphate or monophosphate. Syn. *synthetase.*

li·ga·tion (lye·gay′shun) *n.* The operation of tying, especially arteries, veins, or ducts, with some form of knotted ligature. —**li·gate** (lye′ gate) *v.*

lig·a·ture (lig′uh·chur, ·choor) *n.* 1. A cord or thread for tying vessels. 2. The act of tying or binding; ligation. 3. A wire or other material used to secure an orthodontic attachment to an arch wire or to bind teeth together temporarily.

light, *n.* Electromagnetic radiations that give rise to the sensation of vision when the rays impinge upon the retina.

light adaptation. The disappearance of dark adaptation; the chemical processes by which the eyes, after exposure to a dim environment, become accustomed to bright illumination, which initially is perceived as quite intense and uncomfortable.

light difference. 1. The difference between the two eyes in respect to their sensitivity to light. 2. The smallest difference in illumination which can be distinguished by the eyes. Abbreviated, L.D.

light·en·ing (lite′un·ing) *n.* The sinking of the

fetus into the pelvic inlet with an accompanying descent of the uterus.

light·er·man's bottom (lite′ur·munz). Inflammation of the bursa over the tuberosity of the ischium; due to prolonged sitting. Syn. *weaver's bottom.*

light·head·ed (lite′hed″id) *adj.* Dizzy, delirious, disordered in the head; faint. —**light·head·ed·ness** (lite″hed′id·nis) *n.*

lightning pains. Lancinating pains coming on and disappearing with lightninglike rapidity and most commonly felt in the legs. They may come in bouts lasting several hours or days. They are characteristic of tabes dorsalis, but occur occasionally in other forms of neuropathy and radiculopathy.

light reflex. 1. A cone of light on the anterior and inferior part of the tympanic membrane, with its apex directed toward the umbo. 2. A circular area of light reflected from the retina during retinoscopic examination or from any light source. 3. The contraction of the pupil in response to light. Syn. *Whytt's reflex.*

light sense. *In ophthalmology,* the faculty of perceiving light and recognizing gradations of its intensity.

light sense tester. Any instrument used to test the sensitivity of the eye to light.

lig·ne·ous (lig′nee·us) *adj.* Woody, or having a woody texture.

ligneous thyroiditis. RIEDEL'S DISEASE.

lig·ni·fi·ca·tion (lig″ni·fi·kay′shun) *n.* The process by which the cell wall of a plant acquires greater rigidity by deposition of lignin.

lig·nin (lig′nin) *n.* A modification of cellulose, constituting the greater part of the weight of most dry wood. A substance deposited in the cell walls of plants.

lig·ro·in (lig′ro·in) *n.* A liquid fraction obtained from petroleum; used as a solvent.

Lil·li·pu·tian hallucination (lil′i·pew′shun). A false visual perception in which all objects and persons appear diminutive, often seen in febrile or intoxicated states, psychomotor seizures, and in manic-depressive illness. Syn. *microptic hallucination.*

limb, *n.* 1. One of the extremities attached to the trunk and used for prehension or locomotion. 2. An elongated limblike structure, as one of the limbs of the internal capsule.

lim·ber·neck (lim′bur·neck) *n.* An avian type of botulism; a disease caused by *Clostridium botulinum* toxin and characterized by muscular incoordination, weakness, and death.

lim·bic (lim′bick) *adj.* 1. Pertaining to or of the nature of a limbus or border; circumferential; marginal. 2. Pertaining to the limbic system or lobes of the brain.

limbic cortex, lobe, or **system.** A ring of cerebral cortex, composed of archipallium and paleopallium, which includes the paraterminal gyrus and parolfactory area, the gyrus cinguli, part of the gyrus parahippocampalis, and uncus. It is the oldest portion of the cortex which has its evolutionary rudiment in the reptiles, amphibians, and fish. Now thought to control various emotional and behavioral patterns.

lim·bus (lim′bus) *n.,* pl. **lim·bi** (·bye) A border; the circumferential edge of any flat organ or part.

¹**lime**, *n.* CALCIUM OXIDE.

²**lime**, *n.* The fruit of *Citrus aurantifolia;* its juice is antiscorbutic.

li·men (lye'mun) *n.,* pl. **lim·i·na** (lim'i·nuh) 1. A boundary line. 2. THRESHOLD.

limen na·si (nay'zye) The boundary line between the osseous and the cartilaginous portions of the nasal cavity.

li·mes (lye'meez) *n.,* pl. **li·mi·tes** (·mi·teez) Limit, boundary.

limes death. The least amount of diphtheria toxin which, when mixed with one unit of antitoxin and injected into a guinea pig weighing 250 g, kills within 5 days. Symbol, L_+.

limes zero. The greatest amount of diphtheria toxin which causes no local edema when mixed with one unit of antitoxin and injected into a guinea pig weighing 250 g. Symbol, L_0.

limina. Plural of *limen.*

lim·i·nal (lim'i·nul) *adj.* Pertaining to the limen or threshold, especially pertaining to the lowest limit of perception to a sensory stimulus.

limit dextrinosis. Glycogenosis caused by a deficiency of amylo-1,6-glucosidase (debrancher enzyme), with abnormal storage of excessively branched glycogen in liver, heart, and muscle in various combinations depending on which organs are enzyme deficient; manifested clinically by moderate to marked hepatomegaly and varying degrees of skeletal weakness and cardiomegaly. Involvement of erythrocytes results in high levels of blood glycogen. Syn. *type III of Cori, Forbes' disease.*

Limnatis ni·lo·ti·ca (nye·lot'i·kuh). A widely distributed species of leech which produces internal hirudiniasis in man.

li·mo·nite (lye'mo·nite, lim'o·) *n.* Ferric oxide, of the approximate formula $2Fe_2O_3.3H_2O$; a yellow powder.

li·moph·i·sis (li·mof'thi·sis, lye·) *n.* Wasting of the body, due to starvation; INANITION.

¹**limp**, *n.* An abnormal gait resulting from one or a combination of malfunctions of musculoskeletal structures pertinent to locomotion, or pain in a joint or other lower extremity structure.

²**limp**, *adj.* Floppy, flaccid; HYPOTONIC (1).

limy bile syndrome. Opacification of the gallbladder or common duct on a plain abdominal x-ray film, due to excessive calcium salts in the bile.

lin·a·mar·in (lin''uh·mär'in) *n.* The toxic cyanogenetic glycoside, $C_{10}H_{17}NO_6$, of linseed.

Lincocin. Trademark for the antibiotic substance lincomycin.

lin·co·my·cin (lin·ko·migh'sin) *n.* Methyl 6,8-dideoxy-6-(1-methyl-4-propyl-L-2-pyrrolidinecarboxamido)-1-thio-D-*erythro*-α-D-*galacto*-octopyranoside, $C_{18}H_{34}N_2O_6S$, an antibiotic produced by *Streptomyces lincolnensis.* Its spectrum of action is limited to gram-positive bacteria, especially cocci.

linc·tus (link'tus) *n.* A syrupy preparation, usually containing sugar, of a medicinal that will alleviate irritation of the mucous membrane of the throat.

lin·dane (lin'dane) *n.* The gamma isomer of 1,2,3,4,5,6-hexachlorocyclohexane, $C_6H_6Cl_6$, known also as benzene hexachloride, of a purity of not less than 99%; a powerful insecticide.

line, *n.* 1. Extension of dimension having length, but neither breadth nor thickness. 2. *In anatomy,* anything resembling a mathematical line in having length without breadth or thickness; a boundary or guide mark. 3. *In genetics,* lineage; the succession of progenitors and progeny. 4. *Obsol.* The 1/12 part of an inch.

lin·ea (lin'ee·uh) *n.,* pl. **lin·e·ae** (·ee·ee) LINE.

linea al·ba (al'buh) [NA]. A tendinous raphe extending in the median line of the abdomen from the pubes to the xiphoid process; it is formed by the blending of the aponeuroses of the oblique and transverse muscles of the abdomen.

lineae. Plural of *linea* (= LINE).

lineae al·bi·can·tes (al·bi·kan'teez). Glistening white lines seen in the skin, especially that of the anterior abdominal wall, after reduction from extreme distention, as in pregnancy; produced by rupture of the elastic fibers.

lin·e·al (lin'ee·ul) *adj.* 1. Of or pertaining to a line of descent or lineage. 2. Being in a direct line of descent. 3. Linear.

linea ni·gra (nigh'gruh). A dark pigmented line often present in pregnant women and extending from the pubes upward in the median line.

lin·e·ar (lin'ee·ur) *adj.* Pertaining to or resembling a line or lines.

linear correlation. A correlation between two variables in which the regression equation is represented by a straight line; a relationship that can be described graphically by a straight line.

linear nevus. A nevus verrucosus of linear shape.

linear osteotomy. Simple surgical division of a bone.

line of demarcation. A line of division between healthy and gangrenous tissue.

line of fixation. An imaginary line drawn from the object viewed through the center of rotation of the eye.

line of occlusion. An imaginary line formed by the opposing arches of teeth when they are in maximum contact.

line of sight. An imaginary line drawn from the object viewed to the center of the pupil.

lingu-, lingua-, lingui-, linguo-. A combining form meaning *tongue, lingual.*

lin·gua (ling'gwuh) *n.* TONGUE.

lin·gual (ling'gwul) *adj. & n.* 1. Of or pertaining to the tongue. 2. Toward or nearest the tongue. 3. Either the inferior or superior intrinsic longitudinalis muscle of the tongue.

lingual bar. A metal bar on the lingual side of the mandibular arch, connecting the two or more parts of a mandibular removable partial denture.

lingual goiter. A mass of thyroid tissue, at the upper end of the original thyroglossal duct, near the foramen cecum of the tongue.

lingual occlusion. An occlusion where the line of a tooth is internal.

lingual septum. The vertical median partition of

the tongue which divides the muscular tissue into halves.

lingual titubation. Stammering; stuttering.

lingual tonsil. Accumulations of lymphatic tissue more or less closely associated with crypts which serve also as ducts of the mucous glands of the base of the tongue.

lingua ni·gra (nigh'gruh). BLACK, HAIRY TONGUE.

lingua pli·ca·ta (pli·kay'tuh). FISSURED TONGUE.

Linguatula ser·ra·ta (se·ray'tuh). A tongue worm found in the nose or paranasal sinuses of dogs and other carnivores; rarely infests man.

lin·gu·la (ling'gew·luh) *n.*, pl. **lingu·lae** (·lee) 1. LINGULA CEREBELLI. 2. A tonguelike structure. **—lingu·lar** (·lur) *adj.*

lingula ce·re·bel·li (serr·e·bel'eye) [NA]. The portion of the vermis of the cerebellum attached to the superior medullary velum.

lingula of the mandible. The prominent, thin process of bone partly surrounding the mandibular foramen.

lin·gu·lec·to·my (ling"gew·leck'tuh·mee) *n.* Surgical removal of the lingula of the upper lobe of the left lung.

lin·guo·dis·tal (ling"gwo·dis'tul) *adj.* Distally and toward the tongue, as the inclination of a tooth.

lin·guo·gin·gi·val (ling"gwo·jin'ji·vul, ·jin·jye'vul) *adj.* Pertaining to the tongue and the gingiva.

lin·i·ment (lin'i·munt) *n.* A liquid intended for application to the skin by gentle friction.

li·nin (lye'nin) *n.* 1. A strongly purgative principle obtainable from *Linum catharticum*, or purging flax. 2. *In biology*, the substance of the achromatic network of the nucleus of a cell.

li·ni·tis (li·nigh'tis, ·lye·nigh'tis) *n.* GASTRITIS.

linitis plas·ti·ca (plas'ti·kuh). Infiltrating, poorly differentiated carcinoma of the stomach involving all coats of the wall. Syn. *leather-bottle stomach.*

link·age (link'ij) *n.* 1. *In chemistry*, the lines used in structural formulas to represent valency connections between the atoms: a single line represents a valency of one, a double line a valency of two. 2. *In genetics*, the association of genes located in the same chromosome.

linkage law. Different gene pairs tend to segregate together if they are located on the same pair of homologous chromosomes. Linked genes may be separated with a frequency which varies from 0 to 50%, depending chiefly upon the relative linear distances between them.

lin·o·le·ic acid (lin"o·lee'ick, li·no'lee·ick). 9,12-Octadecadienoic acid, $C_{17}H_{31}COOH$, an unsaturated acid containing two double bonds, occurring in the glycerides of linseed and other oils. Syn. *linolic acid.*

lin·ono·pho·bia (lin"on·o·fo'bee·uh) *n.* Morbid fear of string.

lin·seed, *n.* The dried ripe seed of *Linum usitatissimum;* it contains 30 to 40% of a fixed oil, together with wax, resin, tannin, gum, and protein. Linseed is demulcent and emollient; infusions of the whole seed have been used in respiratory infections, and the whole seed is sometimes employed as a laxative. Syn. *flaxseed.*

linseed oil. The fixed oil obtained from linseed (oil that has been boiled or treated with a drier must not be used medicinally); used mostly in liniments and cerates, occasionally given for its laxative effect.

lint, *n.* A loosely woven or partly felted mass of broken linen fibers, made by scraping or picking linen cloth. It was once much used as a dressing for wounds.

lin·tin (lin'tin) *n.* Absorbent cotton rolled, or compressed into sheets; used for dressing wounds.

lip, *n.* 1. One of the two fleshy folds surrounding the orifice of the mouth. 2. One of the labia majora or labia minora. 3. A projecting margin; rim.

lip-, lipo- A combining form meaning (a) *fat, fatty;* (b) *lipid.*

lip·ac·i·de·mia (lip·as"i·dee'mee·uh) *n.* The presence of fatty acids in the blood.

lip·a·ro·trich·ia (lip"uh·ro·trick'ee·uh) *n.* Abnormal oiliness of the hair.

lip·a·rous (lip'uh·rus) *adj.* Fat; obese.

li·pase (lye'pace, lip'ace) *n.* A fat-splitting enzyme contained in the pancreatic juice, in blood plasma, and in many tissues.

li·pa·su·ria (lip"ay·syoo'ree·uh, lye"pay·) *n.* The presence of lipase in the urine.

li·pec·to·my (li·peck'tuh·mee) *n.* Excision of fatty tissue.

li·pe·mia, li·pae·mia (li·pee"mee·uh) *n.* The presence of a fine emulsion of fatty substance in the blood. Syn. *lipidemia, lipoidemia.* **—lipe·mic, li·pae·mic** (li·pee'mick) *adj.*

lipemia ret·i·na·lis (ret"i·nay'lis). Fatty infiltration of the retina and its blood vessels in hyperlipemic states.

lip·id (lip'id, lye'pid) *n.* Any one of a group of fats and fatlike substances having in common the property of insolubility in water and solubility in the fat solvents. Included are fats, fatty acids, fatty oils, waxes, sterols, and esters of fatty acids containing other groups such as phosphoric acid (phospholipids) and carbohydrates (glycolipids). Syn. *lipin.*

lip·ide (lip'ide, ·id, lye'pid) *n.* LIPID.

lipid granulomatosis. HAND-SCHÜLLER-CHRISTIAN DISEASE.

lipid histiocytosis. 1. Any collection of lipid-containing histiocytes. 2. NIEMANN-PICK DISEASE.

li·pid·ic (li·pid'ick) *adj.* 1. Of or pertaining to a lipid; having the nature of a lipid.

lipid nephrosis. *Obsol.* A chronic renal disease chiefly of children, characterized clinically by severe proteinuria, edema, hypoalbuminemia, hypercholesterolemia, and normal blood pressure, and associated with glomerular basement membrane thickening.

lip·i·dol·y·sis (lip"i·dol'i·sis) *n.* LIPOLYSIS.

lip·i·do·sis (lip"i·do'sis) *n.*, pl. **lipido·ses** (·seez) The generalized deposition of fat or fat-containing substances in cells of the reticuloendothelial system.

lipid pneumonia. 1. Pneumonia due to aspiration of oily substances, particularly kerosene, mineral oil, or cod-liver oil; more common in children or in adults when the cough reflex is impaired. 2. The deposition of cholesterol and other lipids in chronically inflamed pulmonary tissue.

lipid proteinosis. A hereditary disorder characterized by extracellular deposits of phospholipid-protein conjugate involving various areas of the body including the skin and air passages.

lipid storage disease. Any of a group of rare diseases, including Gaucher's disease, Niemann-Pick disease, and the amaurotic familial idiocies; characterized by an accumulation of large, lipid-containing cells throughout the viscera and nervous system. They occur primarily in childhood.

Lipiodol. The trademark for an iodized poppy seed oil used as a contrast medium for roentgenologic work.

lipo- A combining form meaning *lack, absence.*

lipo·blast (lip′o·blast) *n.* A formative fat cell, small or moderate in size, polyhedral, and having numerous tiny droplets of fat in its cytoplasm. —**lipo·blas·tic** (lip″o·blas′tick) *adj.*

lipo·blas·to·sis (lip″o·blas·to′sis) *n.* Multiple lipomas in subcutaneous and visceral fat deposits. Syn. *systemic multiple lipomas.*

lip·o·ca·ic (lip″o·kay′ick) *n.* A substance, probably a hormone, found in the pancreas which prevents deposition of lipids in the liver.

lipo·chon·dro·dys·tro·phy (lip″o·kon′dro·dis′truh·fee) *n.* MUCOPOLYSACCHARIDOSIS.

lipo·chon·dro·ma (lip″o·kon·dro′muh) *n.* Chondroma containing fat cells.

lipo·chrome (lip′o·krohm) *n.* 1. A readily soluble carotenoid pigment giving a blue color with sulfuric acid. 2. LIPOFUSCIN.

lipo·cyte (lip′o·site) *n.* A specialized cell for fat storage. Syn. *adipocyte.*

lipo·dys·tro·phy (lip″o·dis′truh·fee) *n.* A disturbance of fat metabolism in which the subcutaneous fat disappears over some regions of the body, but is unaffected in others.

lipo·fi·bro·ma (lip″o·figh·bro′muh) *n.* A benign connective tissue tumor composed of adipose and fibrous tissue.

lipo·fi·bro·myx·o·ma (lip″o·figh″bro·mick·so′muh) *n.* A benign mesodermal mixed tumor, containing fatty tissue, fibrous tissue, and mucoid or myxomatous tissue.

lipo·fi·bro·sar·co·ma (lip″o·figh″bro·sahr·ko′muh) *n.* A malignant tumor whose parenchyma is composed of anaplastic fibrous and adipose tissue cells.

lipo·fus·cin (lip″o·fus′in, ·few′sin) *n.* One of a group of at least partly insoluble lipid pigments occurring in cardiac and smooth muscle cells, in macrophages and in parenchyma and interstitial cells of various organs; characterized by sudanophilia, Nile blue staining, fatty acid, glycol, and ethylene reactions, slow reduction of diammine silver, osmic acid, and ferric ferricyanide.

lipo·gen·e·sis (lip″o·jen′e·sis) *n.* The formation or deposit of fat. —**lipogen·ic** (·ick) *adj.*

li·pog·e·nous (li·poj′e·nus) *adj.* Fat-producing.

lipo·gran·u·lo·ma (lip″o·gran·yoo·lo′muh) *n.* A nodule of fatty tissue, consisting of a center of degenerated and necrotic fat associated with granulomatous inflammation.

lipo·he·mar·thro·sis, lipo·hae·mar·thro·sis (lip″o·hee″mahr·thro′sis) *n.,* pl. **lipohemarthro·ses, lipohaemarthro·ses** (·seez) The presence of blood and lipids in the joint cavity following injury.

lip·oid (lip′oid, lye′poid) *adj. & n.* 1. Resembling fat or oil. 2. Having the character of a lipid; lipidic. 3. Lipid, particularly one of the intracellular lipids which contain nitrogen. The chemists have officially adopted the term lipid, but many histologists still use the term lipoid.

lip·oi·do·sis (lip″oy·do′sis) *n.,* pl. **lipoido·ses** (·seez) LIPIDOSIS.

lipoid pneumonia. LIPID PNEUMONIA.

li·pol·y·sis (li·pol′i·sis) *n.,* pl. **lipoly·ses** (·seez) The hydrolysis of fat. —**lipo·lytic** (lip″o·lit′ick) *adj.*

lipolytic enzyme. An enzyme that hydrolyzes fats to glycerin and fatty acids, as pancreatic lipase.

li·po·ma (li·po′muh, lye·) *n.,* pl. **lipomas, lipoma·ta** (·tuh) A benign tumor whose parenchyma is composed of mature adipose tissue cells. —**li·pom·a·tous** (·pom′uh·tus), **lipoma·toid** (·toid) *adj.*

li·po·ma·to·sis (li·po″muh·to′sis, lye·) *n.,* pl. **lipomato·ses** (·seez) 1. Multiple lipomas. 2. A general deposition of fat; obesity.

lipo·mel·a·not·ic (lip″o·mel·uh·not′ick) *adj.* Pertaining both to fat and melanin.

lipomelanotic reticular hyperplasia. LIPOMELANOTIC RETICULOSIS.

lipomelanotic reticulosis. A form of lymph-node hyperplasia characterized by preservation of the architectural structure, inflammatory exudate, and hyperplasia of the reticulum cells which show phagocytosis of hemosiderin, melanin, and occasionally fat. It is often secondary to an extensive dermatitis. Syn. *lipomelanotic reticular hyperplasia, dermatopathic lymphadenitis.*

lipo·me·nin·go·cele (lip″o·me·ning′go·seel) *n.* The association of lobules of adipose tissue with a meningocele.

lipo·my·e·lo·me·nin·go·cele (lip″o·migh″e·lo·me·ning′go·seel) *n.* The association of masses of adipose tissue with a myelomeningocele.

lipo·myo·he·man·gi·o·ma, lipo·myo·hae·man·gi·o·ma (lip″o·migh″o·he·man″jee·o′muh) *n.* A benign hamartomatous tumor whose parenchyma is composed of adipose tissue, muscle, and blood vessels.

lipo·my·o·ma (lip″o·migh·o′muh) *n.* A benign hamartomatous tumor whose parenchyma is composed of adipose tissue and muscle.

lipo·myo·sar·co·ma (lip″o·migh″o·sahr·ko′muh) *n.* A malignant tumor whose parenchyma is composed of anaplastic adipose tissue and muscle cells.

lipo·myx·o·ma (lip″o·mick·so′muh) *n.* A benign tumor whose parenchyma is composed of adipose tissue and mucinous connective tissue elements.

lipo·myxo·sar·co·ma (lip″o·mick″so·sahr·ko′muh) *n.* A malignant tumor whose parenchyma is composed of anaplastic adipose tissue and mucinous connective-tissue cells.

lipo·pe·nia (lip'o·pee'nee·uh) *n.* Abnormal diminution of fat in tissues.

lipo·phage (lip'o·faje, ·fahz) *n.* A cell which has taken up fat in its cytoplasm.

lipophagic granuloma. A granuloma whose macrophages contain fat derived from the breakdown of adipose tissue in the area.

lipo·pha·gy (lip'o·fay'jee, li·pof'uh·jee) *n.* The destruction of adipose tissue, associated with cellular elements which ingest products of fat breakdown.

lipo·plas·tic (lip'o·plas'tick) *adj.* Producing adipose tissue.

lipoplastic lymphadenopathy. Lymph node enlargement due to an increment in adipose tissue, largely in the hilum.

lipo·poly·sac·cha·ride (lip''o·pol''ee·sack'uh·ride) *n.* A compound of a lipid with a polysaccharide.

lipo·pro·tein (lip''o·pro'tee·in, ·teen) *n.* One of a group of conjugated proteins consisting of a simple protein combined with a lipid. A lipoprotein may be classified according to its physical properties or density as alpha-lipoprotein, containing more protein and having high density; beta-lipoprotein, containing more lipid compared to protein and having low density; or omega-lipoprotein, containing the largest amount of lipids and appearing as chylomicra in the serum.

lipo·sar·co·ma (lip''o·sahr·ko'muh) *n.* A malignant tumor whose parenchyma is composed of anaplastic adipose tissue cells. —**liposarco·ma·tous** (·tus) *adj.*

lipo·sol·u·ble (lip'o·sol'yoo·bul) *adj.* Soluble in fats.

lipo·trop·ic (lip'o·trop'ick) *adj.* 1. Having an affinity for lipids, particularly fats and oils. 2. Having a preventive or curative effect on the deposition of excessive fat in abnormal sites.

lipotropic factor. A substance that reduces the amount of liver fat; more specifically, choline or any compound, or compounds, which metabolically can give rise to choline. Syn. *lipotropia.*

lipo·vac·cine (lip''o·vack'seen, ·vack'seen') *n.* A vaccine with a fatty or oily menstruum.

lip·ping. The perichondral growth of osteophytes which project beyond the margin of the joint in degenerative joint disease.

lip·pi·tude (lip'i·tewd) *n.* LIPPITUDO.

lip·pi·tu·do (lip''i·tew'do) *n.* A condition of the eyes marked by ulcerative marginal blepharitis; a state of being blear-eyed.

Lip·schütz body (lip'shuᵉts) Eosinophilic nuclear inclusion, granular or amorphous, designated as type A, found in cells infected with such viruses as herpes simplex, herpes zoster, cytomegalovirus, and yellow fever.

li·pu·ria (li·pew'ree·uh) *n.* The presence of fat in the urine; ADIPOSURIA.

liq·ue·fa·cient (lick''we·fay'shunt) *n.* An agent capable of producing liquefaction.

q·ue·fac·tion (lick''wi·fack'shun) *n.* 1. The change to a liquid form, usually of a solid

tissue to a fluid or semifluid state. 2. Condensation of a gas to a liquid or the conversion of a solid to a liquid.

liquefaction necrosis. Tissue death in which the remains are converted to a liquid state.

liq·ue·fac·tive (lick''wi·fack'tiv) *adj.* Pertaining to, causing, or characterized by liquefaction.

li·ques·cent (li·kwes'unt) *adj.* Becoming liquid.

liq·uid (lick'wid) *n.* A fluid or substance that flows readily. A state of matter intermediate between a solid and a gas, shapeless and fluid, taking the shape of the container and seeking the lowest level.

liq·uo·gel (lick'wo·jel) *n.* A gel which, when melted, yields a sol of low viscosity.

li·quor (lye'kwor, lick'wor; in senses 3 and 4, lick'ur) *n.* 1. Any of certain medicinal solutions, usually including aqueous solutions of nonvolatile substances, except those solutions which belong to the class of syrups, infusions, or decoctions. 2. In Latin anatomical terms, a body fluid. 3. Any of various liquids occurring in nature or, more usually, in the preparation of certain man-made products, as dye liquor, mother liquor. 4. A distilled alcoholic drink.

liquor am·nii (am'nee·eye). AMNIOTIC FLUID.

Lis·franc's amputation (lees·frahⁿ') Partial amputation of the foot by disarticulation of the metatarsal bones from the tarsus.

lisp, *n. & v.* 1. A speech defect consisting in the substitution of interdental spirant sounds (th, th) for sibilants (s, z). 2. Any of various other speech defects or affectations, especially those reminiscent of baby talk. 3. To speak with a lisp.

lis·sen·ce·pha·lia (lis''en·se·fay'lee·uh) *n.* Smallness of the brain and failure of sulcal formation, resulting in a smooth brain.

lis·ter·el·lo·sis (lis'tur·el·o'sis) *n.,* pl. **listerello·ses** (·seez) LISTERIOSIS.

Lis·te·ria (lis·teer'ee·uh) *n.* A genus of bacteria of the family Corynebacteriaceae. Its members are small, non-spore-forming, gram-positive rods, motile by means of a single terminal flagellum. —**lis·te·ric** (·rick) *adj.*

Listeria mono·cy·tog·e·nes (mon''o·sigh·toj'e·neez). One cause of sporadic cases of purulent meningitis in man, granulomatosis infantasepticum, septicemia, and less commonly, mononucleosis and conjunctivitis.

lis·te·ri·o·sis (lis·teer''ee·o'sis) *n.,* pl. **listerio·ses** (·seez) Infection of animals and man with the gram-positive bacillus *Listeria monocytogenes;* the protean manifestations include meningitis, lymphadenopathy, disseminated granulomas, respiratory symptoms, and ill-defined acute febrile illness; it can produce abortion and fetal or neonatal death.

Lis·ter·ism (lis'tur·iz·um) *n.* A general name for the antiseptic and aseptic treatment of wounds according to the principles of Joseph Lister.

li·ter, li·tre (lee'tur) *n.* The metric unit of volume, representing 0.001 cubic meter or 1000 cubic centimeters. Formerly defined as the volume occupied by 1 kg of pure water at 4°C and 760 mm pressure. It is equal to 1.056 United States quarts. Abbreviated, l.

lith-, litho- A combining form meaning *stone, calculus.*

-lith A combining form meaning *stone, calculus.*

lith·a·gogue (lith'uh-gog) *n.* Any agent that is supposed to expel calculi from the urinary bladder.

lith·arge (lith'ahrj, li-thahrj') *n.* LEAD MONOXIDE.

li·he·mia, li·thae·mia (li-theem'ee-uh) *n.* HYPERURICEMIA.

lith·ia (lith'ee-uh) *n.* Li₂O. Lithium oxide. Lithia water is a mineral water containing lithium salts in solution.

li·thi·a·sis (li-thigh'uh-sis) *n.,* pl. **lithia·ses** (-seez) The formation of calculi in the body. **—lithia·sic** (-sick) *adj.*

lith·ic (lith'ick) *adj.* 1. Pertaining to calculi. 2. Pertaining to lithium.

lithic acid. URIC ACID.

lith·i·co·sis (lith·i·ko'sis) *n.* Silicosis or other pneumoconiosis occurring in stonecutters.

lith·i·um (lith'ee-um) *n.* Li = 6.941. A soft, silver-white metal belonging to the alkali group. It is the lightest solid element, having a density of 0.534. Salts of lithium have been used like salts of other alkali metals; under certain conditions they are toxic; now widely used in the treatment of hypomanic and manic states.

lithium carmine (Orth's). Contains 2.5 to 5.0 g of carmine in 100 ml of saturated aqueous lithium carbonate solution; used to stain histologic sections, the nuclei being stained bright red, and as a vital stain.

litho·di·al·y·sis (lith''o·dye·al'i·sis) *n.* 1. The solution of calculi in the urinary bladder. 2. The breaking of a vesical calculus previous to its removal.

litho·gen·e·sis (lith''o·jen'e·sis) *n.* The formation of calculi or stones. **—litho·gen·et·ic** (·je·net'ick), **li·thog·e·nous** (li·thoj'e·nus) *adj.*

lith·oid (lith'oid) *adj.* Resembling a stone.

li·thol·a·paxy (li·thol'uh·pack''see, lith'o·luh·) *n.* The operation of crushing a urinary calculus in the bladder by means of the lithotrite, and then removing the fragments by irrigation, a procedure now performed by a transurethral approach. Syn. *lithotrity.*

litho·ne·phri·tis (lith''o·ne·frye'tis) *n.* Inflammation of the kidney, associated with the presence of renal calculi.

litho·ne·phrot·o·my (lith''o·ne·frot'uh·mee) *n.* Lithotomy performed by means of an incision into the kidney parenchyma or the renal pelvis; renal lithotomy.

lith·o·pe·di·on (lith''o·pee'dee·on) *n.* A retained fetus that has become calcified.

li·thot·o·mist (li·thot'uh·mist) *n.* 1. A surgeon who performs lithotomies. 2. Formerly, an individual who cut for stone in the urinary bladder.

li·thot·o·my (li·thot'uh·mee) *n.* The removal of a calculus, usually vesical, through an operative incision.

lithotomy forceps. A special type of forceps for removing a stone from the urinary bladder or ureter.

litho·trip·sy (lith''o·trip'see) *n.* The operation of crushing calculi in the urinary bladder.

lith·o·trite (lith'o·trite) *n.* An instrument for crushing a vesical calculus. **—lith·o·trit·ic** (lith''o·trit'ick) *adj.*

lith·u·re·sis (lith''yoo·ree'sis) *n.* Voiding of small calculi with the urine; gravel urine.

lit·mus (lit'mus) *n.* A blue pigment obtained from *Roccella tinctoria,* a lichen; used as an acid-base indicator.

litmus milk. Milk that contains litmus; used as an indicator in bacteriology.

Lit·ten's sign DIAPHRAGMATIC SIGN.

lit·ter (lit'ur) *n.* 1. A stretcher, basket, or bed with handles, used for carrying the sick or injured. 2. In animals, the group of young brought forth at one birth.

Little's disease Cerebral palsy; especially the spastic diplegic type, considered by Little to be due to perinatal asphyxia and prematurity.

littoral cells. The cells that line lymph sinuses in lymphatic tissue, or the sinusoids of bone marrow. They form a type of endothelium once thought to be phagocytic.

Lit·tré's glands (lee·trey') URETHRAL GLANDS.

live-born, *adj.* Born in such a state that acts of life are manifested after the extrusion of the whole body.

li·ve·do (li·vee'do) *n.* A mottled discoloration of the skin.

livedo re·tic·u·la·ris (re·tick''yoo·lair'is). CUTIS MARMORATA.

liv·er, *n.* The largest glandular organ in the body, situated directly beneath the diaphragm mainly on the right side of the abdominal cavity. It is encapsulated and consists of two principal lobes: a larger right and a smaller left. Its specific functions are many and include secretion of bile, storage of glycogen and fat, protein breakdown, and detoxification. It receives nutrients and oxygen for cellular metabolism via the hepatic portal circulatory system. The gall bladder lies within the cystic fossa, a depression on its inferior surface. Comb. form *hepat(o)-.*

liver breath. FETOR HEPATICUS.

liver failure. Severe inability of the liver to carry out its normal functions or the demands made upon it, as evidenced by such clinical phenomena as severe jaundice, disturbed mental functioning including coma, and abnormal levels of blood ammonia, bilirubin, alkaline phosphatase, glutamic oxaloacetic transaminase, lactic dehydrogenase, and reversal of the albumin/globulin ratio.

liver flap. ASTERIXIS.

liver fluke. A trematode that lodges in the intrahepatic biliary passages, most frequently *Clonorchis sinensis,* rarely *Fasciola hepatica.*

liv·id (liv'id) *adj.* Of a pale lead color; black and blue; discolored, as flesh from contusion or from hyperemia. **—li·vid·i·ty** (li·vid'i·tee) *n.*

li·vor (lye'vor, ·vur) *n.* 1. LIVIDITY. 2. LIVOR MORTIS.

livor mor·tis (mor'tis). Mottled purple-red discoloration of the dependent parts of the body after death, related to pooling of blood in those regions. Syn. *cadaveric lividity.*

L.M.A. Abbreviation for *left mentoanterior* position of the fetus.

L.M.P. Abbreviation for *left mentoposterior* position of the fetus.

L.O.A. Abbreviation for *left occipitoanterior* position of the fetus.

Loa (lo'uh) *n.* A genus of filarial worms.

load, *n. & v.* 1. A supported mass, weight, or force. 2. Something given to a patient to test a physiologic process. 3. To place a weight or physical stress on something. 4. To stress a process or to weight a test or experimental situation in order to observe or to influence the outcome.

loading test. *In medicine,* the administration of a substance to a patient to test his capacity for handling that substance, as the administration of phenylalanine to carriers of phenylketonuria, or of xylose for the detection of intestinal malabsorption.

Loa loa. A species of filaria that invades human subcutaneous tissues; the eye worm.

lo·bar (lo'bur, bahr) *adj.* Of or pertaining to a lobe.

lobar bronchus. Any bronchus which originates in a primary bronchus and through its branches, the segmental bronchi, ventilates a lobe of a lung; the right superior, right middle, right lower, left superior, or left lower.

lobar pneumonia. Pneumonia involving one or more lobes of the lung, usually pneumococcal pneumonia; characterized by abrupt onset with chill, fever, pleuritic pain, cough, and dyspnea. The pathologic changes are of hyperemia, hepatization, and finally, resolution.

lobar sclerosis. Gliosis and atrophy of a lobe of the cerebrum, resulting in mental and neurologic deficits; applied particularly to the hardening and shrinkage seen in the brains of infants and children who suffered prolonged intrauterine or neonatal hypoxia.

lo·bate (lo'bate) *adj.* Arranged in lobes.

lobe, *n.* 1. A more or less rounded part or projection of an organ, separated from neighboring parts by fissures and constrictions. 2. A division or part of a tooth formed from a separate point of the beginning of calcification.

lo·bec·to·my (lo·beck'tuh·mee) *n.* Excision of a lobe of an organ or gland; specifically, the excision of a lobe of the lung or a frontal or temporal lobe of the brain.

lo·be·lia (lo·bee'lee·uh, lo·beel'yuh) *n.* The leaves and tops of *Lobelia inflata;* contains several alkaloids including lobeline. It has been used as an expectorant.

lo·be·line (lo'be·leen, ·lin, lo·bee') *n.* 1. A mixture of alkaloids obtained from lobelia; these have been separated into alpha-, beta-, and gamma-forms. 2. Alpha-lobeline, $C_{22}H_{27}NO_2$, an alkaloid from lobelia having emetic, respiratory, and vasomotor actions similar to those of nicotine.

lo·bot·o·my (lo·bot'uh·mee) *n.* Surgical sectioning of brain tissue, particularly of the frontal lobe for the relief of mental disorders.

Lob·stein's disease (lohp'shtine) OSTEOGENESIS IMPERFECTA.

lobster-claw deformity. BIDACTYLY.

lobular carcinoma. A form of breast cancer.

lobular pneumonia. BRONCHOPNEUMONIA.

lob·ule (lob'yool) *n.* A small lobe or a subdivision of a lobe. —**lob·u·lar** (lob'yoo·lur), **lob·u·lat·ed** (lob'yoo·lay·tid) *adj.*

lobuli. Plural of *lobulus.*

lob·u·lus (lob'yoo·lus) *n.,* pl. **lobu·li** (·lye) [NA]. LOBULE.

lobulus an·si·for·mis (an"si·for'mis). ANSIFORM LOBULE.

lo·cal (lo'kul) *adj.* Limited to a part or place; not general.

local anaphylaxis. A reaction at the site of injections, dependent upon the union in the tissues of the circulating precipitin and its specific antigen, as edema, induration, and necrosis caused by repeated subcutaneous injections of horse serum into rabbits.

local anesthesia. Anesthesia produced in a local area usually by infiltration technique.

local asphyxia. Stagnation or diminution of the circulation in a part, as the fingers, hands, toes, or feet; often used in reference to Raynaud's disease.

local immunity. Immunity confined to a given tissue or area of the body. Syn. *tissue immunity.*

lo·cal·iza·tion (lo"kul·i·zay'shun) *n.* 1. The determination of the site of a lesion or process. 2. The limitation or restriction of a process to a circumscribed place. —**lo·cal·ize** (lo'kul·ize) *v.*

lo·cal·ized (lo'kul·ize'd) *adj.* Confined to a particular situation or place.

localized pericarditis. A form of pericarditis characterized by localized white areas, the so-called milk spots.

lo·cal·iz·er (lo'kul·eye"zur) *n.* An instrument used in roentgenographic examination of the eye for localizing opaque foreign bodies.

local Shwartzman phenomenon. SHWARTZMAN PHENOMENON (1).

lo·chia (lo'kee·uh, lock'ee·uh) *n.* The discharge from the uterus and vagina during the first few weeks after labor. —**lo·chi·al** (lo'kee·ul, lock'ee·ul) *adj.*

lochia al·ba (al'buh). The whitish or yellowish flow that takes place after the seventh day after labor.

lochia cru·en·ta (kroo·en'tuh). The sanguineous flow of the first few days after labor. Syn. *lochia rubra.*

lochia ru·bra (roo'bruh). LOCHIA CRUENTA.

lochia se·ro·sa (se·ro'suh). The serous discharge taking place about the fifth day after labor.

lo·chio·col·pos (lo"kee·o·kol'pos) *n.* Distention of the vagina by retained lochia.

lo·chio·cyte (lo'kee·o·site) *n.* A decidual cell found in the lochia.

lo·chio·me·tra (lo"kee·o·mee'truh) *n.* A retention of lochia in the uterus.

lo·chio·me·tri·tis (lo"kee·o·me·trye'tis) *n.* PUERPERAL METRITIS.

lo·chi·or·rhea, lo·chi·or·rhoea (lo"kee·o·ree'uh) *n.* An abnormal flow of the lochia.

lo·chi·os·che·sis (lo"kee·os'ke·sis) *n.* Suppression or retention of the lochia.

lo·cho·me·tri·tis (lo"ko·me·trye'tis, lock"o·) *n.* PUERPERAL METRITIS.

locked bite. Interdigitation of the teeth in such a manner that normal excursions of the mandible are restricted or prevented while the teeth are in occlusion.

lock finger. A peculiar affection of the fingers in which they suddenly become fixed in a flexed position, due to the presence of a fibrous constriction of the tendon sheath or a nodular enlargement in the tendon.

lock·jaw, *n.* TRISMUS.

lo·co disease (lo'ko) A poisoning produced in livestock by eating plants which take up selenium from the soil; the symptoms of the disease are loss of flesh, disordered vision, delirium, convulsive movements, and stupor, often terminating fatally.

lo·co·mo·tion (lo"kuh·mo'shun) *n.* The act of moving from place to place. —**locomo·tive** (·tiv), **locomo·tor** (·tur) *adj.*

locomotor ataxia. TABES DORSALIS.

loco weed. Those species of *Astragalus* which contain selenium.

loc·u·la·tion (lock"yoo·lay'shun) *n.* The formation of loculi in tissue. —**loc·u·lat·ed** (lock'yoo-lay·tid), *adj.*

loc·u·lus (lock'yoo·lus) *n.*, pl. **locu·li** (·lye) A small space or compartment. —**locu·lar** (·lur), **locu·late** (·late) *adj.*

lo·cum te·nens (lo'kum ten'enz) A physician who temporarily acts as a substitute for another physician.

lo·cus (lo'kus) *n.*, pl. **lo·ci** (·sigh) 1. Place, site. 2. *In genetics*, the position on a chromosome occupied by a particular gene.

Loeffler's disease Fibroplastic parietal endocarditis, characterized by progressive congestive heart failure, eosinophilia, and multiple embolic systemic infarct.

Loeffler's pneumonia or **eosinophilia** LOEFFLER'S SYNDROME.

Loeffler's syndrome Transient pulmonary infiltration by eosinophils associated with peripheral blood eosinophilia and minimal or no symptoms; sometimes associated with parasitic infections in which their lodging in the lungs causes inflammatory reactions. Syn. *eosinophilic pneumonitis.*

log-, logo- A combining form meaning (a) *word, speech;* (b) *thought, reason.*

-logia A combining form meaning (a) *a condition involving the faculty of speech or of reasoning;* (b) *-logy, a field of study.*

logo·ma·nia (log"o·may'nee·uh) *n.* Logorrhea so excessive as to be a form of a manic state; new words may be invented to keep up the garrulity.

log·op·a·thy (log·op'uth·ee) *n.* Any disorder of speech.

logo·pe·dics, logo·pae·dics (log"o·pee'dicks) *n.* The study, knowledge, and treatment of defective speech.

log·or·rhea, log·or·rhoea (log"o·ree'uh) *n.* Excessive, uncontrollable, or abnormal talkativeness or loquacity; may be exceedingly rapid and even incoherent.

-logy A combining form meaning (a) *a field of study;* (b) *discourse, treatise.*

lo·i·a·sis (lo·eye'uh·sis) *n.*, pl. **loia·ses** (·seez) A filariasis of tropical Africa, caused by the filaria *Loa*, acquired from bites by *Chrysops dimidiata* and *C. silacea*, and characterized by diurnal periodicity of microfilariae in the blood and transient cutaneous swelling caused by migrating adult worms. The eye may be involved.

loin, *n.* The lateral and posterior region of the body between the false ribs and the iliac crest.

lol·ism (lol'iz·um, lo'liz·um) *n.* Poisoning by the seeds of *Lolium temulentum* (darnel ryegrass).

Lomotil. Trademark for diphenoxylate hydrochloride with atropine sulfate, an antidiarrheal drug combination.

long-acting thyroid stimulator. A circulating gamma globulin whose action resembles that of thyroid-stimulating hormone of the pituitary, found in the serum of some patients with Grave's disease, occasionally in exophthalmos without other evidence of Grave's disease, and in pretibial myxedema. It is probably produced by lymphocytes and may represent an autoantibody to a thyroid antigen. Abbreviated, LATS.

long bone. A bone in which the length markedly exceeds the width.

lon·gev·i·ty (lon·jev'i·tee) *n.* Long life; length of life.

lon·gi·ma·nous (lon"ji·may'nus, ·man'us, lon·jim'uh·nus) *adj.* Long-handed.

lon·gi·ped·ate (lon"ji·ped'ate, ·pee'date) *adj.* Long-footed.

lon·gis·si·mus (lon·jis'i·mus) *adj. & n.* 1. Longest; applied to muscles, as longissimus thoracis. 2. The middle part of the erector spinae muscle.

lon·gi·tu·di·nal (lon"ji·tew'di·nul) *adj.* 1. Lengthwise; in the direction of the long axis of a body. 2. Over a protracted period of time, as of a study of population growth.

longitudinal arch of the foot. The anteroposterior arch formed by the tarsal and metatarsal bones, consisting of the inner, or medial, longitudinal arch formed by the calcaneus, the talus, the navicular, three cuneiform bones, and the first three metatarsals, and the outer, or lateral, longitudinal arch formed by the calcaneus, the cuboid, and the fourth and fifth metatarsals.

longitudinal duct of the epoophoron. DUCTUS EPOOPHORI LONGITUDINALIS.

longitudinal fissure of the cerebrum. The deep fissure that divides the cerebrum into two hemispheres. Syn. *interhemispheric fissure.*

lon·gi·tu·di·na·lis (lon"ji·tew'di·nay'lis) *n.* Either of the longitudinal intrinsic muscles of the tongue: the inferior or the superior.

long-term care. Medical care providing symptomatic treatment or maintenance and rehabilitative services for patients of all age groups in a variety of settings.

long-term memory. 1. Memory store in which the rate of loss is relatively low and where information is held without active rehearsal. Syn. *secondary memory.* 2. Generally, anything retained for more than a very brief period of time, from minutes to years, sometimes thought of as a person's total store of knowledge.

lon·gus (long'gus) *adj. & n.* 1. Long. 2. A long muscle.

loop, *n.* 1. A bend in a cord or cordlike structure. 2. A platinum wire, in a handle, with its extremity bent in a circular form; used to transfer bacterial cultures.

loop of Henle The U-shaped section of a uriniferous tubule which is formed by a descending and an ascending limb.

L.O.P. Abbreviation for *left occipitoposterior* position of the fetus in utero.

loph·o·dont (lof′o·dont, lo′fo·) *adj.* Having the crowns of the molar teeth formed in crests or ridges.

lo·phot·ri·chous (lo·fot′ri·kus) *adj.* Pertaining to microorganisms characterized by a tuft of cilia or flagella at each pole.

lo·quac·i·ty (lo·kwas′i·tee) *n.* Volubility of speech; talkativeness; a condition frequently excessive in various mental disorders.

Lo·rain-Lé·vi syndrome (loh·ræn′, ley·vee′) PITUITARY DWARFISM.

lor·do·sis (lor·do′sis) *n.*, pl. **lordo·ses** (-seez) Forward curvature of the lumbar spine; spinal curvature in the sagittal plane which is concave to the dorsal aspect. —**lor·dot·ic** (-dot′ick) *adj.*

L organisms. Forms derived from various bacteria which may or may not revert to the parent strains, occurring spontaneously or favored by penicillin and other agents, pleomorphic, lacking cell walls, and growing in minute colonies.

Loridine. Trademark for the antibiotic substance cephaloridine.

lo·tio (lo′shee·o, lo′tee·o) *n.* LOTION.

lo·tion (lo′shun) *n.* Any of a class of liquid medicinal preparations, either suspensions or dispersions, intended for local application.

loupe (loop) *n.* A magnifying lens.

loup·ing ill (læwp′ing, lo′ping) An enzootic and sometimes epizootic disease of sheep; a form of encephalomyelitis caused by a group B encephalitis virus and transmitted by the tick *Ixodes ricinus.* The virus is infectious also for monkeys, mice, horses, and cattle. Infected animals display ataxia. Syn. *ovine encephalomyelitis, trembling ill.*

louse (læwce) *n.*, pl. **lice.** A small, wingless, dorsoventrally flattened insect which lacks true metamorphosis. An ectoparasite of birds and mammals, it is medically important as a vector of disease and as a producer of irritating dermatitis.

louse-borne typhus. EPIDEMIC TYPHUS.

lousy (læwz′ee) *adj.* Infested with lice. —**lous·i·ness,** *n.*

love object. 1. Any person or object that regularly excites or receives a person's affection or love. 2. *In psychoanalysis,* the person or object with which libido is concerned, and which stimulates the instinctual activity generated by it. Syn. *libidinal object.*

lower brachial plexus paralysis. Weakness of the small hand muscles and flexors of the wrist resulting in claw hand, and ulnar-type sensory loss, due to injury to the eighth cervical and first thoracic roots or the lower trunk of the brachial plexus; usually caused by birth injury; the prognosis is favorable. Syn. *Klumpke's paralysis.*

lower extremity. In human anatomy, the ex-

tremity comprising the hip, thigh, leg, ankle, and foot.

lower motor neuron. An efferent neuron which has its cell body located in the anterior gray column of the spinal cord or in the brainstem nuclei and its axon passing by way of a peripheral nerve to skeletal muscle. Syn. *final common pathway.*

lower motor neuron disease, lesion, or **paralysis.** An injury to the cell bodies or axons of lower motor neurons, characterized by flaccid paralysis of the muscle(s), diminished or absent reflexes, absence of pathological reflexes, reaction of degeneration (about two weeks after injury), and progressive muscle atrophy.

lower nephron nephrosis or **syndrome.** ACUTE TUBULAR NECROSIS.

lower uterine segment. The isthmus of the uterus which expands as pregnancy progresses, and whose muscle fibers are stretched passively during labor, together with the cervix, allowing the upper uterine musculature to retract and thus to expel the fetus.

low forceps. An obstetric forceps applied to the fetal head when it is well within the lower portion of the pelvic canal.

low myopia. Myopia of less than 2 diopters.

low-salt syndrome. A clinical syndrome characterized by a low serum sodium concentration, occurring acutely in heat exhaustion or water intoxication; and chronically in cardiac or renal disease, especially with prolonged restriction of sodium chloride intake and diuretic therapy. There are postural hypotension, tachycardia, nausea, vomiting, drowsiness, muscle cramps, azotemia, oliguria, convulsions, and coma.

low-tension pulse. A pulse sudden in its onset, short, and quickly declining. It is easily obliterated by pressure.

lox·ia (lock′see·uh) *n.* TORTICOLLIS.

Lox·os·ce·les (lock·sos′e·leez) *n.* A genus of spiders that includes the poisonous brown recluse, *Loxosceles reclusa,* of south central United States, and the larger *L. laeta* of South America, both of which are often found in human dwellings.

lox·os·ce·lism (lock·sos′e·liz·um) *n.* The clinical state resulting from the bite of the brown recluse spider, which includes pain and vesiculation at the bite site, ischemic changes in the affected area, and systemic complaints.

lox·ot·ic (lock·sot′ick) *adj.* Slanting; twisted.

loz·enge (loz′inj) *n.* A solid dosage form containing one or more medicinal agents and, usually, flavor, sugar, and a demulcent substance, for therapeutic application in the throat and bronchial area.

LPN Abbreviation for *licensed practical nurse.*

L. R. C. S. Licentiate of the Royal College of Surgeons.

L. R. C. S. E. Licentiate of the Royal College of Surgeons of Edinburgh.

L. R. C. S. I. Licentiate of the Royal College of Surgeons of Ireland.

L. R. F. P. S. Licentiate of the Royal Faculty of Physicians and Surgeons.

L. S. A. 1. Abbreviation for *left sacroanterior*

position of the fetus. 2. Licentiate of the Society of Apothecaries.

LSD Abbreviation for *lysergic acid diethylamide.*

L. S. P. Abbreviation for *left sacroposterior* position of the fetus.

Lu Symbol for *lutetium.*

lu·cent (lew'sunt) *adj.* 1. Luminous. 2. Translucent; readily transmitting rays, as x-rays. —**lu·cen·cy** (lew'sun·see) *n.*

lucid interval. *In neurology* and *psychiatry,* a transitory return of the normal state of consciousness following the initial loss of consciousness, sometimes observed in cerebral trauma, particularly in cases of temporal or parietal fracture with rupture of the middle meningeal artery and epidural hematoma.

lu·cif·er·ase (lew·sif'ur·ace, ·aze) *n.* An oxidative enzyme that catalyzes the reaction between oxygen and luciferin to produce luminescence.

lu·cif·er·in (lew·sif'ur·in) *n.* An organic substrate found in luminescent organisms which when oxidized in the presence of the enzyme luciferase emits light, as in fireflies and glow-worms.

lu·cif·u·gal (lew·sif'yoo·gul) *adj.* Fleeing from, or avoiding, light.

Lu·cio leprosy or **phenomenon** (loo'syo) An unusual form of severe lepromatous leprosy occurring in Mexico and in Central and South America, characterized by diffuse cutaneous infiltration, later with vesiculation, ulceration, and necrosis, and with necrotizing lesions of blood vessels.

Lück·en·schä·del (lick'un·shay"dul, Ger. lu^ek'^en·she^y·d^el) *n.* CRANIOLACUNIA.

Lud·wig's angina (loot'vi^kh) A indurated cellulitis of the submandibular space, often rapidly progressive, and usually caused by hemolytic streptococci.

Luer syringe A glass syringe for intravenous and hypodermic injections with a mechanism to attach the needle securely.

lu·es (lew'eez) *n.* SYPHILIS. —**lu·et·ic** (lew·et'ick) *adj.*

lu·e·tin (lew'e·tin) *n.* An extract of killed cultures of several strains of the *Treponema pallidum;* once used in skin tests for syphilis.

Lu·gol's solution (lu^e·goh'l') STRONG IODINE SOLUTION.

luke·warm (lewk"wawrm') *adj.* Tepid; about the temperature of the body, approximately 37°C.

lum·ba·go (lum·bay'go) *n.* 1. Backache in the lumbar or lumbosacral region. 2. AZOTURIA (2).

lum·bar (lum'bur, ·bahr) *adj.* Pertaining to the loins.

lumbar enlargement. Broadening of the spinal cord starting at the level of the ninth and maximal at the level of the twelfth thoracic vertebra. Syn. *lumbar intumescence.*

lum·bar·i·za·tion (lum"bur·i·zay'shun) *n.* A condition in which the first segment of the sacrum is partially or completely separate from the remainder of the sacrum.

lumbar puncture. Puncture of the spinal canal, in the subarachnoid space usually between the third and fourth lumbar vertebrae, for the removal of cerebrospinal fluid, especially for

diagnostic purposes, or for the introduction of medication. Syn. *spinal tap.*

lumbar vertebrae. The five vertebrae associated with the lower part of the back.

lum·bo·co·los·to·my (lum"bo·ko·los'tuh·mee) *n.* Colostomy in the left lumbar region.

lum·bo·cos·tal (lum"bo·kos'tul) *adj.* Pertaining to the loins and ribs, as lumbocostal arch.

lum·bo·dor·sal (lum"bo·dor'sul) *adj.* Pertaining to the lumbar region of the back.

lum·bo·in·gui·nal (lum"bo·ing'gwi·nul) *adj.* Pertaining to the lumbar and inguinal regions.

lum·bo·is·chi·al (lum"bo·is'kee·ul) *adj.* Pertaining to the ischium and the lumbar part of the vertebral column.

lum·bo·sa·cral (lum"bo·say'krul) *adj.* Pertaining to the lumbar vertebrae and to the sacrum.

lum·bo·ver·te·bral (lum"bo·vur'te·brul) *adj.* Pertaining to the lumbar region and the vertebrae.

lum·bri·cal (lum'bri·kul) *adj.* & *n.* 1. Pertaining to, or resembling, an earthworm or *Lumbricus.* 2. Any of four small muscles in the hand and foot.

lu·men (lew'min) *n.,* pl. **lu·mi·na** (·mi·nuh), **lumens** 1. The space inside of a tube, as the lumen of a thermometer, blood vessel, or duct. 2. The unit of flux of light: the flux in a unit of solid angle from a source having a uniform luminous intensity of one candela.

lu·mi·nal, lu·me·nal (lew'mi·nul) *adj.* Of or pertaining to a lumen (1).

Luminal. A trademark for phenobarbital, a sedative and hypnotic.

lu·mi·nance (lew'mi·nunce) *n.* The amount of light emitted from a source and projected on a measuring surface; also called brightness, although, technically, brightness is a subjective quality of light as measured by the eye.

lu·mi·nes·cence (lew"mi·nes'unce) *n.* An emission of light without a production of heat sufficient to cause incandescence. It is encountered in certain animals, as some protozoa and fireflies.

lu·mis·ter·ol (lew·mis'tur·ol) *n.* The first product obtained in the irradiation of ergosterol with ultraviolet light; further irradiation produces calciferol (vitamin D_2).

lump, *n.* 1. A small mass; a protuberant part. 2. Any localized swelling or tumor.

lu·na·cy (lew'nuh·see) *n. In legal medicine,* mental disorder in which the individual is not legally responsible; insanity.

lu·nar (lew'nar) *adj.* 1. Pertaining to the moon. 2. Pertaining to silver (*luna* of the alchemists).

lu·nate (lew'nate) *n.* One of the carpal bones.

lu·na·tic (lew'nuh·tick) *n.* A psychotic person.

lu·na·to·ma·la·cia (lew"nuh·to·ma·lay'shuh) *n.* KIENBÖCK'S DISEASE.

lu·nel·la (lew·nel'uh) *n.* HYPOPYON.

lung, *n.* The organ of respiration, in which venous blood is relieved of carbon dioxide and oxygenated by air drawn through the trachea and bronchi into the alveoli. There are two lungs, a right and a left, the former consisting of three, the latter of two, lobes. The lungs are situated in the thoracic cavity, and are enveloped by the pleura.

lung fluke. PARAGONIMUS WESTERMANI.

lu·nu·la (loo'new·luh) *n.*, pl. **lunu·lae** (·lee) [NA]. 1. The white, semilunar area of a nail near the root. 2. The thin, crescentic area of a semilunar valve of the heart, on either side of the nodule.

lu·pine (lew'pin, ·pine, ·peen) *n.* A plant of the genus *Lupinus*. One or more poisonous alkaloids have been found in various species of the genus. The bruised seeds of *L. albus* have been used as an external application to ulcers.

lu·poid (lew'poid) *adj.* Resembling lupus.

lu·pus (lew'pus) *n.* 1. LUPUS ERYTHEMATOSUS. 2. Any chronic progressive ulcerative skin lesion. 3. LUPUS VULGARIS.

lupus er·y·the·ma·to·sus (err''i·theem''uh·to'sus, ·them'). A disease of unknown causation and variable manifestations, ranging from a skin disorder (discoid lupus erythematosus) to a generalized disorder involving the skin and viscera (systemic lupus erythematosus).

lupus erythematosus body. A mass of altered nuclear material found in a lupus erythematosus cell.

lupus erythematosus cell. A polymorphonuclear leukocyte which has ingested nuclear material from another cell which has been denatured in a specific way by the action of a substance occurring in the blood and body fluids of patients with systemic lupus erythematosus and, occasionally, other diseases. Syn. *L.E. cell.*

lupus per·nio (pur'nee·o). SARCOIDOSIS.

lupus vul·gar·is (vul·gair'is). True tuberculosis of the skin; a slow-developing, scarring, and deforming disease, often asymptomatic, often involving the face, and occurring in a wide variety of appearances. Syn. *tuberculosis luposa.*

Lusch·ka's bursa (loosh'kah) PHARYNGEAL BURSA.

Luschka's glands or **ducts** Aberrant bile ducts in the wall of the gallbladder.

lute, *n.* A pasty substance which hardens when dry; used sometimes to make joints waterproof in laboratory apparatus.

lu·te·al (lew'tee·ul) *adj.* Of or pertaining to the corpus luteum or its principle.

lu·te·in (lew'tee·in) *n.* 1. A yellow dihydroxy-α-carotene, $C_{40}H_{56}O_2$, first isolated from egg yolk, but widely distributed in nature. Syn. *xanthophyll.* 2. A dried, powdered preparation of corpus luteum.

lu·tein·iza·tion (lew''tee·in·i·zay'shun) *n.* The acquisition by ovarian follicle cells of the characteristics of lutein cells following release of the ovum they surround.

luteinizing hormone. An adenohypophyseal hormone which stimulates both epithelial and interstitial cells in the ovary, where together with the follicle-stimulating hormone it induces follicular maturation and formation of corpora lutea. In the male, where it acts only on the interstitial cells of the testis, it is more appropriately called interstitial cell-stimulating hormone (ICSH). Abbreviated, L.H. Syn. *corpus luteum-stimulating hormone, metakentrin, pituitary B gonadotropin.*

Lutembacher's syndrome. An atrial septal defect associated with congenital mitral stenosis.

lu·te·o·ma (lew''tee·o'muh) *n.*, pl. **luteomas, luteoma·ta** (·tuh) An ovarian tumor made up of cells resembling those of the corpus luteum. Syn. *luteinized granulosa-cell carcinoma, lutenoma, luteinoma, luteoblastoma, struma ovarii luteinocellulare, lipid-cell tumor of the ovary.*

luteotropic hormone. PROLACTIN. Abbreviated, LTH.

lux (lucks) *n.*, pl. **lux, luxes** A unit of illumination equivalent to one lumen per square meter.

lux·a·tion (luck·say'shun) *n.* 1. A dislocation, especially a complete dislocation of a joint. 2. The partial or complete separation of a tooth from its socket by mechanical force.

lux·u·ri·ant (lug·zhoor'ee·unt) *adj.* Growing to excess, exuberant; specifically referring to the abnormal growth of certain body cells, as in granulation tissue.

LVH Left ventricular hypertrophy.

ly·can·thro·py (lye·kan'thruh·pee) *n.* The delusion of being a wolf or some other wild beast, seen in schizophrenic patients. **—ly·can·throp·ic** (lye'kan·throp'ick) *adj.;* **ly·can·thrope** (lye'kun·thrope) *n.*

ly·co·per·don·o·sis (lye''ko·pur''dun·o'sis) *n.* A respiratory disease caused by inhalation of large quantities of spores from the mature puffball mushroom, *Lycoperdon.*

Lycopodium, *n.* The large type genus of the evergreen plant family Lycopodiaceae. *Lycopodium saururus* is the source of the alkaloids sauroxine and saururine; the spores of *Lycopodium clavatum* (lycopodium) have various uses.

ly·co·rex·ia (lye''ko·reck'see·uh) *n.* A wolfish or ravenous appetite.

lye, *n.* 1. An alkaline solution obtained by leaching wood ashes. 2. A solution of sodium or potassium hydroxide.

ly·go·phil·ia (lye''go·fil'ee·uh) *n.* Morbid love of dark places.

ly·ing-in. 1. PARTURITION. 2. PUERPERIUM (1).

Lyme arthritis. An acute, transient, epidemic form of arthritis, accompanied by fever and a skin lesion resembling an insect bite; presumably due to a transmissible, possibly arthropod-borne agent which has not been identified. It has been observed near Lyme, Connecticut beginning in 1974.

lymph·ad·e·nec·to·my (lim·fad''e·neck'tuh·mee) *n.* Excision of a lymph node.

lymph·ad·e·ni·tis (lim·fad''e·nigh'tis) *n.* Inflammation of the lymph nodes.

lymph·ad·e·noid (lim·fad'e·noid) *adj.* Resembling a lymph node.

lymphadenoid goiter. STRUMA LYMPHOMATOSA.

lymph·ad·e·no·ma (lim·fad''e·no'muh) *n.*, pl. **lymphadenomas, lymphadenoma·ta** (·tuh) Tumorlike enlargement of a lymph node; it probably exists in two forms, the neoplastic and the hyperplastic.

lymph·ad·e·no·ma·to·sis (lim·fad''e·no''muh·to'sis) *n.* A malignant lymphoma.

lymph·ad·e·nop·a·thy (lim·fad''e·nop'uth·ee) *n.* 1. Lymph node enlargement in response to any disease. 2. Any disease of the lymph nodes.

lymph·ad·e·no·sis (lim·fad″e·no′sis) *n.*, pl. **lymphadeno·ses** (·seez) Hyperplasia or neoplasia affecting the lymph nodes.

lym·pha·gogue (lim′fuh·gog) *n.* An agent that stimulates the flow of lymph.

lym·phan·gi·ec·ta·sia (lim·fan″jee·eck·tay′zhuh, ·zee·uh) *n.* LYMPHANGIECTASIS.

lym·phan·gi·ec·ta·sis (lim·fan″jee·eck′tuh·sis) *n.* Dilatation of the lymphatic vessels. —**lym·phangi·ec·tat·ic** (·eck·tat′ick) *adj.*

lym·phan·gi·ec·to·my (lim·fan″jee·eck′tuh·mee) *n.* Excision of a pathologic lymphatic channel, as in surgery for cancer.

lym·phan·gio·en·do·the·li·o·ma (lim·fan″jee·o·en″do·theel·ee·o′muh) *n.* A tumor composed of a congeries of lymphatic vessels, between which are many large mononuclear cells presumed to be endothelial cells.

lym·phan·gio·fi·bro·ma (lim·fan″jee·o·figh·bro′muh) *n.* A benign tumor whose parenchyma contains both lymphangiomatous and fibromatous elements.

lym·phan·gio·gram (lim·fan″jee·o·gram) *n.* A radiographic representation of lymph nodes and lymph vessels produced by lymphangiography.

lym·phan·gi·og·ra·phy (lim·fan″jee·og′ruh·fee) *n.* The process of radiographic visualization of lymph channels and lymph nodes by injection of radiopaque contrast media into afferent lymphatic channels.

lym·phan·gi·o·ma (lim·fan″jee·o′muh) *n.*, pl. **lymphangiomas, lymphangioma·ta** (·tuh) A benign, abnormal collection of lymphatic vessels forming a mass. Syn. *simple lymphangioma.*

lym·phan·gio·plas·ty (lim·fan″jee·o·plas′tee, lim·fan″jee·o·plas′tee) *n.* Replacement of lymphatics by artificial channels.

lym·phan·gio·sar·co·ma (lim·fan″jee·o·sahr·ko′muh) *n.* A sarcoma whose parenchymal cells form vascular channels resembling lymphatics; often associated with preexisting lymphedema.

lym·phan·gi·tis (lim″fan·jye′tis) *n.*, pl. **lymphan·git·i·des** (·jit′i·deez) Inflammation of a lymphatic vessel or vessels. —**lymphan·git·ic** (·jit′ick) *adj.*

lym·phat·ic (lim·fat′ick) *adj. & n.* 1. Pertaining to lymph. 2. A vessel conveying lymph.

lymphatic leukemia. LYMPHOCYTIC LEUKEMIA.

lym·phat·i·cos·to·my (lim·fat″i·cos′tuh·mee) *n.* Formation of an opening into a lymphatic trunk, as the thoracic duct.

lymphatic tissue. Tissue consisting of networks of reticular and collagenous fibers and lymphocytes.

lym·pha·to·cele (lim·fat′o·seel) *n.* LYMPHANGIOMA.

lymph·ede·ma, lymph·oe·de·ma (lim″fe·dee′muh) *n.* Edema due to obstruction of lymph vessels.

lymph nodes. Masses of lymphatic tissue 1 to 25 mm long, often bean-shaped, intercalated in the course of lymph vessels, more or less well organized by a connective-tissue capsule and trabeculae into cortical nodules and medul-

lary cords which form lymphocytes, and into lymph sinuses through which lymph filters, permitting phagocytic activity of reticular cells and macrophages. Syn. *lymph glands.*

lymph nodule. A small mass of dense lymphatic tissue in which new lymphocytes are formed.

lym·pho·blast (lim′fo·blast) *n.* A blast cell, considered a precursor or early form of a lymphocyte. —**lym·pho·blas·tic** (lim′fo·blas′tick) *adj.*

lymphoblastic leukemia. A form of lymphocytic leukemia in which the cells are poorly differentiated but recognizably of the lymphocytic series; associated with an acute course, if untreated.

lym·pho·blas·to·ma (lim″fo·blas·to′muh) *n.* A type of malignant lymphoma whose parenchyma is composed of lymphoblasts.

lym·pho·blas·to·sis (lim″fo·blas·to′sis) *n.* An excessive number of lymphoblasts in peripheral blood; occasionally found also in tissues.

lym·pho·cyte (lim′fo·site) *n.* A leukocyte found in the lymphoid tissue, blood, and lymph, characterized by a round, centrally located nucleus, cytoplasm showing various degrees of basophilia due to the presence of free ribosomes, and a lack of specific granules. Two major classes, B and T lymphocytes, are active in the immune response. —**lym·pho·cyt·ic** (lim″fo·sit′ick) *adj.*

lymphocytic choriomeningitis. An acute viral meningitis due to a specific virus endemic in mice; characterized clinically by the syndrome of aseptic meningitis, and a short, benign course with usual recovery.

lymphocytic leukemia. A form of leukemia, acute or chronic, in which the predominating cell type belongs to the lymphocytic series. Syn. *lymphoid leukemia, lymphogenous leukemia.*

lym·pho·cy·toid (lim″fo·sigh′toid) *adj.* Resembling a lymphocyte.

lym·pho·cy·to·ma (lim″fo·sigh·to′muh) *n.*, pl. **lymphocytomas, lymphocytoma·ta** (·tuh) A type of malignant lymphoma in which the predominant cell type closely resembles mature lymphocytes. Syn. *pseudolymphoma.*

lymphocytoma cu·tis (kew′tis). A benign collection of lymphocytes, with or without germinal centers, in the dermis. Syn. *Spiegler-Fendt sarcoid, lymphadenosis benigna cutis.*

lym·pho·cy·to·pe·nia (lim″fo·sigh″to·pee′nee·uh) *n.* Reduction of the absolute number of lymphocytes per unit volume of peripheral blood. Syn. *lymphopenia.*

lym·pho·cy·toph·thi·sis (lim″fo·sigh·tof′thi·sis) *n.* SWISS TYPE AGAMMAGLOBULINEMIA.

lym·pho·cy·to·poi·e·sis (lim″fo·sigh″to·poy·ee′sis) *n.*, pl. **lymphocytopoie·ses** (·seez) The genesis of lymphocytes.

lym·pho·cy·to·sis (lim″fo·sigh·to′sis) *n.*, pl. **lymphocyto·ses** (·seez) An abnormally large number of lymphocytes in peripheral blood.

lym·pho·ep·i·the·li·o·ma (lim″fo·ep″i·theel·ee·o′muh) *n.* A poorly differentiated squamous cell carcinoma of the nasopharynx whose parenchymal cells resemble elements of the reticuloendothelial system. —**lymphoepithelioma·tous** (·tus) *adj.*

lym·pho·gen·ic (lim-fo-jen'ick) *adj.* LYMPHOGENOUS.

lym·phog·e·nous (lim-foj'e·nus) *adj.* 1. Producing lymph. 2. Produced or spread in the lymphatic system.

lym·pho·gran·u·lo·ma (lim″fo-gran″yoo·lo'muh) *n.*, pl. **lymphogranulomas, lymphogranuloma·ta** (·tuh) HODGKIN'S DISEASE.

lym·pho·gran·u·lo·ma·to·sis (lim″fo-gran-yoo·lo″muh·to'sis) *n.*, pl. **lymphogranulomato·ses** (·seez) HODGKIN'S DISEASE.

lymphogranuloma ve·ne·re·um (ve·neer'ee·um). A systemic infectious disease, due to a member of the psittacosis-lymphogranuloma group of agents, transmitted by sexual contact and characterized by genital ulceration, regional lymphadenitis, and constitutional symptoms. Abbreviated, LGV.

lym·pho·his·tio·cyt·ic (lim″fo·his″tee·o·sit'ick) *adj.* Involving both lymphocytes and histiocytes.

lym·phoid (lim'foid) *adj.* Resembling or pertaining to lymphocytes, lymph nodes, or lymph.

lym·pho·ma (lim·fo'muh) *n.*, pl. **lymphomas, lymphoma·ta** (·tuh) Any neoplasm, usually malignant, of the lymphatic tissues.

lym·pho·ma·toid (lim·fo'muh·toid) *adj.* Resembling a malignant lymphoma.

lym·pho·ma·to·sis (lim″fo·muh·to'sis) *n.*, pl. **lymphomato·ses** (·seez) 1. Involvement of multiple body sites by malignant lymphoma. 2. A disease of animals, especially chickens, characterized by widespread involvement of the viscera by malignant lymphoma.

lym·pho·mono·cy·to·sis (lim″fo·mon″o·sigh·to'sis) *n.*, pl. **lymphomonocyto·ses** (·seez) An increase in both lymphocytes and monocytes.

lym·pho·pe·nia (lim″fo·pee'nee·uh) *n.* 1. LYMPHOCYTOPENIA. 2. A reduction in the amount of lymph.

lym·pho·poi·e·sis (lim″fo·poy·ee'sis) *n.*, pl. **lymphopoie·ses** (·seez) 1. LYMPHOCYTOPOIESIS. 2. Lymph production. —**lymphopoi·et·ic** (·et′ick) *adj.*

lym·pho·pro·lif·er·a·tive (lim″fo·pro·lif'ur·uh·tiv) *adj.* Characterized by proliferation—benign, malignant, or undetermined—of lymphoid tissues.

lymphoproliferative disease or **syndrome.** Any condition featured by a lymphoproliferative response by host tissues; included are the malignant lymphomas.

lym·pho·re·tic·u·lo·sis (lim″fo·re·tick·yoo·lo'sis) *n.* 1. NODULAR LYMPHOMA. 2. Reticuloendothelial hyperplasia in lymphatic organs, especially lymph nodes.

lym·phor·rhage (lim'fuh·rij) *n.* 1. A flow of lymph from a ruptured lymphatic vessel. 2. An aggregation of lymphocytes, usually seen in muscle tissue.

lym·phor·rhea, lym·phor·rhoea (lim″fo·ree'uh) *n.* LYMPHORRHAGE (1).

lym·pho·sar·co·ma (lim″fo·sahr·ko'muh) *n.* A malignant lymphoma composed of anaplastic lymphoid cells resembling lymphocytes or lymphoblasts, according to the degree of differentiation. Syn. *lymphocytic sarcoma.*

lym·pho·sar·co·ma·to·sis (lim″fo·sahr·ko·muh·

to'sis) *n.* Diffuse involvement of various anatomic sites by lymphosarcoma.

lymph·uria (lim·few'ree·uh) *n.* The presence of lymph in the urine.

lyo·chrome (lye'o·krome) *n.* FLAVIN.

lyo·en·zyme (lye'o·en'zime) *n.* EXTRACELLULAR ENZYME.

lyo·gel (lye'o·jel) *n.* A gel rich in liquid.

lyo·phile (lye'o·file, ·fil) *adj.* Pertaining to the dispersed phase of a colloidal system when there is strong affinity between the dispersion medium and the dispersed phase.

lyo·phil·ic (lye'o·fil'ick) *adj.* LYOPHILE.

lyophilic colloid. A colloid capable of combining with, or attracting to it, the dispersion medium.

ly·oph·i·li·za·tion (lye·off″i·li·zay'shun) *n.* The process of rapidly freezing a substance (pollen, blood plasma, antitoxin, serum) at an unusually low temperature, and then quickly dehydrating the frozen mass in a high vacuum. —**ly·oph·i·lized** (lye·off'i·lize′d) *adj.*

lyo·phobe (lye'o·fobe) *adj.* Pertaining to the dispersed phase of a colloidal system when there is lack of strong affinity between the dispersed phase and the dispersion medium.

lyo·sorp·tion (lye'o·sorp'shun) *n.* The preferential adsorption of the solvent constituent of a solution or of the dispersing medium of a colloidal system.

ly·sate (lye'sate) *n.* The product of lysis.

lyse (lize) *v.* To cause or undergo lysis (1).

ly·ser·gic acid (lye·sur'jick) The tetracyclic moiety, $C_{16}H_{16}N_2O_2$, of many ergot alkaloids and obtained from these on hydrolysis.

lysergic acid di·eth·yl·am·ide (lye·deth″il·am′ide). *N,N-*Diethyl-d-lysergamide, $C_{20}H_{25}N_3O$, a synthetic compound structurally related to ergot alkaloids but differing from these in being a very potent psychotogen. Abbreviated, LSD.

ly·sig·e·nous (lye·sij'e·nus) *adj.* Formed by the breaking down of adjoining cells; used especially of some intercellular spaces.

ly·sin (lye'sin) *n.* A substance, especially an antibody, capable of causing lysis.

ly·sine (lye'seen, ·sin) *n.* α, ε-Diaminocaproic acid, $NH_2(CH_2)_4CHNH_2COOH$, an amino acid present in many proteins. The hydrochloride salt is used to produce systemic acidosis and increase responsiveness to mercurial diuretics.

ly·sis (lye'sis) *n.*, pl. **ly·ses** (·seez) 1. Disintegration or dissolution, as of cells, bacteria, or tissue. 2. Gradual decline in the manifestations of a disease, especially an infectious disease, or of fever. 3. Loosening of or detachment from adhesions.

ly·so·gen·e·sis (lye″so·jen'e·sis) *n.* The production of lysins or lysis. —**lysogen·ic** (·jen'ick) *adj.*

ly·so·ki·nase (lye″so·kigh'nace, ·naze) *n.* Any substance of the fibrinolytic system which activates the plasma activators.

ly·so·some (lye'so·sohm) *n.* A cytoplasmic body bound by a single membrane, present in most types of cells but especially abundant in the liver and kidney, that contains various hydrolytic enzymes whose pH optima are acid. —**ly·so·so·mal** (lye″so·so′mul) *adj.*

ly·so·zyme (lye′so·zime) *n.* An enzyme present in the tears (as well as in other secretions) which has a hydrolytic action on certain bacterial cell walls (composed of specific polysaccharide units); can induce pinocytosis. It has been isolated in the granules of intestinal Paneth cells and may play a role in the regulation of intestinal flora. Syn. *muramidase.*

ly·so·zy·mu·ria (lye″so·zye·mew′ree·uh) *n.* The presence of lysozyme in the urine.

lys·sa (lis′uh) *n. Obsol.* RABIES.

lys·soid (lis′oid) *adj.* Resembling rabies.

lys·so·pho·bia (lis″o·fo′bee·uh) *n.* 1. CYNOPHO-BIA (2). 2. Morbid fear of becoming insane.

lyt·ic (lit′ick) *adj.* Pertaining to or causing lysis.

M

M Roman numeral for one thousand.
M. An abbreviation for (a) *mass*; (b) *molar*; (c) *misce*, mix.
m, m. Abbreviation for *meter*.
m- In chemistry, symbol for *meta-*.
MA, M.A. Abbreviation for *mental age*.
M.A. Master of Arts.
ma, mA Abbreviation for *milliampere*.
ma·ca·cus ear (muh·kah′kus, muh·kay′kus). An ear with a prominent auricular (Darwin's) tubercle.
*Mc·Ar·dle's syndrome or **disease** Glycogenosis caused by a deficiency of the muscle phosphorylase, with abnormal accumulation of glycogen in skeletal muscle, manifested clinically by temporary weakness and cramping of muscles after exercise, and no rise in blood lactic acid during exercise. Muscle fibers are destroyed to a variable degree. Syn. *myophosphorylase deficiency glycogenesis, type V of Cori*.
Mc·Bur·ney's incision A short diagonal incision in the lower right quadrant, used for appendectomy, in which the muscle fibers are separated rather than cut.
McBurney's point A point halfway between the umbilicus and the anterior superior iliac spine, a point of extreme tenderness in appendicitis, and usually the approximate location of the base of the appendix.
McBurney's sign. A sign for acute appendicitis in which the area of maximum tenderness is over McBurney's point.
Mac·Cal·lum's patch An irregular area of endocardial thickening on the posterior surface of the left atrium, usually representing the effects of rheumatic fever.
McCarthy's resectoscope A modification of the cystoscope for use in transurethral surgery. Syn. *McCarthy's electrotome*.
Mace, *n.* A lacrimatory agent consisting of a methylchloroform solution of chloroacetophenone, used in riot control.
mac·er·ate (mas′ur·ate) *v.* To soften a solid or a

tissue, or remove therefrom certain constituents, by steeping in a fluid. **—mac·er·a·tive** (mas′ur·ay″tiv) *adj.*
mac·er·a·tion (mas″ur·ay′shun) *n.* 1. The act or process of macerating. 2. *In obstetrics.* the changes undergone by a dead fetus as it is retained in utero, characterized by reddening, loss of skin, and distortion of features.
machinery murmur. A continuous murmur; usually used to describe the rumbling murmur of patent ductus arteriosus or other arteriovenous communication.
M'Naghten rule The formula for criminal responsibility still widely in use in the United States that holds a person not responsible for a crime if the accused "was laboring under such a defect of reason from the mind as not to know the nature and quality of the act; or, if he did know it, that he did not know that he was doing what was wrong."
Mac·Neal's tetrachrome stain A blood stain containing eosin, methylene azure A, methylene blue, and methylene violet in methyl alcohol; it is used like Wright's stain.
M.A.C.P. Master of the American College of Physicians.
macr-, macro- A combining form meaning (a) *large, great*; (b) *long, length*.
mac·ren·ceph·a·ly (mack″ren·sef′uh·lee) *n.* MEGALENCEPHALY. **—macrencepha·lous** (·lus), **mac·ren·ce·phal·ic** (·se·fal′ick) *adj.*
mac·ro·am·y·lase (mack″ro·am′i·lace, ·laze) *n.* An amylase of abnormally large size occurring in the blood serum of patients with macroamylasemia.
mac·ro·am·y·la·se·mia (mack″ro·am″i·lay·see″mee·uh) *n.* The presence of high-molecular-weight amylase molecules in the serum.
mac·ro·an·gi·op·a·thy (mack″ro·an″jee·op′uh·thee) *n.* Any disease of the larger blood vessels.
mac·ro·blast (mack′ro·blast) *n.* PRONORMOBLAST.
mac·ro·ble·phar·ia (mack″ro·ble·făr′ee·uh) *n.* Abnormal largeness of the eyelid.
mac·ro·bra·chia (mack″ro·bray′kee·uh) *n.* Excessive development of the arms.

*Names beginning with Mc or M' are alphabetized as if spelled Mac. . . . .

mac·ro·ce·phal·ic (mack″ro-se-fal′ick) *adj.* Having an abnormally large head.

mac·ro·ceph·a·ly (mack″ro-sef′uh-lee) *n.* Abnormal largeness of the head; megalocephaly.

mac·ro·chei·lia (mack″ro-kigh′lee-uh) *n.* 1. Relatively large size of the lips as a normal human variation. 2. Enlargement of the lips resulting from disease.

mac·ro·chei·ria (mack″ro-kigh′ree-uh) *n.* Abnormal enlargement of the hands.

mac·ro·cra·nia (mack″ro-kray′nee-uh) *n.* Disproportionately large head size compared with face size.

mac·ro·cyst (mack′ro-sist) *n.* 1. A cyst visible to the naked eye. 2. A very large cyst.

mac·ro·cyte (mack′ro-site) *n.* An erythrocyte having either a diameter or a mean corpuscular volume (MCV), or both, exceeding by more than two standard deviations that of the mean normal, as determined by the same method on the blood of healthy persons of the patient's age and sex group. Syn. *macronormocyte.* —**mac·ro·cyt·ic** (mack″ro-sit′ick) *adj.*

macrocytic anemia. Any anemia characterized by the presence in the blood of abnormally large erythrocytes (MCV greater than 100 $\mu\mu^3$), with or without megaloblastic bone marrow changes.

mac·ro·cy·to·sis (mack″ro-sigh-to′sis) *n.* The presence of macrocytes, or abnormally large erythrocytes, in the blood as determined microscopically or by measurement of cell volume.

mac·ro·dac·ty·ly (mack″ro-dack′til-ee) *n.* Abnormally large size of the fingers or toes; DACTYLOMEGALY.

mac·ro·don·tia (mack″ro-don′chee-uh) *n.* The condition of having abnormally large teeth. Syn. *megalodontia.* —**mac·ro·dont** (mack′ro-dont) *adj.*

mac·ro·fol·lic·u·lar (mack″ro-fol·ick′yoo-lur) *adj.* Having large follicles.

mac·ro·gam·ete (mack″ro-gam′eet) *n.* A relatively large, nonmotile reproductive cell of certain protozoans and thallophytes, comparable to an ovum of the metazoans.

mac·ro·gen·i·to·so·mia (mack″ro-jen″i-to-so′mee-uh) *n.* Excessive bodily development, especially of the external genitalia.

mac·rog·lia (ma·krog′lee-uh) *n.* Obsol. ASTROCYTES.

mac·ro·glob·u·lin (mack″ro-glob′yoo-lin) *n.* GAMMA-M GLOBULIN.

mac·ro·glob·u·li·ne·mia, mac·ro·glob·u·li·nae·mia (mack″ro-glob″yoo-lin·ee·mee-uh) *n.* 1. A disorder of the hemolytopoietic system characterized by proliferation of cells of the lymphocytic and plasmacytic series and the presence of abnormally large amounts of macroglobulin in the blood. 2. A marked increase in blood macroglobulins.

mac·ro·glos·sia (mack″ro-glos′ee-uh) *n.* Enlargement of the tongue.

mac·ro·gnath·ic (mack″ro-nath′ick, -nay′thick, mack″rog-) *adj.* Having long jaws; prognathous. —**mac·rog·na·thism** (ma-krog′nuh-thiz″um) *n.*

mac·ro·gy·ria (mack″ro-jye′ree-uh) *n.* A congenital condition of excessively large convolutions of the brain, often associated with retardation.

mac·ro·mas·tia (mack″ro-mas′tee-uh) *n.* Abnormal enlargement of the breast.

mac·ro·me·lia (mack″ro-mee′lee-uh) *n.* Abnormally large size of arms or legs.

ma·crom·e·lus (ma·krom′e·lus) *n.* An individual having excessively large limbs.

mac·ro·mol·e·cule (mack″ro-mol′e·kyool) *n.* A very large molecule, as of a protein, polysaccharide, rubber, or synthetic polymer.

mac·ro·my·e·lo·blast (mack″ro-mye′e·lo-blast) *n.* An excessively large myeloblast.

mac·ro·nu·cle·us (mack″ro-new′klee-us) *n.* The vegetative or trophic nucleus of protozoa as contrasted with the micronucleus which is reproductive in function.

mac·ro·nych·ia (mack″ro-nick′ee-uh) *n.* Excessive size of the nails.

mac·ro·phage (mack′ro-faij) *n.* A phagocytic cell belonging to the reticuloendothelial system; important in resistance to infection and in immunological responses. It has the capacity for accumulating certain aniline dyes, as trypan blue or lithium carmine, in its cytoplasm in the form of granules.

mac·ro·po·dia (mack″ro-po′dee-uh) *n.* Abnormally large size of the foot or feet. Syn. *pes gigas, sciapody.*

mac·ro·poly·cyte (mack″ro-pol′ee-site) *n.* An unusually large, neutrophilic leukocyte with six or more lobes in the nucleus.

mac·ro·pro·so·pia (mack″ro-pruh-so′pee-uh) *n.* Abnormal enlargement of the face.

ma·crop·sia (ma·krop′see-uh) *n.* A disturbance of vision in which objects seem larger than they are. Syn. *megalopia.*

mac·ro·scop·ic (mack″ro-skop′ick) *adj.* Large enough to be seen by the naked eye; gross; not microscopic.

mac·ros·mat·ic (mack″roz-mat′ick) *adj.* Possessing a highly developed sense of smell.

mac·ro·so·mia (mack″ro-so′mee-uh) *n.* GIGANTISM.

mac·ro·throm·bo·cy·to·path·ia (mack″ro-throm″bo·sigh″to-path′ee-uh) *n.* A platelet disorder characterized by thrombocytopenia, giant platelets with abnormal structure, prolonged bleeding time, and defective adherence of platelets to glass.

Ma·cruz index The ratio of P wave duration to P-R segment duration in the electrocardiogram, used as a criterion of atrial enlargement.

mac·u·la (mack′yoo-luh) *n.,* pl. **mac·u·lae** (·lee) 1. In general, a spot. 2. [NA] MACULA LUTEA. 3. A circumscribed corneal scar or opacity. 4. MACULE.

macula com·mu·nis (kom-yoo′nis). The thickening in the medial wall of the auditory vesicle, which divides to form the maculae, cristae, and spiral organ (of Corti) of the internal ear.

macula cor·ne·ae (kor′nee-ee). A permanent corneal opacity from an ulcer or keratitis.

macula den·sa (den′suh). A thickening of the epithelium of the ascending limb of the loop of Henle, at the level of attachment to the vascular pole of the renal corpuscle.

maculae. Plural of *macula.*

macula lu·tea (lew′tee·uh) [BNA]. The yellow spot of the retina; the point of clearest vision.

macular corneal dystrophy. A heredodegenerative disease of the eye, characterized by irregular gray opacities with a diffuse cloudiness of the corneal stroma between the opacities, as well as involvement of the periphery, resulting usually in severe early impairment of vision; transmitted as a recessive trait.

macular degeneration or **dystrophy.** Pathologic changes of the macula lutea, occurring bilaterally at any age, characterized by spots of pigmentation, a moth-eaten appearance or other alterations, and producing a reduction or loss of central vision; may be hereditary, traumatic, senile, or atherosclerotic.

macular dysplasia. A congenital macular defect which may show pigmentation or abnormality of the retinal vessels; rarely, the macula is absent; usually due to intrauterine choroiditis.

macular vision. CENTRAL VISION.

mac·ule (mack′yool) n. A small, circumscribed, discolored spot on the skin; especially, one not perceptibly raised above the surrounding level.

mac·u·lo·an·es·thet·ic (mack″yoo·lo·an″is·thet′ick) *adj.* Having the appearance of a macule and being insensitive to pain in the affected area; said of certain leprous lesions.

mac·u·lo·pap·ule (mack″yoo·lo·pap′yool) n. A small, circumscribed, discolored elevation of the skin; a macule and papule combined. —**maculopap·u·lar** (·yoo·lur) *adj.*

mad, *adj.* 1. Insane. 2. Affected with rabies; rabid.

mad·a·ro·sis (mad″uh·ro′sis) n. Loss of the eyelashes or eyebrows. —**mad·a·rot·ic** (·rot′ick), **mad·a·rous** (mad′uh·rus) *adj.*

Ma·de·lung′s deformity (mah′de·loong) A congenital or developmental deformity of the wrist characterized by palmar angulation of the distal end of the radius and dorsal dislocation of the head of the ulna.

mad·i·dans (mad′i·danz, ·dance) *adj.* Weeping, oozing.

mad·ness n. Mental disorder.

ma·du·ra foot (ma·dew′ruh, mad′yoo·ruh) MYCETOMA.

mad·u·ro·my·co·sis (mad″yoo·ro·migh·ko′sis) n. MYCETOMA.

ma·fe·nide (may′fe·nide) n. α-Amino-*p*-toluenesulfonamide, $C_7H_{10}N_2O_2S$, an antibacterial drug. Syn. *sulfbenzamine.*

Maf·fuc·ci′s syndrome (maf·fooch′ee) Cutaneous hemangiomas associated with enchondromatosis.

ma·gen·bla·se (mah′gun·blah″zeh) n. In *radiology,* the bubble of gas in the fundus of the stomach, usually seen in erect films of the chest or abdomen beneath the left hemidiaphragm.

ma·gen·stras·se (mah′gun·shtrah″seh) n. GASTRIC CANAL.

mag·got, n. A fly larva, especially one of the kinds that live on decaying animal matter.

magical thinking. In *psychiatry,* a person's confusion of imagining with doing, wish with fulfilment, cause with effect, or symbol with event. So called by analogy to certain magical beliefs and practices, it is commonly observed in dreams and in children's thinking as well as in a variety of mental disorders.

mag·ma (mag′muh) n. 1. Any pulpy mass; a paste. 2. In *pharmacy,* a more or less permanent suspension of a precipitate in water.

mag·ne·sia (mag·nee′zhuh, ·shuh, ·zee·uh) n. Magnesium oxide, MgO.

mag·ne·site (mag′ne·site) n. Native magnesium carbonate; sometimes used as a substitute for plaster of Paris.

mag·ne·sium (mag·nee′zhum, ·zee·um, ·shum) n. Mg = 24.305. A bluish white metal of the group of elements to which calcium and barium belong. Abundantly distributed throughout inorganic and organic nature and essential to life; certain of its salts are used in medicine. —**magne·sic** (·zick, ·sick) *adj.*

magnesium carbonate. Basic or normal hydrated magnesium carbonate, $(MgCO_3)_4$·$Mg(OH)_2$·$5H_2O$ or $MgCO_3$·H_2O. Exists in two densities: light and heavy magnesium carbonate. Used as an antacid and laxative.

magnesium hydroxide. $Mg(OH)_2$. A white powder, used as an antacid and cathartic. Syn. *magnesium hydrate.*

magnesium oxide. MgO. Obtained by calcining magnesium carbonate. Exists in two densities: light and heavy. Used as an antacid and laxative and as a dusting powder.

magnesium sulfate. $MgSO_4$·$7H_2O$. Epsom salt, an active cathartic, especially useful in inflammatory affections; has central depressant action when administered intravenously.

magnesium trisilicate. Approximately $2MgO$·$3SiO_2$ with varying amounts of water. Almost insoluble in water; reacts slowly with acid. Used as an antacid and absorbent.

mag·net, n. 1. A variety of iron ore or mineral, as lodestone, that attracts iron. 2. Any body having the power to attract iron. —**mag·net·ic,** *adj.*

magnetic field. The portion of space around a magnet in which its action can be felt.

mag·ne·tism, n. 1. The power possessed by a magnet to attract or repel other masses. 2. ANIMAL MAGNETISM.

mag·ne·to·car·di·og·ra·phy (mag″ne·to·kahr″dee·og′ruh·fee) n. Measurement of the magnetic field of the heart.

mag·ne·to·ther·a·py (mag·nee″to·therr′uh·pee, mag′ne·to·) n. The treatment of diseases by magnets or magnetism.

mag·ni·fi·ca·tion, n. 1. Apparent enlargement; the production of an image larger than that produced by the naked eye. 2. A ratio, usually expressed in diameters or in degrees of arc subtended, between the dimensions of an image produced by an optical instrument and the dimensions of the object. 3. Exaggeration.

mag·no·cel·lu·lar (mag″no·sel′yoo·lur) *adj.* Having large cell bodies; said of various nuclei of the central nervous system.

¹mag·num (mag′num) *adj.* Large, as in foramen magnum.

²magnum, *n.* CAPITATE.

maid·en·head, *n.* HYMEN; the intact hymen of a virgin.

ma·ieu·sio·ma·nia (migh·yoo″see·o·may′nee·uh, may·) *n.* PUERPERAL PSYCHOSIS.

ma·ieu·sio·pho·bia (migh·yoo″see·o·fo′bee·uh, may·) *n.* Morbid fear of childbirth.

maim, *v.* To mutilate or disable; to commit mayhem, especially by destroying or crippling a limb.

maize oil. CORN OIL.

Ma·joc·chi's disease or **purpura** (mah,yoh′kee) PURPURA ANNULARIS TELANGIECTODES.

ma·jor (may′jur) *adj.* Larger, greater.

major amputation. Any amputation through the long bones of the upper or lower extremities; disarticulation at the hip joint or shoulder girdle.

major calices. The primary divisions of the renal pelvis; derived from the embryonic pole tubules, usually two or three in number.

major cross match. See *cross matching.*

major duodenal papilla. A small elevation of the mucosa of the medial wall of the second part of the duodenum where the common bile duct and the main pancreatic duct empty.

major histocompatibility complex. The human chromosomal segment situated on a pair of autosomes not yet identified, which determines the major leukocyte antigens and certain other characteristics of lymphocytes. Abbreviated, MHC

major operation. An extensive, relatively difficult, potentially dangerous surgical procedure, frequently involving a major cavity of the body, or requiring general anesthesia; one which demands of the surgeon a special degree of experience and skill.

major surgery. MAJOR OPERATION.

make, *n.* In electricity, the establishing of the flow of an electric current.

mal- A prefix meaning *wrong, abnormal, bad, badly.*

mal, *n.* Sickness, disease.

ma·la (may′luh) *n.* [NA alt.]. CHEEK. NA alt. *bucca.*

mal·ab·sorp·tion (mal″ub·sorp′shun) *n.* Defective absorption of nutritive substances from the alimentary canal.

malabsorption syndrome. A syndrome in which intestinal malabsorption of fat results in bulky, loose, foul-smelling stools high in fatty acid content, as well as failure to gain or loss of weight, weakness, anorexia, and vitamin deficiencies with their accompanying symptoms. This syndrome is common to a number of different diseases, including infantile celiac disease, nontropical and tropical sprue, cystic fibrosis of the pancreas, and other specific enzyme deficiencies, as well as obstruction of digestive and absorptive pathways as in Whipple's disease, Hirschsprung's disease, giardiasis, and tuberculous and lymphomatous infiltration of mesenteric nodes.

ma·la·cia (ma·lay′shee·uh, ·shuh) *n.* Abnormal softening of part of an organ or structure.

mal·a·co·pla·kia, mal·a·ko·pla·kia (mal″uh·ko·play′kee·uh) *n.* The accumulation of histiocytes containing Michaelis-Gutmann calcospherules to produce soft, pale elevated plaques, usually in the urinary bladder of middle-aged women.

maladie de Roger VENTRICULAR SEPTAL DEFECT.

mal·ad·just·ment (mal″uh·just′munt) *n.* A state of faulty or inadequate conformity to one's environment, due to the inability to adjust one's desires, attitudes, or feelings to social requirements. —**maladjust·ed** (·id) *adj.*

mal·a·dy (mal′uh·dee) *n.* Disease, illness.

mal·aise (mal·aiz′) *n.* A general feeling of illness or discomfort.

malakoplakia. MALACOPLAKIA.

mal·align·ment (mal″uh·line′munt) *n.* Improper alignment, as of fragments of a fractured bone, or of teeth.

ma·lar (may′lur) *adj. & n.* 1. Pertaining to the cheek or to the zygoma. 2. ZYGOMATIC BONE.

ma·lar·ia (muh·lār′ee·uh) *n.* An infectious febrile disease produced by several species of the protozoan genus *Plasmodium,* transmitted from host to host by the bite of an infected anopheline mosquito. It is characterized by paroxysms of severe chills, fever, and sweating, splenomegaly, anemia, and a chronic relapsing course. —**malar·i·al** (·ee·ul) *adj.*

malarial nephropathy. Nephrotic syndrome associated with quartan malaria. Soluble immune-complex injury has been postulated as a cause of the glomerular alterations. Syn. *quartan malarial nephropathy.*

ma·lar·i·ol·o·gist (muh·lār″ee·ol′uh·jist) *n.* An expert in the diagnosis, treatment, and control of malaria.

mal·ar·tic·u·la·tion (mal″ahr·tick″yoo·lay′shun) *n.* 1. Defective production of speech sounds. 2. Defective positioning of joint surfaces.

Malassezia furfur. PITYROSPORUM FURFUR.

mal·as·sim·i·la·tion (mal″uh·sim″i·lay′shun) *n.* Defective assimilation.

Malayan filariasis. Filariasis of man caused by *Brugia malayi,* occurring in southeast Asia, transmitted by mosquitoes of the genera *Mansonia* and *Anopheles.* Lymphadenopathy, lymphadenitis, and elephantiasis, principally of the lower limbs, occur.

mal de mer (mal duh mehr) SEASICKNESS.

mal·de·vel·op·ment (mal″de·vel′up·munt) *n.* Faulty development.

male, *adj. & n.* 1. Of or pertaining to the sex that produces small motile gametes, as spermatozoa, which fertilize ova. 2. Of instruments or connecting tubes, having a protuberance which fits into a corresponding (female) part in order to function. 3. An individual of the male sex. Symbol, ⬜. ♂. 4. *In botany,* a plant having stamens only.

ma·le·ate (mal′ee·ate) *n.* Any salt or ester of maleic acid.

ma·le·ic acid (ma·lee′ick, ma·lay′ick). *cis*-Ethylene carboxylic acid, HOOCCH=CHCOOH. A dibasic acid, the *cis*-isomer of fumaric acid. Does not occur in nature.

male pseudohermaphroditism. Androgyny; a condition simulating hermaphroditism in which the individual has external sexual characteristics of female aspect, but has testes (usually undescended). Syn. *pseudohermaphroditismus masculinus.*

male Turner's syndrome. ULLRICH-TURNER SYNDROME.

mal·for·ma·tion, *n.* An abnormal development or formation of a part of the body; deformity.

mal·func·tion, *n. & v.* 1. Failure to function normally or properly. 2. To function abnormally or improperly.

mal·ic acid (mal'ick, may'lick). Hydroxysuccinic acid, $HOOCCH_2CHOHCOOH$, a dibasic hydroxy acid found in apples and many other fruits. Exists in two optically active isomers and a racemic form. The acid and various of its salts have been used medicinally.

ma·lig·nant (muh·lig'nunt) *adj.* 1. Endangering health or life. 2. Specifically, characterizing the progressive growth of certain tumors which if not checked by treatment spread to distant sites, terminating in death. —**malignan·cy** (·nun·see) *n.*

malignant acanthosis nigricans. Acanthosis nigricans associated with visceral adenocarcinoma.

malignant adenoma. A tumor with cytologic features of an adenoma which gives rise to local or distant metastases.

malignant disease. 1. Any disease in a particularly violent form, threatening to produce death in a short time. 2. CANCER.

malignant edema. 1. An acute toxemic infection of ungulates usually caused by *Clostridium septicum.* 2. An inflammatory edema in humans caused by *Clostridium* species.

malignant exophthalmos. Rapidly progressive severe exophthalmos in hyperthyroidism.

malignant freckle. LENTIGO MALIGNA.

malignant glaucoma. Glaucoma attended with violent pain and rapidly leading to blindness. Generally occurs following ocular surgery for glaucoma.

malignant hypertension. The accelerated phase of essential hypertension, with papilledema, retinal hemorrhages and exudates, higher and less labile blood pressure levels, progressive cardiac, renal and vascular disease, and encephalopathy. Syn. *accelerated hypertension.*

malignant mixed mesodermal tumor. A tumor whose parenchyma is composed of anaplastic cells resembling two or more derivatives of the mesoderm.

malignant pustule. A localized skin lesion of anthrax.

malignant transformation. A permanent genetic change in a somatic cell, which may be induced by physical, chemical, or viral means, resulting in formation of a cancer cell.

ma·lin·ger (muh·ling'gur) *v.* To feign or exaggerate illness or incapacity in order to avoid work or other responsibilities. —**malinger·er** (·ur) *n.*

mal·lea·ble (mal'ee·uh·bul) *adj.* Capable of being beaten or rolled into thin sheets. —**malle·a·bil·i·ty** (mal''ee·uh·bil'i·tee) *n.*

mallear prominence. The bulge on the medial surface of the tympanic membrane overlying the lateral process of the malleus.

mal·le·a·tion (mal''ee·ay'shun) *n.* A spasmodic ticlike action of the hands, consisting in regularly striking any near object.

mal·lei (mal'ee·eye) 1. Plural of *malleus.* 2. Genitive singular of *malleus;* of or pertaining to the malleus. 3. Of or pertaining to malleus (glanders).

mal·le·in (mal'ee·in) *n.* A protein concentrate of *Actinobacillus mallei,* used in a skin test for the diagnosis of glanders, analogous to the tuberculin test.

mal·leo·in·cu·dal (mal''ee·o·ing'kew·dul, ·in'kew·dul) *adj.* Pertaining to the malleus and the incus.

mal·le·o·lar (mal·lee'uh·lur) *adj.* 1. Pertaining to a malleolus. 2. MALLEAR.

mal·le·o·lus (ma·lee'o·lus) *n.,* pl. & genit. sing. **malleo·li** (·lye) A part or process of bone having a hammerhead shape.

Mal·leo·my·ces (mal''ee·o·mye'seez) *n.* ACTINOBACILLUS.

Malleomyces mallei. Obsol. PSEUDOMONAS MALLEI.

Malleomyces pseudomallei. PSEUDOMONAS PSEUDOMALLEI.

mal·leo·my·rin·go·plas·ty (mal''ee·o·mi·ring'go·plas·tee) *n.* A method of reestablishing an effective sound-conducting method when the tympanic membrane and the handle of the malleus have been destroyed, by reconstructing the tympanic membrane from adherent fascial layers covering the temporalis muscle and the handle of the malleus, incorporating a shaped bone graft between the layers.

mal·le·ot·o·my (mal''ee·ot'um·ee) *n.* 1. Incision or division of the malleus. 2. Division of the ligaments attached to the malleoli.

mallet finger. A deformity marked by undue flexion of the last phalanx.

mal·le·us (mal'ee·us) *n.,* pl. & genit. sing. **mal·lei** (·ee·eye) 1. [NA] One of the ossicles of the internal ear, having the shape of a hammer. 2. *In veterinary medicine,* GLANDERS. Adj. *malleal, mallear.*

Mal·lo·ry bodies Oval acidophilic hyalin inclusion bodies of cytoplasm of hepatic cells, observed in Laennec's cirrhosis.

Mallory's triple stain. A stain which differentially colors different tissue components; contains acid fuchsin, orange G, and aniline blue dyes.

Mallory-Weiss syndrome Painless hematemesis secondary to lacerations of the distal esophagus and esophagogastric junction, involving only the mucosa and submucosa, usually a result of prolonged violent vomiting, coughing, or hiccuping.

mal·nu·tri·tion (mal''new·trish'un) *n.* Defective nutrition. —**mal·nour·ish** (·nur'ish) *v.*

mal·oc·clu·sion (mal''uh·kloo'zhun) *n.* Any deviation from a physiologically normal occlusion of the teeth.

ma·lon·ic acid (ma·lo'nick, ·lon'ick). Propanedioic acid, $HOOCCH_2COOH$, a dibasic acid found in many plants and obtainable from malic acid by oxidation.

mal·o·nyl (mal'o·nil, ·neel) *n.* $—COCH_2CO—$ The bivalent radical of malonic acid.

mal·pigh·i·an (mal·pig'ee·un) *adj.* Discovered

described by Marcello Malpighi, Italian anatomist, 1628–1691.

malpighian corpuscle or **body.** 1. A lymph nodule of the spleen. 2. RENAL CORPUSCLE.

mal·po·si·tion (mal″puh·zish′un, mal″po-) n. An abnormal position of any part or organ, as of the fetus.

mal·pos·ture (mal·pos′chur) n. Faulty posture.

mal·prac·tice (mal·prak′tis) n. Improper or injurious medical or surgical treatment, through carelessness, ignorance, or intent.

mal·pre·sen·ta·tion (mal″prez″un·tay′shun, ·pree″zen·tay′shun) n. Abnormal position of the child at birth, making delivery difficult or impossible.

mal·re·duc·tion (mal″re·duck′shun) n. Faulty or incomplete reduction of a fracture.

malt, n. Grain, commonly of one or more varieties of barley, which has been soaked, made to germinate, and dried. The germinated grains contain diastase, dextrin, maltose, and proteins. Malt has been used as a nutrient and digestant.

Mal·ta fever. BRUCELLOSIS.

malt·ase (mawl′tace, ·taze) n. An enzyme found in the saliva and pancreatic juice which converts maltose into dextrose.

Mal·thu·sian·ism (mal·thoo′zhun·iz·um, mawl·, ·zee·un·) n. The theory that in the absence of such checks as epidemics and war, population tends to increase more rapidly than the food supply. —**Malthusian,** adj.

malt·ose (mawl′toce) n. 4-(α-D-Glucopyranosido)-D-glucopyranose, $C_{12}H_{22}O_{11}.H_2O$, a reducing disaccharide representing 2 molecules of D-glucose joined by α-glycosidic linkage, and yielding 2 molecules of D-glucose on hydrolysis. It does not appear to exist free in nature, being a product of enzymatic hydrolysis of starch by diastase, as in malt. It exists in 2 forms, α-maltose and β-maltose. Syn. *maltobiose, malt sugar.*

malt·os·uria (mawl″to·sue′ree·uh) n. The presence of maltose in the urine.

mal·um (mal′um, mah′lum, may′lum) n. DISEASE.

malum cox·ae (kock′see). Hip joint disease.

malum coxae se·ni·lis (se·nigh′lis). Hypertrophic arthritis of the hip joint in the aged.

mal·un·ion (mal·yoon′yun) n. Incomplete or faulty union of the fragments of a fractured bone.

nam·e·lon (mame′e·lon, ·lun) n. One of the three elevations on the incisal edge of a recently erupted or little-worn incisor tooth.

namillary body. Either of the two small, spherical masses of gray matter in the interpeduncular space at the base of the brain. They receive projections from the hippocampus by means of the fornix and relay them to the anterior nucleus of the thalamus via the mamillothalamic tract and to the tegmentum of the pons and medulla oblongata via the mamillotegmental bundle.

namm-, mammo- A combining form meaning *mamma* or *breast.*

nam·ma (mam′uh) n., pl. **mam·mae** (·mee) The breast; the milk-secreting gland.

mam·mal (mam′ul) n. An individual of the class Mammalia.

mam·mal·gia (ma·mal′jee·uh) n. Pain in the mammary gland; mastalgia.

Mam·ma·lia (ma·may′lee·uh) n.pl. The class of vertebrates that includes all animals that have hair and suckle their young. —**mamma·li·an** (·lee·un) adj.

mam·ma·ry (mam′uh·ree) adj. Pertaining to the mammae.

mammary dysplasia. A group of common pathologic conditions in the breasts of women during sexual maturity. Included are adenosis of breast, cystic disease, and mastodynia. Syn. *chronic cystic mastitis.*

mammary gland. A gland that secretes milk.

mam·mec·to·my (ma·meck′tum·ee) n. MASTECTOMY.

mam·mi·form (mam′i·form) adj. Shaped like a breast or nipple.

mammill-, mammillo-. See *mamill-.*

mammilla. MAMILLA.

Mam·mil·lar·ia (mam″i·lăr′ee·uh) n. A genus of cacti. The mescal or peyote cactus, once assigned to this genus, is now properly designated *Lophophora williamsii.*

mammillary. MAMILLARY.

mammillated. MAMILLATED.

mammillation. MAMILLATION.

mammilliform. MAMILLIFORM.

mammilliplasty. MAMILLIPLASTY.

mammillitis. MAMILLITIS.

mammillotegmental. MAMILLOTEGMENTAL.

mammillothalamic. MAMILLOTHALAMIC.

mam·mo·gen (mam′uh·jin, ·jen″) n. PROLACTIN. —**mammogen·ic** (mam″o·jen′ick) adj.

mam·mo·gram (mam′o·gram) n. A radiographic depiction of the breast.

mam·mog·ra·phy (ma·mog′ruh·fee) n. Radiographic examination of the breast, occasionally performed with a contrast medium injected into the ducts of the mammary gland, usually without.

mam·mo·plas·ty (mam′o·plas·tee) n. Any plastic surgery operation altering the shape of the breast.

mam·mose (mam′oce, ma·moce′) adj. Having full or abnormally large breasts.

mam·mot·o·my (ma·mot′um·ee) n. MASTOTOMY.

Man·chu·ri·an fever. EPIDEMIC HEMORRHAGIC FEVER.

Mandelamine. Trademark for methenamine mandelate, a salt of methenamine and mandelic acid used as a urinary antibacterial agent.

man·del·ic acid (man·del′ick, ·dee′lick) Alphahydroxyphenylacetic acid, $C_6H_5CH(OH)COOH$, a urinary antiseptic; usually used in the form of one of its salts.

man·di·ble (man′di·bul) n. The lower jawbone.

mandibul-, mandibulo-. A combining form meaning *mandible, mandibular.*

man·dib·u·lar (man·dib′yoo·lur) adj. Of or pertaining to the mandible.

mandibular arch. The first visceral arch, including the maxillary process. Syn. *oral arch.*

mandibular canal. The canal in the mandible

which transmits the inferior alveolar vessels and nerve.

mandibular foramen. The aperture of the inferior dental or alveolar canal in the ramus of the mandible; it transmits the inferior dental or alveolar vessels and nerve to the lower jaw.

mandibular fossa. The fossa in the temporal bone that receives the condyle of the mandible.

mandibular gland. SUBMANDIBULAR GLAND.

mandibular nerve. A motor (masticator nerve) and somatic sensory nerve, attached to the trigeminal nerve, which innervates the tensor tympani, tensor veli palatini, mylohyoid, anterior belly of the digastric, and muscles of mastication, the lower teeth, the mucosa of the anterior two-thirds of the tongue, the floor of the mouth, the cheek and the skin of the lower portion of the face, and the meninges.

man·dib·u·lec·to·my (man-dib″yoo-leck′tum-ee) *n.* Surgical removal of the mandible.

man·drel (man′dril) *n.* A shank or shaft that fits into a dental handpiece and which holds a cup, disk, or stone for polishing or grinding.

man·drin (man′drin) *n.* A guide or stylet.

ma·neu·ver (muh·new′vur) *n.* Skillful procedure or manual method.

man·ga·nese (mang′guh·neece, ·neez, man′guh·) *n.* Mn = 54.9380. A brittle, hard, grayish-white metal resembling iron in its properties. Manganese salts have been used in medicine, but proof of their value is lacking.

mange (mainj) *n.* Infestation of the skin of mammals by mange mites which burrow into the epidermal layer of the skin; characterized by multiple lesions in the skin with vesiculation and papule formation accompanied by intense itching.

mange mite. Any species of the Sarcoptoidea.

-mania A combining form designating *obsession, abnormal preoccupation,* or *compulsion.*

mania a po·tu (ah po′too, ay po′tew) PATHOLOGIC INTOXICATION.

ma·ni·ac (may′nee·ack) *n.* 1. A psychotic person with violent or destructive tendencies. 2. A person with a mania for something. **—ma·ni·a·cal** (muh·nigh′uh·kul) *adj.*

manic-depressive illness, reaction, or **psychosis.** One of a group of psychotic reactions, fundamentally marked by severe mood swings from normal to elation or to depression or alternating, and a tendency to remission and recurrence. Illusions, delusions, and hallucinations are often associated with the change of affect, but milder forms are often observed. The manic type is characterized by elation or irritability, overtalkativeness, flight of ideas, and increased motor activity; the depressive type exhibits outstanding depression of mood, mental and motor retardation, and inhibition. Marked mixture of these phases is the mixed type; continuous alternation of phases is the circular type.

manifest hyperopia. The amount of hyperopia represented by the strongest convex lens that a person will accept without paralysis of the accommodation; may be facultative or absolute. Symbol, Hm.

man·i·kin (man′i·kin) *n.* 1. A model of the body; made of plaster, papier-mâché, or other material, and showing, by means of movable parts, the relations of the organs. 2. A model of a term fetus; used for the teaching of obstetrics.

ma·nip·u·la·tion (muh·nip″yoo·lay′shun) *n.* The use of the hands in a skillful manner, as reducing a dislocation, returning a hernia into its cavity, or changing the position of a fetus.

man·na (man′uh) *n.* The concrete, saccharine exudation of the flowering ash, *Fraxinus ornus;* contains mannitol, sugar, mucilage, and resin. Has been used as a mild laxative.

man·ni·tol (man′i·tol) *n.* D-Mannitol, $HOCH_2(CHOH)_4CH_2OH$; a hexahydric alcohol from manna and other plant sources. Hypertonic solutions are administered intravenously to promote diuresis. Sometimes used to measure the rate of glomerular filtration, and as an irrigating fluid in transurethral resection of the prostate; in pharmacy used as a diluent and excipient. Syn. *manna sugar, mannite.*

ma·nom·e·ter (ma·nom′e·tur) *n.* An instrument for measuring the pressure of liquids and gases. **—mano·met·ric** (man″uh·met′rick) *adj.*

manometric block. A partial or complete obstruction to the free flow of cerebrospinal fluid as measured usually by pressure on the abdomen or jugular veins during a lumbar or cisternal puncture or both.

ma·nom·e·try (ma·nom′e·tree) *n.* Use of manometers.

Man·so·nia (man·so′nee·uh) *n.* A genus of mosquitoes which are important as vectors of human disease. Species of *Mansonia,* subgenus *Mansonioides,* are the principal carriers of *Wuchereria malayi,* and also are carriers of *Wuchereria bancrofti.*

man·tle, *n.* 1. An enveloping layer. 2. The portion of brain substance that includes the convolutions, corpus callosum, and fornix.

Man·toux test (mahⁿ·too′) Any intradermal test for tuberculin hypersensitivity.

ma·nu·bri·um (ma·new′bree·um) *n.,* pl. **manu·bria** (·bree·uh) 1. A handlike process. 2. MANUBRIUM STERNI. **—manubri·al** (·ul) *adj.*

manubrium ster·ni (stur′nigh) [NA]. The upper segment of the sternum.

man·u·duc·tion (man″yoo·duck′shun) *n.* Operation performed by the hands in surgical and obstetric practice.

ma·nus (man′us) *n.,* pl. & genit. sing. **manus** (man′oos, man′us) HAND.

manus ca·va (kay′vuh). Excessive concavity of the palm of the hand.

manus cur·ta (kur′tuh). CLUBHAND.

manus ex·ten·sa (eck·sten′suh). Clubhand with a backward deviation.

manus flexa (fleck′suh). Clubhand with a forward deviation.

manus val·ga (val′guh) Clubhand with ulnar deviation.

manus va·ra (vair′uh, vahr′uh) Clubhand with radial deviation.

many·plies (men′ee·plize) *n.* OMASUM.

MAO Abbreviation for *monoamine oxidase.*

maple bark disease. CONIOSPORIOSIS.

maple syrup urine disease. A hereditary metabolic disorder in which there is a deficiency of branched-chain keto acid decarboxylase with abnormally high concentrations of valine, leucine, isoleucine, and the presence of alloisoleucine in blood, urine, and cerebrospinal fluid; manifested clinically by the aromatic maple syruplike odor of urine noted shortly after birth. In the severe infantile form, in which the enzyme deficiency is nearly complete, there is protracted vomiting and hypertonicity and, unless treated by diet, severe mental retardation, seizures, and death. In the intermittent form, the enzyme activity is decreased to about 10 to 20% of normal, and the above symptoms occur usually only with infection or trauma; the patient may die in status epilepticus unless treated by diet. Syn. *branched-chain ketoaciduria.*

ma·ran·tic (muh·ran'tick) *adj.* 1. Pertaining to marasmus. 2. Pertaining to slowed circulation.

marantic endocarditis. Nonbacterial thrombotic endocarditis, usually associated with neoplasm or other debilitating diseases.

marantic thrombosis. Thrombosis, usually of a cerebral sinus, associated with a wasting disease.

marantic thrombus. A thrombus occurring in an area of retarded blood flow, as the atria.

marasmic kwashiorkor. Kwashiorkor in which there is caloric deficiency as well as protein deficiency.

ma·ras·mus (muh·raz'mus) *n.* Chronic severe wasting of the tissues of the body, particularly in children, resulting in loss of subcutaneous fat, inelastic, wrinkled skin, loss of muscle tissue and strength, growth failure, lethargy, and often acidosis and hypoproteinemia; may be due to chronic severe malnutrition or defective absorption or utilization of a good food supply. —**maras·mic** (·mick) *adj.*

marble bone. 1. OSTEOPETROSIS. 2. The osteopetrotic form of lymphomatosis in chickens.

mar·ble·iza·tion (mahr''bul·eye·zay'shun, ·i·zay'shun) *n.* The condition of being marked or veined like marble.

Mar·burg virus A large arbovirus transmitted by green monkeys, *Cercopithecus aethiops,* to man; reported in 1968 in Marburg and Frankfurt, West Germany.

marc, *n.* The residue remaining after the extraction of the active principles from a vegetable drug, or after the extraction of the juice or oil from fruits.

march albuminuria. Proteinuria associated with long walks or runs.

marche à pe·tit pas (mahrsh ah p'tee pah') A slow, shuffling, short-stepped uncertain gait, associated with a slightly flexed posture and a loss of adaptive movements; observed usually in the aged and senile.

march fracture. A fracture usually of the metatarsal bones, without obvious trauma, as a result of marching, running, etc.

march hemoglobinuria. A paroxysmal hemoglobinuria noted sometimes after strenuous marching.

Mar·chia·fa·va-Bi·gna·mi disease (mar''kyah.fah'vah, been·nyah'mee) A disease of unknown cause, observed almost exclusively in alcoholic men and characterized by a degeneration of the middle portion of the corpus callosum and, in advanced cases, of the central portions of the anterior and posterior commissures, the superior cerebellar peduncles and centrum ovale. The clinical manifestations are variable and may include coma, dementia, seizures, focal neurologic signs and a frontal lobe syndrome. Syn. *primary degeneration of the corpus callosum.*

Marchiafava-Micheli syndrome PAROXYSMAL NOCTURNAL HEMOGLOBINURIA.

Mar·fan's syndrome (mar·fahn') 1. A heritable disorder of connective tissue, clinically manifested by skeletal changes such as abnormally long, thin extremities (dolichostenomelia), spidery fingers and toes (arachnodactyly), as well as high-arched palate, defects of the spine and chest, redundant ligaments and joint capsules; by ocular changes including subluxation of the lens, cataract, coloboma, enlarged cornea, strabismus and nystagmus; and by congenital heart disease, particularly weakness of the media of the ascending aorta causing diffuse dilatation and dissection. Chemically there may be an altered ratio of chondroitin sulfate to keratosulfate in costal cartilage, decreased serum mucoproteins, and increased urinary excretion of hydroxyproline. Transmitted as a simple Mendelian dominant with a high degree of penetrance. 2. DENNIE-MARFAN SYNDROME.

mar·ga·ri·to·ma (mahr''guh·ri·to'muh) *n.* A true primary cholesteatoma formation in the auditory canal.

mar·gin (mahr'jin) *n.* The boundary or edge of a surface. —**margin·al** (·ul) *adj.*

marginal blepharitis. Inflammation of the hair follicles and sebaceous glands along the margins of the lids.

marginal gingiva. The unattached gingiva that surrounds a tooth; it lies occlusally or incisally to the floor of the gingival sulcus and forms its soft tissue wall.

marginal keratitis. An inflammation around the periphery of the cornea. Syn. *annular keratitis.*

mar·gin·ation (mahr''ji·nay'shun) *n.* 1. Adhesion of leukocytes to the walls of capillaries in the early stage of inflammation. 2. The establishment or finishing of a dental cavity preparation or restoration.

mar·gino·plas·ty (mahr'ji·no·plas'tee) *n.* Plastic surgery of the marginal portion of the eyelid.

mar·go (mahr'go) *n.,* genit. **mar·gi·nis** (mahr'ji·nis), pl. **margi·nes** (·neez) MARGIN.

Ma·rie-Bam·ber·ger disease HYPERTROPHIC PULMONARY OSTEOARTHROPATHY.

Marie's ataxia MARIE'S HEREDITARY CEREBELLAR ATAXIA.

Marie-Strümpell encephalitis A focal imflammatory lesion of the brain observed in an infant with acute hemiplegia. In the light of current knowledge, the lesion probably represented acute necrotizing hemorrhagic encephalitis.

marihuana. MARIJUANA.

mar·i·jua·na (măr″i·wah′nuh) n. A relatively crude preparation of cannabis used most often for smoking; a mood-altering or mildly hallucinogenic drug.

Mar·jo·lin's ulcer (mar·zhoh·lăn′) An ulcer due to malignant change in an indolent ulcer or in a scar.

mark·er. A gene or gene-associated genetic element which is identifiable in individuals possessing it.

mar·mo·ri·za·tion (mahr″mo·ri·zay′shun) n. MARBLEIZATION.

Ma·ro·teaux-La·my syndrome (mah·roh·to′, lah·mee′) Mucopolysaccharidosis VI, transmitted as an autosomal recessive, characterized chemically by the excessive excretion of chondroitin sulfate B in the urine, and clinically by an appearance similar to that seen in the more common Hurler's syndrome, including marked skeletal changes and corneal opacities, but normal intellectual development.

mar·row (măr′o) n. 1. A fatty or soft substance occupying certain cavities; MEDULLA. 2. Specifically, bone marrow: the soft tissues contained in the medullary canals of long bones and in the interstices of cancellous bone.

marsh gas. The gaseous products, chiefly methane, formed from decaying, moist organic matter in marshes and mines.

Marsh's test A test for arsenic or antimony in which the metal is dissolved in dilute acid, reduced to arsine or stibine in the presence of zinc, and then deposited as metal on a cold surface. Potassium hypochlorite will dissolve arsenic but leave antimony.

mar·su·pi·al·iza·tion (mahr·sue″pee·ul·eye·zay′shun) n. An operation for pancreatic, hydatid, and other cysts when extirpation of the cyst walls and complete closure are not possible. The cyst is evacuated and its walls sutured to the edges of the wound, leaving the packed cavity to close by granulation. The procedure has been used also in cases of extrauterine pregnancy when the placenta cannot be removed. **—marsupial·ize** (mahr·sue′pee·ul·ize) v.

mas·cu·line (mas′kew·lin) adj. Having the appearance or qualities of a male. **—mas·cu·lin·i·ty** (mas″kew·lin′i·tee) n.

masculine pelvis. A pelvis resembling the normal male pelvis; an android pelvis.

mas·cu·lin·ize (mas′kew·lin·ize) v. To induce male secondary sex characteristics in a female or in a sexually immature animal. **—masculin·iza·tion** (mas″kew·lin·eye·zay′shun) n.

mas·cu·lin·o·ma (mas″kew·lin·o′muh) n. ADRENOCORTICOID ADENOMA OF THE OVARY.

mas·cu·lin·ovo·blas·to·ma (mas″kew·lin·o″vo·blas·to′muh) n. ADRENOCORTICOID ADENOMA OF THE OVARY.

mask, n. 1. A bandage applied to the face. 2. A gauze shield, fitted with tapes, to enclose the mouth and nose during surgical operations. 3. An apparatus for covering the nose and mouth in giving anesthetics.

mask face. An immobile, expressionless face, with flattened and smoother than usual features, seen in pseudobulbar palsy and in par-

kinsonism. In the latter disorder there may be near-normal voluntary movements of the face and an exaggerated frozen smile, but blinking, spontaneous smiling, and other associated involuntary movements are infrequent.

mask·ing, n. In audiometry, the use of a sound stimulus to interfere with the perception of one ear while testing the other.

mask of pregnancy. Irregularly shaped, brownish patches of varying size which frequently appear on the face and neck during pregnancy; CHLOASMA (1).

mas·o·chism (maz′uh·kiz·um, mas·o·) n. Pleasure derived from physical or psychological pain inflicted by oneself or by others, often unconsciously invited but sometimes sought consciously as in flagellation; a sexual component is always present; and in moral masochism there is an implication of punishment for some feeling of guilt. Masochistic tendencies exist to some extent in many human relationships and to a larger degree in most psychiatric disorders. It is the opposite of sadism but the two conditions tend to coexist in the same individual. **—maso·chist** (-kist) n.; **masochis·tic** (maz″uh·kis′tick) adj.

mass, n. 1. That essential property of matter which is responsible for inertia and weight. 2. A relatively solid or bulky piece of any substance or part of any object. 3. A cohesive medicinal substance that may be formed into pills. 4. (In attributive use) Space-occupying (as: mass lesion).

mas·sage (muh·sahzh′) n. The act of rubbing, kneading, or stroking the superficial parts of the body with the hand or with an instrument, for therapeutic purposes such as modifying nutrition, restoring power of movement, breaking up adhesions, or improving the circulation.

mas·se·ter (ma·see′tur) n. A muscle of mastication, arising from the zygomatic arch, and inserted into the mandible.

mas·seur (ma·sur′) n. 1. A man who practices massage. 2. An instrument used for mechanical massage.

mas·seuse (ma·suhz′, ·soos′) n. A woman who practices massage.

mass lesion. Any space-occupying lesion in the central nervous system, particularly the brain, such as an abscess, hematoma, or tumor.

Mas·son body (mah·sohn′) Fibrin and macrophages in the pulmonary alveoli in organizing pneumonia of any cause, originally thought to be associated with rheumatic pneumonitis.

mas·so·ther·a·py (mas″o·therr′uh·pee) n. Treatment by massage.

mass reflex. Exaggerated withdrawal reflexes accompanied by profuse sweating, piloerection, and automatic emptying of the bladder and occasionally of the rectum; observed in patients with transection of the spinal cord during the stage of heightened reflex activity.

mast-, masto- A combining form meaning (a) breast; (b) mastoid.

mas·tal·gia (mas·tal′juh, ·jee·uh) n. Pain in the breast. Syn. mastodynia (1).

mast cell A type of connective tissue cell associated with the formation and storage of heparin, histamine, and other pharmacologically active substances. It is characterized by numerous large, basophil, metachromatic granules.

mast-cell tumor. MASTOCYTOMA.

mas·tec·to·my (mas-teck'tuh-mee) *n.* Excision, or amputation, of the breast.

Master's two-step test TWO-STEP TEST.

mas·ti·cate (mas'ti-kate) *v.* To chew. —**mas·ti·ca·tion** (mas''ti-kay'shun) *n.*

mas·ti·ca·tor (mas'ti-kay''tur) *adj.* Of or pertaining to chewing or mastication.

mas·ti·ca·to·ry (mas'ti-kuh-to''ree) *adj. & n.* 1. For or pertaining to mastication. 2. A medicinal preparation to be chewed but not swallowed; used for its local action in the mouth.

masticatory system. The functional unit of mastication composed of the teeth, their surrounding and supporting structures, the jaws, the temporomandibular joints, the muscles which are attached to the mandible, lip and tongue muscles, and the vascular and nervous systems for these tissues.

mas·ti·tis (mas-tye'tis) *n.* Inflammation of the breast.

mas·to·cy·to·ma (mas''to-sigh-to''muh) *n.* A local proliferation of mast cells forming a tumorous nodule, seen most commonly in dogs, less frequently in cats, oxen, and men.

mas·to·cy·to·sis (mas''to-sigh-to'sis) *n.* Excessive proliferation of mast cells, either local (mastocytoma) or systemic.

mas·to·dyn·ia (mas''to-din'ee-uh) *n.* 1. A pain in the breast. Syn. *mastalgia.* 2. A type of mammary dysplasia in which pain and tenderness are prominent symptoms.

mas·toid (mas'toid) *adj. & n.* 1. Breast-shaped, as the mastoid process of the temporal bone. 2. The mastoid portion of the temporal bone.

mastoid air cell. MASTOID CELL.

mas·toid·al·gia (mas''toy-dal'jee-uh) *n.* Pain in, or over, the mastoid process.

mastoid antrum. The pneumatic space between the epitympanic recess and the mastoid cells.

mastoid cell. One of the compartments in the mastoid part of the temporal bone, connected with the mastoid antrum and lined with a thin mucous membrane. Syn. *mastoid air cell.*

mas·toid·ec·to·my (mas''toy-deck'tuh-mee) *n.* Exenteration of the mastoid cells.

mastoid foramen. A small foramen behind the mastoid process; it transmits a small artery from the dura mater and a vein opening into the lateral sinus.

mas·toid·i·tis (mas''toid-eye'tis) *n.*, pl. **mastoid·it·i·des** (·it'i-deez) Inflammation of the mastoid cells.

mas·toid·ot·o·my (mas''toy-dot'uh-mee) *n.* Incision into mastoid cells or the mastoid antrum.

mastoid process. The blunt inferior projection of the mastoid part of the temporal bone; it may be described as nipple-shaped.

mas·to·pa·ri·etal (mas''to-puh-rye'uh-tul) *adj.* PARIETOMASTOID.

mas·top·a·thy (mas-top'uth-ee) *n.* Any disease or pain of the mammary gland.

mas·to·pexy (mas'to-peck''see) *n.* Surgical fixation of a pendulous breast.

mas·to·pla·sia (mas''to-play'zhuh, ·zee-uh) *n.* 1. Hyperplasia of breast tissue. 2. MASTODYNIA (2).

mas·to·plas·ty (mas'to-plas''tee) *n.* Plastic surgery on the breast.

mas·tot·o·my (mas-tot'uh-mee) *n.* Incision of the breast.

mas·tous (mas'tus) *adj.* Having large breasts.

mas·tur·bate (mas'tur-bate) *v.* To manipulate the genitalia, usually producing an orgasm. —**mas·tur·ba·tion** (mas''tur-bay'shun) *n.*

match, *v.* To supply as nearly exact a counterpart as possible of a desired object, through comparison of the characteristics of that object with possible sources of counterparts, as the selection of blood donors whose erythrocytes have the same antigens as those of the recipient.

mate, *v.* To pair for breeding; to copulate.

ma·te·ria al·ba (ma-teer'ee-uh al'buh) A soft, cheeselike, white deposit on the necks of teeth and adjacent gums, made up of epithelial cells, leukocytes, bacteria, and molds.

materia med·i·ca (med'i-kuh) 1. The science that treats of the sources, properties, and preparation of medicinal substances. 2. A treatise on these substances.

ma·ter·nal (muh-tur'nul) *adj.* Pertaining to a mother.

maternal mortality rate. The number of deaths reported as due to puerperal causes in a calendar year per 100,000 live births reported in the same year and place.

ma·ter·ni·ty (muh-tur'ni-tee) *n.* 1. Motherhood. 2. PARTURITION.

mat·ri·cide (mat'ri-side) *n.* 1. The murder of one's own mother. 2. A person who murders his own mother.

ma·trix (may'tricks) *n.*, pl. **mat·ri·ces** (mat'riseez), **matrixes** 1. A mold; the cavity in which anything is formed. 2. That part of tissue into which any organ or process is set, as the matrix of a nail. 3. GROUND SUBSTANCE. 4. An arrangement of mathematical elements in rows and columns for special algebraic evaluation. *Adj. matrical.*

mat·ter, *n.* 1. Any material or substance, described as having three states of aggregation, solid, liquid, or gaseous. 2. PUS.

mat·u·ra·tion (match''oo-ray'shun, mat''yoo·) *n.* 1. The process of coming to full development. 2. The final series of changes in the growth and formation of the germ cells. It includes two divisions of the cell body but only one division of the chromosomes, with the result that the number of chromosomes in the mature germ cell is reduced to one-half (haploid, n) the original number (diploid, 2n). The term also includes the cytoplasmic changes which occur in the preparation of the germ cell for fertilization. 3. The achievement of emotional and intellectual maturity.

ma·ture (muh-tewr') *adj. & v.* 1. Fully developed, full grown, ripe. 2. To become ripe, to attain full development.

mature cataract. A cataract in which the whole

lens is opaque, of a dull gray or amber color, and in which the opacity has advanced to the anterior capsule and no shadow is thrown by the iris on the lens with focal illumination. Such a cataract is suitable for extraction.

ma·tur·i·ty (muh·tewr'i·tee) *n.* 1. The state of being mature. 2. The period of life when the organs of reproduction become and remain best capable of functioning. 3. The stage between adolescence or youth and old age or senescence.

maturity-onset diabetes. Diabetes mellitus which develops later in life, characterized by more gradual development and less severe symptoms than juvenile-onset diabetes.

ma·tu·ti·nal (muh·tew'ti·nul) *adj.* Occurring in the morning, as matutinal nausea.

max·il·la (mack·sil'uh) *n.,* pl. & genit. sing. **max·il·lae** (-ee) The bone of the upper jaw.

max·il·lary (mack''si·lerr·ee) *adj.* Of or pertaining to the maxilla.

maxillary antrum. MAXILLARY SINUS.

maxillary nerve. A somatic sensory nerve, attached to the trigeminal nerve, which innervates the meninges, the skin of the upper portion of the face, the upper teeth, and the mucosa of the nose, palate, and cheeks.

maxillary sinus. The paranasal sinus in the maxilla. Syn. *antrum of Highmore.*

max·il·lo·fa·cial (mack·sil''o·fay'shul) *adj.* Pertaining to the maxilla and the face.

max·il·lo·lac·ri·mal (mack·sil''o·lack'ri·mul) *adj.* Pertaining to the maxilla and the lacrimal bone.

max·il·lo·man·dib·u·lar (mack·sil''o·man·dib' yoo·lur) *adj.* Pertaining to the maxillae and the mandible.

max·il·lo·tur·bi·nal (mack·sil''o·tur'bi·nul) *n.* INFERIOR NASAL CONCHA.

max·i·mal (mack'si·mul) *adj.* Pertaining to the maximum; highest; greatest.

max·i·mum, *n.,* pl. **maxi·ma** (-muh) The greatest possible degree or amount of anything; the highest point attained or attainable by anything.

maximum breathing capacity. The greatest amount of air which can be voluntarily breathed during a 10-to-30-second period, and expressed as liters of air per minute. It is a test of many factors, including patient cooperation, his physical state, muscular function and lung compliance. Adequately performed, it is a reliable test of the ventilatory capacity of the thoracic bellows. Abbreviated, MBC.

May-Hegg·lin anomaly. Inclusions of basophilic RNA (Doehle bodies) in the cytoplasm of the granulocytes and marked variation in the size and shape of the platelets, inherited as an autosomal dominant trait.

may·hem (may'hem) *n. In legal medicine,* the willful, malicious, and usually permanent depriving of a person, by violence, of any limb, member, or organ, or causing any mutilation of the body.

¹maz-, mazo- A combining form meaning *breast.*

²maz-, mazo- A combining form meaning *placenta, placental.*

maze, *n.* A network of paths, blind alleys, and compartments; used in intelligence tests and in experimental psychology for developing learning curves.

ma·zo·pla·sia (may''zo·play'zhuh) *n.* MASTODYNIA (2).

Maz·zi·ni test A rapid cardiolipin slide flocculation test for syphilis.

M. B. *Medicinae Baccalaureus.* Bachelor of Medicine.

MBC Abbreviation for *maximum breathing capacity.*

M. C., M. Ch. *Magister Chirurgiae,* Master of Surgery.

mcg An abbreviation for *microgram.*

MCH Abbreviation for *mean corpuscular hemoglobin.*

MCHC Abbreviation for *mean corpuscular hemoglobin concentration.*

M-component. A single homogeneous (monoclonal) species of immunoglobulin; may be found in excess in benign or in malignant forms of hypergammaglobulinemia.

M-component hypergammaglobulinemia. A form of hypergammaglobulinemia characterized by a single, prominent, more or less narrow band occurring anywhere from the slow gamma (γ) to the fast alpha (α_1) region of the electrophoretic strip; associated clinically with neoplasia of the plasma cell, lymphoid, and reticuloendothelial cell series in such diseases as multiple myeloma, Waldenström syndrome leukemia, lymphoma, and carcinoma, but also found in apparently normal individuals.

MCV Abbreviation for *mean corpuscular volume.*

M.D. *Medicinae Doctor,* Doctor of Medicine.

M.D.S. Master of Dental Surgery.

mean, *adj. & n.* 1. Midway between extremes. 2. A point or value midway between two extremes, commonly of mathematical terms.

mean corpuscular hemoglobin. An expression, in absolute terms, of the average content of hemoglobin of the individual erythrocyte, calculated from the equation

$$MCH = \frac{hemoglobin\ [(g/100\ ml) \times 10]}{erythrocyte\ count\ (10^6/mm^3)}$$

and stated in picograms (10^{-12} g) per cell. Normal values are 28 to 32 pg. Abbreviated, MCH.

mean corpuscular hemoglobin concentration. An expression, in absolute terms, of the average hemoglobin concentration per unit volume (per 100 ml) of packed erythrocytes, calculated from the equation

$$MCHC = \frac{hemoglobin\ [(g/100\ ml) \times 100]}{hematocrit}$$

and stated in grams per 100 ml of packed red cells, or in percent. Normal values for adults are 32 to 36%. Abbreviated, MCHC.

mean corpuscular volume. An expression, in absolute terms, of the average volume of the individual erythrocyte, calculated from the equation

$$MCV = \frac{hematocrit\ (percent) \times 10}{erythrocyte\ count\ (10^6/mm^3)}$$

and stated in cubic micrometers per cell. Normal values are 82 to 92 μm^3, or 80 to 96 μm^3, depending on methods used. Abbreviated, MCV.

mea·sle (mee'zul) *n.* CYSTICERCUS.

mea·sles (mee'zulz) *n.* 1. An acute infectious viral disease, characterized by a fine dusty rose-red, maculopapular eruption and by catarrhal inflammation of the conjunctiva and of the air passages. After a period of incubation of nearly two weeks, the disease begins with coryza, cough, conjunctivitis, and the appearance of Koplik spots on the oral mucous membranes; on the third or fourth day chills and fever and dusky rose-red maculopapular eruptions appear, arranged in the form of crescentic groups, at times becoming confluent, usually appearing first on the face or behind the ears. In three or four days, the eruption gradually fades and is followed by a branny desquamation. The symptoms are worse at the height of the eruption. The disease affects principally the young, is exceedingly contagious, and one attack of the vaccine usually confers immunity. Central nervous system involvement may occur. Syn. *rubeola.* 2. Plural of *measle;* CYSTICERCI.

measles encephalitis. Acute disseminated encephalomyelitis as a result of measles.

measles immune globulin. A sterile solution of globulins from the blood plasma of human donors; used for passive immunization against measles.

measles virus vaccine. A vaccine prepared from measles virus. Two principal types are available: live attenuated measles virus vaccine, and inactivated measles virus vaccine. Both vaccines produce active immunity against measles, although only the live attenuated vaccine is in current use.

mea·sly (meez'lee) *adj.* 1. Infected with measles; spotted with measles. 2. Containing cysticerci; said of pork.

meat-, meato-. A combining form meaning *meatus.*

me·a·ti·tis (mee''ay·tigh'tis, mee''uh·) *n.* Inflammation of the wall of a meatus.

me·a·tot·o·my (mee''uh·tot'um·ee) *n.* Incision into and enlargement of a meatus.

me·a·tus (mee·ay'tus) *n.,* L. pl. & genit. sing. **meatus** An opening or passage. —**mea·tal** (·tul) *adj.*

meatus acu·sti·cus ex·ter·nus (a·koos'ti·kus ecks·tur'nus) [NA]. EXTERNAL ACOUSTIC MEATUS.

meatus acusticus in·ter·nus (in·tur'nus) [NA]. INTERNAL ACOUSTIC MEATUS.

meatus na·si com·mu·nis (nay'zye kom·ew'nis) [BNA]. The portion of each nasal cavity adjacent to the nasal septum.

meatus ure·thrae (yoo·ree'three). The orifice or external ostium of the urethra.

mec·a·myl·a·mine (meck''a·mil'uh·meen) *n.* $N,2,3,3$-Tetramethyl-2-norbornanamine, $C_{11}H_{21}N$, a ganglionic blocking agent used, as the hydrochloride salt, for treatment of hypertension.

me·chan·i·cal (me·kan'i·kul) *adj.* Caused by or pertaining to gross physical forces as opposed to chemical, electrical, or other forces.

mechanical fragility. The susceptibility to breakage of erythrocytes when mechanically agitated under standard conditions as with glass beads in a flask.

mechanical ileus. Obstruction of the intestines by extrinsic pressure or internal blockage, due to a variety of causes.

mech·a·nism (meck'uh·niz·um) *n.* 1. An aggregation of parts arranged in a mechanical way to perform a specific function. 2. A series or combination of processes by which a given change in the state of matter or energy is brought about.

mech·a·no·re·cep·tor (meck''uh·no·re·sep'tur) *n.* A specialized structure of sensory nerve terminals which responds to mechanical stimuli such as pressure or touch.

mech·a·no·ther·a·py (meck''uh·no·therr'uh·pee) *n.* Treatment of injury or disease by mechanical means. —**mechanothera·pist** (·pist) *n.*

me·chlor·eth·a·mine hydrochloride (meck''lor·eth'uh·meen). 2,2'-Dichloro-*N*-methyldiethylamine hydrochloride, $C_5H_{11}Cl_2N \cdot HCl$; white, crystalline, hygroscopic powder. A cytotoxic drug used for the treatment of various neoplastic diseases. Syn. *mustine hydrochloride, nitrogen mustard* (1).

me·cism (mee'siz·um) *n.* A condition marked by abnormal lengthening of one or more parts of the body.

Meckel's diverticulum DIVERTICULUM ILEI.

mec·li·zine (meck'li·zeen) *n.* 1-(*p*-Chloro-α-phenylbenzyl)-4-(*m*-methylbenzyl)piperazine, $C_{25}H_{27}ClN_2$, an antinauseant drug used as the hydrochloride salt.

me·com·e·ter (me·kom'e·tur) *n.* An instrument resembling calipers with attached scales used in measuring fetuses or newborn infants.

mecon-, mecono-. A combining form meaning *opium.*

me·co·nal·gia (mee''ko·nal'jee·uh, meck''on·al'jee·uh) *n.* Pain or neuralgia when the use of opium is discontinued.

me·con·ic (me·kon'ick, ·ko'nick) *adj.* 1. Pertaining to or derived from opium. 2. Pertaining to the meconium.

meconic acid. 3-Hydroxy-4-oxo-1,4-pyran-2,6-dicarboxylic acid, $C_7H_4O_7$, a dibasic acid occurring in opium.

me·co·ni·or·rhea (me·ko'nee·o·ree'uh, meck''o·nigh'o·) *n.* An excessive discharge of meconium.

me·co·ni·um (me·ko'nee·um) *n.* The pasty, greenish mass, consisting of mucus, desquamated epithelial cells, bile, lanugo hairs, and vernix caseosa, that collects in the intestine of the fetus. It forms the first fecal discharge of the newborn and is not wholly expelled until the third or fourth day after birth.

meconium ileus. Intestinal obstruction caused by inspissation of the meconium due to deficiency of trypsin production, occurring in the newborn with cystic fibrosis of the pancreas.

me·cys·ta·sis (me·sis'tuh·sis) *n.* A process in which a muscle increases in length but maintains its original degree of tension. —**mecy·stat·ic** (mes''i·stat'ick) *adj.*

medi-, medio-. A combining form meaning *middle, medial, median,* or *intermediate.*

me·di·a (mee'dee-uh) *n.* 1. TUNICA MEDIA; the middle coat of a vein, artery, or lymph vessel. 2. Plural of *medium.*

me·di·ad (mee'dee·ad) *adv.* Toward the median plane or line.

me·di·al (mee'dee·ul) *adj.* 1. Internal, as opposed to lateral (external); toward the midline of the body. 2. Of or pertaining to the tunica media or middle coat of a blood vessel.

medial aperture of the fourth ventricle. MEDIAN APERTURE OF THE FOURTH VENTRICLE.

medial arteriosclerosis or calcinosis. Calcification of the middle coat of the small- and medium-sized muscular arteries. Syn. *Mönckeberg's arteriosclerosis.*

medial geniculate body. A nuclear mass just lateral to the posterior thalamic zone which receives auditory impulses from the inferior colliculus and relays them to the superior temporal (Heschl's) gyri via the auditory radiation.

medial lemniscus. A lemniscus arising in the nucleus gracilis and nucleus cuneatus, crossing almost immediately as internal arcuate fibers, and terminating mainly in the posterolateral ventral nucleus of the thalamus.

medial ligament. The ligament on the medial side of the ankle joint, attached to the tibia at the medial malleolus and consisting of a part, an anterior and posterior tibiotalar part, a tibiocalcaneal part, and a tibionavicular part. Syn. *deltoid ligament.*

medial longitudinal fasciculus. One of two heavily medullated bundles close to the midline, just ventral to the central gray matter and extending from the upper spinal cord to the rostral end of the midbrain.

medial malleolus. A process on the internal surface of the lower extremity of the tibia. Syn. *internal malleolus.*

medial meniscus. The articular disk in the knee joint between the medial condyles of the tibia and femur; a crescentic fibrocartilaginous disk attached to the margin of the medial condyle of the tibia, resting on and serving to deepen the tibia's medial articular surface. Syn. *internal semilunar cartilage.*

medial necrosis of aorta. MEDIONECROSIS AORTAE IDIOPATHICA CYSTICA.

medial vestibular nucleus. A nucleus in the floor of the fourth ventricle medial and lateral to the ala cinerea.

me·di·an (mee'dee·un) *adj. & n.* 1. Situated or placed in the middle of the body or in the middle of a part of the body, as the arm. 2. That value on the numerical scale of classification in a frequency distribution below which and above which half the observations fall.

median aperture of the fourth ventricle. An aperture in the posterior central portion of the fourth ventricle through which cerebrospinal fluid passes into the subarachnoid space. Syn. *foramen of Magendie.*

median bar. Contracture of the vesical neck, or constriction of the prostatic urethra, caused by prostatic hyperplasia (glandular bar) or by overgrowth of connective tissue across the posterior lip of the vesical orifice or of the vesical trigone (fibrous bar).

median laryngotomy. Incision of the larynx through the thyroid cartilage; THYROTOMY.

median lethal dose. That dose of an injurious agent (drug, virus, radiation) given to a population of animals or man, that 50 percent will die within a specific time period. Symbol, LD 50, LD_{50}.

median nasal process. The entire region between the olfactory sacs and below the frontonasal sulcus of the embryo. It forms the bridge, mobile septum, and anterior portion of the cartilaginous septum of the nose, the philtrum of the lip, and the premaxillary portion of the upper jaw.

median plane. A plane that bisects a structure in the anteroposterior direction, dividing it into right and left halves.

median rhomboidal glossitis. A congenital anomaly of the tongue in which an oval or rhomboidal area, devoid of papillae and sometimes elevated, is found on the dorsal surface anterior to the circumvallate papillae.

me·di·as·ti·nal (mee"dee·as·tye'nul) *adj.* Of or pertaining to a mediastinum.

mediastinal emphysema. Accumulation of air in the tissues of the mediastinum.

me·di·as·ti·ni·tis (mee"dee·as''ti·nigh'tis) *n.* Inflammation of the tissues of the mediastinum.

me·di·as·ti·no·per·i·car·di·tis (mee·dee·as·tigh''no·perr'i·kahr·dye'tis) *n.* 1. Combined inflammation of the mediastinum and the pericardium. 2. POLYSEROSITIS.

me·di·as·tino·scope (mee"dee·as·tin'o·skope) *n.* An instrument for examining the mediastinum through a skin incision.

me·di·as·ti·nos·co·py (mee"dee·as''ti·nos'kuh·pee) *n.* Examination of the mediastinum using the mediastinoscope.

me·di·as·ti·not·o·my (mee"dee·as''ti·not'um·ee) *n.* Incision into the mediastinum.

me·di·as·ti·num (mee"dee·as·tye'num) *n.,* pl. **mediasti·na** (·nuh) 1. A partition separating adjacent parts. 2. [NA] The space left in the middle of the chest between the two pleurae, divided into the anterior, middle, posterior, and superior mediastinum.

¹me·di·ate (mee'dee·ate) *v.* To function as an interposed action in a chain of actions, as adrenocorticotrophin mediates the hypothalamic regulation of cortisol secretion.

²me·di·ate (mee'dee·ut) *adj.* Indirect; performed through something interposed.

mediate auscultation. Listening with the aid of a stethoscope interposed between the ear and the part being examined.

mediate percussion. INDIRECT PERCUSSION.

me·di·a·tor (mee'dee·ay''tur) *n.* An agent, such as a hormone, that mediates a chemical reaction or a process of a particular type.

med·i·ca·ble (med'i·kuh·bul) *adj.* 1. Amenable to cure. 2. Specifically, amenable to drug therapy.

med·i·cal (med'i·kul) *adj.* 1. Pertaining to medicine. 2. Pertaining to the nonsurgical treatment of disease.

medical center. 1. A medical clinic usually serving a discrete geographical area. 2. A group of medical facilities, incorporating all the medical specialities, and possessing the capacity for medical education, and the diagnosis, care, and treatment of patients.

medical examiner. 1. A professionally qualified physician duly authorized and charged by a governmental unit, such as a municipality, county, or state, to determine facts concerning causes of death, particularly when not occurring under natural circumstances, and to testify thereto in courts of law. Such a physician now frequently replaces or works with a coroner, who may not be a physician, or a coroner's jury of laymen. 2. An officer of a corporation or bureau, whose duty is to determine facts relating to injuries and deaths alleged to have occurred, to place responsibility on the part of the corporation or other agency, and to make recommendations as to compensation. In certain cases, as in life insurance applications, the examiner is charged with passing upon the state of health.

medical history. An account of the past and present medical status of a patient.

me·dic·a·ment (me·dick'uh·munt, med'i·kuh·munt) n. A medicinal substance used for the treatment of disease.

med·i·cant (med'i·kunt) n. MEDICATION (3).

Medicare. Popular designation for 1965 amendments to the U.S. Social Security Act, providing hospitalization and certain other benefits to qualified people, most of them over age 65.

med·i·cate (med'i·kate) v. 1. To impregnate with medicine. 2. To treat with a medicine.

med·i·cat·ed (med'i·kay·tid) adj. Containing a medicinal substance.

med·i·ca·tion (med''i·kay'shun) n. 1. Impregnation with a medicine. 2. Treatment by medicines; the administration of medicines. 3. A medicine or combination of medicines administered.

me·dic·i·nal (me·dis'i·nul) adj. Pertaining to, due to, or having the nature of medicine.

med·i·cine (med'i·sin) n. 1. Any substance used for treating disease. 2. The science of treating disease; the healing art. 3. In a restricted sense, that branch of the healing art dealing with internal diseases, which can be treated by a physician rather than by a surgeon.

med·i·co·le·gal (med''i·ko·lee'gul) adj. Pertaining both to medicine and law.

med·i·co·psy·chol·o·gy (med''i·ko·sigh·kol'uh·jee) n. The study of mental diseases in relation to medicine.

med·i·co·sta·tis·tic (med''i·ko·stuh·tis'tick) adj. Pertaining to medical statistics.

med·i·co·sur·gi·cal (med''i·ko·sur'ji·kul) adj. Pertaining conjointly to medicine and surgery.

me·dio·car·pal (mee''dee·o·kahr'pul) adj. Between the two rows of carpal bones.

me·dio·dor·sal (mee''dee·o·dor'sul) adj. Both median and dorsal; on the median line of the back.

me·dio·fron·tal (mee''dee·o·frun'tul, ·fron'tul)

adj. Pertaining to the middle of the forehead.

me·dio·lat·er·al (mee''dee·o·lat'ur·al) adj. Pertaining to the median plane and one side.

me·dio·ne·cro·sis (mee''dee·o·ne·kro'sis) n. Necrosis occurring in the tunica media of an artery.

medionecrosis aor·tae id·io·path·i·ca cys·ti·ca (ay·or'tee id''ee·o·path'i·kuh sis'ti·kuh) Degeneration of the muscle and elastic fibers of the aorta. Syn. *medial necrosis of aorta.*

me·dio·plan·tar (mee''dee·o·plan'tahr, ·tur) adj. Pertaining to the midsole.

me·dio·su·pe·ri·or (mee''dee·o·sue·peer'ee·ur) adj. Toward the middle and above.

me·dio·tar·sal (mee''dee·o·tahr'sul) adj. Pertaining to the middle articulations of the tarsal bones.

Med·i·ter·ra·nean anemia or **disease.** THALASSEMIA.

Mediterranean fever. BRUCELLOSIS.

me·di·um (mee'dee·um) n., pl. **me·dia** (·dee·uh) 1. That in which anything moves or through which it acts. 2. *In microbiology,* any substrate on which microorganisms are cultivated.

me·di·us (mee'dee·us) adj. & n. 1. Middle. 2. The middle finger.

MEDLARS A computerized system to aid in the search and retrieval of articles published in medical and related journals, based on the citations in Index Medicus, and made available through the U.S. National Library of Medicine.

me·dul·la (me·dul'uh) n., pl. & genit. sing. **medul·lae** (·ee) 1. A fatty or soft substance occupying certain cavities; MARROW. 2. The central part of certain organs as distinguished from the cortex. 3. MEDULLA OBLONGATA.

medulla ob·lon·ga·ta (ob''long·gay'tuh, ·gah'tuh) [NA]. The most caudal part of the brain and extending from the pons to the spinal cord.

med·ul·lary (med'yoo·lerr·ee, med'uh·, me·dul'ur·ee) adj. 1. Pertaining to a medulla. 2. Pertaining to or resembling marrow. 3. Pertaining to the spinal cord or medulla oblongata.

medullary canal. The cavity of a long bone, containing the marrow.

medullary carcinoma. A form of poorly differentiated adenocarcinoma, usually of the breast, grossly well circumscribed, gray-pink and firm. Syn. *encephaloid carcinoma.*

medullary cords. 1. The primary invaginations of the germinal epithelium of the embryonic gonad that differentiate into rete testis and seminiferous tubules or into rete ovarii. Syn. *primary cords, testis cords.* 2. The cords of dense, lymphatic tissue separated by sinuses in the medulla of a lymph node.

medullary cystic disease of the kidney. A slowly progressive familial disease characterized by multiple renal medullary cysts, usually located at the corticomedullary junction, in association with interstitial fibrosis; it appears clinically in childhood as a salt-wasting syndrome with anemia and uremia. Syn. *familial juvenile nephronophthisis.*

medullary plate. NEURAL PLATE.

medullary rays. Raylike extensions of medullary substance of the kidney projected from the base of the medullary pyramid into the cortex. Syn. *cortical rays.*

medullary sponge kidney. A congenital condition characterized by bilateral cystic dilatations of the papillary collecting ducts; occasionally renal calculi or pyelonephritis develop.

medullary syndrome. Any clinical complex or disorder resulting from involvement of the motor and sensory pathways and of the cranial nerve nuclei within the medulla oblongata.

medullary tractotomy. Surgical incision of the spinothalamic tract in the medulla or of the descending or spinal root of the trigeminal nerve. Syn. *bulbar tractotomy.*

medulla spi·na·lis (spye-nay′lis) [NA]. SPINAL CORD.

med·ul·lat·ed (med″uh-lay-tid, med′yoo-, me-dul′ay-tid) *adj.* MYELINATED.

med·ul·la·tion (med″uh-lay′shun, med″yoo-) *n.* MYELINIZATION.

med·ul·li·za·tion (med″uh-lye-zay′shun, med″yoo-li-zay′shun) *n.* Conversion into marrow, as the replacement of bone tissue in the course of osteitis.

med·ul·lo·blas·to·ma (med″uh-lo-blas-to′muh, med″yoo-lo-, me-dul′o-) *n.* A malignant brain tumor with a tendency to spread in the meninges; most common in the cerebellum of children. The cells are small, with scanty cytoplasm, dense spheroid or oval nuclei, many mitoses, and a tendency to form pseudorosettes.

med·ul·lo·ep·i·the·li·o·ma (med″uh-lo-ep″i-theel-ee-o′muh) *n. Obsol.* 1. EPENDYMOMA. 2. A locally invasive tumor of the eye arising from the ciliary epithelium or iris.

meg-, mega- A combining form meaning (a) *large, extended, enlarged;* (b) *unit one million times as large as* a specified unit of measure.

mega·blad·der (meg″uh-blad′ur) *n.* MEGALOCYSTIS.

mega·car·dia (meg″uh-kahr′dee-uh) *n.* MEGALOCARDIA.

mega·ce·cum, mega·cae·cum (meg″uh-see′kum) *n.* A cecum with a markedly distended lumen.

mega·co·lon (meg′uh-ko″lun) *n.* Hypertrophy and dilatation of the colon, usually first seen in childhood, associated with prolonged constipation and consequent abdominal distention.

mega·co·ni·al (meg″uh-ko′nee-ul) *adj.* Pertaining to or characterized by large mitochondria or particles seen in certain cells with the electron microscope.

megacystis syndrome. A large, thin walled urinary bladder with poor muscular development, often associated with ureteral reflux; usually congenital in origin.

mega·dont (meg′uh-dont) *adj.* Having abnormally large teeth; MACRODONT.

mega·du·o·de·num (meg″uh-dew-o-dee′num, dew-od′e-num) *n.* Idiopathic dilatation of the duodenum.

mega·dyne (meg″uh-dine) *n.* A million dynes.

mega·esoph·a·gus, mega·oe·soph·a·gus (meg″uh-e-sof′uh-gus) *n.* A markedly dilated esophagus.

mega·gna·thus (meg″uh-naith′us) *n.* An individual having an abnormally large jaw.

mega·karyo·blast (meg″uh-kār′ee-o-blast) *n.* An immature, developing megakaryocyte. It is a large cell with nongranular, deeply basophilic cytoplasm, and a nucleus showing a fine chromatin structure and numerous nucleoli.

mega·karyo·cyte (meg″uh-kār′ee-o-site) *n.* A giant cell of bone marrow, 30 to 70μm, containing a large, irregularly lobulated nucleus; the progenitor of blood platelets. The cytoplasm contains fine azurophil granules. —**mega·karyo·cyt·ic** (-kār″ee-o-sit′ick) *adj.*

mega·karyo·cy·to·pe·nia (meg″uh-kār″ee-o-sigh″to-pee′nee-uh) *n.* MEGAKARYOPHTHISIS.

mega·karyo·cy·to·sis (meg″uh-kār″ee-o-sigh-to′sis) *n.* Excessive numbers of megakaryocytes.

mega·karyo·phthi·sis (meg″uh-kār-ee-off′thi-sis, -kār″ee-o-thigh′sis) *n.* A scarcity of megakaryocytes in the bone marrow.

meg·al·er·y·the·ma (meg″ul-err-ith-ee′muh) *n.* ERYTHEMA INFECTIOSUM.

meg·a·lo·blast (meg′ul-o-blast) *n.* A large erythroblast with a characteristic nuclear pattern formed in marrow in vitamin B₁₂ or folic acid deficiency. —**meg·a·lo·blas·tic** (meg″ul-o-blas′tick) *adj.*

megaloblastic anemia. Any anemia characterized by the presence of megaloblasts in the bone marrow, usually associated with macrocytosis in the peripheral blood.

meg·a·lo·blas·toid (meg″ul-o-blas′toid) *adj.* Resembling a megaloblast.

meg·a·lo·car·dia (meg″ul-o-kahr′dee-uh) *n.* Enlargement of the heart.

meg·a·lo·ceph·a·ly (meg″ul-o-sef′uh-lee) *n.* 1. The condition of having a head whose maximum fronto-occipital circumference is greater than two standard deviations above the mean for age and sex. 2. LEONTIASIS OSSEA. —**megalo·ce·phal·ic** (-se-fal′ick) *adj.*

meg·a·lo·cor·nea (meg″ul-o-kor′nee-uh) *n.* An enlarged cornea.

meg·a·lo·cys·tis (meg″uh-lo-sis′tis) *n.* Abnormal enlargement of the urinary bladder.

meg·a·lo·cyte (meg′ul-o-site) *n.* A large, nonnucleated, red blood corpuscle, usually oval, derived from a megaloblast. —**meg·a·lo·cyt·ic** (meg″ul-o-sit′ick) *adj.*

meg·a·lo·gas·tria (meg″ul-o-gas′tree-uh) *n.* Abnormal enlargement of the stomach.

meg·a·lo·ma·nia (meg″ul-o-may′nee-uh) *n.* A delusion of personal greatness; the patient is pathologically preoccupied with or expresses in words or actions ideas of exalted attainment, power, or wealth, a symptom common in schizophrenia and other psychoses. —**megalo·man·ic** (-man′ick) *adj.;* **megalo·ma·ni·ac** (-may′nee-ack) *n.*

meg·a·lo·mas·tia (meg″ul-o-mas′tee-uh) *n.* MACROMASTIA.

meg·a·lo·me·lia (meg″ul-o-mee′lee-uh) *n.* Excessive enlargement of one or more limbs.

meg·al·on·y·cho·sis (meg″uh-lon-i-ko′sis) *n.* Universal, noninflammatory hypertrophy of the nails.

meg·a·lo·pe·nis (meg″ul·o·pee′nis) *n.* Abnormally large penis; MACROPHALLUS.

meg·a·loph·thal·mos, meg·a·loph·thal·mus (meg″ul·off·thal′mus) *n.* Excessive largeness of the eyes.

meg·a·lo·splanch·nic (meg″ul·o·splank′nick) *adj.* Possessing large viscera, especially a large liver.

meg·a·lo·ure·ter (meg″ul·o·yoo·ree′tur) *n.* A greatly enlarged ureter.

-megaly A combining form designating *abnormal enlargement.*

mega·nu·cle·us (meg″uh·new′klee·us) *n.* MACRONUCLEUS.

mega·pros·o·pous (meg″uh·pros′uh·pus) *adj.* Having an unusually large face.

mega·ure·ter (meg″uh·yoo·ree′tur, ·yoo·ree′tur) *n.* MEGALOURETER.

mega·volt (meg′uh·vohlt) *n.* A unit equal to 1 million volts.

me·glu·mine (me·gloo′meen, meg′loo·meen) *n.* *N*-Methylglucamine, $C_7H_{17}NO_5$, a crystalline base; used to prepare salts of certain acidic radiopaque and therapeutic substances.

me·grim (mee′grim) *n. Obsol.* MIGRAINE.

Mei·bo·mi·an cyst (migh·bo′mee·un) CHALAZION.

mei·bo·mi·a·ni·tis (migh·bo″mee·uh·nigh′tis) *n.* Inflammation of tarsal glands.

Meigs's syndrome (megz) Ovarian fibroma with ascites and hydrothorax.

mei·o·sis (migh·o′sis) *n.,* pl. **meio·ses** (·seez) The nuclear changes which take place in the last two cell divisions in the formation of the germ cells. The chromosomes separate from one another once but the cell body divides twice with the result that the nucleus of the mature egg or sperm contains the reduced (haploid) number of chromosomes. In addition, by mechanisms such as crossing-over, chromosomal segments are exchanged between chromatids and genetic variation is achieved. Syn. *reduction division.* —**mei·ot·ic** (migh·ot′ick) *adj.*

Meiss·ner's corpuscle (mice′nur) An ovoid end organ connected with one or more myelinated nerve fibers which lose their sheaths as they enter a surrounding capsule, make several spiral turns, and break up into a complex network of branches. Found in the dermal papillae especially of the volar surfaces of the fingers and toes.

Meissner's plexus SUBMUCOUS PLEXUS.

¹mel-, melo- A combining form meaning *limb, extremity.*

²mel-, melo- A combining form meaning *cheek.*

me·lal·gia (me·lal′jee·uh) *n.* Pain or neuralgia in the extremities.

melan-, melano- A combining form meaning (a) *black, dark;* (b) *pertaining to melanin.*

mel·an·cho·lia (mel″un·ko′lee·uh) *n.* Severe depression, usually of psychotic proportion. —**melan·chol·ic** (·kol′ick), *adj.;* **melan·cho·li·ac** (·ko′lee·ack) *n.*

mel·an·choly (mel′un·kol·ee) *n.* 1. Dejection, gloom, sadness. 2. MELANCHOLIA.

mel·an·idro·sis (mel″uh·ni·dro′sis, me·lan″i·) *n.*

A form of chromhidrosis in which the sweat is dark-colored or black.

mel·a·nif·er·ous (mel″uh·nif′ur·us) *adj.* Containing melanin.

mel·a·nin (mel′uh·nin) *n.* A group of black or dark-brown pigments produced by many kinds of cells. Occurs naturally in the choroid coat of the eye, the skin, hair, cardiac muscle, pia mater, adrenal medulla, and nervous tissue. Chemically, melanins are polymers of indole-5,6-quinone, which may be derived from 3,4-dihydroxyphenylalanine, from epinephrine, from homogentisic acid, or from *p*-phenylenediamine.

mel·a·nism (mel′uh·nizum) *n.* Abnormal deposition of dark pigment (melanin) in tissues, in organs, or in the skin.

mel·a·nize (mel′uh·nize) *v.* To form and deposit melanin in a tissue or organ. —**mel·a·ni·za·tion** (mel″uh·nigh·zay′shun) *n.*

mel·a·no·am·e·lo·blas·to·ma (mel″uh·no·am″e·lo·blas·to′muh) *n.* Ameloblastoma in which melanin is found.

mel·a·no·blast (mel′uh·no·blast) *n.* 1. The precursor of all melanocytes and melanophores. 2. *In biology,* an immature pigment cell, of neural crest origin, in certain vertebrates. 3. *In medicine,* the mature melanin-elaborating cell.

mel·a·no·blas·to·ma (mel″uh·no·blas·to′muh) *n.* A malignant melanoma.

mel·a·no·car·ci·no·ma (mel″uh·no·kahr·si·no′muh) *n.* A malignant melanoma.

mel·a·no·cyte (mel′uh·no·site, me·lan′o·) *n.* A fully differentiated melanin-forming cell; a cell which synthesizes melanosomes.

melanocyte–stimulating hormone. A substance found in the pituitary gland which causes darkening of human skin and nevi, formation of new pigmented nevi, and pigmentary changes in fish and amphibia, where it has been called intermedin. Abbreviated, MSH. Syn. *melanophore hormone, melanophore-dilating principle.*

mel·a·no·cy·to·ma (mel″uh·no·sigh·to′muh) *n.* 1. Any benign tumor of melanocytes. 2. A benign, heavily pigmented tumor of melanocytes arising at the optic disk.

mel·a·no·cy·to·sis (mel″uh·no·sigh·to′sis) *n.* An excessive number of melanocytes.

mel·a·no·der·ma (mel″uh·no·dur′muh) *n.* Any abnormal darkening of the skin, either diffuse or in patches, and either by accumulation of melanin or by deposition of other substances as, for example, silver salts in argyria. —**mela·noder·mic** (·mick) *adj.*

mel·a·no·der·ma·ti·tis (mel″uh·no·dur″muh·tigh′tis) *n.* Any inflammatory skin disease accompanied by increased skin pigmentation.

mel·a·no·ep·i·the·li·o·ma (mel″uh·no·ep·i·theel·ee·o′muh) *n.* A malignant melanoma.

me·lano·gen (me·lan′o·jin) *n.* A colorless precursor which is transformed into melanin. Patients, especially those with widespread melanomas, may excrete urine containing melanogen; on standing, the urine becomes dark brown or black.

mel·a·no·gen·e·sis (mel″uh·no·jen′e·sis) *n.* The formation of melanin.

mel·a·no·glos·sia (mel″uh·no·glos′ee·uh) *n.*
BLACKTONGUE.

mel·a·no·ma (mel″uh·no′muh) *n.* 1. A malignant
tumor whose parenchyma is composed of
anaplastic melanocytes. 2. Any tumor, benign
or malignant, of melanocytes.

mel·a·no·ma·to·sis (mel″uh·no″muh·to′sis) *n.*
Widespread distribution of melanoma.

mel·a·no·nych·ia (mel″uh·no·nick′ee·uh) *n.*
Blackening of the fingernails or toenails.

mel·a·no·phage (mel″uh·no·faje) *n.* A cell, unrelated to the pigment-producing cells, which
contains phagocytized melanin.

mel·a·no·phore (mel″uh·no·fore, me·lan′o·) *n.* A
type of melanocyte which participates with
other pigment cells in the rapid color changes
of certain animals; rearrangement of melanosomes within the cell is probably responsible.

mel·a·no·pla·kia (mel″uh·no·play′kee·uh) *n.*
Pigmentation of the mucous membrane of the
mouth, usually in patches and occasionally
with leukoplakia superimposed.

mel·a·nor·rha·gia (mel″uh·no·ray′jee·uh) *n.* MEL-
ENA.

mel·a·no·sar·co·ma (mel″uh·no·sahr·ko′muh) *n.*
A malignant melanoma.

mel·a·no·sis (mel″uh·no′sis) *n.* Dark-brown or
brownish-black pigmentation of surfaces by
melanins or, in some instances, by hematogenous pigments. —**mel·a·not·ic** (mel″uh·not′-
ick) *adj.*

**melanosis cir·cum·scrip·ta pre·blas·to·ma·to·sa
of Du·breuilh** (sur″kum·skrip′tuh pree·blas″-
to·muh·to′suh) LENTIGO MALIGNA.

melanosis co·li (ko′lye). Brown-black pigmentation of mucosa of the colon in innumerable,
approximated, minute foci.

melanosis iri·dis (irr′i·dis, eye′ri·dis). Abnormal
melanotic pigmentation of the iris.

mel·a·no·some (mel″uh·no·sohm) *n.* A discrete,
melanin-containing organelle, ovoid, about
0.2 nm. in diameter; membrane-bound and
has longitudinally arranged fibers on which
the pigment is located.

melanotic freckle. LENTIGO MALIGNA.

melanotic sarcoma. A malignant melanoma.

melanotic whitlow. A malignant melanoma of
the nail bed.

mel·a·not·ri·chous (mel″uh·not′ri·kus) *adj.*
Black-haired.

mel·a·nu·ria (mel″uh·new′ree·uh) *n.* The presence of black pigment in the urine, the result
of oxidation of melanogens. —**melanu·ric**
(·rick) *adj.*

me·las·ma (me·laz′muh) *n.* MELANODERMA.

mel·a·to·nin (mel″uh·to′nin) *n. N*-acetyl-5-meth-
oxytryptamine, $C_{13}H_{16}O_2N_2$, a compound secreted by the pineal gland which has been
found to inhibit the estrous cycle.

me·le·na, me·lae·na (me·lee′nuh) *n.* The discharge of stools colored black by altered
blood.

me·le·nic, me·lae·nic (me·lee′nick) *adj.* Pertaining to, or marked by, melena.

meli- A combining form meaning *sugar.*

meli·bi·ose (mel″i·bye′oce, ·oze) *n.* A disaccharide, $C_{12}H_{22}O_{11}$, resulting from hydrolysis of
raffinose and also occurring naturally; it may
be hydrolyzed to glucose and galactose.

mel·i·oi·do·sis (mel″ee·oy·do′sis) *n.* A disease
characterized by infectious granulomas similar to glanders; it is primarily a disease of
rodents but is occasionally communicable to
man. This disease has been observed in Ma-
laysia, Indochina, and Ceylon and is caused
by *Pseudomonas pseudomallei.*

me·li·tis (me·lye′tis) *n.* Inflammation of the
cheek.

mel·i·tu·ria (mel″i·tew′ree·uh) *n.* The presence of
any sugar in urine.

Mel·kers·son-Ro·sen·thal syndrome A disease of
unknown cause, usually beginning in childhood or adolescence characterized by recurrent peripheral facial paralysis, swelling of the
face and lips, and deep furrows in the tongue.
May be hereditary.

melo·ma·nia (mel″o·may′nee·uh) *n.* A psychotic
disorder marked by an inordinate devotion to
music. —**melomani·ac** (·ack) *n.*

me·lom·e·lus (me·lom′e·lus) *n.* An individual
with one or more rudimentary accessory
limbs attached to a limb.

melo·rhe·os·to·sis (mel″o·ree″os·to′sis) *n.* A very
rare condition of unknown cause in which
certain bones, or parts of bones, undergo
asymmetrical or local enlargement and sclerotic changes, typically confined to the bones
of one extremity, with distortion of affected
bone, limitation of movement in the joints
between the bones, and marked pain. Syn.
Léri type of osteopetrosis.

me·los·chi·sis (me·los′ki·sis) *n.* A facial cleft,
usually a transverse one.

me·lo·tus (me·lo′tus) *n.* An individual showing
congenital displacement of the ear, which lies
on the cheek.

mel·pha·lan (mel′fuh·lan) *n.* L-3-*p*-[Bis(2-chloro-
ethyl)amino]-phenylalanine, $C_{13}H_{18}Cl_2N_2O_2$,
an antineoplastic drug.

mem·ber, *n.* A part of the body, especially a
projecting part, as the upper or lower extremity.

mem·bra·na (mem·bray′nuh) *n.,* pl. & genit.
sing. **membra·nae** (·nee) MEMBRANE.

membrana tym·pa·ni (tim′puh·nigh) [NA]. TYM-
PANIC MEMBRANE.

mem·brane (mem′brane) *n.* A thin layer of tissue
surrounding a part, separating adjacent cavities, lining a cavity, or connecting adjacent
structures.

mem·bra·nous (mem′bruh·nus) *adj.* Pertaining
to or characterized by a membrane or membranes.

membranous cataract. A cataractous lens, flattened in the anteroposterior direction, consisting of lens capsule, variable amounts of
proliferated lens epithelium, and fibrous tissue; may be unilateral or bilateral, and is often
due to intrauterine iritis and associated with
other anomalies of the eye. Syn. *pseudoapha-
kia.*

membranous glomerulonephritis. A form of glomerulonephritis characterized clinically by
proteinuria or nephrotic syndrome which
usually follows a benign course. The charac-

teristic lesions of the glomerular basement membrane are seen by the electron microscope and consist of subendothelial or intramembranous electron-dense deposits interspersed with a thickened basement membrane. Proliferation of endocapillary cells is absent. Syn. *epimembranous nephropathy.*

membranous labyrinth. Those membranous canals corresponding to the shape of the osseous labyrinth, suspended in the perilymph, and containing endolymph.

membranous pneumocyte. SQUAMOUS ALVEOLAR CELL.

membranous semicircular canals. Three loop-shaped tubes in the membranous labyrinth of the ear lying at right angles to one another and communicating with the utricle. The superior (frontal) semicircular canal and the posterior (sagittal) semicircular canal lie in the vertical plane, making a right angle which opens laterally. The lateral or horizontal canal lies in the horizontal plane. Syn. *semicircular ducts.*

mem·brum (mem′brum) *n.*, pl. **mem·bra** (·bruh) MEMBER.

membrum mu·li·e·bre (mew′lee·ee′bree) CLITORIS.

membrum vi·ri·le (vi·rye′lee) PENIS.

mem·o·ry (mem′uh·ree) *n.* 1. That faculty of mind by which ideas and sensations are recalled. 2. The mental process of recalling and reproducing that which has been learned and retained. 3. The capacity of an object to resume its original shape after being deformed, as, for example, a plastic IUD after being stretched during insertion.

men-, meno- A combining form meaning *menses.*

men·ac·me (me·nack′mee) *n.* The period of a woman's life during which menstruation persists.

menadiol sodium diphosphate. Tetrasodium 2-methyl-1,4-naphthalenediolbis(dihydrogenphosphate), $C_{11}H_8Na_4O_8P_2.6H_2O$, a water-soluble prothrombogenic compound having the actions and uses of menadione. Syn. *sodium menadiol phosphate.*

men·a·di·one (men′uh·dye′ohn) *n.* 2-Methyl-1,4-naphthoquinone, $C_{11}H_8O_2$; practically insoluble in water but soluble in vegetable oils. Has vitamin-K activity in promoting synthesis of prothrombin and possibly other clotting factors in blood; used for the treatment of conditions characterized by hypoprothrombinemia. Syn. *menaphthone, vitamin K_3.*

men·ar·che (me·nahr′kee) *n.* The time when menstruation starts.

Mendelian ratio The approximate numerical relation between various types of progeny in crosses involving sharply contrasted characters that conform to Mendel's law of heredity; the typical ratios for the F_2 generation are 3:1 for one pair of characters, 9:3:3:1 for two pairs.

Men·del·ism (men′duh·liz·um) *n.* The body of knowledge growing out of the application of Mendel's laws; this knowledge refers to all inheritance through the chromosomes. —**Men·de·lian** (men·dee′lee·un) *adj.*

Mendel's laws The laws of heredity, concerning the way in which the hereditary units, the genes, pass from one generation to the next by way of the germ cells. In neo-Mendelian terms the principles may be stated as follows: Genes segregate at the time of maturation, with the result that a mature germ cell gets either the maternal or the paternal gene of any pair (first law). Genes of different pairs segregate independently of one another, provided they are located on different pairs of chromosomes (second law). If they are located on the same pair of chromosomes, they are linked and consequently segregate in larger or smaller blocks depending mainly on their relative distances apart on the chromosome, that is, on the percentage of crossing over (a discovery made after Mendel's time).

Men·del·son's syndrome Postoperative chemical pneumonitis caused by silent aspiration of gastric contents.

Mé·né·tri·er's disease (mey·ney·tree·ey′) Diffuse giant hypertrophic gastritis, benign, of unknown etiology. Symptoms include vomiting, diarrhea, weight loss, excessive mucus secretion, and hypoproteinemia.

Men·go virus. A strain of encephalomyocarditis virus, belonging to the picornavirus group.

Mé·nière's syndrome or **disease** (mey·nyehr′) A disease of the internal ear characterized by deafness, vertigo, and tinnitus, frequently accompanied by nausea, vomiting, and nystagmus. An allergic mechanism for some cases has been suggested but not proven. Syn. *endolymphatic hydrops, labyrinthine hydrops* or *syndrome.*

mening-, meningo-. A combining form meaning (a) *meninx, meninges;* (b) *membrane, membranous.*

me·nin·ge·al (me·nin′jee·ul) *adj.* Pertaining to the meninges.

me·nin·ge·or·rha·phy (me·nin′jee·or′uh·fee) *n.* 1. Suture of membranes. 2. Suture of the meninges of the brain or spinal cord.

meninges [NA]. Plural of *meninx.*

meningi-, meningio-. See *mening-.*

me·nin·gio·blas·to·ma (me·nin′jee·o·blas·to′muh) *n.* MENINGIOMA.

me·nin·gi·o·ma (me·nin′jee·o′muh) *n.* A tumor derived from arachnoidal cells or dural fibroblasts, arranged in various patterns, involving the meninges or other central nervous system structures, and usually confined to local growth. Syn. *arachnothelioma, dural endothelioma, meningeal fibroblastoma, meningioblastoma, meningiothelioma.*

me·nin·gi·o·ma·to·sis (me·nin′jee·o′muh·to′sis) *n.* Multiple meningiomas.

me·nin·gism (me·nin′jiz·um, men′in·) *n.* A condition in which there are signs and often symptoms of meningeal irritation, particularly nuchal rigidity, suggesting meningitis, but no evidence of this on examination of the cerebrospinal fluid; associated with many acute febrile illnesses in childhood.

men·in·gis·mus (men′′in·jiz′mus) *n.* MENINGISM.

men·in·gi·tis (men′′in·jye′tis) *n.*, pl. **menin·git·i·des** (·jit′i·deez) 1. Any inflammation of the membranes of the brain or spinal cord. Meningitides may be classified according to the causative agent, as tuberculous meningitis, pneumococcal meningitis. 2. LEPTOMENINGITIS. **—mening·it·ic** (·jit′ick) adj.

men·in·gi·to·pho·bia (men″in·jit″o·fo′bee·uh) n. 1. A morbid fear of meningitis. 2. A pseudomeningitis due to fear of that disease.

meningo-. See mening-.

me·nin·go·ar·te·ri·tis (me·ning′go·ahr″tur·eye′tis) n. Inflammation of the arteries of the meninges.

me·nin·go·cele (me·ning′go·seel) n. A protrusion of the cerebral or spinal meninges through a defect in the skull or vertebral column, forming a cyst filled with cerebrospinal fluid.

me·nin·go·cer·e·bral (me·ning′go·serr′e·brul) adj. Pertaining to the cerebrum and the meninges.

me·nin·go·cer·e·bri·tis (me·ning′go·serr″e·brigh′tis) n. MENINGOENCEPHALITIS.

me·nin·go·coc·ce·mia (me·ning′go·kock·see′mee·uh) n. 1. The presence of meningococci in the blood. 2. A clinical disorder consisting of fever, skin hemorrhages, varying degrees of shock and meningococci in the blood.

me·nin·go·coc·cus (me·ning′go·kock′us) n., pl. **meningococ·ci** (·sigh) Common name for Neisseria meningitidis. **—meningococ·cal** (·ul), **me·ningococ·cic** (·sick) adj.

me·nin·go·cor·ti·cal (me·ning′go·kor′ti·kul) adj. Pertaining to the meninges and the cortex of the cerebral hemispheres.

me·nin·go·cyte (me·ning′go·site) n. A flattened epithelioid cell lining a subarachnoid space, which may become phagocytic.

me·nin·go·en·ceph·a·li·tis (me·ning″go·en·sef″uh·lye′tis) n. Inflammation of the brain and its membranes. **—meningoencepha·lit·ic** (·lit′ick) adj.

me·nin·go·en·ceph·a·lo·cele (me·ning″go·en·sef′uh·lo·seel) n. Hernia of the brain and its meninges through a defect in the skull.

me·nin·go·en·ceph·a·lo·my·e·li·tis (me·ning″go·en·sef″uh·lo·migh″e·lye′tis) n. Combined inflammation of the meninges, brain, and spinal cord.

me·nin·go·en·ceph·a·lop·a·thy (me·ning″go·en·sef″uh·lop′uth·ee) n. Disease of the brain and meninges.

me·nin·go·my·e·li·tis (me·ning″go·migh″e·lye′tis) n. Inflammation of the spinal cord and its meninges.

me·nin·go·my·e·lo·cele (me·ning″go·migh′e·lo·seel) n. A protrusion of a portion of the spinal cord and membranes through a defect in the vertebral column.

men·in·gop·a·thy (men″ing·gop′uth·ee) n. Any disease of the cerebrospinal membranes.

me·nin·go·ra·chid·i·an (me·ning″go·ra·kid′ee·un) adj. Pertaining to the spinal cord and its membranes.

me·nin·go·ra·dic·u·lar (me·ning″go·ra·dick′yoo·lur) adj. Pertaining to the meninges and nerve roots (cranial or spinal).

me·nin·gor·rha·gia (me·ning″go·ray′jee·uh) n. Obsol. Hemorrhage from the meninges.

me·nin·go·the·li·o·ma (me·ning″go·theel·ee·o′muh) n. MENINGIOMA. **—meningotheli·om·a·tous** (·om″uh·tus) adj.

me·nin·go·the·li·um (me·ning″go·theel′ee·um) n. The epithelial cells of the arachnoid; the meningocytes. **—meningotheli·al** (·ul) adj.

me·nin·go·vas·cu·lar (me·ning″go·vas′kew·lur) adj. Involving both the meninges and the cerebral blood vessels.

me·ninx (me′ninks, men′inks) n., pl. **me·nin·ges** (me·nin′jeez) A membrane, especially one of the brain or spinal cord; the meninges covering the brain and spinal cord consist of the dura mater, pia mater, and arachnoid.

menisc-, menisco- A combining form meaning (a) crescentic, sickle-shaped, semilunar; (b) meniscus, semilunar cartilage.

men·is·cec·to·my (men″i·seck′tuh·mee) n. The surgical excision of a meniscus or semilunar cartilage.

menisci. Plural and genitive singular of meniscus.

men·is·ci·tis (men″i·sigh′tis) n. An inflammation of any interarticular cartilage; specifically, of the semilunar cartilages of the knee joint.

me·nis·co·cyte (me·nis′ko·site) n. A sickle-shaped erythrocyte.

me·nis·co·cy·to·sis (me·nis″ko·sigh·to′sis) n. SICKLE CELL ANEMIA.

me·nis·cus (me·nis′kus) n., L. pl. & genit. sing. **menis·ci** (·skye, ·sigh), 1. A crescent-shaped interarticular wedge of fibrocartilage found especially in the sternoclavicular, acromioclavicular, and knee joints. 2. A concavoconvex lens (positive meniscus) or a convexoconcave lens (negative meniscus). 3. The curved surface of a column of liquid.

Menkes' syndrome KINKY HAIR DISEASE.

meno·lip·sis (men″o·lip′sis) n. The retention or absence of the menses.

meno·me·tror·rha·gia (men″o·mee″tro·ray′jee·uh, ·met″ro·) n. Uterine bleeding of excessive amount at the time of menstruation, plus irregular uterine bleeding at other times.

menopausal syndrome. CLIMACTERIC.

meno·pause (men′o·pawz) n. The physiologic cessation of menstruation, usually between the forty-fifth and fifty-fifth years. **—menopaus·ic** (men″o·pawz′ick), **menopaus·al** (·ul) adj.

meno·pla·nia (men″o·play′nee·uh) n. A discharge of blood occurring at the menstrual period, but derived from some part of the body other than the uterus; vicarious menstruation, as in endometriosis.

men·or·rha·gia (men″o·ray′jee·uh) n. An excessive menstrual flow. Syn. hypermenorrhea. **—menor·rhag·ic** (·raj′ick) adj.

men·or·rhal·gia (men″o·ral′jee·uh) n. Pelvic pain at menstrual periods other than characteristic midline cramp; characteristic of endometriosis.

men·or·rhea, men·or·rhoea (men″o·ree′uh) n. The normal flow of the menses.

me·nos·ta·sis (me·nos′tuh·sis) n. Suppression of the menstrual flow.

meno·stax·is (men″o·stack′sis) n. Prolonged menstruation.

mens (menz, mence) n., genit. **men·tis** (men′ti) MIND.

men·ses (men'seez) *n.pl.* The recurrent monthly discharge of blood from the genital canal of a woman during reproductive years.

men·stru·al (men'stroo-ul) *adj.* Of or pertaining to menstruation.

men·stru·ant (men'stroo-unt) *adj. & n.* 1. Subject to, or capable of, menstruating. 2. A girl or woman who menstruates.

men·stru·ate (men'stroo-ate) *v.* To discharge the products of menstruation.

men·stru·a·tion (men''stroo-ay'shun) *n.* A periodic discharge of a sanguineous fluid from the uterus, occurring during the period of a woman's sexual maturity from puberty to the menopause.

men·stru·um (men'stroo-um) *n.* A solvent, commonly one that extracts certain principles from entire plant or animal tissues.

men·su·al (men'shoo-ul, men'sue-ul) *adj.* Monthly.

men·su·ra·tion (men''shoo-ray'shun, men''sue-) *n.* The act or process of measuring.

¹**men·tal**, *adj.* 1. Pertaining to the mind, psyche, or inner self, as in mental health. 2. Pertaining to the intellectual or cognitive functions, as distinct from the affective and conative, as in mental test. 3. Imaginary or unreal, as when a pain is said to be merely mental.

²**men·tal**, *adj.* Pertaining to the chin. Syn. *genial.*

mental age. 1. The degree of mental development of an individual in terms of the chronological age of the average individual of equivalent mental ability. 2. Specifically, a score, derived from intelligence tests, expressed in terms of the age at which an average individual attains that score. An adult whose score is the equivalent of that of an average child of 12 has a mental age of 12. Abbreviated, MA.

mental deficiency. 1. A defect of intelligence, the degree of which may be indicated by the intelligence quotient for the specific test employed; graded as mild (I.Q. 70 to 85), moderate (I.Q. 50 to 69), and severe (I.Q. below 50). In the United States, the presently preferred term is mental retardation, although some authorities seek to make a distinction between the two terms on the basis of a demonstrable organic lesion in mental deficiency, and the implication that deficiency is a nonremediable state. 2. *In civil law,* the condition as defined by statute, frequently divided into three grades: idiocy, the lowest, imbecility, the intermediate; and morority, the highest.

mental disorders. Related psychiatric conditions, divided into two major groups: (a) Those in which there is a primary impairment of brain function, generally associated with an organic brain syndrome upon which diagnosis is based; the psychiatric picture is characterized by impairment of intellectual functions, including memory, orientation, and judgment, and by shallowness and lability of affect. Additional disturbances, such as psychosis, neurosis, or behavioral reactions, may be associated with these disorders but are secondary to the diagnosis. (b) Those conditions which are more directly the result of the individual's difficulty in adapting to his environment, and in which any associated impairment of brain function is secondary to the psychiatric disturbance.

mental healing. The use of suggestion or faith in the attempt to cure illness, particularly physical illness.

mental health. A relatively enduring state of being in which an individual has effected an integration of his instinctual drives in a way that is reasonably satisfying to himself as reflected in his zest for living and his feeling of self-realization. For most individuals, mental health also implies a large degree of adjustment to the social environment as indicated by the satisfaction derived from their interpersonal relationships as well as their achievements.

men·ta·lis (men-tay'lis) *n.* A muscle of the lower lip.

men·tal·i·ty (men-tal'i-tee) *n.* 1. Mental endowment, capacity, or power; intellect. 2. Outlook, ways of thinking.

mental retardation. Subnormal intellectual functioning, often present since birth or apparent in early life; may be primary (hereditary or familial), without demonstrable organic brain lesion or known prenatal cause, or secondary, due to brain tissue anomalies, chromosomal disorder, prenatal, maternal, or postnatally acquired infections, intoxication or trauma, prematurity, disorders of growth, nutrition, or metabolism, degenerative diseases, tumor, or following major psychiatric disorders or associated with psychosocial (environmental) deprivation; classified as borderline, mild, moderate, severe, and profound. Syn. *mental subnormality.*

mental vaginismus. Painful spasm of the vagina due to extreme aversion to the sexual act; PSYCHOLOGIC DYSPAREUNIA.

men·ta·tion (men-tay'shun) *n.* The mechanism of thought; mental activity.

men·thol (men'thol) *n.* p-Menthan-3-ol, $C_{10}H_{19}OH$, an alcohol obtained from peppermint or other mint oils or prepared synthetically. Used externally for its antipruritic, anesthetic, or antiseptic effects.

men·ti·cide (men'ti-side) *n.* BRAINWASHING.

mento- *In anatomy,* a combining form meaning *chin.*

men·to·an·te·ri·or (men''to-an-teer'ee-ur) *adj.* With the chin pointing anterior; usually referring to the position of the child's face during parturition.

men·to·pa·ri·etal (men''to-puh-rye'e-tul) *adj.* Pertaining to the chin and the parietal bone.

men·to·pos·te·ri·or (men''to-pos-teer'ee-ur) *adj.* With the chin pointing backward; usually referring to the position of the child's face during parturition.

men·tum (men'tum) *n.,* pl. **men·ta** (·tuh) CHIN.

me·per·i·dine (me-perr'i-deen, ·din, mep'ur-) *n.* Ethyl 1-methyl-4-phenylisonipecotate, $C_{15}H_{21}NO_2$, a narcotic analgesic; used as the hydrochloride salt. Syn. *isonipecaine, pethidine.*

me·phen·e·sin (me-fen'e-sin) *n.* 3-o-(Tolyloxy)-

1,2-propanediol, $C_{10}H_{14}O_3$, a skeletal muscle relaxant.

me·phen·y·to·in (me·fen′ee·to″in) *n.* 5-Ethyl-3-methyl-5-phenylhydantoin, $C_{12}H_{14}N_2O_2$, an anticonvulsant drug effective in generalized seizures. Syn. *methoin.*

me·phit·ic (me·fit′ick) *adj.* Foul or noxious; stifling, as mephitic gangrene, necrosis of bone associated with the evolution of offensive odors.

Mephyton. A trademark for phytonadione or vitamin K_1, a prothrombogenic vitamin.

me·pro·ba·mate (me·pro′buh·mate, ·pro·bam′) *n.* 2-Methyl-2-*n*-propyl-1,3-propanediol dicarbamate, $C_9H_{18}N_2O_4$, a tranquilizer with anticonvulsant, muscle relaxant, and sedative actions.

meq, mEq Abbreviation for *milliequivalent.*

mer-, mero- A combining form meaning (a) *part, segment;* (b) *partial.*

me·ral·gia (me·ral′jee·uh) *n.* Neuralgic pain in the thigh.

meralgia par·es·thet·i·ca (păr″es·thet′i·kuh) A neuropathy characterized by pain, paresthesias, and sensory disturbances in the area supplied by the lateral femoral cutaneous nerve; usually due to compression of the nerve where it enters the thigh beneath the inguinal ligament, at the level of the anterior superior iliac spine. Syn. *Roth-Bernhardt's disease.*

mer·am·au·ro·sis (merr·am″aw·ro′sis, merr″uh·maw·ro′sis) *n.* Partial amaurosis.

M:E ratio. MYELOID:ERYTHROID RATIO.

mer·bro·min (mur·bro′min) *n.* The disodium salt of 2′,7′-dibromo-4′-(hydroxymercuri)fluorescein, an organomercurial antibacterial agent applied topically.

mer·cap·tan (mur·kap′tan) *n.* 1. An organic compound of the general formula RSH, representing an alcohol ROH, in which oxygen is replaced by sulfur. Syn. *thio alcohol, thiol.* 2. Ethyl mercaptan, C_2H_5SH.

mer·cap·to·pu·rine (mur·kap″to·pew′reen) *n.* 6-Mercaptopurine, $C_5H_4N_4S$, the mercapto analogue of 6-aminopurine or adenine; a cytotoxic agent useful for the treatment of acute leukemia.

mercuri-. A combining form meaning (a) *mercury;* (b) *mercuric.*

mer·cu·ri·al (mur·kew′ree·ul) *adj. & n.* 1. Pertaining to or caused by mercury. 2. Any preparation of mercury or its salts.

mer·cu·ri·al·ism (mur·kew′ree·ul·iz·um) *n.* Poisoning due to absorption of mercury.

mer·cu·ric (mur·kew′rick) *adj.* Pertaining to, or containing, mercury in the bivalent state.

mercuric chloride. MERCURY BICHLORIDE.

mercuric oxide, red. HgO. Orange-red, crystalline powder; has been used locally as an antiseptic.

mercuric oxide, yellow. HgO. Yellow powder, more finely subdivided than red mercuric oxide; used locally as an antibacterial agent, especially for infections of the eye.

Mercurochrome. Trademark for merbromin, an organomercurial antibacterial agent applied topically.

Mercurophen. Trademark for sodium hydroxymercuri-*o*-nitrophenolate, an organomercurial antibacterial agent applied topically.

mer·cu·ro·phyl·line (mur′kew·ro·fil′een, ·in) *n.* The sodium salt of 3-{[3-(hydroxymercuri)-2-methoxypropyl]carbamoyl}-1,2,2-trimethyl-cyclopentanecarboxylic acid, and theophylline, in approximately molecular proportions; a mercurial diuretic administered orally or intramuscularly.

mer·cu·rous (mur·kew′rus, mur′kew·rus) *adj.* Pertaining to, or containing, mercury in the univalent state.

mercurous chloride. HgCl. White powder, insoluble in water; occasionally used as a cathartic. Syn. *calomel, mild mercurous chloride.*

mer·cu·ry (mur′kew·ree) *n.* Hg = 200.59. A shining, silver-white, liquid, volatile metal, having a specific gravity of 13.55. Forms two classes of compounds: (a) mercurous, in which the metal is univalent, and (b) mercuric, in which it is bivalent. Mercuric salts are more soluble and more poisonous than the mercurous. Mercury in the form of its salts was formerly used as a purgative and cholagogue, as an alterative in chronic inflammations, as an antisyphilitic, an antiphlogistic, an intestinal antiseptic, a disinfectant, a parasiticide, a caustic, and an astringent. Absorption of mercury in sufficient quantity causes poisoning, characterized by a coppery taste in the mouth, ptyalism, loosening of the teeth, sponginess of the gums; in more severe cases, ulceration of the cheeks, necrosis of the jaws, marked emaciation; at times neuritis develops, and a peculiar tremor.

mercury bichloride. Mercuric chloride, $HgCl_2$; white crystals or powder, soluble in water. Now used only as a germicide and disinfectant. Syn. *corrosive sublimate.*

mer·er·ga·sia (merr″ur·gay′zhuh, ·zee·uh) *n.* 1. Partial or subnormal ability to function physically or mentally. 2. *In psychobiology,* Meyer's term for a partial disturbance of the personality, as a neurotic or psychoneurotic reaction. Syn. *cacergasia.* **—mer·er·gas·tic** (·gas′tick) *adj.*

me·rid·i·an (me·rid′ee·un) *n.* A great circle surrounding a sphere and intersecting the poles.

meridians of the eye. Lines drawn around the globe of the eye and passing through the poles of the vertical axis (vertical meridian), or through the poles of the transverse axis (horizontal meridian).

me·rid·i·o·nal (me·rid′ee·uh·nul) *adj.* Of or pertaining to a meridian.

meridional aniseikonia. Aniseikonia in which one image is larger than the other in one meridian.

mer·in·tho·pho·bia (merr″in·tho·fo′bee·uh, merin′tho·) *n.* A morbid fear of being tied up.

me·ris·tic (me·ris′tick) *adj.* Pertaining to, or divided into, segments.

mero·blas·tic (merr″o·blas′tick) *adj.* Dividing only in part, referring to an egg in which the cleavage divisions are confined to the animal pole, owing to the presence of a large amount of yolk.

mero·crine (merr′o·krin, ·krine) *adj.* Pertaining

to glands in which the act of secretion leaves the cell itself intact, for example, in salivary and pancreatic glands.

mero·mi·cro·so·mia (merr″o·mye″kro·so′mee·uh) *n.* Abnormal smallness of some part of the body.

me·ro·pia (me·ro′pee·uh) *n.* Obscuration of vision.

me·ros·mia (me·roz′mee·uh, me·ros′) *n.* Partial loss of the sense of smell in that certain odors are not perceived.

mero·zo·ite (merr″o·zo′ite) *n.* Any one of the segments resulting from the splitting up of the schizont in the asexual form of reproduction of sporozoa.

mer·sal·yl (mur′sah·lil, ·leel, mur·sal′il) *n.* Sodium *o*-[3-(hydroxymercuri)-2-methoxypropyl] carbamoyl]phenoxyacetate, introduced as a mercurial antisyphilitic but now used as a parenterally administered diuretic; the available preparation contains also theophylline and is called mersalyl and theophylline injection.

Merthiolate. Trademark for thimerosal, a bacteriostatic and fungistatic agent.

Meruvax. A trademark for live rubella virus vaccine.

mer·y·cism (merr′i·siz·um) *n.* RUMINATION (2).

mes-, meso- A prefix and combining form meaning (a) *mid-, middle, medial;* (b) *medium, moderate, intermediate;* (c) *mesentery;* (d) *mesodermal.*

mes·an·gi·al (mes·an′jee·ul) *adj.* Pertaining to or involving the mesangium.

mes·an·gi·um (mes·an′jee·um) *n.* The suspensory structure of the renal glomerulus, consisting of a network of sponge fibers and associated cells, which attaches to the hilus of the glomerulus supporting the capillary loops in the fashion of a mesentery.

Mesantoin. Trademark for mephenytoin, an anticonvulsant drug.

mes·aor·ti·tis (mes″ay·or·tye′tis) *n.* Inflammation of the middle coat of the aorta.

mes·ar·te·ri·tis (mes″ahr″te·rye′tis) *n.* Inflammation of the middle coat of an artery.

mes·cal (mes·kal′) *n.* 1. The cactus *Lophophora williamsii,* a potential intoxicant. Syn. *peyote.* 2. An intoxicant spirit distilled from Mexican pulque.

mescal buttons. The dried tops from the cactus *Lophophora williamsii;* capable of producing inebriation and hallucinations.

mes·ca·line (mes′kuh·leen) *n.* 3,4,5-Trimethoxyphenethylamine, $C_{11}H_{17}NO_3$, an alkaloid present in mescal buttons; produces unusual psychic effects and visual hallucinations.

mes·en·ce·phal·ic (mez·en″se·fal′ick, mes″en·) *adj.* Of or pertaining to the mesencephalon.

mes·en·ceph·a·li·tis (mez″en·sef′uh·lye′tis, mes″) *n.* Inflammation of the mesencephalon.

mes·en·ceph·a·lon (mez″en·sef′uh·lon, mes″) *n.,* genit. **mesencepha·li** (·lye) The part of the brain developed from the middle cerebral vesicle and consisting of the tectum and cerebral peduncles, and traversed by the cerebral aqueduct. Syn. *midbrain.*

mes·en·chy·mal (me·seng′ki·mul, mes″in·kye′

mul, mez″) *adj.* Of or pertaining to mesenchyme.

mes·en·chyme (mes′in·kime, mez′) *n.* The portion of the mesoderm that produces all the connective tissues of the body, the blood vessels, and the blood, the entire lymphatic system proper, and the heart; the nonepithelial portions of the mesoderm.

mes·en·chy·mo·ma (mes″in·kigh·mo′muh, ·ki·mo′muh) *n.* 1. A tumor, benign or malignant, whose parenchyma is composed of cells resembling those of the embryonic mesenchyme. 2. A tumor, benign or malignant, whose parenchyma is composed of cells resembling those of the mesenchyme with its derivatives. Syn. *mixed mesenchymal tumor, mixed mesodermal tumor.*

mes·en·ter·ec·to·my (mes″en·tur·eck′tum·ee) *n.* Excision of a mesentery or a part of it.

mes·en·ter·ic (mes″un·terr′ick, mez″) *adj.* Of or pertaining to a mesentery.

mesenteric arteries. See Table of Arteries in the Appendix.

mesenteric lymphadenitis. Inflammation of the mesenteric lymph nodes.

mes·en·ter·i·co·meso·col·ic (mes·en·terr″i·ko·mes·o·ko′lick, ·kol′ick) *adj.* Pertaining to the mesentery and the mesocolon.

mesenteric recess. A recess in the primitive gastric mesentery, formed by an invagination of the peritoneum on the right side, that separates the definitive gastric mesentery from the caval mesentery and gives rise to the omental bursa, its vestibule, and the infracardiac bursa.

mes·en·ter·io·pexy (mes″un·terr′ee·o·peck″see) *n.* MESOPEXY.

mes·en·teri·or·rha·phy (mes″un·terr″ee·or′uh·fee) *n.* Surgical repair of a mesentery.

mes·en·ter·i·pli·ca·tion (mes″un·terr″i·pli·kay′shun) *n.* Mesenteriorrhaphy; reduction of folds of redundant mesentery by overlapping and suture.

mes·en·ter·i·tis (mes″en·ter·eye′tis) *n.* Inflammation of a mesentery.

mes·en·tery (mes′un·terr″ee, mez′) *n.* 1. Any of the peritoneal folds attaching certain organs, especially the intestine, to the abdominal wall. 2. Specifically, that which attaches the small intestine to the posterior abdominal wall.

mes·en·tor·rha·phy (mes″en·tor′uf·ee, mez″un·) *n.* Suture of a mesentery.

me·si·al (mee″zee·ul, ·see·ul, mes′ee·ul) *adj.* 1. MEDIAL. 2. *In dentistry,* toward the sagittal plane along the curve of a dental arch.

mesial drift. The tendency of teeth in proximal contact to move toward the midline as their contact areas become worn.

mesial occlusion. The occlusion occurring when a tooth is more anterior than normal.

mesio-. *In dentistry,* a combining form meaning *mesial.*

me·sio·buc·cal (mee″zee·o·buck′ul, mee″see·o·) *adj.* Pertaining to the mesial and buccal aspects of the teeth.

me·sio·buc·co·oc·clu·sal (mee″zee·o·buck″o·uh·kloo′zul) *adj.* Pertaining to the mesial, buccal, and occlusal surfaces of a tooth.

me·sio·clu·sion (mee″zee·o·klew′zhun) *n.* Any malocclusion in which the mandible is anterior to its normal relationship with the maxilla; the mesial groove of the mandibular first permanent molar articulates anteriorly to the mesiobuccal cusp of the maxillary first permanent molar.

me·sio·dis·tal (mee″zee·o·dis′tul) *adj.* Pertaining to the mesial and distal surfaces of a tooth.

me·sio·gres·sion (mee″zee·o·gresh′un) *n.* The location of teeth anterior to their normal position.

me·sio·in·ci·sal (mee″zee·o·in·sigh′zul) *adj.* Pertaining to the mesial and incisal surfaces of a tooth.

me·sio·la·bi·al (mee″zee·o·lay′bee·ul) *adj.* Pertaining to the mesial and labial surfaces of a tooth.

me·sio·lin·gual (mee″zee·o·ling′gwul) *adj.* Pertaining to the mesial and lingual aspects of a tooth.

me·sio·lin·guo·oc·clu·sal (mee″zee·o·ling″gwo·uh·kloo′zul) *adj.* Pertaining to the mesial, lingual, and occlusal surfaces of a tooth.

me·sio·oc·clu·sal (mee″zee·o·uh·kloo′zul) *adj.* Pertaining to the mesial and occlusal surfaces of a tooth.

me·sio·ver·sion (mee″zee·o·vur′zhun) *n.* Greater than normal proximity of a tooth to the median plane of the face along the dental arch.

mes·mer·ism (mez′mur·iz·um) *n.* Hypnotism induced by animal magnetism, a supposed force passing from operator to man.

meso-. 1. See *mes-.* 2. (italicized) *In chemistry,* a combining form designating (a) an optical isomer that does not rotate polarized light because of internal compensation of its chiral centers; (b) a middle position of a substituent group in certain organic compounds; (c) a porphyrin or other pyrrole derivative in which one or more vinyl groups have been converted to ethyl by hydrogenation; (d) an intermediate hydrated form of an inorganic acid.

meso·ap·pen·di·ci·tis (mes″o·uh·pen″di·sigh′tis) *n.* Inflammation of the mesoappendix.

meso·ap·pen·dix (mes″o·uh·pen′dicks) *n.* [NA]. The mesentery of the vermiform appendix.

meso·bil·i·fus·cin (mes″o·bil·i·fus′in) *n.* Either of two isomeric substances, each containing two pyrrole rings but not of definitely known structure, obtained as products of hydrolytic cleavage of mesobilirubinogen when the latter is prepared by reduction of bilirubin. They contribute significantly to the color of normal feces.

meso·blast (mez′o·blast, mes′) *n.* 1. The mesoderm during its early development. 2. MESODERM. —**meso·blas·tic** (mez″o·blas′tick) *adj.*

meso·ce·cum (mes″o·see′kum, mez″) *n.* The mesentery that in some cases connects the cecum with the right iliac fossa.

meso·co·lon (mes″o·ko′lun, mez″) *n.* The mesentery connecting the colon with the posterior abdominal wall. It may be divided into ascending, descending, and transverse portions. In the adult the transverse portion persists. —**meso·co·lic** (·ko′lick, ·kol′ick) *adj.*

meso·derm (mez′o·durm, mes′) *n.* The third germ layer, lying between the ectoderm and entoderm. It gives rise to the connective tissues, muscles, urogenital system, vascular system, and the epithelial lining of the coelom. —**meso·der·mal** (mez″o·dur′mul, mes′) *adj.*

meso·di·a·stol·ic (mez″o·dye″uh·stol′ick, mes′o·) *adj.* Of or pertaining to the middle of ventricular diastole.

meso·du·o·de·num (mes″o·dew″o·dee′num, ·dew·od′e·num, mez′) *n.* That part of the mesentery that sometimes connects the duodenum with the posterior wall of the abdominal cavity. Normally in man the true duodenum has no mesentery in its fully developed state.

meso·gas·ter (mez′o·gas″tur, mes′o·) *n.* The primitive mesentery of the stomach.

meso·glia (me·sog′lee·uh) *n. Obsol.* A type of ameboid phagocyte found in the neuroglia, probably of mesodermal origin.

meso·morph (mez′o·morf, mes′) *n.* In the somatotype, an individual exhibiting relative predominance of mesomorphy.

meso·mor·phy (mez′o·mor·fee, mes′) *n.* Component II of the somatotype, representing relative predominance of somatic structures or the bony and muscular framework of the body, derived from mesoderm. Mesomorphs tend toward massive strength and heavy muscular development. The counterpart on the behavioral level is somatotonia. —**meso·morph·ic** (mez″o·mor′fick, mes′) *adj.*

meso·neph·ric (mes″o·nef′rick) *adj.* Of or pertaining to the mesonephros.

mesonephric duct. The duct of the mesonephros or embryonic kidney; becomes the excretory duct of the testis and gives rise to the ureteric bud in both sexes. Syn. *Wolffian duct.*

mesonephric rests. Fetal rests of a mesonephric duct.

meso·ne·phro·ma (mes″o·nef·ro′muh) *n.* Any of a variety of rare tumors supposed to be, but not proved to be, derived from mesonephros (Wolffian body), and occurring in the genital tract. Included are extrauterine adenomyomas, cystic or solid tumors of the ovary situated near the hilus, and tumors resembling the adenomyosarcoma of the kidney. Syn. *teratoid adenocystoma.*

mesonephroma ova·rii (o·vair′ee·eye). A malignant tumor of the ovary which microscopically contains structures resembling the primitive mesonephros.

meso·neph·ros (mes″o·nef′ros) *n.*, pl. **mesoneph·roi** (·roy) The middle kidney of higher vertebrates; functional in the embryo, it is replaced by the metanephros. Syn. *Wolffian body.*

meso·pexy (mes′o·peck″see) *n.* The surgical fixation of a mesentery.

me·sor·chi·um (me·sor′kee·um) *n.*, pl. **mesor·chia** (·kee·uh) The mesentery of the fetal testis by which it is attached to the mesonephros; represented in the adult by a fold between testis and epididymis.

meso·rec·tum (mes″o·reck′tum, mez′o·) *n.* The narrow fold of the peritoneum connecting the upper part of the rectum with the sacrum.

meso·sal·pinx (mes″o·sal′pinks, mez″) *n.*, pl.

meso·sal·pin·ges (·sal·pin′jeez) The upper part of the broad ligament that forms the mesentery of the uterine tube. —**meso·sal·pin·ge·al** (·sal·pin′jee·ul, ·sal·pin·jee′ul) adj.

meso·sig·moid (mez″o·sig′moid, mes″o·) n. SIGMOID MESOCOLON.

meso·ten·don (mes″o·ten′don, mez″o·) n. The fold of synovial membrane extending to a tendon from its synovial tendon sheath.

meso·the·li·o·ma (mes″o·theel″ee·o′muh) n. A primary tumor, either benign or malignant, composed of cells similar to those forming the lining of the peritoneum, pericardium, or pleura. Syn. celioma, celothelioma.

meso·the·li·um (mes″o·theel′ee·um, mez″) n., pl. **mesothe·lia** (·ee·uh) 1. The lining of the wall of the primitive body cavity situated between the somatopleure and splanchnopleure. 2. The simple squamous epithelium lining the pleural, pericardial, peritoneal, and scrotal cavities. —**mesotheli·al** (·ul) adj.

meso·tho·ri·um (mes″o·tho′ree·um) n. Either of the radioactive disintegration products, mesothorium-1 ($MsTh_1$) and mesothorium-2 ($MsTh_2$), formed from thorium and ultimately converted to radiothorium.

mes·ova·ri·um (mes″o·vair′ee·um) n., pl. **mesova·ria** (·ree·uh) A peritoneal fold connecting the ovary and the broad ligament. —**mesovarian** (·un) adj.

messenger RNA. A single-stranded ribonucleic acid which arises from, and is complementary to, the double-stranded DNA. It passes from the nucleus to the cytoplasm where its information is translated into protein structure. Abbreviated, mRNA.

mes·tra·nol (mes′truh·nol) n. 17α-Ethynyl-3-methoxy-1,3,5(10)-estratrien-17β-ol, $C_{21}H_{26}O_2$, an estrogen; used principally, in combination with a progestogen, to inhibit ovulation and control fertility.

met-, meta- 1. A prefix signifying (a) behind, beyond, distal to; (b) between, among; (c) change, transformation; (d) after, post-; (e) subsequent in development or evolution. 2. (italicized) In chemistry, a prefix indicating the relationship of two atoms in the benzene ring that are separated by one carbon atom in the ring, i.e., the 1,3-position; also any benzene derivative in which two substituents have such a relationship. Symbol, m-. 3. In chemistry, a prefix designating an acid containing one less molecule of water than the parent acid, commonly designated the ortho-acid; as metaphosphoric acid, HPO_3, from orthophosphoric acid, H_3PO_4.

metabolic alkalosis. Alkalosis in which the tendency to an increased blood pH results either from the addition to body fluids of excess alkali by injection or ingestion or from excessive loss of acid, usually by vomiting or gastric aspiration. Physiological compensation is by pulmonary retention of carbon dioxide via hypoventilation and accelerated renal excretion of sodium bicarbonate.

metabolic craniopathy. STEWART-MOREL-MORGAGNI SYNDROME.

metabolic ileus. Ileus resulting from interference with the function of the smooth muscle of the intestine, due to metabolic disturbances.

metabolic pigment. A pigment, such as melanin, formed by the metabolic action of cells.

me·tab·o·lism (me·tab′o·liz·um) n. The sum total of all synthetic (anabolic) and degradative (catabolic) biochemical reactions in the body.

me·tab·o·lite (me·tab′o·lite) n. A product of metabolic change.

me·tab·o·lize (me·tab′o·lize) v. To transform by metabolism, to subject to metabolism.

met·a·bol·o·gy (met″uh·bol′uh·jee) n. Study of the metabolic processes.

meta·car·pal (met″uh·kahr′pul) adj. Pertaining to the metacarpus, or to a bone of it.

meta·car·pec·to·my (met″uh·kahr·peck′tum·ee) n. Excision of a metacarpal bone.

meta·car·po·pha·lan·ge·al (met″uh·kahr″po·fuh·lan′jee·ul) adj. Pertaining to the metacarpus and the phalanges.

meta·car·pus (met″uh·kahr′pus) n., pl. & genit. sing. **metacar·pi** (·pye) The part of the hand between the carpus and the phalanges; it contains five bones.

meta·cer·car·i·a (met″uh·sur·kâr′ee·uh) n., pl. **metacercar·i·ae** (·ee·ee) An encysted, maturing stage of a trematode in the tissues of an intermediate host, often representing the infectious part of a parasite's life cycle.

meta·chro·ma·sia (met″uh·kro·may′zee·uh, ·zhuh) n. 1. The property exhibited by certain pure dyestuffs, chiefly basic dyes, of coloring certain tissue elements in a different color, usually of a shorter wavelength absorption maximum, than most other tissue elements. 2. The assumption of different colors or shades by different substances when stained by the same dye. —**metachro·mat·ic** (·mat′ick) adj.

metachromatic granules. 1. Granules which take on a color different from that of the dye used to stain them. 2. VOLUTIN GRANULES.

metachromatic leukodystrophy. A heredodegenerative disease due to a deficiency of the enzyme aryl sulfatase A, with increase in sulfated lipids which are normally degraded to cerebrosides; excess cerebroside sulfatides are responsible for metachromasia in cerebral white matter, peripheral nerves, liver and kidney, associated with progressive neurological disease. The disease usually has its onset between 1 and 4 years of age, but variant forms occur in childhood and occasionally in adult life. Variant forms due to other sulfatase deficiencies occur. Autosomal recessive transmission is usual. Abbreviated, MLD. Syn. sulfatide lipidosis.

metachromatic stain. A stain which changes apparent color when absorbed by certain cell constituents, as mucin staining red instead of blue with toluidine blue.

meta·chro·ma·tism (met″uh·kro′muh·tiz·um) n. METACHROMASIA.

me·tach·ro·nous (me·tack′ruh·nus) adj. Occurring or beginning at different times.

meta·cone (met′uh·kone) n. The outer posterior (distobuccal) cusp of an upper molar tooth.

meta·co·nid (met″uh·ko′nid, kon′id) n. The inner anterior (mesiolingual) cusp of a lower molar tooth.

meta·cre·sol (met″uh·kree′sole, ·sol) n. The meta form of cresol, $C_6H_4(CH_3)OH$, a colorless liquid obtained from coal tar. A more powerful germicide than phenol, but less toxic.

meta·cy·e·sis (met″a·sigh·ee′sis) n. EXTRAUTERINE PREGNANCY.

meta·drom·ic (met″uh·drom′ick, ·dro′mick). adj. FESTINATING.

Meta·gon·i·mus (met″uh·gon′i·mus) n. A genus of digenetic trematodes.

Metagonimus yo·ko·ga·wai (yo·ko·gah·wah′eye). A species of trematode found most commonly in the Far East which infects the small intestine of man, dogs, cats, pigs, and mice, producing a mild diarrhea.

met·al (met′ul) n. An elementary substance, or mixture of such substances, usually characterized by hardness, malleability, ductility, fusibility, luster, and conduction of heat and electricity.

metal fume fever. A febrile influenza-like occupational disorder following the inhalation of finely divided particles and fumes of metallic oxides. Syn. *brass chills, brass founder's ague, galvo, metal ague, zinc chills, spelter shakes, Teflon shakes, Monday fever.*

me·tal·lic (me·tal′ick) adj. 1. Of, pertaining to, or resembling metal. 2. *In physical diagnosis,* referring to a sound similar to that produced by metal, high-pitched, short in duration, and with overtones; a form of tympany.

metallo-, metalo-. A combining form meaning *metal, metallic.*

met·al·loid (met′uh·loid) n. & adj. 1. An element which has metallic properties in the free state but which behaves chemically as an amphoteric or nonmetallic element. 2. Characteristic of or pertaining to a metalloid.

me·tal·lo·phil·ia (me·tal″o·fil′ee·uh) n. The property exhibited by certain tissue elements of binding metal ions, presumably by chelation, which are then identified by inorganic chemical reactions or by binding of dyestuffs which form colored pigments with the bound metal.

met·al·lo·pho·bia (met″uh·lo·fo′bee·uh, me·tal″o·) n. A morbid fear of metals or metallic objects.

me·tal·lo·por·phy·rin (me·tal″o·por′fi·rin, met″uh·lo·) n. A compound formed by the combination of a porphyrin with a metal such as iron, copper, cobalt, nickel, silver, tin, zinc, manganese, or magnesium. Heme is a metalloporphyrin in which a porphyrin is combined with iron.

me·tal·lo·pro·tein (me·tal″o·pro′tee·in, ·teen) n. A protein enzyme containing metal as an inherent portion of its molecule.

me·talo·phil (me·tal′o·fil) n. Any of the reticular cells which stain with metallic salts, as silver carbonate. It may be a fixed or ameboid cell or a monocyte of peripheral blood.

meta·mer (met′uh·mur) n. One of two or more compounds having the same number and kind of atoms but with a different distribution of the component radicals.

meta·mere (met′uh·meer) n. One of the linear series of more or less similar segments of the body of many animals.

me·tam·er·ism (me·tam′ur·iz·um) n. 1. *In zoology,* the repetition of more or less similar parts or segments (metameres) in the body of many animals, as exhibited especially by the Annelida, Arthropoda, and Vertebrata. 2. *In chemistry,* the relationship existing between two or more metamers.

meta·mor·phic (met″uh·mor′fick) adj. Pertaining to metamorphosis.

meta·mor·phop·sia (met″uh·mor·fop′see·uh) n. A visual disturbance in which the image is distorted.

meta·mor·pho·sis (met″uh·mor·fuh·sis, ·mor·fo′sis) n., pl. **metamorpho·ses** (·seez) 1. A structural change or transformation; usually associated with growth and development of an organism through successive stages, such as egg, larva, pupa, adult. 2. *In pathology,* a retrogressive change.

meta·my·e·lo·cyte (met″uh·migh′e·lo·site) n. A cell of the granulocytic series intermediate between the myelocyte and granular leukocyte, having a full complement of specific granules and an indented, bean-shaped (juvenile) nucleus. Syn. *metagranulocyte, juvenile cell.*

Metandren. A trademark for methyltestosterone, a crystalline androgen.

meta·neph·ric (met″uh·nef′rick) adj. Of or pertaining to the metanephros.

metanephric blastema. The caudal end of the nephrogenic cord.

meta·neph·rine (met″uh·nef′reen) n. An inactive metabolite of epinephrine (3-*O*-methylepinephrine) which is excreted in the urine, where its measurement is used as a test for pheochromocytoma.

meta·neph·ro·gen·ic (met″uh·nef″ro·jen′ick) adj. Capable of forming, or giving rise to, the metanephros.

meta·neph·ros (met″uh·nef′ros) n., pl. **metanephroi** (·roy) The definitive or permanent kidney of reptiles, birds, and mammals. It develops from the caudal part of the nephrogenic cord in association with the ureteric bud from the mesonephric duct.

meta·phase (met′uh·faze) n. 1. The middle stage of mitosis when the chromosomes lie nearly in a single plane at the equator of the spindle, forming the equatorial plate. It follows the prophase and precedes the anaphase. 2. The middle stage of the first (metaphase I) or second (metaphase II) meiotic division.

Metaphen. Trademark for nitromersol, an organomercurial antibacterial agent used topically.

meta·phos·phor·ic acid (met″uh·fos·for′ick). HPO_3. A clear, viscous liquid or glasslike solid; the commercial product, prepared in stick-form, contains about 17% Na_2O. Used as a reagent.

me·taph·y·se·al (me·taf″i·see′ul, met″uh·fiz′ee·ul) adj. Pertaining to a metaphysis.

metaphyseal aclasis. MULTIPLE HEREDITARY EXOSTOSES.

metaphyseal chondrodysplasia. METAPHYSEAL DYSOSTOSIS.

metaphyseal dysostosis. A very rare condition in which the roentgenographic appearance of the metaphyses is unique, being largely cartilaginous and irregularly calcified. Many metaphyses appear enlarged and the radiolucent space between the epiphysis and the shaft is markedly widened.

metaphyseal dysplasia. A possibly hereditary condition in which the ends of the long bones become markedly widened, with thin cortices, as a result of failure to become remodeled during endochondral osteogenesis.

me·taph·y·sis (me·taf′i·sis) *n.*, pl. **metaphy·ses** (·seez) 1. The region of growth between the epiphysis and diaphysis of a bone. Syn. *epiphyseal plate.* 2. The growing end of the diaphysis.

me·taph·y·si·tis (met″uh·fi·sigh′tis, me·taf′i·) *n.* Inflammation of a metaphysis.

meta·pla·sia (met″uh·play′zee·uh, ·zhuh) *n.* Transformation of one form of adult tissue to another, such as replacement of respiratory epithelium by stratified squamous epithelium. —**meta·plas·tic** (·plas′tick) *adj.*

me·ta·pla·sis (me·tap′luh·sis) *n.* Fulfilled growth and development seen in the stage between anaplasis and cataplasis.

meta·pro·tein (met″uh·pro′tee·in, ·teen) *n.* An intermediate product of acid or alkaline hydrolysis of a protein. Soluble in weak acids and alkalis, insoluble in water.

meta·ram·i·nol (met″uh·ram′i·nol) *n. l*-α-(1-Aminoethyl)-*m*-hydroxybenzyl alcohol, $C_9H_{13}NO_2$, a sympathomimetic amine; used as the bitartrate salt.

me·tas·ta·size (me·tas′tuh·size) *v.* To be transferred to another part of the body by metastasis.

metastasizing struma. An apparently benign goiter which gives rise to metastases.

metastatic abscess. A visceral or brain abscess complicating pyemia or septic embolism.

metastatic calcification. Pathologic calcification associated with high serum calcium levels and chiefly involving the lungs, stomach, and kidneys.

metastatic ophthalmia. A type of suppurative endophthalmitis caused by blood-borne infectious agents which localize in the intraocular structures, producing an exudate which collects in the vitreous chamber.

metastatic parotitis. Parotitis secondary to disease elsewhere; it occurs in infectious disease and usually goes on to suppuration. Syn. *symptomatic parotitis.*

Meta·stron·gy·lus (met″uh·stron′ji·lus) *n.* A genus of nematode parasites.

Metastrongylus elon·ga·tus (ee″long·gay′tus). A species of nematode common to hogs, occasionally to sheep and cattle, which infects the respiratory tract and produces a pneumonitis and bronchitis often fatal in young animals. A few cases of human infection have been reported.

meta·tar·sal·gia (met″uh·tahr·sal′jee·uh) *n.* Pain and tenderness in the metatarsal region.

meta·tar·sec·to·my (met″uh·tahr·seck′tum·ee) *n.* Excision of a metatarsal bone.

metatarsus ab·duc·tus (ab·duck′tus). A congenital deviation of the fore part of the foot away from the midline of the body, the heel remaining in a neutral or slightly valgus position. At birth there is no bone deformity, the deviation of the metatarsals being produced by soft-tissue contracture. In older persons bone deformity may develop due to secondary adaptation.

metatarsus ad·duc·to·va·rus (a·duck″to·vair′us). A congenital deformity of the foot; a deviation of the fore part of the foot toward the midline of the body, associated with an elevation of its inner border, the heel remaining in a neutral or slightly valgus position. It is caused by soft tissue contracture with bony deformity, occurs only in older cases and is due to secondary adaptation.

metatarsus ad·duc·tus (a·duck′tus). A congenital deviation of the fore part of the foot toward the midline of the body, the heel remaining in a neutral or slightly valgus position. At birth there is no bone deformity, the deviation of the metatarsals being produced by soft-tissue contracture. In older persons bone deformity may develop due to secondary adaptation.

me·tath·e·sis (me·tath′e·sis) *n.*, pl. **metathe·ses** (·seez) A chemical reaction in which there is an exchange of radicals or elements of the type AB + CD = AD + CB with no change in valence. —**meta·thet·ic** (meth·thet′ick) *adj.*

Meta·zoa (met″uh·zo′uh) *n.pl.* 1. A subdivision of the animal kingdom which includes all the multicellular forms, and so stands in contrast to the Protozoa. 2. In another classification, a subdivision including all multicellular forms except the Porifera (sponges). —**metazo·an** (·un) *adj. & n.*; **metazo·al** (·ul) *adj.*

Metch·ni·koff′s theory (m°etch′n°i·kuf) A theory of development of inflammation and immunity as manifestations of phagocytosis.

met·em·pir·ic (met″em·pirr′ick) *adj.* Not derived from experience, but implied or presupposed by it.

met·en·ceph·a·lon (met″en·sef′uh·lon) *n.* The cephalic part of the rhombencephalon, giving rise to the cerebellum and pons.

me·te·or·ism (mee′tee·ur·iz·um) *n.* Gaseous distention of the abdomen or intestine; tympanites.

me·te·o·rol·o·gy (mee″tee·ur·ol′uh·jee) *n.* The science that deals with the atmosphere and various atmospheric phenomena, including weather and weather forecasting.

-meter. A combining form designating *an instrument for measuring or recording* the specified kind of phenomena.

me·ter, *n.* 1. The basic unit of length in the metric system, originally established as the distance between two scratches on a bar of platinum-iridium alloy kept at the International Bureau of Weights and Measures, near Paris; later defined as 1650763.73 wavelengths, in vacuo, of a specified radiation of the krypton atom of mass 86. Abbreviated, m, m. 2. An instrument for measuring and recording quantities, as of the flow of electricity, liquids, or gases, of intensity of radiation, etc.

meth·a·cho·line chloride (meth″uh·ko′leen, ·lin). (2-Hydroxypropyl)trimethylammonium chloride acetate, $C_8H_{18}ClNO_2$, a parasympathomimetic drug employed mainly in the management of disorders of the cardiovascular system. The salt is usually administered subcutaneously; for oral administration methacholine bromide is used.

meth·a·done (meth′uh·dohn) n. 6-(Dimethylamino)-4,4-diphenyl-3-heptanone, $C_{21}H_{27}NO$, a narcotic analgesic used also for maintenance treatment of heroin addiction; employed as the hydrochloride salt.

meth·al·len·es·tril (meth″uh·le·nes′tril) n. β-Ethyl-6-methoxy-α,α-dimethyl-2-naphthalenepropionic acid, $C_{18}H_{22}O_3$, an orally effective, nonsteroid estrogen.

meth·am·phet·a·mine (meth″am·fet′uh·meen, ·min) n. Deoxyephedrine or N, α-dimethylphenethylamine, $C_{10}H_{15}N$, a central stimulant and pressor drug; used as the hydrochloride salt. Syn. *desoxyephedrine, methylamphetamine.*

meth·a·nal (meth′uh·nal) n. FORMALDEHYDE.

meth·ane (meth′ane) n. The first member, CH_4, of the homologous series of paraffins having the general formula C_nH_{2n+2}. A colorless, odorless, inflammable gas. Syn. *marsh gas.*

meth·a·no·ic acid (meth″uh·no′ick). FORMIC ACID (1).

meth·a·nol (meth′uh·nol, ·nole) n. METHYL ALCOHOL.

meth·an·the·line bromide (meth·anth′e·leen, ·in). Diethyl(2-hydroxyethyl)methylammonium bromide   xanthene-9-carboxylate, $C_{21}H_{26}BrNO_3$, a parasympatholytic drug with the antisecretory and antispasmodic actions of anticholinergic drugs.

meth·a·qua·lone (meth″uh·kway′lone, me·thack′wuh·lone) n. 2-Methyl-3-o-tolyl-4(3H)-quinazolinone, $C_{16}H_{14}N_2O$, a nonbarbiturate sedative and hypnotic.

Methedrine. A trademark for methamphetamine hydrochloride, a central stimulant drug.

met·hem·al·bu·min (met′heem·al·bew′min, ·hem·, ·al′bew·min) n. A product of the combination of hematin and serum albumin, comparable to methemoglobin. Syn. *pseudomethemoglobin. Fairley's pigment.*

met·hem·al·bu·mi·ne·mia (met″heem·al·bew″mi·nee′mee·uh, ·al″bew·) n. Methemalbumin in the plasma.

met·heme (met′heem) n. HEMATIN.

met·he·mo·glo·bin (met″hee′muh·glo′bin) n. The oxidized form of hemoglobin, in which the iron atom is trivalent, and which is not able to combine reversibly with oxygen. Syn. *ferrihemoglobin.*

met·he·mo·glo·bi·ne·mia, met·hae·mo·glo·bi·ne·mia (met·hee″muh·glo·bi·nee′mee·uh) n. 1. An excess of methemoglobin in the blood. 2. Any of several hereditary enzyme or hemoglobin abnormalities resulting in elevated methemoglobin levels and characterized clinically by cyanosis.

met·he·mo·glo·bin·uria, met·hae·mo·glo·bin·
uria (met·hee″muh·glo·bi·new′ree·uh) n. The presence of methemoglobin in the urine.

me·the·na·mine (meth·ee′nuh·meen, ·min, meth′in·uh·meen″) n. Hexamethylenetetramine, $(CH_2)_6N_4$, a urinary tract antiseptic. Syn. *hexamine.*

meth·ene (meth′een) n. 1. The first member, CH_2, of the ethylene (alkene) series of unsaturated hydrocarbons. It has never been isolated. 2. The hydrocarbon radical —CH_2—. Syn. *methylene.*

meth·e·nyl (meth′e·nil) n. The trivalent radical, $CH\equiv$. Syn. *methine, methyne.*

Methergine. Trademark for methylergonovine, an oxytocic agent used as the maleate salt.

meth·i·cil·lin (meth″i·sil′in) n. 2,6-Dimethoxyphenylpenicillin, $C_{17}H_{20}N_2O_6S$, a semisynthetic penicillin antibiotic; used as the sodium salt.

meth·im·a·zole (meth·im′uh·zole, me·thigh′muh·zole) n. 1-Methyl-2-imidazolethiol, $C_4H_6N_2S$, a thyroid inhibitor drug.

methiodal sodium. SODIUM METHIODAL.

me·thi·o·nine (me·thigh′o·neen, ·nin) n. DL-2-Amino-4-(methylthio)butyric acid, $CH_3S(CH_2)_2CHNH_2COOH$, an amino acid essential for growth of animals as it furnishes both labile methyl groups and sulfur necessary for normal metabolism. May be useful for prevention and treatment of certain types of liver damage.

methionine malabsorption syndrome. A hereditary metabolic disorder in which there appears to be a defect in the transport of methionine across the intestinal and renal tubular epithelium, with high urinary excretion of methionine and α-hydroxybutyric acid resulting from the conversion by *Escherichia coli* of unabsorbed methionine in the colon; manifested clinically by an offensive urinary odor, unpigmented hair, seizures, mental retardation, and episodes of fever, hyperpnea, and edema. Syn. *oasthouse urine disease.*

meth·o·car·ba·mol (meth″o·kahr′buh·mol, ·kahr·bam′ol) n. 2-Hydroxy-3-o-methoxyphenoxypropyl carbamate, $C_{11}H_{15}NO_5$, a skeletal muscle relaxant.

meth·od, n. The manner of performance of any act or operation, as a surgical procedure, a maneuver, a treatment, or a test.

meth·o·trex·ate (meth″o·treck′sate) n. Principally 4-amino-10-methylfolic acid, $C_{20}H_{22}N_8O_5$, with related compounds; an antineoplastic drug that functions as a folic acid antagonist. Used also in the treatment of psoriasis.

me·thoxy·flu·rane (me·thock″see·floo′rane) n. 2,2-Dichloro-1,1-difluoroethyl methyl ether, $CHCl_2CF_2OCH_3$, a colorless liquid; used as a general anesthetic.

meth·yl (meth′il) n. The univalent hydrocarbon radical CH_3—.

methyl alcohol. CH_3OH. A colorless, toxic liquid, obtained by destructive distillation of wood and by synthesis. Syn. *carbinol. methanol. wood alcohol.*

meth·yl·ate (meth′i·late) n. & v. 1. A compound formed from methyl alcohol by substitution of the hydrogen of the hydroxyl by a base. 2. To introduce a methyl group into a compound. —**meth·yl·at·ed** (meth′il·lay·tid) *adj.*

meth·yl·a·tion (meth″il·lay′shun) *n.* The process of introducing a methyl group into a compound.

meth·yl·ben·zene (meth″il·ben′zeen) *n.* TOLUENE.

meth·yl·benz·etho·ni·um chloride (meth″il·benz′eth·o′nee·um). Benzyldimethyl (2-[2-(*p*-1,1,3,3-tetramethylbutylcresoxy)ethoxy]ethyl)ammoniumchloride, $C_{28}H_{44}ClNO_2·H_2O$, a quaternary ammonium salt with surface-active and disinfectant properties; used especially for bacteriostasis of urea-splitting organisms causing ammonia dermatitis.

meth·yl·cel·lu·lose (meth″il·sel′yoo·loce) *n.* A methyl ether of cellulose, occurring as a grayish-white fibrous powder, swelling in water to produce a clear to opalescent, viscous, colloidal solution. Used in the treatment of chronic constipation because it imparts bulk and blandness to the stool. Used in pharmacy to produce stable dispersions.

methyl chloride. Chloromethane, CH_3Cl, a gas that may be compressed to a liquid which volatilizes rapidly and produces localized freezing; has been used as a local anesthetic.

meth·yl·do·pa (meth″il·do′puh) *n.* L-3-(3,4-Dihydroxyphenyl)-2-methylalanine, $C_{10}H_{13}NO_4$, an antihypertensive agent. Syn. *alpha methyldopa.*

meth·yl·ene (meth′i·leen) *n.* The bivalent hydrocarbon radical, $—CH_2—$.

methylene blue. 3,7-Bis(dimethylamino)phenazathionium chloride, $C_{16}H_{18}ClN_3S.3H_2O$, occurring as dark green crystals or a crystalline powder with a bronzelike luster but forming deep blue solutions. Used as an antidote to cyanide poisoning and, formerly, as a urinary antiseptic; an ingredient of many biologic staining solutions. Syn. *methylthionine chloride.*

methylene blue O. TOLUIDINE BLUE O.

meth·y·lep·sia (meth″i·lep′see·uh) *n.* 1. Abnormal desire for intoxicating drink. 2. Hyperexcitability in an alcohol-intoxicated individual.

meth·yl·er·go·no·vine (meth″il·ur″go·no′veen) *n.* N-[1-(Hydroxymethyl)propyl]-D-lysergamide, $C_{20}H_{25}N_3O_2$, an oxytocic drug with the actions and uses of ergonovine; employed as the maleate salt.

meth·yl·gly·ox·al (meth″il·glye·ock′sal) *n.* CH_3COCHO. The aldehyde of pyruvic acid, capable of transformation into glycogen by the liver.

methyl hydrate. METHYL ALCOHOL.

methyl hydride. CH_4. METHANE.

meth·yl·mer·cap·tan (meth″il·mur·kap′tan) *n.* Methanethiol, CH_3SH, a gas of disagreeable odor produced in the intestinal tract by decomposition of certain proteins; also occurs in coal tar.

methyl meth·ac·ryl·ate (meth·ack′ri·late). The methyl ester of methacrylic acid, $CH_2=C(CH_3)COOCH_3$, a liquid that polymerizes readily to form thermoplastic substances called acrylics.

meth·yl·mor·phine (meth″il·mor′feen, ·fin) *n.* CODEINE.

meth·yl·par·a·ben (meth″il·păr′uh·ben) *n.* Methyl *p*-hydroxybenzoate, $HOC_6H_4·COOCH_3$, an antifungal preservative.

meth·yl·phen·i·date (meth″il·fen′i·date) *n.* Methyl α-phenyl-2-piperidineacetate, $C_{14}H_{19}NO_2$, a central nervous system stimulant used in the treatment of various types of depression; employed as the hydrochloride salt.

meth·yl·phe·nol (meth″il·fee′nol) *n.* CRESOL.

meth·yl·pred·nis·o·lone (meth″il·pred·nis′uh·lone) *n.* 11β,17,21-Trihydroxy-6α-methylpregna-1,4-diene-3,20-dione, $C_{22}H_{30}O_5$. An adrenocortical steroid with the actions and uses of prednisolone; used also in the form of its 21-acetate and 21-(sodium succinate).

meth·yl·pu·rine (meth″il·pew′reen, ·rin) *n.* Any compound in which one or more methyl radicals have been introduced into the purine nucleus. Among the more important compounds of this type are caffeine, theobromine, and theophylline.

methyl red. *p*-Dimethylaminoazobenzene-*o*-carboxylic acid, $C_{15}H_{15}N_3O_2$, violet crystals; used as an indicator in titrating weak bases.

methyl red test. A test for the differentiation of Enterobacteriaceae, such as the aerogenes group and the colon group of bacteria, performed by incubating the bacteria in a special medium and testing with methyl red indicator.

meth·yl·ros·an·i·line chloride (meth″il·ro·zan′il·een, ·lin). Hexamethylpararosaniline chloride, $C_{25}H_{30}ClN_3$, usually with more or less pentamethylpararosaniline chloride and tetramethylpararosaniline chloride; a dye mixture used as an antibacterial, antifungal, and anthelmintic agent and also as a biological stain. Crystal violet, gentian violet, and methyl violet are frequently used as synonyms for methylrosaniline chloride but the substances are not absolutely identical, differing in the specific methylpararosanilines present and in their proportions.

methyl salicylate. $C_6H_4(OH)COOCH_3$. A colorless, oily liquid, identical with the essential constituent of wintergreen oil; used externally as a counterirritant and in histology as a clearing agent.

meth·yl·tes·tos·ter·one (meth″il·tes·tos′tur·ohn) *n.* 17β-Hydroxy-17-methylandrost-4-en-3-one, $C_{20}H_{30}O_2$, an orally effective androgenic steroid hormone.

methyl theobromine. CAFFEINE.

meth·yl·thi·o·nine chloride (meth″il·thigh′o·neen, ·nin). METHYLENE BLUE.

meth·y·pry·lon (meth″i·prye′lon) *n.* 3,3-Diethyl-5-methyl-2,4-piperidinedione, $C_{10}H_{17}NO_2$, a nonbarbiturate sedative and hypnotic.

meth·y·ser·gide (meth″i·sur′jide) *n.* N-[1-(Hydroxymethyl) propyl]-1-methyl-D-lysergamide, a homologue of methylergonovine; used as the bimaleate salt for prophylactic management of migraine headache.

Meticorten. A trademark for prednisone, an anti-inflammatory adrenocortical steroid.

me·top·ic (me·top'ick, me·to'pick) *adj.* 1. Pertaining to the forehead; frontal. 2. Pertaining to a cranium having a frontal suture; characterized by metopism.

metopic suture. The frontal suture, present in infancy, between the two vertical halves of the frontal bone; especially the inferior part or all of it when it persists in the adult skull.

met·o·pism (met'o·piz·um) *n.* The condition of having a metopic suture: a frontal suture that persists beyond infancy.

¹metr-, metro- A combining form meaning (a) *uterus, uterine;* (b) *mother, maternal.*

²metr-, metro- A combining form meaning *measure or distance.*

me·tral·gia (me·tral'jee·uh, ·juh) *n.* Pain of uterine origin. Syn. *metrodynia.*

me·tra·pec·tic (mee''truh·peck'tick, met''ruh·) *adj.* Pertaining to a disease which is transmitted through the mother but which she herself escapes (such as hemophilia).

me·tra·to·nia (mee''truh·to'nee·uh, met''ruh·) *n.* Atony of the uterus.

me·tra·tro·phia (mee''truh·tro'fee·uh, met''ruh·) *n.* Atrophy of the uterus.

Metrazol. A trademark for pentylenetetrazol, a central nervous system stimulant.

me·tre (mee'tur) *n.* METER.

me·trec·ta·sia (mee''treck·tay'zee·uh, ·zhuh, met''reck·) *n.* Enlargement of the nonpregnant uterus.

me·trec·to·pia (mee''treck·to'pee·uh, met''reck·) *n.* Displacement of the uterus.

me·tre·mia, me·trae·mia (me·tree'mee·uh) *n.* Hyperemia of the uterus.

me·treu·ryn·ter (mee''troo·rin'tur, met''roo·) *n.* An inflatable bag for dilating the cervical canal of the uterus.

me·treu·ry·sis (mee·troo'ri·sis) *n.* Dilatation of the uterine cervix with the metreurynter.

me·tria (mee'tree·uh) *n.* 1. Any uterine affection. 2. Any inflammatory condition during the puerperium.

met·ric (met'rick) *adj.* 1. Of or pertaining to the metric system. 2. Of or for measurement.

metric system. A decimal system of weights and measures based on the meter as the unit of length, the kilogram as the unit of mass, and the liter as the unit of capacity, the last representing 0.001 cubic meter or 1000 cubic centimeters.

me·tri·tis (me·trye'tis) *n.* Inflammation of the uterus, involving the endometrium and myometrium. **—me·trit·ic** (me·trit'ick) *adj.*

metro-. See *metr-.*

me·tro·cele (mee'tro·seel) *n.* Hernia of the uterus.

me·tro·clyst (mee'tro·klist) *n.* An instrument for giving uterine douches.

me·tro·col·po·cele (mee''tro·kol'po·seel, met''ro·) *n.* Protrusion or prolapse of the uterus into the vagina, with prolapse of the anterior vaginal wall.

me·tro·cys·to·sis (mee''tro·sis·to'sis, met''ro·) *n.* 1. The formation of uterine cysts. 2. The condition giving rise to uterine cysts.

me·tro·dy·na·mom·e·ter (mee''tro·dye''nuh·mom'e·tur) *n.* An instrument for measuring uterine contractions.

me·trog·ra·phy (me·trog'ruh·fee) *n.* Radiography of the uterus through the injection of contrast media into the uterine cavity; UTEROGRAPHY.

me·trol·o·gy (me·trol'uh·jee) *n.* The science that deals with methods of measurement and units of measure.

me·tro·ma·la·cia (mee''tro·ma·lay'shee·uh, met''ro·) *n.* Softening of the tissues of the uterus.

met·ro·ni·da·zole (met''ro·nigh'duh·zole, ·nid'uh·zole) *n.* 1-(2-Hydroxyethyl)-2-methyl-5-nitroimidazole, $C_6H_9N_3O_3$, a systemic trichomonacide.

me·tro·pa·ral·y·sis (mee''tro·puh·ral'i·sis, met''ro·) *n.* Uterine paralysis, usually that which may occur immediately following childbirth.

me·tro·path·ia hem·or·rhag·i·ca (mee''tro·path'ee·uh hem'o·raj'i·kuh) Abnormal uterine bleeding, now generally considered to be of endocrine origin.

me·trop·a·thy (me·trop'uth·ee) *n.* Any uterine disease. **—me·tro·path·ic** (mee''tro·path'ick, met''ro·) *adj.*

me·tro·phle·bi·tis (mee''tro·fle·bye'tis, met''ro·) *n.* Inflammation of the veins of the uterus.

me·tro·plas·ty (mee'tro·plas''tee, met'ro·) *n.* Plastic surgical repair of the uterus.

me·trop·to·sis (mee''tro·to'sis, mee''tro·to'sis) *n.* PROLAPSE OF THE UTERUS.

me·tror·rha·gia (mee''tro·ray'jee·uh, met''ro·) *n.* Uterine hemorrhage independent of the menstrual period. Syn. *intermenstrual flow, polymenorrhea.*

me·tror·rhex·is (mee''tro·reck'sis) *n.* Rupture of the uterus.

me·tro·sal·pin·gi·tis (mee''tro·sal''pin·jye'tis) *n.* Inflammation of the uterus and oviducts.

me·tro·sal·pin·gog·ra·phy (mee''tro·sal''ping·gog'ruh·fee) *n.* HYSTEROSALPINGOGRAPHY.

me·tro·scope (mee'tro·skope) *n.* An instrument for examining the uterus.

me·tro·stax·is (mee''tro·stack'sis) *n.* Slight but persistent uterine hemorrhage.

me·tro·ste·no·sis (mee''tro·ste·no'sis) *n.* Abnormal contraction of the cavity of the uterus.

me·tro·tome (mee'tro·tome, met'ro·tome) *n.* An instrument for incising the uterine neck.

Metycaine. Trademark for piperocaine, an ester local anesthetic used as the hydrochloride salt.

me·tyr·a·pone (me·tirr'uh·pone) *n.* 2-Methyl-1,2-di-3-pyridyl-1-propanone, $C_{14}H_{14}N_2O$, a diagnostic aid for determining pituitary function. Metyrapone blocks 11β-hydroxylation of steroids in the adrenal cortex and causes a compensatory increase in secretion of corticotropin by the normal pituitary as a result of which there is increased urinary excretion of 17-hydroxycorticoids and 17-ketogenic steroids; the quantity excreted is an index of pituitary function. Syn. *mepyrapone, methopyrapone.*

Meu·len·gracht diet A high calorie, vitamin-rich diet for the treatment of bleeding peptic ulcer.

mev Million electron volts.

mev·a·lon·ic acid (mev''uh·lon'ick). 3,5-Dihydroxy-2-methylvaleric acid, $C_6H_{12}O_4$, a precursor in the biosynthesis of cholesterol and of vitamin A.

Mex·i·can hat cell. TARGET CELL.

Mey·er·hof cycle or **scheme** (migh'ur·hofe) A series of enzymatic reactions which have been shown to occur in a variety of animal, plant, and microbial tissues, whereby glucose (or glycogen or starch) is converted to pyruvic acid. Syn. *Embden-Meyerhof scheme.*

Mey·er-Over·ton theory A theory that the degree of anesthetic activity of a compound is correlated with a high oil/water distribution ratio of the anesthetic.

Mg Symbol for magnesium.

mg, mg. Abbreviation for *milligram.*

mg %, mg. %. MILLIGRAMS PERCENT.

mgh, mgh. MILLIGRAM-HOUR; an older method of expressing radium dosage (exposure) obtained by the application of one milligram of radium element for one hour.

mho (mo) *n.* The unit of electric conductance; the reciprocal of the ohm.

Mi·a·na or **Mi·a·neh fever** (mee·ah·ney') RELAPSING FEVER.

mi·ca (migh'kuh) *n.* 1. A crumb. 2. A silicate mineral occurring in the form of thin, shining, transparent scales.

mi·celle (mi·sel', migh·sel') *n.* 1. *Obsol.* One of the fundamental submicroscopic structural units of protoplasm. 2. Originally, a highly hydrated and charged colloidal aggregate such as phospholipids dispersed in aqueous media and detergents. 3. More, broadly, any unit of structure composed of an aggregate or oriented arrangement of molecules, as in cellulose and rubber. —**mi·cel·lar** (migh·sel'ur, mi·) *adj.*

Mi·cha·e·lis constant (Ger. mikh·ah·ey'lis) The substrate concentration, in moles per liter, at which an enzymic reaction proceeds at one-half the maximal velocity. Symbol, K_m.

Mi·cha·e·lis-Gut·mann bodies or **calcospherules** (goot'mahn) Basophilic and often concentrically laminated bodies, which may contain iron and calcium, seen in malacoplakia.

Michel clip. A type of skin clip for closing incisions.

micr-, micro- A combining form meaning (a) *small, minute,* as in microinfarct, microwave; (b) *undersized, abnormally small,* as in microcyte, microcephalic; (c) *pertaining to minute objects or quantities,* as in microscope, microanalysis; (d) *microscopic,* as in microanatomy; (e) *one one-millionth,* as in microgram.

micra. A plural of *micron* (= ²MICROMETER).

mi·cra·cous·tic (migh''kruh·koos'tick) *adj.* Pertaining to or adapted to the hearing of very faint sounds.

mi·cren·ceph·a·ly (migh''kren·sef'uh·lee) *n.* The condition of having an abnormally small brain. —**micrencepha·lous** (·lus) *adj.*

mi·cro·ab·scess (migh''kro·ab'ses) *n.* A very small abscess.

mi·cro·aero·phil·ic (migh''kro·ay''ur·o·fil'ick) *adj.* Pertaining to microorganisms which require free oxygen for their growth, but which

thrive best when the oxygen is less in amount than that in the atmosphere.

mi·cro·anat·o·my (migh''kro·uh·nat'uh·mee) *n.* MICROSCOPIC ANATOMY. —**microanato·mist** (·mist) *n.*

mi·cro·an·eu·rysm (migh''kro·an'yoo·riz·um) *n.* Aneurysmal dilatation of a capillary, characteristic of diabetic retinopathy, but also seen in the conjunctiva in patients with other diseases.

mi·cro·an·gi·op·a·thy (migh''kro·an''jee·op'uh·thee) *n.* Any disease of small blood vessels (precapillaries, capillaries, arterioles, or venules).

mi·cro·ar·te·rio·gram (migh''kro·ahr·teer'ee·o·gram) *n.* Radiographic visualization of minute arterial branches, usually on material obtained at surgical operations or autopsies. —**microar·te·rio·graph·ic** (·teer''ee·o·graf'ick) *adj.;* **microar·te·ri·og·ra·phy** (·teer''ee·og'ruh·fee) *n.*

mi·cro·au·di·phone (migh''kro·aw'di·fone) *n.* An instrument for rendering very slight sounds audible.

mi·crobe (migh'krobe) *n.* Microorganism; especially, bacterium. —**mi·cro·bi·al** (migh·kro'bee·ul), **mi·cro·bic** (migh·kro'bick) *adj.*

mi·cro·bi·cide (migh·kro'bi·side) *n.* An agent that destroys microbes. Syn. *germicide.* —**mi·cro·bi·ci·dal** (migh·kro''bi·sigh'dul) *adj.*

mi·cro·bi·in·ert (migh''kro·bi·nurt') *adj.* Unable to support microbial growth because of absence of necessary nutrients. —**microbinert·ness** (·nis) *n.*

mi·cro·bi·ol·o·gy (migh''kro·bye·ol'uh·jee) *n.* The biology of microorganisms. —**micro·bi·o·log·ic** (·bye''uh·loj'ick) *adj.;* **micro·bi·ol·o·gist** (bye·ol'uh·jist) *n.*

mi·cro·bi·o·ta (migh''kro·bye·o'tuh) *n.* The totality of microorganisms normally found in a given area or habitat.

mi·cro·bi·ot·ic (migh''kro·bye·ot'ick) *adj.* Pertaining to microscopic forms of life.

mi·cro·blast (migh'kro·blast) *n.* 1. An immature blood cell. 2. A small, nucleated, red blood cell. 3. A small, anaplastic leukocyte having the other characteristics of blast cells, but found in the peripheral blood.

mi·cro·body (migh'kro·bod''ee) *n.* PEROXISOME.

mi·cro·bra·chia (migh''kro·bray'kee·uh) *n.* Abnormally (congenital) small arms.

mi·cro·brachy·ce·pha·lia (migh''kro·brack''ee·se·fay'lee·uh) *n.* Brachycephalia combined with microcephaly.

mi·cro·bu·ret (migh''kro·bew·ret') *n.* An apparatus for delivering or measuring small quantities of liquids or gases.

mi·cro·cal·cu·lus (migh''kro·kal'kew·lus) *n.,* pl. **microcalcu·li** (·lye) A concretion of extremely small size; especially, a small focus of renal tubular calcification.

mi·cro·cal·o·rie (migh''kro·kal'uh·ree) *n.* A small calorie; for practical purposes, the quantity of heat necessary to raise the temperature of 1 g of water from 15° to 16°C.

mi·cro·car·dia (migh''kro·kahr'dee·uh) *n.* Congenital smallness of the heart.

mi·cro·cav·i·ta·tion (migh″kro·kav·i·tay′shun) *n.* The presence of minute cavities in a tissue or organ.

mi·cro·ceph·a·lus (migh″kro·sef′uh·lus) *n.*, *pl.* **microcepha·li** (·lye) An individual with an unusually small head.

mi·cro·ceph·a·ly (migh″kro·sef′uh·lee) *n.* A condition characterized by a small head whose circumference is less than two standard deviations below mean for age and sex; may be due to congenital hypoplasia of the cerebrum or be the consequence of severe brain damage in early life; often associated with mental retardation, but may be seen in pituitary dwarfs of normal intelligence. —**micro·ce·phal·ic** (·se·fal′ick), **micro·ceph·a·lous** (·sef′uh·lus) *adj.*

mi·cro·chei·lia (migh″kro·kigh′lee·uh) *n.* Abnormal smallness of the lips.

mi·cro·chem·is·try (migh″kro·kem′is·tree) *n.* 1. The study of chemical reactions, using small quantities of materials, frequently less than 1 mg or 100 μl, and often requiring special small apparatus and microscopical observation. 2. The chemistry of individual cells and minute organisms. —**microchem·i·cal** (·i·kul) *adj.*

mi·cro·chi·ria (migh″kro·kigh′ree·uh) *n.* Abnormal smallness of the hand.

mi·cro·cir·cu·la·tion (migh″kro·sur′kew·lay′shun) *n.* The flow of blood or lymph in the vessels of the microcirculatory system.

mi·cro·cir·cu·la·to·ry system (migh″kro·sur′kew·luh·tor·ee). The portion of a blood or lymphatic circulatory system which is made up of minute vessels; especially, the system of arterioles, precapillaries, capillaries, and venules, including that part of the vasculature in which exchange of nutrients, wastes, and other substances occurs between tissues and blood.

Mi·cro·coc·ca·ce·ae (migh″kro·cock·ay′see·ee) *n.pl.* A family of bacteria containing the genera *Micrococcus*, *Gaffkya*, *Sarcina*, and *Staphylococcus*.

Mi·cro·coc·cus (migh″kro·kock′us) *n.* A genus of bacteria of the family Micrococcaceae.

micrococcus, *n.*, *pl.* **micrococ·ci** (migh″kro·cock′sigh). A bacterium of the genus *Micrococcus* or any similar small coccus.

Micrococcus al·bus (al′bus) STAPHYLOCOCCUS EPIDERMIDIS.

Micrococcus aureus. STAPHYLOCOCCUS AUREUS.

Micrococcus gonorrheae. NEISSERIA GONORRHOEAE.

Micrococcus in·tra·cel·lu·la·ris meningitidis (in″truh·sel·yoo·lair′is). NEISSERIA MENINGITIDIS.

Micrococcus lan·ce·o·la·tus (lan″see·o·lay′tus). STREPTOCOCCUS PNEUMONIAE.

Micrococcus melitensis. BRUCELLA MELITENSIS.

Micrococcus meningitidis. NEISSERIA MENINGITIDIS.

Micrococcus pneumoniae. STREPTOCOCCUS PNEUMONIAE.

Micrococcus py·og·e·nes (pye·oj′e·neez). 1. STAPHYLOCOCCUS AUREUS. 2. STAPHYLOCOCCUS EPIDERMIDIS.

mi·cro·co·lon (migh″kro·ko′lun) *n.* An abnormally small colon.

mi·cro·cor·nea (migh″kro·kor′nee·uh) *n.* Abnormal smallness of the cornea.

mi·cro·crys·tal·line (migh″kro·kris′tuh·lin) *adj.* Composed of crystals of microscopic size.

mi·cro·cu·rie (migh″kro·kew′ree) *n.* The amount of a radioactive substance which undergoes 3.7×10^4 disintegrations per second; equivalent to one-millionth of a curie. Symbol, μCi.

mi·cro·cyst (migh″kro·sist) *n.* A cyst of small size. —**mi·cro·cys·tic** (migh″kro·sis′tic) *adj.*

mi·cro·cyte (migh″kro·site) *n.* 1. An erythrocyte having either a diameter or a mean corpuscular volume (MCV), or both, more than two standard deviations below the mean normal, determined by the same method on the blood of healthy persons of the patient's age and sex group. 2. A cell of the microglia. —**mi·cro·cyt·ic** (migh″kro·sit′ick) *adj.*

microcytic anemia. Any anemia in which the erythrocytes are smaller than normal.

mi·cro·cy·to·sis (migh″kro·sigh·to′sis) *n.* A condition of the blood characterized by a preponderance of microcytes, as observed microscopically or determined by measurement of cell volume.

mi·cro·dac·ty·ly (migh″kro·dack′ti·lee) *n.* Abnormal smallness of one or more fingers or toes. —**microdacty·lous** (·lus) *adj.*

mi·cro·dis·sec·tion (migh″kro·di·seck′shun) *n.* Dissection with the aid of a microscope.

mi·cro·don·tia (migh″kro·don′chee·uh) *n.* The condition of having one or more abnormally small teeth. —**mi·cro·dont** (migh″kro·dont) *adj.*

mi·cro·drep·a·no·cyt·ic (migh″kro·drep′uh·no·sit′ick, ·drep·an″o·) *adj.* Both microcytic and drepanocytic.

microdrepanocytic disease. SICKLE CELL THALASSEMIA.

mi·cro·drep·a·no·cy·to·sis (migh″kro·drep′uh·no·sigh·to′sis) *n.* SICKLE CELL THALASSEMIA.

mi·cro·elec·tro·pho·ret·ic (migh″kro·e·lec″tro·fo·ret′ick) *adj.* Pertaining to electrophoresis of minute quantities of solutions.

mi·cro·en·ceph·a·ly (migh″kro·en·sef′ul·ee) *n.* MICRENCEPHALY.

mi·cro·far·ad (migh″kro·far′ad) *n.* The one-millionth part of a farad.

mi·cro·fi·bril (migh″kro·figh′bril) *n.* An extremely fine fibril. —**microfi·bril·lar** (·bri·lur) *adj.*

mi·cro·fi·lar·ia (migh″kro·fi·lâr′ee·uh) *n.*, *pl.* **microfilar·i·ae** (·ee·ee). The embryonic or prelarval forms of filarial worms; slender motile forms, 150 to 300 μm in length, found in the blood stream and tissues. On ingestion by the proper blood-sucking insects the microfilariae pass through developmental stages in the body of the host and become infective larvae.

mi·cro·fol·lic·u·lar (migh″kro·fol·ick′yoo·lur) *adj.* Characterized by very small follicles.

microfollicular adenoma. A thyroid adenoma whose follicles are very small.

mi·cro·frac·ture (migh″kro·frack″chur) *n.* A minute fracture, usually clinically and radiographically obscure.

mi·cro·gam·ete (migh″kro·gam′eet, ·ga·meet′) *n.* A male reproductive cell in certain Protozoa, corresponding to the sperm cell in Metazoa.

mi·cro·gen·e·sis (migh″kro·jen′e·sis) *n.* Abnormally small development of a part.

mi·cro·ge·nia (migh″kro·jee′nee·uh) *n.* Abnormal smallness of the chin.

mi·cro·gen·i·tal·ism (migh″kro·jen′i·tul·iz·um) *n.* Having extremely undersized genital organs.

mi·crog·lia (migh·krog′lee·uh) *n.* Small neuroglial cells of the central nervous system having long processes and exhibiting ameboid and phagocytic activity under pathologic conditions. —**microg·li·al** (·lee·ul) *adj.*

mi·cro·gli·o·ma·to·sis (migh·krog″lee·o″muh·to′sis, migh″kro·glye″o·) *n.* A brain tumor composed largely, or entirely, of metalophil cells representing varying stages from primitive reticulum cells to mature microglia; it is similar to, or identical with, reticulum-cell sarcoma elsewhere in the body.

mi·cro·glos·sia (migh″kro·glos′ee·uh) *n.* Abnormal smallness of the tongue.

mi·cro·gram (migh′kro·gram) *n.* One one-thousandth of a milligram. Abbreviated, mcg. Symbol, μg. Syn. *gamma.*

mi·cro·graph (migh′kro·graf) *n.* 1. A pantographic device for enabling one to draw sketches on a very small scale. 2. An instrument that magnifies the vibrations of a diaphragm and records them on a moving photographic film.

mi·cro·graph·ia (migh″kro·graf′ee·uh) *n.* Very small handwriting; particularly the tendency to write smaller than during a state of normal health, seen in certain cerebral disorders, such as parkinsonism.

mi·crog·ra·phy (migh·krog′ruh·fee) *n.* 1. A description of structures studied under the microscope. 2. MICROGRAPHIA.

mi·cro·gy·ria (migh″kro·jye′ree·uh, ·jirr′ee·uh) *n.* Abnormal smallness of the convolutions of the brain.

mi·crohm (migh′krome) *n.* One one-millionth of an ohm.

mi·cro·in·cin·er·a·tion (migh″kro·in·sin″uh·ray′shun) *n.* Reduction of small quantities of organic substances to ash by application of heat.

mi·cro·in·farct (migh″kro·in′fahrkt) *n.* A very small infarct, usually detected only by microscopic examination. —**micro·in·farc·tion** (in·fahrk′shun) *n.*

mi·cro·in·va·sion (migh″kro·in·vay′zhun) *n.* Invasion by tumor, especially a squamous cell carcinoma of the uterine cervix, a very short distance into the tissues beneath the point of origin.

mi·cro·ker·a·tome (migh″kro·kerr′uh·tome) *n.* A small keratome used in microsurgery of the cornea.

mi·cro·li·ter (migh′kro·lee′tur) *n.* A millionth of a liter, or a thousandth of a milliliter.

mi·cro·lith (migh′kro·lith) *n.* A microscopic calculus.

mi·cro·li·thi·a·sis (migh″kro·li·thigh′uh·sis) *n.* The presence of numerous very minute calculi.

microlithiasis al·ve·o·la·ris pul·mo·num (al″vee·o·lair′is pool·mo′num). A rare form of pulmonary calcification of uncertain cause in which many minute, spherical, concentrically calci-fied bodies (calcospherites or microliths), and osseous nodules of larger size are found; may simulate pulmonary tuberculosis on radiologic examination.

mi·cro·ma·nia (migh″kro·may′nee·uh) *n.* A delusional state in which the patient believes himself diminutive in size and mentally inferior.

mi·cro·ma·nip·u·la·tion (migh″kro·ma·nip′yoo·lay′shun) *n.* Manipulation of minute objects under a microscope; use of a micromanipulator. —**micro·ma·nip·u·la·tive** (·nip′yoo·luh·tiv, ·lay·tiv) *adj.*

mi·cro·ma·nip·u·la·tor (migh″kro·ma·nip′yoo·lay·tur) *n.* A device for moving exceedingly fine instruments, under the magnification of a microscope, for dissection of cells or for other operations involving minute objects.

mi·cro·ma·nom·e·ter (migh″kro·muh·nom′e·tur) *n.* A manometer for measuring very small differences of pressure, as in the gasometric determination of the metabolic activity of minute quantities of tissue.

mi·cro·mas·tia (migh″kro·mas′tee·uh) *n.* Abnormal smallness of the breasts. Syn. *micromazia.*

mi·cro·me·lia (migh″kro·mee′lee·uh) *n.* Abnormal smallness of the limbs.

mi·cro·mel·ic (migh″kro·mel′ick, ·mee′lick) *adj.* Having abnormally small limbs.

mi·cro·me·lus (migh·krom′e·lus) *n.* An individual with abnormally small limbs.

¹mi·crom·e·ter (migh·krom′e·tur) *n.* An instrument designed for measuring distances, or apparent diameters; used with a microscope or telescope. —**microme·try** (·tree) *n.*

²mi·cro·me·ter (migh′kro·mee′tur) *n.* The one-thousandth part of a millimeter, or the one-millionth part of a meter. Symbol, μm.

mi·cro·meth·od (migh′kro·meth″ud) *n.* A method of laboratory examination in which very small quantities of the substances to be examined are used.

mi·cro·mi·cron (migh″kro·migh′kron) *n. Obsol.* The millionth part of a micron. Symbol, μμ.

mi·cro·mil·li·me·ter (migh″kro·mil′i·mee·tur) *n. Obsol.* NANOMETER.

mi·cro·mo·to·scope (migh″kro·mo′tuh·skope) *n.* An apparatus for photographing and exhibiting motile microorganisms.

mi·cro·my·e·lia (migh″kro·migh·ee′lee·uh) *n.* Abnormal smallness of the spinal cord.

mi·cro·my·e·lo·blast (migh″kro·migh′e·lo·blast) *n.* An extremely small myeloblast.

mi·cron (migh′kron) *n.* pl. **microns, mi·cra** (·kruh) ²MICROMETER. Symbol, μ.

mi·cro·nod·u·la·tion (migh″kro·nod″yoo·lay′shun) *n.* The presence of very small nodules in a tissue or organ. —**micro·nod·u·lar** (·nod′yoo·lur) *adj.*

mi·cro·nu·cle·us (migh″kro·new′klee·us) *n.,* pl. **micronu·clei** (·klee·eye). 1. A small or minute nucleus. 2. The reproductive nucleus of protozoa as contrasted with the macronucleus. 3. NUCLEOLUS.

mi·cro·nu·tri·ent (migh″kro·new′tree·unt) *n.* A vitamin or mineral occurring in traces essential for growth, development, and health.

mi·cro·nych·ia (migh″kro·nick′ee·uh) *n.* The presence of one or more abnormally small nails which in every other respect seem normal.

mi·cro·or·chism (migh″kro·or′kiz·um) *n.* Congenital hypoplasia of the testes; when severe, it may be associated with the eunuchoid state.

mi·cro·or·gan·ism (migh″kro·or′gun·iz·um) *n.* A microscopic organism, either animal or plant, especially a bacterium or protozoan. —**micro·organ·ic** (·or·gan′ick) *adj.*

mi·cro·pap·u·lar (migh″kro·pap′yoo·lur) *adj.* Having or pertaining to very small papules.

mi·cro·pe·nis (migh″kro·pee′nis) *n.* MICROPHALLUS.

mi·cro·phage (migh′kro·faij) *n.* 1. A neutrophil granulocyte in tissues. 2. A small phagocyte.

mi·cro·pha·kia (migh″kro·fay′kee·uh) *n.* A congenital or developmental anomaly in which there is an abnormally small crystalline lens.

mi·cro·phal·lus (migh″kro·fal′us) *n.* Abnormal smallness of the penis. Syn. *micropenis*.

mi·cro·pho·bia (migh″kro·fo′bee·uh) *n.* 1. Morbid fear of microbes. 2. Morbid fear of small objects.

mi·cro·phone (migh′kro·fone) *n.* An instrument in which sounds modulate an electric current which can be amplified so that the sounds become audible.

mi·cro·pho·nia (migh″kro·fo′nee·uh) *n.* Weakness of voice.

mi·cro·pho·no·scope (migh″kro·fo′nuh·skope) *n.* A binaural stethoscope with a membrane in the chestpiece to accentuate the sound.

mi·cro·pho·to·graph (migh″kro·fo′tuh·graf) *n.* 1. A photograph of microscopic size. 2. *Erron.* PHOTOMICROGRAPH.

mi·croph·thal·mia (migh″krof·thal′mee·uh) *n.* MICROPHTHALMUS (1).

mi·croph·thal·mus (migh″krof·thal′mus) *n.* 1. A condition in which the eyeball is abnormally small. Syn. *microphthalmia, nanophthalmus, nanophthalmos, nanophthalmia*. 2. A person manifesting such a condition.

mi·cro·phys·ics (migh″kro·fiz′icks) *n.* A branch of science that deals with elementary particles, atoms, and molecules.

mi·cro·phyte (migh′kro·fite) *n.* Any microscopic plant, especially one that is parasitic.

mi·cro·pi·pet (migh″kro·pye·pet′, ·pi·pet′) *n.* 1. A small pipet with a fine-pointed tip used in microinjection. 2. A pipet for measuring very small volumes.

mi·cro·po·dia (migh″kro·po′dee·uh) *n.* Abnormal smallness of the feet.

mi·cro·pro·jec·tion (migh″kro·pro·jeck′shun) *n.* The projection of the image of microscopic objects on a screen.

mi·cro·pro·so·pia (migh″kro·pro·so′pee·uh) *n.* Congenital abnormal smallness of the face.

mi·crop·sia (migh·krop′see·uh) *n.* Disturbance of visual perception in which objects appear smaller than their true size.

mi·crop·tic (migh·krop′tick) *adj.* Pertaining to, or affected with, micropsia.

mi·cro·pus (migh·kro·pus, migh·kro′pus) *n.* MICROPODIA.

mi·cro·pyle (migh′kro·pile) *n.* A minute opening in the investing membrane of many ova, permitting entrance of the sperm.

mi·cro·ra·di·og·ra·phy (migh″kro·ray″dee·og′ruh·fee) *n.* Radiography using a special photographic emulsion so that enlargement (of the order of 100 times) does not reveal silver grains in the emulsion, thereby permitting great magnification of the original image of a very small object.

mi·cro·res·pi·rom·e·ter (migh″kro·res″pi·rom′e·tur) *n.* An apparatus for measuring the respiratory activity of minute amounts of tissue. —**microrespi·ro·met·ric** (·ro·met′rick) *adj.*

mi·cror·rhi·nia, mi·cro·rhi·nia (migh″kro·rye′nee·uh) *n.* Congenital smallness of the nose.

mi·cro·ruth·er·ford (migh″kro·ruh′thur·furd) *n.* A unit equivalent to one one-millionth of a rutherford or 1 disintegration per second. Symbol, μrd.

mi·cro·scel·ous (migh″kro·skel′us, migh·kros′ke·lus) *adj.* Having abnormally small legs.

mi·cro·scope (migh′kruh·skope) *n.* An apparatus through which minute objects are rendered visible. It consists of a lens, or group of lenses, by which a magnified image of the object is produced.

mi·cro·scop·ic (migh″kro·skop′ick) *adj.* 1. Extremely small; too small to be readily visible to the naked eye. 2. MICROSCOPICAL; pertaining to or done with a microscope.

mi·cro·scop·i·cal (migh″kro·skop′i·kul) *adj.* 1. Pertaining to or done with a microscope. 2. MICROSCOPIC; too small to be readily visible to the naked eye.

microscopic anatomy. The branch of anatomy that deals with the minute structure of tissues; HISTOLOGY.

mi·cros·co·py (migh·kros′kuh·pee) *n.* The use of the microscope; examination with the microscope.

mi·cros·mat·ic (migh″kroz·mat′ick) *adj.* Having a poorly developed sense of smell. Man is classified as a micrasmatic animal.

mi·cro·some (migh′kro·sohm) *n.* A small cytoplasmic body composed of fragments of endoplasmic reticulum and associated ribosomes.

mi·cro·so·mia (migh″kro·so′mee·uh) *n.* Abnormal smallness of the whole body. Syn. *dwarfism, nanosomia*.

mi·cro·spec·trog·ra·phy (migh″kro·speck·trog′ruf·ee) *n.* Spectrographic methods applied to the study of the composition of minute samples, as, for example, of protoplasm.

mi·cro·sphero·cyte (migh″kro·sfeer′o·site) *n.* A characteristically small, spheroidal erythrocyte observed in hereditary spherocytosis.

mi·cro·sphero·cy·to·sis (migh″kro·sfeer″o·sigh·to′sis) *n.* The presence of microspherocytes in the peripheral blood.

mi·cro·sphyx·ia (migh″kro·sfick′see·uh) *n.* Weakness of the pulse.

mi·cro·spo·ro·sis (migh″kro·spo·ro′sis) *n.* Dermatophytosis caused by a species of *Microsporum*.

Mi·cros·po·rum (migh·kros′puh·rum, migh″kro·spor′um) *n.* A genus of dermatophytes which attack only the hair and the skin.

Microsporum au·dou·i·ni (o·doo′i·nigh) A species of fungus responsible for epidemic tinea capitis in children; slow growing, producing few spores, with very little growth on polished rice; not found in animals.

Microsporum can·is (kan´is, kay´nis) A species of fungus that causes sporadic tinea capitis in children, generally through contact with infected cats and dogs; grows well on polished rice and other media, with abundant macroconidia and yellow-orange pigmentation of the agar.

Microsporum gyp·se·um (jip´see·um) A worldwide soil-inhabiting fungus, fast growing with numerous macroconidia, which produces tinea corporis and tinea capitis in man and animals exposed to soil.

mi·cro·stetho·scope (migh´kro·steth´uh·skope) *n.* A stethoscope which amplifies the sounds heard.

mi·cro·sto·mia (migh´kro·sto´mee·uh) *n.* Abnormal smallness of the mouth.

mi·cro·sur·gery (migh´kro·sur´juh·ree) *n.* Surgery in which a microscope and minute surgical instruments are employed, often on structures as small as an ovum or single living cell.

mi·cro·the·lia (migh´kro·theel´ee·uh) *n.* Congenital hypoplasia of the nipple of the breast.

mi·cro·tia (migh·kro´shee·uh) *n.* Abnormal smallness of one or both external ears.

mi·cro·tome (migh´kro·tome) *n.* An instrument for making thin sections of tissues for microscopical examination, the tissues usually being embedded in a supporting matrix.

mi·crot·o·my (migh·krot´uh·mee) *n.* The cutting of thin sections of tissue or other substances for microscopic study. **—microto·mist,** *n.*

mi·cro·trau·ma (migh´kro·trow´´muh, ·traw´´muh) *n.* A minor or insignificant injury, in itself not recognized as harmful, which if occurring repeatedly will give rise to an obvious lesion or disorder.

mi·cro·tu·bule (migh´kro·tew´bewl) *n.* Any of the hollow, tubular filaments, composed of repeating subunits of the globular protein tubulin, which play various important structural roles in prokaryotic and eukaryotic cells. Microtubules make up centrioles and cilia, contribute as elements of the cytoskeleton to the formation and maintenance of distinctive, nonsymmetrical cell shapes (as in the axons of neurons), and constitute the distinctive aster and spindle seen in mitosis.

Mi·cro·tus (migh·kro´tus) *n.* A genus of field voles of the Orient that may transmit leptospirosis and rat-bite fever.

mi·cro·unit (migh´kro·yoo´´nit) *n.* A unit of minute measurements; the one-millionth part of an ordinary unit.

mi·cro·vas·cu·la·ture (migh´kro·vas´kew·luh·chur) *n.* The sum of minute vessels in a region, part, organ, or organism.

mi·cro·vil·lus (migh´kro·vil´us) *n.,* pl. **microvil·li** (·eye) Any of the free cell surface evaginations which, depending upon cell location, may be absorptive or secretory in function.

mi·cro·volt (migh´kro·vohlt) *n.* One one-millionth of a volt.

mi·cro·wave (migh´kro·wave) *n.* An electromagnetic wave having a wavelength between a few tenths of a millimeter and about 30 centimeters, the limits being to some degree arbitrary.

mi·cro·zo·on (migh´´kro·zo´on) *n.,* pl. **micro·zoa** (·zo´uh) A microscopic animal.

mi·cro·zoo·sper·mia (migh´´kro·zo´´uh·spur´mee·uh) *n.* Abnormally small living sperms in the semen.

mic·tu·rate (mick´tew·rate) *v.* To urinate.

mic·tu·ri·tion (mick´´tew·rish´un) *n.* URINATION.

mid-. A combining form meaning *middle*.

mid·ax·il·la (mid´´ack·sil´uh) *n.* The center of the axilla. **—mid·ax·il·lary** (mid·ack´si·lerr·ee) *adj.*

mid·brain, *n.* MESENCEPHALON.

mid·cla·vic·u·lar (mid´´kla·vick´yoo·lur) *adj.* Pertaining to or passing through the middle of the clavicle.

midclavicular line. A vertical line parallel to, and midway between, the midsternal line and a vertical line drawn downward through the outer end of the clavicle.

middle cerebellar peduncle. One of the bands of white matter joining the pons and the cerebellum. Syn. *pontocerebellar tract, brachium pontis.*

middle clinoid process. Usually a small tubercle situated behind the lateral end of the tuberculum sellae. In some skulls it is not present and in others it is large and joins with the anterior clinoid process.

middle cranial fossa. One of the three fossae into which the interior base of each side of the cranium (right and left) is divided; it is deeply concave on a much lower level than the anterior cranial fossa, and lodges the temporal lobe of the cerebrum.

middle ear. The tympanic cavity with associated structures, including the tympanic membrane, the ossicles, the auditory tube, and the mastoid antrum and cells.

middle lobe syndrome. Atelectasis, bronchiectasis, or chronic pneumonitis of the right middle lobe, presumably due to enlarged usually calcified lymph nodes compressing the right middle lobe bronchus. Syn. *Brock's syndrome.*

middle mediastinum. The division of the mediastinum that contains the heart and pericardium, the ascending aorta, the superior vena cava, the bifurcation of the trachea, the pulmonary trunk and pulmonary veins, and the phrenic nerves.

mid·epi·gas·tric (mid´´ep·i·gas´trick) *adj.* Transversely bisecting the epigastrium.

mid forceps. An obstetric forceps applied when the fetal head is engaged, but has not yet become visible at the introitus and rotated to the occiput anterior position.

mid·fron·tal (mid´frun´tul) *adj.* Pertaining to the middle of the forehead.

midge, *n.* An insect of those Diptera which comprise the families of Ceratopogonidae and Chironomidae; small, delicate forms usually smaller than mosquitoes. The genus *Culicoides* is the most important medically.

midg·et, *n.* An individual who is abnormally small, but otherwise normal.

mid·gut, *n.* The middle portion of the embryonic digestive tube, opening ventrally into the yolk sac.

mid·line, *n.* Any line that bisects a figure symmetrically, as for example the intersection of the median plane with the surface of the body or with structures within the body.

mid·pain, *n.* MITTELSCHMERZ.

mid·riff, *n.* 1. The diaphragm. 2. Loosely, the upper part of the abdomen.

mid·wife, *n.* A trained or experienced person, especially a woman, who attends women in labor and delivery.

mid·wife·ry (mid'wīf'ee-, ·wye·free, ·fur·ee) *n.* The practice of a midwife; practical obstetrics.

mi·graine (migh'grain) *n.* Recurrent paroxysmal vascular headache; varied in intensity, frequency, and duration; commonly unilateral in onset and often associated with nausea and vomiting; may be preceded by or associated with sensory, motor, or mood disturbances; often familial. Syn. *sick headache.* **—migrain·ous** (·us) *adj.*

mi·grate (migh'grate) *v.* To wander; to shift from one site to another. **—mi·grant** (migh'grunt), **mi·gra·to·ry** (migh'gruh·tor·ee) *adj.;* **mi·gra·tion** (migh·gray'shun) *n.*

migration inhibitory factor. A soluble protein released by sensitized lymphocytes exposed to the proper antigen, which concentrates macrophages at the site of antigen-lymphocyte interaction.

migration of leukocytes. The passage or diapedesis of leukocytes through the vessel wall into the connective tissues; one of the phenomena of inflammation.

migratory pneumonia. Pneumonic infection which seems to shift from one part of the lung to another. Syn. *creeping pneumonia.*

Mi·ku·licz cell (mee'koo·litch) A large round or oval phagocytic cell with vacuolated cytoplasm and a small pycnotic nucleus, characteristic of rhinoscleroma.

Mikulicz operation A multiple-staged enterectomy for obstructive disease of the colon.

Mikulicz's disease or **syndrome** Salivary and lacrimal gland enlargement from any of a variety of causes, including tuberculosis, sarcoidosis, and malignant lymphoma.

mil·dew, *n.* Any of various minute fungi parasitic on plants, also found on dead vegetable substances such as textiles.

Miles' operation A one-stage, radical, abdominoperineal resection of the rectum for carcinoma.

milia. Plural of *milium.*

mil·i·a·ria (mil''ee·ãr'ee·uh, ·air'ee·uh) *n.* An acute inflammatory disease of the sweat glands, characterized by lesions of the skin consisting of vesicles and papules, which may be accompanied by a prickling or tingling sensation. It occurs especially in summer and in the tropics, often in the folds of the skin. Syn. *prickly heat, heat rash.*

miliaria pro·fun·da (pro·fun'duh). The skin reaction seen in the sweat-retention syndrome. The skin is uniformly studded with many discrete normal skin-colored papules located around a sweat pore. There are no subjective symptoms.

miliaria pus·tu·lo·sa (pus''tew·lo'suh). A pustu-

lar dermatitis occurring when another dermatitis is complicated by sweat retention.

mil·i·ary (mil'ee·ãr''ee, ·air''ee, mil'yuh·ree) *adj.* 1. Of the size of a millet seed, 0.5 to 1.0 mm., as miliary aneurysm, miliary tubercle. 2. Characterized by the formation of numerous lesions the size of a millet seed distributed rather uniformly throughout one or more organs, especially as in miliary tuberculosis.

miliary abscess. A minute embolic abscess.

miliary fever. A febrile illness associated with profuse sweating and characterized by papular, vesicular, and other eruptions attributed to the blockage of the sweat glands.

miliary tubercles. Tubercles of uniform size, approximating the millet seed, 1.0 to 2.0 mm. in diameter, distributed rather uniformly throughout an organ or series of organs.

Milibis. Trademark for glycobiarsol, an antiamebic drug.

mi·lieu (mee·lyuh', mee·lyoo') *n.,* pl. **mi·lieux** (·lyuh', ·lyoo'), **milieus** Environment, surroundings.

milieu in·té·rieur (an·tay·ryur') Claude Bernard's concept, now fundamental for modern physiology, postulating that the living organism exists not so much in its gaseous or aqueous external environment (milieu extérieur) as within its aqueous internal environment. Formed by circulating liquid, the blood plasma, interstitial fluid, and lymph, this milieu intérieur bathes all tissue elements, and is the medium in which all elementary exchanges of nutrient and waste materials take place. Its stability is the primary condition for independent existence of the organism, and the mechanisms by which stability is achieved ensure maintenance of all conditions necessary to the life of tissue elements.

milieu therapy. *In psychiatry,* the treatment of a mental disorder or maladjustment by making substantial changes in a patient's immediate life circumstances and environment in a way that will enhance the effectiveness of other forms of therapy. Within a hospital setting, this may involve pleasant physical surroundings, recreational facilities, and the staff. Syn. *situation therapy.*

mil·i·um (mil'ee·um) *n.,* pl. **mil·ia** (·ee·uh) A minute epidermal cyst, thought to represent either epidermal inclusion cyst formation or blockage of a pilosebaceous opening.

milk, *n. & v.* 1. The white fluid secreted by the mammary gland for the nourishment of the young. It is composed of carbohydrates, proteins, fats, mineral salts, vitamins, antibodies. 2. Any white fluid resembling milk, as coconut milk. 3. A suspension of certain metallic oxides, as milk of magnesia, iron, bismuth, etc. 4. To express milk from the mammary gland, manually or mechanically. 5. To press a finger along a compressible tube or duct in order to squeeze out the contents.

milk abscess. A mammary abscess occurring during lactation.

milk-alkali syndrome. Hypercalcemia without hypercalcuria or hypophosphaturia, normal or slightly elevated alkaline phosphatase, renal insufficiency with azotemia, mild alkalosis, conjunctivitis, and calcinosis complicating the prolonged excessive intake of milk and soluble alkali. Syn. *Burnett's syndrome, milk-drinker's syndrome.*

milk corpuscle. 1. The detached, fat-drop filled, distal portion of a glandular cell of the mammary gland, constricted off from the rest of the cell body in apocrine secretion. It breaks down, freeing milk globules. 2. A milk globule.

milk factor. A filtrable, noncellular agent in the milk and tissues of certain strains of inbred mice; transmitted from the mother to the offspring by nursing. It seems to be an essential factor in the genesis of mammary cancer in these strains. Syn. *Bittner milk factor.*

milk fever. 1. A fever during the puerperium, once thought to be due to a great accumulation of milk in the breasts, but now generally believed to be due to actual puerperal infection. 2. PARTURIENT PARESIS.

milk leg. PHLEGMASIA ALBA DOLENS.

Milk·man's syndrome or **disease** Decreased tubular reabsorption of phosphate, resulting in osteomalacia which gives a peculiar transverse striped appearance (multiple pseudofractures) to the bones in roentgenograms. Syn. *Looser-Milkman syndrome.*

milk of magnesia. A suspension of magnesium hydroxide containing 7 to 8.5% of $Mg(OH)_2$; used as an antacid and laxative.

milk plaques. MILK SPOTS.

milk sickness. An acute disease of human beings, characterized by weakness, anorexia, constipation, and vomiting due to ingestion of milk or flesh of animals which have a disease called trembles.

milk spots. Patches of thickening and opacity of the epicardium, found post mortem, usually over the right ventricle; of common occurrence in persons who have passed middle life. Syn. *soldier's patches* or *spots, milk plaques.*

milk sugar. LACTOSE.

milk teeth. DECIDUOUS TEETH.

Mil·ler-Ab·bott tube A long, double-lumen, balloon-tipped rubber tube, inserted usually through a nostril and passed through the pylorus; used to locate and treat obstructive conditions of the small intestine.

milli- A combining form meaning *a thousand* or *a thousandth.*

mil·li·am·me·ter (mil″ee-am′mee-tur) *n.* An ammeter which records electric current in milliamperes. Used in measuring currents passing through the filament circuits of roentgenray tubes.

mil·li·am·pere (mil″ee-am′peer) *n.* One one-thousandth of an ampere. Abbreviated, ma.

mil·li·bar (mil′i-bahr) *n.* A unit of atmospheric pressure, the one-thousandth part of a bar. Abbreviated, mb.

mil·li·cu·rie (mil′i-kew·ree) *n.* The amount of a radioactive substance which undergoes 3.7 × 10[7] disintegrations per second, equivalent to one-thousandth of a curie. Abbreviated, mCi.

millicurie-hour. A dosage unit of radon; the amount of radiation emitted by a millicurie of

radon multiplied by time of treatment in hours.

mil·li·equiv·a·lent (mil″ee-e-kwiv′uh-lunt) *n.* One one-thousandth of an equivalent, in specified weight units, of a chemical element, ion, radical, or compound. Abbreviated, meq, mEq.

mil·li·gram (mil′i-gram) *n.* One one-thousandth of a gram. Abbreviated, mg, mg.

milligram-hour. An exposure unit for radium therapy; the amount of radiation emitted by a milligram of radium multiplied by the time of treatment in hours. Abbreviated, mgh, mgh.

milligrams percent. *In biochemistry,* indicating milligrams of a substance per 100 ml of blood. Symbol, mg %, mg. %.

mil·li·li·ter (mil′i-lee″tur) *n.* The one one-thousandth part of a liter, equivalent to a cubic centimeter. Abbreviated, ml, ml.

mil·li·me·ter (mil′i-mee″tur) *n.* One one-thousandth of a meter. Abbreviated, mm, mm.

mil·li·mi·cron (mil″i-migh′kron) *n.* NANOMETER. Abbreviated, mμ.

mil·li·mol (mil′i-mol, -mole) *n.* One one-thousandth of a gram molecule. —**mil·li·mo·lar** (mil″i-mo′lur) *adj.*

mil·li·nor·mal (mil″i-nor′mul) *adj.* Containing a thousandth part of the quantity designated as normal, as a millinormal solution.

mil·li·os·mol (mil″ee-oz′mol, -mole) *n.* The concentration of an ion in a solution expressed as milligrams per liter divided by atomic weight. In univalent ions, milliosmolar and milliequivalent values are identical; in divalent ions, 1 milliosmol equals 2 milliequivalents. —**milli·os·mo·lar** (-oz′mo′lur) *adj.*

mil·li·pede, mil·le·pede (mil′i·peed) *n.* Wingless, vermiform arthropods with two pairs of legs on each body segment. Some species are incriminated as hosts of *Hymenolepis diminuta.*

mil·li·ruth·er·ford (mil″i·ruth′thur·furd) *n.* A unit of radioactivity representing 10[3] disintegrations per second. Abbreviated, mrd.

mil·li·volt (mil′i·vohlt) *n.* One one-thousandth of a volt.

Millon's reagent. A solution, prepared by dissolving metallic mercury in concentrated nitric acid, that produces a red color with proteins containing tyrosine and also with phenols.

mil·pho·sis (mil·fo′sis) *n.* Baldness of the eyebrows.

Mil·roy's disease Familial chronic lymphedema of the lower extremities with onset at birth.

Miltown. A trademark for meprobamate, a tranquilizer drug.

mi·me·sis (mi·mee′sis, migh·mee′sis) *n.* 1. Mimicry, as of an organic disease. 2. The assumption or imitation of the symptoms of one disease by another disease.

mi·met·ic (mi·met′ick, migh-) *adj.* 1. Characterized by or pertaining to mimesis; false, pseudo-. 2. Pertaining to facial expression.

mim·ic (mim′ick) *adj.* MIMETIC.

mim·ma·tion (mim·ay′shun) *n.* The unduly frequent use of the sound of the letter M in speech.

Minamata disease Organic mercurial poisoning

from consumption of contaminated fish and shellfish, resulting in constriction of visual fields, ataxia, dysarthria, tremors, mental changes, salivation, sweating, and various signs of extrapyramidal dysfunction.

mind (mine'd) *n*. 1. The sum total of the neural processes which receive, code, and interpret sensations, recall and correlate stored information, and act on it. 2. The state of consciousness. 3. The understanding, reasoning, and intellectual faculties and processes considered as a whole, often as contrasted with body or with feeling. 4. *In psychiatry*, the psyche, or the conscious, subconscious, and unconscious considered together.

mind cure. MENTAL HEALING.

min·er·al, *n*. *& adj*. 1. An inorganic chemical compound found in nature, especially one that is solid. 2. Pertaining to, or having characteristics of, a mineral.

mineral balance. The state of dynamic equilibrium in the body, maintained by physiologic processes, between the outgo and intake of any mineral or of any particular mineral constituent such as iron, calcium, or sodium.

min·er·al·iza·tion (min''ur·uh·li·zay'shun, ·lye·zay'shun) *n*. Deposition of mineral substances, under either normal or pathologic conditions.

mineral jelly. PETROLATUM.

min·er·alo·cor·ti·coid (min''ur·uh·lo·kor'ti·koid) *n*. An adrenal cortical steroid hormone, such as aldosterone, that primarily regulates mineral metabolism and, indirectly, fluid balance.

mineral oil. A mixture of liquid hydrocarbons obtained from petroleum. When refined to meet U.S.P. standards, it is sometimes known as white mineral oil. The refined oil is sometimes used as a vehicle for medicinal agents to be applied externally, and sometimes for its mechanical action in alleviating constipation. Syn. *liquid petrolatum*.

mineral water. Water naturally or artificially impregnated with sufficient inorganic salts to give it special properties.

miniature fluorography. FLUOROGRAPHY.

min·im (min'im) *n*. A unit of volume in the apothecaries' system; it equals 1/60 fluidram or about 1 drop (of water). Abbreviated, min. Symbol, ♏.

min·i·mal (min'i·mul) *adj*. The least or smallest; extremely minute.

minimal air. The small amount of air left in the alveoli of an excised or collapsed lung.

minimal brain dysfunction syndrome. A complex of learning and behavioral disabilities seen primarily in children of near average to above average intelligence, exhibiting also deviations of function of the central nervous system. The impairment may involve perception, conceptualization, language, memory, and control of attention, impulse, and motor function. Multiple causes, particularly pre- and perinatal disturbances, have been cited. Similar symptoms may complicate the problem of children with more severe brain disease such as epilepsy or blindness.

min·i·mum, *n*., pl. **min·i·ma** (·muh) The least quantity or amount; the lowest intensity or level.

minimum lethal dose. 1. That amount of an injurious agent (drug, virus, radiation) which is the average of the smallest dose that kills and the largest dose that fails to kill, when each of a series of animals is given a different dose under controlled conditions. Because of its general lack of accuracy, this measurement has been largely abandoned in favor of *median lethal dose*. Abbreviated, MLD. 2. Formerly, the quantity of a toxin which will kill a guinea pig of 250 g weight in from 4 to 5 days.

Min·ne·so·ta multiphasic personality inventory. An empirical scale of an individual's personality based mainly on his own yes-or-no responses to a questionnaire of 550 items; designed to provide scores on all the more important personality traits and adaptations, and including special validating scales which measure the individual's test-taking attitude and degree of frankness. Abbreviated, MMPI.

mi·nor (migh'nur) *adj*. *& n*. 1. Less; lesser; smaller. 2. An individual under legal age; one under the authority of parents or guardians.

minor calices. The 4 to 13 cuplike divisions of the major calices; derived from tubules of the second, third, and fourth orders, each receiving one or more of the renal papillae.

minor cross match. See *cross matching*.

minor lip. LABIUM MINUS.

minor operation. An operation which does not threaten life; one in which there is little or no danger.

minute ventilation or **volume.** The total volume of air breathed in a minute.

mio-, meio- A combining form meaning (a) *reduced, rudimentary*; (b) *contraction, constriction*.

mio·car·dia (migh''o·kahr'dee·uh) *n*. Diminution of the volume of the heart during systole.

mi·o·sis (migh·o'sis) *n*. 1. Constriction of the pupil of the eye. 2. Specifically, abnormal contraction of the pupil below 2 mm.

mi·ot·ic (migh·ot'ick) *adj*. *& n*. 1. Pertaining to, or characterized by, miosis. 2. Causing contraction of the pupil. 3. Any agent that causes contraction of the pupil of the eye.

mire (meer) *n*. The object on the arc of the ophthalmometer whose reflection from the cornea is employed in determining the amount of corneal astigmatism.

mir·ror, *n*. 1. A polished surface for reflecting light or forming images of objects placed in front of it. 2. (*Attributive use only*) In a bilaterally symmetrical system, reflecting or imitating the other of a pair, as mirror movements of an infant's hands; in an asymmetrical system reversed or backward (as: mirror writing).

mirror vision. The visualization of objects or written words in reverse, as if reflected in a mirror.

mirror writing. Writing in which the letters appear backward, as if seen in a mirror; a not uncommon trait in children first learning to write, but also seen when a person is forced to write with the nondominant hand, following paralysis of the dominant hand.

mis-, miso- A combining form meaning *hatred, hating.*

mis·an·thro·py (mis·san'thruh·pee, mi·zan') *n.* An aversion to society; hatred of mankind. —**mis·an·thrope** (mis'un·throp, miz') *n.;* **mis·an·throp·ic** (mis''un·throp'ick) *adj.*

mis·car·riage (mis·kār'ij) *n.* Expulsion of the fetus before it is viable. —**miscar·ry** (·ee) *v.*

mis·ce·ge·na·tion (mis''e·je·nay'shun) *n.* Intermarriage or interbreeding of different human races.

mis·ci·ble (mis'i·bul) *adj.* Capable of mixing or dissolving in all proportions.

mi·sog·a·my (mi·sog'uh·mee) *n.* Aversion to marriage. —**misoga·mist** (·mist) *n.*

mi·sog·y·ny (mi·soj'i·nee) *n.* Hatred of women. —**misogy·nist** (·nist) *n.*

mi·sol·o·gy (mi·sol'uh·jee, migh·sol') *n.* Unreasoning aversion to intellectual or literary matters, or to argument or speaking.

miso·ne·ism (mis''o·nee'iz·um) *n.* Hatred or horror of novelty or change. —**misone·ist** (·ist) *n.*

miso·pe·dia (mis''o·pee'dee·uh) *n.* Morbid hatred of all children, but especially of one's own.

miso·psy·chia (mis''o·sigh'kee·uh) *n.* Morbid disgust with life; hatred of living.

missed abortion. A condition of pregnancy in which a fetus weighing less than 500 g dies in utero with failure of expulsion for an extended period of time.

mist. Abbreviation for *mistura* [L.], mixture.

mite, *n.* Any representative of a large group of small arachnids, which together with the larger ticks constitute the order Acarina.

mite-borne typhus. TSUTSUGAMUSHI DISEASE.

mi·ti·cide (migh'ti·side) *n.* A substance destructive to mites. —**mi·ti·ci·dal** (migh''ti·sigh'dul) *adj.*

mit·i·gate (mit'i·gate) *v.* To allay, make milder; to moderate.

mi·tis (migh'tis) *adj.* Mild.

mi·to·car·cin (migh''to·kahr'sin) *n.* An antineoplastic antibiotic obtained from *Streptomyces.*

mi·to·chon·dria (migh''to·kon'dree·uh, mit''o') *n.,* sing. **mitochondri·on** (·un) Cytoplasmic organelles in the form of granules, short rods, or filaments which are present in all cells. The fine structure consists of external and internal membrane systems; the inner membrane is folded to form cristae extending into the mitochondrial matrix. Mitochondria supply energy to the cell by stepwise oxidation of substrates. They store the energy in ATP. —**mitochondri·al** (·ul) *adj.*

mitochondrion. Singular of *mitochondria.*

mi·to·gen (migh'to·jin, ·jen) *n.* Any substance which induces mitosis.

mitogenetic radiation. A kind of radiation said to be produced in cells and tissues, which induces or is induced by the process of mitosis. Syn. *Gurvich radiation.*

mi·to·gen·ic (migh''to·jen'ick) *adj.* Promoting mitosis.

mi·to·my·cin (migh''to·migh'sin) *n.* A complex of related antibiotic substances (mitomycin A, mitomycin B, mitomycin C) produced by *Streptomyces caespitosus (griseovinaceseus).*

Mitomycin C, $C_{15}H_{18}N_4O_5$, is a potent antineoplastic agent.

mitoses. Plural of *mitosis.*

mi·to·sis (migh·to'sis, mi·) *n.,* pl. **mito·ses** (·seez) 1. Nuclear division; usually divided into a series of stages: prophase, metaphase, anaphase, and telophase. 2. The division of the cytoplasm and nucleus.

mi·tot·ic (migh·tot'ick, mi·) *adj.* Of or pertaining to mitosis.

mitotic index. The number of dividing cells per thousand cells; used in the estimation of the rate of growth of a tissue.

mi·tral (migh'trul) *adj.* 1. Resembling a bishop's miter. 2. Pertaining to the atrioventricular valve of the left side of the heart.

mitral commissurotomy. An operation for the relief of mitral stenosis, commonly a valvulotomy.

mitral insufficiency or **incompetence.** MITRAL REGURGITATION.

mi·tral·iza·tion (migh''truh·li·zay'shun, ·lye·zay'shun) *n.* Changes in the radiographic outline of the heart seen in mitral stenosis.

mitral regurgitation. Imperfect closure of the mitral valve during the cardiac systole, permitting blood to reenter the left atrium. Syn. *mitral insufficiency, mitral incompetence.*

mitral stenosis or **obstruction.** Obstruction to the flow of blood through the mitral valve, usually due to narrowing of the valve orifice.

mitral valve. A heart valve containing two cusps, situated between the left atrium and left ventricle. Syn. *left atrioventricular valve, bicuspid valve.*

mi·troid (migh'troid) *adj.* Shaped like a miter cap.

Mi·tsu·da reaction or **test** LEPROMIN TEST.

mit·tel·schmerz (mit'ul·shmehrts) *n.* Pain or discomfort in the lower abdomen of women occurring midway in the intermenstrual interval, thought to be secondary to the irritation of the pelvic peritoneum by fluid or blood escaping from the point of ovulation in the ovary.

mixed infection. Concurrent infection with more than one type of organism. Syn. *multiple infection.*

mixed laterality. The tendency, when there is a choice, to prefer to use parts of one side of the body for certain tasks and parts of the opposite side for others, as when a person prefers to use the right eye for sighting, the left hand for writing, and the right foot for kicking.

mixed leukocyte culture test. A matching test to measure the degree of histocompatibility between two individuals by mixing peripheral blood leukocytes of the recipient with the donor's leukocytes treated with mitomycin C; the response of the recipient's leukocytes to those of the donor's being measured as a function of the incorporation of radioactive thymidine into the cells of the recipient; the reactive cells are lymphocytes.

mixed tumor. A tumor whose parenchyma is composed of two or more tissue types or cell types.

mixo·sco·pia (mick''so·sko'pee·uh) *n.* A form of

sexual perversion in which the orgasm is excited by the sight of coitus. —**mixo·scop·ic** (·skop'ick) adj.

mix·ture, n. 1. In pharmacy, a preparation made by incorporating insoluble ingredients in a liquid vehicle, usually with the aid of a suitable suspending agent so that the insoluble substances do not readily settle out. 2. An aqueous solution containing two or more solutes.

Mi·ya·ga·wa·nel·la (mee"yuh·gah"wuh·nel'uh) n. A genus of the family Chlamydiaceae that includes the causative agents of psittacosis (Miyagawanella psittaci), ornithosis (M. ornithosis), and lymphogranuloma (M. lymphogranulomatosis).

mks. Meter-kilogram-second, a system of units based on the meter as the unit of length, the kilogram as the unit of mass, and the second as the unit of time.

ml, ml. Abbreviation for milliliter.

MLD. Abbreviation for (a) metachromatic leukodystrophy; (b) minimum lethal dose.

mm, mm. Abbreviation for millimeter.

MMPI. Abbreviation for Minnesota multiphasic personality inventory.

Mn Symbol for manganese.

M'Naghten. Listed as if spelled MacNaghten.

mnem-, mnemo- A combining form meaning memory.

mne·mas·the·nia (nee"mas·theen'ee·uh) n. Weakness of memory not due to organic disease.

mne·mo·der·mia (nee"mo·dur'mee·uh) n. Pruritis and discomfort of the skin hours and days after the cause of the symptoms has been removed and recovery well established, usually stimulated by scratching or rubbing, sometimes by heat and other stimuli.

mne·mon·ic (ne·mon'ick) adj. & n. 1. Aiding memory. 2. Pertaining to memory. 3. A mnemonic device; any combination of letters, words, pictures, or the like, to help one remember the facts they represent.

mne·mon·ics (ne·mon'icks) n. 1. The science of cultivation of the memory by systematic methods. 2. Any technique which makes recall more effective.

MNS blood group. A major erythrocyte antigen system defined at first by reactions to immune rabbit sera designated anti-M and anti-N, broadened later to include reactions to sera designated anti-S, anti-s, and certain others.

Mo Symbol for molybdenum.

mo·bil·i·ty (mo·bil'i·tee) n. The condition of being movable.

mo·bi·lize (mo'bi·lize) v. 1. To render movable, as an ankylosed part. 2. To free, make accessible, as an organ during surgical operation. 3. To release or liberate in the body, as for example glycogen stored in the liver. —**mo·bi·li·za·tion** (mo"bi·li·zay'shun) n.

Möbius' syndrome 1. Congenital, usually bilateral, paralysis of the facial muscles, associated often with abducent paralysis as well as of the oculomotor nerves, but also defects in hearing, musculoskeletal anomalies and mental deficit; presumably due to a lack of nerve cells in the motor nuclei of the brainstem. Syn. congenital facial diplegia, congenital oculofacial paralysis, infantile nuclear aplasia. 2. OPHTHALMOPLEGIC MIGRAINE.

mo·dal·i·ty (mo·dal'i·tee) n. A form of sensation, such as touch, pressure, vision, or audition.

mode, n. That value in a series of observations which occurs most frequently. —**mo·dal** (mo'dul) adj.

mod·el, n. 1. The form or material pattern of anything to be made, or already existing. 2. CAST (2).

mod·er·a·tor, n. A substance, such as water or graphite, used to reduce the velocity of nuclear particles, especially to slow down neutrons to a thermal equilibrium state and thus to promote a chain reaction.

mo·dus (mo'dus) n. Mode, method.

modus ope·ran·di (op"uh·ran'dye, ·dee) One's method of doing something.

Moenckeberg. See Mönckeberg.

mogi·graph·ia (moj"i·graf'ee·uh) n. Obsol. WRITER'S CRAMP.

mogi·la·lia (moj"i·lay'lee·uh) n. Obsol. Difficult or painful speech, as stammering or stuttering.

moi·e·ty (moye'tee) n. A part or portion, especially of a molecule, generally complex, having a characteristic chemical or pharmacological property.

moist, n. Damp; slightly wet; characterized by the presence of fluid.

moist gangrene. The invasion of necrotic tissue by microorganisms with resultant putrefaction.

mol (mol, mole) n. ²MOLE.

mo·lal (mo'lul) adj. Pertaining to moles of a solute per 1000 g of solvent.

¹mo·lar (mo'lur) adj. 1. Pertaining to masses, in contradistinction to molecular. 2. Pertaining to moles of solute in a definite volume of solution, usually 1 liter. Abbreviated, M. —**mo·lar·i·ty** (mo·lãr'i·tee) n.

²molar, n. & adj. 1. A molar tooth. 2. Serving to grind or pulverize.

mo·lar·i·form (mo·lãr'i·form) adj. Shaped like a molar tooth.

molar pregnancy. Gestation in which the ovum has been converted into a fleshy tumor mass or mole.

molar solution. A solution which contains a gram-molecular weight or mole of reagent in 1000 ml of solution.

molar teeth. Multicuspidate, usually multi-rooted, teeth used for crushing, grinding, or triturating food. In the human primary dentition there are two in each quadrant immediately distal to the canine; in the permanent dentition, three, distal to the premolars.

¹mold, mould, n. Any of those fungi which form slimy or cottony growths on foodstuffs, leather, etc.

²mold, mould, n. & v. 1. A cavity or form in which a thing is shaped. 2. To make conform to a given shape, as the fetal head in its passage through the birth canal.

¹mole, n. 1. A mass formed in the uterus by the maldevelopment of all or part of the embry or of the placenta and membranes. 2. A fleshy, pigmented nevus.

²**mole,** *n.* The weight of a chemical in mass units, usually grams, numerically equal to its molecular weight.

mo·lec·to·my (mo·leck'tuh·mee) *n.* Surgical removal of a mole, usually a pigmented nevus of the skin.

mo·lec·u·lar (mo·leck'yoo·lur) *adj.* 1. Pertaining to or consisting of molecules. 2. Individual, piecemeal.

molecular biology. The study of the relationship between the properties of specific molecules and the structure and function of living things in which these molecules occur.

molecular layer of the cerebellum. The outermost layer of the cerebellar cortex, made up of neuroglia, a few small ganglion cells, and a reticulum of myelinated and unmyelinated nerve fibers.

molecular layer of the retina. One of the two layers, inner and outer, of the retina made up of interlacing dendrites. Syn. *plexiform layer.*

molecular sieve chromatography. GEL FILTRATION CHROMATOGRAPHY.

molecular volume. The volume of one gram molecule of substance; in the gaseous state under the same conditions of temperature and pressure, the molecular volumes of all substances are equal.

molecular weight. The weight of a molecule of any substance, representing the sum of the weights of its constituent atoms. Abbreviated, M.W.

mol·e·cule (mol'e·kyool) *n.* 1. A minute mass of matter. 2. The smallest quantity into which a substance can be divided and retain its characteristic properties; or the smallest quantity that can exist in a free state.

moli·la·lia (mol''i·lay'lee·uh) *n. Obsol.* MOGILALIA.

mol·li·ti·es (mo·lish'ee·eez) *n.* Softness.

mol·lus·coid (mol·us'koid) *adj.* Resembling molluscum contagiosum.

mol·lus·cum (muh·lus'kum, mol·us') *n.,* pl. **mol·lus·ca** (·kuh) Any skin disease in which soft, globoid masses occur. —**mollus·cous** (·kus) *adj.*

molluscum bodies. The ovoid or spheroidal keratin bodies formed in the epithelium by the development of the inclusion bodies of molluscum contagiosum. They are much larger than the epithelial cells originally invaded by the virus of molluscum contagiosum.

molluscum con·ta·gi·o·sum (kon·tay''jee·o'sum). A viral, often venereal disease of the skin, characterized by one or more discrete, waxy dome-shaped nodules with frequent umbilication; molluscum bodies are found in the infected epidermal cells.

molluscum se·ba·ce·um (se·bay'shee·um, ·see·um). KERATOACANTHOMA.

molt, moult, *v. & n.* 1. To shed skin, feathers, or hair periodically, with the seasons or in stages of growth. 2. An instance of such shedding.

mo·lyb·de·num (mo·lib'de·num, mol''lib·dee'num) *n.* Mo = 95.94. A hard, silvery-white metallic element, with a density of about 10.2.

mo·lyb·dic (mo·lib'dick) *adj.* Containing or pertaining to hexavalent molybdenum.

mo·lys·mo·pho·bia (mo·liz''mo·fo'bee·uh) *n.* Abnormal dread of infection or contamination.

mo·ment, *n.* 1. The tendency or a measure of the tendency to move a body, especially about a point or axis; defined as the product of the force involved and the perpendicular distance from the line of action of the force to the point or axis of rotation. 2. The arithmetic mean of the deviations of the observations in a frequency distribution from any selected value, each raised to the same power. First power for first moment, second power for second moment, etc.

mo·men·tum (mo·men'tum) *n. In physics,* the mass of a body multiplied by its linear velocity.

mon-, mono- A combining form meaning (a) *single, one, alone;* (b) in chemistry, the presence of *one atom* or *group* of that to the name of which it is attached.

mo·nad (mo'nad, mon'ad) *n.* 1. A univalent element or radical. 2. Any of the small flagellate protozoa. 3. In meiosis, one of the elements of the tetrad produced by the pairing and splitting of homologous chromosomes. Each monad is separated into a different daughter cell as the result of the two meiotic divisions.

mon·am·ine (mon·am'een, ·in) *n.* MONOAMINE.

mon·ar·thric (mon·ahr'thrick) *adj.* Pertaining to one joint.

mon·ar·thri·tis (mon''ahr·thrigh'tis) *n.* Arthritis affecting only a single joint.

mon·ar·tic·u·lar (mon''ahr·tick'yoo·lur) *adj.* Pertaining to one joint; MONARTHRIC.

mon·as·ter (mon·as'tur) *n.* 1. The chromosomes in the equatorial plate at the end of the prophase of mitosis; the "mother-star." 2. The single aster formed in an aberrant type of mitosis, in which the chromosomes are doubled but the cell body does not divide.

mon·ath·e·to·sis (mon''ath·e·to'sis) *n.* Athetosis affecting one limb or side.

mon·atom·ic (mon''uh·tom'ick) *adj.* 1. Having but one atom of replaceable hydrogen, as a monatomic acid. 2. Having only one atom, as a monatomic molecule. 3. Having the combining power of one atom of hydrogen, as a monatomic radical. 4. Formed by the replacement of one hydrogen atom in a compound by a radical, as a monatomic alcohol.

Möncke·berg's arteriosclerosis or **sclerosis** (mœnk'e·behrk) MEDIAL ARTERIOSCLEROSIS.

Mon·dor's disease or **syndrome** (mohn·dohr') Thrombophlebitis of an isolated venous segment, chiefly affecting the thoracoepigastric vein, where it may be mistaken for lymphatic permeation by breast cancer.

Mon·go·li·an (mong·go'lee·un) *adj.* 1. Pertaining to Mongolia or to Mongols. 2. MONGOLOID.

Mongolian idiocy. DOWN'S SYNDROME.

Mongolian spot. A focal bluish-grey discoloration of the skin of the lower back, also aberrantly on the face, present at birth and fading gradually.

mon·gol·ism (mong'guh·liz·um) *n.* DOWN'S SYNDROME.

mon·gol·oid (mong'guh·loid) *adj.* 1. Characteristic of the eastern and northern Asian and native American races of man. 2. Having physical characteristics associated with Down's syndrome.

mo·nil·e·thrix (mo·nil'e·thricks) *n.* A congenital defect of the hair characterized by dryness and fragility and by nodes which give it a beaded appearance. Syn. *moniliform hair, beaded hair.*

Mo·nil·ia (mo·nil'ee·uh) *n.* CANDIDA. —**monil·i·al** (-ee·ul) *adj.*

mon·i·li·a·sis (mon"i·lye'uh·sis) *n.,* pl. **monilia·ses** (-seez) CANDIDIASIS.

Mo·nil·i·for·mis (mo·nil'i·for'mis) *n.* A genus of acanthocephalan worms.

mo·nil·i·id (mo·nil'ee·id) *n.* CANDIDID.

mon·i·tor (mon'i·tur) *n. & v.* 1. A person or an apparatus whose function is to give continuous or periodic reports based on scanning or measurements, as of a health or security hazard. 2. To determine periodically or continuously the amount of ionizing radiation or radioactive contamination in an occupied area, or in or on personnel, as a safety measure for health protection.

mono-. See *mon-.*

mono·ac·id (mon"o·as'id) *adj.* 1. Having one replaceable hydroxyl group (OH), as a monoacid base. 2. Capable of uniting directly with a molecule of a monobasic acid, with half a molecule of a dibasic acid, etc.

mono·am·ine (mon"o·am'een, -in) *n.* An amine containing one amino group.

monoamine oxidase inhibitor. Any drug, such as isocarboxazid and tranylcypromine, that inhibits monoamine oxidase and thereby leads to an accumulation of the amines on which the enzyme normally acts. Abbreviated, MAOI.

mono·am·ni·ot·ic (mon"o·am"nee·ot'ick) *adj.* Having a single amnion.

mono·bal·lism (mon"o·bal'iz·um) *n.* Ballism confined to one limb.

mono·ba·sic (mon"o·bay'sick) *adj.* Having one hydrogen which can be replaced by a metal or positive radical, as a monobasic acid.

mono·blast (mon'o·blast) *n.* The progenitor of the monocytes found in bone marrow. The nucleus has a finely granular to lacy chromatin structure, nucleoli are present, the cytoplasm shows more gray-blue than other blast cells, and may have pseudopods.

mono·blep·sia (mon"o·blep'see·uh) *n.* 1. A condition in which either eye has a better visual power than both together. 2. The form of color blindness in which but one color can be perceived.

mono·bra·chi·us (mon"o·bray'kee·us) *n. & adj.* 1. An individual lacking one arm congenitally. 2. Characterizing a one-armed condition, congenital or acquired.

mono·car·di·an (mon"o·kahr'dee·un) *adj.* Having a heart with a single atrium and ventricle.

mono·car·dio·gram (mon"o·kahr'dee·o·gram) *n.* VECTORCARDIOGRAM.

mono·cel·lu·lar (mon"o·sel'yoo·lur) *adj.* UNICELLULAR.

mono·chord (mon'o·kord) *n.* A device once used

for testing hearing, particularly for the higher tones of speech.

mono·cho·rea (mon"o·ko·ree'uh) *n.* Chorea confined to a single part of the body.

mono·cho·ri·on·ic (mon"o·kor·ee·on'ick) *adj.* Having a common chorion, as monochorionic twins.

mono·chro·ma·sia (mon"o·kro·may'zee·uh, ·zhuh) *n.* TOTAL COLORBLINDNESS.

mono·chro·ma·sy (mon"o·kro'muh·see) *n.* Monochromasia (= TOTAL COLORBLINDNESS).

mono·chro·mat·ic (mon"o·kro·mat'ick) *adj.* 1. Pertaining to or possessing one color or substantially one wavelength of light. 2. *In optics,* having no variation in hue and saturation, and varying only in brightness.

mono·chro·ma·tism (mon"o·kro'muh·tiz·um) *n.* TOTAL COLORBLINDNESS.

mono·clin·ic (mon"o·klin'ick) *adj.* Applied to crystals in which the vertical axis is inclined to one, but is at a right angle to the other, or lateral, axis.

mono·clo·nal (mon"o·klo'nul) *adj.* Pertaining to a single group, or clone, of cells, thus involving an identical cell product.

monoclonal gammopathy. M-COMPONENT HYPERGAMMAGLOBULINEMIA.

mono·coc·cus (mon"o·kock'us) *n.,* pl. **monococci** (-sigh) A coccus occurring singly, not united in chains, pairs, or groups.

mono·crot·ic (mon"o·krot'ick) *adj.* Having a single beat or impulse; having a single crested wave.

mon·oc·u·lar (mon·ock'yoo·lur) *adj.* 1. Pertaining to or affecting only one eye, as monocular diplopia; performed with one eye only, as monocular vision. 2. Having a single ocular or eyepiece, as a monocular microscope.

monocular diplopia. Diplopia with a single eye; usually due to hysteria, double pupil, beginning cataract, or subluxated lens.

mono·cy·e·sis (mon"o·sigh·ee'sis) *n.* Pregnancy with but one fetus.

mono·cys·tic (mon"o·sis'tick) *adj.* Composed of, or containing, but one cyst.

mono·cyte (mon'o·site) *n.* A large, mononuclear leukocyte with a more or less deeply indented nucleus, slate-gray cytoplasm, and fine, usually azurophilic granulation; the same as, or related to, the large mononuclear cell, transitional cell, resting wandering cell, clasmatocyte, endothelial leukocyte, or histiocyte of other classifications. It is the precursor of macrophages. —**mono·cyt·ic** (mon"o·sit'ick) *adj.*

monocytic leukemia. A form of leukemia in which the predominant cell type belongs to the monocytic series. Two types are differentiated on the basis of the predominant cell present in the peripheral blood; Naegeli (myelomonocytic) type, and the Schilling type.

mono·cy·to·ma (mon"o·sigh·to'muh) *n.* A tumor whose parenchyma is composed of monocytes, usually anaplastic.

mono·cy·to·pe·nia (mon"o·sigh"to·pee'nee·uh) *n.* Diminution in the number of monocytes per unit volume of peripheral blood.

mono·cy·to·sis (mon″o·sigh·to′sis) n. Increase in the number of monocytes per unit volume of peripheral blood.

mono·dac·tyl·ism (mon″o·dack′ti·liz·um) n. The presence of only one toe or finger on the foot or hand.

mono·di·plo·pia (mon″o·di·plo′pee·uh) n. MONOCULAR DIPLOPIA.

mo·nog·a·my (muh·nog′uh·mee) n. Marriage with only one person at a time.

mono·gas·tric (mon″o·gas′trick) adj. Having one stomach.

mono·ger·mi·nal (mon″o·jur′mi·nul) adj. Having or developing from a single ovum, as twins with but one chorionic sac.

mo·nog·o·ny (mo·nog′uh·nee) n. AGAMOGENESIS; asexual reproduction. —**monogo·nous** (·nus) adj.

mono·graph (mon′uh·graf) n. 1. A detailed documented treatise written about a single subject or a limited area of study or inquiry. 2. The standards of purity and strength, tests, assay, and other requirements officially specified by a pharmacopeia or formulary for a drug or drug dosage form.

mono·hy·drate (mon″o·high′drate) n. A compound containing one molecule of water of hydration. —**monohy·drat·ed** (·dray·tid) adj.

mono·hy·dric (mon″o·high′drick) adj. Containing one replaceable hydrogen atom as a monohydric alcohol or a monohydric acid.

mono·ide·ism (mon″o·eye·dee′iz·um) n. A mental condition marked by the domination of a single idea; persistent and complete preoccupation with one idea, seldom complete. May be induced by suggestion or hypnosis, wherein an elementary idea or image is left isolated and is not synthesized or associated with other ideas or impressions.

mono·lep·sis (mon″o·lep′sis) n. The transfer of the characteristics of one parent to a child.

mono·lob·u·lar (mon″o·lob′yoo·lur) adj. Pertaining to a single lobule.

mono·ma·nia (mon″o·may′nee·uh) n. A form of mental disorder in which the patient's thoughts and actions are dominated by one subject or one idea, as in paranoid states. —**monoma·ni·ac** (·nee·ack) n.; **mono·ma·ni·a·cal** (·ma·nigh′uh·kul) adj.

mono·mel·ic (mon″o·mel′ick) adj. Pertaining to one limb.

mono·mer (mon′uh·mur) n. The simplest molecular form of a substance.

mono·mer·ic (mon″o·merr′ick) adj. 1. Consisting of a single piece or segment. 2. Consisting of or pertaining to a monomer.

mono·mo·lec·u·lar (mon″o·mo·leck′yoo·lur) adj. 1. Pertaining to or consisting of one molecule. 2. Composed of many molecules arranged in one molecule thickness.

mono·mor·phous (mon″o·mor′fus) adj. Having a single form or the same appearance; not polymorphous.

mono·neph·rous (mon″o·nef′rus) adj. Pertaining or limited to one kidney.

mono·neu·ral (mon″o·new′rul) adj. 1. Pertaining to a single nerve. 2. Receiving branches from but one nerve; said of muscles.

mono·neu·ri·tis (mon″o·new·rye′tis) n. Neuritis affecting a single nerve.

mono·neu·rop·a·thy (mon″o·new·rop′uh·thee) n. Neuropathy affecting a single nerve.

mono·nu·cle·ar (mon″o·new′klee·ur) adj. Having only one nucleus.

mononuclear cell. 1. Any cell with a single nucleus. 2. A lymphocyte, monocyte, plasma cell, or histiocyte.

mono·nu·cle·ate (mon″o·new′klee·ate, ·ut) adj. MONONUCLEAR.

mono·nu·cle·o·sis (mon″o·new″klee·o′sis) n. 1. A condition of the blood or tissues in which there is an increase in the number of monocytes above the normal. 2. INFECTIOUS MONONUCLEOSIS.

mono·nu·cle·o·tide (mon″o·new′klee·o·tide) n. A product obtained by hydrolytic decomposition of nucleic acid; it is a compound of phosphoric acid, a pentose, and a purine or pyridine base such as guanine, adenine, cytosine, or uracil.

mono·oxy·gen·ase (mon″o·ock′si·je·nace, ·naze) n. Any of a group of enzymes which catalyzes the insertion of one oxygen atom into an organic substrate with reduction of the second oxygen atom to water.

mono·pa·re·sis (mon″o·pa·ree′sis, ·păr′e·sis) n. Weakness of all the muscles of one limb, whether arm or leg.

mono·pha·gia (mon″o·fay′jee·uh) n. 1. Desire for a single article of food. 2. The eating of a single daily meal.

mo·noph·a·gism (muh·nof′uh·jiz·um) n. Habitual eating of a single article of food.

mono·pha·sia (mon″o·fay′zhuh, ·zee·uh) n. A form of aphasia in which speech is limited to a single syllable, word, or phrase.

mono·pha·sic (mon″o·fay′zick) adj. Having a single phase.

mono·pho·bia (mon″o·fo′bee·uh) n. Abnormal dread of being alone.

mon·oph·thal·mia (mon″off·thal′mee·uh) n. Congenital absence of one eye. Syn. unilateral anophthalmia.

mono·phy·let·ic (mon″o·figh·let′ick) adj. Pertaining to, or derived from, a single original ancestral type.

mono·phy·odont (mon″o·figh′o·dont) adj. Having but a single set of teeth, the permanent ones.

mono·ple·gia (mon″o·plee′jee·uh) n. Paralysis of all the muscles of a single limb. It is designated as brachial or crural, when affecting the arm or the leg, respectively, and as central or peripheral, according to the seat of the causal lesion.

mono·po·dia (mon″o·po′dee·uh) n. The condition of having but one lower limb.

mono·pus (mon″o·pus) n. An individual with congenital absence of one foot or leg.

mon·or·chid (mon·or′kid) n. A person who has but one testis, or in whom only one testis has descended into the scrotum.

mon·or·chid·ism (mon·or′kid·iz·um) n. Congenital absence of one testis. —**monorchid,** adj.

mono·sac·cha·ride (mon″o·sack′uh·ride, ·rid) n. A carbohydrate which cannot be hydrolyzed to a simpler carbohydrate, hence called a simple sugar; chemically, a polyhydric alcohol having reducing properties associated with an actual or potential aldehyde or ketone group. It may contain 3 to 10 carbon atoms, and on this basis be classified as a triose, tetrose, pentose, hexose, heptose, octose, nonose, or decose. A diose, glycolaldehyde, is by some classed as a monosaccharide, but does not exhibit the characteristic properties of the class.

mono·so·di·um glutamate (mon″o·so′dee-um). Monosodium L-glutamate, HOOCCH-NH₂CH₂CH₂COONa, used intravenously for symptomatic treatment of hepatic coma in which there is a high blood level of ammonia. It imparts a meat flavor to foods. Abbreviated, MSG. Syn. *sodium glutamate.*

Mono·spo·ri·um (mon″o·spor′ee-um) *n.* A genus of the Fungi Imperfecti. The species *Monosporium apiospermum* and *M. scleriotiale* have been isolated in cases of white-grained mycetoma.

Mono·spot test. A commercial agglutination test to detect heterophile antibodies in patients suspected of having infectious mononucleosis.

mon·os·tot·ic (mon″os·tot′ick) *adj.* Involving only one bone.

mono·stra·tal (mon″o·stray′tul) *adj.* Arranged in a single layer or stratum.

mono·symp·to·mat·ic (mon″o·simp″tuh·mat′ick) *adj.* Having but a single symptom.

mono·syn·ap·tic (mon″o·si·nap′tick) *adj.* Involving only one synapse.

mono·ther·mia (mon″o·thur′mee·uh) *n.* Lack of normal diurnal variation in body temperature.

mon·ot·ic (mon·o′tick, mon·ot′ick) *adj.* Pertaining to or affecting but one of the ears.

mo·not·o·cous (mo·not′uh·kus) *adj.* Producing one young at a birth.

mon·ox·ide (muh·nock′side, mon·ock′) *n.* 1. An oxide containing a single oxygen atom. 2. A popular name for carbon monoxide.

mono·zy·got·ic (mon″o·zye·got′ick, ·go′tick) *adj.* Developed from a single fertilized egg or zygote, as identical twins.

Mon·ro's foramen INTERVENTRICULAR FORAMEN.

mons pu·bis (pew′bis) [NA]. The eminence of the lower anterior abdominal wall above the superior rami of the pubic bones.

mon·ster, *n.* A fetus (rarely an adult) which, through congenital faulty development, is incapable of properly performing the vital functions, or which, owing to an excess or deficiency of parts, differs markedly from the normal type of the species; TERATISM.

mon·stri·cide (mon′stri·side) *n.* The killing of a monster.

mon·strip·a·ra (mon·strip′uh·ruh) *n.* A woman who has given birth to one or more monsters.

mon·stros·i·ty (mon·stros′i·tee) *n.* 1. The condition of being a monster. 2. MONSTER.

mons ve·ne·ris (ven′e·ris) The mound of Venus; MONS PUBIS.

Mont·gom·ery's glands Apocrine sweat glands in the areola of the nipple of the breast.

Montgomery's tubercles The elevations due to the apocrine sweat glands in the areola of the nipple which appear more prominent during pregnancy and lactation.

mon·tic·u·lus (mon·tick′yoo·lus) *n.* 1. A small elevation. 2. MONTICULUS CEREBELLI.

monticulus ce·re·bel·li (serr″e·bel′eye) The prominent central portion of the superior vermis of the cerebellum including the culmen and declive.

moon face. Rounded, full facies characteristic of hyperadrenocorticism.

Moon's molars Maldevelopment of the first molar teeth in congenital syphilis; the cusps are so deformed that they resemble a mulberry.

moral idiocy, imbecility, or **insanity.** Inability to understand moral principles and values and to act in accordance with them, apparently without impairment of the reasoning and intellectual faculties. Once used for medicolegal purposes, the concept pertains to aspects of psychopathic and sociopathic personality disturbances.

Morax-Axenfeld conjunctivitis Chronic conjunctivitis caused by *Moraxella lacunata.*

Mo·rax·el·la (mor″ack·sel′uh) *n.* A genus of bacteria, family Brucellaceae.

Moraxella lac·u·na·ta (lack″yoo·nay′tuh) A nonmotile, gram-negative, short rod bacterium, occurring singly, in pairs, or in short chains; the type species of its genus. Syn. *Morax-Axenfeld bacillus.*

mor·bid (mor′bid) *adj.* 1. PATHOLOGIC. 2. Unwholesome; unhealthy.

morbid anatomy. PATHOLOGIC ANATOMY.

morbid hunger syndrome. KLEINE-LEVIN SYNDROME.

mor·bid·i·ty (mor·bid′i·tee) *n.* 1. The quality or state of being diseased. 2. The conditions inducing disease. 3. The ratio of the number of sick individuals to the total population of a community.

morbidity rate. The number of cases of a disease for a certain number of the population in a given time interval.

mor·bil·li (mor·bil′eye, ·ee) *n.* MEASLES.

mor·bil·li·form (mor·bil′i·form) *adj.* Resembling measles or the fine dusky rose-red, confluent maculopapular eruption seen in measles.

mor·bus (mor′bus) *n.* genit. **mor·bi** (·bye) DISEASE.

morbus cu·cul·la·ris (kew″kuh·lair′is, kuk″yoo·lair′is) Whooping cough; PERTUSSIS.

morbus di·vi·nus (di·vye′nus). EPILEPSY.

morbus gal·li·cus (gal′i·kus). SYPHILIS.

morbus mac·u·lo·sus neo·na·to·rum (mack″yoo·lo′sus nee″o·nay·to′rum). HEMORRHAGIC DISEASE OF THE NEWBORN.

morbus mag·nus (mag′nus) Recurrent GENERALIZED SEIZURES.

morbus major Grand mal epilepsy; recurrent GENERALIZED SEIZURES.

morbus med·i·co·rum (med·i·ko′rum) An abnormal or excessive tendency to seek the advice of physicians, as for imaginary diseases.

morbus mi·ser·i·ae (mi·zerr′ee·ee). Any disease due to poverty and neglect.

morbus re·gi·us (ree′jee·us) JAUNDICE.

mor·cel·la·tion (mor″se·lay′shun) *n.* A procedure whereby a solid tissue is reduced to fragments.

mor·da·cious (mor·day'shus) *adj.* Biting, pungent.

mor·dant (mor'dunt) *n. & v.* 1. A substance, such as alum, phenol, aniline, that fixes the dyes used in coloring materials or in staining tissues and bacteria. 2. To treat with a mordent.

mor·ga·gni·an (mor·gah'nee·un) *adj.* Described by or associated with Giovanni Battista Morgagni, Italian anatomist and pathologist, 1682–1771.

morgagnian cyst. A vesicle derived from the paramesonephric duct attached to the oviduct or head of the epididymis.

morgue, *n.* 1. A place where unknown dead are exposed for identification. 2. A place where dead bodies are stored pending disposition or for autopsy.

mo·ria (mo'ree·uh) *n.* 1. A dementia characterized by talkativeness and silliness. 2. Abnormal desire to joke.

mor·i·bund (mor'i·bund) *adj.* In a dying condition.

morning sickness. Nausea and vomiting, usually in the early part of the day; a common symptom of pregnancy from about the end of the first month, usually ceasing by the end of the third month.

mo·ron (mo'ron) *n.* A mentally defective person with a mental age roughly between 7 and 12 years, or, if a child, an I.Q. between 50 and 69.

mo·ron·i·ty (mo·ron'i·tee) *n.* The condition of being a moron.

Mo·ro reflex, reaction, or **response** The startle reflex observed in normal infants from birth through the first few months, consisting in abduction and extension of all extremities with extension and fanning of all digits except for flexion of thumbs and index fingers, followed by flexion and adduction of the extremities as in an embrace; may be elicited by altering the equilibrium or the plane between the child's head and trunk, or by a loud noise. Consistent failure to respond may indicate diffuse central nervous system damage, while asymmetric responses are seen in palsies of both central and peripheral origin. The presence of the reflex after six months of age usually indicates cerebral cortical disturbance.

mor·phea (mor'fee·uh) *n.* Scleroderma in which the changes are limited to local areas of the skin and associated subcutaneous tissue. Syn. *circumscribed scleroderma.*

mor·phine (mor'feen, -fin, mor·feen') *n.* $C_{17}H_{19}NO_3 \cdot H_2O$. The principal and most active alkaloid of opium; a narcotic analgesic used in the form of the hydrochloride and sulfate salts, especially the latter.

mor·phin·ism (mor'fi·niz·um) *n.* 1. Morphine addiction. 2. Morphine poisoning.

mor·pho·gen·e·sis (mor'fo·jen'e·sis) *n.* The morphologic transformations including growth, alterations of germinal layers, and differentiation of cells and tissues during development. Syn. *topogenesis.* —**morpho·ge·net·ic** (·je·net'ick), **morpho·gen·ic** (·jen'ick) *adj.*

mor·phol·o·gy (mor·fol'uh·jee) *n.* The branch of biology which deals with structure and form. It includes the anatomy, histology, and cytology of the organism at any stage of its life history. —**mor·pho·log·ic** (mor'fuh·loj'ick), **morpholog·i·cal** (·i·kul) *adj.;* **mor·phol·o·gist** (mor·fol'uh·jist) *n.*

mor·phom·e·try (mor·fom'e·tree) *n.* The measurement of the forms of organisms.

Morquio-Brailsford disease MORQUIO'S SYNDROME.

Mor·quio's syndrome (mor'kyo) Mucopolysaccharidosis IV, transmitted as an autosomal recessive characterized chemically by the presence of large amounts of keratosulfate in urine, and clinically by severe, distinctive bone changes, including dwarfism due to shortening of the spine and kyphoscoliosis, moderate shortening of the extremities and protruding sternum; the facies is typical with broad mouth, prominent maxilla, short nose, and widely spaced teeth. Clouding of the cornea usually appears later than in Hurler's syndrome, and there may be aortic regurgitation. Mental impairment is variable, but neurologic symptoms frequently result from spinal cord and medullary compression. Syn. *Brailsford-Morquio syndrome, familial osteochondrodystrophy.*

mors, *n.,* genit. **mor·tis** DEATH.

mor·sal (mor'sul) *adj.* Pertaining to the cutting or grinding portion of a tooth; OCCLUSAL.

mor·sus (mor'sus) *n.* A bite or sting.

mor·tal (mor'tul) *adj.* 1. Liable to death or dissolution. 2. Causing death; fatal.

mor·tal·i·ty (mor·tal'i·tee) *n.* 1. The quality of being mortal. 2. DEATH RATE.

mor·tar (mor'tur) *n.* A bowl-shaped vessel of porcelain, iron, glass, or other material; used for pulverizing and mixing substances by means of a pestle.

mor·ti·fi·ca·tion (mor''ti·fi·kay'shun) *n.* 1. GANGRENE. 2. NECROSIS.

Mor·ton's metatarsalgia A specific clinical type of metatarsalgia characterized by severe pain between the heads of the third and fourth metatarsal bones and due to retrogressive changes at the point of union of the digital branches from the medial and lateral plantar nerves.

Morton's syndrome A condition characterized by tenderness at the head of the second metatarsal bone, callosities beneath the second and third metatarsals, and hypertrophy of the second metatarsal, due to a short first metatarsal bone.

Morton's toe. A painful condition of one or more toes and metatarsalgia characterized by hyperextension deformity at the metatarsophalangeal joint and flexion contracture of the proximal interphalangeal joint.

mor·tu·ary (mor'choo·err''ee) *adj. & n.* 1. Pertaining to death or burial. 2. MORGUE. 3. A funeral home.

mor·u·la (mor'yoo·luh, mor'oo·luh) *n.* A type of solid blastula, without a blastocoele but having central cells not reaching the free surface.

Frequently used, incorrectly, for the late cleavage stage of the mammalian ovum.

mo·sa·ic (mo-zay'ick) *n.* 1. A pattern made on a surface by the assembly and arrangement of many small pieces. 2. *In genetics,* an individual with adjacent cells of different genetic constitution, as a result of mutation, somatic crossing-over, chromosome elimination, or chimera formation. 3. *In embryology,* an egg in which the cells of the early cleavage stages have already a type of cytoplasm which determines its later fate.   4. In plant pathology, infection with a virus which produces a characteristic spotting, as in tobacco mosaic disease.

mosaic bone. Microscopically, bone appearing as though formed of small pieces fitted together, due to cement lines indicating regional alternating periods of osteogenesis and osteoclasis; characteristic of Paget's disease.

mo·sa·i·cism (mo-zay'i-siz-um) *n. In genetics,* the presence of cells with differing genetic constitution in the same individual.

Mosch·co·witz's disease or **syndrome** THROMBOTIC THROMBOCYTOPENIC PURPURA.

Mo·sen·thal test A test for kidney function in which the variability of specific gravity of the urine is measured through a 24-hour period of controlled dietary intake.

mos·qui·to (muh-skee'to) *n.* Any insect of the subfamily Culicinae of the Diptera. Various species are vectors of important diseases such as filariasis, malaria, dengue, and yellow fever.

mosquito forceps. HALSTED'S FORCEPS (1).

Moss's groups A superseded classification of the ABO group in which type IV = O, III = B, II = A, I = AB.

mossy foot. CHROMOBLASTOMYCOSIS.

¹moth·er, *n.* 1. A female parent. 2. The source of anything.

mother cell. 1. The cell from which daughter cells are formed by cell division; PARENT CELL. 2. A chromophobe cell of the adenohypophysis.

mother yaw. The primary lesion of yaws. Syn. *maman pian.*

mo·tile (mo'til) *adj.* Able to move; capable of spontaneous motion, as a motile flagellum. **—mo·til·i·ty** (mo·til'i·tee) *n.*

mo·tion, *n.* 1. The act of changing place; movement. 2. An evacuation of the bowels; the matter evacuated.

motion sickness. A syndrome characterized by nausea, vertigo, and vomiting; occurs in normal persons as the result of random multidirectional accelerations of a ship, airplane, train, or automobile.

mo·to·neu·ron (mo''to·new'ron) *n.* A motor neuron.

mo·tor, *n. & adj.* 1. That which causes motion. 2. Pertaining to any activity or behavior involving muscular movement, as motor response. 3. Pertaining to the innervation of muscles, especially voluntary muscles; efferent, as motor neuron, motor impulse.

motor agraphia. *Obsol.* The agraphia characteristic of Broca's aphasia.

motor alexia. *Obsol.* Loss of the ability to read aloud, while understanding of written or printed words is preserved.

motor amusia. *Obsol.* Loss of the power of singing or otherwise reproducing music, while comprehension of musical notes or sounds is preserved.

motor aphasia. BROCA'S APHASIA.

motor apraxia. A division of the apractic syndromes, now largely abandoned, which included those syndromes thought to be due to affection of motor association cortex rather than of an ideation area or pathways connecting it with motor association cortex.

motor area. The area of cerebral cortex from which isolated movements can be evoked by electrical stimuli of minimal intensity. It includes the precentral convolution, containing the Betz cells (Brodmann's area 4) and extends anteriorly into area 6, and posteriorly into sensory areas 1, 2, and 3.

motor ataxia. Inability to coordinate the muscles which becomes apparent only on body movement.

motor cell. A motor neuron.

motor cortex. MOTOR AREA.

motor end plate. An area of specialized structure beneath the sarcolemma where a motor nerve fiber makes functional contact with a muscle fiber.

motor neuron. See *lower motor neuron, upper motor neuron.*

motor paralysis. The loss of voluntary control of skeletal muscle, due to interruption at any point in the motor pathway from the cerebral cortex to, and including, the muscle fiber.

motor point. A point on the skin over a muscle at which electric stimulation will cause contraction of the muscle. Syn. *Ziemssen's point.*

motor speech area. The cerebral cortical area located in the triangular and opercular portions of the inferior frontal gyrus. In right-handed and most left-handed individuals it is more developed on the left side. Syn. *Brodmann's area 44, Broca's area.*

mot·tling, *n.* Variability of coloration without distinct pattern.

mou·lage (moo-lahzh') *n.* A mold or cast made directly from any portion of the body, used especially to show a surface lesion or defect.

mound·ing (mæwn'ding) *n.* The rising in a lump of wasting, degenerating muscle fibers when struck by a slight, firm blow.

mound of Venus. MONS PUBIS.

moun·tain fever. 1. ROCKY MOUNTAIN SPOTTED FEVER. 2. COLORADO TICK FEVER.

mouse·pox. A disease of mice caused by a virus very similar to vaccinia which may be latent in many stocks of laboratory mice, but which may result in edema and necrosis leading to a loss of limbs or the tail, and in addition may lead to conjunctivitis, pneumonia, mastitis, and hepatitis. Syn. *infectious ectromelia.*

mouse tapeworm. HYMENOLEPIS DIMINUTA.

mouse-tooth forceps. A dressing forceps with interlocking fine teeth at the tips of the blades.

mouth, *n.* 1. The commencement of the alimentary canal; the cavity in which mastication takes place. In a restricted sense, the aperture between the lips. 2. The entrance to any cavity or canal.

mouth-to-mouth breathing or **insufflation.** A first-aid method of artificial respiration in which the operator places his or her mouth tightly over the patient's and forces air into the lungs in a regular breathing rhythm, allowing passive expiration; the patient's head is kept well back, and the nostrils must be blocked during insufflation.

mouth-wash, *n.* A solution for rinsing the teeth and mouth.

move-ment, *n.* 1. The act or process of moving. 2. Bowel movement, defecation.

movement disorder. DYSKINESIA.

moving-boundary electrophoresis. A method of electrophoresis applicable to dissolved substances; used in the study of biologic mixtures in their natural state. It separates, isolates, and defines the homogeneity of various components of the mixture.

moxa (mock′suh) *n.* A combustible material which in Japan has been applied to the skin and ignited for the purpose of producing an eschar or counterirritant effect. It is made with the down of dried leaves of several species of *Artemisia.* Artificial moxa is made from cotton saturated with niter.

mox-i-bus-tion (mock″si-bus′chun) *n.* The application and combustion of moxa.

m.p. Abbreviation for *melting point.*

M protein. Surface protein of group A streptococci which determines their type specificity and is important as a virulence factor.

M. R. C. P. Member of the Royal College of Physicians.

M. R. C. P. E. Member of the Royal College of Physicians of Edinburgh.

M. R. C. P. I. Member of the Royal College of Physicians of Ireland.

M. R. C. S. Member of the Royal College of Surgeons.

M. R. C. S. E. Member of the Royal College of Surgeons of Edinburgh.

M. R. C. S. I. Member of the Royal College of Surgeons of Ireland.

M. R. C. V. S. Member of the Royal College of Veterinary Surgeons.

mRNA Abbreviation for *messenger RNA.*

MS Abbreviation for (a) *multiple sclerosis;* (b) *mitral stenosis.*

M.S. Master of Science.

M. Sc. Master of Science.

MSG Abbreviation for *monosodium glutamate.*

M substance. M PROTEIN.

muc-, muci-, muco-. A combining form meaning (a) *mucus;* (b) *mucin;* (c) *mucosa.*

Mu-cha-Ha-ber-mann's disease (moo′khah, hah′bur-mahⁿ) PITYRIASIS LICHENOIDES ET VARIOLIFORMIS ACUTA.

mu chain, μ chain. The heavy chain of the I_gM immunoglobulin molecule.

mu-cic acid (mew′sick). Tetrahydroxyadipic acid, $C_6H_{10}O_8$, a dibasic acid resulting from oxidation of D-galactose or from carbohydrates yielding this sugar. Syn. *galactosaccharic acid.*

mu-cif-er-ous (mew-sif′e-rus) *adj.* Producing or secreting mucus.

mu-ci-lage (mew′si-lij) *n. In pharmacy.* a solution of a gum in water. Mucilages (mucilagines) are employed as applications to irritated surfaces, particularly mucous membranes, as excipients for pills and tablets, and to suspend insoluble substances. The most important are acacia mucilage and tragacanth mucilage. —**mu-ci-lag-i-nous** (mew″si-laj′i-nus) *adj.*

mu-cin (mew′sin) *n.* A mixture of glycoproteins that forms the basis of mucus. It is soluble in water and precipitated by alcohol or acids.

mu-cino-gen (mew-sin′o-jen) *n.* The antecedent principle from which mucin is produced.

mu-ci-no-sis (mew″si-no′sis) *n.* Collections of mucinous material in the skin, with papule and nodule formation in some cases; usually associated with myxedema.

mu-cin-ous (mew′si-nus) *adj.* Resembling or pertaining to mucin.

mucinous carcinoma. A carcinoma whose parenchymal cells produce mucin.

mu-cip-a-rous (mew-sip′uh-rus) *adj.* Secreting or producing mucus.

mu-co-buc-cal (mew″ko-buck′ul) *adj.* Pertaining to the oral mucosa and the cheeks.

mu-co-cele (mew′ko-seel) *n.* A cystic structure filled with mucus; may affect certain viscera which have become obstructed or it may develop without relationship to a recognizable normal structure.

mu-co-col-pos (mew″ko-kol′pos) *n.* A collection of mucus in the vagina.

mu-co-cu-ta-ne-ous (mew″ko-kew-tay′nee-us) *adj.* Pertaining to a mucous membrane and the skin, and to the line where these join.

mucocutaneous junction. The point of transition from skin to mucous membrane at the body orifices.

mucocutaneous lymph node syndrome. An illness of uncertain etiology affecting young children, characterized by high fever, conjunctivitis, strawberry tongue, and nonsuppurative cervical lymphadenitis, followed by characteristic desquamation of the skin of the fingertips. Syn. *Kawasaki disease.*

mu-co-en-ter-i-tis (mew″ko-en″tur-eye′tis) *n.* Inflammation of the mucous membrane of the intestine.

mu-co-epi-der-moid (mew″ko-ep″i-dur′moid) *adj.* Having both mucous and epidermal characteristics.

mucoepidermoid tumor. A usually benign tumor of salivary glands which contains both mucin-producing elements and squamous epithelium.

mu-co-gin-gi-val (mew″ko-jin′ji-vul, -jin-jye′vul) *adj.* Pertaining to mucosa and gingiva.

mu-co-hem-or-rhag-ic (mew″ko-hem″o-raj′ick) *adj.* Related to, or accompanied by, mucus and blood.

mu-coid (mew′koid) *adj. & n.* 1. Resembling mucus. 2. Any of a group of glycoproteins, differing from true mucins in their solubilities and precipitation properties. They are found in cartilage, in the cornea and crystalline lens, in white of egg, and in certain cysts and ascitic fluids.

mu·co·i·tin·sul·fu·ric acid (mew·ko″i·tin·sul·few′rick). A component of the mucin of saliva; on hydrolysis, yields sulfuric acid, glucuronic acid, glucosamine, and acetic acid.

mu·co·lyt·ic (mew″ko·lit′ick) adj. Dissolving, liquefying, or dispersing mucus.

mu·co·me·tria (mew″ko·mee′tree·uh) n. An accumulation of mucus in the uterine cavity.

mu·co·peri·os·te·um (mew″ko·perr″ee·os′tee·um) n. Periosteum with a closely associated mucous membrane.

mu·co·poly·sac·cha·ride (mew″ko·pol″ee·sack′uh·ride, ·rid) n. A polysaccharide containing an amino sugar as well as uronic acid units.

mu·co·poly·sac·cha·ri·do·sis (mew″ko·pol″ee·sack″uh·ri·do′sis) n. One of several inborn errors in the metabolism of mucopolysaccharides, differentiated on the basis of clinical, genetic, and biochemical findings thus far into six types: MPS I, Hurler's syndrome; MPS II, Hunter's syndrome; MPS III, Sanfilippo's syndrome; MPS IV, Morquio's syndrome; MPS V, Scheie's syndrome; MPS VI, Maroteaux-Lamy's syndrome. May also include MPS VII, a variant of metachromatic leukodystrophy.

mu·co·pro·tein (mew″ko·pro′tee·in, ·teen) n. A glycoprotein, particularly one in which the sugar component is chondroitinsulfuric or mucoitinsulfuric acid.

mu·co·pu·ru·lent (mew″ko·pewr′yoo·lunt) adj. Containing mucus mingled with pus, as mucopurulent sputum.

mu·co·pus (mew′ko·pus″) n. A mixture of mucus and pus.

Mu·cor (mew′kore) n. A genus of the order Mucorales.

Mu·co·ra·ce·ae (mew″ko·ray′see·ee) n.pl. A fungus family in the Mucorales order characterized by thalluses without ramifications or segments.

Mu·co·ra·les (mew″ko·ray′leez) n.pl. An order of the nonseptate class of lower fungi, the Phycomycetes, which includes such genera as Mucor, Rhizopus, and Absidia.

mu·cor·my·co·sis (mew″kor·migh·ko′sis) n. An acute, usually fulminant infection by fungi of the order Mucorales, including such genera as Absidia, Rhizopus, and Mucor, often associated with underlying disease such as diabetes mellitus, leukemia, or lymphoma. Invasion may be of the brain, lungs, or gastrointestinal tract. Ophthalmoplegia and meningoencephalitis are the most common manifestations.

mu·co·sa (mew·ko′suh, ·zuh) n., pl. **muco·sae** (·see, ·zee), **mucosas** MUCOUS MEMBRANE. —**muco·sal** (·sul, ·zul) adj.

mu·co·sal·pinx (mew″ko·sal′pinks) n. Accumulation of mucoid material in a uterine tube.

mu·co·san·guin·e·ous (mew″ko·sang·gwin′ee·us) adj. Consisting of mucus and blood.

mu·co·se·rous (mew″ko·seer′us) adj. Mucous and serous; containing mucus and serum.

mu·co·si·tis (mew″ko·sigh′tis) n. Inflammation of mucous membranes.

mu·cos·i·ty (mew·kos′i·tee) n. The quality or

condition of being mucous or covered with mucus.

mu·co·stat·ic (mew″ko·stat′ick) adj. 1. Arresting the secretion of mucus. 2. Descriptive of the normal, relaxed condition of the mucosal tissues covering the jaws when not in function.

mu·cous (mew′kus) adj. Of or pertaining to mucus; secreting mucus, as a mucous gland; depending on the presence of mucus, as mucous rales.

mucous colitis. IRRITABLE COLON.

mucous membrane. The membrane lining those cavities and canals communicating with the air. It is kept moist by the secretions of various types of glands.

mucous patch. CONDYLOMA LATUM.

mucous plug. 1. The mass of inspissated mucus which occludes the cervix uteri during pregnancy and is discharged at the beginning of labor. 2. Mucous material obstructing a bronchus.

mucous vaginitis. Vaginitis with a profuse mucoid discharge.

mu·co·vis·ci·do·sis (mew″ko·vis″i·do′sis) n. CYSTIC FIBROSIS OF THE PANCREAS.

mu·cro·nate (mew′kro·nate, ·nut) adj. Tipped with a sharp point.

Mu·cu·na (mew·kew′nuh) n. A genus of leguminous herbs. The hairs of the pods of Mucuna pruriens (Stizolobium pruritum), called cowage or cowitch, were formerly used as a vermifuge and counterirritant.

mu·cus (mew′kus) n. The viscid liquid secreted by mucous glands, consisting of water, mucin, inorganic salts, epithelial cells, leukocytes, etc., held in suspension. Adj. mucous.

Muehr·cke lines. Parallel, paired white bands in the fingernails and toenails of patients with chronic hypoalbuminemia; possibly a sign of mild protein deficiency.

mu·lat·to (mew·lat′o) n. 1. A person having one white and one black parent. 2. Any person with mixed Negro and Caucasian ancestry.

mulberry mass. MORULA.

mu·li·e·bria (mew″lee·ee′bree·uh, ·eb′ree·uh) n.pl. The female genitals.

mull, v. 1. To mix dental amalgam by hand following trituration in order to produce a smoother mass. 2. To reduce a relatively coarse solid to a fine powder by rubbing it, usually in a semifluid dispersion medium, on a flat surface with the flattened area of a piece of glass, stone, or metal.

mül·le·ri·an (mew·leer′ee·un, ·lerr′) adj. 1. Discovered by or associated with Johannes Müller, German anatomist and physiologist, 1801–1858. 2. Pertaining to the müllerian (paramesonephric) duct and its derivatives.

müllerian duct. PARAMESONEPHRIC DUCT.

müllerian duct cyst. A congenital cyst arising from vestiges of the müllerian ducts.

Müller's fibers Modified neuroglial cells that traverse perpendicularly the layers of the retina, and connect the internal and external limiting membranes.

mult·an·gu·lar (mul·tang′gyoo·lur) n. MULTANGULUM.

mul·tan·gu·lum (mul·tang'gyoo·lum) n. A bone with many angles.

multi- 1. A combining form meaning *many, much.* 2. *In medicine,* a combining form meaning *affecting many parts.*

mul·ti·cel·lu·lar (mul''ti·sel'yoo·lur) adj. Having many cells.

mul·ti·cen·tric (mul''ti·sen'trick) adj. Having many centers.

Multiceps multiceps. A species of tapeworm occurring in the small intestine of dogs and wolves. The larval stage develops in the brain and spinal cord of sheep, goats, cattle, horses, and has also been found in man.

mul·ti·cos·tate (mul''ti·kos'tate) adj. Having many ribs.

mul·ti·cus·pid (mul''ti·kus'pid) adj. & n. 1. Having several cusps, as the molar teeth. 2. A tooth that has several cusps. —**multicus·pi·date** (·pi·date) adj.

mul·ti·cys·tic kidney (mul''ti·sis'tick) A congenital anomaly in which one kidney is replaced by a mass of cysts, with atresia or absence of the associated ureter. There is little or no renal parenchyma and there may be an admixture of such mesodermal derivatives as cartilage.

mul·ti·den·tate (mul''ti·den'tate) adj. Having many teeth or toothlike processes.

mul·ti·dig·i·tate (mul''ti·dij'i·tate) adj. Having many digits or digitate processes.

mul·ti·fac·to·ri·al (mul''ti·fack·to'ree·ul) adj. Pertaining to an inheritance pattern dependent upon the interaction of multiple genetic and environmental factors.

mul·ti·fa·mil·i·al (mul''ti·fa·mil'ee·ul) adj. Affecting several successive generations of a family, as certain diseases.

mul·ti·fid (mul'ti·fid) adj. Divided into many parts.

mul·ti·fo·cal (mul''ti·fo'kul) adj. Having, arising from, or pertaining to many discrete locations or collections.

mul·ti·glan·du·lar (mul''ti·glan'dew·lur) adj. Pertaining to several glands, as multiglandular secretions, a mixture of secretions from two or more glands; PLURIGLANDULAR.

mul·ti·grav·i·da (mul''ti·grav'i·duh) n. A woman who has had one or more previous pregnancies. —**multi·grav·id·i·ty** (·gra·vid'i·tee) n.

mul·ti·in·fec·tion (mul''tee·in·feck'shun) n. MIXED INFECTION.

mul·ti·lo·bar (mul''ti·lo'bahr, ·bur) adj. Composed of many lobes.

mul·ti·lo·bate (mul''ti·lo'bate) adj. MULTILOBAR.

mul·ti·lob·u·lar (mul''ti·lob'yoo·lur) adj. Having many lobules.

multilobular cirrhosis. Portal cirrhosis in which several lobules are surrounded by fibrotic portal spaces; the usual form of the disease.

mul·ti·loc·u·lar (mul''ti·lock'yoo·lur) adj. Containing or consisting of many loculi or compartments.

mul·ti·mam·mae (mul''ti·mam'ee) n. POLYMASTIA; the presence of more than two breasts in a human being.

mul·ti·nod·u·lar (mul''ti·nod'yoo·lur) adj. Having many nodules.

mul·ti·nu·cle·ar (mul''ti·new'klee·ur) adj. Having two or more nuclei.

mul·ti·nu·cle·ate (mul''ti·new'klee·ate, ·ut) adj. MULTINUCLEAR. —**multinucle·at·ed** (·ay·tid) adj.

mul·tip·a·ra (mul·tip'uh·ruh) n. A woman who has already borne one or more children. —**multipa·rous** (·rus) adj.; **mul·ti·par·i·ty** (mul''ti·păr'i·tee) n.

mul·ti·par·tite (mul''ti·pahr'tite) adj. Divided into many parts.

mul·ti·pha·sic (mul''ti·fay'zick) adj. Having numerous phases or facets.

mul·ti·ple, adj. Manifold; affecting many parts at the same time, as multiple sclerosis; repeated two or more times.

multiple alleles. Alleles numbering more than two for a single locus.

multiple endocrine adenomatosis. Hereditary hyperplasia or neoplasia of two or more endocrine glands, usually with increased function. The parathyroid glands, pancreatic islet cells, and pituitary gland are the most frequently affected; transmitted as an autosomal dominant trait.

multiple hereditary exostoses. A common heritable disorder of connective tissue, transmitted as a dominant and usually discovered in childhood or adolescence, in which ossified projections capped by proliferating cartilage arise from the cortex of bone within the periosteum, commonly in metaphyseal regions. Syn. *diaphyseal aclasis, hereditary deforming chondrodysplasia.*

multiple idiopathic hemorrhagic sarcoma. A mesodermal tumor characterized by the occurrence of multiple bluish-red or brown nodules and plaques, usually on the extremities. In the early granulomatous lesions, which occasionally involute spontaneously, tumor is not evident; in later stages, the histologic picture resembles angiosarcoma or fibrosarcoma. Syn. *Kaposi's sarcoma, sarcoma cutaneum telangiectaticum multiplex, multiplex angiosarcoma.*

multiple myeloma. A neoplasm that results from a progressive, uncontrolled proliferation of plasma cells in bone marrow. Its clinical manifestations include tumor formation, skeletal and renal disease, abnormal synthesis of immunoglobulins, and bone marrow dysfunction.

multiple neuritis. POLYNEURITIS.

multiple personality. A personality capable of dissociation into several or many other personalities at the same time, whereby the delusion is entertained that the one person is many separate persons; a symptom in schizophrenic patients.

multiple pregnancy. Gestation with two or more fetuses present within the uterus.

multiple sclerosis. A common disease of young adults, characterized clinically by episodes of focal disorder of the optic nerves, spinal cord, and brain, which remit to a varying extent and recur over a period of many years; and pathologically by the presence of numerous, scattered, sharply defined demyelinative lesions (plaques) in the white matter of the central nervous system. Syn. *insular sclerosis, disseminated sclerosis, sclérose en plaques.*

mul·ti·plex (mul'ti-plecks) *adj.* Multiple.

mul·ti·plic·i·ty (mul'ti-plis'i-tee) *n.* 1. The state or quality of being multiple. 2. Increase, reproduction.

mul·ti·po·lar (mul''ti-po'pul'ar) *adj.* Having more than one pole, as multipolar nerve cells, those having more than one process.

mul·ti·pol·yp·oid (mul''ti-pol'i-poid) *adj.* Having more than one polyp.

mul·ti·sep·tate (mul''ti-sep'tate) *adj.* Divided by more than one septum, as in the case of various fungus conidia.

mul·ti·sys·tem (mul'ti-sis''tum) *adj.* Involving more than one of the major body systems.

mul·ti·va·lent (mul''ti-vay'lunt, mul·tiv'uh-lunt) *adj.* 1. Capable of combining with more than one atom of a univalent element. 2. POLYVALENT.

mum·mi·fi·ca·tion (mum''i-fi-kay'shun) *n.* 1. The change of a part into a hard, dry mass. 2. DRY GANGRENE.

mum·mi·fied (mum'i-fide) *adj.* Dried, as mummified pulp, the condition of the dental pulp when it is affected by dry gangrene.

mumps, *n.* An acute communicable viral disease, usually manifest by painful enlargement of the salivary glands, but frequently invading other tissues, notably testes, pancreas, and meninges. Syn. *epidemic parotitis.*

Mun·chau·sen syndrome (mun'chaw-zun) A personality disorder in which the patient describes dramatic but false symptoms or simulates acute illness, happily undergoing numerous examinations, hospitalizations, and diagnostic or therapeutic manipulations, and upon discovery of the real nature of his case, often leaves without notice and moves on to another hospital.

Münch·mey·er's disease (muᵉnᶜh'migh·ur) Myositis ossificans of a progressive nature.

mun·dif·i·cant (mun-dif'ick-unt) *adj.* & *n.* 1. Having the power to cleanse, purge, or heal. 2. A cleansing, purging, or healing agent.

mu·ral (mew'rul) *adj.* Pertaining to, or located in or on, the wall of a cavity.

mural thrombus. A thrombus attached to the wall of a blood vessel or mural endocardium. Syn. *lateral thrombus.*

mu·rex·ide (mew'reck'side) *n.* Ammonium purpurate, $C_8H_8N_6O_6$, a purple coloring matter resulting from uric acid by treatment with nitric acid and neutralization with ammonia.

mu·ri·at·ic (mew''ree·at'ick) *adj.* Pertaining to brine.

mu·rine (mew'rine, ·rin, mew·reen') *adj.* Of, resembling, or pertaining to mice, especially to the genus *Mus;* or to mice and rats of the family Muridae in general.

murine typhus. A relatively mild, acute, febrile illness of worldwide distribution caused by *Rickettsia typhi,* characterized by headache, macular rash, and myalgia; a natural infection of rats, sporadically transmitted to man by the flea. Syn. *endemic typhus, urban typhus, shop typhus, flea-borne typhus, rat typhus.*

mur·mur, *n.* A benign or pathologic blowing or roaring sound heard on auscultation, especially having a cardiac or vascular origin.

Murphy's sign 1. A sign for cholecystitis in which pressure is applied over the gallbladder; inspiration produces pain and arrest of respiration as the descending diaphragm causes the inflamed gallbladder to impinge against the examining hand. 2. Punch tenderness at the costovertebral angle in perinephric abscess.

Mur·ray Valley encephalitis An acute viral encephalomyelitis, confined to Australia and New Guinea, and occurring predominantly in children. Syn. *Australian X disease.*

Mus·ca (mus'kuh) *n.* A genus of flies of the family Muscidae.

mus·cae vol·i·tan·tes (mus'ee vol''i·tan'teez, mus'kee) FLOATERS.

mus·ca·rine (mus'kuh·reen, ·rin, mus·kay'reen) *n.* A poisonous alkaloid obtained from certain mushrooms, as *Amanita muscaria;* a quaternary ammonium compound, the cation of which is trimethyl(tetrahydro-4-hydroxy-5-methylfurfuryl)ammonium, $(C_9H_{20}NO_2)+$, a parasympathomimetic drug which mimics certain effects of acetylcholine, having the same action as postganglionic cholinergic nerve impulses on endocrine glands, smooth muscle, and heart.

mus·ca·rin·ism (mus'kuh·ri·niz·um) *n.* Mushroom poisoning.

mus·ci·cide (mus'i·side) *n.* An agent which is poisonous or destructive to flies.

mus·cle, *n.* 1. A tissue composed of contractile fibers or cells. Classified by microscopical appearance as nonstriated (smooth) or striated; by volitional control as voluntary or involuntary; by location in the body as skeletal, cardiac, or visceral. 2. A contractile organ composed of muscle tissue, effecting the movements of the organs and parts of the body; particularly, that composed of a belly of skeletal muscle tissue attached by tendons to bone on either side of a joint effecting movements at the joint by contraction of the belly drawing the more movable attachment, the insertion, toward the more fixed attachment, the origin.

muscle-contraction headache. Any headache or sensation of tightness, constriction or pressure, associated with sustained contraction of head and neck muscles in the absence of permanent structural changes, and usually associated with emotional tension; the headache varies widely in intensity, frequency, and duration; frequently suboccipital.

muscle of Hall. ISCHIOBULBOSUS.

muscul-, musculo-. A combining form meaning *muscle* or *muscular.*

mus·cu·lar (mus'kew·lur) *adj.* 1. Of or pertaining to muscles. 2. Having well-developed muscles. —**mus·cu·lar·i·ty** (mus''kew·lar'i·tee) *n.*

muscular artery. DISTRIBUTING ARTERY.

muscular atrophy. A loss of muscle bulk due to a lesion involving either the cell body or axon of the lower motor neuron, or secondary to aging, disuse, deficiency states, or to a variety of degenerative, toxic, inflammatory, vascular, or metabolic disorders of the muscle fibers themselves.

muscular dystrophy. A hereditary, progressive degeneration of muscle. See *pseudohypertrophic infantile muscular dystrophy.*

muscular irritability. The inherent capacity of a muscle to respond or its capacity to respond to threshold or suprathreshold stimuli by contraction.

mus·cu·la·ris (mus″kew·lair′is) *n.* 1. The muscular layer of a tubular or hollow organ. 2. MUSCULARIS MUCOSAE.

muscularis mu·co·sae (mew·ko′see). The single or double thin layer of smooth muscle in the deep portion of some mucous membranes, as in most of the digestive tube.

muscular tension. The state present when muscles are passively stretched or actively contracted.

mus·cu·la·ture (mus′kew·luh·chur, ·tewr) *n.* The muscular system of the body, or a part of it.

musculi. Plural and genitive singular of *musculus.*

musculo-. See *muscul-.*

mus·cu·lo·apo·neu·rot·ic (mus″kew·lo·ap″o·new·rot′ick) *adj.* Composed of muscle and of fibrous connective tissue in the form of a membrane.

mus·cu·lo·cu·ta·ne·ous (mus″kew·lo·kew·tay′nee·us) *adj.* Pertaining to or supplying the muscles and skin.

mus·cu·lo·fas·cial (mus″kew·lo·fash′ee·ul) *adj.* Consisting of both muscular and fascial elements, as in an amputation flap.

mus·cu·lo·fi·brous (mus″kew·lo·figh′brus) *adj.* Pertaining to a tissue which is partly muscular and partly fibrous connective tissue.

mus·cu·lo·mem·bra·nous (mus″kew·lo·mem′bruh·nus) *adj.* Composed of muscular tissue and membrane.

mus·cu·lo·phren·ic (mus″kew·lo·fren′ick) *adj.* Pertaining to or supplying the muscles of the diaphragm.

mus·cu·lo·skel·e·tal (mus″kew·lo·skel′e·tul) *adj.* Pertaining to or composed of the muscles and the skeleton.

musculospiral groove or **sulcus.** RADIAL SULCUS.

mus·cu·lo·ten·di·nous (mus″kew·lo·ten′di·nus) *adj.* Composed of muscular and tendinous fibers.

musculus longissimus tho·ra·cis (tho·ray′sis) [NA]. The longissimus thoracis muscle.

mush·room, *n.* Any of numerous fleshy fungi of the Basidiomycetes.

musical agraphia. Loss of ability to write musical notes.

musical alexia. Loss of ability to read music.

musical deafness. 1. SENSORY AMUSIA. 2. TONE DEAFNESS.

mu·si·co·ma·nia (mew″zi·ko·may′nee·uh) *n.* Monomania for, or insane devotion to, music.

mu·si·co·ther·a·py (mew″zi·ko·therr′uh·pee) *n.* The use of music in the treatment of diseases, particularly of mental disorders.

mus·si·ta·tion (mus″i·tay′shun) *n.* Movement of the lips as if speaking but without making speech sounds; frequently observed in silent reading.

mus·tard, *n.* 1. A plant of the genus *Brassica.* 2. The dried seed of *Brassica alba* or *B. nigra.* The powdered seed of the latter is used as a rubefacient.

mustard gas. Bis (2-chloroethyl) sulfide, $(ClC_2H_4)_2S$, an oily liquid with deadly vesicant action; has been used as a chemical warfare agent. Syn. *yperite.*

mu·ta·gen (mew′tuh·jen) *n.* Any substance or agent causing a genetic mutation. —**mu·ta·gen·ic** (mew″tuh·jen′ick) *adj.;* **mu·ta·gen·e·sis** (mew″tuh·jen′e·sis) *n.*

mu·tant (mew′tunt) *adj. & n.* 1. Having undergone or resulting from mutation. 2. An individual with characteristics different from those of the parental type due to a genetic constitution that includes a mutation.

mu·ta·ro·ta·tion (mew″tuh·ro·tay′shun) *n.* A change in optical rotation of solutions of certain sugars occurring while standing and continuing until equilibrium between the isomeric forms present in the solution is attained.

mu·tase (mew′tace, ·taze) *n.* 1. An enzyme that simultaneously catalyzes the oxidation of one molecule and reduction of another molecule of the substrate. 2. An enzyme that catalyzes the apparent migration of a phosphate group from one to another hydroxyl group of the same molecule.

mu·ta·tion (mew·tay′shun) *n.* 1. A change of small or moderate extent, which represents a definite stage in the gradual evolution of an organism, such as may be recognized in a series of fossils from successive geologic strata. 2. A change in the characteristics of an organism produced by an alteration of the hereditary material. The alteration in the germ plasm may involve an addition of one or more complete sets of chromosomes, the addition or loss of a whole chromosome, or some change within a chromosome, ranging from a gross rearrangement, loss or addition of a larger or smaller section, down through minute rearrangements to a change at a single locus. The latter are gene mutations, or simply mutation in the restricted use of the term.

mute (mewt) *adj.* Unable to speak.

mu·ti·late (mew′ti·late) *v.* To maim or disfigure; to deprive of a member or organ. —**mu·ti·la·tion** (mew″ti·lay′shun) *n.*

mut·ism (mewt′iz·um) *n.* The condition or state of being speechless.

mut·ton-fat (keratic) precipitates. Large clumps of yellowish epithelial cells deposited upon the endothelial surface of the cornea that indicate chronic types of uveitis.

muz·zle, *n.* The projecting jaws and nose of an animal; a snout.

M. W. Abbreviation for *molecular weight.*

M waves. Microwaves of atrial fibrillation, occurring at a rate of about 40,000 per minute.

my. Abbreviation for *myopia.*

my-, myo- A combining form meaning *muscle.*

my·al·gia (migh·al′juh, ·jee·uh) *n.* Pain in the muscles. —**myal′gic** (·jick) *adj.*

my·as·the·nia (migh″as·theen′ee·uh) *n.* 1. Muscular weakness from any cause. 2. Specifically, myasthenia gravis. —**my·as·then·ic** (migh"as-thenn'ick, ·theen'ick) adj.

myasthenia grav·is (grav'is). A disorder, characterized by a fluctuant weakness of certain voluntary skeletal muscles, particularly those innervated by the bulbar nuclei, affecting women twice as often as men, and sometimes associated with hyperthyroidism or, in the older age group, with carcinoma, as well as with thymic hyperplasia or with thymic tumor. Recent evidence suggests an autoimmune basis for this disorder resulting in a decreased number of acetylcholine receptors and a simplification of the junctional folds in the postsynaptic membrane of the motor end plate.

myasthenic crisis. Profound muscular weakness and respiratory paralysis observed in myasthenia gravis, due to lack of or to insufficient treatment with anticholinesterase drugs.

myasthenic reaction. In electromyography, the reaction observed in myasthenia gravis, in which there is a rapid reduction in the amplitude of compound muscle action potentials evoked during repetitive stimulation of a peripheral nerve at a rate of 3 per second (decrementing response) and reversal of the response by neostigmine.

myasthenic syndrome. A special form of myasthenia, observed most often in association with oat-cell carcinoma of the lung and affecting the muscles of the trunk, pelvic, and shoulder girdles predominantly. Unlike myasthenia gravis, a single stimulus of nerve may yield a low amplitude muscle action potential, whereas stimulation at the rate of 50 per second yields an increase in amplitude of action potentials (incrementing response). Syn. Eaton-Lambert syndrome.

myc-, myco- 1. A combining form meaning (a) fungus, fungous; (b) funguslike in appearance, moldlike. 2. See muc-.

my·ce·li·um (migh·see'lee·um) n., pl. **myce·lia** (·lee·uh) The vegetative filaments of fungi, usually forming interwoven masses. —**mycelial** (·ul) adj.

mycet-, myceto- A combining form meaning fungus.

my·ce·tis·mus (migh"se·tiz'mus) n. Fungus poisoning, including mushroom poisoning.

my·ce·to·gen·ic (migh·see"to·jen'ick, migh·set" o·) adj. Produced or caused by fungi.

my·ce·to·ma (migh"se·to'muh) n. A chronic infection, usually of the feet, by various fungi or by Nocardia or Streptomyces, resulting in swelling and sinus tracts. Syn. maduromycosis.

Mycifradin. A trademark for the antibiotic neomycin, used as the sulfate salt.

My·co·bac·te·ri·a·ce·ae (migh"ko·back·teer"ee·ay'see·ee) n.pl. A family of the order Actinomycetales; contains one genus, Mycobacterium.

my·co·bac·te·ri·o·sis (migh"ko·back·teer·ee·o' sis) n. A mycobacterial infection.

My·co·bac·te·ri·um (migh"ko·back·teer'ee·um) n. A genus of rod-shaped, aerobic bacteria of the family Mycobacteriaceae. Species of this genus are rarely filamentous and occasionally branch but produce no conidia. They are gram-positive, and stain with difficulty, but are acid-fast. —**mycobacterium**, pl. **mycobacteria**, com. n.

Mycobacterium bo·vis (bo'vis). The principal cause of cattle tuberculosis and, rarely, the cause of human tuberculosis as well; acid-fast rods.

Mycobacterium lep·rae (lep'ree). The causative organism of leprosy; formerly called Bacillus leprae.

Mycobacterium paratuberculosis. The causative agent of a chronic enteritis of cattle, sheep, and deer, nonpathogenic for man.

Mycobacterium phlei (flee'eye). A species of Mycobacterium found in soil and water.

Mycobacterium tuberculosis. A species of acid-fast bacteria; the principal cause of tuberculosis in man. Syn. Bacillus tuberculosis.

my·co·ci·din (migh"ko·sigh'din) n. An antibiotic substance extracted from a mold of the Aspergillaceae family. It is active, in vitro, against Mycobacterium tuberculosis.

my·coid (migh'koid) adj. Resembling, or appearing like, a fungus; fungoid.

my·col·o·gy (migh·kol'uh·jee) n. The science of fungi.

my·coph·thal·mia (migh"koff·thal'mee·uh) n. Ophthalmia due to a fungus.

My·co·plas·ma (migh"ko·plaz'muh) n. A genus of minute microorganisms that lack rigid cell walls, give rise to small colonies on media enriched with body fluids such as serum, and include nonpathogens and pathogens of man and animals.

Mycoplasma ar·thri·ti·dis (ahr·thrit'i·dis). A species of Mycoplasma thought to be the causative agent of murine arthritis.

Mycoplasma my·coi·des (migh"koy'deez). The causative agent of bovine pleuropneumonia.

Mycoplasma pneu·mo·ni·ae (new·mo'nee·ee). The causative agent of primary atypical pneumonia of man, often resulting in the appearance of cold agglutinins for human type O red blood cells or of Streptococcus MG in the infected individual.

my·co·sis (migh·ko'sis) n., pl. **myco·ses** (·seez) Any infection or disease caused by a fungus.

mycosis fun·goi·des (fung·goy'deez). A form of malignant lymphoma, with special cutaneous manifestations, characterized by eczematoid areas, infiltrations, nodules, tumors, and ulcerations. Syn. granuloma fungoides.

mycosis fungoides d'em·blée (dahm·blay') The presence of mycosis fungoides without previous erythema or plaques.

Mycostatin. Trademark for the antibiotic substance nystatin, used as an antifungal agent for the treatment of infections caused by Candida (Monilia) albicans.

my·cos·ter·ol (migh·kos'tur·ol, ·ole) n. Any sterol occurring in yeast or fungi.

my·cot·ic (migh·kot'ick) adj. 1. Of or pertaining to mycosis. 2. Fungoid; resembling a fungus in appearance.

mycotic aneurysm. A localized abnormal dilatation of a vessel due to destruction of all or part of its wall by microorganisms.

mycotic keratitis. 1. KERATOMYCOSIS. 2. DENDRITIC KERATITIS.

my·cot·i·za·tion (migh-kot"i-zay'shun) n. Superimposition of a mycotic infection on a nonfungous lesion; secondary mycosis.

my·co·tox·i·co·sis (migh"ko-tock"si-ko'sis) n. 1. Poisoning due to a bacterial or fungal toxin. 2. Poisoning from a fungus which is ingested either by itself or in food contaminated by the fungus.

myc·tero·pho·nia (mick"tur-o-fo'nee-uh) n. A nasal quality of the voice.

my·de·sis (migh-dee'sis) n. 1. PUTREFACTION. 2. A discharge of pus from the eyelids.

myd·ri·at·ic (mid"ree-at'ick) adj. & n. 1. Producing mydriasis; dilating the pupil. 2. An agent that dilates the pupil, such as eucatropine hydrochloride.

my·ec·to·my (migh-eck'tuh-mee) n. Excision of a portion of muscle.

my·ec·to·py (migh-eck'tuh-pee) n. The displacement of a muscle.

myel-, myelo- A combining form meaning (a) marrow; (b) spinal cord; (c) myelin.

my·el·en·ceph·a·lon (migh"e-len-sef'uh-lon) n. The caudal part of the embryonic hindbrain, from which the medulla oblongata develops.—**my·el·en·ce·phal·ic** (-se-fal'ick) adj.

my·el·ic (migh-el'ick) adj. Pertaining to the spinal cord.

my·e·lin (migh'e-lin) n. 1. The white, fatty substance forming a sheath of some nerves. Syn. white substance of Schwann. 2. A complex mixture of lipids extracted from nervous tissue; it is doubly refractile and contains phosphatides and cholesterol.

my·e·li·nat·ed (migh'e-li-nay'tid) adj. Provided with a myelin sheath; medullated.

my·e·li·ni·za·tion (migh"e-li-ni-zay'shun) n. The process of elaborating or accumulating myelin during the development, or regeneration of nerves.

my·e·li·noc·la·sis (migh"e-li-nock'luh-sis) n. DEMYELINATION; destruction of the myelin.

my·e·lino·gen·e·sis (migh"e-lin-o-jen'e-sis) n. MYELINIZATION.

my·e·lin·ol·y·sis (migh"e-lin-ol'i-sis) n. Disintegration of myelin.

my·e·li·nop·a·thy (migh"e-li-nop'uth-ee) n. Any disease of the myelin.

my·e·li·no·sis (migh"e-li-no'sis) n. Decomposition of fat with the formation of myelin.

myelin sheath. The short (750 μm) segment of myelin which surrounds the axon and which is enveloped by a Schwann cell plasma membrane.

my·e·li·tis (migh"e-lye'tis) n. 1. Inflammation of the spinal cord. 2. Inflammation of the bone marrow. —**my·e·lit·ic** (-lit'ick) adj.

myelo-. See myel-.

my·e·lo·blast (migh'e-lo-blast) n. The youngest of the precursor cells of the granulocytic series, having a nucleus with a finely granular or homogeneous chromatin structure and nucleoli and intensely basophilic cytoplasm. Syn. granuloblast.

my·e·lo·blas·te·mia, my·e·lo·blas·tae·mia (migh"e-lo-blas-tee'mee-uh) n. Presence of myeloblasts in the circulating blood.

my·e·lo·blas·tic (migh"e-lo-blas'tick) adj. Originating from, or characterized by, the presence of myeloblasts.

my·e·lo·blas·to·ma (migh"e-lo-blas-to'muh) n. A malignant tumor composed of poorly differentiated granulocytes. Syn. granulocytic sarcoma.

my·e·lo·blas·to·sis (migh"e-lo-blas-to'sis) n. Diffuse proliferation of myeloblasts, with involvement of blood, bone marrow, and other tissues and organs.

my·e·lo·cele (migh'e-lo-seel) n. Spina bifida, with protrusion of the spinal cord.

my·e·lo·cys·to·cele (migh"e-lo-sis'to-seel) n. A hernial protrusion, in spina bifida, in which there is accumulation of fluid in the central canal of the spinal cord.

my·e·lo·cys·tog·ra·phy (migh"e-lo-sis-tog'ruh-fee) n. The demonstration of an intramedullary spinal cord cyst by scanning or radiography after percutaneous puncture of the cyst and injection into it of an isotope-labeled substance or contrast material, such as opaque material or air.

my·e·lo·cyte (migh'e-lo-site) n. 1. A granular leukocyte, precursor in the stage of development intermediate between the promyelocyte and metamyelocyte. The staining reactions of the granules differentiate myelocytes into neutrophilic, eosinophilic, and basophilic types. 2. Any cell concerned in development of granular leukocytes. —**my·e·lo·cyt·ic** (migh"e-lo-sit'ick) adj.

my·e·lo·cy·to·ma (migh"e-lo-sigh-to'muh) n. A malignant plasmacytoma.

my·e·lo·cy·to·sis (migh"e-lo-sigh-to'sis) n. Myelocytes in the blood.

my·e·lo·dys·pla·sia (migh"e-lo-dis-play'zhuh, -zee-uh) n. Defective development of the spinal cord, especially in its lumbosacral portion.

my·e·lo·en·ceph·a·li·tis (migh"e-lo-en-sef'uh-lye'tis) n. Inflammation of both spinal cord and brain.

my·e·lo·fi·bro·sis (migh"e-lo-figh-bro'sis) n. Fibrosis of the bone marrow. It may be a primary disorder of unknown cause, or a complication of bone marrow injury.

my·e·lo·gen·e·sis (migh"e-lo-jen'e-sis) n. MYELINIZATION.

my·e·lo·gen·ic (migh"e-lo-jen'ick) adj. Produced in, or by, bone marrow.

my·e·log·e·nous (migh"e-loj'e-nus) adj. 1. MYELOGENIC. 2. Pertaining to cells produced in bone marrow.

myelogenous leukemia. GRANULOCYTIC LEUKEMIA.

my·e·lo·gram (migh'e-lo-gram) n. 1. A radiograph of the spinal canal, made after the injection of a contrast medium into the subarachnoid space. 2. A differentiated count of nucleated cells of bone marrow.

my·e·log·ra·phy (migh"e-log'ruh-fee) n. Radiographic demonstration of the spinal subarachnoid space, after the introduction of contrast media such as air, Pantopaque, or absorbable contrast material.

my·e·loid (migh'e·loid) *adj.* Pertaining to bone marrow.

myeloid:erythroid ratio. The ratio of leukocytes of the granulocytic series to nucleated erythrocyte precursors in an aspirated sample of bone marrow. The limits of normal are 0.6:1 to 2.7:1. Syn. *M:E ratio.*

myeloid leukemia. GRANULOCYTIC LEUKEMIA.

myeloid metaplasia. The occurrence of hemopoietic tissue in areas of the body where it is not normally found.

myeloid tissue. Red bone marrow consisting of reticular cells attached to argyrophile fibers which form wide meshes containing scattered fat cells, erythroblasts, myelocytes, and mature myeloid elements.

my·e·lo·li·po·ma (migh''e·lo·li·po'muh) *n.* A choristoma, usually of the adrenal gland, composed of adipose tissue and hemopoietic cells.

my·e·lo·lym·pho·cyte (migh''e·lo·lim'fo·site) *n.* A small lymphocyte formed in the bone marrow.

my·e·lo·ma (migh''e·lo'muh) *n.* A malignant plasmacytoma.

my·e·lo·ma·la·cia (migh''e·lo·ma·lay'shee·uh) *n.* Infarction or softening of the spinal cord.

my·e·lo·ma·to·sis (migh''e·lo·muh·to'sis) *n.* A malignant plasmacytoma.

my·e·lo·ma·tous (migh''e·lo'muh·tus, ·lom'uh·tus) *adj.* Pertaining to or caused by myeloma.

my·e·lo·men·in·gi·tis (migh''e·lo·men''in·jye'tis) *n.* Inflammation of the spinal cord and its meninges.

my·e·lo·men·in·go·cele (migh''e·lo·me·ning'go·seel) *n.* Spina bifida with protrusion of a meningeal sac containing elements of the spinal cord or cauda equina.

my·e·lo·mere (migh'e·lo·meer) *n.* An embryonic segment of the spinal cord.

my·e·lo·mono·cyte (migh''e·lo·mon'o·site) *n.* 1. A monocyte developing in the bone marrow. 2. A blood cell having characteristics of both the monocytic and granulocytic series, seen in the Naegeli type of monocytic leukemia. —**myelo·mono·cyt·ic** (·mon''o·sit'ick) *adj.*

myelomonocytic leukemia. The Naegeli type of monocytic leukemia.

my·e·lo·neu·ri·tis (migh''e·lo·new·rye'tis) *n.* Polyneuritis combined with myelitis.

my·e·lo·pa·ral·y·sis (migh''e·lo·puh·ral'i·sis) *n.* SPINAL PARALYSIS.

my·e·lo·path·ic (migh''e·lo·path'ick) *adj.* Pertaining to disease of the spinal cord, or of myeloid tissue.

my·e·lop·a·thy (migh''e·lop'uth·ee) *n.* Any disease of the spinal cord, or of myeloid tissues.

my·e·lo·pe·tal (migh''e·lop'e·tul) *adj.* Moving toward the spinal cord.

myelophthisic anemia. An anemia associated with space-occupying disorders of the bone marrow. Syn. *myelopathic anemia, myelosclerotic anemia, osteosclerotic anemia.*

my·e·lo·phthi·sis (migh''e·lo·thigh'sis) *n.* 1. Loss of bone marrow due to replacement by other tissue, notably fibrous tissue or bone. 2. Spinal

cord atrophy in tabes dorsalis. —**myelo·phthis·ic** (·thiz'ick), **myelophthis·i·cal** (·i·kul) *adj.*

my·e·lo·plast (migh'e·lo·plast) *n.* A leukocyte of the bone marrow.

my·e·lo·ple·gia (migh''e·lo·plee'juh, ·jee·uh) *n.* SPINAL PARALYSIS.

my·e·lo·poi·e·sis (migh''e·lo·poy·ee'sis) *n.* The process of formation and development of the blood cells in the bone marrow.

my·e·lo·pro·lif·er·a·tive disorders or **syndrome** (migh''e·lo·pro·lif'ur·uh·tiv). Proliferation of one or more bone marrow elements without definite evidence of neoplasia, accompanied by extramedullary hemopoiesis and immature cells in the peripheral blood.

my·e·lo·ra·dic·u·li·tis (migh''e·lo·ra·dick''yoo·lye'tis) *n.* Inflammation of the spinal cord and roots of the spinal nerves.

my·e·lo·ra·dic·u·lo·dys·pla·sia (migh''e·lo·ra·dick''yoo·lo·dis·play'zhuh, ·zee·uh) *n.* Congenital abnormality of the spinal cord and roots of the spinal nerves.

my·e·lo·ra·dic·u·lop·a·thy (migh''e·lo·ra·dick'' yoo·lop'uth·ee) *n.* Disease of the spinal cord and roots of the spinal nerves.

my·e·lor·rha·gia (migh''e·lo·ray'jee·uh) *n.* Hemorrhage into the spinal cord.

my·e·lo·sar·co·ma (migh''e·lo·sahr·ko'muh) *n.* A malignant plasmacytoma.

my·e·los·chi·sis (migh''e·los'ki·sis) *n.* Complete or partial failure of the neural plate to form a neural tube, resulting in a cleft spinal cord.

my·e·lo·scin·to·gram (migh''e·lo·sin'tuh·gram) *n.* A graphic presentation of the distribution of a radioactive tracer introduced into the subarachnoid space.

my·e·lo·scin·tog·ra·phy (migh''e·lo·sin·tog'ruh·fee) *n.* A technique of introducing a radioactive tracer substance into the spinal subarachnoid space and then of determining the distribution of the radioactive substance by means of a scintiscanner.

my·e·lo·scle·ro·sis (migh''e·lo·skle·ro'sis) *n.* 1. Multiple sclerosis of the spinal cord. 2. MYELOFIBROSIS.

my·e·lo·scle·rot·ic (migh''e·lo·skle·rot'ick) *adj.* Of or pertaining to myelophthisis or to myelofibrosis.

myelosclerotic anemia. MYELOPHTHISIC ANEMIA.

my·e·lo·sis (migh''e·lo'sis) *n.* 1. MYELOCYTOSIS. 2. A malignant plasmacytoma. 3. GRANULOCYTIC LEUKEMIA.

my·e·lo·sup·pres·sive (migh''e·lo·suh·pres'iv) *adj.* Tending to suppress the development of white blood cells and platelets. —**myelosuppres·sion** (·shun) *n.*

my·en·ta·sis (migh·en'tuh·sis) *n.* The extension or stretching of a muscle.

my·en·ter·ic (migh''en·terr'ick) *adj.* Pertaining to the muscular coat of the intestine.

myenteric plexus. A visceral nerve plexus situated between the circular and longitudinal muscle layers of the digestive tube. Syn. *Auerbach's plexus.*

my·en·ter·on (migh·en'tur·on) *n.* The muscular coat of the intestine.

my·es·the·sia (migh''es·theezh'uh, ·theez'ee·uh) *n.* The perception or sensibility of impressions coming from the muscles, as of touch, contraction, or direction of movement.

my·ia·sis (migh·eye′uh·sis) *n.* Invasion or infection of a body area or cavity by the larvae of flies.

myl-, mylo- A combining form meaning *molar.*

Myleran. Trademark for busulfan, an antineoplastic drug.

mylo-. See *myl-.*

my·lo·hy·oid (migh″lo·high′oid) *adj.* Pertaining to the region of the lower molar teeth and the hyoid bone.

myo-. See *my-.*

myo·ar·chi·tec·ton·ic (migh″o·ahr″ki·teck·ton′ick) *adj.* Pertaining to the structure and arrangement of muscle fibers.

myo·blast (migh′o·blast) *n.* A cell which develops into a muscle fiber. —**myo·blas·tic** (migh″o·blas′tick) *adj.*

myo·blas·to·ma (migh″o·blas·to′muh) *n.* GRANULAR CELL MYOBLASTOMA.

myo·car·di·al (migh″o·kahr′dee·ul) *adj.* Of or pertaining to the myocardium.

myocardial insufficiency. HEART FAILURE.

myo·car·di·op·a·thy (migh″o·kahr·dee·op′uth·ee) *n.* Any disease of the myocardium; cardiomyopathy.

myo·car·di·tis (migh″o·kahr·dye′tis) *n.* Inflammation of the myocardium.

myo·car·di·um (migh″o·kahr′dee·um) *n.,* pl. **myocar·dia** (·dee·uh) The muscular tissue of the heart.

myo·car·do·sis (migh″o·kahr·do′sis) *n.* 1. Any noninflammatory disease of the myocardium. 2. MYOCARDIOPATHY; CARDIOMYOPATHY.

Myochrysine. Trademark for gold sodium thiomalate, an antirheumatic drug.

myo·clo·nia (migh″o·klo′nee·uh) *n.* MYOCLONUS.

myo·clon·ic (migh″o·klon′ick) *adj.* Pertaining to or characterized by myoclonus.

myoclonic epilepsy. The association of myoclonus with epilepsy. Included under this title are several seizure states, some relatively benign (idiopathic epilepsy) and others which are associated with intellectual deterioration and a variety of abnormalities of the nervous system.

myoclonic status. A state lasting on the order of an hour or more during which myoclonic seizures occur continually.

myo·clo·nus (migh″o·klo′nus, migh·ock′luh·nus) *n.* Exceedingly abrupt, shocklike contractions of muscles, irregular in rhythm and amplitude and usually asynchronous or asymmetrical in distribution.

myo·cyte (migh′o·site) *n.* A muscle cell.

myo·cy·tol·y·sis (migh″o·sigh·tol′i·sis) *n.* 1. Destruction of muscle cells. 2. Disappearance of cardiac muscle cells without cellular reaction to the loss.

myo·dys·to·nia (migh″o·dis·to′nee·uh) *n.* Any abnormal condition of muscle tone.

myo·dys·tro·phy (migh″o·dis′truh·fee) *n.* Degeneration of muscles.

myo·ede·ma (migh″o·e·dee′muh) *n.* Edema of a muscle.

myo·elas·tic (migh″o·e·las′tick) *adj.* Pertaining to the layer of intimately interrelated smooth muscle cells and elastic fibers in bronchi and bronchioles.

myo·ep·i·the·li·al (migh″o·ep·i·theel′ee·ul) *adj.* Of or pertaining to myoepithelium.

myo·ep·i·the·li·o·ma (my″o·ep·i·theel″ee·o′muh) *n.* A slow-growing sweat-gland tumor appearing as a solitary or rarely multiple, firm, well-circumscribed intracutaneous nodule usually less than 2 cm in diameter. The two types of cells found are the secretory and the myoepithelial cells.

myo·ep·i·the·li·um (my″o·ep·i·theel′ee·um) *n.* Collectively, the smooth muscle cells of ectodermal origin.

myo·fa·cial (migh″o·fay′shul) *adj.* Pertaining to the face and related muscles.

myofacial pain-dysfunction syndrome. A unilateral facial pain aggravated by mandibular movement and associated with tenderness of the head and neck muscles and sometimes of the temporomandibular joint on the affected side. The symptoms are presumably related to dysfunction of the temporomandibular joint.

myo·fas·ci·al (migh″o·fash′ee·ul) *adj.* Pertaining to the fasciae of muscles, as myofascial inflammation.

myo·fas·ci·tis (migh″o·fa·sigh′tis) *n.* Musculoskeletal pain of obscure nature; probably due to inflammation of muscle and fascia at its insertion on bone.

myo·fi·ber (migh′o·figh″bur) *n.* MYOFIBRIL.

myo·fi·bril (migh″o·figh′bril, ·fib′ril) *n.* A fibril found in the cytoplasm of muscle. —**myo·fi·bril·lar** (migh″o·figh′bril·ur) *adj.*

myo·fi·bro·ma (migh″o·figh·bro′muh) *n.* LEIOMYOMA.

myo·fi·bro·sar·co·ma (migh″o·figh″bro·sahr·ko′muh) *n.* Leiomyosarcoma with rich fibromatous component.

myo·fi·bro·si·tis (migh″o·figh″bro·sigh′tis) *n.* MYOSITIS.

myo·fil·a·ment (migh″o·fil′uh·munt) *n.* One of the filaments constituting the fine structure of a myofibril, seen by means of the electron microscope.

myo·ge·lo·sis (migh″o·je·lo′sis) *n.* A hardened region in a muscle; specifically, hard nodules localized at the origin of a muscle.

myo·gen (migh′o·jen) *n.* Collectively, the water-soluble proteins of muscle, largely located in the sarcoplasm and consisting of various enzymes.

myo·gen·ic (migh″o·jen′ick) *adj.* 1. Of muscular origin, as myogenic contraction vs. in contrast to neurogenic contraction. 2. Giving rise to muscle.

my·og·e·nous (migh·oj′e·nus) *adj.* MYOGENIC (1).

myo·glo·bin (migh′o·glo″bin) *n.* Myohemoglobin, muscle hemoglobin; the form of hemoglobin occurring in red or mixed muscle fibers. It differs somewhat from blood hemoglobin in showing a displacement of the spectral absorption bands toward the red, a higher oxygen affinity, and a hyperbolic dissociation curve, a smaller Bohr effect, a lower affinity for carbon monoxide, and a lower molecular weight. It serves as a short-time oxygen store, carrying the muscle from one contraction to the next.

myo·glo·bin·uria (migh″o·glo′bi·new′ree·uh) *n.* The presence of free myoglobin in the urine, seen in Haff disease, trauma, ischemia, and other primary lesions of striated muscle which result in muscle necrosis.

myo·gram (migh′o·gram) *n.* The recording made by a myograph.

myo·graph (migh′o·graf) *n.* An instrument for recording muscular contractions. —**myo·graph·ic** (migh″o·graf′ick) *adj.*

myo·he·mo·glo·bin (migh″o·hee′muh·glo″bin) *n.* MYOGLOBIN.

my·oid (migh′oid) *adj.* Musclelike; resembling muscle.

myoid cells. Polygonal cells, cytologically similar to smooth muscle cells, found in the seminiferous tubules of laboratory rodents; believed to be responsible for the rhythmic contractions observed in the seminiferous tubules of these species.

myo·ki·nase (migh″o·kigh′nace, ·naze, ·kin′ace, migh·ock′i·nace) *n.* An enzyme present in muscle tissue which enables myosin to bring about the reaction by which two moles of adenosine diphosphate yield one mole of adenylic acid and one mole of adenosine triphosphate. It also facilitates the action of hexokinase in catalyzing the reaction between glucose or fructose and adenosine triphosphate by which glucose 6-phosphate or fructose 6-phosphate and adenosine diphosphate are formed.

myo·ki·ne·si·og·ra·phy (migh″o·ki·nee″zee·og′ruh·fee) *n.* 1. A method of recording graphically the movement of muscle either in vivo or in vitro. 2. Specifically, a method for studying muscle action during walking; it reveals disturbances in neuromuscular activity and coordination.

myo·ky·mia (migh″o·kigh′mee·uh, ·kim′ee·uh) *n.* A state of almost continuous fasciculations, which impart a rippling appearance to the overlying skin. It may be transitory or persistent and limited to one muscle or universal, and may be associated with muscle cramps and myotonic-like contractions. Syn. *live flesh, myoclonia fibrillaris multiplex.*

myo·li·po·ma (migh″o·li·po′muh) *n.* A benign tumor whose parenchyma is composed of adipose and smooth muscle tissue.

my·ol·o·gy (migh·ol′uh·jee) *n.* The science of the nature, structure, functions, and diseases of muscles.

my·o·ma (migh·o′muh) *n.* 1. A leiomyoma of the uterus. 2. Any tumor derived from muscle. —**my·om·a·tous** (migh·om′uh·tus) *adj.*

myo·ma·la·cia (migh″o·ma·lay′shee·uh) *n.* Degeneration, with softening, of muscle tissue.

myomalacia cor·dis (kor′dis) Softening of a portion of the heart muscle, usually resulting from myocardial infarction.

my·o·ma·to·sis (migh·o″muh·to′sis) *n.* The presence of multiple leiomyomas, usually uterine.

my·o·mec·to·my (migh″o·meck′tuh·mee) *n.* Excision of a uterine or other myoma.

myo·me·tri·tis (migh″o·me·trye′tis) *n.* Inflammation of the uterine muscular tissue.

myo·me·tri·um (migh″o·mee′tree·um) *n.* The uterine muscular structure. —**myometri·al** (·ul) *adj.*

myo·neu·ral (migh″o·new′rul) *adj.* 1. Pertaining to both muscle and nerve. 2. Pertaining to nerve endings in muscle tissue.

myoneural junction. The point of junction of a motor nerve with the muscle which it innervates. Syn. *neuromuscular junction.*

myo·pal·mus (migh″o·pal′mus) *n.* Twitching of the muscles.

myo·pa·ral·y·sis (migh″o·puh·ral′i·sis) *n.* Paralysis of a muscle or muscles.

myo·pa·re·sis (migh″o·pa·ree′sis, ·păr′e·sis) *n.* Slight paralysis of muscle.

myo·path·ic (migh″o·path′ick) *adj.* Of or pertaining to disease of the muscles.

myopathic facies. A peculiar facial appearance in patients with myopathies, especially myotonic dystrophy. The brow shows no wrinkling, the face is expressionless or glum, the cheeks are sunken, the lower lip droops. Enophthalmos may be present.

myopathic nystagmus. Nystagmus due to defects or disease of one or more of the extraocular muscles; may be congenital or acquired, as in myasthenia gravis.

my·op·a·thy (migh·op′uth·ee) *n.* Any disease of the muscles.

my·ope (migh′ope) *n.* A person affected with myopia.

myo·peri·car·di·tis (migh″o·perr″i·kahr·dye′tis) *n.* A combination of pericarditis and myocarditis.

my·o·pia (migh·o′pee·uh) *n.* Nearsightedness; an optical defect, usually due to too great length of the anteroposterior diameter of the globe, whereby the focal image is formed in front of the retina. Abbreviated, my. —**my·op·ic** (migh·op′ick, ·o′pick) *adj.*

myo·plas·ty (migh′o·plas·tee) *n.* Plastic surgery on a muscle or group of muscles.

my·o·por·tho·sis (migh″o·por·tho′sis) *n.* The correction of myopia.

my·or·rha·phy (migh·or′uh·fee) *n.* Suture of a muscle.

myo·sar·co·ma (migh″o·sahr·ko′muh) *n.* A sarcoma derived from muscle.

myo·scle·ro·sis (migh″o·skle·ro′sis) *n.* FIBROUS MYOSITIS.

my·o·sin (migh·o′sin, migh′uh·sin) *n.* One of the principal contractile proteins occurring in muscle, comprising up to one-half of the total muscle protein. It combines reversibly with actin to form actomyosin, and as such is responsible for the birefringent, contractile, and elastic properties of muscle. It is closely associated with the enzyme adenosine triphosphatase (ATPase). Its coagulation with ATP after death is the cause of rigor mortis.

my·o·si·tis (migh″o·sigh′tis) *n.* Inflammation of muscle, usually voluntary muscle. —**myo·sit·ic** (·sit′ick) *adj.*

myositis os·sif·i·cans (os·if′i·kanz) Myositis with formation of bone.

myo·stat·ic (migh″o·stat′ick) *adj.* Pertaining to a muscle of fixed length in relaxation, as in myostatic contracture.

myo·su·ture (migh'o·sue"chur) *n.* Suture of a muscle; myorrhaphy.

myo·syn·o·vi·tis (migh"o·sin'o·vye'tis) *n.* Inflammation of synovial membranes and surrounding musculature.

myo·tac·tic (migh"o·tack'tick) *adj.* Pertaining to the sense of touch of muscle.

my·o·ta·sis (migh·ot'uh·sis) *n.* Stretching of a muscle.

myo·tat·ic (migh"o·tat'ick) *adj.* Of or pertaining to myotasis.

myo·ten·di·nous (migh"o·ten'di·nus) *adj.* Pertaining to both muscle and tendon, especially the junction of the two.

myo·ten·o·si·tis (migh"o·ten"o·sigh'tis) *n.* Inflammation of a muscle and its tendon.

myo·te·not·o·my (migh"o·te·not'um·ee) *n.* Surgical division of muscles and tendons.

myo·tome (migh'o·tome) *n.* 1. An instrument for performing myotomy. 2. The part of a somite that differentiates into skeletal muscle.

my·ot·o·my (migh·ot'uh·mee) *n.* Division or cutting (dissection) of a muscle, particularly through its belly.

myo·to·nia (migh"o·to'nee·uh) *n.* Continued contraction of muscle, despite attempts at relaxation, characteristic of certain diseases such as myotonia congenita, myotonic dystrophy, and paramyotonia of von Eulenberg.

myotonia ac·qui·si·ta (ack"wi·sigh'tuh, a·kwiz'i·tuh). A form of myotonia which does not become evident until adult years and which may be an expression of a rare, recessive form of congenital myotonia, of hypothyroidism, or of myotonic dystrophy. Syn. *myotonia tarda.*

myotonia con·gen·i·ta (kon·jen'i·tuh). A familial disorder of muscle, usually inherited as an autosomal dominant trait, and rarely as a recessive trait, with onset in infancy or childhood, characterized by lack of relaxation of skeletal muscles after initial forceful contraction, often aggravated by cold or emotional stress, and hypertrophy of skeletal muscles. Syn. *Thomsen's disease.*

myotonia par·a·dox·i·ca (păr·uh·dock'si·kuh). A form of myotonia in which the first voluntary movements in a series are less likely to be followed by myotonic spasm than later ones.

myo·ton·ic (migh"o·ton'ick) *adj.* Of or characterized by myotonia.

myotonic dystrophy. A hereditary disease, transmitted as an autosomal dominant, characterized by lack of normal relaxation of muscles after contraction, slowly progressive muscular weakness and atrophy, especially of the face, neck, and distal muscles of the limbs, cataract formation, early baldness, gonadal atrophy, abnormal glucose tolerance curve, and frequently mental deficiency.

myotonic reaction. *In electromyography,* the high frequency, repetitive discharges which wax and wane in amplitude and frequency, producing a "dive-bomber" sound on the audiomonitor. This electrical picture is also seen following voluntary contraction or electrical stimulation of the muscle via its motor nerve.

my·ot·o·nus (migh·ot'uh·nus) *n.* Muscle tone; the slight resistance that normal muscle offers to passive movement. This state has no electrical counterpart.

my·ot·ro·phy (migh·ot'ruh·fee) *n.* Nutrition of muscle.

myr·ia·gram (mirr'ee·uh·gram) *n.* Ten thousand grams.

myr·ia·li·ter (mirr'ee·uh·lee"tur) *n.* Ten thousand liters.

myr·in·ga (mi·ring'guh) *n.* TYMPANIC MEMBRANE.

myr·in·gec·to·my (mirr"in·jeck'tuh·mee) *n.* MYRINGODECTOMY.

myr·in·go·my·co·sis (mi·ring"go·migh·ko'sis) *n.* An infection of the eardrum due to fungi, usually as the result of spread from the external auditory canal; an otomycosis.

myr·in·go·plas·ty (mi·ring'go·plas"tee) *n.* A plastic operation to close perforations in the tympanic membrane. —**myr·in·go·plast·ic** (mi·ring"go·plas'tick) *adj.*

myr·in·go·tome (mi·ring'go·tome) *n.* An instrument used in incising tympanic membrane.

myr·in·got·o·my (mirr"in·got'uh·mee) *n.* Incision of the tympanic membrane for the drainage of fluid or pus in the treatment of otitis media. Syn. *paracentesis of the tympanum, tympanotomy.*

my·ris·tic acid (mi·ris'tick, migh·ris'tick). Tetradecanoic acid, $CH_3(CH_2)_{12}COOH$, a fatty acid occurring in the glycerides of many fats.

myrrh (mur) *n.* A gum resin obtained from *Commiphora molmol, C. abyssinica,* or other species of *Commiphora.* Contains a volatile oil, a resin myrrhin, and a gum. Has been used as a local protective agent.

Mysoline. Trademark for primidone, an anticonvulsant drug used for control of generalized and psychomotor seizures.

my·so·pho·bia (migh"so·fo'bee·uh) *n.* Abnormal dread of contamination or dirt.

my·ta·cism (migh'tuh·siz·um) *n.* Excessive or faulty use of the sound of *m.* and its substitution for other sounds.

mytho·ma·nia (mith"o·may'nee·uh) *n.* A pathologic tendency to lie or to exaggerate; a condition seen in certain psychiatric patients.

mytho·pho·bia (mith"o·fo'bee·uh) *n.* A morbid dread of stating what is not absolutely correct.

myt·i·lo·tox·in (mit"i·lo·tock'sin) *n.* A neurotoxic principle found in certain mussels.

myt·i·lo·tox·ism (mit"i·lo·tock'siz·um) *n.* Poisoning from eating mussels with paralysis of the central and peripheral nervous system.

myx-, myxo- A combining form meaning (a) *mucus, mucous;* (b) *mucin, mucinous.*

myx·ad·e·ni·tis (mick·sad"'e·nigh'tis) *n.* Inflammation of a mucous gland.

myx·ede·ma (mick"se·dee'muh) *n.* A condition due to inadequacy of thyroid hormone, characterized by hypometabolism, cold sensitivity, dry, coarse skin, hair loss, mental dullness, anemia, and slowed reflexes. —**myxedematous** (·tus) *adj.*

myx·id·i·o·cy (mick·sid'ee·uh·see) *n.* CRETINISM.

myxo·ad·e·no·ma (mick"so·ad·e·no'muh) *n.* An adenoma of a mucous gland.

myxo·chon·dro·fi·bro·sar·co·ma (mick"so·kon"dro·figh"bro·sahr·ko'muh) *n.* A sarcoma whose parenchyma consists of anaplastic myxoid, chondroid, and fibrous elements.

myxo·chon·dro·ma (mick″so·kon·dro′muh) *n.* A benign tumor whose parenchymal cells are myxoid and chondroid.

myxo·chon·dro·sar·co·ma (mick″so·kon″dro·sahr·ko′muh) *n.* CHONDROMYXOSARCOMA.

myxo·cyte (mick′so·site) *n.* A large cell, polyhedral or stellate, found in mucous tissue.

myxo·fi·bro·ma (mick″so·figh·bro′muh) *n.* A benign fibroma with a myxomatous component.

myxo·fi·bro·sar·co·ma (mick″so·figh″bro·sahr·ko′muh) *n.* A malignant tumor composed of myxosarcomatous and fibrosarcomatous elements.

myxo·gli·o·ma (mick″so·glye·o′muh) *n.* A gelatinous form of glioma.

myx·oid (mick′soid) *adj.* Like mucus; MUCOID.

myxo·li·po·ma (mick″so·li·po′muh) *n.* 1. A benign tumor whose parenchyma contains myxoid and adipose tissue cells. 2. LIPOSARCOMA.

myxo·lipo·sar·co·ma (mick″so·lip″o·sahr·ko′muh) *n.* A sarcoma whose parenchyma is composed of anaplastic myxoid and adipose tissue cells.

myx·o·ma (mick·so′muh) *n.* A benign tumor whose parenchyma is composed of mucinous connective tissue.

myx·o·ma·to·sis (mick″so·muh·to′sis) *n.* 1. A viral disease of rabbits producing fever, myxomatous skin masses, and mucoid swelling of the mucous membranes. 2. The presence of numerous myxomas.

myx·om·a·tous (mick·som′uh·tus) *adj.* Like or pertaining to myxomas.

Myxo·my·ce·tes (mick″so·migh·see′teez) *n.pl.* A class of fungi, known as the slime molds, none of which is pathogenic to man; resemble protozoa in some respects.

myxo·neu·ro·ma (mick″so·new·ro′muh) *n.* A neuroma, or more often a neurofibroma, with a myxomatous component, occurring in peripheral nerves.

myx·or·rhea (mick″so·ree′uh) *n.* A copious mucous discharge.

myxo·sar·co·ma (mick″so·sahr·ko′muh) *n.* A sarcoma whose parenchyma is composed of anaplastic myxoid cells. —**myxosar·com·a·tous** (·kom′uh·tus, ·ko′muh·tus) *adj.*

myxo·vi·rus (mick″so·vye′rus) *n.* A member of a group of ether-sensitive, hemagglutinating RNA viruses, including the influenza, mumps, Newcastle, and parainfluenza viruses; so named because of a special affinity for mucins.

N Symbol for nitrogen.

N, _N_ Abbreviation for _normal (3)._

n 1. Symbol for a unit of neutron dosage corresponding to the roentgen. 2. Symbol for refractive index. 3. Symbol for the prefix _nano-._

N- In chemistry, symbol for _normal._

NA Abbreviation for _Nomina Anatomica._

N. A. Abbreviation for _numerical aperture._

Na Symbol for sodium.

Na·bo·thi·an cyst (na·bo′thee·un) Cystic distention of the mucous (Nabothian) glands of the uterine cervix.

Nabothian follicle. NABOTHIAN CYST.

Nabothian glands Mucous glands of the cervix of the uterus.

na·cre·ous (nay′kree·us, nack′ree·us) _adj._ Resembling nacre or mother-of-pearl.

N. A. D. No appreciable disease.

NAD Abbreviation for _nicotinamide adenine dinucleotide._

NADP Abbreviation for _nicotinamide adenine dinucleotide phosphate._

NADP⁺ Symbol for the oxidized form of nicotinamide adenine dinucleotide phosphate.

Nae·ge·le pelvis (ney′ge·leʰ) An obliquely contracted pelvis with ankylosis of one sacroiliac synchondrosis, underdevelopment of the associated sacral ala, and other distorting defects producing an obliquely directed conjugata vera.

Nae·ge·li type leukemia (ney′ge·lee) A variety of monocytic leukemia in which the cells bear certain resemblances to the granulocytic series.

Naff·zig·er's operation Excision of the superior and lateral walls of the orbit for the relief of progressive exophthalmos.

Naffziger's test or **sign** 1. Pressure on the jugular veins increases the intraspinal tension which increases the pain in cases of herniated disk. 2. Pressure on the anterior scalene muscles at the root of the neck causes tingling in the hand in the scalenus anterior syndrome.

nail, _n._ 1. The horny structure covering the dorsal aspect of the terminal phalanx of each finger and toe. It consists of intimately united, horny epithelial cells probably representing the stratum corneum of the epidermis. Comb. form onych(o)-. 2. A metallic (usually stainless steel or vitallium) elongated rod with one sharp and one blunt end, used in surgery to anchor bone fragments. Syn. _pin._

nail bed. Vascular tissue, corresponding to the corium and the germinative layer of the skin, on which a nail rests.

nail biting. A nervous habit or neurotic reaction chiefly in children and adolescents, manifested by the habit of biting the fingernails down to the quick.

nail fold. The fold of skin bounding the sides and proximal portion of a nail.

nail-patella syndrome. A genetic disorder involving tissues of both ectodermal and mesodermal origin, characterized by defects in the nails ranging from complete anonychia to longitudinal ridging, hypoplastic or absent patellae, abnormalities of the elbows, iliac horns and a wide spectrum of other bone, joint, skin, eye, and renal abnormalities. Inherited as an autosomal dominant. Syn. _Fong's lesion._

nal·i·dix·ic acid (nal′′i·dick′sick). 1-Ethyl-1,4-dihydro-7-methyl-4-oxo-1, 8-naphthyridine-3-carboxylic acid, $C_{12}H_{12}N_2O_3$, an antibacterial agent used clinically for treatment of urinary tract infections caused by gram-negative organisms.

nal·or·phine (nal′ur·feen, nal·or′feen) _n._ N-Allylmorphine, $C_{19}H_{21}NO_3$, a derivative of morphine used, as the hydrochloride salt, principally to counteract severe respiratory depression from overdosage with narcotics and to diagnose addiction to narcotics.

na·nism (nay′niz·um, nan′iz·um) _n._ Abnormal smallness from arrested development; DWARFISM.

nano- A combining form meaning (a) _dwarfed_ or _undersized;_ (b) _the one-billionth_ (10^{-9}) _part of_ the unit adjoined. Symbol, n

na·no·ceph·a·lus (nay′′no·sef′ul·us, nan′′o·) _n._ A fetus with a dwarfed head.

na·no·gram (nay′no·gram) _n._ One billionth

(10^{-9}) of a gram. Abbreviated, ng Syn. *millimicrogram.*

na·noid (nay'noid, nan'oid) *adj.* Dwarflike.

na·nom·e·lus (nay-nom'e-lus, nan-) *n.* An individual characterized by undersized limbs.

na·no·me·ter (nay'no-mee-tur) *n.* A unit of length equal to one billionth (10^{-9}) of a meter, or to 10 angstroms; the one thousandth part of a micrometer. Abbreviated, nm

na·no·sec·ond (nay'no-seck''und) *n.* One billionth (10^{-9}) of a second. Syn. *millimicrosecond.*

na·no·so·ma (nay''no-so'muh, nan''o-) *n.* DWARFISM.

na·no·so·mus (nay''no-so'mus, nan''o-) *n.* An individual with a dwarfed body.

na·nus (nay'nus, nan'us) *n.* DWARF (1). —**nanous,** *adj.*

na·palm (nay'pahm, -pahlm) *n.* An aluminum soap, prepared from naphthenic acids and the fatty acids of coconut oil, used for producing gels of gasoline for incendiary munitions.

nape, *n.* The back of the neck; NUCHA.

na·pex (nay'pecks) *n.* That portion of the scalp just below the occipital protuberance.

na·phaz·o·line (nuh-faz'o-leen, naf-az'o-leen) *n.* 2-(1-Naphthylmethyl)-2-imidazoline, $C_{14}H_{14}N_2$, a sympathomimetic drug; used, as the hydrochloride salt, locally on nasal or ocular mucous membranes for its vasoconstrictor action.

naphth-, naphtho-. A combining form meaning *pertaining to naphthalene or its ring structure.*

naph·tha (naf'thuh) *n.* 1. Formerly, any strong-smelling, inflammable, volatile liquid. 2. A mixture of low-boiling hydrocarbons distilled from petroleum and bituminous shale.

naph·tha·lene (naf'thuh-leen) *n.* The hydrocarbon, $C_{10}H_8$, a constituent of coal tar; formerly used locally as an antiseptic. Used as a moth repellent and insecticide.

naph·tho·qui·none (naf''tho-kwi-nohn') *n.* Either of two compounds, $C_{10}H_6O_2$, derived from naphthalene: 1,4-naphthoquinone (α-naphthoquinone), derivatives of which have vitamin-K activity, or 1,2-naphthoquinone (β-naphthoquinone), used as a reagent.

na·pi·form (nay'pi-form, nap'i-) *adj.* Turnip-shaped.

NAPNAP National Association of Pediatric Nurse Associates and Practitioners.

nar·cis·sism (nahr-sis'iz-um, nahr'si-siz-um) *n. In psychoanalysis,* fixation of the libido upon one's self. Some degree of self-love is considered healthy; excessive self-love, however, interferes in one's relations with others. —**nar·cis·sis·tic** (nahr''si-sis'tick) *adj.;* **nar·cis·sist** (nahr-sis'ist, nahr'si-sist) *n.*

nar·co·anal·y·sis (nahr''ko-uh-nal'uh-sis) *n.* The induction of a quickly reversible sleep by intravenous injections of amobarbital or thiopental sodium during which a trained interrogator elicits memories and feelings not expressed in the patient's wakeful state because of either willful or unconscious resistance; used in the treatment of neuroses and psychophysiologic disorders and occasionally in the investigation of suspected criminals.

nar·co·lep·sy (nahr'ko-lep''see) *n.* A disorder of sleep mechanism, closely related if not identical with REM sleep, characterized by (1) uncontrollable attacks of drowsiness or sleep in the daytime, (2) cataplectic attacks of loss of muscular power, occurring without warning or during some emotional experience, (3) sleep paralysis, and (4) vivid nocturnal or hypnagogic hallucinations. —**nar·co·lep·tic** (nahr''ko-lep'tick) *adj.*

nar·co·ma (nahr-ko'muh) *n.* Stupor from the use of a narcotic. —**narcoma·tous** (-tus) *adj.*

nar·co·ma·nia (nahr''ko-may'nee-uh) *n.* A pathologic craving for narcotics (medicinal or psychologic). —**narcoma·ni·ac** (-ni·ack) *n.*

nar·co·sis (nahr-ko'sis) *n.* A state of profound stupor, unconsciousness, or arrested activity produced by drugs. Adj. & n. *narcotic.*

narcosis therapy. Prolonged sleep as a treatment for certain types of mental disorders, usually induced by drugs such as barbiturates or phenothiazines. Syn. *sleep therapy.*

nar·co·syn·the·sis (nahr''ko-sin'thi-sis) *n.* Psychotherapeutic treatment originally employed in acute combat cases under partial anesthesia as with amobarbital sodium or thiopental sodium, in which abreaction plays an important role in the therapeutic results.

nar·co·ther·a·py (nahr''ko-therr'up-ee) *n.* NARCOANALYSIS.

nar·cot·ic (nahr-kot'ick) *adj.* & *n.* 1. Pertaining to or producing narcosis. 2. A drug that in therapeutic doses diminishes sensibility, relieves pain, and produces sleep, but in large doses causes stupor, coma, or convulsions. 3. Any drug, with properties similar to morphine, identified as a narcotic drug by federal law. 4. An individual addicted to the use of narcotics.

nar·co·tism (nahr'kuh-tiz-um) *n.* 1. Narcotic poisoning. 2. Narcotic addiction.

nar·co·tize (nahr'kuh-tize) *v.* To put under the influence of a narcotic; to render unconscious through a narcotic.

nares [NA]. NOSTRILS; plural of *naris.*

narrow-angle glaucoma. Increased intraocular tension due to a block of the angle of the anterior chamber from contact of the iris with the trabecula; begins acutely with extreme eye pain, hyperemia, and sudden visual loss and may resolve spontaneously, medically, or surgically; however, it may become chronic due to repeated acute attacks with the formation of synechial and gradual permanent closure of the angle. May be primary or secondary.

nas-, naso-. A combining form meaning *nose, nasal.*

na·sal (nay'zul) *adj.* & *n.* 1. Of or pertaining to the nose. 2. With reference to the eye and its appendages: medial; situated on the side nearer the nose.

nasal area. The ventrolateral thickened ectoderm of the frontonasal process from which the olfactory placode arises.

nasal canal. 1. NASOLACRIMAL CANAL. 2. An occasional canal found in the posterior portion of the nasal bone; it gives passage to nasal nerves.

nasal cavity. One of the pair of cavities between the anterior nares and nasopharynx.

nasal concha. Any of the three or four medial projections of thin bone from the lateral wall of the nasal cavity, covered by mucous membrane and designated according to position as supreme, superior, middle, and inferior. The supreme nasal concha is inconstant and, when present, is situated above the superior nasal concha.

nasal cycle. Alternating congestion and decongestion of the nasal airways, first one side becoming hyperemic and showing increasing mucosal gland secretion, then the other.

nasal field. 1. NASAL AREA. 2. The medial half of the field of vision, as contrasted with the temporal field.

nasal fossa. 1. OLFACTORY PIT. 2. NASAL CAVITY.

nasal glioma. Heterotopic glial tissue in the nose.

nasal hemianopsia. Loss of the nasal half of the field of vision.

nasal polyp. 1. A sessile or pedunculated polypoid mass of edematous connective tissue covered by epithelium and including glands and inflammatory exudate, projecting from the nasal mucosa into the nasal cavity. 2. Any polypoid tumor in the nasal cavity.

nasal reflex. Sneezing induced by stimulation of the nasal mucosa.

nasal septum. The septum between the two nasal cavities.

nasal voice. A peculiar, muffled timbre of the voice, especially marked in cases of perforated palate.

nas·cent (nas'unt, nay'sunt) adj. 1. Characterizing an atom or simple compound at the moment of its liberation from chemical combination, when it may have greater activity than in its usual state. 2. Coming into being.

na·sio·al·ve·o·lar (nay"zee·o·al·vee'ul·ur) adj. Pertaining to, or connecting, the nasion and the alveolar point.

na·si·on (nay'zee·on, nay'see·on) n. In craniometry, the point where the sagittal plane intersects the frontonasal suture.

na·si·tis (nay·zigh'tis, ·sigh'tis) n. RHINITIS.

naso-. See nas-.

na·so·al·ve·o·lar (nay"zo·al·vee'uh·lur) adj. Pertaining to the nose and a tooth socket.

na·so·an·tral (nay"zo·an'trul) adj. Pertaining to the nose and the maxillary sinus (antrum).

na·so·cil·i·ary (nay"zo·sil'ee·err·ee) adj. Pertaining to a nerve distributed to the nose, the ethmoid sinuses, and the eyeball.

na·so·fa·cial (nay"zo·fay'shul) adj. Pertaining to the nose and the face.

na·so·fron·tal (nay"zo·frun'tul, ·fron'tul) adj. Pertaining to the nasal and the frontal bones.

nasofrontal duct. The duct between the frontal sinus and the middle meatus of the nose. Syn. frontonasal duct.

na·so·gas·tric (nay"zo·gas'trick) adj. Pertaining to the nose and the stomach; used to describe tubes inserted through the nose to end in the stomach.

na·so·la·bi·al (nay"zo·lay'bee·ul) adj. Pertaining to the nose and lip.

na·so·lac·ri·mal (nay"zo·lack'ri·mul) adj. Pertaining to the nose and the lacrimal apparatus.

nasolacrimal canal. The bony canal that lodges the nasolacrimal duct.

nasolacrimal duct. The membranous duct lodged within the nasolacrimal canal; it gives passage to the tears from the lacrimal sac to the inferior meatus of the nose.

na·so·max·il·lary (nay"zo·mack'sil·err·ee) adj. Pertaining to the nasal and maxillary bones.

na·so·men·tal (nay"zo·men'tul) adj. Pertaining to the nose and the chin.

na·so·oc·cip·i·tal (nay"zo·ock·sip'i·tul) adj. Pertaining to the nose and the occiput.

na·so·oral (nay"zo·or'ul) adj. Pertaining to the nose and the mouth.

na·so·or·bit·al (nay"zo·or'bi·tul) adj. Pertaining to the nose and the orbit.

na·so·pal·a·tine (nay"zo·pal'uh·tine, ·tin) adj. Pertaining to both the nose and the palate.

na·so·pal·pe·bral (nay"zo·pal'pe·brul) adj. Pertaining to the nose and the eyelids.

na·so·pha·ryn·ge·al (nay"zo·fa·rin'jee·ul) adj. Of or pertaining to the nasopharynx.

na·so·phar·yn·gi·tis (nay"zo·făr"in·jye'tis) n. Inflammation of the nasal passages and pharynx.

na·so·pha·ryn·go·scope (nay"zo·fa·ring'go·skope) n. An electrically lighted instrument for inspecting the nasopharynx.

na·so·phar·yn·gos·co·py (nay"zo·făr"ing·gos'kup·ee) n. Inspection of the nasopharynx.

na·so·phar·ynx (nay"zo·făr'inks) n. The space behind the choanae and above a horizontal plane through the lower margin of the palate. Syn. epipharynx. —**nasopha·ryn·ge·al** (·fa·rin'jee·ul) adj.

na·so·scope (nay'zuh·skope) n. An instrument for examining the nasal cavity.

na·sos·co·py (nay·zos'kup·ee) n. Inspection of the nasal cavity.

na·so·spi·na·le (nay"zo·spye·nay'lee, ·nah'lee) n. In craniometry, a point located in the sagittal plane where it meets a line joining the lowest points on the nasal margins. If this falls within the substance of the anterior nasal spine, a point on the left side wall of the nasal spine is used for taking measurements.

na·so·tra·che·al (nay"zo·tray'kee·ul) adj. Pertaining to the nasal cavity and the trachea.

nasotracheal tube. A tube or catheter inserted into the trachea by way of the nasal cavity and pharynx.

na·so·tur·bi·nal (nay"zo·tur'bi·nul) n. The ridge-like elevation midway between the anterior extremity of the middle turbinate and the roof of the nose in most lower mammals. In man its rudimentary homologue is the agger nasi.

na·sus (nay'sus, ·zus) n., genit. **na·si** (nay'zye) [NA]. NOSE.

¹na·tal (nay'tul) adj. Of or pertaining to birth.

²natal, adj. Pertaining to the nates or buttocks; GLUTEAL.

na·tal·i·ty (nuh·tal'i·tee, nay·) n. 1. In medical statistics, birth rate. 2. Birth.

na·tant (nay'tunt) adj. Swimming or floating on the surface of a liquid.

na·tes (nay'teez) n.pl. BUTTOCKS.

National Formulary. A formulary previously

published by the American Pharmaceutical Association, now the property of USPC; it is officially recognized by the Federal Food, Drug, and Cosmetic Act. Abbreviated, NF

National Health Service. In Great Britain, a government agency under the Ministry of Health, charged with providing health services for the entire population, such as hospitalization, preventive medicine, family medical, dental, and nursing services, medicines, and appliances; it is financed by the national government. Abbreviated, N.H.S.

National Institutes of Health. A division of the U. S. Department of Health, Education and Welfare that is devoted to research in public health and the diseases of man. Abbreviated, NIH.

na·tive, adj. 1. Of indigenous origin or growth. 2. Occurring in its natural state; not artificially prepared or altered.

native albumin. Any albumin occurring normally in the tissues.

native immunity. Resistance inherent in the genetic, anatomic, and physiologic attributes of the body, as contrasted with that mediated by operation of specific antibodies or by specific cellular immunity.

native protein. A protein in its original state; a protein which has not been altered in composition or properties.

natr-, natro-. A combining form meaning sodium or natron.

na·tre·mia (na·tree'mee·uh) n. 1. Sodium in the blood. 2. HYPERNATREMIA.

na·tri·um (nay'tree·um) n. SODIUM.

na·tri·ure·sis (nay'tri·yoo·ree'sis) n. The excretion of excessive amounts of sodium in the urine.

na·tri·uret·ic (nay''tree·yoo·ret'ick, nat''ree·) n. & adj. 1. A medicinal agent which inhibits reabsorption of cations, particularly sodium, from urine. 2. Pertaining to, or characterized by, a natriuretic.

na·tron (nay'tron, ·trun, nat'run) n. Native sodium carbonate, $Na_2CO_3 \cdot 10H_2O$.

nat·u·ral, adj. 1. Not abnormal or artificial. 2. Of or pertaining to nature.

natural antibody. An antibody which is not acquired following specific infection or immunization but arises as a result of cross-reacting antigenic stimuli; for example, an isohemagglutinin.

natural childbirth. A form of childbirth in which psychological, physiological, and emotional aspects are emphasized in order to educate the patient for labor and, when possible, to reduce or eliminate the use of drugs; popular term. The expectant mother is prepared for natural childbirth by gaining an understanding of the anatomy and physiology of the labor process and by a regimen of exercises.

natural resistance. NATIVE IMMUNITY.

natural selection. Darwin's theory of evolution, according to which organisms tend to produce progeny far above the means of subsistence; a struggle for existence ensues which results in the survival of those with favorable variations. Since the favorable variations accumulate as

the generations pass, the descendants tend to diverge markedly from their ancestors, and to remain adapted to the conditions under which they live.

na·tur·o·path (nay'chur·o·path) n. A person who professes to heal the sick without drugs or surgery, exclusively by the use of natural remedies such as light, heat, cold, water, and fruits. —**na·tur·op·a·thy** (nay''chur·op'uth·ee) n.

nau·sea (naw'zhuh, ·zee·uh) n. A feeling of discomfort in the region of the stomach, with aversion to food and a tendency to vomit.

nau·se·ant (naw'zee·unt, ·zhee·unt) adj. & n. 1. Producing nausea. 2. Any agent that produces nausea.

nau·se·ate (naw'zee·ate, ·zhee·ate) v. To induce nausea in (someone).

nau·seous (naw'shus, naw'zee·us) adj. Producing nausea.

na·vel (nay'vul) n. UMBILICUS.

na·vic·u·lar (na·vick'yoo·lur) adj. & n. 1. Boat-shaped. 2. A tarsal bone.

navicular abdomen. SCAPHOID ABDOMEN.

navicular cells. In exfoliative cytology, glycogen-filled, boat-shaped squamous epithelial cells prominent in the cervical exfoliated cells of pregnant women.

navicular disease. NAVICULARTHRITIS.

navicular fossa. 1. VESTIBULAR FOSSA OF THE VAGINA. 2. The dilated distal portion of the urethra in the glans penis.

na·vic·u·lar·thri·tis (na·vick''yoo·lahr·thrigh'tis) n. Inflammation of the distal sesamoid bone in the horse; causes chronic lameness due to incomplete extension of the joint. Syn. navicular disease.

na·vic·u·lo·cu·boid (na·vick''yoo·lo·kew'boid) adj. Pertaining to the navicular and cuboid bones, as naviculocuboid ligament.

na·vic·u·lo·cu·ne·i·form (na·vick''yoo·lo·kew-nee'i·form) adj. Pertaining to the navicular and cuneiform bones.

NCA Abbreviation for neurocirculatory asthenia.

NCI National Cancer Institute, one of the National Institutes of Health.

N.D.A. National Dental Association.

Ne Symbol for neon.

ne-, neo- A combining form meaning (a) new, newly formed; (b) phylogenetically recent; (c) young, immature; (d) a new chemical compound related to the one to whose name it is prefixed.

near point. The punctum proximum; the point nearest the eye at which an object can be seen distinctly.

near-sight, n. MYOPIA.

near·sight·ed, adj. Affected with myopia. —**nearsighted·ness,** n.

ne·ar·thro·sis (nee''ahr·thro'sis) n., pl. **nearthroses** (·seez) 1. PSEUDARTHROSIS. 2. An artificial joint constructed surgically in the shaft of a long bone.

neb·u·la (neb'yoo·luh) n., pl. **nebu·lae** (·lee), **nebulas** 1. A faint, grayish opacity of the cornea. 2. A spray; a liquid intended for use in an atomizer.

neb·u·lize (neb'yoo·lize) v. To convert into

spray or vapor. —**neb·u·li·za·tion** (neb″yoo·lye·zay′shun) n.

neb·u·liz·er (neb′yoo·lye″zur) n. ATOMIZER.

Ne·ca·tor (ne·kay′tur) n. A genus of nematode hookworms.

Necator amer·i·ca·nus (uh·merr″i·kay′nus). A species of hookworm widely distributed in tropical America, southern U.S., Africa, southern Asia, Melanesia, and Polynesia; causes necatoriasis.

ne·ca·to·ri·a·sis (ne·kay″tur·eye′uh·sis, nek″uh·to·rye′uh·sis) n. Infection of man with the American hookworm, *Necator americanus*, whose infective larvae enter the skin usually at the interdigital regions and may produce a ground itch and vesicular lesions. The adult parasite is found in the small intestine and during the larval migration to the intestine damage to the lungs is commonly incurred.

neck, n. 1. The constricted portion of the body connecting the head with the trunk. 2. The narrow portion of any structure serving to join its parts. 3. The area of junction of the crown and root of a tooth.

necr-, necro- A combining form meaning *pertaining to death.*

nec·ro·bac·il·lo·sis (neck″ro·bas″i·lo′sis) n. A disease of animals caused by species of *Sphaerophorus.*

nec·ro·bi·o·sis (neck″ro·bye·o′sis) n. Physiologic death of a cell or group of cells, in contrast to necrosis or pathologic death of cells, and to somatic death or death of the entire organism. —**necrobi·ot·ic** (·ot′ick) adj.

necrobiosis li·poi·di·ca (li·poy′di·kuh). A cutaneous disease, characterized by multiple yellow to red plaques generally on the extremities, occurring mostly in women, and in about half of the cases in people with diabetes mellitus. There is connective-tissue necrosis with an accumulation of macrophages containing lipids. Syn. *Oppenheim-Urbach disease, necrobiosis lipoidica diabeticorum.*

necrobiosis lipoidica di·a·bet·i·co·rum (dye″uh·bet·i·ko′rum). NECROBIOSIS LIPOIDICA.

necrobiotic atrophy. Atrophy resulting from slow disintegration and loss of cells by necrobiosis.

nec·ro·cy·to·sis (neck″ro·sigh·to′sis) n. Death of cells.

nec·ro·cy·to·tox·in (neck″ro·sigh″to·tock′sin) n. A toxin produced by the death of cells.

nec·ro·gen·ic (neck″ro·jen′ick) adj. Originating from dead substances.

ne·crol·y·sis (ne·krol′i·sis) n. Dissolution or disintegration of dead tissue. —**nec·ro·lyt·ic** (neck″ro·lit′ick) adj.

nec·ro·ma·nia (neck″ro·may′nee·uh) n. 1. A morbid desire for death. 2. NECROPHILISM.

nec·ro·mi·me·sis (neck″ro·mi·mee′sis, ·migh·mee′sis) n. 1. A delusional state in which the patient believes himself to be dead. 2. Simulation of death by a deluded person.

nec·ro·pha·gic (neck″ro·fay′jick, ·faj′ick) adj. 1. NECROPHAGOUS. 2. Pertaining to the eating of carrion. —**necropha·gia** (·fay′jee·uh, ·fay′juh) n.

ne·croph·a·gous (ne·krof′uh·gus) adj. Eating or subsisting on carrion, or putrid meat.

nec·ro·phile (neck′ro·file) n. A person affected with necrophilism.

nec·ro·phil·ia (neck″ro·fil′ee·uh) n. NECROPHILISM. —**necrophil·ic** (·ick) adj.

ne·croph·i·lism (ne·krof′il·iz·um) n. 1. Unnatural pleasure in dead bodies and in being in their presence. 2. Sexual perversion in which dead bodies are violated; sexual desire for a corpse.

ne·croph·i·lous (ne·krof′il·us) adj. Subsisting on dead matter; said of certain bacteria.

nec·ro·pho·bia (neck″ro·fo′bee·uh) n. 1. Abnormal dread of dead bodies. 2. Thanatophobia; extreme dread of death.

nec·rop·sy (neck′rop·see) n. AUTOPSY.

ne·crose (ne·kroze′, ·kroce′, neck′roze) v. To undergo necrosis or tissue death.

ne·cro·sis (ne·kro′sis) n. The pathologic death of a cell or group of cells in contact with living cells.

ne·crot·ic (ne·krot′ick) adj. Pertaining to, undergoing, or causing necrosis.

necrotic myelitis or **myelopathy.** NECROTIZING MYELITIS.

nec·ro·tize (neck′ro·tize) v. 1. To undergo necrosis; to become necrotic. 2. To affect with necrosis, to produce necrosis.

necrotizing arteritis. 1. POLYARTERITIS NODOSA. 2. Any process which involves necrosis of arteries.

necrotizing myelitis or **myelopathy.** A rare disorder of the spinal cord, which may be acute or subacute in onset, characterized by a hemorrhagic necrosis of tissue like that of necrotizing hemorrhagic leukoencephalitis. The subacute variety is also called *Foix-Alajouanine syndrome.*

necrotizing papillitis. PAPILLARY NECROSIS.

necrotizing ulcerative gingivitis. Vincent's infection involving the gingivae. Syn. *trench mouth, Vincent's gingivitis.*

nec·ro·zoo·sper·mia (neck″ro·zo″o·spur′mee·uh) n. A condition in which spermatozoa are present but are immobile and without evidence of life.

nee·dle, n. 1. A sharp-pointed steel instrument, used for puncturing or for sewing tissue; of various shapes, sizes, and edges, the sewing needle has an eye for carrying suture material through the parts. 2. A hollow needle, usually attached to a syringe, for injection or aspiration.

needle biopsy. The securing of biopsy material by means of a hollow needle.

needle forceps. NEEDLE HOLDER.

needle holder. A handle, usually in the form of a self-locking forceps, for grasping and using a surgical needle.

need·ling, n. Discission with a needle, as of a cataract, to afford entrance to the aqueous humor and cause swelling and softening of the lens for either aspiration or absorption.

neg·a·tive, adj. 1. Indicating or expressing denial, contradiction, or opposition; in psychiatry, resisting suggestions or advice or reacting with hostility. 2. Indicating failure of response, as to drugs or other therapy. 3. Indicating absence of the entity or condition tested for. **4.** Included in a class or range opposite or complementary to that conceived as fundamental or primary, or to that conventionally termed positive, as negative integer, negative pressure, negative pole. Symbol, −. **5.** Tending or serving to subtract, retard, or decrease, as negative feedback. **6.** Of images (visual, photographic, etc.), having light and dark, or complementary colors, reversed.

negative feeling. 1. Aversion, antipathy; coldness. 2. Hostility, antagonism; destructive urge.

negative phase. The temporary lessening of the amount of antibody in the serum immediately following a second inoculation of antigen.

negative pressure. 1. Pressure less than atmospheric pressure. 2. The force of suction.

neg·a·tiv·ism (neg'uh·tiv·iz·um) n. Indifference, opposition, or resistance to suggestions or commands of another person who is in a position to give these; persistent refusal, without apparent or objective reasons, to do as suggested or asked, seen normally in late infancy and early childhood, but also in adults who feel "pushed around"; in its most pathologic form, is seen in the catatonic form of schizophrenia as markedly reduced activity, with patients ignoring even inner stimuli.

neg·li·gence (neg'li·junce) n. In legal medicine, an act of commission or omission in the care of patients which, without regard to circumstances, violates a statute or is obviously opposed to the dictates of accepted medical practices.

NeGram. Trademark for nalidixic acid, an antibacterial agent used for treatment of urinary tract infections caused by gram-negative organisms.

Ne·gri bodies (ne'gree) Acidophil inclusion bodies in the cytoplasm of nerve cells, considered diagnostic of rabies; found most often in large cells of the hippocampus and Purkinje cells of the cerebellum, but not limited to these locations.

Neis·se·ria (nigh·seer'ee·uh, nigh·serr'ee·uh) n. A genus of gram-negative cocci of the family Neisseriaceae.

Neisseria cat·ar·rha·lis (kat''uh·ray'lis, ·ral'is). A species of bacteria found in the respiratory tract; generally not pathogenic.

Neisseria fla·ves·cens (fla·ves'enz). A species of bacteria found in the spinal fluid in rare instances of clinical meningitis, and on the mucous membranes of the respiratory tract.

Neisseria gon·or·rhoe·ae (gon''o·ree'ee). The bacterium that causes gonorrhea; the type species of its genus.

Neisseria men·in·git·i·dis (men''in·jit'i·dis). The species of bacteria that causes epidemic cerebrospinal meningitis. Syn. Diplococcus intracellularis meningitidis, Neisseria intracellularis.

Neisseria sic·ca (sick'uh). A species of bacteria forming dry, crenated colonies on simple media, found in mucous membranes of the respiratory tract, and generally nonpathogenic.

Nélaton's line A line between the tuberosity of the ischium and the anterior superior iliac spine. In dislocated hip, the tip of the greater trochanter is above this line.

Nel·son's syndrome Skin hyperpigmentation resulting from secretion of melanocyte-stimulating hormone by a pituitary adenoma developing after adrenalectomy for Cushing's disease; adrenocorticotropic hormone is also secreted.

nem, n. A unit of nutrition representing the calorific value of 1 gram of breast milk of standard composition; equivalent to approximately ⅔ calorie.

nem-, nema-, nemo- A combining form meaning filament, filamentous, threadlike.

nem·a·line (nem'uh·line, ·lin) adj. Threadlike.

nemaline myopathy. A familial muscular disorder characterized by generalized weakness and skeletal muscular atrophy from the time of birth; there are abnormal rod-shaped structures seen microscopically in affected muscle fibers. The inheritance appears to be autosomal dominant with variable expression of the gene.

Nem·a·thel·min·thes (nem''uh·thel·min'theez, nee''muh·) n.pl. The phylum of the roundworms, which includes the true roundworms or nematodes, the hair snakes, and acanthocephalan worms.

Nem·a·to·da (nem''uh·to'duh, nee''muh·) n.pl. A class of the phylum Nemathelminthes; the true roundworms. Members of the class are bilaterally symmetrical, unisexual, without a proboscis, and have a body cavity not lined with epithelium.

nem·a·tode (nem''uh·tode, nee''muh·) n. Any worm of the class Nematoda.

nem·a·tol·o·gy (nem''uh·tol'uh·jee, nee''muh·) n. That portion of the science of parasitology concerned with the study of nematode worms.

Nembutal. Trademark for the barbiturate, pentobarbital, commonly used as the sodium salt.

neo·ars·phen·a·mine (nee''o·ahrs·fen'uh·meen, ·in) n. Chiefly sodium 3,3'-diamino-4,4'-dihydroxyarsenobenzene-N-methylenesulfoxylate, $C_{13}H_{13}As_2N_2NaO_4S$, formerly used for the treatment of spirochetal and some other diseases.

neo·blas·tic (nee''o·blas'tick) adj. Pertaining to, or of the nature of, new tissue.

neo·cer·e·bel·lum (nee''o·serr''e·bel'um) n. Phylogenetically the most recent part of the cerebellum; consists of the middle portions of the vermis and their large lateral extensions. Practically all of the cerebellar hemispheres fall into this subdivision. It receives cerebral cortex impulses via the corticopontocerebellar tract. —neocerebel·lar (·lur) adj.

neo·cor·tex (nee''o·kor'tecks) n. That part of the cerebral cortex which is phylogenetically the most recent in development; it includes all of the cortex except the olfactory portions, the hippocampal regions, and the piriform areas. Syn. isocortex, neopallium.

neo·cys·tos·to·my (nee''o·sis·tos'tum·ee) n. A surgical procedure whereby a new opening is made into the urinary bladder.

neo·dym·i·um (nee''o·dim'ee·um) n.

Nd = 144.24. A rare-earth metal occurring in cerium and lanthanum minerals.

neo·gen·e·sis (nee″o·jen′e·sis) *n.* Growth of tissues or production of a metabolite from a generically different substrate. —**neo·ge·net·ic** (·je·net′ick) *adj.*

neo·ki·net·ic (nee″o·ki·net′ick) *adj.* Pertaining to the motor nervous mechanism that regulates voluntary muscular control; the most recently developed nervous system.

ne·ol·o·gism (nee·ol′uh·jiz·um) *n.* 1. A new word-coinage or unconventional vocabulary innovation. 2. The use of such a coinage or innovation, either rationally to represent a new idea, method, or object, or in disordered neurologic states such as delirium, or in mental disorders such as schizophrenia when the patient wishes to express a highly complex meaning related to his conflicts.

neo·mem·brane (nee″o·mem′brane) *n.* A new or false membrane.

neo·mor·phism (nee″o·mor′fiz·um) *n. In biology,* the development of a new form.

neo·my·cin (nee″o·migh′sin) *n.* An antibiotic substance isolated from cultures of *Streptomyces fradiae;* a polybasic compound. It is active against a variety of gram-positive and gram-negative bacteria. The sulfate, administered orally, is used as an intestinal antiseptic in surgery of the large bowel and anus; the salt is used for topical application in treatment or prevention of susceptible infections of the skin and the eye.

ne·on (nee′on) *n.* Ne = 20.179. A chemically inert, gaseous element occurring, in small amounts, in air.

neo·na·tal (nee″o·nay′tul) *adj.* Pertaining to a newborn infant.

neonatal impetigo. A form of bullous impetigo, occurring in the newborn, usually due to staphylococcal, but occasionally to streptococcal, infection. Syn. *pemphigus neonatorum.*

neonatal mortality rate. The number of deaths reported among infants under one month of age in a calendar year per 1,000 live births reported in the same year and place.

neo·nate (nee′o·nate) *n.* A newborn infant; specifically, an infant from birth through its 28th day.

neo·na·ti·cide (nee″o·nay′ti·side) *n.* 1. The murder of a newborn. 2. The murderer of a newborn.

neo·na·tol·o·gy (nee″o·na·tol′uh·jee) *n.* The study and science of the newborn up to 2 months of age postnatally. —**neonatolo·gist** (·jist) *n.*

neo·na·to·rum (nee″o·nay·to′rum) Genitive plural of *neonatus;* of the newborn.

neo·na·tus (nee″o·nay′tus) L. *adj. & n.,* pl. & genit. sing. **neona·ti** (·tye), genit. pl. **neo·na·to·rum** (·nay·to′rum) NEWBORN.

neo·ol·ive (nee″o·ol′iv) *n.* The olive with the exception of its small medial portion which is part of the paleo-olive.

neo·pal·li·um (nee″o·pal′ee·um) *n.* The cerebral cortex with the exception of the rhinencephalon. —**neopalli·al** (·ul) *adj.*

ne·oph·il·ism (nee·off′il·iz·um) *n.* Morbid or undue desire for novelty.

neo·pho·bia (nee″o·fo′bee·uh) *n.* Dread of new scenes or of novelties.

neo·phre·nia (nee″o·fren′ee·uh, ·free′nee·uh) *n.* Any psychosis of childhood.

neo·pla·sia (nee″o·play′zhuh, ·zee·uh) *n.* 1. Formation of tumors or neoplasms. 2. Formation of new tissue.

neo·plasm (nee′o·plaz·um) *n.* An aberrant new growth of abnormal cells or tissues; a tumor. —**neo·plas·tic** (nee″o·plas′tick) *adj.*

neo·prene (nee′o·preen) *n.* Generic name for synthetic rubber made by polymerization of 2-chloro-1,3-butadiene. Neoprene vulcanizates are markedly resistant to oils, greases, chemicals, sunlight, ozone, and heat.

neo·stig·mine (nee″o·stig′meen, ·min) *n.* (m-Hydroxyphenyl)trimethylammonium ion, a quaternary ammonium cation with anticholinesterase activity; used as the bromide ($C_{12}H_{19}BrN_2O_2$) or methylsulfate ($C_{13}H_{22}N_2O_6S$) salts for prevention and treatment of postoperative abdominal distention and urinary retention, symptomatic control of myasthenia gravis, as an antidote for excessive curarization with skeletal muscle relaxants, and other conditions.

neo·stri·a·tum (nee″o·strye·ay′tum) *n.* The caudate nucleus and putamen combined; the phylogenetically new part of the corpus striatum.

Neo-Synephrine. Trademark for phenylephrine, a sympathomimetic amine used as the hydrochloride salt to maintain blood pressure and as a local vasoconstrictor.

neo·vas·cu·lar (nee″o·vas′kew·lur) *adj.* Pertaining to newly formed vessels.

neo·vas·cu·lar·i·za·tion (nee″o·vas′kew·lur·i·zay′shun, ·eye·zay′shun) *n.* 1. New formation of blood vessels in abnormal tissues such as tumors, or in abnormal positions as in diabetic retinopathy. 2. REVASCULARIZATION.

neo·vas·cu·la·ture (nee″o·vas′kew·luh·chur) *n.* A newly formed collection of blood vessels, usually representing an abnormality.

neph·a·lism (nef′ul·iz·um) *n.* Total abstinence from alcoholic liquors.

neph·e·lom·e·ter (nef″e·lom′e·tur) *n.* An apparatus for ascertaining the number of bacteria in a suspension, or the turbidity of a fluid.

neph·e·lom·e·try (nef″e·lom′e·tree) *n.* The determination of the degree of turbidity of a fluid. —**nephe·lo·met·ric** (·lo·met′rick) *adj.*

nephr-, nephro- A combining form meaning *kidney, renal.*

ne·phral·gia (ne·fral′juh, ·jee·uh) *n.* Pain in a kidney. —**nephral·gic** (·jick) *adj.*

ne·phrec·ta·sia (nef″reck·tay′zhuh, ·zee·uh, nee″freck·) *n.* Dilatation of a kidney.

ne·phrec·to·mize (ne·freck′tuh·mize) *v.* To remove a kidney.

ne·phrec·to·my (ne·freck′tuh·mee) *n.* Excision of a kidney.

neph·ric (nef′rick) *adj.* Pertaining to the kidney; RENAL.

ne·phrit·ic (ne·frit′ick) *adj.* 1. Pertaining to or

affected with nephritis. 2. Pertaining to or affecting the kidney.

ne·phri·tis (ne-frye'tis) *n.*, pl. **ne·phrit·i·des** (ne-frit'i-deez) Inflammation of the kidney.

neph·ri·to·gen·ic (nef''ri-to-jen'ick, ne-frit''o-) *adj.* Producing nephritis; said especially of certain strains of streptococci.

nephro-. See *nephr-*.

neph·ro·ab·dom·i·nal (nef''ro-ab-dom'i-nul) *adj.* Pertaining to the kidneys and abdomen.

neph·ro·blas·to·ma (nef''ro-blas-to'muh) *n.* WILMS'S TUMOR.

neph·ro·cal·ci·no·sis (nef''ro-kal''si-no'sis) *n.* Renal calcinosis, marked by radiologically detectable deposits of calcium throughout the renal parenchyma.

neph·ro·cap·sec·to·my (nef''ro-kap-seck'tum-ee) *n.* NEPHROCAPSULECTOMY.

neph·ro·cap·sul·ec·to·my (nef''ro-kap''sue-leck'tum-ee) *n.* Excision of the renal capsule.

neph·ro·cap·su·lot·o·my (nef''ro-kap''sue-lot'um-ee) *n.* Incision of the renal capsule.

neph·ro·car·ci·no·ma (nef''ro-kahr''si-no'muh) *n.* Carcinoma of the kidney.

neph·ro·car·di·ac (nef''ro-kahr'dee-ack) *adj.* Pertaining to the kidney and the heart.

neph·ro·col·ic (nef''ro-kol'ick) *adj.* Pertaining to the kidneys and the colon.

neph·ro·co·lo·pexy (nef''ro-kol'o-peck-see, -ko'luh-) *n.* The surgical anchoring of a kidney and the nearby part of the colon.

neph·ro·co·lop·to·sis (nef''ro-ko''lop-to'sis) *n.* Downward displacement of a kidney and the colon.

neph·ro·cyst·an·as·to·mo·sis (nef''ro-sis''tan-as''tuh-mo'sis) *n.* The surgical formation of an opening between the renal pelvis and the urinary bladder.

neph·ro·cys·ti·tis (nef''ro-sis-tigh'tis) *n.* Inflammation of both the urinary bladder and kidney.

neph·ro·gen·e·sis (nef''ro-jen'e-sis) *n.* 1. Formation of a kidney. 2. Formation of a nephron or nephrons.

neph·ro·gen·ic (nef''ro-jen'ick) *adj.* 1. Having the ability to produce kidney tissue. 2. Of renal origin.

nephrogenic cord. The longitudinal, cordlike mass of mesenchyme derived from the mesomere or nephrostomal plate of the mesoderm, from which develop the functional parts of the pronephros, mesonephros, and metanephros.

nephrogenic diabetes insipidus. Diabetes insipidus that is unresponsive to vasopressin, because of inability of the renal tubules to resorb water; it is usually congenital, inherited as a sex-linked trait with variable expression in females, but may occur in chronic renal insufficiency.

neph·ro·gram (nef'ro-gram) *n.* Delineation of the kidney parenchyma by radiographic means. —**neph·ro·graph·ic** (nef''ro-graf'ick) *adj.*

nephrographic phase. That early portion of a radiographic contrast study of the kidneys (excretory or arteriographic) in which the renal parenchyma is opacified.

neph·roid (nef'roid) *adj.* Kidney-shaped, reniform, resembling a kidney.

neph·ro·lith (nef'ro-lith) *n.* KIDNEY STONE. —**neph·ro·lith·ic** (nef''ro-lith'ick) *adj.*

neph·ro·li·thi·a·sis (nef''ro-li-thigh'uh-sis) *n.* The formation of renal calculi, or the disease state characterized by their presence.

neph·ro·li·thot·o·my (nef''ro-li-thot'um-ee) *n.* An incision of the kidney for the removal of a calculus.

ne·phrol·o·gy (ne-frol'uh-jee) *n.* The scientific study of the kidney, including its diseases. —**nephrolo·gist,** *n.*

ne·phrol·y·sin (ne-frol'i-sin, nef''ro·lye'sin) *n.* A toxic substance capable of disintegrating kidney cells.

ne·phrol·y·sis (ne-frol'i-sis) *n.* 1. The disintegration of the kidney by the action of a nephrolysin. 2. The operation of loosening a kidney from surrounding adhesions. —**neph·ro·lyt·ic** (nef''ro-lit'ick) *adj.*

ne·phro·ma (ne-fro'muh) *n.*, pl. **nephromas, nephroma·ta** (-tuh) 1. Any kidney tumor. 2. RENAL CELL CARCINOMA.

neph·ro·meg·a·ly (nef''ro-meg'uh-lee) *n.* Kidney enlargement.

neph·ron (nef'ron) *n.* The renal unit, consisting of the glomerular capsule, its glomerulus, and the attached uriniferous tubule.

neph·ro·noph·thi·sis (nef''ro-nof'thi-sis) *n.* 1. Loss of renal substance. 2. An idiopathic kidney disease, often familial, characterized by loss of renal substance with cyst formation, anemia, and uremia.

ne·phrop·a·thy (ne-frop'uth-ee) *n.* 1. Any disease of the kidney. 2. NEPHROSIS (2). —**neph·ro·path·ic** (nef''ro-path'ick) *adj.*

neph·ro·pexy (nef'ro-peck''see) *n.* Surgical fixation of a floating or ptotic kidney.

neph·rop·to·sis (nef''rop-to'sis) *n.* Inferior displacement of the kidney.

neph·ro·py·e·li·tis (nef''ro-pye''e-lye'tis) *n.* PYELONEPHRITIS.

neph·ro·py·e·lo·plas·ty (nef''ro-pye'e-lo-plas''tee) *n.* A plastic operation on the pelvis of the kidney.

ne·phror·rha·phy (ne-fror'uh-fee) *n.* 1. The stitching of a floating kidney to the posterior wall of the abdomen or to the loin. 2. Suturing a wound in a kidney.

neph·ros (nef'ros) *n.*, pl. **neph·roi** (-roy) KIDNEY.

neph·ro·scle·ro·sis (nef''ro-skle-ro'sis) *n.* Scarring of renal tubules, interstitium, and glomeruli due to arteriosclerotic changes in renal arteries or arterioles; systemic hypertension and sometimes renal failure may be clinically associated.

neph·ro·sid·er·o·sis (nef''ro-sid''ur-o'sis) *n.* The accumulation of hemosiderin in the kidneys.

ne·phro·sis (ne-fro'sis) *n.* 1. NEPHROTIC SYNDROME. 2. *In pathology,* degenerative or retrogressive renal lesions, distinct from inflammation (nephritis) or vascular involvement (nephrosclerosis), especially as applied to tubular lesions (tubular nephritis). Syn. *nephropathy, nephrodystrophy.*

ne·phro·so·ne·phri·tis (ne-fro''so-ne-frye'tis) *n.* A

renal disease having features of nephrosis and nephritis.

ne·phros·to·gram (nef·ros'to·gram) n. The radiographic depiction of a nephrostomy.

ne·phros·to·my (ne·fros'tum·ee) n. The formation of a fistula leading through the renal parenchyma to the pelvis of a kidney.

ne·phrot·ic (ne·frot'ick) adj. Pertaining to or affected by nephrosis.

nephrotic syndrome. Marked proteinuria, hypoproteinemia, anasarca, and hyperlipemia accompanied by normal blood pressure, resulting from any agent damaging the basement membrane of the renal glomerulus.

neph·ro·to·mo·gram (nef"ro·to'muh·gram) n. Radiographic depiction of the kidney by means of tomography and intravenous urography.

neph·ro·to·mog·ra·phy (nef"ro·to·mog'ruh·fee) n. A roentgenologic technique combining intravenous urography and sectional radiography.

ne·phrot·o·my (ne·frot'um·ee) n. Incision of the kidney.

neph·ro·tox·ic (nef"ro·tock'sick) adj. 1. Pertaining to nephrotoxin. 2. Injurious to the kidney cells; NEPHROLYTIC.

neph·ro·tox·in (nef"ro·tock'sin) n. A cytotoxin that damages the cells of the kidney.

neph·ro·tu·ber·cu·lo·sis (nef"ro·tew·bur"kew·lo'sis) n. Disease of the kidney due to the tubercle bacillus.

neph·ro·ure·ter·al (nef"ro·yoo·ree'tur·ul) adj. Pertaining to the kidney and ureter.

neph·ro·ure·ter·ec·to·my (nef"ro·yoo·ree"tur·eck'tum·ee) n. The excision of a kidney and whole ureter at one operation.

nep·tu·ni·um (nep·tew'nee·um) n. Np = 237.0482. An element, atomic number 93, obtained by bombarding ordinary uranium with neutrons. Undergoes transformation into plutonium.

nerve, n. A bundle of nerve fibers, usually outside the brain or spinal cord; the nerve fibers are held together by connective tissue called endoneurium inside the nerve bundle and perineurium, the enclosing sheath. A collected bundle of nerve fibers within the brain and spinal cord is usually called a nerve tract.

nerve block. The interruption of the passage of impulses through a nerve, as by chemical, mechanical, or electric means.

nerve cell. 1. NEURON. 2. The CELL BODY of a neuron.

nerve deafness. Deafness due to lesion of the vestibulocochlear nerve.

nerve decompression. Surgical relief of the fibrous or bony constriction of a nerve.

nerve ending. The termination of a nerve at the periphery or in the central nervous system.

nerve fiber. The long process of a neuron, usually the axon. Myelinated nerve fibers have a thick layer of myelin surrounding the nerve fiber; unmyelinated nerve fibers contain very little myelin.

nerve gas. Any of a group of chemical compounds, of potential utility as war gases, having a rapid, profound, cumulative, and only slowly reversible effect on the central, peripheral, and parasympathetic nervous system. They act by inhibiting cholinesterase; the effects may be counteracted with atropine. The compounds are mostly derivatives of organic esters of phosphoric acid.

nerve grafting. The transplantation of a portion of a nerve to reestablish the continuity of a severed nerve.

nerve impulse. A transient physicochemical change in the membrane of a nerve fiber which sweeps rapidly along the fiber to its termination, where it causes excitation of other nerves, muscle, or gland cells, depending on the connections and functions of the nerve.

nerve-sheath tumor. NEURILEMMOMA.

nerve tracing. A method used by chiropractors for locating nerves and studying their diseases, dependent on the patient's reports about areas of tenderness or pain when adjoining areas are pressed upon by the operator.

nerve tract. A bundle of nerve fibers having the same general origin and destination within the nervous system; as a rule, all fibers of a nerve tract serve the same or a very similar function.

nervi. Plural and genitive singular of nervus.

ner·von (nur'von) n. A cerebroside occurring in brain tissue; its characteristic fatty acid is nervonic acid. —**ner·von·ic** (nur·von'ick) adj.

nervonic acid. cis-15-Tetracosenic acid, $C_{23}H_{45}COOH$, an unsaturated acid combined in the cerebroside nervon.

ner·vos·i·ty (nur·vos'i·tee) n. Nervousness.

ner·vous, adj. 1. Of or pertaining to the nerves, as: nervous system, nervous tissue. 2. Affecting or involving a nerve or nerves, as: nervous diseases. 3. Originating in or affected by the nerves; neurogenic. 4. Loosely, psychogenic; pertaining to mental or emotional disorders. 5. In a state of nervousness, afflicted with nervousness. 6. Loosely, NEUROTIC.

nervous breakdown. A nonspecific, nonmedical term for any emotional or mental disorder, particularly of sudden onset, and when characterized by a predominantly depressive mood.

nervous diarrhea. Diarrhea as a manifestation of a psychophysiologic disorder.

nervous exhaustion. A state of fatigue and discomfort from emotional causes.

nervous headache. PSYCHOGENIC HEADACHE.

nervous irritability. The property of a nerve to respond to stimuli by conducting impulses.

ner·vous·ness, n. Excessive excitability of the nervous system, characterized by lack of mental poise, restless, impulsive, or purposeless activity, an uncomfortable awareness of self, and a variety of somatic symptoms such as tremors, fatigue, weight loss, weakness, sleeplessness.

nervous system. 1. The entire nervous apparatus of the body, including the brain, brainstem, spinal cord, cranial and peripheral nerves, and ganglions. 2. A functional or anatomic subsystem of this nervous apparatus, as: autonomic nervous system, central nervous system.

ner·vus (nur'vus) *n.*, pl. & genit. sing. **ner·vi** (·vye), genit. pl. **ner·vo·rum** (nur·vo'rum) [NA]. NERVE.

nervus in·ter·me·di·us (in·tur·mee'dee·us) [NA]. The intermediate branch of the seventh cranial or facial nerve.

nesidi-, nesidio- A combining form meaning *islets of the pancreas.*

ne·sid·i·ec·to·my (ne·sid''ee·eck'tum·ee) *n.* Surgical excision of an islet-cell tumor of the pancreas, or of pancreatic tissue for islet-cell hyperplasia.

ne·sid·io·blas·to·ma (ne·sid''ee·o·blas·to'muh) *n.* ISLET-CELL TUMOR.

ness·ler·ize (nes'lur·ize) *v.* To test with Nessler's reagent. —**ness·ler·iza·tion** (nes''lur·i·zay'shun) *n.*

Ness·ler's reagent An aqueous solution of potassium iodide, mercuric chloride, and potassium hydroxide, used in testing for ammonia.

nes·ti·at·ria (nes''tee·at'ree·uh, ·ay'tree·uh) *n.* Treatment by fasting.

nes·tis (nes'tis) *n.* 1. Fasting. 2. JEJUNUM.

net·tle rash. URTICARIA.

Neu·hau·ser's sign 1. The bubbly appearance of inspissated meconium seen in roentgenograms of the abdomen of newborns, often a pathognomonic sign of meconium ileus. 2. Absence of adenoid tissue on a lateral roentgenographic view of the nasopharynx, seen in neonates with agammaglobulinemia.

neur-, neuro- A combining form meaning *neural, nervous, nerve.*

neu·ral (new'rul) *adj.* Pertaining to nerves or nervous tissue.

neural arc. A nerve circuit consisting of two or more neurons, the receptor and the effector, with intercalated neurons between them.

neural arch. 1. VERTEBRAL ARCH. 2. *In comparative anatomy,* the dorsal loop of the typical vertebra including the neural canal.

neural canal. *In embryology,* VERTEBRAL CANAL.

neural crest. A band of ectodermal cells on either side of the neural tube which is the primordium of the cranial, spinal, and autonomic ganglions. Syn. *ganglionic crest.*

neural ectoderm. That part of the ectoderm destined to form the neural tube and neural crest. Syn. *neuroblast.*

neu·ral·gia (new·ral'juh) *n.* Severe, sharp, stabbing, paroxysmal pain along the course of a nerve; not associated with demonstrable neurologic signs or structural changes in the nerve. The pain is usually brief; tenderness is often present at the points of exit of the nerve, and the paroxysm can be produced by contact with specific areas (trigger zones). Various forms of neuralgia are named according to their anatomic situation. —**neural·gic** (·jick) *adj.*

neu·ral·gi·form (new·ral'ji·form) *adj.* Resembling neuralgia.

neural lamina. The lateral portion of the neural arch of a vertebra.

neural leprosy. TUBERCULOID LEPROSY.

neural lymphomatosis. A form of the avian leukosis complex affecting primarily the sciatic nerve.

neural plate. The thickened ectodermal plate overlying the head process that differentiates into the neural tube.

neural tube. The embryonic tube formed from the ectodermal neural plate that differentiates into brain and spinal cord.

neur·a·min·ic acid (nur''a·min'ick). An acid, $C_9H_{17}NO_8$, the aldol condensation product of pyruvic acid and *N*-acetyl-D-mannosamine, regarded as the parent acid of a family of widely distributed acyl derivatives known as sialic acids.

neur·amin·i·dase (newr''a·min'i·dace, ·am'in·) *n.* A bacterial enzyme specific for neuraminic acid glycosides, whose action is to split sialic acid from the polymer.

neur·aprax·ia (newr''uh·prack'see·uh, ·ay·prack') *n.* Paralysis due to impairment of peripheral nerve function without anatomic interruption of the nerve. Recovery is spontaneous, complete, and rapid.

neur·as·the·nia (newr''as·theen'ee·uh) *n.* A group of symptoms formerly considered an important neurosis and ascribed to debility or exhaustion of the nerve centers. —**neuras·then·ic** (·then'ick) *adj.*

neurasthenic neurosis. A neurotic disorder, formerly considered an important neurosis, characterized by chronic complaints of easy fatigability, lack of energy, weakness, various aches and pains, and sometimes exhaustion. Most patients with these complaints are now included in the categories of anxiety neurosis or depression.

neur·ax·is (newr·ack'sis) *n.* 1. The cerebrospinal axis; NEURAL TUBE. 2. *Obsol.* AXON.

neur·ec·ta·sis (newr·eck'tuh·sis) *n.* Nerve stretching.

neu·rec·to·my (new·reck'tum·ee) *n.* Excision of a part of a nerve.

neur·ec·to·pia (newr''eck·to'pee·uh) *n.* Displacement or anomalous distribution of a nerve.

neur·en·ter·ic (newr''en·terr'ick) *adj.* Pertaining to the embryonic neural canal and the intestinal tube.

neurenteric cyst. A cystic epithelium-lined tumor of embryonic origin, resulting from the failure of entodermal tissue to separate from the primitive notochordal plate. The cyst may develop at any point between the lung or gut and the center of the spinal chord, most often in close relation to the lower cervical and upper thoracic portions of the cord.

neur·ex·er·e·sis (newr''eck·serr'e·sis, ·se·ree'sis) *n.* The surgical extraction, or avulsion, of a nerve.

neu·ri·a·try (new·rye'uh·tree) *n. Obsol.* The study and treatment of nervous diseases; neurology.

neu·ri·lem·ma, neu·ri·lema (new''ri·lem'uh) *n.* Any of the supporting structures of the nerve fiber, until recently not distinguished from one another. —**neurilem·mal** (·ul) *adj.*

neu·ri·lem·mo·ma, neu·ri·lem·o·ma (new''ri·lem·o'muh) *n.* A solitary encapsulated benign tumor which originates in the peripheral, cranial, and autonomic nerves, and which is composed of Schwann cells in a collagenous matrix. Syn. *schwannoma, neurinoma.*

neu·rine (new'reen, ·rin) n. Trimethylvinyl-ammonium hydroxide, $(CH_3)_3N(OH)CH=CH_2$, a product of putrefaction of choline formed in brain, cadavers, and bile.

neu·ri·no·ma (new''ri·no'muh) n. 1. NEURILEMMOMA. 2. NEUROFIBROMA.

neu·rite (new'rite) n. Obsol. AXON.

neu·ri·tis (new·righ'tis) n., pl. **neu·rit·i·des** (new-rit'i·deez) An inflammatory disorder of a nerve or nerves, with loss or impairment of motor, sensory, and reflex function in the part supplied. —**neurit·ic** (·rit'ick) adj.

neu·ro·abi·ot·ro·phy (new''ro·ay''bye·ot'ruh·fee, ·ab''ee·ot') n. ABIOTROPHY (1).

neu·ro·anas·to·mo·sis (new''ro·uh·nas''tuh·mo'sis, ·an''us·tuh·) n. Surgical anastomosis of nerves.

neu·ro·anat·o·my (new''ro·uh·nat'uh·mee) n. The anatomy of the nervous system. —**neuro·anato·mist** (·mist) n.

neu·ro·ar·thri·tism (new''ro·ahr'thri·tiz·um) n. A disease with both neurologic and joint manifestations.

neu·ro·ar·throp·a·thy (new''ro·ahr·throp'uth·ee) n. A neuropathic joint disease; joint disease related to disease of the nervous system, as Charcot's joint.

neu·ro·as·tro·cy·to·ma (new''ro·as''tro·sigh·to'muh) n. 1. A tumor composed of neurons and glial cells, mainly astrocytes. 2. GANGLIONEUROMA.

neu·ro·bi·ol·o·gy (new''ro·bye·ol'uh·jee) n. Biology of the nervous system.

neu·ro·blast (new'ro·blast) n. A formative cell of a neuron, derived from ectoderm of the neural plate.

neu·ro·blas·to·ma (new''ro·blas·to'muh) n. A malignant neoplasm composed of primitive neuroectodermal cells, originating in any site in the autonomic nervous system, most commonly in the adrenal medulla of children. Spontaneous remissions may occur. Syn. *sympathicoblastoma.*

neuroblastoma sym·pa·thet·i·cum (sim''puh·thet'i·kum). NEUROBLASTOMA.

neu·ro·blas·to·ma·to·sis (new''ro·blas''to·muh·to'sis) n. 1. Diffuse involvement by neuroblastoma, primary and metastatic. 2. NEUROFIBROMATOSIS.

neu·ro·ca·nal (new''ro·kuh·nal') n. The vertebral canal, containing the spinal cord, cauda equina, and their coverings.

neu·ro·chem·is·try (new''ro·kem'is·tree) n. The chemistry of nervous tissue.

neu·ro·cir·cu·la·to·ry (new''ro·sur'kew·luh·tor''ee) adj. Pertaining to both the nervous and the circulatory systems.

neurocirculatory asthenia. A form of anxiety neurosis characterized by dyspnea, palpitation, chest pain, fatigue, and faintness. Syn. *soldier's heart.* Abbreviated, NCA.

neu·ro·cra·ni·um (new''ro·kray'nee·um) n. The portion of the cranium which forms the brain case.

neu·ro·cu·ta·ne·ous (new''ro·kew·tay'nee·us) adj. 1. Pertaining to the skin and nerves. 2. Pertaining to the innervation of the skin.

neurocutaneous syndrome. Any heritable disorder or embryologic defect involving both the nervous system and skin, but frequently also other tissues such as bones and the viscera, exemplified by tuberous sclerosis, Hippel-Lindau disease, Sturge-Weber disease, and neurofibromatosis. Syn. *neuroectodermal dysplasia.*

neu·ro·cyte (new'ro·site) n. Obsol. NERVE CELL.

neu·ro·cy·tol·y·sis (new''ro·sigh·tol'i·sis) n. Destruction of nerve cells.

neu·ro·der·ma·ti·tis (new''ro·dur''muh·tigh'tis) n. A skin disorder characterized by localized, often symmetrical, patches of pruritic dermatitis with lichenification, occurring in patients of nervous temperament.

neurodermatitis cir·cum·scrip·ta (sur''kum·skrip'tuh). LICHEN CHRONICUS SIMPLEX.

neurodermatitis dis·sem·i·na·ta (di·sem''i·nay'tuh). Atopic dermatitis in which psychogenic factors are important.

neu·ro·der·ma·to·sis (new''ro·dur''muh·to'sis) n. A disease of the skin which is presumed to have a psychogenic component or basis.

neu·ro·der·ma·tro·phia (new''ro·dur''ma·tro'fee·uh) n. Atrophy of the skin resulting from neuropathy.

neu·ro·di·as·ta·sis (new''ro·dye·as'tuh·sis) n. Stretching of nerves; neurectasis.

neu·ro·ec·to·derm (new''ro·eck'to·durm) n. The ectoderm which gives rise to neuroepithelium. —**neuro·ec·to·der·mal** (·eck''to·dur'mul) adj.

neu·ro·ef·fec·tor (new''ro·e·feck'tur) adj. Pertaining to or involving an efferent nerve and the organ, muscle, or gland innervated.

neu·ro·elec·tro·ther·a·peu·tics (new''ro·e·leck''tro·therr·uh·pew'ticks) n. The treatment of nervous affections by means of electricity.

neu·ro·en·do·crine (new''ro·en'duh·krin, ·en'do·krine) adj. Pertaining to the nervous and endocrine systems in anatomic or functional relationship; as the hypothalamic nuclei and the hypophysis constitute a neuroendocrine apparatus.

neu·ro·ep·i·the·li·o·ma (new''ro·ep''i·theel·ee·o'muh) n. A tumor resembling primitive medullary epithelium, containing cells of small cuboidal or columnar form with a tendency to form true rosettes, occurring in the retina, where it is also described as a glioma of the retina or retinocytoma, in the central nervous system, and occasionally in peripheral nerves. Syn. *diktyoma, esthesioneuroblastoma, esthesioneuroepithelioma.*

neu·ro·ep·i·the·li·um (new''ro·ep·i·theel'ee·um) n., pl. **neuroepithe·lia** (·lee·uh) The highly specialized epithelial structures constituting the terminations of the nerves of special sense, as the rod and cone cells of the retina, the olfactory cells of the nose, the hair cells of the internal ear, and the gustatory cells of the taste buds. —**neuroepitheli·al** (·ul) adj.

neu·ro·fi·bril (new''ro·figh'bril) n. A fibril of a nerve cell, usually extending from the processes and traversing the cell body, seen by light microscopy after silver or methylene blue staining of fixed tissues. —**neurofibril·lar** (·ur), **neurofibril·lary** (·err·ee) adj.

neu·ro·fi·bro·ma (new"ro·figh·bro'muh) n. A benign, slowly growing, relatively circumscribed but nonencapsulated neoplasm originating in a nerve and composed principally of Schwann cells. The intercellular matrix contains collagen fibrils and a nonorganized mucoid or myxomatous component. The tumor is usually solitary, but may be multiple in patients with neurofibromatosis. Syn. *perineural fibroma, myxofibroma of nerve sheath, neurofibromyxoma.*

neu·ro·fi·bro·ma·to·sis (new"ro·figh·bro'muh·to'sis) n. A hereditary disease characterized by presence of neurofibromas in the skin or along the course of peripheral nerves. Syn. *von Recklinghausen's disease.*

neu·ro·fi·bro·sar·co·ma (new"ro·figh"bro·sahr'ko'muh) n. A malignant tumor composed of interlacing bundles of anaplastic spindle-shaped cells which resemble those of nerve sheaths.

neu·ro·fil·a·ment (new"ro·fil'uh·munt) n. A structure of indefinite length and about 10 μm in diameter, found throughout the neuron, from the farthest reaches of the dendrites to the tip of the axon. Refined ultrastructural techniques have shown that the neurofilament is a tubular rather than a solid structure.

neu·ro·gas·tric (new"ro·gas'trick) adj. Pertaining to the nerves and the stomach.

neu·ro·gen·e·sis (new"ro·jen'e·sis) n. The formation of nerves.

neu·ro·gen·ic (new"ro·jen'ick) adj. 1. Of nervous-tissue origin, as neurogenic tumors. 2. Stimulated by nerves, as neurogenic muscular contractions. 3. Caused or affected by a dysfunction, trauma, or disease of nerves or the nervous system, as neurogenic shock, neurogenic bladder. 4. Pertaining to neurogenesis.

neurogenic arthropathy. CHARCOT'S JOINT.

neurogenic bladder. A urinary bladder in a state of dysfunction due to lesions of the central or peripheral nervous system.

neurogenic shock. NEUROPATHIC SHOCK.

neu·rog·e·nous (new·roj'e·nus) adj. NEUROGENIC.

neu·rog·li·a (new·rog'lee·uh) n. 1. The supporting cells of the central nervous system, consisting of the macroglia (astrocytes and oligodendrocytes), which have an ectodermal origin, and the microglia, the exact origin of which is still not settled. —**neurog·li·al** (·lee·ul) adj.

neu·rog·li·o·ma (new·rog"lee·o'muh) n. A tumor composed of neuroglial tissue; a glioma.

neu·rog·li·o·sis (new·rog"lee·o'sis) n. A condition of multiple neurogliomas developing diffusely throughout the nervous system.

neu·ro·his·tol·o·gy (new"ro·his·tol'uh·jee) n. The histology of the nervous system.

neu·ro·hu·mor (new"ro·hew'mur) n. Obsol. NEUROTRANSMITTER. —**neurohumor·al** (·ul) adj.

neu·ro·hy·poph·y·se·al (new"ro·high·pof"i·see'ul, ·high"po·fiz'ee·ul) adj. Pertaining to the neurohypophysis.

neu·ro·hy·poph·y·sis (new"ro·high·pof'i·sis) n. The posterior, neural portion of the hypophysis, which develops as a downward evagination of the neural ectoderm from the floor of the diencephalon and secretes antidiuretic hormone and oxytocin which are produced in the hypothalamus; consists of a main body, the neural lobe or infundibular process, and a stalk, the neural stalk or infundibulum, by which the hypophysis is attached to the hypothalamus. Some classifications also include the pars intermedia. Syn. *posterior pituitary, posterior lobe of the hypophysis.*

neu·roid (new'roid) adj. Resembling a nerve or nerve substance.

neu·ro·in·duc·tion (new"ro·in·duck'shun) n. SUGGESTION (2).

neu·ro·lath·y·rism (new"ro·lath'ur·iz·um) n. LATHYRISM.

neu·ro·lem·ma (new"ruh·lem'uh) n. NEURILEMMA.

neu·ro·lept·an·al·ge·sia (new"ro·lep"tan·al·jee'zee·uh) n. NEUROLEPTOANALGESIA.

neu·ro·lep·tic (new"ro·lep'tic) adj. & n. 1. Of drug actions: tending to result in overall improvement of patients with mental process. 2. A drug that by its characteristic actions and effects is useful in the treatment of mental disorders, especially psychoses.

neu·ro·lep·to·an·al·ge·sia (new"ro·lep"to·an'ul·jee'zee·uh) n. A state of altered consciousness produced by a combination of one or more neuroleptic drugs with an analgesic, allowing certain surgical procedures to be carried out on a wakeful subject.

neu·rol·o·gist (new·rol'uh·jist) n. A person versed in neurology, usually a physician who specializes in the diagnosis and treatment of disorders of the nervous system and the study of its functioning.

neu·rol·o·gy (new·rol'uh·jee) n. The study of the anatomy, physiology, and pathology of the nervous system and treatment of its disorders. —**neu·ro·log·ic** (new"ruh·loj'ick) adj.

neu·ro·lo·pho·ma (new"ro·lof·o'muh, ·luh·fo'muh) n. Any tumor derived from cells of neural crest origin, including neuromas, schwannomas, melanomas, and apudomas.

neu·ro·lu·es (new"ro·lew'eez) n. NEUROSYPHILIS.

neu·ro·lym·pho·ma·to·sis (new"ro·lim"fo·muh·to'sis) n. Involvement of nerves by malignant lymphoma.

neu·rol·y·sin (new·rol'i·sin, new"ro·lye'sin) n. A cytolysin having action upon nerve cells.

neu·rol·y·sis (new·rol'i·sis) n. 1. Stretching of a nerve to relieve anatomical tension. 2. Surgical release of a nerve from harmful fibrous adhesions. 3. Destruction or disintegration of nerve tissue.

neu·ro·ma (new·ro'muh) n. Any tumor of the nervous system, as originally described by Virchow. These tumors have since been classified into special groups on a histologic basis —**neu·rom·a·tous** (new·rom'uh·tus, ·ro'muh·tus) adj.

neu·ro·ma·toid (new·ro'muh·toid) adj. Resembling a neuroma.

neu·ro·mech·a·nism (new"ro·meck'uh·niz·um) n. The correlated structure and function of the nervous system in relation to a bodily activity.

neu·ro·mere (new'ro·meer) n. An embryonic segment of the brain or spinal chord.

neu·ro·mi·me·sis (new″ro·mi·mee′sis, ·migh·mee′ sis) *n.* A group of phenomena seen in hysterical neurosis resembling neurologic disease. —**neuromi·met·ic** (·met′ick) *adj.*

neu·ro·mus·cu·lar (new″ro·mus′kew·lur) *adj.* Pertaining to both nerves and muscles.

neuromuscular junction. MYONEURAL JUNCTION.

neu·ro·my·e·li·tis (new″ro·migh·e·ligh′tis) *n.* The conjunction of peripheral nerve and spinal cord inflammation.

neuromyelitis op·ti·ca (op′ti·kuh). A clinical syndrome characterized by simultaneous or successive involvement of the optic nerves and spinal cord; usually a form of mulitple sclerosis, sometimes of another demyelinating disease. Syn. *Devic's disease.*

neu·ron (new′ron) *n.* The complete nerve cell, including the cell body, axon, and dendrites; specialized as a conductor of impulses. —**neu·ro·nal** (new′run·ul, new·ro′nul) *adj.*

neu·rone (new′rone) *n.* NEURON.

neu·ro·ne·vus (new″ro·nee′vus) *n.* **1.** A variety of intradermal nevus largely composed of nevus cells possessing neural characteristics. **2.** A single neurofibroma.

neuron pathway. The successive neurons over which a given impulse is thought to be transmitted.

neu·ro·noph·a·gia (new″ro″no·fay′jee·uh) *n.* The removal of injured or diseased nerve cells by phagocytes.

neu·ro·oph·thal·mol·o·gy (new″ro·off″thal·mol′ uh·jee) *n.* The neurologic aspects of ophthalmology; the study of the physiology and diseases of the visual system as related to the nervous system. —**neuroophthalmolo·gist** (·jist) *n.*; **neuro·oph·thal·mo·log·ic** (·off·thal″mo·loj′ ick) *adj.*

neu·ro·pa·ral·y·sis (new″ro·puh·ral′i·sis) *n.* Paralysis or trophic disturbance due to a lesion of the nerve, or the nucleus of the nerve, that supplies the muscle or dermatome involved. —**neuro·par·a·lyt·ic** (·pär″il·lit′ick) *adj.*

neu·ro·path·ic (new″ro·path′ick) *adj.* **1.** Characterized by a diseased or imperfect nervous system. **2.** Depending upon, or pertaining to, nervous disease. **3.** Originating in or caused by disease or dysfunction of nerves or the nervous system.

neuropathic shock. A widespread, serious reduction of tissue perfusion due to spinal cord injury, primary autonomic insufficiency, or intoxication with certain drugs, such as anesthetics and ganglion-blocking agents. Syn. *neurogenic shock.*

neu·ro·pa·thol·o·gy (new″ro·pa·thol′uh·jee) *n.* That part of pathology concerned with diseases of the nervous system. —**neuro·patho·log·ic** (·path·uh·loj′ick) *adj.*

neu·rop·a·thy (new·rop′uth·ee) *n.* Any noninflammatory disease of peripheral nerves.

neu·ro·phar·ma·col·o·gy (new″ro·fahr″muh·kol′ uh·jee) *n.* The science dealing with the action of drugs on the nervous system.

neu·ro·phys·i·ol·o·gy (new″ro·fiz·ee·ol′uh·jee) *n.* The physiology of the nervous system. —**neu·rophys·i·o·log·ic** (·ee·o·loj′ick) *adj.*; **neurophysiolo·gist** (·jist) *n.*

neu·ro·pil (new′ro·pil) *n.* Areas of the central nervous system that contain a feltwork of intermingled and interconnected processes of neurons; in these areas most of the synaptic junctions occur.

neu·ro·plasm (new′ro·plaz·um) *n.* The protoplasm filling the interstices of the fibrils of nerve cells.

neu·ro·plas·ty (new′ro·plas″tee) *n.* A plastic operation on the nerves.

neu·ro·pore (new′ro·pore) *n.* The anterior or posterior terminal aperture of the embryonic neural tube before complete closure occurs (about the 20- to 25-somite stage).

neu·ro·psy·chi·a·try (new″ro·sigh·kigh′uh·tree) *n.* The branch of medical science dealing with both nervous and mental diseases. —**neuro·psychia·trist** (·trist) *n.*; **neuro·psy·chi·at·ric** (·sigh″kee·at′rick) *adj.*

neu·ro·psy·chol·o·gy (new″ro·sigh·kol′uh·jee) *n. Obsol.* A system of psychology based on neurology.

neur·op·ti·co·my·e·li·tis (newr·op″ti·ko·migh″e· ligh′tis) *n.* NEUROMYELITIS OPTICA.

neu·ro·ra·di·ol·o·gy (new″ro·ray″dee·ol′uh·jee) *n.* A subspecialty of radiology dealing with the roentgenology of neurologic disease. —**neuro·ra·dio·log·ic** (·dee·o·loj′ick) *adj.*

neu·ro·re·lapse (new″ro·re·laps′) *n.* Subacute syphilitic meningitis, becoming symptomatic during a period of inadequate treatment of early syphilis.

neu·ro·ret·i·ni·tis (new″ro·ret·i·nigh′tis) *n.* Inflammation of both the optic nerve and the retina.

neu·ro·ret·i·nop·a·thy (new″ro·ret″i·nop′uth·ee) *n.* Any lesion of the retina not due to inflammation.

neu·ror·rha·phy (new·ror′uh·fee) *n.* The operation of suturing a divided nerve.

neu·ro·sar·co·ma (new″ro·sahr·ko′muh) *n.* A sarcoma having features suggesting a nervous system origin.

neu·ro·se·cre·tion (new″ro·se·kree′shun) *n.* **1.** The secretory activity of nerve cells. **2.** The product of secretory activity of nerve cells. —**neurosecre·to·ry** (·tuh·ree) *adj.*

neu·ro·sis (new·ro′sis) *n.,* pl. **neuro·ses** (·seez) **1.** *In psychiatry,* one of the two major categories of emotional maladjustments, classified according to the predominant symptom or defense mechanism. Anxiety is the chief symptom, and though there is no gross disorganization of personality in relation to external reality, there may be some impairment of thinking and judgment. A neurosis usually represents an attempt at resolving unconscious emotional conflicts in a way that diminishes the individual's effectiveness in living. **2.** *Obsol.* A nervous disorder.

neu·ro·skel·e·tal (new″ro·skel′e·tul) *adj.* Pertaining to nervous and skeletal muscular tissues.

neu·ro·spasm (new′ro·spaz·um) *n.* Spasm or twitching of a muscle due to or associated with a neurologic disorder.

Neu·ros·po·ra (new·ros′pur·uh) *n.* A generic name for one of the fungi, more commonly known as the bread mold, which is used as a bioassay organism in enzyme studies.

neu·ro·sthe·nia (new″ro-sthee′nee·uh) n. *Obsol.* Marked nervous excitement. **—neuro·sthen·ic** (·sthen′ick) adj.

neu·ro·sur·geon (new″ro-sur′jun) n. A physician who specializes in surgery of the central and peripheral nervous system.

neu·ro·sur·gery (new″ro-sur′jur·ee) n. Surgery of the nervous system. **—neurosur·gi·cal** (·ji·kul) adj.

neu·ro·syph·i·lis (new″ro-sif′i·lis) n. Syphilitic infection of the nervous system.

neu·ro·ther·a·py (new″ro-therr′up·ee) n. The treatment of nervous diseases.

neu·rot·ic (new·rot′ick) adj. & n. 1. Pertaining to or affected with a neurosis. 2. An individual affected with a neurosis.

neu·rot·i·ca (new·rot′i·kuh) n.pl. *Obsol.* Functional nervous disorders.

neurotic excoriation. Excoriation from scratching of the skin in response to psychogenic pruritis.

neu·rot·i·cism (new·rot′i·siz·um) n. A neurotic condition, character, or trait.

neu·roti·za·tion (newr″uh·tye·zay′shun, ·tiz·ay′) n. *Obsol.* 1. The regeneration of a divided nerve. 2. Surgical implantation of a nerve into a paralyzed muscle. 3. Providing an anatomic structure with a nerve supply.

neu·rot·me·sis (new″rot·mee′sis) n. A condition in which the connective-tissue structures and nerve constituents have been interrupted. In the regeneration of new nerve fibers, the new axons and connective tissue grow in misdirected confusion, preventing spontaneous regeneration of the nerve trunk.

neur·otol·o·gy (new″ro-tol′uh·jee) n. The branch of medical science dealing with the structure and functions of the internal ear, its nervous connections with the brain, and its central pathways within the brain.

neu·ro·tome (new′ro·tome) n. 1. An instrument for the division or dissection of a nerve. 2. One of the segments of the embryonic neural tube. Syn. *neuromere.*

neu·rot·o·my (new·rot′um·ee) n. The surgical division or dissection of some or all of the fibers of a nerve.

neu·ro·tox·ic (new″ro-tock′sick) adj. Harmful to nerve tissue. **—neuro·tox·ic·i·ty** (·tock·sis′i·tee) n.

neu·ro·tox·in (new″ro-tock′sin) n. A toxin capable of damaging nerve tissue.

neu·ro·trans·mit·ter (new″ro-trans·mit′ur) n. A chemical agent produced by a nerve cell, usually at the nerve ending, that reacts with a receptor on a neighboring cell or a cell at some distant site, and produces a response in the receptor cell, as, for example, acetylcholine, norepinephrine, vasopressin.

neu·ro·trau·ma (new″ro-traw′muh, ·trow′muh) n. Trauma to nervous tissue.

neu·ro·trip·sy (new″ro-trip″see) n. The crushing of a nerve.

neu·ro·troph·ic (new″ro-trof′ick, ·tro′fick) adj. Pertaining to the influence of nerves upon

nutrition and maintenance of normal condition in tissues.

neurotrophic arthritis. CHARCOT'S JOINT.

neurotrophic atrophy. Atrophy of muscle and overlying tissue as a result of separation of these tissues from their nerve supply, as seen in the chronic sensory neuropathies.

neurotrophic ulcer. Destruction of skin and underlying tissue as a result of separation of these tissues from their nerve supply, as seen in the chronic sensory neuropathies.

neu·ro·tro·pic (new″ro·tro′pick, ·trop′ick) adj. Having an affinity for, or localizing in, nervous tissue.

neu·rot·ro·pism (new·rot′ro·piz·um) n. An affinity for nervous tissue, said of certain chemicals, toxins, and viruses.

neu·ro·tu·bule (new″ro·tew′bewl) n. An elongated type of microtubule measuring 20 to 26 nm in transverse diameter, observed by electron microscopy in the axon, dendrites, and perikaryon of nerve cells.

neu·ro·vas·cu·lar (new″ro·vas′kew·lur) adj. Pertaining to both the nervous and vascular structures.

neurovisceral lipidosis. 1. FAMILIAL NEUROVISCERAL LIPIDOSIS. 2. FUCOSIDOSIS.

neutr–, neutro– A combining form meaning *neutral.*

neu·tral (new′trul) adj. 1. Inert, inactive; on neither one side nor the other. 2. Neither alkaline nor acid. **—neutral·i·ty** (new·tral′i·tee) n.

neu·tral·iza·tion (new″truh·li·zay′shun, ·lye·zay′ shun) n. 1. That process or operation which counterbalances or cancels the action of an agent. 2. *In medicine,* the process of checking the functioning of any agent that produces a morbid effect. 3. *In microbiology,* rendering innocuous a toxin or virus by combining it with its corresponding antitoxin or specific antibody. 4. *In chemistry,* a change of medium to that which is neither alkaline nor acid.

neu·tral·ize (new′truh·lize) v. To render neutral; render inert; to counterbalance an action or influence.

neutral stain. A compound produced by the interaction of an acid and a basic dye. It may give a stain differing from that imparted by either component.

neu·tri·no (new·tree′no) n. A hypothetical atomic particle having the mass of the electron but without an electric charge.

neu·tro·clu·sion (new″truh·klew′zhun) n. Occlusion in which the mesiobuccal cusp of the upper first molar interdigitates with the buccal groove of the lower first molar.

neu·tron (new′tron) n. An atomic nuclear particle with mass = 1 and charge = 0. A constituent of all atomic nuclei except $^1H_1$. (Isotopes differ from one another solely by the number of neutrons in their nuclei.) Free neutrons with various kinetic energies are produced in various nuclear reactions.

neutron capture. A form of nuclear reaction in which a neutron is absorbed by an atomic nucleus.

neutron capture therapy. A technique of internal radiation of an organ or tumor by the administration of a stable compound with an affinity for the organ or tumor and for neutron capture. The area is radiated with neutrons, the stable compound in the target cells becoming radioactive and subsequently undergoing radioactive decay resulting in intense local radiation.

neu·tro·pe·nia (new″tro·pee′nee·uh) *n.* A decrease below normal in the number of neutrophils per unit volume of peripheral blood.

neu·tro·phil (new′truh·fil) *n. & adj.* 1. NEUTROPHIL LEUKOCYTE. 2. Any histologic element which, according to Ehrlich's theory, will bind the neutral eosin-azure-methylene blue complex. 3. Stained readily by neutral dyes. —**neu·tro·phil·ic** (new″truh·fil′ick) *adj.*

neutrophil granules. Granules which take up simultaneously both a basic and an acid dye, assuming a combination tint.

neu·tro·phil·ia (new″tro·fil′ee·uh) *n.* 1. An affinity for neutral dyes. 2. An increase of neutrophil leukocytes in the blood or tissues.

neutrophil leukocyte. A highly motile and phagocytic (antimicrobial) leukocyte having numerous fine granules which do not stain definitely either blue (basic dye) or red (acid dye). Its polymorphous nucleus may be ribbonlike, bandlike, or segmented, having two to seven lobules. It has two classes of cytoplasmic granules, one lysosomal, the other smaller and specific.

nevi. Plural of *nevus.*

ne·vi·form (nee′vi·form) *adj.* NEVOID.

ne·vo·car·ci·no·ma, nae·vo·car·ci·no·ma (nee″vo·kahr·si·no′muh) *n.* A malignant melanoma.

ne·void, nae·void (nee′void) *adj.* 1. Nevuslike. 2. Associated with nevi.

nevoid cyst. A cyst whose walls contain a congeries of blood vessels.

ne·vo·mel·a·no·ma, nae·vo·mel·a·no·ma (nee″vo·mel·uh·no′muh) *n.* A malignant melanoma.

ne·vose, nae·vose (nee′voze, ·voce) *adj.* Spotted; having nevi.

ne·vo·xan·tho·en·do·the·li·o·ma, nae·vo·xan·tho·en·do·the·li·o·ma (nee″vo·zan″tho·en″do·theel·ee·o′muh) *n.* JUVENILE XANTHOGRANULOMA.

ne·vus, nae·vus (nee′vus) *n.,* pl. **ne·vi, nae·vi** (·vye) 1. Any lesion containing melanocytes. 2. *In dermatology,* a cutaneous hamartoma; a birthmark.

nevus ac·ne·i·for·mis uni·lat·e·ra·lis (ack″nee·i·for′mis yoo″ni·lat·ur·ay′lis). NEVUS COMEDONICUS.

nevus ara·ne·us (uh·ray′nee·us) SPIDER NEVUS.

nevus cell. MELANOCYTE.

nevus com·e·do·ni·cus (kom″e·do′ni·kus, ·don′i·kus). A unilateral verrucous nevus with hard follicular accretions simulating comedones of acne. Syn. *nevus acneiformis unilateralis, nevus follicularis.*

nevus flam·me·us (flam′ee·us) PORT-WINE NEVUS.

nevus fus·co·cae·ru·li·us oph·thal·mo·max·il·la·ris of Ota (fus″ko·se·roo′lee·us off·thal′mo·mack″si·lair′is) An aberrant Mongolian spot in the region of the eye and upper jaw.

nevus li·po·ma·to·des (li·po″muh·to′deez) An

elevated pigmented nevus with connective tissue and fat hypertrophy.

nevus pel·li·nus (pel·eye′nus) A markedly hairy nevus which has the appearance of pelt or fur.

nevus pig·men·to·sus (pig″men·to′sus). PIGMENTED NEVUS.

nevus pi·lo·sus (pi·lo′sus) HAIRY NEVUS.

nevus se·ba·ce·us (se·bay′see·us). A single lesion formed by an aggregate of sebaceous glands, usually as a linear streak, most often present since birth on the scalp and face. Syn. *Jadassohn's nevus.*

nevus spi·lus (spye′lus) A smooth, flat, pigmented nevus devoid of hair.

nevus uni·us lat·e·ra·lis (yoo′nee·us lat″ur·ay′lis). *Error.* Nevus unius lateris (= NEVUS VERRUCOSUS).

nevus uni·us lat·e·ris (yoo·nigh′us lat′ur·is, yoo′nee·us) NEVUS VERRUCOSUS.

nevus vas·cu·lo·sus (vas″kew·lo′sus). STRAWBERRY MARK.

nevus ver·ru·co·sus (verr″oo·ko′sus, verr′yoo·). A warty brown skin lesion often of linear shape, which is present at birth or appears in early life.

new·born, *adj. & n.* 1. Born recently; said of human infants less than a month old, especially of those only a few days old. 2. A newborn infant.

New·cas·tle disease. An acute, highly contagious, virus disease of fowls characterized by pneumonia and encephalomyelitis. This virus can cause mild follicular conjunctivitis in humans. Syn. *avian pneumoencephalitis, avian pseudoplague, Philippine fowl disease.*

Newcastle virus. An RNA, hemagglutinating myxovirus responsible for Newcastle disease.

nex·us (neck′sus) *n.,* pl. **nexuses** A tying or binding together, as the grouping of several causes which bring about an infectious disease; interlacing.

NF Abbreviation for *National Formulary.*

ng Abbreviation for *nanogram.*

NHLI National Heart and Lung Institute, one of the Institutes of Health.

N hormone. The factor or factors in adrenocortical secretions having nitrogen-retaining, or protein-anabolic, as well as androgenic activity. Syn. *nitrogen hormone.*

N.H.S. Abbreviation for *National Health Service.*

Ni Symbol for nickel.

NIA National Institute on Aging, one of the National Institutes of Health.

ni·a·cin (nigh′uh·sin) *n.* 3-Pyridinecarboxylic acid, $C_6H_5NO_2$, a component of the vitamin B complex; a specific for the treatment of pellagra. Syn. *nicotinic acid.*

ni·a·cin·a·mide (nigh″uh·sin′uh·mide, ·sin·am′ide) *n.* Nicotinic acid amide, $C_6H_6N_2O$; has the vitamin action of niacin but lacks its vasodilator effect. Syn. *nicotinamide.*

NIAID National Institute of Allergy and Infectious Diseases, one of the National Institutes of Health.

NIAMD National Institute of Arthritis and Metabolic Disease, former name of the NIAMDD.

NIAMDD National Institute of Arthritis, Meta

bolic and Digestive Diseases, one of the National Institutes of Health.

niche (nitch, neesh) *n.* RECESS.

NICHHD National Institute of Child Health and Human Development, one of the National Institutes of Health.

nick·el, *n.* Ni = 58.70. A metal of silver-white luster, with a density of 8.9, resembling iron in physical properties.

Nick·er·son-Kveim test. KVEIM TEST.

nick·ing, *n.* 1. Notching. 2. Localized constrictions of retinal veins. 3. Incising of the ventral muscles of the base of a horse's tail, causing the tail to be carried higher.

Ni·co·la's operation An operation for relief of habitual dislocation of the shoulder, by transplant of the long head of the biceps.

Nic·ol prism (nick'ul) A prism prepared from two obliquely bisected parts of a rhombohedron of calcite; used for production and analysis of polarized light.

nic·o·tin·am·ide (nick'uh-tin'uh-mide) *n.* Nicotinic acid amide, $C_6H_6N_2O$; has the vitamin action of nicotinic acid but lacks its vasodilator effect. Syn. *niacinamide.*

nicotinamide adenine dinucleotide. A nucleotide composed of one molecule each of adenine and nicotinamide, and two molecules each of D-ribose and phosphoric acid. It is a coenzyme for numerous hydrogenase reactions. Abbreviated, NAD. Syn. *nadide, diphosphopyridine nucleotide.*

nicotinamide adenine dinucleotide phosphate. A nucleotide composed of one molecule each of adenine and nicotinamide, two molecules of D-ribose, and three molecules of phosphoric acid. It is a coenzyme for oxidation of glucose 6-phosphate to 6-phosphogluconic acid in erythrocytes and is, like nicotinamide adenine dinucleotide, a coenzyme for many other dehydrogenase reactions. Abbreviated, NADP. Syn. *triphosphopyridine nucleotide.*

nic·o·tine (nick'uh-teen) *n.* 1-Methyl-2-(3-pyridyl)pyrrolidine, $C_{10}H_{14}N_2$, a colorless, liquid alkaloid in the leaves of the tobacco plant; a toxic substance responsible for many of the effects of tobacco.

nicotine stomatitis. Chronic inflammation and hyperkeratosis around the minor palatal salivary glands; caused by irritation from smoking.

nic·o·tin·ic acid (nick"o·tin'ick). 3-Pyridinecarboxylic acid, $C_6H_5NO_2$, a component of the vitamin B complex; a specific for the treatment of pellagra. Syn. *niacin.*

nic·ta·tion (nick·tay'shun) *n.* The act of blinking.

nic·ti·tate (nick'ti·tate) *n.* To blink, or blink repeatedly. —**nic·ti·tat·ing** (·tay·ting) *adj. & n.;* **nic·ti·ta·tion** (nick"ti·tay'shun) *n.*

nictitating membrane. The third eyelid of such vertebrates as reptiles and birds, represented vestigially in the human eye by the semilunar fold of the conjunctiva.

ni·da·tion (nigh·day'shun, ni·) *n.* The implantation of the fertilized ovum in the endometrium (decidua) of the pregnant uterus.

NIDR National Institute of Dental Research, one of the Institutes of Health.

ni·dus (nigh'dus) *n.,* pl. **ni·di** (·dye) 1. A locus of production or accumulation, such as a focus of infection or a site at which crystallization or precipitation is initiated. 2. A nestlike structure. —**ni·dal** (·dul) *adj.*

NIEHS National Institute of Environmental Health Sciences, one of the National Institutes of Health.

Nie·mann-Pick disease (nee'mahⁿ) A hereditary sphingolipidosis due to the deficiency of an enzyme which catalyzes the hydrolysis of phosphorylcholine from sphingomyelin, resulting in an abnormal accumulation of that substance; manifested in early life by anemia; enlargement of liver, spleen, and lymph nodes; and various neurologic deficits including retinal degeneration and mental retardation.

Niemann-Pick lipid SPHINGOMYELIN.

night blindness. The condition of reduced dark adaptation, resulting temporarily from vitamin A deficiency or permanently from retinitis pigmentosa or other peripheral retinal diseases. Syn. *nyctalopia.*

night cry. A shrill cry uttered during sleep; usually of psychic origin, but in a child sometimes symptomatic of a physical disorder.

night·mare, *n.* A terrifying anxiety dream due to the bursting forth of repressed sexual or aggressive impulses or the fear of death. It is characterized by feelings of helplessness, oppression, or suffocation, and usually awakens the sleeper.

night pain. Pain, usually in the hip or knee, occurring during muscular relaxation of the limb in sleep; often a symptom of disease of the joints.

night palsy. Numbness of the extremities, sometimes with weakness, occurring during the night, or on waking in the morning, due to positional compression of a part during sleep.

night·shade, *n.* Any of various plants of the family Solanaceae.

night sweat. Drenching perspiration occurring at night or whenever the patient sleeps, in the course of pulmonary tuberculosis or other febrile diseases.

night terrors. NIGHTMARE.

night vision. Vision at light intensities below the threshold at which cones are activated, using the rods and rhodopsin.

NIGMS National Institute of General Medical Sciences, one of the National Institutes of Health.

ni·gri·cans (nig'ri·kanz, nigh'gri·) *adj.* Black or blackish.

ni·gro·re·tic·u·lar (nigh"gro·re·tick'yoo·lur) *adj.* Pertaining to the substantia nigra and to the reticular formation.

ni·gro·ru·bral (nigh"gro·roo'brul) *adj.* Pertaining to the substantia nigra and to the red nucleus.

ni·gro·sine (nigh'gro·seen, ·sin) *n.* Any one of several black or dark blue aniline dyes; variously used in bacteriologic and histologic techniques.

ni·gro·stri·a·tal (nigh"gro·strye·ay'tul) *adj.* Pertaining to the substantia nigra and the corpus striatum.

NIH Abbreviation for *National Institutes of Health.*

ni·hil·ism (nigh'ul-iz-um, -hil-iz-um) *n.* 1. *In medicine,* pessimism in regard to the efficacy of treatment, particularly the use of drugs; therapeutic nihilism. 2. *In psychiatry,* the content of delusions encountered in depressed or melancholic states. The patient insists that his inner organs no longer exist, and that his relatives have passed away.

nik·eth·a·mide (nick-eth'uh-mide, -mid) *n.* N,N-Diethylnicotinamide, $C_{10}H_{14}N_2O$; stimulates medullary centers. Used, parenterally, as an analeptic, and for its respiratory stimulant effects.

NIMH National Institute of Mental Health, one of the National Institutes of Health.

NINDS National Institute of Neurological Diseases and Stroke, one of the National Institutes of Health.

Ninhydrin. Trademark for triketohydrindene hydrate, a reagent that gives a color reaction with proteins and amino acids.

niph·ablep·sia (nif"a-blep'see-uh) *n.* SNOW BLINDNESS.

nipho·typh·lo·sis (nif"o-tif-lo'sis) *n.* SNOW BLINDNESS.

nip·pers, *n.pl.* 1. An instrument for cutting the cuticle or nail. 2. A small bone-trimming forceps.

nip·ple, *n.* The conical projection in the center of the mamma, containing the outlets of the milk ducts.

Nissl bodies or **granules** Clumps of chromophil substance which represent stocks of rough endoplasmic reticulum in nerve cell cytoplasm. Their staining reactions (basophilia) are due to the ribosomes; CHROMOPHIL GRANULES.

Nissl reaction or **degeneration** AXONAL REACTION.

Nissl substance The chromophil substance of nerve cells.

ni·sus (nigh'sus) *n.* 1. Any strong effort or struggle. 2. The periodic desire for procreation manifested in the spring season by certain species of animals. Syn. *nisus formativus.* 3. The contraction of the diaphragm and abdominal muscles for the expulsion of feces, urine, or a fetus.

nit, *n.* The egg or the larva of a louse.

ni·ter, ni·tre (nigh'tur) *n.* SALTPETER.

nitr-, nitro-. A combining form designating (a) *the presence of the monovalent radical* NO_2; (b) *combination with nitrogen.*

ni·trate (nigh'trate) *n.* A salt or ester of nitric acid.

nitric acid. A liquid containing about 70% HNO_3, the remainder being water; has a characteristic, highly irritating odor and is very caustic and corrosive. Used externally as an escharotic.

ni·trite (nigh'trite) *n.* A salt or ester of nitrous acid.

ni·tri·tu·ria (nigh"tri-tew'ree-uh) *n.* The presence of nitrates or nitrites, or both, in the urine when voided.

ni·tro·cel·lu·lose (nigh"tro-sel'yoo-loce) *n.* Any nitrate ester, or mixture of nitrate esters, of cellulose.

ni·tro·fur·an·to·in (nigh"tro-few-ran'to-in) *n.* 1-[(5-Nitrofurfurylidene)amino]hydantoin, $C_8H_6N_4O_5$, a urinary antibacterial drug.

ni·tro·fur·a·zone (nigh"tro-few'ruh-zone) *n.* 5-Nitro-2-furaldehyde semicarbazone, $C_6H_6N_4O_4$, an antibacterial drug used topically.

ni·tro·gen (nigh'truh-jin) *n.* N = 14.0067. A nonmetallic element existing free in the atmosphere, of which it constitutes about 77 percent by weight. A colorless, odorless gas, incapable of sustaining life. Chemically relatively inert, but an important constituent of all animal and vegetable tissues.

nitrogen balance or **equilibrium.** The difference between the nitrogen excreted and the nitrogen taken into the body, excluding respiratory nitrogen.

nitrogen dioxide. NO_2. A toxic gas resulting from the decomposition of nitric acid.

nitrogen lag. The time elapsing between the ingestion of a protein and the appearance in the urine of an amount of nitrogen equal to that taken in.

nitrogen mustard. 1. MECHLORETHAMINE HYDROCHLORIDE. 2. Any of a series of nitrogen analogs of bis(2-chloroethyl) sulfide, the chemical warfare agent known as mustard gas. Several nitrogen mustards, including mechlorethamine hydrochloride, melphalan (L-phenylalanine mustard), and uracil mustard, are useful antineoplastic agents.

ni·trog·e·nous (nigh-troj'e-nus) *adj.* Containing nitrogen.

ni·tro·glyc·er·in (nigh"tro-glis'ur-in) *n.* Glyceryl trinitrate or glonoin, $C_3H_5(NO_3)_3$, an oily liquid which is explosive but when suitably dispersed may be handled safely. A prompt-acting coronary vasodilator usually administered sublingually.

ni·tro·hy·dro·chlo·ric acid (nigh"tro-high"druh-klor'ick). A mixture of 1 volume of nitric acid and 4 volumes of hydrochloric acid; has been used, well diluted, as a choleretic. Syn. *nitromuriatic acid, aqua regia.*

ni·tro·mer·sol (nigh"tro-mur'sol) *n.* 4-Nitro-3-hydroxymercuri-*o*-cresol anhydride, $C_7H_5HgNO_3$, an organomercurial antibacterial agent used topically.

ni·tro·prus·side (nigh"tro-prus'ide) *n.* Any salt containing the anion $[Fe(CN)_5NO]^{2-}$; a nitroferricyanide.

nitros-, nitroso-. A combining form signifying *combination with nitrosyl,* the univalent radical —NO.

ni·trous (nigh'trus) *adj.* 1. Containing nitrogen in a lower valence state than in corresponding nitric compounds. 2. Pertaining to or derived from nitrous acid.

nitrous oxide. A colorless gas, N_2O, used to produce anesthesia which consists mainly of moderate analgesia and minimum amnesia in dentistry and in surgery. Syn. *hyponitrous oxide, laughing gas, nitrogen monoxide.*

NK Nomenklatur Kommission; a committee appointed to revise the BNA. The recommendations of this committee, published in 1935, have not been widely adopted.

N.L.N. National League of Nursing.

nm Abbreviation for *nanometer*.

No. *Numero.* number, to the number of.

noble gases. The inert gases, helium, neon, argon, krypton, xenon, and radon, so called because they do not generally combine with other elements.

No·car·dia (no-kahr'dee-uh) *n.* A genus of aerobic branching organisms of the family Actinomycetaceae.

Nocardia as·ter·oi·des (as''tur·oy'deez) A species of *Nocardia* which is aerobic and acidfast; causes pulmonary, brain, and subcutaneous lesions, usually without granules.

Nocardia ma·du·rae (ma·dew'ree) A species of *Nocardia* which is one of the causes of whitegrained mycetoma.

Nocardia mi·nu·tis·si·ma (migh''new·tis'i·muh). A species of *Nocardia* associated with chronic infection of the stratum corneum known as erythrasma.

Nocardia so·ma·li·en·sis (so·mah·lee·en'sis) A species of *Nocardia* which is one of the causes of white-grained mycetoma.

Nocardia ten·u·is (ten'yoo·is) A species of *Nocardia* which is the causative agent of trichomycosis axillaris.

no·car·di·o·sis (no·kahr''dee·o'sis) *n.* Infection by certain species of *Nocardia*.

noci- A combining form meaning *pain*.

no·ci·cep·tor (no''si·sep'tur) *n.* A high-threshold receptor which responds to stimuli such as burning, crushing, cutting, or pressure sufficiently intense to cause tissue damage. —**noci·cep·tive** (-tiv) *adj.*

no·ci·per·cep·tion (no''si·pur·sep'shun) *n.* Perception of pain.

noct-, nocti-, nocto-, noctu- A combining form meaning *night*.

noc·tam·bu·la·tion (nock·tam''bew·lay'shun) *n.* SLEEPWALKING.

noc·ti·pho·bia (nock''ti·fo'bee·uh) *n.* Morbid fear of night or darkness.

noc·tu·ria (nock·tew'ree·uh) *n.* Frequency of urination at night. Syn. *nycturia*.

noc·tur·nal (nock·tur'nul) *adj.* 1. Occurring or becoming manifest at night. 2. Of animals, active at night.

nocturnal emission. Involuntary seminal discharge occurring during sleep in physiologically normal males beginning with puberty.

nocturnal enuresis. Involuntary urination at night during sleep, by a person in whom bladder control may normally be expected to be present; bed-wetting.

nocturnal pollution. NOCTURNAL EMISSION.

noc·u·ous (nock'yoo·us) *adj.* Injurious, noxious; poisonous.

nodal rhythm. JUNCTIONAL RHYTHM.

node, *n.* 1. A knob or protuberance. 2. A point of constriction. 3. A small, rounded organ. —**nod·al** (no'dul) *adj.*

node of Keith and Flack SINOATRIAL NODE.

node of Ran·vier (rahⁿv·yay') The region, in a myelinated nerve, of a local constriction in the myelin sheath at varying intervals on both central and peripheral axons. At each node, the axis cylinder is also constricted. Electron microscopy reveals that the node is formed by the end of one Schwann cell and the beginning of another.

node of Virchow-Troisier SIGNAL NODE.

no·dose (no'dose) *adj.* Characterized by nodes or protuberances; jointed or swollen at intervals.

no·dos·i·ty (no·dos'i·tee) *n.* 1. The character or state of being nodose. 2. NODE.

nod·u·lar (nod'yoo·lur) *adj.* Of or like a nodule; characterized by nodules.

nodular goiter. ADENOMATOUS GOITER.

nodular hidradenoma. MYOEPITHELIOMA.

nodular lymphoma. A variety of malignant lymphoma in which the anaplastic cells grow in such a fashion as to produce nodules superficially resembling the follicles of normal lymph nodes; it is associated with a better prognosis than that of the diffuse form. Syn. *Brill-Symmers disease, follicular lymphoma, giant follicular lymphoblastoma* or *lymphoma, lymphoreticulosis*.

nodular salpingitis. A form of salpingitis marked by formation of solid nodules.

nodular subepidermal fibrosis. DERMATOFIBROMA.

nod·u·la·tion (nod''yoo·lay'shun) *n.* The formation of nodules or the state of being nodular. —**nod·u·lat·ed** (nod'yoo·lay·tid) *adj.*

nod·ule (nod'yool) *n.* 1. A small node. 2. A small aggregation of cells. 3. *In dermatology.* one of the primary skin lesions, a circumscribed solid elevation of varying size but larger than a papule, which is of the order of 1 cm or less.

noduli. Plural of *nodulus*.

noduli Aran·tii (a·ran'shee·eye, ·tee·eye) NODULES OF THE SEMILUNAR VALVES.

no·du·lus (nod'yoo·lus, no'dew·lus) *n.,* pl. **nodu·li** (·lye). 1. NODULE. 2. [NA] One of the anterior subdivisions of the vermis of the cerebellum.

no·dus (no'dus) *n.,* pl. & genit. sing. **no·di** (·dye) NODE.

nodus lym·pha·ti·cus (lim·fat'i·kus), pl. **nodi lymphati·ci** (·sigh) [NA]. LYMPH NODE.

no·e·ma·ta·chom·e·ter (no·ee'muh·ta·kom'e·tur) *n.* An apparatus for estimating the time taken in recording a simple perception.

no·e·mat·ic (no·e·mat'ick) *adj.* Pertaining to thought or to any mental process.

no·e·sis (no·ee'sis) *n. In pyschology.* the cognitive process; perception, understanding, and reasoning. —**no·et·ic** (no·et'ick) *adj.*

Noludar. Trademark for methyprylon, a nonbarbiturate sedative and hypnotic.

no·ma (no'muh) *n.* Spreading gangrene beginning in the mucous membranes, most frequently in the mouth, but also the nose, external auditory canals, genitalia, or anus, usually following an infectious disease such as measles, and seen most frequently in children under conditions of poor hygiene and nutrition; generally regarded as a malignant form of infection by fusospirochetal organisms. Noma of the mouth is also known as gangrenous stomatitis.

no·mad·ic (no·mad′ick) *adj.* Spreading; wandering; loose.

no·men·cla·ture (no′min·klay″chur, no·meng′kluh·chur) *n.* A systematic arrangement of the distinctive names employed in any science.

No·mi·na An·a·to·mi·ca (nom′i·nuh an″uh·tom′i·kuh, no′mi·nuh). The international anatomical nomenclature in Latin. A revision of the Basle Nomina Anatomica, approved originally in Paris in 1955. Abbreviated, NA.

nom·i·nal (nom′i·nul) *adj.* 1. Pertaining to names. 2. In name only; formal, token.

nominal aphasia. ANOMIA.

nomo·gram (nom′o·gram) *n.* NOMOGRAPH.

nomo·graph (nom′o·graf) *n.* A graph on which appear graduated lines for all variables in a formula, arranged in such a manner that the value of one variable can be read on the appropriate line from a knowledge of the values of the other variables.

nomo·top·ic (nom″o·top′ick) *adj.* Occurring at the usual site.

¹non- A prefix meaning *not*.

²non- A combining form meaning *ninth. nine, nine times.*

non·ab·sorb·able (non″ub·sor′buh·bul) *adj.* Not absorbable.

non·ad·her·ent (non″ad·heer′unt) *adj.* Not connected to an adjacent organ or part.

no·nan (no′nun) *adj.* Having an exacerbation or recurring every ninth day.

non·aque·ous (non″ay′kwee·us, ·ack′wee·us) *adj.* Not consisting of, or pertaining to, water; said of organic solvents.

non·ar·tic·u·lar (non″ahr·tick′yoo·lur) *adj.* Not pertaining to joints.

nonarticular rheumatism. FIBROSITIS.

non·bac·te·ri·al gastroenteritis. An acute illness characterized by nausea, vomiting, and diarrhea, generally assumed to be caused by as yet unknown viruses. Syn. *winter vomiting disease.*

non·chro·maf·fin (non·kro′muh·fin, ·kro·maf′in) *adj.* Not chromaffin; not involving chromaffin cells.

nonchromaffin paraganglioma. CHEMODECTOMA.

nonchromaffin paraganglioma of the middle ear. GLOMUS JUGULARE TUMOR.

non com·pos men·tis (non kom′pus men′tis) Of unsound mind.

non·con·duc·tor (non″kun·duck′tur) *n.* Any substance not transmitting electricity or heat.

non·de·form·ing, *adj.* Not deforming.

non·dis·junc·tion (non″dis·junk′shun) *n.* 1. The failure of homologous material to separate at meiosis. 2. The failure of sister chromosomes to separate in an ordinary mitosis.

non·dom·i·nant (non″dom′i·nunt) *adj.* Not dominant.

non·en·cap·su·lat·ed (non″en·kap′sue·lay′tid) *adj.* Not encapsulated.

nonencapsulated sclerosing tumor. A small, well-differentiated papillary thyroid carcinoma with marked stromal fibrosis.

nonendemic goitrous cretinism. Cretinism as a result of defective synthesis of thyroid hormone due to defects in the trapping of iodide by the thyroid, iodide organification, cou-

pling, deiodinase activity, or the production of an abnormal serum iodoprotein.

non·equil·i·bra·to·ry (non″e·kwil′i·bruh·tor″ee, ·ee″kwi·lib′) *adj.* 1. Not pertaining to equilibrium. 2. Pertaining to or characterized by disequilibrium.

nonequilibratory ataxia. Disturbance of coordination involving the extremities and sparing equilibrium; usually due to a lesion of one or both cerebellar hemispheres, or of deep sensory pathways.

nonfluent aphasia. Aphasia in which speech is sparse, produced slowly with great effort, poorly articulated, agrammatical, and telegraphic in quality; due to a lesion in Broca's area.

non·gran·u·lar (non″gran′yoo·lur) *adj.* Not granular.

non·i·grav·i·da (no″ni·grav′i·duh, non″i·) *n.* A woman pregnant for the ninth time.

non·ion·ic (non″eye·on′ick) *adj.* Not ionic.

no·nip·a·ra (no·nip′uh·ruh, non·ip′) *n.* A woman who has been in labor nine times.

nonlipid histiocytosis. LETTERER-SIWE DISEASE.

nonlipid reticuloendotheliosis. LETTERER-SIWE DISEASE.

non·lu·et·ic (non″lew·et′ick) *adj.* Not due to syphilitic infection.

non·med·ul·la·ted (non″med′uh·lay″tid, ·me·dul′) *adj.* UNMYELINATED.

non·mo·tile (non·mo′til) *adj.* Not motile; not having the power of active motion.

non·my·e·li·nat·ed (non″migh′e·lin·ay″tid) *adj.* UNMYELINATED.

non·opaque (non″o·pake′) *adj.* Radiolucent or relatively permeable to x-rays; not opaque.

nonossifying fibroma. A common benign tumor of bone, exhibiting no osteogenic tendencies, usually found in the shaft of long bones, and histologically characterized by whorls of spindle-shaped connective-tissue cells.

non·os·teo·gen·ic (non″os·tee·o·jen′ick) *adj.* Not producing bone.

nonosteogenic fibroma. NONOSSIFYING FIBROMA.

non·ovu·la·to·ry (non″o′vyoo·luh·tor″ee) *adj.* Not ovulatory; not pertaining to ovulation.

non·patho·gen (non″path′o·jin) *n.* An organism or substance that is not pathogenic. —**non·patho·gen·ic** (non″path″o·jen′ick) *adj.*

non·pa·thog·no·mic (non″path″ug·nom′ick, ·no′mick) *adj.* NONPATHOGNOMONIC.

non·pro·tein (non″pro′tee·in, ·teen) *adj.* Not derived from protein, as nonprotein nitrogen; not containing protein, as nonprotein fraction of an extract.

nonprotein nitrogen. The fraction of nitrogen in the blood, tissues, urine, and excreta not precipitated by the usual protein precipitants such as sodium tungstate. Abbreviated, N.P.N.

non·pu·ru·lent (non·pewr′yoo·lunt) *adj.* NONPYOGENIC.

non·pyo·gen·ic (non″pye·o·jen′ick) *adj.* Not inducing the formation of pus.

non·re·frac·tive (non″re·frack′tiv) *adj.* Not possessing properties permitting the refraction of light rays.

non-REM sleep. NREM SLEEP.

non·re·straint (non″re′straint′) *n. In psychiatry,* the treatment of a psychotic, particularly a manic individual, without any forcible means of compulsion.

non·seg·ment·ed (non″seg′men·tid) *adj.* Not segmented.

non·spe·cif·ic (non″spe·sif′ick) *adj.* 1. Not attributable to any one definite cause, as a disease not caused by one particular microorganism, or an immunity not conferred by a specific antibody. 2. Of medicines or therapy, not counteracting any one causative agent.

nonspecific immunity. Resistance not assignable to specific antibodies or specific cellular immunity, and including such factors as genetics (innate immunity), age, sex, or hormonal factors.

nonspecific inflammation. Simple inflammation, as opposed to granulomatous inflammation.

nonspecific protein therapy. Treatment which recognizes that stock and autogenous vaccines may owe a part of their value in disease therapy to nonspecific effects; for example, peptone, milk, normal serum, etc., have been employed to replace bacterial products.

nonspecific urethritis. An acute nongonococcal urethritis with a urethral discharge and dysuria; common as a venereal infection; *Chlamidia* and *Mycoplasma* have been implicated in some cases.

non·spo·rog·e·nous (non″spo·roj′e·nus) *adj.* Not sporogenous; not producing spores.

non·stri·at·ed (non″strye′ay·tid) *adj.* Not striated; smooth.

non·sup·pu·ra·tive (non″sup′yoo·ray″tiv) *adj.* Uninfected; surgically clean; not forming pus.

non·sur·gi·cal (non″sur′ji·kul) *adj.* Not surgical; without surgical operation.

non·throm·bo·cy·to·pe·nic (non″throm″bo·sigh·to·pee′nick) *adj.* Not thrombocytopenic.

non·un·ion (non″yoon′yun) *n.* Failure of union; especially, failure of fractured bone ends to unite firmly.

non·ve·ne·re·al (non″ve·neer′ee·ul) *adj.* Not venereal.

nonvenereal syphilis. 1. Syphilis not acquired during sexual intercourse. 2. BEJEL.

non·vi·a·ble (non″vye′uh·bul) *adj.* Not viable; incapable of surviving.

non·vi·su·al·iza·tion (non″vizh″yoo·ul·i·zay′shun, ·eye·zay′shun) *n.* Failure of an excretory organ to opacify roentgenographically after administration of radiopaque contrast materials which normally opacify that organ.

noo·psy·che (no′o·sigh″kee) *n.* Mental or reasoning processes.

N.O.P.H.N. National Organization for Public Health Nursing.

nor- A prefix indicating (a) *removal from a parent compound of a radical* (often methyl) *to form another compound;* (b) *a compound of normal structure isomeric with another compound having the same name but without the prefix,* as norleucine and leucine.

nor·epi·neph·rine (nor·ep″i·nef′reen, ·rin) *n.* α-(Aminomethyl)-3,4-dihydroxybenzyl alcohol, $C_8H_{11}NO_3$, a demethylated epinephrine. The levorotatory isomer (levarterenol) is formed at sympathetic nerve endings as a mediator of functional activity; it is probably the postulated sympathin E. Therapeutically it is useful for maintenance of blood pressure in acute hypotensive states caused by surgical and nonsurgical trauma, central vasomotor depression, and hemorrhage; the bitartrate salt is commonly employed. Syn. *arterenol, noradrenaline.*

nor·eth·in·drone (nor·eth′in·drone) *n.* 17α-Ethinyl-19-nortestosterone, $C_{20}H_{26}O_2$, a potent, orally active progestogen that produces clinical effects similar to those of progesterone; also used, in combination with an estrogen, as an oral contraceptive.

nor·ethy·no·drel (nor″e·thigh′no·drel, ·eth′i·no·) *n.* 17-Hydroxy-19-nor-17α-pregn-5(10)-en-20-yn-3-one, $C_{20}H_{26}O_2$, a progestogen; used principally, in combination with the estrogen mestranol, to inhibit ovulation and control fertility.

nor·leu·cine (nor·lew′seen, ·sin) *n.* 2-Aminohexanoic acid, $C_6H_{13}NO_2$, an amino acid.

Norlutin. Trademark for norethindrone, an orally active progestogen.

norm, *n.* A standard representing the average, typical, or acceptable.

nor·ma (nor′muh) *n.,* pl. **nor·mae** (·mee) *In anatomy,* a view or aspect, essentially of the skull.

nor·mal, *adj.* 1. Conforming to some ideal norm or standard; pertaining to the central values of some homogeneous group, as that which is typical of or acceptable to a majority or dominant group; average, common, mean, median, standard, typical, usual, ideal, modal. 2. *In medicine and psychology,* "healthy," i.e., lacking observable or detectable clinical abnormalities, deficiencies, or diseases; also, pertaining to or describing a value or measurement obtained in an ideal group by a particular method, i.e., a value which in itself is not significant of disease; pertaining to the normal variability of an individual's anatomical, physiological, and psychological pattern within the parameters of age, sex, social and physical anthropological factors, population or segment thereof to which the individual belongs, and variability in time, activity, etc. Normal variability frequently is used to cover the values falling within some range, usually the 95-percent range of some factor or factors (mental, physical, emotional, social) measured in a random or selected sample of population or even an individual by standardized methods and recording system during many observations. 3. *In chemistry,* referring to solutions containing the equivalent weight of a substance, in grams, in a liter. Abbreviated, N. 4. *In mathematics,* pertaining to a right angle, i.e., in a perpendicular line or plane.

nor·mal·cy (nor′mul·see) *n.* The condition or state of being normal (1,2).

normal distribution. *In statistics,* a frequency distribution, specified by its mathematical form and two constants, the mean and the standard deviation. This distribution is continuous and bell-shaped; 95 percent of the area covered by the distribution curve lies within two standard deviations below and two above the mean. This distribution describes adequately some individual biological measurements and many random sample measurements.

nor·mal·i·ty (nor-mal'i-tee) *n.* The quality or state of being normal.

normal saline solution. SODIUM CHLORIDE IRRIGATION; a sterile solution of 0.9 g of sodium chloride in 100 ml of purified water. Isotonic with body fluids; variously used as a physiological salt solution but not to be employed parenterally, for which purpose sodium chloride injection is used. Syn. *normal salt solution.*

normal tremor. A tremor present in all muscle groups of the body that persists throughout the waking state and sleep. It is so fine that it cannot be recognized by the naked eye and requires special instruments to be detected. It ranges in frequency between 8 and 13 Hz, the usual rate being 10 Hz in adults and somewhat slower in children and in the elderly. Syn. *physiologic tremor.*

normo-. A combining form meaning *normal.*

nor·mo·blast (nor'mo-blast) *n.* 1. The smallest of the nucleated precursors of the erythrocyte, and of slightly larger size than the adult erythrocyte. It has almost a full complement of hemoglobin and shows a small, centrally placed chromatic and pyknotic nucleus. It is usually considered that a single normoblast gives rise to a single erythrocyte. 2. In some terminologies, any nucleated cell of the erythrocytic series.

nor·mo·chro·mic (nor'mo-kro'mick) *adj.* Pertaining to or characterizing blood in which the erythrocytes have a mean corpuscular hemoglobin (MCH) or color index and a mean corpuscular hemoglobin concentration (MCHC) or saturation index within (plus or minus) two standard deviations of the mean normal as determined by the same method on the blood of healthy persons of the same age and sex group.

normochromic anemia. A type of anemia in which the hemoglobin content of the red blood cell is normal.

nor·mo·cyte (nor'mo-site) *n.* An erythrocyte having both a diameter and a mean corpuscular volume (MCV) within (plus or minus) two standard deviations of the mean normal determined by the same method on the blood of healthy persons of the same age and sex group. **—nor·mo·cyt·ic** (nor'mo-sit'ick) *adj.*

normocytic anemia. Anemia in which the erythrocytes are of normal size.

nor·mo·cy·to·sis (nor'mo-sigh-to'sis) *n.* A normal state of the cells of the blood.

nor·mo·gly·ce·mia (nor'mo-glye-see'mee-uh) *n.* Normal concentration of glucose in the blood.

nor·mo·ka·le·mic (nor'mo-ka-lee'mick) *adj.* Having normal blood potassium levels; not hyperkalemic or hypokalemic.

nor·mo·re·flex·ia (nor'mo-re-fleck'see-uh) *n.* The state of having reflexes of the usual strength.

nor·mo·ten·sive (nor'mo-ten'siv) *adj.* Pertaining

to or having normal blood pressure; not hypertensive or hypotensive.

nor·mo·ther·mia (nor'mo-thur'mee-uh) *n.* A state of normal temperature.

nor·mo·vo·le·mia (nor'mo-vo-lee'mee-uh) *n.* The blood volume found in normal healthy individuals.

North American blastomycosis. A primary pulmonary infection, due to *Blastomyces dermatitidis,* that frequently disseminates to the skin and other organs. Syn. *Gilchrist disease.*

North Asian tick-borne rickettsiosis. Infection caused by *Rickettsia siberica* occurring in Siberia, Mongolia, Central Asia, and Armenia, closely related to boutonneuse fever and Rocky Mountain spotted fever.

nor·trip·ty·line (nor-trip'ti-leen) *n.* 5-(3-Methylaminopropylidene)-10,11-dihydro-5*H*-dibenzo[*a,d*]cycloheptene, $C_{19}H_{21}N$, an antidepressant and tranquilizing drug; used as the hydrochloride salt.

Nor·we·gian itch. A severe variety of scabies; has been seen in many countries, including the United States; scabies crustosa.

nos·ca·pine (nos'kuh-peen) *n.* An alkaloid, $C_{22}H_{23}NO_7$, from opium; used as a nonaddicting antitussive. Syn. *narcotine.*

nose, *n.* The prominent organ in the center of the face; the upper part (regio olfactoria) constitutes the organ of smell, the lower part (regio respiratoria) the beginning of the respiratory tract, in which the inspired air is warmed, moistened, and deprived of impurities.

nose·bleed, *n.* A hemorrhage from the nose. Syn. *epistaxis.*

no·se·ma·to·sis (no-see'muh-to'sis) *n.* ENCEPHALITOZOONOSIS.

noso-. A combining form meaning *disease.*

nos·o·co·mi·al (nos'o-ko'mee-ul) *adj.* 1. Pertaining to a hospital. 2. Of disease, caused or aggravated by hospital life.

no·sog·e·ny (no-soj'e-nee) *n.* The development of diseases; PATHOGENESIS. **—noso·ge·net·ic** (nos'o-je-net'ick) *adj.*

no·sol·o·gy (no-sol'uh-jee) *n.* The science of the classification of diseases. **—no·so·log·ic** (nos'o-loj'ick, no"so-), **nosolog·i·cal** (-i-kul) *adj.*

noso·ma·nia (nos'o-may'nee-uh) *n.* 1. NOSOPHOBIA. 2. A delusion that one is suffering from disease; extreme HYPOCHONDRIASIS.

no·som·e·try (no-som'e-tree) *n.* The calculation of morbidity rates.

noso·phil·ia (nos'o-fil'ee-uh) *n.* Love of sickness, a desire to be ill.

noso·pho·bia (nos'o-fo'bee-uh) *n.* An exaggerated fear of disease.

Nosopsyllus fas·ci·a·tus (fash'ee-ay'tus). A species of rat fleas which may transmit plague.

nos·tal·gia (nos-tal'juh, -jee-uh) *n.* 1. A strong desire to return to things or conditions of the past. 2. HOMESICKNESS. **—nostal·gic** (-jick) *adj.*

nos·to·ma·nia (nos'to-may'nee-uh) *n.* A pathologic degree of nostalgia, particularly of homesickness.

nos·top·a·thy (nos-top'uth-ee) *n.* Pathogenic homecoming, as observed in veterans discharged from military service or others who have spent a considerable length of time in institutions such as hospitals or prisons. The situational factor of returning home represents a major psychological stress which precipitates illness. The stress may be a fear of assuming adult responsibilities, a reaction against a dependency situation, guilt feelings, or difficulties in controlling instinctual rivalry.

nos·to·pho·bia (nos″to·fo′bee·uh) *n.* A fear of returning home.

nos·tril (nos′tril) *n.* One of the external orifices of the nose.

nos·trum (nos′trum) *n.* A quack medicine; a secret medicine.

not-, noto- A combining form meaning *back, dorsal.*

notalgia par·es·thet·i·ca (păr″es·thet′i·kuh) A sensory disturbance of the region supplied by the posterior branches of the lumbar nerves; occurs occasionally in vertebral lesions.

no·ta·tion (no·tay′shun) *n.* A system of symbols to indicate in brief form more extensive ideas or data.

notch, *n.* A deep indentation; incisure. **—notched,** *adj.*

notched teeth. Teeth with irregular incisal edges due to imperfect fusion or hypoplasia of the developmental lobes.

no·ten·ceph·a·lus (no″ten·sef′ul·us) *n. Obsol.* An individual with occipital encephalocele, or more usually hydrencephalocele.

no·ti·fi·a·ble (no″ti·fye′uh·bul) *adj.* Pertaining to a disease which must by law be reported to health authorities.

no·to·chord (no′tuh·kord) *n.* An elongated cord of cells enclosed in a structureless sheath, which is the primitive axial skeleton of the embryo. It serves as a focal axis about which the vertebral bodies develop and persists as the nuclei pulposi of the intervertebral disks. Syn. *chorda dorsalis.* **—no·to·chord·al** (no″tuh·kor′dul) *adj.*

notochordal canal. A canal formed by a continuation of the primitive pit into the head process of mammals. It perforates the entoderm and opens into the yolk sac, thus forming a temporary connection between yolk sac and amnion.

Novatrin. A trademark for homatropine methylbromide.

Novatropine. A trademark for homatropine methylbromide.

no·vo·bi·o·cin (no″vo·bye′o·sin) *n.* An antibiotic, $C_{31}H_{36}N_2O_{11}$, produced by *Streptomyces niveus* (known also as *S. spheroides*). Used as the calcium or sodium salt for treatment of staphylococcic infections.

Novocain. A trademark for procaine hydrochloride.

nox·ious (nock′shus) *adj.* Harmful, deleterious; poisonous.

NP In U.S. Army medicine, neuropsychiatric.

Np Symbol for neptunium.

NPD No pathologic diagnosis.

NPH Iletin. Trademark for NPH insulin or isophane insulin suspension.

NPH insulin. *Neutral Protamine Hagedorn* insu-

lin; a preparation of isophane insulin with intermediate duration of action developed Hagedorn; consists of crystals containing i sulin, protamine, and zinc, suspended in buffered medium of pH 7.2. Syn. *isopha insulin suspension.*

N.P.N. Abbreviation for *nonprotein nitrogen.*

n-rays, *n.pl.* A nonexistent form of radiant e ergy once considered to have a variety properties such as ability to pass through th metals and to increase the luminosity of pho phorescent bodies. Syn. *Blondot's rays.*

NREM sleep The phases of sleep in which n ther rapid eye movements nor dreams occ the first four stages of the normal sleep cyc

nu·bile (new′bil) *adj.* Marriageable; of an age childbearing. **—nu·bil·i·ty** (new·bil′i·tee) *n.*

nu·cha (new′kuh) *n.* The nape of the neck. **—n chal** (·kul) *adj.*

nuchal ligament. An elastic ligament extendi from the external occipital protuberance the spinous process of the seventh cervi vertebra.

nuchal rigidity. Stiffness of the neck and resi ance to passive movements, particula flexion, usually accompanied by pain a spasm on attempts at motion; recogniz widely as the most common sign, after ea infancy, of meningeal irritation, notably meningitis and bleeding into the subarac noid space.

Nuck's canal or **diverticulum** (ncck) CANAL NUCK.

Nuck's hydrocele A hydrocele resulting fro incomplete disappearance, in the female, the vaginal process of the peritoneum.

nucle-, nucleo-. A combining form meani *nucleus* or *nuclear.*

nu·cle·ar (new′klee·ur) *adj.* Pertaining to, constituting, a nucleus.

nuclear cap. A small mass of chromophilic m ter on one side of a cell nucleus.

nuclear cataract. A cataract beginning in t nucleus of the lens.

nuclear energy. Energy released in reactio involving the nucleus of an atom, especially quantities sufficient to be of interest in en neering or in astrophysics.

nuclear fission. *In chemistry and physics,* t splitting of certain heavy nuclei into two lar fragments, accompanied by the emission neutrons and the release of large amounts energy.

nuclear medicine. The branch of medicine th deals with the use of radioisotopes in diagr sis and therapy.

nuclear ophthalmoplegia. Inability to move t eye due to a lesion of the nuclei of origin of t motor nerves of the eyeball.

nuclear paralysis. Paralysis from lesions of t nuclei of origin of the nerves.

nuclear reactor. An apparatus in which nucle fission may be sustained in a self-supporti chain reaction. It includes fissionable mater such as uranium or plutonium (referred to fuel) and generally a moderating mater such as carbon or heavy water; also, a refle tor to conserve escaping neutrons, and provision for heat removal. Syn. *pile.*

nuclear sclerosis. Hardening of the nucleus lentis associated with aging of the ocular lens, which also becomes less pliable, loses its normal clarity, and enlarges. Nuclear sclerosis can give rise to myopia, and in advanced cases can lead to nuclear cataract.

nu·cle·ase (new'klee·ace, ·aze) *n.* An enzyme capable of splitting nucleic acids to nucleotides, nucleosides, or the components of the latter.

nu·cle·at·ed (new'klee·ay'tid) *adj.* Possessing a nucleus.

nuclei. Plural and genitive singular of *nucleus.*

nu·cle·ic acid (new·klee'ick). One of a group of compounds found in nuclei and cytoplasm, which on complete hydrolysis yields pyrimidine and purine bases, a pentose sugar, and phosphoric acid.

nu·cle·ide (new'klee·ide) *n.* A compound of nuclein with some metal, as iron, copper, silver, mercury, etc.

nu·cle·i·form (new'klee·i·form, new·klee') *adj.* Resembling a nucleus.

nu·cle·in (new'klee·in) *n.* Any one of a group of ill-defined complexes of protein and nucleic acid occurring in the nuclei of cells. On hydrolysis, they yield simple proteins and nucleic acid.

nu·cle·in·ic acid (new''klee·in'ick). NUCLEIC ACID.

nu·cleo·cap·sid (new''klee·o·kap'sid) *n.* The structure of a virus, composed of the capsid, or the protein coat, and the enclosed viral nucleic acid.

nu·cleo·cy·to·plas·mic (new''klee·o·sigh''to·plaz'mick) *adj.* Pertaining to both the nucleus and cytoplasm of a cell.

nucleocytoplasmic ratio. The ratio of the measured cross-sectional area or the estimated volume of the nucleus of a cell to its cytoplasm.

nu·cle·of·u·gal (new''klee·off'yoo·gul, new''klee·o·few'gul) *adj.* Moving away from a nucleus.

nucleoli. Plural of *nucleolus.*

nu·cle·o·loid (new·klee'uh·loid) *adj.* Resembling a nucleolus.

nu·cle·on (new'klee·on) *n.* An atomic nuclear particle; a proton or a neutron.

nu·cle·on·ics (new''klee·on'icks) *n.* The study of atomic nuclei, including the application of nuclear science in all fields of specialization; nuclear technology.

nu·cleo·phil·ic (new''klee·o·fil'ick) *adj.* Having an affinity for atomic nuclei whereby a bond is formed when an ion or molecule (called the nucleophilic agent) donates a pair of electrons to an electrophilic ion or molecule.

nu·cleo·plasm (new'klee·o·plaz·um) *n.* The protoplasm of the nucleus. Syn. *karyoplasm.*

nu·cleo·pro·te·id (new''klee·o·pro'tee·id) *n.* NUCLEOPROTEIN.

nu·cleo·pro·tein (new''klee·o·pro'tee·in, ·teen) *n.* A protein constituent of cell nuclei, consisting of nucleic acid and a basic protein, which on hydrolysis yields purine and pyrimidine

bases, phosphoric acid, and a pentose sugar, in addition to the protein.

nu·cleo·sid·ase (new''klee·o·sigh'dace, ·daze, ·o'si·dace) *n.* An enzyme that catalyzes the hydrolysis of a nucleoside into its component pentose and purine or pyrimidine base.

nu·cleo·side (new'klee·o·side) *n.* A glycoside resulting from the removal of phosphate from a nucleotide. It is a combination of a sugar (pentose) with a purine or pyrimidine base.

nu·cleo·tide (new'klee·o·tide) *n.* An ester of phosphoric acid and a pentose sugar linked to a pyrimidine or purine base; a phosphorylated nucleoside. The basic structural unit of a nucleic acid.

nu·cleo·tox·in (new''klee·o·tock'sin) *n.* 1. A toxin derived from cell nuclei. 2. Any toxin affecting the nuclei of cells. —**nucleotox·ic** *adj.*

nu·cle·us (new'klee·us) *n.,* pl. & genit. sing. **nu·clei** (·klee·eye) 1. The differentiated central protoplasm of a cell; its trophic center. 2. A collection of nerve cells in the central nervous system concerned with a particular function. 3. A stable and characteristic complex of atoms to which other atoms may be attached. 4. The center around which the mass of a crystal aggregates. 5. The core of an atom consisting of protons, neutrons, and alpha particles.

nucleus am·bi·gu·us (am·big'yoo·us) [NA]. A column of cells lying in the lateral half of the reticular formation whose cells give origin to efferent fibers of the glossopharyngeal, vagus, and accessory nerves. Syn. *ambiguus nucleus.*

nucleus cu·ne·a·tus (kew·nee·ay'tus) [NA]. CUNEATE NUCLEUS.

nucleus len·tis (len'tis) [NA]. The nucleus of the lens; the harder central portion of the crystalline lens of the eye.

nucleus pul·po·sus (pul·po'sus), pl. **nuclei pulpo·si** (·sigh) [NA]. The pulpy body at the center of an intervertebral disk; a remnant of the notochord.

nucleus ru·ber (roo'bur) [NA]. RED NUCLEUS.

nu·clide (new'klide) *n.* A species of atom characterized by the constitution of its nucleus, in particular by the number of protons and neutrons in the nucleus.

nud·ism (new'diz·um) *n.* 1. *In psychiatry,* a more or less complete intolerance of clothing; a pathologic tendency to remove the clothing. 2. The practice or cult of those who profess to believe in the benefits of society in which clothes are discarded.

nui·sance, *n. In legal medicine,* that which is noxious, offensive, or capable of causing distress; applied to persons or things.

nul·lip·a·ra (nuh·lip'ur·uh) *n.* A woman who has never borne a child. —**nullipa·rous** (·rus) *adj.;* **nul·li·par·i·ty** (nul''i·păr'i·tee) *n.*

numb, *adj.* Of a part of the body: anesthetic; having deadened sensation.

numb·ness, *n.* Partial or local anesthesia with torpor; deficiency of sensation.

nu·mer·i·cal aperture. A mathematical expression of the resolving power of a microscope objective; specifically, the product of the sine of one-half the angle of aperture of the lens and the refractive index of the medium in front of the lens.

num·mu·lar (num'yoo-lur) *adj.* 1. Resembling a coin in form, as nummular sputum. 2. Resembling rouleaux or rolls of coin.

nummular dermatitis. Coin-shaped patches of vesicular dermatitis, usually affecting the extensor surfaces of the forearms and legs.

nummular erythema. Discoid lesions of tinea corporis.

nummular sputum. Sputum containing small, round, flattened masses of heavy material resembling coins.

num·mu·la·tion (num''yoo·lay'shun) *n.* The aggregation of blood cells into coinlike rolls or rouleaux.

Numorphan. Trademark for the semisynthetic narcotic analgesic oxymorphone, used as the hydrochloride salt.

nun·na·tion (nuh·nay'shun) *n.* The frequent, or abnormal, use of the *n* sound.

Nupercaine. A trademark for dibucaine, a local anesthetic used as the base and as the hydrochloride salt.

¹nurse, *n.* 1. One who cares for a sick person under supervision of a physician. 2. One who cares for an infant or young child; nursemaid.

²nurse, *v.* 1. To suckle (an infant). 2. Of an infant: to take milk from the breast. 3. To care for (a sick person).

nurse corps. The nurses in the Armed Services, who have ranks, titles, and status as officers in those services.

nurse-maid's elbow. PULLED ELBOW.

nurse's aide. A worker in a hospital or other medical facility who assists nurses in nonspecialized tasks of patient care, such as bathing, feeding, making beds, taking weights and temperatures.

nurses' registry. An office listing nurses available for general or special services.

nurs·ing, *n.* 1. Care for the ill and infirm. 2. The practice and profession of ¹nurses (1).

nurs·ling, *n.* A nursing infant; an infant that has not been weaned.

nu·ta·tion (new·tay'shun) *n.* Nodding or oscillation.

nut·meg liver. Chronic passive hyperemia of the liver; named for the resemblance of the cut surface of such a liver to the cut surface of a nutmeg.

nu·tri·ent (new'tree·unt) *adj. & n.* 1. Affording nutrition. 2. A substance that affords nutrition.

nutrient artery. An artery that supplies blood to a bone.

nu·tri·lite (new'tri·lite) *n.* A substance which, in small amounts, functions in the nutrition of microorganisms.

nu·tri·ment (new'tri·munt) *n.* Anything that nourishes.

nu·tri·tion (new·trish'un) *n.* 1. The sum of the processes concerned in the growth, maintenance, and repair of the living body as a whole, or of its constituent parts. 2. Especially, those processes most directly involved in the intake, metabolism, and utilization of food; nourishment. —**nutri·tion·al** (·ul) *adj.*

nutritional anemia. Anemia associated with nutritional deficiencies, usually of iron.

nutritional edema. Edema occurring in starvation or in a poorly nourished state. Syn. *famine edema, hunger edema.*

nu·tri·tious (new·trish'us) *adj.* Nourishing; rich in nutritive substances.

nu·tri·tive (new'tri·tiv) *adj.* 1. Of or pertaining to nutrition. 2. Providing nourishment.

nux vom·i·ca (nucks''vom'i·kuh) The seed of *Strychnos nux-vomica,* an Indian tree of the Loganiaceae. It contains the alkaloid strychnine, for the effects of which nux vomica were formerly used in medicine.

nyct-, nycto- A combining form meaning *night.*

nyc·tal·gia (nick·tal'jee·uh) *n.* Pain which occurs chiefly during the night or during sleep.

nyc·ta·lope (nick'tuh·lope) *n.* One who cannot see well in reduced light.

nyc·ta·lo·pia (nick''tuh·lo'pee·uh) *n.* NIGHT BLINDNESS.

nyc·ta·pho·nia (nick''tuh·fo'nee·uh, nikt''a·) *n.* A conversion type of hysterical neurosis in which there is loss of the voice during the night only.

nyc·ter·ine (nick'tur·ine, ·een, ·in) *adj.* 1. Occurring in the night. 2. Obscure.

nyc·te·ro·hem·er·al (nick''tuh·ro·hem'ur·ul) *adj.* NYCTOHEMERAL.

nyc·to·hem·er·al (nick''to·hem'ur·ul) *adj.* Pertaining to day and night, as in circadian rhythm.

nyc·to·phil·ia (nick''to·fil'ee·uh) *n.* Preference for night or darkness.

nyc·to·pho·nia (nick''to·fo'nee·uh) *n.* A conversion type of hysterical neurosis in which there is loss of the voice during the day in one who is capable of speaking during the night.

nyc·to·typh·lo·sis (nick''to·tif·lo'sis) *n.* NIGHT BLINDNESS.

Nydrazid. A trademark for isoniazid, a tuberculostatic drug.

ny·li·drin (nye'li·drin, nil'i·drin) *n.* 1-(*p*-Hydroxyphenyl)-2-(1-methyl-3-phenylpropylamino)propanol, $C_{19}H_{25}NO_2$, a peripheral vasodilator; used as the hydrochloride salt.

nymph, *n.* The immature stage of an insect during which the wing pads first appear and the reproductive organs have not developed to the functional stage.

nymph-, nympho- A combining form signifying (a) *nymphae, labia minora;* (b) *female sexuality.*

nym·phec·to·my (nim·feck'tum·ee) *n.* Surgical removal of one or both labia minora of the vulva.

nym·phi·tis (nim·fye'tis) *n.* Inflammation of the labia minora.

nym·pho·lep·sy (nim'fo·lep''see) *n.* Ecstasy of an erotic type.

nym·pho·ma·nia (nim''fo·may'nee·uh) *n.* Excessive sexual desire on the part of a woman. Syn. *hysteromania.* —**nymphoma·ni·ac** (·nee·ack) *adj. & n.*

nym·phot·o·my (nim·fot'um·ee) *n.* Incision of one or both of the labia minora.

nystagm-, nystagmo-. A combining form meaning *nystagmus.*

nys·tag·mi·form (nis·tag′mi·form) *adj.* Resembling nystagmus.

nys·tag·mo·graph (nis·tag′mo·graf) *n.* An apparatus for recording the movements of the eyeball in nystagmus.

nys·tag·mog·ra·phy (nis″tag·mog′ruf·ee) *n.* The study and recording of the movements of the eyeballs in nystagmus.

nys·tag·moid (nis·tag′moid) *adj.* Resembling nystagmus.

nys·tag·mus (nis·tag′mus) *n.* An oscillatory movement of the eyeballs. It may be congenital, acquired, physiologic, or pathologic; due to neurogenic, myopathic, labyrinthine, or ocular causes.

nys·ta·tin (nis′tuh·tin, nis′tat·in) *n.* An antibiotic substance, $C_{46}H_{77}NO_{19}$, produced by *Streptomyces noursei;* used as an antifungal agent for the treatment of infections caused by *Candida* (*Monilia*) *albicans*.

O

O Symbol for oxygen.

O. Abbreviation for (a) *oculus,* eye; (b) *octarius,* pint; (c) *occiput.*

o- *In chemistry,* symbol for ortho-.

O agglutinin. An agglutinin specific for the somatic antigens of a microorganism.

O antigen. The thermostable, somatic antigen of the enteric and related gram-negative bacilli.

oast-house urine disease METHIONINE MALAB-SORPTION SYNDROME.

oat-cell carcinoma. A poorly differentiated carcinoma, usually of the lung, in which the anaplastic cells bear a fancied resemblance to oats.

oath of Hip·poc·ra·tes (hi·pock′ruh·teez). HIPPO-CRATIC OATH.

ob·ce·ca·tion, ob·cae·ca·tion (ob″se·kay′shun) *n.* Partial blindness.

ob·duc·tion (ob·duck′shun) *n.* A postmortem examination; an autopsy; a necropsy.

obese (o·beece′) *adj.* Extremely fat; corpulent.

obe·si·ty (o·bee′si·tee, o·bes′i·tee) *n.* An increase of body weight due to accumulation of fat, 10 to 20 percent beyond the normal range for the particular age, sex, and height.

obex (o′becks) *n.* The thin triangular lamina formed by the meeting of the taeniae choroideae of the fourth ventricle over the caudal limit of the cavity.

ob·fus·ca·tion (ob″fus·kay′shun) *n.* 1. Mental confusion. 2. The act of causing mental confusion or the clouding of an issue to confuse the listener.

ob·jec·tive, *adj. & n.* 1. Pertaining to an object or to that which is contemplated or perceived, as distinguished from that which contemplates or perceives. 2. Pertaining to those relations and conditions of the body perceived by another, as objective signs of disease. 3. The lens or lens system in a compound microscope which is nearest the object and produces the primary inverted magnified image.

objective sign. *In medicine,* a sign which can be detected by someone other than the patient himself.

ob·late (ob′late, ob·late′) *adj.* Having a form or shape that is flattened or depressed at th[e] poles.

ob·li·gate (ob′li·gate, ·gut) *adj.* Able to live onl[y] in the way specified, as an obligate anaerob[e;] an organism that can live only anaerobically.

obligate aerobe. An organism dependent upo[n] free oxygen at all times.

obligate parasite. A parasite incapable of livin[g] without a host.

oblig·a·to·ry (o·blig′uh·tor″ee) *adj.* 1. Require[d;] necessary. 2. OBLIGATE.

oblique (o·bleek′, o·blike′) *adj. & n.* 1. Not direc[t;] aslant; slanting. 2. *In botany,* unequal-side[d.] 3. *In anatomy,* an oblique muscle, as the exter[nal] or internal oblique of the abdomen, or th[e] superior or inferior oblique of the eye. Se[e] Table of Muscles in the Appendix. —**oblique·ly** (·lee) *adv.*

oblique diameter of the pelvic inlet. The line, o[r] the length of the line, joining the iliopectine[al] eminence to the sacroiliac articulation on th[e] opposite side.

oblique facial cleft. An embryonic fissure be[·]tween the maxillary and frontonasal pro[·]cesses.

oblique fissure. A fissure separating the superio[r] and inferior lobes of the left lung and th[e] superior and middle lobes of the right lun[g] from the inferior lobe of that lung.

ob·liq·ui·ty (ob·lick′wit·ee) *n.* The state of bein[g] oblique.

oblit·er·a·tion (uh·blit″ur·ay′shun, o·blit″) *[n.]* 1. The complete removal of a part by diseas[e] or surgical operation; extirpation. 2. Co[m]plete closure of a lumen. 3. The complete los[s] of memory or consciousness of certain event[s.] —**oblit·er·a·tive** (o·blit′ur·uh·tiv, ·ay·tiv) *adj.*

ob·mu·tes·cence (ob″mew·tes′unce) *n.* The con[·]dition of becoming or keeping silent.

ob·nu·bi·la·tion (ob·new″bi·lay′shun) *n.* Menta[l] clouding; may precede loss of consciousnes[s.]

ob·ses·sion, *n.* An idea or emotion that persist[s] in an individual's mind in spite of any con[·]scious attempts to remove it; an imperativ[e] idea, as seen in the psychoneurotic disorder[s.] —**obsession·al, ob·ses·sive,** *adj.*

obsessive-compulsive neurosis. A neurotic disorder in which anxiety relates to unwanted thoughts and repetitive impulses to perform acts against which the individual usually fights and which he may consider abnormal, inappropriate, or absurd, but which he cannot control and by which he is dominated. The acts often become organized into rituals, and include such forms as touching, counting, hand-washing, and excessive neatness; inability to control the acts or being prevented from performing them often produces extreme distress and anxiety.

obsessive-compulsive personality. An individual who is generally characterized by chronic, excessive concern with adherence to standards of conscience or of conformity resulting in inhibited, rigid, over-dutiful behavior, the inability to relax, and the performance of an inordinate amount of work. This behavioral disturbance may eventually lead to an obsessive-compulsive neurosis.

ob·so·les·cent (ob″suh·les′unt) *adj.* Becoming obsolete. **—obsoles·cence** (·unce) *n.*

obstetric forceps. A large, double-bladed traction forceps; the blades are demountable and are applied separately before interlocking at the handles, in order to fit the fetal head. Employed in difficult labor or to facilitate delivery.

ob·ste·tri·cian (ob″ste·trish′un) *n.* One who practices obstetrics.

ob·stet·rics (ob·stet′riks) *n.* The branch of medicine concerning the care of women and their offspring during pregnancy and parturition, with continued care of the women during the puerperium.

ob·sti·pa·tion (ob″sti·pay′shun) *n.* Intractable constipation.

ob·struc·tion, *n.* 1. The state of being occluded or stenosed, applied especially to hollow viscera, ducts, and vessels. 2. The act of occluding or blocking. 3. An obstacle. **—obstruc·tive,** *adj.;* **ob·struct,** *v.*

obstructive anosmia. See *anosmia.*

obstructive atelectasis. Atelectasis caused by occlusion or obstruction of a bronchus, ascribed to subsequent absorption of the trapped air and collapse of the alveoli. Syn. *absorption atelectasis.*

obstructive emphysema. Overdistention of the lung due to partial obstruction of the air passages, which permits air to enter the alveoli but which resists expiration of the air.

obstructive hydrocephalus. Increased volume of cerebrospinal fluid in the ventricular system caused by a blocking of the fluid's passage from the brain ventricles, where it is produced, to the subarachnoid space, where it is absorbed. Obstruction may occur at the interventricular foramens, in the cerebral aqueduct, at the median and lateral apertures of the fourth ventricle, or may be due to arachnoiditis. Syn. *internal hydrocephalus, noncommunicating hydrocephalus.*

obstructive jaundice. Jaundice due to interference with the outflow of bile by mechanical obstruction of the biliary passages, as by gallstones, tumor, or fibrosis.

ob·stru·ent (ob′stroo·unt) *adj. & n.* 1. Obstructive, tending to obstruct. 2. Something which tends or serves to obstruct.

ob·tund (ob·tund′) *v.* To blunt or make dull; lessen, as to obtund sensibility. **—ob·tun·da·tion** (ob″tun·day′shun) *n.*

ob·tun·dent (ob·tun′dunt) *adj. & n.* 1. Tending to obtund sensibility. 2. A remedy that relieves or overcomes irritation or pain.

ob·tu·ra·tion (ob″tew·ray′shun, ob″tur·ay′shun) *n.* 1. The closing of an opening or passage. 2. A form of intestinal obstruction in which the lumen of the intestine is occupied by its normal contents or by foreign bodies. **—ob·tu·rate** (ob′tew·rate) *v.*

ob·tu·ra·tor (ob′tew·ray″tur, ob′tur·) *adj. & n.* 1. Characterizing that which closes or stops up, as the obturator membrane. 2. Pertaining to various structures associated directly or indirectly with the obturator membrane, as the obturator foramen, obturator muscles. 3. Any obturator muscle. 4. A solid wire or rod contained within a hollow needle or cannula. Obturators may be bayonet-pointed for piercing tissues, or obliquely faced at the end for fitting, exactly, large aspirating needles. The term includes the metal carriers within urethroscopes and cystoscopes. 5. An appliance that closes a cleft or fissure of the palate.

obturator canal. A gap in the obturator membrane which closes the obturator foramen in the hipbone; it gives passage to the obturator nerve and vessels.

obturator foramen. The large oval opening between the ischium and the pubis, anterior, inferior, and medial to the acetabulum, partly closed in by a fibrous membrane; it gives passage to the obturator vessels and nerves.

obturator hernia. A rare hernia through the obturator canal; occurs principally in women. Syn. *pelvic hernia.*

obturator membrane. 1. The fibrous membrane closing the obturator foramen of the pelvis. 2. The thin membrane between the crura and foot plate of the stapes.

ob·tuse (ob·tewce′) *adj.* 1. Blunt. 2. Of angles, greater than 90°.

ob·tu·sion (ob·tew′zhun) *n.* The blunting or weakening of normal sensation and perception.

occipit-, occipito-. A combining form meaning *occiput, occipital.*

oc·cip·i·tal (ock·sip′i·tul) *adj.* Of or pertaining to the occiput.

occipital eye field. The region (Brodmann's areas 17, 18, and 19) around the calcarine fissure of the occipital lobe where stimulation produces conjugate deviation of the eyes to the opposite side, with stimulation above the fissure resulting in turning of the eyes downward and to the opposite side, while stimulation below the calcarine fissure produces upward movements to the opposite side.

oc·cip·i·tal·ize (ock·sip′i·tul·ize) *v.* To incorporate with the occipital bone; to fuse the atlas with the occipital bone.

occipital lobe. One of the lobes of the cerebrum, a triangular area at the occipital extremity, bounded medially by the parieto-occipital fissure and merging laterally with the parietal and the temporal lobes.

occipital sinus. A sinus of the dura mater running in the attached margin of the falx cerebelli from the foramen magnum to the confluence of the sinuses.

occipito-. See *occipit-*.

oc·cip·i·to·an·te·ri·or (ock·sip″i·to·an·teer′ee·ur) *adj.* Having the occiput directed toward the front, as the occipitoanterior position of the fetus in the uterus.

oc·cip·i·to·ax·i·al (ock·sip″i·to·ack′see·ul) *adj.* Pertaining to the occipital bone and the axis.

oc·cip·i·to·cer·vi·cal (ock·sip″i·to·sur′vi·kul) *adj.* Pertaining to the occiput and adjacent cervical regions.

oc·cip·i·to·fron·tal (ock·sip″i·to·frunt′ul) *adj.* Pertaining to the occiput and forehead, the epicranius (occipitofrontalis) muscle, or the occipital and frontal bones.

oc·cip·i·to·mas·toid (ock·sip″i·to·mas′toid) *adj.* Of or pertaining to the occipital bone and the mastoid process of the temporal bone.

oc·cip·i·to·men·tal (ock·sip″i·to·men′tul) *adj.* Of or pertaining to the occiput and the chin.

oc·cip·i·to·pa·ri·e·tal (ock·sip″i·to·pa·rye′e·tul) *adj.* Pertaining to the occipital and parietal bones or lobes.

oc·cip·i·to·pon·tine (ock·sip″i·to·pon′teen, ·tine) *adj.* Pertaining to the occipital lobe of the cerebrum and to the pons.

oc·cip·i·to·pos·te·ri·or (ock·sip″i·to·pos·teer′ee·ur) *adj.* Having the occiput directed backward, as the occipitoposterior position of the fetus in the uterus.

oc·cip·i·to·tem·po·ral (ock·sip″i·to·tem′puh·rul) *adj.* Pertaining to the occipital and temporal regions, lobes, or bones.

oc·cip·i·to·tha·lam·ic (ock·sip″i·to·tha·lam′ick) *adj.* Of or pertaining to the occipital lobe and the thalamus.

oc·ci·put (ock′si·put) *n.* The back part of the head.

oc·clude (uh·klewd′) *v.* To obstruct, stop up; to close; to bring into occlusion.

occlus-, occluso- A combining form meaning *occlusion, occlusal.*

oc·clu·sal (uh·klew′zul) *adj.* 1. Pertaining to the masticatory surfaces of the teeth or to the plane in which they lie. 2. Of or pertaining to occlusion. —**occlusal·ly** (·ee) *adv.*

occlusal trauma. Injury to the periodontium associated with abnormal or damaging forces of occlusion.

oc·clu·sio (ock·lew′zee·o) *n.* Closure; obliteration.

oc·clu·sion (uh·klew′zhun) *n.* 1. A closing or shutting up. 2. The state of being closed or shut. 3. The absorption, by a metal, of gas in large quantities, as of hydrogen by platinum. 4. The relationship of the masticatory surfaces of the maxillary teeth to the masticatory surfaces of the mandibular teeth when the jaws are closed. 5. *In neurophysiology*, the deficit in muscular tension when two afferent nerves that share certain motoneurons in the central nervous system are stimulated simultaneously, as compared to the sum of tensions when the two nerves are stimulated separately.

occlusion rim. An occluding device made on a temporary or permanent artificial denture base for the development of maxillomandibular relation records and for the arrangement of teeth. Syn. *record rim.*

oc·clu·sive (uh·klew′siv) *adj.* Closing or shutting up, as an occlusive surgical dressing.

oc·clu·som·e·ter (ock″lew·zom′e·tur, ·som′e·tur) *n.* GNATHODYNAMOMETER.

oc·cult (uh·kult′, ock′ult) *adj.* Hidden; concealed; not evident, as an occult disease the nature of which is not readily determined, or occult blood.

occult blood. Blood not visible on gross inspection of body products such as feces, and detected only by laboratory tests.

occult blood test. A test for blood not apparent on ordinary inspection of the material concerned.

occupational acne. Acne artificialis acquired from regular exposure to acnegenic materials in certain industries.

occupational dermatosis. Dermatosis resulting from chemicals or irritations characteristically encountered in an occupation.

occupational disease. Any disease, organic or functional, arising from the particular toxic substances, characteristic hazards, or frequently repeated mechanical operations of a particular industry, trade, or occupation.

occupational medicine. The branch of medicine which deals with the relationship of people to their occupation, for the purpose of the prevention of disease and injury and the promotion of optimal health, productivity, and social adjustment.

occupational neurosis. Any neurotic disorder manifested by inability to use those parts of the body commonly employed in one's occupation, such as a writer's inability to write due to cramps or painful feeling of fatigue in the hand. The occupation is not the cause of the neurosis, but only an outlet for it.

occupational therapy. 1. The use of selected occupations for therapeutic purposes. 2. The teaching of trades and arts as a means for the rehabilitation of patients handicapped physically or mentally.

och·le·sis (ock·lee′sis) *n.* A morbid condition produced by or exacerbated by crowding.

och·lo·pho·bia (ock″lo·fo′bee·uh) *n.* Morbid fear of crowds.

ochrom·e·ter (o·krom′e·tur) *n.* An instrument for measuring the capillary blood pressure, which records the force or pressure required to blanch a finger.

ochro·no·sis (o″kruh·no′sis) *n.* A blue or brownish blue pigmentation of cartilage and connective tissue, especially around joints, by a melanotic pigment. The condition is frequently accompanied by alkaptonuria and occurs in those who have had phenol, in large quantities, applied to skin or mucous membrane for a long time. A disturbed metabolism of aromatic compounds is associated with this condition. —**ochro·not·ic** (·not'ick) *adj.*

ochronotic osteoarthritis. A rare degenerative arthropathy associated with the diseased cartilage of ochronosis, accompanied by alkaptonuria.

OCP. Oral contraceptive pill(s).

oct-, octa-, octo- A combining form meaning *eight* or *eighth.*

oc·ta·meth·yl py·ro·phos·phor·am·ide (ock''meth'ul pye''ro·fos''for·am'ide). Bis[bisdimethylaminophosphonous]anhydride, $C_8H_{24}N_4O_3P_2$, a systemic insecticide and also a potent anticholinesterase agent, with selective action on peripheral cholinesterase; has been employed in treating myasthenia gravis. Abbreviated, OMPA.

oc·tan (ock'tan) *adj.* Returning or recurring every eighth day, as an octan fever.

oc·tane (ock'tane) *n.* C_8H_{18}. The eighth member of the paraffin or marsh gas series.

oc·ta·ri·us (ock·tār'ee·us) *n.* An eighth part of a gallon; a pint. Abbreviated, O.

oc·ta·va·lent (ock''tuh·vay'lunt) *adj.* Having a valence of eight.

oc·ti·grav·i·da (ock''ti·grav'id·uh) *n.* A woman pregnant for the eighth time.

Octin. Trademark for isometheptene, an antispasmodic and vasoconstrictor drug used as the hydrochloride or mucate salt.

oc·tip·a·ra (ock·tip'ur·uh) *n.* A woman who has been in labor eight times.

octo-. See *oct-.*

oc·to·roon (ock''tuh·roon') *n.* A person with one quadroon and one white parent.

oc·tyl (ock'til) *n.* The radical C_8H_{17}—.

ocul-, oculo- A combining form meaning *eye* or *ocular.*

oc·u·lar (ock'yoo·lur) *adj.* Of or pertaining to the eye.

ocular, *n.* EYEPIECE.

ocular adnexa. ADNEXA OCULI.

ocular crisis. 1. Any sudden disturbance of eye function. 2. Sudden intense eye pain, tearing, and photophobia.

ocular dominance. EYE DOMINANCE.

ocular headache. A headache that results from organic disease or impaired function of ocular structures.

ocular image. The image that reaches consciousness through the eye; determined by the retinal image, also by the anatomic and physiologic modification imposed upon it before it reaches the brain.

ocular micrometer. EYEPIECE MICROMETER.

ocular motor apraxia. Inability to move the eyes horizontally voluntarily or on command with preservation of reflex eye movements, and lateral rotational jerky thrusts of the head to compensate for the deficiency of eye movements. The congenital form (Cogan's syndrome) is usually seen in boys, who may also have difficulties in reading and in coordination; in the acquired, adult form, compensatory head turning is rarely seen since there is usually an associated apraxia of head turning.

The anatomic basis of the condition is not known.

ocular nystagmus. To-and-fro movements of the eyes when central vision is defective, making fixation difficult or impossible, observed when vision has been deficient since birth or before fixation was achieved (shimmering nystagmus), or when vision becomes impaired due to spending a long time in poorly lit surroundings, as may occur in miners.

oc·u·len·tum (ock''yoo·len'tum) *n.* An ointment for use in the eye.

oculi. Plural and genitive singular of *oculus.*

oc·u·list (ock'yoo·list) *n.* OPHTHALMOLOGIST.

oc·u·lo·au·ric·u·lo·ver·te·bral (ock''yoo·lo·aw·rick''yoo·lo·vur'te·brul) *adj.* Pertaining to the eyes, the ears, and the vertebral column.

oc·u·lo·car·di·ac (ock''yoo·lo·kahr'dee·ack) *adj.* Pertaining to the eyes and the heart.

oculocardiac reflex. Bradycardia or termination of cardiac arrhythmia in response to eyeball pressure; due to the association of the fifth cranial and the vagus nerve. This means of vagal stimulation is employed in the electroencephalographic diagnosis of breath-holding spells, but may be a dangerous maneuver in that retinal detachment may occur.

oc·u·lo·ceph·a·lo·gy·ric (ock''yoo·lo·sef''uh·lo·jye'rick) *adj.* Pertaining to rotatory movements of the eyes and the head.

oculocephalogyric reflex. The associated movements of the eye, head, and body in the process of focusing visual attention upon an object.

oc·u·lo·cer·e·bro·re·nal (ock''yoo·lo·serr''e·bro·ree'nul) *adj.* Pertaining to the eyes, cerebrum, and kidneys.

oc·u·lo·cu·ta·ne·ous (ock''yoo·lo·kew·tay'nee·us) *adj.* Pertaining to both the eyes and skin, as certain congenital or hereditary disorders.

oc·u·lo·den·to·dig·i·tal (ock''yoo·lo·den''to·dij'i·tul) *adj.* Pertaining to the eyes, teeth, and digits, usually the fingers.

oc·u·lo·fa·cial (ock''yoo·lo·fay'shul) *adj.* Pertaining to the eyes and face.

oc·u·lo·gas·tric (ock''yoo·lo·gas'trick) *adj.* Pertaining to the eyes and the stomach.

oc·u·lo·glan·du·lar (ock''yoo·lo·glan'dew·lur) *adj.* Pertaining to the eyes and lymph nodes.

oc·u·lo·gy·ra·tion (ock''yoo·lo·jye·ray'shun) *n.* Movement of the eyeballs. —**oculo·gy·ric** (·jye' rick), **oculo·gy·ral** (·jye'rul) *adj.*

oculogyric crisis or **spasm.** Involuntary tonic spasm of extraocular muscles, lasting minutes to hours, resulting usually in conjugate upward deviation of the eyes, but sometimes in forced conjugate movement in other directions, seen as a sequel of postencephalitic parkinsonism.

oc·u·lo·mo·tor (ock''yoo·lo·mo'tur) *adj.* Pertaining to the movement of the eye, or to the oculomotor nerve.

oculomotor nerve. The third cranial nerve, whose motor fibers arise from nuclei in the central gray matter at the level of the superior colliculus and supply the levator palpebrae superioris and all extrinsic eye muscles except the lateral rectus and superior oblique, and whose parasympathetic component goes to the ciliary ganglion, from which short fibers pass to the ciliary and sphincter pupillae muscles.

oculomotor paralysis. Paralysis of the oculomotor nerve, with pupillary mydriasis and areflexia, ptosis, and external deviation of the eye.

oc·u·lo·my·co·sis (ock″yoo·lo·migh·ko′sis) n. Any disease of the eye or its appendages due to a fungus.

oc·u·lo·pha·ryn·ge·al (ock″yoo·lo·fa·rin′jee·ul) adj. Involving the eyes and the pharynx.

oc·u·lo·phren·i·co·re·cur·rent (ock″yoo·lo·fren′i·ko·ree·kur′unt) adj. Pertaining to the recurrent laryngeal and phrenic nerves associated with Horner's syndrome.

oc·u·lo·pu·pil·lary (ock″yoo·lo·pew′pi·ler″ee) adj. Of or pertaining to the pupil of the eye, or to the pupil in relation to the eye as a whole.

oc·u·lo·sen·so·ry (ock″yoo·lo·sen′suh·ree) adj. Pertaining to stimuli to the eye.

oc·u·lo·zy·go·mat·ic (ock″yoo·lo·zye″go·mat′ick) adj. Pertaining to the eye and the zygoma.

oc·u·lus (ock′yoo·lus) n., pl. **oc·u·li** (·lye) EYE. Abbreviated, O.

oculus cae·si·us (see′zee·us) GLAUCOMA.

oculus dex·ter (decks′tur) The right eye. Abbreviated, O. D.

oculus sin·is·ter (sin′is·tur, si·nis′tur) The left eye. Abbreviated, O. S.

OD, O.D. Abbreviation for *overdose.*

O. D. Abbreviation for *oculus dexter,* right eye.

odax·es·mus (o″dack·sez′mus) n. Biting the tongue, lip, or cheek during a convulsion.

odont-, odonto- A combining form meaning (a) *tooth;* (b) *odontoid.*

odon·tal·gia (o″don·tal′juh, ·jee·uh) n. TOOTHACHE. —**odontal·gic** (·jick) adj.

odon·tec·to·my (o″don·teck′tuh·mee) n. Surgical removal of a tooth.

odon·tex·e·sis (o·don″teck·see′sis) n. Removal of deposits such as salivary calculi from the teeth.

-odontia A combining form designating a *condition* or a *treatment of the teeth.*

odon·tic (o·don′tick) adj. Pertaining to teeth.

odon·ti·a·sis (o·don·tye′uh·sis) n. DENTITION; the cutting of teeth.

odon·ti·tis (o·don·tye′tis) n. Inflammation associated with a tooth or teeth.

odonto-. See *odont-.*

odon·to·at·lan·tal (o·don″to·ut·lan′tul) adj. ATLANTOAXIAL.

odon·to·blast (o·don′to·blast) n. One of the cells covering the dental papilla or dental pulp, concerned with the formation of the dentin. —**odon·to·blas·tic** (o·don″to·blas′tick) adj.

odontoblastic process. The cytoplasmic process of an odontoblast which lies in a dentinal tubule. Syn. *Tomes's fiber.*

odon·to·blas·to·ma (o·don″to·blas·to′muh) n. AMELOBLASTIC ODONTOMA.

odon·to·cele (o·don′to·seel) n. A dentoalveolar cyst.

odon·to·cla·sis (o·don″to·klay′sis, o″don′tock′luh·sis) n. The process of resorption of the dentin of a tooth.

odon·to·clast (o·don′to·klast) n. A multinuclear cell, morphologically identical to an osteoclast, which is associated with resorption of tooth roots.

odontogenesis imperfecta. DENTINOGENESIS IMPERFECTA.

odon·to·gen·ic (o·don″to·jen′ick) adj. 1. Pertaining to odontogeny. 2. Originating in tissues associated with teeth.

odontogenic cyst. A cyst originating in tissues associated with teeth; of two main types, dentigerous and radicular.

odontogenic fibroma. A benign tumor formed from the mesenchymal derivatives of the tooth germ, which usually develops at the apex of a tooth.

odontogenic myxoma. A myxoma of the jaws, considered to be of dental origin, and usually seen in young individuals.

odon·tog·e·ny (o″don·toj′e·nee) n. The origin and development of teeth.

odon·tog·ra·phy (o″don·tog′ruf·ee) n. The descriptive anatomy of the teeth. —**odon·to·graph·ic** (o·don″to·graf′ick) adj.

odon·toid (o·don′toid) adj. 1. Resembling a tooth; toothlike. 2. Pertaining to the dens of the axis, as: odontoid ligament.

odon·tol·o·gist (o″don·tol′uh·jist) n. DENTIST.

odon·tol·o·gy (o″don·tol′uh·jee) n. A branch of science dealing with the formation, development, and abnormalities of the teeth.

odon·to·lox·ia (o·don″to·lock′see·uh) n. Irregularity or obliquity of the teeth.

odon·tol·y·sis (o″don·tol′i·sis) n. The loss of calcified tooth substance by dissolution.

odon·to·ma (o″don·to′muh) n., pl. **odontomas, odontoma·ta** (·tuh) A benign tumor representing a developmental excess, composed of mesodermal or ectodermal tooth-forming tissue, alone or in association with the calcified derivatives of these structures.

odon·to·pho·bia (o·don″to·fo′bee·uh) n. Morbid fear of teeth (usually animals' teeth).

odon·to·plas·ty (o·don′to·plas″tee) n. The reshaping of a tooth by grinding to produce a more desirable contour in the management of a periodontal problem.

odon·to·pri·sis (o·don″to·prye′sis, o″don·top′ri·sis) n. BRUXISM.

odon·to·scope (o·don′tuh·skope) n. A dental mirror used for inspecting the teeth.

odon·tot·o·my (o″don·tot′uh·mee) n. The cutting into a tooth.

odor, n. Any stimulus, usually chemical in nature, which adequately results in a sensation of smell; a scent or fragrance. —**odor·ous** (·us) adj.

odor·if·er·ous (o″dur·if′ur·us) adj. Emitting an odor.

odor·im·e·try (o″dur·im′e·tree) n. The measuring of the effect of odors upon the nasal sensory organs.

odor-of-sweaty-feet syndrome. An inborn error of short-chain fatty acid metabolism, clinically characterized by apparent normality at birth, followed by anorexia, weakness, lethargy, and an unusual odor suggestive of sweaty feet within the first few weeks of life, and severe acidosis and seizures terminally. Butyric and hexanoic acids are found in the exhaled air, blood, and urine. Considered to be an autosomal recessive disorder.

odyn-, odyno- A combining form meaning *pain.*

odyn·a·cou·sis (o·din″uh·koo′sis) *n.* Hypersensitivity to noise, to the point of being painful.

-odynia A combining form designating *a painful condition.*

odyno·pha·gia (o·din″o·fay′juh, ·jee·uh) *n.* 1. Painful swallowing. 2. DYSPHAGIA.

odyno·pho·bia (o·din″o·fo′bee·uh) *n.* Abnormal dread of pain.

oedema. EDEMA.

oed·i·pal (ed′i·pul, ee′di·pul) *adj.* Pertaining to the Oedipus complex.

Oed·i·pus complex (ed′i·pus, ee′di·pus) *In psychoanalytic theory,* the attraction and attachment of the child to the parent of the opposite sex, accompanied by feelings of envy and hostility toward the parent of the child's sex, whose displeasure and punishment the child so fears that he represses his feelings. Applied by Freud originally to the male child, the Electra complex referring to the female.

Oe·soph·a·gos·to·mum (ee·sof″uh·gos′to·mum) *n.* A genus of nematodes parasitic in the intestines, particularly the cecum, of ruminants, monkeys, and apes; rarely infects man.

Oes·tri·dae (es′tri·dee) *n.pl.* A family of botflies and warble flies. **—oestrid,** *adj. & n.*

of·fi·cial, *adj.* Of medicines: recognized by, and conforming to the standards of, the United States Pharmacopeia or the National Formulary.

off·spring, *n.* A lineal descendent from a known line of forebears.

Oha·ra's disease TULAREMIA.

ohm, *n.* 1. The unit of electric resistance, equal to one thousand million (10^9) units of resistance of the centimeter-gram-second system of electromagnetic units. 2. The international ohm, the resistance of a column of mercury 106.3 cm long and weighing 14.4521 g at 0° C.

ohm-am·me·ter (ome″am′e·tur, ·am′ee·tur) *n.* A combined ohmmeter and ammeter.

ohm·me·ter (ome′mee·tur) *n.* An apparatus for measuring electric resistance in ohms.

-oid A suffix meaning *like* or *resembling.*

oi·kol·o·gy (oy·kol′uh·jee) *n.* 1. The science of the home. 2. ECOLOGY.

oi·ko·pho·bia (oy″ko·fo′bee·uh) *n.* Morbid fear of home, or of a house.

oil, *n.* A liquid, generally viscous, obtained from animal, vegetable, or mineral sources but sometimes synthesized; miscible with water but miscible with many organic solvents. Most oils are nonvolatile (fixed oils), but some volatilize slowly (volatile oils). The chemical composition of oils varies greatly. **—oily,** *adj.*

oi·no·ma·nia (oy″no·may′nee·uh) *n. Obsol.* A form of mental disorder characterized by an irresistible craving for, and consequent indulgence in, alcoholic drink.

oint·ment, *n.* A semisolid preparation used for a protective and emollient effect or as a vehicle for the local or endermic administration of medicaments. Ointment bases are composed of various mixtures of fats, waxes, animal and vegetable oils, and solid and liquid hydrocarbons, or, in the so-called washable or water-soluble bases, there may be from 50 to 75% of water incorporated into an emulsified product.

-ol *In organic chemistry,* a suffix designating (a) an *alcohol* or a *phenol,* both characterized by the presence of the OH group; (b) loosely, *oil.*

old tuberculin. A broth culture of tubercle bacilli, sterilized by heat, filtered, and concentrated by evaporation. Abbreviated, O.T., T.O.

Old World hookworm. ANCYLOSTOMA DUODENALE.

ole-, oleo- A combining form meaning (a) *oil;* (b) *olein, oleic.*

ole·ag·i·nous (o″lee·aj′i·nus) *adj.* Oily.

ole·an·do·my·cin (o″lee·an″do·migh′sin) *n.* A basic antibiotic, $C_{35}H_{61}NO_{12}$, elaborated by strains of *Streptomyces antibioticus;* used in the treatment of infections due to strains of staphylococci and other gram-positive organisms resistant to penicillin, tetracyclines, and other established antibiotics.

ole·ate (o′lee·ate) *n.* 1. A salt of oleic acid. 2. A pharmaceutical preparation made by a solution of medicinal ingredients in oleic acid.

ole·cra·nar·thri·tis (o″lee·kray″nahr·thrye′tis, o·leck″ra) *n.* Inflammation of the elbow joint.

ole·cra·nar·throp·a·thy (o″le·kray″nahr·throp′uth·ee, o·leck″ran·ahr·) *n.* A disease of the elbow joint.

olec·ra·non (o·leck′ruh·non, o″le·kray′non) *n.* The large process at the upper extremity of the ulna. **—olecra·nal** (·nul) *adj.*

ole·fin (o′le·fin, ol′e·fin) *n.* Any member of the ethylene series of hydrocarbons; unsaturated compounds of the general formula C_nH_{2n}.

ole·ic acid (o·lee′ick, o′lee·ick) An unsaturated acid, $CH_3(CH_2)_7CH=CH(CH_2)_7COOH$, present as a glyceride in most fats and fixed oils.

ole·in (o′lee·in) *n.* Glyceryl oleate, $(C_{17}H_{33}COO)_3C_3H_5$, the chief constituent of olive oil and occurring in varying amounts in most other fixed oils. Syn. *triolein.*

oleo-. See *ole-.*

oleo·gran·u·lo·ma (o″lee·o·gran″yoo·lo′muh) *n.* A granuloma resulting from deposits, usually injected, of lipid material.

oleo·res·in (o″lee·o·rez′in) *n.* A substance consisting chiefly of a mixture of an oil, either fixed or volatile, and a resin, sometimes with other active constituents, extracted from plants by means of a volatile solvent.

oleo·ther·a·py (o″lee·o·therr′uh·pee) *n.* The treatment of disease by the administration of oils. Syn. *eleotherapy.*

oleo·tho·rax (o″lee·o·tho′racks) *n.* A condition in which a lung is compressed in the treatment of tuberculosis by injections of sterile oil.

oleo·vi·ta·min (o″lee·o·vye′tuh·min) *n.* A solution of a vitamin in oil.

ole·um (o′lee·um) *n.,* pl. **olea** (o′lee·uh) 1. OIL. 2. Fuming sulfuric acid; a solution of sulfur trioxide in concentrated sulfuric acid.

ol·fac·tion (ol·fack'shun, ohl·) *n.* 1. The function of smelling. 2. The sense of smell.

ol·fac·tom·e·ter (ol''fack·tom'e·tur, ohl'') *n.* An instrument for determining the power of smell.

ol·fac·to·ry (ol·fack'tur·ee, ohl·) *adj.* Of or pertaining to olfaction or the sense of smell.

olfactory area. ANTERIOR PERFORATED SUBSTANCE.

olfactory aura. A sudden disagreeable sensation of smell preceding or characterizing an epileptic attack.

olfactory bulb. The enlarged distal end of either olfactory tract situated on each side of the longitudinal fissure upon the undersurface of each anterior lobe of the cerebrum.

olfactory esthesioneuroepithelioma. A rare neuroepithelioma occurring in the nasal cavity of adults, which may infiltrate the paranasal sinuses.

olfactory lobe. An area on the inferior surface of the frontal lobe of the brain and demarcated from the lateral surface of the pallium by the rhinal sulcus. The anterior portion includes the olfactory tract and bulb and the posterior portion includes the anterior perforated substance and other olfactory structures of the anteromedial portion of the temporal lobe, collectively known as the piriform lobe.

olfactory nerve or **nerves.** The first cranial nerve; a plexiform group of sensory nerve fibers, consisting of axons that originate in the olfactory cells of the nasal mucosa, traverse the cribriform plate of the ethmoid bone and end in the glomeruli of the olfactory bulb.

olfactory pit. A pit formed about the olfactory placode in the embryo by the growth of the median and lateral nasal processes; the anlage of part of the nasal cavity. Syn. *nasal pit.*

olfactory region. The area on and above the superior conchae and on the adjoining nasal septum where the mucous membrane has olfactory epithelium and olfactory (Bowman's) glands.

olfactory sulcus. A well-defined anteroposterior groove on the medial orbital gyrus for the passage of the olfactory tract.

olfactory tract. A narrow band of white substance originating in the olfactory bulb and extending posteriorly in the olfactory sulcus toward the anterior perforated substance where it divides into lateral and medial olfactory striae.

olig-, oligo- A combining form meaning (a) *few, scant;* (b) *deficiency.*

ol·ig·e·mia, ol·i·gae·mia (ol''ig·ee'mee·uh) *n.* A state in which the total quantity of the blood is diminished.

ol·ig·er·ga·sia (ol''i·gur·gay'zhuh, ·zee·uh) *n.* MENTAL DEFICIENCY.

ol·ig·hid·ria (ol''ig·hid'ree·uh, ·high'dree·uh, ol''ig·id'ree·uh) *n.* OLIGOHIDRIA.

oligo-. See *olig-.*

ol·i·go·am·ni·os (ol''i·go·am'nee·os) *n.* OLIGOHYDRAMNIOS.

ol·i·go·blast (ol'i·go·blast) *n.* The precursor cell of the oligodendrocyte.

ol·i·go·blen·nia (ol''i·go·blen'ee·uh) *n.* A deficient secretion of mucus.

ol·i·go·cho·lia (ol''i·go·ko'lee·uh) *n.* A deficiency of bile.

ol·i·go·chro·ma·sia (ol''i·go·kro·may'zhuh, ·zee·uh) *n.* A decreased amount of hemoglobin in the erythrocytes, which present a pale appearance.

ol·i·go·chro·me·mia (ol''i·go·kro·mee'mee·uh) *n.* Deficiency of hemoglobin in the blood.

ol·i·go·chy·lia (ol''i·go·kigh'lee·uh) *n.* Deficiency of chyle.

ol·i·go·cy·the·mia (ol''i·go·sigh·theem'ee·uh) *n.* A reduction in the total quantity of erythrocytes in the body. **—oligocy·the·mic** (·theem'ick, ·themm'ick) *adj.*

ol·i·go·dac·rya (ol''i·go·dack'ree·uh) *n.* Deficiency of the tears.

ol·i·go·dac·tyl·ia (ol''i·go·dack·til'ee·uh) *n.* Congenital deficiency of fingers or toes.

ol·i·go·den·dro·blas·to·ma (ol''i·go·den''dro·blas·to'muh) *n.* A glial tumor similar to the oligodendroglioma, but composed of somewhat larger cells showing more cytoplasm, larger nuclei with less dense chromatin, and mitotic figures.

ol·i·go·den·dro·cyte (ol''i·go·den'dro·site) *n.* A cell of the oligodendroglia.

ol·i·go·den·dro·cy·to·ma (ol''i·go·den''dro·sigh·to'muh) *n.* OLIGODENDROGLIOMA.

ol·i·go·den·drog·lia (ol''i·go·den·drog'lee·uh) *n.* Small supporting cells of the nervous system, located about the nerve cells and between nerve fibers (interfascicular oligodendrocytes) and characterized by spheroidal or polygonal cell bodies and fine cytoplasmic processes with secondary divisions. **—oligodendrog·li·al** (·lee·ul) *adj.*

ol·i·go·den·dro·gli·o·ma (ol''i·go·den''dro·glye·o'muh, ·den·drog''lee·o'muh) *n.* A slowly growing glioma mainly of the cerebrum, rarely of septum pellucidum, fairly large and well defined, with a tendency to focal calcification. Microscopically, most of the cells are small, with richly chromatic nuclei and scanty, poorly staining cytoplasm without processes. Syn. *oligodendrocytoma, oligodendroma.*

ol·i·go·den·dro·gli·o·ma·to·sis (ol''i·go·den·drog''lee·o''muh·to'sis) *n.* Diffuse dissemination of oligodendroglioma tumor tissue through the leptomeninges and, sometimes, also into the ependymal lining of the cerebral ventricles.

ol·i·go·den·dro·ma (ol''i·go·den·dro'muh) *n.* OLIGODENDROGLIOMA.

ol·i·go·don·tia (ol''i·go·don'chee·uh) *n.* Congenital deficiency of teeth.

ol·i·go·dy·nam·ic (ol''i·go·dye·nam'ick, ·di·nam'ick) *adj.* 1. Active in very small quantities. 2. Pertaining to the toxic or other effect of very small quantities of a substance, as a metal, on cells or organisms.

oligodynamic action. Toxicity of heavy metals in very dilute solution for algae and other microorganisms.

ol·i·go·ga·lac·tia (ol''i·go·ga·lack'tee·uh, ·shee·uh) *n.* Deficiency in the secretion of milk.

ol·i·go·graph·ia (ol''i·go·graf'ee·uh) *n.* Oligologia as manifested in writing.

ol·i·go·hid·ria (ol″i·go·hid′ree·uh) *n.* Deficiency of perspiration.

ol·i·go·hy·dram·ni·os (ol″i·go·high·dram′nee·os) *n.* Deficiency of the amniotic fluid.

ol·i·go·hy·dru·ria (ol″i·go·high·droor′ee·uh) *n.* Urine with a relative diminution of water; highly concentrated urine.

ol·i·go·la·lia (ol″i·go·lay′lee·uh) *n.* Oligologia in speech.

ol·i·go·lo·gia (ol″i·go·lo′jee·uh, ·lo′juh) *n.* Fewness of words; a condition in which a person says or writes less than might normally be expected, given his personality, education, and the specific circumstances. Syn. *oligophasia.*

ol·i·go·men·or·rhea (ol″i·go·men″o·ree′uh) *n.* Abnormally infrequent menstruation.

ol·i·go·phos·pha·tu·ria (ol″i·go·fos″fuh·tew′ree·uh) *n.* A decrease in the amount of phosphates in the urine.

ol·i·go·phre·nia (ol″i·go·free′nee·uh) *n.* Mental deficiency. **—oligo·phren·ic** (·fren′ick) *adj.*

ol·i·gop·nea, ol·i·gop·noea (ol″i·gop·nee′uh, ol″i·gop′nee·uh) *n.* Respiration diminished in depth or frequency.

ol·i·go·pty·a·lism (ol″i·go·tye′uh·liz·um, ol″i·gop·) *n.* Deficient secretion of saliva.

ol·i·go·py·rene (ol″i·go·pye′reen) *adj.* Of sperm cells, having only a part of the full complement of chromosomes.

ol·i·go·ria (ol″i·gor′ee·uh) *n.* An abnormal apathy or indifference to persons or to environment, as in a depressed state.

ol·i·go·sac·cha·ride (ol″i·go·sack′ur·ide) *n.* Any carbohydrate of a class comprising disaccharides, trisaccharides, tetrasaccharides, and, according to some authorities, pentasaccharides; so named because they yield on hydrolysis a small number of monosaccharides.

ol·i·go·si·al·ia (ol″i·go·sigh·al′ee·uh, ·ay′lee·uh) *n.* Deficiency of saliva.

ol·i·go·sper·mia (ol″i·go·spur′mee·uh) *n.* Scarcity of spermatozoa in the semen; specifically, less then 20 million per ml.

ol·i·go·trich·ia (ol″i·go·trick′ee·uh) *n.* Scantiness or thinness of hair.

ol·i·gu·ria (ol″ig·yoo′ree·uh) *n.* A diminution in the quantity of urine excreted; specifically, less then 400 ml in a 24-hour period.

ol·i·va·ry (ol′i·verr·ee) *adj.* 1. Olive-shaped. 2. Pertaining to the olivary nucleus.

olivary nucleus. A conspicuous convoluted gray band opening medially, dorsal to the pyramids, occupying the entire upper two-thirds of the medulla oblongata, the cells of which give rise to most of the fibers of the olivocerebellar tract.

ol·ive, *n.* 1. The oil tree, *Olea europaea,* of the Oleaceae. Its fruit yields olive oil, a fixed oil which consists chiefly of olein and palmitin, and is used as a nutritive food; in medicine as a laxative; as an emollient external application to wounds or burns, and as an ingredient of liniments and ointments. 2. OLIVARY NUCLEUS. 3. An oval eminence on the anterior, ventrolateral surface of the medulla oblongata; it marks the location of the olivary nucleus, which lies just beneath the surface.

ol·i·vo·cer·e·bel·lar (ol″i·vo·serr·e·bel′ur) *adj.* Pertaining to the olivary nucleus and the cerebellum.

ol·i·vo·pon·to·cer·e·bel·lar (ol″i·vo·pon″to·serr·e·bel′ur) *adj.* Pertaining to the olivary nucleus, pons, and cerebellum.

olivopontocerebellar atrophy, ataxia, or **degeneration.** A heredodegenerative disease occurring in the middle and later decades of life; causes ataxia, hypotonia, and dysarthria. It is characterized pathologically by degeneration of the middle cerebellar white matter, and the pontine, arcuate, and olivary nuclei.

ol·i·vo·spi·nal (ol″i·vo·spye′nul) *adj.* Pertaining to the olivary nucleus and the spinal cord.

Ol·lier's disease (o^hl·yey′) ENCHONDROMATOSIS.

olo·pho·nia (ol″o·fo′nee·uh) *n.* Abnormal speech due to a structural defect of the vocal organs.

om-, omo- A combining form meaning *shoulder.*

-oma A suffix designating a *tumor* or *neoplasm.*

oma·gra (o·may′gruh, o·mag′ruh) *n.* Gout in the shoulder.

omar·thral·gia (o″mahr·thral′juh) *n.* Pain in the shoulder joint.

omar·thri·tis (o″mahr·thrigh′tis) *n.* Inflammation of the shoulder joint.

oma·sum (o·may′sum) *n.* The third compartment of the stomach of a ruminant. Syn. *manyplies, psalterium.*

om·bro·pho·bia (om″bro·fo′bee·uh) *n.* A morbid fear of rain.

oment-, omento-. A combining form meaning *omentum.*

omen·tal (o·men′tul) *adj.* Of or pertaining to an omentum.

omental bursa. The large irregular space lined with peritoneum, lying dorsal to the stomach and lesser omentum, and communicating with the general peritoneal cavity through the epiploic foramen. Syn. *lesser peritoneal cavity, lesser sac.*

omental hernia. A hernia which contains only omentum.

omental sac. The sac formed between the ascending and descending portions of the greater omentum.

omen·tec·to·my (o″men·teck′tum·ee) *n.* Excision of an omentum or any part of it.

omen·ti·tis (o″men·tye′tis) *n.* Inflammation of an omentum.

omen·to·cele (o·men′to·seel) *n.* A hernia containing omentum only.

omen·to·pexy (o·men′to·peck″see) *n.* The surgical operation of suspending the greater omentum, by suturing it to the abdominal wall.

omen·tor·rha·phy (o″men·tor′uh·fee) *n.* Suture of an omentum.

omen·tot·o·my (o″men·tot′um·ee) *n.* Surgical incision of an omentum.

omen·tum (o·men′tum) *n.,* pl. **omen·ta** (·tuh), Apron; a fold of the peritoneum connecting abdominal viscera with the stomach.

om·niv·o·rous (om·niv′ur·us) *adj.* Subsisting on a wide variety of food; applied mainly to animals that feed on both animal and vegetable matter.

omo-. See *om-.*

omo·hy·oid (o″mo·high′oid) adj. Pertaining conjointly to the scapula and the hyoid bone.

omo·pha·gia (o″mo·fay′jee·uh) n. The practice of eating raw foods.

omphal-, omphalo- A combining form meaning *navel, umbilicus.*

om·pha·lec·to·my (om″fuh·leck′tum·ee) n. Excision of the navel.

om·phal·ic (om·fal′ick) adj. Pertaining to the umbilicus.

om·pha·li·tis (om″fuh·lye′tis) n. Inflammation of the umbilicus.

om·pha·lo·cele (om·fal′o·seel, om′fuh·lo·) n. A hernia into the umbilical cord, caused by a congenital midline defect.

om·pha·lo·mes·en·ter·ic (om″fuh·lo·mes″un·terr′ick, ·mez″un·) adj. Pertaining conjointly to the umbilicus and mesentery.

om·pha·lop·a·gus (om″fuh·lop′uh·gus) n. Conjoined twins united at the abdomen.

om·pha·lo·prop·to·sis (om″fuh·lo·prop·to′sis) n. Abnormal protrusion of the navel.

om·pha·los (om′fuh·los) n., pl. **om·pha·li** (·lye) UMBILICUS.

om·pha·lo·site (om·fal′o·site, om′fuh·lo·site) n. The parasitic member of asymmetric uniovular twins. The parasite has no heart, or only a vestigial one, deriving its blood supply from the placenta of the more or less normal twin (autosite).

om·pha·lo·tome (om·fal′o·tome) n. An instrument for dividing the umbilical cord.

om·pha·lot·o·my (om·fuh·lot′um·ee) n. The cutting of the umbilical cord.

om·pha·lo·trip·sy (om′fuh·lo·trip″see) n. Separation of the umbilical cord by a crushing instrument.

onan·ism (o′nuh·niz·um) n. 1. Incomplete coitus; COITUS INTERRUPTUS. 2. MASTURBATION. **—onan·ist** (·ist) n.

On·cho·cer·ca (onk″o·sur′kuh) n. A genus of filarial worms.

Onchocerca vol·vu·lus (vol′vew·lus) A species of filarial worm which infects man, forming fibrous nodular tumors with encapsulation of the adult worms in the subcutaneous connective tissue, and often causing severe ocular disease when microfilariae invade the tissues of the eye.

on·cho·cer·ci·a·sis (onk″o·sur·sigh′uh·sis, ·kigh′uh·sis) n. Infection with the filarial worm *Onchocerca volvulus*; produces tumors of the skin, papular dermatitis, and ocular complications in humans. Syn. *river blindness* (in western equatorial Africa).

on·cho·cer·co·ma (onk″o·sur·ko′muh) n. The fibrous nodular lesion of onchocerciasis which contains the adult worms (*Onchocerca*), usually located at a site at which a bone is close to the surface.

on·cho·cer·co·sis (onk″o·sur·ko′sis) n. ONCHOCERCIASIS.

on·cho·der·ma·ti·tis (onk″o·dur″muh·tigh′tis) n. The cutaneous manifestations of onchocerciasis.

onco-, oncho- A combining form meaning (a) *tumor;* (b) *bulk, volume;* (c) *hooked, curved.*

on·co·cyte (onk′o·site) n. One of the columnar cells with granular eosinophilic cytoplasm found in salivary and certain endocrine glands, nasal mucosa, and other locations. They represent dedifferentiation of parenchymal cells and may occur singly or in aggregates (oncocytomas).

on·co·cy·to·ma, on·ko·cy·to·ma (onk″o·sigh·to′muh) n. A benign tumor whose parenchyma is composed of large, finely granular eosinophilic cells (oncocytes); it occurs almost exclusively in the salivary glands.

on·co·gen·e·sis (onk″o·jen′e·sis) n. The process of tumor formation. **—oncogen·ic** (·ick) adj.

on·col·o·gist (ong·kol′uh·jist) n. A specialist in oncology.

on·col·o·gy (ong·kol′uh·jee) n. The study or science of neoplastic growth.

on·col·y·sis (ong·kol′i·sis) n. The destruction or lysis of neoplastic cells, particularly those of carcinoma.

on·co·lyt·ic (ong″ko·lit′ick) adj. & n. 1. Pertaining to or causing oncolysis. 2. An agent that effects oncolysis.

On·co·me·la·nia (onk″o·me·lay′nee·uh) n. A genus of amphibious snails.

Oncomelania hu·pen·sis (hew·pen′sis). A species of snail found in the Yangtze basin; one of the intermediate hosts of *Schistosoma japonicum.*

Oncomelania hy·dro·bi·op·sis (high″dro·bye·op′sis). A species of snail found in Leyte and other Philippine Islands; an intermediate host of *Schistosoma japonicum.*

on·com·e·ter (ong·kom′e·tur) n. An instrument for measuring variations in the volume of an organ, as of the kidney or spleen, or of an extremity. **—oncome·try** (·tree) n. **on·co·met·ric** (onk″o·met′rick) adj.

on·co·sis (ong·ko′sis) n. Any condition marked by the development of tumors.

on·co·sphere (onk′o·sfeer) n. The hexacanth embryo of tapeworms.

on·cot·ic (ong·kot′ick, on·) adj. 1. Pertaining to oncosis. 2. Pertaining to anything that increases volume or pressure.

oncotic agent. A substance, such as human serum albumin or dextran, that may be used to increase colloidal osmotic pressure and expand plasma volume.

oncotic pressure. 1. The osmotic pressure exerted by colloids in a solution. 2. The pressure exerted by plasma proteins. Syn. *colloidal osmotic pressure.*

-one A suffix in organic chemistry signifying a ketone or certain other compounds that contain oxygen, as a lactone or sulfone.

oneir-, oneiro- A combining form meaning *dream.*

onei·ro·dyn·ia (o·nigh″ro·din′ee·uh) n. Disquietude of the mind during sleep; somnambulism and nightmare.

onei·rol·o·gy (o″nigh·rol′uh·jee) n. The science, or scientific view, of dreams.

onei·ron·o·sus (o″nigh·ron′uh·sus) n. Disorder manifesting itself in dreams; morbid dreaming.

onei·ros·co·py (o″nigh·ros′kup·ee) n. Dream interpretation; diagnosis of a mental state by the analysis of dreams.

onio·ma·nia (o″nee·o·may′nee·uh) n. An irresistible impulse for buying, usually beyond one's needs.

onkocytoma. ONCOCYTOMA.

on·o·mato·ma·nia (on″o·mat″o·may′nee·uh) n. An irresistible impulse to repeat certain words.

on·o·mato·pho·bia (on″o·mat″o·fo′bee·uh) n. Pathological fear of hearing certain names or words.

on·o·mato·poi·e·sis (on″o·mat″o·poy·ee′sis) n. 1. The formation of words in imitation of a sound. 2. *In psychiatry*, the extemporaneous formation of words on the basis of sound association; frequently a symptom of schizophrenia.

-ont A combining form meaning *cell* or *organism*.

ont-, onto- A combining form meaning (a) *existence, existential*; (b) *an individual being, organism*.

on·to·anal·y·sis (on″to·uh·nal′i·sis) n. A branch of psychiatry that combines psychoanalysis with existentialism. —**onto·an·a·lyt·ic** (·an·uh·lit′ick) adj.

on·tog·e·ny (on·toje′e·nee) n. The origin and development of the individual organism from fertilized egg to adult, as distinguished from phylogeny, the evolutionary history of the race or group to which the individual belongs. —**on·to·ge·net·ic** (·to·je·net′ick) adj.

onych-, onycho- A combining form meaning *nail* or *claw*.

on·y·cha·tro·phia (on″i·kuh·tro′fee·uh) n. 1. Atrophy of nails. 2. Failure of development of the nail.

on·ych·aux·is (on″i·kawk′sis) n. Hypertrophy of the nail.

on·y·chec·to·my (on″i·keck′tuh·mee) n. Excision of a fingernail or toenail.

onych·ia (o·nick′ee·uh) n. Inflammation of the nail matrix.

on·y·cho·cryp·to·sis (on″i·ko·krip·to′sis) n. Ingrowing of a nail. Syn. *unguis incarnatus*.

on·y·cho·dys·tro·phy (on″i·ko·dis′truh·fee) n. Any distortion of a nail; a symptom seen in several diseases.

on·y·cho·gry·po·sis (on″i·ko·grye·po′sis, ·gri·) n. A thickened, ridged, and curved condition of a nail.

on·y·cho·hel·co·sis (on″i·ko·hel·ko′sis) n. Ulceration of a nail.

on·y·cho·het·ero·to·pia (on″i·ko·het″ur·o·to′pee·uh) n. An anomaly consisting of the presence of abnormally situated nails, as on the lateral aspect of the terminal phalanges. Most often occurs on the little finger.

on·y·chol·y·sis (on″i·kol′i·sis) n. A slow process of loosening of a nail from its bed, beginning at the free edge and progressing gradually toward the root.

on·y·cho·ma (on″i·ko′muh) n. A tumor of the nail bed.

on·y·cho·ma·de·sis (on″i·ko·muh·dee′sis) n. Spontaneous separation of a nail from its bed, beginning at the proximal end and progressing rapidly toward the free edge until the nail plate falls off; defluvium unguium.

on·y·cho·ma·la·cia (on″i·ko·ma·lay′shee·uh, ·shuh) n. Abnormally soft nails.

on·y·cho·my·co·sis (on″i·ko·migh·ko′sis) n. A disease of the nails due to fungi.

on·y·cho·os·teo·dys·pla·sia (on″i·ko·os″tee·o·dis·play′zhuh, ·zee·uh) n. NAIL-PATELLA SYNDROME.

on·y·chop·a·thy (on″i·kop′uth·ee) n. Any disease of the nails. —**ony·cho·path·ic** (·ko·path′ick) adj.

on·y·cho·pha·gia (on″i·ko·fay′jee·uh) n. NAIL BITING.

on·y·choph·a·gist (on″i·kof′uh·jist) n. A person addicted to biting his fingernails.

on·y·chop·to·sis (on″i·kop·to′sis) n. Downward displacement of the nails.

on·y·chor·rhex·is (on″i·ko·reck′sis) n. Longitudinal striation of the nail plate, with or without the formation of fissures.

on·y·cho·schiz·ia (on″i·ko·skiz′ee·uh) n. An ungual dystrophy consisting of lamination on the nail in two or more superimposed layers.

on·y·cho·sis (on″i·ko′sis) n. Any deformity or disease of the nails.

on·y·chot·il·lo·ma·nia (on″i·kot″il·lo·may′nee·uh) n. The neurotic picking at a nail until it is permanently altered.

on·y·chot·o·my (on″i·kot′uh·mee) n. Surgical incision into a fingernail or toenail.

on·y·chot·ro·phy (on″i·kot′ruh·fee) n. Nourishment of the nails.

oo- A combining form meaning *egg, ovum*.

oo·cyst (o′o·sist) n. The encysted zygote in the life history of some sporozoa.

oo·cyte (o′o·site) n. An egg cell before the completion of the maturation process. Its full history includes its origin from an oogonium, a growth period, and the final meiotic divisions.

oo·gen·e·sis (o″o·jen′e·sis) n. The process of the origin, growth, and formation of the ovum in its preparation for fertilization. —**oo·ge·net·ic** (·je·net′ick) adj.

oo·go·ni·um (o″o·go′nee·um) n., pl. **oogo·nia** (·nee·uh) 1. A cell which, by continued division, gives rise to oocytes. 2. An ovum in a primary follicle immediately before the beginning of maturation.

oo·ki·nete (o″o·kigh′neet, ·ki·neet′) n. The elongated, motile zygote in the life history of some sporozoan parasites; as that of the malaria parasite as it bores through the epithelial lining of the mosquito's intestine, in the wall of which it becomes an oocyst. —**oo·ki·net·ic** (·ki·net′ick) adj.

oophor-, oophoro- A combining form meaning *ovary, ovarian*.

oo·pho·rec·to·my (o″uh·fo·reck′tuh·mee, o·off″o·) n. Excision of an ovary.

oo·pho·ri·tis (o″uh·fo·rye′tis, o·off″uh·rye′tis) n. Inflammation of an ovary.

ooph·o·ro·cys·tec·to·my (o·off″ur·o·sis·teck′tuh·mee) n. Removal of an ovarian cyst.

ooph·o·ro·cys·to·sis (o·off″ur·o·sis·to′sis) n. The formation of ovarian cysts.

ooph·o·ro·hys·ter·ec·to·my (o·off″ur·o·his·tur·eck′tuh·mee) n. Removal of the uterus and ovaries.

ooph·o·ro·pex·y (o-off'ur·o·peck"see) n. Surgical fixation of an ovary.

ooph·o·ro·plas·ty (o-off'ur·o·plas"tee) n. Plastic surgery on the ovary.

ooph·o·ro·sal·pin·gec·to·my (o-off"ur·o·sal"pin·jeck'tum·ee) n. Excision of an ovary and oviduct.

ooph·o·ro·sal·pin·gi·tis (o-off"ur·o·sal"pin·jye'tis) n. Inflammation of an ovary and oviduct.

oo·phor·rha·phy (o'uh·for'uh·fee) n. Operation of suturing an ovary to the pelvic wall.

oothec-, ootheco- A combining form meaning *ovary, ovarian.*

opac·i·fy (o·pas'i·fye) v. 1. To make opaque. 2. To become opaque. —**opac·i·fi·ca·tion** (o·pas"i·fi·kay'shun) n.

opac·i·ty (o·pas'i·tee) n. 1. The condition of being opaque. 2. An opaque spot, as opacity of the cornea or lens.

opal·es·cent (o"puh·les'unt) adj. Showing a play of colors; reflecting light; iridescent. —**opalescence** (·unce) n.

opaque (o·pake') adj. Impervious to light or to other forms of radiation, as: opaque to x-rays.

opei·do·scope (o·pye'duh·scope) n. An instrument for projecting the vibrations of the voice visually onto a screen.

open, adj. 1. Exposed to the air, as an open wound. 2. Interrupted, as an open circuit, one through which an electric current cannot pass.

open-angle glaucoma. Increased intraocular tension, which is insidious in onset, bilateral, and slowly progressive, with visual loss occurring only when the disease is well advanced, due to diminished aqueous outflow but with the angle open and the aqueous in free contact with the trabecula.

open chest cardiac massage. Direct manual compression of the heart; usually done in the operating room where the thoracic cavity is opened. Syn. *direct cardiac massage.*

opening snap. A brief heart sound related to the sudden opening of a heart valve, usually the mitral valve. Abbreviated, O. S.

open reduction. In surgery, a reduction performed after making an incision through the soft parts in order to expose the fracture or dislocation.

op·er·a·ble (op'ur·uh·bul) adj. Admitting of an operation with reasonable expectation of favorable results; pertaining to a condition where operation is not contraindicated. —**op·er·a·bil·i·ty** (op"ur·uh·bil'i·tee) n.

op·er·ant (op'ur·unt) adj. In psychology, pertaining to or characterizing behavior or response to a stimulus recognized by its effect on the organism (experimental animal or human subject); the stimulus may or may not be identifiable.

operant conditioning or **learning.** A form of learning in which the subject, human or animal, is taught to make a response or perform a task voluntarily, and this, in turn, determines whether or not the conditioning is reinforced. Syn. *instrumental conditioning, reinforced conditioning.*

op·er·a·tion (op"uh·ray'shun) n. 1. The mode of action of anything. 2. Anything done or performed, especially with instruments. 3. In surgery, a procedure in which the method follows a definite routine. —**operation·al** (·ul), **op·er·a·tive** (op'uh·ruh·tiv) adj.; **op·er·ate** (op'uh·rate) v.

op·er·a·tor (op'ur·ay"tur) n. 1. One who performs a surgical operation. 2. One who gives treatments, especially those involving mechanotherapy. 3. The proximal portion of an operon which provides the site for recognition by a repressor protein.

oper·cu·late (o·pur'kew·lut, ·late) adj. Having an operculum.

oper·cu·lum (o·pur'kew·lum) n., pl. **opercu·la** (·luh). 1. A lid or cover; a valve. 2. One of the convolutions overlying the crown of a partially erupted tooth, specifically, over a lower third molar. —**opercu·lar** (·lur) adj.

op·er·on (op'ur·on) n. A genetic unit consisting of two or more adjacent cistrons which are coordinately regulated via an operator site and whose transcription is initiated at a promotor site.

ophi·a·sis (o·fye'uh·sis) n. Alopecia areata in which the baldness progresses in a serpentine form about the hair margin. Usually seen in children.

ophid·io·pho·bia (o·fid"ee·o·fo'bee·uh) n. Morbid fear of snakes.

ophid·ism (o'fid·iz·um) n. Poisoning from snake venom.

oph·io·phobe (off'ee·o·fobe, o'fee·o·fobe) n. A person who has an unusual dread of snakes.

oph·ry·o·sis (off"ree·o'sis) n. Spasm of the muscles of the eyebrow.

ophthalm-, ophthalmo- A combining form meaning *eye.*

oph·thal·ma·gra (off"thal·may'gruh, ·mag'ruh) n. Sudden pain in the eye.

oph·thal·mal·gia (off"thal·mal'juh, ·jee·uh) n. Neuralgia of the eye.

oph·thal·mec·chy·mo·sis (off"thal·meck"i·mo'sis) n. An effusion of blood into the conjunctiva.

oph·thal·mec·to·my (off"thal·meck'tum·ee) n. Excision, or enucleation, of an eye.

oph·thal·mia (off·thal'mee·uh) n. Inflammation of the eye, especially when the conjunctiva is involved.

ophthalmia neonatorum. Conjunctivitis in the newborn, which may be from bacterial, viral, or chemical causes.

oph·thal·mic (off·thal'mick) adj. Pertaining to the eye.

ophthalmic nerve. A somatic sensory nerve, a division of the trigeminal nerve, which innervates the skin of the forehead, the upper eyelids, the anterior portion of the scalp, the orbit, the eyeball, the meninges, the nasal mucosa, the frontal, ethmoid, and sphenoid air sinuses.

oph·thal·mi·tis (off"thal·migh'tis) n. Inflammation of the eye. —**ophthal·mit·ic** (·mit'ick) adj.

ophthalmo-. See *ophthalm-.*

oph·thal·mo·blen·nor·rhea (off·thal"mo·blen·or·ee'uh) n. Blennorrhea of the conjunctiva.

oph·thal·mo·cen·te·sis (off·thal″mo·sen·tee′sis) n. Surgical puncture of the eye. Syn. *paracentesis oculi*.

oph·thal·mo·dy·na·mom·e·ter (off·thal″mo·dye″nuh·mom′e·tur, ·din″uh·) n. An instrument which measures the pressure necessary to cause pulsation and collapse the retinal arteries.

oph·thal·mo·dy·na·mom·e·try (off·thal″mo·dye″nuh·mom′e·tree) n. Measurement of the systolic and diastolic blood pressure in the retinal circulation by means of an ophthalmodynamometer.

oph·thal·mo·dyn·ia (off·thal″mo·din′ee·uh) n. Pain referred to the eye.

oph·thal·mo·fun·do·scope (off·thal″mo·fun′duh·skope) n. OPHTHALMOSCOPE.

oph·thal·mog·ra·phy (off″thal·mog′ruh·fee) n. Descriptive anatomy of the eye.

oph·thal·mo·gy·ric (off·thal″mo·jye′rick) adj. OCULOGYRIC.

oph·thal·mo·ico·nom·e·ter, oph·thal·mo·ei·ko·nom·e·ter (off·thal″mo·eye″kuh·nom′e·tur) n. A complex apparatus for the detection and measurement of aniseikonia.

oph·thal·mo·ico·nom·e·try (off·thal″mo·eye″kuh·nom′e·tree) n. Measurement of the retinal image with an ophthalmoiconometer.

oph·thal·mo·lith (off·thal′mo·lith) n. A calculus of the eye or lacrimal duct.

oph·thal·mol·o·gist (off″thal·mol′uh·jist) n. One skilled or specializing in ophthalmology.

oph·thal·mol·o·gy (off″thal·mol′uh·jee) n. The science of the anatomy, physiology, diseases, and treatment of the eye. —**oph·thal·mo·log·ic** (off·thal″mo·loj′ick) adj.

oph·thal·mo·ma·la·cia (off·thal″mo·ma·lay′shee·uh) n. Abnormal softness or subnormal tension of the eye.

oph·thal·mom·e·ter (off″thal·mom′e·tur) n. 1. An instrument for measuring refractive errors, especially astigmatism. 2. An instrument for measuring the capacity of the chambers of the eye. 3. An instrument for measuring the eye as a whole.

oph·thal·mo·my·co·sis (off·thal″mo·migh·ko′sis) n. Any disease of the eye or its appendages due to a fungus.

oph·thal·mo·my·ia·sis (off·thal″mo·migh·eye′uh·sis). n. Invasion of the eyes by fly larvae, such as those belonging to the family Oestridae.

oph·thal·mo·my·ot·o·my (off·thal″mo·migh·ot′uh·mee) n. Division of a muscle or muscles of the eye.

oph·thal·mo·neu·ri·tis (off·thal″mo·new·rye′tis) n. OPTIC NEURITIS.

oph·thal·mo·neu·ro·my·e·li·tis (off·thal″mo·new″ro·migh″e·lye′tis) n. NEUROMYELITIS OPTICA.

oph·thal·mop·a·thy (off″thal·mop′uth·ee) n. Any disease of the eye.

oph·thal·mo·pho·bia (off·thal″mo·fo′bee·uh) n. Morbid dislike of being stared at.

oph·thal·moph·thi·sis (off·thal″mof·thi·sis, off·thal″mo·tye′sis, off·thal″mo·thigh′sis) n. Shrinking of the eyeball.

oph·thal·mo·plas·ty (off·thal″mo·plas′tee) n. Plastic surgery of the eye or accessory parts.

—**oph·thal·mo·plas·tic** (off·thal″mo·plas′tick) adj.

oph·thal·mo·ple·gia (off·thal″mo·plee′jee·uh) n. Paralysis of the muscles innervated by the third, fourth, and sixth cranial nerves; may be supranuclear, internuclear, or due to a lesion of individual ocular motor nerves or their nuclei; may be external, internal, or complete. —**ophthalmople·gic** (·jick) adj.

oph·thal·mor·rha·gia (off·thal″mo·ray′jee·uh) n. Hemorrhage from the eye.

oph·thal·mor·rhea (off·thal″mo·ree′uh) n. A watery or sanguineous discharge from the eye.

oph·thal·mor·rhex·is (off·thal″mo·reck′sis) n. Rupture of the eyeball.

oph·thal·mos (off·thal′mos) n. EYE.

oph·thal·mo·scope (off·thal″muh·skope) n. An instrument for examining the interior of the eye. It consists essentially of a mirror with a hole in it, through which the observer looks, the concavity of the eye being illuminated by light reflected from the mirror into the eye through the pupil and seen by means of the rays reflected from the eye ground back through the hole in the mirror. The ophthalmoscope is fitted with lenses of different powers that may be revolved in front of the observing eye, and these neutralize the ametropia of either the patient's or the observer's eye, thus rendering clear the details of the fundus of the eye. A wide variety of ophthalmoscopes exist, some offering special features, both for direct and indirect ophthalmoscopy.

oph·thal·mos·co·py (off″thal·mos′kuh·pee) n. The examination of the interior of the eye by means of an ophthalmoscope. —**oph·thal·mo·scop·ic** (off·thal″mo·skop′ick) adj.

oph·thal·mo·so·nom·e·try (off·thal″mo·so·nom′e·tree) n. A method employing ultrasound for assessing ophthalmic arterial pulsation by applying the transducer over the lid of the closed eye.

oph·thal·mo·spin·ther·ism (off·thal″mo·spin′thur·iz·um) n. A condition of the eye in which there is a visual impression of luminous sparks.

oph·thal·mos·ta·sis (off″thal·mos′tuh·sis) n. Fixation of the eye during an operation upon it.

oph·thal·mo·syn·chy·sis (off·thal″mo·sing′ki·sis) n. Effusion into the interior chambers of the eye.

oph·thal·mot·o·my (off″thal·mot′um·ee) n. The dissection or incision of the eye.

oph·thal·mo·to·nom·e·try (off″thal·mo·to·nom′e·tree) n. Measurement of intraocular tension.

oph·thal·mo·tro·pom·e·try (off″thal·mo·tro·pom′e·tree) n. The measurement of the movement of the eyeballs.

-opia, -opy A combining form meaning *a defect of the eye.*

opi·ate (o′pee·ut, ·ate) n. 1. A preparation of opium. 2. Any narcotic or synthetic analgesic. 3. Anything that quiets uneasiness or dulls the feelings.

opio·ma·nia (o″pee·o·may′nee·uh) n. An uncontrollable desire for opium; opium habit. —**opiomani·ac** (·ack) n.

opio·pha·gia (o″pee·o·fay′jee·uh) *n.* The eating of opium.

opio·phile (o′pee·o·file) *n.* An addict of opium; an opium smoker or eater.

opisth-, opistho- A combining form meaning (a) *posterior, dorsal;* (b) *backward.*

opis·the·nar (o·pis′thi·nahr) *n.* The back of the hand.

opis·tho·cra·ni·on (o·pis″tho·kray′nee·on) *n. In craniometry,* the point, wherever it may lie in the sagittal plane on the occipital bone, which marks the posterior extremity of the longest diameter of the skull, measured from the glabella.

opis·thog·na·thism (o″pis·thog′nuh·thiz·um, ·tho′nuh·thiz·um, op″is·) *n.* Recession of the lower jaw.

opis·tho·po·reia (o·pis″tho·po·rye′uh) *n.* Involuntary walking backward in an attempt to go forward; occurs occasionally in postencephalitic parkinsonism.

opis·thor·chi·a·sis (o·pis″thor·kigh′uh·sis, op″is·) *n.* Infection of the liver with the fluke *Opisthorchis felineus.*

Op·is·thor·chis (op″is·thor′kis, o″pis·) *n.* A genus of trematodes or flukes.

Opisthorchis fe·lin·e·us (fe·lin′ee·us, fe·lye′nee·us). A species of fluke naturally parasitic to cats, dogs, foxes, and hogs, and accidentally in man. Produces hepatic lesions and extensive hyperplasia of the biliary ducts.

Opisthorchis vi·ver·ri·ni (viv″ur·eye′nye). A natural parasite of civet, dog and cat, and an important human infection in northern Thailand.

opis·thot·o·nus, opis·thot·o·nos (op″is·thot′uh·nus) *n.* A postural abnormality characterized by hypertension of the back and neck muscles, with retraction of the head, and arching forward of the trunk. It is seen in its most dramatic forms in cases of severe meningeal irritation, particularly bacterial meningitis, but also in advanced states of decerebration and spasticity due to various causes. —**opisthotonoid** (·noid), **opis·tho·ton·ic** (o·pis″tho·ton′ick) *adj.*

opi·um (o′pee·um) *n.* The air-dried juice from unripe capsules of *Papaver somniferum,* or its variety *album.* It contains a number of alkaloids, of which morphine is the most important, since it represents the chief properties of the drug. Crude opium contains 5 to 15% morphine, 2 to 8% narcotine, 0.1 to 2.5% codeine, 0.5 to 2.0% papaverine, 0.15 to 0.5% thebaine, 0.1 to 0.4% narceine, and lesser amounts of cryptopine, laudanine, and other alkaloids. Opium acts as a narcotic, dulls pain and discomfort, and produces deep sleep. The drug is used for the relief of pain of all forms except that due to cerebral inflammation. Used in the form of a standardized powder (10% morphine), extract (20% morphine), and tincture (1% morphine).

opo·ceph·a·lus (op″o·sef′uh·lus) *n.* A fetus with cyclopia, arrhinia, agnathia, and synotia; a form of cyclotia.

O point. The point of the apex cardiogram at the maximum inward motion of the cardiac apex,

occurring at the time of opening of the mitral valve.

op·pi·la·tion (op″i·lay′shun) *n.* Obstruction; a closing of the pores. —**op·pi·la·tive** (op′i·lay·tiv) *adj.*

op·po·nens (op·o′nenz) *adj.* Opposing; applied to certain muscles that bring one part opposite another.

ops- A combining form meaning *sight, vision.*

-ops *In botany and zoology,* a combining form meaning *-eyed.*

-opsia A combining form designating a *condition of vision.*

op·sig·e·nes (op·sij′e·neez) *n.pl.* Body tissues which come into use long after birth, as the wisdom teeth.

op·sino·gen (op·sin′o·jen) *n.* A substance producing an opsonin. —**opsi·nog·e·nous** (op″si·noj′e·nus) *adj.*

op·so·clo·nus (op″so·klo′nus) *n.* Rapid, conjugate oscillations of the eyes in a horizontal, rotatory, or vertical direction, made worse by voluntary movement or the need to fixate the eyes, and usually associated with widespread myoclonus of diverse causes.

op·so·ma·nia (op″so·may′nee·uh) *n.* Intense craving for dainties or some special food. —**opsoma·ni·ac** (·nee·ack) *n.*

opsonic action. The effect produced upon susceptible microorganisms and other cells by opsonins, which renders them vulnerable to phagocytes.

op·so·nin (op′suh·nin, op·so′nin) *n.* Any of various substances, including some complement components and specific antibodies, that facilitate phagocytosis of microbial organisms; these substances may be increased by immunization. —**op·son·ic** (op·son′ick) *adj.*

op·so·no·cy·to·phag·ic (op″suh·no·sigh″to·fay′jick, ·faj′ick) *adj.* Pertaining to the phagocytic activity of blood containing serum opsonins and homologous leukocytes.

op·so·no·ther·a·py (op″suh·no·therr′up·ee) *n.* The treatment of disease by increasing the opsonic action of the blood.

opt-, opto- A combining form meaning *optic* or *vision* or *eye.*

op·tes·the·sia (op″tes·theezh′uh, ·theez′ee·uh) *n.* Visual sensibility.

op·tic (op′tick) *adj.* Pertaining to the eye.

op·ti·cal (op′ti·kul) *adj.* 1. OPTIC. 2. Pertaining to light and the science of optics.

optical activity. The ability of a substance to rotate the plane of vibration of polarized light. It is characteristic of compounds having an asymmetric atom, usually of carbon.

optical index. A constant applied to objectives for purposes of comparison, taking into account the focal length or magnifying power of the lens and also the numerical aperture.

optic atrophy. Atrophy of the optic nerve. On funduscopic examination, the optic disk appears starkly white and sharply demarcated.

optic canal. The channel at the apex of the orbit, the anterior termination of the optic groove, just beneath the lesser wing of the sphenoid bone; it gives passage to the optic nerve and ophthalmic artery.

optic chiasma. The commissure anterior to the hypophysis where there is a partial decussation of the fibers in the optic nerves.

optic cup. The double-walled cup formed by invagination of the optic vesicle which differentiates into pigmented and sensory layers of the retina.

optic disk. The circular area in the retina that is the site of the convergence of fibers from the ganglion cells of the retina to form the optic nerve.

op·ti·cian (op·tish'un) *n.* A maker of optical instruments or lenses.

optic nerve. The second cranial nerve; the sensory nerve that innervates the retina.

optic neuritis. Acute impairment of vision in one eye or both, which may be affected simultaneously or successively, and which may recover spontaneously or leave the patient with a scotoma or scotomas, or even blindness. Usually due to demyelinative disease, sometimes to a toxic or nutritional disorder.

optic neuromyelitis. NEUROMYELITIS OPTICA.

op·ti·co·chi·as·mat·ic (op''ti·ko·kigh''az·mat'ick) *adj.* Pertaining to the optic nerves and optic chiasma.

op·ti·co·cil·i·ary (op''ti·ko·sil'ee·err·ee) *adj.* Pertaining to the optic and ciliary nerves.

op·ti·co·fa·cial (op''ti·ko·fay'shul) *adj.* Pertaining to the optic and facial nerves.

op·ti·co·pu·pil·lary (op''ti·ko·pew'pil·err·ee) *adj.* Pertaining to the optic nerve and the pupil.

op·tics (op'ticks) *n.* That branch of physics treating of the laws of light, its refraction and reflection, and its relation to vision.

optic tract. A band of nerve fibers running around the lateral side of a cerebral peduncle from the optic chiasma to the lateral geniculate body and midbrain.

optic vesicle. The embryonic evagination of the diencephalon from which are derived the pigment and sensory layers of the retina.

op·ti·mal (op'ti·mul) *adj.* Most desirable or satisfactory.

op·ti·mum (op'ti·mum) *n.* The amount or degree of something, such as temperature, that is most favorable, desirable, or satisfactory for some end or purpose.

Optochin. Trademark for ethylhydrocupreine, a pneumococcidal agent.

op·to·ki·net·ic (op''to·kigh·net'ick) *adj.* Of or pertaining to eye movements associated with movement of objects in the visual field.

optokinetic nystagmus. Nystagmus which occurs in normal individuals when a succession of moving objects traverses the field of vision, or when the individual moves past a succession of stationary objects. Syn. *train nystagmus.*

op·tom·e·ter (op·tom'e·tur) *n.* An instrument for determining the power of vision, especially the degree of refractive error that is to be corrected.

op·tom·e·trist (op·tom'e·trist) *n.* One who measures the degrees of visual powers, without the aid of a cycloplegic or mydriatic; a refractionist.

op·tom·e·try (op·tom'e·tree) *n.* Measurement of the visual powers.

op·to·my·om·e·ter (op''to·migh·om'e·tur) *n.* An instrument for measuring the strength of the extrinsic muscles of the eye.

op·to·type (op'to·tipe) *n.* A test type used in determining the acuity of vision.

¹ora (o'ruh) *n.* MARGIN.

²ora. Plural of *os* (L., mouth).

orad (or'ad) *adv.* Toward the mouth, or the oral region.

oral (or'ul) *adj.* Pertaining to the mouth.

oral candidiasis. An infection in the mouth by *Candida albicans,* occurring frequently in young infants.

oral character. A Freudian term applied to persons who, during the developmental period, have undergone an unusual degree of oral stimulation through poor feeding habits and otherwise and who thereby have laid the basis for a particular type of character, usually characterized by a general attitude of carefree indifference and by dependence on a mother or mother substitute to provide for their needs throughout life with little or no effort of their own.

oral erotic stage. *In psychoanalysis,* the first, or receptive, part of the oral phase of psychosexual development, dominated by sucking and lasting for the first 6 to 9 months of life.

oral personality. An individual who is mouth-centered far beyond the age when the oral phase should have been passed, and who exhibits oral erotism and sadism in disguised and sublimated forms.

oral physiotherapy. The procedures practiced by the individual to maintain mouth hygiene and properly stimulate the soft tissues surrounding the teeth.

ora ser·ra·ta (se·ray'tuh) [NA]. The serrated margin of the sensory portion of the retina, behind the ciliary body.

or·bic·u·lar (or·bick'yoo·lur) *adj.* Circular; applied to circular muscles, as the orbicular muscle of the eye (orbicularis oculi) or of the mouth (orbicularis oris).

or·bic·u·la·ris (or·bick''yoo·lair'is) *n.* An orbicular muscle.

orbicularis ocu·li (ock'yoo·lye). The ring muscle of the eye.

orbicularis oris (o'ris). The ring muscle of the mouth.

or·bit, *n.* The bony cavity containing the eye, which is formed by parts of the frontal, sphenoid, ethmoid, nasal, lacrimal, maxillary, and palatal bones.

or·bi·tal (or'bi·tul) *adj. & n.* 1. Of or pertaining to an orbit. 2. Any of certain fibers of smooth muscle bridging the inferior orbital fissure. 3. Any one of the permissible modes of motion of an electron in an atom or molecule.

orbital cellulitis. An infection of the orbit usually associated with acute sinusitis and characterized by conjunctival edema and proptosis with subsequent motion limitation and diplopia.

or·bi·ta·le (or''bi·tah'lee, ·tay'lee) *n.,* pl. **orbi·ta·lia** (·tay'lee·uh, ·tal'ee·uh) *In craniometry,* the lowest point on the inferior margin of the orbit, used in conjunction with the poria to orient the skull on the Frankfort horizontal plane.

or·bi·to·nom·e·ter (or″bi·to·nom′e·tur) *n.* A device used to measure the resistance to pressure of the eye into the orbit in cases of exophthalmic goiter.

or·bi·to·nom·e·try (or″bi·to·nom′e·tree) *n.* The measurement of the resistance of the globe of the eye to retrodisplacement.

or·bi·tot·o·my (or″bi·tot′um·ee) *n.* Incision into the orbit.

or·ce·in (or′seen, or·see′in) *n.* A brownish red crystalline powder, containing many components, obtained by oxidation of orcinol; insoluble in water, soluble in alcohol. Used in microscopy as a stain.

or·ches·tro·ma·nia (or·kes″tro·may′nee·uh) *n. Obsol.* SYDENHAM'S CHOREA.

orchi-, orchio-, orchid-, orchido-, orch- A combining form meaning *testis.*

or·chi·al·gia (or″kee·al′juh, -jee·uh) *n.* Testicular pain.

or·chic (or′kick) *adj.* Pertaining to the testis.

or·chi·dec·to·my (or″ki·deck′tum·ee) *n.* ORCHIECTOMY.

or·chi·di·tis (or″ki·digh′tis) *n.* ORCHITIS.

or·chi·dop·a·thy (or″ki·dop′uth·ee) *n.* Disease of a testis.

or·chi·do·pexy (or′ki·do·peck″see, or·kid′o·) *n.* ORCHIOPEXY.

or·chi·dot·o·my (or″ki·dot′um·ee) *n.* Incision into a testis.

or·chi·ec·to·my (or″kee·eck′tum·ee) *n.* Surgical removal of one or both testes; castration.

or·chi·epi·did·y·mi·tis (or″kee·ep″i·did″i·migh′ tis) *n.* Inflammation of both testis and epididymis.

or·chio·ca·tab·a·sis (or″kee·o·ka·tab′uh·sis) *n.* The normal descent of the testis into the scrotum.

or·chio·cele (or′kee·o·seel) *n.* 1. A complete scrotal hernia. 2. A tumor of the testis. 3. Herniation of a testis. 4. A testis retained in the inguinal canal.

or·chi·op·a·thy (or″kee·op′uth·ee) *n.* Any disease of the testis.

or·chio·pexy (or′kee·o·peck″see) *n.* Surgical fixation of a testis, as in a plastic operation for relief of an undescended testis.

or·chio·plas·ty (or′kee·o·plas″tee) *n̄.* Plastic surgery of a testis.

or·chi·tis (or·kigh′tis) *n.* Inflammation of the testis. **—orchit·ic** (·kit′ick) *adj.*

or·ci·nol (or′si·nol) *n.* 5-Methylresorcinol, C_7H_8-$O_2.H_2O$, a constituent of many species of lichens, variously used as a reagent.

or·der, *n.* 1. Systematic arrangement. 2. *In biology,* the taxonomic group below a class and above a family.

or·der·ly, *n.* A male hospital attendant.

Oreton. A trademark for certain preparations or derivatives of the androgen testosterone.

orex·is (o·reck′sis) *n.* The aspect of mental functioning or of an act which pertains to feeling, desire, impulse, volition, or purposeful striving as contrasted with its cognitive or intellectual aspect.

orf, *n.* A pox virus disease of sheep and goats that is transmittable to humans, characterized by red vesicular or pustular lesions on the lips, oral mucosa, udder, and feet. Syn. *ecthyma contagiosum.*

or·gan, *n.* A differentiated part of an organism adapted for a definite function.

or·gan·elle (or·guh·nel′) *n.* A specialized structure or part of a cell presumably having a special function or capacity, as a mitochondrion. **—organel·lar** (·ur) *adj.*

or·gan·ic, *adj.* 1. Of or pertaining to organs; having organs. 2. Of or pertaining to living organisms. 3. *In chemistry,* of or pertaining to compounds of carbon. 4. Physical, as contrasted with mental, emotional, or psychogenic, particularly as applied to any disorder for which there is a known or hypothesized impairment of structure, biochemistry, or physiology. 5. Pertaining to foods grown and produced without the use of artificial fertilizers or pesticides.

organic acid. Commonly, any acid containing the carboxyl group —COOH.

organic brain syndrome or disorder. Any nervous disorder either known to have a physical cause or presumed, because it produces physical symptoms, to have one.

organic disease. A disease associated with recognizable structural changes in the organs or tissues of the body.

or·gan·i·cism (or·gan′i·siz·um) *n.* HOLISM.

or·ga·ni·za·tion, *n.* 1. The systematic interrelationships of structurally and functionally differentiated parts to form an integrated whole. 2. A part of the repair process occurring in an injury that has destroyed tissue; the ingrowth of capillaries and fibroblasts into thrombi or blood clots.

or·ga·nize, *v.* 1. To make organic, to form into an organism; to induce to form or develop. 2. To induce or undergo organization (2).

or·ga·niz·er, *n. In embryology,* the region of the dorsal lip of the blastopore, comprising chordamesoderm, that is self-differentiating and capable of inducing the formation of medullary plate in the adjacent ectoderm; the primary organizer. A second-grade (or higher) organizer, coming into play after the laying down of the main axis of the body induced by the primary organizer is completed, is any part of the embryo which exerts a morphogenetic stimulus on an adjacent part or parts, as in the induction of the lens by the optic vesicle. Syn. *organization center.*

organizing pneumonia. Pneumonia in which the healing process is characterized by organization and cicatrization of the exudate rather than by resolution and resorption. Syn. *unresolved pneumonia.*

or·ga·no·ax·i·al (or″guh·no·ack′see·ul) *adj.* Rotated around the long axis of the organ, as in organoaxial volvulus.

or·gano·gel (or·gan′o·jel) *n.* A gel in which the dispersion medium is an organic liquid.

or·gan·oid (or′guh·noid) *adj.* Resembling an organ.

organoid tumor. A tumor in which the components are so arranged as to resemble the general structure of an organ, as an adenoma.

or·ga·nol·o·gy (or″guh·nol′uh·jee) *n.* The science that treats of the organs of plants and animals.

or·ga·no·meg·a·ly (or″guh·no·meg′uh·lee) *n.* SPLANCHNOMEGALY.

or·gano·mer·cu·ri·al (or·gan′o·mur·kew′ree·ul, or″guh·no·) *n.* An organic compound or substance containing mercury.

or·ga·nos·co·py (or″guh·nos′kuh·pee) *n.* The examination of an organ with a special lens system, such as a cystoscope, esophagoscope, or laryngoscope.

or·ga·no·ther·a·py (or″guh·no·therr′up·ee) *n.* The treatment of diseases by administration of animal organs or their extracts.

or·ga·no·troph·ic (or″guh·no·trof′ick, ·tro′fick) *adj.* Pertaining to the nutrition of living organs.

or·ga·not·ro·pism (or″guh·no·tro′piz·um, or″guh·not′ruh·piz·um) *n.* Ehrlich's theory that certain substances manifest a definite chemical affinity for certain components of cells.

or·gasm (or′gaz·um) *n.* The intense, diffuse, and subjectively pleasurable sensation experienced during sexual intercourse or genital manipulation, culminating, for the male, in seminal ejaculation and for the female, in myotonia with uterine contractions, warm suffusion, and pelvic throbbing sensations.

or·gas·mo·lep·sy (or·gaz′mo·lep″see) *n.* A sudden loss of muscle tone during sexual orgasm, accompanied by a transitory loss of consciousness.

ori·en·ta·tion (or″ee·en·tay′shun) *n.* 1. *In psychology,* the act of determining one's relation to the environment or a specified aspect of it, such as time, person, or place. 2. The process of helping a person or persons to find their way about in a new situation; orientation program. 3. *In chemistry,* the relative positions of atoms or groups of atoms in certain molecules.

or·i·fice (or′i·fis) *n.* An opening, an entrance to a cavity or tube. **—or·i·fi·cial** (or″i·fish′ul) *adj.*

or·i·gin, *n.* 1. The beginning or starting point of anything. 2. *In anatomy,* the end of attachment of a muscle which remains relatively fixed during contraction of the muscle.

Orinase. Trademark for tolbutamide, an orally effective hypoglycemic drug.

or·ni·thine (or′ni·theen, ·thin) *n.* α,δ-Diaminovaleric acid, $NH_2(CH_2)_3CHNH_2COOH$; an amino acid occurring in the urine of some birds, but not found in native proteins; an intermediate in the Krebs-Henseleit cycle of urea formation.

ornithine trans·car·ba·myl·ase (trans″kahr′bam·i·lace, kahr·bam′il·lace, ·laze). The enzyme that catalyzes carbamylation of ornithine to form citrulline, which is the first step in the biochemical synthesis of arginine.

or·ni·tho·sis (or′ni·tho′sis) *n.* Psittacosis contracted from birds other than parrots and parakeets.

oro- A combining form meaning *mouth* or *oral.*

oro- See *orrho-.*

oro·an·tral (or″o·an′trul) *adj.* Pertaining to the mouth and the maxillary sinus.

oro·fa·cial (or″o·fay′shul) *adj.* Of or pertaining to the mouth and face.

oro·na·sal (or″o·nay′zul) *adj.* Involving the mouth and the nose.

oro·phar·ynx (or″o·far′inks) *n.* The oral pharynx, situated below the level of the lower border of the soft palate and above the larynx, as distinguished from the nasopharynx and laryngeal pharynx. **—oro·pha·ryn·ge·al** (or″o·fa·rin′jee·ul) *adj.*

or·phen·a·drine (or·fen′uh·dreen) *n.* 2-(*p*-Chloro-α-methyl-α-phenylbenzyloxy)-*N,N*-dimethylethylamine, $C_{18}H_{23}NO$, an antispasmodic and antitremor drug; used as the citrate and hydrochloride salts.

orrho-, oro- A combining form meaning *serum.*

or·rho·men·in·gi·tis (or″o·men″in·jye′tis) *n.* Inflammation of a serous membrane.

or·rhos (or′os) *n.* SERUM; WHEY.

or·ris·root, *n.* A powder from certain varieties of iris; used in various cosmetics, toothpastes, etc. It is a common sensitizer, both by contact and by inhalation.

orth-, ortho- A combining form meaning (a) *straight;* (b) *direct;* (c) *normal.*

or·the·sis (orth·ee′sis) *n.* An orthopedic brace or device.

orthi-, orthio- *In craniometry,* a combining form meaning *steep* or *upright.*

ortho- 1. See *orth-.* 2. *In chemistry,* a prefix indicating adjacent relationship of two carbon atoms of the benzene ring, such as the 1,2-position; also any benzene derivative in which two substituents occur at adjacent carbon atoms in the ring. Symbol, *o-.* 3. *In chemistry,* a prefix indicating an acid in fully hydrated or hydroxylated form or, sometimes, in the highest hydrated or hydroxylated form that is stable.

or·tho (orth′o) *adj.* 1. Of or pertaining to two positions in the benzene ring that are adjacent. 2. Of or pertaining to the state in which the atomic nuclei of a diatomic molecule spin in the same direction.

or·tho·cho·rea (orth″o·ko·ree′uh) *n.* Choreic movements in the erect posture.

or·tho·chro·mat·ic (orth″o·kro·mat′ick) *adj.* 1. *In photography,* correct in the rendering of tones or colors. 2. Of photographic emulsions, not sensitive to red, able to be developed under a red safelight. 3. Having staining characteristics of a normal type.

or·tho·chro·mic (orth″o·kro′mick) *adj.* ORTHOCHROMATIC.

or·tho·cre·sol (orth″o·kree′sol) *n.* One of the isomers of cresol, $CH_3C_6H_4OH$. It has the weakest germicidal activity of the three isomers.

or·tho·dac·ty·lous (orth″o·dack′ti·lus) *adj.* Having straight digits.

or·tho·di·a·gram (orth″o·dye′uh·gram) *n.* A manual tracing of the fluoroscopic image of the heart.

or·tho·don·tics (orth″o·don′ticks) *n.* The branch of dentistry concerned with the treatment and prevention of malocclusion. —**orthodontic,** *adj.*

or·tho·don·tist (orth"o·don'tist) *n.* A specialist in the field of orthodontics.

or·tho·gen·e·sis (orth"o·jen'e·sis) *n.* The doctrine that phylogenetic evolution takes place according to system in certain well-defined and limited directions, and not by accident in many directions. —**or·tho·ge·net·ic** (·je·net'ick) *adj.*

or·tho·gen·ic (orth"o·jen'ick) *adj.* 1. Of or pertaining to orthogenesis. 2. Pertaining to the training and social habilitation of children who behave retardedly because of emotional disturbances.

or·tho·grade (orth'o·grade) *adj.* Walking or standing in the upright position.

or·thom·e·ter (or·thom'e·tur) *n.* An instrument for measuring the relative degree of protrusion of the eyes. Syn. *exophthalmometer.*

or·tho·pe·dic, or·tho·pae·dic (orth"uh·pee'dick) *adj.* Pertaining to orthopedics, as orthopedic surgery.

or·tho·pe·dics, or·tho·pae·dics (orth"uh·pee'dicks) *n.* That branch of surgery concerned with corrective treatment of deformities, diseases, and ailments of the locomotor apparatus, especially those affecting limbs, bones, muscles, joints, and fasciae, whether by apparatus, manipulation, or open operation; originally devoted to the correction and treatment of deformities in children.

or·tho·pe·dist (orth"uh·pee'dist) *n.* One who practices orthopedic surgery; a specialist in orthopedics.

or·thop·nea (or"thup·nee'uh, or·thop'nee·uh) *n.* A condition in which there is difficulty in breathing except when sitting or standing upright. —**orthopne·ic** (·nee'ick) *adj.*

or·tho·praxy (orth'o·prack·see) *n.* Correction of the deformities of the body.

or·tho·psy·chi·a·try (orth"o·sigh·kigh'uh·tree) *n.* Corrective psychiatry; an approach to the study and treatment of behavior which, placing an emphasis on the prevention and early treatment of behavior disorders, involves the collaboration of psychiatry, psychology, pediatrics, social services, and schools to promote healthy emotional growth and development.

or·thop·tics (or·thop'ticks) *n.* The science of rendering visual reactions and responses right and efficient, usually by some form of exercise or training, as for amblyopia or strabismus.

or·tho·scope (orth'uh·skope) *n.* 1. An instrument for examination of the eye through a layer of water, whereby the curvature and hence the refraction of the cornea is neutralized, and the cornea acts as a plane medium. 2. An instrument used in drawing the projections of skulls.

or·tho·sis (orth·o'sis) *n.* The straightening of a deformity.

or·tho·stat·ic (or"tho·stat'ick) *adj.* Pertaining to, or caused by, standing upright.

orthostatic albuminuria. Proteinuria present only when the patient is in the erect posture.

orthostatic hypotension syndrome. PRIMARY ORTHOSTATIC HYPOTENSION.

orthostatic purpura. Purpura which develops in the lower extremities after prolonged standing.

or·tho·stat·ism (orth"o·stat'iz·um) *n.* The erect standing posture of the normal body.

or·tho·tast (orth'o·tast) *n.* A device for straightening curvatures of long bones. It has also been used as a tourniquet.

or·tho·ther·a·py (orth"o·therr'up·ee) *n.* The treatment of disorders of posture.

or·thot·ics (or·thot'icks) *n.* The science of orthopedic appliances and their use.

or·thot·o·nus, or·thot·o·nos (or·thot'un·us) *n.* Tonic spasm in which the body lies rigid and straight. —**or·tho·ton·ic** (orth"o·ton'ick) *adj.*

or·tho·to·pia (orth"uh·to'pee·uh) *n.* The natural or normal position of a part or organ.

or·tho·top·ic (orth"o·top'ick) *adj.* In the natural or normal position.

or·tho·volt·age (orth·o·vohl'tij) *n.* Roentgen radiation produced by voltages of 200 to 500 kilovolts.

O.S. Abbreviation for (a) *oculus sinister,* left eye; (b) *opening snap.*

Os Symbol for osmium.

¹os (oce, oss) *n.,* genit. *oris* (o'ris), pl. *ora* (o'ruh) MOUTH.

²os (oss) *n.,* genit. sing. **os·sis** (oss'is), pl. **os·sa** (·uh), genit. pl. **os·si·um** (oss'ee·um) BONE.

osa·zone (o'suh·zone) *n.* A compound formed by reaction of a sugar with phenylhydrazine in the presence of acetic acid; used in the identification of sugars.

os cal·cis (kal'sis) CALCANEUS (1).

os·cil·la·tion (os"i·lay'shun) *n.* A swinging or vibration; also any tremulous motion. —**os·cil·la·to·ry** (os'i·luh·tor·ee) *adj.*

os·cil·la·tor (os'i·lay'tur) *n.* A mechanical or electronic device that produces electrical vibration; used in physical therapy.

os·cil·lo·graph (os'i·lo·graf, os·i'lo·graf) *n.* An apparatus for recording oscillations. —**os·cil·lo·graph·ic** (os'i·lo·graf'ick) *adj.*; **oscil·log·ra·phy** (log'ruh·fee) *n.*

os·cil·lom·e·ter (os"i·lom'e·tur) *n.* An instrument for measuring oscillations, as those seen in taking blood pressures. —**os·cil·lo·met·ric** (os"i·lo·met'rick) *adj.*

os·cil·lom·e·try (os"i·lom'e·tree) *n.* Measurement or detection of oscillations of any type, especially circulatory.

os·cil·lop·sia (os"il·op'see·uh) *n.* Illusory movement of the environment, in which stationary objects seem to move up or down or from side to side. It may be associated with parietoocciptal lesions, with severe nystagmus of any type due to lesions involving the vestibular nuclei, or with labyrinthine lesions.

os·cil·lo·scope (os·il'uh·skope) *n.* A cathode-ray vacuum tube so constructed as to portray visually the deflections or oscillations of electromotive forces as a function of time. Syn. *cathode-ray oscilloscope.*

os·ci·ta·tion (os"i·tay'shun) *n.* YAWNING.

os·cu·la·tion (os"kew·lay'shun) *n.* 1. Anastomosis of vessels. 2. Kissing.

os·cu·lum (os"kew·lum) *n.* A small aperture.

Osgood-Schlat·ter disease A traction avulsion

of the tibial tubercle apophysis of chronic nature.

-osis A suffix designating (a) *a process*, as osmosis; (b) *a state*, as narcosis; (c) *a diseased condition of*, as nephrosis; (d) *a disease caused by*, as mycosis; (e) *an increase in*, as leukocytosis.

Osler-Rendu-Weber disease HEREDITARY HEMORRHAGIC TELANGIECTASIA.

Os·ler's disease POLYCYTHEMIA VERA.

Osler's febrile polyneuritis. GUILLAIN-BARRÉ DISEASE.

Osler's nodes Painful red indurated areas in the pads of the fingers or toes in bacterial endocarditis.

Osler-Vaquez disease POLYCYTHEMIA VERA.

os·mat·ic (oz·mat″ick) *adj.* Characterized by a sense of smell.

os·mic acid (oz′mick, os′mick). Osmium tetroxide, OsO₄, employed as a histologic stain and reagent, almost universally used as a primary or secondary fixative in electron microscopy; has been used internally, in the form of the potassium salt, in rheumatic affections and in epilepsy.

os·mics (oz′micks) *n.* The study of olfaction.

os·mi·dro·sis (oz″mi·dro′sis) *n.* BROMHIDROSIS.

os·mio·phil·ic (oz″mee·o·fil′ick) *adj.* Having an affinity for osmium tetroxide or osmic acid.

os·mi·um (oz′mee·um, os′) *n.* Os = 190.2. A heavy metallic element, with a density of 22.48, belonging to the platinum group. —**os·mic** (oz′mick, os′) *adj.*

osmo-. A combining form meaning *osmosis*.

os·mo·dys·pho·ria (oz″mo·dis·fo′ree·uh) *n.* Intolerance of certain odors.

os·mol (oz′mol, ·mole) *n.* The quantity of a solute, existing in solution as molecules and/or ions, commonly stated in grams, that is osmotically equivalent to one mole of an ideally behaving nonelectrolyte. —**os·mo·lal** (oz·mo′lul) *adj.*; **os·mo·lal·i·ty** (oz″mo·lal′i·tee) *n.*

os·mo·lar (oz·mo′lur) *adj.* Of or pertaining to the osmotic property of a solution containing one or more molecular or ionic species, quantitatively expressed in osmol units. —**os·mo·lar·i·ty** (oz″mo·lăr′i·tee) *n.*

os·mol·o·gy (oz·mol′uh·jee) *n.* That part of physical science treating of osmosis.

os·mom·e·ter (oz·mom′e·tur) *n.* An instrument for testing the sense of smell; an olfactometer.

os·mom·e·ter (oz·mom′e·tur) *n.* An apparatus for measuring osmotic pressure.

os·mo·pho·bia (oz″mo·fo′bee·uh) *n.* An abnormal fear of odors.

os·mo·re·cep·tors (oz″mo·re·sep′turz) *n.* Structures in the hypothalamus which respond to changes in osmotic pressure of the blood by regulating the secretion of the neurohypophyseal antidiuretic hormone (ADH).

os·mo·sis (oz·mo′sis, os·) *n.* The passage of a solvent through a membrane from a dilute solution into a more concentrated one.

os·mot·ic (oz·mot′ick, os·) *adj.* Pertaining to osmosis, particularly to osmotic pressure.

osmotic diuretic. A substance producing diuresis because of the osmotic effect of the unab-

sorbed fraction in the renal tubules with resulting loss of water.

osmotic fragility. The susceptibility of erythrocytes to lysis when placed in hypotonic saline solutions.

osmotic pressure. The pressure developed when two solutions of different concentrations of the same solute are separated by a membrane permeable to the solvent only.

os·phre·si·ol·o·gy (os·free″zee·ol′o·jee) *n.* The science of the sense of smell and its organs, and of odors.

os·pu·bis (pew′bis) [NA]. The pubic bone; PUBIS.

ossa. Plural of *os* (L., bone).

os·se·lit (os′e·lit) *n.* A hard nodule on the inner aspect of a horse's knee. Inflammation of the periosteum at the distal end of the third metacarpal, or at the proximal end of the first phalanx, or both, results in new bone growth.

os·seo·car·ti·lag·i·nous (os″ee·o·kahr·ti·laj′i·nus) *adj.* Pertaining to or composed of both bone and cartilage.

os·seo·fi·brous (os″ee·o·figh′brus) *adj.* Pertaining to or composed of both bone and fibrous tissue.

os·seo·lig·a·men·tous (os″ee·o·lig″uh·men′tus) *adj.* Pertaining to the bones and ligaments.

os·seo·mu·coid (os″ee·o·mew′koid) *n.* A mucin or glycoprotein obtained from bone.

os·se·ous (os′ee·us) *adj.* Bony; composed of or resembling bone.

osseous cochlea. OSSEOUS COCHLEAR CANAL.

osseous cochlear canal. The bony canal in which the cochlear duct is housed.

osseous labyrinth. The portion of the petrous part of the temporal bone that surrounds the internal ear. It consists of the vestibule, osseous semicircular canals, and cochlea.

osseous semicircular canals. The bony parts of the labyrinth of the ear that house the membranous semicircular canals; three loop-shaped canals in the petrous portion of the temporal bone, the anterior semicircular canal, the posterior semicircular canal, and the lateral or horizontal semicircular canal. They lie at right angles to one another and communicate with the vestibule.

os·si·cle (os′i·kul) *n.* A small bone; particularly, one of three small bones in the tympanic cavity: the malleus, incus, and stapes.

os·sic·u·lar (os·ick′yoo·lur) *adj.* Of or pertaining to ossicles.

os·sic·u·lec·to·my (os″i·kew·leck′tuh·mee) *n.* The removal of one or more of the ossicles of the middle ear.

os·sic·u·lot·o·my (os″i·kew·lot′um·ee, os·ick″yoo·) *n.* Surgical incision involving the tissues about the ossicles of the ear.

os·sif·ic (os·if′ick) *adj.* Producing bone.

os·si·fi·ca·tion (os″i·fi·kay′shun) *n.* The formation of bone; the conversion of tissue into bone.

os·si·form (os′i·form) *adj.* Bonelike.

os·si·fy (os′i·figh) *v.* To turn into bone.

ossifying fibroma. A benign tumor of bone derived from bone-forming connective tissue, seen particularly in the vertebral column, which microscopically appears as vascularized connective tissue interspersed with fibrous bone trabeculae. Syn. *osteogenic fibroma, fibrous osteoma.*

ost-, oste-, osteo- A combining form meaning *bone.*

os·tal·gia (os·tal'jee·uh) *n.* Pain in a bone. Syn. *ostealgia.* —**ostal·gic** (·jick) *adj.*

os·tal·gi·tis (os''tal·jigh'tis) *n.* Inflammation of a bone attended by pain.

os·tec·to·my (os·teck'tum·ee) *n.* Excision of a bone or a portion of a bone.

os·te·itis (os''tee·eye'tis) *n.* Inflammation of bone. —**oste·it·ic** (·it'ick) *adj.*

osteitis con·den·sans il·ii (kun·den'sanz il'ee·eye). A disease of unknown origin characterized by low back pain bilaterally, accompanied by an oval or triangular area of sclerotic opaque bone adjacent to the sacroiliac joints in the ilium.

osteitis cys·ti·ca (sis'ti·kuh). Osseous lesions originally described in sarcoidosis but also seen in normal individuals and in association with other diseases. The phalanges of fingers and toes appear on roentgenograms to have cysts. They represent replacement of bone and marrow by sarcoid nodules. Syn. *Jüngling's disease, osteitis tuberculosa multiplex cystoides.*

osteitis de·for·mans (de·for'manz). PAGET'S DISEASE (2).

osteitis fibrosa. *Informal.* OSTEITIS FIBROSA CYSTICA.

osteitis fi·bro·sa cys·ti·ca (figh·bro'suh sis'ti·kuh). Generalized skeletal demineralization due to an increased rate of bone destruction resulting from hyperparathyroidism, occasionally complicated by large osteoporotic areas resembling cysts. Syn. *von Recklinghausen's disease, Engel-Recklinghausen disease, osteitis fibrosa generalisata.*

osteitis fibrosa cystica dis·sem·i·na·ta (di·sem''i·nay'tuh, ·nah'tuh). FIBROUS DYSPLASIA (1).

osteitis fibrosa disseminata. FIBROUS DYSPLASIA (1).

osteitis fibrosa gen·er·al·i·sa·ta (jen''ur·al·i·zay'tuh, ·sah'tuh). OSTEITIS FIBROSA CYSTICA.

osteitis fra·gil·i·tans (fra·jil'i·tanz). OSTEOGENESIS IMPERFECTA.

osteitis pubis. Inflammation in the pubic symphysis.

os·tem·bry·on (os·tem'bree·on) *n.* An ossified fetus.

osteo-. See *ost-.*

os·te·o·an·eu·rysm (os''tee·o·an'yoo·riz·um) *n.* 1. ANEURYSMAL BONE CYST. 2. The telangiectatic, pulsating form of osteogenic sarcoma.

os·te·o·ar·threc·to·my (os''tee·o·ahr·threck'tum·ee) *n.* Surgical excision or partial excision of the bony portion of a joint.

os·te·o·ar·thri·tis (os''tee·o·ahr·thrigh'tis) *n.* DEGENERATIVE JOINT DISEASE.

os·te·o·ar·throp·a·thy (os''tee·o·ahr·throp'uth·ee) *n.* Any disease of bony articulations.

os·te·o·ar·thro·sis (os''tee·o·ahr·thro'sis) *n.* DEGENERATIVE JOINT DISEASE.

os·te·o·ar·throt·o·my (os''tee·o·ahr·throt'um·ee) *n.* Surgical excision or partial excision of the bony portion of a joint.

os·te·o·blast (os'tee·o·blast) *n.* Any one of the

cells of mesenchymal origin concerned in the formation of bony tissue. —**os·te·o·blas·tic** (os''tee·o·blast'ick) *adj.*

os·te·o·blas·to·ma (os''tee·o·blas·to'muh) *n.* 1. A benign tumor of bone, composed of osteoblasts, osteoid and immature bone. It is painless, chiefly affects children and young adults, and is most commonly found in the ilia, the vertebrae, or the medulla of long bones. 2. *Obsol.* OSTEOGENIC SARCOMA.

os·te·o·camp·sia (os''tee·o·kamp'see·uh) *n.* Curvature of a bone without fracture, as in osteomalacia.

os·te·o·car·ti·lag·i·nous (os''tee·o·kahr''ti·laj'i·nus) *adj.* Pertaining to or composed of both bone and cartilage.

os·te·o·chon·dral (os''tee·o·kon'drul) *adj.* Composed of both bone and cartilage.

os·te·o·chon·dri·tis (os''tee·o·kon·drigh'tis) *n.* 1. Inflammation of both bone and cartilage. 2. OSTEOCHONDROSIS.

osteochondritis de·for·mans cox·ae ju·ve·ni·lis (de·for'manz kock'see joo·ve·nigh'lis). Osteochondrosis of the head of the femur.

osteochondritis deformans juvenilis. Osteochondrosis of the head of the femur.

osteochondritis dis·se·cans (dis'e·kanz). A joint affection characterized by partial or complete detachment of a fragment of articular cartilage and underlying bone. Syn. *osteochondrosis dissecans.*

os·te·o·chon·dro·dys·pla·sia (os''tee·o·kon''dro·dis·play'zhuh, ·zee·uh) *n.* Abnormal development of bony and cartilaginous structures.

os·te·o·chon·dro·dys·tro·phy (os''tee·o·kon''dro·dis'truh·fee) *n.* MORQUIO'S SYNDROME.

os·te·o·chon·dro·ma (os''tee·o·kon·dro'muh) *n.* 1. A benign hamartomatous tumor originating in bone or cartilage, occasionally from one structure, which histologically contains both bone and cartilage. 2. EXOSTOSIS CARTILAGINEA.

os·te·o·chon·dro·ma·to·sis (os''tee·o·kon·dro''muh·to'sis) *n.* MULTIPLE HEREDITARY EXOSTOSES.

os·te·o·chon·dro·myx·o·ma (os''tee·o·kon''dro·mick·so'muh) *n.* An osteochondroma with myxoid component.

os·te·o·chon·dro·myxo·sar·co·ma (os''tee·o·kon''dro·mick''so·sahr·ko'muh) *n.* An osteosarcoma with a significant myxosarcomatous element.

os·te·o·chon·dro·sar·co·ma (os''tee·o·kon''dro·sahr·ko'muh) *n.* An osteosarcoma with a significant chondrosarcomatous element.

os·te·o·chon·dro·sis (os''tee·o·kon·dro'sis) *n.* A process involving ossification centers chiefly during periods of rapid growth, characterized by avascular necrosis followed by slow regeneration.

osteochondrosis deformans tib·i·ae (tib'ee·ee). Nonrachitic bowing of the legs seen in very young, and less frequently in older, children which usually improves spontaneously. Syn. *Blount-Barber syndrome.*

osteochondrosis dissecans. OSTEOCHONDRITIS DISSECANS.

os·te·oc·la·sis (os''tee·ock'luh·sis) *n.* 1. The fra-ture of a long bone without resort to open operation, for the purpose of correcting deformity. 2. The destruction of bony tissue; the resorption of bone.

os·te·o·clas·to·ma (os''te·o·klas·to'muh) *n.* GIANT-CELL TUMOR.

os·te·o·cyte (os'te·o·site) *n.* BONE CELL.

os·te·o·den·tin (os''te·o·den'tin) *n.* A tissue intermediate in structure between bone and dentin.

os·te·o·der·ma·to·plas·tic (os''te·o·dur''muh·to·plast'ick) *adj.* Pertaining to the formation of osseous tissue in dermal structures.

os·te·o·di·as·ta·sis (os''te·o·dye·as'tuh·sis) *n.* Separation of bone (as an epiphysis) without true fracture, or of two normally contiguous bones.

os·te·o·dyn·ia (os''te·o·din'ee·uh) *n.* A pain in a bone.

os·te·o·dys·tro·phy (os''te·o·dis'truh·fee) *n.* Any defective bone formation, as in rickets or dwarfism.

os·te·o·fi·bro·chon·dro·ma (os''te·o·figh''bro·kon·dro'muh) *n.* An osteochondroma with a significant fibrous element.

os·te·o·fi·bro·li·po·ma (os''te·o·figh''bro·li·po'muh) *n.* A benign tumor with bony, fibrous, and fatty components.

os·te·o·fi·bro·ma (os''te·o·figh·bro'muh) *n.* A benign tumor with fibrous and osseous components.

os·te·o·fi·bro·sar·co·ma (os''te·o·figh''bro·sahr·ko'muh) *n.* An osteogenic sarcoma with a prominent fibrosarcomatous element.

os·te·o·fi·bro·sis (os''te·o·figh·bro'sis) *n.* Fibrosis of bone; a change involving mainly the red bone marrow.

os·te·o·gen·e·sis (os''te·o·jen'e·sis) *n.* The development of bony tissues; ossification; the histogenesis of bone.

osteogenesis im·per·fec·ta (im·pur·feck'tuh), a dominantly heritable disease characterized by hypoplasia of osteoid tissue and collagen, resulting in bone fractures with minimal trauma, hypermotility of joints, blue sclerae, and a hemorrhagic tendency.

osteogenesis imperfecta con·gen·i·ta (kon·jen'i·tuh). A more severe form of osteogenesis imperfecta with onset of multiple fractures in utero and autosomal recessive inheritance in some cases.

osteogenesis imperfecta cys·ti·ca (sis'ti·kuh). A rare form of osteogenesis imperfecta in which cystic changes of bone are found radiographically.

osteogenesis imperfecta tar·da (tahr'duh). Osteogenesis imperfecta in which fractures do not occur until later childhood.

os·te·o·gen·ic (os''te·o·jen'ick) *adj.* Pertaining to osteogenesis, as osteogenic layer, the deep layer of periosteum from which bone is formed.

osteogenic sarcoma. A malignant tumor principally composed of anaplastic cells of mesenchymal derivation. Syn. *osteosarcoma.*

os·te·o·hal·i·ste·re·sis (os''te·o·hal''i·ste·ree'sis) *n.* A loss of the mineral constituents of bone frequently resulting in softening and deformity of the bone.

os·te·o·hy·per·troph·ic (os''te·o·high''pur·trof'ick) *adj.* Pertaining to overgrowth of bone.

os·te·oid (os'te·oid) *adj. & n.* 1. Resembling bone. 2. Of or pertaining to bone. 3. The young hyalin matrix of true bone in which the calcium salts are deposited.

os·te·ol·o·gy (os''te·ol'uh·jee) *n.* The science of anatomy and structure of bones.

os·te·ol·y·sis (os''te·ol'i·sis) *n.* 1. Resorption of bone. 2. Degeneration of bone. —**os·te·o·lyt·ic** (os''te·o·lit'ick) *adj.*

os·te·o·ma (os''te·o'muh) *n.* 1. A benign bony tumor seen particularly in the membrane bones of the skull and exhibiting a tendency to extend into the orbit or paranasal sinuses. 2. Loosely, a nonneoplastic or neoplastic lesion such as a hyperostosis, a fibrous dysplasia, or an exostosis (osteochondroma). —**osteoma·toid** (·toid) *adj.*

os·te·o·ma·la·cia (os''te·o·muh·lay'shee·uh) *n.* Failure of ossification due to a decrease in the amount of available calcium from any of multiple causes. Syn. *adult rickets.* —**osteomala·cial** (·shee·ul), **osteomala·cic** (·sick) *adj.*

os·te·o·ma·to·sis (os''te·o''muh·to'sis) *n.* The presence of multiple osteomas.

os·te·om·e·try (os''te·om'e·tree) *n.* The study of the proportions and measurements of the skeleton. —**os·te·o·met·ric** (os''te·o·met'rick) *adj.*

os·te·o·my·e·li·tis (os''te·o·migh''e·lye'tis) *n.* Inflammation of the marrow and hard tissue of bone, usually caused by a bacterial infection. —**osteomye·lit·ic** (·lit'ick) *adj.*

os·te·o·ne·cro·sis (os''te·o·ne·kro'sis) *n.* Necrosis of bone.

os·te·o·ne·phrop·a·thy (os''te·o·nef·rop'uth·ee) *n.* Any of a variety of syndromes involving bone changes accompanying renal disease.

os·te·o·path (os'te·o·path) *n.* One who practices osteopathic medicine.

os·te·op·a·thy (os''te·op'uth·ee) *n.* 1. A school of healing which teaches that the body is a vital mechanical organism whose structural and functional integrity are coordinate and interdependent, the abnormality of either constituting disease. Its major effort in treatment is in manipulation, but medicine, surgery, and the specialties are also utilized. 2. Any disease of bone. —**os·te·o·path·ic** (os''te·o·path'ick) *adj.*

os·te·o·pe·di·on, os·te·o·pae·di·on (os''te·o·pee'dee·un) *n.* LITHOPEDION.

os·te·o·pe·nia (os''te·o·pee'nee·uh) *n.* Any condition presenting less bone than normal.

os·te·o·peri·os·ti·tis (os''te·o·perr''ee·os·tigh'tis) *n.* Combined inflammation of bone and its periosteum.

os·te·o·pe·tro·sis (os''te·o·pe·tro'sis) *n.* A disorder of bone in which sclerosis obliterates the marrow, leading to bone marrow failure which may cause early death. Clinical features include optic atrophy, deafness, hepatosplenomegaly, and characteristic excess density of bones on x-ray. Syn. *Albers-Schönberg disease.* —**osteope·trot·ic** (·trot'ick) *adj.*

os·te·oph·thi·sis (os''te·off'thi·sis) *n.* Wasting of the bones.

os·te·o·phyte (os'te·o·fite) *n.* A bony outgrowth.

os·teo·phy·to·sis (os″tee·o·fye·to′sis) *n.* A condition characterized by the presence of osteophytes. —**osteo·phyt·ic** (·fit′ick) *adj.*

os·teo·plaque (os′tee·o·plack) *n.* A layer of bone; a flat osteoma.

os·teo·plas·tic (os″tee·o·plas′tick) *adj.* 1. Pertaining to the formation of bone tissue. 2. Pertaining to reparative operations upon bone.

osteoplastic amputation. An amputation in which there is a portion of bone fitted to the amputated bone end.

osteoplastic flap. A flap of skin and underlying bone, commonly of scalp and skull, raised for the purpose of exploring the underlying structures.

os·teo·plas·ty (os′tee·o·plas″tee) *n.* Plastic operations on bone.

os·teo·poi·ki·lo·sis (os″tee·o·poy″ki·lo′sis) *n.* A bone affection of unknown cause, giving rise to no symptoms and discovered by chance on roentgenographic examination when ellipsoidal dense foci are seen in all bones. Syn. *osteopathia condensans disseminata.*

os·teo·po·ro·sis (os″tee·o·po·ro′sis) *n.* Deossification with absolute decrease in bone tissue, resulting in enlargement of marrow and haversian spaces, decreased thickness of cortex and trabeculae, and structural weakness. —**osteopo·rot·ic** (·rot′ick) *adj.*

os·teo·pul·mo·nary arthropathy (os″tee·o·pool″muh·nerr·ee, ·pul′muh·) HYPERTROPHIC PULMONARY OSTEOARTHROPATHY.

os·teo·ra·dio·ne·cro·sis (os″tee·o·ray″dee·o·ne·kro′sis) *n.* Bone necrosis due to irradiation, usually by roentgen or gamma rays.

os·teo·sar·co·ma (os″tee·o·sahr·ko′muh) *n.* OSTEOGENIC SARCOMA. —**osteosarcoma·tous** (·tus) *adj.*

os·teo·scle·ro·sis (os″tee·o·skle·ro′sis) *n.* 1. Abnormal increased density of bone, occurring in a variety of pathologic states. 2. OSTEOPETROSIS. —**osteoscle·rot·ic** (·rot′ick) *adj.*

os·te·o·sis (os″tee·o′sis) *n.* Metaplastic bone formation.

os·teo·stix·is (os″tee·o·stick′sis) *n.* Surgical puncturing of a bone.

os·teo·su·ture (os′tee·o·sue″chur, os″tee·o·sue′chur) *n.* Suture of bone.

os·teo·syn·o·vi·tis (os″tee·o·sin″o·vye′tis, ·sigh″no·vye′tis) *n.* Synovitis complicated with osteitis of adjacent bones.

os·teo·syn·the·sis (os″tee·o·sin′thi·sis) *n.* Fastening the ends of a fractured bone together by mechanical means, such as a plate.

os·teo·ta·bes (os″tee·o·tay′beez) *n.* Bone degeneration beginning with the destruction of the cells of the bone marrow, which disappears in parts and is replaced by soft gelatinous tissue; later the spongy bone diminishes, and lastly the compact bone.

os·teo·tome (os′tee·o·tome) *n.* An instrument for cutting bone; specifically, an instrument somewhat similar to a chisel but without the beveled edge, used for cutting long bones, generally with the aid of a surgical mallet.

os·teo·to·moc·la·sis (os″tee·ot″o·mock′luh·sis, os″tee·o·to·) *n.* The correction of a pathologically curved bone by forcible bending following partial division by an osteotome.

os·te·ot·o·my (os″tee·ot′um·ee) *n.* 1. The division of a bone. 2. Making a section of a bone for the purpose of correcting a deformity.

os·teo·tribe (os′tee·o·tribe) *n.* A bone rasp.

os·te·ot·ro·phy (os″tee·ot′ruh·fee) *n.* Nutrition of bony tissue.

osteotympanic conduction. BONE CONDUCTION.

ostia. Plural of *ostium.*

os·ti·um (os′tee·um) *n.,* genit. **os·tii** (os′tee·eye), pl. **os·tia** (os′tee·uh) A mouth or aperture. —**osti·al** (·ul) *adj.*

ostium ute·ri (yoo′tur·eye) [NA]. The opening of the cervix of the uterus into the vagina.

os·to·my (os′tuh·mee) *n. Informal.* A surgical procedure in which parts of the intestinal or urinary tract are removed from the patient, and an artifical opening or stoma is constructed through the abdominal wall to allow for the passage of urine or feces.

os·treo·tox·ism (os″tree·o·tock′sizm) *n.* Poisoning from eating diseased or contaminated oysters.

os ute·ri (yoo′tur·eye). OSTIUM UTERI.

os uteri ex·ter·num (ecks·tur′num). OSTIUM UTERI.

os uteri in·ter·num (in·tur′num). The juncture of the lower end of the isthmus uteri with the endocervical canal.

OT, O.T. 1. *In anatomy,* old term, in opposition to BNA or NA term. 2. An abbreviation for *original tuberculin* and *old tuberculin.*

ot-, oto- A combining form meaning *ear.*

otal·gia (o·tal′jee·uh) *n.* EARACHE. —**otal·gic** (·jick) *adj.*

otan·tri·tis (o″tan·trye′tis) *n.* Inflammation of the mastoid antrum.

othe·ma·to·ma, othae·ma·to·ma (oat·hee″muh·to′muh, o·theem′uh·) *n.* Hematoma of the external ear, usually the pinna.

ot·hem·or·rha·gia, ot·haem·or·rha·gia (oat″hem·o·ray′juh, ·jee·uh, o·theem′o·) *n.* Hemorrhage from the ear.

-otic A suffix meaning *pertaining to* or *causing the process* or *condition* that is usually designated by a noun ending in *-osis,* as osmotic, narcotic, mycotic, leukocytotic.

otic (o′tick) *adj.* Pertaining to the ear.

otic ganglion. The nerve ganglion immediately below the foramen ovale of the sphenoid bone, medial to the mandibular nerve; it receives preganglionic fibers from the inferior salivatory nucleus of the ninth cranial nerve by way of the minor petrosal nerve and sends postganglionic parasympathetic fibers to the parotid gland.

oti·co·din·ia (o″ti·ko·din′ee·uh) *n. Obsol.* Vertigo from ear disease.

oti·tis (o·tye′tis) *n.,* pl. **otit·i·des** (o·tit′i·deez) Inflammation of the ear. —**otit·ic** (o·tit′ick) *adj.*

otitis ex·ter·na (ecks·tur′nuh). Inflammation of the external ear.

otitis in·ter·na (in·tur′nuh). Inflammation of the internal ear.

otitis lab·y·rin·thi·ca (lab·i·rin′thi·kuh). Inflammation of the labyrinth of the inner ear.

otitis mas·toi·dea (mas·toy'dee·uh). Inflammation confined to the mastoid cells.

otitis me·dia (mee'dee·uh). Inflammation of the middle ear.

otitis par·a·sit·i·ca (păr·uh·sit'i·kuh). Inflammation of the ear caused by a parasite.

otitis scle·rot·i·ca (skle·rot'i·kuh). Inflammation of the inner ear with hardening of the tissues.

oto·blen·nor·rhea, oto·blen·nor·rhoea (o''to·blen''o·ree'uh) n. Any discharge of mucus from the ear.

oto·ceph·a·lus (o''tuh·sef'ul·us) n. A fetus characterized by a union or close approach of the ears, by absence of the lower jaw, and an ill-developed mouth. —**otoceph·a·ly** (·lee) n.

oto·clei·sis (o''to·klye'sis) n. Occlusion of the ear.

oto·co·nia (o''to·ko'nee·uh) n., sing. **otoco·ni·um** (·nee·um) Crystals of calcium carbonate, 1 to 5 μm long, contained in the soft substance over the two maculae acusticae. Syn. statoconia.

oto·dyn·ia (o''to·din'ee·uh) n. Pain in the ear.

oto·gen·ic (oto·jen'ick) adj. Originating or arising within the ear.

oto·lar·yn·gol·o·gist (o''to·lăr''ing·gol'uh·jist) n. A person skilled in the practice of otology, rhinology, and laryngology.

oto·lar·yn·gol·o·gy (o''to·lăr''ing·gol'uh·jee) n. A specialty including otology, rhinology, laryngology, and surgery of the head and neck.

oto·lith (o'to·lith) n. One of the calcareous concretions within the membranous labyrinth of the ear, especially the large ear stones of fishes.

otol·o·gist (o·tol'uh·jist) n. A person skilled in otology.

otol·o·gy (o·tol'uh·jee) n. The science of the ear, its anatomy, functions, and diseases. —**oto·log·ic** (o''tuh·loj'ick), **otolog·i·cal** (·i·kul) adj.

oto·my·as·the·nia (o''to·migh''as·theen'ee·uh) n. 1. Weakness of the muscles of the ear. 2. Defective hearing due to a paretic condition of the tensor tympani or stapedius muscle.

oto·my·co·sis (o''to·migh·ko'sis) n. Infection of the external auditory meatus and of the ear canal, from which a number of fungi and bacteria can be isolated, but with the weight of evidence favoring the bacteria as the prime agents and the fungi as secondary.

oto·pha·ryn·ge·al (o''to·fa·rin'jee·ul) adj. Pertaining to the ear and the pharynx.

oto·plas·ty (o'to·plas''tee) n. Plastic surgery of the external ear.

oto·pol·y·pus (o''to·pol'i·pus) n. A polyp occurring in the ear.

oto·py·or·rhea, oto·py·or·rhoea (o''to·pye''o·ree'uh) n. A purulent discharge from the ear.

oto·rhi·no·lar·yn·gol·o·gy (o''to·rye''no·lăr·ing·gol'uh·jee) n. The study of diseases of the ear, nose, and throat.

oto·rhi·nol·o·gy (o''to·rye·nol'uh·jee) n. Literally, the study of diseases of the ears and the nose only.

otor·rha·gia (o''to·ray'jee·uh) n. A discharge of blood from the external auditory meatus.

otor·rhea, otor·rhoea (o''to·ree'uh) n. A discharge from the external auditory meatus.

oto·sal·pinx (o''to·sal'pinks) n., pl. **oto·sal·pin·ges** (·sal·pin'jeez) Obsol. AUDITORY TUBE.

oto·scle·ro·sis (o''to·skle·ro'sis) n. A pathologic change in the middle and inner ear resulting in the laying down of new bone around the oval window, the cochlea, or both, and causing progressive impairment of hearing. —**otoscle·rot·ic** (·rot'ick) adj.

oto·scope (o'tuh·skope) n. An apparatus designed for examination of the ear and for rendering the tympanic membrane visible.

otos·co·py (o·tos'kuh·pee) n. Visualization of the auditory canal and tympanic membrane by means of the otoscope. —**oto·scop·ic** (o''tuh·skop'ick) adj.

otot·o·my (o·tot'uh·mee) n. 1. Dissection of the ear. 2. Incision of any of the tissues of the external auditory meatus or the ear proper.

oto·tox·ic (o''to·tock'sick) adj. Having harmful effects on the ear, especially on its neural parts. —**oto·tox·ic·i·ty** (·tock·sis'i·tee) n.

oua·ba·in (wah·bah'in, ·bay'in, wah'bah·in) n. $C_{29}H_{44}O_{12}.8H_2O$, a steroidal glycoside obtained from seeds of Strophanthus gratus and other sources; used clinically for its digitalis-like action.

Ouch·ter·lony technique. Double diffusion in agar wherein solutions of antibodies interact with antigens so as to give readily observable lines of precipitation.

ou·la (oo'luh) n. GINGIVA.

ounce, n. A unit of measure and weight.

-ous 1. A general adjective-forming suffix meaning having or pertaining to. 2. In chemistry, a suffix indicating the lower of two valences assumed by an element.

out·flow, n. In neurology, the transmission of efferent impulses, particularly of the autonomic nervous system; these are divided into thoracolumbar and craniosacral outflows.

out·growth, n. Growth or development from a preexisting structure or state.

out·let of the pelvis. The lower aperture of the pelvic canal.

out·pa·tient, n. A patient who comes to the hospital or clinic for diagnosis or treatment but who does not occupy a bed in the institution.

out·pouch·ing, n. EVAGINATION.

out·put, n. Energy or matter leaving a structure or system of structures.

ova. Plural of ovum.

oval (o'vul) adj. Egg-shaped.

ova·le malaria (o·vay'lee). A benign form of malaria occurring in Africa due to Plasmodium ovale, characterized by mild recurring tertian paroxysms, and similar to vivax malaria. Red blood cells and trophozoites are both at times oval in shape.

ovalo·cy·to·sis (o·val''o·sigh·to'sis, o''vuh·lo·) n. ELLIPTOCYTOSIS.

oval window. An oval opening in the medial wall of the middle ear, closed by the foot plate of the stapes. Syn. vestibular window.

ovari-, ovario-. A combining form meaning ovary or ovarian.

ovari·al·gia (o·văr''ee·al'juh, ·jee·uh) n. Neuralgic pain in the ovary.

ovar·i·an (o·văr'ee·un, o·vair') adj. Pertaining to the ovaries.

ovarian agenesis. Failure of development of the ovaries.

ovarian dwarfism. GONADAL DYSGENESIS.

ovarian follicle. The functional unit of oogenesis and ovulation in the ovary, consisting of an oocyte or ovum with its accessory structures. In the primary follicles the growing oocyte is enveloped in increasing layers of follicular cells; the subsequent vesicular follicles develop a fluid-filled cavity which (in humans and many animals) displaces the ovum eccentrically. At this stage the follicles produce estrogenic hormones and a few of them progress to the fully mature (graafian follicle) stage, ready for ovulation.

ovarian insufficiency. Deficiency of ovarian function, either primary or secondary, which can result in either amenorrhea, oligomenorrhea, or abnormal dysfunctional uterine bleeding; a clinical term.

ovarian pregnancy. Gestation within the ovary.

ovari·ec·to·my (o-vâr''ee-eck'tum-ee) n. Excision of an ovary; oophorectomy.

ovar·io·cele (o-vâr'ee-o-seel) n. Hernia of an ovary.

ovar·io·cen·te·sis (o-vâr''ee-o-sen-tee'sis) n. Puncture of an ovary or of an ovarian cyst.

ovar·io·cy·e·sis (o-vâr''ee-o-sigh-ee'sis) n. OVARIAN PREGNANCY.

ovar·io·gen·ic (o-vâr''ee-o-jen'ick) adj. Arising in the ovary.

ovar·io·hys·ter·ec·to·my (o-vâr''ee-o-his-tur-eck'tum-ee) n. Surgical removal of one or both ovaries and the uterus.

ovar·i·ot·o·my (o-vâr''ee-ot'um-ee) n. Removal of an ovary; oophorectomy.

ovar·io·tu·bal (o-vâr''ee-o-tew'bul) adj. Pertaining to an ovary and oviduct.

ova·ri·tis (o''vuh-righ'tis) n., pl. **ova·rit·i·des** (·rit'i-deez) OOPHORITIS.

ova·ry (o'vur-ee) n. One of a pair of glandular organs which contains and releases ova. It consists of a fibrous framework or stroma, in which are embedded the ovarian follicles, and is surrounded by a serous covering derived from the peritoneum.

over·bite, n. The extent to which the upper anterior teeth overlap the lower when the dentition is in centric occlusion.

over·com·pen·sa·tion, n. In psychiatry, a conscious or unconscious mental process in which real or fictitious physical, psychologic, or social deficiencies produce exaggerated correction.

over·cor·rec·tion, n. In optics, an aberration of a lens causing the light rays passing the central zones to focus at a point nearer to the lens than rays passing the outer zone.

over·de·pen·den·cy, n. A behavioral trait or pattern characterized by seeking support and guidance (advice, decision making) far beyond that sought normally by an individual of a particular age, sex, and social status with average or near-average intelligence.

over·de·ter·mi·na·tion, n. In psychoanalysis, the state of having more than one cause, applied especially to behavior disorders and dreams. **—over·de·ter·mined,** adj.

over·growth, n. Hypertrophy or hyperplasia.

over·jet, n. The extent to which the upper incisors project in front of the lower incisors when the dentition is in centric occlusion.

over·ly·ing, adj. & n. 1. Positioned or resting above or on. 2. A cause of death in infants sleeping with adults; suffocation occurs when one of the adults lies upon the child.

over·max·i·mal (o''vur-mack'si-mul) adj. Beyond the normal maximum, as the overmaximal contraction of a muscle.

over·pro·tec·tion, n. Paying more attention to an infant or child than is necessary for its own safety and well-being; usually implying excessive physical contact with the child, preventing independent behavior or competition by the child with its peers, and forcing the child to act more infantile or dependent than his physical and intellectual development require.

over·reach, v. To strike the toe of the hindfoot against the heel or shoe of the forefoot; said of a horse.

over·rid·ing, adj. 1. Characterizing a fracture in which broken ends or fragments of the bone slip past each other, with overlapping due to muscular contraction. 2. Characterizing toes which overlap.

over·strain, v. & n. 1. To strain to excess. 2. Excessive strain and fatigue resulting from effort beyond capacity.

overt, adj. Evident; manifest, outward.

over·weight, adj. Exceeding normal weight, usually connoting an excess of more than 10 percent.

ovi-, ovo-. A combining form meaning egg or ovum.

ovi·duct (o'vi-dukt) n. The duct serving to transport the ovum from the ovary to the exterior, or to an organ such as the uterus. In mammals, the oviduct is also called the uterine or fallopian tube. **—ovi·du·cal** (o''vi-dew'kul), **ovi·duc·tal** (·duck'tul) adj.

ovi·fi·ca·tion (o''vi-fi-kay'shun) n. The production of ova.

ovi·form (o'vi-form) adj. Egg-shaped; oval.

ovig·e·nous (o-vij'e-nus) adj. Producing ova, as the ovigenous layer, the outer layer of the ovary, in which the follicles containing the ova are situated.

ovine (o'vine) adj. 1. Pertaining to or derived from sheep. 2. Sheeplike.

ovip·a·rous (o-vip'ur-us) adj. Producing eggs; bringing forth young in the egg stage of development. **—ovipa·ra** (·uh) n.pl.

ovi·po·si·tion (o''vi-puh-zish'un) n. The act of laying or depositing eggs by the females of oviparous animals. **—ovi·pos·it** (o''vi-poz'it) v.

ovoid (o'void) adj. Egg-shaped.

ovo·tes·tic·u·lar (o''vo-tes-tick'yoo-lur) adj. Pertaining to or characterized by an ovotestis or ovotestes.

ovo·tes·tis (o''vo-tes''tis) n., pl. **ovotes·tes** (·teez) Ovarian and testicular tissues combined in the same gonad.

ovu·lar (o'vyoo-lur) adj. Of or pertaining to an ovule or ovum.

ovu·la·tion (o''vyoo-lay'shun, ov''yoo·) n. The

maturation and discharge of the ovum. —**ovu·late** (o'vyoo·late) v.; **ovu·la·to·ry** (o'vyoo·luh·to''ree), **ovu·la·tion·al** (o''vyoo·lay'shun·ul) adj.

ovum (o'vum) n., pl. **ova** (o'vuh) 1. [NA] A female germ cell; an egg cell; a cell which is capable of developing into a new member of the same species, in animals usually only after maturation and fertilization. The human ovum is a large, spheroidal cell containing a large mass of cytoplasm and a large nucleus (germinal vesicle), within which is a nucleolus (germinal spot). 2. The early embryo from the time of fertilization until the bilaminar blastodisk is formed.

oxa-. In chemistry, a combining form indicating the presence of oxygen in place of carbon.

ox·a·cil·lin (ock''suh·sil'in) n. 5-Methyl-3-phenyl-4-isoxazolylpenicillin, $C_{19}H_{19}N_3O_5S$, a semisynthetic penicillin antibiotic; used as the sodium salt.

oxal-, oxalo-. A combining form meaning oxalic or oxalate.

ox·al·ace·tic acid (ock''sul·a·see'tick). OXALOACETIC ACID.

ox·a·late (ock'suh·late) n. Any salt or ester of oxalic acid.

ox·a·le·mia, ox·a·lae·mia (ock''suh·lee'mee·uh) n. An excess of oxalates in the blood.

ox·al·ic acid (ock·sal'ick) Ethanedioic acid, $HOOCCOOH·2H_2O$, found in many plants and vegetables. Used as a reagent.

ox·a·lism (ock'sul·iz·um) n. Poisoning by oxalic acid or an oxalate.

ox·alo·ace·tic acid (ock''sul·o·a·see'tick, ock·sal''o·). Ketosuccinic acid, $HOOCCH_2COCOOH$, a participant in the citric acid metabolic cycle. Syn. oxalacetic acid.

ox·a·lo·sis (ock·suh·lo'sis) n. A rare autosomal recessive metabolic error resulting in impaired glyoxylic acid metabolism with consequent overproduction of oxalic acid and deposition of calcium oxalate in body tissues; in type I, there is hyperoxaluria and hyperglycoxaluria, while in type II there is hyperoxaluria and hyper-L-glyceric-aciduria. Both types are characterized clinically by renal calculi, nephrocalcinosis, and renal insufficiency.

ox·al·uria (ock''suh·lew'ree·uh) n. The presence of oxalic acid or oxalates in the urine.

ox·i·dant (ock'sid·unt) n. An oxidizing agent.

ox·i·dase (ock'si·dace, ·daze) n. Any enzyme which promotes an oxidation reaction.

ox·i·da·tion (ock''si·day'shun) n. 1. An increase in positive valence of an element (or a decrease in negative valence) occurring as a result of the loss of electrons. Each electron so lost is taken on by some other element, thus accomplishing a reduction of that element. 2. Originally, the process of combining with oxygen. —**ox·i·da·tive** (ock'si·day''tiv) adj.

ox·ide (ock'side) n. A binary compound of oxygen and another element or radical.

ox·i·dize (ock'si·dize) v. To produce an oxidation or increase in positive valence (or decrease in negative valence) through the loss of electrons. The oxidizing agent is itself reduced

in the reaction; that is, it takes on the electrons which have been liberated by the element being oxidized.

ox·ime (ock'seem) n. Any compound resulting from the action of hydroxylamine upon an aldehyde or ketone; the former yields an oxime having the general formula $RCH=NOH$, called aldoxime; the latter yields an oxime of the general formula $R_2C=NOH$, called ketoxime.

ox·im·e·ter (ock·sim'e·tur) n. 1. A photoelectric instrument for measuring the degree of oxygen saturation in a fluid, such as blood. 2. An instrument for measurement of oxygen in a given space, as in an incubator or oxygen tent. —**oxime·try** (·tree) n.

ox·tri·phyl·line (ocks''trye·fil'een, ocks''tri·fil'een) n. Choline theophyllinate, $C_{12}H_{21}N_5O_3$, a drug having the diuretic, myocardial stimulating, vasodilator, and bronchodilator actions of theophylline.

oxy- A combining form meaning (a) sharp, pointed, as in oxycephaly; (b) keen, abnormally acute, as in oxyopia; (c) quick, hastening, as in oxytocic; (d) acid, as in oxyphil; (e) containing oxygen or additional oxygen, as in oxysteroid; (f) containing hydroxyl, as in oxytetracycline.

oxy·a·phia (ock''see·ay'fee·uh, ·af'ee·uh) n. 1. Marked or abnormal acuteness of the sense of touch. 2. Extreme sensitivity to touch.

oxy·blep·sia (ock''see·blep'see·uh) n. Acuteness of vision.

Oxycel. Trademark for an absorbable oxidized cellulose material used in surgical hemostasis.

oxy·ceph·a·ly (ock''see·sef'ul·ee) n. A condition in which the head is roughly conical in shape; caused by premature closure of the coronal or lambdoid sutures, or both, which induces compensatory development in the region of the bregma. It is also caused by artificial pressure on the frontal and occipital regions of the heads of infants to alter the shape. Syn. acrocephaly. —**oxy·ce·phal·ic** (·se·fal'ick) adj.

oxy·chro·ma·tin (ock''see·kro'muh·tin) n. That part of the chromatin having an affinity for acid dyes.

oxy·ci·ne·sis (ock''see·sigh·nee'sis, ·si·nee'sis) n. Excessive movements, particularly of the limbs, observed in the manic phase of manic-depressive illness.

oxy·es·the·sia (ock''see·es·theezh'uh, ·theez'ee·uh) n. HYPERESTHESIA.

ox·y·gen (ock'si·jin) n. O = 15.9994. A colorless, tasteless, odorless gas, constituting one-fifth of the atmosphere, eight-ninths of water, and about one-half the crust of the globe; it supports combustion, and is essential to life of animals. It combines with most elements, and is carried by the blood from the lungs to the tissues.

ox·y·gen·ase (ock'si·ji·naze, ·nace) n. An enzyme that makes it possible for atmospheric oxygen to be utilized by the organism or in the system in which it occurs.

ox·y·gen·ate (ock'si·ji·nate) v. To combine a substance with oxygen, either by chemical reaction or by mixture. —**oxygen·a·tion** (ock''si·ji·nay'shun) n.

oxygen capacity. The maximum amount of oxygen absorbed by a given amount of blood when it is equilibrated with an excess of oxygen, expressed in volume percent (per 100 ml).

oxygen debt or **deficit**. The volume of oxygen required in addition to the resting oxygen consumption during the period of recovery from intense muscular exertion; it reflects the quantity of excess lactic acid produced during the anaerobic work period, and is required to oxidize this excess as well as to replenish stores of adenosine triphosphate and phosphocreatine that were depleted. Syn. *recovery oxygen*.

oxygen saturation. Oxygen content divided by oxygen capacity expressed in volume percent.

oxygen tent. A transparent airtight chamber, enclosing the patient's head and shoulders, in which the oxygen content can be maintained at a higher than normal atmospheric level.

oxy·geu·sia (ock″si·gyoo′see·uh, ·joo′see·uh) *n*. Marked acuteness of the sense of taste.

oxy·hem·a·tin (ock″see·hem′uh·tin, ·hee′muh·tin) *n*. $C_{34}H_{32}N_4O_7Fe$. The coloring matter of oxyhemoglobin; on oxidation, it yields hematinic acid; on reduction, hematoporphyrin.

oxy·hem·a·to·por phy·rin (ock″see·hem″uh·to·por′fi·rin) *n*. A pigment sometimes found in urine; it is related to hematoporphyrin.

oxy·he·mo·glo·bin (ock″si·hee′muh·glo″bin) *n*. Hemoglobin combined with oxygen.

oxy·la·lia (ock″si·lay′lee·uh, ·lal′ee·uh) *n*. Rapid speech.

oxy·mor·phone (ock″see·mor′fone) *n*. 14-Hydroxydihydromorphinone, $C_{17}H_{19}NO_4$, a semisynthetic narcotic analgesic; used as the hydrochloride salt.

oxy·ner·von (ock″see·nur′von) *n*. A cerebroside occurring in brain tissue; its characteristic acid is oxynervonic acid.

oxy·ner·von·ic acid (ock″see·nur·von′ick). An unsaturated acid, $HOC_{23}H_{44}COOH$, the hydroxy derivative of nervonic acid; a component of oxynervon.

ox·yn·tic (ock·sin′tick) *adj*. Secreting acid; formerly applied to the parietal cells of the stomach.

oxy·opia (ock″see·o′pee·uh) *n*. Unusual acuity of vision.

oxy·os·mia (ock″see·oz′mee·uh) *n*. 1. Marked or abnormal sensitivity to smell. 2. Sensitivity to odors to a pathologic extent.

oxy·phen·bu·ta·zone (ock″si·fen·bew′tuh·zone) *n*. 4-Butyl-1-(*p*-hydroxyphenyl)-2-phenyl-3,5-pyrazolidinedione, $C_{19}H_{20}N_2O_3$, a metabolite of phenylbutazone that is used as an antiarthritic and anti-inflammatory drug.

oxy·phil (ock′si·fil) *adj*. ACIDOPHILIC (1).

oxy·pho·nia (ock″see·fo′nee·uh) *n*. Shrillness of voice.

oxy·ste·roid (ock″see·sterr′oid, ·steer′oid) *n*. A steroid having an oxygen atom, thereby forming an alcohol or a ketone group, at some specified position; for example, an 11-oxysteroid has the oxygen atom present at the number 11 carbon atom of the steroid nucleus.

ox·yt·a·lan fibers (ock·sit′uh·lan) Acid-resistant connective-tissue fibers morphologically similar to elastin, but resistant to elastase digestion and not stained by the usual specific elastin stains.

oxy·tet·ra·cy·cline (ock″see·tet″ruh·sigh′kleen) *n*. A broad-spectrum antibiotic substance, $C_{22}H_{24}N_2O_9$, produced by the growth of the soil fungus *Streptomyces rimosus*, or by any other means. It represents tetracycline in which a hydrogen atom is replaced by a hydroxyl group, and is active against a number of gram-negative bacteria, rickettsias, and several viruses.

oxy·to·cia (ock″si·to′shee·uh, ·see·uh) *n*. Rapid childbirth.

oxy·to·cic (ock″si·to′sick) *adj. & n*. 1. Hastening parturition. 2. A drug that hastens parturition.

ox·y·to·cin (ock″si·to′sin) *n*. An octapeptide, obtained from extracts of the posterior lobe of the pituitary gland and also by synthesis, that is the principal uterine-contracting and lactation-stimulating hormone of the gland. Syn. *alpha-hypophamine*.

oxy·uri·a·sis (ock″see·yoo·rye′uh·sis) *n*. ENTEROBIASIS.

Oxy·uri·dae (ock″see·yoor′i·dee) *n.pl*. A family of nematode intestinal parasites, including the human pinworm *Enterobius vermicularis*. —**oxy·urid** (ock″see·yoor′id) *adj. & n*.

Oxy·uris (ock″see·yoor′is) *n*. A genus of nematodes, including the horse pinworm, *Oxyuris equi*, and formerly also the human pinworm (*O. vermicularis*, now designated *Enterobius vermicularis*).

oz. Symbol for avoirdupois ounce.

oze·na, ozae·na (o·zee′nuh) *n*. A disease of the nasal mucosa of uncertain origin, characterized by chronic inflammation with subsequent atrophy, sclerosis, and crusting. Syn. *atrophic rhinitis*.

ozone (o′zone) *n*. O_3. An allotropic form of oxygen, the molecule of which consists of three atoms; a common constituent of the atmosphere. It is a powerful oxidizing agent and is used as a disinfectant, as for swimming pools.

ozon·ide (o′zo·nide) *n*. A compound of ozone with certain unsaturated organic substances. Such derivatives of fixed oils have been applied locally to infected areas for the bactericidal effect of the nascent oxygen released by the oils.

ozo·sto·mia (o″zo·sto′mee·uh) *n*. A foul odor of the breath of oral origin; halitosis.

P

P Symbol for (a) phosphorus; (b) premolar.

P. Abbreviation for (a) *pharmacopeia;* (b) *position;* (c) *punctum proximum,* near point.

P₂ 1. S₂P. 2. Symbol for the second heart sound as heard in the second interspace at the left sternal border.

³²P. Symbol for phosphorus 32; radiophosphorus.

PA A posteroanterior projection of x-rays; as those passing from back to front of an anatomic part.

PABA Abbreviation for *para-aminobenzoic acid.*

pab·u·lum (pab′yoo·lum) *n.* Food; any nutrient.

Pac·chi·o·ni·an bodies (pack″ee·o′nee·un) ARACHNOID GRANULATIONS.

pace·mak·er, *n.* 1. Any substance or object that influences the rate at which a process or reaction occurs. 2. Any body part that serves to establish and maintain a rhythmic activity. 3. Specifically, the sinoatrial node, a subsidiary center, or an electrical device functioning to stimulate and pace the heart.

pa·chom·e·ter (pa·kom′e·tur) *n. In ophthalmology,* an instrument for measuring the thickness of the cornea.

pachy- A combining form meaning (a) *thick, thickness;* (b) *coarse;* (c) *dura mater.*

-pachy A combining form designating *a condition involving thickening of a part or parts.*

pachy·ac·ria (pack″ee·ack′ree·uh) *n.* ACROPACHYDERMA.

pachy·bleph·a·ron (pack″ee·blef′ur·on) *n.* Chronic thickening and induration of the eyelids.

pachy·bleph·a·ro·sis (pack″ee·blef″uh·ro′sis) *n.* PACHYBLEPHARON.

pachy·ceph·a·ly (pack″ee·sef′uh·lee) *n.* Unusual thickness of the walls of the skull. **—pachy·ceph·a·lous** (·lus) *adj.*

pachy·chei·lia, pachy·chi·lia (pack″i·kigh′lee·uh) *n.* Increased thickness of one or both lips.

pachy·dac·tyl·ia (pack″ee·dack·til′ee·uh) *n.* Abnormal thickness of the fingers.

pachy·dac·ty·ly (pack″ee·dack′ti·lee) *n.* PACHYDACTYLIA.

pachy·der·ma (pack″i·dur′muh) *n.* PACHYDERMIA.

pachy·der·ma·to·cele (pack″i·dur′muh·to·seel) *n.* A manifestation of von Recklinghausen's neurofibromatosis, taking the form of an overgrowth of subcutaneous tissue, sometimes reaching enormous size. Syn. *plexiform neuroma, elephantiasis neurofibromatosa.*

pachy·der·ma·to·sis (pack″i·dur″muh·to′sis) *n.* RHINOPHYMA.

pachy·der·ma·tous (pack″i·dur′muh·tus) *adj.* Abnormally thick-skinned.

pachy·der·mia (pack″i·dur′mee·uh) *n.* 1. Abnormal thickening of the skin. 2. ELEPHANTIASIS. **—pachyder·mi·al** (·mee·ul), **pachyder·mic** (·mick) *adj.*

pachydermia la·ryn·gis (la·rin′jis). Extensive thickening of the mucous membrane of the larynx, particularly the posterior commissure.

pachy·glos·sia (pack″ee·glos′ee·uh) *n.* Abnormal thickness of the tongue.

pachy·gy·ria (pack″i·jye′ree·uh) *n.* A variety of cerebral malformation characterized by a reduction in the number secondary gyri and an increased depth of the gray matter underlying the smooth part of the cortex. Syn. *lissencephalia, agyria.*

pachy·lep·to·men·in·gi·tis (pack″ee·lep″to·men″in·jye′tis) *n.* Combined inflammation of the pia-arachnoid and dura mater.

pachy·lo·sis (pack″i·lo′sis) *n.* A thick, dry, harsh, and scaly skin, especially of the legs.

pachy·men·in·gi·tis (pack″ee·men″in·jye′tis) *n.* Inflammation of the dura mater. **—pachy·menin·git·ic** (·jit′ick) *adj.*

pachymeningitis ex·ter·na (ecks·tur′nuh). *Obsol.* EPIDURAL ABSCESS.

pachymeningitis in·ter·na hem·or·rha·gi·ca (in·tur′nuh hem·o·ray′ji·kuh). *Obsol.* Chronic SUBDURAL HEMATOMA.

pachy·men·in·gop·a·thy (pack″ee·men″ing·gop′uth·ee) *n.* Disease of the dura mater.

pachy·me·ninx (pack″ee·mee′ninks) *n.* DURA MATER.

pachy·o·nych·ia (pack″ee·o·nick′ee·uh) *n.* Thickening of the nails. Syn. *pachonychia.*

pachyonychia con·gen·i·ta (kon''jen'i·tuh). An ectodermal defect characterized by dystrophic changes of the nails, palmar and plantar hyperkeratosis, anomalies of the hair, follicular keratosis of the knees and elbows, and dyskeratosis of the cornea.

pachy·o·tia (pack''ee·o'shuh, ·shee·uh) n. Abnormal thickness of the external ears.

pachy·pel·vi·peri·to·ni·tis (pack''ee·pel''vi·perr''i·to·nigh'tis) n. Pelvic peritonitis with a fibrous deposit over the uterus.

pachy·peri·os·to·sis (pack''ee·perr''ee·os·to'sis) n. Pathologic alteration of the long bones in which the periosteum is greatly thickened.

pachy·peri·to·ni·tis (pack''ee·perr''i·to·nigh'tis) n. Inflammation, usually chronic, of the peritoneum associated with peritoneal thickening.

pa·chyp·o·dous (pa·kip'uh·dus) adj. Having thick feet.

pachy·rhine (pack'i·rine) adj. Having a thick or unusually broad and flat nose.

pachy·sal·pin·go·ova·ri·tis (pack''ee·sal·pin''go·o''vuh·rye'tis) n. Inflammation of the ovary and oviduct with thickening of the parts.

pachy·tene (pack'i·teen) n. The stage in the first meiotic prophase in which tetrads are formed.

pachy·vag·i·ni·tis (pack''ee·vaj''i·nigh'tis) n. Vaginitis accompanied by thickening of the vaginal walls.

pac·i·fi·er (pas'i·figh''ur) n. Any article, such as a rubber nipple, placed in the mouths of irritable or teething children to quiet them.

pa·cin·i·an corpuscle (pa·sin'ee·un) The largest and most widely distributed of the encapsulated sensory receptors. It differs from other encapsulated organs mainly in the greater development of its perineural capsule, which consists of a large number of concentric lamellae. Syn. *corpuscle of Vater-Pacini.*

pack, *n. & v.* 1. An assemblage of equipment used for a medical procedure, usually of a surgical nature. 2. TAMPON. 3. A dressing or blanket, dry or wet, hot or cold, placed on or wrapped around the body or a part of the body. 4. To fill a cavity; to produce tamponade.

pack·er, *n.* A tapered surgical instrument equipped with a point ending in a shoulder, for inserting gauze or other dressings into a cavity; used generally in conjunction with an aural, vaginal, or other speculum.

Pad·gett's dermatome An instrument for cutting uniform thickness of skin of any desired calibration in large sheets for grafting purposes.

page·ism (pay'jiz·um) n. *In psychiatry,* the fantasy of a masochistic male that he is the slave or page of a dominating woman.

pag·et·oid (paj'e·toid) adj. Simulating Paget's disease.

Paget's cancer. PAGET'S DISEASE (1).

Paget's cells. Large epithelial cells with clear cytoplasm, associated with a certain type of breast cancer (Paget's disease (1)) or apocrine gland cancer of the skin (Paget's disease (3)).

Paget-Schroetter's syndrome Acute venous thrombosis with obstruction occurring in the upper extremity of an otherwise healthy person. Syn. *axillary vein thrombosis.*

Paget's disease 1. A breast carcinoma involving the nipple or areola and the larger ducts, whose cells are large and have clear cytoplasm (Paget's cells). Syn. *morbus Pageti papillae, Paget's cancer.* 2. A simultaneous osseous hyperplasia and accelerated deossification, resulting in weakness and deformity of various bones. Syn. *osteitis deformans.* 3. A skin cancer associated with apocrine glands, whose parenchyma is composed of Paget's cells.

pa·go·pha·gia (pay''go·fay'jee·uh) n. Compulsive eating of ice.

pa·go·plex·ia (pay''go·pleck'see·uh) n. Numbness from cold; FROSTBITE.

-pagus A combining form designating *a pair of conjoined twins joined at a* (specified) *site.*

-pagy A combining form designating the state of *conjoined twins joined at a* (specified) *site.*

pain, *n.* 1. A localized or diffuse abnormal sensation ranging from discomfort to agony; caused by stimulation of functionally specific peripheral nerve endings. It serves as a physiologic protective mechanism. —**pain·ful** (·ful), **pain·less** (·lus) adj.

pain spots. Small areas of skin overlying the endings of either very small myelinated (delta) or unmyelinated (C) nerve fibers whose stimulation, depending on the intensity and duration, results in the sensation of either pain or itching.

painter's colic. Colic due to lead poisoning.

painter's palsy. LEAD POLYNEUROPATHY.

pain threshold. The lowest limit of perceiving the sensation of pain.

pal·a·tal (pal'uh·tul) adj. Pertaining to the palate.

palatal bar. A bar of metal extended across a portion of the hard palate for the purpose of joining and strengthening the two sections of a maxillary partial denture.

palatal myoclonus. A rhythmic movement, 30 to 60 per second, of the soft palate, and sometimes the pharynx, facial muscles, diaphragm, vocal cords and even the shoulder muscles. The lesions producing this state are situated in the central tegmental tract, inferior olivary nucleus, or olivocerebellar tract.

palatal nystagmus. PALATAL MYOCLONUS.

palatal reflex. 1. Elevation of the soft palate in response to touch. 2. Swallowing produced by irritation of the palate.

pal·ate (pal'ut) n. The roof of the mouth.

pa·lat·ic (pa·lat'ick) adj. PALATAL.

pal·a·tine (pal'uh·tine) adj. & n. 1. PALATAL. 2. The palatine bone. See Table of Bones in the Appendix.

palatine arches. The palatoglossal and palatopharyngeal arches.

palatine tonsil. The aggregation of lymph nodules between the palatine arches.

palato-. A combining form meaning *palate, palatal, palatine.*

pal·a·to·glos·sal (pal''uh·to·glos'ul) adj. Pertaining to the palate and the tongue.

palatoglossal arch. A fold formed by the projection of the palatoglossal muscle covered by mucous membrane.

pal·a·to·glos·sal muscle. PALATOGLOSSUS.

pa·la·to·glos·sus (pal''uh·to·glos'us) *n.* The muscle within the anterior pillar of the fauces; it connects the soft palate with the tongue.

pal·a·to·max·il·lary (pal''uh·to·mack'si·lerr·ee) *adj.* Pertaining to the palate and the maxilla.

pal·a·to·na·sal (pal''uh·to·nay'zul) *adj.* Pertaining to the palate and the nose.

pal·a·to·pha·ryn·ge·al (pal''uh·to·fa·rin'jee·ul, ·fär''in·jee'ul) *adj.* Pertaining conjointly to the palate and the pharynx.

palatopharyngeal arch. A fold formed by the projection of the palatopharyngeal muscle covered by mucous membrane.

pal·a·to·pha·ryn·ge·us (pal''uh·to·fa·rin'jee·us) *n.* The muscle in the palatopharyngeal arch, connecting the soft palate with the lateral wall of the pharynx below.

pal·a·to·plas·ty (pal''uh·to·plas''tee) *n.* Plastic surgery of the palate.

pal·a·to·ple·gia (pal''uh·to·plee'jee·uh) *n.* Paralysis of the soft palate.

pal·a·to·pter·y·goid (pal''uh·to·terr'i·goid) *adj.* Pertaining to the palate bone and pterygoid processes of the sphenoid bone; PTERYGO-PALATINE.

pal·a·tor·rha·phy (pal''uh·tor'uh·fee) *n.* Suture of a cleft palate.

pal·a·tos·chi·sis (pal''uh·tos'ki·sis) *n.* CLEFT PALATE.

pa·la·tum (pa·lay'tum, pa·lah'tum) *n.,* genit. **pala·ti** (·tye), pl. **pala·ta** (·tuh) PALATE.

palatum du·rum (dew'rum) [NA]. HARD PALATE.

palatum fis·sum (fis'um). CLEFT PALATE.

palatum mo·bi·le (mo'bi·lee). SOFT PALATE.

paleo-, palaeo- A combining form meaning (a) *ancient;* (b) *primitive, phylogenetically early.*

pa·leo·cer·e·bel·lum (pay''lee·o·serr·e·bel'um) *n.* Phylogenetically old parts of the cerebellum; the anterior lobe, composed of lingula, central lobule, and culmen, and the posterior part of the posterior lobe, composed of uvula, tonsils, and paraflocculus.

pa·leo·ki·net·ic (pay''lee·o·ki·net'ick, ·kigh·net'ick) *adj.* Pertaining to the motor activities of the older nervous system, represented in mammals by the basal ganglia and brainstem, which are the structures concerned with postural static and automatic movements.

pa·le·on·tol·o·gy (pay''lee·on·tol'uh·jee) *n.* The science and study of fossil remains.

pa·leo·ol·ive (pay''lee·o·ol'iv) *n.* The accessory nuclei and the most medial portion of the main nucleus which phylogenetically, is the oldest part of the olive.

pa·leo·pal·li·um (pay''lee·o·pal'ee·um) *n.* The lateral olfactory lobe, or piriform lobe of lower forms; in the higher mammals, especially in man, it forms the uncus and adjacent anterior part of the parahippocampal gyrus.

pa·leo·pa·thol·o·gy (pay''lee·o·pa·thol'uh·jee) *n.* A branch of pathology dealing with diseases of ancient times demonstrated in human and animal remains.

paleostriatal syndrome. JUVENILE PARALYSIS AGITANS.

pa·leo·stri·a·tum (pay''lee·o·strye·ay'tum) *n.* GLOBUS PALLIDUS; the phylogenetically old part of the corpus striatum. —**paleostria·tal** (·tul) *adj.*

pa·leo·thal·a·mus (pay''lee·o·thal'uh·mus) *n.* The nuclei of the midline of the thalamus, together with some of the intralaminar nuclei.

pali-, palin- A prefix indicating *repetition* or *recurrence.*

pal·i·ki·ne·sia (pal''i·ki·nee'zhuh, ·zee·uh, ·kigh·nee') *n.* Constant and involuntary repetition of movements.

pal·i·ki·ne·sis (pal''i·ki·nee'sis, ·kigh·nee'sis) *n.* PALIKINESIA.

pal·i·la·lia (pal''i·lay'lee·uh) *n.* Pathologic repetition of words or phrases.

pal·in·dro·mia (pal''in·dro'mee·uh) *n.* The recurrence or worsening of a disease; RELAPSE. —**palin·drom·ic** (·drom'ick) *adj.*

palindromic rheumatism. An acute arthritis and periarthritis occurring in multiple, afebrile, irregularly spaced attacks lasting only a few hours or days and disappearing completely; characterized by swelling, redness, and disability of usually only one joint. It attacks adults of either sex. The cause is not known.

pal·in·gen·e·sis (pal''in·jen'e·sis) *n.* The development of characteristics during ontogeny which are regarded as inherited from ancestral species.

pal·in·op·sia (pal''i·nop'see·uh) *n.* The perseveration or recurrence of a visual image after the exciting stimulus object has been removed; a phenomenon of uncertain mechanism which occurs in a defective but not blind homonymous visual field.

pal·ir·rhea, pal·ir·rhoea (pal''i·ree'uh) *n.* 1. The recurrence of a mucoid discharge. 2. REGURGITATION.

pal·la·di·um (pa·lay'dee·um) *n.* Pd = 106.4. A silver-white, fairly ductile, hard metal, with a density of 12.02, belonging to the platinum group of metals.

pall·an·es·the·sia (pal''an·es·theezh'uh, ·theez'ee·uh) *n.* Absence of pallesthesia or vibration sense.

pall·es·the·sia, pall·aes·the·sia (pal''es·theezh'uh, ·theez'ee·uh) *n.* The sense of vibration, involving sensations like those imparted by a vibrating tuning fork.

pal·li·a·tion (pal''ee·ay'shun) *n.* Alleviation; the act of soothing or moderating, without really curing. —**pal·li·ate** (pal'ee·ate) *v.*

pal·li·a·tive (pal'ee·uh·tiv, ·ay·tiv) *adj. & n.* 1. Having a relieving or soothing, but not curative, action. 2. A drug that relieves or soothes the symptoms of a disease without curing it.

pal·li·dal (pal'i·dul) *adj.* Of or pertaining to the globus pallidus.

pal·li·do·hy·po·tha·lam·ic (pal''i·do·high''po·thuh·lam'ick) *adj. Obsol.* Pertaining to the pallidum and the hypothalamus, with reference to the connections once believed to exist between them.

pal·li·doid·o·sis (pal''i·doy·do'sis) *n.* VENEREAL SPIROCHETOSIS.

pal·li·dot·o·my (pal''i·dot'uh·mee) *n.* The surgical destruction of the globus pallidus for the treatment of movement disorders such as parkinsonism.

pal·li·dum (pal'i·dum) *n.* The globus pallidus, the medial pale portion of the lenticular nucleus of the brain. —**palli·dal** (·dul) *adj.*

pal·li·um (pal'ee·um) *n.,* pl. **pal·lia** (·ee·uh), **palliums** The cerebral cortex and superficial white matter of a cerebral hemisphere.

pal·lor (pal'ur) *n.* Paleness, especially of the skin and mucous membranes.

palm (pahm) *n.* The volar or flexor surface of the hand; the hollow of the hand.

pal·ma (pal'muh) *n.,* pl. **pal·mae** (·mee) PALM.

pal·ma·ris (pal·mair'is) *n.,* pl. **palma·res** (·eez) One of two muscles, palmaris longus and palmaris brevis, inserted into the fascia of the palm.

pal·ma·ture (pal'muh·chur, pahl') *n.* Union of the fingers; may be congenital or due to burns, wounds, or other trauma.

pal·mi·ped (pal'mi·ped) *adj.* Having webbed feet.

pal·mi·tate (pal'mi·tate) *n.* A salt or ester of palmitic acid.

palmitic acid. Hexadecanoic acid, $CH_3(CH_2)_{14}COOH$, a saturated acid occurring in the glycerides of many fats and oils. Syn. *cetic acid.*

pal·mi·tin (pal'mi·tin) *n.* Glyceryl tripalmitate or glyceryl palmitate, $C_{51}H_{98}O_6$, a solid ester of glycerin and palmitic acid occurring in many fats. Syn. *tripalmitin.*

pal·mo·men·tal (pal″mo·men'tul, pahl') *adj.* Pertaining to the palm of the hand and the mentalis muscle.

pal·mo·plan·tar (pal″mo·plan'tur, pahl″mo·) *adj.* Pertaining to both the palms of the hands and the soles of the feet.

pal·mus (pal'mus) *n.,* pl. **pal·mi** (·migh) Twitching or jerkiness.

pal·pa·ble (pal'puh·bul) *adj.* 1. Capable of being touched or palpated. 2. Evident.

pal·pa·tion (pal·pay'shun) *n.* Examination by touch for purposes of diagnosis; application of the hand or fingers to a part, or insertion of a finger into a body orifice, to detect characteristics and conditions of local tissues or of underlying organs or tumors. —**pal·pate** (pal'pate) *v.;* **pal·pa·to·ry** (pal'puh·to'ree) *adj.*

pal·pa·to·per·cus·sion (pal'puh·to·pur·kush'un) *n.* Combined palpation and percussion.

palpatory percussion. Direct percussion with the purpose of obtaining diagnostically relevant information by tactile rather than auditory means.

pal·pe·bra (pal'pe·bruh, pal·pee'bruh) *n.,* pl. genit. sing. **palpe·brae** (·bree) EYELID. —**palpe·bral** (·brul) *adj.*

palpebral fissure. The space between the eyelids extending from the outer to the inner canthus.

palpebral fold. A fold formed by the reflection of the conjunctiva from the eyelids onto the eye. There are two folds, the superior and the inferior.

palpebral ligament. A fibrous band running from the extremities of the tarsal plates to the wall of the orbit. There is one medial palpebral ligament and one lateral palpebral ligament for each eye.

pal·pe·brate (pal'pe·brate) *adj. & v.* 1. Furnished with eyelids. 2. To wink, blink repeatedly.

pal·pe·bra·tion (pal″pe·bray'shun) *n.* 1. Blinking; nictation. 2. Excessive winking as a form of tic.

pal·pi·tate (pal'pi·tate) *v.* To flutter, tremble, or beat abnormally fast; applied especially to rapid rate of the heart.

pal·pi·ta·tion (pal″pi·tay'shun) *n.* 1. A fluttering or throbbing, especially of the heart, often associated with a rapid heart rate or irregular heart rhythm. 2. Any heart action that produces a disagreeable awareness in the patient.

pal·sy (pawl'zee) *n.* Paralysis or weakness; used to designate special types, such as cerebral palsy or Erb's palsy. —**pal·sied** (·zeed) *adj.*

pa·lu·dal (pal'yoo·dul, pa·lew'dul) *adj.* 1. Pertaining to swamps or marshes. 2. MALARIAL.

pal·u·dism (pal'yoo·diz·um) *n.* MALARIA.

pam·a·quine (pam'uh·kween, ·kwin) *n.* 8-{[4-(Diethylamino)-1-methylbutyl]amino}-6-methoxyquinoline, $C_{19}H_{29}N_3O$, an antimalarial drug; used as the pamoate salt.

pam·pin·i·form (pam·pin'i·form) *adj.* Having the form of a tendril.

pampiniform plexus. A network of veins in the spermatic cord in the male, and in the broad ligament near the ovary in the female.

pan- A combining form meaning *all, every;* in medicine, *general, affecting all or many parts.*

pan·a·cea (pan″uh·see'uh) *n.* A cure-all; a quack remedy.

pan·ac·i·nar (pan·as'i·nur) *adj.* 1. Involving all acini. 2. Involving all pulmonary alveoli, applied especially to a variety of emphysema.

pan·ag·glu·ti·nin (pan″uh·gloo'ti·nin) *n.* Any agglutinating antibody which agglutinates cells of various types; the apparent lack of specificity indicates that it reacts with cell antigens common to cells of different types.

pan·a·ris (pan'uh·ris, pa·när'is) *n.* PARONYCHIA.

pan·a·ri·ti·um (pan″uh·rish'ee·um) *n.* PARONYCHIA.

pan·ar·te·ri·tis (pan″ahr·te·rye'tis) *n.* 1. Inflammation of all the coats of an artery. 2. Inflammation of several arteries at the same time; POLYARTERITIS.

pan·ar·thri·tis (pan″ahr·thrigh'tis) *n.* Inflammation of many joints.

pan·at·ro·phy (pan·at'ruh·fee) *n.* 1. Atrophy affecting every part of a structure. 2. Atrophy affecting every part of the body.

pan·car·di·tis (pan″kahr·dye'tis) *n.* Inflammation of the entire heart, involving endocardium, myocardium, and pericardium.

pan·chrome stain (pan'krome). A stain for blood which is a modification by Pappenheim of the Giemsa stain.

Pancoast's tumor A tumor of the superior pulmonary sulcus.

Pancoast syndrome The clinical picture of a superior pulmonary sulcus (thoracic inlet) tumor, including ipsilateral Horner's syndrome and brachial motor sensory disturbances due to involvement of the cervical sympathetic chain and brachial plexus; there is usually local bone invasion and destruction. Syn. *Hare's syndrome.*

pan·col·ec·to·my (pan″kol·eck′tuh·mee, ·ko·leck′) *n.* Surgical removal of the entire colon.

pancre-, pancreo-. A combining form meaning *pancreas, pancreatic.*

pan·cre·as (pan′kree·us, pang′kree·us) *n.,* genit. **pan·cre·a·tis** (pan·kree′uh·tis), pl. **pancrea·ta** (·tuh) A compound racemose gland, 6 to 8 inches in length, lying transversely across the posterior wall of the abdomen. Its right extremity, the head, lies in contact with the duodenum; its left extremity, the tail, is in close proximity to the spleen. It secretes a limpid, colorless fluid which contains the enzymes necessary for the digestion of proteins, fats, and carbohydrates. The secretion is conveyed to the duodenum by the pancreatic duct or ducts. It furnishes several important internal secretions, including glucagon and insulin, from the islets of the pancreas.

pan·cre·a·tec·to·my (pan″kree·uh·teck′tuh·mee) *n.* Excision of the pancreas.

pan·cre·at·ic (pan″kree·at′ick) *adj.* Pertaining to the pancreas.

pancreatic amylase. An enzyme in pancreatic juice that hydrolyzes starch to maltose. Syn. *amylopsin, pancreatic diastase.*

pancreatic diabetes. 1. DIABETES MELLITUS. 2. Diabetes mellitus due to pancreatic disease.

pancreatic diarrhea. Diarrhea due to deficiency of pancreatic digestive enzymes; characterized by the passage of large, greasy stools having a high fat and nitrogen content.

pancreatic fistula. 1. An external opening from the pancreas to the skin of the abdominal wall following the drainage of a pancreatic cyst or other gastric or duodenal operation. 2. An internal opening from the pancreas to the jejunum, duodenum, stomach, or gallbladder, to overcome the formation of an external fistula.

pancreatic infantilism. Growth retardation associated with the chronic undernutrition of infantile celiac disease.

pancreatic islet or **island.** ISLET OF THE PANCREAS.

pancreatic juice. The secretion of the pancreas; a thick, transparent, colorless, odorless fluid, of a salty taste, and strongly alkaline, containing proteolytic, lipolytic, and amylolytic enzymes.

pancreatic lipase. An enzyme in pancreatic juice that catalyzes the splitting of fats. Syn. *steapsin.*

pan·cre·at·i·co·du·o·de·nal (pan″kree·at′i·ko·dew″o·dee′nul, ·dew·od′e·nul) *adj.* Pertaining to the pancreas and the duodenum.

pan·cre·at·i·co·du·o·de·nec·to·my (pan″kree·at′i·ko·dew″o·de·neck′tuh·mee) *n.* DUODENOPANCREATECTOMY.

pan·cre·at·i·co·du·o·de·nos·to·my (pan″kree·at′i·ko·dew″o·de·nos′tuh·mee) *n.* PANCREATODUODENOSTOMY.

pan·cre·at·i·co·en·ter·os·to·my (pan″kree·at′i·ko·en″tur·os′tuh·mee) *n.* Anastomosis of the pancreatic duct or a pancreatic fistulous tract with the small intestine.

pan·cre·at·i·co·gas·tros·to·my (pan″kree·at′i·ko·gas·tros′tuh·mee) *n.* Anastomosis of a pancreatic fistulous tract with the pyloric portion of the stomach.

pan·cre·at·i·co·je·ju·nos·to·my (pan″kree·at′i·ko·jej″oo·nos′tuh·mee) *n.* Anastomosis of the pancreatic duct with the jejunum.

pan·cre·at·i·co·li·thot·o·my (pan″kree·at′i·ko·li·thot′uh·mee) *n.* The surgical removal of a stone in the pancreatic duct.

pan·cre·at·i·co·splen·ic (pan″kree·at′i·ko·splen′ick) *adj.* Pertaining to the pancreas and the spleen.

pan·cre·a·tin (pan′kree·uh·tin) *n.* A substance containing enzymes, principally pancreatic amylase (amylopsin), trypsin, and pancreatic lipase (steapsin), derived from the fresh pancreas of the hog, *Sus scrofa* var. *domesticus,* or of the ox, *Bos taurus;* it is a cream-colored amorphous powder with a faint odor. Used for its enzymatic action in various forms of digestive failure but of doubtful activity.

pan·cre·a·ti·tis (pan″kree·uh·tye′tis) *n.,* pl. **pancrea·tit·i·des** (·tit′i·deez) Inflammation of the pancreas, acute or chronic. —**pancrea·tit·ic** (·tit′ick) *adj.*

pan·cre·a·to·du·o·de·nos·to·my (pan″kree·uh·to·dew″o·de·nos′tuh·mee) *n.* The anastomosis of a portion of the pancreas, especially a fistulous tract into the duodenum.

pan·cre·a·to·en·ter·os·to·my (pan″kree·uh·to·en″tur·os′tuh·mee) *n.* Anastomosis of the pancreatic duct with some part of the small intestine.

pan·cre·a·tog·e·nous (pan″kree·uh·toj′e·nus) *adj.* Arising in the pancreas.

pan·cre·a·to·li·pase (pan″kree·uh·to·lye′pace) *n.* Lipase found in the pancreatic juice.

pan·cre·ato·lith (pan″kree·at′o·lith) *n.* A calculus of the pancreas.

pan·cre·a·to·li·thec·to·my (pan″kree·uh·to·li·theck′tuh·mee, pan″kree·at′o·) *n.* Surgical removal of a pancreatic calculus.

pan·cre·a·to·li·thot·o·my (pan″kree·uh·to·li·thot′uh·mee, pan″kree·at′o·) *n.* Surgical removal of calculus from the pancreas.

pan·cre·a·tol·y·sis (pan″kree·uh·tol′i·sis) *n.* Destruction of the pancreas. —**pancre·ato·lyt·ic** (·at″o·lit′ick) *adj.*

pan·cre·a·tot·o·my (pan″kree·uh·tot′uh·mee) *n.* Incision of the pancreas.

pan·cre·op·a·thy (pan″kree·op′uth·ee) *n.* Any disease of the pancreas.

pan·cy·to·pe·ni·a (pan″sigh·to·pee′nee·uh) *n.* Reduction of all three formed elements of the blood: erythrocytes, leukocytes, and blood platelets.

pan·de·mi·a (pan·dee′mee·uh) *n.* A widespread epidemic; one affecting the majority of inhabitants of an area.

pan·dem·ic (pan·dem′ick) *adj. & n.* 1. Epidemic over a wide geographic area, or even worldwide. 2. A widespread or worldwide epidemic.

pan·dic·u·la·tion (pan·dick″yoo·lay′shun) *n.* The act of stretching the limbs, especially on waking from sleep, accompanied by yawning.

Pan·dy's reagent (pahn′dee) A saturated aqueous solution of phenol used in testing for spinal-fluid protein.

Pandy's test A test for protein in which 1 ml of Pandy's reagent is placed in a test tube and one drop of spinal fluid is added. If increased protein is present, a bluish-white ring or cloud is formed.

pan·en·ceph·a·li·tis (pan"en·sef"uh·lye'tis) *n.* 1. Generalized inflammation of the brain, involving both gray and white matter. 2. Specifically, SUBACUTE SCLEROSING PANENCEPHALITIS.

pan·en·do·scope (pan·en'duh·skope) *n.* A modification of the cystoscope, utilizing a Foroblique lens system, permitting adequate visualization of both the urinary bladder and the urethra.

pan·es·the·sia, pan·aes·the·sia (pan"es·theezh'uh, ·theez'ee·uh) *n.* CENESTHESIA. — **panes·thet·ic, panaes·thet·ic** (·thet'ick) *adj.*

Pa·neth cells (pah'net) Coarsely granular secretory cells found in the intestinal glands of the small intestine.

pang, *n.* A momentary, sharp pain; sudden distress.

pan·gen·e·sis (pan·jen'e·sis) *n.* Darwin's comprehensive theory of heredity and development, according to which all parts of the body give off gemmules which aggregate in the germ cells. During development, they are sorted out from one another and give rise to parts similar to those of their origin.

pan·glos·sia (pan·glos'ee·uh) *n.* Excessive or psychotic garrulity.

pan·hem·a·to·pe·nia, pan·haem·a·to·pe·nia (pan·hem"uh·to·pee'nee·uh, ·hee"muh·to·) *n.* PANCYTOPENIA.

pan·hi·dro·sis (pan"hi·dro'sis) *n.* Generalized perspiration.

pan·hy·grous (pan·high'grus) *adj.* Damp as to the entire surface.

pan·hy·po·go·nad·ism (pan"high"po·go'nad·iz·um) *n.* Underdevelopment of all parts of the genital apparatus.

pan·hy·po·pi·tu·i·ta·rism (pan"high"po·pi·tew'i·ta·riz·um) *n.* Complete absence of all pituitary secretions.

pan·hy·po·pi·tu·i·tary dwarfism (pan"high"po·pi·tew'i·terr"ee) Pituitary dwarfism with deficiencies of all pituitary hormones.

pan·hys·ter·ec·to·my (pan"his"tur·eck'tuh·mee) *n.* Total excision of the uterus, including the cervix, body, and associated soft tissue.

pan·hys·tero·col·pec·to·my (pan"his"tur·o·kol·peck'tuh·mee) *n.* Complete removal of the uterus and vagina.

pan·hys·tero·oo·pho·rec·to·my (pan"his"tur·o·o·off"uh·reck'tuh·mee) *n.* Excision of the entire uterus and one or both ovaries.

pan·hys·tero·sal·pin·gec·to·my (pan"his"tur·o·sal"pin·jeck'tuh·mee) *n.* Excision of the entire uterus and the oviducts.

pan·hys·tero·sal·pin·go·oo·pho·rec·to·my (pan"his"tur·o·sal·ping"go·o·off"uh·reck'tuh·mee) *n.* Excision of the uterus, oviducts, and ovaries.

pan·ic, *n.* An extreme anxiety attack which may lead to total inaction or more often to precipitate and unreasonable acts; a state of mind frequently spreading rapidly to others in the same situation.

pan·im·mu·ni·ty (pan"i·mew'ni·tee) *n.* General immunity to disease or infection.

pan·lob·u·lar (pan·lob'yoo·lur) *adj.* Involving all lobules; applied especially to a variety of pulmonary emphysema.

pan·me·tri·tis (pan"me·trye'tis) *n.* Widespread inflammation of the entire uterus, often accompanied by cellulitis of the broad ligaments.

pan·mne·sia (pan·nee'zhuh, ·zee·uh) *n.* A potential remembrance of all impressions.

Panmycin. A trademark for the antibiotic substance tetracycline and certain of its salts.

pan·my·e·lop·a·thy (pan"migh·e·lop'uth·ee) *n.* MYELOPROLIFERATIVE DISORDER.

pan·my·e·lo·phthi·sis (pan"migh"e·lo·thigh'sis, ·tee'sis) *n.* A general wasting of the bone marrow.

pan·my·e·lo·tox·i·co·sis (pan·migh"e·lo·tock"si·ko'sis) *n.* A toxic condition in which all elements of the bone marrow are affected.

pan·my·o·si·tis (pan"migh·o·sigh'tis) *n.* Generalized muscular inflammation.

pan·nic·u·li·tis (pan"nick·yoo·lye'tis) *n.* Inflammation of the panniculus adiposus, especially abdominal.

pan·ni·cu·lus (pa·nick'yoo·lus) *n.,* pl. **pannicu·li** (·lye) A membrane or layer.

panniculus adi·po·sus (ad·i·po'sus) [NA]. The layer of subcutaneous fat.

pan·nus (pan'us) *n.,* pl. **pan·ni** (·nigh) 1. Vascularization and connective-tissue deposition beneath the epithelium of the cornea. 2. CHLOASMA. 3. Connective tissue overgrowing the articular surface of a diarthrodial joint.

pan·o·pho·bia (pan"o·fo'bee·uh) *n.* PANTOPHOBIA.

pan·oph·thal·mia (pan"off·thal'mee·uh) *n.* PANOPHTHALMITIS.

pan·os·te·i·tis (pan"os·tee·eye'tis) *n.* An inflammation of all parts of a bone.

pan·oti·tis (pan"o·tye'tis) *n.* A diffuse inflammation of all parts of the ear, usually beginning in the middle ear.

pan·phle·bi·tis (pan"fle·bye'tis) *n.* 1. Inflammation of all the coats of a vein. 2. Inflammation of several veins simultaneously.

pan·pho·bia (pan·fo'bee·uh) *n.* PANTOPHOBIA.

pan·scle·ro·sis (pan"skle·ro'sis) *n.* Complete hardening of a part or tissue.

pan·si·nus·itis (pan"sigh·nuh·sigh'tis) *n.* Inflammation of all the paranasal sinuses.

Panstrongylus me·gis·tus (me·jis'tus). A species of bug that transmits *Trypanosoma cruzi* in South America.

pan·sys·tol·ic (pan·sis·tol'ick) *adj.* Pertaining to the entire phase of systole; HOLOSYSTOLIC.

pant, *v.* To breathe hard or to breathe in a labored and spasmodic manner.

pan·ta·pho·bia (pan"tuh·fo'bee·uh) *n.* Total absence of fear.

pan·ther·a·pist (pan·therr'uh·pist) *n.* A person who treats on the basis of any available remedial agent from any system of therapy.

pan·to·graph (pan'to·graf) *n.* 1. An instrument for the mechanical copying of diagrams, maps, or other drawings upon the same scale, or upon an enlarged or a reduced scale. 2. An apparatus for graphically recording the contour of the chest. 3. An apparatus used in dental reconstructive treatment to determine the path of movement of the patient's mandibular condyles. —**pan·to·graph·ic** (pan''to·graf'ick) *adj.*

pan·to·mime (pan'tuh·mime) *n.* An expressive sequence of actions or movements unaccompanied by speech, often involving exaggerated or symbolic gestures, and usually for the purpose of conveying information or telling or enacting a story. In medicine, frequently employed as a means of communication by patients suffering from motor aphasia or otherwise incapable of communicating through speech. **pan·to·mim·ic** (pan''tuh·mim'ick) *adj.*

Pantopaque. Trademark for iophendylate injection, a radiopaque diagnostic agent.

pan·to·pho·bia (pan''to·fo'bee·uh) *n.* An abnormal fear of everything, including the unknown.

Pantopon. Trademark for a preparation containing all the alkaloids of opium in the form of hydrochlorides, and in the relative proportion in which they occur in the whole gum.

pan·to·som·a·tous (pan''to·som'uh·tus, ·so'muh·tus) *adj.* Involving the entire body. Syn. *pantasomatous.*

pan·to·then·ic acid (pan''to·thenn'ick) $D(+)$-N-$(\alpha,\gamma$-Dihydroxy-β,β-dimethylbutyryl)-β-alanine, $C_9H_{17}NO_5$, widely distributed in animal and plant tissues; a component of coenzyme A and a member of the vitamin-B complex. Essential for nutrition of some animal species, but little is known about its importance in human nutrition. Syn. *chick antidermatitis factor, filtrate factor, pantoyl-β-alanine.*

pan·trop·ic (pan·trop'ick) *adj.* POLYTROPIC; having affinity for or affecting many tissues; applied to viruses.

pa·nus (pay'nus) *n.* 1. An inflamed, nonsuppurating lymph node. 2. LYMPHOGRANULOMA VENEREUM.

pan·uve·itis (pan''yoo''vee·eye'tis) *n.* An inflammation affecting the entire uveal tract simultaneously.

pan·zo·ot·ic (pan''zo·ot'ick) *adj.* Affecting many species of animals.

pap A soft, semisolid food.

pa·pa·in (pa·pay'in) *n.* An enzyme preparation obtained from the juice of the fruit and leaves of *Carica papaya.* Popularly used as a digestant for protein foods; also employed externally for treatment of inflammatory processes. A special preparation of proteolytic enzymes from *Carica papaya* is used internally for reduction of soft tissue inflammation and edema associated with traumatic injury and localized inflammations.

Pa·pa·ni·co·laou classes (pa^h·pa^h·nee·koh·law') A system of classifying exfoliated cells, as seen in stained smears, into six groups, as follows: Class O, inadequate for diagnosis; Class I, absence of atypical or abnormal cells (negative); Class II, cytology atypical, but no evidence of malignancy (negative); Class III, cytology suggestive of malignancy, but not conclusive (suspicious); Class IV, cytology strongly suggestive of malignancy (positive); Class V, cytology conclusive for malignancy (positive).

Pa·pa·ver (pa·pay'vur, pa·pav'ur) *n.* A genus of herbs of the Papaveraceae; the poppy.

pa·pav·er·ine (pa·pav'ur·een, ·in, pa·pay'vur·) *n.* An alkaloid, $C_{20}H_{21}NO_4$, obtained from opium, belonging to the benzyl isoquinoline group (it is not a morphine derivative). Relaxes smooth muscle; has weak analgesic activity. Generally used as the hydrochloride salt.

pa·paw (pa·paw', pah'paw) *n.* 1. The seed of the tree *Asimina triloba;* has been used as an emetic. 2. PAPAYA.

pa·pa·ya (pa·pah'yuh, pa·pay'uh) *n.* Melon tree; papaw; *Carica papaya,* a tree of the Passifloraceae. The unripe fruit yields a milky juice containing papain.

pa·pil·la (pa·pil'uh) *n.,* pl. & genit. sing. **papil·lae** (·ee) A small, nipplelike eminence.

papilla of Vater MAJOR DUODENAL PAPILLA.

pap·il·lary (pap'i·lerr·ee) *adj.* Pertaining to, having, or resembling a papilla or papillae.

papillary adenoma. An adenoma whose parenchymal cells form papillary processes.

papillary carcinoma. A carcinoma with finger-like outgrowths, a pattern commonly seen in transitional-cell carcinoma of the urinary tract.

papillary cystadenoma lym·pho·ma·to·sum (lim''fo·ma·to'sum). A benign tumor of salivary glands, especially the parotid gland; it is usually cystic, composed of a double layer of eosinophilic cells and has a pronounced lymphoid stroma. Syn. *Warthin's tumor.*

papillary hidradenoma. A benign sweat-gland tumor occurring most commonly on the labia majores and perineum of women.

papillary layer. The zone of fine-fibered connective tissue within and immediately subjacent to the papillae of the corium.

papillary muscles. The muscular eminences in the ventricles of the heart from which the chordae tendineae arise.

papillary necrosis. Renal necrosis occurring in the medulla, particularly in the papillary portion, and affecting one or more papillae in one or both kidneys. It is associated most commonly with urinary tract obstruction, acute pyelonephritis, diabetes mellitus, analgesic abuse, and sickling disorders. Syn. *necrotizing papillitis, medullary necrosis.*

papillary process. A short, rounded process extending inferiorly from the caudate lobe of the liver behind the portal fissure. In the fetus, it is large and is in contact with the pancreas.

papillary varix. A benign cutaneous tumor consisting of a single dilated blood vessel; occurs after middle age. Syn. *angioma senile, Cayenne-pepper spot.*

pap·il·late (pap'i·late, ·pil'ut) *adj.* Having small papillary or nipplelike projections.

pap·il·lec·to·my (pap''i·leck'tuh·mee) *n.* Surgical removal of a papilla or papillae.

pa·pil·le·de·ma, pa·pil·loe·de·ma (pa·pil''e·dee'

muh, pap''i·le·) n. Edema of the optic disk.

pap·il·lif·er·ous (pap''i·lif'ur·us) adj. Bearing or containing papillae, as a papilliferous cyst.

pa·pil·li·form (pa·pil'i·form) adj. Shaped like a papilla.

pap·il·li·tis (pap''i·lye'tis) n. 1. Inflammation of a papilla. 2. OPTIC NEURITIS. 3. Inflammation of a renal papilla.

pap·il·lo·ma (pap''i·lo'ma) n., pl. **papillomas, papilloma·ta** (·tuh) A growth pattern of epithelial tumors in which the proliferating epithelial cells grow outward from a surface, accompanied by vascularized cores of connective tissue, to form a branching structure.

pap·il·lo·mac·u·lar (pap''i·lo·mack'yoo·lur) adj. Pertaining to the optic disk and macula.

pap·il·lo·ma·to·sis (pap''i·lo''muh·to'sis) n. The widespread formation of papillomas; the state of being affected with multiple papillomas.

pap·il·lom·a·tous (pap''i·lom'uh·tus) adj. Characterized by or pertaining to a papilloma or papillomas.

pap·il·lo·ret·i·ni·tis (pap''i·lo·ret''i·nigh'tis) n. Inflammation of the optic disk and retina.

pa·po·va·vi·rus (pa·po''vuh·vye'rus) n. A member of a group of ether-resistant deoxyribonucleic acid viruses, including the Shope papilloma, the human papilloma (wart), the polyoma, and the simian virus 40 (SV_{40}).

Pap·pen·hei·mer bodies Iron-containing granules sometimes found in the cytoplasm of some normoblasts and erythrocytes, particularly after splenectomy.

pap·pus (pap'us) n. The fine downy hair first appearing on the cheeks and chin.

Pap smear A vaginal smear prepared for the study of exfoliated cells.

Pap test. PAPANICOLAOU'S TEST.

pap·u·la·tion (pap''yoo·lay'shun) n. The stage, in certain eruptions, marked by papule formation.

pap·ule (pap'yool) n. A solid circumscribed elevation of the skin varying from less than 0.1 cm to 1 cm in diameter. —**pap·u·lar** (·yoo·lur) adj.

pap·u·lo·er·y·the·ma·tous (pap''yoo·lo·err''i·theem'uh·tus) adj. Having a papular eruption superimposed on a generalized erythema.

pap·u·lo·ne·crot·ic (pap''yoo·lo·ne·krot'ick) adj. Papule formation with a tendency to central necrosis; applied especially to a variety of skin tuberculosis.

pap·u·lo·pus·tu·lar (pap''yoo·lo·pus'tew·lur) adj. Characterized by both papules and pustules.

pap·u·lo·sis (pap''yoo·lo'sis) n. A condition involving multiple papules.

pap·u·lo·squa·mous (pap''yoo·lo·skway'mus) adj. Characterized by both papules and scales.

pap·u·lo·ve·sic·u·lar (pap''yoo·lo·ve·sick'yoo·lur) adj. Characterized by both papules and vesicles.

pap·y·ra·ceous (pap''i·ray'shus, ·see·us) adj. Resembling paper, as the papyraceous plate of the ethmoid bone; papery.

par-, para- A prefix signifying (a) near; (b) beside, adjacent to; (c) closely resembling, almost; (d) beyond; (e) remotely or indirectly related to;

(f) faulty or abnormal condition; (g) associated in an accessory capacity.

para (păr'uh) n. A woman giving birth or having given birth for the time or number of times specified by the following numeral, as: para I (for the first time = primapara), para II (for the second time = secundipara).

para-. A prefix signifying (a) the relationship of two atoms in the benzene ring that are separated by two carbon atoms in the ring, i.e., the 1, 4-position; (b) a benzene derivative in which two substituents have such a relationship. Symbol, p-.

-para A combining form designating a woman as having given (single or multiple) birth for the (specified) time or number of times, as: primipara (for the first time), secundipara (for the second time).

para-ami·no·ben·zo·ic acid (păr''uh·a·mee''no·ben·zo'ick). $NH_2C_6H_4COOH$, an off-white, crystalline powder; has been used as an antirickettsial drug. Abbreviated, PABA

para-ami·no·hip·pu·ric acid (păr''uh·a·mee''no·hi·pew'rick). Aminohippuric acid or p-aminobenzoylaminoacetic acid, $C_9H_{10}N_2O_3$, used intravenously as the sodium salt to determine renal function. Abbreviated, PAH, PAHA.

para-ami·no·sal·i·cyl·ic acid (păr''uh·a·mee''no·sal''i·sil'ick). 4-Aminosalicylic acid or 4-amino-2-hydroxybenzoic acid, $NH_2C_6H_3OH·COOH$, a tuberculostatic drug. Abbreviated, PAS, PASA.

para-am·y·loi·do·sis (păr''uh·am''i·loy·do'sis) n. A type of amyloidosis which has some, but not all, of the characteristics of classic amyloidosis. Syn. atypical amyloidosis.

para-an·al·ge·sia (păr''uh·an''al·jee'zee·uh) n. Analgesia of the lower extremities.

para-an·es·the·sia, para-an·aes·the·sia (păr''uh·an''es·theezh'uh, ·theez'ee·uh) n. Anesthesia of the lower extremities.

para-aor·tic (păr''uh·ay·or'tick) adj. Adjacent to the aorta.

paraaortic bodies. Small masses of chromaffin tissue scattered along the abdominal aorta; they are macroscopic in size in the fetus and in infancy, but are microscopic in later life.

para-bi·o·sis (păr''uh·bye·o'sis) n., pl. **parabio·ses** (·seez) The experimental fusing together of two individuals or embryos so that the effects of one partner upon the other may be studied. —**parabi·ot·ic** (·ot'ick) adj.

para·blep·sia (păr''uh·blep'see·uh) n. False or perverted vision.

para·bu·lia (păr''uh·bew'lee·uh) n. Abnormality of volitional action; particularly the sudden and seemingly inexplicable substitution of one action or its motive by another, as seen in schizophrenia.

par·ac·an·tho·ma (pa·rack''an·tho'muh, păr''uh·kan·) n. A tumor whose parenchyma consists of cells resembling those of the prickle-cell layer of the skin.

para·ca·ri·nal (păr''uh·ka·rye'nul) adj. Beside a carina, especially the urethral carina.

para·ce·cal (păr''uh·see'kul) adj. Adjacent to the cecum.

Paracelsian method. The use of chemical agents alone in treating disease.

para·cen·te·sis (păr″uh·sen·tee'sis) *n.*, pl. **para-cente·ses** (·seez) Puncture; especially the puncture or tapping of a fluid-filled space by means of a hollow needle or trochar, to draw off the contained fluid.

paracentesis of the bladder. The puncture of the urinary bladder with a vesical trocar for the relief of obstruction or to provide constant drainage.

paracentesis of the chest. The insertion of a needle or trocar into the pleural cavity for the relief of pleural effusion.

para·cen·tral (păr″uh·sen'trul) *adj.* Situated near the center.

para·chro·ma·tism (păr″uh·kro'muh·tiz·um) *n.* False, or incorrect, perception of color, not true color blindness, which it may approach more or less completely.

parachute deformity. A congenital deformity of the mitral valve in which the valve resembles a parachute.

par·ac·me (păr·ack'mee) *n.* 1. The degeneration or decadence of a group of organisms after they have reached their acme of development. 2. The period of decline or remission of a disease.

Para·coc·cid·i·oi·des (păr″uh·kock·sid″ee·oy'deez) *n.* Blastomyces. —**paracoccidioi·dal** (·dul) *adj.*

para·co·li·tis (păr″uh·ko·lye'tis) *n.* Inflammation of the tissue adjacent to the colon.

para·co·lon (păr″uh·ko'lun) *n.* A group of bacteria intermediate between the *Escherichia-Aerobacter* genera and the *Salmonella-Shigella* group. Culturally, these organisms may be confused with the non-lactose-fermenting pathogenic bacteria found in the intestinal tract. Some of the paracolon bacilli probably produce disease.

para·col·pi·tis (păr″uh·kol·pye'tis) *n.* Inflammation of the connective tissue about the vagina.

para·con·dy·lar (păr″uh·kon'di·lur) *adj.* Situated alongside a condyle or a condylar region.

para·cone (păr'uh·kone) *n.* The mesiobuccal cusp of an upper molar tooth.

para·co·nid (păr″uh·ko'nid) *n.* The mesiolingual cusp of a lower molar tooth.

par·a·cu·sia (păr″uh·kew'zhuh, ·zee·uh) *n.* Any perversion of the sense of hearing.

paracusia acris (ay'kris, ack'ris). Excessively acute hearing, rendering the person intolerant of sounds.

paracusia du·pli·ca·ta (dew·pli·kay'tuh). A condition in which all or only certain sounds are heard double.

paracusia lo·ca·lis (lo·kay'lis). Difficulty in estimating the direction of sounds, met with in unilateral deafness, or when the two ears hear unequally.

paracusia ob·tu·sa (ob·tew'suh). Difficulty in hearing.

paracusia Wil·li·sii (wi·lis'ee·eye). A condition of deafness in which the hearing is better in a noisy place, as in a train or factory.

para·cy·e·sis (păr″uh·sigh·ee'sis) *n.* Extrauterine pregnancy.

para·cys·tic (păr″uh·sis'tick) *adj.* Situated near, or alongside, the urinary bladder.

para·cys·ti·tis (păr″uh·sis·tye'tis) *n.* Inflammation of the connective tissue surrounding the urinary bladder.

para·cyt·ic (păr″uh·sit'ick) *adj.* Lying among cells.

par·ad·e·ni·tis (păr″ad·e·nigh'tis) *n.* Inflammation of the tissues about a gland.

para·den·tal (păr″uh·den'tul) *adj.* 1. Near, or beside, a tooth. 2. Associated with dental practice.

para·did·y·mis (păr″uh·did'i·mis) *n.*, pl. **para·di·dy·mi·des** (·di·dim'i·deez) The atrophic remains of the paragenital tubules of the mesonephros, which separate from the mesonephric duct and lie near the convolutions of the epididymal duct. Syn. *organ of Giraldes.*

para·diph·the·ri·al (păr″uh·dif·theer'ee·ul) *adj.* Remotely or indirectly resembling diphtheria, as the membrane covering the pharynx in infectious mononucleosis.

para·dis·tem·per (păr″uh·dis·tem'pur) *n.* Hard Pad.

para·dox·ia sex·u·a·lis (păr″uh·dock'see·uh secks″yoo·ay'lis) Sexual activity occurring outside what is usually regarded as the reproductive period, that is, before puberty or in the senile years.

par·a·dox·ic (păr″uh·dock'sick) *adj.* Paradoxical.

par·a·dox·i·cal (păr″uh·dock'si·kul) *adj.* Contrary to the usual or normal kind.

paradoxical embolus. An embolus, usually a venous thrombus, which is transported to the peripheral arterial circulation through a cardiac septal defect or patent ductus arteriosus with a right-to-left shunt, usually a patent foramen ovale. Syn. *crossed embolus.*

paradoxical pupillary reaction or **reflex.** Any response of the pupil to a stimulus contrary to the expected one; such responses include dilation of the pupil on exposure to light or constriction when light is withdrawn (as may occur in certain pathologic states or suggest functional exhaustion), convergence and associated dilation of the pupil with near vision or constriction with distant vision, dilation of the pupil by epinephrine following destruction of the superior cervical ganglion, and dilation of the pupil in response to pain in the lower part of the body.

para·du·o·de·nal (păr″uh·dew″o·dee'nul, ·dew·od'e·nul) *adj.* On either side of the duodenum.

para·dys·en·tery (păr″uh·dis'un·terr·ee) *n.* 1. A mild form of dysentery. 2. Dysentery due to *Shigella flexneri.*

para·ep·i·lep·sy (păr″uh·ep'i·lep″see) *n.* Obsol. An abortive epileptic attack, consisting only of the aura. Consciousness is not lost.

paraesophageal cyst. A bronchogenic cyst intimately connected with the esophageal wall, containing cartilage, and usually filled with a mucoid material and desquamated epithelial cells.

par·af·fin (păr'uh·fin) *n.* 1. Any saturated hydrocarbon having the formula C_nH_{2n+2}. These compounds constitute the paraffin series. Syn.

alkane. 2. A purified mixture of solid hydrocarbons obtained from petroleum; variously used to impart hardness or stiffness to protective agents, such as ointment bases, suppositories, or bandages.

par·af·fin·oma (păr″uh·fĭ·no′muh) *n.* A nodular mass of inflammatory, granulation, or scar tissue, due to injection of paraffin into the tissues.

para·form·al·de·hyde (păr″uh·for·mal′de·hide) *n.* A solid polymer, $(CH_2O)_n$, of formaldehyde, or, more properly, a mixture of polyoxymethylenes, formed when solutions of formaldehyde are allowed to evaporate; has been used as a convenient form for generating small quantities of formaldehyde gas for disinfecting purposes. Syn. *paraform, trioxymethylene.*

para·gam·ma·cism (păr″uh·gam′uh·siz·um) *n.* Inability to pronounce the hard *g* and *k*, other consonants being substituted.

para·gan·glia (păr″uh·gang′glee·uh) *n.*, sing. **paragangli·on** (·on) Groups of chromaffin cells scattered along the ventral surface of the aorta, especially in the fetus.

para·gan·gli·o·ma (păr″uh·gang′glee·o′muh) *n.* A tumor derived from elements that form part of the chemoreceptor system. It originates in the middle ear from the glomus jugulare and consists of a group of cells situated in the adventitia of the jugular bulb or along the ramus tympanicus of the glossopharyngeal nerve.

para·gan·gli·on·ic (păr″uh·gang′glee·on′ick) *adj.* Pertaining to the paraganglia and their secretions.

para·gan·gli·ons (păr″uh·gang′glee·unz) *n.pl.* PARAGANGLIA.

para·gen·i·tal (păr″uh·jĕn′i·tul) *adj.* In the vicinity of a genital organ.

para·geu·sia (păr″uh·gew′see·uh, ·joo′see·uh) *n.* Perversion or impairment of the sense of taste. **—parageu·sic** (·sick) *adj.*

par·ag·glu·ti·na·tion (păr″uh·gloo·ti·nay′shun) *n.* Agglutination of colon bacilli and cocci with the serum of patients infected with or recovering from infection with dysentery bacilli. The property of paragglutination disappears when the bacteria are subcultured.

para·glos·sa (păr″uh·glos′uh) *n.* Swelling of the tongue; a hypertrophy of the tongue, usually congenital.

para·glos·sia (păr″uh·glos′ee·uh) *n.* Inflammation of the muscles and connective tissues under the tongue.

pa·rag·na·thous (pa·rag′nuth·us, păr″ug·nath′us) *adj.* 1. Having upper and lower jaws of equal length, their tips falling together, as in certain birds. 2. Pertaining to or characteristic of a paragnathus.

pa·rag·na·thus (pa·rag′nuth·us, păr″ug·nath′us) *n.* 1. An individual having a supernumerary jaw. 2. A parasitic fetus or part attached to the jaw laterally.

para·gom·pho·sis (păr″uh·gom·fo′sis) *n.* Impaction of the fetal head in the pelvic canal.

par·a·gon·i·mi·a·sis (păr″uh·gon″i·migh′uh·sis) *n.*, pl. **paragonimia·ses** (·seez) Infection by species of the genus *Paragonimus,* especially *P. westermani.*

Par·a·gon·i·mus (păr″uh·gon′i·mus) *n.* A genus of trematode worms.

Paragonimus wes·ter·mani (wes·tur·man′eye). Species of lung flukes which in the adult stage cause tissue destruction, inflammation, and hemorrhage.

para·gran·u·lo·ma (păr″uh·gran″yoo·lo′muh) *n.* In the Jackson-Parker classification, variety of Hodgkin's disease said to be its least aggressive form.

para·graph·ia (păr″uh·graf′ee·uh) *n.* 1. Perverted writing; a form of aphasia in which letters or words are misplaced or improperly used. 2. A loss of ability to express ideas in writing or to write from dictation, as the result of a brain lesion. **—paragraph·ic** (·ick) *adj.*

para·he·mo·phil·ia, para·hae·mo·phil·ia (păr″uh·hee″mo·fĭl′ee·uh, ·hem″o·) *n.* A hemorrhagic disorder characterized by a deficiency of Factor V. Syn. *Owren's disease.*

para·hep·a·ti·tis (păr″uh·hep″uh·tye′tis) *n.* Inflammation of structures about or near the liver.

para·hip·po·cam·pal gyrus (păr″uh·hip″o·kam′pul). A gyrus of the medial portion of the temporal lobe, continuous caudally with the cingulate gyrus above the lingual gyrus below and lying between the hippocampal sulcus and the anterior part of the collateral sulcus.

para·hor·mone (par″uh·hor′mone) *n.* Any substance which, like carbon dioxide in its effect on the respiratory center, exerts a hormone-like regulatory influence on some organ but which is not synthesized by a specific organ adapted to that purpose, as hormones are.

para·hyp·no·sis (păr″uh·hip·no′sis) *n.* Disturbances of sleep, such as somnambulism or night terrors.

para·in·flu·en·za (păr″uh·in″floo·en′zuh) *n.* A condition similar to or due to influenza.

parainfluenza virus. An RNA virus of the paramyxovirus group; a common cause of respiratory infection, particularly croup.

para·ker·a·to·sis (păr″uh·kerr″uh·to′sis) *n.* Incomplete keratinization of epidermal cells characterized by retention of nuclei of cells attaining the level of the stratum corneum; the normal condition of the topmost epithelial cells of mucous membranes. **—parakera·tot·ic** (·tot′ick) *adj.*

para·la·lia (păr″uh·lay′lee·uh, ·lal′ee·uh) *n.* Disturbance of the faculty of speech, characterized by distortion of sounds, or the habitual substitution of one sound for another.

par·al·de·hyde (păr·al′de·hide) *n.* Paracetaldehyde, $(CH_3CHO)_3$, a colorless liquid with an unpleasant taste. Used as a rapidly acting hypnotic and anticonvulsant but is potentially hazardous as it may be completely oxidized to acetic acid.

para·lex·ia (păr″uh·leck′see·uh) *n.* DYSLEXIA. **—paralex·ic** (·sick) *adj.*

par·al·ge·sia (păr″al·jee′zee·uh) *n.* Painful paresthesia. **—paralge·sic** (·zick) *adj.*

par·al·lax (păr′uh·lacks) *n.* The apparent displacement of an object, caused by a change in the position of the observer, or by looking at the object alternately first with one eye and then with the other. —**par·al·lac·tic** (păr″uh-lack′tick) *adj.*

par·al·lel·om·e·ter (păr″uh-lel-om′e-tur) *n.* An instrument used for paralleling attachments and abutments for dental prostheses.

para·lo·gia (păr″uh-lo′jee-uh) *n.* Difficulty in thinking logically; false reasoning.

pa·ral·o·gism (puh-ral′o-jiz-um) *n.* *In logic*, the error of considering effects or unrelated phenomena as the cause of a condition. —**pa·ral·o·gis·tic** (puh-ral″o-jis′tick) *adj.*

para·lu·te·in cells (păr″uh-lew′tee-in). The epithelioid cells of the corpus luteum, derived from the theca interna of the ovarian follicle. Syn. *theca lutein cells.*

pa·ral·y·sis (puh-ral′i-sis) *n.*, pl. **paraly·ses** (-seez) Loss of muscle function or of sensation. Paralyses may be classified according to etiology, as alcoholic or lead; according to part involved, as facial or palatal; according to muscle tone, as flaccid or spastic; according to distribution, as monoplegic or hemiplegic, or according to some other characteristic, as ascending or crossed. Certain types of paralysis are often called palsies; partial paralysis is called paresis.

paralysis ag·i·tans (aj′i-tanz). PARKINSON'S DISEASE.

para·lys·sa (păr″uh-lis′uh) *n.* A South American form of rabies, caused by the bite of a rabid vampire bat.

par·a·lyt·ic (păr″uh-lit′ick) *adj. & n.* 1. Pertaining to, or affected with, paralysis. 2. A person affected with paralysis.

paralytic abasia. Inability to walk or stand because of organic paralysis of the legs.

paralytic aphonia. Inability to produce sounds because of paralysis of vocal folds.

paralytic bladder. ATONIC BLADDER.

paralytic bulbar poliomyelitis. Poliomyelitis affecting chiefly the medulla oblongata and pons, involving motor cranial nuclei and frequently affecting respiratory and circulatory centers.

paralytic bulbospinal poliomyelitis. Both paralytic bulbar and paralytic spinal poliomyelitis.

paralytic dislocation. Dislocation of a joint, most commonly the hip, from paralysis of one group of muscles, usually with overpull by the opposing group.

paralytic ileus. ADYNAMIC ILEUS.

paralytic poliomyelitis. A form of poliomyelitis characterized by muscle weakness or paralysis. Conventionally subdivided, on the basis of the anatomic structures predominantly involved, into spinal, bulbospinal, bulbar, and encephalitic types.

paralytic rabies. A form of rabies confined largely to the spinal cord, or, in dogs, to the spinal cord and brainstem. The chief manifestation in humans is ascending paralysis, with little or no excitation and other signs of brain involvement. In dogs there is also no excitation, but there is usually hydrophobia. The commonest vector of the human infection is the vampire bat. Syn. *dumb rabies.*

paralytic spinal poliomyelitis. A form of paralytic poliomyelitis involving principally the anterior horns of the gray matter of the spinal cord, caused by one or more of the poliomyelitis viruses (type I, Brunhilde; II, Lansing; III, Leon), and producing paralysis of muscle groups, particularly the limbs. Syn. *epidemic paralysis.*

par·a·ly·zant, par·a·ly·sant (păr″uh-lye″zunt, puh-ral′i-zunt) *adj. & n.* 1. Causing paralysis. 2. Something which causes paralysis.

par·a·lyz·er (păr″uh-lye′zur) *n.* 1. Anything that will produce paralysis. 2. Any agent that will inhibit a chemical reaction.

para·mag·net·ic (păr″uh-mag-net′ick) *adj.* Pertaining to or characterizing the property of any substance, excluding iron and certain other materials that attract a magnetic field very strongly, which tends to move to the strongest part of a nonuniform magnetic field. —**para·mag·net·ism** (-uh-mag-ne-tiz-um) *n.*

para·ma·nia (păr″uh-may′nee-uh) *n.* The pleasure or satisfaction derived from complaining; a common neurotic symptom.

para·mas·ti·tis (păr″uh-mas-tye′tis) *n.* Inflammation of the connective tissue about the mammary gland.

para·mas·toid (păr″uh-mas′toid) *adj.* In the vicinity of the mastoid process.

para·mas·toid·itis (păr″uh-mas″toid-eye′tis) *n.* Inflammation of the squamous portion of the temporal bone, from extension following mastoiditis.

para·me·di·al (păr″uh-mee′dee-ul) *adj.* Situated near a medial structure.

paramedian lobule. A rounded lobule on the inferior surface of the cerebellum, medial to the ansiform lobule and lateral to the tonsilla.

para·me·nia (păr″uh-mee′nee-uh) *n.* Difficult or disordered menstruation.

para·men·tal (păr″uh-men′tul) *adj.* Adjacent to the chin or mandible.

para·meso·neph·ric (păr″uh-mes″o-nef′rick) *adj.* Situated near a mesonephric duct.

paramesonephric duct. An embryonic genital duct. In the female, the anlage of the oviducts, uterus, and vagina; in the male, it degenerates, leaving the appendix testis.

pa·ram·e·ter (puh-ram′e-tur) *n.* 1. A constant to which a value is fixed or assigned and by which other values or functions in a given case or system may be defined, such as the definition of an event by the three parameters of space and the parameter of time. 2. *In psychology*, any constant that defines or enters into the equation for some psychological event, such as rate of learning. 3. *In psychiatry*, the difference or variation of a technique of psychoanalysis used for a particular patient or psychiatric disorder, from the theory or model set forth by S. Freud.

para·me·tri·al (păr″uh-mee′tree-ul) *adj.* Pertaining to the tissues about the uterus.

para·met·ric (păr″uh-met′rick) *adj.* Pertaining to or in terms of a parameter.

para·me·trism (păr″uh-mee′triz-um) *n.* Painful spasm of the smooth muscular fibers of the broad ligaments of the uterus.

para·me·tri·tis (păr″uh·me·trye′tis) *n.* Inflammation of the connective tissue about the uterus. —**para·me·trit·ic** (·trit′ick) *adj.*

para·me·tri·um (păr″uh·mee′tree·um) *n.*, pl. **parame·tria** (·tree·uh) The connective tissue surrounding the uterus.

para·me·trop·a·thy (păr″uh·me·trop′uth·ee) *n.* Disease of the parametrium.

para·mim·ia (păr″uh·mim′ee·uh) *n.* A form of aphasia characterized by the faulty use of gestures, inappropriate to the sense expressed.

par·am·ne·sia (păr″am·nee′zhuh, ·zee·uh) *n.* Distortion of memory, in which experiences and fantasies are confused; more frequently responsible for erroneous testimony than mere forgetting.

para·mo·lar (păr″uh·mo′lur) *n.* A usually peg-shaped, occasionally molariform, supernumerary tooth occurring next to the mesiobuccal aspect of a second or third molar.

para·mor·phine (păr″uh·mor′feen, ·fin) *n.* THEBAINE.

para·mor·phism (păr″uh·mor′fiz·um) *n. In chemistry,* a change of molecular structure without alteration of chemical constitution, as when a mineral changes from one modification to another. —**paramor·phic** (·fick) *adj.*

para·mu·sia (păr″uh·mew′zhuh, ·zee·uh) *n.* AMUSIA.

par·am·y·loid (pa·ram′i·loid) *n.* An atypical amyloid.

para·my·oc·lo·nus mul·ti·plex (păr″uh·migh·ock′luh·nus, ·migh″o·klo′nus mul′ti·plecks). The name applied by Friedreich, in 1881, to a disorder of unknown cause, predominating in adult life and distinguished by abrupt, irregular, asymmetric clonic contractions of the muscles of the limbs and to a lesser extent of the trunk.

para·myo·to·nia con·gen·i·ta (păr″uh·migh″o·to′nee·uh kon·jen′i·tuh). A heredofamilial condition characterized by recurrent myotonia and muscular weakness on exposure to cold, transmitted as a dominant trait and considered to be a variety of the hyperkalemic form of periodic paralysis. Syn. *von Eulenburg's disease.*

para·na·sal (păr″uh·nay′zul) *adj.* Located next to, or near, the nasal cavities.

paranasal sinuses. Air cavities lined by mucous membrane which communicate with the nasal cavity; the ethmoid, frontal, sphenoid, and maxillary sinuses.

para·neo·plas·tic (păr″uh·nee·o·plas′tick) *adj.* Pertaining to changes in tissue structure believed either to presage cancer or to resemble it superficially.

para·ne·phri·tis (păr″uh·ne·frye′tis) *n.* 1. Inflammation of the adrenal gland. 2. Inflammation of the connective tissue adjacent to the kidney.

para·neu·ral (păr″uh·new′rul) *adj.* Beside or near a nerve.

pa·ran·gi (pa·ran′jee, pa·rang′ghee) *n.* YAWS.

par·a·noia (păr″uh·noy′uh) *n.* A rare form of paranoid psychosis characterized by the slow development of a complex internally logical system of persecutory or grandiose delusions, which is often based on the misinterpretation

of an actual event. The delusional thinking is isolated from much of the normal stream of consciousness, the remaining personality being intact despite a chronic course. The patient generally considers himself superior, possessing unique or even divine gifts. —**pa·ra·noi·ac** (păr″uh·noy′ack) *adj. & n.*

par·a·noid (păr′uh·noid) *adj.* 1. Resembling paranoia. 2. Characteristic of a paranoid personality.

para·noid·ism (păr′uh·noy·diz·um) *n.* The condition of being paranoid.

paranoid personality. An individual characterized by the tendency to be hypersensitive, rigid, extremely self-important, and jealous, to project hostile feelings so that he always is or easily becomes suspicious of others and is quick to blame them or attribute evil motives to them. This behavior may interfere with his ability to maintain any satisfactory interpersonal relations.

paranoid type of schizophrenia. A form of schizophrenia in which delusions of persecution or of grandeur or both, hallucinations, and ideas of reference predominate and sometimes are systematized. The patient is often more intact and less bizarre in other areas, but generally is hostile, grandiose, excessively religious, and sometimes hypochondriacal.

par·a·no·mia (păr″uh·no′mee·uh) *n.* ANOMIA.

par·an·tral (păr·an′trul) *adj.* Situated near an air sinus, as an accessory air cell of a mastoid sinus.

para·nu·cle·us (păr″uh·new′klee·us) *n.* 1. A small spherical body lying in the cytoplasm of a cell near the nucleus, and perhaps extruded by the latter. 2. A mitochondrial aggregation of a spermatid, which becomes drawn out to form the envelope of the axial filament. Syn. *nebenkern.* —**paranucle·ar** (·ur), **paranucle·ate** (·ate) *adj.*

para·os·ti·al (păr″uh·os′tee·ul) *adj.* Adjacent to an ostium; used to describe atherosclerotic plaques associated with that portion of a coronary artery adjacent to the ostium.

para·pan·cre·at·ic (păr″uh·pan″kree·at′ick) *adj.* Situated beside or near the pancreas.

para·pa·re·sis (păr″uh·pa·ree′sis) *n.* Partial paralysis or weakness of the lower extremities. —**parapa·ret·ic** (·ret′ick) *adj.*

para·pa·tel·lar (păr″uh·pa·tel′ur) *adj.* Adjacent to the knee cap.

para·per·tus·sis (păr″uh·pur·tus′is) *n.* An acute respiratory infection said to resemble mild pertussis, caused by *Bordetella parapertussis.*

para·pha·ryn·ge·al (păr″uh·fa·rin′jee·ul) *adj.* Adjacent to the pharynx.

par·a·pha·sia (păr″uh·fay′zhuh, ·zee·uh) *n.* Aphasic inability to use vocabulary items in relation to objective reality according to their conventional meanings; a pathological tendency to use "the wrong word," often observed in Wernicke's aphasia. —**parapha·sic** (·zick) *adj.*

para·phe·mia (păr″uh·fee′mee·uh) *n.* BROCA'S APHASIA.

pa·ra·phia (pa·ray′fee·uh, pa·raf′ee·uh) *n.* Abnormality of the sense of touch.

para·phil·ia (păr″uh·fil′ee·uh) *n.* SEXUAL DEVI-ATION. —**paraphil·i·ac** (·ee·ack) *adj. & n.*

para·phi·mo·sis (păr″uh·figh·mo′sis, ·fi·mo′sis) *n.*
1. Retraction and constriction, especially of the prepuce behind the glans penis. Syn. *Spanish collar.* 2. Spastic ectropion from contraction of the palpebral part of the orbicularis oculi muscle. Syn. *paraphimosis palpebrae, paraphimosis oculi, paraphimosis orbicularis.*

paraphimosis or·bic·u·la·ris (or·bick″yoo·lair′is). PARAPHIMOSIS (2).

paraphimosis pal·pe·brae (pal′pe·bree). PARA-PHIMOSIS (2).

para·pho·bia (păr″uh·fo′bee·uh) *n.* A slight degree of phobia; phobia which can be controlled or overcome by effort.

para·pho·nia (păr″uh·fo′nee·uh) *n.* Any abnormal condition of the voice.

pa·raph·o·ra (pa·raf′uh·ruh) *n.* 1. Slight mental derangement or distraction. 2. Unsteadiness due to intoxication.

para·phra·sia (păr″uh·fray′zhuh, ·zee·uh) *n.* PARAPHASIA.

para·phre·nia (păr″uh·free′nee·uh) *n.* A term introduced by Kraepelin to describe certain disorders now classed as paranoia or schizophrenia.

para·phre·ni·tis (păr″uh·fre·nigh′tis) *n.* Inflammation of the tissues adjacent to the diaphragm.

pa·raph·y·se·al (puh·raf″i·see′ul, păr″uh·fiz′ee·ul) *adj.* Pertaining to a paraphysis.

pa·raph·y·sis (puh·raf′i·sis) *n.*, *pl.* **paraphy·ses** (·seez) 1. *In biology,* one of sterile filaments among reproductive bodies of various kinds in certain cryptogams. 2. A vestigial structure derived from the roof plate of the telencephalon and presumed to give rise to a colloid cyst of the third ventricle. Syn. *paraphyseal body* or *cyst.*

para·plasm (păr′uh·plaz·um) *n.* 1. HYALOPLASM. 2. A malformed substance.

para·plas·tic (păr″uh·plas′tick) *adj.* 1. Of the nature of paraplasm. 2. Having morbid formative powers. 3. Misshapen.

para·ple·gia (păr″uh·plee′jee·uh) *n.* Paralysis of the lower limbs.

para·ple·gic (păr″uh·plee′jick) *adj. & n.* 1. Affected with or pertaining to paraplegia. 2. An individual afflicted with paraplegia.

para·ple·gi·form (păr″uh·plee′ji·form, ·plej′i·form) *adj.* Resembling paraplegia.

para·pneu·mo·nia (păr″uh·new·mo′nee·uh, ·nyuh) *n.* A disease clinically similar to pneumonia.

par·ap·o·plexy (păr·ap′o·pleck″see) *n.* A masked or slight form of cerebrovascular accident.

para·prax·ia (păr″uh·prack′see·uh) *n.* APRAXIA.

para·prax·is (păr″uh·prack′sis) *n.* APRAXIA.

para·proc·ti·tis (păr″uh·prock·tye′tis) *n.* Inflammation of the connective tissue about the rectum.

para·pros·ta·ti·tis (păr″uh·pros″tuh·tye′tis) *n.* Inflammation of tissues surrounding the prostate gland.

para·pro·tein (păr″uh·pro′tee·in, ·teen) *n.* 1. Any plasma protein, usually a globulin, which has

one or more characteristics unlike those of normal plasma proteins. 2. A modified protein, such as paracasein, which differs slightly from the native protein, as detected by one or more of the standard characterization tests.

para·pro·tein·emia, para·pro·tein·ae·mia (păr″uh·pro″teen·ee′mee·uh) *n.* The presence in the blood plasma of paraprotein.

para·pso·ri·a·sis (păr″uh·suh·rye′uh·sis) *n.*, *pl.* **parapsoria·ses** (·seez) Any of a group of rare skin diseases characterized by red, scaly lesions resembling lichen planus or psoriasis. All types are resistant to treatment and usually present no subjective symptoms.

parapsoriasis en plaques (ahn plack) Parapsoriasis in which the lesions develop as plaques.

parapsoriasis gut·ta·ta (guh·tay′tuh). Parapsoriasis with scaly, droplike lesions.

para·psy·chol·o·gy (păr″uh·sigh·kol′uh·jee) *n.* The study of psi phenomena (extrasensory perception and psychokinesis), i.e., the relationships between persons and events which seem to occur without the intervention of the physical senses or physical power.

para·rec·tal (păr″uh·reck′tul) *adj.* Beside, or near, the rectum.

par·ar·rhyth·mia (păr″uh·rith′mee·uh) *n.* A dual cardiac rhythm, such as parasystole, in which the independence of the two pacemakers does not result from a disturbance of normal conduction. —**pararrhyth·mic** (·mick) *adj.*

para·sa·cral (păr″uh·say′krul) *adj.* Beside, or near, the sacrum.

para·sag·it·tal (păr″uh·saj′i·tul) *adj.* Parallel and lateral to the median (midsagittal) plane.

para·sal·pin·gi·tis (păr″uh·sal″pin·jye′tis) *n.* Inflammation of the tissues around an oviduct.

para·se·cre·tion (păr″uh·se·kree′shun) *n.* An abnormality of secretion; any substance abnormally secreted.

para·sel·lar (păr″uh·sel′ur) *adj.* Adjacent to the sella turcica.

para·sex·u·al·i·ty (păr″uh·seck″shoo·al′i·tee) *n.* Any sexual perversion.

parasit-, parasito-. A combining form meaning *parasite, parasitic.*

par·a·site (păr′uh·site) *n.* 1. An organism that lives, during all or part of its existence, on or in another organism, its host, at whose expense it obtains nourishment and, in some cases, other benefits necessary for survival. 2. *In teratology,* a fetus or fetal parts attached to or included in another fetus. —**par·a·sit·ic** (păr″uh·sit′ick) *adj.*

par·a·sit·emia (păr″uh·si·tee′mee·uh) *n.* The presence of parasites, especially malarial forms, in circulating blood.

parasitic blepharitis. Marginal blepharitis caused by lice and/or mites.

parasitic fetus. A more or less completely formed fetus that is attached to its autosite.

par·a·sit·i·cide (păr″uh·sit′i·side) *n.* An agent capable of destroying parasites, especially the parasites living around or in the skin.

par·a·sit·i·za·tion (păr″uh·si·tye·zay′shun, ·sigh·ti-) *n.* Infection with a parasite.

para·sit·ize (păr″uh·si·tize, ·sigh·tize) *v.* To infect or infest as a parasite.

parasito-. See *parasit-*.

par·a·si·tol·o·gy (păr″uh·sigh·tol′uh·jee, ·si·tol′) *n.* The science and study of organisms that obtain nourishment at the expense of the host on or in which they live. —**parasitolo·gist** (·jist) *n.*

par·a·si·to·pho·bia (păr″uh·sigh″to·fo′bee·uh) *n.* An abnormal fear of parasites.

par·a·si·to·sis (păr″uh·sigh·to′sis) *n.*, pl. **parasito·ses** (·seez) Infestation or infection with parasites.

para·small·pox (păr″uh·smawl′pocks) *n.* A mild form of smallpox.

para·spa·di·as (păr″uh·spay′dee·us) *n.* An acquired condition in which the urethra opens on one side of the penis.

para·spasm (păr′uh·spaz·um) *n.* Spasm involving the lower extremities, as in spastic paraplegia.

para·sprue (păr′uh·sproo″) *n.* A mild form of sprue.

para·ster·nal (păr″uh·stur′nul) *adj.* Beside or near the sternum, as parasternal line. —**para·sternal·ly** (·lee) *adv.*

para·stri·ate (păr″uh·strye′ate) *adj.* Adjacent to the striate area (= VISUAL PROJECTION AREA).

parastriate area. The visual association area of the occipital cortex immediately surrounding the visual projection area. Syn. *Brodmann's area 18.*

para·sym·pa·thet·ic (păr″uh·sim″puh·thet′ick) *adj.* Pertaining to the craniosacral portion of the autonomic nervous system.

parasympathetic nervous system. The craniosacral division of the autonomic nervous system, consisting of preganglionic nerve fibers carried in certain cranial and sacral nerves, outlying ganglions and postganglionic nerve fibers; in general, innervating the same structures and generally having a regulatory function opposite to that of the sympathetic nervous system.

para·sym·pa·tho·lyt·ic (păr″uh·sim″puh·tho·lit′ick) *adj.* Blocking the action of parasympathetic nerve fibers.

para·sym·pa·tho·mi·met·ic (păr″uh·sim″puh·tho·mi·met′ick) *adj.* Of drugs, having an effect similar to that produced when the parasympathetic nerves are stimulated.

para·sys·to·le (păr″uh·sis′toh·lee) *n.* An arrhythmia characterized by two concurrent independent regular cardiac pacemakers, usually with one normal and one ectopic focus. —**para·sys·tol·ic** (·sis·tol′ick) *adj.*

para·tax·ia (păr″uh·tack′see·uh) *n.* 1. Behavior characterized by maladjustment of emotions and desires. 2. A mode of personal experience in which persons, objects, events or other phenomena are seen as separate, in watertight compartments, without relationship to other aspects of one's personality and having only a highly idiosyncratic significance. —**paratax·ic** (·ick) *adj.*

para·tax·is (par″uh·tack′sis) *n.* PARATAXIA.

para·ten·on (păr″uh·ten′un, ·ten′on) *n.* The connective tissue that occupies the interstices of fascial compartments containing tendons and their sheaths.

para·te·re·sio·ma·nia (păr″uh·te·ree″see·o·may′nee·uh) *n.* A mania for observing, or seeing new sights; uncontrollable inquisitiveness; compulsive peeping.

paraterminal gyrus. GYRUS PARATERMINALIS.

Parathion. Trade name for *O,O*-diethyl-*O-p*-nitrophenyl thiophosphate, a liquid insecticide having pronounced cholinesterase-inhibiting action.

para·thy·mia (păr″uh·thigh′mee·uh) *n.* Disturbance of mood in which the emotions are out of harmony with the real situation.

para·thy·reo·pri·val (păr″uh·thigh″ree·o·prye′vul) *adj.* PARATHYROPRIVAL.

par·a·thy·roid (păr″uh·thigh′roid) *adj. & n.* 1. Adjacent to the thyroid gland. 2. Of or pertaining to the parathyroid glands. 3. PARATHYROID GLAND.

para·thy·roid·ec·to·my (păr″uh·thigh″roy·deck′tuh·mee) *n.* Excision of a parathyroid gland.

parathyroid hormone. A polypeptide hormone in parathyroid glands that regulates blood calcium levels.

parathyroid osteodystrophy. Pathologic states in bone associated with hyperparathyroidism, principally including osteitis fibrosa, cysts, and giant-cell tumors; observed most commonly in the hands, clavicles, long bones, and skull. Syn. *parathyroid osteitis.*

para·thy·ro·pri·val (păr″uh·thigh″ro·prye′vul) *adj.* Pertaining to loss of function or removal of the parathyroid glands.

para·to·nia (păr″uh·to′nee·uh) *n.* Uneven resistance of the limbs to passive movement observed in demented and stuporous patients. Syn. *gegenhalten.*

para·ton·sil·lar (păr″uh·ton′si·lur) *adj.* Near, or around, the tonsil, as paratonsillar abscess.

para·tra·che·al (păr″uh·tray′kee·ul) *adj.* In the vicinity of the trachea.

para·tra·cho·ma (păr″uh·tra·ko′muh) *n.* INCLUSION CONJUNCTIVITIS.

para·tri·cho·sis (păr″uh·tri·ko′sis) *n.* A condition in which the hair is either imperfect in growth or develops in abnormal places.

para·trip·sis (păr″uh·trip′sis) *n. Obsol.* 1. A rubbing or chafing. 2. A retardation of catabolic processes.

para·troph·ic (păr″uh·trof′ick) *adj.* Obtaining nourishment from living organic matter.

pa·rat·ro·phy (pa·rat′ruh·fee) *n.* Perverted or abnormal nutrition.

para·tu·bal (păr″uh·tew′bul) *adj.* In the vicinity of a uterine tube.

para·tu·ber·cu·lo·sis (păr″uh·tew·bur″kew·lo′sis) *n.* JOHNE'S DISEASE.

para·ty·phoid fever (păr″uh·tye′foid). A disease of man resembling typhoid fever and caused by *Salmonella* species other than *Salmonella typhi*; the most common etiologic agents are *Salmonella schottmülleri* and *Salmonella typhimurium.*

para·um·bil·i·cal (păr″uh·um·bil′i·kul) *adj.* In the region of the umbilicus.

para·ure·thral (păr″uh·yoo·ree′thrul) *adj.* Beside the urethra.

paraurethral duct. A duct of a paraurethral gland.

paraurethral glands. Small vestigial glands opening into the posterior wall of the female urethra close to its orifice. The homologue of the distal prostatic glands of the male. Syn. *Skene's glands* or *tubules.*

para·uter·ine (păr″uh·yoo′tur·ine, ·in) *adj.* Beside or adjacent to the uterus.

para·vac·cin·ia (păr″uh·vack·sin′ee·uh) *n.* A poxlike viral disease (unrelated to vaccinia) affecting the udders of cows and transmissible to humans (and back to other cows) in the process of milking.

para·va·gi·nal (păr″uh·vaj′i·nul, ·va·jye′nul) *adj.* Beside the vagina.

para·vag·i·ni·tis (păr″uh·vaj″i·nigh′tis) *n.* Inflammation of the connective tissue surrounding the vagina.

para·vas·cu·lar (păr″uh·vas′kew·lur) *adj.* Adjacent to a blood vessel or vessels.

para·ven·tric·u·lar (păr″uh·ven·trick′yoo·lur) *adj.* Situated in the vicinity of the third ventricle.

para·ver·te·bral (păr″uh·vur′te·brul) *adj.* Occurring or situated near the spinal column, as paravertebral sympathetic nerve block.

para·ves·i·cal (păr″uh·ves′i·kul) *adj.* Situated near the urinary bladder.

para·vi·ta·min·o·sis (păr″uh·vye″tuh·min·o′sis) *n.*, pl. **paravitamino·ses** (·seez) 1. A disease associated indirectly with a vitamin deficiency. 2. A disease mimicking vitamin deficiency but not due to avitaminosis.

par·ax·i·al (păr·ack′see·ul) *adj.* 1. Lying near the axis of the body. 2. Referring to the space or rays closely surrounding the principal axis of a lens system.

paraxial mesoderm. The medial part of the mesoderm forming a plate-like mass that eventually segments to form the somites.

parchment crackling. The peculiar sound elicited by pressure on the cranial bones of children in diseases where localized thinning (craniotabes) occurs, such as in rickets.

parchment skin. Atrophy of the skin.

par·ec·ta·sis (păr·eck′tuh·sis) *n.* Excessive stretching or dilatation.

par·e·gor·ic (păr″e·gor′ick) *n.* Camphorated opium tincture, a preparation of opium, camphor, benzoic acid, anise oil, glycerin, and diluted alcohol; used mainly for its antiperistaltic action.

pa·ren·chy·ma (pa·renk′i·muh) *n.* The components of an organ or tissue which confer its distinctive function, as contrasted with the stroma, the supporting and nutritive framework. It is often epithelial although it need not be. **—parenchy·mal** (·mul), *adj.*

par·en·chym·a·ti·tis (păr″eng·kim″uh·tye′tis, pa·renk″i·muh·) *n.* Inflammation of the parenchyma of organs.

par·en·chym·a·tous (păr″un·kim′uh·tus, păr″eng·) *adj.* Consisting of or pertaining to parenchyma.

parenchymatous jaundice. HEPATOCELLULAR JAUNDICE.

parenchymatous mastitis. Inflammation of the proper glandular substance of the breast.

par·ent (păr′unt) *n.* 1. One who begets young in

sexual reproduction. 2. PARENT CELL. 3. *In radiochemistry,* a radioactive nuclide, the disintegration of which gives rise to either a radioactive or stable nuclide, called the daughter. 4. The compound or substance from which another compound or substance is derived. 5. A main trunk or stem from which smaller branches are derived.

par·en·ter·al (pa·ren′tur·ul) *adj.* Outside the intestine; not via the alimentary tract, as a subcutaneous, intravenous, intramuscular, or intrasternal injection. **—parenter·al·ly** (·ul·ee) *adv.*

parent figure. 1. A person who represents within one's emotional life the essential but not necessarily ideal attributes of a father or mother and who is the object of the attitudes and responses, such as respect and love, usually associated with the relationship of a child to his parents. 2. A mature person with whom one identifies and who functions like a parent in providing protection, discipline, love, and comfort.

parent image. 1. The mental picture a child or adult has formed of his parents at an earlier stage. 2. PRIMORDIAL IMAGE.

par·ep·i·thym·ia (păr″ep·i·thim′ee·uh, ·thigh′mee·uh) *n.* An abnormal or perverted desire or craving.

par·er·ga·sia (păr″ur·gay′zhuh, ·zee·uh) *n. In psychiatry,* Meyer's term for psychoses manifesting withdrawal, deep regression, delusions, and hallucinations, as schizophrenia and paranoia.

pa·re·sis (pa·ree′sis, păr′e·sis) *n.*, pl. **pare·ses** (·seez) 1. A slight paralysis; incomplete loss of muscular power; weakness of a limb. 2. GENERAL PARALYSIS.

par·es·the·sia, par·aes·the·sia (păr″es·theezh′uh, ·theez′ee·uh) *n.* Abnormal sensations such as tingling, prickling, burning, tightness, pulling and drawing feelings, or a feeling of a band or girdle around the limb or trunk; occurs with disease of the peripheral nerves, roots, or posterior columns of the spinal cord. **—pares·thet·ic, paraes·thet·ic** (·thet′ick) *adj.*

pa·ret·ic (pa·ret′ick) *adj.* Pertaining to, involving, or affected with paresis.

paretic gait. A disorder of gait attributable to weakness of the legs and characterized by shortness of steps, inability to lift the feet, and widening of base of varying degree.

pa·reu·nia (pa·roo′nee·uh, păr·yoo′nee·uh) *n.* COITUS.

par·fo·cal (pahr·fo′kul) *adj.* Pertaining to microscopical oculars and objectives that are so constructed or so mounted that, in changing from higher to lower magnification, the image remains in focus; in changing from lower to higher magnification, only an adjustment with the fine focus control is required to maintain focus.

par·hi·dro·sis (păr″hi·dro′sis) *n.* Any abnormal secretion of sweat.

pa·ri·es (păr′ee·eez) *n.*, genit. **pa·ri·e·tis** (pa·rye′e·tis), pl. **pari·e·tes** (·teez) An enveloping or investing structure or wall.

pa·ri·e·tal (puh·rye′e·tul) *adj. & n.* 1. Forming or

situated on a wall, as the parietal layer of the peritoneum. 2. Pertaining to, or in relation with, the parietal bone of the skull. 3. The parietal bone. See Table of Bones in the Appendix.

parietal cell. One of the cells found in the fundic glands of the stomach. Their function is supposedly the secretion of hydrochloric acid. Syn. *acid cell, delomorphous cell, oxyntic cell.*

parietal eminence. The rounded part of the parietal bone. This is sometimes bosselated, due to rickets.

parietal lobe. The cerebral lobe above the lateral cerebral sulcus and behind the central sulcus.

parietal lobules. Subdivisions of the parietal lobe of the cerebrum.

parietal pericardium. The outer wall of the pericardial cavity; it consists of the fibrous pericardium and the parietal serous pericardium.

parietal pleura. The portion of the pleura lining the internal surface of the thoracic cavity.

parietal thrombus. A thrombus adherent to the wall of a vessel or a cardiac chamber, not entirely occupying the lumen. Syn. *lateral thrombus.*

parietes. Plural of *paries.*

parieto-. A combining form meaning *parietal.*

pa·ri·e·to·fron·tal (puh-rye''e·to·frun'tul) *adj.* Pertaining to both the parietal and the frontal bones or lobes; frontoparietal.

pa·ri·e·to·mas·toid (puh-rye''e·to·mas'toid) *adj.* Pertaining to the parietal bone and the mastoid portion of the temporal bone; mastoparietal.

pa·ri·e·to·oc·cip·i·tal (puh-rye''e·to·ock·sip'i·tul) *adj.* Pertaining to the parietal and occipital bones or lobes.

parietooccipital sulcus or **fissure.** The upper limb of the calcarine fissure between the precuneus of the parietal lobe and the cuneus of the occipital lobe.

pa·ri·e·to·squa·mo·sal (puh-rye''e·to·skway·mo'sul) *adj.* Pertaining to the parietal bone and the squamous portion of the temporal bone.

pa·ri·e·to·tem·po·ral (puh-rye''e·to·tem'puh·rul) *adj.* Pertaining to the parietal and temporal bones or to the parietal and temporal lobes of the cerebrum.

Pa·ri·naud's conjunctivitis (pah·ree·no') LEPTO-TRICHAL CONJUNCTIVITIS.

Parinaud's syndrome 1. Conjunctivitis associated with palpable preauricular lymph nodes. 2. Conjugate paralysis of upward gaze, indicative of a lesion or compression of the corpora quadrigemina of the midbrain, especially the superior colliculi, as from a pineal tumor.

¹par·i·ty (păr'i·tee) *n.* Similarity approaching equality; equivalence.

²parity, *n.* The status of a woman with regard to the number of times she has given birth.

par·kin·so·nian (pahr''kin·so'nee·un) *adj.* Pertaining to parkinsonism.

parkinsonian crisis. Sudden severe exacerbation of tremor, rigidity, and dyskinesia in a patient with idiopathic or postencephalitic parkinsonism, accompanied by acute anxiety and its clinical manifestations, and usually the result of psychological stress or sudden withdrawal of antiparkinsonian drugs. In the postencephalitic cases, it may be accompanied by an oculogyric crisis.

parkinsonian mask. The immobile or masklike facies that characterizes parkinsonism.

par·kin·son·ism (pahr'kin·sun·iz·um) *n.* A clinical state characterized by a rhythmic, 3 to 4 per second tremor, poverty of movement (akinesia), rigidity of the muscles, and an impairment or loss of postural reflexes. It may occur in middle or late life from unknown causes, such as idiopathic parkinsonism or paralysis agitans, or as a sequel to encephalitis lethargica or to poisoning with phenothiazine drugs or haloperidol.

Par·kin·son's disease A disease of unknown cause, characterized by an expressionless face, infrequency of blinking, poverty and slowness of voluntary movement, rigidity of muscles, rhythmic 3 to 4 per second tremor most prominent in repose, stooped posture, loss of postural reflexes and festinating gait. Syn. *paralysis agitans, idiopathic parkinsonism.*

par·o·dyn·ia (păr''o·din'ee·uh) *n.* Difficult parturition.

pa·role (pa·role') *n.* In psychiatry, the conditional release of a patient from a mental hospital prior to formal discharge so that he may be returned to the hospital, if necessary, without again going through commitment.

par·ol·fac·to·ry (păr''ol·fack'tur·ee, păr''ohl·) *adj.* Situated near the olfactory area.

parolfactory sulcus. Either of the sulci on the medial surface of the frontal lobe which delimit the parolfactory area; specifically, the anterior parolfactory sulcus, which separates the parolfactory area from the superior frontal gyrus, or the posterior parolfactory sulcus, which separates it from the gyrus paraterminalis.

par·o·ni·ria (păr''o·nigh'ree·uh, ·nirr'ee·uh) *n.* Morbid dreaming; a nightmare.

par·o·nych·ia (păr''o·nick'ee·uh) *n.* A suppurative inflammation about the margin of a nail.

par·on·y·cho·my·co·sis (pa·ron''i·ko·migh·ko'sis) *n.* A fungous infection around the nails.

par·on·y·cho·sis (puh·ron''i·ko'sis) *n.* 1. A diseased condition of the structures about the nails. 2. Growth of a nail in unusual places.

par·ooph·o·ri·tis (păr''o·off''uh·rye'tis) *n.* 1. Inflammation of the epoophoron (parovarium). 2. Inflammation of the tissues about the ovary.

par·ooph·o·ron (păr''o·off'uh·ron) *n.* A vestigial, caudal group of mesonephric tubules located in or about the broad ligament of the uterus, homologous with the male paradidymis. They usually disappear in the adult.

par·oph·thal·mia (păr''off·thal'mee·uh) *n.* Inflammation about the eye.

par·op·sia (păr·op'see·uh) *n.* Disordered or false vision.

par·op·tic (păr·op'tick) *adj.* Pertaining to colors produced by the diffraction of light rays.

par·o·ra·sis (păr''o·ray'sis) *n.* Any perversion of vision or color perception; generally a hallucination.

par·o·rex·ia (păr″o·reck′see·uh) *n.* A perverted appetite; PICA.

par·os·mia (păr·oz′mee·uh) *n.* A perversion of the sense of smell, or the smelling of odors not actually there (olfactory hallucination).

par·os·ti·tis (păr″os·tye′tis) *n.* Inflammation of the tissue adjacent to the periosteum.

par·os·to·sis (păr″os·to′sis) *n.* The abnormal formation of bone outside the periosteum, or in the connective tissue surrounding the periosteum.

par·ot·ic (pa·ro′tick, ·rot′ick) *adj.* Situated near, or about, the ear.

par·otid (pa·rot′id) *adj.* 1. Situated near the ear, as the parotid gland. 2. Pertaining to, or affecting, the parotid gland.

parotid duct. The duct of the parotid gland. It passes horizontally across the lateral surface of the masseter muscle, pierces the buccinator muscle, and opens into the oral vestibule opposite the second upper molar tooth.

par·ot·i·dec·to·my (pa·rot″i·deck′tuh·mee) *n.* Excision of a parotid gland.

parotid gland. The salivary gland in front of and below the external ear. It is a compound racemose serous gland.

par·ot·i·do·scle·ro·sis (pa·rot′i·do·skle·ro′sis) *n.* Fibrous induration of the parotid gland.

par·o·ti·tis (păr″o·tye′tis) *n.* 1. Inflammation of the parotid gland, as in mumps. —**paro·tit·ic** (·tit′ick) *adj.*

par·ous (păr′us) *adj.* Having given birth one or more times.

par·o·var·i·an (păr″o·văr′ee·un) *adj.* 1. Situated near the ovary. 2. Pertaining to the epoophoron (parovarium).

parovarian cyst. A cyst of mesonephric origin arising between the layers of the mesosalpinx, adjacent to the ovary.

par·o·var·i·ot·o·my (păr″o·văr″ee·ot′uh·mee) *n.* Excision of a parovarian cyst.

par·o·var·i·um (păr″o·văr′ee·um) *n.* EPOOPHORON.

par·ox·ysm (păr′uck·siz·um) *n.* 1. The periodic increase or crisis in the progress of a disease; a sudden attack, a sudden reappearance or increase in the intensity of symptoms. 2. A spasm, fit, convulsion, or seizure. 3. A sudden, usually uncontrollable outburst of emotion, as of crying and laughter. 4. *In electroencephalography,* a burst of electrical activity such as spikes, or spikes and waves, denoting cerebral dysrhythmia or epileptic discharges. —**par·ox·ys·mal** (păr″uck·siz′mul) *adj.*

paroxysmal hemoglobinuria. A form of hemoglobinuria characterized by repeated acute attacks; it can occur in malaria.

paroxysmal nocturnal hemoglobinuria. A rare disease in which attacks of hemolysis usually occur during sleep; associated with intramuscular thrombosis and its complications.

parrot fever. PSITTACOSIS.

Par·ry's disease HYPERTHYROIDISM.

pars (pahrs) *n.,* genit. **par·tis** (pahr′tis), pl. **par·tes** (pahr′teez) A part.

pars ca·ver·no·sa ure·thrae (kav″ur·no′suh yoo·ree′three) [BNA] PARS SPONGIOSA URETHRAE MASCULINAE.

pars cri·co·pha·ryn·gea mus·cu·li con·stric·to·ris pha·ryn·gis in·fe·ri·o·ris (krye″ko·fa·rin′jee·uh mus′kew·lye kon·strick·to′ris fa·rin′jis in·feer·ee·o′ris) [NA]. The portion of the inferior constrictor muscle of the pharynx which arises from the cricoid cartilage.

pars flac·ci·da mem·bra·nae tym·pa·ni (flack′si·duh mem·bray′nee tim′puh·nigh) [NA]. The small triangular upper portion of the tympanic membrane; it is thin and lax.

pars in·ter·me·dia (in″tur·mee′dee·uh). 1. The posterior portion of the adenohypophysis, between the pars distalis and the neurohypophysis; sometimes classified as part of the neurohypophysis. 2. The nervus intermedius, the intermediate part of the facial nerve.

pars·ley (pahrs′lee) *n. Petroselinum crispum,* a plant of the Umbelliferae, containing a volatile oil. From the seed an oily liquid, termed apiol, is obtained. Various parts of the plant have been used as medicinals.

pars ner·vo·sa (nur·vo′suh). INFUNDIBULAR PROCESS.

pars spon·gi·o·sa ure·thrae mas·cu·li·nae (spon·jee·o′suh yoo·ree′three mas·kew·lye′nee) [NA]. The portion of the male urethra lying within the corpus spongiosum.

partes. Plural of *pars.*

par·the·no·gen·e·sis (pahrth″e·no·jen′e·sis) *n.* A modification of sexual reproduction, in which the organism develops from an unfertilized egg. It occurs chiefly in certain insects, crustacea, and worms. —**partheno·ge·net·ic** (·je·net′ick) *adj.*

par·the·no·pho·bia (pahrth″e·no·fo′bee·uh) *n.* Fear of virgins or girls.

partial pressure. In a mixture of gases, the pressure exerted by one of the gases is said to be the partial pressure of that gas. In such a mixture, the partial pressures of the gases are exerted independently of each other and the total pressure exerted is the sum of the partial pressures.

partial thromboplastin. Any of several lipid-rich clot accelerators dependent upon factors VIII, IX, and XII for maximum acceleration of clotting.

par·ti·cle (pahr′ti·kul) *n.* 1. A small portion or piece of substance. 2. One of the elementary components of atoms and molecules, as the neutron, proton, and electron.

par·tic·u·late (pahr·tick′yoo·lut) *adj.* Composed of particles.

par·ti·tion (pahr·tish′un) *n.* The distribution of a substance or ions between two immiscible liquids, or between a liquid and a gas.

par·tu·ri·ent (pahr·tew′ree·unt) *adj.* 1. In labor; giving birth. 2. Pertaining to parturition.

parturient paresis. A disease of cows, occurring shortly after calving, characterized by motor and sensory nervous paralysis, circulatory collapse, and hypocalcemia. Syn. *milk fever* (2).

par·tu·ri·fa·cient (pahr·tew″ri·fay′shunt) *adj. & n.* 1. Promoting labor. 2. An agent that induces labor.

par·tu·ri·om·e·ter (pahr·tew″ree·om′e·tur) *n.* An instrument to determine the progress of labor by measuring the expulsive force of the uterus.

par·tu·ri·tion (pahr″tew-rish′un) *n.* The process of giving birth to young.

par·tus (pahr′tus) *n.*, accus. **par·tum** (pahr′tum) The bringing forth of offspring; labor.

pa·ru·lis (pa·roo′lis) *n.*, pl. **pa·ru·li·des** (·li·deez) A subperiosteal abscess arising from dental structures; a gumboil.

par·um·bil·i·cal (păr″um·bil′i·kul) *adj. & n.* PARAUMBILICAL.

parvi- A combining form meaning *small, little;* sometimes used instead of the more common *micro-*.

par·vi·cel·lu·lar (pahr″vi·sel′yoo·lur) *adj.* Pertaining to, or composed of, small cells.

par·vi·loc·u·lar (pahr″vi·lock′yoo·lur) *adj.* Pertaining to small loculi.

par·vo·vi·rus (pahr″vo·vye′rus) *n.* Any of various small viruses associated with adenoviruses, upon which they may depend for replication in hosts other than their natural ones. Though parvoviruses have been suspected as agents of slow infections and are known to cause specific diseases in laboratory animals, none has yet been identified as pathogenic for humans.

par·vule (pahr′vyool) *n.* A small pill or pellet; a granule.

PAS Abbreviation for (a) *para-aminosalicylic acid;* (b) *periodic acid Schiff* (reaction).

PASA Abbreviation for *para-aminosalicylic acid.*

Pasch·en bodies (pahsh′en) Aggregates of small-pox virus, often called elementary bodies, which form the characteristic inclusions seen in smallpox (Guarnieri bodies).

pas·sage, *n.* 1. A channel or lumen. 2. The act of passing from one place to another. 3. The introduction of an instrument into a cavity or channel. 4. An evacuation of the bowels.

pas·sion, *n.* 1. An intense emotion of the mind; fervid desire, overpowering emotion. 2. A specific intense excitement, as rage or ardent affection. 3. Pain; suffering. 4. Sexual excitement or love. **—passion·al** (·ul), **passion·ate** (·ut) *adj.*

pas·sive, *adj.* Not active; not performed or produced by active efforts, but by causes from without.

passive-aggressive personality. An individual whose behavior pattern is characterized by aggressiveness and hostility expressed quietly by such reactions as stubbornness, pouting, procrastination, inefficiency, "doing nothing," or passive obstructionism; a character disorder.

passive anaphylaxis. The elicitation of anaphylaxis by the temporary sensitization of an animal with antibodies and the injection of the corresponding sensitizing antigen.

passive congestion. Hyperemia of a part as the result of impairment of return of venous blood.

passive cutaneous anaphylaxis. The vascular reaction at the site of intradermally injected antibody when 3 hours later the specific antigen, usually mixed with Evans blue dye, is injected intravenously.

passive-dependent personality. An individual whose behavioral pattern is characterized by a lack of self-confidence, indecisiveness, and a tendency to cling to and seek support from others; a character disorder.

passive exercise. The moving of parts of the body by another without voluntary help or hindrance by the patient.

passive general anaphylaxis. The introduction of systemic anaphylaxis by the intravenous administration of antibody followed some 48 hours later by the injection of the specific antigen.

passive immunity. 1. Immunity conferred through the parenteral injection of antibodies prepared in the lower animals or other human beings. 2. Immunity acquired by the child in utero by the placental transfer of antibodies from the mother.

passive motion or **movement.** Movement effected by some outside agency.

passive reduction. A form of closed reduction accomplished without manipulative force, but rather by steady traction or the pull of gravity.

passive transfer test. A method of demonstrating skin-sensitizing antibodies in the blood of an allergic patient, performed by sensitizing a local area of the skin of a nonallergic individual by the intracutaneous injection of the serum of that patient and then challenging the prepared site with corresponding allergen.

pas·siv·ism (pas′i·viz·um) *n.* A form of sexual perversion in which one person submits to the will of another in anomalous erotic acts. **—passiv·ist** (·vist) *n.*

pas·ta (pas′tuh) *n.* PASTE.

paste, *n.* An ointmentlike preparation of one or more medicinal substances, such as zinc oxide, coal tar, starch, or sulfur, in a hydrogel or fatty base. Pastes are generally intended for dermatologic use; they are less greasy and better absorbed than ointments.

pas·tern (pas′turn) *n.* The part of a horse's leg between the fetlock joint and the coronet of the hoof.

pastern bone. The first phalanx (great pastern bone) or second phalanx (small pastern bone) of a horse's foot.

pastern joint. The articulation between the proximal and second phalanges (great and small pastern bones) of any leg of a horse.

Pasteur effect The inhibition of fermentation when anaerobic conditions are replaced by abundant oxygen supply.

Pas·teu·rel·la (pas″tur·el′uh) *n.* A genus of bipolar staining rods, oxidase-positive and nonmotile, which includes *Pasteurella multocida* and other species causing disease in animals. Formerly this genus included the organisms responsible for plague and other diseases; these are now assigned to the genus *Yersinia.*

Pasteurella mul·to·ci·da (mul·to′si·duh). A species of small, gram-negative, nonmotile, rod-shaped bacteria, normal inhabitants of the upper respiratory tracts of mammals and birds; the cause of hemorrhagic septicemia in cattle and other animals, a variety of other diseases in mammals, birds, and occasionally man; and occurring as a secondary invader in chicken cholera.

Pasteurella pes·tis (pes'tis). YERSINIA PESTIS.

Pasteurella tularensis. FRANCISELLA TULARENSIS.

pas·teu·rel·lo·sis (pas''tur·el·o'sis) *n.*, pl. **pasteurello·ses** (-seez) Any of several diseases of animals that are associated with organisms in the genus *Pasteurella*, such as shipping fever.

pas·teur·iza·tion (pas''tur·i·zay'shun) *n.* Heat treatment to kill some but not all of the microorganisms in a particular material. In the pasteurization of milk, heating the milk to 62°C for 30 minutes will kill the significant pathogens but leave many harmless bacteria alive. —**pas·teur·ize** (pas'tur·ize) *v.*

Pasteur treatment The original treatment of rabies introduced by Pasteur in which the virus, attenuated by variable periods of drying infected rabbit spinal cords, was administered in doses of progressively increasing virulence during the long incubation period of the disease.

pas·til (pas'til) *n.* 1. A small mass composed of aromatic substances and employed in fumigation. 2. TROCHE. 3. A paper disk, chemically coated, which changes color on exposure to x-rays; used to determine the dosage.

pas·tille (pas·teel', -til') *n.* PASTIL.

past pointing A test in which the patient is asked to point at a fixed object. In cerebellar and labyrinthine disease, there is deviation or past pointing toward the involved side.

patch graft. *In vascular surgery,* a graft of synthetic material or living vein to close and repair a partial defect in the wall of an artery or large vein.

patch test. A test in which material is applied and left in contact with intact skin surface for 48 hours in order to demonstrate tissue sensitivity.

pate, *n.* The crown or top of the head.

pa·tel·la (pa·tel'uh) *n.*, L. pl. & genit. sing. **patellae** (-ee) A sesamoid bone in front of the knee, developed in the tendon of the quadriceps femoris muscle; the kneecap. —**patel·lar** (-ur) *adj.*

patellar clonus. Clonic contraction and relaxation of the quadriceps femoris muscle in response to sharp firm pressure against the upper margin of the patella or on eliciting the patellar reflex; observed with lesions of the corticospinal tract.

patellar reflex. Contraction of the quadriceps femoris muscle with extension of the leg at the knee in response to a quick tap against the patellar tendon. Syn. *knee jerk, quadriceps reflex.*

pa·tel·lec·to·my (pat''el·eck'tuh·mee) *n.* The surgical removal or excision of a patella.

¹pa·tent (pay'tunt, pat'unt) *adj.* Open; exposed, noticeable. —**pa·ten·cy** (pay'tun·see, pat'un· see) *n.*

²pat·ent (pat'unt) *n.* An assignment by a government to an inventor or discoverer of a useful process, composition, formula, machine, or device of the exclusive right, for a specific period of time, to manufacture, use, or sell the product of his invention or discovery or to assign to or license others with that right.

patent ductus arteriosus. A congenital anomaly in which the fetal ductus arteriosus persists after birth.

patent foramen ovale. Persistence of the fetal foramen ovale after birth, usually a functional patency. An anatomic patency is frequent at autopsy without functional patency in life.

pa·ter·nal (puh·tur'nul) *adj.* Pertaining to a father. —**pater·ni·ty** (-ni·tee) *n.*

paternity test. The determination of the blood groups of an identified mother, an identified child, and a putative father in order to determine hereditary blood characters and to establish the probability of paternity or nonpaternity.

path-, patho- A combining form meaning (a) *disease;* (b) *pathologic.*

-path A combining form designating (a) *specialist in a* (specified) *type of medical treatment;* (b) *individual suffering from a* (specified) *sickness or disease.*

path, *n. In neurology,* a nerve fiber pathway.

path·er·ga·sia (path''ur·gay'zhuh, ·zee·uh) *n. In psychiatry,* a term applied by Adolf Meyer to personality maladjustments associated with organic or structural changes in the body or with gross functional disturbances.

pa·thet·ic (puh·thet'ick) *adj.* 1. Pertaining to or causing feelings. 2. *Obsol.* Pertaining to or designating the fourth cranial (trochlear) nerve.

-pathia A combining form meaning *disease, affection.*

-pathic A combining form meaning (a) *affected by, depending on, pertaining to,* or *originating in* or *caused by disease of a* (specified) *kind or part;* (b) *affected in a* (specified) *way.*

patho-. See *path-.*

patho·gen (path'uh·jen, path'o·jin) *n.* Any agent which is capable of producing disease; usually applied to living agents.

patho·gen·e·sis (path''o·jen'e·sis) *n.* The origin and course of development of disease. —**patho·ge·net·ic** (-je·net'ick) *adj.*

patho·gen·ic (path''uh·jen'ick) *adj.* 1. Producing or capable of producing disease. 2. Pertaining to pathogenesis. —**patho·ge·nic·i·ty** (path''o·je·nis'i·tee) *n.*

path·og·nom·ic (path''ug·nom'ick, ·no'mick) *adj.* PATHOGNOMONIC.

patho·log·ic (path''uh·loj'ick) *adj.* 1. Of or pertaining to pathology. 2. Pertaining to or caused by disease.

patho·log·i·cal (path''uh·loj'i·kul) *adj.* PATHOLOGIC.

pathologic anatomy. The study of the changes in structure caused by disease. Syn. *morbid anatomy.*

pathologic fracture. A fracture that occurs at the site of a local disease in a bone (as metastatic carcinoma) without significant external violence.

pathologic intoxication. An unusual reaction to alcoholic intoxication, characterized by an outburst of irrational, combative, and destructive behavior, which terminates when the patient falls into a deep stupor and for which he later has no memory.

pathologic lying or **mendacity.** Persistent habitual lying without external need or actual advantage, involving both falsifications of real events and development of fantasies. The individual may have complete insight, or the condition may be part of a neurosis, organic brain syndrome, personality disorder, or psychosis.

pathologic physiology. PATHOPHYSIOLOGY.

pa·thol·o·gist (pa·thol'uh·jist) n. A person trained and experienced in the study and practice of pathology.

pathologist's wart. TUBERCULOSIS VERRUCOSA.

pa·thol·o·gy (pa·thol'uh·jee) n. 1. The branch of biological science which deals with the nature of disease, through study of its causes, its process, and its effects, together with the associated alterations of structure and function. 2. Laboratory findings of disease, as distinguished from clinical signs and symptoms. 3. *Erron.* DISEASE.

patho·mi·me·sis (path"o·mi·mee'sis) n. Imitation of the symptoms and signs of a disease; occurs in the conversion type of hysterical neurosis and in malingering.

patho·pho·bia (path"o·fo'bee·uh) n. Exaggerated dread of disease.

patho·phor·ic (path"o·for'ick) adj. Carrying or transmitting disease, said of certain insects.

patho·phys·i·ol·o·gy (path"o·fiz"ee·ol'uh·jee) n. The study of disordered functions or of functions modified by disease. —**pathophysi·o·log·ic** (·uh·loj'ick), **pathophysiolog·i·cal** (·i·kul) adj.

patho·psy·chol·o·gy (path"o·sigh·kol'uh·jee) n. The branch of science dealing with mental processes, particularly as manifested by abnormal cognitive, perceptual, and intellectual functioning, during the course of mental disorders.

pa·tho·sis (pa·tho'sis) n., pl. **patho·ses** (·seez) A diseased condition, abnormality, or pathologic finding.

path·way, n. In neurophysiology, a course along nerve fibers which an impulse travels either from the periphery to the center (afferent pathway) or from the center to the effector organ (efferent pathway).

pa·tient (pay'shunt) n. A person under medical care or receiving health care services.

pat·ri·cide (pat'ri·side) n. 1. Murder of one's own father. 2. One who murders his own father.

pat·ri·lin·e·al (pat"ri·lin'ee·ul) adj. Pertaining to descent through the male line.

pat·ten (pat'un) n. A metal support serving as a high sole and attached to the shoe on the sound leg, to prevent weight bearing in hip disease and to permit the employment of traction apparatus on the affected leg.

pat·tern, n. 1. A comparatively fully realized model or form proposed or accepted for copying. 2. A functional integration of elements, perceived simultaneously or successively, which together form a design or unit; the parts are separately distinguishable but together form a perceived whole. Syn. *gestalt.* 3. A functional integration of distinguishable elements which operate or respond as a unit, as

an action, behavioral, motor, neural, social, or thought pattern. 4. A form, usually of wax, from which a mold is made for casting a dental restoration or appliance.

pat·tern·ing, n. 1. Behavior, or the development or imposition thereof, in imitation of a model or in response to a whole set of stimuli. 2. Therapeutic maneuvers and exercises, involving one or more external parts or the whole of the body, imposed on a patient or carried out by him purposefully, and utilizing reflex patterns and various sensory stimuli, designed to facilitate voluntary neuromuscular activity.

pat·u·lous (pat'yoo·lus) adj. Expanded; open; loose. —**patulous·ness** (·nus) n.

Paul-Bun·nell test A test for the presence of heterophil antibodies in the serum produced in infectious mononucleosis and other diseases.

pau·lo·car·dia (paw"lo·kahr'dee·uh) n. 1. A subjective sensation of intermission or momentary stoppage of the heartbeat. 2. An abnormally long interval between heartbeats.

paunch, n. 1. The abdominal cavity and its contents. 2. RUMEN.

pause, n. A temporary stop or rest.

pau·si·me·nia (paw"si·mee'nee·uh) n. MENOPAUSE.

Pau·tri·er's microabscess (po·tree·ey') A small group of atypical cells occurring in the lower epidermis of patients with mycosis fungoides or reticulum-cell sarcoma of the skin.

pave·ment·ing, n. A stage in the process of tissue inflammation in which the bloodstream in the capillaries becomes slowed, the leukocytes gravitating out of the central current to become adherent to the vessel walls.

pa·vex, pa·vaex (pay'vecks) n. A positive-negative pressure apparatus for passive exercise in the treatment of thromboangiitis obliterans or other peripheral vascular disease.

Pav·lov·i·an conditioning (pav·lov'ee·un, ·lo'vee·un) CONDITIONING (1).

Pav·lov's pouch (pah'vluf) A small portion of stomach, completely separated from the main stomach, but retaining its vagal nerve branches, but which communicates with the exterior; used in the long-term investigation of gastric secretion and particularly in the study of conditioned reflexes.

pa·vor (pay'vur, pav'or) n. Fright; fear.

pavor noc·tur·nus (nock·tur'nus). Night terror; differing from a nightmare in that it is not recalled on awakening.

Pb Symbol for lead.

PBI Abbreviation for *protein-bound iodine.*

PCB Abbreviation for *polychlorinated biphenyl.*

PCG Abbreviation for *phonocardiogram.*

P.D. Doctor of Pharmacy.

Pd Symbol for palladium.

peanut oil. Refined foil obtained from seed kernels of one or more cultivated varieties of *Arachis hypogaea;* used as a vehicle for injections. Syn. *arachis oil.*

pearl, n. 1. A rounded aggregation of squamous epithelial cells, concentrically arranged, also in sites of certain carcinomas and also in sites of epithelial union of embryonically open hiatuses, e.g., palatine raphe. Syn. *epithelial pearl.* **2.** PERLE. **3.** A mucous cast of a bronchus or bronchiole in the sputum of asthmatic patients. Syn. *Laennec's perle.*

pearly, *adj.* Resembling a pearl in color or appearance.

pearly tumor. CHOLESTEATOMA.

peat, *n.* The product of the spontaneous decomposition of plants, especially swamp plants, in many cases mixed with sand, loam, clay, lime, iron pyrites, or ocher.

pec·ten (peck'tin) *n.* **1.** *Obsol.* PUBIS. **2.** The middle third of the anal canal. **3.** A body part which is more or less comblike in structure, as pecten of the pubic bone.

pec·te·no·sis (peck''te·no'sis) *n.* Induration of the middle third of the anal canal.

pec·tin (peck'tin) *n.* A purified carbohydrate product obtained from the inner portion of the rind of citrus fruits, or from apple pomace; consists chiefly of partially methoxylated polygalacturonic acids. Used as a demulcent and as an emulsifying and thickening agent.

pec·ti·nate (peck'ti·nate) *adj.* Arranged like the teeth of a comb.

pec·tin·e·al (peck·tin'ee·ul) *adj.* **1.** Comb-shaped. **2.** Pertaining to the pecten or pubic bone.

pectineal line. 1. The line on the posterior surface of the femur, running downward from the lesser trochanter and giving attachment to the pectineus muscle. **2.** PECTEN OF THE PUBIC BONE.

pec·ti·ne·us (peck·tin'ee·us) *n.* A muscle arising from the pubis and inserted on the femur.

pec·to·ral (peck'tuh·rul) *adj.* Pertaining to the chest, as the pectoral muscles (pectorales), which connect the arm and the chest.

pectoral fascia. Deep fascia around the pectoralis major muscle on the anterior aspect of the thorax.

pec·to·ra·lis (peck''to·ray'lis, ·rah'lis) *n.,* pl. **pec·tora·les** (·leez) Either of two muscles, major and minor, on the anterior aspect of the chest.

pectoralis fascia. PECTORAL FASCIA.

pectoralis major. The larger muscle of the anterior thoracic wall.

pectoralis minor. The smaller and deeper muscle of the anterior thoracic wall.

pec·to·ril·o·quy (peck''to·ril'uh·kwee) *n.* Exaggerated bronchophony, in which there is distinct transmission of articulate speech on auscultation over the lung; indicative of cavitation or consolidation.

pec·tus (peck'tus) *n.,* genit. **pec·to·ris** (peck'to·ris) The chest or breast.

pectus car·i·na·tum (kăr·i·nay'tum). PIGEON BREAST.

pectus ex·ca·va·tum (ecks·kuh·vay'tum). FUNNEL CHEST.

¹ped-, paed-, pedo-, paedo- A combining form meaning *child.*

²ped-, pedi-, pedo-, paedo- A combining form meaning *foot, pedal, hoof.*

-ped, -pede A combining form meaning *having a* (specified) *number or kind of feet.*

ped·at·ro·phy, paed·at·ro·phy (pe·dat'ruh·fee) *n.* **1.** Any wasting disease of childhood. **2.** Mesenteric lymphadenitis associated with tuberculous infection.

ped·er·as·ty, paed·er·as·ty (ped'ur·as''tee, pee'dur·) *n.* **1.** Sexual intercourse between man and boy. **2.** Specifically, sodomy between man and boy. —**peder·ast, paeder·ast,** *n.*

pedi·al·gia (ped''ee·al'jee·uh, pee''dee·) *n.* Pain in the foot.

pe·di·at·ric, pae·di·at·ric (pee''dee·at'rick) *adj.* Of or pertaining to pediatrics.

pe·di·a·tri·cian, pae·di·a·tri·cian (pee''dee·uh·trish'un) *n.* A physician specializing in pediatrics.

pe·di·at·rics, pae·di·at·rics (pee''dee·at'ricks) *n.* The branch of medicine that deals with the growth and development of the child through adolescence and with the care, treatment, and prevention of diseases, injuries, and defects of children.

pe·di·at·rist, pae·di·at·rist (pee''dee·at'rist, pe·dye'uh·trist) *n.* PEDIATRICIAN.

ped·i·cle (ped'i·kul) *n.* A slender process serving as a foot or stem, as the pedicle of a tumor, or a narrow connection, as the pedicle of a vertebra.

pedicle flap. A type of flap that provides its blood supply through a narrow base, or pedicle; used when length is required to fill a remote defect, or on a movable part which can be approximated to the donor site.

pedicle graft. PEDICLE FLAP.

pe·dic·ter·us, pae·dic·ter·us (pe·dick'tur·us) *n.* PHYSIOLOGIC JAUNDICE OF THE NEWBORN.

pe·dic·u·lar (pe·dick'yoo·lur) *adj.* Of or pertaining to lice.

¹pe·dic·u·la·tion (pe·dick''yoo·lay'shun) *n.* The development or formation of a pedicle.

²pediculation, *n.* Infestation with lice; PEDICULOSIS.

pe·dic·u·li·cide (pe·dick'yoo·li·side) *n.* An agent that destroys lice.

Pe·dic·u·loi·des (pi·dick''yoo·loy'deez) *n.* A genus of mites.

pe·dic·u·lo·pho·bia (pe·dick''yoo·lo·fo'bee·uh) *n.* Abnormal dread of infestation with lice.

pe·dic·u·lo·sis (pe·dick''yoo·lo'sis) *n.* A skin disease due to infestation by lice, characterized by intense pruritis and cutaneous lesions.

pediculosis cap·i·tis (kap'i·tis). Infestation of the scalp with the species *Pediculus humanus* var. *capitis.*

pediculosis cor·po·ris (kor'puh·ris). Infestation of the skin of the body with the species *Pediculus humanus* var. *corporis.*

pediculosis pal·pe·bra·rum (pal''pe·brair'um). Lice infesting the eyebrows and the eyelashes.

pediculosis pu·bis (pew'bis). An infestation of the pubic hair with *Phthirius pubis,* the crab louse; may spread over the body and involve the axillas, eyebrows, and eyelashes.

pe·dic·u·lous (pe·dick'yoo·lus) *adj.* Infested with lice; lousy.

Pe·dic·u·lus (pe·dick'yoo·lus) *n.* A genus of lice, species of which produce dermatitis and transmit diseases, such as typhus fever, trench fever, and relapsing fever.

Pediculus hu·ma·nus cap·i·tis (hew·may'nus kap'i·tis). HEAD LOUSE.

Pediculus humanus cor·po·ris (kor'puh·ris). BODY LOUSE.

ped·i·cure (ped'i·kewr) *n.* Care of the feet.

ped·i·gree (ped'i·gree) *n.* A register or chart showing ancestral history; used by geneticists to assist in the analysis of Mendelian inheritance.

pe·di·tis (pe·dye'tis) *n.* An inflammation of the pedal bone of a horse.

pe·do·don·tia, pae·do·don·tia (pee''do·don'chee·uh) *n.* PEDODONTICS.

pe·do·don·tics, pae·do·don·tics (pee''do·don'ticks) *n.* The branch of dentistry that is concerned with the dental care and treatment of children.

pe·do·don·tist, pae·do·don·tist (pee''do·don'tist) *n.* A dentist who specializes in pedodontics.

pe·do·don·tol·o·gy, pae·do·don·tol·o·gy (pee''do·don·tol'uh·jee) *n.* PEDODONTICS.

pe·dol·o·gist, pae·dol·o·gist (pee·dol'uh·jist) *n.* A specialist in the study of children.

pe·dol·o·gy, pae·dol·o·gy (pee·dol'uh·jee) *n.* The science, or sum of knowledge, regarding childhood, its psychologic as well as physiologic aspects.

¹**pe·dom·e·ter, pae·dom·e·ter** (pee·dom'e·tur) *n.* An instrument for weighing and measuring a newborn child. —**pedome·try, paedome·try** (·tree) *n.*

²**pe·dom·e·ter** (ped·om'e·tur) *n.* An instrument that registers the number of footsteps in walking. —**pedome·try** (·tree) *n.*

pe·dop·a·thy (ped·op'uth·ee) *n.* Any disease of the foot.

pe·do·phil·ia, pae·do·phil·ia (pee''do·fil'ee·uh) *n.* 1. Fondness for children. 2. Love of children by adults for sexual purposes.

pe·do·pho·bia, pae·do·pho·bia (pee''do·fo'bee·uh) *n.* Abnormal dislike or fear of children.

pe·dun·cle (pe·dunk'ul, ped'unk·ul, pee'dunk·ul) *n.* 1. A narrow part acting as a support. 2. Any of various bands of nerve fibers connecting various parts of the cerebellum, medulla oblongata, pons, and other parts of the brain. —**pe·dun·cu·lar** (pe·dunk'yoo·lur) *adj.*

pe·dun·cu·lat·ed (pe·dunk'yoo·lay·tid) *adj.* Having a peduncle.

pe·dun·cu·lot·o·my (pe·dunk''yoo·lot'uh·mee) *n.* Surgical interruption of the cerebral peduncles, either unilaterally or bilaterally, for the relief of involuntary movement disorders.

Peet's operation Supradiaphragmatic removal of the sympathetic nerves and ganglions for the relief of hypertension.

peg, *n.* 1. A pointed pin of wood, metal, or other material. 2. A wooden leg.

Peganone. Trademark for ethotoin, an anticonvulsant used in the management of grand mal epilepsy.

peg teeth. HUTCHINSON'S TEETH.

pe·la·da (pe·lah'duh) *n.* Alopecia areata of the scalp.

pel·age (pel'ij) *n.* The hairy covering of the body.

pel·a·gism (pel'uh·jiz·um) *n.* SEASICKNESS.

Pel-Ebstein disease, fever, or **syndrome** Cyclic fever occasionally associated with malignant lymphoma.

Pelger's anomaly A hereditary anomaly of granulocytes characterized by small neutrophilic leukocytes in the peripheral blood with no more than one or two nuclear lobes and unusually coarse nuclear chromatin. Syn. *Pelger-Huët anomaly.*

pel·i·o·sis (pel''ee·o'sis, pee''lee·) *n.* PURPURA. —**peli·ot·ic** (·ot'ick) *adj.*

peliosis he·pa·tis (hep'uh·tis). A condition in which small spaces throughout the liver are filled with fluid or clotted blood; seen rarely in patients dead of tuberculosis, or other diseases.

peliosis rheu·mat·i·ca (roo·mat'i·kuh). SCHÖNLEIN'S PURPURA.

Pe·li·zae·us-Merz·bach·er disease (pe²·lee·tse²·ōōs, mehrts'ba^kh·ur) A slowly progressive X-linked recessive genetic disease characterized pathologically by extensive cerebral and cerebellar demyelination and clinically by various signs, including nystagmus, ataxia, spasticity, and dementia starting in early infancy. Some heterozygous females develop symptoms.

pell- A combining form meaning *skin.*

pel·la·gra (pe·lag'ruh, pe·lay'gruh) *n.* A syndrome due to a deficiency of niacin or tryptophan, with a characteristic symmetric dermatitis of the exposed parts, stomatitis, glossitis, diarrhea, and, in later stages, dementia. —**pel·lag·rous** (·lag'rus) *adj.*

pel·la·grin (pe·lag'rin) *n.* A person afflicted with pellagra.

Pel·le·gri·ni-Stie·da disease (pel·le·gree'nee, shtee'dah) Posttraumatic calcification of the medial collateral ligament of the knee.

pel·let (pel'it) *n.* A small pill.

pel·le·tier·ine (pel''e·teer'een, ·in, pel''e·tye'reen, *n.* An alkaloid or mixture of alkaloids from pomegranate bark; formerly used, mostly as the tannate salt, as a taeniafuge. Syn. *punicine.*

pel·li·cle (pel'i·kul) *n.* 1. A thin membrane, or cuticle. 2. A film on the surface of a liquid. 3. A thin brown or gray film of salivary proteins that forms on teeth within minutes after being cleaned. —**pel·lic·u·lar** (pe·lick'yoo·lur) **pellic·u·lous** (·lus), **pellicu·late** (·late) *adj.*

pel·lic·u·la (pe·lick'yoo·luh) *n.* EPIDERMIS.

pel·lu·cid (pe·lew'sid) *adj.* Transparent; translucent; not opaque.

pe·loid (pee'loid) *n.* Generic term for mineral or vegetable muds used in physical therapy.

pe·lop·sia (pe·lop'see·uh) *n.* Illusions of abnormal nearness of objects; may occur in psychomotor seizures.

pel·ta·tin (pel·tay'tin) *n.* Either of two related constituents identified as α-peltatin and β-peltatin, obtained from the rhizome and root of *Podophyllum peltatum.* β-Peltatin, $C_{22}H_{22}O_8$, contains a methoxyl (OCH_3) group in place of a hydroxyl (OH) group in α-peltatin, $C_{21}H_{20}O_8$; both are related to podophyllotoxin. Both are active, when applied topically, against certain wartlike neoplasms.

pelv-, pelvo-. A combining form meaning *pelvis.*

pelves. Plural of *pelvis.*

pel·vi·ab·dom·i·nal (pel''vee·ab·dom'i·nul) *adj.* Pertaining to the pelvic and the abdominal cavities.

pel·vic (pel'vick) *adj.* Of or pertaining to the pelvis.

pelvic canal. The cavity of the true pelvis from inlet to outlet.

pelvic cavity. 1. The cavity within the bony pelvis including both false and true pelves. 2. *In obstetrics*, the cavity of the true pelvis from inlet to outlet, containing the pelvic viscera.

pelvic girdle. The two hipbones united at the pubic symphysis; they support the trunk on the lower extremities.

pelvic hammock. A canvas sling, generally attached to an overhead bed frame, used to suspend the lower part of the trunk and pelvis in pelvic fractures.

pelvic hernia. OBTURATOR HERNIA.

pelvic index. The relation of the anteroposterior diameter to the transverse diameter of the pelvis.

pelvic inflammatory disease. Inflammation of the internal female genital tract; characterized by abdominal pain, fever, and tenderness of the cervix. It may be caused by any of a variety of microorganisms including *Neisseria gonorrhoeae*. Abbreviated, PID.

pelvic inlet. INLET OF THE PELVIS.

pelvic inlet index. The ratio of the sagittal diameter, or conjugata vera of the pelvic inlet, taken between the points where the sagittal plane cuts the sacral promontory and the posterior edge of the superior surface of the symphysis pubis, to the transverse diameter, taken between the points on the arcuate lines that lie farthest lateral from the midline, at right angles to the conjugata vera. When multiplied by 100, values of the index are classified as: platypellic, x-89.9; mesatipellic, 90.0-94.9; dolichopellic, 95.0-x.

pelvic lipomatosis. Fat deposits in the pelvis producing compression and distortion of the bladder, rectum, ureters, and pelvic veins; a rare condition of unknown etiology usually seen in middle-aged men.

pelvic outlet. OUTLET OF THE PELVIS.

pelvic plexus. INFERIOR HYPOGASTRIC PLEXUS.

pel·vi·ec·ta·sis (pel″vee·eck′tuh·sis) *n.* Distention of the renal pelvis by urine, with little or no calyceal distention; HYDROPELVIS.

pel·vi·en·ceph·a·lom·e·try (pel″vee·en·sef″uh·lom′e·tree) *n.* Measurement of the maternal pelvis and fetal skull by means of radiographic examination.

pel·vi·fem·o·ral (pel″vi·fem′ur·ul) *adj.* Pertaining to the pelvic girdle and the thighs.

pel·vim·e·ter (pel·vim′e·tur) *n.* An instrument for measuring the pelvic dimensions.

pel·vim·e·try (pel·vim′e·tree) *n.* The measurement of the dimensions of the pelvis. Average measurements of the adult female pelvis covered by the soft parts, in centimeters, are as follows:

Between iliac spines	26
Between iliac crests	29
External conjugate diameter	20¼
Internal conjugate diagonal	12¾
True conjugate, estimated	11
Right diagonal	22
Left diagonal	22
Between trochanters	31
Circumference of pelvis	90

pel·vio·lith·ot·o·my (pel″vee·o·li·thot′uh·mee). Removal of a kidney stone from the renal pelvis. Syn. *pyelolithotomy.*

pel·vi·ot·o·my (pel″vee·ot′uh·mee) *n.* 1. Incision of the renal pelvis. 2. PELVISECTION.

pel·vi·rec·tal (pel″vi·reck′tul) *adj.* Pertaining to the pelvis and the rectum.

pel·vis (pel′vis) *n.*, L. pl. **pel·ves** (-veez) 1. A basin or basin-shaped cavity, as the pelvis of the kidney. 2. [NA] The bony ring formed by the two hipbones and the sacrum and coccyx. 3. The cavity bounded by the bony pelvis. The cavity consists of the true pelvis and the false pelvis, which are separated by the iliopectineal line. The entrance of the true pelvis, corresponding to this line, is known as the inlet or superior strait; the outlet or inferior strait is bounded by the symphysis pubis, the tip of the coccyx, and the two ischia.

pel·vi·sec·tion (pel″vi·seck′shun) *n.* A cutting through of one or more of the bones of the pelvis.

pelvis major [NA]. FALSE PELVIS.

pelvis minor [NA]. TRUE PELVIS.

pel·vo·cal·i·ec·ta·sis (pel″vo·kal″ee·eck′tuh·sis) *n.* Dilatation of the pelvis and calyces of the kidney.

pel·vo·cal·y·ce·al, pel·vo·cal·i·ce·al (pel″vo·kal″i·see′ul) *adj.* Pertaining to the pelvis and calyces of the kidney.

pem·phi·goid (pem′fi·goid) *n.* A skin disease resembling pemphigus.

pem·phi·gus (pem′fi·gus) *n.* An acute or chronic disease of the skin characterized by the appearance of bullae which develop in crops or continuous succession. —**pemphi·goid** (·goid) *adj.*

pemphigus er·y·the·ma·to·sus (err″i·theem′uh·to′sis, ·themm″). A form of pemphigus foliaceus, either its beginning or an abortive case. Syn. *Senear-Usher syndrome.*

pemphigus fo·li·a·ce·us (fo″lee·ay′shee·us, ·see·us). A type of pemphigus characterized by crops of flaccid blebs which recur and rupture, producing a marked scaliness and generalized exfoliation.

pemphigus veg·e·tans (vej′e·tanz). A form of pemphigus vulgaris in which the denuded areas are covered by warty epidermis, rather than healing normally. These verrucous outgrowths may include small pustules.

pemphigus vul·ga·ris (vul·gair′is). A form of pemphigus, usually chronic, characterized by flaccid bullae involving the skin and oral mucosa; they rupture and leave enlarging denuded areas of epithelium.

pen·al·ge·sia (pen″al·jee′zee·uh) *n.* Reduction in the number of pain and touch spots in the skin.

pen·du·lar (pen′dew·lur) *adj.* Resembling the swinging of a pendulum.

pen·du·lous (pen′dew·lus) *adj.* 1. Hanging down loosely. 2. Swinging freely; pendular.

pe·nec·to·my (pee·neck′tuh·mee) *n.* Surgical removal of the penis.

pen·e·trance (pen'e·trunce) n. The percentage of organisms having a given genetic constitution which show the corresponding hereditary character.

pen·e·trat·ing, adj. Entering beyond the surface, as a penetrating wound that pierces the wall of a cavity or enters an organ.

pen·e·tra·tion, n. 1. The act of penetrating or piercing into. 2. The focal depth of a microscope or lens. 3. The entrance of the penis into the vagina.

-penia A combining form meaning deficiency.

pen·i·cil·la·mine (pen"i·sil'uh·meen, -sil·am'een) n. D-3-Mercaptovaline, $C_5H_{11}NO_2S$, a degradation product of penicillin that chelates heavy metals and is used therapeutically to promote excretion of copper in Wilson's disease. It also reduces urinary cystine concentration and may be used for treatment of cystinuria.

pen·i·cil·late (pen"i·sil'ate) adj. Ending in a tuft of hairs.

pen·i·cil·lin (pen"i·sil'in) n. Generic name for a large group of antibiotic substances derived from several species of Penicillium; some are obtained from cultures of the fungus, while others are prepared by biosynthetic manipulation of 6-aminopenicillanic acid produced by the fungus. The penicillins are 6-carboxamido derivatives of 3,3-dimethyl-7-oxo-4-thia-1-azabicyclo[3.2.0]heptane-2-carboxylic acid. The general formula for penicillins is $C_9H_{11}N_2O_4SR$, where R is the radical in the 6-carboxamido group that characterizes specific penicillins; for example, in penicillin G (benzyl penicillin), R is benzyl $(C_6H_5CH_2-)$, and in penicillin V (phenoxymethyl penicillin) it is phenoxymethyl $(C_6H_4OCH_2-)$. Penicillin G, the first member of the group, continues to be the most widely used; it is employed mainly in the form of its potassium, benzathine, and procaine salts. Penicillin O and its salts, phenoxymethyl penicillin (penicillin V) and its potassium salt, and phenethicillin and its potassium salt are basic variants of penicillin that are used clinically. Methicillin, oxacillin, ampicillin, nafcillin, and cloxacillin are semisynthetic penicillins, certain of which are resistant to penicillinase.

pen·i·cil·lin·ase (pen"i·sil'i·nace) n. Any enzyme, found in many bacteria, which antagonizes the antibacterial action of penicillin by hydrolyzing the β-lactam ring.

penicillin N. D-(4-Amino-4-carboxybutyl) penicillin, an antibiotic produced by Cephalosporium salmosynnematum. Syn. synnematin.

penicillin sensitivity test. A test to determine what bacteria are inhibited by penicillin. The usual method is to place a disk of penicillin in an agar plate. The growth of penicillin-sensitive bacteria will be inhibited in the area around the disk where the penicillin has diffused into the agar. More accurately, serial dilutions of penicillin are incubated with cultures in test tubes.

penicillin V. Phenoxymethyl penicillin (see penicillin), characterized by stability in acid, including gastric fluid; used in the form of the

acid and as the potassium and calcium salts.

pen·i·cil·li·o·sis (pen"i·sil"ee·o'sis) n., pl. **penicil·lio·ses** (·seez) Lesions of the ear, skin, and occasionally lungs, presumed to be caused by certain species of Penicillium.

Pen·i·cil·li·um (pen"i·sil·ee·um) n. A genus of fungi of the Ascomycetes in which the fruiting organs have a brushlike form. The species Penicillium chrysogenum, P. citrinum, P. claviforme, P. gladioli, P. griseofulvum, P. notatum, P. patulum, P. puberulum, P. spinulosum, and P. stoloniferum are used in the production of antibiotics. Some species are also common allergens.

pe·nile (pee'nile) adj. Of or pertaining to the penis.

penile reflex. Contraction of the bulbocavernosus muscle in response to a moderate tap against the dorsum of the penis.

penile strabismus. PEYRONIE'S DISEASE.

pe·nil·lic acid (pe·nil'ick). Any one of the dicarboxylic acids resulting when a penicillin is subjected to a mild acid treatment; the penillic acids are isomeric with the corresponding penicillins.

pe·nis (pee'nis) n. The male organ of copulation. Its essential parts consist of the corpus spongiosum penis enclosing the urethra and forming the glans, and the two corpora cavernosa, all covered by fascia and skin.

penis envy. In psychoanalysis, literally the envy of the young female child for the penis which she does not possess, or which she thinks she has lost (thus forming a part of the castration complex). More generally, the wish by a female for male attributes and advantages, considered by many to play a significant role in the development of the female character. The wish for a penis may be replaced normally by the wish for a child.

pen·nate (pen'ate) adj. Featherlike; comparable in structure to the arrangement of barbs on the shaft of a feather.

pe·no·scro·tal (pee"no·skro'tul) adj. Pertaining to the penis and the scrotum, or at the junction or angle between the two.

pent-, penta- A combining form meaning five.

pen·ta·dac·tyl (pen"tuh·dack'til) adj. Having five fingers or toes upon each hand or foot.

pen·ta·eryth·ri·tyl tetranitrate (pen"tuh·e·rith'ri·til). 2,2-Bis(hydroxymethyl)-1,3-propanediol tetranitrate, $C(CH_2ONO_2)_4$, a coronary vasodilator used in management of angina pectoris.

pen·ta·lo·gy (pen·tal'uh·jee) n. A combination of five related symptoms or defects that are characteristic of a disease or syndrome.

pen·tam·i·dine (pen·tam'i·deen, ·din) n. A diamidine, 4,4'-(pentamethylenedioxy)dibenzamidine, $C_{19}H_{24}N_4O_2$, used as the dimethylsulfonate and isethionate salts in treatment of African trypanosomiasis and kala azar.

Pen·tas·to·ma (pen·tas'tuh·muh, pen"tuh·sto'muh) n. A genus of the Pentastomida. Pentastoma najae has been reported to infect the upper respiratory tract of man.

pen·ta·stome (pen'tuh·stome) n. Any member of the Pentastomida.

Pen·ta·stom·i·da (pen"tuh·stom'i·duh) *n.pl.* A class of arthropods, known as tongue worms, which infect humans; includes the genera *Linguatula, Armillifer, Pentastoma,* and *Porocephalus.*

pen·taz·o·cine (pen·taz'o·sin, ·seen) *n.* 1,2,3,4,5,6-Hexahydro-6,11-dimethyl-3-(3-methyl-2-butenyl)-2,6-methano-3-benzazocin-8-ol, $C_{19}H_{27}NO$, a synthetic narcotic analgesic.

Penthrane. Trademark for methoxyflurane, a general anesthetic.

pen·to·bar·bi·tal sodium (pen"to·bahr'bi·tol, ·tal). Sodium 5-ethyl-5-(1-methylbutyl)barbiturate, $C_{11}H_{17}N_2NaO_3$, a short- to intermediate-acting barbiturate; used as a hypnotic and sedative drug. Syn. *sodium pentobarbitone* (Brit.).

pen·to·lin·i·um tartrate (pen"to·lin'ee·um). 1,1'-Pentamethylenebis(1-methylpyrrolidinium hydrogen tartrate), $C_{15}H_{32}N_2 \cdot 2C_4H_5O_6$, a ganglionic blocking agent used in the management of hypertension.

pen·tose (pen'toce, ·toze) *n.* Any one of a class of carbohydrates containing five atoms of carbon.

pen·tos·uria (pen"to·sue'ree·uh) *n.* The presence of pentose in the urine.

Pentothal. PENTOBARBITAL SODIUM.

pen·tyl·ene·tet·ra·zol (pen"ti·leen·tet'ruh·zol, ·zole) *n.* 6,7,8,9-Tetrahydro-5*H*-tetrazoloazepine, $C_6H_{10}N_4$, a central nervous system stimulant used as an analeptic.

Pen·zoldt's test (pen'tso^hlt) 1. A test for urinary glucose using alkaline sodium diazobenzosulfonate. 2. A test for gastric absorption using potassium iodide and testing for iodine in saliva. 3. An *ortho*-nitrobenzaldehyde test for acetone.

peo·til·lo·ma·nia (pee"o·til'o·may'nee·uh) *n.* The nervous habit of constantly pulling the penis; not an act of masturbation.

pep·per, *n.* The dried, unripe fruit of various species of *Piper;* formerly used as a stimulant, carminative, and counterirritant.

pep·per·mint, *n.* The dried leaves and flowering tops of *Mentha piperita.* Preparations or derivatives of peppermint, such as the oil and spirit, are used as flavors and, sometimes, for carminative action.

Pep·per syndrome or **type** Neuroblastoma with liver metastasis.

pep·sin (pep'sin) *n.* 1. The proteinase of gastric juice, derived from its zymogen precursor pepsinogen elaborated and secreted by the chief cells of the gastric mucosa. 2. A preparation containing proteinase obtained from the glandular layer of the fresh stomach of the hog and sometimes used medicinally for supposed protein digestant action.

pep·sin·o·gen (pep·sin'o·jen) *n.* The antecedent substance or zymogen of pepsin, present in the cells of the gastric glands, which during digestion is converted into pepsin.

pep·tic (pep'tick) *adj.* 1. Pertaining to pepsin. 2. Pertaining to digestion.

peptic ulcer. A sharply circumscribed loss of tissue, involving chiefly the mucosa, submucosa, and muscular layer in areas of the diges-

tive tract exposed to acid-pepsin gastric juice, particularly the lower esophagus, stomach, and first portion of the duodenum.

pep·ti·dase (pep'ti·dace, ·daze) *n.* An enzyme that splits peptides to amino acids.

pep·tide (pep'tide) *n.* A compound of two or more amino acids containing one or more peptide groups, —CONH—. An intermediate between the amino acids and peptones in the synthesis of proteins.

pep·to·nu·ria (pep"to·new'ree·uh) *n.* The presence of peptones in the urine.

per- A prefix signifying (a) *throughout, completely, thoroughly, over,* or *very, extremely;* (b) in chemistry, *the highest valence of a series.*

per·acute (pur"a·kewt') *adj.* Very acute; said of pain or disease.

per anum (pur ay'num) By way of or through the anus, as in the administration of drugs or nutrient substances.

Perazil. A trademark for chlorcyclizine, an antihistaminic drug used as the hydrochloride salt.

per·cent, per cent, *n.* An expression, when preceded by a number, of the proportion of a specific article, object, or substance in 100 parts of the entire system.

per·cen·tile (pur·sen'tile, ·til) *n.* Any of the values of a variable which separate the entire distribution into 100 groups of equal frequency.

per·cep·tion (pur·sep'shun) *n.* Recognition in response to sensory stimuli; the mental act or process by which the memory of certain qualities of an act, experience, or object is associated with other qualities impressing the senses, thereby making possible recognition and interpretation of the new sensory data.

perceptual disorder or **dysfunction.** Any disturbance, usually chronic, of the process of perception, most often involving sight or hearing.

per·co·la·tion (pur"kuh·lay'shun) *n.* The process of extracting the soluble constituents of a substance by allowing a suitable solvent to pass through a column of the powdered substance placed in a long, conical vessel, the percolator. **—per·co·late** (pur'kuh·late) *n. & v.*

Percorten. A trademark for the salt-regulating adrenocortical steroid deoxycorticosterone, used as the acetate ester.

per·cus·si·ble (pur·kus'i·bul) *adj.* Capable of detection by percussion.

per·cus·sion (pur·kush'un) *n.* The act of striking or firmly tapping the surface of the body with a finger or a small hammer to elicit sounds, or vibratory sensations, of diagnostic value. **—per·cuss** (pur·kuss') *v.*

per·cu·ta·ne·ous (pur"kew·tay'nee·us) *adj.* Performed through the skin.

per·fec·tion·ism (pur·feck'shun·iz·um) *n.* The practice of attempting to achieve perfection in all activities of life, no matter how trivial.

per·fo·rans (pur'fo·ranz) *adj.* Penetrating or perforating; a term applied to a muscle, artery, or nerve perforating a part.

¹per·fo·rate (pur'fuh·rut) *adj.* In biology, pierced with small holes.

²per·fo·rate (pur'fuh·rate) *v.* To pierce through.

—**per·fo·rat·ed** (·ray″tid) *adj.*; **per·fo·rat·ing** (·ray″ting) *adj.*

per·fo·ra·tion (pur″fuh·ray′shun) *n.* 1. The act or occurrence of piercing or boring into a part, especially into the wall of a hollow organ or viscus. 2. A hole made through a part or wall of a cavity, produced by a variety of means.

per·fo·ra·tor (pur′fuh·ray″tur) *n.* An instrument for perforating, especially one for performing craniotomy on the fetus.

per·fri·ca·tion (pur″fri·kay′shun) *n.* INUNCTION; rubbing with an ointment.

per·fus·ate (pur·few′zate) *n.* The fluid that is introduced in perfusion (3).

per·fu·sion (pur·few′zhun) *n.* 1. A pouring of fluid. 2. The passage of a fluid through spaces. 3. The introduction of fluids into tissues by their injection into blood vessels, usually veins. —**per·fuse** (·fuze′) *v.*

peri- A prefix signifying *about, beyond, around, near*; especially, *enclosing a part* or *affecting the tissues around a part.*

peri·ac·i·nar (perr″ee·as′i·nur) *adj.* Around an acinus.

peri·ad·e·ni·tis (perr″ee·ad″e·nigh′tis) *n.* Inflammation of the tissues that surround a gland or lymph node.

peri·ad·ven·ti·tial (perr″ee·ad″ven·tish′ul) *adj.* Around the adventitial coat of a blood vessel.

peri·anal (perr″ee·ay′nul) *adj.* Situated or occurring around the anus.

peri·an·gi·itis (perr″ee·an″jee·eye′tis) *n.* Inflammation of the outer coat of or the tissues surrounding a blood or lymphatic vessel.

peri·aor·ti·tis (perr″ee·ay″or·tye′tis) *n.* Inflammation of the tissues surrounding the aorta.

peri·api·cal (perr″ee·ap′i·kul, ·ay′pi·kul) *adj.* Around an apex, particularly the apex of a tooth.

periapical granuloma. A localized mass of chronic granulation tissue formed in response to infection and occurring at the apex of a tooth; often contains islands of epithelial cells (epithelial rests).

peri·ap·pen·di·ci·tis (perr″ee·uh·pen″di·sigh′tis) *n.* Inflammation of the tissue around the vermiform process, or of the serosal region of the vermiform appendix.

peri·aq·ue·duc·tal (perr″ee·ack″we·duck′tul) *adj.* Around the cerebral aqueduct.

peri·are·o·lar (perr″ee·a·ree′uh·lur) *adj.* Around an areola, usually of the breast.

peri·ar·te·ri·al (perr″ee·ahr·teer′ee·ul) *adj.* Surrounding an artery.

peri·ar·te·ri·o·lar (perr″ee·ahr·teer″ee·o′lur) *adj.* Around an arteriole.

peri·ar·te·ri·tis (perr″ee·ahr·te·rye′tis) *n.* Inflammation of the adventitia of an artery and the periarterial tissues.

periarteritis nodosa. POLYARTERITIS NODOSA.

peri·ar·thri·tis (perr″ee·ahr·thrigh′tis) *n.* Inflammation of the tissues about a joint.

peri·ar·tic·u·lar (perr″ee·ahr·tick′yoo·lur) *adj.* About a joint.

peri·au·ric·u·lar (perr″ee·aw·rick′yoo·lur) *adj.* Around the external ear.

peri·ax·i·al (perr″ee·ack′see·ul) *adj.* Surrounding an axis.

peri·blep·sis (perr″i·blep′sis) *n.* The wild look of a patient in delirium.

peri·bron·chi·al (perr″i·bronk′ee·ul) *adj.* Surrounding or occurring about a bronchus.

peri·bron·chi·o·lar (perr″i·bronk″ee·o′lur, ·brong·kigh′o·lur) *adj.* Surrounding or occurring about a bronchiole.

peri·bron·chi·o·li·tis (perr″i·bronk″ee·o·lye′tis) *n.* Inflammation of the tissues around the bronchioles.

peri·bron·chi·tis (perr″i·brong·kigh′tis) *n.* Inflammation of the tissues around bronchi; a subacute bronchopneumonia.

peri·bur·sal (perr″i·bur′sul) *adj.* Around a bursa.

peri·cal·i·ce·al, peri·cal·y·ce·al (perr″i·kal″i·see′ul) *adj.* Around a kidney calix.

peri·can·a·lic·u·lar (perr″i·kan″uh·lick′yoo·lur) *adj.* Occurring around a canaliculus or canaliculi.

pericanalicular fibroadenoma of the breast. A glandular type of benign breast tumor with large amounts of connective tissue which is often arranged concentrically around the multiplied ductules.

peri·cap·il·lary (perr″i·kap′i·lerr·ee) *adj.* Surrounding a capillary.

peri·car·di·ac (perr″i·kahr′dee·ack) *adj.* PERICARDIAL.

peri·car·di·a·co·phren·ic (perr″i·kahr·dye″uh·ko·fren′ick) *adj.* Pertaining to the pericardium and diaphragm.

peri·car·di·al (perr″i·kahr′dee·ul) *adj.* Pertaining to the pericardium; situated around the heart.

pericardial cavity. A space within the pericardium between the serous layer of the pericardium and the epicardium of the heart and roots of the great vessels.

peri·car·di·ec·to·my (perr″i·kahr″dee·eck′tuh·mee) *n.* Excision of a part of the pericardium.

peri·car·dio·cen·te·sis (perr″i·kahr″dee·o·sen·tee′sis) *n.* Puncture of the pericardium.

peri·car·dio·phren·ic (perr″i·kahr″dee·o·fren′ick) *adj.* Pertaining to the pericardium and the diaphragm. Syn. *pericardiacophrenic.*

peri·car·dio·pleu·ral (perr″i·kahr″dee·o·ploor′ul) *adj.* Pertaining to the pericardium and to the pleura.

peri·car·di·or·rha·phy (perr″i·kahr″dee·or′uh·fee) *n.* The suturing of a wound in the pericardium.

peri·car·di·ot·o·my (perr″i·kahr″dee·ot′uh·mee) *n.* Incision of the pericardium.

peri·car·di·tis (perr″i·kahr·dye′tis) *n.*, pl. **pericar·dit·i·des** (·dit′i·deez) Inflammation of the pericardium, acute or chronic, of varied etiology with or without effusion or constriction —**peri·car·dit·ic** (·dit′ick) *adj.*

peri·car·di·um (perr″i·kahr′dee·um) *n.*, genit. **pericar·dii** (·dee·eye), pl. **pericar·dia** (·dee·uh) The closed membranous sac enveloping the heart. Its base is attached to the central tendon of the diaphragm; its apex surrounds, for a short distance, the great vessels arising from the base of the heart. The sac normally contains from 5 to 20 g of clear, serous liquid. The part in contact with the heart (visceral pericardium) is termed the epicardium; the other is the parietal pericardium.

peri·ca·val (perr″i·kay′vul) *adj.* Around one of the caval vessels, usually the inferior vena cava.

peri·ce·cal, peri·cae·cal (perr″i·see′kul) Surrounding the cecum.

peri·ce·ci·tis, peri·cae·ci·tis (perr″i·se·sigh′tis) *n.* Inflammation of the serosa of the cecum and the tissues surrounding the cecum.

peri·ce·men·ti·tis (perr″i·see″men·tye′tis, ·sem′en·) *n.* PERIODONTITIS.

peri·cha·reia (perr″i·ka·rye′uh) *n.* Sudden vehement or abnormal rejoicing; seen in certain psychotic brain disorders.

peri·chol·an·gio·lit·ic (perr″i·ko·lan″jee·o·lit′ick) *adj.* Pertaining to or involving inflammation of tissues around the smaller biliary passages.

peri·chol·an·gi·tis (perr″i·kol″an·jye′tis, ·ko′lan·) *n.* Inflammation of the tissues surrounding the bile ducts or interlobular bile capillaries. —**pericholan·git·ic** (·jit′ick) *adj.*

peri·cho·le·cys·tic (perr″i·kol″e·sis′tick, ·ko′le·) *adj.* Around the gallbladder.

peri·cho·le·cys·ti·tis (perr″i·kol″e·sis·tye′tis, ·ko′le·) *n.* Inflammation of the serosa and tissues around the gallbladder.

peri·chon·dri·tis (perr″i·kon·drye′tis) *n.* Inflammation of perichondrium. —**perichon·drit·ic** (·drit′ick) *adj.*

peri·chon·dri·um (perr″i·kon′dree·um) *n.,* pl. **perichon·dria** (·dree·uh) The fibrous connective tissue covering cartilage, except articular surfaces. —**perichon·dral** (·drul) *adj.*

peri·coc·cyg·e·al (perr″i·kock·sij′ee·ul) *adj.* Around the coccyx.

peri·co·lic (perr″i·ko′lick, ·kol′ick) *adj.* Surrounding or about the colon.

peri·co·li·tis (perr″i·ko·lye′tis) *n.* Inflammation of the peritoneum or tissues around the colon.

peri·con·chal (perr″i·kong′kul) *adj.* Surrounding the concha of the ear.

peri·cor·ne·al (perr″i·kor′nee·ul) *adj.* Surrounding the cornea.

peri·cor·o·nal (perr″i·kor′uh·nul) *adj.* 1. Around a tooth crown. 2. Around the corona of the glans penis.

peri·cor·o·ni·tis (perr″i·kor″o·nigh′tis) *n.* Inflammation of the tissue surrounding the coronal portion of the tooth, usually a partially erupted third molar.

peri·cos·tal (perr″i·kos′tul) *adj.* Around a rib.

peri·cra·ni·um (perr″i·kray′nee·um) *n.* The periosteum on the outer surface of the cranial bones. —**pericrani·al** (·ul) *adj.*

peri·cys·tic (perr″i·sis′tick) *adj.* 1. Surrounding a cyst. 2. Surrounding a bladder, either the gallbladder or the urinary bladder.

peri·cys·ti·tis (perr″i·sis·tye′tis) *n.* 1. Inflammation surrounding a cyst. 2. Inflammation of the peritoneum or other tissue surrounding the urinary bladder.

peri·cyte (perr″i·site) *n.* A cell which is enclosed within the basal membrane of the endothelial cell and which forms a portion of the capillary wall; its functions are presently unknown.

peri·den·drit·ic (perr″i·den·drit′ick) *adj.* Surrounding a dendrite.

peri·den·tal (perr″i·den′tul) *adj.* Surrounding a tooth or its root; periodontal.

peri·di·ver·tic·u·li·tis (perr″i·dye″vur·tick″yoo·lye′tis) *n.* Inflammation of the tissues surrounding a diverticulum, particularly of the gastrointestinal tract.

peri·duc·tal (perr″i·duck′tul) *adj.* Around a duct.

peri·du·o·de·ni·tis (perr″i·dew″o·de·nigh′tis, ·dew·od″e·nigh′tis) *n.* Inflammation of the tissues surrounding the duodenum.

peri·du·ral (perr″i·dew′rul) *adj.* EPIDURAL; especially outside the dura mater of the spinal cord.

peri·en·ceph·a·li·tis (perr″ee·en·sef″uh·lye′tis) *n.* Inflammation of the pia mater and the cortex of the brain; MENINGOENCEPHALITIS.

peri·en·ter·ic (perr″ee·en·terr′ick) *adj.* Situated around the enteron; PERIVISCERAL.

peri·en·ter·i·tis (perr″ee·en″tur·eye′tis) *n.* Inflammation of the intestinal peritoneum.

peri·epi·did·y·mi·tis (perr″ee·ep″i·did·i·migh′tis) *n.* Inflammation around the epididymis.

peri·epi·glot·tic (perr″ee·ep″i·glot′ick) *adj.* Around the epiglottis.

peri·esoph·a·ge·al, peri·oesoph·a·ge·al (perr″ee·e·sof″uh·jee′ul) *adj.* Situated or occurring just outside of, or around, the esophagus.

peri·esoph·a·gi·tis, peri·oesoph·a·gi·tis (perr″ee·e·sof″uh·jye′tis) *n.* Inflammation of the tissues that surround the esophagus.

peri·fis·tu·lar (perr″i·fis′tew·lur) *adj.* Around or about a fistula.

peri·fol·lic·u·lar (perr″i·fol·ick′yoo·lur) *adj.* Surrounding a follicle.

peri·fol·lic·u·li·tis (perr″i·fol·ick″yoo·lye′tis) *n.* Inflammation around the hair follicles.

peri·fu·nic·u·lar (perr″i·few·nick′yoo·lur) *adj.* Around the spermatic cord.

peri·gas·tric (perr″i·gas′trick) *adj.* Surrounding, or in the neighborhood of, the stomach.

peri·gas·tri·tis (perr″i·gas·trye′tis) *n.* Inflammation of the serosa of the stomach.

peri·gen·i·tal (perr″i·jen′i·tul) *adj.* Around the genitalia.

peri·glan·du·lar (perr″i·glan′dew·lur) *adj.* Pertaining to the tissue surrounding a gland.

peri·glot·tic (perr″i·glot′ick) *adj.* Situated around the base of the tongue and the epiglottis.

peri·gnath·ic (perr″i·nath′ick, ·nay′thick) *adj.* Situated about the jaws.

peri·he·pat·ic (perr″i·he·pat′ick) *adj.* Surrounding, or occurring around, the liver.

peri·hep·a·ti·tis (perr″i·hep″uh·tye′tis) *n.* Inflammation of the peritoneum and tissues surrounding the liver.

peri·her·ni·al (perr″i·hur′nee·ul) *adj.* Around or surrounding a hernia.

peri·hi·lar (perr″i·high′lur) *adj.* Around a hilus.

peri·hy·poph·y·se·al (perr″i·high·pof″i·see′ul, ·high′po·fiz″ee·ul) *adj.* Around or near the hypophysis.

peri·je·ju·ni·tis (perr″i·jee″joo·nigh′tis, ·jej″oo·nigh′tis) *n.* Inflammation of the peritoneal coat or tissues around the jejunum.

peri·kar·y·on (perr″i·kăr′ee·on) *n.* 1. The cytoplasmic mass surrounding the nucleus of a cell; especially, the cell body of a neuron exclusive of the nucleus. 2. The CELL BODY of a neuron.

peri·ke·rat·ic (perr″i·ke·rat′ick) adj. PERICORNE-AL.

peri·ky·ma·ta (perr″i·kigh′muh·tuh) n., sing. **perikyma** Transverse, wavelike grooves on the enamel surface of a tooth, thought to be the external manifestations of the incremental lines of Retzius, which are continuous around the tooth and usually lie parallel to each other and to the cementoenamel junction.

peri·lab·y·rin·thi·tis (perr″i·lab″i·rin·thigh′tis) n. Inflammation in the osseous labyrinth of the internal ear.

peri·la·ryn·ge·al (perr″i·la·rin′jee·ul) adj. Situated, or occurring, around the larynx.

peri·lar·yn·gi·tis (perr″i·lăr″in·jye′tis) n. Inflammation of the areolar tissue surrounding the larynx.

peri·len·tic·u·lar (perr″i·len·tick′yoo·lur) adj. Around a lens.

peri·lymph (perr′i·limf) n. The fluid separating the membranous from the osseous labyrinth of the internal ear.

peri·lym·phan·gi·tis (perr″i·lim′fan·jye′tis) n. Inflammation of the tissues surrounding a lymphatic vessel.

peri·lym·phat·ic (perr″i·lim·fat′ick) adj. 1. Pertaining to the perilymph. 2. Situated or occurring about a lymphatic vessel.

perilymphatic space Any of the small, irregular cavities filled with perilymph, between the membranous and bony labyrinths of the internal ear.

peri·mac·u·lar (perr″i·mack′yoo·lur) adj. Around the macula of the retina.

peri·mas·ti·tis (perr″i·mas·tye′tis) n. Inflammation of the fibroadipose tissues around the mammary gland.

pe·rim·e·ter (pe·rim′e·tur) n. 1. Circumference or border. 2. An instrument for measuring the extent of the field of vision. It consists ordinarily of a flat, narrow, metal plate bent in a semicircle, graduated in degrees, and fixed to an upright at its center by a pivot, on which it is movable. Variously colored disks are moved along the metal plate, and the point noted at which the person, looking directly in front of him, distinguishes the color.

peri·met·ric (perr″i·met′rick) adj. Pertaining to perimetry.

peri·me·tri·tis (perr″i·me·trye′tis) n. Inflammation of the tissues about the uterus. —**perime·trit·ic** (·trit′ick) adj.

peri·me·tri·um (perr″i·mee′tree·um) n., pl. **perime·tria** (·tree·uh) The serous covering of the uterus.

peri·me·tro·sal·pin·gi·tis (perr″i·mee″tro·sal″pin·jye′tis) n. A collective name for periuterine inflammations.

pe·rim·e·try (pe·rim′e·tree) n. The measuring of the field of vision.

peri·my·e·li·tis (perr″i·migh″e·lye′tis) n. 1. Inflammation of the pia mater of the spinal cord; MENINGOMYELITIS. 2. Inflammation of the endosteum.

peri·my·o·si·tis (perr″i·migh″o·sigh′tis) n. Inflammation of the connective tissues around muscle.

per·i·my·si·um (perr″i·mis′ee·um, ·miz′ee·um) n.,

pl. **perimy·sia** (·ee·uh) The connective tissue enveloping bundles of muscle fibers. —**peri·mysi·al** (·ul) adj.

peri·na·tal (perr″i·nay′tul) adj. Pertaining to the period of viable pregnancy and neonatal life; in medical statistics the period begins when the fetus attains a weight of 500 g and ends after 28 days of neonatal life.

per·i·ne·al (perr″i·nee′ul) adj. Pertaining to the perineum.

perineal body A wedge-shaped mass of intermingled fibrous and muscular tissue situated between the anal canal and the vagina; in the male, the mass lies between the anal canal and the bulb of the corpus spongiosum penis.

perineal hernia A hernia passing through the pelvic diaphragm to appear as a rectal hernia, vaginal hernia, or bladder hernia.

perineal prostatectomy The removal of the prostate by a U-shaped or V-shaped incision in the perineum, using a special prostatic retractor or a modification.

per·i·neo·plas·ty (perr″i·nee′o·plas″tee) n. Plastic operation upon the perineum.

per·i·neo·rec·tal (perr″i·nee′o·reck′tul) adj. Pertaining to the perineum and the rectum.

per·i·neo·r·rha·phy (perr″i·nee·or′uh·fee) n. Suture of the perineum, usually for the repair of a laceration occurring during labor or for the repair of episiotomy.

per·i·neo·scro·tal (perr″i·nee′o·skro′tul) adj. Relating to the perineum and scrotum.

per·i·ne·ot·o·my (perr″i·nee·ot′uh·mee) n. Incision through the perineum; in gynecologic surgery, an incision into and repair of the perineum for the purpose of enlarging the introitus.

per·i·neo·va·gi·nal (perr″i·nee″o·vaj′i·nul, ·va·jye′nul) adj. Pertaining to the perineum and vagina.

per·i·neo·va·gi·no·rec·tal (perr″i·nee″o·vaj′i·no·reck′tul) adj. Relating to the perineum, vagina, and rectum.

peri·neph·ric (perr″i·nef′rick) adj. Situated or occurring around a kidney.

perinephric abscess An abscess in the region immediately surrounding the kidney.

peri·ne·phri·tis (perr″i·ne·frye′tis) n. Inflammation of the tissues surrounding a kidney. —**peri·ne·phrit·ic** (·frit′ick) adj.

per·i·ne·um (perr″i·nee′um) n., genit. **peri·nei** (·nee′eye), pl. **peri·nea** (·nee·uh) 1. [NA] The portion of the body included in the outlet of the pelvis, bounded in front by the pubic arch, behind by the coccyx and sacrotuberous ligaments, and at the sides by the tuberosities of the ischium. In the male it is occupied by the anal canal, membranous urethra, and root of the penis; in the female by the anal canal, urethra, root of the clitoris, and vaginal orifice; in both sexes by the muscles, fasciae vessels, and nerves of these structures. 2. The region between the anus and the scrotum in the male; between the anus and the posterior commissure of the vulva in the female.

peri·neu·ral (perr″i·new′rul) adj. Situated around nervous tissue or a nerve.

peri·neu·ri·tis (perr''i·new·rye'tis) *n.* Inflammation of the perineurium.

peri·neu·ri·um (perr''i·new'ree·um) *n.*, pl. **perineu·ria** (·ree·uh) The connective-tissue sheath investing a fasciculus or primary bundle of nerve fibers. —**perineuri·al** (·ul) *adj.*

peri·neu·ro·nal (perr''i·new'ruh·nul, ·new·ro'nul) *adj.* Around a neuron or neurons.

peri·ne·void (perr''i·nee'void) *adj.* Surrounding a nevus.

peri·nu·cle·ar (perr''i·new'klee·ur) *adj.* Surrounding a nucleus.

peri·oc·u·lar (perr''ee·ock'yoo·lur) *adj.* Surrounding the eye.

pe·ri·od (peer'ee·ud) *n.* Duration; measure of time. The space of time during which anything is in progress or an event occurs.

pe·ri·od·ic (peer''ee·od'ick) *adj.* Recurring at more or less regular intervals.

peri·od·ic acid (pur''eye·od'ick) A colorless, crystalline acid, $HIO_4.2H_2O$, used as an oxidizing agent.

periodic disease. FAMILIAL MEDITERRANEAN FEVER.

pe·ri·od·ic·i·ty (peer''ee·uh·dis'i·tee) *adj.* Recurrence at regular intervals.

periodic paralysis. A symptom complex, observed in families as an autosomal dominant trait, manifested by recurrent attacks of flaccid muscular weakness which develop abruptly, often on rest after exercise, exposure to cold, or dietary provocation, and which last a few hours to several days. The recognized forms are the hypokalemic, normokalemic, hyperkalemic, and the type associated with hyperthyroidism.

periodic somnolence syndrome. KLEINE-LEVIN SYNDROME.

peri·odon·tal (perr''ee·o·don'tul) *adj.* 1. Surrounding a tooth, as the periodontal ligament, which covers the cement of a tooth. 2. Pertaining to the periodontium or to periodontics.

periodontal ligament. The connective tissue that surrounds the root of a tooth and attaches it to the alveolar bone; it is continuous with the connective tissue of the gingiva.

periodontal membrane. PERIODONTAL LIGAMENT.

periodontal space. The radiolucent space on a dental radiograph which represents the periodontal ligament.

peri·odon·tics (perr''ee·o·don'ticks) *n.* The branch of dentistry dealing with the science and treatment and prevention of periodontal disease.

peri·odon·tist (perr''ee·o·don'tist) *n.* A person who specializes in periodontics.

peri·odon·ti·tis (perr''ee·o·don·tye'tis) *n.* Inflammation of the periodontium.

peri·odon·ti·um (perr''ee·o·don'chee·um) *n.*, pl. **periodon·tia** (·chee·uh) The investing and supporting tissues surrounding a tooth; namely, the periodontal ligament, the gingiva, the cementum, and the alveolar bone.

peri·odon·to·cla·sia (perr''ee·o·don''to·klay'zhuh, ·zee·uh) *n.* Any periodontal disease that results in the destruction of the periodontium.

peri·odon·tol·o·gy (perr''ee·o·don·tol'uh·jee) *n.*

The science and study of the periodontium and periodontal diseases.

peri·odon·to·sis (perr''ee·o·don·to'sis) *n.*, pl. **periodonto·ses** (·seez) A degenerative disturbance of the periodontium, characterized by degeneration of connective-tissue elements of the periodontal ligament and by bone resorption.

peri·om·phal·ic (perr''ee·om·fal'ick) *adj.* Around, or near, the umbilicus.

peri·onych·ia (perr''ee·o·nick'ee·uh) *n.* Inflammation around the nails.

peri·onych·i·um (perr''ee·o·nick'ee·um) *n.*, pl. **perionych·ia** (·ee·uh) The border of epidermis surrounding an entire nail. Syn. *paronychium.*

peri·ooph·o·ri·tis (perr''ee·o·off''ur·eye'tis) *n.* Inflammation of the peritoneum, the ovary, and the adjacent connective tissues.

peri·ooph·oro·sal·pin·gi·tis (perr''ee·o·off''ur·o·sal''pin·jye'tis) *n.* Inflammation of the tissues surrounding an ovary and oviduct.

peri·ople (perr'ee·o''pul) *n.* The outer layer of horny tissue of the hoof secreted by the perioplic ring. It extends downward over the wall of the hoof, acting as an impervious protective covering. —**peri·op·lic** (·op'lick) *adj.*

peri·op·tom·e·try (perr''ee·op·tom'e·tree) *n.* The measurement of the limits of the visual field.

peri·oral (perr''ee·o'rul) *adj.* Surrounding the mouth; circumoral.

peri·or·bit (perr''ee·or'bit) *n.* The periosteum within the orbit. —**periorbit·al** (·ul) *adj.*

peri·or·bi·ti·tis (perr''ee·or''bi·tye'tis) *n.* Inflammation of the periorbit.

peri·os·te·al (perr''ee·os'tee·ul) *adj.* Pertaining to or involving the periosteum.

periosteal bone. Membrane bone formed by the periosteum.

periosteal elevator. A surgical instrument designed to separate and preserve the periosteum in osteotomy.

peri·os·te·um (perr''ee·os'tee·um) *n.*, pl. **perios·tea** (·tee·uh) A fibrous membrane investing the surfaces of bones, except at the points of tendinous and ligamentous attachment and on the articular surfaces, where cartilage is substituted.

peri·os·ti·tis (perr''ee·os·tye'tis) *n.* Inflammation of periosteum. —**perios·tit·ic** (·tit'ick) *adj.*

peri·os·to·sis (perr''ee·os·to'sis) *n.*, pl. **periosto·ses** (·seez) Abnormal bone formation on the exterior of a bone.

peri·otic (perr''ee·o'tick, ·ot'ick) *adj.* 1. Situated about the ear. 2. Of or pertaining to the parts immediately about the internal ear.

peri·pachy·men·in·gi·tis (perr''i·pack''ee·men''in·jye'tis) *n.* EPIDURAL ABSCESS.

peri·pan·cre·a·ti·tis (perr''i·pang''kree·uh·tye'tis) *n.* Inflammation of the tissues around the pancreas.

peri·pap·il·lary (perr''i·pap'i·lerr·ee) *n.* Occurring or situated around the circumference of a papilla, and especially of the optic disk.

peri·pha·ryn·ge·al (perr''i·fa·rin'jee·ul) *adj.* Surrounding the pharynx.

pe·riph·er·al (pe·rif'e·rul) *adj.* 1. Pertaining to or located at a periphery. 2. Located at or involving a noncentral or outer area or portion.

3. Pertaining to, or located at or near, the surface of the body or of an organ.

peripheral anosmia. See *anosmia.*

peripheral blood. 1. Blood in the systemic circulation; excludes blood in the bone marrow. 2. Occasionally used to designate blood not in the pulmonary circulation and cardiac chambers.

peripheral nerve. Any nerve which is a component of the peripheral nervous system.

peripheral vision. Vision in which the image falls upon parts of the retina outside the macula lutea, less distinct than central vision but important normally in the appreciation of the environment not directly looked at or in lesions involving the macula lutea. Syn. *indirect vision.*

pe·riph·er·y (pe·rif'ur·ee) *n.* 1. Circumference. 2. The external surface.

peri·phle·bi·tis (perr''i·fle·bye'tis) *n.* Inflammation of the tissues surrounding a vein or of the adventitia of a vein. —**periphle·bit·ic** (·bit'ick) *adj.*

peri·pleu·ri·tis (perr''i·ploo·rye'tis) *n.* Inflammation of the tissues outside the parietal pleura.

peri·po·ri·tis (perr''i·po·rye'tis) *n.* MILIARIA PUSTULOSA.

peri·por·tal (perr''i·por'tul) *adj.* Surrounding the portal vein and its branches.

peri·proc·tal (perr''i·prock'tul) *adj.* Surrounding the anus or rectum.

peri·proc·ti·tis (perr''i·prock·tye'tis) *n.* Inflammation of the connective tissue about the rectum or anus.

peri·pros·tat·ic (perr''i·pros·tat'ick) *adj.* Situated or occurring around the prostate.

peri·pros·ta·ti·tis (perr''i·pros''tuh·tye'tis) *n.* Inflammation of the tissue situated around the prostate.

peri·py·lo·ric (perr''i·pye·lo'rick, ·pi·lo'rick) *adj.* Surrounding the pylorus.

peri·rec·tal (perr''i·reck'tul) *adj.* About the rectum.

peri·re·nal (perr''i·ree'nul) *adj.* Around a kidney.

peri·sal·pin·gi·tis (perr''i·sal''pin·jye'tis) *n.* Inflammation of the peritoneal covering of a uterine tube.

peri·sig·moid·itis (perr''i·sig''moid·eye'tis) *n.* Inflammation of the tissues, especially the peritoneum, covering the sigmoid flexure of the colon.

peri·si·nus·itis (perr''i·sigh''nuh·sigh'tis) *n.* Inflammation of the tissues around a sinus, especially a sinus of the dura mater.

peri·si·nus·oi·dal (perr''i·sigh''nuh·soy'dul) *adj.* Around a sinusoid.

perisinusoidal space. The space in the liver that is bounded on one side by the endothelium of the sinusoids and on the other by the walls of the liver cells. Syn. *space of Disse.*

peri·sple·nic (perr''i·splee'nick, ·splen'ick) *adj.* Situated near the spleen.

peri·sple·ni·tis (perr''i·sple·nigh'tis) *n.* Inflammation of the peritoneum covering the spleen.

peri·spon·dyl·ic (perr''i·spon·dil'ick) *adj.* Around a vertebra.

peri·spon·dy·li·tis (perr''i·spon''di·lye'tis) *n.* In-

flammation of the tissues around the vertebrae.

peri·stal·sis (perr''i·stal'sis, ·stahl'sis) *n.,* pl. **peri·stal·ses** (·seez') A progressive wave of contraction seen in tubes, such as the gastrointestinal tract, provided with longitudinal and transverse muscular fibers. It consists in a narrowing and shortening of a portion of the tube, which then relaxes, while a distal portion becomes shortened and narrowed. By means of this movement the contents of this tube are forced toward the opening. —**peristal·tic** (·tick') *adj.*

peri·staph·y·li·tis (perr''i·staf''i·lye'tis) *n.* Inflammation of the tissues surrounding the uvula.

peri·sta·sis (perr''i·stay'sis, pe·ris'tuh·sis) *n.* 1. An early stage of vascular change in inflammation, chiefly characterized by increased amounts of blood in the affected part, with decreased blood flow. 2. Environment. —**peri·stat·ic** (perr''i·stat'ick) *adj.*

peri·stri·ate area (perr''i·strye'ate). The visual association area of the occipital cortex surrounding the parastriate area and extending to the borders of the occipital lobe; the second concentric area around the visual cortex. Syn. *Brodmann's areas 18 and 19.*

peri·syn·o·vi·al (perr''i·si·no'vee·ul) *adj.* Situated or occurring around a synovial membrane.

per·i·ten·din·e·um (perr''i·ten·din'ee·um) *n.,* pl. **peritendin·ea** (·ee·uh) The white, fibrous sheath covering the fiber bundles of tendons.

peri·ten·di·ni·tis (perr''i·ten''di·nigh'tis) *n.* Inflammation of the sheath and tissues around a tendon.

peri·ten·on (perr''i·ten'un, ·on) *n.* 1. The sheath of a tendon. 2. PERITENDINEUM.

peri·the·li·o·ma (perr''i·theel''ee·o'muh) *n.* HEMANGIOPERICYTOMA.

peri·the·li·um (perr''i·theel'ee·um) *n.,* pl. **perithe·lia** (·lee·uh) The connective tissue accompanying the capillaries and smaller vessels. —**peri·theli·al** (·ul) *adj.*

peri·thy·roid·itis (perr''i·thigh''roy·dye'tis) *n.* Inflammation of the tissue surrounding the thyroid gland.

pe·rit·o·my (pe·rit'uh·mee) *n.* 1. *In ophthalmology,* the incision into the conjunctiva at the corneal scleral margin and the undermining of this half-moon-shaped segment to divide or remove the vessels of a superficial vascularized keratitis; often performed as a preliminary to enucleation and in preparation for a corneal transplant. 2. CIRCUMCISION.

peri·to·ne·al, peri·to·nae·al (·i·to·nee'ul) *adj.* Pertaining to or affecting the peritoneum.

peritoneal cavity. A space between the visceral and parietal layers of the peritoneum.

peri·to·ne·al·iza·tion (perr''i·to·nee''ul·i·zay'shun) *n.* The process of covering with peritoneum.

peri·to·ne·al·ize (perr''i·to·nee'uh·lize) *v.* To cover with peritoneum by operative procedures.

peri·to·neo·cen·te·sis (perr''i·to·nee''o·sen·tee'sis) *n.* Puncture of the peritoneal cavity, as for the removal of ascitic fluid.

peri·to·neo·peri·car·di·al (perr''i·to·nee''o·perr''i·

kahr′dee·ul) *adj.* Pertaining to the peritoneum and the pericardium.

peri·to·neo·pexy (perr″i·to·nee′o·peck″see) *n.* Fixation of the uterus by the vaginal route in the treatment of retroflexion of this organ.

peri·to·neo·scope (perr″i·to·nee′uh·skope) *n.* A long slender endoscope equipped with sheath, obturator, biopsy forceps, a sphygmomanometer bulb and tubing, scissors, and a syringe; introduced into the peritoneal cavity through a small incision in the abdominal wall permitting visualization of the gas-inflated peritoneal cavity for diagnosis of abdominal and pelvic tumors, biliary disease, and other intra-abdominal diseases. Syn. *laparoscope.*

peri·to·ne·os·co·py (perr″i·to·nee·os′kuh·pee) *n.* A method of examining the peritoneal cavity by means of a peritoneoscope.

peri·to·ne·ot·o·my (perr″i·to·nee·ot′uh·mee) *n.* Incision into the peritoneum.

peri·to·ne·um (perr″i·to·nee′um) *n.,* genit. **perito·nei** (·nee′eye), L. pl. **perito·nea** (·nee′uh) The serous membrane lining the interior of the abdominal cavity and surrounding the contained viscera.

peri·to·ni·tis (perr″i·to·nigh′tis) *n.* Inflammation of the peritoneum.

peri·ton·sil·lar (perr″i·ton′si·lur) *adj.* About a tonsil.

peritonsillar abscess. An abscess forming in acute tonsillitis around one or both faucial tonsils; quinsy.

peri·ton·sil·li·tis (perr″i·ton″si·lye′tis) *n.* Inflammation of the tissues surrounding a tonsil.

peri·tra·che·al (perr″i·tray′kee·ul) *adj.* Surrounding the trachea.

peri·trich·i·al (perr″i·trick′ee·ul) *adj.* Surrounding a hair follicle.

pe·rit·ri·chous (pe·rit′ri·kus) *adj.* Having flagella distributed over the entire body surface; said of certain microorganisms.

peri·trun·cal (perr″i·trunk′ul) *adj.* Perivascular and peribronchial conjointly.

peri·tub·al (perr″i·tew′bul) *adj.* 1. Around a uterine tube. 2. Around a tube.

peri·typh·li·tis (perr″i·tif·lye′tis) *n.* 1. Inflammation of the peritoneum surrounding the cecum and vermiform appendix. 2. PERICECITIS. —**perityph·lit·ic** (·lit′ick) *adj.*

peri·um·bil·i·cal (perr″ee·um·bil′i·kul) *adj.* Surrounding or near the umbilicus.

peri·un·gual (perr″i·ung′gwul) *adj.* Around a nail.

peri·ure·ter·i·tis (perr″i·yoo·ree″tur·eye′tis) *n.* Inflammation of the tissues around a ureter. Syn. *paraureteritis.*

peri·ure·thral (perr″i·yoo·ree′thrul) *adj.* Surrounding the urethra.

peri·ure·thri·tis (perr″i·yoo″re·thrigh′tis) *n.* Inflammation of the connective tissue about the urethra.

peri·uter·ine (perr″i·yoo′tur·in, ·ine) *adj.* About the uterus.

peri·uvu·lar (perr″i·yoo′vew·lur) *adj.* Situated near the uvula.

peri·va·gi·nal (perr″i·vaj′i·nul, ·vuh·jye′nul) *adj.* About the vagina.

peri·vas·cu·lar (perr″i·vas′kew·lur) *adj.* About a vessel.

perivascular foot. The expanded pedicle of a neuroglial cell process attaching it to a blood vessel.

perivascular spaces of Virchow-Robin Fluid-filled spaces between the adventitia of the blood vessels of the brain substance and the pial limiting membrane, lined with endothelial cells, connecting with the subarachnoid space.

peri·vas·cu·li·tis (perr″i·vas″kew·lye′tis) *n.* Inflammation of the perivascular sheaths and surrounding tissues.

peri·ve·nous (perr″i·vee′nus) *adj.* Investing a vein; occurring around a vein.

peri·ven·tric·u·lar (perr″i·ven·trick′yoo·lur) *adj.* Around a ventricle, usually of the brain or heart.

peri·ver·te·bral (perr″i·vur′te·brul) *adj.* Around a vertebra or vertebrae.

peri·ves·i·cal (perr″i·ves′i·kul) *adj.* Situated about or surrounding the urinary bladder.

peri·ve·sic·u·lar (perr″i·ve·sick′yoo·lur) *adj.* Occurring around a seminal vesicle or vesicles.

peri·ve·sic·u·li·tis (perr″i·ve·sick″yoo·lye′tis) *n.* Inflammation around a seminal vesicle.

peri·vis·cer·al (perr″i·vis′ur·ul) *adj.* Surrounding a viscus or viscera.

peri·vi·tel·line (perr″i·vi·tel′ine, ·in) *adj.* Surrounding the vitellus or yolk.

peri·vul·var (perr″i·vul′vur) *adj.* Around the vulva.

peri·xe·ni·tis (perr″i·ze·nigh′tis) *n.* FOREIGN-BODY REACTION.

perle (purl) *n.* 1. A soft capsule for administration of a volatile or unpleasant liquid medicine. 2. A thin glass globule that contains a volatile liquid to be inhaled, and that is crushed prior to use.

per·lèche (pur·lesh′) *n.* An inflammatory condition occurring at the angles of the mouth with resultant fissuring. In some instances, it appears to be due to overclosure of the mouth in edentulous patients or extreme wearing away of the teeth. Syn. *angular stomatitis.*

Perls's reaction (pehrlss) A method of demonstrating hemosiderin in tissues.

permanent teeth. The 32 adult teeth of the second, or permanent, dentition; there are 8 incisors, 4 canines, 8 premolars, and 12 molars.

per·man·ga·nate (pur·mang′guh·nate) *n.* A salt of permanganic acid.

per·man·gan·ic acid (pur″mang·gan′ick). A monobasic acid, $HMnO_4$, obtained only in solution.

per·me·abil·i·ty (pur″mee·uh·bil′i·tee) *n. In physiology,* the property of membranes which permits transit of molecules and ions.

per·me·able (pur′mee·uh·bul) *adj.* Affording passage; pervious.

per·me·ation (pur″mee·ay′shun) *n.* The process of permeating or passing through; specifically, the extension of a malignant tumor, especially carcinoma, by continuous growth through lymphatics.

Permutit. Trademark for certain synthetic solid substances used to exchange a component ion, such as sodium, for other ions, such as calcium and magnesium, present in water or an aqueous solution in contact with the solid.

per·ni·cious (pur-nish'us) *adj.* Highly destructive; of intense severity; potentially fatal.

pernicious anemia. A megaloblastic, macrocytic anemia resulting from lack of vitamin B_{12} secondary to gastric atrophy and loss of intrinsic factor necessary for vitamin B_{12} absorption, and accompanied by degeneration of the posterior and lateral columns of the spinal cord.

pernicious anemia of pregnancy. A megaloblastic anemia of pregnancy due to folic acid deficiency.

pernicious vomiting. Vomiting occasionally occurring in pregnancy and becoming so prolonged and excessive as to threaten life.

per·nio (pur'nee·o) *n.*, pl. **per·ni·o·nes** (pur''nee·o'neez) CHILBLAIN.

per·ni·o·sis (pur''nee·o'sis) *n.* Any dermatitis resulting from chilblain.

pero- A combining form meaning *malformed, stunted, defective.*

pe·ro·bra·chi·us (peer''o·bray'kee·us) *n.* A developmental defect in which the forearms and hands are malformed or wanting.

pe·ro·chi·rus, pe·ro·chei·rus (peer''o·kigh'rus) *n.* Congenital absence or stunted growth of the hand.

pe·ro·cor·mus (peer''o·kor'mus) *n.* Congenital defect of the trunk.

pe·ro·dac·tyl·ia (peer''o·dack·til'ee·uh) *n.* Defective development of the fingers or toes.

pe·ro·dac·ty·lus (peer''o·dack'ti·lus) *n.* An individual having congenitally defective and partially absent fingers or toes.

pe·ro·me·lia (peer''o·mee'lee·uh) *n.* Teratic malformation of the limbs.

pe·rom·e·lus (pe·rom'e·lus) *n.* An individual with congenitally deficient, stunted, or misshapen limbs.

per·o·ne·al (perr''o·nee'ul) *adj.* Pertaining to the fibular side of the leg.

peroneal artery. A large branch of the posterior tibial artery which descends close to the fibula through the calf of the ankle, with branches to the heel, ankle, and deep muscles of the calf.

peroneal muscular atrophy. A chronic familial polyneuropathy usually inherited as an autosomal dominant (or occasionally X-linked dominant, or recessive) trait with onset during late childhood or adolescence. It is characterized by distal muscle atrophy beginning in the feet and legs and later involving the hands. Syn. *Charcot-Marie-Tooth disease.*

peroneal sign. In tetany, tapping the fibular side of the leg over the peroneal nerve results in eversion and dorsiflexion of the foot.

peroneo-. A combining form meaning *peroneal* or *peroneus.*

pe·ro·nia (pe·ro'nee·uh) *n.* Mutilation; malformation.

pe·ro·pla·sia (peer''o·play'zhuh, ·zee·uh) *n.* A malformation due to abnormal development.

pe·ro·pus (peer'o·pus) *n.* An individual with congenitally malformed feet.

per·oral (pur·o'rul) *adj.* Passed or performed through the mouth.

per os (pur oce, os) By way of, or through, the mouth, as in the administration of medicines.

pe·ro·sis (pe·ro'sis) *n.*, pl. **pero·ses** (·seez) 1. The condition of abnormal or defective formation. 2. Rotation or torsion of the metatarsus of chickens and turkeys associated with either choline, biotin, or manganese deficiency.

per·os·se·ous (pur·os'ee·us) *adj.* Through bone.

per·ox·i·dase (pur·ock'si·dace, ·daze) *n.* A conjugated, nonporphyrin enzyme, found largely in plant tissues and to a lesser extent in animal tissues, which catalyzes reactions in which hydrogen peroxide is an electron acceptor, i.e., of the following type: $AH_2 + H_2O_2 \rightarrow A + 2H_2O$.

peroxidase stain. Any method for detecting peroxidase activity in tissues by means of providing a peroxide and a substance, usually benzidine, which produces a color when oxidized. Chiefly used to differentiate cells of the granulocytic series from other leukocytes.

per·ox·ide (pur·ock'side) *n.* That oxide of any base which contains the most oxygen. —**per·ox·i·da·tion** (pur·ock''si·day'shun) *n.*

per·ox·i·some (pur·ock'si·sohm) *n.* Any of a group of membrane-bound subcellular particles, formed in the cytoplasm of many types of cells, that contain a variety of enzymes, especially relatively high proportions of catalase, D-amino acid oxidase, and other oxidases.

per·pen·dic·u·lar (pur''pun·dick'yoo·lur) *adj.* At right angles to any given line or plane; at right angles to the horizontal plane.

per·phen·a·zine (pur·fen'uh·zeen) *n.* 2-Chloro-10-{3-[4-(2-hydroxyethyl)piperazinyl]propyl}phenothiazine, $C_{21}H_{26}ClN_3OS$, a tranquilizer and antiemetic drug.

per pri·mam (pur prye'mum) HEALING BY FIRST INTENTION.

per rectum By way of the rectum.

persecution complex. PARANOIA.

per·sev·er·a·tion (pur·sev''ur·ay'shun) *n.* Involuntary, pathological repetition of words or some activity.

per·so·na (pur·so'nuh) *n.* In the analytic psychology of C. Jung, the personality "mask" or facade that each person presents to the outside world.

per·son·al, *adj.* Pertaining to a person, as personal equation, the peculiar difference of individuals in their relation to various orders of stimuli.

per·son·al·i·ty, *n.* 1. The totality of traits and the habitual modes of behavior of the individual as they impress others; the physical and mental qualities peculiar to the individual, which have social connotations. Regarded by psychoanalysts as the resultant of the interaction of the instincts and the environment. 2. In psychiatry, an individual with a certain basic personality pattern which resists efforts at change by either the person himself or others.

personality disorders. *In psychiatry,* a group of disorders characterized by pathological trends in personality structure, with minimal subjective anxiety; in most instances, manifested by a lifelong pattern of abnormal action or behavior (often recognizable by the time of adolescence or earlier) rather than by psychotic, neurotic, or mental disturbances.

personality formation. *In psychoanalysis,* the arrangement of the basic constituents of personality.

personality pattern disturbance. *In psychiatry,* an abnormal pattern of behavior that can rarely if ever be altered therapeutically in its inherent structure; said of more or less cardinal or arch personality types.

per·sorp·tion (pur·sorp'shun) *n.* Direct passage of intact substances through a surface of the body.

per·spi·ra·tion (pur''spi·ray'shun) *n.* 1. The secretion of sweat. 2. SWEAT (2). —**per·spi·ra·to·ry** (pur·spye'ruh·tor·ee) *adj.*

per·spire (pur·spire') *v.* To sweat.

per·sua·sion (pur·sway'zhun) *n. In psychiatry,* a largely intellectual therapeutic approach, directed toward influencing the patient, his attitudes, behavior, or goals.

Per·thes' disease (pehr'tess) OSTEOCHONDRITIS DEFORMANS JUVENILIS.

per·tur·ba·tion (pur''tur·bay'shun) *n.* 1. Restlessness or disquietude; great uneasiness. 2. Abnormal variation in or deviation from the regularity of certain characteristic properties, as in the motions of atoms or planets when a field of force varying with time is applied.

per·tus·sal (pur·tus'ul) *adj.* Resembling or pertaining to pertussis.

per·tus·sis (pur·tus'is) *n.* A highly infectious inflammatory disease of the air passages, due to *Bordetella pertussis,* characterized at its height by paroxysmal explosive coughing ending in a loud whooping inspiration. Syn. *whooping cough.*

Peruvian bark. CINCHONA.

Peruvian wart. VERRUCA PERUVIANA.

per·ver·sion (pur·vur'zhun) *n.* 1. The state of being turned away from the normal or correct. 2. *In psychopathology,* SEXUAL DEVIATION. —**per·vert** (pur·vurt') *v.;* **per·vert** (pur'vurt) *n.*

per·vi·ous (pur'vee·us) *adj.* PERMEABLE.

pes (peece, pace) *n.,* genit. **pe·dis** (ped'is), pl. **pe·des** (ped'eez) A foot or footlike structure.

pes an·se·ri·nus (an·se·rye'nus) 1. The radiate branching of the facial nerve after its exit from the facial canal. 2. The junction of the tendons of the sartorius, gracilis, and semitendinosus muscles at their insertion on the medial aspect of the knee. 3. The distinctive plexiform arrangement of lipoblasts seen in liposarcoma, resembling a goose's foot.

pes ca·vus (kay'vus). A foot deformity characterized by a high plantar arch with retraction of the toes at the metatarsal phalangeal joints and flexion at the interphalangeal joints. Observed frequently in Friedreich's ataxia and peroneal muscular atrophy.

pes con·tor·tus (kon·tor'tus). TALIPES.

pes pedunculi. CRUS OF THE CEREBRUM.

pes pla·no·val·gus (play''no·val'gus). FLATFOOT.

pes pla·nus (play'nus). FLATFOOT.

pes·sa·ry (pes'uh·ree) *n.* 1. An appliance of varied form placed in the vagina for uterine support or contraception. 2. Any suppository or other form of medication placed in the vagina for therapeutic purposes.

pest, *n.* 1. An annoying, destructive, or infectious organism; often, large numbers of such organisms, as a cockroach or rat pest. 2. A plague; pestilence; in the old medical literature, any major epidemic. 3. BUBONIC PLAGUE.

pest·house, *n.* A hospital for persons sick with pestilential diseases.

pes·ti·cide (pes'ti·side) *n.* A substance destructive to pests, especially to insects.

pes·ti·lence (pes'ti·lunce) *n.* 1. Any epidemic contagious disease. 2. Infection with the plague organism *Yersinia pestis.* —**pes·ti·len·tial** (pes''ti·len'shul) *adj.*

pes·tis (pes'tis) *n.* Pest or plague.

pes·tle (pes'ul, pes'tul) *n.* The device for mixing or powdering substances in a mortar.

-petal A combining form meaning *moving toward, seeking.*

pe·te·chia (pe·tee'kee·uh, pe·teck'ee·uh) *n.,* pl. **pete·chi·ae** (·kee·ee) A minute, rounded spot of hemorrhage on a surface such as skin, mucous membrane, serous membrane, or on a cross-sectional surface of an organ. —**pete·chi·al** (·kee·ul) *adj.*

peth·i·dine (peth'i·deen, ·din) *n.* Meperidine, an analgesic drug used as the hydrochloride salt.

pet·i·ole (pet'ee·ole) *n.* A stem or stalk.

pe·tit mal (pe·tee' mal', puh·tee') ABSENCE ATTACK.

petit mal epilepsy. A form of epilepsy characterized by recurrent absence attacks.

petit mal triad. A concept originally proposed by Lennox, but now abandoned, that absence, and myoclonic and akinetic seizures constitute a petit mal triad.

petr-, petri-, petro- A combining form meaning (a) *stone;* (b) *petroleum;* (c) *pertaining to the petrous portion of the temporal bone.*

pet·ri·fac·tion (pet''ri·fack'shun) *n.* The process of changing to stone, as petrifaction of the fetus.

Pe·tri plate or **dish** (pee'tree, Ger. pey'tree) PLATE (3).

pé·tris·sage (pay''tri·sahzh') *n.* Kneading massage.

pet·ro·bas·i·lar (pet''ro·bas'i·lur) *adj.* Pertaining to the petrous part of the temporal bone and the basilar part of the occipital bone.

pet·ro·la·tum (pet''ro·lay'tum) *n.* A purified, semisolid mixture of hydrocarbons obtained from petroleum. Occurs as a yellowish to light amber, unctuous mass. Used as a bland, protective dressing and as a base for ointments. Syn. *petroleum jelly, yellow petrolatum.*

pe·tro·le·um (pe·tro'lee·um) *n.* A complex mixture of hydrocarbons consisting chiefly of paraffins and cycloparaffins or of cyclic aromatic hydrocarbons, with small amounts of benzene hydrocarbons, sulfur, and oxygenated compounds. Occurs as a dark-yellow to brown or greenish-gray, oily liquid.

petroleum benzin. Benzin, usually a purified grade.

petroleum ether. Benzin, usually a purified grade.

petroleum jelly. PETROLATUM.

pet·ro·mas·toid (pet''ro·mas'toid) *n.* Pertaining to the petrous and mastoid portions of the temporal bone.

pet·ro·oc·cip·i·tal (pet''ro·ock·sip'i·tul) *adj.* Pertaining to the petrous portion of the temporal bone and to the occipital bone.

pe·tro·sa (pe·tro'suh) *n.*, pl. **petro·sae** (·see) PETROUS PART OF THE TEMPORAL BONE. —**petro·sal** (·sul) *adj.*

pet·ro·si·tis (pet''ro·sigh'tis) *n.* Inflammation of the petrous portion of the temporal bone, usually from extension of a mastoiditis or from middle ear disease.

pet·ro·squa·mous (pet''ro·skway'mus) *adj.* Pertaining to the petrous and squamous portions of the temporal bone.

pet·rous (pet'rus, pee'trus) *adj.* Stony; of the hardness of stone.

petrous part of the temporal bone. The pyramidal dense portion of the temporal bone which projects medially.

pe·trox·o·lin (pe·trock'so·lin) *n.* A liquid or solid preparation made with a vehicle or base composed of light liquid petrolatum with soft ammonia soap and alcohol and containing medicinal substances. Petroxolins were used as externally applied dermatologic agents.

Peutz–Je·ghers syndrome (poehts, jay'gurz) Familial gastrointestinal polyposis associated with mucocutaneous melanin pigmentation of mouth, hands, and feet. Syn. *hereditary multiple polyposis.*

pex·is (peck'sis) *n.* FIXATION.

-pexy In surgery, a combining form meaning *fixation.*

Pey·er's patches or **glands** (pye'ur) AGGREGATE FOLLICLES.

pe·yo·te (pay·o'tee) *n.* MESCAL (1).

Pey·ro·nie's disease (peh·roh·nee') A condition of unknown etiology characterized by the development of plaques or masses of dense fibrous tissue in the fascia about the corpus cavernosum of the penis, resulting in deformity of the penis. Syn. *fibrous cavernitis, penile strabismus, penis plasticus.*

Pfan·nen·stiel's incision (pfah'n'en·shteel) A low transverse incision through the skin, subcutaneous tissue, and fascia, separating the rectus muscles in the midline vertically, placed below the pubic hair line above the mons pubis, thus making an inconspicuous scar.

Pfaund·ler–Hurler syndrome (pfaownd'lur) HURLER'S SYNDROME.

Pfeif·fer·el·la (figh''fur·el'uh) *n.* ACTINOBACILLUS.

pH A symbol, introduced by Sørensen, to express hydrogen-ion concentration. It signifies the logarithm, on the base 10, of the reciprocal of the hydrogen-ion concentration. A pH above 7 represents alkalinity in an aqueous medium; below 7, acidity.

Ph¹ Symbol for Philadelphia chromosome.

phac-, phaco- A combining form meaning *lens.*

pha·ci·tis (fa·sigh'tis) *n.* Inflammation of the lens of the eye.

phaco-. See *phac-.*

phaco·an·a·phy·lax·is (fack''o·an''uh·fi·lack'sis)

n. Allergic reaction to crystalline lens protein. —**phacoanaphy·lac·tic** (·lack'tick) *adj.*

phaco·cele (fack'o·seel) *n.* Displacement of the crystalline lens from its proper position; herniation of the lens.

phaco·cyst (fack'o·sist) *n.* The capsule of the crystalline lens.

phaco·cys·tec·to·my (fack''o·sis·teck'tuh·mee) *n.* Excision of a part of the capsule of the crystalline lens.

pha·co·emul·si·fi·ca·tion (fay''ko·e·mul'si·fi'kay' shun) *n.* Extracapsular dissolution of a cataract using ultrasonic energy.

phac·oid (fack'oid, fay'koid) *adj.* Lens-shaped.

pha·col·y·sis (fa·kol'i·sis) *n.* 1. Dissolution or disintegration of the crystalline lens. 2. An operation for the relief of high myopia, consisting in discission of the crystalline lens followed by extraction. —**phaco·lyt·ic** (fack''o·lit'ick) *adj.*

pha·co·ma, pha·ko·ma (fa·ko'muh) *n.*, pl. **phaco·mas, phacoma·ta** (·tuh), **phakomas, phakoma·ta** (·tuh) 1. A lens-shaped retinal hamartoma, occurring in tuberous sclerosis. 2. Any of the hamartomatous masses occurring in familial neurocutaneous diseases such as Hippel-Lindau disease or tuberous sclerosis.

pha·co·ma·to·sis, pha·ko·ma·to·sis (fay''ko·muh·to'sis, fack''o·) *n.*, pl. **phacomato·ses, phakoma·to·ses** (·seez) A term applied by van der Hoeve (1920) to particular forms of neurocutaneous abnormality, which are often present in minor degree at birth and later evolved as quasineoplastic disorders. The latter include tuberous sclerosis, neurofibromatosis, and cutaneous angiomatosis with central nervous system abnormalities.

phaco·met·e·ce·sis (fack''o·met''e·see'sis) *n.* PHACOCELE.

pha·com·e·ter (fa·kom'e·tur) *n.* LENSOMETER.

phaco·pla·ne·sis (fack''o·pla·nee'sis) *n.* Displacement of the crystalline lens of the eye from the posterior to the anterior chamber and back again.

phaco·scle·ro·sis (fack''o·skle·ro'sis) *n.* Hardening of the crystalline lens.

phaco·scope (fack'o·skope) *n.* An instrument for observing the accommodative changes of the crystalline lens. —**pha·cos·co·py** (fa·kos'kuh·pee) *n.*

phaco·sco·tas·mus (fack''o·sko·taz'mus) *n.* Clouding of the crystalline lens.

phag-, phago- A combining form meaning (a) *eating, feeding;* (b) *phagocyte.*

phage (faij, fahzh) *n.* BACTERIOPHAGE.

-phage, -phag A combining form meaning *eater* or *that which ingests;* used especially to designate a *phagocyte.*

phag·e·de·na, phag·e·dae·na (faj''e·dee'nuh) *n.* A rapidly spreading destructive ulceration of soft parts. —**phage·den·ic, phage·daen·ic** (·den'ick) *adj.*

-phagia A combining form designating a *condition involving eating or swallowing.*

phago·cyte (fag'o·site) *n.* A cell having the property of engulfing and digesting foreign or other particles or cells harmful to the body. Fixed phagocytes include the cells of the reticuloendothelial system and fixed macrophages (histiocytes). Free phagocytes include the leukocytes and free macrophages. —**phago·cy·tal** (fag″o·sigh′tul), **phago·cyt·ic** (·sit′ick) adj.

phago·cyt·ize (fag′o·si·tize) v. To consume by enveloping and digesting; to subject to phagocytosis.

phago·cy·tol·y·sis (fag″o·sigh·tol′i·sis) n. Destruction or dissolution of phagocytes. —**phago·cy·to·lit·ic** (·sigh′to·lit′ick) adj.

phago·cy·to·sis (fag″o·sigh·to′sis) n., pl. **phagocy·to·ses** (·seez) Ingestion of foreign or other particles by certain cells. —**phago·cy·tose** (fag″o·sigh′toze) v.

phago·dy·na·mom·e·ter (fag″o·dye″nuh·mom′e·tur) n. An apparatus for estimating the force exerted in chewing.

phago·ma·nia (fag″o·may′nee·uh) n. An insatiable craving for food.

phago·some (fag′o·sohm) n. A single-membrane body in the cytoplasm, the result of either phagocytosis.

phago·ther·a·py (fag″o·therr′uh·pee) n. Treatment by superalimentation; overfeeding.

-phagous A combining form meaning eating or subsisting on.

phakomatosis. PHACOMATOSIS.

phal·a·cro·sis (fal″uh·kro′sis) n. BALDNESS.

pha·lan·ge·al (fa·lan′jee·ul) adj. Pertaining to a phalanx or phalanges.

phal·an·gec·to·my (fal″an·jeck′tuh·mee) n. Surgical excision of a phalanx of a finger or toe.

phalanges. Plural of phalanx.

phal·an·gi·tis (fal″an·jye′tis) n. Inflammation of a phalanx.

pha·lan·gi·za·tion (fa·lan″ji·zay′shun) n. A plastic operation in which a metacarpal bone is separated from its fellows and surrounded with skin, thus forming a substitute for a finger or thumb.

pha·lan·go·pha·lan·ge·al (fa·lang″go·fuh·lan′jee·ul) adj. Pertaining to the successive phalanges of the digits, as in phalangophalangeal amputation, removal of a finger or toe at an interphalangeal joint.

pha·lanx (fay′lanks, fal′anks) n., genit. **pha·lan·gis** (fa·lan′jis), pl. **phalan·ges** (·jeez) 1. One of the bones of the fingers or toes. 2. One of the delicate processes of the headplate of the outer rod of Corti projecting beyond the inner rod.

phal·lic (fal′ick) adj. Pertaining to the penis or phallus.

phallic symbol. In psychoanalysis, any form resembling or suggestive of a penis, as a snake, obelisk, tower, or pencil; often employed in dreams and other mental processes to disguise sexual wishes.

phallic urethra. UROGENITAL TUBE.

phal·lo·plas·ty (fal′o·plas″tee) n. Plastic construction or repair of the penis.

phal·lus (fal′us) n., pl. **phal·li** (·lye), **phalluses** 1. The penis, or an analogous organ in certain invertebrates and nonmammalian vertebrates. 2. The indifferent embryonic structure derived from the genital tubercle that, in the male, differentiates into the penis, and, in the female, into the clitoris. —**phal·li·form** (·i·form), **phal·loid** (·oid) adj.

-phane A combining form designating a substance having a (specified) form or appearance.

phan·ero·gam (fan′ur·o·gam) n. A plant which bears seeds. —**phanero·gam·ic** (·gam′ick) adj.

phan·ero·gen·ic (fan″ur·o·jen′ick) adj. Having a known cause.

phan·ero·ma·nia (fan″ur·o·may′nee·uh) n. A compulsive tendency to handle some external part or growth, such as a pimple, a hair, or a hangnail.

phan·er·o·sis (fan″ur·o′sis) n., pl. **phanero·ses** (·seez) The act of passing from a transparent to a visible state.

phan·tasm (fan′taz·um) n. 1. An illusive perception of an object that does not exist. 2. An illusion or a hallucination. —**phan·tas·mic** (fan·taz′mick) adj.

phan·tas·ma·to·mo·ria (fan·taz″muh·to·mo′ree·uh) n. Childishness, or dementia, with absurd fancies or delusions.

phan·tas·mo·sco·pia (fan·taz″mo·sko′pee·uh) n. The seeing of phantasms; hallucinations involving ghosts.

phan·tom (fan′tum) n. 1. An image formed in the mind; a thing or person which takes the place of the real object in a given situation, such as in an experiment. 2. The outward manifestation of a thing or person after the essential or substantive element has been lost. 3. In radiology, an object made of substances with densities similar to tissue which simulates tissues in absorbing and scattering radiation and permits determination of the dose of radiation delivered to the surface of and within the simulated tissues through measurements within ionization chambers placed within the phantom material. Also used to establish and check radiographic and other imaging techniques.

phantom limb, sensations, or **pain.** A psychological phenomenon frequently occurring in amputees: the patient feels sensations, and often pain, in the missing limb.

phantom odontalgia. Pain felt in the space from which a tooth has been removed.

phantom pregnancy. PSEUDOCYESIS.

phantom tumor. A swelling simulating a tumor; produced usually by the contraction of a muscle or by gaseous distention of the intestine.

phar·ma·cal (fahr′muh·kul) adj. Pertaining to pharmacy.

phar·ma·ceu·tic (fahr″muh·sue′tick) adj. Pertaining to pharmacy.

phar·ma·ceu·ti·cal (fahr″muh·sue′ti·kul) adj. & n. 1. PHARMACEUTIC. 2. A medicinal drug.

phar·ma·cist (fahr′muh·sist) n. One engaged in the practice of pharmacy; an apothecary.

pharmaco- A combining form meaning drug.

phar·ma·co·dy·nam·ics (fahr″muh·ko·dye·nam′icks, ·di·nam′icks) n. The science of the action of drugs. —**pharmacodynam·ic** (·ick) adj.

phar·ma·co·ge·net·ics (fahr″muh·ko·je·net′icks) n. The discipline that deals with genetically determined variations in drug responses.

phar·ma·cog·no·sy (fahr″muh·kog′nuh·see) n. The science of crude natural drugs.

phar·ma·col·o·gist (fahr″muh·kol′uh·jist) n. One versed in pharmacology.

phar·ma·col·o·gy (fahr″muh·kol′uh·jee) n. The

science of the nature and properties of drugs, particularly their actions. **—pharma·co·log·ic** (·ko·loj'ick), **pharmacologic·al** (·ul) adj.

phar·ma·co·ma·nia (fahr''muh·ko·may'nee·uh) n. 1. An abnormal craving for medicines, or for self-medication. 2. An abnormal desire to administer medications.

phar·ma·co·pe·ia, phar·ma·co·poe·ia (fahr'' muh·ko·pee'uh) n. A book containing a selected list of medicinal substances and their dosage forms, providing also a description and the standards for purity and strength for each. **—pharmacope·ial, pharmacopoe·ial** (·ul) adj.

phar·ma·co·pho·bia (fahr''muh·ko·fo'bee·uh) n. Abnormal dislike or fear of medicine.

phar·ma·co·psy·cho·sis (fahr''muh·ko·sigh·ko' sis) n. Any organic brain syndrome associated with ingestion of a drug, alcohol, or poison.

phar·ma·co·ther·a·py (fahr''muh·ko·therr'uh·pee) n. The treatment of disease by means of drugs.

phar·ma·cy (fahr'muh·see) n. 1. The art and science of preparing and dispensing drugs used for the prevention, diagnosis, or treatment of disease. 2. A place where drugs are compounded and dispensed.

pharyng-, pharyngo- A combining form meaning *pharynx, pharyngeal.*

phar·yn·gal·gia (fār''ing·gal'jee·uh) n. Pain in the pharynx.

phar·yn·ge·al (fa·rin'jee·ul, ·jul, fār''in·jee'ul) adj. Pertaining to the pharynx.

pharyngeal bursa. A small pit caudal to the pharyngeal tonsil, resulting from the ingrowth of epithelium along the course of the degenerating tip of the notochord.

pharyngeal bursitis. Purulent or mucopurulent inflammation of a pharyngeal bursa.

pharyngeal pouch. One of a series of five paired lateral sacculations of the embryonic pharynx corresponding to the ectodermal grooves between the pharyngeal arches.

pharyngeal tonsil. ADENOID (3).

phar·yn·gec·to·my (fār''in·jeck'tuh·mee) n. Excision of a part of the pharynx.

phar·yn·ge·us (fa·rin'jee·us) L. adj. PHARYNGEAL.

phar·yn·gism (fār'in·jiz'um) n. PHARYNGISMUS.

phar·yn·gis·mus (fār''in·jiz'mus) n. Spasm of the pharynx.

phar·yn·gi·tis (fār''in·jye'tis) n., pl. **pharyn·git·i·des** (·jit'i·deez) Inflammation of the pharynx. **—pharyn·git·ic** (·jit'ick) adj.

pharyngitis sic·ca (sick'uh). The atrophic form of pharyngitis characterized by a very dry state of the mucous membrane.

pha·ryn·go·cele (fa·ring'go·seel) n. A hernia or pouch of the pharyngeal mucosa projecting through the pharyngeal wall.

pha·ryn·go·con·junc·ti·val (fa·ring''go·kon''junk·tye'vul) adj. Of or pertaining to the pharynx and the conjunctiva.

pharyngoconjunctival fever. An epidemic disease of children, caused by an adenovirus, and characterized by fever, pharyngitis, conjunctivitis, rhinitis, and cervical lymphadenopathy.

pha·ryn·go·dyn·ia (fa·ring''go·din'ee·uh) n. Pain referred to the pharynx.

pha·ryn·go·epi·glot·tic (fa·ring''go·ep''i·glot'ick)

adj. Pertaining to the pharynx and the epiglottis.

pha·ryn·go·esoph·a·ge·al, pha·ryn·go·oesoph·a·ge·al (fa·ring''go·e·sof''uh·jee'ul) adj. Pertaining to the pharynx and esophagus.

pha·ryn·go·glos·sal (fa·ring''go·glos'ul) adj. Pertaining conjointly to the pharynx and the tongue.

pha·ryn·go·ker·a·to·sis (fa·ring''go·kerr''uh·to' sis) n. Thickening of the mucous lining of the pharynx with formation of a tough and adherent exudate.

pha·ryn·go·la·ryn·ge·al (fa·ring''go·la·rin'jee·ul) adj. Pertaining both to the pharynx and to the larynx.

pha·ryn·go·lar·yn·gi·tis (fa·ring''go·lār''in·jye'tis) n. Simultaneous inflammation of the pharynx and larynx.

pha·ryn·go·lith (fa·ring'go·lith) n. A calcareous concretion in the walls of the pharynx.

phar·yn·gol·o·gy (fār''ing·gol'uh·jee) n. The science of the pharyngeal mechanism, functions, and diseases.

phar·yn·gol·y·sis (fār''ing·gol'i·sis) n. PHARYNGOPLEGIA.

pha·ryn·go·max·il·lary (fa·ring''go·mack'si·lerr·ee) adj. Pertaining to the pharynx and the maxilla.

pha·ryn·go·my·co·sis (fa·ring''go·migh·ko'sis) n. Disease of the pharynx due to the action of fungi.

pha·ryn·go·na·sal (fa·ring''go·nay'zul) adj. Pertaining to the pharynx and the nose, as pharyngonasal cavity.

pha·ryn·go·pal·a·tine (fa·ring''go·pal'uh·tine) adj. PALATOPHARYNGEAL.

pha·ryn·go·pa·ral·y·sis (fa·ring''go·puh·ral'i·sis) n. PHARYNGOPLEGIA.

phar·yn·gop·a·thy (fār''ing·gop'uth·ee) n. Any disease of the pharynx.

pha·ryn·go·plas·ty (fa·ring''go·plas'tee) n. Reconstruction of the pharynx by surgery.

pha·ryn·go·ple·gia (fa·ring''go·plee'juh, ·jee·uh) n. Paralysis of the muscles of the pharynx.

pha·ryn·go·rhi·ni·tis (fa·ring''go·rye·nigh'tis) n. Pharyngitis with rhinitis; inflammation of the pharyngeal and nasal mucosa.

pha·ryn·gor·rha·gia (fa·ring''go·ray'juh, ·jee·uh) n. Hemorrhage from the pharynx.

pha·ryn·gor·rhea, pha·ryn·gor·rhoea (fa·ring''go·ree'uh) n. A mucous discharge from the pharynx.

pha·ryn·go·scope (fa·ring'go·skope) n. An instrument for use in examining the pharynx. **—phar·in·gos·co·py** (fār''ing·gos'kuh·pee) n.

pha·ryn·go·spasm (fa·ring'go·spaz·um) n. Spasmodic contraction of the pharynx. **—phar·yn·go·spas·mod·ic** (fa·ring''go·spaz·mod'ick) adj.

phar·yn·got·o·my (fār''ing·got'uh·mee) n. Incision into the pharynx.

pha·ryn·go·ton·sil·li·tis (fa·ring''go·ton''si·lye'tis) n. Inflammation of the pharynx and the tonsils.

pha·ryn·go·xe·ro·sis (fa·ring''go·ze·ro'sis) n. Dryness of the pharynx.

phar·ynx (fār'inks) n., genit. **pha·ryn·gis** (fa·rin'jis), pl. **pharyn·ges** (·jeez) The musculomembranous tube situated back of the nose, mouth, and larynx, and extending from the base of the skull to a point opposite the sixth cervical vertebra, where it becomes continuous with the esophagus. It is lined by mucous membrane, covered in its upper part with pseudo-stratified ciliated epithelium, in its lower part with stratified squamous epithelium.

phase, *n.* 1. The condition or stage of a disease or of biologic, chemical, physiologic, and psychologic functions at a given time. 2. A solid, liquid, or gas which is homogeneous throughout and physically separated from another phase by a distinct boundary. 3. A stage or interval in a periodic or developmental cycle.

phase microscope. A microscope that permits visualization of the parts of an object by converting phase differences in light transmitted through the object into amplitude differences, thereby providing contrast perceivable by the eye.

-phasia, -phasy A combining form meaning *speech disorder.*

pha·sic (fay'zick) *adj.* Pertaining to a phase; having phases.

phasic sinus arrhythmia. Cyclic speeding of the heart rate during inspiration with a slowing during expiration; occasionally the waxing and waning of the heart rate is independent of respiration.

phas·mid (faz'mid) *n.* A minute sensory organ the presence or absence of which determines membership in the complementary nematode subclasses Phasmidia and Aphasmidia; thought to be an olfactory receptor.

-phemia A combining form meaning *speech disorder.*

phen-, pheno- A combining form meaning (a) *light, bright;* (b) *appearing, manifest;* (c) *derivation from benzene.*

phe·nac·e·tin (fe·nas'e·tin) *n.* p-Acetophenetidide, $C_2H_5OC_6H_4NHCOCH_3$, an antipyretic and analgesic drug. Syn. *acetophenetidin.*

phe·nate (fee'nate) *n.* A salt of phenol (1).

phen·az·o·pyr·i·dine (fen·az''o·pirr'i·deen) *n.* 2,6-Diamino-3-phenylazopyridine, $C_{11}H_{11}N_5$, a urinary analgesic drug; used as the hydrochloride salt.

Phenergan. Trademark for promethazine, an antihistaminic drug used as the hydrochloride salt.

phen·go·pho·bia (fen''go·fo'bee·uh) *n.* A morbid fear of daylight.

phe·nin·da·mine (fe·nin'duh·meen, ·min) *n.* 2,3,4,9-Tetrahydro-2-methyl-9-phenyl-1*H*-indeno-[2,1-c]pyridine, $C_{19}H_{19}N$; an antihistaminic drug used as the tartrate salt.

phen·in·di·one (fen''in·dye'ohn) *n.* 2-Phenyl-1,3-indandione, $C_{15}H_{10}O_2$, an anticoagulant.

phen·met·ra·zine (fen·met'ruh·zeen) *n.* 3-Methyl-2-phenylmorpholine, $C_{11}H_{15}NO$, a sympathomimetic drug used as an anorexiant; employed as the hydrochloride salt.

phe·no·bar·bi·tal (fee''no·bahr'bi·tol) *n.* 5-Ethyl-5-phenylbarbituric acid, $C_{12}H_{12}N_2O_3$, a long-acting sedative and hypnotic barbiturate. Syn. *phenobarbitone.*

phe·no·copy (fee'no·kop''ee) *n.* An experimen-

tally produced effect on the body which copies the appearance of genetic effects, e.g., tanning produced by ultraviolet light which duplicates hereditary pigmentation.

phe·no·din (fee'no·din) *n.* HEMATIN.

phe·nol (fee'nol) *n.* 1. Hydroxybenzene or phenyl hydroxide, C_6H_5OH, colorless to light pink crystals. Used as a disinfectant, topical anesthetic, escharotic, and antipruritic. Syn. *carbolic acid.* 2. Any hydroxy derivative of aromatic hydrocarbons that has the OH group directly attached to the ring.

phenol coefficient. A number which indicates the germicidal efficiency of a compound relative to phenol.

phe·nol·phthal·ein (fee''nol·thal'een, ·thal'ee·in) *n.* 3,3-Bis(p-hydroxyphenyl)phthalide, $C_{20}H_{14}O_4$, a white or faintly yellowish powder; a cathartic drug, also used as an indicator of acidity or alkalinity.

phe·nol·phthal·in (fee''nol·thal'in) *n.* 4',4''-Dihydroxytriphenylmethane-2-carboxylic acid, $C_{20}H_{16}O_4$; used as a reagent for detecting the presence of blood.

phe·nol·sul·fon·phthal·ein (fee''nol·sul''fon·thal'een, ·ee·in) *n.* 4,4'-(3*H*-2,1-Benzoxathiol-3-ylidene)diphenol S,S-dioxide, $C_{19}H_{14}O_5S$, a bright to dark red crystalline powder. Used as a diagnostic aid, by intramuscular or intravenous injection, to determine kidney function. Syn. *phenol red.*

phenolsulfonphthalein test. A test for kidney function based upon the ability of the kidneys to excrete phenolsulfonphthalein which has been injected intravenously or intramuscularly. From 50 to 70% of the injected P.S.P. is normally excreted in the urine within 2 hours. Abbreviated, P.S.P.

phe·nol·uria (fee''nol·yoo'ree·uh) *n.* The presence of phenols in the urine.

phe·nom·e·non (fe·nom'e·nun, ·non) *n.,* pl. **phe·nome·na** (·nuh) An event or manifestation.

-phenone A combining form meaning *an aromatic ketone that contains a phenyl or substituted phenyl group attached to an acyl group,* as in acetophenone and benzophenone.

phe·no·pho·bia (fee''no·fo'bee·uh) *n.* Fear of daylight.

phe·no·thi·a·zine (fee''no·thigh'uh·zeen, ·zin) *n.* Thiodiphenylamine, $C_{12}H_9NS$, a veterinary anthelmintic drug. Derivatives of phenothiazine are important drugs used in human and veterinary medicine.

phe·no·type (fee'no·tipe) *n.* 1. The sum total of visible traits which characterize the members of a group. 2. The visible expression of genotype. —**phe·no·typ·ic** (fee''no·tip'ick) *adj.;* **phe·notyp·i·cal·ly** (·i·kuh·lee) *adv.*

phe·noxy·ben·za·mine (fe·nock''see·ben'zuh·meen) *n.* N-(2-Chloroethyl)-N'-(1-methyl-2-phenoxyethyl)benzylamine, $C_{18}H_{22}ClNO$, an adrenergic blocking agent used as the hydrochloride salt as a peripheral vasodilator.

phen·tol·a·mine (fen·tol'uh·meen) *n.* m-[N-(2-Imidazolin-2-ylmethyl)-p-toluidino]phenol, $C_{17}H_{19}N_3O$, an adrenergic blocking drug used in the diagnosis of pheochromocytoma; employed as the hydrochloride and mesylate salts.

phen·yl (fen′il, fee′nil) n. The univalent radical C_6H_5—. —**phe·nyl·ic** (fe·nil′ick) adj.

phen·yl·al·a·nine (fen″il·al′uh·neen) n. α-Amino-β-phenylpropionic acid, $C_6H_5CH_2$·$CH(NH_2)COOH$, an amino acid essential in human nutrition.

phen·yl·al·a·ne·mia, phen·yl·al·a·nin·ae·mia (fen″il·al″uh·ni·nee′mee·uh) n. HYPERPHENYL-ALANINEMIA.

L-phenylalanine mustard. MELPHALAN.

phen·yl·bu·ta·zone (fen″il·bew′tuh·zone) n. 4-Butyl-1,2-diphenyl-3,5-pyrazolidinedione, $C_{19}H_{20}N_2O_2$, an analgesic, antipyretic, and anti-inflammatory drug.

phen·yl·cin·cho·nin·ic acid (fen″il·sing″ko·nin′ick). CINCHOPHEN.

phen·yl·eph·rine (fen″il·ef′reen, -rin) n. l-m-Hydroxy-α-[(methylamino)methyl]benzyl alcohol, $C_9H_{13}NO_2$, a sympathomimetic amine used as a vasoconstrictor; employed as the hydrochloride salt.

phen·yl·eth·yl·bar·bi·tu·ric acid (fen″il·eth″il·bahr″bi·tew′rick). PHENOBARBITAL.

phen·yl·hy·dra·zine (fen″il·high′druh·zeen) n. Hydrazinobenzene, $C_6H_5NHNH_2$, variously used as a reagent, especially in reactions involving aldehydes and ketones. It is a hemolysin, a property once used therapeutically.

phe·nyl·ic acid (fe·nil′ick). PHENOL.

phen·yl·ke·to·nu·ria (fen″il·kee″to·new′ree·uh) n. 1. The presence of phenylketone in the urine. 2. A hereditary (autosomal recessive) metabolic disorder in which there is a deficiency of phenylalanine hydroxylase, resulting in increased amounts of phenylalanine in the blood and of excess phenylpyruvic and other acids in the urine; characterized clinically in the typical untreated case by mental retardation, eczema, fair hair, and occasionally seizures; mentally normal untreated cases occur; transmitted as an autosomal recessive trait. Abbreviated, PKU. —**phenylketonu·ric** (·rick) adj.

phenyl·mer·cu·ric (fen″il·mur·kew′rick) adj. Signifying the monovalent organomercurial cation $C_6H_5Hg^+$, which forms salts (acetate, borate, chloride, nitrate) that have antiseptic, germicidal, and fungicidal action.

phen·yl·pro·pa·nol·amine (fen″il·pro″puh·nol′uh·meen, ·min) n. 1-Phenyl-2-aminopropanol, $C_9H_{13}NO$, a sympathomimetic amine used mainly as a bronchodilator; employed as the hydrochloride salt.

phen·yl·pro·pyl·meth·yl·amine (fen″il·pro″pil·meth′il·uh·meen) n. N,β-Dimethylphenethylamine, $C_{10}H_{15}N$, a sympathomimetic amine used locally, as the base or hydrochloride salt, to shrink nasal mucosa.

phen·yl·py·ru·vic acid (fen″il·pye·roo′vick, ·pi·roo′vick). A metabolic product, $C_6H_5CH_2COCOOH$, of phenylalanine; the state of mental deficiency known as phenylketonuria is characterized by excretion of the acid.

phenylpyruvic amentia or **oligophrenia.** Mental retardation in phenylketonuria.

phen·yl·thio·urea (fen″il·thigh″o·yoo·ree′uh) n. Phenylthiocarbamide, $C_6H_5NHCSNH_2$, a compound of interest in genetics research because it is bitter to most persons but tasteless to others; non-tasting is recessively inherited.

pheo-, phaeo- A combining form meaning brown, brownish.

pheo·chro·mo·blas·to·ma, phaeo·chro·mo·blas·to·ma (fee″o·kro″mo·blas·to′muh) n. A pheochromocytoma made up of less well differentiated cells.

pheo·chro·mo·cy·to·ma (fee″o·kro″mo·sigh·to′muh) n., pl. **pheochromocytomas, pheochromo·cyto·ma·ta** (·tuh) A tumor of the sympathetic nervous system, found most often in the adrenal medulla but occasionally in other sites such as paraganglia and in the thorax. It is made up largely of pheochromocytes, or chromaffin cells, with a strong affinity for taking up chrome salts. May be accompanied by the adrenal-sympathetic syndrome of spasmodic or persistent hypertension.

phe·re·sis (fe·ree′sis) n. The removal from a donor's blood of one or more of its components, followed by return of the remainder to the donor.

Ph.G. Graduate in Pharmacy; German Pharmacopoeia.

Phialophora ver·ru·co·sa (verr″yoo·ko′suh). A species of fungus which is one of the causative agents of chromoblastomycosis.

phil-, philo- A combining form meaning (a) love of or loving; (b) affinity for or having an affinity for.

-phil, -phile A suffix designating a substance having an affinity for, as acidophil, having an affinity for acid stains.

Phil·a·del·phia chromosome. A number 22 chromosome with a deletion of the long arm found in the hematopoietic cells of many patients with chronic granulocytic leukemia. Symbol, Ph^1.

-philia A combining form meaning (a) craving for, abnormal tendency toward; (b) affinity for.

phil·i·a·ter (fil′ee·ay″tur, fi·lye′uh·tur) n. 1. A student of medicine. 2. A dabbler in medicine.

-philic A combining form meaning (a) having an affinity for; (b) loving.

philo·ne·ism (fil′o·nee′iz·um) n. Abnormal love of novelty.

philo·pat·ri·do·ma·nia (fil″o·pat″ri·do·may′nee·uh) n. Abnormal homesickness.

-philous A combining form meaning (a) having an affinity for; (b) loving.

phil·trum (fil′trum) n., pl. **phil·tra** (·truh) The depression on the surface of the upper lip immediately below the septum of the nose.

phi·mo·sis (figh·mo′sis, fi·mo′sis) n., pl. **phimo·ses** (·seez) Elongation of the prepuce and constriction of the orifice, so that the foreskin cannot be retracted to uncover the glans penis. —**phi·mot·ic** (·mot′ick) adj.

phleb-, phlebo- A combining form meaning vein, venous.

phleb·an·gi·o·ma (fleb·an″jee·o′muh) n. A venous aneurysm.

phleb·ar·te·ri·ec·ta·sia (fleb″ahr·teer″ee·eck·tay′

zee·uh, ·zhuh) *n.* General arterial and venous dilation.

phleb·ar·te·rio·di·al·y·sis (fleb''ahr·teer''ee·o·dye·al'i·sis) *n.* ARTERIOVENOUS FISTULA.

phleb·ec·ta·sia (fleb''eck·tay'zee·uh, ·zhuh) *n.* Dilatation of a vein; varicosity. —**phlebec·tat·ic** (·tat'ick) *adj.*

phleb·ec·ta·sis (fle·beck'tuh·sis) *n.* PHLEBECTASIA.

phle·bec·to·my (fle·beck'tuh·mee) *n.* Excision of a vein or a portion of a vein.

phleb·ec·to·pia (fleb''eck·to'pee·uh) *n.* The displacement, or abnormal position, of a vein.

phleb·ex·er·e·sis (fleb''eck·serr'e·sis) *n.* Excision of a vein.

phle·bis·mus (fle·biz'mus) *n.* Persistent overdistention of a vein, usually caused by obstruction.

phle·bi·tis (fle·bye'tis) *n.,* pl. **phle·bit·i·des** (·bit'i·deez) Inflammation of a vein, with or without infection and thrombus formation. —**phle·bit·ic** (fle·bit'ick) *adj.*

phlebo·car·ci·no·ma (fleb''o·kahr''si·no'muh) *n.* Extension of carcinoma to the walls of a vein.

phle·boc·ly·sis (fle·bock'li·sis, fleb''o·klye'sis) *n.* The intravenous injection of a large quantity of any solution.

phlebo·gram (fleb'o·gram) *n.* 1. A radiograph of a vein after the intravascular injection of a radiopaque material. Syn. *venogram.* 2. A tracing or recording of the venous pulse.

phlebo·graph (fleb'o·graf) *n.* An instrument for recording the venous pulse.

phle·bog·ra·phy (fle·bog'ruh·fee) *n.* 1. The radiographic imaging with x-rays of a vein or veins following intravenous injection of a radiopaque substance. 2. Recording of venous pulsations.

phlebo·lith (fleb'o·lith) *n.* A calculus in a vein. —**phlebo·lith·ic** (fleb''o·lith'ick) *adj.*

phlebo·li·thi·a·sis (fleb''o·li·thigh'uh·sis) *n.* The formation of pheboliths.

phlebo·ma·nom·e·ter (fleb''o·ma·nom'e·tur) *n.* An apparatus for the direct measurement of venous pressure.

phlebo·phle·bos·to·my (fleb''o·fle·bos'tuh·mee) *n.* An operation in which an anastomosis is made between veins.

phlebo·plas·ty (fleb'o·plas''tee) *n.* Plastic operation for the repair of veins.

phleb·or·rha·gia (fleb''o·ray'jee·uh) *n.* A venous hemorrhage.

phle·bor·rha·phy (fle·bor'uh·fee) *n.* Suture of a vein.

phleb·or·rhex·is (fleb''o·reck'sis) *n.* Rupture of a vein.

phlebo·scle·ro·sis (fleb''o·skle·ro'sis) *n.* 1. Sclerosis of a vein. 2. Chronic phlebitis.

phle·bos·ta·sis (fle·bos'tuh·sis) *n.* 1. Temporary removal of some blood from the general circulation by compression of the veins in the extremities. Syn. *bloodless phlebotomy.* 2. Slowing or cessation of venous blood flow.

phlebo·ste·no·sis (fleb''o·ste·no'sis) *n.* Constriction of a vein.

phlebo·throm·bo·sis (fleb''o·throm·bo'sis) *n.* Formation or presence of a thrombus in a vein without associated inflammation.

phlebo·tome (fleb'uh·tome) *n.* A cutting instrument used in phlebotomy.

Phle·bot·o·mus (fle·bot'uh·mus) *n.* A genus of small bloodsucking sandflies of the family Psychodidae. The species *Phlebotomus argentipes* transmits the flagellates of kala-azar in India, *P. chinensis* in China; *P. papatasii* is the vector of pappataci fever, phlebotomus sandfly fever of the Balkans. *P. verrucarum* is the vector for *Bartonella bacilliformis,* the causative agent of bartonellosis, or Carrión's disease (Oroya fever and verruca peruviana).

phlebotomus fever. An acute viral infection characterized by fever, headache, ocular pain, conjunctivitis, leukopenia, and malaise, followed by complete recovery. Occurs during the hot dry season in the Mediterranean area, Asia Minor, and India, where the vector fly, *Phlebotomus papatasii,* exists. Syn. *pappataci fever, sandfly fever.*

phle·bot·o·my (fle·bot'uh·mee) *n.* The opening of a vein for the purpose of letting blood. —**phlebo·mist** (·mist) *n.*

phlegm (flem) *n.* 1. A viscid, stringy mucus, secreted by the mucosa of the air passages. 2. One of the four humors of the Hippocratic formulation of general pathology.

phleg·ma·sia (fleg·may'zhuh) *n.* INFLAMMATION.

phlegmasia al·ba do·lens (al'buh do'lenz) A painful swelling of the leg usually seen post partum, due to femoral vein thrombophlebitis or lymphatic obstruction. Syn. *milk leg.*

phleg·mat·ic (fleg·mat'ick) *adj.* 1. Of the nature of phlegm or related to phlegm. 2. Characterized by an apathetic, sluggish, dull temperament.

phleg·mon (fleg'mon, ·mun) *n.* Pyogenic inflammation with infiltration and spread in the tissues; seen with invasive organisms which produce hyaluronidases and fibrinolysins. —**phleg·mon·ous** (·mun·us) *adj.*

phlo·rhi·zin (flo·rye'zin, flor'i·zin) *n.* A glycoside, $C_{21}H_{24}O_{10}$, obtained from the bark and root of certain fruit trees; used experimentally to produce glycosuria in animals. Syn. *phlorizin, phloridzin, phlorrhizin.*

phlox·ine (flock'seen, ·sin) *n.* A red acid dye of the xanthine series; used as a counterstain with blue nuclear dyes.

phlox·ino·phil·ic (flock''sin·o·fil'ick) *adj.* Having an affinity for phloxine.

phlyc·te·na (flick·tee'nuh) *n.,* pl. **phlyc·te·nae** (·nee) A vesicle. —**phlyc·te·nar** (flick'te·nur), **phlyc·te·nous** (·nus) *adj.*

phlyctenular conjunctivitis. PHLYCTENULAR KERATOCONJUNCTIVITIS.

phlyc·te·nule (flick'te·newl) *n.* A minute phlyctena; a little vesicle or blister. —**phlyc·ten·u·lar** (flick·ten'yoo·lur) *adj.*

phlyc·ten·u·lo·sis (flick·ten''yoo·lo'sis) *n.* The presence of phlyctenules.

-phobe. A combining form meaning (a) *resisting, avoiding;* (b) *one having a phobia.*

-phobia A combining form meaning *fear* or *dread.*

pho·bia (fo'bee·uh) *n.* A disproportionate, obsessive, persistent, and unrealistic fear of an external situation or object, symbolically taking the place of an internal unconscious conflict. —**pho·bic** (·bick) *adj.*

pho·bo·pho·bia (fo″bo·fo′bee·uh) *n.* An abnormal dread of being afraid or of developing a phobia.

pho·co·me·lia (fo″ko·mee′lee·uh) *n.* Absence or markedly imperfect development of arms and forearms, thighs and legs, but with hands and feet present. —**phocome·lic** (·lick) *adj.*

Pho·ma (fo′muh) *n.* A genus of fungi whose species may act as common allergens and as laboratory contaminants.

phon-, phono- A combining form meaning (a) *sound;* (b) *speech, voice.*

pho·nal (fo′nul) *adj.* Pertaining to the voice or to sound.

phon·as·the·nia (fo″nas·theen′ee·uh) *n.* Weakness of voice, especially that resulting from bodily exhaustion.

pho·na·tion (fo·nay′shun) *n.* The production of vocal sound. —**pho·nate** (fo′nate) *v.;* **pho·na·to·ry** (fo′nuh·tor″ee) *adj.*

pho·neme (fo′neem) *n.* 1. A speech sound or range of sounds as a structural and functional unit in the sound system of a particular language. 2. An auditory hallucination of hearing speech.

pho·net·ic (fo·net′ick) *adj.* 1. Pertaining to speech sounds. 2. Pertaining to phonetics.

pho·net·ics (fo·net′icks) *n.* The analysis and description of speech sounds in terms of the processes by which they are produced (articulatory phonetics), the physical properties of the sounds themselves (acoustic phonetics), and the relation of these properties to the articulatory and auditory processes.

-phonia, -phony A combining form meaning (a) *sound;* (b) *vocal or speech disorder.*

pho·ni·at·rics (fo″nee·at′ricks) *n.* The study and treatment of the voice.

phon·ic (fon′ick) *adj.* 1. Of or pertaining to the voice. 2. Of or pertaining to phonics.

phon·ics (fon′icks) *n.* 1. The science of sound. 2. The methodology of teaching reading by the association of letters with phonemes, as opposed to the association of word·configurations with spoken words or with concepts.

phonic spasm. A spasm of the laryngeal muscles occurring on attempting to speak, usually a component of a conversion reaction, but also seen in professional singers and speakers due to faulty voice production.

pho·nism (fo′niz·um) *n.* A form of synesthesia in which there is a sensation of sound or hearing, due to the effect of sight, touch, taste, or smell, or even to the thought of some object, person, or general conception.

phono-. See *phon-.*

pho·no·car·dio·gram (fo″no·kahr′dee·o·gram) *n.* A graphic record of heart sounds and murmurs.

pho·no·car·dio·graph (fo″no·kahr′dee·o·graf) *n.* An instrument for recording heart sounds and murmurs. —**phono·car·dio·graph·ic** (·kahr″dee·o·graf′ick) *adj.*

pho·no·car·di·og·ra·phy (fo″no·kahr″dee·og′ruh·fee) *n.* The graphic recording of heart sounds and murmurs.

pho·nol·o·gy (fo·nol′uh·jee) *n.* The analysis and description of speech sounds in terms of the linguistic systems in which they function.

pho·no·mas·sage (fo″no·muh·sahj′) *n.* Stimulation and exercise of the tympanic membrane and ossicular chain, by alternating pressure and suction in the external auditory meatus.

pho·no·my·oc·lo·nus (fo″no·migh·ock′luh·nus, ·migh″o·klo′nus) *n.* A condition in which a sound is heard on auscultation over a muscle, indicating fibrillary contractions which may be so fine that they are not seen on visual inspection.

pho·nop·a·thy (fo·nop′uth·ee) *n.* Any disorder or disease of the voice.

pho·no·pho·bia (fo″no·fo′bee·uh) *n.* 1. A fear of speaking or of one's own voice; may be due to the pain caused by speaking, as in certain organic disorders. 2. Abnormal fear of any sound or noise.

-phor, -phore A combining form meaning *bearer, carrier.*

phor-, phoro- A combining form meaning (a) *carrying, transmission;* (b) *bearing, supporting;* (c) *directing, turning.*

-phoresis A combining form meaning *transmission.*

-phoria A combining form meaning (a) *tendency;* (b) *turning of the visual axis,* as in exophoria.

-phoric A combining form meaning *bearing, carrying.*

pho·rom·e·ter (fo·rom′e·tur) *n.* An instrument for measuring the relative strength of the ocular muscles.

phoro·scope (for′uh·skope) *n.* An apparatus for testing vision, consisting of a trial frame for lenses, fixed to a bench or table.

phoro·tone (for′uh·tone) *n.* An apparatus for exercising the eye muscles.

phose (foze) *n.* Any subjective sensation of light or color, as scintillating scotoma of migraine.

phos·gene (fos′jeen, foz′) *n.* Carbonyl chloride, $COCl_2$, a colorless gas that has been used in chemical warfare.

phosph-, phospho-. A combining form meaning *phosphorous* or *phosphoric.*

phosphataemia. PHOSPHATEMIA.

phos·pha·tase (fos′fuh·tace, ·taze) *n.* An enzyme that catalyzes hydrolysis of esters of phosphoric acid. Numerous phosphatases are known to exist; they play an important role in various metabolic processes, and in bone formation.

phos·phate (fos′fate) *n.* A salt of phosphoric acid.

phos·pha·te·mia, phos·pha·tae·mia (fos″fuh·tee′mee·uh, fos″fay·) *n.* 1. The presence of phosphates in the circulating blood. 2. HYPERPHOSPHATEMIA.

phos·phene (fos′feen) *n.* A subjective, luminous sensation due to stimulation of the retina by stimuli other than light.

phos·phine (fos′feen, ·fin) *n.* 1. Hydrogen phosphide, PH_3, a poisonous gas with a garlicky odor. 2. A substitution compound of PH_3, bearing the same relation to it that an amine does to ammonia.

phos·pho·cre·a·tine (fos″fo·kree′uh·teen, ·tin) *n.* Creatine phosphate, $C_4H_{10}N_3O_5P$, a phosphoric acid derivative of creatine which contains an energy-rich phosphate bond. Phosphocreatine is present in muscle and other tissues, and during the anaerobic phase of muscular contraction it reacts with ADP to form creatine and ATP and makes energy available for the contractile process.

phos·pho·enol·py·ru·vic acid (fos"fo·ee"nol·pye·roo'vick). 2-Phosphoenolpyruvic acid; $CH_2=COP(O)(OH)_2COOH$; a high-energy phosphate formed by dehydration of 2-phosphoglyceric acid; it reacts with adenosine diphosphate to form adenosine triphosphate and enolpyruvic acid.

phos·pho·fruc·to·ki·nase (fos"fo·fruck"to·kigh'nace, ·naze) *n.* Any enzyme that catalyzes the biochemical conversion of fructose 6-phosphate to fructose 1,6-diphosphate.

phos·pho·ga·lac·tose uri·dyl transferase (fos"fo·ga·lack'toce yoo'ri·dil). Galactose 1-phosphate uridyl transferase, an enzyme that catalyzes conversion of galactose 1-phosphate to glucose 1-phosphate. Congenital absence of the enzyme results in galactosemia.

phos·pho·lip·id (fos"fo·lip'id, ·lye'pid) *n.* A type of lipid compound which is an ester of phosphoric acid and contains, in addition, one or two molecules of fatty acid, an alcohol, and a nitrogenous base. They are widely distributed in nature and include such substances as lecithin, cephalin, and sphingomyelin.

phos·pho·ne·cro·sis (fos"fo·ne·kro'sis) *n.* Necrosis of the maxilla and mandible associated with chronic exposure to phosphorus dust. Syn. phossy jaw.

phos·pho·pro·tein (fos"fo·pro'teen, ·tee·in) *n.* A conjugated protein consisting of a compound of protein with a phosphorus-containing substance other than nucleic acid or lecithin.

phos·pho·py·ru·vic acid (fos"fo·pye·roo'vick). An intermediate substance, $CH_2=CO(PO_3·H_2)COOH$, obtained in the breakdown of glycogen to lactic acid and the resynthesis of glycogen from lactic acid.

phos·pho·res·cence (fos"fuh·res'unce) *n.* 1. The continuous emission of light from a substance without any apparent rise in temperature, produced after exposure to heat, light, or electric discharges. 2. The faint green glow of white phosphorus exposed to air, due to its slow oxidation. 3. *In radiology,* the emission of radiation by a substance as a result of previous absorption of radiation of shorter wavelength. —**phosphores·cent** (·unt) *adj.;* **phospho·resce** (·res').

phos·pho·ric (fos·fo'rick) *adj.* 1. PHOSPHORESCENT. 2. Of or pertaining to compounds containing phosphorus in the +5 valence state.

phosphoric acid. H_3PO_4. Orthophosphoric acid, a liquid of a syrupy consistency that contains 85% of H_3PO_4.

phos·pho·rism (fos'fuh·riz·um) *n.* Chronic phosphorus poisoning.

phos·pho·rous (fos·fo'rus) *adj.* Of or pertaining to compounds containing phosphorous in the +3 valence state.

phosphorous acid. A yellow, crystalline acid, H_3PO_3, used as a reducing agent and as a reagent.

phos·pho·rus (fos'fuh·rus) *n.* P = 30.9738. A nonmetallic element occurring in two allotropic forms, white or yellow phosphorus and amorphous or red phosphorus; the density of the former is about 1.82, and of the latter about 2.19.

phosphorus 32. A radioactive isotope of phosphorus, which emits beta rays, used in the form of sodium phosphate for locating tumors and in treating polycythemia vera and leukemia; radiophosphorus. Symbol, ^{32}P.

phos·pho·ryl·ase (fos"for·i·lace, fos·for'i·lace, ·laze) *n.* An enzyme widely distributed in animals, plants, and microorganisms. It catalyzes the formation of glucose 1-phosphate (Cori ester) from glycogen and inorganic phosphate.

phos·pho·ryl·ation (fos"for·i·lay'shun) *n.* The esterification of compounds with phosphoric acid. —**phos·pho·ryl·ate** (fos·for'i·late) *v.*

phos·pho·tung·state (fos"fo·tung'state) *n.* A salt of phosphotungstic acid.

phos·pho·tung·stic acid (fos"fo·tung'stick). Approximately $P_2O_5·24WO_3·25H_2O$. A white or yellowish-green crystalline acid used as a reagent.

phos·sy jaw (fos'ee). PHOSPHONECROSIS.

phot-, photo- A combining form meaning (a) *light;* (b) *photon;* (c) *photographic.*

phot (fote, fot) *n.* A unit of illumination equivalent to one lumen per square centimeter.

pho·tal·gia (fo·tal'jee·uh) *n.* Pain arising from too great intensity of light.

pho·tes·the·sia, pho·taes·the·sia (fo"tes·theezh'uh, ·theez'ee·uh) *n.* 1. Sensitiveness to light. 2. PHOTOPHOBIA.

pho·tic (fo'tick) *adj.* Pertaining to light.

photic driving. *In electroencephalography,* the production of occipital rhythmic activity by intermittent flashing light present.

photic epilepsy. PHOTOGENIC EPILEPSY.

pho·tism (fo'tiz·um) *n.* A form of synesthesia in which there is a visual sensation, as of color or light, produced by hearing, taste, smell, touch, or temperature, or even by the thought of some object, person, or general conception.

photo-. See *phot-.*

pho·to·chem·i·cal (fo"to·kem'i·kul) *adj.* Pertaining to chemical action produced directly or indirectly by means of radiation.

pho·to·chem·is·try (fo"to·kem'is·tree) *n.* The study of chemical reactions produced directly or indirectly by means of radiation.

pho·to·chro·mat·ic (fo"to·kro·mat'ick) *adj.* 1. Pertaining to colored light. 2. Pertaining to color photography.

pho·to·chro·mo·gen (fo"to·kro'muh·jen) *n.* An atypical pathogenic mycobacterium that produces pigment when grown in light.

pho·to·chro·mo·gen·ic (fo"to·kro"muh·jen'ick) *adj.* Producing color in response to a light stimulus.

pho·to·co·ag·u·la·tion (fo"to·ko·ag"yoo·lay'shun) *n.* Coagulation of tissue by a controlled and intense beam of light; used in ophthalmology.

pho·to·col·or·im·e·ter (fo″to·kul″ur·im′e·tur) *n.* PHOTOELECTRIC COLORIMETER.

pho·to·der·ma·ti·tis (fo″to·dur·muh·tye′tis) *n.* Any skin eruption brought on by exposure to light.

pho·to·dyn·ia (fo′to·din′ee·uh) *n.* Pain arising from too great intensity of light.

pho·to·dys·pho·ria (fo″to·dis·fo′ree·uh) *n.* PHOTOPHOBIA.

photoelectric colorimeter. A colorimeter for determining the concentration of the colored component of a solution, consisting of one or more combinations of calibrated filters and photoelectric cells for measurement of the color.

pho·to·elec·tric·i·ty (fo″to·e·leck″tris′i·tee) *n.* Electricity produced under the influence of light or other radiations, such as ultraviolet and x-rays. When irradiated by such radiations, certain metals give off photoelectrons. —**photo·elec·tric** (·e·leck′trick) *adj.*

pho·to·flu·o·rog·ra·phy (fo″to·floo″ur·og′ruh·fee) *n.* The process combining x-ray and photography to produce minature films, as of the chest; a photograph of the fluorescing screen is made.

pho·to·gene (fo′to·jeen) *n.* A retinal impression; an afterimage.

pho·to·gen·ic (fo″to·jen′ick) *adj.* 1. Produced or caused by light. 2. Emitting or producing light. 3. Aesthetically suitable for being photographed.

photogenic epilepsy. A form of reflex epilepsy induced by flicker or intermittent light; the attacks are usually of the myoclonic type, but may be generalized.

pho·to·graph (fo′tuh·graf) *n. & v.* 1. A picture obtained by photography. 2. To obtain a picture by photography.

pho·to·ki·net·ic (fo″to·ki·net′ick) *adj.* Causing movement by means of the energy of light.

pho·tol·y·sis (fo·tol′i·sis) *n.,* pl. **photoly·ses** (·seez) Decomposition by the action of light.

pho·to·lyte (fo′to·lite) *n.* A substance that is decomposed by the action of light.

pho·to·ma·nia (fo″to·may′nee·uh) *n.* 1. The increase of maniacal symptoms under the influence of intense light. 2. An abnormal desire for light.

pho·tom·e·ter (fo·tom′e·tur) *n.* 1. An instrument for measuring the intensity of light. 2. An instrument for testing the sensitiveness of the eye to light, by determining the minimum illumination in which the object is visible. —**pho·to·met·ric** (fo″to·met′rick) *adj;* **photomet·ri·cal·ly** (·ri·kuh·lee) *adv.*

pho·tom·e·try (fo·tom′e·tree) *n.* The measurement of the intensity of light.

pho·to·mi·cro·graph (fo″to·migh′kro·graf) *n.* A photograph of a minute or microscopic object, usually made with the aid of a microscope, and magnified to sufficient size for observation with the naked eye. —**photo·mi·crog·ra·phy** (·migh·krog′ruh·fee) *n.*

pho·to·mo·tor (fo″to·mo′tur) *adj.* Pertaining to a muscular response to light stimuli, as the constriction of the pupil.

pho·to·mul·ti·pli·er tube (fo″to·mul′ti·plye·ur). A

vacuum-tube device that converts signals into electrons and amplifies them through a multiple-stage process.

pho·ton (fo′ton) *n.* A quantum or discrete quantity of energy of visible light or any other electromagnetic radiation.

pho·ton·o·sus (fo·ton′uh·sus) *n.,* pl. **photono·si** (·sigh) A diseased condition arising from continued exposure to intense or glaring light, as snow blindness.

pho·to·par·es·the·sia, pho·to·par·aes·the·sia (fo″to·păr″es·theezh′uh, ·theez′ee·uh) *n.* Defective, or perverted, retinal sensibility.

pho·to·pho·bia (fo″to·fo′bee·uh) *n.* 1. Abnormal intolerance of or sensitivity to light. 2. Abnormal fear of light. —**photopho·bic** (·bick) *adj.*

pho·toph·thal·mia (fo″toff·thal′mee·uh) *n.* ACTINIC KERATOCONJUNCTIVITIS.

pho·top·sia (fo·top′see·uh) *n.* Subjective sensations of sparks or flashes of light occurring in certain pathologic conditions of the optic nerve, the retina, or the brain. —**photop·tic** (·tick) *adj.*

phot·op·tom·e·try (fo″to·tom′e·tree) *n.* The measurement of the perception of light.

pho·to·re·cep·tors (fo″to·re·sep′turz) *n.* The rods and cones of the retina.

pho·to·ret·i·ni·tis (fo″to·ret″i·nigh′tis) *n.* SUN BLINDNESS.

pho·to·scan (fo′to·skan) *n.* A rectilinear recording, made with photographic technique, of the distribution of radioactivity over a body part.

pho·to·sen·si·tiv·i·ty (fo″to·sen″si·tiv′i·tee) *n.* 1. The capacity of an organ or organism to be stimulated to activity by light, or to react to light. 2. The absorption of a certain portion of the spectrum by a chemical system. —**photo·sen·si·tive** (·sen′si·tiv) *adj.*

pho·to·sen·si·ti·za·tion (fo″to·sen″si·ti·zay′shun) *n.* The development in the skin or mucous membrane of abnormally high reactivity to ultraviolet radiation or natural sunlight; may be produced by the ingestion of such substances as fluorescent dyes, endocrine products, certain drugs, or heavy metals.

pho·to·syn·the·sis (fo″to·sin′thi·sis) *n.* The process by which simple carbohydrates are synthesized from carbon dioxide and water by the chloroplasts of living plant cells in the presence of light. —**photo·syn·thet·ic** (·sin·thet′ick) *adj.*

pho·to·ther·a·py (fo″to·therr′uh·pee) *n.* Treatment of disease with light rays.

pho·tu·ria (fo·tew′ree·uh) *n.* The passage of phosphorescent urine.

phren-, phreno- A combining form meaning (a) *mind;* (b) *brain;* (c) *diaphragm;* (d) *phrenic nerve.*

phren·as·the·nia (fren″as·theen′ee·uh) *n.* MENTAL DEFICIENCY. —**phrenas·then·ic** (·thenn′ick) *adj. & n.*

phren·em·phrax·is (fren″em·frack′sis) *n.* Crushing of a phrenic nerve with a hemostat to produce temporary paralysis of the diaphragm.

-phrenia A combining form meaning *mental disorder.*

phren·ic (fren'ick) *adj.* 1. Pertaining to the diaphragm. 2. Pertaining to the mind.

phren·i·cec·to·my (fren''i·seck'tuh·mee) *n.* Resection of a section of a phrenic nerve or removal of an entire phrenic nerve.

phrenic nerve. A nerve, arising from the third, fourth, and fifth cervical (cervical plexus) segments of the cord. It innervates the diaphragm.

phren·i·co·esoph·a·ge·al, phren·i·co·oesoph·a·ge·al (fren''i·ko·e·sof''uh·jee'ul) *adj.* Pertaining to the diaphragm and the esophagus.

phren·i·co·ex·er·e·sis (fren''i·ko·eck·serr'e·sis) *n.* Avulsion of a phrenic nerve.

phren·i·cot·o·my (fren''i·kot'uh·mee) *n.* Surgical division of a phrenic nerve in the neck for the purpose of causing a one-sided paralysis of the diaphragm, with consequent immobilization and compression of a diseased lung.

phren·i·co·trip·sy (fren''i·ko·trip'see) *n.* Crushing of a phrenic nerve.

phre·ni·tis (fre·nigh'tis) *n.* 1. *Obsol.* Inflammation of the brain. 2. Inflammation of the diaphragm. —**phre·nit·ic** (·nit'ick) *adj.*

phreno·col·ic (fren''o·kol'ick, ·ko'lick) *adj.* Pertaining to the diaphragm and the colon.

phreno·gas·tric (fren''o·gas'trick) *adj.* Pertaining conjointly to the stomach and the diaphragm.

phreno·he·pat·ic (fren''o·he·pat'ick) *adj.* Pertaining to the diaphragm and the liver.

phre·nol·o·gy (fre·nol'uh·jee) *n.* A pseudoscience based on the theory that the various faculties of the mind occupy distinct and separate areas in the brain cortex, and that the predominance of certain faculties can be ascertained from modifications of the parts of the skull overlying the areas where these faculties are located.

phreno·ple·gia (fren''o·plee'jee·uh) *n.* Paralysis of the diaphragm.

phren·o·sin (fren'o·sin) *n.* A complex lipid obtained chiefly from white matter of the central nervous system, and containing sphingosine, cerebronic acid, and a sugar, usually galactose.

phreno·spasm (fren'o·spaz·um) *n.* ACHALASIA (1).

phreno·splen·ic (fren''o·splen'ick) *adj.* Pertaining to the diaphragm and the spleen.

phron·e·mo·pho·bia (fron''e·mo·fo'bee·uh) *n.* An abnormal fear of thinking or of having an embarrassing thought.

phryg·i·an cap (frij'ee·un). The x-ray appearance of the gallbladder where kinking exists between the fundus and the body; named for its resemblance to the hats of the inhabitants of ancient Phrygia.

phryno·der·ma (frin''o·dur'muh, frye''no·) *n.* Dryness of the skin with follicular hyperkeratosis; due to vitamin A deficiency.

phthal-, phthalo-. A combining form meaning *origin from or relationship to phthalic acid.*

phthal·ic acid (thal'ick) *o*-Benzenedicarboxylic acid, $C_6H_4(COOH)_2$, derivatives of which are used in various syntheses, including some of medicinal importance.

phthal·yl·sul·fa·thi·a·zole (thal''il·sul''fuh·thigh'uh·zole) *n.* 4'-(2-Thiazolylsulfamoyl)phthalanilic acid, $C_{17}H_{13}N_3O_5S_2$, a relatively insoluble sulfonamide sparingly absorbed from the gastrointestinal tract; used as an intestinal antibacterial drug.

phthi·o·ic acid (thigh·o'ick). A cyclic fatty acid produced by *Mycobacterium tuberculosis.*

phthi·ri·a·sis, phtheiriasis (thigh·rye'uh·sis) *n., pl.* **phthiria·ses, phtheiria·ses** (·seez) Pediculosis pubis; infestation by the pubic louse *Phthirius pubis.*

phthi·rio·pho·bia (thirr''ee·o·fo'bee·uh, thigh'' ree·o·) *n.* An abnormal dread of lice.

Phthir·i·us (thirr'ee·us) *n.* A genus of true lice.

Phthirius pu·bis (pew'bis). A species of louse that infests the human pubic region; the crab louse.

phthis·i·ol·o·gy (tiz''ee·ol'uh·jee, thiz'') *n.* The study or science of tuberculosis.

phthis·io·pho·bia (tiz''ee·o·fo'bee·uh, thiz''ee·o·) *n.* Abnormal fear of tuberculosis.

phthi·sis (tye'sis, thigh'sis) *n., pl.* **phthi·ses** (·seez) 1. Tuberculosis, especially pulmonary tuberculosis. 2. Any disease characterized by emaciation and loss of strength. —**phthis·ic** (tiz'ick), **phthis·i·cal** (·i·kul) *adj.*

phthisis bul·bi (bul'bye). OPHTHALMOPHTHISIS.

Phy·co·my·ce·tes (figh''ko·migh·see'teez) *n.pl.* A class of fungi, with a generally nonseptate mycelium and in which asexual spores are formed endogenously in a saclike structure. This group includes the common black bread mold and water mold.

phy·co·my·co·sis (figh''ko·migh·ko'sis) *n.* Infection of man and of animals caused by members of the class of Phycomycetes, including mucormycosis and the subcutaneous phycomycosis of Africa caused by *Basidiobolus meristosporus.*

phy·lax·is (fi·lack'sis) *n.* The activity of the body in defending itself against infection.

phyll-, phyllo-. A combining form meaning (a) *leaf, leaflike;* (b) *chlorophyll.*

phyl·lo·er·y·thrin (fil''o·err'i·thrin) *n.* A porphyrin pigment resulting from degradation of chlorophyll, found in the bile of ruminants, in bovine gallstones, and in dog feces; claimed to be identical with cholemetin.

phyl·loid (fil'oid) *adj.* Leaflike.

phy·lo·ge·net·ic (figh''lo·je·net'ick) *adj.* Of or pertaining to phylogeny.

phy·log·e·ny (figh·loj'e·nee) *n.* The origin and development of a group or species of organisms; the evolution of the species.

phy·ma (figh'muh) *n., pl.* **phymas, phyma·ta** (·tuh) 1. A tumor or new growth of varying size, composed of any of the structures of the skin or subcutaneous tissue. 2. A localized plastic exudate larger than a tubercle; a circumscribed swelling of the skin. —**phyma·toid** (·toid) *adj.*

phy·ma·to·sis (figh''muh·to'sis) *n., pl.* **phymato·ses** (·seez) Any disease characterized by the formation of phymas or nodules.

phys·a·lif·e·rous (fis''uh·lif'e·rus, figh''suh·) *adj.* PHYSALIPHOROUS.

phy·sal·i·phore (fi·sal'i·fore) *n.* PHYSALIPHOROUS CELL. —**phy·sa·liph·o·rous** (fis''uh·lif'uh·rus, figh''suh·) *adj.*

physaliphorous cell. The large vacuolated cell found in chordomas, usually surrounded by mucinous material similar to the content of the vacuoles.

Phy·sa·lop·tera (figh″suh·lop′te·ruh) *n.* A genus of nematode worms of the family Physalopteridae.

physi-, physio- A combining form meaning (a) *natural;* (b) *physical;* (c) *physiological.*

physi·an·thro·py (fiz″eye·an′thruh·pee, fiz″ee·) *n.* The study of the constitution of man, his diseases, and their remedies.

phys·i·at·rics (fiz″eye·at′ricks, fiz″ee·) *n.* PHYSICAL MEDICINE.

phys·i·at·rist (fiz″ee·at′rist, fiz·eye′uh·trist) *n.* A physician specializing in physical medicine.

phys·ic (fiz′ick) *n. & v.* 1. The science of medicine and therapeutics. 2. A drug, especially a cathartic. 3. To administer a medicine. 4. To purge.

phys·i·cal (fiz′i·kul) *adj. & n.* 1. Pertaining to nature; pertaining to the body or material things. 2. Pertaining to physics. 3. *Informal.* A physical examination.

physical allergy. The response of some individuals to various physical factors, as cold, heat, sunlight, or mechanical irritation, manifested by urticaria, edema, and varying systemic reactions.

physical diagnosis. The part of a physician's clinical study of a patient which utilizes inspection, palpation, percussion, auscultation, and mensuration, including the employment of scopes and other instrumental aids, to assess the patient's physical status or detect his physical abnormalities. It is the counterpart of history-taking and laboratory tests.

physical medicine. A consultative, diagnostic, and therapeutic medical specialty, coordinating and integrating the use of physical and occupational therapy and physical reconditioning in the professional management of the diseased and injured.

physical sign. An objective sign manifested by a patient, or one detected by the physician on inspection, palpation, percussion, auscultation, mensuration, or combinations of these methods.

physical therapist. An individual professionally trained in the utilization of physical agents for therapeutic purposes.

physical therapy. The treatment of disease and injury by physical means, such as light, heat, cold, water, electricity, massage, and exercise.

phy·si·cian (fi·zish′un) *n.* A person who is authorized to practice medicine.

physician's assistant. A person who is trained and authorized to provide medical services under the responsibility and supervision of a physician.

phys·i·cist (fiz′i·sist) *n.* A person skilled in physics.

phys·i·co·chem·i·cal (fiz″i·ko·kem′i·kul) *adj.* Pertaining to the application of the theory and methodology of physics to the study of chemical systems.

phys·i·co·py·rex·ia (fiz″i·ko·pye·reck′see·uh) *n.* Artificial fever produced by physical means for its therapeutic effect.

phys·ics (fiz′icks) *n.* The science of the phenomena and laws of nature, especially that treating of the properties of matter and of the forces governing it.

phys·io·chem·i·cal (fiz″ee·o·kem′i·kul) *adj.* BIOCHEMICAL.

phys·i·og·no·my (fiz″ee·og′nuh·mee) *n.* 1. The countenance; FACIES (1). 2. The science of determining character by a study of the face. 3. PHYSIOGNOSIS.

phys·i·og·no·sis (fiz″ee·og·no′sis) *n.* Diagnosis of disease based on facial characteristics and expression.

phys·i·o·log·ic (fiz″ee·uh·loj′ick) *adj.* 1. Pertaining to physiology. 2. Pertaining to natural or normal functional processes in living organisms, as opposed to those that are pathologic. 3. In normal or natural state or quantity, as opposed to pharmacologic.

physiologic age. Age as judged by the functional development.

phys·i·o·log·i·cal (fiz″ee·uh·loj′i·kul) *adj.* PHYSIOLOGIC.

physiological availability. The extent to which the active ingredient of a nutrient or drug dosage can be absorbed and made available in the body in a physiologically active state. Syn. *bioavailability, biological availability.*

physiological dead space. A calculated expression of the anatomical dead space plus whatever degree of overventilation or underperfusion is present. It reflects the relationship between ventilation to pulmonary capillary perfusion. The formula is: physiological dead space = tidal volume × [(arterial P_{CO_2} − expired P_{CO_2} / arterial P_{CO_2})].

physiologic anemia. 1. A relative hypochromic microcytic anemia occurring normally in most infants about the third month of life, regardless of the nutritional status of the mother during pregnancy, and representing a normal physiologic adjustment to improved oxygenation of arterial blood. 2. Normocytic normochromic anemia occurring during pregnancy.

physiologic death. Death of a cell as part of a normal physiologic process, such as maturation of the epidermis.

physiologic hyperbilirubinemia. Physiologic elevation of the concentration of bilirubin in the serum of neonates.

physiologic jaundice of the newborn. The yellowness of skin and sclera and hyperbilirubinemia frequently seen in newborn infants the first 5 days of life and clearing within 7 to 14 days, due to incomplete development of glucuronyl transferase mechanism resulting in a decreased ability to conjugate bilirubin with glucuronic acid. The condition is usually mild and self-limiting, though in premature infants the hyperbilirubinemia may be more severe, last longer, and more frequently result in kernicterus.

physiologic murmur. INNOCENT MURMUR.

physiologic psychology. A branch of psychology that investigates the structure and functions of the nervous system and bodily organs in their relationship to behavior.

phys·i·ol·o·gist (fiz″ee·ol'uh·jist) *n.* A person skilled in physiology.

phys·i·ol·o·gy (fiz″ee·ol'uh·jee) *n.* The science that studies the functions of living organisms or their parts, as distinguished from morphology.

phys·io·path·o·log·ic (fiz″ee·o·path'uh·loj'ick) *adj.* 1. Pertaining to both physiology and pathology. 2. Involving a pathological modification of normal function. 3. PATHOPHYSIOLOG·IC.

phys·io·ther·a·py (fiz″ee·o·therr'uh·pee) *n.* PHYS·ICAL MEDICINE.

phy·sique (fi·zeek') *n.* Physical structure or organization; body build.

phy·so·hem·a·to·me·tra, phy·so·haem·a·to·me·tra (figh″so·hem″uh·to·mee'truh, ·hee″muh·to·) *n.* An accumulation of gas, or air, and blood in the uterus, as in decomposition of retained menses, or placental tissue.

phy·so·hy·dro·me·tra (figh″so·high'dro·mee'truh) *n.* An accumulation of gas and fluid in the uterus.

phy·so·me·tra (figh″so·mee'truh) *n.* Distention of the uterus with gas.

phy·so·pyo·sal·pinx (figh″so·pye″o·sal'pinks) *n.* Pyosalpinx with formation of gas in the uterine tube.

phy·so·stig·mine (figh″so·stig'meen, ·min) *n.* An alkaloid, $C_{15}H_{21}N_3O_2$, obtained from the seeds of *Physostigma venenosum*; a cholinergic drug that functions by inhibiting cholinesterase and has diverse clinical uses. Employed as the base and as the salicylate and sulfate salts. Syn. *eserine*.

phy·tan·ic acid (fye·tan'ick). 3,7,11,15-Tetramethylhexadecanoic acid, a fatty acid found in the tissues of some patients with Refsum's disease.

phy·tic acid (figh'tick). Inositolhexaphosphoric acid, or 1,2,3,4,5,6-cyclohexanehexolphosphoric acid, $C_6H_6[OPO·(OH)_2]_6$, a constituent of cereal grains. By combining with ingested calcium, it may prevent absorption of the latter.

phy·to·be·zoar (figh″to·bee'zo·ur) *n.* A bezoar or ball of vegetable fiber sometimes found in the stomach.

phy·to·chem·is·try (figh″to·kem'is·tree) *n.* The chemistry of plants and their constituents.

phy·to·hem·ag·glu·ti·nin (figh″to·hee″muh·glew'ti·nin, ·hem'uh·) *n.* A lectin which agglutinates cells and is mitogenic for lymphocytes. Abbreviated, PHA.

phy·to·na·di·one (figh″to·na·dye'ohn) *n.* 2-Methyl-3-phytyl-1,4-naphthoquinone, $C_{31}H_{46}O_2$, occurring in green plants but usually prepared by synthesis; used therapeutically to promote prothrombin formation. Syn. *phylloquinone, 3-phytylmenadione, vitamin K_1*.

phy·toph·a·gous (figh·tof'uh·gus) *adj.* 1. Plant-eating. 2. Vegetarian.

phy·to·phar·ma·col·o·gy (figh″to·fahr″muh·kol'uh·jee) *n.* The branch of pharmacology concerned with the effects of drugs on plant growth. —**phytopharma·co·log·i·cal** (·ko·loj'i·kul) *adj.*

phy·to·pho·to·der·ma·ti·tis (figh″to·fo″to·dur·muh·tye'tis) *n.* Any skin eruption brought on by certain plants and mediated by exposure to light.

phy·to·pneu·mo·co·ni·o·sis (figh″to·new″mo·ko″nee·o'sis) *n.* Pulmonary fibrosis due to inhalation of vegetable dust particles.

phy·to·sis (figh·to'sis) *n.*, *pl.* **phy·to·ses** (·sees) 1. Any disease due to the presence of vegetable parasites. 2. The production of disease by vegetable parasites. 3. The presence of vegetable parasites.

phy·tos·ter·ol (figh·tos'tur·ole, figh″to·steer'ole, ·ol) *n.* Any sterol occurring in a plant oil or fat.

phy·to·throm·bo·ki·nase (figh″to·throm″bo·kigh'nace, ·kin'ace, ·aze) *n.* A thrombokinase prepared from yeast or plant extracts.

phy·to·tox·ic (figh″to·tock'sick) *adj.* 1. Pertaining to a phytotoxin. 2. Pertaining to or describing a substance poisonous to plants.

phy·to·tox·in (figh″to·tock'sin) *n.* A toxin derived from a plant, such as ricin or crotin.

pia (pye'uh, pee'uh) *n.* PIA MATER. —**pi·al** (·ul) *adj.*

pia-arach·noid (pye″uh·uh·rack'noid) *n.* The pia mater and arachnoid considered as one structure. Syn. *leptomeninx*.

pia ma·ter (pye'uh may·tur, pee'uh mah'tur) The vascular membrane enveloping the surface of the brain and spinal cord, and consisting of a plexus of blood vessels held in a fine areolar tissue.

pi·a·rach·noid (pye″uh·rack'noid) *n.* PIA-ARACH·NOID.

pi·as·tre·ne·mia, pi·as·tre·nae·mia (pye·as″tre·nee'mee·uh) *n.* THROMBOCYTOSIS.

pi·ca (pye'kuh, pee'kuh) *n.* 1. A desire for strange foods; may occur as a result of emotional disturbance, malnutrition, or during pregnancy. 2. A craving to eat strange articles, as hair, dirt, or sand; the undue persistence or recurrence in later life of the infantile tendency of bringing everything to the mouth.

¹Pick's disease A form of dementia, often familial, characterized pathologically by severe cerebral atrophy usually restricted to the frontal and temporal lobes with less frequent extension to the parietal lobes. Microscopically, there is diffuse loss of neurones, particularly in the outer layers of the cortex, and ballooning of preserved neurones, which frequently contain argentophilic (Pick) bodies within the cytoplasm. Glial proliferation is prominent, and basal ganglions are frequently involved. Syn. *circumscribed cerebral atrophy*.

²Pick's disease 1. Recurrent or progressive ascites with little or no edema; postmortem examination shows constrictive pericarditis and atypical cirrhosis of the liver. 2. CONSTRICTIVE PERICARDITIS. 3. POLYSEROSITIS.

³Pick's disease NIEMANN-PICK DISEASE.

Pick·wick·i·an syndrome (pick·wick'ee·un) Marked obesity with alveolar hypoventilation, hypoxia, cyanosis, carbon dioxide retention, reduced vital capacity, secondary polycythemia, and somnolence; named for the corpulent, somnolent young man in Dickens' "Pickwick Papers."

pico- A combining form signifying the *one trillionth* (10^{-12}) *part* of the unit adjoined.

pi·co·cu·rie (pye'ko·kew''ree) *n.* One trillionth (10^{-12}) of a curie; the same as a micromicrocurie, a quantity of a radioactive substance resulting in 3.7×10^{-2} nuclear disintegrations per second. Abbreviated, pCi.

pi·co·gram (pye'ko·gram) *n.* One trillionth (10^{-12}) of a gram. Abbreviated, pg.

pi·cor·na·vi·rus (pye·kor''nuh·vye'rus) *n.* A member of a group of small, ether-resistant RNA viruses including the enteroviruses of poliomyelitis, Coxsackie and echoviruses, the rhinoviruses, and those of nonhuman origin such as foot-and-mouth disease and encephalomyocarditis.

pi·co·sec·ond (pye'ko·seck''und) *n.* One trillionth (10^{-12}) of a second.

pic·rate (pick'rate) *n.* A salt of picric acid.

pic·ric acid (pick'rick) TRINITROPHENOL.

pic·ro·tox·in (pick''ro·tock'sin) *n.* A glycoside, $C_{30}H_{34}O_{13}$, obtained from the seed of the East Indian woody vine *Anamirta cocculus;* a powerful central nervous system stimulant used to counteract depression from overdosage with barbiturates. Syn. *cocculin.*

PID Abbreviation for *pelvic inflammatory disease.*

pie·bald·ism (pye'bawl·diz·um) *n.* A distinctively patterned hypomelanosis of skin and usually hair (white forelock), inherited as an autosomal dominant trait.

pie·dra (pee·ay'druh) *n.* A nodular growth on the hair of the scalp, beard, or mustache. The type known as black piedra is found in tropical regions and is caused by the fungus *Piedraia hortai,* which infests only the hair shafts of the scalp. White piedra, a rarer form, occurs in temperate regions and is caused by the fungus *Trichosporon cutaneum,* which infests the hair of the beard and mustache. Syn. *tinea nodosa, Beigel's disease.*

Pierre Ro·bin syndrome (pyehr roh^{bæn'}) ROBIN SYNDROME.

pi·esom·e·ter (pye''e·som'e·tur) *n.* PIEZOMETER.

pi·ezom·e·ter (pye''e·zom'e·tur) *n.* 1. An apparatus for measuring the degree of compression of gases or fluids. 2. An apparatus for testing the sensitiveness of the skin to pressure. 3. A simple liquid manometer.

pi·geon breast or **chest.** A chest with a prominent sternum; may be congenital and associated with other malformations; may be due to rickets or obstructed infantile respiration. Syn. *chicken breast, pectus carinatum.*

pigeon-breeder's lung. BIRD-BREEDER'S LUNG.

pigeon-toed, *adj.* Walking with the feet turned in.

pig·ment (pig'munt) *n.* 1. A dye; a coloring matter. 2. Any organic coloring matter of the body. 3. Any paintlike medicinal applied externally to the skin. **—pig·men·tary** (pig'mun·terr''ee) *adj.;* **pig·ment·ed** (pig'men·tid) *adj.*

pig·men·ta·tion (pig''men·tay'shun) *n.* Deposition of or discoloration by pigment.

pigmented nevus. A pigmented mole, varying in color from light fawn to blackish, sometimes hairy, frequently papillary and hyperkeratotic, characterized by clear cells, melanocytes, and intermediate forms.

pigmented purpuric lichenoid dermatitis. A form of capillaritis, usually of the lower extremities, though the upper extremities and trunk may be involved, characterized by elevated papules which become purpuric or telangiectatic or pigmented in varying shades. Its course is chronic, leading to lichenification. Syn. *Gougerot-Blum disease.*

pil-, pilo- A combining form meaning *hair.*

pil. Abbreviation for *pilula,* pill.

pi·lar (pye'lur) *adj.* Pertaining to the hair or a hair.

pile, *n.* HEMORRHOID.

pi·le·ous (pye'lee·us, pil'ee·us) *adj.* Pertaining to hair; hairy.

piles, *n.pl.* HEMORRHOIDS.

pili. Plural and genitive singular of *pilus.*

pi·li·a·tion (pye''lee·ay'shun, pil''ee·) *n.* The formation and production of hair.

pi·li·form (pye'li·form) *adj.* Having the appearance of hair; FILIFORM.

pili in·car·na·ti (in·kahr·nay'tye). Ingrown hairs.

pill, *n.* A small, solid dosage form, of a globular, ovoid, or lenticular shape, containing one or more medicinal substances.

pil·lion (pil'yun) *n.* a temporary leg prosthesis.

pill-rolling tremor. A parkinsonian tremor which takes the form of flexion-extension of the fingers, combined with adduction-abduction of the thumb.

pi·lo·car·pine (pye''lo·kahr'peen, ·pin) *n.* An alkaloid, $C_{11}H_{16}N_2O_2$, obtained from various species of *Pilocarpus* (jaborandi); a cholinergic agent that also has ganglionic stimulant activity and is a physiological antagonist of atropine. It contracts the pupil, increases the flow of saliva and perspiration, and stimulates peristalsis; used clinically for these effects as the hydrochloride or nitrate salt.

pi·lo·cys·tic (pye''lo·sis'tick) *adj.* Pertaining to encysted tumors containing hair.

pi·lo·erec·tion (pye''lo·e·reck'shun) *n.* Erection of the hair.

pi·lo·mo·tor (pye''lo·mo'tur) *adj.* Causing movement of the hair, as the pilomotor muscles.

pi·lo·ni·dal (pye''lo·nigh'dul) *adj.* Pertaining to or containing an accumulation of hairs in a cyst.

pilonidal abscess. An abscess in the sacrococcygeal area within, or resulting from, a pilonidal cyst or sinus.

pilonidal cyst. A hair-containing cavity, in the dermis or subcutaneous tissues, usually connected to the skin surface by a sinus tract; commonly in the sacrococcygeal region. Syn. *sacrococcygeal cyst.*

pilonidal fistula. A form of pilonidal disease characterized by a hair-containing sinus tract emerging on the skin from the subcutaneous tissues, with or without an associated cavity (cyst).

pi·lose (pye'loce) *adj.* Hairy; covered with hair.

pi·lo·se·ba·ceous (pye''lo·se·bay'shus) *adj.* Pertaining to the hair follicles and sebaceous glands, as the pilosebaceous apparatus, the hair follicle and its attached oil gland.

pi·lo·sis (pye·lo'sis) *n.* The abnormal or excessive development of hair.

pi·los·i·ty (pye·los'i·tee) *n.* The state of being pilose or hairy.

pil·ule (pil'yool) *n.* A small pill.

pi·lus (pye'lus, pil'us) *n.,* pl. & genit. sing. **pi·li** (·lye), genit. pl. **pi·lo·rum** (pi·lo'rum) 1. [NA] A hair. 2. *In biology,* a fine, slender, hairlike body.

pimel-, pimelo- A combining form meaning *fat, fatty.*

pim·e·lo·pte·ryg·i·um (pim''i·lo·te·rij'ee·um) *n.* A fatty outgrowth on the conjunctiva.

pim·e·lor·thop·nea, pim·e·lor·thop·noea (pim''e·lor·thop'nee·uh) *n.* Orthopnea due to obesity.

pim·e·lu·ria (pim''e·lew'ree·uh) *n.* The excretion of fat in the urine; LIPURIA.

pim·ple, *n.* A small pustule or papule.

pince·ment (pance·mahn') *n.* In massage, a pinching or nipping of the tissues.

pinch graft. A small, full-thickness graft lifted from the donor area by a needle and cut free with a razor. Many such small deep grafts are fitted together to cover the defect.

pine, *n.* 1. Any tree of the genus *Pinus.* 2. Loosely, any of various other kinds of coniferous trees.

pi·ne·al (pin'ee·ul, pye'nee·ul) *adj.* Pertaining to the pineal body, or epiphysis cerebri.

pineal body. A small cone-shaped structure attached to the roof of the third ventricle between the superior colliculi. Syn. *epiphysis cerebri.*

pi·ne·al·ec·to·my (pin''ee·ul·eck'tuh·mee, pye'' nee·) *n.* Surgical removal of the pineal body.

pi·ne·a·lo·ma (pin''ee·uh·lo'muh, pye''nee·) *n.,* pl. **pinealomas, pinealoma·ta** (·tuh) An uncommon, usually small, frequently invasive tumor of the pineal body composed of varying proportions of large, round cells with well defined cell membranes, a pale cytoplasm and conspicuous nuclei and small, darkly stained cells, presumably lymphocytes, distributed along the vascular stroma of the tumor. Syn. *pinealcytoma, pineal germinoma, pineal seminoma, pineal tumor.*

pineal syndrome. A rare syndrome due to a pinealoma or other pathological condition in or about the pineal body, resulting in increased intracranial pressure and associated neurologic disturbances, an inability to look upward (Parinaud's syndrome) and slightly dilated pupils which react in accommodation but not to light.

pin·guec·u·la (ping·gweck'yoo·luh) *n.,* pl. **pingue·cu·lae** (·lee) A small, slightly elevated yellowish-white patch situated in the conjunctiva, within the interpalpebral fissure, between the cornea and the canthus of the eye; it is the result of the elastotic degeneration of collagen of the connective tissue of the conjectiva.

pin·guid (ping'gwid) *adj.* FAT (2); UNCTUOUS.

pi·ni·form (pye'ni·form, pin'i·form) *adj.* Shaped like a pinecone.

pink·eye, *n.* 1. A contagious, mucopurulent con-

junctivitis occurring especially in horses. 2. CATARRHAL CONJUNCTIVITIS.

pink puffer. A person with emphysema, marked dyspnea, debility, and hyperinflation of the lungs.

pin·na (pin'uh) *n.,* L. pl. & genit. sing. **pin·nae** (·ee), The projecting part of the external ear; AURICLE (1). —**pin·nal** (·ul) *adj.*

pi·no·cy·to·sis (pin''o·sigh·to'sis, pye''no·) *n.,* pl. **pinocyto·ses** (·seez) A type of absorption by cells in which the cellular membrane invaginates to form a saccular structure that engulfs extracellular fluid and is then closed at the membrane so that the saccule remains as a vesicle or vacuole (pinosome) within the cell.

pint, *n.* The eighth part of a gallon; 16 fluidounces. Symbol, 0. (octarius). Abbreviated, pt.

pin·ta (pin'tuh, peen'tah) *n.* A disease of the skin seen most frequently in tropical America, characterized by dyschromic changes and hyperkeratosis in patches of the skin; caused by the spirochete *Treponema carateum,* which is morphologically identical with the spirochetes of syphilis and of yaws. Syn. *carate, mal del pinto, piquite, purupuru, quitiqua.*

pin·tid (pin'tid) *n.* The characteristic red macular skin eruption of the secondary stage of pinta.

pin·worm, *n.* Any of various oxyurid worms inhabiting the intestinal tracts of mammals, notably *Enterobius vermicularis,* the human pinworm.

pi·per·a·zine (pi·perr'uh·zeen, pip'ur·) *n.* Hexahydropyrazine, $C_4H_{10}O_2$, used in the form of various of its salts (adipate, citrate, tartrate) for treatment of infections caused by certain roundworms. Formerly used for treatment of gout.

pip·er·i·do·late (pip''ur·i·do'late, pi·perr''i·do' late, pye·perr'') *n.* 1-Ethyl-3-piperidyl diphenylacetate, $C_{21}H_{25}NO_2$, an anticholinergic agent used for treatment of spastic disorders of the upper gastrointestinal tract; employed as the hydrochloride salt.

pip·er·o·caine (pip'ur·o·kane) *n.* 3-(2-Methylpiperidino)propyl benzoate, $C_{16}H_{23}NO_2$, a local anesthetic used as the hydrochloride salt.

pip·et, pi·pette (pi·pet', pye·pet') *n.* A graduated open glass or plastic tube used for measuring or transferring definite quantities of liquids.

pip·to·nych·ia (pip''to·nick'ee·uh) *n.* Shedding of the nails.

pir·i·form, pyr·i·form (pirr'i·form, pye'ri·form) *adj.* & *n.* 1. Pear-shaped. 2. PIRIFORMIS.

pir·i·for·mis (pirr'i·for'mis) *n.* A muscle arising from the front of the sacrum and inserted into the greater trochanter of the femur.

Pi·ro·goff's amputation (pɣi·rah·gohf') An osteoplastic operation for amputation of the foot, resembling Syme's amputation, in which part of the calcaneus is retained.

pi·ro·plas·mo·sis (pye''ro·plaz·mo'sis) *n.,* pl. **pi·roplasmo·ses** (·seez) BABESIOSIS. —**piroplas·mot·ic** (·mot'ick) *adj.*

pi·si·form (pye'si·form) *adj.* & *n.* 1. Pea-shaped. 2. A small bone on the inner and anterior aspect of the carpus.

pi·so·ha·mate (pye"so·hay'mate) *adj.* Pertaining to the pisiform and hamate bones.

pis·tol-shot sound. A loud sound heard on auscultation over the peripheral arteries with each pulsation in aortic regurgitation, severe anemia, hyperthyroidism, arteriovenous fistula, and other conditions; due to rapid arterial distention and collapse. Syn. *Traube's sign.*

pit, *n.* 1. A depression, as the pit of the stomach; the armpit. 2. A sharp, pointed depression in the enamel of a tooth; normally occurring where several developmental grooves join. 3. A microscopic tubular depression in the surface of the mucosa.

pitch, *n.* The quality of sound that depends upon the frequency of the vibrations that produce the sound.

Pitocin. Trademark for oxytocin injection, an oxytocic posterior pituitary hormone preparation.

pi·tom·e·ter (pi·tom'e·tur) *n.* An instrument that records the rate of flow of liquids.

Pitressin. Trademark for antidiuretic hormone injection.

pit·ting, *n.* 1. The formation of pits; in the nails, a consequence and sign of psoriasis. 2. The preservation for a short time of indentations on the skin made by pressing with the finger; seen in pitting edema.

pitting edema. Edema of such degree that the skin can be temporarily indented by pressure with the fingers.

pi·tu·i·tary (pi·tew'i·terr"ee) *adj. & n.* 1. Secreting mucus or phlegm. 2. Pertaining to the hypophysis or pituitary gland. 3. PITUITARY GLAND.

pituitary apoplexy. Hemorrhage into a pituitary adenoma, characterized by the acute onset of ophthalmoplegia, bilateral amaurosis, drowsiness or coma, with either subarachnoid hemorrhage or pleocytosis and elevated protein in the cerebrospinal fluid.

pituitary B gonadotropin. LEUTINIZING HORMONE.

pituitary dwarfism. Stunted growth due to primary growth hormone deficiency, but frequently associated with deficiency of thyrotropic and adrenocorticotropic hormones as detected by appropriate tests and with gonadotropin deficiency which is usually not demonstrable in childhood. The condition may be characterized clinically only by growth failure after the first few years of life, or there may be a childish face, high-pitched voice, small hands and feet, delayed sexual maturation and underdeveloped genitalia, and in older individuals, deficient subcutaneous fat with loose wrinkled skin and precocious senility. The condition may also be secondary to destructive pituitary lesions as from tumor, infection, trauma, or aneurysm.

pituitary gland. A small, rounded, bilobate endocrine gland, averaging about 0.5 g in weight, which lies in the sella turcica of the sphenoid bone, is attached by a stalk, the infundibulum, to the floor of the third ventricle of the brain at the hypothalamus, and consists of an anterior lobe, the adenohypophysis, which pro-

duces and secretes various important hormones, including several which regulate other endocrine glands, and a less important posterior lobe, the neurohypophysis, which holds and secretes antidiuretic hormone and oxytocin produced in the hypothalamus. Syn. *hypophysis* (NA).

Pituitrin. A trademark for posterior pituitary injection, a preparation of mixed posterior pituitary hormones.

pit·y·ri·a·sis (pit"i·rye'uh·sis) *n.* A fine, branny desquamation of the skin.

pityriasis lichenoides et var·i·o·li·for·mis acu·ta (văr"ee·o'li·for'mis a·kew'tuh). A noncommunicable, acute, or subacute skin eruption characterized by vesicles and pustules that form crusts and later scars. Syn. *Mucha-Habermann's disease.*

pityriasis ro·sea (ro'zee·uh). An idiopathic self-limited skin disease of the trunk, usually acute; characterized by pale red patches with fawn-colored centers. Syn. *pityriasis circinata, herpes tonsurans maculosus.*

pityriasis rubra pi·la·ris (pi·lair'is). A chronic, mildly inflammatory skin disease in which firm, acuminate papules form at the mouths of the hair follicles with horny plugs in these follicles. By coalescence scaly patches are formed. Syn. *lichen ruber acuminatus.*

pityriasis versicolor. TINEA VERSICOLOR.

Pit·y·ro·spo·rum (pit"i·ro·spo'rum, ·ros'puh·rum) *n.* A genus of fungi which is yeastlike in character, belonging to the Cryptococcaceae.

Pityrosporum ovale (o·vay'lee). A species of fungus found in the hair follicles and on the skin in seborrheic dermatitis; of unknown pathogenicity.

pivot joint. A synovial joint in which movement is limited to rotation; the movement is uniaxial, and in the longitudinal axis of the bones.

pK The negative logarithm of the dissociation constant of an acid or a base; it is equivalent to the hydrogen-ion concentration (expressed in pH units) at which there is an equimolecular concentration of the acidic and basic components of any given buffer system.

PKU Abbreviation for *phenylketonuria* (2).

pla·ce·bo (pla·see'bo) *n.* A preparation, devoid of pharmacologic effect, given for psychological effect, or as a control in evaluating a medicinal believed to have pharmacologic activity.

pla·cen·ta (pluh·sen'tuh) *n.*, L. pl. & genit. sing. **placen·tae** (·tee), E. pl. **placentas** The organ on the wall of the uterus to which the embryo is attached by the umbilical cord. Developed from the chorion of the embryo and the decidua basalis of the uterus, it performs the functions of nutrition, respiration, and excretion, as well as secretion of estrogen, progesterone, and other hormones. At term the average human placenta weighs about ⅙ as much as the fetus, and is about 2 cm thick at its center and 15 cm in diameter.

placenta ac·cre·ta (a·kree'tuh). A placenta that has partially grown into the myometrium (cleavage zone in basal decidua incompletely developed or absent with chorionic villi in direct contact with the myometrium).

placenta cir·soi·dea (sur·soy'dee·uh). A placenta in which the umbilical vessels have a varicose arrangement.

placenta fe·nes·tra·ta (fen·e·stray'tuh). An irregular, four-sided variety of placenta with an opening near the center.

placenta in·cre·ta (in·kree'tuh). A placenta that has grown into the uterine myometrium at all contact areas with no intervening decidua.

placental barrier. The tissues intervening between the maternal and the fetal blood of the placenta, which prevent or hinder certain substances or organisms from passing from mother to fetus.

placental polyp. A uterine polyp composed of retained placental fragments.

placenta pre·via (pree'vee·uh). A placenta superimposed upon and about the os uteri internum, which may produce serious hemorrhage before or during labor.

placenta previa cen·tra·lis (sen·tray'lis). A condition in which the center of the placenta is directly above the os uteri internum.

placenta previa mar·gi·na·lis (mahr·ji·nay'lis). A condition in which the edge of the placenta meets, but does not overlap, the os uteri internum.

placenta previa par·ti·a·lis (pahr·shee·ay'lis). A condition in which the edge of the placenta overlies, but does not completely obstruct, the os uteri internum.

placenta suc·cen·tu·ri·a·ta (suck"sen·tew"ree·ay'tuh). An anomalous formation in which one or more accessory lobules are developed in the membrane at a greater or lesser distance from the margin of the placenta, but connected with the latter by vascular channels. Syn. *accessory placenta.*

plac·en·ta·tion (plas"en·tay'shun) *n.* Formation and mode of attachment of the placenta.

plac·en·ti·tis (plas"en·tye'tis) *n.,* pl. **placen·tit·i·des** (·tit'i·deez) Inflammation of the placenta.

plac·en·tog·ra·phy (plas"en·tog'ruh·fee) *n.* Radiography of the placenta after delivery, using a contrast medium.

pla·cen·to·ther·a·py (pla·sen"to·therr'uh·pee) *n.* The remedial use of biological preparations derived from the placenta of animals.

Placidyl. Trademark for ethchlorvynol, a sedative-hypnotic with short duration of action.

plac·ode (plack'ode) *n.* A platelike epithelial thickening, frequently marking, in the embryo, the anlage of an organ or part. —**pla·co·dal** (pla·ko'dul) *adj.*

plagi-, plagio- A combining form meaning *oblique.*

pla·gio·ceph·a·ly (play"jee·o·sef'uh·lee) *n.* A type of strongly asymmetric cranial deformation, in which the anterior portion of one side and the posterior portion of the opposite side of the skull are developed more than their counterparts, so that the maximum length of the skull is not in the midline but on a diagonal. Due to a number of causes, such as prenatal, developmental (disordered sequence of suture closure), mechanical (intentional or unintentional). Syn. *wry-head.* —**plagiocephalous** (·lus), **plagio·ce·phal·ic** (·se·fal'ick) *adj.*

plague (plaig) *n.* 1. Any contagious, malignant, epidemic disease. 2. An acute disease of rodents due to *Yersinia pestis,* transmitted to humans through the bite of infected fleas, or by inhalation. The human disease is usually divided into three clinical forms: bubonic, septicemic, and pneumonic.

plana. Plural of *planum.*

Planck's constant The constant *h,* which has the value 6.624×10^{-27} erg second, used in mathematical expressions of the quantum theory.

plane, *n.* 1. Any flat, smooth surface, especially any assumed or conventional surface, whether tangent to the body or dividing it. 2. A level in any development, process, or existence. —**pla·nar** (play'nur) *adj.*

planes of anesthesia. Subdivisions of the stages of surgical anesthesia, based on Guedel's classification (1937) of the clinical signs of the stages of general anesthesia. The first plane is marked by loss of the eyelid reflex, the second plane by cessation of eyeball movements, the third plane by beginning of intercostal paralysis, and the fourth plane by complete intercostal paralysis and purely diaphragmatic respiration.

plani-, plano- A combining form meaning *flat* or *level.*

pla·ni·gram (play'ni·gram, plan'i·) *n.* Radiographic depiction of structure at a particular depth, made by planigraphy; TOMOGRAM.

pla·nig·ra·phy (pla·nig'ruh·fee) *n.* SECTIONAL RADIOGRAPHY.

pla·nim·e·ter (pla·nim'e·tur) *n.* An instrument which measures the area of a plane surface by tracing the periphery.

plan·ing (play'ning) *n.* A method of plastic surgery, whereby skin, hardened by freezing, is abraded by means of a burr, sandpaper, or rotating steel-wire brush, to permanently remove scars, pock marks, and superficial skin blemishes.

pla·no·con·cave (play"no·kon'kave, ·kon·kave') *adj.* Concave on one surface and flat on the opposite side.

pla·no·con·ic (play"no·kon'ick) *adj.* Having one side flat and the other conical.

pla·no·con·vex (play"no·kon'vecks, ·kun·vecks') *adj.* Plane on one side and convex on the other.

plano·ma·nia (plan"o·may'nee·uh) *n.* An abnormal desire for wandering; an impulse to throw off social restraints and live in the wilds.

Pla·nor·bis (pla·nor'bis) *n.* A genus of freshwater snails, species of which act as intermediate hosts of the flukes causing schistosomiasis in man.

pla·no·val·gus (play"no·val'gus) *n.* The type of flat foot in which the heel, viewed from behind, is lateral to ankle joint; there is no convexity.

plan·ta (plan'tuh) *n.,* pl. & genit. sing. **plan·tae** (·tee) The sole of the foot.

plan·tar (plan'tur, ·tahr) *adj.* Pertaining to the sole of the foot.

plantar aponeurosis. A thick sheet of dense fibrous connective tissue radiating from the medial portion of the undersurface of the tuberosity of the calcaneus toward the heads of the metatarsal bones.

plantar fascia. PLANTAR APONEUROSIS.

plantar fasciitis. An inflammatory process, usually secondary to trauma or chronic strain, involving the plantar fascia, most commonly at its attachment to the calcaneus.

plantar flexion. Bending the foot or toes downward, toward the sole; opposed to dorsiflexion. —**plan·tar·flex** (plan'tur-flecks) v.

plantar reflex. Flexion of the toes in response to stroking of the outer surface of the sole, from heel to little toe.

plantar wart. VERRUCA PLANTARIS.

plan·ta·tion (plan-tay'shun) n. The insertion of a tooth or other material in the human body.

pla·num (play'num) n., pl. **ple·na** (-nuh) A plane, or level surface.

plaque (plack) n. 1. A patch, or an abnormal flat area on any internal or external body surface. 2. A localized area of atherosclerosis. 3. An area of psoriasis.

Plaquenil. Trademark for hydroxychloroquine, used as the sulfate salt for the treatment of malaria, lupus erythematosus, and rheumatoid arthritis.

plasm (plaz'um) n. 1. PLASMA. 2. A part of the substance of a cell.

plas·ma (plaz'muh) n. 1. The fluid portion of blood or lymph, composed of a mixture of many proteins in a crystalloid solution and corresponding closely to the interstitial fluid of the body. 2. *In nuclear technology,* an electrically neutral gaseous mixture of ions, electrons, and neutral particles formed when matter exists at temperatures of 100 million degrees or more.

plas·ma·blast (plaz'muh-blast) n. The stem cell of the plasmacytes. Syn. *lymphoblastic plasma cell.*

plasma cell. The antibody-producing leukocyte into which a B lymphocyte differentiates upon stimulation by antigen.

plasma cell myeloma. A malignant plasmacytoma.

plas·ma·cyte (plaz'muh-site) n. PLASMA CELL. —**plas·ma·cyt·ic** (-sit'ick) adj.

plasmacytic leukemia. A type of leukemia characterized by anaplastic plasma cells in the peripheral blood.

plas·ma·cy·toid (plaz''muh-sigh'toid) adj. Resembling a plasma cell.

plasmacytoid lymphocyte. PLASMA CELL.

plas·ma·cy·to·ma (plaz''muh-sigh-to'muh) n. Any benign or malignant tumor of plasma cells.

plas·ma·cy·to·sis (plaz''muh-sigh-to'sis) n. 1. An increase in the number of plasmacytes in the spleen, lymph nodes, bone marrow, kidney, or liver. 2. An increase in the number of plasmacytes in the peripheral blood.

plas·ma·lem·ma (plaz''muh-lem'uh) n. PLASMA MEMBRANE.

plas·mal·o·gen (plaz-mal'uh-jen) n. One of a group of phosphatides in which the fatty acid

at the α' position is replaced by an α, β-unsaturated ether.

plasma membrane. A metabolically active, trilaminar sheet that encloses the cytoplasm and limits the cell, providing selective permeability and containing receptor molecules which form linkages with outside substances. Syn. *plasmalemma, cell membrane.*

plas·ma·pher·e·sis, plas·ma·phaer·e·sis (plaz''muh-fe·ree'sis, -ferr'e·sis) n. The withdrawal of blood from a donor to obtain plasma, its components, or the nonerythrocytic formed elements of blood, followed by return of the erythrocytes to the donor.

plasmat-, plasmato- A combining form meaning (a) *protoplasm*; (b) *cytoplasm*; (c) *plasma.*

plas·ma·ther·a·py (plaz''muh-therr'uh·pee) n. Treatment by the intravenous injection of blood plasma.

plas·mat·ic (plaz·mat'ick) adj. Pertaining to plasma.

plas·min (plaz'min) n. A proteolytic enzyme, present in inactive form as plasminogen, occurring in plasma, and responsible for slow digestion and lysis of fibrin clots. Syn. *fibrinolysin.*

plas·min·o·gen (plaz·min'o·jen) n. The inactive form of plasmin; when blood is shed over injured tissues, it is converted to plasmin.

plas·mino·geno·pe·nia (plaz·min''o·jen'o·pee'nee·uh) n. A deficiency of plasmin.

Plasmochin. A trademark for the antimalarial drug pamaquine, used as the pamoate salt.

plasmodia. Plural of plasmodium.

plas·mo·di·al (plaz·mo'dee·ul) adj. Pertaining to or resembling a plasmodium.

plas·mo·di·cide (plaz·mo'di·side) n. An agent that kills malaria parasites.

Plas·mo·di·um (plaz·mo'dee·um) n. A genus of protozoa that cause malaria in birds, lower animals, and man. —**plasmodium,** pl. **plasmodia,** com. n.

Plasmodium fal·cip·a·rum (fal·sip'uh·rum) The species of *Plasmodium* that is the etiologic agent of falciparum malaria.

Plasmodium ma·la·ri·ae (ma·lair'ee·ee). The species of *Plasmodium* that is the etiologic agent of quartan malaria.

Plasmodium ova·le (o·vay'lee). The species of *Plasmodium* that causes ovale malaria, characterized by an oval distortion of the red blood cells.

Plasmodium vi·vax (vye'vacks). The species of *Plasmodium* that causes vivax or benign tertian malaria.

plas·mol·y·sis (plaz·mol'i·sis) n., pl. **plasmoly·ses** (-seez) Shrinkage of a cell or its contents, due to withdrawal of water by osmosis when subjected to a hypertonic salt solution. —**plas·mo·lyt·ic** (plaz''mo·lit'ick) adj.

plas·moph·a·gous (plaz·mof'uh·gus) adj. Pertaining to certain organisms that decompose organic matter.

plas·mo·trop·ic (plaz''mo·trop'ick) adj. Producing excessive hemolysis in the liver, spleen, and bone marrow.

plas·ter (plas'tur) n. 1. A substance intended for external application, made of such material and of such consistency as to adhere to the skin. 2. Calcined gypsum or calcium sulfate.

plaster of Paris. Dried calcium sulfate; used in making bandages and casts to provide mechanical support or to immobilize various parts of the body, and also in various dental procedures.

plaster of Paris cast. A mixture of gypsum and water which becomes hard upon drying; when incorporated into gauze as a binder it may be used to immobilize body parts, such as fractured bones, arthritic joints, or the spine.

plaster of Paris jacket. A casing applied by winding plaster of Paris bandages over padding, so as to encase the body in a hard mold from armpits to groin; used to immobilize the spine.

plas·tic (plas'tick) *adj. & n.* 1. Formative; concerned with building up tissues, restoring lost parts, repairing or rectifying malformations or defects, etc., as plastic surgery, plastic operation, plastic repair. 2. Capable of being molded. 3. Any material of high molecular weight, as acrylics and polystyrene, obtained by various chemical processes, that is solid in its finished state but at some stage of its manufacture or processing can be shaped by flow. 4. Made of or pertaining to plastic.

plas·tic·i·ty (plas·tis'i·tee) *n.* The quality or state of being plastic.

plas·ti·ciz·er (plas'ti·sigh"zur) *n.* A substance incorporated in an organic formulation or substance to maintain it in a flexible or plastic condition, preventing or retarding cracking or development of brittleness.

plastic surgeon. A surgeon who specializes in plastic surgery.

plastic surgery. Operative repair of defects or deformities, usually involving transference of tissue.

plas·tid (plas'tid) *n.* 1. A hypothetical elementary organism; a cytode. 2. Any of certain small cytoplasmic bodies in plant cells, regarded as centers of certain metabolic activities of the cells.

-plasty A combining form meaning *plastic surgery.*

-plasy. See *-plasia.*

plat-, platy- A combining form meaning *broad, flat.*

plate, *n.* 1. A flattened part, especially a flattened process of bone. 2. A thin piece of metal or some other substance to which artificial teeth are attached. 3. *In microbiology,* a shallow, cylindrical, covered culture dish; also such a dish containing solid cultural medium suitable for the growth of microorganisms; a petri dish. 4. *In orthopedics,* a metallic device used with screws or bolts for internal fixation of bone. 5. ARTIFICIAL DENTURE.

pla·teau (pla·to') *n.,* pl. **plateaus, plateaux** 1. A period, state, or stretch of relative stability, often in contrast to normally prevailing cyclical or fluctuating change. 2. In operating Geiger counter tubes, the voltage range over which the number of impulses recorded is nearly constant.

plate·let, *n.* BLOOD PLATELET.

plate·let·phe·re·sis, platelet pheresis (plait'lit·fe·ree'sis) *n.* The removal from a donor of a quantity of blood platelets, followed by the return to him of the remaining portions of the donated blood.

plat·i·num (plat'i·num) *n.* Pt = 195.09. A silver-white metal occurring natively or alloyed with other metals; density, approximately 21.4. It is fusible only at very high temperatures, and is insoluble in all acids except nitrohydrochloric. Platinum forms two types of compounds: platinous, in which it is divalent, and platinic, in which it is tetravalent. It is no longer used medicinally.

plat·onych·ia (plat'o·nick'ee·uh) *n.* A dystrophy of the nail; consisting of a modification of its greatest curvature, which, instead of being transverse, as normally, is lengthwise.

platy·ba·sia (plat'i·bay'see·uh) *n.* A developmental deformity of the skull and axis in which the base of the skull is flattened, having a basal angle of more than 152°.

platy·ce·phal·ic (plat'i·se·fal'ick) *adj.* Having a skull with a relatively flat vertex. —**platy·ceph·a·ly** (·sef'uh·lee) *n.*

Platy·hel·min·thes (plat'i·hel·minth'eez) *n.pl.* A phylum of flatworms characterized by bilaterally symmetrical, many-celled, leaf-shaped bodies lacking a body cavity and usually containing both sexual elements. Includes the medically important classes Trematoda and Cestoda.

platy·mor·phia (plat'i·mor'fee·uh) *n.* A flatness in the formation of the eye and shortening of the anteroposterior diameter, resulting in hyperopia.

platy·pel·lic (plat'i·pel'ick) *adj.* 1. Of a pelvis: having a transverse diameter considerably greater than the anteroposterior diameter. Specifically, having a pelvic-inlet index of 89.9 or less.

pla·tys·ma (pla·tiz'muh) *n.,* pl. **platysma·ta** (·tuh), **platysmas** A subcutaneous muscle in the neck, extending from the face to the clavicle.

plea·sure principle. *In psychoanalysis,* the instinctive endeavor to escape from pain, discomfort, or unpleasant situations; the desire to obtain the greatest possible gratification with the smallest possible effort.

pled·get (plej'it) *n.* A small, flattened compress usually of cotton or gauze.

-plegia A combining form meaning *paralysis.*

-plegic A combining form meaning (a) *paralyzed;* (b) *pertaining to paralysis.*

plei·ot·ro·pism (plye·ot'ro·piz·um) *n.* The occurrence of multiple effects produced by a given gene. —**plei·o·trop·ic** (·o·trop'ick) *adj.*

pleo·co·ni·al (plee"o·ko'nee·ul) *adj.* Of, pertaining to, or characterized by more than the usual number of mitochondria or particles seen in certain muscle cells with the electron microscope.

pleo·cy·to·sis (plee"o·sigh·to'sis) *n.,* pl. **pleocyto·ses** (·seez) Increase of cells in the cerebrospinal fluid.

pleo·mor·phic (plee"o·mor'fick) *adj.* Pertaining to or characterized by pleomorphism.

pleo·mor·phism (plee″o·mor′fiz·um) *n.* Marked difference in size, shape, or other morphological features, among individuals of a single kind or class, as among bacteria of a particular species or cells of a given type. Mesomorphism in cells may include variation in nuclear characteristics and is seen especially in dysplastic or anaplastic cells, but also in such normal cells as trophoblasts.

pleo·mor·phous (plee″o·mor′fus) *adj.* Pertaining to or characterized by pleomorphism.

ple·o·nasm (plee′o·naz·um) *n.* Any malformation marked by superabundance or excessive size of certain organs or parts. —**ple·o·nas·tic** (plee″o·nas′tick) *adj.*

ple·o·nex·ia (plee″o·neck′see·uh) *n.* Excessive desire to have or possess; abnormal greed.

ple·on·os·te·o·sis (plee″on·os″tee·o′sis) *n.* Excessive or premature ossification.

ple·o·no·tus (plee″o·no′tus) *n.* An earlike appendage located on the neck; cervical auricle.

ple·ro·cer·coid (pleer″o·sur′koid) *n.* The second larval stage in the intermediate host of certain cestodes.

ple·si·opia (plee″see·o′pee·uh) *n.* Increased convexity of the crystalline lens, producing myopia.

pleth·o·ra (pleth′uh·ruh) *n.* A state characterized by excess of blood in the body. —**ple·tho·ric** (pleth′uh·rick, ple·tho′rick) *adj.*

ple·thys·mo·gram (ple·thiz′mo·gram) *n.* A record made by a plethysmograph.

ple·thys·mo·graph (ple·thiz′mo·graf) *n.* A device for ascertaining rapid changes in volume of an organ or part, through an increase in the quantity of the blood therein. —**ple·thys·mo·graph·ic** (ple·thiz″mo·graf′ick) *adj.*

pleth·ys·mog·ra·phy (pleth″iz·mog′ruh·fee) *n.* Measurement of volume changes of an extremity or of an organ.

pleur-, pleuro- A combining form meaning (a) *pleura, pleural;* (b) *side, lateral;* (c) *pleurisy.*

pleu·ra (ploor′uh) *n.,* pl. **pleu·rae** (·ree) The serous membrane enveloping the lung and lining the internal surface of the thoracic cavity.

pleu·ra·cot·o·my (ploor″uh·kot′uh·mee) *n.* Incision of the thoracic wall and pleura, usually exploratory. Syn. *thoracotomy.*

pleu·ral (ploor′ul) *adj.* Of or pertaining to the pleura.

pleural cavity. The potential space, included between the parietal and visceral layers of the pleura.

pleu·ral·gia (ploo·ral′jee·uh) *n.* Pain in the pleura or in the side. —**pleural·gic** (·jick) *adj.*

pleural shock. Hypotension, sweating, pallor, and collapse due to pleural irritation, as with a trocar. Syn. *Capp's pleural reflex.*

pleural space. PLEURAL CAVITY.

pleur·apoph·y·sis (ploor″uh·pof′i·sis) *n.* One of the lateral processes of a vertebra, corresponding morphologically to a rib. —**pleur·apo·phys·i·al** (·a·po·fiz′ee·ul), **pleur·apoph·y·se·al** (·a·pof″i·see′ul) *adj.*

pleu·rec·to·my (ploo·reck′tuh·mee) *n.* Excision of any portion of the pleura.

pleu·ri·sy (ploor′i·see) *n.* Inflammation of the pleura. Syn. *pleuritis.*

pleu·rit·ic (ploo·rit′ick) *adj.* Pertaining to, affected with, or of the nature of pleurisy.

pleu·ri·tis (ploo·rye′tis) *n.,* pl. **pleu·rit·i·des** (ploo·rit′i·deez) PLEURISY.

pleu·ro·cen·te·sis (ploor″o·sen·tee′sis) *n.* Puncture of the parietal pleura.

pleu·ro·cu·ta·ne·ous (ploor″o·kew·tay′nee·us) *n.* Pertaining to the parietal pleura and the skin, as a pleurocutaneous fistula.

pleu·ro·dyn·ia (ploor″o·din′ee·uh) *n.* 1. Severe paroxysmal pain and tenderness of the intercostal muscles. 2. EPIDEMIC PLEURODYNIA.

pleu·ro·gen·ic (ploor″o·jen′ick) *adj.* Originating in the pleura.

pleu·rog·e·nous (ploo·roj′e·nus) *adj.* PLEUROGENIC.

pleu·ro·lith (ploor′o·lith) *n.* A calculus in the pleura or the pleural cavity.

pleu·rol·y·sis (ploo·rol′i·sis) *n.* Separation of the parietal pleura from the chest wall.

pleu·ro·peri·car·di·al (ploor″o·perr·i·kahr′dee·ul) *adj.* Pertaining to both pleura and pericardium.

pleu·ro·peri·car·di·tis (ploor″o·perr″i·kahr·dye′tis) *n.* Pleurisy associated with pericarditis.

pleu·ro·peri·to·ne·al (ploor″o·perr·i·to·nee′ul) *adj.* Pertaining to the pleura and the peritoneum.

pleu·ro·pneu·mo·nia (ploor″o·new·mo′nyuh) *n.* 1. Combined pleurisy and pneumonia. 2. An infectious disease of cattle producing pleural and lung inflammation, caused by organisms of the Mycoplasma group.

pleuropneumonia-like organisms. A widely prevalent group of minute, filterable, highly pleomorphic microorganisms belonging to the Mycoplasmataceae; responsible for primary atypical pneumonia in man, for lung disease of cattle and goats, and for mastitis of sheep and goats. Abbreviated, PPLO.

pleu·ro·pul·mo·nary (ploor″o·pul′muh·nerr″ee, ·pool′) *n.* Pertaining to the pleura and lungs.

pleu·rot·o·my (ploo·rot′uh·mee) *n.* Incision into the pleura.

pleu·ro·vis·cer·al (ploor″o·vis′ur·ul) *adj.* Pertaining to the pleura and to the viscera.

plex·ec·to·my (pleck·seck′tuh·mee) *n.* Surgical removal of a plexus.

plexiform neurofibroma or **neuroma.** 1. A diffuse proliferation of nerve fibers and connective tissue elements producing tortuosity and thickening of the affected segment. 2. PACHYDERMATOCELE.

plex·im·e·ter (pleck·sim′e·tur) *n.* 1. A finger, usually the left third finger, held firmly against the skin to receive the stroke in indirect percussion. 2. A small, thin, oblong plate of hard but flexible material, such as ivory or rubber, used for the same purpose.

plex·or (pleck′sur) *n.* A finger, when used to tap the surface of the body in performing percussion. Syn. *plessor.*

plex·us (pleck′sus) *n.,* L. pl. & genit. sing. **plexus,** E. pl. **plexuses** A network of interlacing nerves or anastomosing blood vessels or lymphatics. —**plex·al** (·sul) *adj.*

pli·ca (plye′kuh) *n.,* pl. & genit. sing. **pli·cae** (·see) A fold.

pli·ca·tion (pli·kay'shun) *n.* The state or condition of being folded; the act of folding; any surgical procedure in which folds or tucks are placed in a structure. —**pli·cate** (plye'kate) *v.;* **pli·cate** (plye'kate, ·kut), **pli·cat·ed** (plye'kay·tid) *adj.*

pli·cot·o·my (plye·kot'uh·mee) *n.* Surgical division of the posterior fold of the tympanic membrane.

-ploid. A suffix indicating a given *multiple of* or *relationship to the haploid number of chromosomes,* as diploid, heteroploid.

plomb, plumb (plum) *n.* Any plastic or inert material used to close pathologic cavities in the body, as material inserted extrapleurally to collapse the lung in pulmonary tuberculosis or inert and antiseptic preparations used to pack bone cavities.

plom·bage (plom·bahzh') *n.* The therapeutic use of plastic or inert materials to close pathologic cavities in the body.

plug, *n.* Material that occludes an opening or channel.

plumb. PLOMB.

plum·bic (plum'bick) *adj.* Describing or pertaining to a compound of tetravalent lead.

plum·bism (plum'biz·um) *n.* LEAD POISONING.

Plummer-Vinson syndrome Dysphagia, koilonychia, gastric achlorhydria, glossitis, and hypochromic microcytic anemia, due to an iron deficiency. Syn. *Paterson-Kelly syndrome, sideropenic dysphagia.*

plump·er, *n.* The thickened flange of an artificial denture designed to produce a pleasing contour of the facial outline.

pluri- A combining form meaning *several,* being or having *more than one.*

plurideficiency syndrome. KWASHIORKOR.

plu·ri·de·fi·cient (ploor''i·de·fish'unt) *adj.* Having many deficiencies, usually of one or more vitamins, hormones, or food factors. —**pluride·fi·cien·cy** (·un·see) *n.*

plu·ri·fo·cal (ploor''i·fo'kul) *adj.* MULTIFOCAL.

plu·ri·glan·du·lar (ploor''i·glan'dew·lur) *adj.* Pertaining to more than one gland or to the secretions of more than one gland; MULTIGLANDULAR.

plu·ri·grav·i·da (ploor''i·grav'i·duh) *n.* A woman during her third and subsequent pregnancies; multigravida.

plu·ri·loc·u·lar (ploor''i·lock'yoo·lur) *adj.* Having more than one compartment or loculus; multilocular.

plu·rip·a·ra (ploo·rip'uh·ruh) *n.* A women who has given birth several times.

plu·ri·par·i·ty (ploor''i·păr'i·tee) *n.* The condition of having given birth several times.

plu·rip·o·tent (ploo·rip'uh·tunt) *adj.* Characterizing a cell or embryonic tissue capable of producing more than one type of cell or tissue.

plu·to·ma·nia (ploo''to·may'nee·uh) *n.* 1. The delusion of possessing great wealth. 2. Obsessive greed for wealth.

plu·to·nism (ploo'tuh·niz·um) *n.* A disease caused by exposure to plutonium, manifested in experimental animals by graying of the hair, liver degeneration, and tumor formation.

plu·to·ni·um (ploo·to'nee·um) *n.* Pu = 242. An element, atomic number 94, obtained from neptunium and capable of undergoing fission with release of large amounts of energy.

PMI Abbreviation for *point of maximal impulse* (= APEX IMPULSE).

-pnea, -pnoea A combining form meaning *respiration* or *respiratory condition.*

pneo·car·di·ac reflex (nee''o·kahr'dee·ack). A change in the cardiac rhythm or the blood pressure, due to the inhalation of an irritating vapor.

pneo·dy·nam·ics (nee''o·dye·nam'icks) *n.* The dynamics of respiration.

pneum-, pneumo- A combining form meaning (a) *air, gas;* (b) *pulmonary, lung;* (c) *respiratory, respiration;* (d) *pneumonia.*

pneu·mar·thro·sis (new''mahr·thro'sis) *n.* Air or gas in a joint.

pneumat-, pneumato- A combining form meaning (a) *respiration;* (b) in medicine, *the presence of air or gas in a part.*

pneu·mat·ics (new·mat'icks) *n.* The branch of physics treating of the dynamic properties of air and gases.

pneu·ma·ti·za·tion (new''muh·ti·zay'shun) *n.* The progressive development of, or the state of having, air-filled cavities in bones, lined by a mucous membrane, as the accessory nasal sinuses or mastoid air cells. —**pneu·ma·tize** (new'muh·tize) *v.*

pneumato-. See *pneumat-.*

pneu·ma·to·car·dia (new''muh·to·kahr'dee·uh) *n.* The presence of air or gas in the chambers of the heart.

pneu·ma·to·cele (new'muh·to·seel, new·mat'o·) *n.* 1. Herniation of the lung. 2. A sac or tumor containing gas; especially the scrotum filled with gas.

pneu·ma·to·dysp·nea, pneu·ma·to·dysp·noea (new''muh·to·disp'nee·uh) *n.* Dyspnea due to pulmonary emphysema.

pneu·ma·to·gram (new'muh·to·gram, new·mat'o·) *n.* A tracing showing the frequency, duration, and depth of the respiratory movements.

pneu·ma·tol·o·gy (new''muh·tol'uh·jee) *n.* The science of pulmonary respiration.

pneu·ma·tom·e·ter (new''muh·tom'e·tur) *n.* An instrument for measuring the pressure of the inspired and expired air.

pneu·ma·tom·e·try (new''muh·tom'e·tree) *n.* The measurement of the pressure of the inspired and expired air.

pneu·ma·to·sis (new''muh·to'sis) *n.,* pl. **pneu·mato·ses** (·seez) The presence of air or gas in abnormal situations in the body.

pneumatosis cys·toi·des in·tes·ti·na·lis (sis·toy'deez in·tes·ti·nay'lis). A rare condition characterized by gas-filled cysts in the submucosa or subserosa of the small intestine, usually the terminal ileum.

pneu·ma·tu·ria (new''muh·tew'ree·uh) *n.* The voiding of urine containing free gas.

pneu·ma·type (new'muh·tipe) *n.* Breath picture. The deposit formed upon a piece of glass by the moist air exhaled through the nostrils when the mouth is closed. It is employed in the diagnosis of nasal obstruction.

pneu·mo·an·gi·og·ra·phy (new''mo·an''jee·og'

ruh·fee) n. The outlining of the vessels of the lung by means of a radiopaque material, for roentgenographic visualization.

pneu·mo·ar·throg·ra·phy (new″mo·ahr·throg′ruh·fee) n. Radiographic examination of joints into which air or gas has been injected.
—**pneumo·ar·thro·gram** (·ahr′thro·gram) n.

pneu·mo·bul·bar (new″mo·bul′bur) adj. Pertaining to the lungs and to the respiratory center in the medulla oblongata.

pneu·mo·cen·te·sis (new″mo·sen·tee′sis) n. Puncture of a lung with needle or trocar; usually done to obtain tissue or exudate for diagnostic study, or to establish communication with a cavity.

pneu·mo·ceph·a·lus (new″mo·sef′uh·lus) n. The presence of air or gas within the cranial cavity.

pneu·mo·cho·le·cys·ti·tis (new″mo·kol″e·sis·tye′tis, ·ko′le·) n. Cholecystitis associated with gas in the gallbladder.

pneu·mo·coc·cal (new″mo·kock′ul) adj. Pertaining to or caused by pneumococci.

pneumococcal fever. A febrile illness seen usually in infants with no clinically apparent focus of infection but from whose blood *Streptococcus pneumoniae* can be isolated.

pneu·mo·coc·ce·mia, pneu·mo·coc·cae·mia (new″mo·kock·see′mee·uh) n. The presence of pneumococci in the blood.

pneumococci. Plural of *pneumococcus*.

pneu·mo·coc·cic (new″mo·kock′sick) adj. PNEUMOCOCCAL.

pneu·mo·coc·co·su·ria (new″mo·kock″o·sue′ree·uh) n. The presence of pneumococci in the urine.

pneu·mo·coc·cus (new″mo·kock′us) n., pl. **pneumococ·ci** (·sigh) A common term for *Streptococcus pneumoniae*.

pneu·mo·co·lon (new″mo·ko′lun) n. 1. The presence of air or gas in the colon. 2. Distention of the colon with air as a diagnostic measure.

pneu·mo·co·ni·o·sis, pneu·mo·ko·ni·o·sis (new″mo·ko″nee·o′sis) n. Any disease of the lung caused by the inhalation of dust, especially mineral dusts that produce chronic induration and fibrosis.

pneu·mo·cra·ni·um (new″mo·kray′nee·um) n. PNEUMOCEPHALUS.

Pneu·mo·cyst·is (new″mo·sis′tis) n. A parasite associated with pulmonary infection in hosts with diminished resistance. *Pneumocystis carinii* has received the most attention.

Pneumocystis ca·ri·nii (ka·rye′nee·eye). An extracellular parasite, the taxonomy of which has not been established, consisting of nucleated oval or round organisms 1 to 2 μm in diameter, often with eight cells in a cyst 6 to 9 μm in diameter enclosed in a viscous capsule. It is found in interstitial plasma cell pneumonia of man, and is widely prevalent in animals.

Pneumocystis carinii **pneumonia.** An infection of the lungs associated with *Pneumocystis carinii*, occurring in debilitated premature infants, sometimes in patients with hypogammaglobulinemia or deficiencies of cell-mediated immunity, and in patients receiving immunosuppressive therapy for can-

cer or after organ transplantation; treated by pentamidine isethionate. Syn. *interstitial plasma-cell pneumonia.*

pneu·mo·cys·tog·ra·phy (new″mo·sis·tog′ruh·fee) n. Cystography performed after introduction of air or carbon dioxide into the bladder.
—**pneumo·cys·to·gram** (·sis′to·gram) n.

pneu·mo·der·ma (new″mo·dur′muh) n. Air or gas collected under, or in, the skin.

pneu·mo·en·ceph·a·lo·cele (new″mo·en·sef′uh·lo·seel) n. PNEUMOCEPHALUS.

pneu·mo·en·ceph·a·lo·gram (new″mo·en·sef′uh·lo·gram) n. A radiographic picture of the brain after the replacement of the cerebrospinal fluid with air or gas, which has been injected through a needle into the spinal subarachnoid space.

pneu·mo·en·ceph·a·log·ra·phy (new″mo·en·sef″uh·log′ruh·fee) n. A method of visualizing the ventricular system and subarachnoid pathways of the brain by radiography after removal of spinal fluid followed by the injection of air or gas into the subarachnoid space.

pneu·mo·en·ter·i·tis (new″mo·en″tur·eye′tis) n. Inflammation of the lungs and of the intestine.

pneu·mo·gram (new′mo·gram) n. An x-ray film of an organ inflated with air. Syn. *aerogram*.

pneu·mog·ra·phy (new·mog′ruh·fee) n. 1. The recording of the respiratory excursions. 2. PNEUMORADIOGRAPHY.

pneu·mo·he·mo·peri·car·di·um, pneu·mo·hae·mo·peri·car·di·um (new″mo·hee″mo·perr″i·kahr′dee·um) n. The presence of air and blood in the pericardial cavity.

pneu·mo·he·mo·tho·rax, pneu·mo·hae·mo·tho·rax (new″mo·hee″mo·tho′racks) n. The presence of air or gas and blood in the thoracic cavity.

pneu·mo·hy·dro·peri·car·di·um (new″mo·high″dro·perr″i·kahr′dee·um) n. An accumulation of air and fluid in the pericardial cavity.

pneu·mo·hy·po·der·ma (new″mo·high″po·dur′muh) n. SUBCUTANEOUS EMPHYSEMA.

pneumokoniosis. PNEUMOCONIOSIS.

pneu·mo·lip·i·do·sis (new″mo·lip″i·do′sis) n. LIPID PNEUMONIA (2).

pneu·mo·lith (new′mo·lith) n. A calculus or concretion occurring in a lung.

pneu·mo·li·thi·a·sis (new″mo·li·thigh′uh·sis) n. The occurrence of calculi or concretions in a lung.

pneu·mol·y·sis (new·mol′i·sis) n. PNEUMONOLYSIS.

pneu·mo·me·di·as·ti·num (new″mo·mee″dee·as·tye′num) n. 1. The presence of gas or air in the mediastinal tissues. 2. The instillation of air or gas into the mediastinum as a diagnostic measure.

pneu·mo·my·co·sis (new″mo·migh·ko′sis) n. Any disease of the lungs due to a fungus.

pneumon-, pneumono- A combining form meaning lung.

pneu·mo·nec·to·my (new″mo·neck′tuh·mee) n. Excision of an entire lung.

pneu·mo·nia (new·mo′nyuh, ·nee·uh) n. 1. Inflammation of the lungs associated with exudate in the alveolar lumens. 2. Any of various infectious diseases characterized by pneumonia (1); the most common causative agents include pneumococci (*Streptococcus pneumoniae*), pleuropneumonia-like organisms (*Mycoplasma pneumoniae*), and many viruses.

pneu·mon·ic (new-mon´ick) *adj.* 1. Pertaining to pneumonia. 2. Pertaining to the lungs.

pneumonic plague. An extremely virulent type of plague with lung involvement and a high mortality rate.

pneu·mo·ni·tis (new″mo-nigh´tis) *n.*, pl. **pneumo·nit·i·des** (-nit´i-deez) 1. Inflammation of the lungs. 2. Inflammation of the lungs in which the exudate is primarily interstitial.

pneu·mo·no·cele (new′mo-no-seel) *n.* PNEUMATOCELE.

pneu·mo·no·co·ni·o·sis, pneu·mo·no·ko·ni·o·sis (new″mo-no-ko″nee-o′sis) *n.* PNEUMOCONIOSIS.

pneu·mo·nol·y·sis (new″mo-nol′i-sis) *n.*, pl. **pneu·monoly·ses** (-seez) The loosening of any portion of lung adherent to the chest wall; a form of collapse therapy used in the treatment of pulmonary tuberculosis.

pneu·mo·nop·a·thy (new″mo-nop′uth-ee) *n.* Any abnormality or disease of the lungs.

pneu·mo·no·pexy (new-mo-no-peck″see, -mon´o·) *n.* Fixation of lung tissue to the chest wall.

pneu·mo·nor·rha·phy (new″mo-nor′uh-fee) *n.* Suture of a lung.

pneu·mo·not·o·my (new″mo-not′uh-mee) *n.* Surgical incision of a lung.

pneu·mo·peri·car·di·tis (new″mo-perr″i-kahr-dye′tis) *n.* Pericarditis with the formation of gas in the pericardial cavity.

pneu·mo·peri·car·di·um (new″mo-perr″i-kahr-dee·um) *n.* The presence of air in the pericardial cavity.

pneu·mo·peri·to·ne·um (new″mo-perr″i-to-nee′um) *n.* 1. The presence of air or gas in the peritoneal cavity. 2. Injection of a gas into the peritoneal cavity as a diagnostic or therapeutic measure. Syn. *aeroperitoneum.*

pneu·mo·peri·to·ni·tis (new″mo-perr″i-to-nigh′tis) *n.* Peritonitis with the presence of air or gas in the peritoneal cavity.

pneu·mo·py·elo·gram (new″mo-pye′e-lo-gram) *n.* A pyelogram in which air or gas is used as the contrast medium instead of an opaque solution.

pneu·mo·pyo·peri·car·di·um (new″mo-pye′o-perr″i-kahr′dee·um) *n.* The presence of air or gas and pus in the pericardial cavity.

pneu·mo·ra·chis (new″mo-ray′kis) *n.* A collection of gas in the spinal canal, accidental or by injection of air for diagnostic purposes.

pneu·mo·ra·di·og·ra·phy (new″mo-ray″dee·og′ruh-fee) *n.* Radiography of a region, as of a joint or of the abdomen, following the injection of air into a cavity.

pneu·mo·scle·ro·sis (new″mo-skle-ro′sis) *n.* Fibrosis of the lungs.

pneu·mo·sid·er·o·sis (new″mo-sid″ur-o′sis) *n.* The accumulation of iron-containing material in the lungs.

pneu·mo·tax·is (new″mo-tack′sis) *n.* The control of pulmonary respiration. —**pneumotax·ic** (-ick) *adj.*

pneu·mo·tho·rax (new″mo-tho′racks) *n.* 1. The presence of air or gas in a pleural cavity from trauma or disease. Syn. *aeropleura.* 2. The introduction of air or gas into the pleural cavity for diagnosis or therapy.

pneu·mo·ty·phus (new″mo-tye′fus) *n.* Typhoid fever with pneumonia. Syn. *typhopneumonia.*

pneu·mo·ven·tri·cle (new″mo-ven′tri-kul) *n.* A form of pneumocephalus in which air enters the ventricles of the brain through the accessory sinuses of the skull; sometimes seen as a complication of skull fracture.

pneu·mo·ven·tric·u·log·ra·phy (new″mo-ven-trick″yoo-log′ruh-fee) *n.* A method of depicting the ventricular system of the brain by roentgenography, after cerebrospinal fluid is removed and air injected in appropriate amounts.

pneu·sis (new′sis) *n.* RESPIRATION.

pni·go·pho·bia (nigh″go-fo′bee-uh) *n.* The fear of choking; sometimes accompanies angina pectoris.

Po Symbol for polonium.

p.o. Abbreviation for *per os,* by mouth.

pock, *n.* A pustule of an eruptive fever, especially of smallpox.

pock·et, *n.* 1. *In anatomy,* a blind sac, or sac-shaped cavity. 2. A diverticulum communicating with a cavity.

pod-, podo- A combining form meaning *foot* or *footlike process.*

-pod A combining form meaning (a) *having feet of a particular number or kind;* (b) *foot or part resembling a foot.*

-poda In zoological taxonomy, a combining form meaning *having feet of a* (specified) *number or kind.*

po·dag·ra (po-dag′ruh) *n.* GOUT (1).

po·dal·gia (po-dal′jee-uh) *n.* Pain in the foot.

po·dal·ic (po-dal′ick) *adj.* Pertaining to the feet.

podalic version. The operation of changing the position of the fetus in the uterus in which one or both feet are brought down to the outlet.

pod·ar·thri·tis (pod″ahr-thrye′tis) *n.* Inflammation of the joints of the feet.

pod·ede·ma, pod·oe·de·ma (pod″e-dee′muh) *n.* Edema of the feet.

-podia A combining form meaning *a condition of the feet.*

po·di·a·try (po-dye′uh-tree) *n.* Diagnosis and treatment of disorders of the feet. Syn. *chiropody.* —**podia·trist** (-trist) *n.*

podo·brom·hi·dro·sis (pod″o-brom″hi-dro′sis) *n.* Offensive sweating of the feet.

podo·cyte (pod′o-site) *n.* An epithelial cell of the renal glomerulus, so called because of the footlike processes which attach it to the capillary basement membrane of the glomerular tuft. —**podo·cyt·ic** (pod″o-sit′ick) *adj.*

pod·o·dyn·ia (pod″o-din′ee-uh) *n.* Pain in the foot, especially a neuralgic pain in the heel unattended by swelling or redness.

podo·phyl·lin (pod″o-fil′in) *n.* Podophyllum resin.

podo·phyl·lo·tox·in (pod″o-fil″o-tock′sin) *n.* A crystalline polycyclic substance, $C_{22}H_{22}O_8$, obtained from the rhizome and roots of *Podophyllum peltatum;* has cathartic properties and, when applied topically, is active against certain wartlike neoplasms.

podo·phyl·lum (pod″o·fil′um) *n.* The dried rhizome and roots of the mayapple, *Podophyllum peltatum,* containing podophyllotoxin, α-peltatin, β-peltatin, and other constituents. Used in the form of an extract called podophyllum resin or podophyllin as a cathartic, and, locally, as a cytotoxic agent for the treatment of certain warts.

-podous A combining form meaning *having feet of a* (specified) *number or kind.*

-poiesis A combining form meaning *production, making, forming.*

-poietic A combining form meaning *producing, formative.*

poikilo- A combining form meaning *irregular, abnormal, variable.*

poi·ki·lo·cyte (poy′ki·lo·site, poy·kil′o·) *n.* An erythrocyte of irregular shape.

poi·ki·lo·cy·the·mia, poi·ki·lo·cy·thae·mia (poy″ki·lo·sigh·theem′ee·uh) *n.* The presence of poikilocytes in the blood.

poi·ki·lo·cy·to·sis (poy″ki·lo·sigh·to′sis) *n.,* pl. **poikilocyto·ses** (·seez) Abnormality in shape of circulating erythrocytes.

poi·ki·lo·der·ma (poy″ki·lo·dur′muh) *n.* A skin syndrome characterized by pigmentation, telangiectasia, and, usually, atrophy.

poikiloderma atro·phi·cans vas·cu·la·re (a·trof′i·kanz vas·kew·lair′ee). A widespread or localized disorder of skin characterized by atrophy, pigmentation, telangiectasia, and purpura; usually observed in association with, or as an end result of, other disorders involving the skin, especially dermatomyositis and mycosis fungoides. When observed independently, it is also referred to as Jacobi's type.

poikiloderma of Ci·vatte (see·vaht′) RETICULATED PIGMENTED POIKILODERMA.

poi·ki·lo·der·ma·to·my·o·si·tis (poy″ki·lo·dur″muh·to·migh″o·sigh′tis) *n.* Poikiloderma atrophicans vasculare in association with dermatomyositis.

poi·ki·lo·ther·mal (poy″ki·lo·thur′mul) *adj.* POIKILOTHERMIC.

poi·ki·lo·ther·mic (poy″ki·lo·thur′mick) *n.* Having a body temperature that varies with environmental temperature, usually slightly higher than that of the environment, as in all plants and animals except birds and mammals; COLD-BLOODED. —**poikilother·mism** (·miz·um), **poi·ki·lo·ther·my** (poy′ki·lo·thur″mee, poy·kil′o·) *n.*

poi·ki·lo·ther·mous (poy″ki·lo·thur′mus) *adj.* POIKILOTHERMIC.

poi·ki·lo·throm·bo·cyte (poy″ki·lo·throm′bo·site) *n.* A blood platelet of abnormal shape.

point·ing, *n.* 1. The coming to a point. 2. The stage of abscess formation when the pus has approached the surface at a localized area.

point of maximal impulse. APEX IMPULSE. Abbreviated, PMI.

poi·son (poy′zun) *n.* A substance that in relatively small doses has an action, when it is ingested by, injected into, inhaled or absorbed by, or applied to a living organism, that either destroys life or impairs seriously the functions of one or more organs or tissues.

poi·son·ing, *n.* The abnormal condition caused by a toxic substance.

poison ivy. A North American climbing vine, *Toxicodendron radicans* (also called *Rhus toxicodendron* and *R. radicans*); contains an oleoresin (urushiol) which is sensitizing and causes a form of contact dermatitis.

poison oak. *Toxicodendron quercifolium* (also called *Rhus toxicodendron* Linné but not the *R. toxicodendron* of American authors, which is poison ivy); contains an oil which is sensitizing and causes a contact dermatitis similar to that produced by poison ivy. Western poison oak is the *Toxicodendron diversilobum* (also known as *Rhus diversiloba*).

poi·son·ous, *adj.* Having the properties of a poison.

poisonous snakes. The venom-producing snakes, which belong mainly to four families: Elapidae, the cobras and allies; Hydrophidae, the sea snakes; Crotalidae, the pit vipers; and Viperidae, the true vipers. Most have large, hypodermic-like front fangs by which venom is injected.

poison su·mac (sue′mack). A smooth shrub, *Toxicodendron vernix* (also called *Rhus vernix* and *R. venenata*); contains an oil which is sensitizing and causes eruptions resembling poison-ivy dermatitis.

Pois·son distribution (pwah·sohn″) In *statistics,* a discrete mathematical distribution, often called the law of small numbers, that may be regarded as an approximation of the binomial distribution when p (probability) is small and n (number) large.

po·ker back or **spine.** ANKYLOSING SPONDYLITIS.

po·lar, *adj.* 1. Pertaining to or having a pole. 2. Of chemical compounds: having molecules composed of atoms that share their common electron pairs unequally and thereby effect a separation of positive and negative centers of electricity to form a dipole.

polar bodies or **cells.** The two minute, abortive cells given off successively by the ovum during the maturation divisions. They mark the animal pole.

polar cataract. A cataract in which the opacity is confined to one pole of the lens.

po·lar·im·e·ter (po″lar·im′e·tur) *n.* An instrument for making quantitative studies on the rotation of polarized light by optically active substances.

po·lari·scope (po·lār′i·skope) *n.* An instrument for studying the properties of or for observing substances in polarized light; a polarimeter.

po·lar·i·ty (po·lār′i·tee) *n.* 1. The state or quality of having poles or regions of intensity with mutually opposite qualities. 2. The electrically positive or negative condition of a battery, cell, or other electric device with terminals.

po·lar·iza·tion (po″lur·i·zay′shun) *n.* 1. The act of polarizing or the state of being polarized. 2. A condition produced in light or other transverse wave radiation in which the vibrations are restricted and take place in one plane only (plane polarization) or in curves (circular or elliptic polarization). The plane of polarization is altered or rotated when the light is passed through a quartz crystal or solutions of certain substances (rotatory polarization). 3. The deposit of gas bubbles (hydrogen) on the electronegative plate of a galvanic battery, whereby the flow of the current is impeded. 4. Acquisition of electric charges of opposite sign, as across semipermeable cell membranes in living tissues.

po·lar·ize (po'lur-ize) v. To endow with polarity; to place in a state of polarization.

po·lar·og·ra·phy (po''lur·og'ruh·fee) n. A method of chemical analysis based on the interpretation of the current-voltage curve characteristic of a solution of an electrooxidizable or electroreducible substance when it is electrolyzed with the dropping mercury electrode. —**po·laro·graph·ic** (po·lăr''o·graf'ick, po''lur·o·) adj.

Polaroid. Trademark for a film containing an oriented light-polarizing compound. Used as a substitute for Nicol prisms, in polariscopes, and in eyeglasses to prevent glare.

pole, n. 1. Either extremity of the axis of a body, as of the fetus or the crystalline lens. 2. One of two points at which opposite physical qualities (of electricity or of magnetism) are concentrated, as either of the electrodes of an electrochemical cell, battery, or dynamo.

pole tubule. In embryology, the first two tubules to grow out of the renal pelvis; there is a cranial and a caudal pole tubule.

poli-, polio- A combining form meaning (a) gray; (b) gray substance, gray matter.

po·li·en·ceph·a·li·tis (po''lee·en·sef''uh·lye'tis) n. POLIOENCEPHALITIS.

po·lio (po'lee·o) n. POLIOMYELITIS.

po·lio·dys·tro·phy (po''lee·o·dis'truh·fee) n. Degeneration of gray matter.

po·lio·en·ceph·a·li·tis (po''lee·o·en·sef''uh·lye'tis) n. Inflammation of the gray matter of the brain.

polioencephalitis acu·ta (a·kew'tuh). POLIOENCEPHALITIS.

po·lio·en·ceph·a·lo·me·nin·go·my·e·li·tis (po''lee·o·en·sef''uh·lo·me·nin''go·migh·e·lye'tis) n. Inflammation of the gray matter of the brain and spinal cord and of their meninges.

po·lio·en·ceph·a·lo·my·e·li·tis (po''lee·o·en·sef''uh·lo·migh·e·lye'tis) n. Any inflammation of the gray matter of the brain and spinal cord, more specifically paralytic spinal poliomyelitis with encephalitis.

po·lio·en·ceph·a·lop·a·thy (po''lee·o·en·sef''uh·lop'uth·ee) n. Any disease of the gray matter of the brain.

po·lio·my·el·en·ceph·a·li·tis (po''lee·o·migh''ul·en·sef''uh·lye'tis) n. POLIOENCEPHALO-MYELITIS.

po·lio·my·e·li·tis (po''lee·o·migh''e·lye'tis) n. 1. A common virus disease of man which usually runs an abortive course, characterized by upper respiratory and gastrointestinal symptoms, but which may progress to involve the central nervous system and result in a nonparalytic or paralytic form of the disease,

the latter being the classical form of paralytic spinal poliomyelitis. It is endemic with epidemic flare-ups, but is preventable through immunization. 2. Any inflammation of the gray matter of the spinal cord. —**poliomye·lit·ic** (·lit'ick) adj.

poliomyelitis vaccine. 1. Officially (USP, USPHS), a sterile suspension of inactivated poliomyelitis virus of types 1, 2, and 3; used for active immunization against poliomyelitis. Syn. Salk vaccine. 2. Unofficially and more broadly, any vaccine against poliomyelitis, including preparations of living attenuated poliomyelitis virus, such as Sabin vaccine.

poliomyelitis virus. A small (20 to 25 nm), relatively stable virus which is the causative agent of poliomyelitis. On an immunological basis, three distinct types have been identified, of which the classical prototypes are type 1, Brunhilde; type 2, Lansing; type 3, Leon. Type 1 is the most frequently responsible for the epidemic form of the disease.

po·lio·my·e·lop·a·thy (po''lee·o·migh''e·lop'uth·ee) n. Disease of the gray matter of the spinal cord.

po·li·o·sis (po''lee·o'sis) n. 1. A condition characterized by the absence of pigment in the hair. Syn. canities. 2. Premature graying of the hair.

po·lio·vi·rus (po''lee·o·vye'rus) n. POLIOMYELITIS VIRUS.

Po·lit·zer bag (po'lit·sur) A waterproof bag used to inflate the middle ear. One end is tightly fixed into one nostril while the other is held closed during the act of swallowing water or pronouncing the letter k.

po·lit·zer·i·za·tion (po''lit·sur·i·zay'shun, pol''it·) n. The production of sudden increased air pressure in the nasopharynx to inflate the middle ear, by means of compression by a Politzer bag.

Politzer's test A hearing test in which a tuning fork held in front of the nares will be heard only by the unaffected ear during swallowing.

poll (pole) n. & v. 1. Obsol. The crown and back of the head. 2. Specifically, the vertex or crest between the ears of a quadruped; in cattle, the part from which the horns grow. 3. To cut off the horns of (cattle).

pol·la·ki·u·ria (pol''uh·kee·yoor'ee·uh) n. Abnormally frequent micturition.

pol·len (pol'un) n. The fecundating element of flowering plants.

pol·len·osis (pol''e·no'sis) n. HAY FEVER.

pol·lex (pol'ecks) n., genit. **pol·li·cis** (pol'i·sis), pl. **pol·li·ces** (·seez) THUMB. NA alt. digitus I.

pollex val·gus (val'gus). A thumb abnormally bent toward the ulnar side.

pollex va·rus (vair'us). A thumb abnormally bent toward the radial side.

pol·li·ci·za·tion (pol''i·si·zay'shun) n. 1. The freeing of a webbed thumb. 2. A surgically produced substitution of another digit to replace a thumb. —**pol·li·cize** (pol'i·size) v.

pol·lu·tion, n. 1. The act of defiling or rendering impure, as pollution of drinking water. 2. The discharge of semen without sexual intercourse, as in nocturnal emission.

po·lo·cyte (po'lo·site) n. One of the polar bodies.

po·lo·ni·um (po·lo'nee·um) *n.* Po = 210. The first radioactive element isolated by Pierre and Marie Curie from pitchblende (1898); a product of disintegration of radium. Syn. *radium-F*.

pol·toph·a·gy (pol·tof'uh·jee) *n.* Complete chewing of the food to the consistency of porridge before swallowing it.

po·lus (po'lus) *n.,* pl. & genit. sing. **po·li** (·lye) POLE.

poly- A combining form meaning (a) *multiple, compound, complex;* (b) *various, diverse;* (c) *excessive;* (d) *generalized, disseminated.*

poly·ac·id (pol"ee·as'id) *n.* 1. An acid, such as phosphoric acid, having more than one replaceable hydrogen atom. 2. A complex acid derived from a number of molecules of one or more inorganic acids by elimination of water.

poly·am·ine (pol"ee·am'in, pol"ee·uh·meen') *n.* Any compound having two or more amine groups. —**poly·am·i·no** (·am'i·no, ·uh·mee'no) *adj.*

poly·an·dry (pol'ee·an"dree) *n.* A social state in which the marriage of one woman with more than one man at the same time is lawful.

poly·an·gi·i·tis (pol"ee·an"jee·eye'tis) *n.* An inflammatory process involving multiple vascular channels.

poly·ar·te·ri·tis (pol"ee·ahr"te·rye'tis) *n.* 1. Inflammation of a number of arteries at the same time. 2. POLYARTERITIS NODOSA.

polyarteritis no·do·sa (no·do'suh). A systemic disease characterized by widespread inflammation of small and medium-sized arteries in which some of the foci are nodular; complications of the process such as thrombosis lead to retrogressive changes in the tissues and organs supplied by the affected vessels with a correspondingly diverse array of symptoms and signs. Syn. *periarteritis nodosa, disseminated necrotizing periarteritis.*

poly·ar·thric (pol"ee·ahr'thrick) *adj.* Pertaining to many joints.

poly·ar·thri·tis (pol"ee·ahr·thrye'tis) *n.* Simultaneous inflammation of several joints.

poly·ar·throp·a·thy (pol"ee·ahr·throp'uth·ee) *n.* Disease of several joints.

poly·ar·tic·u·lar (pol"ee·ahr·tick'yoo·lur) *adj.* Pertaining to or affecting several joints.

Pó·lya's operation or **method** (po'yah) Partial resection of the stomach, followed by posterior end-to-side gastrojejunostomy; a type of Billroth II gastric resection.

poly·atom·ic (pol"ee·uh·tom'ick) *adj.* Containing several atoms.

poly·ba·sic (pol"ee·bay'sick) *adj.* Referring to an acid having several hydrogen atoms replaceable by bases.

poly·blast (pol'ee·blast) *n.* A free macrophage of inflamed connective tissue derived from blood-borne monocytes.

poly·bleph·a·ron (pol"ee·blef'uh·ron) *n.* A supernumerary eyelid.

poly·cen·tric (pol"ee·sen'trick) *adj.* Having many centers or nuclear points.

poly·chlo·ri·nat·ed (pol"ee·klo'rin·ay·tid) *adj.* Having chlorine atoms substituted for more than three hydrogen atoms.

polychlorinated biphenyl. 1. Any biphenyl structure with chlorine atoms attached. 2. Originally, any of a class of pesticides with polychlorinated biphenyl residues. Abbreviated, PCB

poly·chon·dri·tis (pol"ee·kon·drye'tis) *n.* Inflammation of cartilage in various parts of the body.

poly·chro·ma·sia (pol"ee·kro·may'zhuh) *n.* POLYCHROMATOPHILIA.

poly·chro·mat·ic (pol"ee·kro·mat'ick) *adj.* 1. Of, pertaining to, or having several colors. 2. POLYCHROMATOPHILIC.

poly·chro·mato·cyte (pol"ee·kro·mat'o·site, ·kro' muh·to·) *n.* A cell that will simultaneously assume the color of different dyes.

poly·chro·mato·phil (pol"ee·kro'muh·to·fil, ·kro· mat'o·fil) *n.* A structure stainable with both acidic and basic dyes.

poly·chro·mato·phil·ia (pol"ee·kro"muh·to·fil' ee·uh) *n.* The presence in the blood of polychromatophilic cells.

poly·chro·mato·phil·ic (pol"ee·kro"muh·to·fil' ick) *adj.* Susceptible to staining with more than one dye.

poly·chrome (pol'ee·krome) *adj.* Of or pertaining to many colors.

polychrome methylene blue. Methylene blue partially oxidized into its lower homologues, the methylene violet and the azures, with an increase in metachromatic properties; prepared by allowing methylene blue to age or by boiling a methylene blue solution with alkali.

poly·chro·mia (pol"ee·kro'mee·uh) *n.* Increased or abnormal pigmentation.

poly·chy·lia (pol"ee·kigh'lee·uh) *n.* Excessive formation of chyle. —**polychy·lic** (·lick) *adj.*

poly·clin·ic (pol"ee·klin'ick) *n.* A hospital in which many types of diseases are treated.

poly·clo·nal (pol"ee·klo'nul) *adj.* Pertaining to or characterizing cells of various differen[t] clones, with the implication that the principa[l] proteins or other products manufactured by these cells are different.

polyclonal gammopathy. DIFFUSE HYPERGAM MAGLOBULINEMIA.

poly·co·ria (pol"ee·ko'ree·uh) *n.* A hereditar[y] anomaly of the eye characterized by the pres[ence] of more than one pupil, each surrounde[d] by a sphincter (true polycoria); the exac[t] mechanism of which is unknown. Simila[r] defects in the periphery of the iris (false poly[·] coria) also occur.

poly·cy·clic (pol"ee·sigh'click, ·sick'lick) *ad[j.]* 1. Describing a molecule that contains two [or] more groupings of atoms in the form of ring[s] or closed chains. 2. *In dermatology,* pertainin[g] to cutaneous lesions exhibiting many confl[u]ent rings or arcs.

poly·cy·e·sis (pol"ee·sigh·ee'sis) *n.* MULTIPL[E] PREGNANCY.

poly·cys·tic (pol"ee·sis'tick) *adj.* Containin[g] many cysts.

polycystic disease or **kidney.** Hereditary bila[t]eral cysts distributed throughout the ren[al] parenchyma, resulting in markedly enlarg[ed] kidneys and progressive renal failure.

poly·cy·the·mia, poly·cy·thae·mia (pol"ee·sig[h·] theem'ee·uh) *n.* A condition characterized an increased number of erythrocytes and erythroblasts.

poly·cy·the·mia hy·per·ton·i·ca (high-pur-ton'i-kuh). GAISBÖCK'S DISEASE.

poly·cy·the·mia ru·bra ve·ra (roo'bruh veer'uh). POLYCYTHEMIA VERA.

poly·cy·the·mia ve·ra (veer'uh). An absolute increase in all marrow-derived blood cells, especially erythrocytes and erythroblasts, of unknown cause. Syn. *erythremia, Osler-Vaquez disease, primary polycythemia.*

poly·dac·tyl·ia (pol''ee-dack-til'ee-uh) n. POLYDACTYLY.

poly·dac·tyl·ism (pol''ee-dack'til-iz-um) n. POLYDACTYLY.

poly·dac·ty·ly (pol''ee-dack'ti-lee) n. The existence of supernumerary fingers or toes.

poly·de·fi·cient (pol''ee-de-fish'unt) adj. PLURIDEFICIENT. —**polydeficien·cy** (·un-see) n.

poly·dip·sia (pol''ee-dip'see-uh) n. Excessive thirst. Syn. *anadipsia.*

poly·don·tia (pol''ee-don'chee-uh) n. POLYODONTIA.

poly·dys·troph·ic (pol''ee-dis-trof'ick) adj. Characterized by or pertaining to many congenital anomalies, especially of connective tissue.

poly·dys·tro·phy (pol''ee-dis'truh-fee) n. The presence of several, usually congenital, structural abnormalities.

poly·elec·tro·lyte (pol''ee-e-leck'tro-lite) n. Any substance of high molecular weight that behaves as an electrolyte, such as proteins.

poly·emia, poly·ae·mia (pol''ee-ee'mee-uh) n. An excess of blood over the normal amount in the body.

poly·es·the·sia, poly·aes·the·sia (pol''ee-es-theezh'uh, ·theez'ee-uh) n. An abnormality of sensation in which a stimulus such as a single touch or pinprick is felt in two or more places at the same time.

poly·es·trus, poly·oes·trus (pol''ee-es'trus) n. In animals, the existence of several estrus periods during each sexual season. —**polyestrous,** adj.

poly·eth·yl·ene (pol''ee-eth'il-een) n. A long-chain plastic polymer containing hundreds of ethylene units per molecule. In the form of flexible tubing and film, a pure form of the plastic is useful in surgical procedures.

poly·ga·lac·tia (pol''ee-ga-lack'tee-uh, ·shee-uh) n. Excessive secretion of milk.

po·lyg·a·mous (po-lig'uh-mus) adj. 1. Having, or allowing, more than one wife or husband at one time, more particularly the former. 2. Having both unisexual and hermaphrodite flowers on one plant. —**polyga·my** (·mee) n.

poly·gas·tria (pol''ee-gas'tree-uh) n. Excessive secretion of gastric juice.

poly·gas·tric (pol''ee-gas'trick) adj. 1. Having several bellies, as certain muscles. 2. Having more than one stomach.

poly·gen·ic (pol''ee-jen'ick) adj. Pertaining to or determined by several different genes.

poly·glan·du·lar (pol''ee-gland'yoo-lur) adj. Pluriglandular; pertaining to or affecting several glands and their secretions.

po·lyg·o·nal (po-lig'uh-nul) adj. Having many angles.

poly·gram (pol'ee-gram) n. The tracing made by a polygraph.

poly·graph (pol'ee-graf) n. An instrument by means of which tracings can be taken simultaneously of the cardiac movements, the arterial or venous pulse, respiration, and skin resistance. Syn. *polysphygmograph.* —**poly·graph·ic** (pol''ee-graf'ick) adj.

poly·gy·ria (pol''i-jye'ree-uh) n. The existence of an excessive number of convolutions in the brain.

poly·he·dral (pol''i-hee'drul) adj. Having many surfaces.

poly·hy·dram·ni·os (pol''ee-high-dram'nee-os) n. An excessive volume of amniotic fluid.

poly·hy·dric (pol''ee-high'drick) adj. 1. In acids, containing more than one replaceable atom of hydrogen. 2. Containing more than one hydroxyl group; polyhydroxy.

poly·hy·droxy (pol''ee-high-drock'see) adj. POLYHYDRIC.

poly·hy·dru·ria (pol''ee-high-droor'ee-uh) n. A large increase in fluid content of the urine.

poly·in·fec·tion (pol''ee-in-feck'shun) n. Infection resulting from the presence of more than one type of organism; mixed infection.

poly·lep·tic (pol''ee-lep'tick) adj. Characterized by numerous remissions and exacerbations.

poly·lob·u·lar (pol''ee-lob'yoo-lur) adj. MULTILOBULAR.

poly·mas·tia (pol''ee-mas'tee-uh) n. The presence of more than two breasts.

poly·me·lia (pol''ee-mee'lee-uh) n. The presence of more than the normal number of limbs.

poly·me·lus (pol''ee-mee'lus) n., pl. **polyme·li** (·lye) An individual having more than the normal number of limbs.

poly·me·nia (pol''ee-mee'nee-uh) n. MENORRHAGIA.

poly·men·or·rhea, poly·men·or·rhoea (pol''ee-men'o-ree'uh) n. METRORRHAGIA.

poly·mer (pol'i-mur) n. The product formed by joining together many small molecules (monomers). A polymer may be formed from units of the same monomer (addition polymer) or different monomers (condensation polymer).

polymer fume fever. A disease similar to metal fume fever, but associated with inhalation of vaporized polymers.

poly·me·ria (pol''ee-meer'ee-uh) n. The presence of extra or supernumerary parts of the body.

poly·mer·ic (pol''i-merr'ick) adj. 1. Exhibiting polymerism. 2. Of muscles, derived from two or more myotomes.

po·lym·er·ism (po-lim'ur-iz-um, pol'i-mur-iz-um) n. 1. The existence of more than a normal number of parts. 2. A form of isomerism in which two or more molecules of a simple compound interact to form larger molecules, called polymers, that have repeating structural units of the simple compound.

po·lym·er·iza·tion (po-lim''ur-i-zay'shun, pol'i-mur-) n. A reaction in which a complex molecule of relatively high molecular weight is formed by the union of a number of simpler molecules, which may or may not be alike; the reaction may or may not involve elimination of a by-product, such as water or ammonia.

po·lym·er·ize (pol·im'ur·ize, pol'i·mur·ize) *v.* To form a compound from several molecules of the same or different simple molecules. The molecular weight of the polymer may be a simple multiple of the molecular weight of the single simple molecule or the product of the molecular weights of the simple molecules less the molecular weight of the eliminated molecule.

poly·meta·car·pal·ism (pol''ee·met''uh·kahr'pul·iz·um) *n.* A developmental anomaly in which the metacarpus contains more than the normal five bones.

poly·mor·phic (pol''ee·mor'fick) *adj.* 1. Having or occurring in several forms, as a substance crystallizing in different forms. 2. *In clinical medicine,* POLYSYMPTOMATIC.

poly·mor·pho·cel·lu·lar (pol''ee·mor''fo·sel'yoo·lur) *adj.* Having cells of many forms.

poly·mor·pho·nu·cle·ar (pol''ee·mor''fo·new'klee·ur) *adj.* Having a nucleus which is lobated, the lobes being connected by more or less thin strands of nuclear substance; for example, the nucleus of a neutrophil leukocyte.

polymorphonuclear leukocyte. The mature neutrophil leukocyte, so-called because of its segmented and irregularly shaped nucleus.

poly·mor·phous (pol''ee·mor'fus) *adj.* POLYMORPHIC.

polymorphous light eruption. An inflammatory dermatosis induced by sunlight presenting pleomorphic or polymorphic clinical patterns.

poly·my·al·gia (pol''ee·migh·al'jee·uh, ·juh) *n.* Pain involving many muscles.

poly·my·oc·lo·nus (pol''ee·migh·ock'luh·nus, ·migh''o·klo'nus) *n.* Generalized myoclonus.

poly·my·op·a·thy (pol''ee·migh·op'uth·ee) *n.* Any disease affecting several muscles at the same time.

poly·my·o·si·tis (pol''ee·migh''o·sigh'tis) *n.* Simultaneous inflammation of many muscles.

poly·myx·in (pol''ee·mick'sin) *n.* A generic term for a group of related polypeptide antibiotic substances derived from cultures of various strains of the spore-forming soil bacterium *Bacillus polymyxa* (*B. aerosporus*); the individual substances are differentiated by affixing A,B,C,D, and E to the name polymyxin. Polymyxin B, the least toxic of the group, is bactericidal against most gram-negative microorganisms; it is used clinically, in the form of the water-soluble sulfate salt, in a variety of infections, especially against *Pseudomonas aeruginosa*.

poly·neu·ral·gia (pol''ee·new·ral'jee·uh, ·juh) *n.* Neuralgia in which many nerves are involved.

poly·neu·ri·tis (pol''ee·new·rye'tis) *n.* Simultaneous inflammatory involvement of multiple nerves, usually symmetrical, as occurs in leprosy and in the Guillain-Barré disease. Syn. *multiple neuritis.* **—polyneu·rit·ic** (·rit'ick) *adj.*

poly·neu·ro·my·o·si·tis (pol''ee·new''ro·migh''o·sigh'tis) *n.* A disease in which there is concurrent polyneuritis and polymyositis.

poly·neu·rop·a·thy (pol''ee·new·rop'uth·ee) *n.* Simultaneous involvement of many peripheral and/or cranial nerves, usually symmetrical and affecting the distal portions of the limbs more than the proximal ones; a result of metabolic disorders (such as diabetes, uremia, or porphyria), intoxications (arsenic or lead), nutritional defects (beriberi or alcoholism) or a remote effect of carcinoma or myeloma.

poly·neu·ro·ra·dic·u·li·tis (pol''ee·new''ro·ra·dick·yoo·lye'tis) *n.* GUILLAIN-BARRÉ DISEASE.

poly·nu·cle·ar (pol''ee·new'klee·ur) *adj.* MULTINUCLEAR.

poly·nu·cle·ate (pol''ee·new'klee·ate) *adj.* MULTINUCLEAR.

poly·nu·cle·o·tid·ase (pol''ee·new''klee·o·tye'dace, ·ot'i·dace) *n.* An enzyme that depolymerizes nucleic acid to form mononucleotides.

poly·nu·cle·o·tide (pol''i·new'klee·o·tide) *n.* A nucleic acid composed of four mononucleotides.

poly·odon·tia (pol''ee·o·don'chee·uh) *n.* The presence of supernumerary teeth.

poly·oma virus (pol''ee·o'muh). A small deoxyribonucleic acid virus normally causing inapparent infection in mice, but experimentally capable of producing parotid and a wide variety of other tumors.

poly·onych·ia (pol''ee·o·nick'ee·uh) *n.* A condition of supernumerary nails on fingers or toes.

poly·opia (pol''ee·o'pee·uh) *n.* A condition in which more than one image of an object is formed upon the retina.

poly·or·chi·dism (pol''ee·or'ki·diz·um) *n.* The presence of more than two testes in one individual.

poly·orex·ia (pol''ee·o·reck'see·uh) *n.* Excessive hunger or appetite; BULIMIA.

poly·or·gano·sil·ox·ane (pol''ee·or''guh·no·sil·ock'sane) *n.* Any synthetic polymer consisting of a chain of alternate links of silicon atoms and oxygen atoms, the two other bonds of the tetravalent silicon atom generally being attached to an organic group. Commonly known as silicones, these substances may be limpid or viscous fluids or semisolid to solid substances. The fluids impart to glass surfaces a water-repellent film.

poly·or·rhomen·in·gi·tis (pol''ee·or''o·men·in·jye'tis) *n.* POLYSEROSITIS.

poly·os·tot·ic (pol''ee·uh·stot'ick) *adj.* Involving more than one bone.

polyostotic fibrous dysplasia. FIBROUS DYSPLASIA (1) involving more than one bone.

poly·o·tia (pol''ee·o'shee·uh) *n.* A congenital defect in which there is more than one auricle on one or both sides of the head.

pol·yp (pol'ip) *n.* 1. A smooth spherical or oval mass projecting from a membranous surface; may be broad-based or pedunculated. 2. The sessile form of a coelenterate.

poly·pa·re·sis (pol''ee·pa·ree'sis, ·păr·e'sis) *n.* GENERAL PARALYSIS.

poly·path·ia (pol''ee·path'ee·uh) *n.* The presence of several diseases at one time, or the frequent recurrence of disease.

pol·yp·ec·to·my (pol''i·peck'tuh·mee) *n.* Surgical excision of a polyp.

poly·pep·ti·dase (pol''ee·pep'ti·dace, ·daze) *n.*

One of the enzymes that hydrolyze proteins and molecular fragments of proteins.

poly·pep·tide (pol″ee-pep′tide) n. A compound containing two or more amino acids united through the peptide linkage —CONH—.

poly·pep·ti·de·mia, poly·pep·ti·dae·mia (pol″ee-pep″ti·dee′mee·uh) n. The presence of polypeptides in the blood.

poly·pha·gia (pol″ee·fay′jee·uh) n. 1. Excessive eating. 2. BULIMIA.

poly·pha·lan·gism (pol″ee·fuh·lan′jiz·um) n. An extra phalanx in a finger or toe.

poly·phar·ma·cy (pol″ee·fahr′muh·see) n. 1. The prescription of many drugs at one time. 2. The excessive use of medication.

poly·pho·bia (pol″ee·fo′bee·uh) n. Abnormal fear of many things.

poly·phy·let·ic (pol″ee·fye·let′ick) adj. Pertaining to origin from many lines of descent.

polyphyletic theory of hemopoiesis. A hypothesis concerning the mode of origin of blood cells which assumes the development of a specific parental cell for each cell type.

poly·phy·odont (pol″i·fye′o·dont) adj. Having more than two successive sets of teeth at intervals throughout life.

polypi. Plural of polypus.

poly·ploid (pol′i·ploid) adj. Having more than the somatic number of whole sets of chromosomes characteristic for the species. —**poly·ploi·dy** (pol′i·ploy·dee) n.

pol·yp·nea, pol·yp·noea (pol″ip·nee′uh) n. Very rapid respiration; panting.

poly·po·dia (pol″i·po′dee·uh) n. The condition of having supernumerary feet.

pol·yp·oid (pol′i·poid) adj. 1. Resembling a polyp. 2. Pertaining to or characterized by polyps.

po·lyp·o·rous (pol·ip′uh·rus) adj. Having many small openings; cribriform.

pol·yp·o·sis (pol″i·po′sis) n., pl. polypo·ses (·seez) The condition of being affected with polyps.

polyposis co·li (ko′lye). Multiple polyps of the large intestine.

polyposis ven·tric·u·li (ven·trick′yoo·lye). Multiple polyps of the gastric mucosa.

poly·pus (pol′i·pus) n., pl. poly·pi (·pye) POLYP.

poly·ra·dic·u·li·tis (pol″ee·ra·dick″yoo·lye′tis) n. GUILLAIN-BARRÉ DISEASE.

poly·ra·dic·u·lo·neu·ri·tis (pol″ee·ra·dick″yoo·lo·new·rye′tis) n. GUILLAIN-BARRÉ DISEASE.

poly·ra·dic·u·lo·neu·rop·a·thy (pol″ee·ra·dick″yoo·lo·new·rop′uth·ee) n. The simultaneous involvement, usually symmetrical, of multiple peripheral nerves and roots.

poly·ri·bo·some (pol″ee·rye′buh·sohm) n. An aggregate of ribosomes.

poly·sac·cha·ride (pol″ee·sack′uh·ride, ·rid) n. A carbohydrate that is formed by the condensation of two or more, usually many, monosaccharides. Examples are cellulose and starch.

poly·sce·lia (pol″ee·see′lee·uh) n. Excess in the number of legs.

poly·scle·ro·sis (pol″ee·skle·ro′sis) n. MULTIPLE SCLEROSIS.

poly·se·ro·si·tis (pol″ee·seer″o·sigh′tis) n. Widespread, chronic, fibrosing inflammation of serous membranes, especially in the upper abdomen. Syn. Pick's disease, multiple serositis, Concato's disease, chronic hyperplastic perihepatitis, polyorrhymenitis.

poly·si·nus·itis (pol″ee·sigh″nuh″sigh′tis) n. Simultaneous inflammation of several air sinuses.

poly·so·mic (pol″ee·so′mick) adj. 1. Having more than two of any given chromosome. 2. Having more than two sets of chromosomes, as tetraploids, hexaploids. 3. POLYPLOID.

poly·so·mus (pol″ee·so′mus) n. A general term embracing all grades of duplicity, triplicity, etc. It includes monochorionic twins, conjoined twins, equal or unequal, placental parasitic twins, and all grades of double monsters.

poly·sor·bate (pol″ee·sor′bate) n. Any of various polyoxyethylene (20) sorbitan fatty acid esters obtained by copolymerizing the appropriate fatty acid ester of sorbitol and its anhydrides with approximately 20 moles of ethylene oxide for each mole of sorbitol and sorbitol anhydrides. The esters are individually identified by appending a number, as polysorbate 40, which is polyoxyethylene 20 sorbitan monopalmitate, and polysorbate 80, which is polyoxyethylene 20 sorbitan mono-oleate. Polysorbates are used as emulsifying, dispersing, and solubilizing agents.

poly·sper·mia (pol″ee·spur′mee·uh) n. 1. The secretion and discharge of an excessive quantity of seminal fluid. 2. Penetration of the ovum by more than one spermatozoon.

poly·sper·my (pol″ee·spur′mee) n. POLYSPERMIA (2).

poly·stich·ia (pol″ee·stick′ee·uh) n. A condition in which the eyelashes are arranged in more than the normal number of rows.

poly·sty·rene (pol″ee·stye′reen) n. A clear, lightweight plastic prepared by polymerization of styrene and used for the manufacture of various molded articles and sheet materials.

poly·sus·pen·soid (pol″ee·suh·spen′soid) n. A colloid system in which there are several phases in different degrees of dispersion.

poly·symp·to·mat·ic (pol″ee·simp″tuh·mat′ick) adj. In clinical medicine, pertaining to a pathological process having manifold symptoms, which may not all occur simultaneously or in the same patient.

poly·syn·dac·tyl·ism (pol″ee·sin·dak′til·iz·um) n. Multiple syndactyly.

poly·the·lia (pol″ee·theel′ee·uh) n. The presence of supernumerary nipples.

poly·trich·ia (pol″ee·trick′ee·uh) n. Excessive development of hair; hypertrichosis.

poly·trop·ic (pol″ee·trop′ick, ·tro′pick) adj. Having affinity for or affecting more than one type of cell; applied to viruses; pantropic.

poly·uria (pol″ee·yoo′ree·uh) n. The passage of an excessive quantity of urine. —**poly·uric** (·yoo′rick) adj.

poly·va·lent (pol″ee·vay′lunt) adj. 1. Of antigens, having many combining sites or determinants. 2. Pertaining to vaccines composed of mixtures of different organisms, and to the resulting mixed antiserum. 3. Of a chemical

poly·vi·nyl·pyr·rol·i·done (pol''ee-vye''nil·pirr·ol'i·dohn) *n.* A synthetic polymer of high molecular weight formed by interactions of formaldehyde, ammonia, hydrogen, and acetylene; has been used as a plasma expander and to retard absorption of certain parenterally administered drugs. Abbreviated, PVP.

po·made (po·maid', po·mahd') *n.* A perfumed ointment, especially one for applying to the scalp.

Pom·pe's disease Generalized glycogenosis caused by a deficiency of the lysosomal enzyme, α-1,4-glucosidase, with abnormal storage of glycogen in skeletal muscles, heart, liver, and other organs. The clinical manifestations include marked weakness, cardiomegaly, and cardiac failure with death usually occurring in the first year. Inheritance is autosomal recessive. Syn. *maltase deficiency, cardiomegalia glycogenica diffusa, idiopathic generalized glycogenosis, type II of Cori.*

pom·pho·lyx (pom'fo·licks) *n.* CHEIROPOMPHOLYX.

Pon·cet's disease (pohn·seh') An atypical form of generalized tuberculosis chiefly characterized by joint manifestations, with associated disease of different viscera; the usual gross features of tuberculosis infection are lacking, although organisms can be demonstrated by animal inoculation.

pon·der·al (pon'dur·ul) *adj.* Of or pertaining to weight.

pons (ponz) *n.,* genit. **pon·tis** (pon'tis), pl. **pon·tes** (pon'teez) 1. A process or bridge of tissue connecting two parts of an organ. 2. [NA] The portion of the brainstem between the midbrain and the medulla oblongata. **—pon·tile** (pon'tile), **pon·tine** (·tine, ·teen) *adj.*

pont-, ponto- A combining form meaning (a) *bridge;* (b) *pons, pontine.*

pon·tic (pon'tick) *n.* The portion of a prosthetic bridge that is between the abutments and serves as the artificial substitute for a lost tooth or teeth. Syn. *dummy.*

pon·to·bul·bar (pon''to·bul'bur) *adj.* Pertaining to the pons and to the medulla oblongata.

Pontocaine. A trademark for the local anesthetic tetracaine, used as the hydrochloride salt.

pon·to·cer·e·bel·lar (pon''to·serr''e·bel'ur) *adj.* Pertaining to the pons and the cerebellum.

pop·lit·e·al (pop·lit'ee·ul, pop''li·tee'ul) *adj.* Pertaining to or situated in the ham, as popliteal artery, popliteal nerve, popliteal space.

popliteal fossa. POPLITEAL SPACE.

popliteal space or region. A diamond-shaped area behind the knee joint.

population pyramid. A graphic method of representing the age structure of populations. Usually each 5-year age group is represented by a horizontal bar with females shown on one side and males on the other side of the vertical central line. Differences in birth rate and longevity result in pyramid patterns which are distinctively different for different countries, depending on living standards, epidemiology, health care, fertility, and other variables.

por-, poro- A combining form meaning (a) *passageway, duct;* (b) *pore, opening;* (c) *cavity, tract.*

por·ad·e·ni·tis (por·ad''e·nigh'tis) *n.* LYMPHOGRANULOMA VENEREUM.

por·ad·e·no·lym·phi·tis (por·ad''e·no·lim·fye'tis) *n.* LYMPHOGRANULOMA VENEREUM.

por·cine (por'sine, ·seen) *adj.* Pertaining to or characteristic of swine.

pore, *n.* 1. A minute opening on a surface. 2. The opening of the duct of a sweat gland.

por·en·ceph·a·li·tis (pore''en·sef·uh·lye'tis) *n.* A term once proposed for encephalitis with a tendency to form cavities in the brain, a pathologic entity now thought not to exist.

por·en·ceph·a·ly (pore''en·sef'uh·lee) *n.* A term introduced by Heschl, in 1869, to designate a congenital defect extending from the surface of the cerebral hemisphere into the subjacent ventricle, now commonly used to designate any cystic cavity in the brain of an infant or child; may be the result of brain tissue destruction of any causation (encephaloclastic porencephaly) or due to maldevelopment (schizencephaly). **—poren·ce·phal·ic** (·se·fal'ick), **poren·ceph·a·lous** (·sef'uh·lus) *adj.*

pore of Kohn ALVEOLAR PORE.

po·rio·ma·nia (po''ree·o·may'nee·uh) *n.* A compulsion to wander or travel, usually in a state of impaired consciousness. **—porioma·ni·ac** (·nee·ack) *n.*

po·ri·on (po'ree·on) *n.,* pl. **po·ria** (·ree·uh) The point of the upper margin of the porus acusticus externus. The two poria and the left orbitale define the Frankfort horizontal plane.

pork tapeworm. TAENIA SOLIUM.

por·nog·ra·phy (por·nog'ruh·fee) *n.* 1. Obscene writing, drawing, photography, and the like. 2. A treatise on prostitution.

po·ro·ceph·a·li·a·sis (po''ro·sef''uh·lye'uh·sis) *n.,* pl. **porocephalia·ses** (·seez) An uncommon infection of the lungs, liver, trachea, or nasal cavities of man with any of the varieties of *Porocephalus.*

po·ro·ker·a·to·sis (po''ro·kerr''uh·to'sis) *n.* A genodermatosis characterized by a collar of elevated hyperkeratosis about an irregular patch of depressed atrophic skin; microscopically, horn plugs or cornoid lamella in the dermis are prominent, but are not necessarily located in the openings of sweat glands as the name "porokeratosis" implies. Syn. *hyperkeratosis excentrica, Mibelli's disease.*

po·ro·ma (po·ro'muh) *n.* A callosity.

po·ro·sis (po·ro'sis) *n.,* pl. **poro·ses** (·seez) Rarefaction; increased roentgen translucency; formation of vacuoles or pores; cavity formation. **—po·rot·ic** (po·rot'ick) *adj.*

po·ros·i·ty (po·ros'i·tee) *n.* The condition or quality of being porous.

por·pho·bi·lin (por''fo·bye'lin) *n.* A product derived from hemoglobin which may be excreted in urine.

por·pho·bi·lin·o·gen (por''fo·bye·lin'o·jen) *n.* A chromogen intermediate in the biosynthesis of porphyrins and heme; found with its precursor, δ-aminolevulinic acid, in the urine in some forms pf porphyria.

por·phyr·ia (por·firr'ee·uh, ·fye'ree·uh) n. 1. An inborn error of metabolism characterized by the presence of increased quantities of porphyrins or their precursors in the blood and other tissues and in feces and urine, abdominal pain, polyneuropathy, convulsions, and psychosis, as well as dark discoloration of the urine on standing in sunlight. 2. Any disturbance of porphyrin metabolism, congenital or acquired, resulting in porphyrinuria.

porphyria cu·ta·nea tar·da he·re·di·ta·ria (kew·tay'nee·uh tahr'duh he·red·i·tair'ee·uh). A hereditary porphyria with constant increased fecal excretion of coproporphyrin and uroporphyrin, characterized clinically by cutaneous lesions and acute attacks of jaundice and abdominal colic. Syn. *porphyria variegata.*

porphyria cutanea tarda symp·to·ma·ti·ca (simp·to·mat'i·kuh). Acquired porphyria appearing in late adulthood, characterized by photosensitivity, cutaneous lesions, and hepatic dysfunction; abdominal pain and neurologic complications do not occur.

porphyria eryth·ro·poi·et·i·ca (e·rith''ro·poy·et'i·kuh). ERYTHROPOIETIC PORPHYRIA.

porphyria he·ma·to·poi·et·i·ca (hee''muh·to·poy·et'i·kuh). ERYTHROPOIETIC PORPHYRIA.

porphyria he·pat·i·ca (he·pat'i·kuh). ACUTE INTERMITTENT PORPHYRIA.

por·phy·rin (por'fi·rin) n. A heterocyclic ring derived from porphin by replacing the eight hydrogen atoms attached to the carbon atoms of the pyrrole rings of porphin by various organic groups. In the center of the ring a metal, such as iron (in heme) or magnesium (in chlorophyll), may or may not be present.

por·phy·rin·uria (por''fi·ri·new'ree·uh) n. The excretion of an abnormal amount of a porphyrin, commonly believed to be uroporphyrin I, in the urine.

por·poise heart (por'pus). A heart with preponderance of the right ventricle.

Por·ro's operation (poh'rro) A cesarian section immediately followed by hysterectomy.

port, n. The area and contour of the beam of radiation directed through the body surface for external radiation therapy.

por·ta (por'tuh) n., pl. & genit. sing. **por·tae** (·tee) The hilus of an organ through which vessels or ducts enter.

por·ta·ca·val (por''tuh·kay'vul) adj. Pertaining to the portal vein and the inferior vena cava.

portacaval shunt. A surgical connection between the portal vein and inferior vena cava.

porta he·pa·tis (hep'uh·tis) [NA]. The transverse fissure of the liver through which the portal vein and hepatic artery enter the liver and the hepatic ducts leave.

por·tal (por'tul) adj. & n. 1. Of or pertaining to the porta hepatis. 2. Pertaining to the portal vein or system. 3. The porta or hilus of an organ.

portal canal or **area.** An interlobular artery, vein, bile duct, nerve, and lymph vessel, and the interlobular connective tissue in which they lie, between the corners of the anatomic lobules of the liver.

portal circulation. The passage of blood by a vein from one capillary bed to a second independent set of capillaries; usually, the passage of the blood from the capillaries of the gastrointestinal tract and red pulp of the spleen into the sinusoids of the liver.

portal cirrhosis. Progressive fibrosis centered in the portal areas of the liver; loosely, LAENNEC'S CIRRHOSIS.

portal hypertension. Portal venous pressure in excess of 20 mmHg, resulting from intrahepatic or extrahepatic portal venous compression or occlusion, and producing in the late stages large variceal collateral veins, splenomegaly, and ascites.

portal space. PORTAL CANAL.

portal system. The portal circulation, usually the hepatic portal vein and its tributaries.

portal triad. The three main structures found in each portal canal: a branch of the hepatic artery and of the portal vein, and a tributary to the common bile duct.

por·ta·re·nal shunt (por''tuh·ree'nul). A surgical connection between the left renal vein and the portal system, usually the splenic vein.

por·tio (por'shee·o, por'tee·o) n., pl. **por·ti·o·nes** (por''shee·o'neez, por''tee·) Portion.

portio va·gi·na·lis cer·vi·cis (vaj·i'·nay'lis sur'vi·sis) The portion of the cervix of the uterus which protrudes into the vagina.

porto-. A combining form meaning *portal.*

por·to·ca·val (por''to·kay'vul) adj. PORTACAVAL.

por·to·gram (por''to·gram) n. The image produced by portography.

por·tog·ra·phy (por·tog'ruh·fee) n. Radiographic depiction of the portal venous system following injection of contrast medium.

por·to·sys·tem·ic (por''to·sis·tem'ick) adj. Pertaining to the portal system.

por·to·ve·no·gram (por''to·vee'no·gram) n. PORTOGRAM.

port-wine nevus, mark, or **stain.** A congenital hemangioma characterized by one or several red to purplish flat or slightly elevated patches, most often on the face. Syn. *nevus flammeus.*

po·rus (po'rus) n., pl. & genit. sing. **po·ri** (·rye) A pore or foramen.

porus acus·ti·cus ex·ter·nus (a·koos'ti·kus eck·stur'nus) The opening of the external acoustic meatus.

po·si·tion (puh·zish'un) n. Place; location; attitude; posture. Abbreviated, P. —**position·al** (·ul) adj.

position of the fetus. The relation of the presenting part of the fetus to the cardinal points. For the vertex, the face, and the breech there are four positions each: a right anterior, a right posterior, a left anterior, and a left posterior. For each of the shoulders there is an anterior and a posterior position. In order to shorten and memorize these positions, the initials of the chief words are made use of, as follows: for vertex presentations the word occiput is abbreviated O., and preceded by the letter R. or L. for right or left, and followed by A. or P.

according to whether the presenting part is anterior or posterior. Thus the initials L.O.A., left occipitoanterior, indicate that the presenting occiput is upon the anterior left side. In the same way are derived the terms L.O.P., R.O.A., R.O.P. For facial presentations, in the same way L.F.A., left frontoanterior, L.F.P., R.F.A., R.F.P. For breech or sacral presentations, L.S.A., L.S.P., R.S.A., R.S.P., and for shoulder or dorsal presentations, L.D.A., L.D.P., R.D.A., R.D.P.

pos·i·tive (poz′i-tiv) *adj.* 1. Indicating or expressing affirmation or confirmation; *in psychiatry,* receptive, responsive; warm; constructive. 2. Of a response to a drug or other therapy, satisfactory or as expected. 3. Of results of a test or experiment, confirming the presence or existence of the entity tested for. 4. Included in that one of two classes or ranges which is conceived as fundamental or primary; opposed to negative, as a positive integer. Symbol, +. 5. Of images (visual, photographic, etc.), corresponding to the subject in distribution of light and dark, or in colors with respect to their complements.

positive lens. Any lens with a positive focal length; it is thicker in the center than around the circumference. There are three types of positive lenses: double convex or biconvex, planoconvex, and converging concavoconvex.

positive pressure breathing. Breathing by introduction of a suitable gas mixture into the lungs at a pressure above the ambient pressure exerted on the external surface of the chest.

pos·i·tron (poz′i-tron) *n.* An elementary particle having the mass of an electron but carrying a unit positive charge. It is evanescent, dissipating itself as radiation as soon as it encounters an electron, which is annihilated with it.

po·sol·o·gy (po-sol′uh-jee) *n.* The branch of medical science that deals with the dosage of medicines.

post- A prefix meaning *after, behind,* or *subsequent.*

post·abor·tal (pohst′′uh-bort′ul) *adj.* Occurring after an abortion.

post·anal (pohst′′ay′nul) *adj.* Situated behind the anus.

post·an·es·thet·ic, post·an·aes·thet·ic (pohst′′an-es-thet′ick) *adj.* Following anesthesia.

post·ap·o·plec·tic (pohst′′ap-o-pleck′tick) *adj.* Occurring after or as a consequence of a cerebral accident.

post·ax·i·al (pohst-ack′see-ul) *adj.* Situated behind the axis: in the arm, behind the ulnar aspect; in the leg, behind the fibular aspect.

post·bra·chi·al (pohst-bray′kee-ul) *adj.* Situated posterior to the arm.

post·cap·il·lary (pohst-kap′i-lerr′′ee) *n.* VENOUS CAPILLARY.

post·car·di·ot·o·my (pohst′′kahr′′dee-ot′uh-mee) *adj.* Occurring after open-heart surgery.

postcardiotomy syndrome. A syndrome of acute nonspecific pericarditis, which may be recurrent, occurring weeks to months following cardiac surgery, cardiac trauma, or myocardial infarction, responding dramatically to corticosteroid therapy; thought to represent sensitivity to antigens from myocardial necrosis. Syn. *postcardiac injury syndrome.*

post·ca·va (pohst-kay′vuh) *n.* INFERIOR VENA CAVA. —**postca·val** (·vul) *adj.*

post·cen·tral (pohst-sen′trul) *adj.* 1. Situated behind a center. 2. Situated behind the central sulcus of the brain.

postcentral gyrus. The cerebral convolution that lies immediately posterior to the central sulcus and extends from the longitudinal fissure above to the posterior ramus of the lateral sulcus.

post·cla·vic·u·lar (pohst′′kla-vick′yoo-lur) *adj.* Situated behind the clavicle.

post·co·i·tal (pohst-ko′it-ul) *adj.* After coitus.

postcoital pill. A high-dose estrogen pill given after coitus to prevent implantation.

post·com·mis·sur·ot·o·my (pohst-kom′′i-shur-ot′uh-mee) *adj.* Following surgical incision of the mitral valve commissure.

post·con·cus·sion syndrome (pohst′′kon′kush′un). Symptoms which follow brain concussion: giddiness and occasional vertigo; headache, insomnia, irritability, fatigability, inability to concentrate, tearfulness, and an intolerance of emotional excitement and crowds. Syn. *minor contusion syndrome.*

post·con·i·za·tion (pohst′′kon-i-zay′shun, ·ko·ni·) *adj.* Occurring after cervical conization.

post·con·nu·bi·al (pohst′′kuh-new′bee-ul) *adj.* Coming on or occurring after marriage.

post·con·vul·sive (pohst′′kun-vul′siv) *adj.* Coming on after a convulsion.

post·cor·di·al (pohst-kor′dee-ul) *adj.* Situated behind the heart.

post·cri·coid (pohst-krye′koid) *adj.* Behind the cricoid cartilage.

post·di·ges·tive (pohst′′di-jes′tiv) *adj.* Occurring after digestion.

post·diph·the·rit·ic (pohst′′dif-the-rit′ick) *adj.* Occurring after or resulting from an attack of diphtheria.

post·en·ceph·a·lit·ic (pohst′′en-sef′′uh-lit′ick) *adj.* Occurring after and presumably as a result of encephalitis.

postencephalitic parkinsonism. The parkinsonian syndrome occurring as a sequel to encephalitis lethargica within a variable period, from days to many years, after the acute process. Clinically distinct, it is characterized by commencing almost exclusively before the age of 40, by a history of varying degrees of lethargy, and very slow but steady evolution of the classical parkinsonian syndrome. Patients frequently exhibit oculogyric and other spasms, tics, breathing arrhythmias, bizarre movements, postures and gaits, and psychopathic behavior. Pathologically, changes in the substantia nigra are demonstrable.

post·ep·i·lep·tic (post′′ep·i·lep′tick) *adj.* Occurring after an epileptic attack.

pos·te·ri·or (pos-teer′ee-ur) *adj. In anatomy* (with reference to the human or animal body as poised for its usual manner of locomotion): hind, in back; situated relatively far in the direction opposite to that of normal locomotion.

posterior atlantooccipital membrane. A broad membrane extending from the posterior surface and cranial border of the posterior arch of the atlas to the posterior margin of the foramen magnum.

posterior chamber. The space between the posterior surface of the iris and the ciliary zonule, the lens, and the vitreous body.

posterior clinoid process. One of the two short bony extensions from the superior angles of the dorsum sellae which give attachment to the tentorium cerebelli.

posterior column. A division of the longitudinal columns of gray matter in the spinal cord.

posterior commissure of the cerebrum. A transverse band of nerve fibers crossing dorsal to the opening of the cerebral aqueduct into the third ventricle.

posterior communicating artery. A vessel which passes from the internal carotid artery to the posterior cerebral artery.

posterior cranial fossa. The lowest in position of the three cranial fossae, lodging the cerebellum, pons, and medulla oblongata. It is formed by the posterior surface of the petrous and inner surface of the mastoid portion of the temporal bone and the inner surface of the occipital bone below the horizontal limb of the confluence of the sinuses.

posterior iter. The aperture through which the chorda tympani nerve enters the tympanum. Syn. *iter chordae posterius.*

posterior mallear fold. 1. A fold on the external surface of the tympanic membrane stretching from the mallear prominence to the posterior portion of the tympanic sulcus of the temporal bone, forming the lower posterior border of the pars flaccida. 2. A fold of mucous membrane on the inner aspect of the tympanic membrane over the lateral ligament of the malleus.

posterior palatal seal. The seal at the posterior border of an upper artificial denture; it is usually established along the junction of the hard and soft palates.

posterior pillar of the fauces. PALATOPHARYNGEAL ARCH.

posterior pituitary. NEUROHYPOPHYSIS.

posterior root ganglion. SPINAL GANGLION.

posterior tubercle. A tubercle at the posterior part of the extremity of the transverse process of certain cervical vertebrae.

postero-. A combining form meaning *posterior.*

pos·ter·o·an·te·ri·or (pos″tur·o·an·teer′ee·ur) *adj.* From the back to the front of the body, as in describing the direction of roentgen rays traversing the patient. Abbreviated, PA.

pos·ter·o·ex·ter·nal (pos″tur·o·ecks·tur′nul) *adj.* Occupying the outer side of a back part, as the posteroexternal column of the spinal cord. —**posteroexter·nad** (·nad) *adv.*

pos·ter·o·in·ter·nal (pos″tur·o·in·tur′nul) *adj.* Occupying the inner side of a back part, as the posterointernal column of the spinal cord. —**posterointer·nad** (·nad) *adv.*

pos·ter·o·lat·er·al (pos″tur·o·lat′ur·ul) *adj.* Situated behind and at the side of a part. —**posterolater·ad** (·ad) *adv.*

pos·ter·o·me·di·al (pos″tur·o·mee′dee·ul) *adj.* Situated posteriorly and toward the midline. —**posteromedi·ad** (·ad) *adv.*

pos·ter·o·su·pe·ri·or (pos″tur·o·sue·peer′ee·ur) *adj.* Situated behind and above a part.

post·erup·tive (pohst″e·rup′tiv) *adj.* Following eruption.

post·esoph·a·ge·al, post·oesoph·a·ge·al (pohst″e·sof″uh·jee′ul, ·ee″so·faj′ee·ul) *adj.* Situated behind the esophagus.

post·fe·brile (pohst·feb′ril, ·fee′bril) *adj.* Occurring after or resulting from a fever.

post·gan·gli·on·ic (pohst″gang″glee·on′ick) *adj.* Situated beyond a ganglion.

post·gas·trec·to·my (pohst″gas·treck′tuh·mee) *adj.* Occurring after or resulting from removal of part or all of the stomach.

post·gle·noid (pohst·glee′noid, ·glen′oid) *adj.* Situated behind the mandibular (glenoid) fossa of the temporal bone.

post·grav·id (pohst·grav′id) *adj.* After pregnancy.

post·hemi·ple·gic (pohst″hem·i·plee′jick) *adj.* Occurring after or following hemiplegia.

post·hem·or·rhag·ic, post·haem·or·rhag·ic (pohst″hem·o·raj′ick) *adj.* Occurring after or resulting from a hemorrhage.

post·he·pat·ic (pohst″he·pat′ick) *adj.* Situated or occurring behind the liver.

posthepatic jaundice. OBSTRUCTIVE JAUNDICE.

post·hep·a·tit·ic (pohst·hep″uh·tit′ick) *adj.* Following or resulting from hepatitis.

post·her·pet·ic (pohst″hur·pet′ick) *adj.* Occurring after or resulting from herpes zoster or herpes simplex.

pos·thi·tis (pos·thigh′tis) *n., pl.* **pos·thit·i·des** (·thit′i·deez) Inflammation of the prepuce.

post·hu·mous (pos′tew·mus) *adj.* 1. Occurring after death. 2. Born after the death of the father, or by cesarean section after the death of the mother. 3. Published after the death of the writer.

post·hyp·not·ic (pohst″hip·not′ick) *adj.* Succeeding the hypnotic state; acting after the hypnotic state has passed off.

post·ic·tal (pohst″ick′tul) *adj.* Following or resulting from a seizure or a stroke.

postictal automatism. A complex semipurposeful act carried out by the patient after an epileptic attack; usually the consequence of postictal confusion.

post·ic·ter·ic (pohst·ick·terr′ick) *adj.* Of or pertaining to the period or condition following jaundice.

post·in·fec·tious (pohst″in·feck′shus) *adj.* Following an infection.

postinfectious psychosis. Psychosis following an acute infectious disease, such as pneumonia or typhoid fever.

post·in·flu·en·zal (pohst″in″floo·en′zul) *adj.* Occurring after or resulting from influenza.

post·mas·tec·to·my (pohst″mas·teck′tuh·mee) *adj.* Occurring after or resulting from surgical removal of the breast.

post·ma·ture (pohst″muh·tewr′) *adj.* 1. Of a fetus, having remained in the uterus beyond the normal length of gestation. 2. Overdeveloped. —**postma·tu·ri·ty** (·tewr′i·tee) *n.*

post·men·ar·che (pohst″me·nahr′kee) *adj.* Occurring after the beginning of menstrual cycles.

post·men·o·pau·sal (pohst″men″uh·paw′zul) *adj.* Occurring after the menopause.

post·men·stru·al (pohst·men′stroo·ul) *adj.* Following menstruation.

post mor·tem (mor′tum) *adv. phrase* After death, as: 2 hours post mortem.).

post·mor·tem (pohst·mor′tum) *adj. & n.* 1. Following death. 2. An examination of the body after death; AUTOPSY.

post·na·sal (pohst″nay′zul) *adj.* Situated behind the nose, or in the nasopharynx.

post·na·tal (pohst·nay′tul) *adj.* Subsequent to birth.

post·ne·crot·ic (pohst″ne·krot′ick) *adj.* 1. Occurring after the death of a tissue or part. 2. Occurring after death.

postnecrotic cirrhosis. Cirrhosis, usually due to toxic agents or viral hepatitis, characterized by necrosis of liver cells, large regenerating nodules of hepatic tissue, the presence of large bands of connective tissue which course irregularly through the liver, and, in some areas, preservation of the normal hepatic architecture.

post·oc·u·lar (pohst·ock′yoo·lur) *adj.* Behind the eye.

post·op·er·a·tive (pohst·op′ur·uh·tiv) *adj.* Occurring after an operation; following closely upon an operation.

postoperative myxedema. Myxedema resulting from total or partial thyroidectomy. Syn. *operative myxedema.*

post·oral (pohst·o′rul) *adj.* Situated behind the mouth; posterior to the first visceral arch.

post·or·bit·al (pohst·or′bi·tul) *adj.* Behind the orbit.

post·par·a·lyt·ic (pohst″păr·uh·lit′ick) *adj.* Following the onset of paralysis.

post·par·tum (pohst·pahr′tum) *adj.* Following childbirth.

postperfusion syndrome. Fever, splenomegaly, lymphadenopathy, lymphocytosis, and eosinophilia occurring 2 to 8 weeks following use of a pump-oxygenator in open-heart surgery; may represent a reaction to the large amount of blood usually administered during such operations.

post·phle·bit·ic (pohst″fle·bit′ick) *adj.* Following or resulting from venous inflammation.

postphlebitic syndrome. The postthrombotic syndrome following thrombophlebitis of deep veins, particularly the ileofemoral vessels.

post·pran·di·al (pohst·pran′dee·ul) *adj.* After a meal.

post·pu·ber·al (pohst·pew′bur·ul) *adj.* Occurring after puberty.

post·ra·di·a·tion (pohst″ray·dee·ay′shun) *adj.* Occurring after exposure to ionizing radiation.

post·re·nal (pohst″ree′nul) *adj.* In the urinary tract, caudal to the kidneys.

post·ro·ta·to·ry (pohst·ro′tuh·tor″ee) *adj.* After rotation, as postrotatory ocular nystagmus.

post·sple·nec·to·my (pohst″sple·neck′tuh·mee) *adj.* Following or resulting from surgical removal of the spleen.

post·ste·not·ic (pohst″ste·not′ick) *adj.* Pertaining to the area beyond an orifice narrowed by disease, or beyond an abnormal constriction of a hollow viscus; usually the area beyond a narrowed heart valve or blood vessel.

post·syn·ap·tic (pohst″si·nap′tick) *adj.* Situated behind or occurring after a synapse.

post·throm·bot·ic (pohst″throm·bot′ick) *adj.* Occurring after or as a result of thrombosis.

postthrombotic syndrome. Chronic venous insufficiency resulting from deep venous thrombosis of the lower extremity, characterized by edema, pain, stasis dermatitis, stasis cellulitis, varicose veins, pigmentation of the skin, and eventually chronic ulceration of the lower leg.

post·trau·mat·ic (pohst″traw·mat′ick) *adj.* Pertaining to any process or event following, or resulting from, traumatic injury.

posttraumatic personality disorder. A disorder resulting from direct injury to the head or brain followed by a brief loss of consciousness; manifested by headache, emotional instability, fatigability, insomnia, and memory defects, but usually no demonstrable organic deficits.

post·tus·sive (pohst·tus′iv) *adj.* Occurring after a cough.

pos·tu·late (pos′tew·late, -lut) *n.* 1. A proposition assumed without proof. 2. A condition that must be fulfilled.

pos·tur·al (pos′tew·rul, pos′chur·ul) *adj.* Pertaining to posture or position; performed by means of a special posture.

postural drainage. Removal of bronchial secretions or of the contents of a lung abscess by the use of gravity and position to drain a specific area of the lung.

pos·ture (pos′chur) *n.* Position or bearing, especially of the body.

post·vac·ci·nal (pohst·vack′si·nul) *adj.* Following, or resulting from, vaccination.

postvaccinal encephalomyelitis. ACUTE DISSEMINATED ENCEPHALOMYELITIS.

post·ves·i·cal (pohst·ves′i·kul) *adj.* Behind the urinary bladder.

po·ta·ble (po′tuh·bul) *adj.* Drinkable; fit to drink.

po·tas·si·um (puh·tas′ee·um) *n.* K = 39.102. A light, malleable metallic element formed into ductile lumps, rods, or spheres, which reacts violently with water. A small amount of potassium is physiologically essential.

potassium bicarbonate. $KHCO_3$, used medicinally as a source of potassium ion, and also as a gastric antacid and to alkalinize urine.

potassium bitartrate. $KHC_4H_4O_6$, used as a saline cathartic. Syn. *cream of tartar, potassium hydrogen tartrate.*

potassium chloride. KCl, used for the treatment of potassium deficiency states.

potassium citrate. $K_3C_6H_5O_7$, used for the treatment of potassium deficiency states; also as a systemic alkalizer, diuretic, and expectorant.

potassium iodide. KI, used mainly as an expectorant and as a source of iodide ion.

potassium nitrate. KNO_3; has some diuretic properties; SALTPETER.

potassium permanganate. $KMnO_4$, used as a disinfectant and cleansing agent; sometimes also as an antidote to certain poisons.

potassium sodium tartrate. COOK(CHOH)$_2$-COONa, used as a saline cathartic. Syn. *Rochelle salt*.

potassium tolerance test. A formerly used test based on the increased rise and duration of the serum potassium in patients with hypoadrenalism as compared to normal after the oral ingestion of a potassium salt.

po·ta·to nose. RHINOPHYMA.

potato tumor. CAROTID-BODY TUMOR.

po·ten·cy (po'tun·see) *n.* 1. Inherent power or strength. 2. Power of the male to perform the sexual act. 3. *In homeopathy*, the degree of dilution of a drug. —**po·tent** (·tunt) *adj.*

po·ten·tial (po·ten'chul) *adj. & n.* 1. Possible or probable. 2. Existing in the form of a capacity or disposition as opposed to being realized or overtly manifested; latent. 3. Any inherent possibility, capacity, or power of a thing or a being. 4. In electricity, a state of tension or of difference in energy capable of doing work. If two bodies of different potential are brought into contact, a current is established between them that is capable of producing electric effects.

po·ten·ti·a·tion (po·ten''shee·ay'shun) *n.* 1. The effect of a substance, when added to another, of making the latter more potent. 2. The effect of combination of two drugs resulting in action greater than the total effect of each used separately. —**po·ten·ti·ate** (·ten'shee·ate) *v.*

po·tion (po'shun) *n.* A drink or draught.

po·to·ma·nia (po''to·may'nee·uh) *n.* DELIRIUM TREMENS.

pot·ter's asthma, consumption, or **rot.** SILICOSIS.

Pott's disease Kyphosis resulting from tuberculous osteitis of the spine.

Pott's fracture Fibular fracture a few inches above the ankle, sometimes accompanied by fracture of the medial malleolus.

Potts' operation The creation of an aortic-pulmonary artery anastomosis as palliative surgery for tetralogy of Fallot, and other forms of cyanotic heart disease.

pouch, *n.* A sac or pocket.

pou·drage (poo·drahzh') *n.* The therapeutic introduction of an irritating powder on a serous surface to stimulate the formation of adhesions for obliteration of the pleural space, or to stimulate the development of a collateral circulation, as in the pericardial space.

poul·tice (pohl'tis) *n.* A soft, semiliquid mass made of some cohesive substance mixed with water, and used for application to the skin for the purpose of supplying heat and moisture or acting as a local stimulant.

pound, *n.* A unit of measure of weight. See Table of Weights and Measures in the Appendix.

pour plate. A bacterial culture in which the culture is incorporated into a medium, poured into a sterile petri dish, and allowed to solidify.

povidone-iodine, *n.* A water-soluble complex of polyvinylpyrrolidone and iodine used topically for prevention and control of cutaneous infections susceptible to iodine.

pow·der, *n.* 1. A group of pharmaceutical preparations of definite formula, consisting of intimate mixtures of finely divided medicinal substances. 2. *In pharmacy*, a single dose of medicine placed in powder paper, dusting powder, douche powder, or other bulk powder to be administered or used internally or externally.

pow·er, *n.* 1. The ability to produce an effect. 2. *In optics*, the magnification given by a lens or prism.

pox, *n.* 1. A vesicular or pustular exanthematic disease, such as smallpox, that may leave pit scars. 2. SYPHILIS.

pox diseases. A group of diseases caused by poxviruses, characterized clinically usually by vesicles, pustules, and crusting and pathologically by ballooning degeneration and necrosis of the epidermis. Diseases such as chickenpox and herpes simplex show similar skin lesions but are caused by a different group of viruses.

pox·vi·rus (pocks'vye'rus) *n.* A member of a group of large, chemically complex DNA viruses, variably stable to ether, which includes those causing smallpox, vaccinia, ectromelia (mousepox), molluscum contagiosum, and infectious myxomatosis.

P.P.D. Abbreviation for *purified protein derivative* of tuberculin.

PPLO Abbreviation for *pleuropneumonia-like organisms.*

p.p.m., ppm Parts per million.

ppt. Abbreviation for *precipitate.*

P-Q interval. P-R INTERVAL.

prac·tice, *v. & n.* 1. To perform the duties of a physician as regards the diagnosis and treatment of disease. 2. The routine application of the principles of medicine to the diagnosis and treatment of disease. 3. Collectively, the patients of a physician.

prac·ti·tion·er (prack·tish'un·ur) *n.* A qualified person engaged in practicing medicine.

praevia. PREVIA.

prag·mat·ag·no·sia (prag''mat·ag·no'see·uh) *n.* Loss of ability to recognize an object formerly known to the patient.

prag·mat·am·ne·sia (prag''mat·am·nee'zhuh, ·zee·uh) *n.* Loss of ability to remember the appearance of an object formerly known.

pran·di·al (pran'dee·ul) *adj.* Of or pertaining to a meal, especially a dinner.

pra·tique (pra·teek') *n.* The bill of health given to incoming vessels by a health officer of a port.

Praus·nitz–Küst·ner reaction (prɑowss'nits, kuᵉst'nur) A reaction of local hypersensitivity produced by intradermal injection of blood serum from a hypersensitive person followed by injection of the appropriate antigen; a method of passive transfer of hypersensitivity. The reaction forms the basis of the passive transfer test.

prax·i·ol·o·gy (prack''see·ol'uh·jee) *n.* 1. The psychology of acts and of deeds. 2. The science of conduct, as of behavior, in relation to values, such as social, moral, or esthetic ones.

pre- A prefix signifying *before.*

pre·ag·o·nal (pree·ag'uh·nul) *adj.* Immediately preceding the death agony.

pre·anal (pree·ay'nul) *adj.* Situated in front of the anus.

pre·an·es·thet·ic, pre·an·aes·thet·ic (pree"an·es·thet'ick) *adj.* Before anesthesia.

pre·aor·tic (pree"ay·or'tick) *adj.* Situated in front of the aorta.

pre·au·ric·u·lar (pree"aw·rick'yoo·lur) *adj.* Situated in front of the auricle.

pre·ax·i·al (pree·ack'see·ul) *adj.* Situated in front of the axis of the body or of a limb.

pre·beta·lipo·pro·tein (pree"bay"tuh·lip"o·pro'tee·in, ·teen) *n.* A lipoprotein which on electrophoretic determination appears before the beta-lipoproteins but behind the alpha-lipoproteins.

pre·beta·lipo·pro·tein·emia (pree·bay"tuh·lip"o·pro"tee·in·ee'mee·uh) *n.* The presence of an excessive amount of prebetalipoproteins in the blood.

pre·can·cer·ous (pree·kan'sur·us) *adj.* Pertaining to any pathological condition of a tissue which is likely to develop into cancer.

pre·cap·il·lary (pree·kap'i·lerr"ee) *n.* A blood vessel intermediate in position and structural characteristics between an arteriole and a true capillary. Syn. *metarteriole, arteriolar capillary.*

pre·cen·tral (pree·sen'trul) *adj.* Situated in front of the central sulcus of the brain.

precentral gyrus. The cerebral convolution that lies between the precentral sulcus and the central sulcus and extends from the superomedial border of the hemisphere to the posterior ramus of the lateral sulcus.

precentral sulcus. A groove separating the other frontal gyri from the precentral gyrus.

pre·cip·i·tant (pree·sip'i·tunt) *n.* 1. Any reagent causing precipitation. 2. Any action or event which triggers an otherwise latent or dormant event, as a loud sudden noise may act as a precipitant for a startle response or for startle epilepsy.

pre·cip·i·tate (pre·sip'i·tut, ·tate) *adj.* Headlong; hasty.

precipitate labor. An abnormally rapid labor with the rate of cervical dilatation greater than 5 cm per hour in nulliparas or 10 cm per hour in multiparas.

pre·cip·i·ta·tion (pre·sip'i·tay·shun) *n.* The process of making substances insoluble by the addition of a reagent, evaporation, freezing, or electrolysis.

pre·cip·i·ta·tor (pre·sip'i·tay"tur) *n.* An apparatus that causes precipitation of particles, especially dust particles in the air, which may be counted. Precipitation may be effected by a difference in electrical potential or by a thermal procedure, using a heated wire.

pre·cip·i·tin (pre·sip'i·tin) *n.* An antibody that causes precipitation when combined with a specific soluble antigen.

pre·cip·i·tin·o·gen (pre·sip"i·tin'uh·jen) *n. In immunology,* an antigen capable of giving rise to precipitating antibodies when it is injected into an animal.

precipitin test or **reaction.** An immunologic test in which the reaction between antigen and antibody results in the formation of a visible complex appearing as a precipitate.

pre·clin·i·cal (pree"klin'i·kul) *adj.* 1. Occurring prior to the period in a disease in which recognized symptoms or signs make diagnosis possible. 2. Pertaining to medical studies undertaken before the study of patients.

pre·coc·cyg·e·al (pree"kock·sij'ee·ul) *adj.* In front of the coccyx.

pre·co·cious (pre·ko'shus) *adj.* Developing at an age earlier than usual.

precocious puberty. The premature development of somatic changes associated with puberty; arbitrarily, before the age of 8 years in girls and 10 years in boys.

pre·coc·i·ty (pre·kos'i·tee) *n.* 1. Early development or maturity; especially great development of the mental faculties at an early age. 2. PRECOCIOUS PUBERTY.

pre·con·scious (pree·kon'shus) *adj.* FORECONSCIOUS.

pre·con·vul·sive (pree"kun·vul'siv) *adj.* Pertaining to the period just prior to the occurrence of an epileptic seizure.

pre·cor·di·al (pree·kor'dee·ul) *adj.* Of or pertaining to the precordium.

precordial lead. An exploring unipolar electrocardiographic electrode placed at standard positions across the precordium, usually designated V_1 to V_6; earlier precordial leads were bipolar and were designated CR, CL, CF.

pre·cor·di·um (pree·kor'dee·um) *n.,* pl. **precor·dia** (·dee·uh) The area of the chest overlying the heart.

pre·cos·tal (pree·kos'tul) *adj.* Situated in front of the ribs.

pre·cox, prae·cox (pree'kocks) *L. adj.* Precocious, developing early.

pre·cur·sor (pree·kur'sur) *n.* Something in a stage of a process or development that precedes a later or definitive stage.

pre·den·tin (pree·den'tin) *n.* Uncalcified dentinal matrix.

pre·di·gest·ed (pree"di·jes'tid) *adj.* Partly digested before being taken into the stomach.

pre·di·ges·tion (pree"di·jes'chun, ·dye·jes'chun) *n.* The partial digestion of food before it is eaten.

pre·dis·pos·ing (pree"di·spo'zing) *adj.* Rendering susceptible, often referring to vulnerability to disease.

pre·dis·po·si·tion (pree"dis·puh·zish'un) *n.* The state of having special susceptibility, as to a disease or condition.

pred·nis·o·lone (pred·nis'uh·lohn) *n.* 11β,17,21-Trihydroxypregna-1,4-diene-3,20-dione, $C_{21}H_{28}O_5$, a glucocorticoid with clinically useful anti-inflammatory action; also used as acetate, butylacetate, sodium phosphate, and succinate esters.

pred·ni·sone (pred'ni·sohn) *n.* 17,21-Dihydroxypregna-1,4-diene-3,11,20-trione, $C_{21}H_{26}O_5$, a glucocorticoid with clinically useful anti-inflammatory action.

pre·dor·mi·tion (pree"dor·mish'un) *n.* The stage

of marked drowsiness and cloudy consciousness immediately preceding deep sleep.

pre·ec·lamp·sia (pree''e·klamp'see·uh) *n.* A toxemia occurring in the latter half of pregnancy, characterized by an acute elevation of blood pressure and usually by edema and proteinuria, but without the convulsions or coma seen in eclampsia. **—preeclamp·tic** (·tick) *adj.*

pre·erup·tive (pree''e·rup'tiv) *adj.* Preceding eruption.

pre·fi·brot·ic (pree''fye·brot'ick) *adj.* Characterizing that stage of an inflammatory process in which the cellular part of the exudate persists while healing is taking place, with associated increase in fibrous tissue.

pre·fron·tal (pree·frun'tul) *adj.* Situated in the anterior part of the frontal lobe of the brain.

prefrontal lobotomy or **leukotomy.** A form of psychosurgery in which the white fibers connecting the prefrontal and frontal lobes with the thalamus are severed.

pre·gan·gli·on·ic (pree''gang·glee·on'ick) *adj.* Situated in front of or preceding a ganglion.

preg·nan·cy (preg'nun·see) *n.* The condition of being pregnant; the state of a woman or any female mammal from conception to parturition. The duration of pregnancy in humans is approximately 280 days from the first day of the last menses or approximately 267 days from conception. To estimate the date of confinement, take the first day of the last menstrual period, count back 3 months, and add 1 year and 7 days.

pregnancy cells. Alpha cells of the adenohypophysis distinguished by their smaller size and finer granules; seen during pregnancy.

pregnancy gingivitis. Changes in the gums seen most frequently during pregnancy; marked by bleeding, hypertrophy of the interdental papillae, inflammation, and, occasionally, a tumorous formation.

pregnancy test. Any procedure, usually biologic or chemical, used to diagnose pregnancy. Biologic tests usually depend upon a significant level of chorionic gonadotropin in the serum or urine.

preg·nant (preg'nunt) *adj.* Having potential offspring (fertilized ovum, viable embryo or fetus) within the uterus or analogous organ; said mainly of mammals or other viviparous animals.

preg·nen·in·o·lone (preg''nen·in'o·lone, preg''neen') *n.* ETHISTERONE.

preg·nen·o·lone (preg·nen'uh·lone, preg·neen') *n.* 3β-Hydroxypregn-5-en-20-one, $C_{21}H_{32}O_2$, a steroid oxidation product of cholesterol and stigmasterol, apparently effective in reducing fatigue and formerly believed of value as an antiarthritic agent.

preg·no·pho·bia (preg''no·fo'bee·uh) *n.* Morbid fear of becoming pregnant.

pre·hal·lux (pree·hal'ucks) *n.* A supernumerary digit attached to the great toe on its medial aspect.

pre·hemi·ple·gic (pree''hem·i·plee'jick) *adj.* Occurring before hemiplegia.

pre·hen·sile (pre·hen'sil, ·sile) *adj.* Adapted for grasping, as the tail of certain species of monkeys.

pre·hen·sion (pree·hen'shun) *n.* The act of grasping or seizing.

pre·he·pat·ic (pree''he·pat'ick) *adj.* 1. In front of the liver. 2. Taking place before the liver is involved, as in certain metabolic activities.

prehepatic jaundice. Jaundice in which there is no apparent liver lesion, as hemolytic jaundice and physiologic hyperbilirubinemia.

pre·ic·ter·ic (pree''ick·terr'ick) *adj.* Before the appearance of jaundice.

pre·in·farc·tion (pree''in·fahrk'shun) *adj.* Occurring as an antecedent of infarction.

pre·in·va·sive (pree''in·vay'siv) *adj.* Before invasion of adjacent tissues; said of malignant changes in cells which are confined to their normal location.

pre·lac·ri·mal (pree·lack'ri·mul) *adj.* Situated in front of the lacrimal sac.

pre·leu·ke·mia, pre·leu·kae·mia (pree''lew·kee'mee·uh) *n.* A variety of abnormal maturation patterns of blood cells which sometimes precede a recognizable leukemia.

pre·lo·co·mo·tion (pree''lo·kuh·mo'shun) *n.* The movements of a child who has not yet learned to walk, which indicate the intention of moving from one place to another but show lack of coordination.

Preludin. Trademark for phenmetrazine, an anorexiant drug used as the hydrochloride salt.

pre·ma·lig·nant (pree''muh·lig'nunt) *adj.* PRECANCEROUS.

pre·ma·ni·a·cal (pree''ma·nigh'uh·kul) *adj.* Previous to, or preceding, a psychotic disorder.

Premarin. Trademark for preparations of conjugated estrogens, chiefly in the form of sodium estrone sulfate.

pre·mar·i·tal (pree''mar'i·tul) *adj.* Occurring before marriage; as of a blood test or sexual relations.

pre·ma·ture (pree''muh·choor', ·tewr', prem'uh·tewr) *adj.* 1. Occurring before the proper time. 2. Born prematurely.

premature beat or **contraction.** A cardiac contraction arising prematurely from a site other than the normal pacemaker in the atrium, ventricle, or atrioventricular node.

premature delivery. Expulsion of the fetus after the twenty-eighth week and before term.

premature ejaculation. Male orgasm prior to or just upon the penetration by the penis of the vagina; common in males who, because of their immature psychosexual development, unconsciously look on coitus as another form of masturbation and self-gratification, as well as in those who, because of unconscious feelings of guilt or inferiority accompanied by the need for self-punishment, lack the confidence to function well sexually.

premature infant. 1. An infant born before the 37th to 38th week of gestation. 2. Formerly, a neonate weighing less than 2500 g at birth.

premature labor. Labor taking place before the normal period of gestation, but when the fetus is viable.

premature senility syndrome. 1. In a child,

HUTCHINSON-GILFORD SYNDROME. 2. In an adult, WERNER'S SYNDROME.

premature ventricular contraction. An ectopic beat of ventricular origin, dependent on and coupled to the preceding beat, and occurring before the next dominant beat.

pre·ma·tur·i·ty (pree″muh·tewr′i·tee) n. 1. The state or fact of being premature. 2. An initial point or area of contact of a tooth with an opposing tooth when it limits the opportunity of maximum intercuspation of the teeth in the jaws in any position.

pre·max·il·la (pree″mack·sil′uh) n. INCISIVE BONE. —**pre·max·il·lary** (pree·mack′si·lerr·ee) adj.

pre·med·i·ca·tion (pree″med·i·kay′shun) n. 1. The administration of drugs before induction of anesthesia, primarily to quiet the patient and to facilitate the administration of the anesthetic. 2. Any drug administered for this purpose. —**pre·med·i·cate** (pree·med′i·kate) v.

pre·men·o·paus·al (pree″men′o·pawz′ul) adj. Before the menopause.

pre·men·stru·al (pree·men′stroo·ul) adj. Preceding menstruation.

pre·mo·lar (pree·mo′lur) adj. & n. 1. In front of (mesial to) the molars. 2. In each quadrant of the permanent human dentition, one of the two teeth between the canine and the first molar; a bicuspid.

pre·mon·i·to·ry (pre·mon′i·to″ree) adj. Giving previous warning or notice, as in premonitory symptoms. Syn. prodromal.

pre·mor·bid (pree·mor′bid) adj. Before the appearance of the signs or symptoms of a disease or disorder.

pre·mo·tor area (pree″mo′tur) The main cortical motor area lying immediately in front of the motor area (Brodmann's area 4) from which it differs histologically by the absence of Betz cells; BRODMANN'S AREA 6.

pre·mu·ni·tion (pree″mew·nish′un) n. An immunity that depends upon a persistent latent infection, such as an immunity in malaria due to long-continued quiescent infection.

pre·nar·co·sis (pree″nahr·ko′sis) n. Preliminary, light narcosis produced prior to general anesthesia; PREMEDICATION.

pre·na·tal (pree·nay′tul) adj. 1. Existing or occurring before birth. 2. Loosely: ANTEPARTUM.

pre·neo·plas·tic (pree″nee·o·plas′tick) adj. Before the development of a definite tumor.

pre·oc·cip·i·tal (pree″ock·sip′i·tul) adj. Situated anterior to the occipital region, as the preoccipital notch, a notch indicating the division between the occipital and temporal lobes of the brain.

prep·a·ra·tion (prep″uh·ray′shun) n. 1. The act of making ready. 2. Anything made ready; especially, in anatomy, any part of the body prepared or preserved for illustrative or other uses. 3. In pharmacy, any compound or mixture made according to a formula.

pre·par·tum (pree·pahr′tum) adj. ANTEPARTUM.

pre·pa·tel·lar (pree″puh·tel′ur) adj. Situated in front of the patella.

pre·pel·vic (pree·pel′vick) adj. In front of the pelvis.

pre·pol·lex (pree·pol′ecks) n. A supernumerary digit attached to the thumb on its radial aspect.

pre·pon·der·ance (pre·pon′dur·unce) n. 1. The state of being greater in amount or force. 2. In electrocardiography, of a cardiac ventricle, superiority over the other in electric force generated; in the normal adult the left ventricular forces are greater than those of the right.

pre·psy·chot·ic (pree″sigh·kot′ick) adj. Of or pertaining to the mental state that precedes or is potentially capable of precipitating a psychotic disorder.

pre·pu·ber·al (pree·pew′bur·ul) adj. Before puberty.

pre·pu·ber·tal (pree″pew′bur·tul) adj. PREPUBERAL.

pre·puce (pree′pewce) n. 1. The foreskin of the penis, a fold of skin covering the glans penis. 2. A similar fold over the glans clitoridis. —**pre·pu·tial** (pree·pew′shul) adj.

pre·pu·cot·o·my (pree″pew·kot′uh·mee) n. An incision into the prepuce; an incomplete circumcision.

pre·py·lo·ric (pree″pye·lo′rick) adj. Placed in front of, or preceding, the pylorus.

pre·rec·tal (pree·reck′tul) adj. Situated in front of the rectum.

pre·re·nal (pree·ree′nul) adj. 1. Situated in front of the kidney. 2. Taking place before the kidney is reached; used especially concerning nitrogen retention in the blood due to decreased blood flow to the kidney, or to increased amounts of nitrogenous metabolites entering the blood.

prerenal uremia. Failure of renal function due to disturbances outside the urinary tract, such as shock, dehydration, hemorrhage, or electrolyte abnormality. Syn. extra renal uremia.

pre·re·pro·duc·tive (pree″ree·pruh·duck′tiv) adj. Pertaining to the period of life preceding puberty.

pre·ret·i·nal (pree·ret′i·nul) adj. Anterior to the internal limiting membrane of the retina.

pre·sa·cral (pree·say′krul) adj. Lying in front of the sacrum.

presby-, presbyo- A combining form meaning old age.

pres·by·at·rics (prez″bee·at′ricks) n. GERIATRICS.

pres·by·car·dia (pres″bi·kahr′dee·uh) n. Involutional aging changes of the myocardium, with associated pigmentation of the heart. It decreases cardiac reserve but rarely produces heart failure itself. Syn. senile heart disease.

pres·by·cu·sis (prez″bi·kew′sis) n. The lessening of the acuteness of hearing that occurs with advancing age.

pres·by·der·ma (prez″bi·dur′muh) n. Cutaneous changes associated with the middle and later years of life.

pres·byo·phre·nia (prez″bee·o·free′nee·uh) n. Senile dementia, especially that variety in which apparent mental alertness is combined with failure of memory, disorientation, and confabulation. —**presbyo·phren·ic** (·fren′ick) adj.

pres·by·o·pia (prez″bee·o′pee·uh) n. The condition of vision commonly seen after the middle forties but beginning in late childhood (after age 8), due to diminished power of accommodation from impaired elasticity of the crystalline lens, whereby the near point of distinct vision is removed farther from the eye so that the individual has difficulties in focusing on near objects and in reading fine print. Abbreviated, Pr. —**presby·opic** (·op′ick, ·o′pick) adj.; **presby·ope** (prez′bee·ope) n.

pres·by·tism (prez′bi·tiz·um) n. PRESBYOPIA.

pre·sca·lene (pree·skay′leen) adj. In front of the scalene muscles; used to refer to lymph nodes in the fat of this region.

pre·schizo·phren·ic (pree″skiz″o·fren′ick, ·skit′so·) adj. Pertaining to symptoms and personality characteristics that usually precede schizophrenia.

pre·scribe (pre·skribe′) v. To write an order for a medication and give instructions concerning its use.

pre·scrip·tion (pre·skrip′shun) n. Written instructions designating the preparation and use of substances to be administered.

pre·se·nile (pree·see′nile) adj. 1. Characterized by or pertaining to a condition occurring in early or middle life that involves characteristics resembling those of old age. 2. Pertaining to presenility.

presenile dementia. 1. Any dementia that has its onset in the presenium. 2. ALZHEIMER'S DISEASE.

pre·se·nil·i·ty (pree″se·nil′i·tee) n. 1. Premature old age or the infirmities associated with it. 2. The period of life immediately preceding old age or the senile state.

pre·se·ni·um (pree·see′nee·um, ·sen′ee·um) n. The period just before the onset of old age.

pres·en·ta·tion (prez″un·tay′shun, pree″zen·) n. 1. In obstetrics, the part of the fetus that is palpated through the cervix uteri at the beginning of labor. The relation of the part of the fetus to the birth canal determines the type of presentation. 2. The rather formal oral report of a patient's history made before a group of physicians or a medical teacher by a medical student or a physician.

pre·ser·va·tive (pre·zur′vuh·tiv) n. Any additive used to prevent or retard spoilage or decay, or other chemical or physical change, as in a medicine or food product.

pre·spas·tic (pree″spas′tick) adj. Occurring at or a stage prior to the manifestation of spasticity.

pres·sor (pres′ur) adj. Producing a rise in blood pressure.

pres·so·re·cep·tor (pres″o·re·sep′tur) n. BARORECEPTOR.

pressor headache. Any headache produced by a sudden rise in systemic blood pressure, as with pheochromocytoma.

pres·so·sen·si·tive (pres″o·sen′si·tiv) adj. Stimulated by changes in blood pressure, as nerve endings in the carotid sinus.

pres·sure, n. Physical or mental force, weight, or tension.

pressure atrophy. The atrophy following prolonged pressure on a part, chiefly the result of local inanition.

pressure palsy or **paralysis.** Flaccid paralysis due to pressure on a nerve.

pressure pulse wave. Arterial expansion produced by ejection of blood from the left ventricle into the aorta; marked changes in contour, which may be palpated and recorded, occur as the pulse wave passes to the periphery.

pressure ulcer. DECUBITUS ULCER.

pre·sump·tive (pre·zum′tiv) adj. 1. Justifying reasonable belief, though not conclusively; based on probable evidence or presumption. 2. Of or pertaining to an embryonic structure, cell, or tissue whose probable later identity in the developed organism is known.

pre·sup·pu·ra·tive (pree″sup′yoo·ruh·tiv) adj. Pertaining to an early stage of inflammation, prior to suppuration.

pre·symp·to·mat·ic (pree″simp·tuh·mat′ick) adj. Pertaining to a state of mental or physical health before a disorder becomes manifest, as a patient with a diabetic type of glucose-tolerance curve but without clinical signs and symptoms of diabetes mellitus.

pre·syn·ap·tic (pree″si·nap′tick) adj. Situated near or occurring before a synapse.

presynaptic membrane. The electrically excitable membrane bounding the axon terminal adjacent to the dendrite.

pre·sys·tol·ic (pree″sis·tol′ick) adj. Preceding a cardiac systole, often used in reference to the time immediately preceding the first heart sound.

presystolic extra sound. The heart sound following atrial contraction, immediately preceding the first heart sound, to which it may sometimes contribute. Syn. *fourth heart sound.*

presystolic thrill. A thrill that can sometimes be felt before the systole when the hand is placed over the apex beat (mitral stenosis).

pre·ter·mi·nal (pree·tur′mi·nul) adj. Just before the end.

pre·ter·nat·u·ral (pree″tur·nach′ur·ul) adj. Abnormal.

pre·thy·roid (pree·thigh′royd) adj. PRETHYROIDEAN.

pre·thy·roi·de·an (pree″thigh·roy′dee·un) adj. In front of the thyroid cartilage or thyroid gland.

pre·tib·i·al (pree·tib′ee·ul) adj. In front of the tibia.

pretibial fever. An acute infectious disease due to *Leptospira autumnalis* with clinical manifestations of fever, headache, leukopenia, and a cutaneous erythematous eruption on the pretibial aspect of the legs. Syn. *Fort Bragg fever.*

pretibial myxedema. Circumscribed deposition of mucinous material in the pretibial skin, occurring during thyrotoxicosis or treatment for thyrotoxicosis. Syn. *circumscribed myxedema.*

pre·trans·fer·ence (pree″trans·fur′unce, ·trans′fur·unce) n. In psychoanalysis, the arousal of feelings in a patient when he perceives the therapist as a primordial parent or as a part of himself.

pre·ure·thri·tis (pree·yoo″re·thrigh′tis) n. Inflammation of the vestibule of the vagina, around the urethral orifice.

prev·a·lence (prev′uh·lunce) n. 1. Frequency of occurrence. 2. PREVALENCE RATE.

prevalence rate. A measure of the prevalence of

a disease in a population; usually expressed as the number of cases of a disease present at a given time per 1,000 or 100,000 population.

pre·ven·tive, *adj.* Done, used, or designed for the purpose of prevention rather than correction or cure, as of disease.

preventive medicine. Any medical activity that seeks to prevent disease, prolong life, and promote physical and mental health and efficiency; especially, the science of the etiology and epidemiology of disease processes, dealing with factors that increase vulnerability, factors that initiate or precipitate a disease, and factors that cause disease progression.

pre·ver·te·bral (pree-vur'te-brul) *adj.* Situated in front of a vertebra or the vertebral column.

pre·ver·tig·i·nous (pree''vur-tij'i-nus) *adj.* Pertaining to a state of vertigo in which the patient has a tendency to fall prone, having the sensation of having been pushed forward.

pre·ves·i·cal (pree-ves'i-kul) *adj.* Situated in front of the urinary bladder.

pre·via, prae·via (pree'vee-uh) *adj.* Coming before, or in front of, as placenta previa.

pre·zo·nu·lar (pree-zo'new-lur, -zon'yoo-lur) *adj.* Pertaining to the posterior chamber of the eye.

pri·a·pism (prye'uh-piz·um) *n.* Abnormal, persistent, painful erection of the corpora cavernosa of the penis unrelated to sexual desire, as seen in blood dyscrasia, sickle cell anemia, or lesions of the central nervous system; impotence may result.

Price-Jones curve The distribution of erythrocyte diameters as shown by their direct measurement in a stained blood film.

prick·le cell. A cell possessing conspicuous intercellular bridges; especially, a cell of the epidermis lying between the basal layer and the granular layer.

prickly heat. MILIARIA.

pri·mal (prye'mul) *adj.* Primordial or fundamental; PRIMARY.

pri·ma·quine (prye'muh·kwin, prim'uh·kween) *n.* 8-(4-Amino-1-methylbutylamino)-6-methoxyquinoline, $C_{15}H_{21}N_3O$, an antimalarial drug used as the diphosphate salt.

pri·ma·ry (prye'merr·ee) *adj.* 1. First in order of time, development, or derivation (initial, original, primordial, embryonic), in importance (main, principal), or in systematic order (basic, fundamental). 2. Not derivative or mediated; direct. 3. *In chemistry,* first or simplest of a series of related compounds, as that resulting from replacement of one of two or more atoms or groups in a molecule by a substituent, or an alcohol or an amine containing the —CH₂OH or —NH₂ group, respectively. 4. *In pathology,* original as opposed to metastatic (secondary), as a primary tumor or infection.

primary alveolar hypoventilation syndrome. A disorder in individuals with normal lungs and chest walls, characterized by an elevated alveolar and arterial carbon dioxide tension, cyanosis, polycythemia, and cor pulmonale. It is a result of a functional abnormality of the medullary respiratory neurons, and is associated with subnormal increases in ventilation

during exercise and following the inhalation of carbon dioxide-enriched gas mixtures.

primary amputation. An amputation performed immediately after injury, during the period of reaction from shock and before the onset of suppuration.

primary amyloidosis. A rare disorder of unknown origin characterized by the deposition in various tissues—heart, tongue, gastrointestinal tract, skeletal muscle—of amyloid, a fibrous protein containing sulfated mucopolysaccharides.

primary atypical pneumonia. 1. An acute respiratory disease caused by infection with *Mycoplasma pneumoniae,* characterized by fever, constitutional symptoms, cough, pulmonary infiltrations, and often prolonged convalescence. 2. Any clinical syndrome simulating primary atypical pneumonia, caused by unknown or known agents, including viruses, bacteria, or rickettsiae.

primary care. The care provided at a person's first contact, in any given episode of illness, with the health care system, leading to a decision as to what must be done and including responsibility for the continuum of care, as: appropriate referral, evaluation and management of symptoms, and subsequent maintenance of health.

primary dentition. 1. The first set of teeth, the DECIDUOUS TEETH, considered collectively and in place in the dental arch. 2. The eruption of the deciduous teeth. Syn. *deciduous dentition.*

primary follicle. The immature ovarian follicle in which the ovum is surrounded by a single layer of follicular cells.

primary lateral sclerosis. Degeneration of the descending motor pathways of the spinal cord with spastic weakness of the extremities, hyperreflexia, and Babinski signs, but without muscular atrophy; a variant or early form of amyotrophic lateral sclerosis.

primary lesion. 1. In syphilis, tuberculosis, cowpox, a chancre. 2. *In dermatology,* the earliest clinically recognizable manifestation of a cutaneous disease, such as a macule, papule, vesicle, pustule, or wheal.

primary lymphopenic immunologic deficiency. A primary decrease in the number of circulating lymphocytes and often also of plasma cells, usually with some deficit in the amount of immunoglobulin present, with deficient cellular and humoral immunity, frequently associated clinically with fungus, *Pneumocystis carinii,* or virus infections, leading to early death; inherited both as an X-linked or autosomal recessive trait. Syn. *Gitlin's syndrome.*

primary orthostatic hypotension. A form of thostatic hypotension with onset in middle or late adult years, associated with extrapyramidal symptoms (tremor, ataxia, rigidity) and frequently accompanied by impotence, atonicity of the urinary bladder, impaired sweating in the lower part of the body, and other signs of deranged autonomic function. Pathologically, there is a degeneration of preganglionic sympathetic neurons. Syn. *primary autonomic insufficiency, Shy-Drager syndrome.*

primary refractory anemia. Normocytic normochromic anemia of unknown causation, usually associated with granulocytopenia and thrombocytopenia, unresponsive to treatment other than blood transfusion. Syn. *aregeneratory anemia, cryptogenic anemia, hypoplastic anemia, progressive hypocythemia.*

primary shock. Shock manifested immediately after an injury.

primary tuberculosis. The reaction to the first implantation of tubercle bacilli in the body. It consists of a caseous focal reaction in the parenchyma of the organ and in the regional lymph node or nodes. Both foci usually run a benign course and undergo healing, often with calcification. The most frequent site is the lung. Syn. *childhood type tuberculosis.*

Pri·ma·tes (prye·may'teez) *n.pl.* The order of mammals that includes human beings, apes, monkeys, and prosimians. **—pri·mate** (prye'mate) *adj. & n.*

pri·mi·done (prye'mi·dohn) *n.* 5-Ethyldihydro-5-phenyl-4,6(1*H*,5*H*)-pyrimidinedione, $C_{12}H_{14}N_2O_2$, an anticonvulsant used primarily for control of generalized and psychomotor seizures.

pri·mip·a·ra (prye·mip'uh·ruh) *n.* A woman who has given birth for the first time. **—primiparous** (·rus) *adj.*; **pri·mi·par·i·ty** (prye''mi·pâr'i·tee) *n.*

pri·mi·ti·ae (prye·mish'ee·ee) *n.pl.* The part of the amniotic fluid discharged before the extrusion of the fetus at birth.

prim·i·tive (prim'i·tiv) *adj.* 1. Undeveloped; undifferentiated; simple; rudimentary. 2. At a very early stage of development; embryonic. 3. Original; underived.

primitive interatrial foramen. FORAMEN PRIMUM.

primitive streak. A dense, opaque band of ectoderm in the bilaminar blastoderm associated with the morphogenetic movements and proliferation of the mesoderm and notochord. It indicates the first trace of the embryo.

pri·mor·di·al (prye·mor'dee·ul) *adj.* Existing in the beginning; first-formed; primitive; original; of the simplest character.

primordial dwarfism. The condition of being of extremely short stature, usually from birth, but with otherwise normal physical proportions, mental and sexual development, endocrine status, and bone age. There may be a definite genetic history, or it may occur sporadically.

primordial image or **parent.** *In analytic psychology*, the archetype, primitive, or original parent; the source of all life; the stage prior to the differentiation of mother and father.

pri·mor·di·um (prye·mor'dee·um) *n.*, pl. **primor·dia** (·dee·uh) The earliest discernible indication of an organ or part, as: acousticofacial primordium; ANLAGE (1).

prin·ceps (prin'seps) *adj.* First; original; main.

prin·ci·ple (prin'si·pul) *n.* 1. A constituent of a compound representing its essential or characteristic properties. 2. A rule or basis of action.

principle of inertia. REPETITION-COMPULSION PRINCIPLE.

P-R interval. The time between the onset of the P wave and the beginning of the QRS complex of the electrocardiogram; represents the duration of impulse conduction from the sinoatrial node to the ventricles.

Priodax. Trademark for iodoalphionic acid, a radiopaque medium for cholecystography.

prism (priz'um) *n.* 1. A solid whose bases or ends are similar plane figures and whose sides are parallelograms. 2. *In optics*, a transparent solid with triangular ends and two converging sides. It disperses white light into its component colors, bends the rays of light toward the side opposite the angle (the base of the prism), and is used to measure or correct imbalance of the ocular muscles.

pris·mat·ic (priz·mat'ick) *adj.* 1. Of or pertaining to a prism. 2. Prism-shaped. 3. Produced by the action of a prism, as prismatic colors.

private antigen. An erythrocyte antigen system, defined by specific antisera, found only in a very small number of people, usually members of a given family. Less than 1 percent of the population has such antigens. Syn. *low incidence factors.*

Privine. Trademark for naphazoline, a vasoconstrictor used topically as the hydrochloride salt.

p.r.n. Abbreviation for *pro re nata.*

pro- A prefix signifying (a) *front, forward*; (b) *prior, before*; (c) *precursor*; (d) *promoting, furthering.*

pro·band (pro'band) *n.* The individual or index case, who is the starting point of a family pedigree or geneological chart. Syn. *propositus.*

probe, *n.* 1. A slender, flexible rod, for exploring or dilating a natural channel, as the lacrimal duct, or for following a sinus or the course of a wound. 2. A stiff rod, usually pointed at one end, used for separating tissues in dissection. 3. An electron stream used to strike a tissue in a scanning electron microscope, generating x-ray spectra which reveal the presence and concentration of various elements. 4. The act of using a probe.

pro·ben·e·cid (pro·ben'e·sid) *n.* p-(Dipropylsulfamoyl)benzoic acid, $C_{13}H_{19}NO_4S$, a substance that inhibits renal tubular excretion of penicillin, aminosalicylic acid, and phenolsulfonphthalein, and also depresses renal tubular resorption of urate, thereby increasing urinary excretion of uric acid. Useful in prolonging the action of penicillin and aminosalicylic acid, and in the treatment of gout.

pro·cain·am·ide (pro''kane·am'ide, pro·kay'nuh·mide) *n.* p-Amino-*N*-[2-(diethylamino)ethyl]-benzamide, $C_{13}H_{21}N_3O$, a cardiac depressant used as the hydrochloride salt for treatment of ventricular and atrial arrhythmias and extrasystoles. Syn. *procaine amide.*

pro·caine (pro'kane) *n.* 2-Diethylaminoethyl p-aminobenzoate, $C_{13}H_{20}N_2O_2$, a local anesthetic used as the hydrochloride salt.

pro·cess (pro'sess, pros'ess) *n.* 1. A course of action or events; a sequence of phenomena, as an inflammatory process. 2. A prominence or outgrowth of tissue, as the spinous process of a vertebra. **3.** *In chemistry,* a method of procedure; reaction; test.

pro·ces·so·ma·nia (pro·ses''o·may'nee·uh) *n.* A mania for litigation.

pro·ces·sus (pro·ses'us) *n.,* pl. & genit. sing. **processus** PROCESS.

pro·chei·lia (pro·kigh'lee·uh) *n.* A condition in which a lip is farther forward than is normal.

pro·chei·lon (pro·kigh'lon) *n.* The prominence in the middle of the upper lip.

pro·chlor·per·a·zine (pro''klor·perr'uh·zeen) *n.* 2-Chloro-10-[3-(4-methyl-piperazinyl)propyl]phenothiazine, $C_{20}H_{24}ClN_3S$, an antiemetic and tranquilizing drug; used as the base and as the edisylate (ethanedisulfonate) and maleate salts.

pro·ci·den·tia (pro''si·den'chee·uh, pros''i·) *n.* **1.** PROLAPSE. **2.** *In gynecology,* PROLAPSE OF THE UTERUS.

pro·co·ag·u·lant (pro·ko·ag'yoo·lunt) *n.* Any of several clotting factors (V to XII) present in normal human plasma. These factors, along with thromboplastin and calcium, accelerate the conversion of prothrombin to thrombin.

pro·cre·ate (pro'kree·ate) *v.* To beget.

pro·cre·a·tion (pro''kree·ay'shun) *n.* The begetting of offspring. **—pro·cre·a·tive** (pro'kree·ay''tiv) *adj.*

proct-, procto- A combining form meaning (a) *anus;* (b) *rectum;* (c) *anus and rectum.*

proc·tag·ra (prock·tag'ruh) *n.* Sudden pain in the anal region.

proc·tal·gia (prock·tal'jee·uh) *n.* Pain in the anus or rectum.

proctalgia fu·gax (few'gacks). Acute severe intermittent pain of the anorectal region, more common at night.

proct·atre·sia (prock''ta·tree'zhuh, ·zee·uh) *n.* An imperforate condition of the anus or rectum.

proct·ec·ta·sia (prock''teck·tay'zhuh, ·zee·uh) *n.* Dilatation of the anus or rectum.

proc·tec·to·my (prock·teck'tuh·mee) *n.* Excision of the anus and rectum, usually through the perineal route.

proc·ten·cli·sis (prock·teng'kli·sis) *n.* Stricture of the rectum or anus.

proct·eu·ryn·ter (prock''tew·rin'tur) *n.* A baglike device for dilating the anus or rectum.

proc·ti·tis (prock·tye'tis) *n.* Inflammation of the anus or rectum.

procto- See *proct-.*

proc·to·cele (prock'to·seel) *n.* The extroversion or prolapse of the mucous coat of the rectum.

proc·to·cly·sis (prock·tock'li·sis) *n.,* pl. **proctocly·ses** (·seez) RECTOCLYSIS.

proc·to·co·li·tis (prock''to·ko·lye'tis) *n.* Inflammation of the rectum and colon.

proc·to·co·lon·os·co·py (prock''to·ko''lun·os'kuh·pee) *n.* Inspection and examination of the interior of the rectum and lower colon.

proc·to·col·po·plas·ty (prock''to·kol'po·plas''tee) *n.* Closure of a rectovaginal fistula.

proc·to·cys·to·plas·ty (prock''to·sis'to·plas''tee) *n.* A plastic operation on the rectum and the urinary bladder for repair of rectovesical fistula.

proc·to·de·um, proc·to·dae·um (prock''to·dee'um) *n.,* pl. **procto·dea, procto·daea** (·dee'uh) A pitlike ectodermal depression formed by the growth of the anal hillocks surrounding the anal part of the cloacal membrane. Upon rupture of the latter, it forms part of the anal canal. Syn. *anal pit.* **—procto·de·al, proctodae·al** (·ul) *adj.*

proc·to·dyn·ia (prock''to·din'ee·uh) *n.* Pain about the anus or in the rectum.

proc·tol·o·gist (prock·tol'uh·jist) *n.* A specialist in diseases of the anus and rectum.

proc·tol·o·gy (prock·tol'uh·jee) *n.* The science of the anatomy, functions, and diseases of the rectum and anus. **—proc·to·log·ic** (prock''to·loj'ik) *adj.*

proc·to·pa·ral·y·sis (prock''to·puh·ral'i·sis) *n.* Paralysis of the external anal sphincter muscle, usually accompanied by fecal incontinence.

proc·to·pexy (prock'to·peck''see) *n.* The fixation of the rectum by anchoring it into the hollow of the sacrum by means of sutures passing externally across the sacrum. Syn. *rectopexy.*

proc·to·phil·ia (prock''to·fil'ee·uh) *n.* A pathological interest in, or liking of, anything connected with the anus.

proc·to·pho·bia (prock''to·fo'bee·uh) *n.* **1.** An abnormal fear of anything to do with the anus or rectum. **2.** An abnormal dread or apprehension of pain in persons with diseases of the rectum.

proc·to·plas·ty (prock'to·plas''tee) *n.* Plastic surgery of the rectum and anus.

proc·tor·rha·phy (prock·tor'uh·fee) *n.* The plaiting of the enlarged and prolapsed rectal walls by suture, to reduce the circumference.

proc·tor·rhea, proc·tor·rhoea (prock''to·ree'uh) *n.* Discharge of mucus through the anus.

proc·to·scope (prock'tuh·skope) *n.* An instrument for inspecting the anal canal and rectum.

proc·tos·co·py (prock·tos'kuh·pee) *n.* Inspection of the anal canal and rectum with a proctoscope.

proc·to·sig·moid·ec·to·my (proc''to·sig''moy''deck'tuh·mee) *n.* The abdominoperineal excision of the anus and rectosigmoid, usually with the formation of an abdominal colostomy.

proc·to·sig·moid·itis (prock''to·sig''moy·dye'tis) *n.* Inflammation of the rectum and sigmoid colon.

proc·to·sig·moid·os·co·py (proc''to·sig''moy·dos'kuh·pee) *n.* Examination of the rectum and sigmoid colon with a sigmoidoscope.

proc·to·spasm (prock'to·spaz·um) *n.* Spasm or tenesmus of the rectum; may extend to the anus.

proc·tos·ta·sis (prock·tos'tuh·sis) *n.* Constipation due to nonresponse of the rectum to the defecation stimulus.

proc·to·ste·no·sis (prock''to·ste·no'sis) *n.* Stricture of the anus or rectum.

proc·tos·to·my (prock·tos'tuh·mee) *n.* The establishment of a permanent artificial opening into the rectum.

proc·tot·o·my (prock·tot'uh·mee) *n.* Incision into the rectum or anus, especially for stricture or imperforate anus; described as external if the incision is below the external sphincter, and internal if above it.

pro·cur·sive (pro·kur'siv) *adj.* Running forward.

procursive epilepsy. A form of epilepsy in which the patient runs at the beginning of the epileptic attack.

pro·cur·va·tion (pro"kur·vay'shun) *n.* Forward inclination of the body.

pro·dro·mal (prod'ro·mul, pro·dro'mul) *adj.* Pertaining to early manifestations or symptoms of a disease; premonitory.

pro·drome (pro'drome) *n.* 1. An early or premonitory manifestation of impending disease, before the specific symptoms begin. 2. AURA.

prod·uct, *n.* 1. Effect; result; that which is produced. 2. *In chemistry,* the compound formed by a reaction.

pro·duc·tive, *adj.* 1. Forming or capable of forming new tissue. 2. Raising mucous or secretion, as a productive cough.

productive cough. A cough in which mucus or secretion is removed from the respiratory tract.

productive inflammation. Inflammation in which there is a considerable multiplication of fibroblasts.

pro·en·zyme (pro·en'zime) *n.* An inactive precursor in a living cell from which an enzyme is formed.

pro·fes·sion·al (pro·fesh'uh·nul) *adj.* 1. Pertaining to a profession. 2. Of or pertaining to the ethical or technical standards of a profession.

pro·file, *n.* 1. An outline or representation of the distinctive features of something. 2. A graph, curve, or other schema presenting quantitatively or descriptively the chief characteristics of something, as of an organ, process, or person.

pro·flu·vi·um (pro·floo'vee·um) *n.,* pl. **proflu·via** (·vee·uh) A flux or discharge.

pro·fun·da (pro·fun'duh) *adj.* Deep-seated; a term applied to certain arteries.

pro·fun·dus (pro·fun'dus) *adj.* Deep-seated; applied to certain muscles and nerves.

pro·gen·er·ate (pro·jen'ur·ut) *n.* An individual endowed with superior faculties; a genius.

prog·e·ny (proj'e·nee) *n.* OFFSPRING; descendants.

pro·ge·ria (pro·jeer'ee·uh) *n.* Premature senility. In a child, HUTCHINSON-GILFORD SYNDROME; in an adult, WERNER'S SYNDROME.

pro·ges·ta·gen (pro·jes'tuh·jin) *n.* Any progestational hormone; PROGESTOGEN.

pro·ges·ta·tion·al (pro"jes·tay'shun·ul) *adj.* Pertaining to the second, or luteal, phase of the menstrual cycle, during which the endometrium changes from the proliferative to the secretory state under the influence of progesterone released from the corpus luteum.

progestational hormone. 1. The natural hormone progesterone, which induces progestational changes of the uterine mucosa. 2. Any derivative or modification of progesterone having similar actions.

pro·ges·ter·one (pro·jes'tur·ohn) *n.* Pregn-4-ene-3,20-dione, $C_{21}H_{30}O_2$, the steroid hormone secreted by the ovary mainly from the corpus luteum. It is essential for nidation of the ovum and maintenance of pregnancy; cessation of its secretion at the end of the menstrual cycle largely determines the time of onset of menstruation. The hormone, now obtained by synthesis, is used for the management of various ovarian disorders.

pro·ges·tin (pro·jes'tin) *n.* Any progestational hormone; a progestogen. The name has been applied specifically to progesterone.

pro·ges·to·gen (pro·jes'to·jin) *n.* Any progestational hormone.

pro·glot·tid (pro·glot'id) *n.* A segment of a tapeworm.

pro·glot·tis (pro·glot'is) *n.,* pl. **proglot·ti·des** (·i·deez). PROGLOTTID.

pro·gnath·ic (pro·nath'ick, ·nay'thick) *adj. In craniometry,* designating a condition of the upper jaw in which it projects anteriorly with respect to the profile of the facial skeleton, when the skull is oriented on the Frankfort horizontal plane; having a gnathic index of 103.0 or more.

prog·na·thism (prog'nuh·thiz·um) *n.* The condition of having projecting jaws.

prog·na·thous (prog'nuth·us) *adj.* PROGNATHIC.

prog·no·sis (prog·no'sis) *n.,* pl. **progno·ses** (·seez) A prediction as to the probable course and outcome of a disease, injury, or developmental abnormality in a patient, based on general knowledge of such conditions, as well as on specific information and exercise of clinical judgment in the particular case. **—prog·nos·tic** (·nos'tick) *adj.*

prog·nos·ti·cate (prog·nos'ti·kate) *v.* To give a prognosis.

pro·go·no·ma (pro"gon·o'muh, pro"guh·no'muh) *n.* A nodular or tumorlike mass containing structures resembling those of ancestral forms of a species, as exemplified in hairy moles.

pro·grav·id (pro·grav'id) *adj.* Pertaining to the second, or luteal, phase of the menstrual cycle, when secretion of progesterone changes the endometrium to the secretory state essential for nidation and maintenance of pregnancy.

pro·gres·sion (pruh·gresh'un) *n.* The act of advancing or moving forward.

pro·gres·sive (pruh·gres'iv) *adj.* Gradually extending; advancing or increasing in complexity or severity.

progressive bulbar paralysis or **palsy.** Progressive symmetrical degeneration of the motor nuclei of the medulla and lower pons, with onset usually in late adult life and occasionally familial, resulting in atrophy, fasciculations, and paralysis of the denervated muscles; related to or associated with progressive spinal muscular atrophy and amyotrophic lateral sclerosis.

progressive cerebral poliodystrophy. Cortical degeneration, usually of infants and children, characterized clinically by myoclonic and generalized seizures, ataxia, choreoathetosis, or spasticity, as well as varying degrees of mental deterioration, and pathologically by widespread severe loss of the neurons of the cerebral cortex, accompanied by astrocytic and microglial proliferation, with relative sparing of the white matter; cause or causes are unknown, but slow virus infection may be present. Syn. *Alpers' disease, poliodystrophia cerebri progressiva infantilis.*

progressive diaphyseal dysplasia. Cortical thickening of the long bones, beginning in the midshaft and progressing toward the epiphyses; it becomes apparent in infancy or early childhood. Syn. *diaphyseal sclerosis, Engelmann's disease.*

progressive familial myoclonic epilepsy. A heredodegenerative disease beginning in childhood or adolescence, characterized by progressively worsening generalized and myoclonic seizures, cerebellar and extrapyramidal disturbances, and dementia; associated with deposits of relatively insoluble polyglucosans (Lafora bodies) in various sites, and transmitted as an autosomal recessive trait. Syn. *Unverricht's disease.*

progressive muscular dystrophy. Chronic progressive wasting and weakness of skeletal musculature, frequently hereditary and usually associated with elevations of serum creatine kinase and electromyographic abnormalities. There are several variants, named after the age of onset, site of initial muscular involvement, and the severity and distribution of apparent hypertrophy and atrophy.

progressive myopia of children. Continuous increase of myopia, due to increasing growth of the eyeball.

progressive pallidal atrophy or **degeneration.** JUVENILE PARALYSIS AGITANS.

progressive pigmentary dermatosis. A form of capillaritis, characterized by a reddish, purpuric, papular eruption; it is seen principally on the legs and is often progressive in character. Syn. *Schamberg's disease.*

progressive spinal muscular atrophy. A chronic slowly progressive wasting of individual muscles, or physiologic groups of muscles, and associated weakness and paralysis, usually symmetrical, but more frequently involving the upper extremities than the lower; due to degeneration of the anterior horn cells of the spinal cord, with consecutive degeneration of the anterior nerve roots and muscles, and, occasionally, involvement of bulbar nuclei. It affects adults primarily and may be caused by infections, toxins, avitaminosis, or familial factors.

progressive subcortical gliosis. A rare form of presenile dementia with an insidious progressive course, characterized pathologically by pronounced subcortical gliosis without severe involvement of the cerebral cortex and no significant myelin loss.

progressive systemic sclerosis. DIFFUSE SCLERODERMA.

pro·gua·nil (pro·gwah'nil) *n.* Chloroguanide, an antimalarial drug used as the hydrochloride salt.

pro·in·su·lin (pro·in'sue·lin) *n.* The precursor of insulin; a single-chain protein, with a molecular weight of approximately 9,000, which is converted to the two-chain insulin molecule by enzyme-catalyzed proteolytic cleavage.

pro·jec·tile (pro·jeck'til, ·tile) *adj.* Hurled or impelled forward with great force.

projectile vomiting. A form of vomiting in which the stomach contents are suddenly and forcefully shot forth out of the mouth to some distance, usually without nausea.

pro·jec·tion (pro·jeck'shun) *n.* 1. The act of throwing forward. 2. A part extending beyond its surroundings. 3. The referring of impressions made on the organs of sense to the position of the object producing them. 4. *In psychology,* the process of unconsciously attributing to other persons or objects one's own qualities or feelings, as a child's assumption that his mother feels as he does. 5. *In psychiatry,* a defense mechanism against feelings of inadequacy or guilt, operating unconsciously, whereby what is emotionally unacceptable to the self is rejected and attributed to others. 6. *In neurology,* the connection of parts of the cerebral cortex (projection area) through projection fibers with subcortical centers which, in turn, are connected with peripheral sense organs.

projection fibers. Fibers joining the cerebral cortex to lower centers, and vice versa.

pro·jec·tive (pro·jeck'tiv) *adj.* Pertaining to or caused by projection.

pro·ki·nase (pro·kigh'nace, ·kin'ace, ·aze) *n.* A proteolytic enzyme found in extracts of the pancreas and demonstrated to pass into the pancreatic secretion.

pro·la·bi·um (pro·lay'bee·um) *n.* 1. The exposed part of the lip. 2. The central prominence of the lip.

pro·lac·tin (pro·lack'tin) *n.* A hormone secreted by the adenohypophysis, which stimulates lactation in the mammalian breast and also promotes functional activity of the corpus luteum. Syn. *lactogenic hormone, luteotropic hormone, mammotropin.*

pro·lapse (pro·laps', pro'laps) *n. & v.* 1. The falling or sinking down of a part or organ; procidentia. 2. To fall or sink down.

prolapse of the uterus. Displacement of the uterus downward, sometimes outside the vulva. Syn. *descensus uteri, prolapsus uteri.*

pro·lap·sus (pro·lap'sus) *n.* PROLAPSE.

prolapsus ani (ay'nigh). Extrusion of the lower division of the intestinal tract through the external sphincter of the anus.

pro·lep·sis (pro·lep'sis) *n.,* pl. **prolep·ses** (·seez) In a periodic or recurrent disease, the return of an attack or paroxysm before the expected time or at progressively shorter intervals. —**prolep·tic** (·tick) *adj.*

pro·lif·er·ate (pro·lif'ur·ate) *v.* To multiply; to generate by increase in number.

pro·lif·er·a·tion (pro·lif''ur·ay'shun) *n.* Rapid and increased production, as of offspring, or of new parts or cells by repeated cell division. —**pro·lif·er·a·tive** (pro·lif'ur·uh·tiv) *adj.*

proliferative arthritis. RHEUMATOID ARTHRITIS.

pro·lif·ic (pro·lif'ick) *adj.* Fruitful; highly productive.

pro·lig·er·ous (pro·lij'ur·us) *adj.* Germinating producing offspring.

pro·line (pro'leen, ·lin) *n.* 2-Pyrrolidinecarboxylic acid, $C_5H_9NO_2$, an amino acid resulting from the hydrolysis of proteins.

pro·lin·uria (pro·lin·yoo'ree·uh) n. The presence of proline in the urine.

pro·li·pase (pro·lye'pace, ·paze) n. Inactive form of steapsin found in pancreatic juice.

pro·lym·pho·cyte (pro·lim'fo·site) n. A cell of the lymphocyte series intermediate in maturity between the lymphoblast and the lymphocyte.

pro·ma·zine (pro'muh·zeen) n. 10-[3-(Dimethylamino)propyl]phenothiazine, $C_{17}H_{20}N_2S$, a drug with antiemetic, tranquilizing, and analgesic-potentiating actions; used as the hydrochloride salt.

pro·mega·karyo·cyte (pro·meg''uh·kǎr'ee·o·site) n. The precursor of the megakaryocyte. It is smaller than the megakaryocyte; the nucleus becomes indented; cytoplasm is lightly basophilic and contains fine granules. Syn. *lymphoid megakaryocyte.*

pro·meg·a·lo·blast (pro·meg'uh·lo·blast) n. The earliest precursor of the abnormal red blood cells in diseases such as pernicious anemia; it is similar to the pronormoblast, but the nuclear chromatin is finer and arranged in a scrollwork pattern.

pro·meth·a·zine (pro·meth'uh·zeen) n. 10-(2-Dimethylaminopropyl)phenothiazine, $C_{17}H_{20}N_2S$, an antihistaminic drug used as the hydrochloride salt.

prom·i·nence (prom'i·nunce) n. 1. A projection, especially on a bone. 2. The state of projecting or standing out.

pro·mono·cyte (pro·mon'o·site) n. 1. An immature monocyte derived from a monoblast. The nucleus is spheroidal or moderately indented, and a nucleolus may be visible. Syn. *young monocyte, premonocyte.* 2. One of the transitional stages between the lymphocyte and monocyte.

prom·on·to·ry (prom'un·to·ree) n. A projecting prominence.

promontory of the sacrum. The prominence formed by the angle between the upper extremity of the sacrum and the last lumbar vertebra.

pro·my·e·lo·cyte (pro·migh'e·lo·site) n. The earliest myelocyte stage derived from the myeloblast; it contains a few granules, some of which may be azurophilic, while others may be characteristic of the type of granulocyte into which the myelocyte develops. In early forms, the nucleus may be covered by the nonspecific granules and still contain small nucleoli.

pro·nate (pro'nate) v. 1. To turn the forearm so that the palm of the hand is down or toward the back. 2. In the foot, to turn the sole outward with the lateral margin of the foot elevated; to evert.

pro·na·tion (pro·nay'shun) n. 1. The condition of being prone; the act of placing in the prone position. 2. The turning of the palm of the hand downward.

pro·na·tor (pro·nay'tur, pro'nay·tur) n. That which pronates, as the pronator teres (musculus pronator teres) and pronator quadratus (musculus pronator quadratus), muscles of the forearm attached to the ulna and radius.

prone, adj. Lying with the face downward.

pro·neph·ros (pro·nef'ros) n., pl. **proneph·roi** (·roy) The primitive or head kidney, derived from the cranial part of the nephrogenic cord. Vestigial in mammalian embryos, its duct, the pronephric duct, is taken over by the mesonephros and called the mesonephric duct. —**proneph·ric** (·rick) adj.

Pronestyl. Trademark for the antiarrhythmic cardiac depressant procainamide, used as the hydrochloride salt.

pro·nor·mo·blast (pro·nor'mo·blast) n. The earliest erythrocyte precursor; a round or oval cell 12 to 19 microns in diameter, with a large nucleus having fine chromatin and nucleoli, with scanty, basophilic cytoplasm without hemoglobin. Syn. *macroblast, rubriblast, prorubricyte, lymphoid hemoblast (of Pappenheim), proerythroblast (of Ferrata), megaloblast (of Sabin).*

Prontosil. Trademark for 2,4-diaminoazobenzene-4'-sulfonamide hydrochloride, the forerunner of the sulfonamide drugs.

proof gallon. A gallon of proof spirit.

proof spirit. A mixture of ethyl alcohol and water containing 50% by volume of C_2H_5OH.

pro·otic (pro·o'tick, ·ot'ick) adj. In front of the ear.

prop·a·gate (prop'uh·gate) v. To produce offspring; to multiply; to extend forward. —**prop·a·ga·tion** (prop''uh·gay'shun) n.

pro·pane (pro'pane) n. The gaseous hydrocarbon $CH_3CH_2CH_3$, occurring in natural gas and in solution in crude petroleum.

pro·pep·sin (pro·pep'sin) n. The zymogen of pepsin, found in the cells of the gastric glands. Syn. *pepsinogen.*

pro·per·din (pro·pur'din, pro'pur·din) n. A macroglobulin of normal plasma capable of killing various bacteria and viruses in the presence of complement and magnesium ions, and involved in the alternate pathway of complement activation.

pro·peri·to·ne·al (pro''perr·i·to·nee'ul) adj. Situated in front of the peritoneum.

pro·phase (pro'faze) n. 1. The first stage of mitosis, in which the chromosomes are organized from nuclear materials as elongate spiremes. 2. The first stage of the first (prophase I) or second (prophase II) meiotic divisions; the first meiotic prophase is further divided into leptotene, zygotene, pachytene, diplotene, and diakinesis.

pro·phy·lac·tic (pro·fi·lack'tick) adj. & n. 1. Pertaining to prophylaxis; tending to prevent disease. 2. Any agent or device that prevents or helps to prevent the development of disease. 3. CONDOM.

pro·phy·lax·is (pro''fi·lack'sis) n., pl. **prophylax·es** (·seez) 1. Prevention of disease; measures preventing the development or spread of disease. 2. *In military medicine,* measures taken to prevent or reduce the harmful effects of chemical agents.

pro·pi·on·ic acid (pro''pee·on'ick) Propanoic acid, CH_3CH_2COOH, used as the acid and in the form of its calcium and sodium salts as a topical fungicide.

pro·plas·ma·cyte (pro·plaz'muh·site) n. 1. The

precursor of the plasmacyte (plasma cell), usually larger than the adult cell, with a nucleus which has a finer chromatin structure and which is not necessarily eccentrically placed. Syn. *lymphoblastic* or *myeloblastic plasma cell.* 2. TÜRK CELL.

pro·pos·i·tus (pro·poz'i·tus) *n.,* pl. **proposi·ti** (·tye) PROBAND.

pro·poxy·phene (pro·pock'see·feen) *n.* (+)-α-4-(Dimethylamino)-3-methyl-1,2-diphenyl-2-butanol propionate, $C_{22}H_{29}NO_2$, an analgesic compound, structurally related to methadone, employed for relief of mild to moderate pain; used as the hydrochloride salt.

pro·pri·etary (pro·prye'e·terr''ee) *n. & adj.* 1. Any chemical, drug, or similar preparation used in the treatment of diseases, if such an article is protected against free competition as to name, product, composition, or process of manufacture, by secrecy, patent, copyright, or any other means. 2. Of or pertaining to a proprietary or a proprietor; protected by copyright or patent; made, marketed, or operated by a person or persons having the exclusive right to do so.

pro·prio·cep·tion (pro''pree·o·sep'shun) *n.* The normal ongoing awareness, mediated by the action of proprioceptors, of the position, balance, and movement of one's own body or any of its parts. —**proprio·cep·tive** (·tiv) *adj.*

pro·prio·cep·tor (pro''pree·o·sep'tur) *n.* A receptor located in a muscle, tendon, joint, or vestibular apparatus, whose reflex function is locomotor or postural.

pro·pri·us (pro'pree·us) *adj.* Individual; special; applied to certain muscles.

prop·tom·e·ter (prop·tom'e·tur) *n.* An instrument for measuring the amount of exophthalmos.

prop·to·sis (prop·to'sis) *n.,* pl. **propto·ses** (·seez) 1. A falling downward or forward. 2. PROLAPSE. 3. EXOPHTHALMOS. —**prop·tot·ic** (·tot'ick) *adj.*

pro·pul·sion (pro·pul'shun) *n.* 1. The act of pushing or driving forward. 2. A leaning and falling forward in walking, as observed in parkinsonism and other disorders of the nervous system. —**propul·sive** (·siv) *adj.*

pro·pyl (pro'pil) *n.* The univalent radical $CH_3CH_2CH_2—$, derived from propane.

propylene glycol. 1,2-Propanediol, $CH_3CHOH·CH_2OH$, used as a solvent vehicle for many medicinals.

pro·pyl·hex·e·drine (pro''pil·heck'se·dreen) *n.* $N,α$-Dimethylcyclohexaneethylamine, $C_{10}H_{21}N$, a volatile sympathomimetic amine used as a nasal decongestant.

pro·pyl·par·a·ben (pro''pil·pär'a·ben) *n.* Propyl *p*-hydroxybenzoate, $C_{10}H_{12}O_3$, an antifungal preservative agent.

pro·pyl·thio·ura·cil (pro''pil·thigh''o·yoor'uh·sil) *n.* 6-Propyl-2-thiouracil, $C_7H_{10}N_2OS$, a thyroid inhibitor used in the treatment of hyperthyroidism.

pro re na·ta (pro ree nay'tuh) According to the circumstances of the case, or when necessary. Abbreviated, p.r.n.

pro·se·cre·tin (pro·se·kree'tin) *n.* The precursor of secretin; it is secreted by the epithelium of the small intestine.

pro·sect (pro·sekt') *v.* To dissect a subject or part for purposes of anatomic teaching or demonstration.

pro·sec·tor (pro·seck'tur) *n.* An individual who prepares subjects for anatomic dissection or to illustrate didactic lectures.

pros·en·ceph·a·lon (pros''en·sef'uh·lon) *n.* The forebrain or anterior brain vesicle of the embryo that subdivides into telencephalon and diencephalon. From it are derived the cerebral hemispheres, olfactory lobes, corpus striatum, and various parts of the thalamus, as well as the third and the lateral ventricles. —**prosen·ce·phal·ic** (·se·fal'ick) *adj.*

pros·o·dy (pros'uh·dee) *n. In phonology,* the system of rhythmic and melodic elements in speech, consisting mainly of modulations in pitch, timing, and loudness, which help to organize the segmental elements and supplement their meaning.

pros·op·ag·no·sia (pros''up·ag·no'see·uh) *n.* A form of visual agnosia characterized by inability to identify a familiar face either by looking at the person or at a picture, even though the patient knows that it is a face and can point to its separate parts.

pros·o·pal·gia (pros''o·pal'jee·uh) *n.* TRIGEMINAL NEURALGIA. —**prosopo·plegic** (·plee'jick, ·plej'ick) *adj.*

proso·pla·sia (pros''o·play'zee·uh, ·zhuh) *n.* 1. Progressive transformation in the direction of higher orders of differentiation, complexity, or function. 2. Abnormal tissue differentiation. 3. CYTOMORPHOSIS. —**proso·plas·tic** (·plas'tick) *adj.*

pros·o·po·di·ple·gia (pros''uh·po·dye·plee'jee·uh) *n.* Bilateral facial paralysis.

pros·o·po·dyn·ia (pros''uh·po·din'ee·uh) *n.* Facial pain; TRIGEMINAL NEURALGIA.

pros·o·po·ple·gia (pros''uh·po·plee'jee·uh) *n.* Peripheral FACIAL PALSY; it may be unilateral (monoplegia facialis) or bilateral (diplegia facialis). —**prosopo·ple·gic** (·plee'jick, ·plej'ick) *adj.*

pros·o·po·va·rus (pros'o·pus vair'us, pros·o'pus) A congenital hemiatrophy of the face and cranium, resulting in marked facial obliquity.

pros·ta·glan·din (pros''tuh·glan'din) *n.* One of several physiologically potent compounds, of ubiquitous occurrence, that have a unique structure containing 20 carbon atoms and are formed from essential fatty acids, and with activities affecting the nervous system, circulation, female reproductive organs, and metabolism. The highest concentration of prostaglandins has been found in normal human semen.

Prostaphlin. A trademark for the sodium salt of oxacillin, a semisynthetic penicillin antibiotic.

pros·ta·ta (pros'tuh·tuh) *n.* [NA]. PROSTATE.

pros·tate (pros'tate) *n.* The organ surrounding the neck of the urinary bladder and beginning of the urethra in the male (prostatic urethra). It consists of two lateral lobes, an anterior and a posterior lobe, and a middle lobe; it is composed of muscular and glandular tissue; a distinct capsule surrounds it. It is the largest auxiliary gland of the male reproductive system and its secretions comprise approximately 40 percent of the semen. —**pros·tat·ic** (pros·tat'ick) *adj.*

pros·ta·tec·to·my (pros"tuh·teck'tuh·mee) *n.* Excision of part or all of the prostate.

prostatic calculus. Calcium phosphate stones of variable size commonly seen in prostatic acini of older men; may be associated with prostatitis.

prostatic sinus. The groove on each side of the urethral crest into which open the ducts of the prostate gland.

pros·ta·tism (pros'tuh·tiz·um) *n.* The condition caused by chronic disorders of the prostate, especially obstruction to urination by prostatic enlargement.

pros·ta·ti·tis (pros"tuh·tye'tis) *n.* Inflammation of the prostate gland. —**prosta·tit·ic** (·tit'ick) *adj.*

pros·ta·to·cys·ti·tis (pros"tuh·to·sis·tye'tis) *n.* Inflammation of the prostate, prostatic urethra, and urinary bladder.

pros·ta·to·gram (pros·tat'o·gram) *n.* A radiograph of the prostate gland, made after injecting a radiopaque substance into the orifices of the tubuloalveolar units through the urethral route.

pros·ta·tog·ra·phy (pros"tuh·tog'ruh·fee) *n.* Radiography of the prostate gland after injecting a radiopaque substance into the orifices of the tubuloalveolar units through the urethral route.

pros·ta·to·lith (pros·tat'o·lith) *n.* PROSTATIC CALCULUS.

pros·ta·to·li·thot·o·my (pros"tuh·to·li·thot'uh·mee, pros·tat'o·) *n.* Removal of a stone or calculus from the prostate gland.

pros·ta·tor·rhea, pros·ta·tor·rhoea (pros"tuh·to·ree'uh) *n.* A thin urethral discharge coming from the prostate gland.

pros·ta·tot·o·my (pros"tuh·tot'uh·mee) *n.* Incision into the prostate gland.

pros·ta·to·ve·sic·u·li·tis (pros"tuh·to·ve·sick"yoo·lye'tis) *n.* Inflammation of the seminal vesicles combined with prostatitis.

pros·the·sis (pros·thee'sis) *n.*, pl. **prosthe·ses** (·seez) 1. Replacement or substitution. 2. An artificial substitute for a missing part, as denture, hand, leg, or eye. —**pros·thet·ic** (·thet'ick) *adj.*

prosthetic group. 1. The group formed by a substance that is combined with a simple protein to form a complex protein, as the chromophoric group in chromoproteins. 2. The group formed by an organic radical not derived from an amino acid, that enters into the complex molecule of a conjugated protein. 3. The nonprotein component, or coenzyme, of certain enzyme systems.

pros·thet·ics (pros·thet'icks) *n.* The branch of surgery that deals with prostheses.

pros·the·tist (pros'the·tist) *n.* An individual who makes artificial limbs, artificial dentures, or external organs or parts.

pros·tho·don·tia (pros·tho·don'chee·uh) *n.* PROSTHODONTICS.

pros·tho·don·tics (pros"tho·don'ticks) *n.* The science and practice of the replacement of missing dental and oral structures.

pros·tho·don·tist (pros"tho·don'tist) *n.* A dentist who specializes in prosthodontics.

Prostigmin. Trademark for neostigmine, a quaternary cholinergic drug used as the bromide and methyl sulfate salts.

pros·ti·tu·tion (pros"ti·tew'shun) *n.* The condition or act of using the body for sexual intercourse promiscuously for pay or other considerations.

pros·trate (pros'trate) *adj. & v.* 1. Lying prone or supine; stretched out. 2. Lacking in vitality, powerless, exhausted, stricken down. 3. To render oneself or another prostrate.

pros·trat·ed (pros'tray·tid) *adj.* Exhausted; stricken down.

pros·tra·tion (pros·tray'shun) *n.* The condition of being prostrated; extreme exhaustion; collapse.

pro·tal (pro'tul) *adj.* CONGENITAL.

pro·ta·mine (pro'tuh·meen, ·min) *n.* One of a group of simple proteins occurring in the sperm of fish, as clupeine, iridine, salmine, or sturine.

protamine sulfate. A water-soluble salt of protamine, a protein prepared from the sperm or mature testes of certain species of fish; because it interacts with heparin to inactivate the latter, protamine sulfate is used as an antidote to overdosage with heparin.

protamine zinc insulin. A preparation of insulin modified by addition of zinc chloride and protamine to produce long duration of action.

pro·ta·no·pia (pro"tuh·no'pee·uh) *n.* A form of partial color blindness in which there is defective red vision; green sightedness. —**prota·nop·ic** (·nop'ick, ·no'pick) *adj.*

¹**pro·te·an** (pro'te·un, pro·tee'un) *adj.* Taking on many shapes or changing form.

²**pro·te·an** (pro'te·an) *n.* One of a group of derived proteins, insoluble products due to the action of water or enzymes.

pro·te·ase (pro'tee·ace, ·aze) *n.* An enzyme that digests proteins.

pro·tec·tive (pruh·teck'tiv) *adj. & n.* 1. Affording defense or immunity; PROPHYLACTIC. 2. A covering or shield that protects. 3. A specific dressing, as oiled silk or rubber, used to prevent ingress of water.

pro·tein (pro'te·in, pro'teen) *n.* One of a group of complex nitrogenous substances of high molecular weight which are found in various forms in animals and plants and are characteristic of living matter. On complete hydrolysis they yield amino acids.

pro·tein·a·ceous (pro"tee·nay'shus, pro"tee·i·nay'shus) *adj.* Of, pertaining to, or characteristic of a protein.

pro·tein·ase (pro'tee·nace, ·naze, pro'tee·i·nace) *n.* One of the subgroups of proteases or proteolytic enzymes which act directly on the native proteins in the first step of their conversion to simpler substances.

protein-bound iodine. Iodine attached to protein; commonly, iodine bound to the protein fraction of the blood; in most instances, it reflects the level of circulating thyroid hormone. Abbreviated, PBI.

pro·tein·emia, pro·tein·ae·mia (pro″tee·nee′mee·uh, ·tee·i·nee′) n. 1. Protein in the blood. 2. HYPERPROTEINEMIA.

protein hydrolysate. An artificial digest of protein derived by acid, enzymatic, or other hydrolysis of casein, lactalbumin, fibrin, or other suitable proteins that supply the approximate nutritive equivalent of the source protein in the form of its constituent amino acids.

pro·tein·o·sis (pro″teen·o′sis, pro″tee·i·no′sis) n. The accumulation of protein in the tissues.

protein quotient. The result of dividing the amount of globulin in the blood plasma by the amount of albumin in it.

pro·tein·uria (pro″tee·new′ree·uh, pro″tee·i·new′ree·uh) n. The presence of protein in the urine.

pro·te·ol·y·sis (pro″tee·ol′i·sis) n. The addition of water to peptide bonds of proteins with resultant fragmentation of the protein molecule. Proteolysis may be enzymatically catalyzed by numerous enzymes, many of which have stereochemically selective points of attack, or it may occur nonenzymatically, especially consequent to the action of mineral acids and heat. —**pro·teo·lyt·ic** (pro″tee·o·lit′ick) adj.

pro·teo·me·tab·o·lism (pro″tee·o·me·tab′uh·liz·um) n. The processes of digestion, absorption, and utilization of proteins. —**proteo·metab·ol·ic** (·met″uh·bol′ick) adj.

pro·teo·pep·tic (pro″tee·o·pep′tick) adj. Pertaining to protein digestion.

pro·te·ose (pro′tee·oce, ·oze) n. One of a group of derived proteins intermediate between native proteins and peptones. Soluble in water, not coagulable by heat, but precipitated by saturation with ammonium or zinc sulfate.

Pro·teus (pro′tee·us) n. A genus of bacteria of the family Enterobacteriaceae composed of lactose-negative rods which decompose urea rapidly and actively deaminate phenylalanine to phenylpyruvic acid. Included are *Proteus vulgaris, P. mirabilis, P. rettgeri,* and *P. morganii.* Normal inhabitants of the intestinal tract, they have significant pathogenicity in such conditions as diarrhea in infants, urinary tract infection, and suppurative lesions.

pro·throm·bin (pro·throm′bin) n. A plasma protein precursor of the proteolytic enzyme thrombin, formed in the liver through the action of vitamin K.

pro·throm·bin·emia, pro·throm·bin·ae·mia (pro·throm″bi·nee′mee·uh) n. An excess of prothrombin in the blood plasma.

pro·throm·bi·no·gen·ic (pro·throm″bi·no·jen′ick) adj. Having the property of causing or promoting the biosynthesis of prothrombin, an effect characteristic of vitamin K and related compounds.

pro·throm·bi·no·pe·nia (pro·throm″bi·no·pee′nee·uh) n. Decrease in the prothrombin content of the blood.

prothrombin time. A widely used one-stage clotting test devised by A. J. Quick based on the time required for clotting to occur after the addition of tissue thromboplastin and calcium to decalcified plasma.

pro·throm·bo·gen·ic (pro·throm″bo·jen′ick) adj. PROTHROMBINOGENIC.

pro·thy·mia (pro·thigh′mee·uh) n. Intellectual alertness.

Pro·tis·ta (pro·tis′tuh) n.pl. A group of organisms which includes the unicellular plants and animals and, on some classifications, the viruses. —**pro·tist** (pro′tist), com. n.

pro·ti·um (pro′tee·um) n. The predominant constituent of ordinary hydrogen; the atom consists of one proton and one electron and therefore has an atomic weight of approximately 1. Symbol, ^{1}H. Syn. *light hydrogen.*

pro·to·chlo·ride (pro″to·klo′ride) n. The first in a series of chloride compounds, containing the fewest chlorine atoms.

pro·to·col (pro′tuh·kol) n. 1. The original notes or records of an experiment, autopsy, or clinical examination. 2. The records from which a document is prepared. 3. The outline or plan for an experiment or experimental procedure.

pro·to·cone (pro′tuh·kone) n. 1. The primitive single cusp of a reptilian tooth. 2. The mesiolingual cusp on an upper molar.

pro·to·co·nid (pro″to·ko′nid, ·kon′id) n. The mesiobuccal cusp on a molar tooth of the lower jaw.

pro·to·di·a·stol·ic (pro″to·dye″uh·stol′ick) adj. 1. Of or pertaining to the first diastolic action in an embryo. 2. Pertaining to the early part of ventricular diastole, that is, immediately following the second heart sound.

protodiastolic gallop. VENTRICULAR GALLOP.

pro·to·elas·tose (pro″to·e·las′toce, ·toze) n. A poorly defined product of the digestion of elastin.

pro·to·fi·bril (pro″to·figh′bril) n. One of the fine filaments, seen under the electron microscope, of which fibrils are composed.

pro·tol·y·sis (pro·tol′i·sis) n., pl. **protoly·ses** (·seez) Any reaction in which a proton (hydrogen ion) is transferred, as: $HCl + H_2O = H_3O^+ + Cl^-$.

pro·ton (pro′ton) n. A subatomic particle identical with the nucleus of the hydrogen atom. It has a positive electric charge numerically equal to the negative charge on the electron, but its mass is over 1,800 times that of the electron. The atomic number of an element is equivalent to, and defined by, the number of protons in its nucleus.

proton-synchrotron, n. A synchrotron in which protons are accelerated to have energies in the billion electron volt range. Syn. *bevatron, cosmotron.*

pro·to·path·ic (pro″to·path′ick) adj. A term used by Henry Head to designate a primitive system of cutaneous sensory nerves and end organs, which, he postulated, mediated painful cutaneous stimuli and extremes of heat and cold. According to this theory, an "epicritic" system of nerves has been developed to amplify and control the more primitive protopathic system.

pro·to·plasm (pro′tuh·plaz·um) n. The viscid material constituting the essential substance of living cells, upon which all the vital functions of nutrition, secretion, growth, reproduction, irritability, and motility depend.

pro·to·plas·mic (pro″tuh·plaz′mick) *adj.* Pertaining to, or composed of, protoplasm.

protoplasmic astrocytes. The astrocytes in the gray matter, characterized by numerous, freely branching protoplasmic processes.

protoplasmic astrocytoma. A rare form of astrocytoma which, in pure form, is found almost exclusively in the cerebral hemispheres. Microscopically, the tumor consists of stellate cells with delicate processes devoid of neurofibrils.

pro·to·plast (pro′tuh·plast) *n.* 1. CELL (1). 2. PROTOPLASM. 3. An osmotically fragile, spherical bacterial cell, consisting of the cytoplasm and the nucleus, but lacking the cell wall.

pro·to·por·phyr·ia (pro″to·por·feer′ee·uh) *n.* The presence of protoporphyrin in red blood cells.

pro·to·por·phy·rin (pro′to·por′fi·rin) *n.* $C_{32}H_{32}N_4(COOH)_2$. Any of the 15 metal-free porphyrins having as substituents 4 methyl, 2 vinyl, and 2 propionic acid (— CH_2CH_2COOH) groups. The particular arrangement of these groups represented by protoporphyrin IX is the one occurring in hemoglobin.

pro·to·por·phy·rin·uria (pro″to·por″fi·ri·new′ree·uh) *n.* The excretion of protoporphyrins in the urine.

pro·to·pro·te·ose (pro″to·pro′tee·oce) *n.* A primary proteose; further digestion changes it into deuteroproteose.

pro·to·spasm (pro′to·spaz·um) *n.* A spasm beginning in a limb or part of a limb and extending to others.

pro·to·ver·a·trine (pro″to·verr′uh·treen) *n.* An ester alkaloid isolated from *Veratrum viride* and *V. album* and subsequently found to consist of protoveratrine A and protoveratrine B. Protoveratrine A is a tetraester and yields, on hydrolysis, protoverine, two moles of acetic acid, and one mole each of 2-methylbutyric acid and methylethylglycolic acid. Protoveratrine B is also a tetraester; on hydrolysis, it yields protoverine, two moles of acetic acid, and one mole each of 2-methylbutyric acid and 2,3-dihydroxy-2-methylbutyric acid. Both protoveratrines possess hypotensive activity.

Pro·to·zo·a (pro″tuh·zo′uh) *n.pl.* The phylum of unicellular animals, subdivided into the subphyla Mastigophora, Sarcodina, Sporozoa, and Ciliophora. —**pro·to·zo·an** (·zo′un) *n.* & *adj.;* **protozo·al** (·ul) *adj.*

pro·to·zo·a·cide (pro″tuh·zo′uh·side) *n.* An agent that will kill protozoa.

pro·to·zo·ol·o·gy (pro″tuh·zo·ol′uh·jee) *n.* The study of protozoa.

pro·to·zo·on (pro″tuh·zo′on) *n.,* pl. **pro·to·zoa** (·zo′uh). Any member of the phylum Protozoa.

pro·trude (pruh·trood′) *v.* To project; to assume an abnormally prominent position, as a tooth that is thrust forward out of line.

pro·tru·sion (pruh·trew′zhun) *n.* The condition of protruding or being thrust forward, as the protrusion of the incisor teeth. —**protru·sive** (·siv) *adj.*

pro·tu·ber·ance (pro·tew′bur·unce) *n.* A knoblike projecting part.

proud flesh. EXUBERANT GRANULATION.

pro·ven·tric·u·lus (pro″ven·trick′yoo·lus) *n.,* pl. **proventric·u·li** (·lye) The glandular stomach of birds.

pro·vi·ta·min (pro·vye′tuh·min) *n.* A precursor of a vitamin. That which assumes vitamin activity upon activation or chemical change within the body, as ergosterol (provitamin D_2), which upon ultraviolet irradiation is converted in part to calciferol (vitamin D_2); or β-carotene, which in the liver is hydrolyzed to vitamin A.

pro·voc·a·tive (pruh·vock′uh·tiv) *adj.* Tending to excite or provoke; arousing signs, symptoms, or reactions.

Pro·wa·zek-Hal·ber·staedt·er bodies (proh^v′ah.zeck, hal′bur·shtet″ur) Homogeneous irregular inclusion bodies that are near the nuclei of epithelial cells of the conjunctival sac; seen in cases of trachoma. Syn. *trachoma bodies.*

prox·i·mal (prock′si·mul) *adj.* 1. Nearer or nearest the point of origin along the course of any asymmetrical structure; nearer the beginning; of a limb or appendage, nearer the attached end. 2. In any symmetrical structure, nearer or nearest the center or midline or median plane. 3. *In dentistry,* of the surface of a tooth, next to the adjacent tooth.

prox·i·mate (prock′si·mut) *adj.* Nearest; immediate, as proximate cause.

proximate cause. The one cause of several causes which is immediately direct and effective.

proximo-. A combining form meaning *proximal.*

prox·i·mo·a·tax·ia (prock″si·mo·uh·tack′see·uh) *n.* Lack of coordination in the muscles of the proximal part of the limbs.

prox·i·mo·buc·cal (prock″si·mo·buck′ul) *adj.* Pertaining to the proximal and buccal surfaces of a tooth.

prox·i·mo·la·bi·al (prock″si·mo·lay′bee·ul) *adj.* Pertaining to the proximal and labial surfaces of a tooth.

prox·i·mo·lin·gual (prock″si·mo·ling′gwul) *adj.* Pertaining to the proximal and lingual surfaces of a tooth.

pro·zone (pro′zone) *n.* The area of the dilution range in which there is an absence or delay of a reaction at a higher concentration of one of the reactants than at a more dilute level.

P-R segment. The interval on the electrocardiogram between the end of the P wave and the beginning of the QRS complex.

prune-belly syndrome. ABDOMINAL MUSCLE DEFICIENCY SYNDROME.

prune-juice sputum. Dark reddish-brown bloody sputum, resembling prune juice.

pru·ri·go (proo·rye′go) *n.* A chronic inflammatory disease of the skin characterized by small, pale papules and severe itching. It usually begins in childhood and is most prominent on the extensor surfaces of the limbs. There are two forms of the disease: prurigo mitis, comparatively mild, and prurigo agria or ferox, severe. —**pru·rig·i·nous** (proo·rij′i·nus) *adj.*

prurigo nod·u·la·ris (nod″yoo·lair′is). A chronic

skin disease which occurs chiefly in women and is characterized by pruritic, nodular, and verrucous lesions. It is regarded as an atypical nodular form of neurodermatitis circumscripta, unrelated to the prurigos. Syn. *lichen obtusus corneus.*

pru·ri·tus (proo·rye'tus) *n.* Itching, an uncomfortable sensation due to irritation of a peripheral sensory nerve; a symptom rather than a disease. **—pru·rit·ic** (·rit'ick) *adj.*

pruritus ani (ay'nigh). A common itching condition in and about the anus, especially in men; may be due to several causes.

pruritus hi·e·ma·lis (high''e·may'lis). Itching related to cold, either from the climate or air-conditioning; dryness is also a factor. Syn. *frost-itch, winter itch.*

pruritus se·ni·lis (se·nigh'lis). The pruritus of the aged, probably caused by a lack of oil in the skin; accompanies the atrophy of the skin in old age.

pruritus vul·vae (vul'vee). Intense or mild itching of the vulva and at times adjacent parts. May lead to atrophy, lichenification, and even malignancy. Etiology is varied.

Prussian blue reaction. Formation of an insoluble dark greenish-blue pigment (Prussian blue) by ferric salts reacting with ferrocyanides; used histochemically for identification of hemosiderin and other iron-bearing pigments.

prus·sic acid (prus'ick). HYDROCYANIC ACID.

psam·mo·ma (sa·mo'muh) *n.,* pl. **psammomas, psammo·ma·ta** (·tuh) A tumor, usually a meningioma, which contains psammoma bodies. **—psammoma·tous** (·tus) *adj.*

psammoma bodies. Concentric laminae of calcium salts that have been laid down in degenerating tumor cells.

psam·mous (sam'us) *adj.* Sandy or sabulous.

psel·lism (sel'iz·um) *n. Obsol.* Stuttering or stammering.

psel·lis·mus mer·cu·ri·a·lis (sel·iz'mus mur·kewr''ee·ay'lis). *Obsol.* The unintelligible, hurried, jerking speech accompanying the tremor of mercury poisoning.

pseud-, pseudo- A prefix meaning (a) *false, deceptively resembling;* (b) in chemistry, *resembling* or *isomeric with.*

pseud·acu·sis (sue''da·kew'sis, ·koo'sis) *n.* A disturbance of hearing in which sounds are perceived as strange or peculiar, being altered in pitch and quality.

pseud·agraph·ia (sue''da·graf'ee·uh) *n.* 1. Incomplete agraphia, in which a person can copy correctly but is unable to write intelligibly or legibly independently. 2. The form of agraphia in which meaningless words are written.

pseud·am·ne·sia (sue''dam·nee'zhuh, ·zee·uh) *n.* A fragmentary type of amnesia with scattered loss of memory for unrelated experiences, usually transient and associated with organic brain disease.

pseud·an·ky·lo·sis (sue·dang''ki·lo'sis) *n.* 1. FIBROUS ANKYLOSIS. 2. EXTRACAPSULAR ANKYLOSIS.

pseud·ar·thro·sis (sue''dahr·thro'sis) *n.* A bony junction that permits abnormal motion, such as a fracture healed by fibrosis or an interspinal articulation that lacks normal rigidity.

pseud·es·the·sia, pseud·aes·the·sia (sue''des·theezh'uh, ·theez'ee·uh) *n.* An imaginary sensation for which there is no corresponding object, as a sensation referred to parts of the body that have been removed by accident or surgical operation.

pseudo-acanthosis nigricans. Acanthosis nigricans sometimes associated with obesity.

pseu·do·ac·ro·meg·a·ly (sue''do·ack''ro·meg'uh·lee) *n.* 1. Enlargement of the face and extremities not due to disease of the hypophysis. 2. HYPERTROPHIC PULMONARY OSTEOARTHROPATHY.

pseu·do·ag·glu·ti·na·tion (sue''do·a·gloo''ti·nay'shun) *n.* Rouleau formation and clumping tendency of erythrocytes simulating true agglutination, occurring as a result of the increased concentration of plasma proteins, particularly fibrinogen.

pseu·do·al·bu·min·uria (sue''do·al·bew''mi·new'ree·uh) *n.* FALSE PROTEINURIA; the presence in the urine of protein derived from blood, pus, or special secretions and mixed with the urine during its transit through the urinary passages.

pseu·do·al·ve·o·lar (sue''do·al·vee'uh·lur) *adj.* Simulating an alveolus or alveolar structure.

pseu·do·ane·mia, pseu·do·anae·mia (sue''do·uh·nee'mee·uh) *n.* Pallor and the appearance of anemia without blood changes to support the diagnosis. Syn. *apparent anemia.*

pseu·do·an·eu·rysm (sue''do·an'yoo·riz·um) *n.* FALSE ANEURYSM.

pseu·do·an·gi·na (sue''do·an·jye'nuh) *n.* A psychophysiologic cardiovascular disorder characterized by pain in the chest at the apex of the heart and at times radiating down the left arm, with no evidence of organic disease.

pseu·do·an·gi·o·ma (sue''do·an·jee·o'muh) *n.* 1. Canalized thrombus of the portal vein. 2. The formation of a temporary angioma, as is sometimes seen in healing stumps.

pseu·do·an·orex·ia (sue''do·an''o·reck'see·uh) *n.* Rejection of food because of dysphagia or gastric distress.

pseu·do·apha·kia (sue''do·a·fay'kee·uh) *n.* MEMBRANOUS CATARACT.

pseu·do·apo·plexy (sue''do·ap'uh·pleck''see) *n.* A condition resembling a cerebrovascular accident, but unaccompanied by cerebral hemorrhage.

pseu·do·ap·pen·di·ci·tis (sue''do·uh·pen''di·sigh'tis) *n.* A condition simulating appendicitis but with no lesion of the vermiform process.

pseu·do·ath·e·to·sis (sue''do·ath''e·to'sis) *n.* Athetoid movements, particularly of the fingers of the outstretched hand, as a result of the loss of proprioceptive sense; seen in such conditions as tabes dorsalis and subacute combined degeneration.

pseu·do·blep·sia (sue''do·blep'see·uh) *n.* A visual hallucination; a distorted visual image.

pseu·do·bul·bar (sue''do·bul'bur) *adj.* Not really bulbar; not concerned with or involving the medulla oblongata.

pseudobulbar palsy or **paralysis.** A weakness or paralysis of the muscle innervated by the motor nuclei of the bulb (the motor nuclei of the fifth, seventh, ninth, tenth, eleventh, and twelfth cranial nerves), due to bilateral interruption of the corticobulbar pathways which project to these nuclei. Clinically, there is impairment of swallowing, articulation and chewing movements, forced laughing or crying, exaggerated facial and jaw jerks, and lack of atrophy and fasciculations of the tongue. Signs of corticospinal tract disease are frequently conjoined. Bilateral lacunar infarction is the commonest cause. Syn. *spastic bulbar palsy* or *paralysis.*

pseu·do·car·ti·lage (sue"do-kahr'ti-lij) *n.* An embryonic type of cartilage in which but little matrix is formed, as that of the notochord.

pseu·do·chan·cre (sue'do-shank"ur) *n.* An indurated sore simulating a chancre.

pseu·do·cho·les·tane (sue"do-kol'e-stane, -ko·les'tane) *n.* COPROSTANE.

pseu·do·cho·les·te·a·to·ma (sue"do-ko·les"tee-uh·to'muh) *n.* A cholesteatoma secondary to epithelial ingrowth from the ear canal in chronic otitis media.

pseu·do·cho·lin·es·ter·ase (sue"do-ko"lin·es'tur-ace, -aze) *n.* An enzyme that catalyzes the hydrolysis of acetylcholine but that differs from cholinesterase in that it is nonspecific and hydrolyzes esters other than choline esters.

pseu·do·chrom·es·the·sia, pseu·do·chrom·aes·the·sia (sue"do·kro"mes·theez'ee·uh, ·theezh'uh) *n.* A form of synesthesia in which each of the vowels of a word (whether seen, heard, or remembered) seems to have a distinct visual tint.

pseu·do·chro·mia (sue"do·kro'mee·uh) *n.* A false or incorrect perception of color.

pseu·do·chy·lous (sue"do·kigh'lus) *adj.* Pertaining to or characterized by a milky fluid, resembling chyle, but containing no fat.

pseu·do·cir·rho·sis (sue"do·si·ro'sis) *n.* A disease resembling cirrhosis, due to obstruction of the hepatic vein or of inferior vena cava, or to pericarditis.

pseu·do·clau·di·ca·tion syndrome (sue"do·klaw·di·kay'shun). Pain on walking, usually in the thigh and buttocks, which is relieved by rest, caused by herniated disk, osteoarthritis, or spinal cord neoplasm, distinguished from intermittent claudication usually by variation in the walk-pain-rest cycle and by location of the pain.

pseu·do·co·arc·ta·tion (sue"do·ko"ahrk·tay'shun) *n.* A condition mimicking coarctation but in which the lumen of the affected structure is not significantly narrowed.

pseu·do·col·loid (sue"do·kol'oid) *n.* A mucoid material, found particularly in ovarian cysts.

pseu·do·col·o·bo·ma (sue"do·kol"o·bo'muh) *n.* A scarcely noticeable fissure of the iris, the remains of the embryonic ocular fissure, which has almost, but not perfectly, closed.

pseu·do·cow·pox (sue"do·kaw'pocks, sue"do·kaow'pocks) *n.* PARAVACCINIA.

pseu·do·cri·sis (sue"do·krye'sis) *n.* A false crisis;

a sudden fall of temperature resembling the crisis of a disease, subsequently followed by a rise of temperature and a continuation of the fever.

pseu·do·croup (sue"do·kroop) *n.* SPASMODIC CROUP.

pseu·do·cryp·tor·chism (sue"do·krip·tor'kiz·um) *n.* The condition in which one or both testes are either in the abdomen or in the inguinal canal, but can be brought down by various nonsurgical techniques, including the application of warmth; a common finding in young boys.

pseu·do·cy·e·sis (sue"do·sigh·ee'sis) *n.* A condition characterized by amenorrhea, enlargement of the abdomen, and other symptoms simulating gestation, due to an emotional disorder.

pseu·do·cyst (sue"do·sist) *n.* A sac-like space or cavity containing liquid, semiliquid, or gas but without a definite lining membrane.

pseu·do·de·cid·ua (sue"do·de·sid'yoo·uh) *n.* DECIDUA MENSTRUALIS.

pseu·do·de·men·tia (sue"do·de·men'shuh) *n.* A condition of apathy resembling dementia, but without the mental degenerative changes.

pseu·do·diph·the·ria (sue"do·dif·theer'ee·uh) *n.* Any membranous formation not due to *Corynebacterium diphtheriae.*

pseu·do·di·ver·tic·u·lum (sue"do·dye"vur·tick'yoo·lum) *n.* A herniation, commonly observed in the large bowel, in which the mucous membrane protrudes through a defect in the muscular layer, producing a pouch the wall of which contains no muscle. Syn. *false diverticulum.*

pseu·do·ede·ma, pseu·do·oe·de·ma (sue"do·e·dee'muh) *n.* A puffy condition simulating edema.

pseu·do·en·do·me·tri·tis (sue"do·en"do·me·trye'tis) *n.* A condition resembling endometritis marked by changes in the blood vessels, hyperplasia of the glands, and atrophy.

pseu·do·frac·ture (sue"do·frack"chur) *n.* A bony defect which in roentgenograms has the appearance of an incomplete fracture with associated periosteal reaction and callus or new bone formation, sometimes observed in osteomalacia.

pseu·do·geus·es·the·sia, pseu·do·geus·aes·the·sia (sue"do·gew"ses·theezh'uh) *n.* COLOR GUSTATION.

pseu·do·geu·sia (sue"do·gew'see·uh) *n.* A false perception, or hallucination, of taste independent of any stimulus, often occurring as an aura in psychomotor epilepsy. Syn. *phantogeusia.*

pseu·do·glob·u·lin (sue"do·glob'yoo·lin) *n.* A protein, one of the class of globulins; distinguished from the euglobulins by its solubility in distilled water, as well as in dilute salt solutions.

pseu·do·gon·or·rhea, pseu·do·gon·or·rhoea (sue"do·gun·uh·ree'uh) *n.* NONSPECIFIC URETHRITIS.

pseu·do·gout syndrome (sue"do·gowt'). A condition characterized by acute attacks of arthritis resembling gout and deposition of calcium pyrophosphate crystals in the articular cartilage. Syn. *chondrocalcinosis.*

pseu·do·gy·ne·co·mas·tia, pseu·do·gy·nae·co·mas·tia (sue″do·jin″e·ko·mas′tee·uh, ·guy″ne·ko·) *n.* Enlargement of the male breast due to excessive adipose tissue, as opposed to glandular hyperplasia.

pseu·do·hal·lu·ci·na·tion (sue″do·ha·lew″si·nay′shun) *n.* A vivid perception without external stimulus (hallucination) recognized by the individual as a hallucinatory, hypnagogic, or hypnopompic experience.

pseu·do·he·mo·phil·ia, pseu·do·hae·mo·phil·ia (sue″do·hee″mo·fil′ee·uh, ·hem″o·) *n.* VASCULAR HEMOPHILIA.

pseu·do·her·maph·ro·dite (sue″do·hur·maf′ro·dite) *n.* An individual with congenitally malformed external genitalia resembling one sex while the gonads are those of the opposite sex. **—pseudoher·maph·ro·dit·ic** (·maf″ro·dit′ick) *adj.*

pseu·do·her·maph·ro·dit·ism (sue″do·hur·maf′ro·dye·tiz·um) *n.* The condition of being a pseudohermaphrodite.

pseudohermaphroditismus mas·cu·li·nus (mas″kew·lye′nus). MALE PSEUDOHERMAPHRODITISM.

pseu·do·hy·dro·ceph·a·lus (sue″do·high″dro·sef′uh·lee·uh) *n.* False hydrocephalus; a condition in which the head appears disproportionately large as compared to the body; commonly seen in infants who are or were premature and small for their gestational age, the head growing at a faster rate than the body.

pseudohypertrophic infantile muscular dystrophy. A progressive hereditary, sex-linked recessive disorder of muscle, affecting chiefly males, beginning in early childhood; characterized by bulky calf and forearm muscles, which are doughy as a result of infiltration of fat and fibrous tissue, and by progressive weakness and atrophy of the thigh, hip, and back muscles, with resulting waddling gait, inability to rise from the supine position without "climbing-up on oneself" (Gower's sign), and lordosis. There is eventual involvement of the shoulder girdle and the muscles of respiration, as well as of the myocardium and esophagus. Syn. *Duchenne's muscular dystrophy.*

pseu·do·hy·per·tro·phy (sue″do·high·pur′truh·fee) *n.* FALSE HYPERTROPHY; increase in the size of an organ resulting from causes other than increased size of one or more of its normal components. **—pseudo·hy·per·troph·ic** (·high″pur·trof′ick) *adj.*

pseu·do·hy·po·na·tre·mia, pseu·do·hy·po·na·trae·mia (sue″do·high″po·na·tree′mee·uh) Low serum sodium concentration due to hyperglycemia or hyperlipemia, which does not mean diminished effective serum osmotic pressure.

pseu·do·hy·po·para·thy·roid·ism (sue″do·high″po·păr″uh·thigh′roy·diz·um) *n.* A condition exhibiting the signs, symptoms, and chemical findings of hypoparathyroidism, but due to an inability of the body to respond to parathyroid hormone, and not to a deficiency thereof.

pseu·do·il·e·us (sue″do·il′ee·us) *n.* ADYNAMIC ILEUS.

pseu·do·iso·chro·mat·ic (sue″do·eye″so·kro·mat′ick) *adj.* Pertaining to the different colors which appear alike to a person who is color-blind.

pseu·do·jaun·dice (sue″do·jawn′dis) *n.* Yellow discoloration of the skin from causes other than hepatic disease.

pseu·do·ker·a·tin (sue″do·kerr′uh·tin) *n.* A keratin that is partly digested by the common proteolytic enzymes, as distinguished from those keratins, classified as eukeratins, which are not digested.

pseu·do·ker·a·to·sis (sue″do·kerr″uh·to′sis) *n.* A condition in which pseudokeratin is present.

pseu·do·leu·ke·mia, pseu·do·leu·kae·mia (sue″do·lew·kee′mee·uh) *n.* Any condition simulating leukemia in the absence of that disease.

pseu·do·li·thi·a·sis (sue″do·li·thigh′uh·sis) *n.* A condition in which symptoms mimic those of a calculus in the biliary or urinary passages but where no stone can be demonstrated.

pseu·do·lo·gia fan·tas·ti·ca (sue″do·lo′jee·uh fan·tas′ti·kuh). A syndrome marked by a single, elaborate fantasy, of which the patient gives full details. The fantasy includes real occurrences added to a fantastic basis.

pseu·do·mal·a·dy (sue″do·mal′a·dee) *n.* An imaginary or simulated illness.

pseu·do·ma·nia (sue″do·may′nee·uh) *n.* 1. A mental disorder in which the patient accuses himself of crimes of which he is innocent. 2. A persistent compulsion for lying. 3. An excited mental state in a conversion type of hysterical neurosis which simulates the true manic phase of manic-depressive illness.

pseu·do·mel·a·no·sis (sue″do·mel·uh·no′sis) *n.* The staining of tissues, usually after death, by dark-brown or black pigments commonly derived from hemoglobin.

pseudomelanosis co·li (ko′lye). 1. Brown to black discoloration of all or a part of the colonic mucosa resulting from accumulations of an iron-containing pigment in mucosal macrophages; the presence of iron has been considered the feature distinguishing the pigment in this condition from that found in melanosis coli, but the distinctions are probably less obvious or even nonexistent. 2. Postmortem brown to black discoloration of all or part of the colonic mucosa due to the action of hydrogen sulfide in the bowel on iron in the mucosa.

pseu·do·mem·brane (sue″do·mem′brane) *n.* FALSE MEMBRANE, as in diphtheria. **—pseudo·mem·bra·nous** (·bruh·nus) *adj.*

pseu·do·men·in·gi·tis (sue″do·men·in·jye′tis) *n.* MENINGISM.

pseu·do·men·stru·a·tion (sue″do·men″stroo·ay′shun) *n.* Bloody vaginal discharge in newborn female infants, ceasing after a few days.

Pseu·dom·o·nas (sue·dom′o·nas, sue″do·mo′nas) *n.* A genus of bacteria of the family Pseudomonadaceae; members are small, motile, aerobic, and gram-negative.

Pseudomonas ae·ru·gi·no·sa (e·rue″ji·no′suh). A species of bacteria pathogenic to man; it is the causative agent of various suppurative infections in man. In the multiplication of *Pseudomonas aeruginosa*, pigments are liberated which give pus a blue-green color. Syn. *Pseudomonas pyocyanea, Bacillus pyocyaneus, blue-pus microbe.*

Pseudomonas pseu·do·mal·lei (sue"do-mal'ee-eye). An organism responsible for septicemia, pyemia, and granulomatous nodules in man and in rodents. Syn. *Malleomyces pseudomallei, Bacillus whitmori.*

pseu·do·mon·gol·ism (sue"do-mong'guh-liz-um) *n.* A congenital disorder in which the child is a partial phenotype of the Down's syndrome; however, the karyotype may have an extra chromosome fragment presumed to represent a partially deleted 21st chromosome, may show mosaicism, or may be normal. —**pseudo-mongol·oid** (-loid) *n. & adj.*

pseu·do·mu·cin (sue"do-mew'sin) *n.* A substance allied to mucin, found in certain cysts. —**pseudomucin·ous** (-us) *adj.*

pseudomucinous cystadenocarcinoma. MUCINOUS CYSTADENOCARCINOMA.

pseudomucinous cystadenoma. MUCINOUS CYSTADENOMA.

pseudomyxoma pe·ri·to·nei (perr"i·to-nee'eye). A widespread implantation in the peritoneal cavity of nodules secondary to mucinous tumors of the ovary or rupture of a mucocele of the appendix. Syn. *gelatinous ascites, gelatinous peritonitis, Werth's tumor.*

pseu·do·nar·co·tism (sue"do·nahr'ko·tiz·um) *n.* A conversion type of hysterical neurosis simulating narcotism.

pseu·do·neo·plasm (sue"do·nee'o·plaz·um) *n.* 1. PHANTOM TUMOR. 2. A temporary swelling, generally of inflammatory origin. —**pseudo-neo·plas·tic** (·nee"o·plas'tick) *adj.*

pseu·do·neu·ro·ma (sue"do·new·ro'muh) *n.* AMPUTATION NEUROMA.

pseudoneurotic type of schizophrenia. A form of schizophrenia in which symptoms usually held to be neurotic tend to mask the basic psychotic disorders.

pseu·do·nu·cle·o·lus (sue"do·new·klee'o·lus) *n.* KARYOSOME (1).

pseu·do·nys·tag·mus (sue"do·nis·tag'mus) *n.* Any of the symptoms resembling nystagmus but without the regular rhythmic movements of true nystagmus.

pseu·do·oph·thal·mo·ple·gia (sue"do·off·thal'mo·plee·jee·uh) *n.* A disorder in which eye movements on command or for following an object are unequally affected or even abolished, or in which the patient cannot fix his eyes on an object in the peripheral field, but in which the eyes may follow a slowly moving object or show full excursions with stimulation of the labyrinths. Syn. *ocular apraxia.*

pseu·do·os·teo·ma·la·cia (sue"do·os'tee·o·ma·lay'shee·uh). Rachitis in which the pelvic basin is distorted so as to resemble in form that of osteomalacia.

pseu·do·pap·il·le·de·ma, pseu·do·pap·il·loe·de·ma (sue"do·pa·pil"e·dee'muh, ·pap'il·) *n.* Apparent swelling of the optic disk, but without elevation of the disk or dilatation of the retinal veins, hyperemia, or enlargement of the blind spot; due to crowding and piling up of the optic nerve fibers and excess glial tissue; seen in extremely hypermetropic eyes, especially in children; may be congenital and familial.

pseu·do·pa·ral·y·sis (sue"do·puh·ral'i·sis) *n.* An apparent motor paralysis that is caused by voluntary inhibition of motor impulses because of pain or other organic or psychic causes.

pseu·do·par·a·site (sue"do·pâr'uh·site) *n.* 1. Any object resembling a parasite. 2. COMMENSAL.

pseu·do·pe·lade (sue"do·pe·lahd') *n.* ALOPECIA CICATRISATA.

pseu·do·ple·gia (sue"do·plee'jee·uh) *n.* Simulated paralysis, observed in hysteria or malingering.

pseu·do·pock·et (sue'do·pock"it) *n.* GINGIVAL POCKET.

pseu·do·pod (sue'do·pod) *n.* PSEUDOPODIUM.

pseu·do·po·di·um (sue"do·po'dee·um) *n.*, pl. **pseudopo·dia** (·dee·uh) 1. A temporary protrusion of a portion of the cytoplasm of an ameboid cell, as an aid to locomotion or for engulfing particulate matter. 2. An irregular projection of the margin of a wheal.

pseu·do·poly·co·ria (sue"do·pol·ee·kor'ee·uh) *n.* The "false" form of polycoria.

pseu·do·poly·po·sis (sue"do·pol·i·po'sis) *n.* An acquired form of polyposis of the colon, secondary to ulcerative colitis or amebic dysentery, in which tufts of mucosa have a pedunculated appearance due to adjacent ulcers or scars.

pseu·do·por·en·ceph·a·ly (sue"do·por"en·sef'uh·lee) *n.* A cavity in the cerebral mantle, usually due to a destructive process, which does not communicate with one of the lateral ventricles.

pseu·do·preg·nan·cy (sue"do·preg'nun·see) *n.* PSEUDOCYESIS.

pseu·do·pseu·do·hy·po·para·thy·roid·ism (sue"do·sue"do·high'po·pâr·uh·thigh'roy·diz·um) *n.* A condition with all the stigmata of pseudohypoparathyroidism, but with normal serum phosphorus and calcium levels.

pseu·dop·sia (sue·dop'see·uh) *n.* Visual hallucination, or error of visual perception.

pseu·do·psy·cho·path·ic (sue"do·sigh"ko·path'ick) *adj.* Of a condition or symptom, seemingly psychopathic but not so in fact.

pseu·do·pte·ryg·i·um (sue"do·te·rij'ee·um) *n.* A false, or cicatricial, pterygium.

pseu·do·pto·sis (sue"do·to'sis, sue"dop·) *n.* A condition resembling ptosis, caused by a fold of skin and fat descending below the edge of the eyelid.

pseu·do·pus (sue'do·pus") *n.* Any fluid resembling a purulent exudate.

pseu·do·ra·bies (sue"do·ray'beez) *n.* 1. A viral disease chiefly affecting cattle and swine, rarely man, transmitted by wild brown rats. Intense pruritus is followed by various central nervous system signs, including bulbar paralysis. Syn. *Aujeszky's disease.* 2. A disease superficially resembling rabies but hysterical in origin.

pseu·do·re·ac·tion (sue"do·ree·ack'shun) *n.* 1. A

localized reaction following intracutaneous inoculation of a test substance, due to irritating impurities contained in the material. 2. In the Schick test for immunity to diphtheria, a reaction to the toxin and the toxoid which fades within 48 hours, indicating immunity to the toxin and hypersensitivity.

pseu·do·re·tar·da·tion (sue″do-ree″tahr′day′shun) n. A state of slow or defective mentation, in which the patient appears to be mentally retarded when in fact he is not; often due to emotional deprivation or depression or large doses of drugs, such as anticonvulsants or neuroleptics, in which sedation is a major side effect.

pseu·do·rick·ets (sue′do-rick″its) n. RENAL RICKETS.

pseu·do·ro·sette (sue″do-ro-zet′) n. An arrangement of cells in a fashion resembling the primitive ependymal canal, but usually lacking the open central space of that canal; usually composed of tumor cells arranged around a blood vessel or around necrotic material.

pseu·do·ru·bel·la (sue″do-roo-bel′uh) n. EXANTHEM SUBITUM.

pseu·do·sci·ence (sue″do-sigh′unce) n. Any system of theories or methods claiming or appearing to be scientific, but clearly fallacious.

pseu·do·scle·re·ma (sue″do-skle-ree′muh) n. Induration of the subcutaneous fat of newborn infants.

pseu·do·scle·ro·sis (sue″do-skle-ro′sis) n. 1. CREUTZFELDT-JAKOB DISEASE. 2. HEPATOLENTICULAR DEGENERATION.

pseu·dos·mia (sue-doz′mee-uh) n. A hallucination of smell; frequently observed in uncinate epilepsy. Syn. *phantosmia.*

pseu·do·strat·i·fied (sue″do-strat′i-fide) adj. Characterizing an epithelium in which the cells all reach the basement membrane, but are of different lengths, with their nuclei lying at different levels, thus producing the appearance of several layers of cells.

pseu·do·ta·bes (sue″do-tay′beez) n. A neuropathy with symptoms like those of tabes dorsalis (lightning pains, sensory ataxia, atonic bladder), but not due to syphilis. Most often observed with diabetes mellitus. —**pseudo·ta·bet·ic** (-ta-bet′ick) adj.

pseu·do·tet·a·nus (sue″do-tet′uh-nus) n. Tonic spasms of muscles simulating tetanus without the presence of *Clostridium tetani.*

pseu·do·tu·ber·cu·lo·sis (sue″do-tew-bur″kew-lo′sis) n. An infection caused by *Yersinia pseudotuberculosis,* occurring in many animals, including rodents and birds, and which in man may produce severe disease with septicemia and sometimes symptoms resembling typhoid fever.

pseu·do·tu·mor (sue″do-tew′mur) n. PSEUDONEOPLASM.

pseudotumor cer·e·bri (serr′e-brye). A syndrome of increased intracranial pressure associated with normal or small cerebral ventricles, of unknown etiology but, in children, sometimes associated with obstruction of the large intracranial sinuses or veins, particularly the lateral sinus. Syn. *benign intracranial hypertension, meningeal hydrops.*

pseu·do·tym·pa·ni·tes (sue″do-tim″puh-nigh′teez) n. A distension of the abdomen similar to tympanites but not due to accumulation of gas; generally appears and disappears rapidly.

pseu·do·ven·tri·cle (sue″do-ven′tri-kul) n. The cavity of the septum pellucidum, called the fifth ventricle of the brain, although not a true one.

pseu·do·xan·tho·ma elas·ti·cum (sue″do-zan-tho′muh e-las′ti-kum). A genodermatosis, usually of recessive inheritance, resulting in deformed and often calcified elastic fibers. There are slightly elevated yellow plaques in the lax skin, accompanied in many cases by degenerative changes in the elastic blood vessels and in the eyes (angioid streaks of the retina).

psi (sigh) adj. Psychological or parapsychological.

psi·lo·cin (sigh′lo-sin) n. 4-Hydroxy-N,N-dimethyltryptamine, $C_{12}H_{16}N_2O$, an active constituent of the hallucinogenic mushroom *Psilocybe mexicana;* a dephosphorylated derivative of psilocybin that is isomeric with bufotenine.

psi·lo·cyb·in (sigh″lo-sib′in, -sigh′bin) n. 4-Phosphoryloxy-N,N-dimethyltryptamine, $C_{12}H_{17}N_2O_4P$, an active constituent of the hallucinogenic mushroom *Psilocybe mexicana.*

psi·lo·sis (sigh-lo′sis) n., pl. **psilo·ses** (-seez) 1. ¹SPRUE. 2. The falling out of the hair. —**psi·lot·ic** (-lot′ick) adj.

psi phenomena. In *parapsychology,* personal experiences or events defying physical explanation, such as clairvoyance, precognition, and telepathy.

psit·ta·co·sis (sit″uh-ko′sis) n., pl. **psittaco·ses** (-seez) Pneumonia and generalized infection of man and birds, usually acquired by man from such birds as parrots, parakeets, lovebirds, ducks, pigeons, and turkeys; caused by members of the family Chlamydiaceae. Syn. *parrot fever.*

pso·as (so′us) n., pl. **pso·ai** (-eye), **pso·ae** (-ee) One of the two muscles, psoas major and psoas minor.

psoas major. The greater psoas muscle, which arises from the bodies and transverse processes of the lumbar vertebrae and is inserted into the lesser trochanter of the femur.

psoas minor. The inconstant smaller psoas muscle, which arises from the bodies and transverse processes of the lumbar vertebrae and is inserted on the pubis.

psoas sign. Flexion of the hip, or pain on hyperextension of the hip due to an inflammatory process in contact with the psoas muscle on that side.

pso·i·tis (so-eye′tis) n. Inflammation of the psoas major muscle.

pso·mo·pha·gia (so″mo-fay′jee-uh) n. Swallowing chunks of food without thorough chewing. —**psomo·phag·ic** (-faj′ick) adj.

pso·ra (so′ruh) n. PSORIASIS.

pso·ra·line (sor′uh-leen, -lin) n. CAFFEINE.

pso·ri·a·si·form (so·rye'uh·si·form, so''rye·as'i·form) *adj.* Like psoriasis.

pso·ri·a·sis (so·rye'uh·sis) *n.* An idiopathic chronic inflammatory skin disease characterized by the development of red patches covered with silvery-white imbricated scales. The disease affects especially the extensor surfaces of the body and the scalp.

psoriasis gut·ta·ta (guh·tay'tuh). PSORIASIS PUNCTATA.

psoriasis punc·ta·ta (punk·tay'tuh). A form of psoriasis in which the lesions consist of minute red papules which rapidly become surmounted by pearly scales.

pso·ri·at·ic (so''ree·at'ick) *adj.* Pertaining to or affected with psoriasis.

psoriatic arthritis or **arthropathy.** Arthritis associated with psoriasis which is either a variant of rheumatoid arthritis or a distinct entity. Inflammatory involvement of the distal interphalangeal joint is frequent.

P. S. P. Abbreviation for *phenolsulfonphthalein.*

psy·cha·go·gy (sigh'kuh·go''jee) *n.* A reeducational, psychotherapeutic procedure that stresses the proper socialization of the individual. —**psy·cha·gog·ic** (sigh''kuh·goj'ick) *adj.*

psy·chal·gia (sigh·kal'jee·uh) *n.* Pains in the head, ascribed by depressed patients to anxiety, or to some psychic rather than physical cause.

psy·cha·lia (sigh·kay'lee·uh) *n.* An abnormal mental state attended by auditory and visual hallucinations.

psych·as·the·nia (sigh''kas·theen'ee·uh) *n.* Any psychoneurotic disorder containing compulsive, obsessive, and phobic tensions. A nervous state characterized by an urge to think, feel, or do something which at the same time is recognized by the patient as being senseless, silly, or irrational. —**psychas·then·ic** (·thenn'ick) *adj.*

psych·atax·ia (sigh''kuh·tack'see·uh) *n.* Impaired power of mental concentration; mental confusion or groping.

psych·au·di·to·ry (sigh·kaw'di·to·ree) *adj.* Pertaining to the conscious or intellectual interpretation of sounds.

psy·che (sigh'kee) *n.* 1. In Greek philosophy, the personification of the life principle. 2. The mind or self as a functional entity, serving to adjust the total organism to the needs or demands of the environment.

psy·che·del·ic (sigh''ke·del'ick, ·deel'ick) *adj.* Pertaining to or producing a psychic state, commonly by use of a hallucinatory drug, in which normally repressed elements are revealed or manifested; mind-revealing or mind-manifesting.

psy·chen·to·nia (sigh''ken·to'nee·uh) *n.* Mental strain or overwork.

psy·chi·at·ric (sigh''kee·at'rick, sick''ee·at'rick) *adj.* Pertaining to psychiatry.

psy·chi·a·trist (sigh·kigh'uh·trist) *n.* A specialist in psychiatry; specifically, a graduate of a medical school, licensed to practice, with postgraduate training in the diagnosis and treatment of mental and emotional disorders.

psy·chi·a·try (sigh·kigh'uh·tree, si·) *n.* The medi-

cal science and specialty that deals with the origins, diagnosis, prevention, and treatment of mental and emotional disorders and, by extension, of many problems of personal adjustment. It also includes special fields such as mental retardation and legal psychiatry.

psy·chic (sigh'kick) *adj.* 1. Pertaining to the psyche. 2. Sensitive to nonphysical forces. 3. Mental.

psychic energizer. Any drug, as a monoamine oxidase inhibitor or an amphetamine, that produces elevation of mood or mental excitement or stimulation, especially in a depressed person.

psychic epilepsy. A form of psychomotor or temporal lobe epilepsy in which the seizure consists mainly or solely of psychic aberrations, such as hallucinations, illusions, cognitive aberrations (feelings of increased reality, familiarity, unfamiliarity, depersonalization), or affective experiences (fear, anxiety).

psy·cho·an·al·ge·sia (sigh''ko·an''ul·jee'zee·uh) *n.* The relief of pain by psychological means, principally by assurance of and explanations to the patient, suggestion, and therapeutic measures, such as music.

psy·cho·anal·y·sis (sigh''ko·uh·nal'i·sis) *n.* 1. The method developed by Sigmund Freud for the exploration and synthesis of patterns in emotional thinking and development; a technique used in the treatment of a wide variety of emotional disorders, particularly the neuroses. Relies essentially upon the free associations of the patient to produce valuable information of which the patient was formerly unaware, by bringing to conscious manipulation ideas and experiences from the unconscious divisions of the psyche. 2. The body of data and theory based on the discoveries of this method; concerned chiefly with the conflict between infantile instinctual striving and parental or social demand, and the manner in which this conflict affects emotional growth, character development, and the formation of mental and emotional disorders.

psy·cho·an·a·lyst (sigh''ko·an'uh·list) *n.* A person who practices psychoanalysis.

psy·cho·an·a·lyt·ic (sigh''ko·an·uh·lit'ick) *adj.* Pertaining to psychoanalysis.

psychoanalytic theory. PSYCHOANALYSIS (2).

psy·cho·bi·ol·o·gy (sigh''ko·bye·ol'uh·jee) *n.* The school of psychology and psychiatry originated by Adolf Meyer in the United States in which the individual is considered not only as a physical organism but as the sum of his environment. Mental disorders, like normal behavioral processes, are considered dynamic adaptive reactions of the individual to stress or conflict, and are the understandable results of the development of the individual. —**psy·cho·bi·o·log·ic** (·bye''uh·loj'ick), **psychobiolog·i·cal** (·i·kul) *adj.*

psy·cho·cor·ti·cal (sigh''ko·kor'ti·kul) *adj.* Pertaining to the cerebral cortex as the seat of the mind.

psy·cho·di·ag·no·sis (sigh''ko·dye''ug·no'sis) *n.* Any procedure or means to discover the factors underlying behavior, particularly disordered or abnormal behavior.

psy·cho·di·ag·nos·tics (sigh"ko·dye"ug·nos'ticks) n. 1. The evaluation of the personality, particularly as furnished by the Rorschach test. 2. PSYCHOGNOSIS (3).

psy·cho·dra·ma (sigh"ko·drah"muh) n. 1. In psychotherapy, the reenactment of events from the patient's life, with the patient as either spectator or actor; a technique for obtaining cathartic relief. 2. A form of group psychotherapy in which the patients act out or dramatize their emotional problems.

psy·cho·dy·nam·ic (sigh"ko·dye·nam'ick) adj. 1. Pertaining to any psychological process which is undergoing change or causing change. 2. Pertaining to psychodynamics. 3. Pertaining to psychoanalysis.

psy·cho·dy·nam·ics (sigh"ko·dye·nam'icks) n. The study of human behavior from the point of view of motivation and drives, depending largely on the functional significance of emotion, and based on the assumption that an individual's total personality and reactions at any given time are the product of the interaction between his genetic constitution and the environment in which he has lived from conception onward.

psy·cho·gal·van·ic reflex (sigh"ko·gal·van'ick). A variation in the electric conductivity of the skin in response to emotional stimuli; due to changes in blood circulation, secretion of sweat, and skin temperature.

psy·cho·gal·va·nom·e·ter (sigh"ko·gal'vuh·nom'e·tur) n. A device for recording electrodermal responses to various mental stimuli which provoke emotional reactions. Its practical application is the lie detector, which indicates the emotional reactions of one who is suppressing the truth.

psy·cho·gen·e·sis (sigh"ko·jen'e·sis) n. 1. The development of mental characteristics. 2. The process by which activities or ideas originate in the mind, or psyche. 3. The production or causation of a symptom or illness by psychic, rather than organic, factors. The origin of psychic activity contributing to a mental disorder. —**psycho·gen·ic** (·jen'ick), **psycho·ge·net·ic** (·je·net'ick) adj.

psychogenic blindness. Blindness of mental or psychic origin; may be a symptom of hysterical type of conversion neurosis.

psychogenic deafness. Any deafness that has 50 percent or more of a psychic factor. Persons so affected do not know they can hear better than they manifest. It must be distinguished from malingering deafness.

psychogenic headache. Headache attributed to tension, anxiety, or a basic personality disorder.

psy·cho·geu·sic (sigh"ko·gew'sick, ·joo'sick) adj. Pertaining to perception of taste.

psy·cho·gno·sis (sigh"kog·no'sis) n., pl. **psycho·gno·ses** (·seez) 1. Diagnosis or recognition of mental and psychic conditions. 2. The study of a person by hypnosis. 3. The study of personality and behavior based on the somatotype, facial expressions, and such other signs as posture, gait, and gestures. —**psychog·nos·tic** (·nos'tick) adj.

psy·cho·graph·ic (sigh"ko·graf'ick) adj. 1. Pertaining to a chart of the personality traits of an individual. 2. In psychiatry, pertaining to the natural history of the mind.

psy·cho·ki·ne·sis (sigh"ko·ki·nee'sis, ·kigh·nee'sis) n. 1. Explosive or impulsive maniacal action; a lack of inhibition of primitive instincts leading to violent and hasty actions. 2. In parapsychology, the postulated direct action of mind on matter without any intermediate physical energy or instrument, as the supposed determination of how the dice shall fall by mere action of the will.

psy·cho·lep·sy (sigh"ko·lep"see) n. A sudden intense, usually short decrease in mental tension or mood level, approaching depression. —**psycho·lep·tic** (sigh"ko·lep'tick) adj.

psy·cho·log·ic (sigh"kuh·loj'ick) adj. 1. Of or pertaining to psychology. 2. PSYCHIC. 3. Emotional.

psy·cho·log·i·cal (sigh"ko·loj'i·kul) adj. PSYCHOLOGIC.

psychological autopsy. The investigation of the psychological and social circumstances which led to suicide or to unnatural death, such as from an accident, and of the manner in which patients contribute to their own deaths.

psychologic dyspareunia. Painful intercourse in the female due to emotional difficulties with no anatomic or pathologic explanation.

psychologic screening. The use of psychologic tests, usually for large groups, as a means of determining general suitability for some specific duty or occupation, such as army service.

psy·chol·o·gist (sigh·kol'uh·jist) n. 1. An individual who has made a professional study of, and usually thereafter professionally engages in, psychology. 2. Specifically, an individual with the minimum professional qualifications set forth by an intraprofessionally recognized psychological association, as the American Psychological Association.

psy·chol·o·gy (sigh·kol'uh·jee) n. The science that studies the functions of the mind, such as sensation, perception, memory, thought, and, more broadly, the behavior of an organism in relation to its environment. 2. The psychological or mental activity characteristic of a person or a situation, as the psychology of surgeons, or the psychology of dying.

psy·cho·math·e·mat·ics (sigh"ko·math"e·mat'icks) n. Mathematics associated with or applied to psychology; specifically, the application of mathematical formulas and procedures to psychology and psychologic tests.

psy·cho·me·tri·cian (sigh"ko·me·trish'un) n. 1. A psychologist who specializes in the administration and interpretation of psychologic tests. 2. A specialist in the mathematical and statistical treatment of psychologic data.

psy·cho·met·rics (sigh"ko·met'ricks) n. The measurement of mental and psychological abilities, potentials, and performance; frequently applied specifically to the measurement of intelligence. 2. PSYCHOMATHEMATICS. —**psychomet·ric** (·rick) adj.

psy·cho·mo·tor (sigh″ko·mo′tur) *adj.* Pertaining to both mental and motor activity, particularly as applied to the development of an infant or a child, to seizures, and to overactivity or underactivity of a confused or delirious patient.

psychomotor development. The progressive acquisition by the infant within a given time period of such motor skills as the ability to turn over at will, sit, crawl, stand, walk, and run, or intellectual skills such as meaningful speech or other ways of communication, of voluntary bladder and bowel control, and of cognitive skills such as the ability to solve problems; in the neurologically and mentally intact child, these developmental milestones are achieved by 3 to 4 years of age, after which there is primarily an increase in cognitive skills due to the child's educational experience.

psychomotor epilepsy. Recurrent multiple psychomotor seizures.

psychomotor seizure. An epileptic attack characterized by an aura which is often a complex hallucination or perceptual illusion, indicating a temporal lobe origin, and by complex semipurposeful activities for which the patient later has no recollection.

psychomotor status. Continuous psychomotor seizures.

psy·cho·neu·ro·log·ic (sigh″ko·new″ruh·loj′ick) *adj.* Pertaining to a condition involving both psychic and organic neural components.

psy·cho·neu·ro·sis (sigh″ko·new·ro′sis) *n.* NEUROSIS (1).

psy·cho·neu·rot·ic (sigh″ko·new·rot′ick) *adj.* NEUROTIC.

psychoneurotic disorder. NEUROSIS (1).

psy·cho·nom·ics (sigh″ko·nom′icks) *n.* 1. PSYCHOLOGY. 2. Psychological development as affected by environmental factors. —**psychonom·ic** (·ick) *adj.*

psy·cho·path (sigh′ko·path) *n.* A morally irresponsible person; one who continually comes in conflict with accepted behavior and the law.

psy·cho·path·ic (sigh″ko·path′ick) *adj.* 1. Pertaining to any mental disorder, particularly any disorder not yet diagnosed or not yet severe. 2. Pertaining to a psychopath.

psychopathic personality. An individual characterized by emotional immaturity with marked defects of judgment, prone to impulsive behavior without consideration of others, and without evidence of learning by experience. Though behavior is generally amoral or antisocial, there is little outward evidence of guilt.

psy·cho·pa·thol·o·gist (sigh″ko·pa·thol′uh·jist) *n.* An individual who specializes in the pathology of mental disease.

psy·cho·pa·thol·o·gy (sigh″ko·pa·thol′uh·jee) *n.* The systematic study of mental diseases.

psy·cho·phar·ma·col·o·gy (sigh″ko·fahr″muh·kol′uh·jee) *n.* The science dealing with the action of drugs on mental function.

psy·cho·phon·as·the·nia (sigh″ko·fo″nas·theen′ee·uh) *n.* A speech difficulty of mental origin.

psy·cho·phys·ics (sigh″ko·fiz′icks) *n.* 1. The study of mental processes by physical methods. 2. The study of the relation of stimuli to the sensations they produce, especially the determination of the differences of stimulus required to produce recognizable differences of sensation; experimental psychology. —**psychophys·i·cal** (·i·kul) *adj.*

psychophysiologic disorders. Symptoms arising from chronic and exaggerated forms of the normal physiologic organic components of emotion but with the subjective awareness of the emotion repressed. If long continued, may lead to structural changes in the affected organs, such as peptic ulcer. These disorders differ from conversion types of hysterical neurosis in that they involve overactivity or underactivity of organs and viscera innervated by the autonomic nervous system, fail to alleviate anxiety, and are physiologic rather than symbolic in origin. Syn. *psychosomatic disorders.*

psy·cho·ple·gic (sigh″ko·plee′jick) *adj. & n.* 1. Pertaining to psychoplegia. 2. A drug that lessens mental excitability and suppresses mental and sensory receptivity.

psy·cho·rhyth·mia (sigh″ko·rith′mee·uh) *n.* A mental condition in which there is involuntary repetition of previous volitional behavior.

psy·cho·sen·so·ry (sigh″ko·sen′suh·ree) *adj.* 1. Perceptual. 2. Imaginary or hallucinatory.

psy·cho·sex·u·al (sigh″ko·seck′shoo·ul) *adj.* Pertaining to the mental and emotional aspects of sexuality as contrasted to the strictly physical or endocrine manifestations.

psy·cho·sis (sigh·ko′sis) *n.,* pl. **psycho·ses** (·seez) In psychiatry, an impairment of mental functioning to the extent that it interferes greatly with an individual's ability to meet the ordinary demands of life, characterized generally by severe affective disturbance, profound introspection, and withdrawal from reality with failure to test and evaluate external reality adequately, formation of delusions or hallucinations, and regression presenting the appearance of personality disintegration. In contrast to organic brain syndromes, there is no impairment of orientation, memory, or intellect, though these may be difficult to examine readily, but differentiation from the neuroses may require long and acute observations. Included in this grouping are the affective disorders, paranoid states, and schizophrenias. A psychotic reaction may also accompany a symptomatic clinical picture, as in chronic brain syndromes associated with senile changes or alcohol intoxication.

psy·cho·so·cial (sigh″ko·so′shul) *adj.* Pertaining to or involving both psychological and social factors.

psychosomatic medicine. The branch of medicine dealing with psychic and physical components as a unit, and the interrelationship between them.

psy·cho·sur·gery (sigh″ko·sur′je·ree) *n.* Treatment of chronic, severe, and medically untreatable mental disorders by surgical interruption or removal of certain areas or pathways in the brain, especially amygdalotomy or prefrontal lobotomy.

psy·cho·ther·a·peu·tics (sigh″ko-therr″uh-pew′ticks) n. PSYCHOTHERAPY.

psy·cho·ther·a·pist (sigh″ko-therr′uh-pist) n. A person professionally trained and engaged in psychotherapy, usually a psychiatrist, clinical psychologist, or psychiatric social worker.

psy·cho·ther·a·py (sigh″ko-therr′uh-pee) n. 1. Treatment of any disease, but particularly emotional maladjustments and mental disorders, by psychological means, i.e., by verbal or nonverbal communication with the patients in distinction to therapy based on physical means. 2. Specifically, treatment of emotional or mental disorders by a psychotherapist. —**psychothera·peu·tic** (·pew′tick) adj.

psy·chot·ic (sigh-kot′ick) adj. & n. 1. Pertaining to, marked by, exhibiting, or caused by psychosis. 2. A psychotic individual.

psychotic depressive reaction. An affective disorder characterized by a depressed mood attributable to or precipitated by some real experience and occurring in an individual with no history of repeated depressions or mood swings.

psy·chot·o·gen (sigh-kot′o-jen) n. Any natural or synthetic substance that is capable of inducing in man a psychotic-like state. —**psy·chot·o·gen·ic** (sigh-kot″o-jen′ick) adj.

psy·cho·to·mi·met·ic (sigh-kot″o-mi-met′ick) adj. 1. Mimicking a psychotic disorder. 2. Pertaining to any drug or compound, such as lysergic acid diethylamide or mescaline, which can induce a psychotic-like state.

psy·cho·trop·ic (sigh″ko-trop′ick) adj. Pertaining to any substance or drug having a special affinity for or effect on the psyche or mind.

psychr-, psychro- A combining form meaning cold.

psy·chral·gia (sigh-kral′jee-uh) n. A painful subjective sense of cold.

psy·chro·es·the·sia, psy·chro·aes·the·sia (sigh″kro-es-theezh′uh, -theez′ee-uh) n. Subjective sensation of cold.

psy·chro·lu·sia (sigh″kro-lew′see-uh, -zee-uh) n. Cold bathing.

psy·chrom·e·ter (sigh-krom′e-tur) n. A hygrometer for determining atmospheric moisture by observing the difference in the indication of two identical thermometers, the bulb of one being kept dry, and the other wet, with a water-soaked wick; both are swung through the air to facilitate evaporation from the wet bulb.

psy·chro·phil·ic (sigh″kro-fil′ick) adj. Cold-loving; applied to microorganisms that develop best at temperatures between 15 and 20°C. Syn. crymophilic.

psy·chro·pho·bia (sigh″kro-fo′bee-uh) n. 1. An abnormal fear of cold. 2. An abnormal sensibility to cold.

psy·chro·phore (sigh′kro-fore) n. An instrument for applying cold to deeply seated parts, as a double-current catheter for applying cold to the posterior part of the urethra.

psy·chro·ther·a·py (sigh″kro-therr′uh-pee) n. The treatment of disease by the application of cold.

Pt Symbol for platinum.

pt. Abbreviation for pint.

PTA Abbreviation for plasma thromboplastin antecedent (= FACTOR XI).

pter-, ptero- A combining form meaning (a) wing; (b) feather.

pter·i·on (terr′ee-on, teer′ee-on) n. In craniometry, the region surrounding the sphenoparietal suture where the frontal bone, parietal bone, squama temporalis, and greater wing of the sphenoid bone come together most closely.

pter·o·yl·glu·tam·ic acid (terr″o-il-gloo-tam′ick) FOLIC ACID.

pte·ryg·i·um (te-rij′ee-um) n., pl. **pteryg·ia** (·ee-uh) 1. A triangular patch of mucous membrane growing on the conjunctiva, usually on the nasal side of the eye. The apex of the patch points toward the pupil, the fan-shaped base toward the canthus. 2. EPONYCHIUM (2). 3. Any fold of skin extending abnormally from one part of the body to another. —**pterygi·al** (·ul) adj.

pterygo-. A combining form meaning pterygoid, pterygoid process.

pter·y·goid (terr′i-goid) adj. 1. Wing-shaped. 2. Pertaining, directly or indirectly, to the pterygoid process of the sphenoid bone.

pterygoid process of the sphenoid bone. A process descending perpendicularly from the point of junction of the body with the greater wing of the sphenoid bone, and consisting of a lateral and a medial plate.

pter·y·go·man·dib·u·lar (terr″i-go-man-dib′yoo-lur) adj. Pertaining to the pterygoid process and the mandible.

pter·y·go·max·il·lary (terr″i-go-mack′si-lerr″ee) adj. Pertaining to the pterygoid process and the maxilla.

pter·y·go·pal·a·tine (terr″i-go-pal′uh-tine, -tin) adj. Situated between the pterygoid process of the sphenoid bone and the palatine bone.

pterygopalatine fossa. The gap between the pterygoid process of the sphenoid bone and the maxilla and palatine bone.

pterygopalatine ganglion. A parasympathetic ganglion located in the pterygopalatine fossa. From it, postganglionic fibers arise which project to the lacrimal gland and to the glands in the mucous membrane of the nose and pharynx.

pter·y·go·spi·nous (terr″i-go-spye′nus) adj. Pertaining to a pterygoid process and the angular spine of the sphenoid bone.

pti·lo·sis (ti-lo′sis) n., pl. **ptilo·ses** (·seez) Falling out of the eyelashes.

pto·maine (to′mane, to″may-een) n. Any of various nitrogenous bases, some of which are poisonous, produced by action of putrefactive bacteria on proteins. Certain ptomaines were formerly believed to cause food poisoning.

pto·sis (to′sis) n., pl. **pto·ses** (·seez) Prolapse, abnormal depression, or falling down of an organ or part; applied especially to drooping of the upper eyelid, as from paralysis of the third cranial nerve. —**ptosed** (toazd), **ptot·ic** (tot′ick) adj.

-ptosis A combining form meaning *a lowered position of an organ.*

pty·al·a·gogue (tye'al·uh·gog) *n.* SIALAGOGUE.

pty·a·lin (tye'uh·lin) *n.* A diastatic enzyme found in saliva, having the property of hydrolyzing starch to dextrin, maltose, and glucose, and hydrolyzing sucrose to glucose and fructose. Syn. *ptyalase, salivary diastase.*

pty·a·lism (tye'uh·liz·um) *n.* SALIVATION.

pty·a·lo·cele (tye'uh·lo·seel) *n.* A cyst containing saliva; usually due to obstruction of the duct of a salivary gland.

pty·a·lo·gogue (tye·al'o·gog) *n.* SIALOGOGUE.

pty·a·log·ra·phy (tye'uh·log'ruh·fee) *n.* Radiography of the salivary glands or their ducts; SIALOGRAPHY.

pty·a·lo·lith (tye'uh·lo·lith) *n.* SALIVARY CALCULUS.

pty·a·lo·li·thi·a·sis (tye'uh·lo·li·thigh'uh·sis) *n.* The formation, or presence, of a salivary calculus.

pty·a·lor·rhea, pty·a·lor·rhoea (tye'uh·lo·ree'uh) *n.* Excessive flow of saliva.

pty·sis (tye'sis) *n.,* pl. **pty·ses** (·seez) The act of spitting.

ptys·ma (tiz'muh) *n.* SALIVA.

ptys·ma·gogue (tiz'muh·gog) *n.* A drug that promotes the secretion of saliva.

Pu Symbol for plutonium.

pub·ar·che (pew·bahr'kee) *n.* The onset of pubic hair growth.

pu·ber·al (pew'bur·ul) *adj.* Pubertal. See *puberty.*

pu·ber·tas (pew'bur·tas) *n.* PUBERTY.

pubertas pre·cox (pree'koks). PRECOCIOUS PUBERTY.

pu·ber·ty (pew'bur·tee) *n.* The period at which the generative organs become capable of exercising the function of reproduction; signalized in the boy by a change of voice and discharge of semen, in the girl by the appearance of the menses. —**puber·tal** (·tul) *adj.*

pu·bes (pew'beez) *n.* 1. [NA] The hairy region covering the pubic bone. 2. The two pubic bones considered together; the portion of the hipbones forming the front of the pelvis.

pu·bes·cence (pew·bes'unce) *n.* 1. Puberty, or the coming on of puberty. 2. Hairiness; the presence of fine, soft hairs. —**pubes·cent** (·unt) *adj.*

pu·bic (pew'bick) *adj.* Pertaining to the pubes.

pubic crest. A crest extending from the pubic tubercle to the medial extremity of the pubis.

pubic region. The lowest of the three median abdominal regions, above the symphysis pubis and below the umbilical region. Syn. *hypogastric region, hypogastrium.*

pubic spine. PUBIC TUBERCLE.

pubic symphysis. SYMPHYSIS PUBIS; the fibrocartilaginous union (synchondrosis) of the pubic bones.

pu·bis (pew'bis) *n.* The pubic bone, the portion of the hipbone forming the front of the pelvis.

pub·lic antigen. An erythrocyte antigen system, defined by specific antiserums, found in virtually all people. More than 99 percent of the population have such antigens. Syn. *high incidence factors.*

public health. 1. The state of health of a population, as that of a state, nation, or a particular community. 2. The art and science dealing with the protection and improvement of community health through organized community effort, including preventive medicine, health education, communicable disease control, and application of the sanitary and social sciences.

public health nurse. COMMUNITY HEALTH NURSE.

pubo-. A combining form meaning *pubis, pubic,* or *pubes.*

pu·bo·ad·duc·tor (pew'bo·a·duck'tur) *adj.* Pertaining to the pubis and the adductor muscles of the hip.

pu·bo·cap·su·lar (pew'bo·kap'sue·lur) *adj.* Pertaining to the os pubis and the capsule of the hip joint.

pu·bo·coc·cyg·e·al (pew'bo·kock·sij'ee·ul) *adj.* Pertaining to the pubic bone and the coccyx.

pu·bo·fem·o·ral (pew'bo·fem'o·rul) *adj.* Pertaining to the os pubis and the femur.

pu·bo·pros·tat·ic (pew'bo·pros·tat'ick) *adj.* Pertaining to the pubic bone and the prostate gland.

pu·bo·rec·ta·lis (pew'bo·reck·tay'lis) *n.* A part of the levator ani muscle.

pu·bo·ves·i·cal (pew'bo·ves'i·kul) *adj.* Pertaining to the pubic bone and the urinary bladder.

pudenda. Plural of *pudendum.*

pu·den·dag·ra (pew'den·dag'ruh, ·day'gruh) *n.* Pain in the genital organs, particularly those of the female.

pu·den·dal (pew·den'dul) *adj.* Of, pertaining to, or situated in the region of the pudendum.

pu·den·dum (pew·den'dum) *n.,* pl. **puden·da** (·duh) The external genital organs, especially of the female.

pu·er·i·cul·ture (pew'ur·i·kul''chur, pew·err'i·) *n.* The specialty of child training.

pu·er·ile (pew'ur·il) *adj.* 1. Characteristic of or similar to that of children. 2. Childish. 3. Of or pertaining to childhood.

pu·er·il·ism (pew'ur·i·liz·um) *n.* Childishness; the reversion particularly in an adult to childlike behavior.

pu·er·i·tia (pew''ur·ish'ee·uh) *n.* SENILE DEMENTIA.

pu·er·pera (pew·ur'pur·uh) *n.,* pl. **puer·per·ae** (·ee) A woman who has recently given birth.

pu·er·per·al (pew·ur'pur·ul) *adj.* Pertaining to, caused by, or following childbirth.

puerperal fever. A febrile state caused by infection of the endometrium and septicemia following delivery. Syn. *childbed fever.*

puerperal metritis. Inflammation of the uterus following childbirth.

puerperal psychosis. Any psychotic reaction in a woman during the postpartum period, usually schizophrenic in nature. Organic or toxic factors may be present.

pu·er·pe·ri·um (pew''ur·peer'ee·um) *n.,* pl. **puerpe·ria** (·ree·uh) 1. The state of having just given birth. 2. The period from delivery to the time when the uterus has regained its normal size, which is about six weeks.

Pu·lex (pew'lecks) *n.* A genus of fleas.

Pulex ir·ri·tans (irr'i·tanz). The human flea; a species which is the intermediate host and transmitter of *Dipylidium caninum* and *Hymenolepis diminuta,* and may spread plague. It is parasitic on the skin of man and also infests hogs, dogs, and other mammals.

pu·li·ca·tio (pew″li·kay′shee·o) *n.* The state of being infested with fleas.

pu·li·cide (pew′li·side) *n.* An agent capable of killing fleas.

pulled elbow. Subluxation, or partial subluxation, of the head of the radius in small children. Syn. *nursemaid's elbow.*

pul·lo·rum disease (puh·lo′rum). A disease of chickens and other birds caused by *Salmonella pullorum.* Syn. *white diarrhea, bacillary white diarrhea.*

pul·mo (pul′mo) *n.,* genit. **pul·mo·nis** (pul·mo′ nis), pl. **pul·mo·nes** (·neez) LUNG.

pulmo- A combining form meaning *lung, pulmonic, pulmonary.*

pul·mo·nary (pul′muh·nerr″ee, pool·) *adj.* Pertaining to, or affecting, the lungs or any anatomic component of the lungs. Syn. *pulmonic.*

pulmonary adenomatosis. Progressive overgrowth of alveolar surfaces by columnar cells of uncertain origin, possibly a form of bronchiolar carcinoma, or an infectious disease.

pulmonary alveolar proteinosis. A condition characterized by gradually progressive dyspnea and hypoxia and a productive cough clinically, diffuse perihilar densities on x-ray, and large groups of alveoli filled with eosinophilic proteinaceous material on pathologic examination.

pulmonary circulation. The circulation of blood through the lungs by means of the pulmonary arteries and veins, for the purpose of oxygenation and release of carbon dioxide. Syn. *lesser circulation.*

pulmonary edema. An effusion of fluid into the air sacs and interstitial tissue of the lungs, producing severe dyspnea; most commonly due to left heart failure. Syn. *Potain's disease.*

pulmonary epithelial cell. SQUAMOUS ALVEOLAR CELL.

pulmonary pleura. The portion of the pleura directly enveloping the lung.

pulmonary stenosis. Narrowing of the orifice of the pulmonary trunk.

pulmonary trunk. The arterial vessel arising from the right ventricle and giving rise to the right and left pulmonary arteries.

pul·mo·nec·to·my (pul″mo·neck′tuh·mee, pool·) *n.* PNEUMONECTOMY.

pul·mon·ic (pul·mon′ick) *adj.* PULMONARY.

pulmonic stenosis. PULMONARY STENOSIS.

pulp, *n.* 1. The soft, fleshy part of fruit. 2. The soft part in the interior of an organ. —**pulp·al** (·ul), **pulp·ar** (·ur) *adj.*

pul·pa (pul′puh) *n.* PULP.

pulpa co·ro·na·le (kor·o·nay′lee) [NA]. The portion of the dental pulp located in the crown portion of the pulp cavity.

pulp cavity. The space within the central part of a tooth which contains the dental pulp and comprises the pulp chamber and a root canal for each root.

pulp chamber. The coronal portion of the central cavity in a tooth.

pulp·ec·to·my (pul·peck′tuh·mee) *n.* Excision or extirpation of a dental pulp.

pulp·i·tis (pul·pye′tis) *n.,* pl. **pulp·it·i·des** (pul·pit′ i·deez) An inflammation of the dental pulp.

pulp of the intervertebral disk. The pulpy body at the center of the intervertebral disk, a remnant of the notochord.

pulp·ot·o·my (pul·pot′uh·mee) *n.* The surgical removal of the pulp of a tooth.

pulp·stone, *n.* DENTICLE (2).

pulpy (pulp′ee) *adj.* Resembling pulp; characterized by the formation of a substance resembling pulp.

pul·sate (pul′sate) *v.* To beat or throb.

pul·sa·tile (pul′suh·til) *adj.* Pulsating; throbbing.

pul·sa·tion (pul·say′shun) *n.* 1. A beating or throbbing; usually rhythmic. 2. PULSE (2).

pulse, *n. & v.* 1. The regularly recurrent palpable wave of distention in an artery due to blood ejected with each cardiac contraction. 2. A single beat or wave in pulsation from any source. 3. To generate, emit, or modulate energy, as electromagnetic radiation, in the form of pulses.

pulse cycle. The period between the beginning and end of a pulse wave.

pulse deficit. The difference between the auscultatory heart rate and the rate of the peripheral pulse determined by palpation.

pulse-echo diagnosis or technique. The use of ultrasonic energy between 1 and 15 megahertz directed into the human body for the purposes of studying alterations of structure. Syn. *ultrasonography.*

pulse·less, *adj.* Devoid of pulse or pulsation.

pulseless disease. AORTIC ARCH SYNDROME.

pulse pressure. The difference between the systolic and diastolic blood pressure.

pulse rate. The number of pulsations of an artery per minute; same as the heart rate.

pulse wave. PRESSURE PULSE WAVE.

pul·sim·e·ter (pul·sim′e·tur) *n.* An instrument for determining the rate or force of the pulse.

pul·sion (pul′shun) *n.* The act of pushing forward.

pulsion diverticulum. Herniation of the mucous membrane through the muscular coat of an organ, usually the pharynx or esophagus, caused by pressure from within.

pul·sus (pul′sus) *n.* PULSE.

pulsus al·ter·nans (awl′tur·nanz). A pulse pattern in which the beats occur at regular intervals but with alternating weak and strong beats; commonly seen with left ventricular failure.

pulsus ce·ler (sel′ur) A pulse that rises and falls quickly.

pulsus celer et al·tus (al′tus) A quick, full, bounding pulse, seen especially in aortic regurgitation.

pulsus deb·i·lis (deb′i·lis). A weak pulse.

pulsus du·rus (dew′rus). A hard, incompressible pulse.

pulsus ir·reg·u·la·ris per·pet·u·us (i·reg″yoo·lair′ is pur·pet′yoo·us). The pulse of atrial fibrillation which is completely irregular in rate and amplitude.

pulsus par·a·dox·us (păr′uh·dock′sus). Fall in the systolic blood pressure during inspiration greater than the normal 3 to 10 mmHg; may be seen with conditions such as cardiac tamponade, severe heart failure, emphysema.

pulsus par·vus (pahr'vus). A pulse small in amplitude.

pulsus tardus. A pulse with a delayed systolic peak.

pul·ta·ceous (pul-tay'shus) *adj.* Having the consistency of pulp; mushy; soft.

pulv. Abbreviation for *pulvis.*

pul·ver·ize (pul'vur·ize) *v.* To reduce a substance to a powder. —**pul·ver·i·za·tion** (pul'vur·i·zay'shun) *n.*

pul·ver·u·lent (pul·verr'yoo·lunt) *adj.* 1. Powdery, dusty, or reducible to a fine powder. 2. Covered with fine powder or dust.

pul·vi·nar (pul·vye'nur) *n.* A nuclear mass forming the posterior portion of the thalamus.

pul·vis (pul'vis) *n.* POWDER.

pum·ice (pum'is) *n.* A substance of volcanic origin, consisting of complex silicates of aluminum, potassium, and sodium; used as an abrasive.

pump, *n.* An apparatus or machine which, by alternate suction and compression, raises or transfers liquids, or which exhausts or compresses gases.

punch, *n.* A surgical instrument for perforating or cutting out a disk or segment of resistant tissue, as cartilage or bone.

punch-drunk, *adj.* Pertaining to or suffering from the punch-drunk state. —**punch-drunkenness,** *n.*

punch-drunk state. A condition caused by repeated cerebral injury, observed in professional boxers; characterized clinically by dysarthria, ataxia, and impairment of cognition and memory; characterized pathologically by neuronal loss in the substantia nigra and the cerebral and cerebellar cortices and fibrillary changes in remaining neurons. Syn. *dementia pugilistica, boxer's encephalopathy.*

puncta. Plural of *punctum.*

punc·tate (punk'tate) *adj.* Dotted; full of minute points.

punctate cataract. A form of congenital cataract in which small opacities, appearing light-blue or gray in color, are scattered throughout the lens. There is no loss of vision.

puncta vas·cu·lo·sa (vas·kew·lo'suh). Minute red spots studding the cut surface of the white central mass of the fresh brain. They are produced by the blood escaping from divided blood vessels.

punc·tic·u·lum (punk·tick'yoo·lum) *n.* A small point.

punc·ti·form (punk'ti·form) *adj.* 1. Having the nature or qualities of a point; seeming to be located at a point, as a punctiform sensation. 2. Of bacterial colonies: very minute.

punc·to·graph (punk'to·graf) *n.* A radiographic instrument for the surgical localization of foreign bodies, as bullets embedded in the tissues.

punc·tum (punk'tum) *n.,* pl. **punc·ta** (·tuh) Point.

punctum lac·ri·ma·le (lack·ri·may'lee) [NA]. LACRIMAL PUNCTUM.

punctum prox·i·mum (prock'si·mum). NEAR POINT. Abbreviated, P., P.p.

punc·ture (punk'chur) *n.* 1. A hole made by the piercing of a pointed instrument. 2. The procedure of making a puncture.

pun·gent (pun'junt) *adj.* Acrid; penetrating; producing a painful sensation.

P.U.O. Pyrexia of unknown origin.

pu·pa (pew'puh) *n.,* pl. **pu·pae** (·pee), **pupas** The stage, usually quiescent, in the life history of some insects, which follows the larval period and precedes the adult imago. —**pu·pal** (·pul) *adj.*

pu·pil (pew'pil) *n.* The aperture in the iris of the eye for the passage of light.

pu·pil·la (pew·pil'uh) *n.,* pl. & genit. sing. **pupil·lae** (·ee) PUPIL.

pu·pil·lary (pew'pi·lerr·ee) *adj.* Of or pertaining to the pupil of an eye.

pupillary reflex. 1. Contraction of the pupil in response to stimulation of the retina by light. Syn. *Whytt's reflex.* 2. Contraction of the pupil on accommodation for close vision and dilatation of the pupil on accommodation for distant vision. 3. CONSENSUAL LIGHT REFLEX. 4. Contraction of the pupil on attempted closure of the eye. Syn. *Westphal-Pilcz reflex, Westphal's pupillary reflex.*

pu·pil·lom·e·ter (pew'pi·lom'e·tur) *n.* An instrument for measuring the pupil of the eye. —**pupillome·try** (·tree) *n.*

pu·pil·lo·sta·tom·e·ter (pew·pil'o·sta·tom'e·tur) *n.* An instrument for measuring the exact distance between the centers of the two pupils.

puppet-head phenomenon. DOLL'S-HEAD PHENOMENON.

pure, *adj.* Free from mixture or contact with that which weakens or pollutes; containing no foreign or extraneous material.

pur·ga·tion (pur·gay'shun) *n.* 1. The evacuation of the bowels by means of purgatives. 2. Cleansing.

pur·ga·tive (pur'guh·tiv) *adj. & n.* 1. Producing purgation. 2. A drug that produces evacuation of the bowel; specifically, a cathartic of moderate potency.

purge (purj) *v. & n.* 1. To cause purgation or catharsis. 2. A purgative or cathartic.

purg·ing (pur'jing) *n.* A condition in which there is rapid and continuous evacuation of the bowels.

pu·ri·fied (pewr'i·fide) *adj.* Cleansed; freed from extraneous matter.

purified protein derivative of tuberculin. A form of dried tuberculin. Abbreviated, P.P.D.

pu·ri·form (pewr'i·form) *adj.* In the form of or resembling pus.

pu·rine (pew'reen, ·in) *n.* A heterocyclic compound, $C_5H_4N_4$, in which a pyrimidine ring is fused to an imidazoline ring. Various derivatives of purine, generically called purines and including adenine, guanine, the xanthines, and uric acid, are widely distributed in nature.

purine bases. Generic term for purine and other bases derived from it, as adenine and guanine, which are components of nucleotides, and also caffeine and theobromine, which are alkaloids.

pu·ri·ty (pewr'i·tee) *n. In optics,* the percentage

contribution to luminous intensity by the dominant wavelength in a beam of light.

Pur·ki·nje cells (poor'kin·yeʰ) Cells of the cerebellar cortex with large, flask-shaped bodies forming a single cell layer between the molecular and granular layers. Their dendrites branch in the molecular layer in a plane at right angles to the long axis of the folia, and their axons run through the granular layer into the white substance to end in the central cerebellar nuclei.

Purkinje fibers The modified cardiac muscle fibers that form the terminal part of the conducting system of the heart.

pu·ro·mu·cous (pew'ro·mew'kus) *adj.* Consisting of mucus mixed with pus; mucopurulent.

pu·ro·my·cin (pew'ro·migh'sin) *n.* An antibiotic substance, $C_{22}H_{29}N_7O_5$, produced by *Streptomyces alboniger*, that has trypanocidal and amebicidal activity.

pur·pu·ra (pur'pew·ruh) *n.* A condition in which hemorrhages occur in the skin, mucous membranes, serous membranes, and elsewhere. The characteristic skin lesions are petechiae, ecchymoses, and vibices.

purpura an·nu·la·ris te·lan·gi·ec·to·des (an·yoo·lair'is te·lan''jee·eck·to'dees). An eruption of purpuric spots, grouped in ring form and accompanied by telangiectasis. Syn. *Majocchi's disease.*

purpura ful·mi·nans (ful'mi·nanz). Rapidly progressive cutaneous and mucosal bleeding as a result of marked disseminated intravascular clotting with overutilization of platelets, factor V, and other clotting factors, occurring in many overwhelming bacterial and viral infections, especially in children, and best treated with the initiating agent, when possible.

purpura hem·or·rhag·i·ca (hem''o·raj'i·kuh, ·ray'ji·kuh). IDIOPATHIC THROMBOCYTOPENIC PURPURA.

purpura hy·per·glob·u·li·ne·mi·ca (high''per·glob''yoo·li·nee'mi·kuh). Hemorrhagic diathesis attributed to elevation of the concentration of globulin in the serum.

purpura ne·crot·i·ca (ne·krot'i·kuh). A condition characterized by enormous ecchymotic skin lesions which in later stages become necrotic and gangrenous.

purpura rheu·mat·i·ca (roo·mat'i·kuh). SCHÖNLEIN'S PURPURA.

purpura se·ni·lis (se·nigh'lis). Purpura of unknown cause that occurs in elderly people.

purpura sim·plex (sim'plecks). A mild form of purpura not associated with well-defined defects of blood-clotting mechanisms or mucous-membrane bleeding; often familial and particularly prone to occur in females.

purpura ur·ti·cans (ur'ti·kanz). Purpura associated with urticaria.

pur·pu·ric (pur·pew'rick) *adj.* Pertaining to or characterized by purpura.

pur·pu·rin·uria (pur''pew·ri·new'ree·uh) *n.* The presence of purpurin in the urine. Syn. *porphyruria.*

purr, *n.* A low-pitched vibratory murmur, like the purring of a cat.

pu·ru·lence (pewr'yoo·lunce) *n.* The quality or state of containing pus.

pu·ru·lent (pewr'yoo·lunt) *adj.* Containing, consisting of, or forming pus.

purulent inflammation. An inflammatory process productive of an exudate rich in neutrophils, which undergoes liquifaction necrosis to produce pus. It is distinguished from suppurative inflammation by the lack of necrosis of fixed tissues, and is exemplified by the exudate often occurring in the common cold.

purulent meningitis. Meningitis due to a pyogenic organism.

pu·ru·loid (pewr'yoo·loid) *adj.* Resembling pus; puriform.

pus, *n.* The product of liquefaction necrosis in an exudate rich in neutrophils, giving a viscous, creamy, pale-yellow or yellow-green fluid.

pustular bacterid. PUSTULOSIS PALMARIS ET PLANTARIS.

pustular psoriasis. 1. A variant form of psoriasis occurring in the course of chronic psoriasis, characterized by shiny, dark-red scaly patches bearing superficial pustules. Oral lesions may occur, and chills and fever may be present at onset. 2. ACRODERMATITIS CONTINUA. 3. IMPETIGO HERPETIFORMIS.

pus·tu·la·tion (pus''tyoo·lay'shun) *n.* The formation of pustules.

pus·tule (pus'tyool) *n.* A small, circumscribed elevation of the skin containing pus. **—pus·tu·lar** (·tyoo·lur) *adj.*

pus·tu·li·form (pus'tyoo·li·form) *adj.* Resembling a pustule.

pus·tu·lo·der·ma (pus''tew·lo·dur'muh) *n.* Any skin disease characterized by the formation of pustules.

pus·tu·lo·sis (pus''tew·lo'sis) *n.* Any condition characterized by the presence of pustules.

pustulosis pal·ma·ris et plan·ta·ris (pal·mair'is et plan·tair'is). A chronic indolent noninfectious dermatitis chiefly of palms and soles, not related to psoriasis. The pustules are sterile, deep-seated, and appear in continuous crops. Syn. *pustular acrodermatitis, pustular bacterid.*

pu·ta·men (pew·tay'mun) *n.* The outer darker part of the lenticular nucleus of the brain. **—pu·tam·i·nal** (pew·tam'i·nul) *adj.*

pu·tre·fac·tion (pew''tre·fack'shun) *n.* The enzymic decomposition of organic matter, especially of proteins, by anaerobic microorganisms, with formation of malodorous substances such as indole and skatole, nitrogenous bases such as cadaverine and putrescine, and many other compounds.

pu·tre·fac·tive (pew''tre·fack'tiv) *adj.* Pertaining to or causing putrefaction.

pu·tre·fy (pew'tre·figh) *v.* 1. To render putrid. 2. To become putrid.

pu·tres·cent (pew·tres'unt) *adj.* Undergoing putrefaction. **—putres·cence** (·unce) *n.*

pu·tres·cine (pew·tres'een, ·in) *n.* 1,4-Diaminobutane or tetramethylenediamine, $NH_2(CH_2)_4NH_2$, a product of decarboxylation of ornithine and also found in putrefying flesh; formerly believed to be responsible for food poisoning, and referred to as a ptomaine.

pu·trid (pew'trid) *adj.* Rotten; characterized by putrefaction.

pu·tro·maine (pew'tro-mane) *n.* A ptomaine developed in putrefactive processes.

PVC. Abbreviation for *premature ventricular contraction.*

PVP Abbreviation for *polyvinylpyrrolidone.*

P wave of the electrocardiogram. The electrocardiographic deflection due to depolarization of the atria.

py-, pyo- A combining form meaning *pus* or *suppuration.*

py·ar·thro·sis (pye''ahr-thro'sis) *n.* Suppuration involving a joint.

pycnosis. PYKNOSIS.

pyel-, pyelo- A combining form meaning *renal pelvis, renal pelvic.*

py·ec·ta·sis (pye''e-leck'tuh-sis) *n.* Dilation of a renal pelvis.

py·eli·tis (pye''e-lye'tis) *n.* Inflammation of the pelvis of a kidney. —**py·elit·ic** (pye''e-lit'ick) *adj.*

pyelitis cys·ti·ca (sis'ti-kuh). A nonspecific chronic inflammatory reaction of the renal pelvis, characterized by numerous minute translucent cysts scattered over the surface of the pelvic mucosa.

py·elo·cys·ti·tis (pye''e-lo-sis-tye'tis) *n.* Inflammation of the pelvis of the kidney and of the urinary bladder.

py·elo·gram (pye''e-lo-gram) *n.* A radiograph of the renal pelvis and ureter, employing contrast material.

py·elog·ra·phy (pye''e-log'ruh-fee) *n.* Radiography of a renal pelvis and ureter, which have been filled with an opaque solution.

py·elo·li·thot·o·my (pye''e-lo-li-thot'uh-mee) *n.* Removal of a renal calculus through an incision into the pelvis of a kidney. Syn. *pelviolithotomy.*

py·elo·ne·phri·tis (pye''e-lo-ne-frye'tis) *n.* The disease process from the immediate and late effects of bacterial and other infections of the parenchyma and the pelvis of the kidney.

py·elo·plas·ty (pye''e-lo-plas''tee) *n.* Plastic repair of the renal pelvis.

py·elo·pli·ca·tion (pye''e-lo-pli-kay'shun) *n.* Reducing an enlarged renal pelvis by plicating or suturing the infolded walls.

py·elos·to·my (pye''e-los'tuh-mee) *n.* Incision into the renal pelvis.

py·elot·o·my (pye''e-lot'uh-mee) *n.* Incision of the renal pelvis.

py·elo·tu·bu·lar (pye''e-lo-tew'bew-lur) *adj.* Pertaining to the renal pelvis and tubules.

py·elo·ure·ter·al (py''e-lo-yoo-ree'tur-ul) *adj.* Pertaining to the renal pelvis and ureter.

py·elo·ure·ter·og·ra·phy (pye''e-lo-yoo-ree''tur-og'ruh-fee) *n.* PYELOGRAPHY.

py·elo·ve·nous (pye''e-lo-vee'nus) *adj.* Pertaining to the renal pelvis and the veins.

py·em·e·sis (pye-em'e-sis) *n.* Vomiting of purulent material.

py·emia, py·ae·mia (pye-ee'mee-uh) *n.* A disease state due to the presence of pyogenic microorganisms in the blood and the formation, wherever these organisms lodge, of embolic or metastatic abscesses. —**py·emic, py·ae·mic** (pye-ee'mick) *adj.*

py·en·ceph·a·lus (pye''en-sef'uh-lus) *n.* Suppuration within the brain; a brain abscess.

pyg-, pygo- A combining form meaning *buttocks.*

py·gal·gia (pye-gal'juh, -jee-uh) *n.* Pain in the buttocks.

pyg·ma·li·on·ism (pig-may'lee-un-iz-um) *n.* The pathological erotic fantasies in which an individual falls in love with a creation of his own.

pyg·my (pig'mee) *n.* An abnormally small person or dwarf.

py·gom·e·lus (pye-gom'e·lus) *n.,* pl. **pygome·li** (-lye) An individual with an accessory limb or limbs attached to the buttock. Syn. *epipygus.*

py·gop·a·gus (pye-gop'uh-gus) *n.* Conjoined twins united in a sacral region.

pyk·nic (pick'nick) *adj.* Pertaining to or characterizing a constitutional body type marked by roundness of contour, amplitude of body cavities, and considerable subcutaneous fat.

pyk·no·dys·os·to·sis, pyc·no·dys·os·to·sis (pick''no-dis''os-to'sis) *n.* A heritable disorder of bone, characterized by short stature, a large skull with absence of knitting of the anterior fontanel, receding chin, shortness of fingers and toes, and fragility of bones. Radiographs show an abnormal thickness of bones, which is responsible for the fractures. Transmitted as an autosomal recessive trait. Syn. *Toulouse-Lautrec disease.*

pyk·no·lep·sy, pyc·no·lep·sy (pick'no-lep-see) *n.* A form of absence attack in which the episodes of unawareness occur very frequently. —**pyk·no·lep·tic** (pick''no-lep'tick) *adj.*

pyk·nom·e·ter, pyc·nom·e·ter (pick-nom'e-tur) *n.* An instrument for the determination of the specific gravity of fluids.

pyk·no·phra·sia, pyc·no·phra·sia (pick''no-fray'zhuh, -zee-uh) *n.* Thickness of speech.

pyk·no·sis, pyc·no·sis (pick-no'sis) *n.* 1. Thickening; inspissation. 2. A degenerative change in cells whereby the nucleus is condensed and shrinks to a dense, structureless mass of chromatin. —**pyk·not·ic, pyc·not·ic** (-not'ick) *adj.*

pyl-, pyle-, pylo- A combining form meaning *portal vein.*

py·le·phle·bec·ta·sis (pye''le-fle-beck'tuh-sis) *n.* Dilation of the portal vein.

py·le·phle·bi·tis (pye''le-fle-bye'tis) *n.* Inflammation of the portal vein, usually secondary to suppuration in tissues drained by its tributaries, or to contiguous tissue suppuration.

py·le·throm·bo·phle·bi·tis (pye''le-throm''bo-fle-bye'tis) *n.* Inflammation and thrombosis of the portal vein.

py·le·throm·bo·sis (pye''le-throm-bo'sis) *n.* Thrombosis of the portal vein.

pylor-, pyloro-. A combining form meaning *pylorus, pyloric.*

py·lo·ral·gia (pye''lo-ral'jee-uh) *n.* Pain in the region of the pylorus.

py·lo·rec·to·my (pye''lo-reck'tuh-mee) *n.* Excision of the pylorus; partial gastrectomy.

py·lo·ric (pye-lo'rick) *adj.* Pertaining to or lying in the region of the pylorus.

pyloric antrum. The portion of the stomach

lying between the body of the stomach and the pyloric canal.

pyloric canal or **channel.** That portion of the stomach lying between the pyloric antrum and the base of the duodenal bulb.

pyloric stenosis. Obstruction (usually congenital) of the pyloric orifice of the stomach caused by hypertrophy of the pyloric muscle.

py·lo·ro·col·ic (pye·lor″o·ko′lick, ·kol′ick) *adj.* Pertaining to or connecting the pyloric end of the stomach and the transverse colon.

py·lo·ro·di·la·tor (pye·lor″o·dye′lay·tur, ·dye·lay′tur) *n.* An appliance for dilating the pyloric orifice of the stomach.

py·lo·ro·du·o·de·nal (pye·lor″o·dew″o·dee′nul, ·dew·od′e·nul) *adj.* Pertaining to the pylorus and the duodenum.

py·lo·ro·gas·trec·to·my (pye·lor″o·gas·treck′tuh·mee) *n.* Resection of the pyloric end of the stomach; pylorectomy.

py·lo·ro·my·ot·o·my (pye·lor″o·migh·ot′uh·mee) *n.* The division, anteriorly, of the pyloric muscle, without incision through the mucosa, for congenital pyloric stenosis in infants. Syn. *Ramstedt's operation, Fredet-Ramstedt operation.*

py·lo·ro·plas·ty (pye·lor″o·plas′tee) *n.* An operation upon the pylorus, for stenosis due to ulcer, which may involve removal of a portion of the pylorus but which, in principle, divides the pylorus on the gastric and duodenal sides transversely, the wound being closed by sutures which convert it into a transverse incision. It provides a larger opening from the stomach to duodenum.

py·lo·ro·sche·sis (pye·lor″o·skee′sis, pye″lo·ros′ki·sis) *n.* Obstruction of the pylorus.

py·lo·ros·co·py (pye″lo·ros′kuh·pee) *n.* Inspection of the pylorus.

py·lo·ro·spasm (pye·lor′o·spaz·um) *n.* Spasm of the pylorus.

py·lo·ro·ste·no·sis (pye·lor″o·ste·no′sis) *n.* Narrowing or stricture of the pylorus.

py·lo·ros·to·my (pye″lo·ros′tuh·mee) *n.* Incision into the pylorus, as in the formation of a gastric fistula.

py·lo·rot·o·my (pye″lo·rot′uh·mee) *n.* An incision into or through the pylorus in the axis of the canal, converting it by sutures from a longitudinal to a transverse wound. Pyloroplasty, Finney's operation, Heineke-Mikulicz operation, gastroduodenostomy are types of pylorotomy.

py·lo·rus (pye·lo′rus, pi·lor′us) *n.,* L. pl. & genit. sing. **pylo·ri** (·rye) 1. [NA] The circular opening of the stomach into the duodenum. 2. The fold of mucous membrane and muscular tissue surrounding the aperture between the stomach and the duodenum. 3. PYLORIC CANAL.

pyo·ar·thro·sis (pye″o·ahr·thro′sis) *n.* PYARTHROSIS.

pyo·cele (pye′o·seel) *n.* A pocketing of pus, as in the scrotum.

pyo·ceph·a·lus (pye″o·sef′uh·lus) *n.* PYENCEPHALUS.

pyo·che·zia (pye″o·kee′zee·uh) *n.* Discharge of pus with or in the stool.

pyo·col·po·cele (pye″o·kol′po·seel) *n.* A suppurating cyst of the vagina.

pyo·col·pos (pye″o·kol′pos) *n.* An accumulation of pus within the vagina.

pyo·cyst (pye′o·sist) *n.* A cyst containing pus.

pyo·cys·tis (pye″o·sis′tis) *n.* Purulent infection in the urinary bladder after diversion of urine inflow.

pyo·der·ma (pye″o·dur′muh) *n.* Any pus-producing skin lesion or lesions, used in referring to groups of furuncles, pustules, or even carbuncles.

pyoderma gan·gre·no·sum (gang″gre·no′sum). A pyogenic dermatosis usually of the trunk, often with large irregular ulcers; usually associated with ulcerative colitis.

pyo·der·ma·to·sis (pye″o·dur″muh·to′sis) *n.* An inflammation of the skin in which pus formation occurs.

pyo·gen (pye′o·jen) *n.* PYOGENIC MICROORGANISM.

pyo·gen·e·sis (pye″o·jen′e·sis) *n.* The formation of pus. —**pyogen·ic** (·ick), **pyo·ge·net·ic** (·je·net′ick), **py·og·e·nous** (pye·oj′e·nus) *adj.*

pyogenic membrane. The lining of an abscess cavity or a fistula tract.

pyogenic microorganism. A microorganism producing pus; usually staphylococci and streptococci, but many other organisms may produce pus.

pyo·he·mo·tho·rax, py·o·hae·mo·tho·rax (pye″o·hee′mo·tho′racks) *n.* Pus and blood in the pleural cavity.

pyo·me·tra (pye″o·mee′truh) *n.* A collection of pus in the uterine cavity.

pyo·me·tri·um (pye″o·mee′tree·um) *n.* PYOMETRA.

pyo·my·o·si·tis (pye″o·migh″o·sigh′tis) *n.* Suppurative myositis.

pyo·ne·phri·tis (pye″o·ne·frye′tis) *n.* Suppurative inflammation of a kidney.

pyo·neph·ro·li·thi·a·sis (pye″o·nef″ro·li·thigh′uh·sis) *n.* The presence of pus and calculi in a kidney.

pyo·ne·phro·sis (pye″o·ne·fro′sis) *n.* Replacement of a substantial portion of the kidney, or all of the kidney, by abscesses. —**pyone·phrot·ic** (·frot′ick) *adj.*

pyo·ovar·i·um (pye″o·o·vār′ee·um) *n.* An ovarian abscess.

pyo·peri·car·di·tis (pye″o·perr″i·kahr·dye′tis) *n.* Purulent pericarditis.

pyo·peri·car·di·um (pye″o·perr″i·kahr′dee·um) *n.* The presence of pus in the pericardium.

pyo·peri·to·ne·um (pye″o·perr″i·to·nee′um) *n.* The presence of pus in the peritoneal cavity.

pyo·peri·to·ni·tis (pye″o·perr″i·to·nigh′tis) *n.* Suppurative inflammation of the peritoneum.

pyo·pha·gia (pye″o·fay′jee·uh) *n.* The swallowing of purulent material.

py·oph·thal·mia (pye″off·thal′mee·uh) *n.* Purulent ophthalmia.

pyo·pneu·mo·peri·car·di·tis (pye″o·new″mo·perr″i·kahr·dye′tis) *n.* Pericarditis complicated by the presence of pus and gas in the pericardium.

pyo·pneu·mo·peri·car·di·um (pye″o·new″mo·

perr·i·kahr'dee·um) *n.* Pus and air or gas in the pericardium.

pyo·pneu·mo·peri·to·ne·um (pye"o·new"mo·perr"i·to·nee'um) *n.* Pus and gas in the peritoneal cavity.

pyo·pneu·mo·peri·to·ni·tis (pye"o·new"mo·perr"i·to·nigh'tis) *n.* Suppurative inflammation of the peritoneum associated with gas in the abdominal cavity.

pyo·pneu·mo·tho·rax (pye"o·new"mo·tho'racks) *n.* The presence of air or gas and pus in the pleural cavity.

pyo·poi·e·sis (pye"o·poy·ee'sis) *n.* Pus formation. —**pyo·poi·et·ic** (·et'ick) *adj.*

py·op·ty·sis (pye·op'ti·sis) *n.* The expectoration of pus or purulent material.

py·or·rhea, py·or·rhoea (pye"o·ree'uh) *n.* 1. A purulent discharge. 2. PYORRHEA ALVEOLARIS.

pyorrhea al·ve·o·la·ris (al"vee·o·lair'is). A periodontal disease in which there is a purulent exudate; periodontitis.

pyo·sal·pin·gi·tis (pye"o·sal"pin·jye'tis) *n.* Purulent inflammation of the uterus or auditory tube.

pyo·sal·pin·go·oo·pho·ri·tis (pye"o·sal·pin"go·o"uh·fo·rye'tis) *n.* Combined suppurative inflammation of an ovary and oviduct.

pyo·sal·pinx (pye"o·sal'pinks) *n.* An accumulation of pus in an oviduct.

pyo·sep·ti·ce·mia, pyo·sep·ti·cae·mia (pye"o·sep"ti·see'mee·uh) *n.* Septicemia coupled with the development of pyemia.

py·o·sis (pye·o'sis) *n.* Suppuration; pus formation.

pyo·stat·ic (pye"o·stat'ick) *adj. & n.* 1. Arresting or checking the formation of pus. 2. An agent arresting the formation of pus.

pyo·tho·rax (pye"o·tho'racks) *n.* EMPYEMA.

pyo·ura·chus (pye"o·yoo'ruh·kus) *n.* The presence of pus in or about the urachus.

pyo·ure·ter (pye"o·yoo·ree'tur, ·yoor·e'tur) *n.* An accumulation of pus in a ureter.

pyr-, pyro- A combining form meaning (a) *fire;* (b) *heat;* (c) *burning sensation;* (d) *fever;* (e) in chemistry, *derived by the action of heat.*

pyr·a·mid (pirr'uh·mid) *n.* 1. Any conical eminence of an organ. 2. A body of the longitudinal nerve fibers of the corticospinal tract on each side of the anterior median fissure of the medulla oblongata. 3. A polyhedron whose base is a polygon and whose other faces are triangular with a common vertex. —**pyr·am·i·dal** (pi·ram'i·dul) *adj.*

pyramidal cell. A nerve cell of the cerebral cortex, somewhat triangular in shape, with one large apical dendrite and several smaller dendrites at the base. The axon is given off from the base of the cell and the upper pointed end of the cell is continued toward the surface of the brain as the apical dendrite.

pyramidal tract. All those fibers which course longitudinally in the pyramid of the medulla oblongata.

pyr·a·mi·dot·o·my (pirr"a·mi·dot'uh·mee) *n.* Sectioning of the pyramidal tract in the medulla.

py·ra·mis (pirr'uh·mis) *n.,* pl. **py·ra·mi·des** (pi·ram'i·deez) PYRAMID.

py·ra·nose (pye'ruh·noce) *n.* The isomeric form of certain sugars and glycosides having a structural analogy to a pyran.

py·rec·tic (pye·reck'tick) *adj.* PYRETIC.

pyr·e·tol·y·sis (pirr"e·tol'i·sis) *n.* 1. Reduction of a fever. 2. A lytic process accelerated by the presence of fever.

py·rex·ia (pye·reck'see·uh) *n.* Elevation of temperature above the normal; fever. —**pyrex·ial** (·see·ul) *adj.*

py·rex·io·pho·bia (pye·reck"see·o·fo'bee·uh) *n.* An abnormal fear of fever.

Pyribenzamine. Trademark for the antihistaminic drug tripelennamine, used as the citrate and hydrochloride salts.

pyr·i·dine (pirr'i·deen, ·din) *n.* A heterocyclic compound, C_5H_5N, first of a series of homologous bases; a colorless liquid with a persistent odor. Used as a solvent and in synthesis; has been used as an antiseptic and germicide.

Pyridium. A trademark for phenazopyridine, a urinary analgesic drug that is used as the hydrochloride salt.

pyr·i·dox·al (pirr"i·dock'sal) *n.* The 4-aldehyde of pyridoxine, an essential component of enzymes concerned with amino acid decarboxylation and with transamination, and therefore with amino acid synthesis.

pyr·i·dox·ine (pirr"i·dock'seen, ·sin) *n.* 5-Hydroxy-6-methyl-3,4-pyridinedimethanol, $C_8H_{11}NO_3$; vitamin B_6. Essential in human nutrition, and used for treatment of a variety of conditions, such as vomiting and nausea of pregnancy, or pyridoxine deficiency; employed as the hydrochloride salt.

pyriform. PIRIFORM.

pyr·i·meth·a·mine (pirr"i·meth'uh·meen) *n.* 2,4-Diamino-5-(*p*-chlorophenyl)-6-ethylpyrimidine, $C_{12}H_{13}ClN_4$, an antimalarial drug.

py·rim·i·dine (pye·rim'i·deen, pi·) *n.* 1. Any six-membered cyclic compound containing four carbon and two nitrogen atoms in the ring, the nitrogen atoms being separated by one carbon atom. To this group belong barbituric acid and its derivatives, the nucleic acid hydrolysis products thymine, uracil, and cytosine, and many other compounds of physiologic or therapeutic importance. 2. 1,3-Diazine, $C_4H_4N_2$.

py·ro·cat·e·chol (pye"ro·kat'e·chole, ·kole, ·kol) *n. o*-Dihydroxybenzene, $C_6H_4(OH)_2$; has been used topically as an antiseptic. Syn. *pyrocatechin, catechol, oxyphenic acid.*

py·ro·gal·lol (pye"ro·gal'ole, ·ol) *n.* 1,2,3-Trihydroxybenzene, $C_6H_3(OH)_3$; has been used topically in the treatment of various skin diseases, especially psoriasis. Syn. *pyrogallic acid.*

py·ro·gen (pye'ro·jen) *n.* Any fever-producing substance; exogenous pyrogens include bacterial endotoxins, especially of gram-negative bacteria; endogenous pyrogen is a thermolabile protein derived from such cells as polymorphonuclear leukocytes which acts on the brain centers to produce fever.

py·ro·gen·ic (pye"ro·jen'ick) *adj.* Producing fever.

py·ro·glob·u·lin (pye"ro·glob'yoo·lin) *n.* A

globulin, abnormally present in blood serum, which coagulates on heating.

py·ro·glos·sia (pye″ro·glos′ee·uh) *n.* A burning sensation of the tongue.

py·rol·y·sis (pye·rol′i·sis) *n.* The decomposition of organic substances by heat. —**py·ro·lyt·ic** (pye″ro·lit′ick) *adj.*

py·ro·ma·nia (pye″ro·may′nee·uh) *n.* A monomania for setting or watching fires. —**pyroma·ni·ac** (·nee·ack) *n.*

py·rom·e·ter (pye·rom′i·tur) *n.* An instrument for measuring high temperatures.

py·ro·nine (pye′ro·neen, ·nin) *n.* A histologic stain, tetraethyldiaminoxanthene, used to indicate the presence of ribonucleic acid.

py·ro·nino·phil·ic (pye″ro·nin″o·fil′ick) *adj.* Having an affinity for pyronine.

py·ro·pho·bia (pye″ro·fo′bee·uh) *n.* An abnormal dread of fire.

py·rop·to·thy·mia (pye·rop″to·thigh′mee·uh) *n.* A form of mental disorder in which the person imagines himself enveloped in flame.

py·ro·punc·ture (pye′ro·punk″chur) *n.* Puncturing with hot needles; ignipuncture.

py·ro·sis (pye·ro′sis) *n.* A substernal or epigastric burning sensation accompanied by eructation of an acrid, irritating fluid; heartburn.

py·ro·tox·in (pye″ro·tock′sin) *n.* A toxic agent generated in the course of the febrile process.

py·rox·y·lin (pye·rock′si·lin) *n.* A product obtained by the action of a mixture of nitric and sulfuric acids on cotton; consists chiefly of cellulose tetranitrate ($C_{12}H_{16}O_6(NO_3)_4$); used as a protective covering in the form of collodion. Syn. *soluble guncotton.*

pyr·role (pirr′ole) *n.* $NHCH=CHCH=CH$. A colorless liquid occurring in bone oil and to a slight extent in coal tar. Many complex natural compounds, such as hemoglobin and chlorophyll, contain pyrrole components in their structure.

py·ru·vate (pye·roo′vate, pi·) *n.* A salt or ester of pyruvic acid.

pyruvate-kinase deficiency. Congenital erythrocytic deficiency of the enzyme catalyzing the conversion of phosphoenolpyruvate to pyruvate, associated with hemolytic anemia.

py·ru·vic acid (pye·roo′vick, pi·) 2-Oxopropanoic acid, $CH_3COCOOH$, which is a normal intermediate in carbohydrate and protein metabolism. Excess quantities of pyruvic acid accumulate in blood and tissues in thiamine deficiency. Syn. *ketopropionic acid.*

py·uria (pye·yoor′ee·uh) *n.* The presence of pus in the urine. —**py·uric** (·yoor′ick) adj.

Q

Qco₂ Symbol for the rate of evolution of carbon dioxide, in microliters given off in 1 hour by 1 mg (dry weight) of tissue.

Qo₂ Symbol for the oxygen consumption in terms of the number of microliters consumed in 1 hour by 1 mg (dry weight) of tissue; by convention, the consumption of oxygen is given a negative value.

q.d.s. Abbreviation for *quater die sumendum,* to be taken four times a day (= q.i.d.).

Q fever An acute infectious disease caused by the filtrable microorganism *Coxiella burnetii,* acquired by inhalation, handling infected material, or drinking contaminated milk; characterized by sudden onset of fever, malaise, headache, and interstitial pneumonitis, but lacking the rash and the agglutinins for *Proteus* bacteria occurring in other rickettsial diseases.

q.h. Abbreviation for *quaque hora;* every hour.

q.2h. Abbreviation for *quaque secunda hora;* every second hour.

q.3h. Abbreviation for *quaque tertia hora;* every third hour.

q.i.d. Abbreviation for *quater in die;* 4 times a day.

q.l. Abbreviation for *quantum libet;* as much as is desired.

q.p. Abbreviation for *quantum placet;* as much as you please.

QRS Q wave, R wave, and S wave.

QRS axis. ELECTRICAL AXIS.

QRS complex of the electrocardiogram. The electrocardiographic deflection representing ventricular depolarization. The initial downward deflection is termed a Q wave; the initial upward deflection, an R wave; and the downward deflection following the R wave, an S wave. Syn. *ventricular depolarization complex.*

QRS interval. The duration of depolarization or excitation of the ventricles, measured from the beginning of Q (or R) wave to the end of S wave of the electrocardiogram; usually 0.10 second or less.

QRS loop. The vectorcardiographic representation of ventricular depolarization.

QRS-T angle. The spatial angle between the mean QRS and T vector axes.

q.s. Abbreviation for *quantum sufficit;* as much as suffices.

Q-T interval. The time from the beginning of the QRS complex to the end of the T wave, representing the time from the beginning of ventricular depolarization to the end of repolarization, i.e., ventricular systole.

qt. Abbreviation for *quart.*

Quaalude. Trademark for the nonbarbiturate sedative and hypnotic, methaqualone.

quack, *n.* A pretender to medical skill; a medical charlatan.

quack·ery (kwack'uh-ree) *n.* The practice of medicine by a quack.

quack·sal·ver (kwack'sal-vur) *n.* A quack or mountebank; a peddler of his own medicines and salves.

qua·dran·gu·lar (kwah-drang'gew-lur) *adj.* Having four angles.

quad·rant (kwah'drunt) *n.* 1. The fourth part of a circle, subtending an angle of 90°. 2. One of the four regions into which the abdomen may be divided for purposes of physical diagnosis. 3. A sector of one-fourth of the field of vision of one or both eyes. —**qua·dran·tic** (kwah-dran'tick) *adj.*

quad·ran·ta·no·pia (kwah"dran-tuh-no'pee-uh) *n.* Loss of vision in about one-quarter of the visual field; may be bitemporal or homonymous, upper or lower.

quad·rate (kwah'drate) *adj.* Square, four-sided.

qua·dra·tus (kwah-dray'tus) *L. adj. & n.,* pl. & genit. sing. **quadra·ti** (-tye) 1. Square. 2. A muscle having four sides.

quadratus lum·bo·rum (lum-bo'rum). A muscle of the back attached to the iliac crest and the twelfth rib.

quadri-, quadru- A combining form meaning *four.*

quad·ri·ceps (kwah'dri·seps) *adj.* Four-headed.

quadriceps fe·mo·ris (fem'o·ris). The large extensor muscle of the thigh.

quad·ri·cus·pid (kwah"dri·kus'pid) *adj.* Having four cusps.

qua·dri·ge·mi·na (kwah″dri·jem′i·nuh) *n.pl.*
CORPORA QUADRIGEMINA.

quad·ri·gem·i·nal (kwah″dri·jem′i·nul) *adj.*
Fourfold; consisting of four parts.

quadrigeminal pulse. A pulse in which a pause
occurs after every fourth beat.

quad·ri·lat·er·al (kwah″dri·lat′ur·ul) *adj.* Having
four sides.

qua·drip·a·ra (kwah·drip′uh·ruh) *n.* A woman
who has given birth four times. —**quadripa·**
rous (·rus) *adj.*

quad·ri·pa·re·sis (kwah″dri·puh·ree′sis, ·păr′uh·
sis) *n.* Weakness of all four limbs.

quad·ri·ple·gia (kwah″dri·plee′jee·uh) *n.* Paralysis affecting the four extremities of the body;
may be spastic or flaccid. —**quadriple·gic,** *adj.*
& *n.*

quad·ri·tu·ber·cu·lar (kwah″dri·tew·bur′kew·lur)
adj. Having four tubercles or cusps.

qua·droon (kwah·droon′) *n.* The offspring of a
white person and a mulatto.

quad·ru·ped (kwah′droo·ped) *n.* A four-footed
animal. —**qua·dru·pe·dal** (kwah·droo′pe·dul,
kwah″droo·ped′ul) *adj.*

quadrupedal extensor reflex. An associated
movement of extension of the flexed arm in
hemiplegia which is sometimes evoked by
causing the patient, when standing or kneel-
ing, to lean forward and throw his weight on
to the observer's supporting hand placed beneath his chest.

quad·ru·ple rhythm (kwah′druh·pul, kwah·droo′
pul) A cardiac cadence in which four sounds
recur in each successive cycle.

quad·ru·plet (kwah′druh·plut, kwah·droo′plut)
n. Any one of four children born at one birth.

qual·i·ta·tive (kwahl′i·tay″tiv) *adj.* Of or pertaining to quality; limited to or concerned with
kind as opposed to degree.

qual·i·ty, *n.* 1. A distinguishing or identifying
characteristic. 2. The value of a variable characteristic as, in radiobiology, the approximate
characterization of radiation with respect to
its penetrating power.

quanta. Plural of *quantum.*

quan·tim·e·ter (kwahn·tim′e·tur) *n.* An instrument for measuring the quantity of x-rays.

quan·ti·ta·tive (kwahn′ti·tay″tiv) *adj.* Of or pertaining to quantity; limited to or concerned
with degree as opposed to kind.

quan·tum (kwahn′tum) *n.,* pl. **quan·ta** (·tuh) An
elementary, particulate unit of energy.

quantum lib·et (lib′it) As much as is desired.
Abbreviated, q.l.

quantum plac·et (plas′it) As much as you please.
Abbreviated, q.p.

quantum suf·fi·cit (suf′i·sit) As much as suffices.
Abbreviated, q.s.

quantum vis As much as you wish. Abbreviated,
q.v.

quar·an·tine (kwahr′un·teen) *n.* 1. The limitation
of freedom of movement of such susceptible
persons or animals as have been exposed to
communicable disease, for a period of time
(formerly usually 40 days) equal to the longest
usual incubation period of the disease to
which they have been exposed. 2. The place of
detention of such persons. 3. The act of de-

taining vessels or travelers from suspected
ports or places for purposes of inspection or
disinfection.

quart, *n.* In the United States, the fourth part of
a gallon; 0.9463 liter. Abbreviated, qt.

quar·tan (kwor′tun, kwahr′tun) *adj.* 1. Recurring at about 72-hour intervals, on the fourth
day. 2. Pertaining to quartan malaria.

quartan malaria or **fever.** A form of malaria
caused by *Plasmodium malariae,* characterized
by paroxysms occurring every 72 hours, that
is, on the first, fourth, and seventh days.

quar·ter, *n.* 1. The part of the horse's hoof between the heel and the toe. 2. The fourth part
of a slaughtered animal.

quar·tip·a·ra (kwor·tip′uh·ruh, kwahr·) *n.* QUA-
DRIPARA. —**quartipa·rous** (·rus) *adj.*

quartz, *n.* A crystalline silicon dioxide, SiO_2;
when pure, in colorless hexagonal crystals.
Used in chemical apparatus and for optical
and electric instruments.

quas·sia (kwahsh′ee·uh, kwahsh′uh) *n.* The
wood of *Picrasma excelsa,* known as Jamaica
quassia, or of *Quassia amara,* known as Suri-
nam quassia. Has been used as a simple bitter
and, in the form of an infusion given as an
enema, for expulsion of seatworms.

qua·ter·na·ry (kwah·tur′nuh·ree, kwah′tur·nerr″
ee) *adj.* 1. Consisting of four elements or substances, as quaternary solutions. 2. Fourth in
order or stage. 3. Characterizing or pertaining
to compounds in which four similar atoms of
a radical, as the hydrogen atoms in the ammonium radical, have been replaced by organic
radicals.

quaternary ammonium compound. Any compound that may be considered a derivative of
an ammonium ion in which the four hydrogen
atoms have been replaced by organic radicals;
many medicinals are compounds of this kind.

quat·tu·or (kwat′oo·or) *n.* Four.

Queck·en·stedt test, sign or **maneuver** (kveck′
en·shtet) Manual compression of the internal
jugular veins with a manometer attached to
the lumbar puncture needle to test for th[e]
patency of the subarachnoid space. Normally
compression causes a prompt rise in the cere[-]
brospinal fluid pressure with rapid return t[o]
resting levels on release of compression; i[n]
partial or total subarachnoid block, this doe[s]
not occur. The maneuver is contraindicate[d]
where increased intracranial pressure is pre[-]
sent or suspected.

Queensland tick typhus fever. Infection cause[d]
by *Rickettsia australis,* occurring in Queens[-]
land, Australia, transmitted by ixodid tick[s]
with marsupial and wild rodent animal host[s]
closely related to boutonneuse fever and t[o]
Rocky Mountain spotted fever.

quellung reaction. Swelling of the capsule of [a]
bacterium when in contact with its antige[n]

quer·ce·tin (kwur′se·tin) *n.* 3,3′,4′,5,7-Pentah[y-]
droxyflavone, $C_{15}H_{10}O_7$, the aglycone [of]
quercitrin, rutin, and other glycosides, four[d]
especially in various rinds and barks, b[ut]
widely distributed in the plant kingdom. H[as]
been used in the expectation of reducing ca[p]
illary fragility. Syn. *flavin, meletin.*

quer·ci·tan·nic acid (kwur"si·tan'ick). The tannic acid from oak bark.

quer·ci·tan·nin (kwur"si·tan'in) n. QUERCITANNIC ACID.

Quey·rat's erythroplasia (keʰ·raʰ') A condition characterized by a circumscribed, erythematous, velvety lesion affecting mucocutaneous junctions or mucosa of the mouth, tongue, vulva, glans penis, or prepuce. Considered precancerous to squamous cell carcinoma.

quick, adj. & n. 1. Manifesting life and movement, as a fetus. 2. An exquisitely tender part, as the bed of a nail.

quick·en·ing, n. The first feeling on the part of the pregnant woman of fetal movements, occurring between the fourth and fifth months of pregnancy.

quick·sil·ver, n. MERCURY.

qui·es·cent (kwye·es'unt) adj. Inactive, latent, dormant.

quin-, quino- A combining form meaning (a) cinchona; (b) quinine.

quin·a·crine (kwin'uh·kreen, ·krin). 6-Chloro-9-{[4-(diethylamino)-1-methylbutyl]amino}-2-methoxyacridine, $C_{23}H_{30}ClN_3O$, formerly an important antimalarial drug but now used in the treatment of giardiasis, tapeworm infections, amebiasis, and a variety of other conditions; employed as the hydrochloride salt. Syn. mepacrine.

Quincke's disease or **edema** (kvink'eʰ) ANGIOEDEMA.

Quincke's pulse CAPILLARY PULSE.

quin·i·dine (kwin'i·deen, ·din) n. An alkaloid, $C_{20}H_{24}N_2O_2$, of cinchona, isomeric with quinine; used, as the gluconate and sulfate salts, for the treatment of cardiac arrhythmias.

qui·nine (kwye'nine, kwi·neen') n. An alkaloid, $C_{20}H_{24}N_2O_2$, of cinchona; used principally as an antimalarial drug, generally as the sulfate salt. Quinine and urea hydrochloride is used as a sclerosing agent.

qui·nin·ism (kwye'ni·niz·um, kwin'i·) n. CINCHONISM.

quin·i·no·der·ma (kwin"i·no·dur'muh) n. A drug dermatitis following the ingestion of quinine or its derivatives.

quin·ism (kwin'iz·um, kwye'niz·um) n. CINCHONISM.

quin·o·line (kwin'o·leen, ·lin) n. 1-Benzazine or benzo[b]pyridine, C_9H_7N, used in organic synthesis and, formerly, as an antimalarial; also a structural unit of quinine and other cinchona alkaloids.

qui·none (kwi·nohn', kwin'ohn) n. 1. Either of two known isomers, $C_6H_4O_2$, ortho- or parabenzoquinone, a benzenoid compound of two internal alternating carbon-carbon double bonds and two carbonyl groups. 2. Any derivative of either quinone defined in 1.

quin·sy (kwin'zee) n. PERITONSILLAR ABSCESS.

quin·tan (kwin'tun) n. & adj. 1. Recurring every fifth day. 2. A quintan fever.

quintan fever. 1. An intermittent fever, the paroxysms of which recur every 96 hours; that is, on the fifth, ninth, thirteenth days. 2. TRENCH FEVER.

quin·tip·a·ra (kwin·tip'uh·ruh) n. A woman who has given birth five times.

quin·tu·plet (kwin'tuh·plit, kwin·tup'lit) n. One of five children who have been born at one birth.

quit·tor, quit·ter (kwit'ur) n. In veterinary medicine, a disease of the collateral cartilages of the equine foot caused by injury and infection, resulting in the formation of a fistulous tract in the region of the coronet over the quarter.

quo·tid·i·an (kwo·tid'ee·un) adj. Recurring every day.

quotidian fever. An intermittent fever, especially malarial, the paroxysms of which recur daily.

quo·tient (kwo'shunt) n. The result of the process of division.

q.v. Abbreviation for (a) quantum vis, as much as you wish; (b) quod vide, which see.

Q wave of the electrocardiogram. The initial negative deflection of the (QRS) ventricular depolarization complex, usually preceding an R wave.

R

R Symbol for (a) electrical resistance; (b) any alkyl radical of the general formula C_nH_{2n+1}, where n is the number of carbon atoms in the molecule.

R. Abbreviation for (a) *Réaumur*; (b) right.

R_f *In chromatography,* a symbol for the ratio of the distance traveled by a substance undergoing diffusion to the distance traveled by the solvent; the ratio is characteristic of the substance.

℞ Symbol for *recipe,* take; used in prescription writing.

r Symbol for roentgen.

Ra Symbol for radium.

rab·bit fever. TULAREMIA.

rab·id (rab'id) *adj.* Affected with rabies; pertaining to rabies.

ra·bies (ray'beez) *n.* An acute viral infection mainly of the central nervous system of a variety of animals, occasionally transmitted to man by the bite of a rabid dog, cat, skunk, fox, raccoon, or bat. Symptoms in man generally appear 2 to 12 weeks after infecting contact, and progress from fever, restlessness, and extreme excitability to hydrophobia (1) (with resultant drooling of saliva), generalized seizures, confusional psychosis, and death. A less common paralytic form, due to spinal cord affection, may replace or accompany the state of excitement.

rabies fixed virus. Pasteur's term for a virus that is so high in virulence for rabbits by successive intracerebral transfers that it will kill the animals in a period of 6 or 7 days.

rabies vaccine. 1. A sterile preparation of killed, fixed virus of rabies obtained from brain tissue of rabbits or from duck embryos that have been infected with fixed rabies virus. The vaccine is used as a prophylactic agent against rabies. 2. One of several living modified rabies virus vaccines, such as the Flury strain.

race, *n.* A breed or strain of a species. Adj. *racial.*

ra·ce·mic (ra·see'mick, ·sem'ick) *adj.* Composed of equal parts of dextrorotatory and levorotatory forms of optical isomers and, therefore, optically inactive.

racemic acid. An optically inactive mixture of dextrorotatory and levorotatory forms of tartaric acid.

ra·ce·mi·za·tion (ray''se·mi·zay'shun, ras''e·) *n.* Conversion of the optically active form of a compound to its racemic form, commonly by heating.

rac·e·mose (ras'e·moce) *adj.* Resembling a bunch of grapes.

rac·e·phed·rine (ras''e·fed'rin) *n.* Racemic ephedrine, a sympathomimetic amine used, as the hydrochloride salt, like ephedrine. Syn. *dl-ephedrine.*

rachi-, rachio-, rhachi-, rhachio- A combining form meaning *vertebral column,* *spinal.*

ra·chi·as·mus (ray''kee·az'mus) *n.* Spasm of the muscles at the back of the neck.

ra·chi·cele (ray'ki·seel) *n.* Hernial protrusion of the contents of the spinal canal in spina bifida. It includes spinal meningocele, myelomeningocele, and myelocystocele (syringomyelocele).

ra·chi·cen·te·sis (ray''ki·sen·tee'sis) *n.* LUMBAR PUNCTURE.

-rachidia, -rrhachidia A combining form meaning *condition of the vertebral column.*

ra·chil·y·sis (ra·kil'i·sis) *n.,* pl. **rachily·ses** (·seez) A method of treating lateral curvature of the spine by mechanical counteraction of the abnormal curves.

ra·chio·camp·sis (ray''kee·o·kamp'sis) *n.* CURVATURE OF THE SPINE.

ra·chio·cen·te·sis (ray''kee·o·sen·tee'sis) *n.* LUMBAR PUNCTURE.

ra·chi·o·dyn·ia (ray''kee·o·din'ee·uh) *n.* Pain in the spinal column.

ra·chi·om·e·ter (ray''kee·om'e·tur) *n.* An instrument used to measure the degree of spinal curvature.

ra·chio·ple·gia (ray''kee·o·plee'jee·uh) *n.* Obsol. SPINAL PARALYSIS.

ra·chio·sco·li·o·sis (ray''kee·o·sko''lee·o'sis) *n.* Lateral curvature of the spine.

ra·chio·tome (ray'kee·o·tome) *n.* A bone-cutting instrument used in operations upon the vertebrae.

ra·chi·o·to·my (ray″kee·ot′uh·mee) n. The operation of cutting into the vertebral column.

ra·chis (ray′kis) n., pl. **rachises**, **rach·i·des** (rack′i·deez) VERTEBRAL COLUMN.

ra·chis·chi·sis (ra·kis′ki·sis) n., pl. **rachischi·ses** (·seez) SPINA BIFIDA.

ra·chit·ic (ra·kit′ick) adj. Affected with, resembling, or produced by rickets.

rachitic rosary or **beads.** The row of nodules appearing on the ribs at the junctions with their cartilages; often seen in rachitic children.

ra·chi·tis (ra·kye′tis) n., pl. **ra·chit·i·des** (ra·kit′i·deez) RICKETS.

rach·i·to·gen·ic (rack″i·to·jen′ick) adj. Producing rickets, as a vitamin-D deficient diet.

ra·cial (ray′shul) adj. Of or pertaining to a race or to races.

racial unconscious. COLLECTIVE UNCONSCIOUS.

ra·clage (rah·klahzh′) n. The destruction of a soft growth by rubbing, as with a brush or harsh sponge.

ra·cle·ment (rah″kluh·mahn′) n. RACLAGE.

RAD Abbreviation for *right axis deviation.*

rad, n. In radiology, the unit of absorbed dose (100 ergs per gram).

ra·dar·ky·mo·gram (ray″dahr·kigh′mo·gram) n. A depiction of wave patterns of muscular contraction during a cardiac cycle produced by radarkymography.

ra·dar·ky·mog·ra·phy (ray″dahr·kigh·mog′ruh·fee) n. Recording of the horizontal movements of the cardiac silhouette as projected on a television monitor scanning a fluoroscopic screen; the recording is made through a radar device which scans the television image.

ra·dec·to·my (ray·deck′tuh·mee) n. Resection of the root of a tooth, in whole or in part.

ra·di·al (ray′dee·ul) adj. 1. Radiating; diverging from a common center. 2. Pertaining to, or in relation to, the radius bone of the forearm, as the radial artery.

radial collateral artery. The anterolateral terminal branch of the deep brachial artery, which descends with the radial nerve through the upper arm supplying the brachial, brachioradialis, and triceps muscles, sends a branch to the rete olecranon, and enters the forearm where it anastamoses with the radial recurrent artery.

ra·di·a·lis (ray″dee·ay′lis) L. adj. Pertaining to the radius; a term applied to various arteries, nerves, and muscles, as flexor carpi radialis.

radial nerve. See Table of Nerves in the Appendix.

radial notch. A depression on the lateral surface of the coronoid process of the ulna for articulation with the head of the radius.

radial reflex. BRACHIORADIALIS REFLEX.

radial sulcus. A spiral groove on the shaft of the humerus indicating the course of the radial nerve. Syn. *musculospiral groove, radial groove.*

ra·di·ant (ray′dee·unt) adj. Emitting rays or occurring in the form of rays.

ra·di·a·tio (ray″dee·ay′shee·o, ray″dee·) n., pl. **radiatio·nes** (·neez) RADIATION (3).

ra·di·a·tion (ray″dee·ay′shun) n. 1. The act of radiating or diverging from a central point, as radiation of light; divergence from a center, having the appearance of rays. 2. The emission and propagation of energy through space or through a material medium in a form having certain characteristics of waves, including the energy commonly described as electromagnetic and that of sound; usually, electromagnetic radiation, classified, according to frequency, as Hertzian, infrared, visible, ultraviolet, x-ray, and gamma ray; also, by extension, such corpuscular emissions as alpha and beta particles and cosmic rays. 3. *In neurology,* certain groups of fibers that diverge after leaving their place of origin. —**ra·di·ate** (ray′dee·ate) v. & adj.

radiation anemia. Aplastic or hypoplastic anemia following excessive exposure to ionizing radiation. Syn. *roentgen-ray anemia.*

radiation burn. A burn resulting from exposure to radiant energy, such as x-ray, radium, or sunlight.

radiation carcinoma. A carcinoma, usually squamous-cell, which is associated with overexposure to radiation.

radiation caries. Demineralization, usually in the cervical areas of the teeth, resembling dental caries and resulting from excessive radiation therapy in the head and neck region.

radiation cataract. IRRADIATION CATARACT.

radiation cystitis. Acute chronic inflammation of the urinary bladder due to radiation therapy; RADIOCYSTITIS.

radiation dermatitis. RADIODERMATITIS.

radiation dosage. The quantity of radiation absorbed; the product of radiation intensity and time also measured as the amount of energy transferred (ergs per gram).

radiation myelitis or **myelopathy.** A delayed, progressive myelopathy that follows heavy exposure of the spinal cord to ionizing radiation.

radiation nephritis. Hypertension with or without renal failure due to glomerular, tubular, vascular, and interstitial damage as a result of excessive renal irradiation.

radiation neuropathy. ACTINONEURITIS.

radiation sickness, poisoning, or **syndrome.** 1. Illness due to the effects of therapeutic irradiation, usually manifested by nausea and vomiting. 2. The effect of radiant energy following the explosion of an atomic bomb; the resultant effects may range from a mild white blood cell depression to rapid death with convulsions.

radiation therapy. The treatment of disease with any type of radiation, most commonly with ionizing radiation, such as x-rays, beta rays, and gamma rays.

¹rad·i·cal (rad′i·kul) adj. 1. Belonging or relating to a root. 2. Going to the root, or attacking the cause, of a disease. 3. Characterizing or involving extreme measures or treatment to remove the main cause of a disease or condition.

²radical, n. 1. A group of atoms that acts as a unit, but commonly does not exist in the free state, as NH_4^+, ammonium, or C_6H_5, phenyl. 2. *Obsol.* The haptophore group of an antibody.

radical cesarean section. Cesarean section followed by hysterectomy; CESAREAN HYSTERECTOMY.

radical mastectomy. Surgical removal of the entire breast and also of adjacent tissue, including the pectoralis minor muscle, part or all of the pectoralis major muscle, and all the lymphatic tissue of chest wall and axilla.

radical mastoidectomy. The complete exenteration of mastoid, epitympanic, perilabyrinthine, and tubal air cells. The tympanic membrane, ossicular chain, middle ear mucous membrane, stapedius muscle, and tensor tympani muscle are also removed.

radices. Plural of *radix*.

rad·i·cle (rad'i·kul) *n.* 1. A little root, as the radicle of a nerve, one of the ultimate fibrils of which a nerve is composed; or radicle of a vein, one of the minute vessels uniting to form a vein. 2. ²RADICAL.

radicul-, radiculo- A combining form meaning *root*, as of a nerve or tooth; specifically, *spinal nerve root or roots*.

ra·dic·u·lar (ra·dick'yoo·lur) *adj.* Pertaining to a root or to a radicle; specifically, pertaining to the roots of the spinal nerves or to those of the teeth.

radicular cyst. A cyst arising from chronic infection of a granuloma about the root of a tooth.

ra·dic·u·lec·to·my (ra·dick''yoo·leck'tuh·mee) *n.* Excision or resection of a spinal nerve root.

ra·dic·u·li·tis (ra·dick''yoo·lye'tis) *n.* Inflammation of a nerve root.

radiculo-. See *radicul-*.

ra·dic·u·lo·my·e·lop·a·thy (ra·dick''yoo·lo·migh'e·lop'uth·ee) *n.* Disease of the spinal cord and roots of the spinal nerves.

ra·dic·u·lo·neu·ri·tis (ra·dick''yoo·lo·new·rye'tis) *n.* Inflammation of a peripheral spinal nerve and its root.

ra·dic·u·lo·neu·rop·a·thy (ra·dick''yoo·lo·new·rop'uth·ee) *n.* Disease of the peripheral spinal nerves and their roots.

ra·dic·u·lop·a·thy (ra·dick''yoo·lop'uth·ee) *n.* Disease of the roots of spinal nerves.

radii. Plural and genitive singular of *radius*.

radio- A combining form meaning (a) *radiation*; (b) *radium*; (c) *radioactive* or *radioactivity*; (d) *the radius*.

ra·dio·ab·la·tion (ray''dee·o·a·blay'shun) *n.* Destruction of tissue by means of radioactive substances.

ra·dio·ac·tin·i·um (ray''dee·o·ack·tin'ee·um) *n.* A radioactive product of actinium. It gives off alpha rays and disintegrates into actinium x.

ra·dio·ac·tive (ray''dee·o·ack'tiv) *adj.* Pertaining to or possessing radioactivity.

ra·dio·ac·tiv·i·ty (ray''dee·o·ack·tiv'i·tee) *n.* The spontaneous decay or disintegration of an unstable atomic nucleus, accompanied by emission of alpha particles, beta particles, or gamma rays.

ra·dio·ar·te·ri·o·gram (ray''dee·o·ahr·teer'ee·o·gram) *n. Obsol.* Radiographic depiction of an artery or series of arteries following injection of a contrast medium.

ra·dio·au·to·gram (ray''dee·o·aw'to·gram) *n.* RADIOAUTOGRAPH.

ra·dio·au·to·graph (ray''dee·o·aw'to·graf) *n.* A direct photographic record of the distribution of a radioactive substance in an organism or tissue section.

ra·dio·au·tog·ra·phy (ray''dee·o·aw·tog'ruh·fee) *n.* The technique of locating and measuring the distribution of radioactive elements in a test material, such as tissue, by means of photographic registration of emanations from the radioactive elements.

ra·dio·bi·ol·o·gy (ray''dee·o·bye·ol'uh·jee) *n.* The study of the scientific principles, mechanisms, and effects of the interaction of ionizing radiation with living matter. —**radio·bio·log·i·cal** (·bye''o·loj'i·kul) *adj.*

ra·dio·car·pal (ray''dee·o·kahr'pul) *adj.* Pertaining to the radius and the carpus.

ra·dio·chem·is·try (ray''dee·o·kem'is·tree) *n.* The branch of chemistry that deals with radioactive phenomena.

ra·dio·co·balt (ray''dee·o·ko'bawlt) *n.* Any radioactive isotope of cobalt, especially that having a mass number of 60 (^{60}C), which has a half-life of 5.2 years and emits a negative beta particle and two gamma rays for each atom of cobalt that decays. In the form of metallic cobalt, its radiation is used in the therapy of malignant tumors.

ra·dio·col·loid (ray''dee·o·kol'oid) *n.* Any colloidal aggregate of radioactive substances.

ra·dio·cur·a·bil·i·ty (ray''dee·o·kewr·uh·bil'i·tee) *n.* The condition of being susceptible to cure or elimination by irradiation; said of cancer cells.

ra·dio·cys·ti·tis (ray''dee·o·sis·tye'tis) *n.* Inflammation of the bladder following radiation therapy; RADIATION CYSTITIS.

ra·di·ode (ray'dee·ode) *n.* An electric attachment for the application of radium.

ra·dio·der·ma·ti·tis (ray''dee·o·dur''muh·tye'tis) *n.* The retrogressive changes occurring in the skin after excessive exposure to ionizing radiation, especially x-rays and gamma rays.

ra·dio·di·ag·no·sis (ray''dee·o·dye''ug·no'sis) *n.* The diagnosis of disease by means of radiography or radioscopy.

ra·di·o·don·tics (ray''dee·o·don'ticks) *n.* The science and practice of radiography of the teeth and associated structures.

ra·di·o·don·tist (ray''dee·o·don'tist) *n.* A specialist in radiodontics.

ra·dio·el·e·ment (ray''dee·o·el'e·munt) *n.* An element that is radioactive.

radio frequency. Any of the electromagnetic frequencies between those of the audible range and the infrared range.

ra·dio·gen·ic (ray''dee·o·jen'ick) *adj.* Pertaining to a substance or state resulting from a radioactive transformation, as radiogenic lead resulting from disintegration of radium, or radiogenic heat produced within the earth by disintegration of radioactive substances.

ra·dio·gold (ray''dee·o·gohld') *n.* Any radioactive isotope of gold, especially that having mass number of 198 (^{198}Au), which has a half-life of 2.70 days and emits a negative beta particle and a gamma ray for each atom of gold that decays. In the form of a colloidal dispersion of the metal it is used, by injection, in the therapy and palliation of neoplastic disease and in the treatment of neoplastic effusions, and also as a tracer in various studies involving gold.

ra·dio·gram (ray"dee·o·gram) n. RADIOGRAPH.

ra·dio·graph (ray"dee·o·graf) n. & v. 1. A photograph made on a sensitive film by projection of x-rays through a part of the body. 2. To make a radiograph.

ra·di·og·ra·pher (ray"dee·og'ruh·fur) n. A person skilled in radiography; an x-ray technician.

ra·di·og·ra·phy (ray"dee·og'ruh·fee) n. The practice or act of making radiographs. —**ra·dio·gra·phic** (ray"dee·o·graf'ick) adj.

ra·dio·hu·mer·al (ray"dee·o·hew'mur·ul) adj. Pertaining to the radius and the humerus.

ra·dio·im·mu·no·as·say (ray"dee·o·im"yoo·no·a·say') n. The quantitative determination of antigen, antibody, or hapten concentration by the introduction of a radioactively labeled complementary substance which can be expected to bind the molecule in question and the subsequent measurement of resulting radioactive immune complex.

ra·dio·io·dine (ray"dee·o·eye'uh·dine, ·din) n. Any radioactive isotope of iodine, especially that having a mass number of 131 (^{131}I), which has a half-life of 8.08 days and emits two negative beta particles and several gamma rays for each atom of iodine that decays. In the form of sodium iodide, it is used, by intravenous or oral administration, in the treatment of hyperthyroidism and carcinoma of the thyroid, and also for various diagnostic purposes.

ra·dio·iron (ray"dee·o·eye'urn) n. Any radioactive isotope of iron, especially that having a mass number of 59 (^{59}Fe), which has a half-life of 45 days and emits two negative beta particles and several gamma rays for each atom of iron that decays. In the form of ferric or ferrous salts, it has been used in the study of iron metabolism.

ra·dio·iso·tope (ray"dee·o·eye'suh·tope) n. A radioactive isotope, commonly of an element which is stable. Although certain isotopes of normally stable elements exist naturally in radioactive form, many are prepared only artificially, as by bombarding an element with neutrons, protons, deuterons, or alpha particles in a nuclear reactor or in an accelerating device such as the cyclotron or cosmotron; the bombarded element may form a radioactive isotope of the same element or of another element. By virtue of its radioactivity, a radioisotope is used either for the effect of its radiations, such use often being diagnostic or therapeutic, or as a tracer added to the stable form of a compound to follow the course of the latter in a particular sequence of reactions in living organisms or even in an inanimate system.

radioisotope camera. Any array (one or more) of radiation counters that visualizes a radioisotope deposition and is fixed in relation to the patient.

radioisotope scanner. Any array (one or more) of radiation counters that visualizes a radioisotope deposition and is movable in relation to the patient.

ra·dio·ky·mog·ra·phy (ray"dee·o·kigh·mog'ruh·fee) n. A method of obtaining a graphic record of movement of the silhouette of an organ or tissue on a single film. Syn. roentgenokymography.

ra·di·ol·o·gist (ray"dee·ol'uh·jist) n. A physician specializing in radiology.

ra·di·ol·o·gy (ray"dee·ol'uh·jee) n. The branch of medicine that deals with radioactive substances, x-rays and other ionizing radiations, and with their utilization in the diagnosis and treatment of disease. —**ra·dio·log·ic** (ray"dee·o·loj'ick) adj.

ra·dio·lu·cent (ray"dee·o·lew'sunt) adj. Partly or wholly transparent to x-rays or other forms of radiation. —**radiolu·cen·cy** (·sun·see) n.

ra·dio·lu·mi·nes·cence (ray"dee·o·lew"mi·nes'unce) n. The luminescence brought about by x- or gamma rays striking a suitable crystalline substance.

ra·di·om·e·ter (ray"dee·om'e·tur) n. An instrument for detecting and measuring radiant energy (normally infrared, visible, or ultraviolet). —**ra·dio·met·ric** (ray"dee·o·met'rick) adj.

ra·dio·mi·met·ic (ray"dee·o·mi·met'ick) adj. Capable of producing in tissue biologic effects similar to those of ionizing radiation.

radiomimetic agent. Any agent, such as the nitrogen mustards, capable of duplicating many of the radiation-induced effects in tissue.

ra·dio·ne·cro·sis (ray"dee·o·ne·kro'sis) n. Destruction or ulceration of tissues caused by radiation.

ra·dio·neu·ri·tis (ray"dee·o·new·rye'tis) n. A form of neuritis due to exposure to radiation.

ra·dio·ni·tro·gen (ray"dee·o·nigh'truh·jin) n. The radioactive isotope of nitrogen, having a mass number of 13 (^{13}N), which has a half-life of 10.1 minutes and emits a positive beta particle for each atom of nitrogen that decays.

ra·dio·nu·clide (ray"dee·o·new'klide) n. A nuclide that is radioactive.

ra·di·o·paque (ray"dee·o·pake') adj. Not transparent to the x-ray; not permitting total passage of radiant energy. —**ra·di·opac·i·ty** (ray"dee·o·pas'i·tee) n.

ra·dio·pa·thol·o·gy (ray"dee·o·puh·thol'uh·jee) n. Study of tissue changes brought about by ionizing radiation.

ra·dio·pel·vim·e·try (ray"dee·o·pel·vim'e·tree) n. A radiographic procedure for making measurements of the maternal pelvis and fetal skull.

ra·dio·phar·ma·ceu·ti·cal (ray"dee·o·fahr"muh·sue'ti·kul) n. In nuclear medicine, a preparation of a radioactive element or compound containing such an element, commonly used for the diagnosis or treatment of disease.

ra·dio·phos·pho·rus (ray"dee·o·fos'fuh·rus) n. The radioactive isotope of phosphorus, having a mass number of 32 (^{32}P), which has a half-life of 14.3 days and emits a negative beta particle for each atom of phosphorus that decays. In the form of sodium phosphate (sodium phosphate P 32) it is used, by intravenous or oral administration, in the treatment of polycythemia vera and as an antineoplastic agent, and in various ways as a diagnostic agent, as in the determination of blood volume, and also as a tracer in various studies involving phosphorus.

ra·dio·prax·is (ray''dee·o·prack'sis) *n.* The use of radiant energy either in therapy or for other purposes.

ra·dio·re·sist·ance (ray''dee·o·re·zis'tunce) *n.* The relative resistance of tissues or organisms to the injurious effects of radiation.

ra·di·os·co·py (ray''dee·os'kuh·pee) *n.* The process of securing an image of an object upon a fluorescent screen by means of radiant energy.

ra·dio·sen·si·tiv·i·ty (ray''dee·o·sen''si·tiv'i·tee) *n.* The sensitivity of tissues or organisms to various types of radiations, such as x-rays or rays from radioactive materials. —**radio·sen·si·tive** (·sen'si·tiv) *adj.*

ra·dio·ster·e·os·co·py (ray''dee·o·sterr''ee·os'kuh·pee, ·steer'') *n.* The application of the principle of the stereoscope, obtaining a viewpoint for the left eye and one for the right by corresponding displacement of the x-ray tube along the plane of the film, and viewing the two radiographs by one of several methods to obtain a third-dimensional effect.

ra·dio·sur·gery (ray''dee·o·sur'jur·ee) *n.* The use of radium in surgical therapy.

ra·dio·ther·a·peu·tic (ray''dee·o·therr''uh·pew'tick) *adj.* Of or pertaining to the therapeutic use of radiant energy.

ra·dio·ther·a·pist (ray''dee·o·therr'uh·pist) *n.* A physician specializing in, or administering, radiotherapy.

ra·dio·ther·a·py (ray''dee·o·therr'uh·pee) *n.* RADIATION THERAPY.

ra·dio·ther·my (ray''dee·o·thur'mee) *n.* 1. Treatment by radiant heat. 2. SHORT-WAVE DIATHERMY.

ra·dio·thy·roid·ec·to·mize (ray''dee·o·thigh''roy·deck'tuh·mize) *v.* To ablate thyroid function by administration of large doses of radioactive iodine.

ra·dio·tox·emia (ray''dee·o·tock·see'mee·uh) *n.* Toxemia induced from overexposure to any radioactive substance.

ra·dio·trans·par·ent (ray''dee·o·trans·pâr'unt) *adj.* Permitting the passage of radiations; used notably in connection with x-rays.

ra·dio·trop·ic (ray''dee·o·trop'ick, tro'pick) *adj.* Reacting predictably to radiation.

ra·dio·ul·nar (ray''dee·o·ul'nur) *adj.* Pertaining to the radius and the ulna.

ra·di·um (ray''dee·um) *n.* Ra = 226. A highly radioactive metallic element; atomic number, 88. Discovered in 1898 by Pierre and Marie Curie, who separated it from pitchblende. Radium and its salts emit continuously alpha particles, beta particles, and gamma rays. As the bromide or chloride salt, it has been used as an irradiation source in the treatment of malignant tumors.

radium needles. Steel or platinum-iridium-walled, needle-shaped containers filled with radium salt and used in radium therapy.

radium therapy. Exposure of a body part to high-voltage radium emanations, usually for their destructive effect on malignant tissues.

ra·di·us (ray''dee·us) *n.,* pl. & genit. sing. **ra·dii** (·dee·eye) *In anatomy,* the outer of the two bones of the forearm.

ra·dix (ray'dicks) *n.,* genit. **ra·di·cis** (ray'di·sis, ray·dye'sis), pl. **radi·ces** (·di·seez, ·dye'seez) ROOT.

ra·don (ray'don) *n.* Rn = 222. A radioactive element, a gas, that is a product of the nuclear disintegration of radium; used as a source of irradiation in the treatment of malignant tumors. Syn. *radium emanation.*

radon seed. A small sealed capillary tube containing radon, suitable for implantation in tissues; the tube may be placed inside a small gold tube.

raf·fi·nase (raf'i·nace) *n.* An enzyme that hydrolyzes raffinose, fructose being produced in the reaction.

raf·fi·nose (raf'i·noce) *n.* A trisaccharide, $C_{18}H_{32}O_{16}.5H_2O$, found in sugar beets, cottonseed meal, and molasses. On complete hydrolysis, it yields glucose, fructose, and galactose.

rage reaction or response. An attack of intense and uncontrollable rage which may be encountered: (1) rarely, as part of the behavioral automatism of a psychomotor seizure; (2) as an episodic reaction without recognizable seizures or other neurologic abnormalities; and (3) in the course of some recognizable acute or chronic neurologic disease, particularly one that involves the anteromedian portions of the temporal lobes, the fornices, or the hypothalamus.

rag·weed, *n.* Any of several species of the genus *Ambrosia;* its pollen is the most important allergen in the central and eastern United States, the pollinating period being from the middle of August to the time of frost.

Raillietina cel·e·ben·sis (sel·e·ben'sis). A species of tapeworm; infections of man have been reported in Tokyo and in Taiwan.

Raillietina dem·e·rar·i·en·sis (dem''e·râr·ee·en'sis) A species of tapeworm; human infections have been reported in Guyana, Cuba, and especially rural Ecuador.

Raillietina qui·ten·sis (kwi·ten'sis). RAILLIETINA DEMERARIENSIS.

Raillietina mad·a·gas·car·i·en·sis (mad''uh·gas·kâr''ee·en'sis). A species of tapeworm that infects man.

railway sickness. MOTION SICKNESS.

railway spine. Traumatic neurosis following concussion injury with spinal symptoms and without demonstrable disease. Frequently compensation or indemnity neurosis play major role.

rake retractor. An instrument shaped like a rake, with sharp or blunt prongs, particularly effective in retracting tissues without slippage.

rale (rahl) *n.* An abnormal sound arising within the lungs or air passages and heard on auscultation over the chest; generally characterized by terms such as coarse, medium, fine, moist, dry.

ra·mal (ray'mul) *adj.* Of or pertaining to a ramus.

rami. Plural and genitive singular of *ramus*.

rami com·mu·ni·can·tes (kom-yoo-ni-kan'teez) [NA]. Plural of *ramus communicans*.

ram·i·fi·ca·tion (ram"i·fi·kay'shun) *n.* 1. The act or state of branching. 2. A branch.

ram·i·fy (ram'i·figh) *v.* To form branches; to branch.

rami·sec·tion (ram"i·seck'shun) *n.* Surgical division of the rami communicantes of the sympathetic nervous system.

rami·sec·to·my (ram"i·seck'tuh·mee) *n.* RAMISECTION.

ra·mose (ray'moce) *adj.* Having many branches; branching.

ra·mous (ray'mus) *adj.* Having many branches; branching.

Ram·stedt operation (rahm'shtet) PYLOROMYOTOMY.

ra·mu·lus (ram'yoo·lus, ray'mew·lus) *n.*, pl. **ramu·li** (·lye) A small branch, or ramus.

ra·mus (ray'mus) *n.*, pl. & genit. sing. **ra·mi** (·migh) 1. A branch, especially of a vein, artery, or nerve. 2. A process of bone projecting like a branch or twig from a large bone, as the ramus of the lower jaw, or the superior or inferior ramus of the pubis.

Ra·na (ray'nuh) *n.* A genus of frogs, species of which are often used as experimental animals and especially in certain pregnancy tests.

ran·cid (ran'sid) *adj.* Having the characteristic odor and taste of fat that has undergone oxidative and/or hydrolytic decomposition. —**ran·cid·i·ty** (ran·sid'i·tee) *n.*

ran·dom mating. A system of breeding in which individuals mate in accordance with the frequency with which they occur in the population; as a first approximation, mating in any human population is of this type.

random sample. A finite number of individuals, cases, or measurements chosen from a larger group in such a manner that each individual, case, or measurement has an equal and independent chance of being selected.

range, *n.* An area or extent over which something varies, or a measure of that extent, as, for example, the difference between the lowest and the highest values in a series of observations.

range of accommodation. The span of clear vision through which the eye can focus (that is, from its far point to its near point).

range paralysis. NEURAL LYMPHOMATOSIS.

ra·nine (ray'nine) *adj.* Pertaining to a ranula or to the region in which a ranula occurs.

ran·u·la (ran'yoo·luh) *n.* A retention cyst of a salivary gland, situated beneath the tongue.

rape, *n.* 1. *In legal medicine,* intimate sexual contact by a male with a female, not his wife, without her valid consent, by compulsion through violence, threats, stealth, or deceit. Laws vary as to whether contact with or penetration of the female genitalia is required to constitute rape; in some laws "without valid consent" means psychologically or physically incapable of resisting the male. Syn. *rape of the first degree.* 2. *In veterinary medicine,* the forcible sexual intercourse of the male while the female is not in heat.

rape oil. The semidrying oil from the seeds of *Brassica campestris, B. napus,* and other species. Used as a food and for industrial purposes. Syn. *colza oil.*

ra·pha·nia (ra·fay'nee·uh) *n.* A disease characterized by spasms of the limbs, attributed to a poison in the seeds of the wild radish which get mixed with grain and thus is ingested over a long period of time.

ra·phe (ray'fee) *n.* A seam or ridge, especially one indicating the line of junction of two symmetric halves.

raphe of the pharynx. A fibrous band in the median line of the posterior wall of the pharynx.

raphe of the scrotum. A medial ridge dividing the scrotum into two lateral halves; it is continuous posteriorly with the raphe of the perineum, anteriorly with the raphe of the penis.

raphe of the tongue. A median furrow on the dorsal surface of the tongue corresponding to the fibrous septum which partially divides it into symmetric halves.

rap·id ejection phase. The period of early cardiac systole, after opening of the aortic valve, during which the largest volume of blood per unit time is discharged by the ventricles.

rapid eye movement. The rapid, conjugate, usually lateral eye movement which characterizes REM sleep. Abbreviated, REM.

rapid filling wave. The outward deflection of the apex cardiogram immediately following the O point, corresponding to the rapid filling phase of ventricular diastole. Abbreviated, RFW.

rap·port (ra·por') *n.* A comfortable, harmonious, trusting, and mutually responsive relationship between two or more people, of which they are aware, and which in special situations, as between patient and physician or psychiatric therapist, or between testee and tester, contributes to the willingness of the patient or subject to be helped.

rap·tus (rap'tus) *n.* 1. Any sudden attack, intense emotion, or seizure. 2. RAPE.

rar·e·fac·tion (rair"e·fack'shun) *n.* The act of rarefying or of decreasing the density of a substance.

rar·e·fy (rair'i·figh, răr'i·figh) *v.* To make less dense or more porous.

ra·sce·ta (ra·see'tuh) *n.pl.* The transverse lines or creases on the palmar surface of the wrist.

rash, *n.* A lay term used for nearly any skin eruption but more commonly for acute inflammatory dermatoses.

ra·sion (ray'zhun) *n.* The scraping of drugs with a file.

Ras·mus·sen's aneurysm (rahs'moo·s*n) Aneurysm of a terminal pulmonary artery in a tuberculous cavity; rupture results in hemorrhage.

ras·pa·to·ry (ras'puh·to"ree) *n.* A rasp or file for trimming rough surfaces or margins of bone or for removing the periosteum.

rasp·ber·ry (raz'berr·ee) *n.* The fruit of *Rubus idaeus,* a plant of the Rosaceae. A syrup is used as a vehicle.

rat, *n.* A rodent that lives in close proximity to man, such as in barns, barns, wharves, ships, and garbage dumps. Feral rats are notorious disease carriers, harboring many varieties of intestinal parasites and being responsible especially for the transmission of bubonic plague, as well as a distinct septic disease, rat-bite fever.

rat-bite fever. One of two distinct diseases contracted from the bite of infected rats or other animals. One (Haverhill fever) is caused by *Streptobacillus moniliformis.* The other (sodoku) is due to *Spirillum minus.*

rate, *n.* The quantity or degree of some property or thing measured or calculated per unit of a reference standard, as the basal metabolic rate, the morbidity rate, or the radioactive decay rate.

rat flea. XENOPSYLLA CHEOPIS.

Rathke's pouch CRANIOBUCCAL POUCH.

Rathke's pouch cyst. Cystic distention of the remnants of the craniobuccal (Rathke's) pouch.

rat-ing, *n.* A systematic, often graded estimate of the qualities or characteristics of a person, process, or thing.

ra-tio (ray'shee-o) *n.* A proportion.

ra-tion (rash'un, ray'shun) *n.* A daily allowance of food or drink. In the armed services, the term usually means the complete subsistence for one man for one day.

ra-tio-nal (rash'un-ul) *adj.* 1. Based upon reason; reasonable. 2. *In therapeutics,* opposed to empirical.

ra-tio-nal-iza-tion (ra''shun-ul-i-zay'shun) *n.* A mode of adjustment to difficult and unpleasant situations; a defense mechanism, operating unconsciously, in which the individual attempts to justify, defend, or make tolerable by plausible means unacceptable attitudes or traits, behavior, feelings, and motives. Not to be confused with conscious misrepresentation or withholding of essential facts.

rat louse. *Polyplax spinulosa,* which carries the organism of murine typhus, *Rickettsia mooseri,* and transmits it to its rat host, but not to man.

rats-bane, *n.* 1. ARSENIC TRIOXIDE. 2. A name given to any rat poison containing arsenic.

rat-tle, *n.* RALE.

rat-tle-snake, *n.* Any snake of the New World pit vipers belonging to the genera *Crotalus* and *Sistrurus.*

rat typhus. MURINE TYPHUS.

Rauwiloid. Trademark for alseroxylon, a fat-soluble alkaloidal fraction from *Rauwolfia serpentina.*

Rau-wol-fia (raw-wol'fee-uh) *n.* A genus of tropical trees and shrubs, mostly poisonous, of the Apocynaceae family. The dried root of *Rauwolfia serpentina,* which contains reserpine and other alkaloids, is used as an antihypertensive and sedative drug.

rau-wol-fine (raw-wol'feen, -fin) *n.* An alkaloid, $C_{20}H_{26}N_2O_3$, from *Rauwolfia serpentina;* ajmaline.

ray, *n.* 1. A beam of light or other radiant energy. 2. A stream of discrete particles, such as alpha rays or beta rays. 3. A radial streak of different color in an organ, as medullary rays of the kidney.

ray fungus. Formerly, any organism of the genus *Actinomyces* or *Nocardia.*

Ray-naud's disease (reh-no') 1. Episodes of Raynaud's phenomenon, usually bilateral, excited by cold or emotion, with normal arterial pulsations and the absence of other primary causal disease. 2. Primary Raynaud's phenomenon, which occurs more commonly in women.

Raynaud's phenomenon Intermittent pallor, cyanosis, or rubor of the fingers or toes, or both, usually induced by cold or by emotion; secondary to many diseases, but often to chronic arterial occlusive disease.

RBC, rbc Abbreviation for (a) *red blood cell;* (b) red blood count.

RBE Abbreviation for *relative biological effectiveness* (of radiation).

R.C.P. Royal College of Physicians.

R.C.S. Royal College of Surgeons.

R.D. Abbreviation for *reaction of degeneration.*

rd Abbreviation for *rutherford.*

R.D.A. The right dorsoanterior position of the fetus.

R.D.P. The right dorsoposterior position of the fetus.

RDS Abbreviation for *respiratory distress syndrome of the newborn.*

re- A prefix signifying *back* or *again.*

re-ac-tant (ree-ack'tunt) *n.* Any substance that reacts chemically with another substance or substances.

re-ac-tion (ree-ack'shun) *n.* 1. A response to stimulus. 2. *In psychiatry,* a behavioral pattern constituting a recognizable clinical disorder. 3. Any chemical change, transformation, or interaction. 4. The state of a system, especially in solution, with reference to the relative proportion of hydrogen and hydroxyl ions, that is, whether neutral, acid, or alkaline. —**re-act** (ree-ackt') *v.*

reaction center. GERMINAL CENTER.

reaction formation. *In psychoanalysis,* a defense mechanism operating unconsciously, characterized by the development of conscious, socially acceptable activity which is the antithesis of repressed or rejected unconscious desires, as excessive prudishness in reaction to strong but repressed erotic wishes.

reaction of degeneration. The electric reaction of denervated muscle, developing about 10 days after and varying with the severity of injury; in mild partial degeneration, faradic stimulation of nerve requires more current than normal and galvanic stimulation of nerve and muscle results in normal responses; in severe partial degeneration, faradic stimulation of nerve produces no contraction while galvanic stimulation of nerve and muscle produces normal reactions; in complete or total degeneration, neither faradic nor galvanic stimulation of nerve produces any response, while galvanic stimulation of muscle results in vermicular contractions. Abbreviated, R.D.

reaction period. The time required for the body to respond to some form of stimulation following application of the stimulus; latent or lag period.

reaction time. The interval between the application of a stimulus and the beginning of the response.

re·ac·ti·vate (ree-ack'ti-vate) v. 1. To make active again, as by the addition of fresh normal serum containing complement to an immune serum which has lost its complement through age or heat. 2. To restore complementary activity to a serum, deprived of one or several of its C' components, by the addition of these components.

re·ac·ti·va·tion (ree-ack"ti-vay'shun) n. Rendering active again, as in the case of the addition of complement or one or several of its components to a serum that has become inactive.

re·ac·tive (ree-ack'tive) adj. Pertaining to or marked by reaction. —**re·ac·tiv·i·ty** (ree"ack-tiv'i-tee) n.

reactive depression. DEPRESSIVE NEUROSIS.

reactive psychosis. PSYCHOTIC DEPRESSIVE REACTION.

reactive schizophrenia. Schizophrenia considered primarily to be due to predisposing or precipitating environmental events, or both; typically manifested by a rapid onset and brief course, with the patient seemingly well before and after the episode.

re·ac·tor (ree-ack'tur) n. 1. A subject that reacts positively to a foreign substance, as in a test for a disease. 2. A subject that reacts to a stimulus in a psychological test. 3. A chemical or organism that reacts. 4. An apparatus in which a chemical or nuclear reaction occurs.

reading epilepsy. A form of sensory epilepsy triggered by reading.

re·a·gent (ree-ay'junt) n. 1. Any substance involved in a chemical reaction. 2. A substance used for the detection or determination of another substance by chemical, microscopical, or other means.

re·a·gin (ree-ay'jin) n. An antibody which occurs in human atopy, such as hay fever and asthma, and which readily sensitizes the skin and other tissues by attaching to mast cells and basophils. When combined with the corresponding antigen, it is responsible for the liberation of histamine and other mediators which cause atopic symptoms. —**re·a·gin·ic** (ree"uh-jin'ick) adj.

reaginic antibody. REAGIN.

real image. An image formed of real foci.

re·al·i·ty principle (ree-al'i-tee). In psychoanalysis, the concept that the pleasure principle is normally modified by the demands of the external environment and that the individual adjusts to these inescapable requirements in a way so that he ultimately secures satisfaction of his instinctual wishes.

reality testing. In psychiatry, the efforts made by a person to achieve balance between the demands and restrictions of his external environment and his needs for self-recognition, usually in some nonthreatening ways such as fantasy or projection; may be a part of normal adjustment or may become all-absorbing as in the regression of a psychosis.

ream·er (ree'mur) n. 1. A surgical instrument used for gouging out holes or enlarging those already made, especially in bone operations. 2. An endodontic instrument with spiral blades used for cleaning and enlarging root canals.

re·am·i·na·tion (ree-am"i-nay'shun) n. The introduction of an amino group into a compound from which an amino group had previously been removed.

re·am·pu·ta·tion (ree-am"pew-tay'shun) n. An amputation upon a member on which the operation has already been performed.

re·an·i·mate (ree-an'i-mate) v. To revive; resuscitate; to restore to life, as a person apparently dead.

Ré·au·mur thermometer (rey'o-mue'r) A thermometer on which the freezing point of water is 0° and the boiling point 80° with an interval of 80 points or degrees.

re·bound, n. 1. In reflex activity, a sudden contraction of a muscle following its relaxation; associated with a variety of forms of reflex activity. Seen most typically following the cessation of an inhibitory reflex. 2. The return to health from illness; vigorous recovery.

rebound phenomenon. The normal tendency of a limb whose movement is being resisted to move in the intended direction when resistance is removed and then to jerk back, or rebound, in the opposite direction. The rebound is exaggerated in spastic limbs and is absent in limbs affected by cerebellar disease.

re·breath·ing, n. The act of respiring air, or air plus other gases, which has already been exhaled.

rebreathing bag. A flexible rubber bag into and from which breathing takes place for therapeutic or experimental purposes; also, such a bag used in the administration of gas anesthesia.

re·cal·ci·fi·ca·tion (ree-kal"si-fi-kay'shun) n. 1. The restoration of lime salts to bone matrix. 2. The addition of a solution of calcium salts to blood or plasma decalcified by an anticoagulant. —**re·cal·ci·fy** (ree-kal'si-fye) v.

recalcification time. RECALCIFIED CLOTTING TIME.

recalcified clotting time. The clotting time of decalcified blood or plasma upon the readdition of calcium ions.

re·cal·ci·trant (re-kal'si-trunt) adj. Resistant to treatment, whether medical or psychiatric; stubborn.

re·call, n. 1. In psychology, the complex mental process of bringing the memory trace or engram of a past experience or of material learned into consciousness. 2. In immunology, ANAMNESTIC RESPONSE.

re·ca·pit·u·la·tion (ree"ka-pit"yoo-lay'shun) n. The summarizing of the main points of a subject; the repetition of the steps of a process.

recent memory. Recall of events that occurred in the relatively immediate past.

re·cep·tac·u·lum (ree"sep-tack'yoo-lum) n., pl. **receptacu·la** (·luh) A receptacle; a small container.

re·cep·tive, adj. Having the quality of, or capacity for, receiving. Specifically, pertaining to the mind, open to impressions, ideas, and suggestions from sources other than oneself.

receptive aphasia. SENSORY APHASIA.

receptive centers. *In physiology and psychophysics*, nerve centers which receive influences that may excite sensations or some kind of activity not associated with conscious perception.

receptive field. The area of the retina where spot illumination continues to yield a response in a particular optic nerve fiber.

re·cep·to·ma (ree″sep·to′muh) *n.* CHEMODECTOMA.

re·cep·tor (re·sep′tur) *n.* 1. A specialized structure of sensory nerve terminals characteristically excited by specific stimuli. 2. A molecular structure at the cell surface or within the cell which is capable of combining with molecules such as toxins, hormones, antigens, immunoglobulins and complement components. 3. *In pharmacology*, a receptor (2) which combines, with varying degrees of specificity, with a drug or other substance resulting in a given alteration of cell function.

re·cess, *n.* A fossa, ventricle, or ampulla; an anatomic depression.

re·ces·sion (re·sesh′un) *n.* The gradual withdrawal of a part from its normal position, as recession of the gums from the necks of teeth.

re·ces·sive (re·ses′iv) *adj. & n.* 1. *In genetics*, characterizing the behavior of an allele which is not expressed in the presence of another (dominant) allele. 2. A recessive character or trait.

recessive character or **trait.** The member of a pair of contrasted traits which fails to manifest itself in the heterozygote.

re·ces·sus (ree·ses′us) *n.*, pl. & genit. sing. **recessus** RECESS.

re·cid·i·va·tion (re·sid″i·vay′shun) *n.* 1. The relapse of a patient recovering from a disease. 2. *In criminology*, a relapsing into crime.

re·cid·i·vism (re·sid′i·viz·um) *n.* The repetition of criminal or delinquent acts; repeated bad behavior.

re·cid·i·vist (re·sid′i·vist) *n.* 1. A patient who returns to a hospital for treatment, especially a mentally ill person who so returns. 2. *In criminology*, a confirmed, relapsed, or habitual criminal.

re·cid·i·vi·ty (res″i·div′i·tee) *n.* The tendency to relapse in illness or to return to hospital or jail.

re·ci·pe (res′i·pee) *v. & n.* 1. The heading of a physician's prescription, signifying *take*. Symbol, ℞. 2. The prescription itself.

re·cip·i·ent (re·sip′ee·unt) *n.* One who receives blood or other tissue from another, the donor.

re·cip·ro·cal (re·sip′ruh·kul) *adj.* 1. Complementary. 2. Mutual and equal.

reciprocal inhibition and desensitization. *In psychiatry*, a form of behavior therapy in which the patient, while made to relax in comfortable surroundings, is gradually exposed to increasing amounts of anxiety-provoking stimuli. In this way the patient can tolerate

these stimuli and may eventually learn to dissociate the anxiety from them.

rec·i·proc·i·ty (res″i·pros′i·tee) *n. In medicine*, the reciprocal recognition among some states of the U.S. of the validity of examinations and licensures for doctors, nurses, and other professional and paraprofessional personnel.

Recklinghausen's disease. VON RECKLINGHAUSEN'S DISEASE.

rec·li·na·tion (reck″li·nay′shun) *n.* An operation for cataract, in which the lens is pushed back into the vitreous chamber. Syn. *couching.*

Re·clus' disease (ruh·kluⁱ) Mammary dysplasia of the cystic disease type.

re·com·bi·na·tion (ree·kom″bi·nay′shun) *n. In radiobiology*, the coming together of two or more ionized or activated atoms, radicals, or molecules.

re·com·po·si·tion (ree·kom″puh·zish′un) *n.* Reunion of parts or constituents after temporary dissolution.

re·com·pres·sion (ree″kum·presh′un) *n.* Resubjection to increased atmospheric pressure; a procedure used in treating caisson workers or divers who develop decompression sickness returning too rapidly to normal atmospheric pressures.

re·con·stit·u·ent (ree″kun·stich′oo·unt) *n.* A medicine which promotes continuous repair of tissue waste or makes compensation for its loss.

re·con·sti·tu·tion (ree·kon″sti·tew′shun) *n.* Continuous repair of progressive destruction of tissues.

re·con·struc·tion (ree″kun·struck′shun) *n.* 1. In medical history taking and psychoanalysis, the integration into a significant whole of facts which are presented first without consciousness of their relationship. 2. Reproduction, usually with enlargement of the form, of an embryo, organ system, or part by assemblage of properly spaced and oriented outlines of serial sections. 3. *In plastic surgery*, the attempt, often by a series of operations, to restore a disfigured, deformed, or deficient part to more normal appearance or function. —**re·construc·tive** (·tiv) *adj.*

re·cov·ery (re·kuv′ur·ee) *n.* Return to a state of rest, equilibrium, or health from a state of fatigue, stress, or illness.

recreation therapy. *In psychiatry*, the use of music, theater, games, and other such group activities which provide the patient relaxation as well as outlets for self-expression and the discharge of aggression and hostility; an adjuvant form of psychotherapy.

rec·re·ment (reck′re·munt) *n.* A substance secreted from a part of the body, as a gland, and again absorbed by the body, as for example saliva or bile. —**rec·re·men·tal** (reck″re·men′tul), **rec·re·men·ti·tial** (reck″re·men·tish′ul), **rec·remen·ti·tious** (·tish′us) *adj.*

re·cru·des·cence (ree″kroo·des′unce) *n.* An increase or recurrence of the symptoms of a disease after a remission or a short intermission. —**recrudes·cent** (·unt) *adj.*

re·cruit·ment (re·kroot′munt) *n.* Involvement of

increasing numbers of motor units in response to increasing strength of stimulus.

recruitment test. The measurement of the span between the threshold of a deafened person's hearing and the level of his discomfort. This span is much shorter when there is loss of perception due to a cochlear defect than when there is loss of conduction.

rect-, recto-. A combining form meaning *rectum, rectal.*

rectal ampulla. The dilated part of the rectum situated just above the anal canal.

rectal columns. ANAL COLUMNS.

rec·tal·gia (reck·tal'jee·uh) *n.* PROCTALGIA.

rectal hernia. A condition in which the small bowel, or other abdominal contents, protrudes through the rectovesical excavation or rectouterine pouch, carrying the anterior rectal wall through the anus.

rectal shelf. BLUMER'S SHELF.

rec·tec·to·my (reck·teck'tuh·mee) *n.* PROCTECTOMY.

rec·ti·fi·ca·tion (reck″ti·fi·kay'shun) *n.* 1. A straightening, as rectification of a crooked limb. 2. The redistillation or fractional distillation of liquids to obtain a product of higher purity or greater concentration of the desired constituent 3. The conversion of alternating to direct current.

rec·ti·lin·ear (reck″ti·lin'ee·ur) *adj.* Describing or characterized by a straight line.

rec·ti·tis (reck·tye'tis) *n.* PROCTITIS.

rec·to·ab·dom·i·nal (reck″to·ab·dom'i·nul) *adj.* Pertaining to the rectum and the abdomen.

rec·to·anal (reck″to·ay'nul) *adj.* Pertaining to the rectum and the anus.

rec·to·cele (reck'to·seel) *n.* Protrusion or herniation of the rectum into the vagina. Syn. *vaginal proctocele.*

rec·toc·ly·sis (reck·tock'li·sis) *n.* The slow instillation of a liquid into the rectum. Syn. *proctoclysis, Murphy drip.*

rec·to·coc·cyg·e·al (reck″to·cock·sij'ee·ul) *adj.* Pertaining to the rectum and the coccyx.

rec·to·co·li·tis (reck″to·ko·lye'tis) *n.* Inflammation of the mucosa of the rectum and colon.

rec·to·co·lon·ic (reck″to·ko·lon'ick) *adj.* Pertaining to the rectum and the colon.

rec·to·cu·ta·ne·ous (reck″to·kew·tay'nee·us) *adj.* Pertaining to both the rectum and the skin.

rec·to·fis·tu·la (reck″to·fis'tew·luh) *n.* A fistula of the rectum.

rec·to·gen·i·tal (reck″to·jen'i·tul) *adj.* Pertaining to the rectum and the genital organs.

rec·to·la·bi·al (reck″to·lay'bee·ul) *adj.* Relating to the rectum and the labia pudenda.

rec·to·per·i·ne·al (reck″to·perr·i·nee'ul) *adj.* Pertaining to the rectum and the perineum.

rec·to·pexy (reck'to·peck″see) *n.* PROCTOPEXY.

rec·to·pho·bia (reck″to·fo'bee·uh) *n.* PROCTOPHOBIA.

rec·to·plas·ty (reck'to·plas″tee) *n.* PROCTOPLASTY.

rec·to·rec·tos·to·my (reck″to·reck·tos'tuh·mee) *n.* Surgical anastomosis between two parts of the rectum.

rec·to·scope (reck'tuh·skope) *n.* PROCTOSCOPE.

—rec·tos·co·py (reck·tos'kuh·pee) *n.*

rec·to·sig·moid (reck″to·sig'moid) *n.* The rectum and sigmoid portion of the colon considered together.

rec·to·sig·moid·ec·to·my (reck″to·sig″moy·deck'tuh·mee) *n.* Surgical excision of the rectum and sigmoid colon.

rec·to·sig·moid·os·co·py (reck″to·sig″moy·dos'kuh·pee) *n.* Inspection of the rectum and sigmoid flexure of the colon with the aid of a sigmoidoscope.

rec·to·ste·no·sis (reck″to·ste·no'sis) *n.* Stenosis of the rectum.

rec·tos·to·my (reck·tos'tuh·mee) *n.* PROCTOSTOMY.

rec·tot·o·my (reck·tot'uh·mee) *n.* PROCTOTOMY.

rec·to·ure·thral (reck″to·yoo·ree'thrul) *adj.* Pertaining to the rectum and the urethra.

rec·to·ure·thra·lis (reck″to·yoo·ree·thray'lis) *n.* A small band of smooth muscle fibers running from the rectum to the membranous part of the urethra in the male.

rec·to·uter·ine (reck″to·yoo'tur·ine) *adj.* Pertaining to the rectum and the uterus.

rectouterine excavation or **fossa.** The portion of the peritoneal cavity between the rectum and the posterior surface of the uterus and vagina. Syn. *pouch of Douglas.*

rectouterine pouch. RECTOUTERINE EXCAVATION.

rec·to·va·gi·nal (reck″to·vaj'i·nul, ·va·jye'nul) *adj.* Pertaining to the rectum and the vagina.

rectovaginal fistula. An opening between the vagina and the rectum.

rectovaginal septum. The tissue forming the partition between the rectum and the vagina.

rec·to·vag·i·no·ab·dom·i·nal (reck″to·vaj″i·no·ab·dom'i·nul) *adj.* Pertaining to or by way of the rectum, vagina, and abdomen; said of a type of combined pelvic examination.

rec·to·ves·i·cal (reck″to·ves'i·kul) *adj.* Pertaining to the rectum and the urinary bladder.

rectovesical excavation. The part of the peritoneal cavity between the urinary bladder and the rectum in the male.

rectovesical fistula. A congenital or acquired opening between the rectum and the urinary bladder.

rec·tum (reck'tum) *n.,* genit. **rec·ti** (·tye), pl. **rec·ta** (·tuh) The lower part of the large intestine, extending from the sigmoid flexure to the anal canal. It begins opposite the third sacral vertebra and passes downward to terminate at the anal canal.

rectum reflex. The mechanism by which feces accumulated in and pressing against the rectum are evacuated, characterized by peristaltic contraction of the rectal musculature and relaxation of the internal and external sphincters of the anus.

rec·tus (reck'tus) *L. adj. & E. n.,* pl. & genit. sing. **rec·ti** (·tye) 1. Straight; forward. 2. Vertical or perpendicular. 3. Any of various muscles that are either rectilinear in shape, or oriented along—or perpendicular to—an axis of the body or of a part.

rectus ab·do·mi·nis (ab·dom'i·nis). The muscle of the anterior abdominal wall which has vertical fibers.

rectus incision. An incision made through the

rectus abdominis muscle or through its sheath.

re·cum·ben·cy (re·kum'bun·see) *n.* The reclining position.

re·cum·bent (re·kum'bunt) *adj.* Leaning back; reclining.

re·cu·per·ate (re·koo'pur·ate, re·kew') *v.* To regain strength or health.

re·cu·per·a·tion (re·koo''pur·ay'shun, re·kew'') *n.* Convalescence; restoration to health.

re·cu·per·a·tive (re·koo'pur·uh·tiv, re·kew'') *adj.* Pertaining to, or tending to, recovery or restoration of health or strength.

re·cur·rence (re·kur'unce) *n.* 1. The return of symptoms or a disease. 2. Reappearance of a neoplasm after apparent complete removal.

re·cur·rent (re·kur'unt) *adj.* 1. Returning. 2. *In anatomy,* turning back in its course.

recurrent summer eruption. HYDROA VACCINIFORME.

re·cur·va·tion (ree''kur·vay'shun) *n.* The act or process of bending backward.

red atrophy. Atrophy complicating chronic hyperemia, especially of the liver.

red blindness. PROTANOPIA.

red blood cell. ERYTHROCYTE. Abbreviated, RBC, rbc.

red bug. CHIGGER.

red degeneration. Red discoloration of a uterine fibromyoma due to degeneration, necrosis, and edema of the tumor.

red diaper syndrome. Red discoloration of soiled diapers after 24 to 36 hours incubation in a diaper receptacle, due to predominance of *Serratia macrescens* in the bowel flora of newborn infants.

red hepatization. A pathologic change in the lungs, usually in pneumococcal lobar pneumonia, in which the lungs have the consistency of the liver and are discolored red.

re·dia (ree'dee·uh) *n.,* pl. **re·di·ae** (·dee·ee) *In parasitology,* the second larval stage of a trematode, which results from the development of a parthenogenetic egg of the first larval stage.

re·dif·fer·en·ti·a·tion (ree·dif''ur·en''shee·ay'shun) *n.* The return to a position of greater specialization in actual and potential functions.

red induration. 1. Fibrosis of the lung associated with deposit of red oxide of iron; pulmonary hemosiderosis. 2. Marked passive hyperemia of the lung.

red infarct. An infarct in which the necrotic focus is swollen, firm, and either bright or dark red, as the result of hemorrhage.

red·in·te·gra·tion (red·in''te·gray'shun) *n.* 1. Complete restoration of a part that has been injured or destroyed; the reestablishing of a whole. 2. *In psychology,* the principle that the recall of a part of an event or a fraction of the stimulus originally resulting in a certain response will revive the event or response as a whole.

red mite. Any member of the genus *Trombicula.*

red muscle. A muscle that appears red in the fresh state; in the fibers of red muscles, the longitudinal striation is more prominent and the transverse striation is somewhat irregular. The red color probably is due to myoglobin and cytochrome.

red nucleus. A large oval nucleus, situated in the midbrain ventral to the cerebral aqueduct, which in the fresh brain has a slightly pink color. It receives fibers from the superior cerebellar peduncle and gives fibers to the rubrospinal tract.

red-out (red'owt) *n.* A condition encountered by flyers as a consequence of centripetal acceleration, causing blood to be driven to the head with resulting severe headache and transient blurring of vision as by a red mist.

re·dox (ree'docks) *n.* An oxidation-reduction reaction, state, or system.

red pulp. The red material consisting of anastomosing, cordlike columns of reticular connective tissue separating the venous sinuses of the spleen.

red pulp cords. RED PULP.

red reflex. The red glow of light seen to emerge from the pupil when the interior of the eye is illuminated, due to the reflected light having passed through the choroid.

red sweat. A peculiar, red perspiration noted in the axillas and genital region, and due to microorganisms which have developed on the hairs of these warm, moist parts.

red thrombus. A thrombus composed principally of erythrocytes and fibrin intimately mixed, commonly formed by clotting of blood in an occluded vessel.

re·duce (re·dewce') *v.* 1. To restore a part to its normal relations, as to reduce a hernia or fracture. 2. *In chemistry,* to bring to the metallic form, deprive of oxygen, or add electrons. 3. To lose weight by dietetic regimen.

re·duc·ible (re·dew'si·bul) *adj.* Capable of being reduced.

reducible hernia. A hernia whose contents can be replaced through the hernial opening.

re·duc·tion (re·duck'shun) *n.* 1. *In chemistry,* an increase in the negative valence of an element (or a decrease in positive valence) occurring as a result of the gain of electrons. Each electron so gained is taken from some other element, thus accomplishing an oxidation of that element. 2. Originally, the process of separation from oxygen, or the combining with hydrogen. 3. The restoration by surgical or manipulative procedures of a dislocated joint or a fractured bone to normal anatomic relationships, or the restoration of an incarcerated hernia to its original location.

re·dun·dant (re·dun'dunt) *adj.* Superfluous; characterized by an excess, as of skin. **—redun·dan·cy** (·dun·see) *n.*

re·du·pli·cat·ed (re·dew'pli·kay·tid) *adj.* Doubled, as reduplicated heart sounds.

re·du·pli·ca·tion (re·dew''pli·kay'shun) *n.* A doubling.

reduplication cyst. Any cyst arising from a duplicated segment of a hollow organ such as intestine or bronchus.

Red·u·vi·i·dae (red''yoo·vye'i·dee, ree''dew·) *n.pl.* A family of the Heteroptera or true bugs, including some 4,000 species, commonly called assassin bugs and kissing bugs. Includes vectors of Chagas' disease, and may cause painful dermatitis at the site of the bite. Syn. *Triatomidae.* —**re·du·vi·id** (re-dew'vee-id) *n. & adj.*

Reed-Frost theory. *In epidemiology,* a theory, intended to cover acute communicable diseases, based on an expression of the probable number of cases at time $T+1$ in terms of known facts at time T. The theory is one that proceeds stepwise in time and does not give a continuous time curve; it is not expected to describe the course of a particular epidemic, but allows the exploration of a variety of epidemiologic principles.

Reed-Stern·berg cell (shtehrn'behrk) An anaplastic reticuloendothelial cell characteristic of Hodgkin's disease, although found in other conditions as well.

re·ed·u·ca·tion (ree-ej″oo·kay'shun) *n.* The development of the processes of adjustment in an individual who has acquired these processes and then lost them.

Reen·stier·na reaction or test (reʸn'steer·nah[h]) ITO-REENSTIERNA TEST.

re·ep·i·the·li·al·iza·tion (ree-ep″i·theel″ee·ul·i·zay'shun) *n.* 1. The regrowth of epithelium over a denuded surface. 2. The placement of epithelium over a denuded surface by surgical means.

re·ep·i·the·lial·ize (ree-ep″i·theel″ee·ul·ize) *v.* To restore an epithelial surface, either surgically or through natural regrowth.

Rees and Eck·er's diluting fluid A sodium citrate-sucrose solution used as a diluent in blood platelet counting.

re·ev·o·lu·tion (ree-ev″uh·lew'shun) *n.* According to J. Hughlings Jackson, a symptom following an epileptic attack, which consists of three stages: suspension of power to understand speech (word deafness), perception of words and echolalia without comprehension, return to conscious perception of speech with continued lack of comprehension.

re·ex·cise (ree-eck·size') *v.* To excise after a previous excision or incomplete excision.

re·ex·ci·ta·tion (ree-eck″si·tay'shun) *n.* Reentrance of the excitation wave into tissue that has recovered from a refractory state.

re·ex·pand (ree″eck·spand') *v.* To expand again following collapse, as of the lungs.

re·fec·tion (re-feck'shun) *n.* 1. Restoration, refreshment, or recovery, especially after fatigue or hunger. 2. The phenomenon of vitamin B-complex synthesis by the bacterial flora of the intestine in certain animals maintained on a diet devoid of the vitamins.

referred pain. Pain whose origin is not in the area in which it is felt; for example, pain felt under the right scapula due to gallbladder disease.

re·fine, *v.* To purify a substance, extract it from raw material, or remove impurities from it.

re·flec·tance (re-fleck'tunce) *n.* The ratio of the light reflected from a surface to that incident upon it. Syn. *reflection coefficient, reflection factor.*

re·flect·ed, *adj.* 1. Cast or thrown back. 2. *In*

anatomy, turned back upon itself, as visceral peritoneum from the surface of an organ to become parietal peritoneum.

re·flec·tion (re-fleck'shun) *n.* 1. A bending or turning back; specifically, the turning back of a ray of light from a surface upon which it impinges without penetrating. 2. In membranes, as the peritoneum, the folds which are made in passing from the wall of the cavity over an organ and back again to the wall which bounds such a cavity.

re·flex (ree'flecks) *n.* A stereotyped involuntary movement or other response of a peripheral organ to an appropriate stimulus, the action occurring immediately, without the aid of the will or without even entering consciousness. —**re·flex·ly,** *adv.*

reflex akinesia. Impairment or loss of reflex action.

reflex arc. The pathway traversed by an impulse during reflex action, extending from a receptor to an effector usually, but not necessarily, via some part of the central nervous system.

reflex arrhythmia. PHASIC SINUS ARRHYTHMIA.

reflex bladder. A urinary bladder whose activity or function is dependent solely upon the primary (simple) reflex arc through the sacral cord, as the result of removal of suprasegmental control secondary to complete transection of the spinal cord, or gross lesions which result in profound disturbance of suprasegmental pathways, comparable to complete transection of the cord. Syn. *automatic bladder, spastic reflex bladder.*

reflex cough. Cough produced by irritation of a remote organ.

reflex epilepsy. Seizures brought about by sensory stimuli such as music, sudden noise (acousticomotor epilepsy), reading, or an object of touch or sight, often with electroencephalographic changes in the sensory projection area corresponding to the trigger zone.

reflex ileus. ADYNAMIC ILEUS.

re·flex·io (re-fleck'see·o) *n.* A bending back, turning back, or reflection.

re·flex·o·gen·ic (re-fleck″so·jen'ick) *adj.* Causing or increasing a tendency to reflex action; producing reflexes.

re·flex·o·graph (re-fleck'so·graf) *n.* An instrument for graphically recording a reflex, such as the knee jerk or calcaneal tendon reflex.

re·flex·om·e·ter (ree″fleck·some'e·tur) *n.* 1. An instrument used to measure the force required to produce a stretch reflex. 2. Any device used to measure the force required to elicit a reflex.

re·flex·o·ther·a·py (re-fleck″so·therr'uh·pee) *n.* A form of therapeutics based on stimulation by manipulation, anesthetization, or cauterization of areas more or less distant from the affected lesion.

re·flux (ree'flucks) *n.* A return flow, as in a reflux condenser, which returns condensate to the original fluid.

reflux esophagitis. Inflammation of the esophagus due to reflux of gastric contents into the esophagus.

re·fract (re-frakt') *v.* 1. To change direction by refraction. 2. To estimate the degree of ametropia, heterophoria, and strabismus present in an eye.

re·frac·ta do·si (re-frack'tuh do'sigh) In divided doses.

re·frac·tile (re-frack'til, -tile) *adj.* REFRACTIVE.

re·frac·tion (re-frack'shun) *n.* 1. The act of refracting or bending back. 2. The deviation of a ray of light from a straight line in passing obliquely from one transparent medium to another of different density. 3. The state of refractive power, especially of the eye; the ametropia, emmetropia, or muscle imbalance present. 4. The act or process of correcting errors of ocular refraction.

re·frac·tion·ist (re-frack'shun·ist) *n.* One who determines the status of ocular refraction.

refraction of the eye. The influence of the ocular media upon a cone or beam of light, whereby a normal or emmetropic eye produces a proper image of the object upon the retina.

re·frac·tive (re-frack'tiv) *adj.* 1. Refracting; capable of refracting or bending back. 2. Pertaining to refraction.

refractive error. A defect of the eye which prevents parallel light rays from being brought to a single focus precisely on the retina.

refractive index. The refractive power of any substance as compared with air. It is the quotient of the angle of incidence divided by the angle of refraction of a ray passing through a substance. Symbol, n.

re·frac·tiv·i·ty (ree"frack·tiv'i·tee) *n.* The power of refraction; the ability to refract.

re·frac·tom·e·ter (ree"frack·tom'e·tur) *n.* 1. An instrument for measuring the refraction of the eye. 2. An instrument for measuring the refractive index of a substance.

re·frac·to·ry (re-frack'tuh·ree) *adj.* 1. Resisting treatment. 2. Resisting the action of heat; slow to melt. 3. Unable to respond to appropriate stimulation, as a muscle or nerve immediately after responding to a stimulation.

refractory megaloblastic anemia. Megaloblastic and macrocytic anemia of unknown cause and unresponsive to therapeutic agents such as vitamin B_{12} and folic acid.

refractory period. *In physiology,* the transient period immediately following effective stimulation of an irritable tissue; especially a tissue subject to the all-or-none law.

refractory rickets. VITAMIN D-REFRACTORY RICKETS.

re·frac·ture (ree·frack'chur) *n.* The breaking again of fractured bones that have united by faulty union.

re·fran·gi·bil·i·ty (re-fran"ji·bil'i·tee) *n.* The capability of undergoing refraction. —**re·fran·gi·ble** (·fran'ji·bul) *adj.*

re·fresh, *v. In surgery,* to give to an old lesion the character of a fresh wound.

re·frig·er·ant (re·frij'ur·unt) *adj. & n.* 1. Cooling; lessening fever or thirst. 2. A coolant; a medicine or agent having cooling properties or lowering body temperature.

re·frig·er·a·tion (re·frij''ur·ay'shun) *n.* The act of lowering the temperature of a body by conducting away its heat to a surrounding cooler substance.

re·frin·gent (re-frin'junt) *adj.* REFRACTIVE.

Ref·sum's syndrome or **disease** An autosomal recessive disorder characterized by visual disturbances, ataxia, neuritic changes, and cardiac damage, associated with high blood levels of phytanic acid. Syn. *heredopathia atactica polyneuritiformis.*

re·fu·sion (re·few'zhun) *n.* Injection of blood into the circulation after its removal from the same patient.

re·gen·er·ate (re·jen'er·ate) *v.* 1. To form anew. 2. To reproduce, after loss. —**regener·a·ble** (·uh·bul) *adj.*

re·gen·er·a·tion (ree·jen''er·ay'shun) *n.* 1. The new growth or repair of structures or tissues lost by disease or by injury. 2. *In chemistry,* the process of obtaining from the by-products or end products of a process a substance which was employed in the earlier part of the process.

re·gen·er·a·tive (ree·jen'er·uh·tiv, ·uh·ray·tiv) *adj.* Pertaining to, promoting, or capable of regeneration.

reg·i·men (rej'i·mun) *n.* A systematic course or plan directed toward the improvement of health, the diagnosis of disease, or the investigation of biologic activities. Such a plan is likely to consider diet, drugs, exercise, and therapeutic or experimental procedures.

re·gio (rej'ee·o, ree'jee·o) *n.,* pl. **re·gi·o·nes** (rej"ee·o'neez, ree"jee·) REGION.

re·gion, *n.* One of the divisions of the body possessing either natural or arbitrary boundaries. —**region·al,** *adj.*

regional anatomy. The study of the anatomy of the body based upon a regional approach.

regional anesthesia. REGIONAL BLOCK ANESTHESIA.

regional block anesthesia. Anesthesia of a region of the body produced by injection of an anesthetic solution into and around the nerve trunks supplying the operative field. The injection may be made at a distance from the site of operation.

regional colitis. GRANULOMATOUS COLITIS.

regional enteritis. A chronic, nonspecific, granulomatous process frequently involving the terminal portion of the ileum, but occasionally extending into the colon or arising in the more proximal portions of the small intestine; characterized clinically by recurrent crampy abdominal pain accompanied by diarrhea, fever, anorexia, and weight loss. Syn. *Crohn's disease.*

regional enterocolitis. REGIONAL ENTERITIS.

regiones. Plural of *regio.*

reg·is·ter (rej'is·tur) *n.* 1. The compass of a voice. 2. A subdivision of the compass of a voice, consisting in a series of tones produced in the same way and of a like character.

reg·is·trar (rej'is·trahr) *n.* 1. An official custodian of records. 2. An officer in charge of hospital registry office. 3. In British hospitals, a resident specialist.

reg·is·tra·tion (rej''is·tray'shun) *n.* 1. The act of recording, as of deaths, births, or marriages. 2. A document certifying an act of registering, as a physician's registration.

reg·is·try (rej'i·stree) n. 1. An office listing nurses available for general or special services. 2. A place or central agency where data can be recorded for processing and subsequent retrieval for analysis.

Regitine. Trademark for phentolamine, an adrenergic blocking drug used as the hydrochloride and mesylate salts.

reg·le·men·ta·tion (reg''le·men·tay'shun) n. The legal restriction or regulation of prostitution, as by compulsory medical inspection.

re·gress, v. 1. To return to a former state. 2. To subside.

re·gres·sion (re·gresh'un) n. 1. The act or process of regressing. 2. FILIAL REGRESSION. 3. In psychology, a mental state and a mode of adjustment to difficult and unpleasant situations, characterized by behavior of a type that had been satisfying and appropriate at an earlier stage of development but which no longer befits the age and social status of the individual. A terminal state in some forms of schizophrenia. 4. In mathematics, the tendency for a group equated in one trait to have a mean value closer to the general mean in a related trait.

re·gres·sive (re·gres'iv) adj. 1. Going back to a former state, the return to infantile patterns of behavior in an adult. 2. Subsiding, said of symptoms.

regressive metaplasia. Transformation in the direction of lower orders of differentiation. Syn. retrogressive atrophy.

reg·u·la·tion (reg''yoo·lay'shun) n. The processes by which a given biological phenomenon is maintained within narrow limits compatible with the survival of the organism.

reg·u·la·tive (reg'yoo·lay''tiv) adj. In embryology, descriptive of development of eggs in which the cells of the early stages can be affected by inducing agents from the surrounding parts; opposed to mosaic development.

re·gur·gi·tant (re·gur'ji·tunt) adj. Flowing backward.

re·gur·gi·ta·tion (re·gur''ji·tay'shun) n. 1. A backflow of blood through a heart valve that is defective. 2. The return of food from the stomach to the mouth without vomiting. —**re·gur·gi·tate** (re·gur'ji·tate) v.

regurgitation jaundice. Jaundice due to resorption of conjugated bilirubin into the blood. It may be hepatocellular or obstructive. Syn. resorptive jaundice.

re·ha·bil·i·ta·tion (ree''ha·bil''i·tay'shun) n. The restoration to a disabled individual of maximum independence commensurate with his limitations by developing his residual capacities. In medicine, it implies prescribed training and employment of many different methods and professional workers. —**re·ha·bil·i·tate** (ree''ha·bil'i·tate) v.

re·ha·la·tion (ree''ha·lay'shun) n. Rebreathing; the inhalation of air that has been inspired previously; sometimes used in anesthesia.

Reh·fuss method REHFUSS TEST MEAL.

Rehfuss test meal A test meal of toast and tea. Specimens of gastric contents are withdrawn at intervals via a stomach tube and tested for acid content.

Rehfuss tube A stomach tube designed for the removal of specimens of gastric contents for analysis after administration of a test meal.

Reilly bodies. The cytoplasmic inclusions of Alder's anomaly.

re·im·plan·ta·tion (ree·im''plan·tay'shun) n. Replantation, as of a tooth.

Reincke's crystals (rine'keh) Rod-shaped crystalloids in the interstitial cells of the testis.

rei·necke salt (rye'ne·kuh). Ammonium reineckate, $NH_4[Cr(NH_3)_2(SCN)_4].H_2O$. Dark-red crystalline powder; used as a reagent, especially for amines.

re·in·fec·tion (ree''in·feck'shun) n. A second infection with the same kind of organism.

reinfection tuberculosis. CHRONIC TUBERCULOSIS.

re·in·force·ment (ree''in·force'munt) n. Augmentation or strengthening by addition, repetition, or any action that contributes to a cumulative result. —**reinforce,** v.

reinforcement of reflexes. Increased myotatic irritability (or other reflex response) when muscular or mental actions are synchronously carried out, or other stimuli are coincidentally brought to bear upon parts of the body other than that concerned in the reflex arc.

re·in·fu·sion (ree''in·few'zhun) n. The reinjection of blood, serum, or cerebrospinal fluid.

re·in·ner·va·tion (ree·in''ur·vay'shun) n. Restoration of motor or sensory function, either spontaneously or by nerve grafting, to a part that had been deprived of its nerve supply.

re·in·oc·u·la·tion (ree''i·nock''yoo·lay'shun) n. Inoculation a second time with the same kind of organism.

re·in·te·gra·tion (ree''in''te·gray'shun) n. In psychiatry, the restoration to harmonious mental functioning after disintegration of the personality by a severe mental disorder, as by a psychosis.

re·in·ver·sion (ree''in·vur'zhun) n. The act of reducing an inverted uterus by the application of pressure to the fundus.

Rei·ter's syndrome or **disease** (rye'tur) The triad of idiopathic nongonococcal urethritis, conjunctivitis, and subacute or chronic polyarthritis; mucocutaneous lesions are common. Syn. arthritis urethritica, idiopathic blennorrheal arthritis, infectious uroarthritis.

re·ju·ve·nes·cence (re·joo''ve·nes'unce) n. A renewal of youth; a renewal of strength and vigor; specifically a restoration of sexual vigor.

re·lapse (re·laps', ree'laps) n. The return of symptoms and signs of a disease after apparent recovery.

relapsing fever. Any of a group of acute arthropod-borne diseases characterized by alternating febrile and afebrile periods; caused by spirochetes, and transmitted by the louse Pediculus humanus, and by ticks of the genus Ornithodorus. Syn. famine fever, spirillum fever, recurrent fever.

relapsing polychondritis. An idiopathic inflammatory disease of cartilage, especially of the ears, trachea, bronchi, larynx, and nose, which tends to recur and to eventuate in deformity; fever, malaise, and polyarthritis are associated; an immunologic basis is suspected.

re·late, v. 1. To enter or put into a relationship; to stand in relationship to another. 2. *In psychology and psychiatry,* to be in or establish a meaningful relationship with another individual or individuals, to interact with one's environment, usually on the basis that such interaction will be of significance.

re·la·tion, n. 1. Interdependence; mutual influence or connection between organs or parts. 2. Connection by consanguinity; kinship. 3. *In anatomy,* the position of parts of the body as regards each other. **—relation·al,** *adj.*

rel·a·tive, *adj.* 1. Connected with or considered in reference to something else, as relative accommodation. 2. Comparative or not absolute, as relative sterility, relative scotoma. 3. Not independent; stemming from another condition or state. 4. Of a magnitude, expressed as the ratio of the specified quantity to another magnitude, as relative humidity. 5. Involving a relative magnitude, as relative lymphocytosis.

relative accommodation. Extent of accommodation possible for any particular degree of convergence.

relative biologic effectiveness of radiation. The inverse ratio of tissue doses of two different types of radiation that produces a particular biologic response under identical conditions.

relative humidity. The amount of water vapor in the air as compared with the total amount the air would hold at a given temperature.

relative hyperopia. A high hyperopia in which distinct vision is possible only when excessive convergence is made.

relative lymphocytosis. Increase of lymphocytes in the differential leukocyte count; not necessarily an increase per unit volume of blood.

relative sterility. Inability to produce a viable child.

re·lax, v. 1. To loosen or make less tense. 2. To become less tense.

re·lax·ant (ree-lack'sunt) *adj.* & *n.* 1. Producing relaxation. 2. An agent that lessens or reduces tension, or produces relaxation. 3. *Obsol.* A laxative.

re·lax·a·tion (ree″lack·say′shun) *n.* A diminution of tension in a part; a diminution in functional activity, as relaxation of the skin or, more specifically, of a muscle.

re·lax·in (re·lack′sin) *n.* A water-soluble hormone found in human serum and the serums of certain other animals during pregnancy; probably acting with progesterone and estrogen, it causes relaxation of pelvic ligaments in the guinea pig.

re·lease phenomenon. Any behavior, motor function, or reflex that appears or is exaggerated as a result of the destruction of nerve tissues that normally serve to inhibit the neurons responsible for the particular function or reflex, as the increased tendon reflexes in limbs with interruption of corticospinal tracts.

release syndrome. A symptom complex that follows release of a part from severe crushing injury.

re·lief, n. The partial removal of anything distressing; alleviation of pain or discomfort.

re·lieve, v. To free from pain, discomfort, or distress; to alleviate.

¹REM Abbreviation for *rapid eye movement.*

²REM, rem Abbreviation for *roentgen equivalent man.*

Remak's reflex Flexion of the toes following irritation of the upper anterior thigh in spinal cord lesions.

re·me·di·al (re·mee′dee·ul) *adj.* 1. Having the nature of a remedy; relieving; curative. 2. Designed to correct a defect or faulty habit.

rem·e·dy, n. Anything used in the treatment of disease.

re·min·er·al·iza·tion (ree·min″ur·ul·i·zay′shun) *n.* The restoration of the mineral content of the body or any part, especially of bone.

re·mis·sion (re·mish′un) *n.* 1. Abatement or subsidence of the symptoms of disease. 2. The period of diminution thereof.

re·mit·tence (re·mit′unce) *n.* Temporary abatement or remission of symptoms. **—remit·tent** (-unt) *adj.*

remittent fever. A paroxysmal fever with exacerbations and remissions, but without return to normal temperature.

re·mote memory. Recall of events that occurred in the relatively distant past.

REM sleep The stage of sleep that follows the deep sleep of stages 3 and 4 and is characterized by bursts of rapid eye movements (REMs), loss of tonic activity of the facial muscles, and desynchronization of the electroencephalogram.

ren-, reni-, reno- A combining form meaning *kidney, renal.*

re·nal (ree′nul) *adj.* Pertaining to the kidney.

renal aminoaciduria. Excess amounts of one or more amino acids in the urine due to defective renal tubular reabsorption; the concentration of the relevant amino acids in the blood is normal or low.

renal anuria. Failure of urine formation due to intrinsic renal disease.

renal autoamputation. The condition in which a kidney is cut off functionally by a diseased or obstructed ureter.

renal calculus. A concretion in the kidney. Syn. *kidney stone.*

renal calix. One of the divisions or subdivisions of the renal pelvis. The major calices are the two or three (rarely four) primary divisions of the pelvis and the minor calices are the cuplike terminal subdivisions, between 4 and 13 in number, each of which receives one or more of the renal papillae.

renal cell carcinoma. A malignant tumor of the kidney whose parenchyma usually consists of large polygonal cells with abundant, often clear, cytoplasm. Syn. *Grawitz's tumor, clear cell carcinoma, hypernephroma.*

renal corpuscle. The glomerulus together with its glomerular capsule in the cortex of the kidney.

renal diabetes. RENAL GLYCOSURIA.

renal dwarfism. Failure to thrive from a certain growth point commonly seen in children with severe chronic renal failure.

renal failure. A reduction in kidney function,

acute or chronic, to a level at which the kidneys are unable to maintain normal biological homeostasis.

renal fascia. The connective-tissue investment of the kidney. There is an anterior and a posterior layer with the kidney and perirenal fat between. The two layers form a pocket; above, below, and laterally they are fused. Syn. *Gerota's fascia.*

renal glycosuria. An anomalous condition characterized by a low renal threshold for sugar together with a normal blood sugar level.

renal hypertension. RENOVASCULAR HYPERTENSION.

renal infantilism. RENAL DWARFISM.

renal insufficiency. A measurable quantitative reduction in renal function, acute or chronic.

renal osteodystrophy. RENAL RICKETS.

renal papillae. The summits of the renal pyramids projecting into the renal pelvis.

renal pelvis. The expansion of the proximal end of the ureter which receives the major and minor calices within the renal sinus.

renal pyramids. The conical masses composing the medullary substance of the kidney.

renal rickets. A metabolic bone disease due to increased bone resorption resulting from the acidosis and secondary hyperparathyroidism of renal insufficiency. Syn. *renal osteodystrophy, pseudorickets, renal osteitis, renal osteitis fibrosa generalista.*

renal sinus. The space surrounded by the mass of the kidney and occupied by the renal pelvis, calices, vessels, and parts of the renal capsule.

renal tubular acidosis. A heritable disorder characterized by the inability to acidify the urine. In the proximal renal tubular type, hyperchloremic acidosis results from incomplete reabsorption of bicarbonate in the proximal tubule and excessive base is lost in the urine; the disease is usually confined to males. In the distal type growth, retardation, rickets, nephrocalcinosis, and renal failure are seen predominantly in females, resulting from the inability of the distal tube to establish an acid urine.

renal tubules. The glandular tubules which elaborate the urine in the kidney.

Ren-du-Osler-Weber disease (rahⁿ-duᵉ') HEREDITARY HEMORRHAGIC TELANGIECTASIA.

renes. Plural of *ren.*

ren·i·form (ren'i·form) *adj.* Kidney-shaped.

re·nin (ree'nin) *n.* A proteolytic enzyme in kidney that acts on renin substrate to liberate angiotensin I.

ren·i·punc·ture (ren''i·punk'chur, ree'ni·punk''chur) *n.* Puncture of the capsule of a kidney.

ren·net (ren'it) *n.* 1. RENNIN. 2. A preparation of the lining of the calf stomach used as a source of rennin.

ren·nin (ren'in) *n.* The milk-coagulating enzyme found in the gastric juice of the fourth stomach of the calf. Syn. *chymosin.*

ren·nin·o·gen (re·nin'o·jen) *n.* The zymogen of rennin, found in the wall of the fourth stomach of the calf. Syn. *prorennin.*

ren·no·gen (ren'o·jen) *n.* RENNINOGEN.

Renografin. A trademark for meglumine diatrizoate in injectable dosage forms suitable for excretory urography, retrograde pyelography, and venography.

re·no·gram (ree'no·gram) *n.* 1. A continuous recording of the level of radioactivity monitored externally over each kidney after the intravenous injection of an appropriate radiopharmaceutical. 2. NEPHROGRAM.

re·no·pri·val (ree''no·prye'vul) *adj.* 1. Without kidneys. 2. Pertaining to or caused by absence of kidneys or kidney function.

renoprival hypertension. Systemic arterial hypertension presumed due to the absence of a renal vasodepressor substance in nephrectomized animals or man.

re·no·re·nal (ree''no·ree'nul, ren''o'·) *adj.* Of or pertaining to both kidneys; affecting one kidney and then the other.

renorenal reflex. The mechanism by which disease or injury of one kidney may produce pain in, or impair the function of, the opposite kidney.

re·no·tro·phic (ree''no·tro'fick, ·trof'ick) *adj.* Having the property of promoting enlargement of the kidneys.

re·no·vas·cu·lar (ree''no·vas'kew·lur) *adj.* Pertaining to the blood vessels of the kidneys.

renovascular hypertension. Systemic arterial hypertension as a result of intrinsic renal vascular disease; it is usually mediated through the renal pressor system.

ren un·gui·for·mis (ung''gwi·for'mis). HORSESHOE KIDNEY.

re·or·ga·ni·za·tion (ree·or''guh·ni·za'shun) *n.* Healing by the development of tissue elements similar to those lost through some morbid process.

reo·vi·rus (ree''o·vye'rus) *n.* A member of a group of hemagglutinating, ether-resistant ribonucleic acid viruses, about 72 millimicrons in diameter, producing distinctive intracytoplasmic inclusion bodies in monkey renal cells; parasitic for human and animal species.

REP, rep Abbreviation for *roentgen equivalent physical.*

rep. Abbreviation for *repetatur;* let it be repeated.

re·pair, *v.* To mend; to restore to a more normal state, artificially as by surgical means, or naturally through the process of healing.

re·par·a·tive (re·pār'uh·tiv) *adj.* Pertaining to or making repairs; repairing.

re·pel·lent, re·pel·lant (re·pel'unt) *adj.& n.* 1. Having a tendency or an action to repel or drive away. 2. A substance that repels, as any one of various chemicals used to repel or kill external parasites, such as mosquitoes, chiggers, or ticks.

re·pel·ler (re·pel'ur) *n.* An instrument used in large-animal obstetrics to push back the fetus so head and limbs can be placed for normal delivery.

re·per·cus·sion (ree''pur·kush'un) *n.* 1. BALLOTTEMENT. 2. A driving in, or dispersion of, a tumor or eruption.

re·per·cus·sive (ree''pur·kus'iv) *adj.* REPELLENT.

rep·e·ti·tion aphasia (rep''e·tish'un). A form of aphasia characterized by a selective disturbance of repetition of speech, though there is normal comprehension of what was said.

re·place·ment, n. In psychiatry, a mental mechanism operating outside of and beyond conscious awareness in which the real object or feeling is replaced by another; as in a phobia, the actual internal but hidden object of fear and dread is replaced by a substitute external one.

replacement fibrosis. Fibrosis that replaces destroyed tissues, in part or wholly.

replacement therapy. Therapy in which a natural body constituent or its synthetic equivalent is used to replace a function which has been destroyed surgically or has ceased naturally.

re·plan·ta·tion (ree″plan·tay′shun) n. 1. The act of planting again. 2. The replacement of teeth that have been extracted or otherwise removed from their alveolar sockets, usually after appropriate treatment such as filling the root canals and planing the roots.

re·ple·tion (re·plee′shun) n. The condition of being, or the act of making, full. —**re·plete** (re·pleet′) adj.

rep·li·ca·tion (rep″li·kay′shun) n. 1. Multiplication of bacteriophage in bacterium; the phage loses its identity after entering bacterium, and shortly before lysis of the bacterium new phages of adult size and consistency appear. 2. The repetition of an experiment under the same conditions to check for possible error due to personal factors of the observer. 3. A folding back of a part; reduplication. —**rep·li·cate** (rep′li·kate) v.

re·po·lar·iza·tion (re·po″lur·i·zay′shun) n. Restoration of the resting or polarized state in a nerve or muscle fiber during recovery from conduction of an impulse or series of impulses.

re·po·si·tion (ree″puh·zish′un) n. The return of an abnormally placed part, organ, or fragment to its proper position.

re·pos·i·to·ry (re·poz′i·tor·ee) adj. & n. 1. Of a drug: prepared in a form that is slowly absorbed and acts over a prolonged period. 2. A receptacle, place, or substance in which something is stored or deposited.

re·pres·sion (re·presh′un) n. 1. In psychiatry, a defense mechanism whereby ideas, feelings, or desires, in conflict with the individual's conscious self-image or motives, are unconsciously dismissed from consciousness. 2. Sometimes, any defense mechanism.

re·pres·sor (re·pres′ur) n. An agent, usually a metabolic end product, which represses the synthesis of the enzymes in the metabolic pathway.

re·pro·duc·tion (ree″pruh·duck′shun) n. A fundamental property of protoplasm by which organisms give rise to other organisms of the same kind.

re·pro·duc·tive (ree″pruh·duck′tiv) adj. Of or pertaining to reproduction.

re·pul·sion (re·pul′shun) n. The act of repelling or driving back or apart.

RER Abbreviation for rough-surfaced endoplasmic reticulum.

RES Abbreviation for reticuloendothelial system.

res·az·u·rin (res·az′yoo·rin) n. So-called diazoresorcinol, a phenoxazine compound, $C_{12}H_7NO_4$; dark-red crystals with a greenish luster. Variously used as a reagent, especially as an oxidation-reduction indicator in the bacteriologic examination of milk.

res·cin·na·mine (re·sin′uh·meen, ·min) n. An alkaloid, $C_{35}H_{42}N_2O_9$, in certain species of Rauwolfia; an antihypertensive and sedative drug.

re·sect (ree·sekt′) v. 1. To cut out a portion of a tissue or organ. 2. To cut away the end of one or more of the bones entering into a joint.

re·sec·tion (ree·seck′shun) n. The operation of cutting out, as the removal of a section or segment of an organ.

re·sec·to·scope (ree·seck′tuh·skope) n. A tubular instrument by means of which small structures may be divided or removed within a body cavity without an opening or incision other than that made by the instrument itself; used especially for prostatectomy.

re·ser·pine (re·sur′peen, ·pin) n. 3,4,5-Trimethoxybenzoyl methyl reserpate, $C_{33}H_{40}N_2O_9$, an alkaloid in certain species of Rauwolfia; an antihypertensive and sedative drug.

re·serve, n. 1. A remainder. 2. A capacity or potentiality retained as an additional store.

reserve-cell carcinoma. OAT-CELL CARCINOMA.

reserve cells. 1. Small undifferentiated epithelial cells at the base of the stratified columnar lining of the bronchial tree. 2. CHROMOPHOBE CELLS.

reserve force. Energy latent within an organism or part over and above that required for normal function.

res·er·voir (rez′ur·vwahr) n. 1. A storage cavity or place. 2. A living organism that supports the growth of an infectious agent although suffering little or no effects from that agent. 3. RESERVOIR HOST.

reservoir host. An animal species on which the parasite depends for its survival in nature and which serves as the source of infection of other species, including man.

res·i·dent, adj. & n. 1. Dwelling in a given place, often as required by regulation or in connection with professional duties. 2. Stable; fixed. 3. A physician serving a major portion of the time in the hospital for further training after an internship. —**resi·dence, resi·den·cy,** n.

resident flora. In surgery, the portion of the cutaneous bacterial flora which is relatively stable, and relatively difficult to remove by washing or destroy by means of antiseptics. It consists principally of staphylococci of low pathogenicity.

re·sid·u·al (re·zid′yoo·ul) adj. Characterizing or pertaining to that which cannot be evacuated or discharged, or which remains.

residual air. RESIDUAL VOLUME.

residual bodies. In the developing spermatid, the anucleate masses that appear in the lumen of tubules after the cytoplasm is shed.

residual cyst. An odontogenic cyst remaining after the loss of the tooth with which it was associated.

residual urine. The urine remaining in the bladder after urination.

residual volume. Air remaining in the lungs after the most complete expiration possible. It is elevated in diffuse obstructive emphysema and during an attack of asthma. Syn. *residual air* or *capacity.*

res·i·due (rez'i-dew) *n.* That which remains after a part has been removed; remainder.

re·sil·ience (re-zil'yunce) *n.* The quality of being elastic or resilient.

re·sil·ient (re-zil'yunt) *adj.* Rebounding; elastic.

res·in (rez'in) *n.* 1. One of a class of vegetable substances exuding from various plants; generally soluble in alcohol and in ether, and insoluble in water. They are composed largely of esters and ethers of organic acids and acid anhydrides. 2. A class of preparations made by extracting resin-containing drugs with alcohol, concentrating the liquid and adding it to water, whereby the resin and other water-insoluble principles precipitate and may be collected and dried. —**resin·ous** (·us) *adj.*

res·in·oid (rez'i-noid) *adj. & n.* 1. Having some of the properties of a resin. 2. A substance which has some of the properties of a resin.

re·sis·tance, *n.* 1. Opposition to force or external impression. 2. In electricity, the opposition offered by a conductor to the passage of the current. Abbreviated, **R.** 3. *In psychiatry,* a defense mechanism characterized by the individual's reluctance to bring repressed material to light and to give up habitual patterns of thinking, feeling, and acting to take on less neurotic and newer modes of adaptation. 4. *In microbiology,* native or acquired immunity. 5. Lack of sensitivity or response to a drug, hormone, or treatment.

re·sis·tant rickets (re-zis'tunt). VITAMIN D-REFRACTORY RICKETS.

res·o·lu·tion (res''uh·lew'shun) *n.* 1. The subsidence of any pathological process, as inflammation, and the return to normal of affected tissues, in some cases occurring by a process of enzymic digestion of an exudate followed by absorption of the products. 2. The ability of the eye or a lens to recognize nearby objects as separate from one another rather than blurred into one apparent object. 3. The separation of an optically inactive mixture of isomers into its optically active components. Syn. *mesotomy.* 4. The analysis of a vector into its component parts. 5. *In psychiatry,* the bringing together or the compromising of opposing views, as in the resolution of emotional conflict.

re·solve, *v.* 1. To return to the normal state after some pathologic process. 2. To separate (something) into its component parts.

re·sol·vent (re-zol'vunt) *adj & n.* 1. Capable of dissipating inflammatory processes or effecting absorption of a neoplasm. 2. An agent capable of these actions.

re·solv·ing power. 1. The capability of a photographic film to make clear the finest details of an object. 2. The capability of a lens to make clear the separation of two closely adjacent objects.

res·o·na·tor (rez'uh·nay''tur) *n.* Any physical body capable of being set into vibration in unison with another vibrating body. The thoracic cage, lung, and other human structures possess this capacity in limited degree.

res·o·nance (rez'uh·nunce) *n.* 1. The attribute of relatively long duration possessed by certain sounds. 2. Normal resonance; in physical diagnosis, the prolonged, nonmusical, composite sound which results from vibration of the normal chest, usually elicited by percussion. 3. *In chemistry,* the phenomenon of a compound simultaneously having the characteristics of two or more structural forms of the compound, thereby providing additional orbital paths for electrons and conferring greater stability on the compound than if it possessed only one of the structures involved. Benzene represents such a resonance hybrid of forms differing only in the alternation of double bonds in the ring.

res·o·nant (rez'uh·nunt) *adj.* Possessing, or capable of producing, resonance.

re·sorb (re-sorb', ·zorb') *v.* 1. To undergo resorption. 2. To dissolve or lyse.

re·sor·cin·ol (re-zor'sin-ole) *n. meta*-Dihydroxybenzene, $C_6H_4(OH)_2$; used in treatment of skin diseases for its antiseptic, keratolytic, exfoliative, and antifungal properties.

re·sorp·tion (re-sorp'shun, -zorp') *n.* The disappearance of all or part of a process, tissue, or exudate by biochemical reactions that may involve dissolution, lysis, absorption, and/or other actions. —**resorp·tive** (·tiv) *adj.*

re·spi·ra·ble (res'pi·ruh·bul, re·spye'ruh·bul) *adj.* Capable of being inspired and expired; capable of furnishing the gaseous interchange in the lungs necessary for life. —**re·spi·ra·bil·i·ty** (res''pi·ruh·bil'i·tee, re·spye''ruh·bil''i·tee) *n.*

res·pi·ra·tion (res''pi·ray'shun) *n.* 1. The physical and chemical processes by which tissues exchange gases with the medium in which they live; generally, aerobic respiration, by which most organisms utilize oxygen in energy-producing reactions and form carbon dioxide and water which is excreted as a waste product; less commonly, anaerobic respiration, by which certain lower organisms can sustain life for some time in the absence of oxygen. 2. The act of breathing with the lungs, consisting of inspiration, or the taking into the lungs of the ambient air, and of expiration, or the expelling of the modified air which contains more carbon dioxide than the air taken in. 3. Transport of respiratory gases (oxygen and carbon dioxide) by the blood.

res·pi·ra·tor (res'pi·ray''tur) *n.* A device or apparatus for producing artificial respiration.

res·pi·ra·to·ry (res'pi·ruh·to·ree, re·spye'ruh·to·ree) *adj.* Pertaining to respiration.

respiratory acidosis. Acidosis in which the tendency to decreased blood pH is due to retention of excessive carbon dioxide in the body. Physiologic compensation is largely by renal retention of sodium bicarbonate.

respiratory alkalosis. Alkalosis in which the tendency to increased blood pH is due to accelerated pulmonary elimination of carbon dioxide. Physiologic compensation is largely by accelerated renal excretion of sodium bicarbonate.

respiratory bronchiole. The last bronchiolar subdivision; one which has pulmonary alveoli in its wall. It is the first portion of the lung capable of gas exchange. NA (pl). *bronchioli respiratorii* (sing. *bronchiolus respiratorius*).

respiratory capacity. 1. VITAL CAPACITY. 2. The ability of the blood to combine with oxygen in the lungs and with the carbon dioxide from the tissues.

respiratory distress syndrome of the newborn. A disease of unknown cause in the first days of life of premature infants characterized by respiratory distress, cyanosis, easy collapsibility of alveoli, and loss of pulmonary surfactant. A hyaline membrane lines the alveoli and alveolar ducts when the disease persists for more than a few hours. Abbreviated, RDS.

respiratory insufficiency. Incompetence of the respiratory processes.

respiratory passage. Any part of the respiratory tract through which breathed air normally passes on its way to and from the lung alveoli. Syn. *airway.*

respiratory quotient. 1. The ratio of the volume of carbon dioxide evolved by respiring cells or tissues to the volume of oxygen consumed in the same time. 2. In respiration, the ratio of the volume of carbon dioxide expired to that of oxygen consumed in a given interval of time. Abbreviated, R.Q.

respiratory system. 1. The system of organs or structures involved in respiration. 2. Specifically, the system of organs and structures involved in breathing, including the respiratory tract, the lungs as a whole, the diaphragm, and the muscles and nerves subserving them.

re·spire, *v.* 1. To move air in and out of the lungs. 2. In animals, to consume oxygen and produce carbon dioxide; in plants, to consume carbon dioxide and produce oxygen.

res·pi·rom·e·ter (res″pi·rom′e·tur) *n.* A device for measurement of several characteristics of respiration.

res·pi·rom·e·try (res″pi·rom′e·tree) *n.* The quantitative study of respiration.

re·sponse, *n.* A change in the state of an organism, organ, tissue, or cell succeeding the application of a stimulus.

re·spon·si·bil·i·ty, *n.* 1. The moral, mental, or legal accountability for one's own acts or those of another. 2. The capacity to differentiate right from wrong. 3. *In legal medicine,* the accountability for professional acts.

¹rest, *n.* 1. Repose; inactivity; cessation of labor or action. 2. A mechanical supportive structure, as: an extension from a dental prosthesis that provides vertical or toothbearing support.

²rest, *n.* 1. Anything remaining or left over. 2. An epithelial remnant persisting after its developmental activity has ceased. Syn. *epithelial debris.*

re·ste·no·sis (ree″ste·no′sis) *n.* Recurrent narrowing, generally referring to the orifice of a heart valve after corrective surgery.

res·ti·form (res′ti·form) *adj.* Corded or cordlike.

resting tremor. A static or parkinsonian tremor, which is maximal in an attitude of repose and which is temporarily diminished by willed movement; with full relaxation, as when the limb is supported against gravity, and with complete rest, as in sleep, the tremor disappears.

resting wandering cell. HISTIOCYTE.

res·ti·tu·tion (res″ti·tew′shun) *n.* 1. The act of restoring. 2. *In obstetrics,* a rotation of the fetal head immediately after its birth. 3. *In psychiatry,* the psychic mechanism whereby the individual seeks to relieve himself of unconscious guilt by benevolent acts which undo, make good, or repair some harm.

rest·less legs. A condition characterized by creeping, crawling, itching, and sometimes pain of the legs and thighs which impels the patient to seek relief by moving the legs or walking. The state is usually benign but may be a prelude to uremic polyneuropathy. Syn. *restless legs of Ekbom, anxietas tibiarum. Wittmaack-Ekbom syndrome.*

res·to·ra·tion (res″to·ray′shun) *n.* 1. The return to a state of health, functioning, or a normal condition. 2. Reconstruction or replacement of a body part. 3. Any structure or appliance that restores or replaces damaged or lost dental parts. —**re·stor·a·tive** (re·stor′uh·tiv) *adj.*

re·stor·a·tive (re·stor′uh·tiv) *n.* A tonic.

re·straint, *n.* 1. Hindrance of any action, physical, moral, or mental. 2. The state of being controlled; confinement.

re·strin·gent (re·strin′junt) *n.* An astringent or styptic.

re·sul·tant (re·zul′tunt) *n.* 1. That which results; the outcome of any process or action. 2. The product or products of a chemical reaction. 3. A single vector equivalent to a set of vectors.

re·su·pi·nate (ree·sue′pi·nate) *adj.* Turned in an abnormal direction.

res·ur·rec·tion·ist (rez″uh·reck′shun·ist) *n.* One who steals dead bodies from the grave as subjects for dissection.

re·sus·ci·ta·tion (re·sus″i·tay′shun) *n.* 1. Restoration to life or consciousness after apparent death. 2. Specifically, restoration of breathing after respiratory arrest or drowning, or of heartbeat after cardiac arrest. —**re·sus·ci·tate** (re·sus′i·tate) *v.*

re·sus·ci·ta·tor (re·sus′i·tay″tur) *n.* A device or apparatus for ventilation of the lungs in resuscitation.

re·su·ture (ree·sue′chur) *n.* Secondary suture; suture of a wound some time after a first suture has been made.

re·tain·er (re·tay′nur) *n.* 1. A dental appliance for holding in position teeth which have been moved orthodontically. 2. Any inlay, crown, clasp, attachment, or other device that provides fixation or stabilization of a fixed or removable dental prosthesis.

re·tar·date (re·tahr′date) *n.* A person with mental retardation.

re·tar·da·tion (ree"tahr·day'shun) *n.* 1. Slow mental or physical functioning. 2. Specifically, MENTAL RETARDATION.

retch, *v.* To make a strong involuntary effort to vomit. —**retch·ing,** *n.*

re·te (ree'tee) *n.,* pl. **re·tia** (·tee·uh) Any network or decussation or interlacing, especially of capillary blood vessels.

re·ten·tion (re·ten'shun) *n.* 1. The act of retaining or holding back, as the holding of urine in the bladder due to some hindrance to urination. 2. The maintenance of orthodontically treated teeth in their reestablished positions until stability of their supporting tissues is established. 3. The fixation and stabilization of a dental prosthesis.

retention cyst. A cyst due to obstruction of outflow of secretion from a gland.

retention defect. RETENTIVE MEMORY DEFECT.

retention enema. Liquid injected into the rectum, the expulsion of which is delayed voluntarily in order to liquefy the rectal contents or provide medication.

retention of urine. A condition in which urine continues to be secreted by the kidneys but is retained in the bladder, as in atonic bladder or other urinary obstruction.

retentive memory defect. An impairment or loss of the ability to retain newly presented information, despite an alert state of mind, and intactness of comprehension and registration as demonstrated by the patient's ability to repeat information immediately after it is presented.

rete ova·rii (o·vair'ee·eye). Vestigial tubules or cords of cells near the hilus of the ovary, corresponding with the rete testis, but not connected with the mesonephric duct.

rete peg. The prolongation of the epidermis between the papillae of the corium; the interpapillary epithelium.

rete tes·tis (tes'tis) [NA]. The network of anastomosing tubules in the mediastinum testis.

retia. Plural of *rete*.

re·tic·u·lar (re·tick'yoo·lur) *adj.* Resembling a net; formed by a network.

reticular degeneration. A process in which intracellular edema of the epidermis causes rupture of the cells with formation of multilocular bullae.

reticular fibers. The delicate, branching connective-tissue fibers forming the reticular framework of lymphatic tissue, myeloid tissue, the red pulp of the spleen, the finest stroma of many glands, and most basement membranes. They differ from collagenous fibers in their response to silver impregnation, in which they are blackened. Syn. *argentaffin fibers, argentophile fibers, lattice fibers, precollagenous fibers.*

reticular formation or substance. Any of those portions of the brainstem core that are characterized structurally by a wealth of cells of various sizes and types, arranged in diverse aggregations and enmeshed in a complicated fiber network. Embedded in this matrix are specific nuclei and tracts.

reticular tissue. Connective tissue in which re-

ticular fibers are the conspicuous element, forming a branching nonelastic network.

re·tic·u·lat·ed (re·tick'yoo·lay"tid) *adj.* Having netlike meshes; formed like a web. —**re·tic·u·la·tion** (re·tick"yoo·lay'shun) *n.*

reticulated pigmented poikiloderma. A variety of Riehl's melanosis, located on the neck as a symmetric, pigmented, telangiectatic, and atrophic erythroderma with retiform arrangement. Causes include sunlight and photodynamic substances in cosmetics. Syn. *poikiloderma reticulare of Civatte. Civatte's poikiloderma.*

re·tic·u·lin (re·tick'yoo·lin) *n.* A protein isolated from the fibers of reticular tissue.

re·tic·u·lo·cyte (re·tick'yoo·lo·site) *n.* 1. An immature erythrocyte. Retention of ribosomes account for the reticulated appearance when stained supravitally with cresyl blue or when viewed by phase microscopy. It is larger than a normal erythrocyte and usually constitutes less than 1 percent (range: 0.5 to 2.5 percent) of the total. There is an increase during active erythrocytopoiesis. In Wright- or Giemsa-stained blood films, these cells appear as polychromatophilic erythrocytes. 2. RETICULUM CELL. —**re·tic·u·lo·cyt·ic** (re·tick"yoo·lo·sit'ick) *adj.*

reticulocytic sarcoma. RETICULUM-CELL SARCOMA.

re·tic·u·lo·cy·to·pe·nia (re·tick"yoo·lo·sigh"to·pee'nee·uh) *n.* Decrease of reticulocytes in the circulating blood.

re·tic·u·lo·cy·to·sis (re·tick"yoo·lo·sigh·to'sis) *n.,* pl. **reticulocyto·ses** (·seez) An excess of reticulocytes in the peripheral blood.

re·tic·u·lo·en·do·the·li·al (re·tick"yoo·lo·en"do·theel·ee·ul) *adj.* Of, pertaining to, or involving the reticuloendothelial system or the reticuloendothelium.

reticuloendothelial granulomatosis. A group of rare diseases characterized by generalized reticuloendothelial hyperplasia with or without intracellular lipid deposition. Included in this group are Letterer-Siwe's disease, Hand-Schüller-Christian disease, and eosinophilic granuloma.

reticuloendothelial system. The macrophage system, which includes all the phagocytic cells of the body, except the granulocytic leukocytes. These cells, diverse morphologically, all have the capacity for the elective storage of certain colloidal dyes. They include the histiocytes and macrophages of loose connective tissue, the reticular cells of lymphatic and myeloid tissues, the microglia, the blood monocytes, the endothelium-like littoral cells lining lymphatic sinuses and sinusoids of bone marrow, the Kupffer cells of hepatic sinusoids, the cells lining the sinusoids of the adrenal and hypophysis, the pulmonary alveolar macrophages (dust cells), and the microglia cells of the central nervous system. Abbreviated, RES. Syn. *system of macrophages.*

re·tic·u·lo·en·do·the·li·o·ma (re·tick"yoo·lo·en"do·theel·ee·o'muh) *n.* RETICULUM-CELL SARCOMA.

re·tic·u·lo·en·do·the·li·o·sis (re·tick"yoo·lo·en"

do·theel·ee·o'sis) n., pl. **reticuloendothelio·ses** (·seez) HISTIOCYTOSIS X.

re·tic·u·lo·en·do·the·li·um (re·tick"yoo·lo·en"do·theel'ee·um) n. The basic tissue that forms the reticuloendothelial system.

re·tic·u·lo·pe·nia (re·tick"yoo·lo·pee'nee·uh) n. RETICULOCYTOPENIA.

re·tic·u·lo·sar·co·ma (re·tick"yoo·lo·sahr·ko'muh) n. RETICULUM-CELL SARCOMA.

re·tic·u·lo·sis (re·tick"yoo·lo'sis) n., pl. **reticulo·ses** (·seez) HISTIOCYTOSIS X.

re·tic·u·lo·the·li·o·ma (re·tick"yoo·lo·theel"ee·o'muh) n. RETICULUM-CELL SARCOMA.

re·tic·u·lo·the·li·um (re·tick"yoo·lo·theel'ee·um) n. RETICULOENDOTHELIUM. —**reticulotheli·al** (·ul) adj.

re·tic·u·lum (re·tick'yoo·lum) n., pl. **reticu·la** (·luh) 1. A fine network. 2. In veterinary medicine, the second division of the ruminant stomach. —**reticu·lose** (·loce) adj.

reticulum cell. A cell of reticular tissue.

reticulum-cell lymphosarcoma. RETICULUM-CELL SARCOMA.

reticulum-cell sarcoma. A type of malignant lymphoma in which the predominant cell type is an anaplastic reticulum cell. Multinucleated cells also occur. Syn. histiocytic sarcoma.

re·tif·ism (ree'ti·fiz·um, re·teef'iz·um) n. A sexual perversion in which a shoe or foot has the same erotic value as the genital organs.

ret·i·form (ret'i·form, ree'ti·) adj. Net-shaped; RETICULAR.

retin-, retino-. A combining form meaning retina, retinal.

ret·i·na (ret'i·nuh) n., L. pl. & genit. sing. **reti·nae** (·nee), E. pl. **retinas** The light-receptive layer and terminal expansion of the optic nerve in the eye. It extends from the point of exit of the nerve forward to the ora serrata. It consists of the following layers, named from behind forward: the pigment layer; the neuroepithelial layer, comprising the layer of rods and cones (bacillary layer), the outer limiting membrane, and the outer nuclear layer; the outer reticular layer (outer granular or plexiform layer), the inner nuclear layer, the inner reticular layer (inner granular or plexiform layer), the ganglionic layer, the nerve fiber layer. These layers are united and supported by neuroglial elements. Adj. retinal.

ret·i·nac·u·lum (ret"i·nack'yoo·lum) n., pl. **retina·cu·la** (·luh) A special fascial thickening that holds back an organ or part.

ret·i·nal (ret'i·nul) adj. & n. 1. Pertaining to or involving the retina. 2. RETINENE.

retinal correspondence. The relationship between corresponding points in the retina of both eyes, simultaneous stimulation of which results in the sensation of one image.

retinal detachment. DETACHMENT OF THE RETINA.

retinal dialysis. A disinsertion of the retina from its attachment to the ora serrata.

retinal dysplasia. A developmental anomaly present at birth involving the inner layer of the neuroectoderm forming the optic vesicle; a consistent finding of trisomy 13 syndrome.

retinal glioma. Neuroepithelioma of the retina.

retinal image. The image of external objects as focused on the retina.

retinal reflex. A round or linear light area reflected from the retina when the retinoscope is employed.

ret·i·nene (ret'i·neen) n. A pigment extracted from the retina, turned yellow by light; the chief carotenoid of the retina, appearing in two forms, retinene$_1$ and retinene$_2$, the aldehydes of vitamin A$_1$ and vitamin A$_2$. Under the influence of light, retinene$_1$ combines with rod opsin to form rhodopsin, and with cone opsin to form iodopsin, while retinene$_2$ combines with rod opsin to form porphyropsin and with cone opsin to form cyanopsin. Syn. retinal.

ret·i·ni·tis (ret"i·nigh'tis) n., pl. **reti·nit·i·des** (·nit'i·deez) Inflammation of the retina.

retinitis exu·da·ti·va (eck·sue·da·tye'vuh). The response of histiocytes and fixed tissues to any subretinal hemorrhage, resulting in the production of a pigmented fibrous nodule containing fat-laden histiocytes; it is not a specific disease. Syn. Coat's disease.

retinitis pig·men·to·sa (pig·men·to'suh). A retinal dystrophy of the outer retinal layers characterized by nyctalopia (night blindness), constriction of the visual field, narrowed retinal arterioles, intraretinal pigmentation, and preservation of good visual acuity until late in the course of the disease; occurs in autosomal dominant, autosomal recessive, or x-linked form and in association with a variety of degenerative disorders, including Laurence-Moon-Biedl syndrome, abetalipoproteinemia, and cerebellospinal degenerations.

retinitis pro·li·fer·ans (pro·lif'ur·anz). Neovascularization of retinal vessels with extension into the vitreous; occurs in diabetic retinopathy and retrolental fibroplasia.

ret·i·no·blas·to·ma (ret"i·no·blas·to'muh) n. A hereditary malignant tumor of the sensory portion of the retina transmitted as an autosomal dominant trait.

ret·i·no·cho·roid·i·tis (ret"i·no·ko"roy·dye'tis) n. Inflammation of the retina and choroid.

ret·i·no·cy·to·ma (ret"i·no·sigh·to'muh) n. Neuroepithelioma of the retina.

ret·i·no·di·al·y·sis (ret"i·no·dye·al'i·sis) n. DISINSERTION (2).

ret·i·no·ic acid (ret"i·no'ick). Vitamin A acid, C$_{20}$H$_{28}$O$_2$, obtained by oxidizing the alcohol group in vitamin A (retinol) to carboxyl. It occurs in two stereoisomeric forms: 9,10-cis-retinoic acid and all-trans-retinoic acid, the latter used for treatment of scaling dermatoses.

ret·i·no·pap·il·li·tis (ret"i·no·pap"i·lye'tis) n. Inflammation of the retina and the optic disk.

ret·i·nop·a·thy (ret"i·nop'uth·ee) n. Any morbid condition of the retina.

ret·i·no·pexy (ret'i·no·peck"see) n. Fixation of a detached retina by operation, or by other methods such as laser, photocoagulation, freezing, or diathermy.

ret·i·nos·chi·sis (ret"i·nos'ki·sis) n., pl. **retinoschi·ses** (·seez) 1. Separation of the retinal layers, with hole formation; usually a degenerative change associated with aging. 2. A congenital anomaly characterized by cleavage of the retina.

ret·i·no·scope (ret′i·nuh·skope) n. An instrument employed in retinoscopy.

ret·i·nos·co·py (ret′i·nos′kuh·pee) n. A method of determining the refraction of the eye by observation of the movements of the shadow phenomena produced and observed by means of a retinoscope.

re·tort (re·tort′) n. A distilling vessel consisting of an expanded globular portion and a long neck.

re·to·the·li·o·ma (ree′′to·theel·ee·o′muh) n. RETICULUM-CELL SARCOMA.

re·to·the·li·o·sar·co·ma (ree′′to·theel′′ee·o·sahr·ko′muh) n. RETICULUM-CELL SARCOMA.

ret·o·the·li·um (ret′′o·theel′ee·um) n. RETICULO-ENDOTHELIUM. —**retotheli·al** (·ul) adj.

re·tract, v. To draw back; to contract; to shorten.

retracted nipple. A nipple below the surrounding level of skin.

re·trac·til·i·ty (ree′′track·til′i·tee) n. The power of retracting or drawing back. —**re·trac·tile** (re·track′til, ·tile) adj.

re·trac·tion, n. The act of retracting or drawing back, as a retraction of the muscles after amputation.

retraction nystagmus. Oscillations of the eyes, which may be horizontal, vertical, or rotatory, accompanied by a drawing of the globes backward into the orbit; may occur spontaneously or on voluntary movements, but usually seen only when there is paresis of upward gaze.

retraction ring. A ridge at the junction of the upper and lower segments of the uterus. Syn. contraction ring.

re·trac·tor, n. 1. A surgical instrument for holding back the edges of a wound to give access to deeper parts or regions. It consists ordinarily of a handle with a right-angle flange. 2. In anatomy, FLEXOR.

retro- A combining form meaning back, backward, or behind.

ret·ro·ac·tion (ret′′ro·ack′shun) n. Reverse action.

ret·ro·an·tero·grade (ret′′ro·an′tur·o·grade) adj. Reversing the usual order of a succession.

ret·ro·bul·bar (ret′′ro·bul′bur) adj. 1. Situated or occurring behind the eyeball. 2. Behind the medulla oblongata.

retrobulbar neuritis or **neuropathy.** Acute impairment of vision in one eye, or in both eyes either simultaneously or successively, due to affection of the optic nerve(s) by demyelinative or nutritional disease or by toxins. The optic disc and retina may appear normal, but if the lesion is near the nerve head there may be swelling of the optic disc (papillitis) and the disc margins may be blurred and surrounded by hemorrhages.

re·tro·cal·ca·ne·al (ret′′ro·kal·kay′nee·ul) adj. Behind the calcaneus.

re·tro·cal·ca·neo·bur·si·tis (ret′′ro·kal·kay′nee·o·bur·sigh′tis) n. ACHILLOBURSITIS.

ret·ro·car·di·ac (ret′′ro·kahr′dee·ack) adj. Posterior to the heart.

ret·ro·ca·val (ret′′ro·kay′vul) adj. Behind a caval vein, usually the inferior vena cava.

ret·ro·ce·cal, ret·ro·cae·cal (ret′′ro·see′kul) adj. Pertaining to the back of the cecum.

ret·ro·cele (ret′ro·seel) n. Persistence of the post-anal part of the embryonic hindgut. Syn. congenital retrocele.

ret·ro·ces·sion (ret′′ro·sesh′un) n. 1. Backward displacement of the entire uterus. 2. Spread of disease from the body surface to deeper areas.

ret·ro·chei·lia (ret′′ro·kigh′lee·uh) n. A condition in which a lip is farther posterior than is normal.

ret·ro·col·ic (ret′′ro·ko′lick, ·kol′ick) adj. Behind the colon.

ret·ro·col·lis (ret′′ro·kol′is) n. Retraction or extension in torticollis.

ret·ro·con·dy·lism (ret′′ro·kon′di·liz·um) n. Posterior deviation of the mandibular condyles.

ret·ro·de·vi·a·tion (ret′′ro·dee′′vee·ay′shun) n. Any backward displacement; a retroflexion or retroversion.

ret·ro·dis·place·ment (ret′′ro·dis·place′munt) n. Backward displacement of a part or organ, especially uterine displacement.

ret·ro·du·o·de·nal (ret′′ro·dew·od′e·nul, ·dew·o·dee′nul) adj. Behind the duodenum.

ret·ro·esoph·a·ge·al, ret·ro·oe·soph·a·ge·al (ret′′ro·e·sof′′uh·jee′ul) adj. Located behind the esophagus.

ret·ro·flex (ret′′ro·flecks) v. To turn back abruptly.

ret·ro·flex·ion (ret′′ro·fleck′shun) n. The state of being bent backward.

ret·ro·gas·se·ri·an (ret′′ro·ga·seer′ee·un) adj. Behind the trigeminal or gasserian ganglion.

ret·ro·gnath·ism (ret′′ro·nath′iz·um) n. Posterior deviation of the mandible.

ret·ro·grade (ret′ro·grade) adj. Going backward; moving contrary to the normal or previous direction or order; characterized by retrogression.

retrograde amnesia. Loss of memory for events that had occurred before the onset of the current injury or illness.

retrograde embolism. An embolism in which the embolus has gone against the normal direction of the bloodstream.

retrograde pyelography or **urography.** Visualization of the renal collecting system by instillation of radiographic contrast medium into the ureters through catheters inserted with the aid of a cystoscope.

re·trog·ra·phy, n. MIRROR WRITING.

ret·ro·gres·sion, n. 1. In biology, the passing from a higher to a lower type of structure in the development of an animal. 2. In medicine, a going backward; degeneration, involution, or atrophy, as of tissue. 3. The subsidence of a disease or its symptoms. 4. In psychology, a return to earlier, more infantile behavior. —**retro·gres·sive** (·gres′iv) adj.

ret·ro·jec·tion (ret′′ro·jeck′shun) n. The washing out of a cavity from within outward.

ret·ro·jec·tor (ret′′ro·jeck′tur) n. An instrument for washing out the uterus.

ret·ro·len·tal (ret′′ro·len′tul) adj. Behind the lens of the eye.

retrolental fibroplasia. An oxygen-induced retinopathy of premature infants.

ret·ro·len·tic·u·lar (ret″ro·len·tick′yoo·lur) *adj.* RETROLENTAL.

ret·ro·lin·gual (ret″ro·ling′gwul) *adj.* Pertaining to the part of the pharynx behind the tongue.

ret·ro·ma·lar (ret″ro·may′lur) *adj.* Behind the zygoma.

ret·ro·mam·ma·ry (ret″ro·mam′uh·ree) *adj.* Behind the breast.

ret·ro·man·dib·u·lar (ret″ro·man·dib′yoo·lur) *adj.* Behind the mandible.

re·tro·max·il·lary (ret″ro·mack′si·lerr·ee) *adj.* Behind the maxilla.

ret·ro·mor·pho·sis (ret″ro·mor′fo·sis, ·mor·fo′sis) *n.* 1. CATABOLISM. 2. Retrograde metamorphosis; METAMORPHOSIS (2).

ret·ro·na·sal (ret″ro·nay′zul) *adj.* Situated behind the nose or nasal cavities; postnasal.

ret·ro·oc·u·lar (ret″ro·ock′yoo·lur) *adj.* Behind the eye.

ret·ro·or·bi·tal (ret″ro·or′bi·tul) *adj.* Behind the orbit.

ret·ro·pa·rot·id (ret″ro·pa·rot′id) *adj.* Behind the parotid gland.

ret·ro·per·i·to·ne·al (ret″ro·perr′i·to·nee′ul) *adj.* Situated behind the peritoneum.

retroperitoneal hernia. A hernia into a recess of the peritoneum, as into a paraduodenal recess.

retroperitoneal space. The space behind the peritoneum, but in front of the vertebral column and lumbar muscles; in it lie the kidneys, the aorta, the inferior vena cava, and the sympathetic trunk.

ret·ro·peri·to·ni·tis (ret″ro·perr′i·tuh·nigh′tis) *n.* Inflammation of the structures in the retroperitoneal space.

ret·ro·pha·ryn·ge·al (ret″ro·fa·rin′jee·ul, ·fār″in·jee′ul) *adj.* Situated behind the pharynx.

ret·ro·phar·yn·gi·tis (ret″ro·fār″in·jye′tis) *n.* Inflammation of the retropharyngeal tissues.

ret·ro·pla·cen·tal (ret″ro·pluh·sen′tul) *adj.* Behind the placenta.

ret·ro·pla·sia (ret″ro·play′zhuh, ·zee·uh) *n.* Retrograde change in a tissue; DEGENERATION.

ret·ro·posed (ret′ro·poazd′) *adj.* Displaced backward.

ret·ro·po·si·tion (ret″ro·puh·zish′un) *n.* Backward displacement of the uterus without flexion or version.

ret·ro·pros·tat·ic (ret″ro·pros·tat′ick) *adj.* Behind the prostate.

ret·ro·pu·bic (ret″ro·pew′bick) *adj.* Behind the pubis.

retropubic prostatectomy. Removal of the prostate by an approach through the prevesical space.

retropubic space. A space lying immediately above the pubis and between the peritoneum and the posterior surface of the rectus abdominis. Syn. *prevesical space, space of Retzius.*

ret·ro·pul·sion (ret″ro·pul′shun) *n.* 1. A driving or turning back, as of the fetal head. 2. An involuntary backward walking or running observed in postencephalitic parkinsonism.

ret·ro·py·ram·i·dal (ret″ro·pi·ram′i·dul) *adj.* Situated behind a pyramid (2).

ret·ro·stal·sis (ret″ro·stal′sis, ·stahl′sis) *n.* REVERSED PERISTALSIS.

ret·ro·tar·sal (ret″ro·tahr′sul) *adj.* Situated behind the tarsus, as the retrotarsal fold of the conjunctiva.

ret·ro·ten·di·nous (ret″ro·ten′di·nus) *adj.* Behind a tendon.

ret·ro·ten·do·achil·lis (ret″ro·ten″do·uh·kil′is) *adj.* Behind the calcaneal tendon.

ret·ro·thy·roid (ret″ro·thigh′roid) *adj.* Behind the thyroid gland.

ret·ro·ton·sil·lar (ret″ro·ton′si·lur) *adj.* Behind a pharyngeal tonsil.

ret·ro·tra·che·al (ret″ro·tray′kee·ul) *adj.* Situated or occurring behind the trachea.

ret·ro·ver·sio·flex·ion (ret″ro·vur″see·o·fleck′shun, ·vur″zho·) *n.* Combined retroversion and retroflexion.

ret·ro·ver·sion (ret″ro·vur′zhun) *n.* A turning back.

ret·ro·vert·ed (ret″ro·vur′tid) *adj.* Tilted or turned backward, as a retroverted uterus.

ret·ro·ves·i·cal (ret″ro·ves′i·kul·) *adj.* Behind the urinary bladder.

re·trude (re·trood′) *v.* To force inward or backward, as in orthodontically repositioning protruding teeth.

re·tru·sion (re·troo′zhun) *n.* 1. The act or process of pressing teeth backward. 2. The condition characterized by the backward or posterior position of the teeth or jaws.

re·un·ion, *n.* In fractures, the securing of union following its interruption by violence or disease.

re·vac·ci·na·tion (ree″vack·si·nay′shun) *n.* Renewed or repeated vaccination.

re·vas·cu·lar·iza·tion (ree·vas″kew·lur·i·zay′shun) *n.* Reestablishment of a blood supply, as after interruption or destruction of the old vessels due to injury or grafting.

rev·e·hent (reve·hunt, re·vee′unt) *adj.* Carrying back.

re·ver·sal, *n.* 1. A turning around, as the reversal of any pathologic process to a state of healing or health. 2. *In psychiatry,* the change of the content or aim of an instinct or mode of behavior into the opposite, as love into hate, or sadism into masochism.

re·verse, *n.* In bandaging, a half-turn employed to change the direction of a bandage.

reversed peristalsis. Peristaltic movement opposite to the normal direction.

reversed Prausnitz-Küstner test An urticarial reaction appearing at an injection site when reagin-containing serum is injected into the skin of a person in whom the allergen is already present; the reaction which appears when Prausnitz-Küstner antibody is administered, not before, but after, the administration of the antigen.

reverse passive anaphylaxis. Hypersensitivity produced when the antigen is injected first, then followed in several hours by the specific antibody, causing shock.

reverse pinocytosis. EMIOCYTOSIS.

re·ver·sion (re·vur′zhun) *n.* The reappearance of long-lost ancestral traits; THROWBACK.

re·vi·tal·iza·tion (ree-vye″tul·i·zay′shun) *n.* The act or process of refreshing.

re·vive, *v.* To return to life after seeming death; to return to consciousness or strength.

re·viv·i·fi·ca·tion (ree-vye″i·fi·kay′shun) *n.* Restoration of life after apparent death.

rev·o·lute (rev′uh-lewt) *adj.* Turned backward or downward.

re·vul·sant (re·vul′sunt) *adj. & n.* 1. Tending to revulsion (2). 2. A revulsive agent.

re·vul·sion (re·vul′shun) *n.* 1. A strong feeling of distaste or dislike. 2. Reduction of local hyperemia or inflammation by means of counterirritation.

re·vul·sive (re·vul′siv) *adj.* 1. Characterized by an altered distribution of blood in one part through congestion or irritation produced elsewhere in the body. 2. Causing revulsion.

Reye's syndrome An acute illness of childhood, which usually follows a respiratory or gastrointestinal viral infection, or varicella. It is characterized clinically by fever, vomiting, disturbance of consciousness progressing to coma, and convulsions, and pathologically by fatty infiltration of the parenchymal cells of the liver and kidneys, and brain swelling.

R. F. A. Right frontoanterior position of the fetus.

R. F. P. Right frontoposterior position of the fetus.

Rh Pertaining to or designating an agglutinogen first found in the red blood cells of the rhesus monkey.

Rh₀(D) antigen. The major antigen of the Rh blood group.

rhabd-, rhabdo- A combining form meaning (a) *stick, rod;* (b) *striped, banded, striated.*

Rhab·di·tis (rab·dye′tis) *n.* A genus of phasmid nematodes a few species of which are parasitic in man but of doubtful pathogenicity.

rhab·do·myo·blast·ic mixed tumor (rab″domigh″o·blas′tick) A malignant mixed mesodermal tumor with a prominent component of anaplastic striated muscle cells.

rhab·do·myo·blas·to·ma (rab″do·migh″o·blas·to′muh) *n.* RHABDOMYOSARCOMA.

rhab·do·my·ol·y·sis (rab″do·migh·ol′i·sis) *n.* Destruction or necrosis of skeletal muscle, often accompanied by myoglobinuria.

rhab·do·my·o·ma (rab″do·migh·o′muh) *n.* A benign tumor, usually hamartomatous, of striated muscle.

rhabdomyoma ute·ri (yoo″tur·eye). SARCOMA BOTRYOIDES.

rhab·do·myo·sar·co·ma (rab″do·migh″o·sahr·ko′muh) *n.* A malignant tumor, usually involving the muscles of the extremities or torso, composed of anaplastic striated muscle cells. Syn. *malignant rhabdomyoma, rhabdomyoblastoma.*

rhab·do·pho·bia (rhab″do·fo′bee·uh) *n.* An unwarranted dread of being beaten; unreasoning fear aroused by the sight of a stick.

rhachi-, rhachio-. See *rachi-.*

rha·cous (rack′us, ray′kus) *adj.* Wrinkled; lacerated; fissured.

rhag·a·des (rag′uh·deez) *n.pl.* Linear cracks or fissures occurring in skin that has lost its elasticity through infiltration and thickening;

observed in syphilis, intertrigo, keratoderma, and other affections.

rha·gad·i·form (ra·gad′i·form) *adj.* Fissured.

rhag·i·o·crin, rhag·i·o·crine (raj′ee·o·krin) *adj.* Characterizing or pertaining to colloid-filled vacuoles in the cytoplasm of secretory cells representing a stage in the development of secretory granules.

rhag·oid (rag′oid) *adj.* Resembling a grape.

Rh antiserums. Antiserums reacting with one or more of the Rh factors.

rha·pon·tic (ra·pon′tick) *adj.* Pertaining to rhubarb.

Rh blood group. The extensive system of erythrocyte antigens originally defined by reactions with the serum of rabbits immunized with the erythrocytes of rhesus monkeys, and recently by antiserums of human origin.

rhe·bo·sce·lia, rhae·bo·sce·lia (ree″bo·see′lee·uh) *n.* The condition of being bowlegged. **—rhebosce·lic, rhaebosce·lic** (·lick) *adj.*

rheg·ma (reg′muh) *n.* 1. A rupture of the walls of a vessel or region, as of the containing membrane of an organ or region, as the coats of the eye, the walls of the peritoneum. 2. The bursting of an abscess.

rheg·ma·tog·e·nous (reg″muh·toj′e·nus) *adj.* 1. Producing rupture, bursting, or fracturing. 2. Producing retinal detachment characterized by a hole or tear.

rhem·bas·mus (rem·baz′mus) *n.* Mental distraction; INDECISION.

rhe·ni·um (ree′nee·um) *n.* Re = 186.2. A metallic element, atomic number 75, of the manganese group; occurs as a minor constituent in many ores.

rheo- A combining form meaning *flow,* as of liquids, or *pertaining to a current.*

rheo·base (ree′o·bace) *n.* The minimum electric potential necessary for stimulation.

rheo·en·ceph·a·log·ra·phy (ree″o·en·sef″uh·log′ruh·fee) *n.* A method of continuous recording of the changes in an electrical current passed through the head for the purpose of demonstrating cerebral blood flow patterns and their pathologic alterations.

rhe·ol·o·gy (ree·ol′uh·jee) *n.* The science of deformation and flow of matter in such a state that it exhibits a tendency to be deformed by the application of force. **—rhe·o·log·ic** (ree″o·loj′ick) *adj.*

rhe·om·e·ter (ree·om′e·tur) *n.* 1. GALVANOMETER. 2. An apparatus for measuring the velocity of the blood current. 3. An apparatus for measuring the flow of viscous materials.

rheo·stat (ree′o·stat) *n.* An apparatus for regulating the amount of electrical current flowing in a circuit by varying the resistance in the circuit.

rhe·os·to·sis (ree″os·to′sis) *n.* OSTEOPETROSIS.

rheo·ta·chyg·ra·phy (ree″o·ta·kig′ruh·fee) *n.* The registration of the curve of variation in electromotive action of muscles.

rheo·taxis (ree″o·tack′sis) *n.* A taxis in which mechanical stimulation by a current of fluid, as of water, is the directing influence to cause movement of an entire organism against the force of the current.

rheo·trope (ree'o-trope) *n.* An apparatus for reversing the direction of an electric current. Syn. *commutator.*

rhe·ot·ro·pism (ree-ot'ruh-piz·um) *n.* A tropism in which mechanical stimulation by a current of fluid, as of water, is the directing influence and causes movement of a part of an organism against the motion of the force of the current.

rheu·mat·ic (roo-mat'ick) *adj.* & *n.* 1. Pertaining to, of the nature of, or affected with rheumatism. 2. A person suffering from rheumatism.

rheumatic arteritis. Diffuse involvement of small cerebral arteries observed in patients with rheumatic heart disease. The vascular lesions and the microinfarcts that accompany them probably represent multiple cerebral emboli.

rheumatic arthritis. 1. Migratory polyarthritis, particularly of the large joints of the extremities, that is completely reversible; occurs during acute rheumatic fever. 2. RHEUMATOID ARTHRITIS.

rheumatic brain disease. 1. RHEUMATIC ARTERITIS. 2. SYDENHAM'S CHOREA.

rheumatic carditis. Inflammation of the heart associated with rheumatic fever.

rheumatic encephalopathy or **encephalitis.** RHEUMATIC BRAIN DISEASE.

rheumatic endocarditis. The endocarditis of acute rheumatic fever, usually involving one or more of the heart valves.

rheumatic fever. A febrile disease occurring as a delayed sequel of infections with beta-hemolytic streptococci, group A; characterized by multiple focal inflammatory lesions of connective tissue, notably in the heart, blood vessels, and joints, with such clinical evidence as carditis, arthritis, and skin rash.

rheumatic myocarditis. Myocarditis characterized by the formation of Aschoff nodules in the myocardium, occurring in acute rheumatic fever.

rheumatic nodules. Subcutaneous nonpainful nodules occurring in rheumatic fever over the extensor tendons of the hands, feet, knees, and elbows, and over the spine, scapula, and skull.

rheumatic pericarditis. An inflammation of the pericardium associated with rheumatic fever.

rheumatic pneumonia. Pneumonia in acute rheumatic fever.

rheumatic pneumonitis. RHEUMATIC PNEUMONIA.

rheumatic purpura. SCHÖNLEIN'S PURPURA.

rheu·ma·tism (roo'muh-tiz·um) *n.* 1. A general term indicating diseases of muscle, tendon, joint, bone, or nerve, that have in common pain and stiffness referable to the musculoskeletal system. 2. RHEUMATIC FEVER.

rheu·ma·toid (roo'muh-toid) *adj.* Resembling rheumatism.

rheumatoid arthritis. A chronic systemic disease of unknown etiology in which symptoms and inflammatory connective-tissue changes predominate in articular and related structures. Pain, limitation of motion, and joint deformity are common. Syn. *atrophic arthritis, chronic infectious arthritis, proliferative arthritis.*

rheumatoid iritis. Inflammation of the iris of the eye in conjunction with rheumatic fever, rheumatoid arthritis, and other collagen diseases.

rheumatoid myositis. Myositis characterized by focal inflammation, lesions occurring in muscles during the course of rheumatoid arthritis.

rheumatoid nodules. Subcutaneous foci of fibrinoid degeneration or necrosis surrounded by mononuclear cells in a regular palisade arrangement, occurring usually in association with rheumatoid arthritis.

rheu·ma·tol·o·gy (roo''muh·tol'uh·jee) *n.* The study of rheumatic diseases. —**rheu·ma·to·log·ic** (·tuh·loj'ick) *adj.*; **rheu·ma·tol·o·gist** (·tol'uh·jist) *n.*

rhex·is (reck'sis) *n.,* pl. **rhex·es** (·seez) Rupture of a blood vessel or of an organ.

Rh factor. Any of a group of erythrocyte antigens originally described by Landsteiner and Weiner in the blood of rhesus monkeys.

Rh genes. The series of allelic genes which determine the various sorts of Rh agglutinogens and Rh blood types. Eight standard genes have been identified (Wiener): R^0, R^1, R^2, R^Z (Rh-positive), and r, r', r'', r^y (Rh-negative).

rhin-, rhino- A combining form meaning (a) *nose, nasal;* (b) *noselike.*

rhi·nal (rye'nul) *adj.* Pertaining to the nose.

rhi·nal·gia (rye·nal'juh, ·jee·uh) *n.* Pain in the nose.

rhi·nan·tral·gia (rye''nan·tral'jee·uh) *n.* Pain in, or referred to, the walls of the cavities of the nose.

rhi·nel·cos (rye·nel'kos) *n.* A nasal ulcer.

rhin·en·ceph·a·lon (rye''nen·sef'uh·lon) *n.* The portions of the central nervous system that receive fibers from the olfactory bulb including the olfactory bulb, tract, tubercle and striae, the anterior olfactory nucleus, parts of the amygdaloid complex and parts of the prepyriform cortex. Syn. *primitive olfactory lobe, olfactory brain.* —**rhin·en·ce·phal·ic** (rye''nen·se·fal'ick) *adj.*

rhi·nen·chy·sis (rye''neng·kigh'sis, rye·neng·ki·sis) *n.* Douching of the nasal passages.

rhi·neu·ryn·ter (rye''new·rin'tur) *n.* A distensible bag or sac which is inflated after insertion into a nostril.

rhin·he·ma·to·ma, rhin·hae·ma·to·ma (rin·hee''muh·to'muh, ·hem''uh·to'muh) *n.* An effusion of blood around the nasal cartilages.

rhin·i·on (rin'ee·on) *n.* In craniometry, the point at the distal end of the internasal suture.

rhi·nism (rye'niz·um) *n.* A nasal quality of the voice.

rhi·ni·tis (rye·nigh'tis) *n.,* pl. **rhi·nit·i·des** (·nit'i·deez) Inflammation of the nasal mucous membrane.

rhinitis sic·ca (sick'uh). OZENA.

rhino-. See *rhin-.*

rhi·no·an·tri·tis (rye''no·an·trye'tis) *n.* Inflammation of the nasal mucous membrane and of the maxillary sinus.

rhi·no·by·on (rye''no·bye'on, rye·no'bee·on) *n.* A nasal plug or tampon.

rhi·no·can·thec·to·my (rye''no·kan·theck'tuh·mee) *n.* Excision of the inner canthus of the eye.

rhi·no·ceph·a·ly (rye″no-sef′uh-lee) n. A form of cyclopia in which the nose is a tubular proboscis situated above the fused orbits.

rhi·no·chei·lo·plas·ty (rye″no-kigh′lo-plas″tee) n. Plastic surgery of the nose and upper lip.

rhi·no·clei·sis (rye″no-klye′sis) n. A nasal obstruction.

rhi·no·cnes·mus (rye″no-k′nez′mus) n. Itching of the nose.

rhi·no·dac·ryo·lith (rye″no-dack′ree-o-lith) n. A calculus in the nasolacrimal duct.

rhi·no·der·ma (rye″no-dur′muh) n. KERATOSIS PILARIS.

rhi·no·dym·ia (rye″no-dim′ee-uh) n. A mild form of diprosopia in which, although there is doubling of the skeletal parts of both nose and upper jaw, the face appears only unusually wide with a broad space between the eyes and thick, wide nose.

rhi·no·dyn·ia (rye″no-din′ee-uh) n. Any pain in the nose.

rhi·nog·e·nous (rye-noj′e-nus) adj. Having its origin in the nose.

rhi·no·ky·pho·sis (rye″no-kigh-fo′sis) n. The condition of having a nose with a prominent bridge.

rhi·no·la·lia (rye″no-lay′lee-uh) n. A nasal tone in the voice.

rhinolalia aper·ta (a-pur′tuh) A nasal tone in the voice due to undue patulousness of the choanae.

rhinolalia clau·sa (klaw′suh) A nasal tone in the voice due to undue closure of the choanae.

rhi·no·lar·yn·gi·tis (rye″no-lār″in-jye′tis) n. Simultaneous inflammation of the mucosa of the nose and larynx.

rhi·no·lar·yn·gol·o·gy (rye″no-lār″in-gol′uh-jee) n. The science of the anatomy, physiology, and pathology of the nose and larynx.

rhi·no·lith (rye′no-lith) n. A nasal calculus.

rhi·no·li·thi·a·sis (rye″no-li-thigh′uh-sis) n. The formation of nasal calculi.

rhi·nol·o·gist (rye-nol′uh-jist) n. A specialist in the treatment of diseases of the nose.

rhi·nol·o·gy (rye-nol′uh-jee) n. The science of the anatomy, functions, and diseases of the nose. —**rhi·no·log·ic** (rye-no-loj′ick) adj.

rhi·no·ma·nom·e·ter (rye″no-ma-nom′e-tur) n. A manometer used for measuring the amount of nasal obstruction.

rhi·no·mi·o·sis (rye″no-migh-o′sis) n. Operative shortening of the nose.

rhi·no·my·co·sis (rye″no-migh-ko′sis) n. The presence of fungi in the mucous membrane and secretion of the nose.

rhi·no·ne·cro·sis (rye″no-ne-kro′sis) n. Necrosis of the nasal bones.

rhi·nop·a·thy (rye-nop′uth-ee) n. Any disease of the nose.

rhi·no·pha·ryn·ge·al (rye″no-fa-rin′jee-ul) adj. Pertaining to the nose and pharynx, or to the nasopharynx.

rhi·no·phar·yn·gi·tis (rye″no-fār″in-jye′tis) n. Inflammation of the nose and pharynx, or of the nasopharynx.

rhi·no·pha·ryn·go·lith (rye″no-fa-ring′go-lith) n. A nasopharyngeal calculus.

rhi·no·phar·ynx (rye″no-fār′inks) n. NASOPHARYNX.

rhi·no·pho·nia (rye″no-fo′nee-uh) n. A nasal tone in the speaking voice.

rhi·no·phy·ma (rye″no-figh′muh) n. A form of acne rosacea of the nose characterized by a marked hypertrophy of the blood vessels, sebaceous glands, and connective tissue, producing a lobulated appearance of the end of the nose. May be markedly disfiguring. Syn. toper's nose, whisky nose.

rhi·no·plas·ty (rye′no-plas″tee) n. A plastic operation upon the nose. This may be accomplished in a variety of ways, such as the so-called Italian method of rotating bone and skin-lined pedicle flap from the forehead, by flaps from the cheeks, by the transplantation of costal cartilage. —**rhi·no·plas·tic** (rye″no-plas′tick) adj.

rhi·no·pol·yp (rye″no-pol′ip) n. A polyp of the nose.

rhi·nor·rha·gia (rye″no-ray′jee-uh) n. Nosebleed, especially a profuse one.

rhi·nor·rha·phy (rye-nor′uh-fee) n. A plastic reduction in the size of the nose, in which redundant nasal tissue is removed by section, followed by approximation and suture of the wound edges.

rhi·nor·rhea, rhi·nor·rhoea (rye″no-ree′uh) n. 1. A mucous discharge from the nose. 2. Escape of cerebrospinal fluid through the nose.

rhi·nos·chi·sis (rye-nos′ki-sis) n. A congenital cleft nose.

rhi·no·scle·ro·ma (rye″no-skle-ro′muh) n. A chronic infectious disease caused by Klebsiella rhinoscleromatis which begins in the nose and may involve adjacent areas, characterized by hard nodules and plaques of inflamed tissue.

rhi·no·scope (rye′nuh-skope) n. An instrument for examining nasal cavities.

rhi·nos·co·py (rye-nos′kuh-pee) n. Examination of the nasal cavities by means of the rhinoscope. —**rhi·no·scop·ic** (rye″no-skop′ick) adj.

rhi·no·si·nus·itis (rye″no-sigh″nuh-sigh′tis) n. Inflammation of the nose and paranasal sinuses.

rhi·no·si·nus·o·path·ia (rye″no-sigh″nus-o-path′ee-uh) n. The diseases of the nose and paranasal sinuses.

rhi·no·spo·rid·i·o·sis (rye″no-spo-rid″ee-o′sis) n. An infection of man and domestic animals, caused by Rhinosporidium seeberi, and characterized by the appearance of polyps on mucous membranes, such as the nose, nasopharynx, conjunctiva, or soft palate.

Rhi·no·spo·rid·i·um (rye″no-spo-rid′ee-um) n. A genus of organisms pathogenic to man not yet precisely classified but thought to be a fungus.

Rhinosporidium see·be·ri (see′bur-eye). The species of Rhinosporidium which is the causative agent of rhinosporidiosis.

rhi·no·ste·no·sis (rye″no-ste-no′sis) n. Permanent constriction of the nose or nasal cavity.

rhi·no·thrix (rye′no-thricks) n. A hair growing in the nostril.

rhi·not·o·my (rye-not′uh-mee) n. Surgical incision of the nose.

rhi·no·vi·rus (rye″no-vye′rus) n. A member of the picornavirus group which is ether-stable, small, and RNA-containing, and etiologically related to the common cold.

rhiz-, rhizo- A combining form meaning *root.*

rhi·zoid (rye'zoid) *adj. & n.* 1. Rootlike; branching irregularly. 2. One of the slender, rootlike filaments which are organs of attachment in many cryptogams. 3. A bacterial plate culture of an irregular branched or rootlike character.

rhi·zo·mel·ic (rye''zo·mel'ick) *adj.* Affecting or pertaining to the roots of the extremities; pertaining to the hip or shoulder joints.

rhi·zo·nych·ia (rye''zo·nick'ee·uh) *n.* The root of a nail.

Rhi·zop·o·da (rye·zop'o·duh) *n.pl.* A class of the Protozoa that includes those amebas, characterized by the possession of pseudopodia, which parasitize man.

rhi·zot·o·my (rye·zot'uh·mee) *n.* Surgical division of any root, as of a nerve. Syn. *radicotomy.*

Rh-negative, *adj.* Designating the absence of $Rh_o(D)$ antigen from the erythrocytes.

rhod-, rhodo- A combining form meaning *red.*

Rhodesian trypanosomiasis or **sleeping sickness.** The more virulent form of trypanosomiasis, caused by *Trypanosoma brucei rhodesiense,* with which humans may be accidentally infected from wild animals by the tsetse fly vectors in tropical East Africa. The clinical course, which may vary greatly in intensity and duration, is divided into two clinical stages: the first or invasive stage, characterized by fever and lymphadenopathy, and the second, by central nervous system involvement.

rho·di·um (ro'dee·um) *n.* Rh = 102.905. A rare metal, atomic number 45, of the platinum group.

rho·dop·sin (ro·dop'sin) *n.* A deep-red pigment contained in the retinal rods, preserved by darkness but bleached by daylight. Syn. *visual purple.*

rhoeb·de·sis (reb·dee'sis) *n.* Absorption, resorption.

RhoGAM. Trademark for $Rh_o(D)$ immune globulin (human), a sterile, concentrated anti-$Rh_o(D)$ antibody solution.

rhomb-, rhombo- A combining form meaning (a) *rhomboid;* (b) *rhombencephalic.*

rhomb·en·ceph·a·lon (rom''ben·sef'uh·lon) *n.,* pl. **rhombencepha·la** (·luh) The most caudal of the three primary brain vesicles of the embryo; it divides into myelencephalon and metencephalon. Syn. *hindbrain.* —**rhomben·ce·phal·ic** (·se·fal'ick) *adj.*

rhom·boid (rom'boid) *adj. & n.* 1. Having a shape similar to that of a rhomb, a quadrilateral figure with opposite sides equal and parallel and oblique angles. 2. RHOMBOIDEUS.

rhom·boi·de·us (rom·boy'dee·us) *n.* Either of the rhomboid muscles, the rhomboideus major (rhomboid major, greater rhomboid,

rhon·chal (ronk'ul) *adj.* RHONCHIAL.

rhonchi. Plural of *rhoncus.*

rhon·chi·al (ronk'ee·ul) *adj.* Pertaining to or caused by rhonchi.

rhon·chus (ronk'us) *n.,* pl. **rhon·chi** (·eye) A coarse rale produced by the passage of air through a partially obstructed bronchus; vi-

brations may be also palpated on the chest wall, as fremitus.

rho·pheo·cy·to·sis (ro''fee·o·sigh·to''sis) *n.* The direct transfer of ferritin particles from macrophages to erythroblasts in the bone marrow.

Rh-positive, *adj.* Designating the presence of $Rh_o(D)$ antigen in erythrocytes.

Rhus (rooce, rus) *n.* A genus of shrubs or small trees of the Anacardiaceae. Poison ivy, poison oak, and poison sumac were formerly classified under this genus.

rhym·ing mania (rye'ming). CLANG ASSOCIATION.

rhy·poph·a·gy (rye·pof'uh·jee) *n.* SCATOPHAGY.

rhy·po·pho·bia (rye''po·fo'bee·uh) *n.* SCATOPHOBIA.

rhy·se·ma (rye·see'muh) *n.* A wrinkle or corrugation.

rhythm, *n.* 1. Action recurring at regular intervals. 2. A method of contraception, in which continence is practiced during the ovulatory phase of the menstrual cycle.

rhyth·mic (rith'mick) *adj.* Pertaining to or having the quality of rhythm, as rhythmic segmentations.

rhyth·mic·i·ty (rith·mis'i·tee) *n.* 1. The property of rhythmic periodicity or recurrence. 2. The property of having rhythmic contractions.

rhythmic nystagmus. Ocular nystagmus in which there is a slow phase in one direction and a rapid recovery; may be physiologic, as in optokinetic nystagmus, or labyrinthine, due to lesions of the vestibular apparatus or its connections.

rhyt·i·dec·tom·y (rit''i·deck'tuh·mee) *n.* Excision of wrinkles for cosmetic purposes.

rhyt·i·do·plas·ty (rit'i·do·plas''tee) *n.* A plastic operation for the removal of skin wrinkles, particularly those of the face and neck, for cosmetic purposes.

rhyt·i·do·sis, rhit·i·do·sis (rit''i·do'sis) *n.* A wrinkling, particularly of the cornea.

rib, *n.* One of the 24 long, flat, curved bones forming the wall of the thorax.

rib cage. The skeletal framework of the chest, made up of the sternum, the ribs, and the thoracic vertebrae. Syn. *thoracic cage.*

rib notching. Indentation of the ribs, such as that occurring in coarctation of the aorta, secondary to dilatation of the intercostal arteries.

ri·bo·des·ose (ri''bo·des'oce, ·oze) *n.* Deoxyribose; a pentose sugar present in deoxyribonucleic acid.

ri·bo·fla·vin (rye''bo·flay'vin, ·flav'in, rib''o·) *n.* 6,7-Dimethyl-9-(D-1'-ributyl)isoalloxazine, $C_{17}H_{20}N_4O_6$, a member of the group of B vitamins; essential in human nutrition. Its deficiency causes characteristic lesions of the tongue, lips, and face, and also certain ocular manifestations. Syn. *vitamin B_2, vitamin G, lactoflavin.*

ri·bo·nu·cle·ase (rye''bo·new'klee·ace, ·aze) *n.* An enzyme present in various body tissues which depolymerizes ribonucleic acid.

ri·bo·nu·cle·ic acid (rye''bo·new·klee'ick) Nucleic acid occurring in cell cytoplasm and the nucleolus, first isolated from plants but later found also in animal cells, containing phosphoric acid, D-ribose, adenine, guanine, cytosine, and uracil. Abbreviated, RNA.

ri·bo·nu·cleo·pro·tein (rye″bo-new″klee-o-pro′tee-in, -teen) n. A nucleoprotein that contains a ribonucleic acid moiety.

ri·bose (rye′boce, -boze) n. D-ribose, HO-CH₂(CHOH)₃CHO; a pentose sugar occurring as a structural component of riboflavin, ribonucleic acid, nicotinamide adenine dinucleotide and other nucleotides.

ri·bo·side (rye′bo-side) n. Any glycoside containing ribose as the sugar component.

ri·bo·some (rye′bo-sohm) n. A flattened, spheroidal, cytoplasmic submicroscopic ribonucleoprotein particle, 150 × 250 Å, which in company with other ribosomes linked by messenger RNA into aggregates termed polyribosomes (or polysomes) synthesizes protein. —**ri·bo·so·mal** (rye″bo-so′mul) adj.

rice, n. A plant, *Oryza sativa*, of the Gramineae; also its seed. Used as a food and, occasionally, as a demulcent.

rice bodies. Small, free white bodies occurring in the synovial cavity of an arthritic joint (most commonly in tuberculous arthritis), composed of compact masses of fibrin, necrotic villi, or cartilage fragments.

rice-water stools. The stools of cholera, in which there is a copious serous exudation containing mucus.

Rich·ter's hernia (rih′tur) A form of enterocele in which only a part of the intestinal wall is situated within the hernial sac.

Rich·ter's syndrome Chronic lymphocytic leukemia complicated terminally by fever, cachexia, dysproteinemia and a pleomorphic type of malignant lymphoma.

ri·cin (rye′sin, ris′in) n. A highly toxic albumin in the seed of *Ricinus communis*.

ric·in·ism (ris′in-iz-um) n. Poisoning from the seeds of *Ricinus communis*. It is marked by hemorrhagic gastroenteritis and icterus.

rick·ets, n. A deficiency disease occurring during skeletal growth, due to concurrent lack of vitamin D and insufficient exposure to ultraviolet radiation (sunshine), resulting in altered calcium and phosphorus metabolism, which is reflected in defective bone growth, and, in severe cases, characteristic skeletal deformities. Syn. *Glisson's disease, infantile osteomalacia, juvenile osteomalacia, rachitis.*

Rick·ett·sia (ri·ket′see-uh) n. A genus of bacteria of the family Rickettsiaceae, causing the spotted fever group of diseases, characterized by intranuclear and intracytoplasmic multiplication in susceptible animal cells, and transmitted to man by ticks, as in Rocky Mountain spotted fever, or by mites, as in rickettsialpox.

rickettsia, n., pl. **rickett·si·ae** (-see-ee), **rickettsias.** A member of the family Rickettsiaceae. —**rickett·si·al** (-see-ul) adj.

Rickettsia aus·tra·lis (aw-stray′lis). The causative agent of Queensland tick typhus fever.

Rickettsia bur·net·ii (bur-net′ee-eye). COXIELLA BURNETII.

Rick·ett·si·a·ce·ae (ri·ket″see-ay′see-ee) n.pl. A family of small, pleomorphic, coccobacillary microorganisms of the order Rickettsiales,

principally obligate intracellular parasites, occurring in arthropods and causing a variety of diseases in animals and in man.

Rickettsia co·no·rii (kon-o′ree-eye). The causative agent of boutonneuse fever.

rick·ett·si·al·pox (ri·ket′see-ul-pocks″) n. A mild, nonfatal, self-limited, acute febrile illness caused by *Rickettsia akari*, which is transmitted from mouse to man by mites. It is characterized by an initial papule at the site of the bite, a week's febrile course, and a papulovesicular rash.

Rickettsia moo·seri (moo′sur-eye). RICKETTSIA TYPHI.

Rickettsia pro·wa·zek·ii (pro-va-zeck′ee-eye). The causative agent of louse-borne epidemic typhus and Brill's disease.

Rickettsia rick·ett·sii (ri-ket′see-eye). The causative agent of Rocky Mountain spotted fever.

Rickettsia ru·mi·nan·ti·um (roo-mi-nan′shee-um). The causative agent of heartwater disease.

Rickettsia si·be·ri·ca (sigh-beer′i-kuh). The causative agent of North Asian tick-borne rickettsiosis.

Rickettsia tsu·tsu·ga·mu·shi (tsoo″tsuh-ga-moo′shee). The causative agent of tsutsugamushi disease. Syn. *Rickettsia orientalis.*

rick·ett·si·o·sis (ri-ket″see-o′sis) n., pl. **rickettsio·ses** (-seez) A disease of man or animals caused by microorganisms in the family Rickettsiaceae.

rick·ety (rick′e-tee) adj. Affected with or distorted by rickets; rachitic.

rid·er's bone. An osseous deposit in the adductor muscles of the leg, from long-continued pressure of the leg against the saddle. Syn. *cavalry bone, cavalryman's osteoma.*

rider's sprain. A sprain of the adductor longus muscle of the thigh, resulting from a sudden effort of the horseman to maintain his seat owing to some unexpected movement of his horse.

ridge, n. An extended elevation or crest.

ridge·ling (rij′ling) n. A domestic animal with cryptorchism.

riding embolus. SADDLE EMBOLUS.

riding of bones. In surgery, the displacement of the fractured ends of bones which are forced past each other by muscular contraction, instead of remaining in end-to-end apposition.

Rie·del's disease or **struma** (ree′del) A form of chronic thyroiditis with irregular localized areas of stony hard fibrosis; in advanced stages the gland is adherent to surrounding structures.

Riedel's lobe A tongue-shaped process extending downward from the costal border of the right lobe of the liver; it occurs infrequently.

Rie·der's cell (ree′dur) An anaplastic leukocyte, considered by some a variety of lymphocyte, by others a type of granulocyte; such cells occur in poorly differentiated acute leukemia.

Riehl's melanosis (reel) An idiopathic inflammatory disease of the skin characterized by hyperpigmentation, chiefly affecting the face.

rif·am·pin (rif′am-pin) n. 3-(4-Methylpiperazinyliminomethyl)rifamycin SV, C₄₃H₅₈N₄O₁₂, a derivative of rifamycin SV active against isoniazid-resistant strains of tubercle bacilli.

Rift Valley fever A toxic generalized febrile illness of short duration characterized by headache, photophobia conjunctivitis, myalgia, anorexia, leukopenia and thrombocytopenia. Caused by a mosquito-borne arbovirus, epizootic in domestic animals and enzootic in wild game in eastern and southern Africa.

Riggs' disease PERIODONTITIS.

right axis deviation. Mean electrical axis of the QRS complex in the frontal plane of greater than 90°. Abbreviated, RAD.

right heart. The part of the heart that furnishes blood to the lungs; the right atrium and right ventricle.

right-to-left shunt. A cardiac defect characterized by flow of deoxygenated blood from the right side of the heart into the left side of the heart or systemic circulation, without passage through the pulmonary circulation.

rig·id (rij′id) *adj.* 1. Stiff, hard, inflexible. 2. Tense, spastic; said of muscles.

ri·gid·i·tas (ri·jid′i·tas) *n.* RIGIDITY.

ri·gid·i·ty (ri·jid′i·tee) *n.* 1. Stiffness; inflexibility; immobility. 2. *In neurology,* a form of hypertonus in which the muscles are continuously or intermittently tense. In contrast to spasticity, the increase in tone has a uniform quality throughout the range of passive movement of the limb. Syn. *lead-pipe rigidity.* 3. *In psychology,* great resistance and reluctance to change, with fixed patterns of behavior.

rig·or (rig′ur) *n.* 1. CHILL. 2. RIGIDITY (1).

rigor mor·tis (mor′tis) Temporary stiffening and rigidity of muscle, particularly skeletal and cardiac, which occurs after death.

RIHSA Radioactive iodine–tagged human serum albumin.

Ri·ley-Day syndrome. FAMILIAL DYSAUTONOMIA.

ri·ma (rye′muh) *n.,* pl. & genit. sing. **ri·mae** (·mee) A chink or cleft. —**ri·mal** (·mul) *adj.*

rima glot·ti·dis (glot′i·dis) [NA]. The space between the true vocal folds.

ri·man·ta·dine (ri·man′tuh·deen) *n.* α-Methyl-1-adamantanemethylamine, $C_{12}H_{21}N$, an antiviral agent.

rima oris (o′ris) [NA]. The line formed by the junction of the lips.

rima pu·den·di (pew·den′dye) [NA]. The fissure between the labia majora.

ri·mose (rye′moce, rye·moce′) *adj. In biology,* marked by many crevices or furrows.

rin·der·pest (rin′dur·pest) *n.* A contagious, epidemic disease of cattle and sometimes sheep and goats in Africa and Asia; caused by a filtrable virus and characterized by fever and ulcerative, diphtheritic lesions of the intestinal tract.

ring, *n.* 1. A circular opening or the structure surrounding it. 2. A cyclic or closed-chain structure.

ring·bin·den (ring·bin′dun) *n.* Abnormal arrangement of myofibrils, best seen in transverse sections as a circular or concentric striated coil entwined about the periphery or penetrating the sarcoplasm at right angles to the usual plane of muscles of aged and prematurely aged individuals, especially in the ex-

traocular muscles where this alteration is occasionally observed in normal younger persons. Syn. *spiral annulet, striated annulet.*

ring bodies. Blue-stained threads arranged in rings and figures of eight, found in the erythrocytes of persons with lead poisoning and other anemias. Syn. *Cabot's rings. Cabot's ring bodies.*

ring·bone. A chronic, hypertrophic osteitis of the pastern or first, second, or third phalanges of the foot in the horse.

ringed hair. A rare form of canities, due to the alternate formation of medulla and no medulla, in which the hairs appear silvery gray and dark in alternating bands. Usually seen in several members of a family. Syn. *pili annulati.*

Ring·er's injection A sterile solution of sodium chloride, potassium chloride, and calcium chloride in sufficient water for injection; used intravenously as a fluid and electrolyte replenisher.

Ringer's lactate solution LACTATED RINGER'S INJECTION.

Ringer's solution A solution of the same composition as Ringer's injection but prepared with recently boiled purified water and not required to be sterile. Used topically as a physiologic salt solution but not to be administered parenterally, for which purpose Ringer's injection should be employed.

ring·worm. An infection of the skin, hair, or nails, with various fungi, producing annular lesions with raised borders. Syn. *tinea.*

Rin·ne's test (rin′eh) A hearing test in which the duration of bone conduction is compared with that of air conduction. Normally air conduction is longer than bone conduction (Rinne positive; symbol, + R). Alteration in this relationship (Rinne negative; symbol, – R) indicates a lesion of the sound-conducting apparatus.

ris·to·ce·tin (ris″to·see′tin) *n.* A mixture of two antibiotics, ristocetin A and ristocetin B, produced by the actinomycete *Nocardia lurida.* Used in infections due to streptococci, enterococci, pneumococci, and staphylococci when the infections are resistant to other antibiotics.

ri·sus (rye′sus) *n.* A grin or laugh.

risus sar·don·i·cus (sahr·don′i·kus). The sardonic grin, a peculiar grinning distortion of the face produced by spasm of the muscles about the mouth; characteristically observed in tetanus.

Ritalin. Trademark for methylphenidate, a central nervous system stimulant used as the hydrochloride in the treatment of various types of depression.

Rit·ter's disease DERMATITIS EXFOLIATIVA NEONATORUM.

rit·u·al (rich′oo·ul) *n.* 1. A ceremony or system of stereotyped and prescribed activities performed periodically and having special significance relating to religion or other code of belief or behavior. 2. An activity considered by an individual to be a routine, but highly significant part of his life, as reading before bedtime, or, for example, the manner in which parents carry out a child's toilet training, regarding the process as inviolate and imbuing it with special significance. 3. *In psychiatry*, any psychomotor activity other than a tic repeatedly performed, in order to relieve anxiety; usually seen in the obsessive-compulsive neurosis.

riz·i·form (riz′i·form) *adj.* Resembling grains of rice.

R.M.A. Right mentoanterior position of the fetus.

R.M.P. Right mentoposterior position of the fetus.

R.N. Abbreviation for *registered nurse*.

Rn Symbol for radon.

RNA Abbreviation for *ribonucleic acid*, nucleic acid occurring in cell cytoplasm and the nucleolus, first isolated from plants but later found also in animal cells, containing phosphoric acid, D-ribose, adenine, guanine, cytosine, and uracil.

RNase Abbreviation for *ribonuclease*.

RNA viruses. Viruses, such as picornaviruses, reoviruses, arboviruses, myxoviruses, viruses of mouse tumors, and plant viruses, as well as those implicated in the avian leukosis complex, in which the nucleic acid core consists of ribonucleic acid.

RNP Abbreviation for *ribonucleoprotein*.

R.O.A. Right occipitoanterior position of the fetus.

roar·ing, *n.* A disease of horses, caused by damage to the recurrent laryngeal nerve resulting in paralysis and atrophy of the muscle controlling the arytenoid cartilage of the larynx; the flaccid cartilage impedes normal inspiration and is responsible for the harsh roaring sound heard during vigorous exercise.

Robaxin. Trademark for methocarbamol, a skeletal muscle relaxant.

ro·bo·rant (rob′o·runt, ro′buh·runt) *adj. & n.* 1. Tonic, strengthening. 2. A strengthening agent.

Ro·chelle salt (rosh·el′) POTASSIUM SODIUM TARTRATE.

Rocky Mountain spotted fever. An acute febrile illness caused by *Rickettsia rickettsii*, transmitted to man by ticks. There is the sudden onset of headache, chills, and fever; a characteristic exanthem occurs on the extremities and trunk. Syn. *American spotted fever*.

Rocky Mountain spotted fever vaccine. A vaccine for prophylactic immunization against Rocky Mountain spotted fever. The original method utilizing killed rickettsiae harvested from ground-infected ticks (the Spencer-Parker vaccine) has been supplanted by a formalized vaccine prepared from rickettsiae grown in the yolk sac of the developing chick.

rod, *n.* 1. Any slender, straight structure or object. 2. One of the rod-shaped photosensitive retinal cells concerned with motion and vision at low degrees of illumination (night vision). 3. A bacterium shaped like a rod.

rod cell. 1. An elongated microglial cell found in the cerebral cortex in various pathologic conditions, especially paresis. 2. BAND CELL. 3. ROD (2).

ro·den·ti·cide (ro·den′ti·side) *n.* A preparation

that is poisonous to, or destroys, rodents; used as an agent against rats or mice.

rodent ulcer. BASAL CELL CARCINOMA.

rods of Corti The columnar cells lining the tunnel of Corti.

roent·gen, rönt·gen (rent′gun) *n. & adj.* 1. The international unit of x- and gamma radiation. 2. The quantity of x- or gamma radiation which results in associated corpuscular emission of 1 electrostatic unit of electrical charge of either sign per 0.001293 g of air under standard conditions. Abbreviated, r. 3. Of or pertaining to x-rays.

roentgen equivalent man. The quantity of radiation which, when absorbed by man, produces a biologic effect equivalent to the absorption by man of 1 roentgen of x- or gamma radiation. Abbreviated, REM, rem.

roentgen equivalent physical. The amount of ionizing radiation which is capable of producing 1.615×10^{12} ion pairs per gram of tissue or that will transfer to tissue 93 ergs per gram. This unit is employed primarily to measure beta radiation. Abbreviated, REP, rep.

roent·gen·o·gram (rent′ge·no·gram) *n.* RADIOGRAPH.

roent·gen·og·ra·phy (rent″ge·nog′ruh·fee) *n.* RADIOGRAPHY. —**roentgen·o·graph·ic** (·o·graf′ick) *adj.*

roent·gen·o·kymo·gram (rent″ge·no·kigh′mo·gram) *n.* Radiographic record of the changes in the size or movements of the heart, or the position of the diaphragm.

roent·gen·ol·o·gist (rent″ge·nol′uh·jist) *n.* A physician specializing in the practice of roentgenology.

roent·gen·ol·o·gy (rent″ge·nol′uh·jee) *n.* The branch of medical science which deals with the diagnostic and therapeutic application of x-rays. —**roentgen·o·log·ic** (·no·loj′ick) *adj.*

roent·gen·os·co·py (rent″ge·nos′kuh·pee) *n.* Examination with x-rays by means of a fluorescent screen. —**roent·gen·o·scope** (rent′ge·no·skope) *n.*

roent·gen·o·ther·a·py (rent″ge·no·therr′uh·pee) *n.* The treatment of disease by means of x-rays.

Ro·ger murmur (roh·zhe′) A harsh holosystolic murmur, usually accompanied by a thrill, heard best parasternally in the third and fourth left intercostal spaces in patients with ventricular septal defect. Syn. *bruit de Roger*.

Roger's disease VENTRICULAR SEPTAL DEFECT.

Ro·ki·tan·sky-Asch·off sinuses (ro·kee·tahn′skee, ahsh′ohf) Small outpouchings of the mucosa of the gallbladder extending through the lamina propria and muscular layer.

ro·lan·dic (ro·lan′dick) *adj.* 1. Described by or named for Luigi Rolando, Italian anatomist, 1773–1831. 2. Pertaining to the central sulcus (fissure of Rolando).

Ro·lan·do's area The motor area of the cerebral cortex.

Rolicton. Trademark for the orally effective non-mercurial diuretic amisometradine.

Ro·ma·nov·sky stains (ruh·mah·nohf′skee) A generic term applied to stains with nearly balanced mixtures of eosin and oxidation products of methylene blue, used as blood stains.

Rom·berg's sign 1. A sign for obturator hernia in which there is pain radiating to the knee. 2. A sign for loss of position sense in which the patient cannot maintain equilibrium when standing with feet together and eyes closed.

ron·geur (rohn·zhur′) n. A bone-cutting forceps.

root, n. 1. The descending axis of a plant. 2. The part of an organ embedded in the tissues, as the root of a tooth. 3. The beginning or proximal portion of a structure, especially one of two bundles of nerve fibers, the posterior and anterior emerging from the central nervous system and joining to form a nerve trunk.

root canal. The cavity within the root of a tooth, which contains pulp, nerves, and vessels.

root canal filling. The closure and filling of the prepared root canal from the apex to the coronal portion of the tooth with an impervious material to prevent subsequent infection.

root canal treatment. The opening, cleansing, and sterilization of a root canal preparatory to root canal filling.

root of the lung. The axis formed by the main bronchus, pulmonary vessels, lymphatics, and nerves in the hilus, connecting the lung with the heart and trachea.

root of the mesentery. The parietal attachment of the mesentery extending from the duodenojejunal flexure to the ileocecal junction.

root of the nail. The small proximal region of the nail plate covered entirely by the nail wall.

root of the nose. The part at the forehead between the eyes, from which emerges the dorsum of the nose.

root of the tongue. The pharyngeal, fixed part of the tongue, posterior to the sulcus terminalis.

R.O.P. Right occipitoposterior position of fetus.

Ror·schach test or **diagnosis** (rohr′shah^kh) A psychologic test in which the subject describes what he sees on a series of 10 standard inkblots of varying designs and colors. The subject's responses indicate personality patterns, special interests, originality of thought, emotional conflicts, deviations of effect, and neurotic or psychotic tendencies.

ro·sa·ce·i·form (ro·zay′shee·i·form) adj. Resembling acne rosacea. Having a dusky red, telangiectatic appearance.

ro·sa·lia (ro·say′lee·uh) n. 1. SCARLET FEVER. 2. MEASLES. 3. ERYTHEMA.

rose ben·gal (beng′gawl). The sodium or potassium salt of 4, 5, 6, 7-tetrachloro-2′, 4′, 5′, 7′-tetraiodofluorescein, used as a bacterial stain and in Lendrum's inclusion-body stain. The rate of disappearance of the dye from the bloodstream following its intravenous administration is a test of liver function.

ro·se·in (ro′zee·in) n. FUCHSIN.

ro·se·o·la (ro·zee′o·luh) n. Any rose-colored eruption.

roseola ty·pho·sa (tye·fo′suh). The eruption of typhoid or typhus fever.

roseola vac·cin·ia (vack·sin′ee·uh). A general rose-colored eruption occurring about 10 days after vaccination. It is of short duration.

rose spots. A red, papular eruption which blanches on pressure, occurring mostly on the abdomen and loins during the first 7 days of typhoid fever. Syn. typhoid roseola, typhoid spots, taches rosées lenticulaires.

ro·sette (ro·zet′) n. Any structure resembling or suggestive of a rose, such as a cluster of cells in a crowded circle.

ros·in (roz′in) n. The residue left after the volatile oil is distilled from turpentine. It consists chiefly of various modifications of anhydrides of abietic acid with varying quantities of hydrocarbons. Used as a component of plasters. Syn. colophony.

ros·tel·lum (ros·tel′um) n. A little beak, especially the hook-bearing portion of the head of certain worms.

ros·tral (ros′trul) adj. 1. Pertaining to or resembling a rostrum. 2. Relatively far advanced in a direction toward the beak, snout, or face (with respect to other parts of the head).

ros·trum (ros′trum) n., pl. **ros·tra** (·truh) A beak; a projection or ridge.

rostrum cor·po·ris cal·lo·si (kor′po·ris ka·lo′sigh) [NA]. The anterior tapering portion of the corpus callosum.

ro·tam·e·ter (ro·tam′e·tur, ro′tuh·mee·tur) n. A device for the measurement of mean flow rate of a liquid or gas.

ro·tate, adj. & v. 1. Wheel-shaped. 2. To undergo or cause rotation.

ro·ta·tion, n. 1. The act of turning about an axis passing through the center of a body, as rotation of the eye, rotation of the head. 2. In dentistry, the operation by which a malturned tooth is turned or twisted into its normal position. 3. In neurophysiology, the phenomenon whereby every third or fourth impulse is carried over the cochlear nerve when the exciting impulse is above 1,800 hertz (cycles per second). 4. In obstetrics, one of the stages of labor, consisting of a rotary movement of the fetal head or other presenting part, whereby it is accommodated to the birth canal. It may be internal, occurring before the birth of the presenting part, or external, occurring afterward.

rotation therapy. A technique of radiation therapy in which either the patient is rotated around a central axis with the radiation beam constant, or the radiation source is revolved about the patient.

ro·ta·to·ry (ro′tuh·tor·ee) adj. 1. Pertaining to or producing rotation. 2. Occurring in or by rotation. 3. Resembling a body in rotation.

rotatory nystagmus. An oscillatory, partial rolling of the eyeball around the visual axis.

Roth's spots (rote) Small white spots surrounded by hemorrhage found in the fundus of the eye in subacute bacterial endocarditis and other conditions.

Ro·tor syndrome Dubin-Johnson syndrome but without hepatic pigmentation.

Rot·ter's test A test for vitamin C deficiency in man, using dichlorophenol-indophenol sodium injected intradermally to color the skin. If decolorization does not occur within 10 minutes, vitamin C deficiency may exist.

rough·age (ruf′ij) n. Food containing indigestible material, such as bran or cellulose, which stimulates intestinal action and promotes peristalsis.

rough-surfaced endoplasmic reticulum. Intracytoplasmic membranes to which granules of ribonucleoprotein (ribosomes) are adherent, seen by electron microscopy. They represent a complex which synthesizes protein and contains it within membranes. Abbreviated, RER.

rou·leau (roo·lo′) n. A column of red blood cells stacked like a roll of coins.

round cell. Generally, any of the particular cells of an inflammatory exudate which have a round nuclear outline, especially lymphocytes, plasma cells, and macrophages.

round-cell carcinoma. 1. Any poorly differentiated carcinoma with round parenchymal cells. 2. A form of poorly differentiated lung carcinoma.

round shoulders. Faulty posture in which drooping of the shoulders and increased convexity of the thoracic spine are conspicuous, the postural abnormalities not being limited to the shoulder girdle and chest.

round window. A round opening in the medial wall of the middle ear, closed by the secondary tympanic membrane. Syn. *cochlear window.*

round·worm. n. A worm of the order Nematoda.

roup (roop) n. An infectious disease of fowls, especially pigeons, characterized by infection of the upper digestive tract and cranial sinuses with the protozoan *Trichomonas gallinae.*

Roux's operation A multistaged operation for excision of the esophagus for carcinoma, in which the esophagus is reattached to the stomach by interposition of a loop of jejunum.

R.Q. Abbreviation for *respiratory quotient.*

R-R interval. The period of the electrocardiogram from one R wave to the next.

R.S.A. Right sacroanterior position of the fetus.

R.S.P. Right sacroposterior position of the fetus.

RSV, RS virus. Abbreviation for *respiratory syncytial virus.*

rubber dam. A thin sheet of rubber attached to a frame and used to isolate a tooth to protect it from moisture and contamination during restorative dentistry procedures.

ru·be·do (roo·bee′do) n. Any diffuse redness of the skin.

ru·be·fa·cient (roo″be·fay′shunt) adj. & n. 1. Causing redness of the skin. 2. Any substance that causes redness of the skin.

ru·be·fac·tion (roo″be·fack′shun) n. 1. Redness of the skin due to the action of an irritant. 2. The act of causing redness of the skin.

ru·bel·la (roo·bel′uh) n. An acute benign viral contagious disease of children and young adults characterized by fever, a pale pink rash, and posterior cervical lymphadenitis. Associated with fetal abnormalities when maternal infection occurs in early pregnancy. Syn. *epidemic roseola, French measles, German measles, röteln, three-day measles.*

rubella syndrome. Infection of the fetus by the mother with rubella virus during early pregnancy, resulting in a wide variety of severe congenital malformations, including cardiovascular defects, microcephaly, cataracts,

deafness, encephalomyelitis, bony changes, and thrombocytopenia.

ru·bel·li·form (roo·bel′i·form) adj. Resembling rubella.

ru·be·o·la (roo·bee′o·luh) n. MEASLES (1).

ru·be·o·sis (roo″bee·o′sis) n. Redness, in particular red discoloration of the skin.

ru·bes·cence (roo·bes′unce) n. The state or quality of redness. **—rubes·cent** (·unt) adj.

ru·bid·i·um (roo·bid′ee·um) n. Rb = 85.4678. An alkali metal, atomic number 37, resembling potassium in appearance.

ru·big·i·nous (roo·bij′i·nus) adj. Rust-colored.

ru·bin (roo′bin) n. BASIC FUCHSIN.

Rubin test A test for patency of the uterine tubes by means of insufflation with carbon dioxide.

ru·bor (roo′bor) n. Redness due to inflammation.

ru·bri·cyte (roo′bri·site) n. BASOPHILIC NORMOBLAST.

ru·bri·uria (roo″bri·yoo′ree·uh) n. Red discoloration of the urine.

ru·bro·bul·bar (roo″bro·bul′bur) adj. Pertaining to the red nucleus and the medulla oblongata.

ru·bro·ol·i·vary (roo″bro·ol′i·verr·ee) adj. Pertaining to the red nucleus and the olive.

ru·bro·spi·nal (roo″bro·spye′nul) adj. Pertaining to the red nucleus and the spinal cord.

ruc·ta·tion (ruck·tay′shun) n. Eructation; BELCHING.

ruc·tus (ruck′tus) n. A belching of gas from the stomach.

ructus hys·te·ri·cus (his·terr′i·kus). Hysterical belching, the gas escaping with a loud, sobbing, gurgling noise.

ru·di·ment (roo′di·munt) n. That which is but partially developed.

ru·di·men·ta·ry (roo″di·men′tuh·ree) adj. Undeveloped; unfinished; incomplete.

rue (roo) n. A plant, *Ruta graveolens*, of the family Rutaceae, yielding a volatile oil consisting chiefly of methyl nonyl ketone, $CH_3COC_9H_{19}$, and acting as a potent local irritant.

ru·fous (roo′fus) adj. Reddish; ruddy.

ru·ga (roo′guh) n., pl. **ru·gae** (·jee, ·gee) A wrinkle, fold, elevation, or ridge, as in the mucosa of the stomach, vagina, and palate.

ru·gi·tus (roo′ji·tus) n. Rumbling of the intestines; borborygmus.

ru·gose (roo′goce) adj. Characterized by many folds.

ru·gos·i·ty (roo·gos′i·tee) n. A condition exhibiting many folds in a tissue or integument.

rule, n. An established guide for action or procedure.

rule of nines. A rule for the estimate of the percentage of body surface area according to which the head and upper extremities each represent 9 percent, the trunk, anterior and posterior, 18 percent, the lower extremities, each 18 percent, and the perineum 1 percent; useful in judging the severity and extent of burns.

ru·men·ot·o·my (roo″me·not′uh·mee) n. A laparotomy in which the rumen is exposed and incised.

ru·mi·nant (roo′mi·nunt) n. A cud-chewing animal, characterized by an arrangement of the forestomach whereby food is regurgitated and remasticated. Ruminants include all even-toed ungulates except swine and hippopotamuses.

ru·mi·na·tion (roo″mi·nay′shun) n. 1. A characteristic of ruminants in which food is regurgitated and remasticated in preparation for true digestion. 2. The voluntary regurgitation of food which has already reached the stomach, remastication, and swallowing a second time; occurs chiefly in emotionally disturbed younger children, and occasionally in mentally retarded and psychiatric patients. Syn. *merycism*. 3. *In psychiatry*, an obsessional preoccupation with a single idea or system of ideas which dominates the mind despite all efforts to dislodge it. Observed in anxiety states and other psychiatric disorders.

rump, n. The region near the end of the backbone; BUTTOCKS.

Rum·pel-Leede phenomenon, sign, or test (room′pel) The production of an abnormally large number of petechiae on the forearm when a tourniquet is applied at slightly above diastolic pressure for 5 to 10 minutes to the upper arm; positive in disorders where there is an increased bleeding tendency due to increased capillary fragility or decreased number of platelets.

run, v. To discharge, as pus or purulent matter from a diseased part.

run-around, n. A paronychia extending completely around a nail.

r unit. ROENTGEN.

ru·pia (roo′pee·uh) n. An eruption on the skin characterized by the formation of large, dirty-brown, stratified, conic crusts that resemble oyster shell; commonly seen in syphilis and psoriasis. —**ru·pi·al** (·pee·ul) adj.

rup·tio (rup′shee·o) n. Rupture of a vessel or organ.

rup·ture (rup′chur) n. 1. A forcible tearing of a part, as rupture of the uterus, rupture of the urinary bladder. 2. HERNIA.

rup·tured, adj. Burst; broken; forcibly torn; affected with hernia.

Rus·sell bodies Hyaline eosinophilic globules 4 to 5 microns in diameter, occurring in the cytoplasm of plasma cells in chronic inflammatory exudates; once considered etiologic agents of disease, they are now thought to be particles of antibody globulin.

Russian tick-borne complex or **encephalitides.** An aggregate of viral diseases of men and animals, widely distributed throughout Europe and Asia, transmitted by ticks of the family Ixodidae; characterized by fever, gastrointestinal disturbances, and hemorrhages or by fever and neurologic manifestations.

rust, n. 1. A product consisting of the oxide, hydroxide, and carbonate of iron, formed on the surface of iron exposed to moist air. 2. Any of a group of parasitic fungi (Uredinales) causing discoloration on plants. They are common allergens.

rut, n. A period of heightened sexual excitement and its accompanying behavior in males, especially that occurring annually in wild ungulates.

ru·the·ni·um (roo·theen′ee·um) n. Ru=101.07. A metallic element, atomic number 44, of the platinum group.

ruth·er·ford (ruth′ur·furd) n. A unit of radioactivity representing 10^6 disintegrations per second. Abbreviated, rd.

ru·tin (roo′tin) n. Quercetin-3-rutinoside, $C_{27}H_{30}O_{16}$, a rhamnoglycoside that occurs in several plants; claimed to decrease capillary fragility in patients with increased fragility. Syn. *eldrin, melin, myrticolorin, phytomelin, violaquercitrin.*

ru·tin·ose (roo′tin·oce, ·oze) n. A disaccharide, $C_{12}H_{22}O_{10}$, produced by enzymic or controlled acid hydrolysis of rutin or hesperidin. Rutinose yields one molecule each of glucose and rhamnose on hydrolysis.

R wave of the electrocardiogram. The initial positive deflection of the QRS complex of the electrocardiogram.

rye smut. ERGOT.

S

S Symbol for sulfur.

S Abbreviation for (a) *signa*, sign; (b) *spherical;* (c) *spherical lens;* (d) smooth variant in bacteria.

S̄, s Symbol for Svedberg sedimentation unit.

S̄ *In electrocardiology,* symbol for spatial vector.

S₁ or **SI.** Symbol for first heart sound.

S₂ or **SII.** Symbol for second heart sound.

S₃ or **SIII.** Symbol for third heart sound.

S₃. VENTRICULAR GALLOP.

S₄ or **SIV.** Symbol for fourth heart sound.

S₄. ATRIAL GALLOP.

S̄ₜ Symbol for Svedberg flotation unit.

s. Abbreviation for (a) *sinister*, left; (b) *semis*, half.

saber tibia or **shin.** Anterior bowing and thickening of the tibia due to periostitis caused by congenital syphilis or yaws.

Sa·be·thes (sa-bee'theez) *n.* A genus of mosquitoes which includes *Sabethes chloropterus*, a species implicated in the transmission of sylvan yellow fever.

Sa·bin-Feld·man dye test. DYE TEST.

Sa·bou·raud's agar or **broth** (sa^h-boo-ro') A liquid medium favorable for the cultivation of fungi, containing 4% glucose or maltose and peptone.

sab·u·lous (sab'yoo-lus) *adj.* Gritty; sandy.

sac, *n.* A pouch; a baglike covering of a natural cavity, or of a hernia, cyst, or tumor.

sacchari-, sacchari-, saccharo- A combining form meaning (a) *sugar;* (b) *saccharine.*

sac·cha·rase (sack'uh-race, -raze) *n.* An enzyme occurring in plants and microorganisms, particularly yeasts, and capable of hydrolyzing disaccharides to monosaccharides; more specifically, the enzyme which is responsible for hydrolysis of sucrose to dextrose and levulose. Syn. *invertase, invertin, sucrase.*

sac·cha·rate (sack'uh-rate) *n.* A salt of saccharic acid.

sac·cha·rat·ed (sack'uh-ray'tid) *adj.* Containing sugar.

saccharated iron oxide. A water-soluble preparation of ferric oxide and sugar; has been used as a nonastringent hematinic. Syn. *soluble ferric oxide, eisenzucker.*

sac·char·eph·i·dro·sis (sack"ur-ef"i-dro'sis) *n.* A form of hyperhidrosis, characterized by the excretion of sugar in the sweat.

sac·char·ic acid (sa-kăr'ick). 1. A product obtained by oxidizing an aldose with nitric acid so that both the aldehyde and primary alcohol groups are converted to carboxyl groups. 2. $HOOC(CHOH)_4COOH$; the saccharic acid obtained by oxidation of D-glucose with nitric acid.

sac·cha·ride (sack'uh-ride) *n.* A compound of a base with sugar; a sucrate.

sac·char·i·fy (sa-kăr'i-fye) *v.* 1. To make sweet. 2. To convert into sugar. —**sac·char·i·fi·ca·tion** (sa-kar"i-fi-kay'shun) *n.*

sac·cha·rim·e·ter (sack"uh-rim'e·tur) *n.* An apparatus for determining the amount of sugar in solutions. It may be in the form of a hydrometer, which indicates the concentration of sugar by the specific gravity of the solution; a polarimeter, which indicates the concentration of sugar by the number of degrees of rotation of the plane of polarization; or a fermentation tube, which indicates the concentration of sugar by the amount of gas formed during fermentation.

sac·cha·rin (sack'uh-rin) *n.* 1,2-Benzisothiazolin-3-one 1,1-dioxide, $C_7H_5NO_3S$, a noncaloric sweetening agent, generally used in the form of sodium saccharin, which is much more soluble in water than is saccharin. Syn. *benzosulfimide, gluside.*

sac·cha·rine (sack'uh-rin, -reen, -rine) *adj.* 1. Having an excessively sweet taste. 2. Like or pertaining to sugar.

saccharin sodium. SODIUM SACCHARIN.

sac·cha·ro·ga·lac·tor·rhea, sac·cha·ro·ga·lac·tor·rhoea (sack"uh-ro-guh-lack"to-ree'uh) *n.* The secretion of milk that contains an excess of sugar.

sac·cha·ro·me·tab·o·lism (sack"uh-ro·me·tab'uh·liz·um) *n.* The metabolism of sugars. —**sac·cha·ro·met·a·bol·ic** (·met"uh·bol'ick) *adj.*

Saccharomyces hom·i·nis (hom'i·nis). *CRYPTOCOCCUS NEOFORMANS.*

sac·cha·ro·my·co·sis (sack"uh·ro·migh·ko'sis) *n.* A pathologic condition due to yeasts or *Saccharomyces.*

sac·char·o·pine (sa·kār'o·peen) *n.* L-*N*-(5-Amino-5-carboxypentyl)glutamic acid, $C_{11}H_{20}N_2O_6$, an intermediate in the synthesis of lysine in *Saccharomyces,* and also an intermediate in the degradation of lysine by mammalian liver.

sac·cha·ro·pi·nu·ria (sack"uh·ro·pi·new'ree·uh) *n.* A rare, inborn error of amino acid metabolism, probably of lysine degradation; clinically associated with mental retardation and chemically characterized by an abnormally large amount of saccharopine in the urine.

sac·cha·ror·rhea, sac·cha·ror·rhoea (sack"uh·ro·ree'uh) *n.* GLYCOSURIA.

sac·cha·rose (sack'uh·roce, ·roze) *n.* 1. SUCROSE. 2. A generic term sometimes applied to disaccharides, less frequently to trisaccharides.

sac·cha·ro·su·ria (sack"uh·ro·sue'ree·uh) *n.* The presence of saccharose in the urine.

sac·cha·rum (sack'uh·rum) *n.* SUCROSE.

sac·ci·form (sack'si·form) *adj.* Resembling a sac.

sac·cu·lar (sack'yoo·lur) *adj.* Sac-shaped.

sac·cu·lat·ed (sack'yoo·lay''tid) *adj.* Divided into small sacs.

sac·cu·la·tion (sack"yoo·lay'shun) *n.* 1. The state of being sacculated. 2. The formation of small sacs.

sac·cule (sack'yool) *n.* 1. A small sac. 2. The smaller of two vestibular sacs of the membranous labyrinth of the ear.

sac·cu·li. Plural of *sacculus.*

sac·cu·lo·coch·le·ar (sack"yoo·lo·kock'lee·ur) *adj.* Pertaining to the saccule of the vestibule and the cochlea.

sac·cu·lus (sack'yoo·lus) *n.,* pl. **sac·cu·li** (·lye) 1. SACCULE (1). 2. [NA] SACCULE (2).

sac·cus (sack'us) *n.,* pl. **sac·ci** (·sigh) SAC.

sacr-, sacro-. A combining form meaning *sacrum, sacral.*

sa·cral (say'krul, sack'rul) *adj.* Of or pertaining to the sacrum.

sa·cral·gia (say·kral'jee·uh) *n.* Pain in the region of the sacrum.

sa·cral·iza·tion (say"krul·i·zay'shun) *n.* Fusion of the sacrum to the fifth and sometimes the fourth lumbar vertebra, leading to proneness to rupture of the disk between the fourth and fifth lumbar vertebrae. —**sa·cral·ize** (say'krul·ize) *v.*

sacral plexus. A nerve plexus usually formed from a small part of the ventral ramus of the fourth lumbar nerve, the ventral rami of the fifth lumbar and first sacral nerves, and part of the ventral rami of the second and third sacral nerves.

sacral promontory. PROMONTORY OF THE SACRUM.

sa·crec·to·my (say·kreck'tuh·mee) *n.* Excision of part of the sacrum.

sa·cro·an·te·ri·or (say"kro·an·teer'ee·ur) *adj.* Of or pertaining to a fetal position with the sacrum directed forward.

sa·cro·coc·cyg·e·al (say"kro·kock·sij'ee·ul, sack"ro·) *adj.* Pertaining to the sacrum and coccyx.

sacrococcygeal fistula. A fistula communicating with a dermoid cyst in the coccygeal region.

sa·cro·cox·al·gia (say"kro·kock·sal'jee·uh, sack"ro·) *n.* SACROILIAC DISEASE.

sa·cro·cox·i·tis (say"kro·kock·sigh'tis, sack"ro·) *n.* SACROILIAC DISEASE.

sa·cro·dyn·ia (say"kro·din'ee·uh, sack"ro·) *n.* Pain in the sacrum.

sa·cro·il·i·ac (sack"ro·il'ee·ack, say"kro·) *adj.* Pertaining to the sacrum and the ilium.

sacroiliac disease. 1. Inflammatory disease of the sacroiliac articulation. 2. Formerly, chronic tuberculous infection of the joint.

sa·cro·lum·bar (say"kro·lum'bur, ·bahr, sack"ro·) *adj.* LUMBOSACRAL.

sa·cro·per·i·ne·al (say"kro·perr''i·nee'ul, sack"ro·) *adj.* Pertaining to the sacrum and the perineum.

sa·cro·pos·te·ri·or (say"kro·pos·teer'ee·ur) *adj.* Characterizing a fetal position with the sacrum directed backward.

sa·cro·pu·bic (say"kro·pew'bick, sack"ro·) *adj.* Pertaining to the sacrum and the pubis.

sa·cro·sci·at·ic (say"kro·sigh·at'ick, sack"ro·) *adj.* Pertaining to the sacrum and the ischium.

sa·cro·spi·na·lis (say"kro·spye·nay'lis, sack"ro·) *n.* ERECTOR SPINAE.

sa·cro·spi·nous (say"kro·spye'nus, sack"ro·) *adj.* Pertaining to the sacrum and the spine of the ischium.

sa·cro·tu·ber·ous (say"kro·tew'bur·us, sack"ro·) *adj.* Pertaining to the sacrum and the ischial tuberosity.

sacrotuberous ligament. A ligament extending from the sacrum, coccyx, and posterior iliac spines to the tuberosity of the ischium.

sa·cro·uter·ine (say"kro·yoo'tur·in, ·ine, sack"ro·) *adj.* Pertaining to the sacrum and the uterus; uterosacral.

sa·cro·ver·te·bral (say"kro·vur'te·brul, sack"ro·) *adj.* Of or pertaining to the sacrum and a vertebra or vertebrae.

sa·crum (say'krum, L. sack'rum) *n.,* genit. **sa·cri** (·krye), pl. **sa·cra** (·kruh) A curved triangular bone composed of five united vertebrae, situated between the last lumbar vertebra above, the coccyx below, and the hipbones on each side, and forming the posterior boundary of the pelvis.

sac·to·sal·pinx (sack"to·sal'pinks) *n.* HYDROSALPINX.

sad·dle, *n.* 1. Any of various structures or surfaces shaped like, or suggestive of, a riding saddle. 2. *In dentistry,* the part of the denture that supports the artificial teeth, or receives support, either from the abutment teeth or the residual ridge, or both.

saddle area. The part of the buttocks surrounding the anus, together with the perineum (2) and the upper inner aspects of the thigh.

sad·dle·back, *n.* LORDOSIS.

saddle block. Sensory loss in the saddle area which occurs in spinal or caudal anesthesia.

saddle embolus. An embolus lodged at the bifurcation of an artery, narrowing or occluding both branches.

sad·dle·nose, *n*. A nose with a depression in the bridge due to loss of the septum.

saddle thrombus. A U- or Y-shaped thrombus straddling the bifurcation of a vessel. Syn. *riding thrombus*.

saddle ulcer. A peptic ulcer which has become elongated so that it partially encircles the lesser curvature of the stomach.

sa·dism (say'diz·um, sad'iz·um) *n*. Sexual perversion in which pleasure is derived from inflicting cruelty upon another. —**sa·dist** (·dist) *n*.; **sa·dis·tic** (sa·dis'tick) *adj*.

sa·do·mas·o·chism (say''do·mas'o·kiz·um, sad''o-) *n*. The coexistence of sadism and masochism, i.e., both aggressiveness and passivity in social and sexual relationships; a strong tendency to hurt others and to invite being hurt.

SAF Abbreviation for *serum accelerator factor* (= FACTOR VII).

safe period. The nonovulatory phase of the menstrual cycle, when conception cannot occur. Since the time of ovulation is variable in different women, the safe period is also variable.

saf·ra·nin (saf'ruh·nin) *n*. SAFRANINE.

safranine (saf'ruh·neen, ·nin) *n*. 2,8-Diamino-3,7-dimethyl-10-phenylphenazonium chloride, a water- and alcohol-soluble basic dye used extensively as a nuclear stain and as a counterstain for gram-negative bacteria.

saf·ra·no·phil (saf'ruh·no·fil) *adj*. Staining readily with safranine.

sage, *n*. SALVIA.

sage·brush, *n*. Any of several members of the genus *Artemisia*; its pollen is among the more important causes of seasonal rhinitis in the Mountain and Pacific states.

sage femme (sahzh fam) MIDWIFE.

sag·it·tal (saj'i·tul) *adj*. 1. Comparable to an arrow, as the sagittal suture. 2. Of or pertaining to the sagittal suture. 3. Of a plane or section through the body, median; bisecting the body into a right and a left half. 4. More broadly, either median (midsagittal) or parallel to the median (parasagittal).

sagittal suture. The site of union between the superior or sagittal borders of the parietal bones.

sa·go (say'go) *n*. A starch derived from the pith of certain East Indian and Malaysian palms; used as a food and as a demulcent.

sago spleen. A spleen in which amyloid is present in the follicles showing on section numerous small glassy areas transmitting the red color of the spleen.

Sah·li method (zah'lee) An acid hematin method for hemoglobin, in which the acid hematin solution is diluted in a special graduated tube by addition of water drop by drop until it matches a glass standard.

sailor's skin. A condition seen in exposed areas of the skin due to chronic actinic exposure. There is pigmentation and keratosis, frequently leading to squamous cell carcinoma. Syn. *farmer's skin*.

Saint Agatha's disease. Any disease of the female breast.

Saint Agnan's disease. RINGWORM.

Saint Aman's disease. PELLAGRA.

Saint Anthony's disease. SYDENHAM'S CHOREA.

Saint Anthony's fire. 1. ERYSIPELAS. 2. ERGOTISM.

Saint Avertin's disease. EPILEPSY.

Saint Blaize's disease. PERITONSILLAR ABSCESS.

Saint Erasmus' disease. COLIC.

Saint Fiacre's disease. HEMORRHOIDS.

Saint Gervasius' disease. RHEUMATISM.

Saint Giles' disease. LEPROSY.

Saint Gothard's disease. ANCYLOSTOMIASIS.

Saint Guy's dance or **disease**. SYDENHAM'S CHOREA.

Saint Ignatius' itch. PELLAGRA.

St. Louis encephalitis A mosquito-borne arbovirus infection of the central nervous system, occurring in central and western United States and in Florida.

Saint Main's evil. SCABIES.

Saint Martin's disease. DIPSOMANIA.

Saint Roch's disease. BUBONIC PLAGUE.

Saint Sebastian's disease. PLAGUE.

Saint Valentine's disease. EPILEPSY.

Saint Vitus' dance. SYDENHAM'S CHOREA.

Saint Zachary's disease. MUTISM.

sal, *n*. 1. SALT. 2. Any substance resembling salt.

sal·ep (sal'ep, suh·lep') *n*. The dried tubers of various species of the genus *Orchis* and the genus *Eulophia*. Used as a food, like sago and tapioca, or as a demulcent.

salicyl-, salicylo-. A combining form meaning *salicylic* or *salicylate*.

sol·i·cyl (sal'i·sil) *n*. 1. The radical, HOC_6H_4CO — of salicylic acid. Syn. *salicylyl*. 2. The radical HOC_6H_4— (*ortho*). 3. The radical $HOC_6H_4CH_2$—.

sal·i·cyl·am·ide (sal''i·sil·am'ide, sal'i·sil'uh·mide) *n*. *o*-Hydroxybenzamide, $HOC_6H_4CONH_2$, an analgesic, antipyretic, and antirheumatic drug.

sa·li·cy·late (sa·lis'i·late, ·lut, sal'i·si·late, sal''i·sil'ate) *n*. A salt or ester of salicylic acid.

sal·i·cyl·azo·sul·fa·pyr·i·dine (sal''i·sil·ay''zo·sul'fuh·pirr'i·deen) *n*. SULFASALAZINE.

sal·i·cyl·ic acid (sal''i·sil'ick) *o*-Hydroxybenzoic acid, HOC_6H_4COOH used topically as a keratoplastic and keratolytic drug, and sometimes for bacteriostatic effect. Its salts, as sodium salicylate, are used mainly as analgesics.

sal·i·cyl·ism (sal'i·sil·iz·um) *n*. A group of symptoms produced by large doses of salicylates; characterized chiefly by tinnitus, dizziness, headache, confusion, nausea, and vomiting.

salicylo-. See *salicyl-*.

sal·i·cyl·uric acid (sal''i·sil·yoo'rick). *o*-$HOC_6H_4CONHCH_2COOH$. A detoxication product of salicylic acid found in the urine.

sal·i·jen·in (sal''i·jen'in, sa·lij'e·nin) *n*. SALICYL ALCOHOL.

sa·lim·e·ter (sa·lim'e·tur) *n*. A hydrometer used to determine the density of salt solutions.

sa·line (say'leen, say'line) *adj. & n*. 1. Saltlike in character. 2. Containing sodium chloride. 3. Any of various salts of the alkalies or of magnesium; used as hydragogue cathartics. Magnesium sulfate and citrate, sodium sulfate, and Rochelle salt are examples.

Salipyrin. A trademark for antipyrine salicylate, an antipyretic and analgesic.

sa·li·va (suh·lye'vuh) *n.* The secretions of the parotid, submandibular, sublingual, and other glands of the mouth. It is opalescent, tasteless, and has a slightly acid pH (6.8). The functions of saliva are to moisten the food and lubricate the bolus, to dissolve certain substances, to facilitate tasting, to aid in deglutition and articulation, and enzymically to begin the digestion of starches, which it converts into maltose, dextrin, and glucose by the action of ptyalin.

sal·i·vant (sal'i·vunt) *adj. & n.* 1. Stimulating the secretion of saliva. 2. A drug that increases the flow of saliva.

sal·i·vary (sal'i·verr·ee) *adj.* 1. Of or pertaining to saliva or the salivary glands. 2. Producing saliva.

salivary calculus. 1. A concretion situated in the duct of a salivary gland. 2. SUPRAGINGIVAL CALCULUS.

salivary fistula. A fistula communicating with a salivary gland or its duct, usually the parotid, with discharge of saliva through an external opening in the skin.

salivary gland. A gland that secretes saliva, as the parotid.

sal·i·va·tion (sal''i·vay'shun) *n.* 1. Increased secretion of saliva in response to the usual stimuli. 2. An excessive secretion of saliva; a condition produced by mercury, pilocarpine, and by nervous disturbances. In severe cases of mercurial salivation, ulceration of the gums and loosening of the teeth may occur. 3. Drooling because of inability to swallow saliva, as in parkinsonism. —**sal·i·vate** (sal'i·vate) *v.*

sal·i·va·tor (sal'i·vay'tur) *n.* An agent causing salivation. —**sal·i·va·to·ry** (sal'i·vuh·to''ree, sal'i·vay'tuh·ree) *adj.*

sal·i·vo·li·thi·a·sis (sal''i·vo·li·thigh'uh·sis) *n.* Presence of a salivary calculus.

Salk vaccine POLIOMYELITIS VACCINE (1).

Sal·mo·nel·la (sal''mo·nel'uh) *n.* A genus of serologically related gram-negative, generally motile, rod-shaped bacteria belonging to the family Enterobacteriaceae. All known species are pathogenic for warm-blooded animals, including man, and cause enteric fevers, acute gastroenteritis, and septicemias. A few species are found in reptiles. —**salmonella,** pl. **salmo·nel·lae** (·ee) *com. n.*

Salmonella chol·e·rae·su·is (kol''e·ree·sue'is). A species of *Salmonella* whose natural host is the pig, where it is a secondary invader in the virus disease, hog cholera, and a primary invader in a diphtheritic form of fibrinous inflammation. In man, it is usually involved in localized lesions with or without septicemia, but may also cause enteric fever or gastroenteritis. Syn. *Salmonella suipestifer.*

Salmonella en·te·rit·i·dis (en''te·rit'i·dis). A species of *Salmonella* causing gastroenteritis in man, isolated also from the horse, hog, mouse, rat, and duck. Syn. *Bacterium enteritidis.*

salmonella fever. A disease similar to typhoid, caused by bacteria of the genus *Salmonella.*

Salmonella hirsch·fel·dii (hursh·fel'dee·eye). A species of *Salmonella* causing enteric fever in man. Syn. *Bacterium paratyphosum* C, *Salmonella paratyphi* C.

Salmonella ora·nien·burg (o·rah'nee·un·burg). A species of *Salmonella* isolated from feces of normal carriers and of persons with food poisoning, and from abscesses; often found in dried-egg products.

Salmonella para·ty·phi A (păr''uh·tye'fye). A species of *Salmonella* which is a natural pathogen of man, causing gastroenteritis and enteric fever.

Salmonella paratyphi B. SALMONELLA SCHOTT-MÜLLERI.

Salmonella paratyphi C. SALMONELLA HIRSCH-FELDII.

Salmonella para·ty·pho·sa (păr''uh·tye·fo'suh). SALMONELLA PARATYPHI A.

Salmonella pul·lo·rum (puh·lo'rum) A species of *Salmonella* causing pullorum disease or bacillary white diarrhea of chicks. Transmission can occur through the egg.

Salmonella schott·mül·leri (shot·mew'lur·eye). A motile species of *Salmonella*; a natural pathogen of man, causing enteric fever; found (rarely) in cattle, sheep, swine, chickens, and lower primates. Syn. *Bacterium paratyphosum* B, *Salmonella paratyphi* B.

Salmonella sui·pes·ti·fer (sue''ee·pes'ti·fur). SALMONELLA CHOLERAESUIS.

Salmonella ty·phi (tye'fye). SALMONELLA TY-PHOSA.

Salmonella ty·phi·mu·ri·um (tye''fi·mew'ree·um). A species of *Salmonella* commonly causing diarrhea in mice, rats, and birds and gastroenteritis in man. The most commonly isolated bacterium in outbreaks of food poisoning in the United States and Great Britain. Syn. *Salmonella aertrycke.*

Salmonella ty·pho·sa (tye·fo'suh). A species of *Salmonella* causing typhoid fever. Syn. *Bacterium typhosum, Eberthella typhosa, Salmonella typhi.*

Sal·mo·nel·le·ae (sal''mo·nel'ee·ee) *n.pl.* A tribe of the family Enterobacteriaceae, including the genera *Salmonella* and *Shigella.*

sal·mo·nel·lo·sis (sal''mo·nel·o'sis) *n.,* pl. **salmonello·ses** (·seez) Infection with an organism of the genus *Salmonella.* It may be food-poisoning, gastroenteritic, typhoidal, or septicemic.

sal·ol (sal'ol) *n.* PHENYL SALICYLATE.

salping-, salpingo- A combining form meaning (a) *auditory tube*; (b) *uterine tube.*

sal·pin·ge·al (sal·pin'jee·ul) *adj.* SALPINGIAN.

sal·pin·gec·to·my (sal''pin·jeck'tuh·mee) *n.* Excision of a uterine tube.

sal·pin·gem·phrax·is (sal''pin·jem·frack'sis) *n.* Closure of the auditory or uterine tube.

sal·pin·gi·an (sal·pin'jee·un) *adj.* Of, pertaining to, or involving the auditory tube or the uterine tube.

sal·pin·gi·tis (sal''pin·jye'tis) *n.* 1. Inflammation of the uterine tube. 2. Inflammation of the auditory tube. —**sal·pin·git·ic** (jit'ick) *adj.*

sal·pin·go·cath·e·ter·ism (sal·ping'go·kath'e·tur·iz·um) *n.* Catheterization of an auditory tube.

sal·pin·go·cele (sal·ping′go·seel) *n.* Hernia of an oviduct.

sal·pin·go·cy·e·sis (sal·ping″go·sigh·ee′sis) *n.* TUBAL PREGNANCY.

sal·pin·go·gram (sal·ping′go·gram) *n.* A radiographic image produced by salpingography.

sal·pin·gog·ra·phy (sal″ping·gog′ruh·fee) *n.* Radiographic demonstration of the uterine tubes after they are filled with a radiopaque liquid.

sal·pin·gol·y·sis (sal″ping·gol′i·sis) *n.* The breaking down of adhesions of a uterine tube.

sal·pin·go·oo·pho·rec·to·my (sal″ping·go·o″o·fo·reck′to·mee) *n.* Excision of a uterine tube and an ovary.

sal·pin·go·oo·pho·ri·tis (sal″ping·go·o″o·fo·rye′tis) *n.* Inflammation of the uterine tubes and the ovaries.

sal·pin·go·ooph·o·ro·cele (sal″ping·go·off′uh·ro·seel) *n.* Hernial protrusion of an ovary and oviduct.

sal·pin·go·pal·a·tine (sal·ping″go·pal′uh·tine) *adj.* Pertaining to the auditory tube and the palate.

sal·pin·go·peri·to·ni·tis (sal·ping″go·perr″i·to·nigh′tis) *n.* Inflammation of the peritoneum and uterine tube.

sal·pin·go·pexy (sal·ping′go·peck″see) *n.* Operative fixation of one or both uterine tubes.

sal·pin·go·pha·ryn·ge·al (sal·ping″go·fa·rin′jee·ul) *adj.* Pertaining to the auditory tube and the pharynx.

sal·pin·go·pha·ryn·ge·us (sal·ping″go·fa·rin′jee·us) *n.* A muscular bundle passing from the auditory tube downward to the constrictors of the pharynx.

sal·pin·go·plas·ty (sal·ping′go·plas″tee) *n.* Surgery of a uterine tube.

sal·pin·gor·rha·phy (sal″ping·gor′uh·fee) *n.* Suture of a uterine tube.

sal·pin·go·sal·pin·gos·to·my (sal·ping″go·sal″ping·gos′tuh·mee) *n.* The operation reuniting an oviduct after removal of an intervening section.

sal·pin·go·scope (sal·ping′go·skope) *n.* NASOPHARYNGOSCOPE.

sal·pin·gos·to·my (sal″ping·gos′tuh·mee) *n.* 1. The operation of making an artificial fistula between a uterine tube and the body surface. 2. Any plastic operation for opening the uterine tube.

sal·pin·got·o·my (sal″ping·got′uh·mee) *n.* The operation of cutting into a uterine tube.

sal·pin·gys·tero·cy·e·sis (sal″pin·jis′tur·o·sigh·ee′sis) *n.* INTERSTITIAL PREGNANCY.

sal·pinx (sal′pinks) *n.,* genit. **sal·pin·gis** (sal·pin′jis), pl. **salpin·ges** (·jeez) 1. AUDITORY TUBE. 2. UTERINE TUBE.

salt, *n.* 1. SODIUM CHLORIDE. 2. *In chemistry,* any of a group of substances that result from the reaction between acids and bases; a compound of a metal or positive radical and a nonmetal or negative radical. 3. A mixture of several salts, especially those occurring in mineral springs.

sal·ta·tion (sal·tay′shun) *n.* 1. Progression or action by jumps or jerks rather than by smoothly controlled movements. 2. SALTATORY CONDUCTION. 3. A genetic mutation resulting in a very significant difference between parent and offspring.

sal·ta·to·ry (sal′tuh·to″ree) *adj.* 1. Characterized by jumping or jerky movements. 2. Progressing in a succession of abrupt changes rather than continuously.

saltatory conduction or **transmission.** The passage of the action potential along myelinated nerve axons by skipping from one node of Ranvier to the next, the active node serving electrotonically to depolarize to the firing level the node ahead without significant activation of internodal segments. This process results in conduction of nerve impulses along myelinated axons 50 times faster than in the fastest unmyelinated nerve fibers.

saltatory spasm. A paroxysmal clonic movement of the lower extremities that causes the patient to leap or jump; the cause is not known, although it is sometimes considered to be a tic.

salting out. A method of decreasing the solubility, and thereby precipitating, certain substances, such as proteins, by adding to their solutions neutral salts, such as sodium chloride.

salt·pe·ter, salt·pe·tre (sawlt·pee′tur) *n.* Potassium nitrate, KNO_3; has some diuretic properties.

sa·lu·bri·ous (sa·lew′bree·us) *adj.* Wholesome; in a state of physical well-being. **—salu·bri·ty** (·bri·tee) *n.*

sal·ure·sis (sal″yoo·ree′sis) *n.* Excretion of salt (specifically, of sodium chloride) in the urine.

sal·u·tary (sal′yoo·terr·ee) *adj.* Promoting health.

sal·vage (sal′vij) *v. & n.* 1. To save through therapeutic or preventive measures, persons, organs, or tissues, that would otherwise be lost. 2. The persons or parts thus saved. 3. The act of salvaging.

salve (sav, sahv) *n.* OINTMENT.

sal·via (sal′vee·uh) *n.* The dried leaves of *Salvia officinalis,* which contain a volatile oil. Formerly used empirically for the treatment of a variety of ailments. Syn. *sage.*

sa·mar·i·um (sa·mâr′ee·um) *n.* Sm (or Sa) = 150.4. A metallic lanthanide, atomic number 62.

sam·bu·cus (sam·bew′kus) *n.* The dried flowers of *Sambucus canadensis,* or of *Sambucus nigra,* which contain a volatile oil, and also eldrin, which is identical with rutin. Sambucus has been used as a diaphoretic and diuretic. Syn. *elder flowers.*

sam·ple, *n.* A specimen or part to show the quality of the whole.

Samp·son's cysts Cystic endometriosis of the ovary.

san·a·to·ri·um (san″uh·to′ree·um) *n.,* pl. **sanatori·ums, sanato·ria** (·ee·uh) An establishment for the treatment of patients with chronic diseases or mental disorders; especially, such a private hospital or place.

san·da·rac (san′duh·rack) *n.* A white, transparent resin produced by *Callitris quadrivalvis,* a tree of North Africa; sometimes employed as a protective in dentistry.

sand flea. *TUNGA PENETRANS.*

sand fly. A fly of the genus *Phlebotomus.*

Sand·hoff's disease. A rare form of G_{M2} gangliosidosis, clinically and pathologically similar to Tay-Sachs disease except for the presence of moderate hepatosplenomegaly and coarse granulations, in bone marrow histiocytes, indicating lipid storage in these organs. It is due to a deficiency of the essential ganglioside-hydrolyzing enzymes hexosaminidase A and hexosaminidase B.

sane, *adj.* Of sound mind; not insane.

San·fi·lip·po's syndrome Mucopolysaccharidosis III, transmitted as an autosomal recessive trait, characterized chemically by excessive amounts of heparitin sulfate in urine, and manifested clinically by a facial appearance similar to that seen in the more common Hurler's syndrome, but otherwise less severe skeletal changes and only slight hepatomegaly. Clouding of the cornea and cardiac abnormalities do not appear. Central nervous system deficit with progressive mental deterioration is pronounced.

sangui-, sanguino- A combining form meaning *blood, sanguineous.*

san·guic·o·lous (sang-gwick'o·lus) *adj.* Living in the blood, as a parasite.

san·guif·er·ous (sang-gwif'ur·us) *adj.* Carrying, or conveying, blood.

san·gui·fi·ca·tion (sang″gwi·fi·kay'shun) *n.* The formation of blood; conversion into blood.

san·gui·na·ria (sang″gwi·nair'ee·uh) *n.* The dried rhizome of *Sanguinaria canadensis,* which contains several alkaloids, including chelerythrine and sanguinarine; has been used as an expectorant. Syn. *bloodroot.*

san·guine (sang'gwin) *adj.* 1. Resembling blood; bloody. 2. Hopeful, active, as sanguine temperament.

san·guin·e·ous (sang-gwin'ee·us) *adj.* Pertaining to the blood; containing blood.

san·guin·o·lent (sang-gwin'o·lunt) *adj.* Tinged with blood.

san·gui·no·pu·ru·lent (sang″gwi·no·pewr'yoo·lunt) *adj.* Pertaining to blood and pus.

san·gui·no·se·rous (sang″gwi·no·seer'us, ·serr'us) *adj.* Pertaining to blood and blood serum.

san·guis (sang'gwis) *n.* BLOOD.

san·gui·suc·tion (sang″gwi·suck'shun) *n.* Abstraction of blood by suction, as by a leech or other parasite.

sa·ni·es (say'nee·eez) *n.* A thin, fetid, greenish, seropurulent fluid discharged from an ulcer, wound, or fistula. —**sani·ous** (·us) *adj.*

san·i·tar·i·an (san″i·tār'ee·un) *n.* A person skilled in sanitary science and matters of public health.

san·i·ta·ri·um (san″i·tār'ee·um) *n.* SANATORIUM.

san·i·tary (san'i·terre·ee) *adj.* Pertaining to health, or to the restoration or maintenance of health, or to the absence of any agent that may be injurious to health.

san·i·ta·tion (san″i·tay'shun) *n.* 1. The act or process of securing a sanitary or healthful condition. 2. The application of sanitary measures.

san·i·tize (san'i·tize) *v.* To make sanitary; to boil instruments, solutions, etc., in order to destroy organisms.

san·i·ty (san'i·tee) *n.* Soundness of mind.

San Joa·quin Valley fever (san wah·keen') COCCIDIOIDOMYCOSIS.

san·ton·i·ca (san·ton'i·kuh) *n.* The dried flower heads of several species of *Artemisia,* which contain santonin. Syn. *wormseed, Levant wormseed.*

san·to·nin (san'to·nin) *n.* A tricyclic constituent, $C_{15}H_{18}O_3$, of the flower heads of certain *Artemisia* species; formerly extensively used as a vermifuge, especially against *Ascaris lumbricoides,* but no longer used because of its potential toxicity.

san·to·nism (san'to·niz·um) *n.* Poisoning produced by santonin.

sap, *n.* Plant juice; the watery solution which circulates through the vascular tissues of a plant.

sa·phe·na (sa·fee'nuh) *n.* SAPHENOUS VEIN.

sa·phe·no·fem·o·ral (sa·fee'no·fem'ur·ul) *adj.* Pertaining to the saphenous and femoral veins.

sa·phe·nous (sa·fee'nus, saf'e·nus) *adj.* 1.See *saphenous vein.* 2. Pertaining to or accompanying a saphenous vein.

saphenous vein. Either of the two main superficial veins of the lower limb: 1. The great saphenous vein, which begins on the dorsum of the foot, ascends medially along the leg and thigh, and drains into the femoral vein just inside the saphenous hiatus of the fascia lata. 2. The small saphenous vein, which ascends from the outer side of the foot along the middle of the back of the leg and drains into the popliteal vein.

sap·id (sap'id) *adj.* 1. Capable of being tasted. 2. Possessing or giving flavor. 3. Palatable.

sa·po (say'po) *n.* SOAP.

sapo-, sapon-, saponi- A combining form meaning *soap, soapy.*

sap·o·gen·in (sap″o·jen'in, sa·poj'e·nin) *n.* The nonsugar or aglycone component of a saponin.

sap·o·na·ceous (sap″o·nay'shus) *adj.* Having the nature of soap.

sa·pon·i·fi·ca·tion (sa·pon″i·fi·kay'shun) *n.* The conversion of an ester into an alcohol and a salt; in particular, the conversion of a fat into a soap and glycerin by means of an alkali. —**sa·pon·i·fy** (sa·pon'i·fye) *v.*

sa·pon·i·form (sa·pon'i·form) *adj.* Soaplike in appearance and consistency.

sap·o·nin (sap'o·nin, sa·po'nin) *n.* 1. A glycoside usually obtained from *Quillaja* or *Saponaria;* used as a detergent, and a foaming and emulsifying agent. 2. Any of a group of glycosidal principles that foam when shaken with water and lyse red blood cells. Saponins are widely distributed in nature. Because they lower surface tension, they form emulsions with oils and resinous substances. Saponins alter the permeability of cell walls and, therefore, are toxic to all organized tissues.

sapo·tox·in (sap″o·tock'sin) *n.* A name sometimes applied to the more toxic saponins.

sap·phism (saf'iz·um) *n.* LESBIANISM.

sapr-, sapro- A combining form meaning

(a) *dead or decaying organic matter;* (b) *putrefaction, putrefactive.*

sa·pre·mia, sa·prae·mia (sa·pree'mee·uh) *n.* The intoxication supposedly produced by absorption of the products of putrefaction. —**sapremic, sapraemic** (·mick) *adj.*

sap·ro·gen (sap'ro·jen) *n.* A putrefactive microorganism.

sap·ro·gen·ic (sap''ro·jen'ick) *adj.* 1. Causing putrefaction. 2. Produced by putrefaction.

sa·proph·a·gous (sa·prof'uh·gus) *adj.* Subsisting on decaying matter.

sap·ro·phyte (sap'ro·fite) *n.* An organism living on dead or decaying organic matter. —**sap·ro·phyt·ic** (sap''ro·fit'ick) *adj.*

sap·ro·zo·ic (sap''ro·zo'ick) *adj.* Living on decaying organic matter; said mainly of animal organisms, as certain protozoans.

sar·a·pus (săr'a·pus) *n.* A flat-footed person.

sarc-, sarco- A combining form meaning (a) *flesh, fleshlike;* (b) *muscle.*

Sar·ci·na (sahr'si·nuh) *n.* A genus of bacteria of the family Micrococcaceae. Cell division occurs in three planes forming cubical groups.

sar·ci·tis (sahr·sigh'tis) *n.* Inflammation of fleshy tissue, especially inflammation of muscle; myositis.

sar·co·bi·ont (sahr''ko·bye'ont) *n.* An organism living on flesh.

sar·co·blast (sahr'ko·blast) *n.* MYOBLAST.

sar·co·cele (sahr'ko·seel) *n.* A tumor of the testis resembling muscle grossly.

Sar·co·cys·tis (sahr''ko·sis'tis) *n.* A group of presumed protozoa of the order Sarcosporidia, with affinity for the striated and cardiac muscles of vertebrate hosts.

Sar·co·di·na (sahr''ko·dye'nuh, ·dee'nuh) *n.pl.* RHIZOPODA.

sar·co·gen·ic (sahr''ko·jen'ick) *adj.* Producing muscle.

sar·co·hy·dro·cele (sahr''ko·high'dro·seel) *n.* A sarcocele complicated with hydrocele of the tunica vaginalis.

sar·coid (sahr'koid) *adj. & n.* 1. Resembling flesh. 2. SARCOIDOSIS.

sar·coid·o·sis (sahr''koy·do'sis) *n.,* pl. **sarcoido·ses** (·seez) A disease of unknown etiology, characterized by granulomatous lesions, somewhat resembling true tubercles, but showing little or no necrosis, affecting lymph nodes, skin, liver, spleen, heart, skeletal muscle, lungs, bones in distal parts of the extremities (osteitis cystica of Jüngling) and other structures, and sometimes by hyperglobulinemia, cutaneous anergy, and hypercalcuria.

sar·co·lem·ma (sahr''ko·lem'uh) *n.* The delicate sheath enveloping a muscle fiber. —**sarcolemmal** (·ul), **sarcolem·mous** (·mus), **sarcolem·mic** (·ick) *adj.*

ʟ-sar·co·ly·sin (sahr''ko·lye'sin) *n.* MELPHALAN.

sar·co·ma (sahr·ko'muh) *n.,* pl. **sarcomas, sarcoma·ta** (·tuh) A malignant tumor whose parenchyma is composed of anaplastic cells resembling those of the supportive tissues of the body.

sarcoma bot·ry·oi·des (bot·ree·oy'deez). A malignant mesenchymoma that forms grapelike structures; most common in the vagina of infants.

sar·co·ma·toid (sahr·ko'muh·toid) *adj.* Suggesting or bearing some resemblance to sarcoma.

sar·co·ma·to·sis (sahr·ko''muh·to'sis) *n.,* pl. **sarcomato·ses** (·seez) The formation of multiple sarcomatous growths in various parts of the body.

sar·co·ma·tous (sahr·ko'muh·tus, sahr·kom'uh·tus) *adj.* Of the nature of, or resembling, sarcoma.

sar·co·mere (sahr'ko·meer) *n.* One of the segments into which a fibril of striate muscle appears to be divided by Z disks.

sar·co·my·ces (sahr''ko·migh'seez) *n.* A fleshy growth of a fungous appearance.

Sar·co·phag·i·dae (sahr''ko·faj'i·dee) *n.pl.* A large cosmopolitan family of the Diptera, commonly known as flesh flies and scavenger flies. They normally deposit their eggs or larvae on the decaying flesh of dead animals, but sometimes also in open wounds and sores of man. The important genera are *Sarcophaga* and *Wohlfahrtia.*

sar·co·plasm (sahr'ko·plaz·um) *n.* The hyaline or finely granular interfibrillar material of muscle tissue. —**sar·co·plas·mic** (sahr''ko·plaz'mick) *adj.*

Sar·cop·tes (sahr·kop'teez) *n.* A genus of minute, rounded, short-legged, flattened mites that cause scabies in man and mange in many kinds of animals.

Sarcoptes sca·bi·ei (skay'bee·eye). The mite that causes scabies in man. Syn. *itch mite, sarcoptic mite.*

sar·cop·tic (sahr·kop'tick) *adj.* Pertaining to scabies or mange.

sarcoptic mange. The form of mange most commonly transmitted to man, caused by mites of the genus *Sarcoptes.*

Sar·cop·toi·dea (sahr''kop·toy'dee·uh) *n.pl.* A superfamily of the parasitic mites; the mange and itch mites of the genus *Sarcoptes* are included.

sar·co·sine (sahr'ko·seen, ·sin) *n.* N-Methylglycine or N-methylaminoacetic acid, CH_3NHCH_2COOH, an amino acid obtained on hydrolysis of certain proteins.

sar·co·si·ne·mia (sahr''ko·si·nee'mee·uh) *n.* An inborn error of metabolism in which there is an increased amount of sarcosine (methylglycine) in plasma and urine due to a deficiency of sarcosine oxidase, and clinically, mental and physical retardation with hypotonia.

Sar·co·spo·rid·ia (sahr''ko·spo·rid'ee·uh) *n.pl.* An order of sporozoa that questionably includes the genus *Sarcocystis.*

sar·co·spo·rid·i·o·sis (sahr''ko·spo·rid''ee·o'sis) *n.,* pl. **sarcosporidio·ses** (·seez) A disease of warm-blooded animals presumed to be caused by sporozoa of the order Sarcosporidia; it is rare in man, but common in lower animals, such as sheep. The parasites usually encyst in striated (skeletal or cardiac) muscle and produce few symptoms.

sar·cous (sahr'kus) *adj.* Pertaining to flesh or muscle.

sa·sa·pa·ril·la (sahr''suh·pa·ril'uh) *n.* The dried root of *Smilax aristolochiaefolia,* or of other species of *Smilax.* The most important principles are at least three saponins: smilasaponin, sarsasaponin, and parillin, which on hydrolysis yield the steroidal sapogenins smilagenin, sarsasapogenin, and parigenin. Sarsaparilla was formerly used in the treatment of chronic rheumatism, skin diseases, and syphilis.

sar·to·ri·us (sahr·to'ree·us) *n.*, pl. **sarto·rii** (·ree-eye) The tailor's muscle, so called from being concerned in crossing one leg over the other.

sas·sa·fras (sas'uh·fras) *n.* The dried bark of the root of *Sassafras albidum*. Contains a volatile oil, and has been used as a mild aromatic and carminative.

sat. Abbreviation for *saturated*.

sat·el·lite (sat'e·lite) *n.* 1. The part of a telomere of a chromosome distal to the secondary constriction. 2. Any secondary or subsidiary body attached to or controlled by a main body.

satellite cell. 1. Any of the cells which encapsulate nerve cells in ganglia. Syn. *capsular cell, amphicyte*. 2. In muscle, a mononuclear cell, lacking contractile substance, which is enclosed within the basement membrane of the muscle fiber and separated from the muscle fiber by plasma membranes. 3. PERICYTE.

satellite phenomenon. The enhancement of growth of one microorganism in proximity to another, for example, that of the growth of *Hemophilus influenzae* around colonies of staphylococci on a plate.

sat·el·lit·osis (sat''e·li·to'sis) *n.*, pl. **satellito·ses** (·sez) *In neuropathology*, a condition in which there is an increase of satellite cells around the nerve cells of the central nervous system in inflammatory and degenerative diseases.

sa·ti·ety (sa·tye'uh·tee, say'shee·uh·tee) *n.* Fullness beyond desire; a condition of gratification beyond desire or need.

satiety center. The region in the ventromedial part of the hypothalamus, near the third ventricle, thought to be concerned with the limitation of food intake.

sat. sol. Abbreviation for *saturated solution*.

sat·u·rat·ed (satch'uh·ray''tid) *adj.* 1. Having all the atoms of molecules linked so that only single bonds exist. 2. Having sufficient substance, either solid or gaseous, dissolved in a solution so that no more of that substance can be dissolved. Abbreviated, sat.

saturated compound. An organic compound with no free valence, and in which there are neither double nor triple bonds.

saturated solution. A solution that normally contains the maximum amount of substance able to be dissolved. Abbreviated, sat. sol.

sat·u·ra·tion (satch'uh·ray'shun) *n. In optics*, the quality of visual sensation that distinguishes between colors of the same dominant wavelength but different purities.

Sat·ur·day night paralysis. DRUNKARD'S ARM PARALYSIS.

sat·ur·nine (sat'ur·nine) *adj.* 1. Pertaining to or produced by lead. 2. Of gloomy nature.

sat·urn·ism (sat'ur·niz·um) *n.* Chronic lead poisoning.

sa·ty·ri·a·sis (sat''i·righ'uh·sis, say''ti·) *n.* Excessive sexual desire in males.

sau·cer·ize (saw'sur·ize) *v.* 1. To convert a cavity or defect into a shallow wound. 2. In chronic osteomyelitis, after removal of diseased bone,

to shape the bone cavity so as to eliminate irregularities and overhanging walls, and thus enable soft parts to fill the cavity completely during the healing process. —**sau·cer·iza·tion** (saw''sur·i·zay'shun) *n.*

sau·na (saow'nuh, saw'nuh) *n.* A type of steam bath originating in Finland. Light whipping of the skin by twigs is an accompaniment.

sau·ria·sis (saw·righ'uh·sis) *n.* ICHTHYOSIS.

sau·ri·o·sis (saw''ree·o'sis) *n.* DARIER'S DISEASE.

Sau·rop·si·da (saw·rop'si·duh) *n.pl.* A superclass of vertebrates comprising the birds and reptiles. —**saurop·sid** (·sid), **sauropsi·dan** (·dun) *n. & adj.*

sau·rox·ine (saw·rock'seen, ·sin) *n.* An alkaloid obtained from the plant *Lycopodium saururus*.

sa·vory (say'vuh·ree) *adj.* Having a pleasant odor or flavor.

Sb Symbol for antimony.

Sc Symbol for scandium.

SCA Abbreviation for *sickle cell anemia*.

scab, *n.* 1. Dried exudate covering an ulcer or wound; crust. 2. A disease of sheep caused by a mite.

sca·bi·cide (skay'bi·side) *n.* Any agent or drug which kills *Sarcoptes scabiei*, the causative organism of scabies.

sca·bies (skay'beez) *n.* A contagious disorder of the skin caused by the mite *Sarcoptes scabiei*; characterized by multiform lesions with intense itching which occurs chiefly at night. The female insect, burrowing beneath the skin to lay eggs, causes the irritation. Syn. *seven-year itch*.

scabies crus·to·sa (krus·to'suh). An extreme form of general scabies of the body resulting in fishscale-like desquamation. Syn. *Boeck's scabies, Norwegian itch*.

sca·bio·pho·bia (skay''bee·o·fo'bee·uh) *n.* Abnormal fear of scabies.

sca·la (skay'luh) *n.*, pl. **sca·lae** (·lee) A subdivision of the cavity of the cochlea; especially, one of the perilymphatic spaces.

scala tym·pa·ni (tim'puh·nigh) [NA]. The perilymphatic space below the osseous spiral lamina and the basilar membrane.

scald (skawld) *n.* The burn caused by hot liquids or vapors.

scalded skin syndrome. TOXIC EPIDERMAL NECROLYSIS.

scald·ing (skawl'ding) *n.* Burning pain in urination.

¹scale, *n.* A visible flake of dead or dying epidermis; squame. —**scaly**, *adj.*

²scale, *n.* 1. A system of measurement based on instruments bearing marks or graduations at regular intervals, as barometric scale, thermometric scale. 2. A system of grading or rating based on tests or other criteria.

sca·lene (skay'leen) *adj.* 1. Having unequal sides, as scalene muscle. 2. Of or pertaining to a scalene muscle.

sca·le·nec·to·my (skay''lee·neck'tuh·mee) *n.* Excision of the scalene muscles, particularly the anterior scalene muscle.

sca·le·not·o·my (skay''lee·not'uh·mee) *n.* Severing of the fibers of a scalene muscle, particularly the anterior scalene muscle.

sca·le·nus (skay·lee'nus) *n.*, pl. **scale·ni** (·nigh)

One of three muscles in the neck, an anterior, medial, and posterior, arising from the transverse processes of the cervical vertebrae, and inserted on the first two ribs.

scalenus anterior syndrome. A symptom complex due to compression of the brachial plexus by the scalenus anterior muscle, characterized by pain and numbness, and often by signs of compression of the subclavian artery. Syn. *Naffziger's syndrome, scalenus anticus syndrome.*

scale·nus an·ti·cus syndrome (an-tye'kus). SCALENUS ANTERIOR SYNDROME.

scal·er (skay'lur) *n.* 1. An instrument for removing calcareous deposits from the teeth. 2. An electronic instrument for counting and recording electrical impulses, as those produced by such detectors of radioactivity as the Geiger-Müller tube and the scintillation probe.

scal·ing, *adj. & n.* 1. Desquamating; producing scales. 2. A pharmaceutical process consisting of drying concentrated solutions of drugs on glass plates.

scaling circuit. A circuit that permits recording of electrical impulses which are produced at a high frequency, by counting only every 2^n or 10^n impulse; such a circuit is employed in a scaler.

scal·pel (skal'pul) *n.* A surgical knife with a short blade, a convex or straight cutting edge, rounded or pointed at the end.

scan, *v. & n.* 1. To observe (an area or volume) systematically, especially by subjecting it to a series of partial observations by a sensory organ or device. 2. The observation, or the record of the observation, made by such an organ or device.

scan·di·um (skan'dee·um) *n.* Sc = 44.9559. A rare metal, atomic number 21, belonging to the aluminum group.

scanning electron microscope. An electron microscope which, by scanning an irregularly contoured surface with a concentrated electron beam, provides a high-resolution image possessing a three-dimensional quality; used for examining and photographing cell and tissue surfaces.

scanning speech. A form of dysarthria, in which speech is slow and words are broken up into syllables, much as verse tends to be pronounced when scanned for meter. Each syllable, after an involuntary pause, may be uttered with less force or more force ("explosive speech") than is natural. Characteristic of lesions of the cerebellum and brainstem.

Scan·zo·ni's maneuver (skahⁿ-tso'nee) Conversion of a posterior vertex presentation to an anterior position by double forceps application.

scaph-, scapho-. A combining form meaning *scaphoid.*

sca·pha (skaf'uh, skay'fuh) *n.* The furrow of the auricle between the helix and antihelix.

scapho·ceph·a·ly (skaf''o·sef'uh·lee) *n.* A condition of the skull characterized by elongation and narrowing and a projecting, keel-like sagittal suture; due to its premature closure. —**scapho·ce·phal·ic** (·se·fal'ick), **scapho·ceph·a·lous** (·sef'uh·lus) *adj.*

scaph·oid (skaf'oid) *adj. & n.* 1. Boat-shaped; CONCAVE. 2. A boat-shaped bone of the carpus.

scaphoid abdomen. A belly characterized by sunken walls, presenting a concavity. Syn. *navicular abdomen.*

scaph·oid·itis (skaf''oy·dye'tis) *n.* Inflammation of the scaphoid bone.

scapul-, scapulo-. A combining form meaning *scapula, scapular.*

scap·u·la (skap'yoo·luh) *n.,* L. pl. & genit. sing. **scapu·lae** (·lee), E. pl. **scapulas** The large, flat, triangular bone forming the back of the shoulder; the shoulder blade.

scap·u·lal·gia (skap''yoo·lal'jee·uh) *n.* Pain in the region of the scapula.

scap·u·lar (skap'yoo·lur) *adj.* Of or pertaining to the scapula.

scap·u·lec·to·my (skap''yoo·leck'tuh·mee) *n.* Surgical removal of a scapula.

scap·u·lo·cos·tal (skap''yoo·lo·kos'tul) *adj.* Of or pertaining to the scapula and the ribs. Syn. *costoscapular.*

scap·u·lo·hu·mer·al (skap''yoo·lo·hew'mur·ul) *adj.* Pertaining to the scapula and the humerus, or to the shoulder joint.

scap·u·lo·pexy (skap'yoo·lo·peck''see) *n.* Fixation of the scapula to the ribs, as in cases of paralysis of scapular muscles.

sca·pus (skay'pus) *n.,* pl. **sca·pi** (·pye) SHAFT.

scar, *n.* A permanent mark resulting from a wound or disease process in tissue, especially the skin.

scar·a·bi·a·sis (skär''uh·bye'uh·sis) *n.* A condition occurring usually in children in which the intestine is invaded by the dung beetle. Characterized by anorexia, emaciation, and gastrointestinal disturbances.

scarf·skin, *n.* EPIDERMIS.

scar·i·fi·ca·tion (skär''i·fi·kay'shun) *n.* The operation of making numerous small, superficial incisions in skin or other tissue. —**scar·i·fy** (skär'i·figh) *v.*

scar·i·fi·ca·tor (skär'i·fi·kay''tur) *n.* An instrument used in scarification, consisting of a number of small lancets operated by a spring.

scar·la·ti·na (skahr''luh·tee'nuh) *n.* SCARLET FEVER. —**scar·la·ti·nal** (·tee'nul), **scar·la·ti·nous** (·teen'us) *adj.*

scar·la·ti·ni·form (skahr''luh·tee'ni·form, ·tin'i·form) *adj.* Resembling scarlet fever.

scarlet fever. An acute contagious febrile disease due to group A hemolytic streptococci, characterized by acute tonsillitis and pharyngitis and a scarlet-red exanthem. Syn. *scarlatina.*

scarlet fever convalescent serum. Human immune serum for scarlet fever. See *human immune serum.*

scarlet fever streptococcus antitoxin. A sterile aqueous solution of antitoxic substances obtained from the blood serum or plasma of a healthy animal which has been immunized against the toxin produced by group A beta hemolytic streptococci. It was formerly used in the treatment of scarlet fever, and occasionally for producing a temporary passive immunity in persons exposed to the infection. It is also used to distinguish the rash of scarlet fever from other rashes.

scarlet fever streptococcus toxin. Toxic filtrates of cultures of *Streptococcus pyogenes* responsible for the characteristic rash of scarlet fever. The toxins are serologically distinct, and are used in the Dick test to establish susceptibility or immunity to scarlet fever.

scarlet fever test. 1. DICK TEST. 2. SCHULTZ-CHARLTON BLANCHING TEST.

scarlet red. The azo dye 1-(4-*o*-tolylazo-*o*-tolylazo)-2-naphthol, $C_{24}H_{20}N_4O$; has been used to stimulate epithelial cell growth in burns, wounds, ulcers.

Scarpa's fascia The deep, membranous layer of the superficial fascia of the lower abdomen.

Scarpa's triangle FEMORAL TRIANGLE.

scat-, scato- A combining form meaning *excrement, feces, fecal.*

scat·ol (skat′ol, -ole) *n.* SKATOLE.

scat·o·lo·gia (skat″o·lo′jee-uh) *n.* SCATOLOGY.

sca·tol·o·gy (ska·tol′uh·jee) *n.* 1. The study of excreta. 2. Preoccupation or obsession with excrement, or with filth and obscenity. **—scat·o·log·ic** (skat″uh·loj′ick), **scatolog·i·cal** (·i·kul) *adj.*

sca·to·ma (ska·to′muh) *n.* A mass of fecal matter in the colon resembling, on palpation, an abdominal tumor.

sca·toph·a·gy (ska·tof′uh·jee) *n.* The eating of filth or excrement.

scato·pho·bia (skat″o·fo′bee·uh) *n.* An abnormal dread of filth or excrement.

scat·ter, *n.* 1. The deflection or deviation of x- or gamma rays due to interaction with matter. 2. *In psychology,* the range of levels through which an individual passes on an intelligence test; specifically, the extent to which the individual tested passes or fails items from widely different levels of ability, as when he does well on verbal and poorly on numerical tests. 3. *In statistics,* the extent to which items in a series are closely grouped about the mean or dispersed over a wide range. **—scat·tered,** *adj.*

scat·ter·ing, *n.* In nuclear science, the change in direction of a particle or photon as a result of a collision with another particle or system.

scav·en·ger (skav′in·jur) *n.* MACROPHAGE.

scavenger cell. MACROPHAGE.

Sc. D. Doctor of Science.

Sc.D.A. Right scapuloanterior position of the fetus.

SC disease. SICKLE CELL–HEMOGLOBIN C DISEASE.

Sc.D.P. Right scapuloposterior position of the fetus.

scent, *n.* An effluvium from any body capable of affecting the olfactory sense; odor; fragrance.

Schamberg's disease PROGRESSIVE PIGMENTARY DERMATOSIS.

Schat·ski ring A diaphragmlike localized narrowing in the lower esophagus, sometimes causing dysphagia.

Schau·mann bodies Concentrically layered structures with a central core of calcite ($CaCO_3$), surrounded by a protein-calcium complex; they occur as cytoplasmic inclusions in the giant cells of sarcoidosis, berylliosis and other diseases.

Scheie's syndrome Mucopolysaccharidosis V transmitted as an autosomal recessive trait characterized chemically by the excretion of excessive amounts of chondroitin sulfate B in the urine, and clinically by a facies similar to that seen in the more common Hurler's syndrome though less coarse, hypertrichosis clouding of the cornea, and aortic valve disease. Stature is usually normal or low-normal and intellect is little impaired if at all.

sche·ma (skee′muh) *n.,* pl. **schema·ta** (·tuh) 1. A simple design to illustrate a complex mechanism. 2. An outline of a subject. **—sche·mat·ic** (skee·mat′ick) *adj.*

sche·mato·gram (skee·mat′uh·gram, skee′muh·to·) *n. In medicine,* the outline of a person or parts of the body, in which details can be filled in, as after a physical examination or autopsy.

sche·mo·graph (skee′mo·graf) *n.* An apparatus for tracing the outline of the field of vision by means of a perimeter.

Scheu·er·mann's disease Osteochondrosis of the vertebrae, associated with kyphosis in adolescents.

Schick test A skin test for immunity to diphtheria performed by the intracutaneous injection of an amount of diluted diphtheria toxin equal to one-fifteenth of the minimal lethal dose. A positive reaction is interpreted on the fifth to seventh day. It consists of local erythema with edema, and indicates the lack of immunity.

Schiff's reagent A solution of acid fuchsin in water decolorized by sulfur dioxide; used in testing for aldehydes, the presence of which causes a blue color.

Schilder's disease A nonfamilial disease of children and young adults, characterized clinically by a progressive dementia, homonymous hemianopia, cortical blindness and deafness, and varying degrees of hemiplegia, quadriplegia and pseudobulbar palsy. The typical lesion is a large, sharply outlined, asymmetrical focus of myelin destruction, often involving an entire lobe or cerebral hemisphere, extending across the corpus callosum to affect the opposite hemisphere. In many cases, the optic nerves, brainstem and spinal cord disclose the typical discrete lesions of multiple sclerosis. Syn. *encephalitis periaxalis diffusa.*

Schiller's test A test using aqueous iodine and potassium iodide solution to delineate areas of squamous epithelium which do not contain glycogen and therefore do not take the stain. It aids in localizing areas of the uterine cervix where biopsy studies should be taken to exclude cancer.

Schil·ling classification, blood count, hemogram, or **method** A system of neutrophilic classification distinguishing myelocytes metamyelocytes, which have an indented nucleus; band cells, with sharply indented T-U-, or V-shaped nuclei; and segmented neutrophils.

Schilling test A test of the absorption of vitamin B_{12} by the gastrointestinal tract following an oral dose tagged with radioactive cobalt. I absorption is below normal, a repeat oral dose of B_{12} with intrinsic factor tests for its specific lack.

Schilling type leukemia Monocytic leukemia in which the cells bear no resemblance to granulocytes.

Schim·mel·busch's disease A variety of mammary dysplasia; CYSTIC DISEASE OF THE BREAST.

schin·dy·le·sis (skin''di·lee'sis) n. pl. **schindyle·ses** (·seez) A synarthrosis in which a plate of one bone is fixed in a fissure of another.

Schiötz tonometer (shyœts) An indentation tonometer to measure intraocular pressure.

-schisis A combining form meaning *cleft, split, fissure, splitting.*

schisto- A combining form meaning *split, fissured, cleft.*

schis·to·ceph·a·lus (skis''to·sef'uh·lus, skis'') n. 1. An individual with a fissured skull. 2. A cleft in any part of the head. —**schisto·ce·phal·ic** (·se·fal'ick) adj.

schis·to·cor·mus (skis''to·kor'mus, shis'') n. An individual having a cleft thorax (schistocormus fissisternalis), neck (schistocormus fissicollis), or abdominal wall (schistocormus fissiventralis).

schis·to·cys·tis (skis''to·sis'tis, shis'') n. EXSTROPHY OF THE BLADDER.

schis·to·cyte (skis''to·site, shis'') n. A fragmented part of an erythrocyte containing hemoglobin.

schis·to·cy·to·sis (skis''to·sigh·to'sis, shis'') n. The presence of large numbers of schistocytes in the blood.

schis·to·glos·sia (skis''to·glos'ee·uh, shis'') n. BIFID TONGUE.

schis·tom·e·lus (skis·tom'e·lus, shis·) n. An individual with a cleft extremity.

schis·tom·e·ter (skis·tom'e·tur, shis·) n. A device for measuring the distance between the vocal folds.

schis·to·pro·so·pia (skis''to·pro·so'pee·uh, shis'') n. A congenital fissure of the face. —**schisto·pros·o·pous** (·pros'o·pus) adj.

schis·to·pros·o·pus (skis''to·pros'o·pus, ·pros·o'pus, shis'') n. An individual having a fissure of the face.

schis·tor·rha·chis, schis·tor·ra·chis (skis·tor'uh·kis, shis·) n. SPINA BIFIDA.

schis·to·sis (shis·to'sis) n. SILICOSIS.

Schis·to·so·ma (shis''to·so'muh, skis'') n. A genus of blood flukes infecting man.

Schistosoma hae·ma·to·bi·um (hee·muh·to'bee·um). A species of flukes the adults of which are found in the vessels of the urinary bladder; common in Africa.

Schistosoma ja·pon·i·cum (ja·pon'i·kum). A species of flukes the adults of which are found in the mesenteric veins; widely distributed in Japan and China.

schis·to·so·mal (shis''to·so'mul) adj. Pertaining to or caused by schistosomes.

Schistosoma man·so·ni (man·so'nigh). A species of flukes the adults of which are found in the mesenteric veins and portal vein; found in parts of Africa, South America, and the West Indies.

schis·to·some (shis''to·sohm, skis') n. A fluke of the genus *Schistosoma.*

schistosome dermatitis. A dermatitis, sometimes occurring after exposure to freshwater lakes of the United States, Canada, Europe, and Asia, resulting from the penetration of the skin by nonhuman schistosome cercariae, with snails as the intermediate hosts and migratory birds and other animals as the definitive hosts. Syn. *swimmer's itch, swamp itch.*

schis·to·so·mi·a·sis (shis''to·so·mye'uh·sis, skis'') n., pl. **schistosomia·ses** (·seez) Disease produced by digenetic trematodes or blood flukes, *Schistosoma mansoni, S. haemotobium,* and *S. japonicum,* the adult worms inhabiting the circulatory system of man and animals in the tropical and subtropical areas of the world, and constituting one of the most prevalent and important diseases of man. Syn. *bilharziasis.*

schis·to·ster·nia (skis''to·stur'nee·uh, shis'') n. A congenital fissure of the sternum.

schis·to·tho·rax (skis''to·tho'racks, shis'') n. A congenital fissure of the thorax.

schis·to·tra·che·lus (skis''to·tray'ke·lus, shis'') n. CERVICAL FISSURE.

schiz-, schizo- A combining form meaning *split or cleft.*

schiz·en·ceph·a·ly (skiz''en·sef'uh·lee) n. A form of developmental porencephaly that is characterized by symmetrically placed clefts in the cerebral cortex.

schizo·af·fec·tive (skit''so·uh·feck'tiv, skiz''o·) adj. Pertaining to psychiatric disorders showing mixtures of schizophrenic and affective or manic-depressive symptoms.

schizoaffective type of schizophrenia. A psychotic disorder in which mental content may be predominantly schizophrenic while mood is markedly excited or depressed.

schizo·ble·phar·ia (skiz''o·ble·fär'ee·uh) n. A fissure of the eyelid.

schizo·cyte (skiz'o·site) n. SCHISTOCYTE.

schizo·gen·e·sis (skiz''o·jen'e·sis) n. Reproduction by fission.

schizo·gnath·ism (skiz''o·nath'iz·um) n. A condition in which either the upper or lower jaw is cleft. —**schizognath·ous** (·us) adj.

schi·zog·o·ny (ski·zog'uh·nee) n. 1. SCHIZOGENESIS. 2. Multiple division in which the contents of the oocyst eventually split into swarm spores. —**schizo·gon·ic** (·schizo·go'nick) adj.

schiz·oid (skit'soid, skiz'oid) adj. & n. 1. Resembling schizophrenia; often applied to individuals who are extremely shy and introverted. 2. A schizoid individual.

schizo·ma·nia (skit''so·may'nee·uh, skiz''o·) n. A schizoaffective type of schizophrenia.

Schizo·my·ce·tes (skiz''o·migh·see'teez) n.pl. A class of fungi; the fission fungi or bacteria.

schiz·ont (skiz'ont) n. A stage in the asexual life cycle of *Plasmodium,* covering the period from beginning of division of nuclear material until the mature merozoites are formed.

schizo·pha·sia (skit''so·fay'zhuh, ·zee·uh, skiz''o·) n. WORD SALAD.

schizo·phre·nia (skit'so·free'nee·uh, ·fren'ee·uh, skiz''o·) n. A group of psychotic disorders, often beginning after adolescence or in young adulthood, characterized by fundamental alterations in concept formations, with misinterpretation of reality, and associated affective, behavioral, and intellectual disturbances in varying degrees and mixtures. These disorders are marked by a tendency to withdraw from reality, ambivalent, constricted, and inappropriate responses and mood, unpredictable disturbances in stream of thought, regressive tendencies to the point of deterioration, and often hallucinations and delusions. Syn. *dementia praecox.* **—schizo·phre·nic** (·fren′ick, ·free′nick) *n. & adj.*

schizo·the·mia (skit″so·theem′ee·uh, skiz′o·) *n.* Interrupting conversational flow with reminiscenses.

schizo·thy·mic (skit″so·thigh′mick, skiz″o·) *adj.* Having a schizoid personality or temperament. **—schizothy·mia** (·mee·uh) *n.*

schizo·type (skit′so·tipe, skiz′o·) *n.* A schizophrenic phenotype.

Schlemm's canal An irregular space or plexiform series of spaces at the sclerocorneal junction in the eye. It drains the aqueous humor from the anterior chamber.

Schmincke's tumor (shmink′e^h) LYMPHOEPITHELIOMA.

Schmorl's nodules The herniation of the intervertebral disk into the end plate of a vertebral body; usually identifiable on x-ray examination.

Schnei·de·ri·an membrane (shnye·deer′ee·un) The mucosa lining the nasal cavities and paranasal sinuses.

Schön·lein's purpura (shœhn′line) A nonthrombocytopenic purpura marked by tenderness and pain of the joints, often with periarticular effusions, mild fever, and erythematous or urticarial exanthema. Syn. *peliosis rheumatica, rheumatic purpura.*

Schüff·ner's dots, granules, or **stippling** (shu^ef nur) Small, round, pink or red-yellow granules that appear in Romanovsky-stained erythrocytes concomitantly with the developing malarial parasite.

Schultz-Charl·ton blanching test (shōolts, charl′tun) *Obsol.* An immunologic skin test of aid in the diagnosis of scarlet fever, performed by the intracutaneous injection of human scarlet fever immune serum. A positive reaction which occurs in scarlet fever consists of blanching of the rash in a zone surrounding the point of injection.

Schwann cell (shva^hn) A cell that ensheaths one or more peripheral axons. The concentric lamellae of the internodal myelin sheath are derived from the plasma membrane of one Schwann cell.

schwan·no·ma (shwah·no′muh, shvah·) *n.,* pl. **schwannomas, schwannoma·ta** (·tuh) NEURILEMMOMA.

Schwartz-Bartter syndrome Dilutional hyponatremia resulting from inappropriate secretion of antidiuretic hormone, seen as a complication of oat-cell bronchogenic carcinoma and occasionally in other carcinomas.

sci·age (see·ahzh′) *n.* A sawing movement in massage, practiced with the ulnar border o with the dorsum of the hand.

sci·as·co·py (sigh·as′kuh·pee) *n.* RETINOSCOPY.

sci·at·ic (sigh·at′ick) *adj.* 1. Pertaining to th ischium. 2. Pertaining to the sciatic nerve.

sci·at·i·ca (sigh·at′i·kuh) *n.* Pain along the cours of the sciatic nerve, dependent upon inflam mation or injury to the nerve or its roots, an most commonly due to a herniated disk of th lower lumbar or upper sacral spine. In addi tion to the pain, there is numbness, tinglin and tenderness along the course of the nerve and eventually loss of the ankle jerk and su perficial sensation in the distribution of the involved root or roots.

sciatic hernia. A hernia through the greater o lesser sciatic notch. Syn. *ischiadic hernia.*

sciatic nerve. A nerve that arises from the sacra plexus, passes out of the pelvis, and extends t the distal third of the thigh where it branche into the tibial and common peroneal nerves. I innervates the skin and muscles of both the foot and the leg.

sci·en·tif·ic, *adj.* 1. Of or pertaining to science 2. In accordance with the principles an methods of science.

sci·e·ro·pia (sigh″e·ro′pee·uh) *n.* Defective vi sion in which all objects appear dark.

scil·la (sil′uh) *n.* SQUILL.

scil·lism (sil′iz·um) *n.* Poisoning produced b squill or its preparations.

scil·lo·ceph·aly (sil″o·sef′uh·lee) *n.* Congenita deformity of the head, in which it is small an conically pointed.

scin·ti·gram (sin′ti·gram) *n.* SCINTISCAN.

scin·til·la·tion (sin′ti·lay′shun) *n.* 1. An emissio of sparks. 2. A subjective visual sensation, a of sparks. 3. Instantaneous emission of ligh from a substance following the absorption c radiant or particulate energy. **—scin·til·lat** (sin′ti·late) *v.;* **scintil·lat·ing** (·lay′ting) *adj.*

scin·ti·scan (sin′ti·skan) *n.* A recording on film o paper of the distribution of a radioactiv tracer in an intact tissue or organ, obtained b an automatic scanning system.

scin·ti·scan·ner (sin′ti·skan″ur) *n.* A directiona scintillation counter which automaticall scans an object or region of the body to deter mine the distribution of a radioactive trace substance and obtain a profile of the radioac tive area, simultaneously recording the infor mation in the form of a scintiscan.

scir·rhous (skirr′us, sirr′us) *adj.* Hard.

scirrhous carcinoma. A form of poorly differen tiated adenocarcinoma in which cords an clusters of anaplastic cells are surrounded b dense collagenous bundles, making the tumo very hard to palpation. Syn. *scirrhus.*

scir·rhus (skirr′us, sirr′us) *n.,* pl. **scir·rhi** (·eye) **scirrhuses** SCIRRHOUS CARCINOMA.

scis·sion (sizh′un) *n.* 1. A splitting or dividing, a of a living cell or a molecule. 2. Fission of the nucleus of an atom.

scis·sor·ing (siz′ur·ing) *n.* The tendency for th legs to cross on standing or lying due to spasr or preponderance of action of the adductors a the hips, seen in spastic diplegia or paraplegia

scis·sors, *n.pl.* An instrument consisting of tw

blades held together on a pivot, and crossing each other so that in closing they cut the object placed between them. The blades may be straight, angular, or curved, blunt, sharp, or probe-pointed.

scissors gait. A spastic gait characteristic of patients with spastic diplegia or paraplegia. The legs are strongly adducted at the thighs, crossing alternately in front of one another with the knees scraping together, resulting in short steps and slow progression.

scis·su·ra (si·sue'ruh) n., pl. **scissu·rae** (·ree) A fissure; a splitting.

scler-, sclero- A combining form meaning (a) *hard, hardness;* (b) *sclerosis, sclerotic;* (c) *sclera, scleral.*

scle·ra (skleer'uh) n., L. pl. & genit. sing. **scle·rae** (·ree) The sclerotic coat of the eye; the firm, fibrous, outer layer of the eyeball, continuous with the sheath of the optic nerve behind and with the cornea in front. —**scle·ral** (·ul) *adj.*

scler·ac·ne (sklerr·ack'nee, skleer·) n. ACNE INDURATA.

scler·ec·ta·sia (sklerr''eck·tay'zhuh, ·zee·uh, skleer''eck·) n. Localized bulging of the sclera.

scle·rec·to·iri·dec·to·my (skle·reck''to·irr''i·deck'tuh·mee) n. Excision of a portion of the sclera and of the iris, for glaucoma.

scle·rec·to·my (skle·reck'tuh·mee) n. Excision of a portion of the sclera.

scler·ede·ma (sklerr''e·dee'muh, skleer'') n. An idiopathic skin disease characterized by diffuse nonpitting edema and induration.

scleredema adul·to·rum (ad·ul·to'rum). A disease of unknown cause characterized by benign spreading swelling and induration of the skin and subcutaneous tissues, sparing the hands and feet; often follows an acute infection.

scleredema neonatorum. A milder form of sclerema neonatorum.

scle·re·ma (skle·ree'muh) n. Sclerosis, or hardening, especially of the skin.

sclerema ne·o·na·to·rum (nee·o·na·to'rum). A life-threatening disease of the newborn of unknown cause, characterized by a waxy-white hardening of the subcutaneous tissue, especially of the legs and the feet, which does not pit on pressure. Most often seen in premature infants or in those who are undernourished, dehydrated, and debilitated.

scle·ren·ce·pha·lia (skleer''en·se·fay'lee·uh) n. Sclerosis of brain tissue.

scle·ri·tis (skle·rye'tis) n. Inflammation of the sclerotic coat of the eye. It may exist alone (simple scleritis or episcleritis), or involve the cornea, iris, or choroid.

sclero-. See *scler-.*

scle·ro·atroph·ic (skleer''o·a·trof'ick) *adj.* Pertaining to fibrosis associated with atrophy.

scle·ro·con·junc·ti·val (skleer''o·kon''junk·tye'vul) *adj.* Pertaining conjointly to the sclerotic coat of the eye and the conjunctiva.

scle·ro·con·junc·ti·vi·tis (skleer''o·kun·junk''ti·vye'tis) n. Simultaneous conjunctivitis and scleritis.

scle·ro·cor·nea (skleer''o·kor'nee·uh) n. The sclera and the cornea regarded as one. Syn. *corneosclera.* —**sclerocor·ne·al** (·nee·ul) *adj.*

sclerocorneal junction. The boundary between the white, opaque sclera and the transparent cornea in the eye.

scle·ro·cys·tic (skleer''o·sis'tick) *adj.* 1. Both hard and cystic. 2. Both fibrous and cystic.

sclerocystic ovaries. The fibrotic ovaries with small cysts found in the Stein-Leventhal syndrome.

scle·ro·dac·tyl·ia (skleer''o·dack·til'ee·uh) n. Thickening and hardening of the fingers which may occur in scleroderma or as a complication of acrosclerosis.

scle·ro·der·ma (skleer''o·dur'muh) n. An increment in collagenous connective tissue in the skin, either focal or diffuse, the latter form associated with similar changes in the viscera. Syn. *elephantiasis sclerosa, scleriasis, dermatosclerosis, chorionitis.*

scle·ro·der·ma·ti·tis (skleer''o·dur''muh·tye'tis) n. Inflammatory thickening and hardening of the skin.

scle·rog·e·nous (skle·roj'e·nus) *adj.* Producing a hard substance.

scle·ro·gy·ria (skleer''o·jye'ree·uh, ·jirr'ee·uh) n. Atrophy and scarring of the convolutions of the cerebral cortex.

scle·roid (skleer'oid) *adj.* Hard or bony in texture.

scle·ro·ker·a·ti·tis (skleer''o·kerr''uh·tye'tis) n. Inflammation of the sclera and cornea.

scle·ro·ma (skle·ro'muh) n., pl. **scleromas, scle·ro·ma·ta** (·tuh) Abnormal hardness or induration of a part.

scle·ro·ma·la·cia (skleer''o·ma·lay'shee·uh) n. Softening of the sclera.

scle·rom·e·ter (skle·rom'e·tur) n. An instrument which measures the hardness of substances.

scle·ro·myx·ede·ma (skleer''o·mick''se·dee'muh) n. Diffuse skin thickening with mucoid deposits in the upper dermis.

scle·ro·nych·ia (skleer''o·nick'ee·uh) n. Induration and thickening of the nails.

scle·ro·nyx·is (skleer''o·nick'sis) n. Operative puncture of the sclera.

scle·ro·plas·ty (skleer''o·plas'tee) n. Plastic surgery on the sclera.

scle·ro·pro·tein (skleer''o·pro'tee·in) n. Any of a class of simple proteins having structural or protective functions, as collagen and keratin, and that are insoluble in aqueous solvents. Syn. *albuminoid.*

scle·ro·sant (skle·ro'sunt, ·zunt) n. A chemical irritant producing an inflammatory reaction and subsequent fibrosis.

scle·rose (skle·roze', ·roce', skleer'oze) v. To affect with sclerosis; to become affected with sclerosis. —**scle·rosed**, *adj.;* **scle·ros·ing**, *adj.*

sclerosing adenomatosis or **adenosis.** A form of mammary dysplasia in which ductular structures are enclaved in fibrous tissue, simulating invading cancerous ductular structures. Syn. *fibrosing adenosis.*

sclerosing hemangioma. A variety of benign histiocytoma, usually seen in the skin, in which capillary channels and fibrosis are prominent.

scle·ro·sis (skle·ro'sis) *n.*, pl. **sclero·ses** (·seez) Hardening, especially of a part by overgrowth of fibrous tissue; applied particularly to hardening of the nervous system from atrophy or degeneration of the nerve elements and hyperplasia of the interstitial tissue; also to a thickening of the coats of arteries, produced by proliferation of fibrous connective tissue and deposit of lipids and calcium salts.

scle·ro·ste·no·sis (skleer″o·ste·no'sis) *n.* Hardening with contracture of a part or closure of an orifice.

scle·ros·to·my (skle·ros'tuh·mee) *n.* Making an artificial opening in the sclera for the relief of glaucoma.

scle·ro·ther·a·py (skleer″o·therr'uh·pee) *n.* Treatment, especially of varicose veins, by injection of chemical agents which cause localized thrombosis and eventual fibrosis and obliteration of the vessels.

scle·rot·ic (skle·rot'ick) *adj. & n.* 1. Hard; indurated. 2. Pertaining to the outer coat of the eye, as the sclerotic coat, or sclera. 3. Pertaining to sclerosis. 4. Related to or derived from ergot. 5. SCLERA.

scle·ro·ti·um (skle·ro'shee·um) *n.*, pl. **sclero·tia** (·shee·uh) A thick mass of mycelium constituting a resting stage in the development of some fungi, as the ergot.

scle·ro·tome (skleer'o·tome) *n.* 1. A knife used in sclerotomy. 2. The fibrous tissue separating successive myotomes in certain of the lower vertebrates. 3. The part of a mesodermal somite which enters into the formation of the vertebrae. —**scle·ro·to·mic** (skleer″o·to'mick, ·tom'ick) *adj.*

scle·rot·o·my (skle·rot'uh·mee) *n.* The operation of incising the sclera.

scle·rous (skleer'us) *adj.* Hard; indurated.

scol·e·coid (skol'e·koid) *adj.* VERMIFORM.

scol·ex (sko'lecks) *n.*, pl. **scol·i·ces** (skol'i·seez, sko'li·), **sco·le·ces** (sko·lee'seez), **scolexes** The head of a tapeworm by means of which it attaches to the intestinal wall.

sco·lio·lor·do·sis (sko″lee·o·lor·do'sis) *n.* Combined scoliosis and lordosis.

sco·li·o·sis (sko″lee·o·o'sis) *n.*, pl. **sco·lio·ses, skolio·ses** (·seez) Lateral curvature of the spine, named according to the location and direction of the convexity, as right thoracic. —**scoli·ot·ic** (·ot'ick) *adj.*

sco·lio·som·e·ter, sco·li·o·som·e·ter (sko″lee·o·som'e·tur) *n.* An instrument for measuring the amount of deformity in scoliosis.

sco·lio·tone (sko'lee·o·tone) *n.* An apparatus for elongating the spine and lessening the rotation in lateral curvature.

-scope A combining form meaning *an instrument for seeing* or *examining.*

sco·po·la (sko'po·luh) *n.* The dried rhizomes of *Scopolia carniolica,* which contain hyoscyamine, scopolamine, and norhyocyamine. It has the actions of belladonna, but is used only as a source of scopolamine and hyoscyamine.

sco·pol·a·mine (sko·pol'uh·meen, ·min, sko″po·lam'in) *n.* An alkaloid, $C_{17}H_{21}NO_4$, from various plants of the Solanaceae. An anticholinergic drug, it resembles atropine in its action

on the autonomic nervous system, but whereas the latter stimulates the central nervous system, scopolamine depresses it. Used, generally as the hydrobromide salt, as a sedative, and also as a mydriatic and cycloplegic.

sco·po·phil·ia (sko″po·fil'ee·uh) *n.* Sexual stimulation derived from looking at the unclad human figure; observed chiefly in normal adolescent and adult males where it takes the aim-inhibited form of "girl watching" or looking at nude or seminude females in magazines or as part of some stage performance, or where it may be sublimated as scientific curiosity; when present to a pathologic degree, it is deviant and called voyeurism. —**scopophil·ic** (·ick) *adj.*

sco·po·pho·bia (sko″po·fo'bee·uh) *n.* Abnormal fear of being seen.

-scopy A combining form meaning *inspection* or *examination.*

scor·a·cra·tia (skor″uh·kray'shee·uh) *n.* Fecal incontinence.

scor·bu·tic (skor·bew'tick) *adj.* Pertaining to or affected with scurvy.

scor·di·ne·ma (skor″di·nee'muh) *n.* Yawning, stretching, and lassitude in the prodromal stage of infectious disease.

scor·pi·on (skor'pee·un) *n.* An arachnid of the order Scorpionida which injects poison by a sting located on the end of the tail. The venom is a neurotoxin similar in action to cobra venom.

scot-, scoto- A combining form meaning *of or pertaining to darkness.*

sco·to·chro·mo·gen (sko″to·kro'muh·jen, skot″o·) *n.* 1. Any microorganism which produces pigment when grown without light as well as with light. 2. A member of group II of the "anonymous" or atypical mycobacteria.

sco·to·din·ia (sko″to·din'ee·uh, skot″o·) *n.* Dizziness and also headache associated with the appearance of black spots before the eyes.

sco·to·gram (sko'to·gram, skot'o·) *n.* An impression made on a photographic plate by a radioactive substance without the intervention of an opaque object.

sco·to·ma (skuh·to'muh, sko·) *n.*, pl. **scotomas, scotoma·ta** (·tuh) An area of absent or depressed vision in the visual field, surrounded by an area of normal or less depressed vision.

sco·to·ma·graph (sco·to'muh·graf) *n.* An instrument for recording the size and shape of a scotoma.

scotomata. A plural of *scotoma.*

sco·tom·e·ter (sko·tom'e·tur) *n.* An instrument for detecting, locating, and measuring scotomas.

sco·to·pho·bia (sko″to·fo'bee·uh, skot″o·) *n.* An abnormal fear of darkness.

sco·to·pia (sko·to'pee·uh) *n.* NIGHT VISION. —**sco·to·pic** (·to'pick, ·top'ick) *adj.*

scour·ing (skowr'ing) *n.* Diarrhea in large domestic farm animals, usually caused by bacteria or viruses.

scours (skowrz) *n.* An infectious diarrhea of large domestic farm animals.

scrap·er (skray'pur) *n.* An instrument used to produce an abrasion.

scrap·ie (scrap'ee, skray'pee) *n.* A virus disease of sheep producing a progressive degenerative disorder of central nervous system neurons; named for the tendency of infected sheep to rub or "scrape" against fences to relieve intense pruritus.

scratch test. A test performed by severing the stratum corneum of the epidermis with a light scratch and placing an allergen upon the site of the scratch.

screen, *n.* A device that cuts off, shelters, or protects.

Scrib·ner shunt. A variety of arteriovenous shunt employing a special tube connection outside the body, so as to permit ready hemodialysis. Syn. *Quinton-Scribner shunt.*

scrof·u·la (skrof'yoo.luh) *n.* Tuberculosis of cervical lymph nodes. —**scrofu·lous** (.lus) *adj.*

scrof·u·lo·der·ma (skrof'yoo.lo.dur'muh) *n.* Lesions of the skin produced by the local action of the *Mycobacterium tuberculosis* by direct extension of some focus of infection beneath the skin, usually on the neck from draining lymph nodes, resulting in ulceration, draining sinuses, and scar formation.

scro·tal (skro'tul) *adj.* Of or pertaining to the scrotum.

scrotal reflex. Slow peristaltic contraction of the dartos muscle in response to stimulation of the perineum or thigh by stroking or by cold application.

scro·tec·to·my (skro.teck'tuh.mee) *n.* Resection of the scrotum or a part of it.

scro·to·plas·ty (skro'to.plas"tee) *n.* Plastic surgery on the scrotum.

scro·tum (skro'tum) *n.,* pl. **scro·ta** (.tuh), **scrotums** The pouch containing the testes, consisting of skin and subcutaneous tissue, dartos, external spermatic fascia, cremasteric fascia, internal spermatic fascia, and parietal tunica vaginalis propria.

scru·ple (skroo'pul) *n.* A unit of apothecaries' weight represented by the symbol ℈, and equal to 20 grains.

scru·pu·los·i·ty (skroo"pew.los'i.tee) *n.* An overprecision, or abnormal conscientiousness as to one's thoughts, words, and deeds. A prominent personality trait in persons predisposed to obsessive-compulsive neurosis and to certain types of schizophrenia.

Scul·te·tus' bandage or binder (skool.te'toos) A short, wide cloth bandage having multiple tails on each end. By overlapping the tails, snug support is obtained, and the bandage can be opened, and closed again, without moving the part.

scurf, *n.* A branlike desquamation of the epidermis, especially from the scalp; DANDRUFF.

scur·vy (skur'vee) *n.* A nutritional disorder caused by deficiency of vitamin C (ascorbic acid); characterized by extreme weakness, spongy gums, and a tendency to develop hemorrhages under the skin, from the mucous membranes, and under the periosteum, and by mental depression and anemia.

scu·tu·late (skew'chuh.late) *adj.* Shaped like a lozenge.

scu·tu·lum (skew'chuh.lum) *n.,* pl. **scutu·la** (.luh) A cup-shaped crust of favus.

scyb·a·lum (sib'uh.lum) *n.,* pl. **scyba·la** (.luh) A mass of abnormally hard fecal matter. —**scyb·a·lous** (.lus) *adj.*

SD Abbreviation for (a) *streptodornase;* (b) *standard deviation.*

Se Symbol for selenium.

seal, *n.* In prosthodontics. POSTERIOR PALATAL SEAL.

sea·sick, *adj.* Afflicted with motion sickness in a watercraft; especially, with motion sickness resulting from the pitching and rolling of a ship in a heavy sea. —**seasick·ness,** *n.*

seat·worm, *n.* ENTEROBIUS VERMICULARIS.

se·ba·ceo·fol·lic·u·lar (se.bay"shee.o.fol.ick'yoo.lur) *adj.* Pertaining to a pilosebaceous apparatus.

se·ba·ceous (se.bay'shus) *adj.* Pertaining to or secreting sebum.

sebaceous cyst. A cyst lined by sebaceous epithelial cells.

sebaceous glands. The glands that secrete sebum, an unctuous material composed primarily of fat.

se·bas·to·ma·nia (se.bas"to.may'nee.uh) *n.* A psychosis, usually schizophrenia, manifested mainly by religiosity.

se·bip·a·rous (se.bip'ur.us) *adj.* Secreting sebum.

se·bo·cys·to·ma·to·sis (see"bo.sis"to.muh.to'sis) *n.* STEATOCYSTOMA MULTIPLEX.

sebo·lith (seb'o.lith) *n.* A calculus in a sebaceous gland.

seb·or·rhea, seb·or·rhoea (seb"o.ree'uh) *n.* A functional disease of the sebaceous glands, characterized by an excessive secretion or disturbed quality of sebum, which collects upon the skin in the form of an oily coating or of crusts or scales.

seborrhea con·ges·ti·va (kon"jes.tye'vuh). CHRONIC DISCOID LUPUS ERYTHEMATOSUS.

seb·or·rhe·ic, seb·or·rhoe·ic (seb"o.ree'ick) *adj.* Pertaining to or characterized by seborrhea.

seborrheic areas. Areas where sebaceous glands are numerous, as the scalp, sides of the nose, chin, center of the chest, back, axillae, and groins.

seborrheic dermatitis. An acute, inflammatory form of dermatitis, occurring usually on oily skin in areas having large sebaceous glands; characterized by dry, moist, or greasy scales and by crusting yellowish patches, remissions, exacerbations, and itching. Syn. *dermatitis seborrheica, eczema seborrheicum.*

seborrheic keratosis. A benign skin tumor composed of squamous and basaloid cells which are arranged in various patterns to produce a brown plaque, studded with yellow collections of keratotic material, giving the lesions a greasy appearance.

se·bum (see'bum) *n.* The secretion of the sebaceous glands, composed of fat, keratohyalin granules, keratin, and cellular debris.

se·cern·ment (se.surn'munt) *n.* SECRETION, especially of a gland.

seco·bar·bi·tal (seck"o.bahr'bi.tol, .tal, see"ko.) *n.* 5-Allyl-5-(1-methylbutyl)barbituric acid, $C_{12}H_{18}N_2O_3$, a short-acting barbiturate used as a sedative and hypnotic, frequently as the sodium derivative (sodium secobarbital). Syn. *quinalbarbitone.*

sec·o·dont (seck'o·dont, see'ko·) *adj.* Possessing molar teeth which have cusps with cutting edges.

sec·ond·ary (seck'un·derr″ee) *adj.* 1. Second in the order of time or development. 2. Second in relation; subordinate; produced by a cause considered primary.

secondary amyloidosis. Amyloidosis that usually follows chronic suppurative inflammatory diseases (tuberculosis, osteomyelitis, bronchiectasis). Amyloid is deposited in fibrous connective tissue, especially in the arterioles, spleen, liver, kidneys, and adrenals.

secondary anemia. Anemia following or resulting from disease outside the blood-forming organs, such as poisoning, hemorrhage, or visceral cancer.

secondary assimilation. Conversion of absorbed food elements into body tissue.

secondary bronchus. Any of the bronchi between the primary bronchi and the bronchioles; a lobar bronchus, segmental bronchus, or any of the small bronchi which derive from segmental bronchi and ventilate portions of the lung segments.

secondary cause. A cause or factor or set of conditions which enhances or adds to the primary cause, as pneumonia may be a secondary cause of death in a patient already fatally ill with another disease.

secondary constriction. Clear areas within a telomere (arm) of a chromosome. Depending upon the presence of a nucleolus, these areas are designated as nucleolar or anucleolar constrictions.

secondary degeneration. Ascending or descending degeneration of nerves or tracts. Syn. *Wallerian degeneration.*

secondary dentition. PERMANENT DENTITION.

secondary infection. Implantation of a new infection upon a preexisting infection.

secondary lesion. A lesion that follows, and is due to, a primary lesion, as the secondary, cutaneous lesions of syphilis or the involvement of mediastinal lymph nodes following pulmonary tuberculosis.

secondary response. An immune response evoked in an organism by a previously encountered antigen, characterized by a lower threshold dosage of antigen and prolonged synthesis of greater amounts of antibody.

secondary sex characters. Differences between males and females not directly concerned with reproduction, as those of voice, distribution of body hair, patterns of adipose tissue, and of skeletal and muscular development.

secondary syphilis. Any of the manifestations of syphilis after the primary chancre heals and before the latent stage begins; skin and mucous membrane lesions predominate. During this period, serologic testing is always reactive.

secondary tympanic membrane. The membrane closing the fenestra cochleae.

second-degree burn. A burn that is more severe than a first-degree burn and is characterized by blistering as well as reddening of the skin, edema, and destruction of the superficial underlying tissues.

second-degree heart block. ATRIOVENTRICULAR BLOCK.

second heart sound. The heart sound complex related primarily to deceleration of blood in the aorta and pulmonary artery following closure of the aortic and pulmonic valves. Symbol, S_2 or SII.

second-set, *adj.* Characterizing a graft to a recipient which has already rejected a graft of the same genetic constitution.

se·cre·ta (se·kree'tuh) *n.pl.* The substances secreted by a gland, follicle, or other organ; the products of secretion.

se·cre·ta·gogue (se·kree'tuh·gog) *n.* A substance promoting or causing secretion, as certain hormones.

se·crete (se·kreet') *v.* To separate; specifically, to secrete from blood, or form out of materials furnished by the blood, various substances. —**secret·ing** (·ing) *adj.*

se·cre·tin (se·kree'tin) *n.* A basic polypeptide hormone produced in the epithelial cells of the duodenum by the contact of acid. It is absorbed from the cells by the blood and excites the pancreas to activity.

se·cre·tin·ase (se·kree'tin·ace) *n.* An enzyme present in blood serum which inactivates the hormone secretin.

se·cre·tion (se·kree'shun) *n.* 1. The act of secreting or forming, from materials furnished by the blood, various substances either eliminated from the body (excretion) or used in carrying on special functions. 2. The substance secreted.

se·cre·tor (se·kree'tur) *n.* A person who secretes demonstrable amounts of the antigen A or B or both in his saliva and gastric juice; a dominant trait.

se·cre·to·ry (se·kree'tuh·ree) *adj.* Pertaining to secretion; performing secretion.

secretory fibers. Centrifugal nerve fibers exciting secretion.

sec·tar·i·an (seck·tair'ee·un, seck·tăr') *n.* One who, in the practice of medicine, follows a dogma, tenet, or principle based on the authority of its promulgator to the exclusion of demonstration and experience.

sec·tile (seck'tile, ·til) *adj.* Capable of being cut.

sec·tion, *n. & v.* 1. A cutting or dividing. 2. A cut or slice. 3. To cut, slice, or divide. —**section·al** (·ul) *adj.*

sectional radiography. The technique of making radiographs of plane sections of objects; its purpose is to show detail in a predetermined plane of the body, while blurring the images of structures in other planes. Syn. *tomography, laminography, planography.*

sec·to·ri·al (seck·to'ree·ul) *adj.* Having cutting edges, as the molar teeth of carnivores.

se·cun·di·grav·i·da (se·kun'di·grav'i·duh) *n.* A woman pregnant the second time. —**secundi·grav·id** (·id) *adj.*

se·cun·dines (seck'un·dine'z, ·deenz, se·kun'

n.pl. The placenta and membranes discharged from the uterus after birth.

sec·un·dip·a·ra (seck"un-dip'uh-ruh, see"kun·) *n.* A woman who has borne two children. —**se·cundip·a·rous** (·rus) *adj.;* **se·cun·di·par·i·ty** (se·kun"di·par'i·tee) *n.*

SED Abbreviation for *skin erythema dose.*

se·da·tion (se·day'shun) *n.* 1. A state of lessened functional activity. 2. The production of a state of lessened activity, or the act of allaying anxiety and irritability, or the amelioration of pain by means of a sedative. —**se·date** (se·date') *v.*

sed·a·tive (sed'uh·tiv) *adj. & n.* 1. Quieting function or activity. 2. Any drug that can be used to calm anxious and disturbed patients and to produce drowsiness.

sed·en·tary (sed'un·terr"ee) *adj.* 1. Occupied in sitting; pertaining to the habit of sitting. 2. Inclined to being physically inactive; pertaining particularly to an occupation or life style in which the individual engages in little physical activity but sits a good part of the time.

sed·i·ment (sed'i·munt) *n.* The material settling to the bottom of a liquid. —**sed·i·men·ta·ry** (sed"i·men'tuh·ree) *adj.*

sed·i·men·ta·tion (sed"i·men·tay'shun) *n.* The process of producing the deposition of a sediment, especially the rapid deposition by means of a centrifugal machine.

sedimentation rate. The rate at which red blood cells settle out of anticoagulated blood.

sed·i·men·tom·e·ter (sed"i·men·tom'e·tur) *n.* An apparatus for recording the sedimentation rate of blood.

seed, *n.* A fertilized and ripened ovule produced by flowering plants, along with reserve nutritive material and protective covering. It is primarily a sporophyte in a resting stage.

seg·ment, *n.* 1. A small piece cut along the radii of anything regarded as circular; a part bounded by a natural or imaginary line. 2. A natural division, resulting from segmentation; one of a series of homologous parts, as a myotome; the part of a limb between two consecutive joints. 3. A subdivision, ring, lobe, somite, or metamere of any cleft or articulated body.

seg·men·tal, *adj.* 1. Of or pertaining to a segment. 2. Made up of segments. 3. Undergoing or resulting from segmentation.

segmental block. Anesthesia producing a block of both the sensory supply of a visceral organ and the somatic nerves of the region of approach.

seg·men·ta·tion (seg"men·tay'shun) *n.* 1. The process of cleavage or cell division, especially as applied to the fertilized ovum and blastomeres. 2. The division of an organism into somites or metameres.

seg·men·tec·to·my (seg"men·teck'tuh·mee) *n.* Surgical removal of a lung segment.

seg·men·tum (seg·men'tum) *n.,* pl. **segmen·ta** (·tuh) SEGMENT.

seg·re·ga·tion (seg"re·gay'shun) *n.* 1. The reappearance of contrasted Mendelian characters in the offspring of heterozygotes. 2. The separation of the paired maternal and paternal genes at meiosis in the formation of gametes. —**seg·re·gate** (seg're·gate) *v.*

seg·re·ga·tor (seg're·gay"tur) *n.* An instrument by means of which urine from each kidney may be secured without admixture.

Seid·litz powders (sed'lits) Two powders, one commonly in a blue paper, containing potassium sodium tartrate and sodium bicarbonate, the other in a white paper, containing tartaric acid. On mixing solutions of the powders, effervescence occurs; the solution is taken for cathartic effect. Syn. *compound effervescent powders.*

sei·es·the·sia, sei·aes·the·sia (sigh"es·theezh'uh, ·theez'ee·uh) *n.* Perception of jarring of the brain.

seis·mo·ther·a·py (size"mo·therr'uh·pee, sice"mo·) *n.* The treatment of disease using mechanical vibration.

Seitz filter (zights) A bacterial filter utilizing a matted asbestos filtering pad or disk, the unit being used with either vacuum or pressure.

sei·zure (see'zhur) *n.* 1. The sudden onset or recurrence of a disease or an attack. 2. Specifically, an epileptic attack, fit, or convulsion.

seizure equivalent. A form of epilepsy, especially in children, characterized by recurrent paroxysms of autonomic and sometimes behavioral disturbances, usually without specific systemic or intracranial disease, but with frequent abnormalities on the electroencephalogram, and responding to adequate anticonvulsant therapy. Common symptoms include headache, abdominal pain, nausea, vomiting, pallor, flushing, dizziness, faintness, fever, chills, and temper outbursts; postictal drowsiness and sleep of varying duration may follow. Other forms of epilepsy may be present. Syn. *convulsive equivalent.*

se·junc·tion (se·junk'shun) *n. In psychology,* the interruption of the continuity of association processes, tending to break up personality.

se·la·pho·bia (see"luh·fo'bee·uh) *n.* Abnormal fear of flashing light or lightning.

se·lec·tion, *n. In biology,* choosing for survival or elimination.

se·lec·tor, *n.* A device for selecting or separating.

se·le·ne (se·lee'nee) *n.,* pl. **sele·nai** (·nay, ·nigh) 1. LUNULA (1). 2. Any object resembling the moon in any of its phases.

se·le·ni·um (se·lee'nee·um) *n.* Se = 78.96. An element, atomic number 34, resembling sulfur and existing in several allotropic forms; it is toxic to humans and animals.

self-abuse, *n.* MASTURBATION.

self-alienation, *n.* The blocking or dissociation of one's own feelings until they seem estranged and depersonalized, and the person considers himself and everything about him unreal.

self-analysis, *n. In psychiatry,* the attempt to gain insight into one's own psychic state and behavior, a practice which, despite Freud's fairly successful one, generally remains rather superficial.

self-fertilization, *n.* The impregnation of the ovules by pollen of the same flower or of the ova by sperm of the same animal.

self-limited, *adj.* Restricted by its own characteristics rather than by external factors; used to designate a disease which runs a definite course in a specific time.

self-retaining catheter. A catheter so constructed that, following its introduction, it will be held in position by mechanisms incorporated in its particular structure.

self-retaining retractor. A special instrument having two retractor arms clamped to a bar and adjusted by means of setscrews. Some are equipped with a third arm for retraction of the pubic portion of the urinary bladder during bladder and prostatic operations.

self-suspension, *n.* Suspension of the body by the head for the purpose of stretching or making extension on the vertebral column.

sel·la (sel'uh) *n.,* pl. & genit. sing. **sel·lae** (·ee) SADDLE. —**sel·lar** (·lur) *adj.*

sella tur·ci·ca (tur'si·kuh) The superior portion of the body of the sphenoid bone that surrounds the hypophyseal fossa. It includes the tuberculum sellae, anterior clinoid processes, and the dorsum sellae with its posterior clinoid processes.

Sel·ye's syndrome (zel'yeh) GENERAL ADAPTATION SYNDROME.

se·man·tic (se·man'tick) *adj.* 1. Pertaining to meaning in language. 2. Pertaining to semantics.

semantic alexia. A form of alexia in which the patient is able to read, but not comprehend, written or printed language.

semantic aphasia. A failure to recognize the full significance of words and phrases apart from their verbal meaning. Although the patient can enumerate many details of what he sees and hears, he fails to integrate them into a general conception.

se·man·tics (se·man'ticks) *n.* 1. The study of meaning in language or in any system of signs or symbols; especially, analysis of signs in terms of what they signify or denote. 2. More broadly, analysis of the interdependencies of language or symbols with anything outside their own system, such as patterns of behavior and thinking.

se·mei·og·ra·phy, se·mi·og·ra·phy (see"migh·og'ruh·fee, see"mee·, sem"ee·) *n.* Description of the signs and symptoms of a disease.

se·mei·ol·o·gy, se·mi·ol·o·gy (see"migh·ol'o·jee, see"mee·, sem"ee·) *n.* SYMPTOMATOLOGY. —**semei·o·log·ic** (·o·loj'ick) *adj.*

se·men (see'mun) *n.,* pl. **semi·na** (sem'i·nuh), **semens** 1. SEED. 2. The fluid produced by the male reproductive organs, carrying the male germ cells or spermatozoa.

semi- A prefix meaning (a) *half;* (b) *partial or partially.*

semi·ca·nal (sem"ee·kuh·nal') *n.* A canal open on one side; a sulcus or groove.

semi·cir·cu·lar (sem"i·sur'kew·lur) *adj.* Having the shape of half a circle.

semicircular canals. See *membranous semicircular canals, osseous semicircular canals.*

semi·co·ma (sem"ee·ko'muh) *n.* A state of impaired consciousness in which the patient can be roused and responds with some purposeful movements to strong stimuli, especially to pain.

semi·com·a·tose (sem"ee·kom'uh·toce, ·ko'muh·) *adj.* Being in a state of semicoma.

semi·con·scious (sem"ee·kon'shus) *adj.* Half conscious; partially conscious.

semi·lu·nar (sem"ee·lew'nur) *adj. & n.* 1. Resembling a half moon in shape. 2. LUNATE.

semilunar cartilage or **fibrocartilage.** Either of the menisci of the knee joint.

semilunar valves. The valves situated between the ventricles and the aorta or the pulmonary trunk.

semi·mem·bra·no·sus (sem"ee·mem"bruh·no'sus) *n.* One of the hamstring muscles, arising from the ischial tuber, and inserted into the tibia.

semi·mem·bra·nous (sem"ee·mem'bruh·nus) *adj.* Partly membranous, applied to a muscle.

sem·i·nal (sem'i·nul) *adj.* Of or pertaining to semen.

seminal duct. The duct of the testis, especially the ductus deferens and the ejaculatory duct.

seminal vesicle. The contorted, branched, saccular, glandular diverticulum of each ductus deferens with which its excretory duct unites to form an ejaculatory duct.

seminal vesiculogram. VESICULOGRAM.

sem·i·na·tion (sem"i·nay'shun) *n.* INSEMINATION.

sem·i·nif·er·ous (sem"i·nif'ur·us, see"mi·) *adj.* Producing or carrying semen.

seminiferous tubule. Any of the tubules of the testes.

sem·i·no·ma (sem"i·no'muh) *n.,* pl. **seminomas, seminoma·ta** (·tuh) A malignant testicular tumor made up of characteristic large, uniform cells with clear cytoplasm which resemble spermatogonia. Syn. *seminal carcinoma, spermatocytoma.*

semi·nor·mal (sem"ee·nor'mul) *adj.* Half normal, as seminormal solution, a solution which contains one-half of an equivalent weight of the active reagent, in grams, in one liter of solution. Symbol, 0.5 *N* or *N*/2.

sem·i·nu·ria (see"mi·new'ree·uh, sem"i·) *n.* The discharge of semen in the urine.

semipermeable membrane. A membrane that permits water and small solute molecules to diffuse freely, but holds back large molecules, salts, and their ions.

semi·pla·cen·ta (sem"ee·pluh·sen'tuh) *n.* A form of placenta in which the maternal and fetal portions are structurally separate.

semi·pro·na·tion (sem"ee·pro·nay'shun) *n.* The assumption of a semiprone or partly prone position; an attitude of semisupination. —**semi·prone** (·prone') *adj.*

semi·pto·sis (sem"ee·to'sis) *n.* Partial ptosis.

se·mis (see'mis) *n.* Half. In prescriptions, abbreviated ss, placed after the sign indicating the measure. Sometimes abbreviated, s.

semi·som·nus (sem"i·som'nus) *n. Obsol.* Partial coma. —**semisom·nous** (·nus) *adj.*

semi·so·por (sem"ee·so'por) *n. Obsol.* Partial coma.

semi·spi·na·lis (sem"ee·spye·nay'lis) *n.* One of the deep longitudinal muscles of the back, attached to the vertebrae.

sem·i·su·pi·na·tion (sem″ee-sue″pi′nay′shun) *n.* A position halfway between supination and pronation.

sem·i·syn·thet·ic (sem″ee-sin-thet′ick) *adj.* Produced by or pertaining to a process of synthesis that involves chemical alteration of a naturally occurring compound, as the synthesis of certain antibiotics from a natural penicillin or a moiety thereof; partly synthetic.

sem·i·ten·di·no·sus (sem″ee-ten″di·no′sus) *n.* One of the hamstring muscles, arising from the ischium and inserted into the tibia.

Senear–Usher syndrome PEMPHIGUS ERYTHEMATOSUS.

se·nec·ti·tude (se·neck′ti·tude) *n.* Old age.

se·nes·cence (se·nes′unce) *n.* The state of being aged. —**se·nes·cent** (se·nes′unt) *adj.*

senescent arthritis. DEGENERATIVE JOINT DISEASE.

Sengstaken–Blakemore tube A large three-lumen rubber tube for the treatment of bleeding from esophageal varices. There is one lumen to each of two balloons and a large central lumen for aspiration of the stomach and for feeding.

se·nile (see′nile, sen′ile) *adj.* 1. Pertaining to, caused by, or characteristic of old age or the infirmities of old age. 2. Afflicted with senile dementia.

senile angioma. PAPILLARY VARIX.

senile dementia. A chronic progressive mental disease of late life characterized by failing memory and loss of other intellectual functions. The most common pathologic state underlying this syndrome is Alzheimer's disease. Syn. *senile psychosis.*

senile freckle. LENTIGO MALIGNA.

senile guttate keratitis. A form of keratitis characterized by small foci of corneal inflammation, occurring in older people.

senile involution. The slowly progressive degenerative changes seen with advanced age, often with loss of muscle and subcutaneous tissues and shrinkage of other organs.

senile keratosis. ACTINIC KERATOSIS.

senile osteoporosis. Osteoporosis in the aged, due to deficient bone matrix formation probably related to deficiency of gonadal hormones and diminished calcium intake. Blood calcium, phosphorus, and phosphatase levels are all normal or low.

senile psychosis or **insanity.** SENILE DEMENTIA.

se·nil·ism (see′nil·iz·um) *n.* Senility, especially when premature, as in progeria.

se·nil·i·ty (se·nil′i·tee) *n.* The state of being senile; physical and mental debility associated with old age.

se·ni·um (see′nee·um) *n.* Old age.

sen·na (sen′uh) *n.* The dried leaflets of *Cassia acutifolia* or of *C. angustifolia* that contain various anthraquinone derivatives; used as a cathartic.

se·no·pia (se·no′pee·uh) *n.* The change of vision in the aged, in which persons formerly myopic acquire what seems to be normal vision because of presbyopia.

sen·sa·tion (sen·say′shun) *n.* 1. The conscious perception caused by stimulation of an afferent nerve or sensory receptor. 2. A feeling or awareness of an emotional state or psychic activity which may arise within the central nervous system, and not necessarily in immediate response to an external stimulus. 3. A bodily feeling, such as pain experienced in the thalamic syndrome, which is the result of stimuli arising from within, and not from outside of the organism. —**sensation·al** (·ul) *adj.*

sense, *n.* 1. Any one of the faculties by which stimuli from the external world or from within the body are received and transformed into sensations. The faculties receiving impulses from the external world are the senses of sight, hearing, equilibrium, touch, smell, and taste, which are the special senses, and the muscular and dermal senses. Those receiving impulses from the internal organs, the visceral senses, are the hunger sense, thirst sense, sexual sense and others. 2. Judgment; understanding; sound reasoning.

sense organ. An association of tissues, including specialized sensory nerve terminals, giving rise to a specific sensation via impulses transmitted along their afferent nerves to the central nervous system, but responding to any adequate stimulus.

sen·si·bil·i·ty (sen″si·bil′i·tee) *n.* 1. The ability to receive, feel, and appreciate physical and psychological impressions. 2. The ability of a nerve or end organ to receive and transmit impulses.

sen·si·bi·liz·er (sen′si·bi·lye″zur) *n.* 1. An agent that renders an enzyme active. 2. *Obsol.* AMBOCEPTOR.

sen·si·ble (sen′si·bul) *adj.* 1. Perceptible by the senses, as by sight or smell. 2. Capable of receiving an impression through the senses; endowed with sensation.

sensible perspiration. Visible drops or beads of sweat.

sen·sim·e·ter (sen·sim′e·tur) *n.* A sensitive galvanometer used to measure skin resistance.

sen·si·tiv·i·ty (sen″si·tiv′i·tee) *n.* 1. The capacity to perceive, appreciate, or transmit sensation. 2. Power to react to a stimulus. 3. The capacity of a person to respond emotionally to changes in his environment, particularly his interpersonal or social relationships; thus frequently used synonymously with hypersensitivity. 4. The degree of change or responsiveness of an organism with respect to some specific factor or substance, as antibiotic sensitivity. —**sen·si·tive** (sen′si·tiv) *adj.*

sensitivity training. The enhancement of an individual's sensitivity to his environment and particularly interpersonal relationships by means of various techniques, usually employed in group therapy sessions (t-groups).

sen·si·ti·za·tion (sen″si·ti·zay′shun) *n.* 1. The coating of cells with antibody so that they may be agglutinated, or lysed if complement is added. 2. A greater response to a later stimulus than to the original one. 3. The process of becoming reactive or hypersensitive, especially to pollens, serums, and other antigens.

sen·si·tiz·er (sen′si·tye″zur) *n. In dermatology,* the secondary irritant which makes the susceptible subject sensitive to the same or other irritant. —**sensi·tize** (·tize) v; **sensitiz·ing** (·zing) adj.

sen·so·ri·mo·tor (sen″suh·ri·mo′tur) adj. Concerned with or pertaining to the perception of sensory impulses and the generation of motor impulses, as sensorimotor centers.

sen·so·ri·neu·ral (sen″suh·ri·new′rul) adj. Of or pertaining to sensory nerves.

sen·so·ry (sen′suh·ree) adj. Pertaining to, or conveying, sensation.

sensory agraphia. Loss of ability to write due to a defect in comprehension of language.

sensory amusia. Amusia characterized chiefly by the loss of the power to comprehend musical sounds; musical deafness.

sensory aphasia. Loosely, any loss of comprehension of spoken and written language, including acoustic and visual verbal agnosias as well as the aphasias closely related to them.

sensory epilepsy. A form of epilepsy in which various disturbances of sensation occur in paroxysms, and may or may not be followed by focal motor or generalized seizures.

sensory paralysis. Loss of sensation due to disease of sensory nerves, pathways, or centers in the nervous system; anesthesia.

sen·su·al (sen′shoo·ul) adj. 1. Of, pertaining to, or affecting the senses or sensory organs. 2. Characterized by sensualism.

sen·su·al·ism (sen′shoo·ul·iz·um) n. The condition or character of one who is controlled by, or lacks control of, the more primitive bodily appetites or emotions.

sen·sus (sen′sus) n. Sense; feeling.

sen·tient (sen′chee·unt) adj. Having sensation; capable of feeling.

sen·ti·ment (sen′ti·munt) n. 1. In psychology, a mental attitude characterized by feeling. 2. An emotional disposition toward some object or objects.

sen·ti·nel node (sen′ti·nul). SIGNAL NODE.

sentinel pile. The thickened wall of the anal pocket at the lower end of an anal fissure.

separation anxiety. The apprehension, fear, or psychosomatic complaints observed in children on being separated from significant persons or familiar surroundings; commonly expressed in school phobias, and often the result of an abnormal symbiotic relationship between the parent, usually the mother, and the child; an extension of the stranger anxiety of the infant.

sep·a·ra·tor (sep′uh·ray″tur) n. 1. Anything that separates, especially an instrument for separating the teeth. 2. PERIOSTEAL ELEVATOR.

sep·sis (sep′sis) n., pl. **sep·ses** (·seez) 1. Poisoning by products of putrefaction. 2. The severe toxic, febrile state resulting from infection with pyogenic microorganisms, with or without associated septicemia.

sept-, septi- A combining form meaning seven.

septa. A plural of septum.

sep·tal (sep′tul) adj. Of or pertaining to a septum.

septal cells. Macrophages in the interalveolar septa of the lung.

septal cyst. A cyst of the septum pellucidum.

septal lines. KERLEY LINES.

sep·tate (sep′tate) adj. Divided into compartments, as by a membrane.

sep·ta·tion (sep·tay′shun) n. 1. Division by a septum. 2. A septum.

sep·tec·to·my (sep·teck′tuh·mee) n. Surgical excision of part of the nasal septum.

sep·tic (sep′tick) adj. 1. Of or pertaining to sepsis. 2. PUTREFACTIVE.

sep·ti·ce·mia, sep·ti·cae·mia (sep″ti·see′mee·uh) n. A clinical syndrome characterized by a severe bacteremic infection, generally involving the significant invasion of the bloodstream by microorganisms from a focus or foci in the tissues, and possibly even with the microorganisms multiplying in the blood. —**septice·mic, septicae·mic** (·mick) adj.

sep·ti·co·phle·bi·tis (sep″ti·ko·fle·bye′tis) n. Inflammation of veins secondary to septicemia.

septic tank. In sewage disposal, a closed chamber through which sewage passes slowly to permit bacterial action.

sep·ti·grav·i·da (sep″ti·grav′i·duh) n. A woman who is pregnant for the seventh time.

sep·ti·me·tri·tis (sep″ti·me·trye′tis) n. Infection of the uterus.

sep·tip·a·ra (sep·tip′uh·ruh) n. A woman who has given birth seven times.

sep·to·mar·gin·al (sep″to·mahr′ji·nul) adj. Relating to the margin of a septum.

¹sep·tom·e·ter (sep·tom′e·tur) n. An instrument for determining the thickness of the nasal septum.

²sep·tom·e·ter (sep·tom′e·tur) n. An apparatus for determining organic impurities in the air

sep·to·plas·ty (sep″to·plas′tee) n. Surgical reconstruction of the nasal septum.

sep·to·tome (sep′to·tome) n. An instrument for cutting the nasal septum.

sep·tot·o·my (sep·tot′uh·mee) n. The operation of cutting the nasal septum.

septula. Plural of septulum.

sep·tu·lum (sep′tew·lum) n., pl. **septu·la** (·luh) A small septum.

sep·tum (sep′tum) n., genit. **sep·ti** (·tye), L. pl. **sep·ta** (·tuh) A partition; a dividing wall between two spaces or cavities.

septum na·si (nay′zye) [NA]. NASAL SEPTUM.

septum pel·lu·ci·dum (pe·lew′si·dum) [NA]. A thin translucent septum forming the internal boundary of the lateral ventricles of the brain and enclosing between its two laminas the so called fifth ventricle.

septum pri·mum (prye′mum). The first in complete interatrial septum of the embryo.

septum rec·to·va·gi·na·le (reck″to·vaj·i·nay′lee [NA]. RECTOVAGINAL SEPTUM.

septum rec·to·ve·si·ca·le (reck″to·ves·i·kay′lee [NA]. The tissue forming a partition between the rectum and the prostate and seminal vesicles and the urinary bladder.

septum se·cun·dum (se·kun′dum). The second incomplete interatrial septum of the embryo containing the foramen ovale; it develops to the right of the septum primum and fuses with it to form the adult interatrial septum.

sep·tu·plet (sep′tuh·plit, sep·tup′lit) n. One o

seven offspring born from a single gestation.

sep·ul·ture (sep'ul·chur) *n.* The disposal of the dead by burial; burial.

se·que·la (se·kwel'uh) *n.*, pl. **seque·lae** (·lee) 1. An abnormal condition following a disease upon which it is directly or indirectly dependent. 2. A complication of a disease.

se·quence (see'kwence) *n.* 1. The order of occurrence, as of symptoms. 2. SEQUELA. —**se·quen·tial** (se·kwen'shul) *adj.*

se·ques·ter (se·kwes'tur) *v.* 1. To separate or to become separated or detached abnormally. 2. To isolate a patient or group of patients. 3. To remove or isolate a constituent of a chemical system, as by binding or chelating. —**sequester·ing,** *adj.*

sequestering agent. Any substance which will inactivate a metallic ion in solution, as by formation of a complex compound, and keep the resulting compound in solution.

sequestra. Plural of *sequestrum.*

se·ques·tra·tion (see''kwes·tray'shun) *n.* 1. The separation of tissue and formation of a sequestrum. 2. The isolation of persons suffering from disease for purposes of treatment or for the protection of others. 3. The pooling of blood in vascular channels, either physiologically, or therapeutically by means of tourniquets.

se·ques·trec·to·my (see''kwes·treck'tuh·mee) *n.* The operative removal of a sequestrum.

Sequestrene. A trademark for ethylenediaminetetraacetic acid and various of its salts.

se·ques·trum (se·kwes'trum) *n.*, pl. **seques·tra** (·truh) A detached or dead piece of bone within a cavity, abscess, or wound. —**seques·tral** (·trul) *adj.*

SER Abbreviation for *smooth-surfaced endoplasmic reticulum.*

ser-, seri-, sero-. A combining form meaning *serum, serous.*

sera. Plural of *serum.*

ser·al·bu·min (seer''al·bew'min, serr') *n.* SERUM ALBUMIN; the albumin fraction of serum.

se·rem·pi·on (se·rem'pee·on) *n.* A form of severe measles occurring especially among children in the West Indies.

se·ri·al (seer'ee·ul) *adj.* 1. Pertaining to, arranged in, or forming a series. 2. Successive.

serial sections. A series of histologic preparations made from a single block of tissue, each succeeding section being immediately adjacent to its predecessor.

ser·i·flux (seer'i·flux, serr') *n.* Any serous or watery discharge, or a disease characterized by such a discharge.

ser·ine (seer'een, serr') *n.* β-Hydroxyalanine or 2-amino-3-hydroxypropanoic acid, HOCH₂CH(NH₂)COOH, an amino acid component of many proteins.

Serobacterin. Trademark for emulsions of killed bacteria which have been sensitized by treatment with a specific immune serum and which more rapidly produce immunity.

se·ro·co·li·tis (seer''o·ko·ly'tis) *n.* Inflammation of the serosa of the colon.

se·ro·cul·ture (see'ro·kul'chur) *n.* A bacterial culture on blood serum.

se·ro·di·ag·no·sis (seer''o·dye''ug·no'sis) *n.* Diagnosis based upon the reactions of blood serum of patients. —**serodiag·nos·tic** (·nos'tick) *adj.*

se·ro·en·ter·i·tis (seer''o·en''tur·eye'tis) *n.* Inflammation of the serosa of the small intestine.

se·ro·fi·brin·ous (seer''o·fye'bri·nus) *adj.* 1. Composed of serum and fibrin, as a serofibrinous exudate. 2. Characterized by the production of a serofibrinous exudate, as a serofibrinous inflammation.

se·ro·group (seer'o·groop) *n.* An arrangement of serotypes with common antigens.

serologic test. 1. Any test on serum for the diagnosis of a specified condition. 2. Any test on serum for the diagnosis of syphilis.

se·rol·o·gist (se·rol'uh·jist) *n.* A person versed in serology.

se·rol·o·gy (se·rol'uh·jee) *n.* 1. The branch of science that deals with the properties, especially immunologic actions, and reactions of serums. 2. *Informal.* SEROLOGIC TEST. —**se·ro·log·ic** (seer''uh·loj'ick), **serolog·i·cal** (·i·kul) *adj.*

se·rol·y·sin (se·rol'i·sin) *n.* A bactericidal substance contained in normal blood serum.

se·ro·ma (se·ro'muh) *n.* An accumulation of blood serum which produces a tumorlike swelling, usually beneath the skin.

se·ro·mem·bra·nous (seer''o·mem'bruh·nus) *adj.* Pertaining to a serous membrane.

se·ro·mu·cous (seer''o·mew'kus) *adj.* Having the nature of or containing both serum and mucus, as a glandular cell which has the characteristics of both a serous cell and a mucous cell.

se·ro·mus·cu·lar (seer''o·mus'kew·lur) *adj.* Of or pertaining to the serous and muscular layers of the digestive tract.

Seromycin. Trademark for cycloserine, an antibiotic compound.

se·ro·neg·a·tive (seer''o·neg'uh·tiv) *adj.* 1. Having a negative serologic test for some condition. 2. Specifically, having a negative serologic test for syphilis.

se·ro·pos·i·tive (seer''o·poz'i·tiv) *adj.* 1. Having a positive serologic test for some condition. 2. Specifically, having a positive serologic test for syphilis.

se·ro·pu·ru·lent (seer''o·pewr'yoo·lunt) *adj.* Composed of serum and pus, as a seropurulent exudate.

se·ro·pus (seer'o·pus') *n.* An exudate which has mixed characteristics of serous and purulent nature.

se·ro·re·ac·tion (seer''o·ree·ack'shun) *n.* A reaction performed with serum.

se·ro·re·sis·tance (seer''o·re·zis'tunce) *n.* Persistent positive serologic reaction for syphilis despite prolonged intensive treatment. —**sero·resis·tant** (·tunt) *adj.*

se·ro·sa (se·ro'suh, ·zuh) *n.*, pl. **serosas, sero·sae** (·see) 1. A serous membrane composed of mesothelium and subjacent connective tissue, lining the pericardial, pleural, and peritoneal cavities and the cavity of the tunica vaginalis testis and covering their contents. 2. The chorion of birds and reptiles. —**sero·sal** (·sul, ·zul) *adj.*

se·ro·sa·mu·cin (se·ro″suh·mew'sin) *n.* A protein resembling mucin found in ascitic fluid.

se·ro·san·guin·e·ous (seer″o·sang·gwin'ee·us) *adj.* Having the nature of, or containing, both serum and blood.

se·ro·si·tis (seer″o·sigh'tis) *n.* Inflammation of a serous membrane.

se·ro·syn·o·vi·tis (seer″o·sin″o·vye'tis, ·sigh″no·) *n.* A synovitis with increase of synovial fluid.

se·ro·ther·a·py (seer″o·therr'uh·pee) *n.* The treatment of disease by means of human or animal serum containing antibodies.

se·ro·to·nin (seer″o·to'nin, serr″) *n.* 5-Hydroxy-tryptamine, $C_{10}H_{12}N_2O$, present in many tissues, especially blood and nervous tissue; stimulates a variety of smooth muscles and nerves, and is postulated to function as a neurotransmitter.

se·ro·type (seer'o·tipe, serr'o·) *n.* A serological type; a type distinguishable on the basis of antigenic composition, used in the subclassification of certain microorganisms, as *Salmonella, Shigella.*

se·rous (seer'us, serr'us) *adj.* 1. Pertaining to, characterized by, or resembling serum. 2. Containing serum. 3. Producing a thin, watery secretion, as a serous gland; may be sero-zymogenic (pancreas) or not (lacrimal glands).

serous atrophy. Loss of lipid from adipose tissue cells accompanied by collection of serous fluid between the shrunken cells, seen in inanition.

serous cystadenocarcinoma. An ovarian tumor, the malignant variant of the serous cystadenoma. Syn. *carcinomatous serous cystoma, papillary serous carcinoma.*

serous cystadenoma. A benign cystic ovarian tumor composed of cylindrical cells resembling those of the uterine tube; the cysts contain clear, watery fluid, and there are often calcific (psammoma) bodies in the wall. Syn. *papillary cystadenoma of ovary, serous cystoma, papillocystoma, psammomatous papilloma.*

serous gland. A gland that secretes a watery, albuminous fluid.

serous inflammation. Inflammation in which the exudate is composed largely of serum.

serous membrane. A delicate membrane covered with flat, mesothelial cells lining closed cavities of the body.

serous otitis media. A common nonpyogenic and often chronic disorder of the middle ear, affecting chiefly children, in which there is an exudate high in protein and in inflammatory cells; may be due to viral infection, allergy, or other factors, and may result in conductive deafness. Syn. *catarrhal otitis media, chronic exudative otitis media, glue ear, secretory otitis media.*

serous pericardium. The thin, smooth lining of the pericardial cavity; its surface is lined with mesothelium. There is a visceral and a parietal portion.

Serpasil. Trademark for reserpine, an antihypertensive and sedative alkaloid.

ser·pens (sur'penz) *adj.* Serpentine, sinuous; creeping.

ser·pen·tar·ia (sur″pen·tār'ee·uh) *n.* The dried rhizome and roots of *Aristolochia serpentaria,* Virginia snakeroot, or of *A. reticulata,* Texas snakeroot; has been used as an aromatic bitter and gastric stimulant.

ser·pig·i·nous (sur·pij'i·nus) *adj.* Progressing from one surface or part to a contiguous one; applied to skin lesions.

serpiginous ulcer. An ulcer which slowly extends in one area while healing in another. Syn. *creeping ulcer.*

ser·rat·ed (serr'ay·tid) *adj.* Having a toothed margin; having a sawlike edge.

Ser·ra·tia (se·ray'shee·uh) *n.* A genus of bacilli commonly found in water, belonging to the family Enterobacteriaceae; about 25 percent of strains are pigmented.

Serratia mar·ces·cens (mahr·ses'enz). A motile, gram-negative organism that occasionally produces a deep red pigment. Found in water, soil, milk, and stools. Long considered a harmless saprophyte, it has recently been incriminated in septicemias, pulmonary disease, hospital epidemics, and even death. Syn. *Bacillus prodigiosus.*

ser·ra·tion (se·ray'shun) *n.* The state or condition of being toothed or having a toothed margin.

ser·ra·tus (se·ray'tus) *L. adj. & n.* 1. SERRATED. 2. A muscle arising or inserted by a series of processes like the teeth of a saw.

Ser·to·li cells (serr'to·lee) The sustentacular cells of seminiferous tubules.

se·rum (seer'um, serr'um) *n.*, pl. **se·ra** (·uh) 1. The cell and fibrinogen-free amber-colored fluid appearing after blood or plasma clots. 2. IMMUNE SERUM. 3. The clear portion of any biologic fluid.

serum accelerator factor. FACTOR VII. ABBREVIATED, SAF.

se·rum·al (seer'um·ul, serr′) *adj.* Of or pertaining to serum.

serum albumin. The chief protein of blood serum and of serous fluids.

serum globulin. The globulin fraction of blood serum; the fraction of serum protein precipitated by half-saturation with ammonium sulfate in contrast to the albumin fraction which is soluble in this salt concentration.

serum hepatitis. A form of viral hepatitis usually transmitted by the parenteral injection of human blood or blood products contaminated with the hepatitis B virus.

serum proteins. The proteins present in the serum from clotted blood, differing from plasma proteins only in the absence of fibrinogen.

serum prothrombin conversion accelerator. FACTOR VII. Abbreviated, SPCA.

serum shock. Anaphylactic shock resulting from the injection of a serum into a sensitive individual.

serum sickness. A syndrome originally observed as a sequel of the administration of foreign serum therapeutically, generally resulting in the occurrence in 8 to 12 days of an urticarial rash, edema, enlargement of lymph nodes, arthralgia, fever, and neuritis in some cases. Immunologically, it is related to the formation of circulating antigen-antibody complexes at moderate antigen excess, and possibly to reaginic antibodies. Similar phenomena are noted with purified protein antigens and with chemicals.

ser·vo·mech·a·nism (sur′′vo-meck′uh-niz·um) n. A means or device for adjusting and controlling the performance of a given system to a desired standard or level through a feedback mechanism.

ser·yl (seer′il, serr′il) n. The univalent radical, $HOCH_2CH-(NH_2)CO-$, of the amino acid serine.

ses·a·me (ses′uh-mee) n. An herb, *Sesamum indicum*, the seeds of which yield sesame oil, a fixed oil used as a vehicle for intramuscular injections.

ses·a·moid (ses′uh-moid) adj. Resembling a sesame seed.

sesamoid bones. Small bones developed in tendons subjected to much pressure.

sesamoid cartilage. One of a pair of small cartilages lying in the aryepiglottic folds; they are constant in some animals and are occasionally found in man.

ses·a·moid·itis (ses′′uh-moy-dye′tis) n. Inflammation of the sesamoid bones which may involve the articular surfaces and cause lameness.

sesqui- A combining form indicating *one and one-half, the proportion of two* (of one radical or element) *to three* (of another).

ses·qui·chlo·ride (ses′′kwi-klo′ride) n. A compound of chlorine and another element containing three atoms of chlorine to two of the other element, as Fe_2Cl_3.

ses·qui·ho·ra (ses′′kwi-ho′ruh) n. An hour and a half.

ses·qui·salt (ses′kwi-sawlt) n. A salt containing one and one-half times as much of the acid as of the radical or base, as $Fe_2(SO_4)_3$.

ses·sile (ses′il, -ile) adj. 1. Attached by a broad base; not pedunculated, as a sessile tumor. 2. Attached, not free moving, as certain invertebrate animals.

set, v. 1. To reduce the displacement in a fracture and apply supporting structures suitably arranged for fixation. 2. To harden or solidify, as a cement, amalgam, or plaster. —**set·ting,** n. & adj.

se·ton (see′tun) n. A thread or bundle of threads, passed through an opening in the skin, once used to provide drainage, produce a fistulous tract, or encourage "healing inflammation."

sev·enth (VIIth) cranial nerve. FACIAL NERVE.

severe combined immunodeficiency. Congenital severe deficiency of lymphocytes and absence of plasma cells with marked hypogammaglobulinemia, deficient cellular and humoral responses to all antigens, and early death; inherited as an X-linked or autosomal recessive trait, or may occur sporadically. Abbreviated, SCID. Syn. *alymphocytosis, Glanzmann and Riniker's lymphocytophthisis.*

se·vip·a·rous (se-vip′uh-rus) adj. SEBIPAROUS; fat-producing.

sew·age (sue′ij) n. The heterogeneous substances constituting the excreta and waste matter of domestic economy and the contents of sewers.

sex-, sexi- A combining form meaning *six*.

sex, n. 1. Either of the two categories, female and male, into which organisms of many species are divided and by the union of whose gametes (ova and spermatozoa) they reproduce. 2. SEXUALITY. 3. *Colloq.* Sexual intercourse; COITUS.

sex chromatin. A condensation of chromatin found in nuclei of cells having more than one X chromosome. It represents the inactive X chromosome and is always equal to the total number of X chromosomes minus one. Syn. *Barr body.*

sex chromosome. A chromosome having a special relation to determining whether a fertilized egg develops into a male or a female; the X chromosome and the Y chromosome. When other conditions are normal, in mammals a fertilized egg with two X's becomes a female; one with the XY combination becomes a male.

sex hormone. Any gonadal hormone, whether estrogenic or androgenic, secreted chiefly by the ovaries and the testes but found also in other tissues.

sexi·dig·i·tal (seck′′si-dij′i·tul) adj. Having six fingers or six toes.

sex-limited, adj. Appearing in, or affecting, one sex only.

sex-linked, adj. Applied to genes located on the X chromosome, and to the characteristics, which may occur in either sex, conditioned by such genes.

sexo·es·thet·ic inversion (seck′′so-es-thet′ick). A variety of sexual deviation in which the individual has the feelings and tastes of, and assumes the habits, manners, and costume of the opposite sex.

sex·ol·o·gy (seck-sol′uh-jee) n. The science or study of sex and sex relations. —**sexo·log·ic** (seck′′so-loj′ick) adj.

sex ratio. The relative number of males and females in the population, usually stated as the number of males per 100 females.

sex reversal. Genetic, developmental, or therapeutic conversion of phenotypic sex.

sex·ti·grav·i·da (secks′′ti-grav′i·duh) n. A woman who is pregnant for the sixth time.

sex·tip·a·ra (secks-tip′uh-ruh) n. A woman who has given birth six times.

sex·tup·let (secks-tup′let) n. One of the six offspring of a single gestation.

sex·u·al (seck′shoo-ul) adj. Pertaining to or characteristic of sex.

sexual deviation. Sexual behavior which is markedly at variance with the generally accepted forms of sexual activities and not part of any more extensive disorder such as schizophrenia or the obsessional neuroses. It includes the various forms and practices of homosexuality, transvestitism, pedophilia, fetishism, and sexual sadism (assault and rape, mutilation).

sexual identity. The chromosomal constitution and, to some extent, the internal genitalia, which make a person biologically a male or a female. This is to be differentiated from gender identity and gender role, which are psychological attributes.

sex·u·al·i·ty (seck"shoo·al'i·tee) *n.* 1. The sum of a person's sexual attributes, behavior, and tendencies. 2. The quality of being sexual, or the degree of a person's sexual attributes, attractiveness, and drives. 3. Excessive preoccupation with sex and sexual functions and behavior. 4. *In psychoanalysis,* the physiological and psychological impulses whose satisfaction affords pleasure, experienced, consciously or unconsciously, even by the infant and young child.

Sé·za·ry cell (sey·zah·ree') An atypical mononuclear cell, recently identified as a T lymphocyte, containing mucopolysaccharide-filled cytoplasmic vacuoles, seen in the peripheral blood in Sézary's syndrome. A peripheral arrangement of granules is also characteristic.

Sézary syndrome or **reticulocytosis** Exfoliative erythroderma with a cutaneous infiltrate of atypical mononuclear cells; similar cells are also present in the peripheral blood. Bone marrow and lymph nodes are normal. It is thought to be related to mycosis fungoides.

SGOT Serum glutamic oxaloacetic transaminase.

SGPT Serum glutamic pyruvic transaminase.

SH Abbreviation and symbol for *sulfhydryl.*

shad·ow, *n.* 1. SHADOW CELL. 2. *In radiology,* the relatively dark outline seen on a developed x-ray film caused by the interposition of an opaque body and the x-ray beam.

shadow cell. 1. A hemolyzed erythrocyte consisting only of stroma. 2. A cell characteristic of pilomatricoma whose well-outlined cytoplasm stains pink with hematoxylin and eosin, but which shows a central unstained "shadow" in place of the nucleus.

shaft, *n.* The trunk of any columnar mass, especially the diaphysis of a long bone.

sha·green patch, plaque, or **spot** (sha·green'). An area of granular, thickened, grayish-green or brown skin found characteristically in tuberous sclerosis. Syn. *sharkskin spot.*

sham rage. A state in which an animal reacts to all stimuli with an expression of intense anger and the signs of autonomic overactivity, produced experimentally by cerebral decortication.

shank, *n.* The leg from the knee to the ankle.

sharp and slow wave complex. *In electroencephalography,* a complex consisting of a spike followed by a slow wave.

sheath, *n.* 1. An envelope; a covering. 2. *In anatomy,* the connective tissue covering an organ or structures such as vessels, muscles, nerves, and tendons. 3. CONDOM. —**sheathed,** *adj.*

shed, *v.* To throw off, cast off.

shed·ding, *n.* 1. Casting off. 2. The natural process of resorption of the roots and the subsequent loss of deciduous teeth.

Shee·han's syndrome Hypopituitarism due to postpartum necrosis of the adenohypophysis.

shell·shock, *n.* 1. WAR NEUROSIS. 2. BLAST INJURY.

shel·tered workshop. A facility for the treatment

of physically, medically, or mentally handicapped ambulatory individuals, where the work, machinery, and tempo are modified so that the handicapped may learn to cope with their jobs successfully.

SH group. SULFHYDRYL.

shi·a·tsu (shee'ah·tsoo) *n.* A therapeutic massage technique, developed in Japan in the 18th century, which involves application of carefully gauged pressure at specific points on the body. The doctrine on which it is based is akin to that of acupuncture.

shield, *n.* 1. A protective structure or apparatus. 2. *In biology,* a protective plate, scute, lorica, or carapace. 3. A structure having the shape of a shield.

shift, *n.* A change of direction or position.

shift to the left. According to Arneth, a marked increase in the percentage of immature neutrophils (those having a single or bilobed nucleus) in the peripheral blood, occurring in granulocytic leukemia, in acute infective diseases, and also in pernicious anemia.

shift to the right. According to Arneth, a marked increase in the percentage of mature neutrophils (those having nuclei with three or more lobes) in the peripheral blood, frequently occurring in diseases of the liver and in pernicious anemia.

Shi·gel·la (shi·ghel'uh, shi·jel'uh) *n.* A genus of nonmotile, gram-negative bacteria of the Enterobacteriaceae which with few exceptions do not produce gas from fermentable substances and do not ferment lactose; the causative agents of bacillary dysentery. They are antigenically related, and are divided into four major subgroups: (A) *Shigella dysenteriae,* (B) *S. flexneri,* (C) *S. boydii,* and (D) *S. sonnei.*

Shigella al·ka·les·cens (al·kuh·les'enz). Formerly classified with the *Shigella,* now regarded as coliform organisms on the basis of antigenic and biochemical characteristics; cause urinary tract infection but doubtfully involved in dysentery.

Shigella am·big·ua (am·big'yoo·uh). Type 2 of *Shigella dysenteriae.* Syn. *Schmitz bacillus. Shigella schmitzii.*

Shigella dys·en·ter·i·ae (dis''en·terr'ee·ee). Subgroup A of *Shigella,* rarely a cause of dysentery in the United States, but involved in highly virulent epidemics elsewhere. In addition to the endotoxin produced by all *Shigella,* type 1 of *S. dysenteriae* elaborates a potent exotoxin which is neurotoxic for laboratory animals.

shig·el·lo·sis (shig''e·lo'sis) *n.,* pl. **shigello·ses** (·seez) BACILLARY DYSENTERY.

shin, *n.* The sharp anterior margin of the tibia and overlying structures.

shin·bone, *n.* TIBIA.

shin·gles, *n.* HERPES ZOSTER.

shin splints. Pain in the anterior tibial compartment of the lower leg brought about by vigorous exercise; caused by ischemia associated with edema secondary to microscopic tears in muscle and connective tissue; considered a mild form of the anterior tibial compartment syndrome.

ship·ping fever. An acute, occasionally sub-acute, septicemic disease in cattle and sheep, probably caused by a combination of virus and *Pasteurella multocida* or *P. hemolytica*.

shiv·er, *n*. A tremor or shaking of the body associated with chill or fear; frequently observed also with rapid rises in temperature as in the onset of fever, when the patient has the cutaneous sensation of being cold although actual body temperature is raised, causing reflex contraction of muscles to produce more body heat.

shock, *n*. 1. The clinical manifestations of defective venous return to the heart with consequent reduction in cardiac output. Manifestations of this circulatory insufficiency include hypotension, a weak thready pulse, tachycardia, restlessness, pallor, and diminished urinary output. Shock may be classified according to mechanism, as cardiogenic, vasogenic, neurogenic, or hypovolemic. Syn. *peripheral circulatory failure*. 2. A physical or emotional trauma. 3. *In physiology*, ELECTRIC SHOCK. 4. The first phase of the alarm reaction in the general adaptation syndrome.

shock organ. The organ or tissue that exhibits the most marked response to the antigen-antibody interaction in hypersensitivity, as the lungs in allergic asthma, or the skin in allergic contact dermatitis.

shock therapy. The treatment of psychiatric patients by inducing coma, with or without convulsions, by means of carbon dioxide or drugs such as insulin or metrazol, or by passing an electric current through the brain.

short-incubation hepatitis. INFECTIOUS HEPATITIS.

short-term memory. Memory store from which information is lost rapidly, usually within 20 to 30 seconds, unless retained through active rehearsal. Syn. *primary memory, immediate memory*.

short-wave diathermy. A process of electrotherapy in which an alternating electric current of extremely high frequency, 10,000 to 100,000 kilohertz per second, at wavelengths of 30 to 3 meters, is run though the body surface for therapeutic heating.

shoul·der, *n*. The region where the arm joins the trunk, formed by the meeting of the clavicle, scapula, humerus, and the overlying soft parts.

shoulder-hand syndrome. A syndrome characterized by pain in the shoulder and arm, limited joint motion, diffuse swelling of the distal part of the upper extremity, atrophy of muscles, cutaneous and subcutaneous structures, and decalcification of underlying bones. The cause is not well understood. It is observed most often following myocardial infarction and self-imposed immobility of the arm. Syn. *hand-shoulder syndrome*.

show, *n*. A bloody discharge from the birth canal prior to labor or to a menstrual flow.

Shrap·nell's membrane PARS FLACCIDA MEMBRANAE TYMPANI.

shreds, *n.pl*. Slender strands of mucus visible grossly in urine, denoting inflammation of the urethra, bladder, or prostate.

shud·der, *n. & v*. 1. A momentary involuntary tremor, caused by fright or disgust, or occurring as a nervous habit. 2. To shake or tremble.

shunt, *n. & v*. 1. A diversion. 2. *In medicine*, an anomalous natural or surgically created anastamosis or channel, diverting flow from one pathway to another or permitting flow from one part or region to another. 3. In electricity, a branch of a circuit parallel with other parts of it, especially one that provides a low-resistance path for the flow of electricity. 4. To divert, shift.

SH virus. The virus (hepatitis virus B) associated with serum hepatitis.

Schwartz·man phenomenon or **reaction** 1. The occurrence of hemorrhage and necrosis at a skin site prepared by the local injection of a bacterial endotoxin when the same or differing material is inoculated intravenously 8 to 24 hours later. Syn. *local Schwartzman phenomenon*. 2. Bilateral cortical renal necrosis and other lesions initiated by intravascular coagulation when both the preparatory and the eliciting materials are administered intravenously. Syn. *generalized Schwartzman phenomenon*.

Si Symbol for silicon.

si·a·go·nag·ra (sigh″uh·go·nag′ruh) *n*. Gouty pain in the maxilla.

sial-, sialo- A combining form meaning *saliva, salivary*.

si·al·a·den (sigh·al′uh·den) *n*. SALIVARY GLAND.

si·al·ad·e·ni·tis (sigh″ul·ad″e·nigh′tis) *n*. Inflammation of a salivary gland.

si·al·ad·e·nog·ra·phy (sigh″ul·ad″e·nog′ruh·fee) *n*. Radiography of the salivary glands.

si·al·a·gogue, si·al·a·gog (sigh·al′uh·gog) *n*. A drug which produces a flow of saliva. —**si·al·a·gog·ic** (sigh″ul·uh·goj′ick) *adj. & n*.

si·al·an·gi·og·ra·phy (sigh″uh·lan″jee·og′ruh·fee) *n*. SIALOGRAPHY.

si·al·a·po·ria (sigh″ul·uh·po′ree·uh) *n*. Deficiency in the amount of saliva.

si·al·ec·ta·sia (sigh″ul·eck·tay′zhuh, ·zee·uh) *n*. A swelling or enlargement of the salivary glands.

si·al·ic (sigh·al′ick) *adj*. Having the nature of saliva.

sialic acid. Any of a family of amino sugars, containing nine or more carbon atoms, that are nitrogen- and oxygen-substituted acyl derivatives of neuraminic acid. As components of lipids, polysaccharides, and mucoproteins, they are widely distributed in bacteria and in animal tissues.

si·a·li·tis (sigh″uh·lye′tis) *n*. 1. SIALADENITIS. 2. Inflammation of a salivary gland or duct.

si·alo·ad·e·nec·to·my (sigh″uh·lo·ad″e·neck′tuh·mee) *n*. Surgical removal of a salivary gland.

si·a·lo·ad·e·ni·tis (sigh″uh·lo·ad″e·nigh′tis) *n*. SIALADENITIS.

si·alo·ad·e·not·o·my (sigh″uh·lo·ad″e·not′uh·mee) *n*. Incision of a salivary gland.

si·alo·an·gi·ec·ta·sis (sigh″uh·lo·an″jee·eck′tuh·sis) *n*. Dilatation of a salivary gland duct.

si·a·lo·an·gi·tis (sigh"uh·lo·an·jye'tis) *n.* Inflammation of a salivary duct.

si·alo·do·chi·tis (sigh"uh·lo·do·kigh'tis) *n.* Inflammation of a salivary duct.

si·alo·do·cho·li·thi·a·sis (sigh"uh·lo·do"ko·li·thigh'uh·sis) *n.* The presence of stones in salivary gland ducts.

si·alo·do·cho·plas·ty (sigh"uh·lo·do'ko·plas"tee) *n.* Plastic surgery of a salivary duct.

si·a·log·e·nous (sigh"uh·loj'e·nus) *adj.* Generating saliva.

si·a·lo·gram (sigh·al'o·gram) *n.* A radiograph of a salivary gland and duct system after the injection of an opaque medium.

si·a·log·ra·phy (sigh"uh·log'ruh·fee) *n.* Radiographic examination of a salivary gland and its duct following injection of an opaque substance into its duct; PTYALOGRAPHY.

si·a·loid (sigh'uh·loid) *adj.* Pertaining to, or like, saliva.

si·a·lo·li·thi·a·sis (sigh"uh·lo·li·thigh'uh·sis) *n.* The occurrence of calcareous concretions in the salivary ducts or glands.

si·a·lo·li·thot·o·my (sigh"uh·lo·li·thot'uh·mee) *n.* Surgical incision into a salivary duct or salivary gland for the removal of a calculus.

si·al·or·rhea, si·al·or·rhoea (sigh"uh·lo·ree'uh, sigh·al'o·) *n.* SALIVATION (2).

si·a·los·che·sis (sigh"uh·los'ke·sis) *n.* Suppression of the secretion of saliva.

si·a·lo·se·mei·ol·o·gy (sigh"uh·lo·see"migh·ol'o·jee) *n.* Diagnosis based upon examination of the saliva.

si·a·lo·ste·no·sis (sigh"uh·lo·ste·no'sis) *n.* Stricture of a salivary duct.

si·a·lo·syr·inx (sigh"uh·lo·sirr'inks) *n.* 1. SALIVARY FISTULA. 2. A syringe for washing out the salivary ducts. 3. A drainage tube for a salivary duct.

Si·a·mese twins (sigh·uh·meez') Viable conjoined twins.

Sia's water test (see'uh) A test for macroglobulins, in which the patient's serum is mixed with distilled water. The formation of a precipitate constitutes a positive reaction.

sib, *n.* 1. *Obsol.* A blood relative. 2. SIBLING. 3. *In cultural anthropology,* a unilateral descent group, as a clan.

sib·i·lant (sib'i·lunt) *adj.* Hissing or whistling.

sibilant rale. A dry, high-pitched, hissing or whistling sound heard most often in bronchiolar spasm or narrowing.

sib·i·la·tion (sib"i·lay'shun) *n.* Pronunciation in which the *s* sound predominates.

sib·i·lis·mus (sib"i·liz'mus) *n.* 1. A hissing sound. 2. SIBILANT RALE.

sib·i·lus (sib'i·lus) *n.* SIBILANT RALE.

sib·ling, *n.* An individual in relation to any other individual having the same parents; a brother or sister.

sibling rivalry. The competition between siblings for the love of one or both parents, or for other recognition or gain which is a rather obvious cover for such competition.

sib·ship, *n.* All the siblings in a family regarded as a single group.

sic·ca (sick'uh) *adj.* Feminine of *siccus;* dry.

sic·cant (sick'unt) *adj. & n.* 1. Drying; tending to make dry. 2. A substance that speeds up drying.

sic·cha·sia (si·kay'zhuh, ·zee·uh) *n.* NAUSEA.

sic·cus (sick'us) *adj.* Dry.

sick, *adj.* 1. Ill; not well. 2. Nauseated.

sick·la·ne·mia (sick"luh·nee'mee·uh) *n.* SICKLE CELL ANEMIA.

sickle cell. A crescent-shaped erythrocyte characteristic of sickle cell anemia. Syn. *drepanocyte.*

sickle cell anemia. A chronic hemolytic and thrombotic disorder in which hypoxia causes the erythrocytes to assume a sickled shape; it occurs in persons (usually blacks) homozygous for sickle cell hemoglobin. Syn. *drepanocythemia, sicklanemia, SS disease.*

sickle cell disease. 1. Any disease resulting wholly or in part from the presence of sickle cell hemoglobin, such as sickle cell anemia, sickle cell–hemoglobin C disease, or sickle cell thalassemia. 2. Specifically, SICKLE CELL ANEMIA.

sickle cell hemoglobin. The hemoglobin found in sickle cell anemia, differing in electrophoretic mobility and other physiochemical properties from normal adult hemoglobin. This hemoglobin is especially common in certain populations inhabiting malarious zones of western and central Africa and its occurrence elsewhere is limited mostly to people with ancestry from these zones. Syn. *hemoglobin S.*

sickle cell–hemoglobin C disease. A disorder of hemoglobin formation in which sickle cell hemoglobin, inherited from one parent, and hemoglobin C, from the other, coexist to the exclusion of normal adult hemoglobin. The clinical disease is usually later in onset and often generally milder than homozygous sickle cell disease. Syn. *hemoglobin SC disease.*

sickle cell thalassemia. A congenital disorder of hemoglobin formation in which sickle cell hemoglobin and one of the forms of thalassemia hemoglobin are present in the erythrocytes.

sickle cell trait. The heterozygous genetic constitution in which there is one gene for normal adult hemoglobin and one for sickle cell hemoglobin. Usually no clinical disease is present, and in malarious areas children with the trait are relatively resistant to the more severe forms of *Plasmodium falciparum* infection, possibly because infected cells are selectively sickled and eliminated from the circulation.

sick·le·mia, sick·lae·mia (sick·lee'mee·uh, sick"ul·ee'mee·uh) *n.* SICKLE CELL ANEMIA.

sick·ness, *n.* Disease; illness.

Sid·bury's syndrome A disorder of fatty acid metabolism characterized by a deficiency of the acyl dehydrogenase specific for oxidation of 4-carbon and 6-carbon fatty acids, resulting in decreased oxidation of *n*-butyric and *n*-hexanoic acids. The clinical picture resembles that seen in isovaleric acidemia, with familial tendency, malodorous sweat, vomiting, acidosis, lethargy, and coma.

side, *n.* The lateral aspect of any body or organ.

side·bone, *n.* Ossification of the lateral cartilages

of the pedal bone in the horse, resulting in lameness.

sider-, sidero- A combining form meaning *iron*.

sid·er·o·cyte (sid'ur·o·site) *n.* An erythrocyte which contains granules of hemosiderin which stain blue with the Prussian blue reaction.

sid·er·o·cy·to·sis (sid''ur·o·sigh·to'sis) *n.* The presence in the peripheral blood of significant numbers of siderocytes.

sid·er·o·dro·mo·pho·bia (sid''ur·o·dro''mo·fo'bee·uh, sid''ur·od''ro·mo·) *n.* Abnormal fear of traveling by railway; fear of trains.

sid·er·o·fi·bro·sis (sid''ur·o·figh·bro'sis) *n.* Fibrosis associated with deposits of iron-bearing pigments.

sid·er·o·pe·nia (sid''ur·o·pee'nee·uh) *n.* Deficiency of iron, especially in the blood. —**side·rope·nic** (·nick) *adj.*

sideropenic dysphagia. PLUMMER-VINSON SYNDROME.

sid·er·o·phage (sid'ur·o·faij) *n.* A macrophage containing granules of iron-containing pigment, especially hemosiderin.

sid·er·oph·i·lin (sid''ur·off'i·lin, sid''ur·o·fil'in) *n.* TRANSFERRIN.

sid·er·o·sil·i·co·sis (sid''ur·o·sil''i·ko'sis) *n.* A pneumoconiosis due to the prolonged inhalation of dusts containing silica and iron.

sid·er·o·sis (sid''ur·o'sis) *n.* 1. The presence or accumulation of stainable iron pigment in the tissues or body fluids or in a particular organ. 2. Pneumoconiosis caused by prolonged inhalation of dust containing iron salt; usually occurring in iron miners and arc welders. Syn. *arc-welder's disease.* —**sider·ot·ic** (·ot'ick) *adj.*

siderosis bul·bi (bul'bye). Degenerative changes in the eyeball resulting from retained ferrous material.

siderotic nodules. Foci of fibrillar material encrusted with iron salts, grossly appearing as brown flecks, usually in spleens with chronic passive hyperemia.

SIDS Abbreviation for *sudden infant death syndrome.*

sig. An abbreviation for (a) *signa,* label it; (b) *signetur,* let it be labeled.

sigh, *n.* A prolonged, deep inspiration followed by a shorter expiration. Syn. *suspirium.*

sight, *n.* 1. The special sense concerned in seeing. 2. That which is seen.

sigmoid-, sigmoido-. A combining form meaning *sigmoid.*

sig·moid (sig'moid) *adj. & n.* 1. Shaped like the letter S. 2. Of or pertaining to the sigmoid colon. 3. SIGMOID COLON.

sigmoid colon. The portion of the colon that extends from the descending colon to the rectum.

sigmoid colostomy. The formation of an artificial anus in the sigmoid colon; SIGMOIDOSTOMY.

sigmoid conduit. A urinary drainage conduit to the skin formed surgically from a defunctionalized segment of the sigmoid colon.

sig·moid·ec·to·my (sig''moy·deck'tuh·mee) *n.* Excision of a part or all of the sigmoid colon.

sigmoid flexure. SIGMOID COLON.

sig·moid·itis (sig''moy·dye'tis) *n.* Inflammation of the sigmoid flexure of the colon.

sigmoid kidney. A congenital anomaly resulting from the fusion of the lower pole of one kidney to the upper pole of the other. Syn. *L-shaped kidney, unilateral fused kidney.*

sigmoid mesocolon. The mesentery of the sigmoid colon.

sig·moi·do·pexy (sig·moy'do·peck''see) *n.* An operation for prolapse of the rectum; fixation of the sigmoid colon by obliterating the intersigmoid fossa and shortening the mesosigmoid by suture, through an abdominal incision.

sig·moi·do·proc·tos·to·my (sig·moy''do·prock·tos'tuh·mee) *n.* Anastomosis of the sigmoid colon with the rectum.

sig·moi·do·rec·tos·to·my (sig·moy''do·reck·tos'tuh·mee) *n.* Formation by surgical means of an artificial anus at the sigmoid colon, at its junction with the rectum; a low colostomy.

sig·moi·do·scope (sig·moy'duh·skope) *n.* An appliance for the inspection, by artificial light, of the sigmoid colon; it differs from the proctoscope in its greater length and diameter.

sig·moid·os·co·py (sig''moy·dos'kuh·pee) *n.* Visual inspection of the sigmoid colon, with the aid of special instruments.

sig·moi·do·sig·moi·dos·to·my (sig·moy''do·sig'moy·dos'tuh·mee) *n.* Surgical anastomosis between two portions of the sigmoid colon.

sig·moid·os·to·my (sig''moy·dos'tuh·mee) *n.* The formation of an artificial anus in the sigmoid colon; SIGMOID COLOSTOMY.

sig·moid·ot·o·my (sig''moy·dot'uh·mee) *n.* Incision into the sigmoid colon.

sig·moi·do·ves·i·cal (sig·moy''do·ves'i·kul) *adj.* Pertaining to the sigmoid colon and the urinary bladder.

sign, *n.* An objective evidence or physical manifestation of disease.

signa. 1. Plural of *signum.* 2. Used in prescriptions to mean "write." Abbreviated, S., sig.

sig·nal node. A metastatic tumor in a supraclavicular lymph node, usually on the left side, and most frequently secondary to primary carcinoma in the abdomen or thorax. Syn. *Ewald's node, sentinel node, Virchow's node.*

signal symptom. The first disturbance of sensation preceding a more extensive seizure, as the aura heralding an attack of epilepsy.

sig·na·ture, *n.* 1. The part of the prescription that is placed on the label, containing directions to the patient. 2. A distinguishing character.

sig·net-ring cell. A cell with a large cytoplasmic vacuole, containing mucin, fat, or glycogen, which pushes the nucleus to one side, making the cell look like a signet ring.

sig·nif·i·cant difference. A difference between two statistical constants, calculated from two separate samples, which is of such magnitude that it is unlikely to have occurred by chance alone. Usually this probability must be less than 0.05 (5%) before a difference is accepted as significant. The smaller the probability, the more significant is the difference.

sig·num (sig'num) *n.,* pl. **sig·na** (·nuh) A mark, sign, or indication.

si·lent, *adj.* 1. *In medicine,* not exhibiting the

usual signs and symptoms of a disorder; characterized by a quiescent state; not manifested clinically. 2. Yielding no response to stimulation. 3. Noiseless.

sil·i·ca (sil'i·kuh) *n.* Silicon dioxide, SiO_2, occurring in nature in the form of quartz, flint, and other minerals.

silica gel. A precipitated and dried silicic acid in the form of granules, used as a dehydrating agent and for absorption of various vapors.

sil·i·cate (sil'i·kate, ·kut) *n.* A salt or ester of silicic acid.

sil·i·ceous, sil·i·cious (si·lish'us) *adj.* 1. Having the nature of, or containing, silicon. 2. Pertaining to silica.

sil·i·cic acid (si·lis'ick). Approximately H_2SiO_3. A white, amorphous powder.

sil·i·co·ma (sil'i·ko'muh) *n.* An abnormal swelling or enlargement of an organ resulting from tissue reaction to injected silicone.

sil·i·con (sil'i·kon) *n.* Si = 28.086. A nonmetallic element, atomic number 14, of the carbon group. It occurs in several allotropic modifications. Like carbon, it forms many complex compounds that are an essential part of the earth's surface.

silicon carbide. A compound of silicon and carbon next to diamond in hardness; used for cutting hard materials, and as an abrasive.

silicon dioxide. SILICA.

sil·i·cone (sil'i·kone) *n.* Any of a class of synthetic polymers having the composition of a polyorganosiloxane; used as an antiflatulent.

sil·i·co·sis (sil'i·ko'sis) *n.*, pl. **silico·ses** (·seez) A chronic pulmonary disease due to inhalation of dust with a high concentration of silica (SiO_2), characterized by widespread fibrosis and clinically by shortness of breath and increased susceptibility to tuberculosis.

sil·i·co·tu·ber·cu·lo·sis (sil''i·ko·tew·bur''kew·lo'sis) *n.* Silicosis with tuberculosis.

silo-filler's disease. Bronchiolitans obliterans and other lung damage caused by nitrogen dioxide and nitric oxide produced by fermentation of fodder in a silo.

sil·ver, silver. Ag = 107.868. A white, soft, ductile, and malleable metal; element number 47. Silver compounds are used in medicine for caustic, astringent, and antiseptic effects, which are characteristic of silver ion.

silver-fork deformity. Displacement of the distal radius and ulna as seen in Colles' fracture.

silver nitrate. $AgNO_3$. In aqueous solution, used locally as an astringent and germicide, and also as a prophylactic against ophthalmia neonatorum. In solid form, sometimes used as an escharotic.

silver picrate. $(NO_2)_3C_6H_2OAg·H_2O$; used locally in treatment of urethritis and vaginitis.

silver protein. A compound of protein and silver used for the germicidal effect of the silver component. Two types of preparations, mild silver protein and strong silver protein, have been used; the former contains more silver than the latter but is milder in its effects, presumably because less of the silver is ionized than in strong silver protein.

Silvol. A trademark for mild silver protein.

sim·i·an (sim'ee·un) *adj.* Apelike; pertaining to or characteristic of apes or monkeys.

simian crease. A single, continuous, transverse palmar crease; said to be characteristic of Down's syndrome, but also seen as a normal variant.

simian hand. SIMIAN CREASE; a hand with a single, continuous transverse palmar crease.

si·mil·i·mum (si·mil'i·mum) *n.* The homeopathic remedy that produces a symptom complex most like that of a given disease.

Sim·monds' disease or **cachexia** Panhypopituitarism with marked insufficiency of the target glands and profound cachexia. Syn. *hypophyseal cachexia, hypopituitary cachexia.*

sim·ple, *adj. & n.* 1. Consisting of or having only one of some component or structural element that is multiple in certain other things of the same class; single. 2. Without elaborations or complications; minimal or fundamental. 3. A medicinal plant, thought of as possessing a single medicinal substance; also, any drug consisting of but one vegetable medicinal ingredient.

simple fracture. A fracture in which the skin is not perforated, from without or within, in such a manner as to expose the fracture site to the environment.

simple goiter. Diffuse thyroid enlargement, either colloid or hyperplastic in type; usually unassociated with constitutional features.

simple inflammation. Inflammation that is not granulomatous. Syn. *nonspecific inflammation.*

simple mastectomy. Surgical removal of the breast only.

simple syrup. SYRUP (2).

Simpson's syndrome A prepuberal endocrine-obesity syndrome characterized by alteration of sexual development and physical habitus, producing a female habitus in boys and accentuated female traits in girls.

Sims's position The patient lies on the left side and chest with the right knee and thigh drawn up and the left arm along the back.

si·mul (sigh'mul, sim'ul) *adv.* At once; at the same time.

sim·u·late, *v.* To take on the appearance of something else; to feign or imitate.

sim·u·la·tion, *n.* 1. The mimicking of one disease or symptom by another. 2. The feigning or counterfeiting of disease; malingering.

Si·mu·li·um (si·mew'lee·um) *n.* A genus of small, robust, humpbacked Diptera with short legs and broad wings, commonly called black flies or buffalo gnats. They are worldwide in distribution. The females are vicious bloodsuckers.

Simulium pe·cu·a·rum (peck·yoo·air'um). A small black fly which is an important scourge of man and cattle in the Mississippi Valley.

Simulium ve·nus·tum (ve·nus'tum). A small black fly of northern New England, New York, the Midwest, and Canada; most bothersome to man in June and July.

si·mul·tag·no·sia (sigh''mul·tag·no'zhuh, ·no'see·uh) *n.* A form of visual agnosia in which the patient is able to perceive parts of a pattern or picture, but fails to recognize the meaning of the whole.

si·nal (sigh'nul) *adj.* Pertaining to or coming from a sinus.

si·na·pis (si·nay'pis) *n.* MUSTARD.

sin·a·pism (sin'uh·piz·um) *n.* The use or application of a mustard plaster.

sin·ci·put (sin'si·put) *n.*, pl. **sincipits, sin·cip·i·ta** (sin·sip'i·tuh) The superior and anterior part of the head. —**sin·cip·i·tal** (sin·sip'i·tul) *adj.*

sin·ew (sin'yoo) *n.* TENDON.

sing·er's node or **nodule.** An inflammatory or fibrous nodule on the free margin of the vocal folds.

single blind experiment or **test.** An experiment in which either the subject or the observer does not know which of several forms of treatment the subject is to receive.

sin·gul·tus (sing·gul'tus) *n.* HICCUP. —**singultous,** *adj.*: **sin·gul·ta·tion** (sing"gul·tay'shun) *n.*

sin·i·grin (sin'i·grin) *n.* Potassium myronate, $KC_{10}H_{16}O_9NS_2 \cdot H_2O$, a glycoside found in black mustard, *Brassica nigra,* which under the influence of myrosin, an albuminous ferment in black mustard, yields allyl isothiocyanate, a powerful rubefacient.

sinistr-, sinistro-. A combining form meaning *left* or *toward the left side.*

sin·is·trad (sin'is·trad, si·nis'trad) *adv.* Toward the left.

sin·is·tral (sin'is·trul, si·nis'trul) *adj. & n.* 1. On the left side. 2. Showing preference for the left hand, eye, or foot for certain acts or functions. 3. A left-handed individual.

sin·is·tral·i·ty (sin"is·tral'i·tee) *n.* 1. The condition, often genetically determined, in which, when there is a choice, the left side of the body is more efficient and hence used more than the right. 2. Specifically, LEFT-HANDEDNESS.

sin·is·tra·tion (sin"is·tray'shun) *n.* 1. A turning to the left. 2. Development of dominance of the right side of the cerebral hemisphere in left-handed persons.

sin·is·trau·ral (sin"is·traw'rul) *adj.* 1. Left-eared; characterizing an individual who prefers to listen with the left ear, as with a telephone receiver, or who depends more on the left ear in binaural hearing. 2. Pertaining to the left ear.

si·nis·tro·car·dia (si·nis"tro·kahr'dee·uh) *n.* Displacement of the heart to the left.

sin·is·tro·cere·bral (sin"is·tro·serr'e·brul) *adj.* 1. Located in the left cerebral hemisphere. 2. Functioning preferentially with the left side of the brain.

sin·is·troc·u·lar (sin"is·trock'yoo·lur) *adj.* Left-eyed; characterizing an individual who uses the left eye in preference to the right one when there is a choice, as when sighting a gun or looking through a telescope.

sin·is·tro·gy·ra·tion (sin"is·tro·jye·ray'shun, si·nis'tro·) *n.* Turning or twisting to the left, as the plane of polarization or a movement of the eye. —**sinistro·gy·ric** (·jye'rick) *adj.*

sin·is·tro·man·u·al (sin"is·tro·man'yoo·ul) *adj.* LEFT-HANDED.

sin·is·tro·ped·al (sin"is·trop'e·dul, sin"is·tro·pee'dul) *adj.* LEFT-FOOTED.

sin·is·tro·tor·sion (sin"is·tro·tor'shun) *n.* A twisting or turning toward the left.

sin·is·trous (sin'is·trus, sin·is'trus) *adj.* Awkward; unskilled.

sino-, sinu-. A combining form denoting *sinus.*

si·no·atri·al (sigh"no·ay'tree·ul) *adj.* Pertaining to the region between the atrium and the sinus venosus.

sinoatrial heart block. Heart block in which the impulses originated in the sinoatrial node are partially or completely prevented from being conducted through the atria.

sinoatrial node. A dense network of Purkinje fibers of the conduction system at the junction of the superior vena cava and the right atrium.

si·no·au·ric·u·lar (sigh"no·aw·rick'yoo·lur) *adj.* SINOATRIAL.

si·no·bron·chi·tis (sigh"no·brong·kigh'tis) *n.* Inflammation of the bronchi and the paranasal sinuses.

si·no·gram (sigh'no·gram) *n.* A radiographic depiction of a natural sinus or acquired sinus tract after the introduction of contrast material.

si·nog·ra·phy (sigh·nog'ruh·fee) *n.* The radiographic demonstration of any sinus by the direct injection of contrast medium.

sin·u·ous (sin'yoo·us) *adj.* Wavy; applied especially to tortuous fistulas and sinuses.

si·nus (sigh'nus) *n.*, L. pl. & genit. sing. **sinus** (sigh'noos, sigh'nus), E. pl. **sinuses** 1. A hollow or cavity; a recess or pocket. 2. A large channel containing blood, especially venous blood. 3. A suppurating tract. 4. A cavity within a bone.

si·nus·al (sigh'nus·ul) *adj.* Of or pertaining to a sinus; SINAL.

sinus arrhythmia. Sinus rhythm with variation of at least 0.12 second between the longest and shortest P-P intervals. P waves and P-R intervals are normal and constant. Phasic sinus arrhythmia accelerates with inspiration and slows with expiration; in nonphasic sinus arrhythmia the irregularity is unrelated to respiration.

sinus bradycardia. Sinus rhythm at a rate of less than 60 beats per minute.

sinus ca·ro·ti·cus (ka·rot'i·kus) [NA]. CAROTID SINUS (1).

si·nus·itis (sigh"nuh·sigh'tis) *n.* Inflammation of a sinus. May affect any of the paranasal sinuses, as ethmoidal, frontal, maxillary, or sphenoid.

sinus of the dura mater. Any endothelially lined, venous blood space situated between the periosteal and meningeal layers of the dura mater. One of the channels by which the blood is conveyed from the cerebral veins, and from some of the veins of the meninges and diploë, into the veins of neck.

sinus of the external jugular vein. The portion of the external jugular vein between two sets of valves in the distal part of the vessel; this area is often dilated.

si·nus·oid (sigh'nuh·soid) *n. & adj.* 1. One of the relatively large spaces or tubes constituting part of the venous circulatory system in the suprarenal gland, liver, spleen, and other viscera. 2. SINUSOIDAL (2).

si·nus·oi·dal (sigh"nuh·soy'dul) *adj.* 1. Varying

in proportion to the sine of an angle or of a time function. 2. Pertaining to a sinus.

si·nus·oid·al current. A symmetrical alternating current, the rise and fall of which describes a sine curve.

si·nus·ot·o·my (sigh"nus-ot'uh-mee) *n.* The production of an artificial opening into a paranasal sinus, to promote drainage.

sinus rhythm. The normal heart rhythm in which the sinoatrial node is the dominant pacemaker.

sinus tachycardia. Sinus rhythm at a rate greater than 100 beats per minute.

sinus ve·no·sus (ve·no'sus). 1. The chamber of the lower vertebrate heart to which the veins return blood from the body. 2. [NA] The vessel in the transverse septum of the embryonic mammalian heart into which open the vitelline and allantoic veins, and the common cardinal veins.

si·phon (sigh'fun) *n.* A tube bent at an angle, one arm of which is longer than the other; used for the purpose of removing liquids from a cavity or vessel, by means of atmospheric pressure.

si·phon·age (sigh'fuh-nij) *n.* The action of a siphon, such as washing out the stomach or drainage of wounds, by the use of atmospheric pressure.

Si·pho·nap·te·ra (sigh"fuh-nap'tur-uh) *n.pl.* An order of insects, commonly called fleas. They have small, hard, laterally compressed bodies without wings, and the mouth parts are adapted for piercing and sucking. They feed exclusively upon the blood of birds and mammals and so become important disease vectors. The important genera are *Ctenocephalides*, *Echidnophaga*, *Pulex*, *Tunga*, and *Xenopsylla*.

Si·phun·cu·la·ta (sigh-funk"yoo-lay'tuh) *n.pl.* A suborder of Anoplura; the sucking lice.

Siphunculina fu·ni·co·la (few"ni-ko'luh, few·nick'o-luh). The common eye fly of India which is responsible for transmitting conjunctivitis.

Sip·py diet. Dietary treatment of peptic ulcer, consisting first of alternate feedings of Sippy's powders and a milk-cream mixture, with progressive addition of bland foods until a standard diet is reached.

Sippy powder. 1. A mixture of precipitated calcium carbonate 23%, sodium bicarbonate 77%; known as Sippy powder No. 1. Syn. *sodium bicarbonate and calcium carbonate powder*. 2. A mixture of magnesium oxide 50%, sodium bicarbonate 50%, known as Sippy powder No. 2. Syn. *sodium bicarbonate and magnesium oxide powder*. Both powders are used as gastric antacids; Sippy powder No. 2 is also mildly laxative.

si·ren·i·form (sigh-ren'i-form) *adj.* Having the form of a siren or sympus.

si·re·no·form (sigh-ren'uh-form) *adj.* SIRENIFORM.

si·re·no·me·lia (sigh"re·no·mee'lee-uh) *n.* The condition of having fused lower extremities.

site, *n.* The place at which something occurs or the space it occupies.

-site. A combining form designating (a) *means or manner of nourishment or life support,* as in

parasite, coinosite, autosite; (b) *fetal parasite,* as in omphalosite.

sit·fast, *n.* A form of dry gangrene that affects horses, resulting from pressure on a circumscribed area of the skin, with firm adherence of the dead tissue to the living tissue below, through its continuity with fibrous elements of the underlying structures.

sito-. A combining form meaning (a) *food,* (b) *grain.*

si·tol·o·gy (sigh-tol'uh-jee) *n.* DIETETICS.

si·to·ma·nia (sigh"to·may'nee-uh) *n.* 1. An abnormal craving for food. 2. Periodic attacks of bulimia.

si·to·pho·bia (sigh"to·fo'bee-uh) *n.* 1. Abnormal aversion to food. 2. Abnormal fear of eating.

si·to·stane (sigh'to-stane, si-tos'tane) *n.* A steroid hydrocarbon, $C_{29}H_{52}$, that may be considered the parent substance of sitosterols.

si·tos·ter·ol (si-tos'tur-ol, sigh"to-steer'ol) *n.* Any one of a group of plant sterols structurally related to sitostane.

si·to·ther·a·py (sigh"to-therr'uh-pee) *n.* DIETOTHERAPY.

sit·u·a·tion, *n.* 1. The more or less fixed position and orientation of an object relative to other objects in an area or space. 2. Position relative to circumstances or environment. 3. A set of circumstances. —**situation·al,** *adj.*

situational crisis. *In psychiatry,* any brief, presumably transient period of psychological stress that represents an individual's reaction to or attempts to cope with a specific set of circumstances. External forces predominate as compared to a developmental crisis.

situational depression. DEPRESSIVE NEUROSIS.

situational psychosis. PSYCHOTIC DEPRESSIVE REACTION.

situation therapy. MILIEU THERAPY.

si·tus (sigh'tus) *n.*, pl. **situs.** 1. Site, location. 2. Position, orientation.

situs in·ver·sus (in-vur'sus). Reversed location or position.

sitz bath. A therapeutic bath in which the patient sits with buttocks and perineal region immersed in warm water.

sixth (VIth) cranial nerve. ABDUCENS NERVE.

Sjö·gren-Lars·son syndrome (shoeh'gre'n", lahr·so'n) Mental deficiency, congenital ichthyosis simplex and spastic diplegia, inherited as an autosomal recessive trait. Patients with a probable variant, Rud's syndrome, also exhibit dwarfism, eunuchoidism, seizures, and polyneuropathies.

Sjögren's syndrome. A symptom complex consisting of keratoconjunctivitis sicca, laryngopharyngitis sicca, rhinitis sicca, xerostomia, enlargement of the parotid gland, and polyarthritis. Syn. *xerodermosteosis.*

skat·ole (skat'ole) *n.* Methylindole, C_9H_9N. A nitrogenous decomposition product of proteins, formed from tryptophan in the intestine. It contributes to the characteristic, disagreeable odor of feces.

skat·ox·yl (skat-ock'sil) *n.* C_9H_9NO. A product of the oxidation of skatole. It occurs as the sulfuric acid ester in the urine in cases of disease of the intestine or in excessive intestinal putrefaction.

skein cell. RETICULOCYTE (1).

ske·lal·gia (ske-lal′jee-uh) *n. Obsol.* Pain in the leg.

skelet-, skeleto-. A combining form meaning *skeleton. skeletal.*

skel·e·tal (skel′e·tul) *adj.* 1. Pertaining to a skeleton. 2. Resembling a skeleton.

skeletal traction. Traction exerted directly upon the long bones themselves by means of pins, wire, tongs, and other mechanical devices which are attached to, or passed through, the bones by operative procedures.

skel·e·ti·za·tion (skel′′e·ti·zay′shun) *n.* The process of converting into a skeleton; gradual wasting of the soft parts, leaving only the skeleton; emaciation.

skel·e·ton (skel′e·tun) *n.* A supporting structure, especially the bony framework supporting and protecting the soft parts of an organism.

skene·itis, ske·ni·tis (skee·nigh′tis) *n.* Inflammation of the paraurethral (Skene's) glands or ducts.

skene's duct PARAURETHRAL DUCT.

skene's glands or **tubules** PARAURETHRAL GLANDS.

skenitis. SKENEITIS.

skew deviation. A maintained deviation of one eye above the other, or hypertropia, which may be fixed or variable for different directions of gaze, seen with lesions in the brainstem and cerebellum, particularly when these are unilateral.

skew foot, *n.* METATARSUS ADDUCTOVARUS.

skia- A combining form meaning *shadow.*

ski·ag·ra·phy (skye·ag′ruh·fee) *n.* RADIOGRAPHY.

ski·as·co·py (skye·as′kuh·pee) *n.* 1. RETINOSCOPY. 2. FLUOROSCOPY.

skin, *n.* The organ that envelops the body, composed of the dermis and epidermis.

skin erythema dose. The least amount of x-ray radiation which will redden the normal skin. Abbreviated, SED.

skin grafting. The application of portions of the skin, either the outer layers or the full thickness, to a granulating wound to promote healing, to fill a defect, or to replace scar tissue for plastic repair.

skin test. Any test, as for immunity or hypersensitivity, in which the test material is introduced into the skin.

skin traction. Traction exerted by direct attachment to the skin, using adhesive plaster or linen or gauze strips cemented to the skin.

skin writing. DERMOGRAPHIA.

skiodan. Trademark for sodium methiodal, a radiopaque contrast medium.

sko·da·ic resonance (sko·day′ick) Tympanitic resonance to percussion in the area above the region of a lung compressed by pleural effusion.

skull, *n.* 1. The entire bony framework of the head, consisting of the cranium and the face. 2. *In embryology.* the neurocranium and visceral cranium.

slake, *v.* 1. To quench or appease. 2. To disintegrate by the action of water.

slap·ping, *n.* 1. *In massage.* percussion movements in which the hands with palms open come down alternately in a sharp series of blows. The movement is carried out chiefly from the wrist. 2. In gait, the striking of the forefoot forcefully due to weakness of the ankle dorsiflexor muscles.

slav·er (slav′ur, slay′vur) *n. & v.* 1. Drivel; saliva, especially that which is discharged involuntarily. 2. To drool, drivel.

sleeping sickness. 1. ENCEPHALITIS LETHARGICA. 2. AFRICAN TRYPANOSOMIASIS.

sleep·less·ness, *n.* INSOMNIA.

sleep paralysis. Transient paralysis with spontaneous recovery, clinically resembling cataplexy and often associated with narcolepsy, occurring on falling asleep (hypnagogic paralysis) or more commonly on awakening (hypnopompic paralysis).

sleep spindle. *In electroencephalography,* the bursts of about 14-per-second waves that occur during sleep.

sleep therapy. NARCOSIS THERAPY.

sleep·walk·ing, *n.* A condition in which an individual walks during sleep. Syn. *somnambulism.* —**sleepwalk·er,** *n.*

slide, *n.* A piece of glass on which objects are examined by use of the microscope.

sliding hernia. A variety of indirect, irreducible inguinal hernia in which a section of a viscus, usually cecum or sigmoid colon, forms one wall of the sac; generally a large scrotal hernia.

sling, *n.* A bandage, usually slung from the neck, to support the arm or wrist.

slipped disk. HERNIATED DISK.

slipped shoulder. A dislocated humerus.

slipping epiphysis. Displacement of the upper femoral epiphysis; of uncertain etiology. It occurs in children.

slit, *n.* A narrow opening; a visceral cleft; the separation between any pair of lips.

slit lamp. An instrument consisting of a light source providing a narrow beam of high intensity and a microscope or binocular magnifier, which makes possible the highly magnified viewing of various parts of the living eye, especially the anterior portions.

slough (sluf) *n. & v.* 1. A mass of necrotic tissue in, or separating from, living tissue, as in a wound or ulcer. 2. To cast off a mass of necrotic tissue. —**slough·ing** (sluf′ing) *n. & adj.*

slow neutron. THERMAL NEUTRON.

sludge, *v. & n.* 1. To agglutinate or precipitate from a liquid, forming a semisolid deposit. 2. The deposit formed.

sludged blood. The intravascular aggregation of erythrocytes associated with decreased blood flow in the involved vascular bed.

Sm Symbol for samarium.

small calorie. CALORIE.

small-cell carcinoma. 1. Any carcinoma with small parenchymal cells. 2. OAT-CELL CARCINOMA.

small intestine. The proximal portion of the intestine, extending from the stomach to the large intestine, and consisting of the duodenum, jejunum, and ileum; it functions primarily in the digestion and absorption of food.

small·pox, *n.* An infectious pox viral disease, characterized by a diphasic severe febrile illness and a generalized vesicular and pustular eruption. It can be prevented by vaccination. Syn. *variola.*

smallpox vaccine. A glycerinated suspension of the vesicles of vaccinia, or cowpox, which have been obtained from healthy vaccinated calves or sheep, used in vaccination to confer lifelong immunity against smallpox. Syn. *virus vaccinum, glycerinated vaccine virus, Jennerian vaccine, antismallpox vaccine.*

smear, *n.* Preparation of secretions or blood or tissue scrapings for microscopical study, made by spreading them on a glass slide or coverslip.

smeg·ma (smeg'muh) *n.* SEBUM. —**smeg·mat·ic** (smeg·mat'ick) *adj.*

smegma cli·to·ri·dis (kli·tor'i·dis) [BNA]. The substance secreted by the sebaceous glands of the clitoris.

smegma prae·pu·tii (pree·pew'shee·eye) [BNA]. The substance secreted by the sebaceous glands of the prepuce.

smell, *n.* 1. The perception of odor, resulting from the adequate stimulation, usually by chemical molecules, of the receptors in the olfactory mucous membrane; a visceral sensation. 2. ODOR.

smell·ing salts. A preparation containing ammonium carbonate and stronger ammonia water, usually scented with aromatic substances.

Smith-Petersen nail A three-flanged nail used to fix fractures of the neck of the femur. It is inserted from just below the greater trochanter, through the neck, and into the head of the femur.

Smith·wick's operation An operation for hypertension; the greater splanchnic nerve and the sympathetic chain from the ninth thoracic through the first lumbar ganglion are resected through a transdiaphragmatic extrapleural incision. Syn. *lumbodorsal splanchnicectomy.*

smoker's cancer. Squamous cell carcinoma of the lip, usually the lower lip, observed in habitual smokers.

smooth muscle. Muscle tissue consisting of spindle-shaped, unstriped muscle cells and found in the walls of viscera and blood vessels.

smooth-surfaced endoplasmic reticulum. Intracytoplasmic membranes devoid of ribosomes, seen by electron microscopy. Abbreviated, SER.

smudge cells. Degenerate leukocytes seen in spreads of blood and bone marrow cells.

smudg·ing (smuj'ing) *n.* A form of defective speech in which the difficult consonants are dropped.

smut, *n.* 1. A fungous disease of plants involving the grains wheat, rye, oats, and corn. 2. A fungus producing such a disease.

Sn Symbol for tin.

snail, *n.* An invertebrate of the order Gastropoda, phylum Mollusca. Important as hosts of many of the flukes.

snake venom. A secretion of the posterior superior labial glands of a poisonous snake, nor-

mally yellowish, sometimes colorless, possessing varying degrees of toxicity. Toxic constituents include neurotoxins, cytolysins, hemolysins, and hemocoagulins.

snap·ping hip. An abnormality caused by the presence of a tendinous band on the surface of the gluteus maximus muscle. Certain movements of the hip cause this band to slip over the greater trochanter.

snapping jaw. A condition characterized by an audible and palpable snap on opening and closing the mouth, usually caused by displacement of the meniscus in the temporomandibular joint.

snare, *n.* An instrument designed to hold a wire loop which can be constricted by means of a mechanism in the handle, and used to remove tonsils, polyps, and small growths having a narrow base or pedicle.

sneeze, *n.* A sudden, noisy, spasmodic expiration through the nose. It is caused by irritation of nasal nerves or overstimulation of the optic nerve by a very bright light.

Snel·len chart A chart for the testing of visual acuity, using letters or numbers for literate patients and letter E's in various positions for small children and illiterates, with the symbols varying in size so that at a distance of 20 feet (or 6 meters) the smallest read normally (and therefore recorded as 20/20 or 6/6) subtends an angle of 5 minutes. If the smallest letter or E the patient can read subtends an angle of 5 minutes at 30 feet, vision is recorded as 20/30 and so forth.

snore, *v.* To breathe during sleep in such a manner as to cause a vibration of the soft palate, thereby producing a rough, audible sound.

snow blindness. Impairment of vision and actinic keratoconjunctivitis, both usually transient, due to exposure of the eyes to the reflection of ultraviolet rays from snow.

snuff·box or **snuffbox space.** ANATOMIST'S SNUFFBOX.

snuf·fles, *n.* Serosanguinous nasal discharge containing spirochetes; one of the early clinical manifestations of congenital syphilis.

soap, *n.* A salt of one or more higher fatty acids with an alkali or metal. Soaps may be divided into two classes, soluble and insoluble. Soluble soaps are detergent and usually are prepared from the alkali metals sodium and potassium. Insoluble soaps are salts of the fatty acids and metals of other groups. Soap (soluble) is used chiefly as a detergent. In constipation, a solution of soap forms a useful enema. In skin conditions, soap is useful not only as a detergent but also because it softens the horny layer of the epidermis and is germicidal. In pharmacy, soap is used as an emulsifying agent when the mixture is intended for external use. Soap is also used in making liniment and plasters.

sob, *n. & v.* 1. A convulsive inspiration due to contraction of the diaphragm and spasmodic closure of the glottis. 2. To inspire convulsively.

so·cial (so'shul) *adj.* 1. Gregarious; growing

near, or together. 2. Of or pertaining to society.

social adaptation. The process whereby an individual or group comes to meet without undue strain the usual demands of society at large, so as to survive and function well.

social deprivation. The condition of lacking or being deprived of certain cultural and educational experiences and opportunities that are deemed essential for normal social and mental development by the majority of the society of which the individual is a member. This may result in pseudoretardation.

so·cial·iza·tion (so'shul·i·zay'shun) *n. In psychology,* the process whereby a child learns to get along with and behave similarly to other people in his group, largely through imitation as well as the pressures of group life; the process of becoming a social being.

socialized medicine. The control, direction, and financing of the medical care of a population by an organized group, a state, or a nation; assumption of legal, administrative, and financial responsibility for the practice of medicine by professional services and for the total care of the patients, with funds derived usually from assessment, philanthropy, and taxation.

social medicine. An approach to the maintenance and advancement of health and the prevention, amelioration, and cure of disease, which has its foundation in the study of man, his heredity, and his environment.

social psychiatry. Psychiatry especially concerned with the study of social influences on the cause and dynamics of emotional and mental illness, the use of the social environment in treatment, and preventive community programs, as well as the application of psychiatry to social issues, industry, law, education, and other such activities and organizations.

social service or **work.** Activity, usually organized and directed by a professionally skilled individual, which seeks to help individuals or groups through their environmental situation.

so·cio·bi·ol·o·gy (so'see·o·bye·ol'uh·jee, so'shee·o·) *n.* The branch of biology dealing with the biological, especially genetic, determinants of social behavior.

so·ci·ol·o·gy (so'see·ol'uh·jee, so'shee·) *n.* The science of mutual relations of people and of society. —**so·cio·log·i·cal** (so'see·o·loj'i·kul, so'shuh·) *adj.*

so·cio·med·i·cal (so'see·o·med'i·kul, so'shee·) *adj.* Pertaining to the relationship between social welfare and medicine.

so·cio·path (so'see·o·path, so'shee·) *n.* An individual with a sociopathic personality disturbance, similar to a psychopathic personality but connoting a pathologic and usually hostile attitude toward society. —**so·cio·path·ic** (so'see·o·path'ick, so'shee·) *adj.*

sociopathic personality disturbance. *In psychiatry,* a personality disorder characterized primarily in terms of the pathologic relationship between the individual and the society and the moral and cultural environment in which he lives, as well as personal discomfort and poor relationships with others. Sociopathic reactions may be symptomatic of severe personality disorders, psychoneurotic or psychotic disorders, or organic brain syndrome, the recognition of which then forms the basic diagnosis.

sock·et, *n.* 1. The concavity into which a movable part is inserted. 2. The space in a jawbone in which a root of a tooth is held.

so·cor·dia (so·kor'dee·uh) *n.* HALLUCINATION.

so·da (so'duh) *n.* SODIUM CARBONATE.

soda lime. A mixture in granular form of calcium hydroxide with sodium hydroxide or potassium hydroxide or both. Used to absorb carbon dioxide in basal metabolism tests, during rebreathing in anesthesia machines, and in oxygen therapy.

sodio-. A combining form meaning *a compound containing sodium.*

so·di·um (so'dee·um) *n.* Na = 22.9898. A metallic element, atomic number 11, of the alkali group of metals, which is light, silver-white, and lustrous when freshly cut, but rapidly oxidizes when exposed to air, becoming dull and gray. It violently decomposes water, forming sodium hydroxide and hydrogen. Sodium ion is of great importance biochemically, and sodium salts are extensively employed medicinally. Sodium ion is the least toxic of the metallic ions, and is therefore the base of choice when it is desired to obtain the effects of various acid ions. The majority of sodium salts occur as white or colorless crystals or as a white, crystalline powder, and are freely soluble in water.

sodium acetate. $CH_3COONa.3H_2O$. Used as a systemic and urinary alkalizer and, formerly, as a diuretic and expectorant.

sodium acetrizoate. Sodium 3-acetylamino-2,4,-6-triiodobenzoate, $C_9H_5I_3NNaO_3$, a radiopaque contrast medium.

sodium acid phosphate. SODIUM BIPHOSPHATE.

sodium alginate. The sodium salt of alginic acid, a gelatinous substance obtained from various seaweeds. Sodium alginate dissolves in cold water to form a mucilage, and is used in pharmaceutical compounding for preparing suspensions.

sodium an·azo·lene (an·az'o·leen). 4-[(4-Anilino-5-sulfo-1-naphthyl)azo]-5-hydroxy-2,7-naphthalenedisulfonic acid trisodium salt, $C_{26}H_{16}N_3Na_3O_{10}S_3$, a diagnostic aid for estimating blood volume and cardiac output and a sensitive stain for the detection of proteins on polyacrylamide gels.

sodium antimony tartrate. ANTIMONY SODIUM TARTRATE.

sodium benzoate. C_6H_5COONa. Used as a diagnostic agent to test for liver function, also as an antimicrobial preservative.

sodium bicarbonate. $NaHCO_3$. Used as a gastric antacid, to combat systemic acidosis, and to alkalinize urine.

sodium biphosphate. $NaH_2PO_4.H_2O$. Used as a urinary acidifier. Syn. *sodium dihydrogen phosphate, monosodium orthophosphate, sodium acid phosphate.*

sodium borate. $Na_2B_4O_7.10H_2O$. A detergent

and emulsifier; also a weak antibacterial and astringent. Syn. *borax, sodium tetraborate.*

sodium bromide. NaBr. Formerly extensively used as a hypnotic, sedative, and antiepileptic drug.

sodium carbonate. Na_2CO_3. The anhydrous and monohydrate forms are used in various chemical and pharmaceutical procedures; sometimes for treatment of scaly skin, and as a detergent.

sodium chloride. NaCl. Comprises over 90 per cent of the inorganic constituents of blood serum; both of its ions are physiologically important. Used medicinally as an electrolyte replenisher.

sodium chloride injection. U.S.P. title for a sterile, isotonic solution of sodium chloride in water for injection, containing 0.9 g of sodium chloride in 100 ml. Used intravenously as a fluid and electrolyte replenisher, also as a solvent for many parenterally administered drugs. Syn. *isotonic sodium chloride injection.*

sodium chloride irrigation. U.S.P. title for a sterile solution of sodium chloride in purified water, containing 0.9 g of sodium chloride in 100 ml. Isotonic with body fluids; variously used as a physiological salt solution but not to be employed parenterally, for which purpose sodium chloride injection is used. Syn. *isotonic sodium chloride solution, normal saline solution, physiological salt solution, physiological sodium chloride solution.*

sodium citrate. $Na_3C_6H_5O_7.2H_2O$. Used to restore bicarbonate reserve of the blood in acidosis, to overcome excessive acidity of urine, and as a mild diuretic and expectorant. Employed also as an anticoagulant for blood to be fractionated or stored.

sodium dehydrocholate. The sodium salt of dehydrocholic acid, used as a choleretic and as a diagnostic agent to determine circulation time.

sodium diatrizoate. Sodium 3,5-diacetamido-2,4,6-triiodobenzoate, $C_{11}H_8I_3N_2NaO_4$, a roentgenographic contrast medium.

sodium fluoride. NaF. Used for fluoridation of water and also applied topically, directly to teeth, to reduce incidence of dental caries.

sodium glucosulfone. *p,p'*-Sulfonyldianiline *N,N'*-diglucoside disodium disulfonate, $C_{24}H_{34}N_2Na_2O_{18}S_3$, a leprostatic drug and suppressant for dermatitis herpetiformis.

sodium glutamate. Monosodium L-glutamate, $HOOCCHNH_2CH_2CH_2COONa$, used intravenously for symptomatic treatment of hepatic coma in which there is a high blood level of ammonia. Imparts a meat flavor to foods. Syn. *monosodium glutamate.*

sodium gold thiosulfate. GOLD SODIUM THIOSULFATE.

sodium hydroxide. NaOH. Occurs as fused masses, small pellets, flakes, or sticks; used as a caustic, and in various chemical and pharmaceutical manipulations. Syn. *caustic soda.*

sodium hy·droxy·di·one suc·ci·nate (high-drock″see-dye′ohn suck′si·nate). Sodium 21-hydroxypregnane-3,20-dione succinate, $C_{25}H_{35}NaO_6$, a steroid that has hypnotic, mild

analgesic, and, possibly, some amnesic action

sodium hypochlorite solution. Contains 5% NaOCl; the solution has the germicidal value of its available chlorine. Used for disinfection of various utensils which are not injured by its bleaching action, such as clinical thermometers, glass, or chinaware. This solution is not suitable for application to wounds; for such use, diluted sodium hypochlorite solution which contains 0.5% NaOCl and is nearly neutral, is employed.

sodium hypophosphite. $NaH_2PO_2.H_2O$. Formerly used as an ingredient of tonic formulations in the erroneous belief that hypophosphite was utilized in synthesis of essential phosphorus compounds in nerve tissue.

sodium iodide. NaI. Used for the therapeutic effects of iodide ion, especially when intravenous administration is indicated, as in thyroid crisis and paroxysm of asthma.

sodium io·do·hip·pur·ate (eye-o″do·hip′yoo-rate). Sodium *o*-iodohippurate, $IC_6H_4CONHCH_2COONa$, a diagnostic agent used for radiography of the urinary tract.

sodium lactate. $CH_3CHOHCOONa$. For medicinal use prepared by neutralizing a solution of lactic acid with sodium hydroxide; used intravenously, in one-sixth molar solution, as a fluid and electrolyte replenisher. Indicated in the treatment of acidosis.

sodium lauryl sulfate. Chiefly $CH_3(CH_2)_{10}CH_2OSO_3Na$. Used as a wetting agent, emulsifying aid, and detergent; not affected by hard water.

sodium liothyronine. LIOTHYRONINE SODIUM.

sodium meth·io·dal (me·thigh′o·dal). Sodium monoiodomethanesulfonate, ICH_2SO_3Na, a radiopaque medium used for intravenous urography or retrograde pyelography.

sodium mor·rhu·ate (mor′oo·ate). A mixture of the sodium salts of the saturated and unsaturated fatty acids occurring in cod liver oil; occurs as a pale, yellowish, granular powder soluble in water. Used as a sclerosing agent for obliteration of varicose veins.

sodium nitrate. $NaNO_3$. Formerly used in the treatment of dysentery. Syn. *Chile saltpeter soda niter.*

sodium perborate. $NaBO_3.4H_2O$. Used as a locally applied anti-infective agent; functions by virtue of decomposition to hydrogen peroxide and release of oxygen.

sodium peroxide. Na_2O_2. The sodium compound analogous to hydrogen peroxide; a powerful oxidizing agent. It has been used for treatment of acne, applied in the form of a paste prepared with liquid petrolatum, or as a soap to remove comedones. Syn. *sodium superoxide.*

sodium phosphate. $Na_2HPO_4.7H_2O$. Used as a mild saline cathartic; also beneficial in the treatment of lead poisoning. Syn. *dibasic sodium phosphate, disodium hydrogen phosphate.*

sodium polystyrene sulfonate. A cation exchange resin that exchanges its sodium for potassium and is used in the treatment of hyperkalemia.

sodium propionate. CH_3CH_2COONa. A salt

with antibacterial and fungicidal properties; used in the control of athlete's foot, tinea cruris, and other mycoses.

sodium pump. An intramembranous active transport system in most resting cells that selectively expels sodium while allowing the simultaneous concentration of potassium within the cell, using energy derived from hydrolysis of adenosine triphosphate. Syn. *sodium-potassium pump.*

sodium ric·i·nate (ris'ĭ-nate). A mixture of the sodium salts of the fatty acids from castor oil, chiefly ricinoleic acid; has been used to detoxify bacterial toxins in various forms of intestinal intoxication. Syn. *sodium ricinoleate.*

sodium salicylate. HOC_6H_4COONa. Used as an analgesic, antirheumatic, and antipyretic.

sodium sulfate. $Na_2SO_4.10H_2O$. In large doses, an efficient hydragogue cathartic; in smaller doses, mildly laxative and diuretic. Syn. *Glauber's salt.*

sodium sulfobromophthalein. SULFOBROMO-PHTHALEIN SODIUM.

sodium suramin. SURAMIN SODIUM.

sodium taurocholate. The sodium salt of taurocholic acid, usually containing also some sodium glycocholate; a constituent of the bile of carnivora; a yellowish-gray powder, soluble in water; used as a choleretic and cholagogue.

sodium thiamylal. THIAMYLAL SODIUM.

sodium thiosulfate. $Na_2S_2O_3.5H_2O$. Used as an antidote, with sodium nitrite, to cyanide poisoning, as a topical application in the treatment of tinea versicolor, and as a prophylactic agent, in foot baths, against ringworm infection. Also used as a reagent. Syn. *sodium hyposulfite.*

so·do·ku (so'do-koo, so·do'koo) n. A disease caused by *Spirillum minus*, usually transmitted by rat bite, and characterized by an indurated ulcer at the site of inoculation, regional lymphadenitis, relapsing fever, and skin rash. Syn. *spirillary rat-bite fever.*

sod·om·ist (sod'um-ist) n. A person who practices sodomy.

sod·om·y (sod'um-ee) n. 1. Sexual intercourse by the anus, usually considered as between males. 2. BESTIALITY (2).

soft cataract. A cataract, occurring especially in the young, in which the cortex of the lens is of soft consistency and milky in appearance, but the nucleus is relatively unaffected.

soft chancre. CHANCROID.

soft diet. A diet consisting of easily consumed, easily digested foods.

soft·en·ing, n. The process of becoming less cohesive, firm, or resistant.

soft palate. The posterior part of the palate which consists of an aggregation of muscles, the tensor veli palatini, levator veli palatini, azygos uvulae, palatoglossus, and palatopharyngeus, and their covering mucous membrane.

soft pulse. A pulse that is readily compressed.

sol, n. A colloidal solution consisting of a suitable dispersion medium, which may be gas, liquid, or solid, and the colloidal substance, the disperse phase, which is distributed throughout the dispersion medium. The disperse phase may be gas, liquid, or solid.

sol. Abbreviation for *solution* (1).

So·la·na·ce·ae (so"luh-nay'see-ee, sol"uh·) n.pl. A family of herbs, shrubs, and trees comprising approximately 75 genera and 1,800 species and including the potato and tomato plants, and also plants from which are derived such drugs as belladonna, hyoscyamus, scopola, and stramonium. **—solana·ceous** (·shus) adj.

So·la·num (so·lay'num) n. A genus of the Solanaceae, including the tomato, potato, bittersweet, and black nightshade.

solar dermatitis. Any skin eruption caused by exposure to the sun, excluding sunburn; it may be plaque-like, eczematous, papular, or erythematous.

so·lar (so'lur) adj. 1. Pertaining to or derived from the sun. 2. Analogous to or resembling the sun.

so·lar·iza·tion (so"lur·i·zay'shun) n. The application of solar or ultraviolet light for therapeutic purposes. **—so·lar·ize** (so'lur·ize) v.

solar plexus. CELIAC PLEXUS.

solar retinitis. Retinal change from the effect of sunlight.

solar therapy. Treatment of disease by exposing the body to the direct rays of the sun. Syn. *heliotherapy.*

soldier's heart. NEUROCIRCULATORY ASTHENIA.

soldier's patches or **spots.** MILK SPOTS.

sole, n. The undersurface of the foot between the heel and the toes.

so·le·al (so'lee-ul) adj. Pertaining to the soleus muscle.

sole·plate, n. END PLATE.

so·le·us (so'lee-us) n., L. pl. & genit. sing. **so·lei** (·lee-eye). A flat muscle of the calf.

sol·id, adj. 1. Firm; dense; not fluid or gaseous. 2. Not hollow.

solid-cell carcinoma. RENAL CELL CARCINOMA.

so·lid·i·fi·ca·tion (suh·lid"i·fi·kay'shun) n. The act of becoming solid.

sol·i·ped (sol'i·ped) n. An animal having a solid, undivided hoof, as the horse, donkey, or zebra.

sol·ip·sism (sol'ip-siz·um) n. The philosophical doctrine that any organism can know only itself and its own conception of its environment, and hence that there is only subjective reality.

sol·i·tary (sol'i·terr"ee) adj. 1. Single. 2. Existing separately; not collected together.

sol·u·bil·i·ty (sol"yoo·bil'i·tee) n. The extent to which a substance (solute) dissolves in a liquid (solvent) to produce a homogeneous system (solution). The degree of solubility is the concentration of a saturated solution at a given temperature.

solubility product. The product of the concentrations (or activities) of the ions of a substance in a saturated solution of the substance, each concentration term being raised to the power equal to the number of ions represented in a molecule of the substance.

sol·u·ble (sol'yoo·bul) adj. Capable of mixing with a liquid (dissolving) to form a homogeneous mixture (solution).

soluble RNA. TRANSFER RNA.

soluble starch. Starch transformed into water-soluble dextrins by heating.

so·lum tym·pa·ni (so'lum tim'puh·nigh) *n.* The floor of the tympanic cavity.

so·lute (sol'yoot, so'lewt) *n.* The dissolved substance in a solution.

so·lu·tion (suh·lew'shun) *n.* 1. A homogeneous mixture of a solid, liquid, or gaseous substance (the solute) in a liquid (the solvent) from which the dissolved substance can be recovered by crystallization or other physical processes. The formation of a solution is not accompanied by permanent chemical change, and is thus commonly considered a physical phenomenon. Abbreviated, sol. 2. *In physical chemistry,* any homogeneous phase consisting of two or more compounds.

solution pressure. The tendency of molecules or ions to leave the surface of a solute and pass into the solvent. It varies in different solute-solvent combinations.

sol·vate (sol'vate) *n.* A compound formed between solute and solvent in a solution.

sol·va·tion (sol·vay'shun) *n.* The process of forming a solvate.

sol·vent (sol'vunt) *n.* 1. The component of a homogeneous mixture which is in excess. 2. A liquid that dissolves another substance (solute) without any change in chemical composition, such as sugar or salt in water. 3. A liquid that reacts chemically with a solid and brings it into solution, such as acids that dissolve metals.

so·ma (so'muh) *n.,* pl. **so·ma·ta** (·tuh), **so·mas** 1. The entire body with the exclusion of the germ cells. 2. The body as contrasted with the psyche. —Adj. *somatic.*

so·mas·the·ni·a (so'mas·theen'ee·uh) *n.* Bodily deterioration and exhaustion.

somat-, somato- A combining form meaning *somatic.*

so·mat·es·the·sia, so·mat·aes·the·sia (so'muh·tes·theezh'uh, ·theez'ee·uh) *n.* SOMESTHESIA. —**somates·thet·ic, somataes·thet·ic** (·thet'ick) *adj.*

so·mat·ic (so·mat'ick) *adj.* 1. Bodily, corporeal. 2. Pertaining to the soma (1). 3. Pertaining to the framework of the body and not to the viscera.

somatic antigen. 1. Any antigen of gram-negative bacteria, located in the cell wall, consisting of complexes of carbohydrate, lipid, and a protein or polypeptide-like material. The carbohydrate determines the somatic O antigen specificity. 2. Any cellular protein or other component that is antigenic, in contrast to extracellular products or structures, such as capsules or flagella, exterior to the cell wall.

somatic death. Death of the whole organism.

somatic nerve. One of the nerves supplying somatic structures, such as voluntary muscles, skin, tendons, joints, and parietal serous membranes.

so·mat·i·co·vis·cer·al (so·mat''i·ko·vis'ur·ul) *adj.* Pertaining to the body and the viscera.

so·ma·tist (so'muh·tist) *n.* A psychiatrist who holds any mental disorder to be of physical origin.

so·ma·ti·za·tion (so''muh·ti·zay'shun) *n. In psychiatry,* the neurotic displacement of emotional conflicts onto the body, resulting in various physical symptoms or complaints this may take the form of a conversion type of hysterical neurosis involving voluntary muscles and the sensory system, or it may express itself as a psychophysiologic disorder involving the autonomic nervous system and the viscera innervated by it. —**so·ma·tize** (so'muh·tize) *v.*

so·ma·tog·e·ny (so''muh·toj'e·nee) *n.* The acquirement of bodily characteristics, especially the acquirement of characteristics due to environment. —**soma·to·gen·ic** (·to·jen'ick) *adj.*

so·ma·tol·o·gy (so''muh·tol'uh·jee) *n.* The study of the development, structure, and functions of the body. —**soma·to·log·ic** (·to·loj'ick) *adj.*

so·ma·to·me·din (so''muh·to·mee'din) *n.* A protein formed in the liver which mediates the effects of growth hormone activity; appears to have anabolic and antilipolytic effects similar to those of insulin.

so·ma·to·meg·a·ly (so''muh·to·meg'uh·lee) *n.* GIGANTISM.

so·ma·tom·e·try (so''muh·tom'e·tree) *n.* Measurement of the human body with the soft parts intact. —**soma·to·met·ric** (·to·met'rick) *adj.*

so·ma·top·a·gus (so''muh·top'uh·gus) *n.* Conjoined twins with their trunks more or less in common.

so·ma·to·path·ic (so''muh·to·path'ick) *adj.* Pertaining to an organic or bodily disorder.

so·ma·to·pleure (so'muh·to·ploor, so·mat'o·) *n.* The body wall composed of ectoderm and somatic mesoderm. —**so·ma·to·pleu·ral** (so''muh·to·ploor'ul) *adj.*

so·ma·to·psy·chic (so''muh·to·sigh'kick) *adj.* Pertaining to both the body and mind.

so·ma·to·sen·so·ry (so''muh·to·sen'suh·ree) *adj.* Pertaining to bodily sensation.

so·ma·to·ther·a·py (so''muh·to·therr'uh·pee) *n. In psychiatry,* the treatment of disease by means such as electric shock, chemotherapy, and other physical means.

so·ma·to·to·nia (so''muh·to·to'nee·uh) *n.* The behavioral counterpart of component II (mesomorphy) of the somatotype, manifested in desire for expenditure of energy through vigorous bodily assertiveness and the enjoyment of muscular activity. —**somato·ton·ic** (·ton'ick) *adj.*

so·ma·to·top·ag·no·sia (so''muh·to·top''ag·no'zhuh, ·zee·uh) *n.* AUTOTOPAGNOSIA.

so·ma·to·top·ic (so''muh·to·top'ick) *adj.* Pertaining to the correspondence between a body part and a particular area of the cerebral cortex, or other region of the brain, to which sensory pathways from the body part are projected, or from which motor pathways to the part take origin.

somatotropic hormone. GROWTH HORMONE. Abbreviated, STH.

so·ma·to·tro·pin (so''muh·to·tro'pin, ·tot'ro·pin) *n.* 1. GROWTH HORMONE. 2. Purified growth hormone extracted from the human pituitary gland, used to stimulate linear growth in patients with growth hormone deficiency.

so·ma·to·type (so''muh·to·tipe, so·mat'o·) *n.* 1. The body type. 2. The quantitative description of the morphological structure of an individual by a series of three numerals representing the primary components: I endomorphy; II mesomorphy; III ectomorphy. On the behavioral level, these are termed viscerotonia, somatotonia, and cerebrotonia.

-some A combining form meaning *body.*

so·mes·the·sia, so·aes·the·sia (so''mes·theezh'uh, ·theez'ee·uh) *n.* Awareness of bodily sensations; consciousness of one's body.

som·es·thet·ic, so·aes·thet·ic (so''mes·thet'ick) *adj.* Pertaining to proprioceptive and tactile sensation.

somesthetic area. The receptive center for proprioceptive or tactile sensation in the postcentral gyrus: Brodmann's areas 1, 2, 3.

som·es·the·to·psy·chic, so·aes·the·to·psy·chic (so''mes·theet''o·sigh'kick, ·es·thet''o·) *adj.* Pertaining to the somesthetopsychic area.

somesthetopsychic area. The somesthetic association area of the parietal cortex: Brodmann's areas 5 and 7.

-somia A combining form designating a *condition of the body or soma,* as nanosomia, macrosomia.

so·mite (so'mite) *n.* A segment of the body of an embryo; one of a series of paired segments of the paraxial mesoderm composed of dermatome, myotome, and sclerotome. —**so·mit·ic** (so·mit'ick) *adj.*

somn-, somno- A combining form meaning *sleep.*

som·nam·bu·la·tor (som·nam'bew·lay''tur) *n.* SOMNAMBULIST.

som·nam·bu·lism (som·nam'bew·liz·um) *n.* 1. SLEEPWALKING. 2. The performance of any fairly complex act while in a sleeplike state or trance. 3. HYPNOTIC SOMNAMBULISM.

som·nam·bu·list (som·nam'bew·list) *n.* One who walks in his sleep.

som·ni·a·tion (som''nee·ay'shun) *n.* Dreaming. —**som·ni·a·tive** (som'nee·uh·tiv, ·ay''tiv) *adj.*

som·ni·fa·cient (som''ni·fay'shunt) *adj. & n.* 1. Producing sleep; HYPNOTIC (1). 2. A medicine producing sleep; HYPNOTIC (3).

som·nif·er·ous (som·nif'ur·us) *adj.* Producing sleep.

som·nif·ic (som·nif'ick) *adj.* Causing sleep.

som·nif·u·gous (som·nif'yoo·gus) *adj.* Driving away sleep.

som·nil·o·quist (som·nil'o·kwist) *n.* A person who talks in his sleep.

som·nil·o·quy (som·nil'uh·kwee) *n.* Talking in one's sleep.

som·nip·a·thy (som·nip'uth·ee) *n.* 1. Any disorder of sleep. 2. HYPNOTIC SOMNAMBULISM.

som·no·cin·e·mat·o·graph (som''no·sin'e·mat'o·graf) *n.* An apparatus for recording movements made during sleep.

som·no·lence (som'nuh·lunce) *n.* Drowsiness; semiconsciousness. —**somno·lent** (·lunt) *adj.*

som·no·len·tia (som''no·len'chee·uh) *n.* 1. The condition of being half awake and unsteady on

one's feet, staggering about as if drunk. 2. SOMNOLENCE.

som·no·les·cent (som''no·les'unt) *adj.* 1. Drowsy. 2. Inducing drowsiness.

som·no·lism (som'nuh·liz·um) *n.* 1. HYPNOTISM. 2. A hypnotic trance.

-somus A combining form designating *an individual with a* (specified) *form or condition of the body.*

son-, sono- A combining form meaning *sound.*

sone, *n.* The unit of loudness.

son·i·ca·tion (son''i·kay'shun) *n.* Disruption with high-frequency sound.

Son·ne dysentery One of the commonest forms of bacterial intestinal infection, occurring often in epidemic form in children, caused by *Shigella sonnei.*

sono·en·ceph·a·lo·gram (son''o·en·sef'uh·lo·gram) *n.* ECHOENCEPHALOGRAM.

sono·gram (son'o·gram) *n.* ECHOGRAM.

so·nog·ra·phy (so·nog'ruh·fee) *n.* The making of a record or an anatomic depiction by means of ultrasound.

so·nom·e·ter (so·nom'e·tur) *n.* An instrument for determining the pitch of sounds and their relation to the musical scale.

so·no·rous (so·no'rus) *adj.* 1. RESONANT. 2. Characterized by a loud sound.

sonorous rale. A low-pitched, resonant, snoring sound heard on auscultation of the lungs in asthma and other bronchiolar diseases.

so·phis·ti·ca·tion (so·fis''ti·kay'shun) *n.* The adulteration or imitation of a substance.

sopho·ma·nia (sof''o·may'nee·uh) *n.* Megalomania in which the patient believes himself to excel in wisdom.

so·por (so'pur) *n.* Sleep, especially the profound sleep symptomatic of an abnormal condition, as in a stupor.

so·po·rif·er·ous (so''puh·rif'ur·us) *adj.* SOPORIFIC.

so·po·rif·ic (so''puh·rif'ick, sop''uh·) *adj. & n.* 1. Producing sleep. 2. NARCOTIC (1, 2).

so·po·rose (so'puh·roce) *adj.* 1. Sleepy; characterized by abnormal sleep; stuporous. 2. COMATOSE.

sor·be·fa·cient (sor''be·fay'shunt) *n. & adj.* 1. A medicine or agent that induces absorption. 2. Absorption-inducing.

sor·bi·tan (sor'bi·tan) *n.* Sorbitol anhydride, $C_6H_{12}O_5$, various fatty acid esters of which, as sorbitan monolaurate and sodium monostearate, are used as surfactants.

sor·bi·tol (sor'bi·tol) *n.* D-Sorbitol or D-glucitol, $C_6H_{14}O_6$, a hexahydric alcohol isomeric with mannitol. Used intravenously as a diuretic; also as a humectant, sweetener, and vehicle for medicinal preparations.

sor·bose (sor'boce, ·boze) *n.* L-Sorbose, $C_6H_{12}O_6$, a ketohexose obtained by oxidative fermentation of D-sorbitol by certain organisms.

sor·des (sor'deez) *n.,* pl. **sordes** Filth, dirt; especially the crusts that accumulate on the teeth and lips in continued fevers, consisting of oral debris, epithelium, food, and microorganisms.

sor·did, *adj. In biology,* of a dull or dirty color.

sore, *adj. & n.* 1. Painful; tender. 2. An ulcer or wound.

sore-head, *n.* 1. AVIAN POX. 2. An allergic dermatitis on the forehead or face of sheep due to microfilariae of the species *Elaeophora schneideri.*

sore throat. Any painful inflammation of the pharynx.

so·ro·ri·a·tion (so-ror″ee·ay′shun) *n.* The development that takes place in the female breasts at puberty.

sor·rel (sor′ul) *n.* A plant of the genus *Rumex,* containing oxalates.

S.O.S. Abbreviation for *si opus sit,* if necessary.

souf·fle (soo′ful, sooff) *n.* A soft blowing sound or murmur heard on auscultation.

¹sound, *n.* An instrument for introduction into a channel or cavity, for determining the presence of constriction, foreign bodies, or other abnormal conditions, and for treatment.

²sound, *n.* 1. The aspect of reality perceived by hearing, consisting objectively of vibrations conveyed to and stimulating the inner ear. 2. Any object of sensation peculiar to the sense of hearing.

South American blastomycosis. A chronic granulomatous disease of the skin and mucous membranes which may involve the lymph nodes and viscera. It is caused by *Blastomyces brasiliensis.*

South American leishmaniasis. AMERICAN MUCOCUTANEOUS LEISHMANIASIS.

soy·bean, *n.* The seed of *Glycine soja (Glycine hispida, Soja hispida),* a legume native to Asia but cultivated in other regions, including the United States, because of the high food value of its seeds. The bean and flour are used in dietetics for their high protein and relatively low carbohydrate content. The enzyme urease is obtained from soybean.

sp. Abbreviation for (a) *spiritus,* spirit; (b) *species.*

spa (spah) *n.* A mineral spring, especially one thought to have medicinal value and visited as a health resort.

space, *n.* 1. A delimited area or region. 2. The realm outside or beyond the earth's atmosphere.

space maintainer. An orthodontic device used in spaces created by the loss of primary teeth to assure space availability for erupting teeth.

space of Dis·se PERISINUSOIDAL SPACE.

space of Retzius RETROPUBIC SPACE.

spaces of Virchow-Robin. PERIVASCULAR SPACES OF VIRCHOW-ROBIN.

spag·y·rism (spaj′i·riz·um) *n.* The Paracelsian, or spagyric, school or doctrine of medicine.

spall·ation (spawl·ay′shun) *n.* The process of bombarding various elements with extremely high-energy protons, deuterons, or alpha particles, whereby extensive alterations of the bombarded nucleus result.

Spanish fly. The beetle *Lytta vesicatoria,* from which the irritant cantharidin is derived, popularly regarded as an aphrodisiac.

Spanish pox. SYPHILIS.

Spanish windlass. 1. An improvised tourniquet consisting of a handkerchief knotted around a limb and tightened by means of a stick which is twisted. 2. A temporary emergency method of making traction upon a splinted extremity, pull being provided by twisting the traction cords with a stick.

spar·a·drap (spar′uh·drap) *n.* A plaster spread on cotton, linen, silk, leather, or paper; adhesive plaster.

spargana. Plural of *sparganum.*

spar·ga·no·sis (spahr″guh·no′sis) *n.,* pl. **sparga·no·ses** (·seez) Infection with sparganum, which is a larval stage of the fish tapeworm *Diphyllobothrium latum.*

spar·ga·num (spahr′guh·num) *n.,* pl. **sparga·na** (·nuh) A general name applied to the plerocercoid larva of *Diphyllobothrium,* especially if the adult form is unknown; also used (with initial capital and italicized) as a generic name.

Sparganum man·so·ni (man·so′nigh). A species of larva seen in the Far East, which is frequently found in the eye. Infection probably follows contact with freshly killed frogs.

Sparganum man·son·oi·des (man·sun·oy′deez). A species of larva that infects mice and has also been reported in the muscles and subcutaneous tissues of man.

Sparganum pro·lif·er·um (pro·lif′ur·um). A species of larva that proliferates in the tissues of the host by branching and budding off large numbers of spargana. The adult form is unknown.

spar·go·sis (spahr·go′sis) *n.* Enlargement or distention, as of the breasts due to accumulation of milk.

Sparine. Trademark for promazine, a drug with antiemetic, tranquilizing, and analgesic-potentiating actions, used as the hydrochloride salt.

spark, *n.* A light flash, usually electric in origin, as that emanating from an electrode through which a current is passing.

spar·te·ine (spahr′tee·een, ·in, spahr′teen) *n.* An alkaloid, $C_{15}H_{26}N_2$, obtained from *Cytisus scoparius;* formerly used, as the sulfate salt, for the treatment of cardiac arrhythmias, as an oxytocic drug for induction of labor at term, and for treatment of uterine inertia following onset of labor.

spasm (spaz′um) *n.* A sudden involuntary muscular contraction.

spas·mod·ic (spaz·mod′ick) *adj.* 1. Of, pertaining to, or affected by spasm. 2. Occurring intermittently or fitfully. 3. Characterized by periodic outbursts of emotional or physical disturbances.

spasmodic croup. A respiratory disorder of young children with sudden onset at night of severe inspiratory dyspnea with crowing stridor and cough, frequently associated with an upper respiratory infection or external irritant.

spasmodic torticollis. Torticollis occurring without other signs of neurological disease and characterized by an intermittent and arrhythmic or continuous spasm of the muscles of the neck, affecting women more than men, beginning in early or middle adult life, and having no known cause. The sternocleidomastoid and trapezius muscles are the muscles of the neck most prominently involved, causing a turning and tilting of the head, which may be slow and smooth, or jerky. Rarely the spasms spread to involve the muscles of the shoulder girdle, back, and limbs. Thought to be a restricted form of dystonia.

spas·mo·lyg·mus (spaz''mo·lig'mus) n. 1. HICCUP. 2. Spasmodic sobbing.

spas·mo·lyt·ic (spaz''mo·lit'ick) n. & adj. ANTISPASMODIC.

spas·mo·phe·mia (spaz''mo·fee'mee·uh) n. STUTTERING.

spas·mo·phil·ia (spaz''mo·fil'ee·uh) n. A morbid tendency to spasms. —**spasmophil·ic** (·ick) adj.

spas·mus (spaz'mus) n. —**SPASM**.

spasmus nic·ti·tans (nick'ti·tanz). WINKING SPASM.

spasmus nu·tans (new'tanz). A specific pendular nystagmus of infants accompanied by head-nodding and occasionally by wry positions of the neck. It affects both sexes, and begins between the fourth and twelfth months of life in most cases, never after the third year. The nystagmus may be horizontal, vertical, or pendular and is more pronounced in or limited to one eye. The cause is unknown and recovery is the rule.

spas·tic (spas'tick) adj. & n. 1. Pertaining to, or characterized by, recurrent and continuous spasms; produced by spasms. 2. Pertaining to spasticity. 3. Extremely tense, easily agitated, anxious; the opposite of calm and relaxed. 4. A person afflicted with spastic paralysis; particularly, a person suffering from a spastic form of cerebral palsy.

spastic bladder. SPASTIC REFLEX BLADDER.

spastic bulbar palsy or **paralysis.** PSEUDOBULBAR PALSY.

spastic colon or **colitis.** IRRITABLE COLON.

spastic diplegia. 1. Spastic paralysis of all four limbs, more marked in the legs; due to cerebral disease. 2. A form of cerebral palsy, due mainly to prenatal or perinatal anoxia, but occasionally to other metabolic disorders of the perinatal period or to malformations or developmental defects; frequently associated with mental retardation and epilepsy. Syn. cerebral spastic diplegia, Little's disease.

spastic ileus. A relatively uncommon form of ileus in which temporary obstruction is caused by segmental spasm of the intestine (the colon especially); seen usually in persons having an extremely nervous makeup, or in such conditions as heavy-metal poisoning, porphyria, or uremia. Syn. dynamic ileus, hyperdynamic ileus.

spas·tic·i·ty (spas·tis'i·tee) n. A state of increased muscular tonus tending to involve the flexors of the arms and extensors of the legs, associated with exaggerated tendon reflexes and a specific two-phased pattern of muscular response to stretch (the "clasp-knife" phenomenon).

spastic paralysis. A condition in which a group of muscles manifest increased tone, exaggerated tendon reflexes, depressed or absent su-

perficial reflexes, and sometimes clonus, due to an upper motor neuron lesion.

spastic paraplegia. Paralysis of the legs with increased muscular tone and hyperactive tendon reflexes, clonus, and Babinski signs; seen in a variety of diseases that involve the corticospinal pathways in the spinal cord.

spastic pseudosclerosis. CREUTZFELDT-JAKOB DISEASE (1).

spatia. Plural of spatium.

spa·tial (spay'shul) adj. Of, pertaining to, or occupying space.

spatial summation. The cumulative effect of spatially distributed, virtually simultaneous stimuli converging on an excitable cell or tissue.

spa·ti·um (spay'shee·um) n., pl. **spa·tia** (·shee·uh) A space.

spat·u·la (spatch'oo·luh) n. A flexible blunt blade; used for mixing or spreading soft materials, or facilitating the mixing of powders in a mortar by scraping. —**spatu·late** (·lut, ·late) adj.

spatulate finger. A particular type of broad finger, flattened at the tip.

spav·in (spav'in) n. Disease of the hock of a horse.

spay, v. To remove the ovaries of (an animal).

SPCA Abbreviation for serum prothrombin conversion accelerator (= FACTOR VII).

spe·cial·ist, n. A physician or surgeon who limits his practice to certain diseases, or to the diseases of a single organ or class, or to a certain type of therapy; in the United States, a diplomate of one of the American specialty boards in medicine, such as the American Board of Surgery.

spe·cial·ty, n. A branch of medicine or surgery pursued by a specialist.

spe·cies (spee'sheez) n., pl. **species** 1. The basic unit of biological taxonomy: For sexually reproducing organisms, a species includes all members of a breeding population together with any other populations that could interbreed freely and productively with it (if geographical, temporal, social, or artificial barriers did not interfere). In the case of asexual organisms, individuals or populations are assigned to species on the basis of similarities—morphological, biochemical, ecological, behavioral, etc.—analogous to those that characterize sexually reproducing species. 2. A specific kind of atomic nucleus, atom, ion, or molecule. 3. A name sometimes applied to certain mixtures of herbs used in making decoctions and infusions. Abbreviated, sp.

spe·cif·ic (spe·sif'ick) adj. & n. 1. Of or pertaining to a species, or to that which distinguishes a thing or makes it of the species to which it belongs. 2. Produced by a certain microorganism, as a specific disease. 3. Particularly adapted to its purpose, as a drug with a specific effect on disease. 4. A medicine that has a distinct remedial influence on a particular disease.

specific activity. The activity of a radioactive

substance expressed on a unit weight or unit volume basis.

specific birth rate. The birth rate calculated for categories such as sex, age of mother, social or economic group of parents, or any other variable or combination of variables.

specific death rate. The death rate calculated for categories such as age, sex, cause, or any other variable or combination of variables.

specific gravity. The measured mass of a substance compared with that of an equal volume of another taken as a standard. For gases, hydrogen or air may be the standard; for liquids and solids, distilled water at a specific temperature. Abbreviated, sp. g., sp. gr.

specific immunity. Immunity directed against a specific antigen or disease, such as that conferred by previous exposure.

spec·i·fic·i·ty (spes″i·fis′i·tee) *n.* The quality of being specific.

specific soluble substance. A soluble, polysaccharide hapten or antigen obtained from the capsule of the pneumococcus; essential for pneumococcal pathogenicity and the basis of the immunological classification of the pneumococci into specific types. Abbreviated, SSS.

spec·i·men (spes′i·mun) *n.* A sample of anything that is selected for diagnosis, examination, study, or testing.

spec·ta·cles, *n.pl.* Framed or mounted lenses for aiding vision where there are optical or muscular defects of the eye.

spec·ti·no·my·cin (speck″ti·no·migh′sin) *n.* A broad-spectrum antibiotic produced by *Streptomyces spectabilis.* Syn. *actinospectocin.*

spec·tral (speck′trul) *adj.* Of or pertaining to a spectrum.

spectro-. A combining form meaning *spectrum, spectral.*

spec·tro·col·or·im·e·ter (speck″tro·kul″ur·im′e·tur) *n.* Combination of spectroscope and ophthalmoscope for the detection of color blindness to one spectral color.

spec·tro·graph (speck′tro·graf) *n.* A spectroscope which records a spectrum on a photographic plate.

spec·tro·pho·tom·e·ter (speck″tro·fo·tom′e·tur) *n.* An apparatus for passing essentially monochromatic radiant energy (visible, ultraviolet, infrared, or other form) through a substance under examination, and measuring the intensity of the transmitted energy. The apparatus includes an energy source, a dispersing device to provide monochromatic radiation, and a sensor that measures the intensity of the incident and transmitted energy. —**spectropho·tom·e·try** (·tree) *n.;* **spectro·pho·to·met·ric** (·fo″to·met′rick) *adj.*

spec·tro·po·lar·im·e·ter (speck″tro·po″lur·im′e·tur) *n.* Combination of a spectrometer and polariscope; used for measuring optical rotation of solutions at different wavelengths.

spec·tro·scope (speck′truh·skope) *n.* An instrument for dispersing radiations by various methods, such as a prism, diffraction gratings, and crystals, and for observing the resultant spectrum. —**spec·tro·scop·ic** (speck″tro·skop′ick) *adj.*

spec·tros·co·py (speck·tros′kuh·pee) *n.* 1. Study of spectra. 2. Use of the spectroscope.

spec·trum (speck′trum) *n.,* L. pl. **spec·tra** (·truh) 1. The series of components or images resulting when a beam of electromagnetic waves (such as electric waves, infrared, visible light, ultraviolet, or x-rays) is dispersed and the constituent waves are arranged according to their frequencies or wavelengths. 2. Figuratively, any series of entities arranged according to the quantitative variation of a given common property; a range.

spec·u·lum (speck′yoo·lum) *n.,* L. pl. **specu·la** (·luh) An instrument for dilating the opening of a cavity of the body in order that the interior may be more easily visible.

speech, *n.* 1. The production of vocal utterances in a language; the activity of speaking. 2. The utterances produced.

speech deafness. 1. AUDITORY APHASIA. 2. AUDITORY VERBAL AGNOSIA.

speech pathologist. A specialist dealing with defects in speech and language.

speech pathology. The science dealing with disorders of speech and language.

speed, *n.* In drug abuse terminology, AMPHETAMINE (2).

spe·le·os·to·my (spee″lee·os′tuh·mee) *n.* CAVERNOSTOMY.

sperm, *n.,* pl. **sperm, sperms** 1. SPERMATOZOON; SPERMATOZOA. 2. Loosely, SEMEN.

sperm-, sperma-, spermi-, spermio-, spermo- A combining form meaning *seed, sperm, semen.*

sper·ma·ce·ti (spur″muh·set′ee, ·see′tee) *n.* A waxy substance obtained from the head of the sperm whale *Physeter macrocephalus.* The chief constituents are cetyl palmitate and cetyl alcohol. Used to impart firmness to ointment bases.

spermat-, spermato-. A combining form meaning (a) *spermatozoa;* (b) *spermatic, seminal.*

sper·ma·ta·cra·sia (spur″muh·tuh·kray′zhuh, ·zee·uh) *n.* Deficiency or decrease of spermatozoa in the semen. Syn. *spermacrasia.*

sper·mat·ic (spur·mat′ick) *adj.* 1. Pertaining to the semen or spermatozoa; conveying semen. 2. Pertaining to the spermatic cord.

spermatic cord. The cord extending from the testis to the deep inguinal ring and consisting of the ductus deferens, the vessels and nerves of the testis and of the epididymis, and the accompanying connective tissue.

sper·ma·tid (spur′muh·tid) *n.* A male germ cell immediately before assuming its final typical form.

sper·ma·to·cele (spur′muh·to·seel, spur·mat′o·) *n.* Cystic dilatation of a duct in the head of the epididymis or in the rete testis. Rupture into the tunica vaginalis testis produces spermatic hydrocele.

sper·ma·to·ce·lec·to·my (spur″muh·to·se·leck′tuh·mee) *n.* Excision of a spermatocele.

sper·ma·to·ci·dal (spur″muh·to·sigh′dul) *adj.* Destructive to spermatozoa.

sper·ma·to·cide (spur′muh·to·side) *n.* An agent that destroys spermatozoa.

sper·ma·to·cys·tec·to·my (spur″muh·to·sis·teck′tuh·mee) *n.* VESICULECTOMY.

sper·ma·to·cys·ti·tis (spur″muh·to·sis·tye′tis) *n.* Inflammation of the seminal vesicles.

sper·ma·to·cys·tot·o·my (spur″muh·to·sis·tot′uh·mee) *n.* Surgical incision of a seminal vesicle.

sper·ma·to·cyte (spur·mat′o·site, spur″muh·to·) *n.* A cell of the last or next to the last generation of cells which divide to form spermatozoa.

sper·ma·to·cy·to·ma (spur″muh·to·sigh·to′muh, spur·mat″o·) *n.* SEMINOMA.

sper·ma·to·gen·e·sis (spur″muh·to·jen′e·sis) *n.* The phenomena involved in the production of spermatozoa, sometimes restricted to denote the process of meiosis in the male.

sper·ma·to·gen·ic (spur″muh·to·jen′ick) *adj.* Producing spermatozoa, as the spermatogenic cells of the testis.

sper·ma·tog·e·nous (spur″muh·toj′e·nus) *adj.* SPERMATOGENIC.

sper·ma·to·go·ni·um (spur″muh·to·go′nee·um) *n., pl.* **spermatogo·nia** (·nee·uh) One of the primitive male germ cells. The primary spermatocytes arise from the last generation of spermatogonia by an increase in size.

sper·ma·toid (spur′muh·toid) *adj.* Resembling a spermatozoon.

sper·ma·tol·y·sin (spur″muh·tol′i·sin, spur″muh·to·lye′sin) *n.* A substance causing dissolution of spermatozoa.

sper·ma·tol·y·sis (spur″muh·tol′i·sis) *n.* The process of dissolution of spermatozoa. —**sperma·to·lyt·ic** (·to·lit′ick) *adj.*

sper·ma·top·a·thy (spur″muh·top′uth·ee) *n.* Disease of the spermatozoa or of their secreting mechanism.

sper·ma·tor·rhea, sper·ma·tor·rhoea (spur″muh·to·ree′uh) *n.* Involuntary discharge of semen without orgasm.

spermatozoa. Plural of *spermatozoon.*

sper·ma·to·zo·on (spur″muh·to·zo′on, spur·mat″o·) *n., pl.* **spermato·zoa** (·zo′uh) The mature male germ cell. —**spermatozo·al** (·ul) *adj.*

sper·ma·tu·ria (spur″muh·tew′ree·uh) *n.* The presence of sperm in the urine.

sperm center. The centrosome which precedes the sperm nucleus as it advances within the egg. In flagellate spermatozoa it arises from the middle piece.

sper·mec·to·my (spur·meck′tuh·mee) *n.* Resection of part of the ductus deferens.

-spermia A combining form meaning (a) *a form or condition of spermatozoa;* (b) *a condition of the semen.*

sper·mi·cide (spur′mi·side) *n.* SPERMATOCIDE.

sper·mine (spur′meen) *n.* N,N′-Bis(3-aminopropyl-1,4-butanediamine, $C_{10}H_{26}N_4$, a constituent of semen and other animal tissues.

sper·mio·gen·e·sis (spur″mee·o·jen′e·sis) *n.* The morphological transformation of spermatids into spermatozoa.

sper·mio·gram (spur′mee·o·gram) *n.* Diagrammatic evaluation of spermatogenic morphology as an aid in the evaluation of infertility.

sper·mo·lith (spur′mo·lith) *n.* A calculus in a ductus deferens or seminal vesicle.

sp. g., sp. gr. Abbreviations for *specific gravity.*

sph. Abbreviation for *spherical* or *spherical lens.*

sphac·e·la·tion (sfas″e·lay′shun) *n.* 1. NECROSIS. 2. GANGRENE. —**sphace·late** (·late) *v.*

sphac·e·lo·der·ma (sfas″e·lo·dur′muh) *n.* Gangrene or ulceration of the skin from any of many different causes.

sphaer-, sphaero-, spher-, sphero-. A combining form meaning *sphere, spherical.*

Sphae·roph·o·rus (sfe·rof′uh·rus) *n.* A genus of the family Bacteroidaceae, by some not differentiated from the genus *Bacteroides,* consisting of pleomorphic gram-negative nonsporulating rods found in the alimentary and urogenital tracts of man and animals, and responsible for gangrenous and purulent infections of man.

Sphaerophorus ne·croph·o·rus (ne·krof′uh·rus). A species of *Sphaerophorus* found in association with septicemia, puerperal infection, or liver abscess.

spha·gi·as·mus (sfay″jee·az′mus) *n.* Spasm of the muscles of the neck in a convulsion.

spha·gi·tis (sfay·jye′tis) *n.* 1. Inflammation of a jugular vein. 2. SORE THROAT.

sphen-, spheno- A combining form meaning (a) *wedge, wedge-shaped;* (b) *sphenoid (bone).*

sphe·no·bas·i·lar (sfee″no·bas′i·lur) *adj.* Of or pertaining to the sphenoid and occipital bones; SPHENO-OCCIPITAL.

sphe·no·ceph·a·lus (sfee″no·sef′uh·lus) *n.* 1. A variety of monster with separated eyes, the ears united under the head, the jaws and mouth distinct, and the sphenoid bone altered in shape. 2. A monster in which the lower jaw is absent or rudimentary, the fauces are occluded, with severe defects in the upper jaw and sphenoid region, and with various degrees of synotia. The upper face is nearly normal. 3. An individual having a wedge-shaped, narrow head, resulting from compensatory enlargement of the anterior fontanel after premature union of the sagittal suture.

sphe·no·ceph·a·ly (sfee″no·sef′uh·lee) *n.* The condition of having a wedge-shaped head.

sphe·no·eth·moid (sfee″no·eth′moid) *adj.* Pertaining to both the sphenoid and the ethmoid bones.

sphe·noid (sfee′noid) *adj. & n.* 1. Wedge-shaped, as the sphenoid bone. 2. The sphenoid bone. See Table of Bones in the Appendix. —**sphe·noi·dal** (sfe·noy′dul) *adj.*

sphenoid air sinus. SPHENOID SINUS.

sphenoid crest. A thin ridge of bone in the median line of the anterior surface of the body of the sphenoid bone.

sphe·noid·i·tis (sfee″noid·eye′tis) *n.* Inflammation of a sphenoid air sinus.

sphe·noid·ot·o·my (sfee″noid·ot′uh·mee) *n.* Incision into the sphenoid air sinus.

sphenoid sinus. A paranasal sinus in the body of the sphenoid bone; there is a right and a left one.

sphe·no·ma·lar (sfee″no·may′lur) *adj.* Pertaining to the sphenoid and zygomatic bones.

sphe·no·man·dib·u·lar (sfee″no·man·dib′yoo·lur) *adj.* Pertaining to the sphenoid and mandibular bones.

sphe·no·max·il·lary (sfee″no·mack′si·lerr·ee)

adj. Pertaining to the sphenoid and maxillary bones.

sphe·no·oc·cip·i·tal (sfee″no-ock·sip′i·tul) *adj.* Of or pertaining to the sphenoid and the occipital bones; SPHENOBASILAR.

sphe·no·pal·a·tine (sfee″no·pal′uh·tine) *adj.* Pertaining to the sphenoid bone and the palate.

sphe·no·pa·ri·e·tal (sfee″no·pa·rye′e·tul) *adj.* Pertaining to the sphenoid and parietal bones.

sphe·no·pe·tro·sal (sfee″no·pe·tro′sul) *adj.* Pertaining to the sphenoid and the petrous portion of the temporal bone.

sphe·no·sis (sfe·no′sis) *n.* The wedging of the fetus in the pelvis.

sphe·no·squa·mo·sal (sfee″no·skway·mo′sul) *adj.* Pertaining to the sphenoid and the squamous portion of the temporal bone.

sphe·no·tem·po·ral (sfee″no·tem′po·rul) *adj.* Pertaining to the sphenoid and the temporal bone.

sphe·no·tre·sia (sfee″no·tree′zhuh, -zee·uh) *n.* A variety of craniotomy in which the basal portion of the fetal skull is perforated.

sphe·no·trip·sy (sfee′no·trip″see) *n.* Crushing of the fetal skull.

sphe·no·zy·go·mat·ic (sfee″no·zye·go·mat′ick) *adj.* Pertaining to the sphenoid and the zygomatic bone.

sphe·res·the·sia, sphe·raes·the·sia (sfeer″es·theezh′uh, -theez′ee·uh) *n.* GLOBUS HYSTERICUS.

spher·i·cal aberration. Unequal refraction of monochromatic light in different parts of a spherical lens, producing faulty images that show lack of sharpness or of flatness, or distortion. Syn. *monochromatic aberration.*

spherical lens. A lens in which the curved surface, either concave or convex, is a segment of a sphere. Abbreviated, S, sph.

sphero·ceph·a·lus (sfeer″o·sef′uh·lus) *n.* A monster with absent or rudimentary lower jaw, occlusion of the fauces, approximation of the ears, lack of the bones of the face, marked deficiencies in the frontal and sphenoid bones, and with a vesicular brain.

sphero·cyte (sfeer′o·site) *n.* An erythrocyte which is spherical rather than biconcave. —**sphero·cyt·ic** (sfeer″o·sit′ick) *adj.*

spherocytic anemia. 1. HEREDITARY SPHEROCYTOSIS. 2. Any anemia characterized by large numbers of spherocytes.

sphero·cy·to·sis (sfeer″o·sigh·to′sis) *n.* 1. A preponderance in the blood of spherocytes. 2. HEREDITARY SPHEROCYTOSIS.

sphe·roid (sfeer′oid, sferr′oid) *n. & adj.* 1. A solid resembling a sphere. 2. SPHEROIDAL.

sphe·roi·dal (sfe·roy′dul) *adj.* Resembling a sphere.

sphe·rom·e·ter (sfe·rom′e·tur) *n.* An instrument for determining the degree of curvature of a sphere or part of a sphere, especially of optical lenses, or of the tools used for grinding them.

sphero·pha·kia (sfeer″o·fay′kee·uh) *n.* A congenital anomaly in which there is a thick spherical ocular lens whose sagittal diameter is increased and equatorial diameter decreased.

spher·ule (sfeer′yool, sferr′yool, -ool) *n.* A minute sphere.

sphinc·ter (sfink′tur) *n.* A muscle surrounding and closing an orifice. —**sphinc·ter·ic** (sfink·terr′ick), **sphinc·ter·al** (sfink′tur·ul) *adj.*

sphincteral achalasia. Failure of relaxation of a gastrointestinal sphincter, practically always at the cardioesophogeal junction.

sphinc·ter·al·gia (sfink″tur·al′jee·uh) *n.* Transient pain in the anal region, due to a spasm of the levator ani muscles. Syn. *proctalgia fugax.*

sphinc·ter·ec·to·my (sfink″tur·eck′tuh·mee) *n.* Oblique blepharotomy for the dilatation of the palpebral fissure, or for blepharospasm.

sphinc·ter·is·mus (sfink″tur·iz′mus) *n.* A spasmodic contraction of the anal sphincter, usually attendant upon fissure or ulcer of the anus, but occasionally occurring independently of such lesion.

sphinc·ter·itis (sfink″tur·eye′tis) *n.* Inflammation of a sphincter, especially the anal sphincter.

sphincter of Od·di (oh′dee) SPHINCTER OF THE HEPATOPANCREATIC AMPULLA.

sphincter of the hepatopancreatic ampulla. The intricate arrangement of smooth muscle about the common bile duct and pancreatic duct in the wall of the duodenum.

sphinc·ter·ol·y·sis (sfink″tur·ol′i·sis) *n.* The operation of freeing the iris in anterior synechia.

sphinc·tero·plas·ty (sfink′tur·o·plas″tee) *n.* A plastic or reparative operation on a sphincter muscle.

sphinc·ter·ot·o·my (sfink″tur·ot′uh·mee) *n.* The operation of incising a sphincter.

sphincter ure·thrae (yoo·ree′three). SPHINCTER URETHRAE MEMBRANACEAE.

sphincter urethrae mem·bra·na·ce·ae (mem″bruh·nay′si·ee). Bundles of voluntary muscle that surround the membranous portion of the urethra in the male; in the female the analogous muscle fibers surround the proximal portion of the urethra.

sphin·go·lip·id (sfing′go·lip′id) *n.* Any lipid, such as a sphingomyelin, that yields sphingosine or one of its derivatives as a product of hydrolysis.

sphin·go·lip·i·do·sis (sfing″go·lip″i·do′sis) *n.* Any one of a group of inherited metabolic disorders characterized by the accumulation of excessive quantities of certain glycolipids and phospholipids in various body tissues. The principal forms include Gaucher's disease, Niemann-Pick disease, metachromatic leukodystrophy, infantile amaurotic familial idiocy (Tay-Sachs disease), familial neurovisceral lipidosis, and angiokeratoma corporis diffusum universale.

sphin·go·my·e·lin (sfing′go·migh′e·lin) *n.* A phospholipid occurring in brain, kidney, liver, and egg yolk. It is composed of choline, sphingosine, phosphoric acid, and a fatty acid.

sphin·go·sine (sfing′go·seen, -sin) *n.* 2-Amino-4-octadecene-1,3-diol, $C_{18}H_{37}NO_2$, a moiety of sphingomyelin, cerebrosides, and certain other phosphatides.

sphygm-, sphygmo- A combining form meaning *pulse.*

sphyg·mic (sfig′mick) *adj.* Pertaining to the pulse.

sphyg·mo·bo·lom·e·ter (sfig″mo·bo·lom′e·tur) *n.*

An instrument for measuring and recording the pulse. —**sphygmobolome·try** (·tree) n.

sphyg·mo·chro·nog·ra·phy (sfig″mo·kro·nog′ruh·fee) n. The registration of the time intervals of the pulse wave.

sphyg·mod·ic (sfig·mod′ick, ·mo′dick) adj. Like the pulse; throbbing, pulsating.

sphyg·mo·dy·na·mom·e·ter (sfig″mo·dye″nuh·mom′e·tur) n. An instrument for measuring the force of the pulse.

sphyg·mo·gram (sfig′mo·gram) n. The tracing made by the sphygmograph.

sphyg·mo·graph (sfig′mo·graf) n. An instrument for recording graphically the pulse wave and the variations in blood pressure. —**sphyg·mo·graph·ic** (sfig″mo·graf′ick) adj.

sphyg·mog·ra·phy (sfig·mog′ruh·fee) n. 1. A description of the pulse and its pathologic variations. 2. The recording of pulse tracings with the sphygmograph.

sphyg·moid (sfig′moid) adj. Resembling the pulse; having the nature of continuous pulsation.

sphyg·mo·ma·nom·e·ter (sfig″mo·ma·nom′e·tur) n. An instrument for measuring the arterial blood pressure. —**sphygmomanome·try** (·tree) n.

sphyg·mo·os·cil·lom·e·ter (sfig″mo·os″i·lom′e·tur) n. A form of sphygmomanometer in which the systolic and diastolic blood pressures are indicated by an oscillating device.

sphyg·mo·pal·pa·tion (sfig″mo·pal·pay′shun) n. The palpation of the pulse.

sphyg·mo·phone (sfig′mo·fone) n. A sphygmograph in which the vibrations of the pulse produce a sound.

sphyg·mo·scope (sfig′mo·skope) n. A pulse pressure recorder in which the force of arterial pressure is made visible.

sphyg·mos·co·py (sfig·mos′kuh·pee) n. 1. The recording of the pulse wave with the sphygmoscope. 2. Examination of the pulse.

sphyg·mo·sys·to·le (sfig″mo·sis′tuh·lee) n. The part of the sphygmogram related to cardiac systole.

sphyg·mo·tech·ny (sfig′mo·teck″nee) n. The art of diagnosis and prognosis by means of the pulse.

sphyg·mo·to·no·graph (sfig″mo·to′nuh·graf) n. An instrument that records pulsations from an inflatable rubber cuff.

sphyg·mo·to·nom·e·ter (sfig″mo·to·nom′e·tur) n. An instrument for measuring the elasticity or tension of the arterial wall.

sphyg·mus (sfig′mus) n. PULSE (1); a pulsation. —**sphygmous**, adj.

sphynx-neck, n. WEBBED NECK.

spi·ca (spye′kuh) n., pl. **spi·cae** (·see). 1. A spike or spur. 2. SPICA BANDAGE.

spica bandage. A bandage with successive turns and crosses, as in a modified figure-of-eight bandage; so-called because it resembles the arrangement of grains in the spike (ear) of certain cereal grasses.

spic·ule (spick′yool) n. 1. A small spike-shaped bone or fragment of bone. 2. A needle-shaped body; a spike. —**spicu·lar** (·lur) adj.

spi·der, n. 1. An arthropod of the order Araneida

of the class Arachnida, characterized by having four pairs of legs, usually eight eyes, and an unsegmented abdomen. 2. (In attributive use) Having a form suggestive of a spider or a spider's web.

spider angioma, SPIDER NEVUS.

spider belly. ARACHNOGASTRIA.

spider burst. SPIDER TELANGIECTASIA.

spider nevus. A type of telangiectasis characterized by a central, elevated, tiny red dot, pinhead in size, from which blood vessels radiate like strands of a spider's web. Syn. nevus araneus, nevus arachnoideus, stellar nevus.

spider telangiectasia. Superficial flat telangiectatic areas of the skin of legs associated with venous dilatation.

Spieg·ler-Fendt sarcoid (shpeeg′lur) LYMPHOCYTOMA CUTIS.

Spiel·mey·er-Vogt disease (shpeel′migh·ur, fohkt) A hereditary disorder of lipid metabolism, transmitted by both dominant and recessive patterns, characterized by the onset between 4 and 10 years of progressive visual loss and eventual blindness, abnormal pigmentation of the retina, convulsions, extrapyramidal disorders of movement and eventual spasticity, psychotic behavior, and progressive dementia. Syn. Batten-Mayou disease, juvenile amaurotic familial idiocy.

Spi·ge·lia (spye·jee′lee·uh) n. A genus of plants of the family Loganiaceae. The rhizome and rootlets of Spigelia marilandica, pinkroot, formerly were used as a vermifuge.

spike, n. In electroencephalography, a transient wave form that is clearly distinguishable from background activity, having a pointed peak at conventional paper speeds and a duration of 20 to 70 msec.

spike and slow wave. In electroencephalography, a pattern consisting of a spike followed by a slow wave.

spike focus. In electroencephalography, a limited region of the scalp, cerebral cortex, or depth of the brain displaying a spike wave form.

spill, n. 1. An overflow, especially that of blood. 2. A form of cellular metastasis in malignant disease.

spill·way, n. The physiologic form or contour of a tooth which provides for the escape of food during mastication; an embrasure or a developmental, occlusal, or supplemental groove. Syn. sluiceway.

spi·lo·ma (spye·lo′muh) n. NEVUS.

spi·lo·pla·nia (spye″lo·play′nee·uh) n. A transient skin erythema.

spi·lus (spye′lus) n. A splotchily colored cutaneous melanocytic nevus.

spin-, spini-, spino-. A combining form meaning spine, spinal, spinous.

spi·na (spye′nuh) n., pl. & genit. sing. **spi·nae** (·nee) SPINE.

spi·na bi·fi·da (bye′fi·duh, bif′i·duh). A congenital defect in the closure of the vertebral canal with hernial protrusion of the meninges of the cord. The hernial sac contains cerebrospinal fluid and sometimes nervous tissue; most common in the lumbosacral region. It may be diagnosed in mid-pregnancy by aspiration of amniotic fluid which is analyzed for elevation of alpha-fetoprotein.

spina bifida oc·cul·ta (ock·ul'tuh). A defect in the closure of the vertebral canal due to incomplete fusion of the posterior arch without hernial protrusion of the meninges, usually asymptomatic and diagnosed only by radiography.

spi·nal (spye'nul) *adj.* 1. Resembling a spine. 2. Pertaining to, or situated near, the vertebral column.

spinal adhesive arachnoiditis. Chronic adhesive arachnoiditis of the spinal cord.

spinal akinesia. Motor impairment due to a lesion of the spinal cord.

spinal anesthesia. 1. Anesthesia due to a lesion of the spinal cord. 2. Anesthesia produced by local anesthetic injected into the spinal subarachnoid space.

spinal apoplexy. A sudden focal neurologic deficit due to infarction of or bleeding into the spinal cord.

spinal ataxia. Motor incoordination due to disease of the posterior columns of the spinal cord.

spinal block. Interference with the flow of cerebrospinal fluid due to blockage of the spinal subarachnoid space.

spinal block syndrome. FROIN'S SYNDROME.

spinal canal. VERTEBRAL CANAL.

spinal cord. The part of the central nervous system contained within the vertebral canal and extending from the medulla oblongata at the level of the foramen magnum to the filum terminale at the level of the first or second lumbar vertebra.

spinal dysraphism. A general term for all manifestations of defective fusion in the dorsal midline whether cutaneous, vertebral, meningeal, or neural.

spinal fluid. CEREBROSPINAL FLUID.

spinal fusion. The fusion of two or more vertebrae, for immobilization of the spinal column. Used in the treatment of spinal deformities, tuberculosis of the spine, and severe arthritis of the spine.

spinal ganglion. Any one of the sensory ganglions, each associated with the dorsal root of a spinal nerve.

spinal hemiplegia. Paralysis of one side of the body due to a lesion of the cervical spinal cord.

spi·na·lis (spye·nay'lis) *n.* A deep muscle of the back attached to the spinous processes of the vertebrae.

spinal man. A patient whose spinal cord has been completely separated from supraspinal influences.

spinal meningitis. Inflammation of the meninges of the spinal cord, usually associated with cerebral meningitis.

spinal nerves. Nerves arising from the spinal cord and exiting through invertebral foramens. There are 31 pairs of spinal nerves: 8 cervical, 12 thoracic, 5 lumbar, 5 sacral, and 1 coccygeal.

spinal paralysis. Paralysis caused by a lesion of the spinal cord.

spinal puncture. LUMBAR PUNCTURE.

spinal reflex. Any reflex mediated through the spinal cord without the necessary participation of more cephalad central nervous system structures.

spinal shock. A condition of flaccid paralysis and suppression of all reflex activity following immediately upon transection of the spinal cord and involving all segments below the lesion. In most cases, reflex activity returns within 1 to 6 weeks but in a small proportion the state of complete areflexia is permanent.

spinal tap. LUMBAR PUNCTURE.

spinal vestibular nucleus. A nucleus dorsolateral to the tractus solitarius the cells of which project to the cerebellum via the juxtarestiform body.

spin·dle *n.* 1. A tapering rod; a fusiform shape. 2. The part of the achromatic figure in mitosis between the centrosomes or asters, consisting of modified cytoplasm and achromatic fibrils. 3. A group of alphalike synchronized waves which appears in the electroencephalograph during periods of light sleep.

spindle cataract. A cataract characterized by a spindle-shaped opacity extending from the posterior to the anterior portion of the lens capsule.

spindle cell. 1. A fibroblast or smooth muscle cell which is spindle-shaped. 2. A fusiform or spindle-shaped cell, typical of certain tumors.

spindle-cell carcinoma. OAT-CELL CARCINOMA.

spindle-cell sarcoma. A malignant connective-tissue tumor composed of spindle-shaped cells.

spine, *n.* 1. A sharp process, especially of bone. 2. VERTEBRAL COLUMN.

spine of the ischium. A pointed eminence on the posterior border of the body of the ischium. It forms the lower border of the greater sciatic notch.

spine of the scapula. The strong, triangular plate of bone attached obliquely to the dorsum of the scapula and dividing it into two unequal parts, the supraspinous and infraspinous fossae.

spi·no·bul·bar (spye"no·bul'bur) *adj.* Pertaining to the spinal cord and the medulla oblongata.

spi·no·cel·lu·lar (spye"no·sel'yoo·lur) *adj.* Pertaining to, or like, prickle cells.

spi·no·cer·e·bel·lar (spye"no·serr"e·bel'ur) *adj.* Pertaining to the spinal cord and the cerebellum.

spi·no·gal·va·ni·za·tion (spye"no·gal"vuh·ni·zay'shun) *n.* An outmoded form of treatment consisting in application of a galvanic current to the spinal column.

spi·no·sal (spye·no'sul) *adj.* Pertaining to or passing through the foramen spinosum of the sphenoid bone.

spi·no·tec·tal (spye"no·teck'tul) *adj.* Pertaining to the spinal cord and the tectum of the mesencephalon.

spi·no·tha·lam·ic (spye"no·tha·lam'ick) *adj.* 1. Pertaining to the spinal cord and the thalamus. 2. Pertaining to a spinothalamic tract.

spi·nous (spye'nus) *adj.* 1. Pertaining to a spine

or a spinelike process. 2. Having spines or sharp processes.

spinous process of a vertebra. The prominent backward projection from the middle of the posterior portion of the arch of a vertebra.

spin·thar·i·con (spin-thăr′i·kon) n. A direct-viewing radiation imaging system, consisting of a collimator with many pinholes and a spark discharge tube.

spin·ther·ism (spin′thur·iz·um) n. Sensation of sparks before the eyes.

spi·nu·lose (spye′new·loce) adj. SPINY.

spi·ny (spye′nee) adj. Having or characterized by spines.

spir-, spiro- A combining form meaning coil, spiral.

spir-, spiro- Combining forms meaning respiration, breathing.

spi·rad·e·no·ma (spye·rad″e·no′muh) n. SWEAT GLAND ADENOMA.

spi·ral (spye′rul) adj. 1. Having the two-dimensional form of something wound in a plane around a center. 2. Having the three-dimensional form of something coiled around an axis; HELICAL.

spiral organ (of Corti) The sensory portion of the cochlear duct; the end organ of hearing.

spi·ril·la Plural of spirillum.

spi·ril·li·ci·dal (spye·ril″i·sigh′dul) adj. Capable of destroying spirilla.

spi·ril·lo·sis (spye″ri·lo′sis, spirr″i·) n. A disease caused by infection with spirilla.

spi·ril·lum (spye·ril′um) n. A genus of spiral bacilli of the family Pseudomonadaceae. —spirillum, pl. spiril·la, com. n.

spirillum fever. RELAPSING FEVER.

Spirillum mi·nus (migh′nus). A causative agent of rat-bite fever.

spir·it, n. 1. An alcoholic solution of a volatile principle, formerly prepared by distillation but now generally prepared by dissolving the volatile substance in alcohol. 2. And distilled liquid. Abbreviated, sp.

spiritus fru·men·ti (froo·men′tye, ·tee) Whiskey.

Spi·ro·chae·ta (spye″ro·kee′tuh) n. A genus of spiral microorganisms of the family Spirochaetaceae, nonpathogenic for man. Formerly included Treponema, Leptospira, and others.

Spi·ro·chae·ta·ce·ae (spye″ro·ke·tay′see·ee) n.pl. A family of spiral microorganisms which includes the genera Spirochaeta, Saprospira, and Cristispira. The family is nonpathogenic for man; a few species of Cristispira are parasites of crustaceans, all other species are free-living forms.

Spirochaeta cuniculi. TREPONEMA CUNICULI.

Spirochaeta ic·ter·og·e·nes (ick″tur·oj′e·neez). LEPTOSPIRA ICTEROHAEMORRHAGIAE.

Spirochaeta ic·tero·hae·mor·rhag·i·ae (ick″tur·o·hem″ur·aj′ee·ee). LEPTOSPIRA ICTEROHAEMORRHAGIAE.

Spi·ro·chae·ta·les (spye″ro·ke·tay′leez) n.pl. An order of spiral microorganisms which includes the families Spirochaetaceae and Treponemataceae.

Spirochaeta mor·sus mu·ris (mor′sus mew′ris) SPIRILLUM MINUS.

spirochaetosis ic·te·ro·hae·mor·rhag·i·ca (ick″

tur·o·hee·mo·raj′i·kuh, ·hem·o·). WEIL′S DISEASE.

spirochetal jaundice. WEIL′S DISEASE.

spi·ro·chete, spi·ro·chaete (spye′ro·keet) n. Any of the spiral microorganisms belonging to the order Spirochaetales. —spi·ro·che·tal, spi·ro·chae·tal (spye″ro·kee′tul) adj.

spi·ro·chet·emia, spi·ro·chae·tae·mia (spye″ro·ke·tee′mee·uh) n. The presence of spirochetes in the blood.

spi·ro·che·ti·cide, spi·ro·chae·ti·cide (spye″ro·keet′i·side) n. An agent that kills spirochetes.

spi·ro·che·tol·y·sis, spi·ro·chae·tol·y·sis (spye″ro·ke·tol′i·sis) n. Destruction of spirochetes by lysis.

spi·ro·chet·osis, spi·ro·chaet·osis (spye″ro·ke·to′sis) n. Any of the diseases caused by infection with one of the spirochetes. —spirochet·ot·ic (·tot′ick) adj.

spi·ro·gram (spye′ro·gram) n. A recorded tracing of the movements and excursion of the chest during respiration.

spi·ro·graph (spye′ro·graph) n. An instrument for registering respiration.

spi·rom·e·ter (spye·rom′e·tur) n. A device for measuring and recording the amount of air inhaled and exhaled. —spi·ro·met·ric (spye″ro·met′rick) adj.

spi·rom·e·try (spye·rom′e·tree) n. The measurement, by means of a spirometer, of inhaled and exhaled air.

spi·ro·no·lac·tone (spye″ro·no·lack′tone) n. 17-Hydroxy-7α-mercapto-3-oxo-17α-pregn-4-ene-21-carboxylic acid γ-lactone 7-acetate, $C_{24}H_{32}O_4S$, a steroid with a lactone ring attached at carbon-17 so that the latter is common to two rings. It is a diuretic drug that blocks the sodium-retaining action of aldosterone.

splanchn-, splanchno- A combining form meaning viscus, viscera, visceral.

splanch·na (splank′nuh) n.pl. 1. The intestines. 2. The viscera.

splanch·nec·to·pia (splank″neck·to′pee·uh) n. The abnormal position or dislocation of a viscus.

splanch·nem·phrax·is (splank″nem·frack′sis) n. Obstruction of a viscus, particularly the intestine.

splanch·nic (splank′nick) adj. Pertaining to, or supplying, the viscera.

splanch·ni·cec·to·my (splank″ni·seck′tuh·mee) n. The surgical excision of the splanchnic nerves.

splanchnic nerve. Any of the two or sometimes three nerves that arise from the thoracic portion of the sympathetic trunk, pierce the diaphragm, and terminate in the prevertebral ganglia of the mesenteric plexuses. These nerves are made up of preganglionic fibers which merely pass through the paravertebral ganglia en route to the celiac and mesenteric ganglia.

splanch·ni·cot·o·my (splank″ni·kot′uh·mee) n. Surgical division of a splanchnic nerve.

splanch·no·cele (splank′no·seel) n. A hernial protrusion of any abdominal viscus.

splanch·no·di·as·ta·sis (splank″no·dye·as′tuh·

sis) n. Displacement or separation of the viscera.

splanch·nog·ra·phy (splank·nog'ruh·fee) n. The descriptive anatomy of the viscera.

splanch·no·lith (splank'no·lith) n. A calculus in a viscus.

splanch·no·li·thi·a·sis (splank"no·li·thigh'uh·sis) n. The condition of having a calculus of the intestine.

splanch·nol·o·gy (splank·nol'uh·jee) n. The branch of medical science pertaining to the viscera.

splanch·no·meg·a·ly (splank"no·meg'uh·lee) n. Abnormal enlargement of a viscus or the viscera.

splanch·no·mi·cria (splank"no·migh'kree·uh) n. Abnormal smallness of a viscus or the visceral organs.

splanch·nop·a·thy (splank·nop'uth·ee) n. Any disease of the viscera.

splanch·no·pleure (splank'no·ploor) n. The wall of the embryonic gut, composed of endoderm and the splanchnic layer of lateral mesoderm. —**splanch·no·pleu·ral** (splank"no·ploor'ul) adj.

splanch·nop·to·sis (splank"nop·to'sis) n. VISCEROPTOSIS.

splanch·no·scle·ro·sis (splank"no·skle·ro'sis) n. A visceral induration.

splanch·nos·co·py (splank·nos'kuh·pee) n. Visual examination of the viscera, as through a peritoneoscope.

splanch·no·so·mat·ic (splank"no·so·mat'ick) adj. Pertaining to the viscera and the body wall.

splanch·not·o·my (splank·not'uh·mee) n. Dissection of the viscera.

splanch·no·tribe (splank'no·tribe) n. An instrument for crushing a segment of the intestine and so occluding its lumen, previous to resecting it.

splay·foot, n. Flatfoot with extreme eversion of the forefoot and tarsus.

spleen, n. One of the abdominal viscera, located immediately below the diaphragm on the left side. It is the largest lymphatic organ of the body and also functions as a producer of erythrocytes.

splen-, spleno-. A combining form meaning spleen, splenic.

sple·nal·gia (sple·nal'jee·uh) n. Pain in the spleen.

sple·nec·to·my (sple·neck'to·mee) n. Excision of the spleen. —**splenecto·mize** (·mize) v.

splen·ec·to·pia (splen"eck·to'pee·uh, splee"neck·) n. Displacement of the spleen.

sple·net·ic (sple·net'ick) adj. 1. Pertaining to the spleen. 2. Having a diseased spleen. 3. Marked by bad temper or sullen humor.

sple·nia. Plural of splenium.

splen·ic (splen'ick, splee'nick) adj. Of or pertaining to the spleen; lienal.

splenic anemia. Anemia associated with chronic passive splenic hyperemia.

splenic artery. The lienal artery. See lienal in the Table of Arteries in the Appendix.

splenic corpuscle or **nodule.** MALPIGHIAN CORPUSCLE (1).

splenic flexure. An abrupt turn of the colon beneath the lower end of the spleen, connecting the descending with the transverse colon.

splenic-flexure syndrome. Left upper quadrant pain, which may radiate to the left shoulder and inner aspect of the left arm; relieved by passage of feces or gas and presumed due to distention or spasmodic contraction of the colon.

splen·i·co·pan·cre·at·ic (splen"i·ko·pan"kree·at'ick) adj. Belonging, or pertaining, to both the spleen and the pancreas.

splenic plexus. A visceral nerve plexus accompanying the splenic artery.

splenic souffle. A murmur said to be audible over the diseased spleen, as in malaria or leukemia.

splenic tumor. A term sometimes applied to an enlarged spleen, not necessarily neoplastic, and usually only hyperplastic or hyperemic.

splen·i·form (splen'i·form, splee'ni·form) adj. Resembling the spleen.

sple·ni·tis (sple·nigh'tis) n. Inflammation of the spleen.

sple·ni·um (splee'nee·um) n., pl. **sple·nia** (·nee·uh) 1. BANDAGE. 2. The rounded posterior extremity of the corpus callosum.

sple·ni·us (splee'nee·us) n., pl. **sple·nii** (·nee·eye) One of two muscles of the back of the neck, splenius capitis and splenius cervicis.

splen·i·za·tion (splen"i·zay'shun) n. The stage of hyperemia and consolidation in pneumonia during which lung tissue grossly resembles the normal spleen or liver.

sple·no·cele (splee'no·seel) n. 1. Hernia of the spleen. 2. A tumor of the spleen.

sple·no·clei·sis (splee"no·klye'sis) n. 1. Irritation of the surface of the spleen causing the production of new fibrous tissue on the spleen. 2. Explantation of a portion of the spleen underneath the rectus abdominis muscle.

sple·no·dyn·ia (splee"no·din'ee·uh, splen"o·) n. Pain in the spleen.

sple·no·gram (splee'no·gram) n. 1. A radiographic depiction of the spleen, usually after contrast medium injection. 2. A differential count of the splenic cellular population.

sple·no·hep·a·to·meg·a·ly (splee"no·hep"uh·to·meg'uh·lee) n. Enlargement of the liver and spleen.

sple·noid (splee'noid) adj. Resembling the spleen.

sple·nol·y·sis (sple·nol'i·sis) n. Destruction of splenic tissue.

sple·no·ma·la·cia (splee"no·ma·lay'shee·uh) n. Softening of the spleen.

sple·no·meg·a·ly (splee"no·meg'uh·lee) n. Enlargement of the spleen.

sple·no·my·e·log·e·nous leukemia (splee"no·migh"e·loj'e·nus). GRANULOCYTIC LEUKEMIA.

sple·nop·a·thy (splee·nop'uth·ee) n. Any disease of the spleen.

sple·no·pexy (splee'no·peck"see) n. Fixation of the spleen to the abdominal wall by means of sutures.

sple·no·pneu·mo·nia (splee"no·new·mo'nyuh) n. The stage of pneumonia producing splenization or hepatization of lung tissue.

sple·no·por·tog·ra·phy (splee"no·por·tog'ruh·fee) n. Roentgenologic demonstration of the splenic and portal vein system by injection of contrast medium into the spleen. —**sple·no·por·to·gram** (·por'to·gram) n.

sple·nop·to·sis (splee"nop·to'sis) n. Downward displacement of the spleen.

splenorenal shunt. An abnormal connection between the splenic vein and the left renal vein; usually it results from a surgical procedure to relieve portal hypertension.

sple·nor·rha·phy (sple·nor'uh·fee) n. Suture of the spleen.

sple·not·o·my (sple·not'uh·mee) n. 1. The operation of incising the spleen. 2. Dissection of the spleen.

sple·no·tox·in (splee"no·tock'sin, splen"o·) n. A cytotoxin with specific action on the cells of the spleen.

splice, v. To overlap and join by suture, as to splice a tendon.

splint, n. 1. A support made of wood, metal, plastic, plaster, or other material for immobilizing the ends of a fractured bone or for restricting the movement of any movable part. 2. *In dentistry,* a device or appliance used to stabilize mobile teeth and redistribute occlusal forces. 3. SPLINT BONE (1).

splint·age (splin'tij) n. The application of splints.

splint bone. A vestigial second or fourth metacarpal or metatarsal of the horse extending, in the forelimb, from the "knee" and, in the hind limb, from the hock, toward the fetlock. 2. FIBULA.

splin·ter hemorrhage. A subungual linear hemorrhage resembling a splinter under the nail; found in patients with bacterial endocarditis and after trauma.

split graft. A free graft of skin using less than full thickness, varying from the very thin epidermal graft to the intermediate split-skin graft and the thick-split graft.

split personality. The type of human being in whom there is a separation of various components of the normal personality unit, and each component functions as an entity apart from the remaining personality structure; observed in hysteria and schizophrenia.

split-skin graft. SPLIT GRAFT.

split·ting, n. A chemical change in which a compound is changed into two or more simpler bodies, as by hydrolysis. 2. A reduplication of the first or second heart sounds due to asynchronous closure of the mitral and tricuspid valves or aortic and pulmonic valves, respectively. 3. *In psychology,* an ego mechanism that precedes, and in some cases determines the type of, repression.

spo·di·o·my·e·li·tis (spo"dee·o·migh"e·lye'tis) n. PARALYTIC SPINAL POLIOMYELITIS.

spodo·gram (spod'o·gram) n. A photograph or diagram picturing the distribution of mineral ash of a cell or tissue section following microincineration.

spondyl-, spondylo- A combining form meaning *vertebra, vertebral.*

spon·dy·lal·gia (spon"di·lal'jee·uh) n. Pain in a vertebra.

spon·dyl·ar·thri·tis (spon"dil·ahr·thrigh'tis) n. Arthritis of the vertebrae.

spon·dyl·ar·throc·a·ce (spon"dil·ahr'throck'uh·see) n. Caries of a vertebra.

spon·dyl·ex·ar·thro·sis (spon"dil·ecks"ar·thro'sis) n. A vertebral dislocation.

spon·dy·li·tis (spon"di·lye'tis) n. Inflammation of the vertebrae. —**spondy·lit·ic** (·lit'ick) adj.

spon·dy·lo·di·dym·ia (spon"di·lo·di·dim'ee·uh) n. The condition of union of conjoined twins united by their vertebrae.

spon·dy·lo·dyn·ia (spon"di·lo·din'ee·uh) n. Pain in a vertebra.

spon·dy·lo·lis·the·sis (spon"di·lo·lis·thees'is) n. Forward displacement of a vertebra upon the one below as a result of bilateral defect in the vertebral arch, or erosion of the articular surface of the posterior facets due to degenerative joint disease or elongation of the pedicle. It occurs most commonly between the fifth lumbar vertebra and the sacrum. —**spondylo·lis·thet·ic** (·thet'ick) adj.

spon·dy·lol·y·sis (spon"di·lol'i·sis) n. A defect or fracture, unilateral or bilateral, through the pars interarticularis of a vertebra which can lead to spondylolisthesis.

spon·dy·lop·a·thy (spon"di·lop'uth·ee) n. Any disease of the vertebrae.

spon·dy·lo·py·o·sis (spon"di·lo·pye·o'sis) n. Suppurative inflammation of one or more vertebrae.

spon·dy·lo·sis (spon"di·lo'sis) n. Vertebral ankylosis. —**spondy·lo·lyt·ic** (·lo·lit'ick) adj.

spon·dy·lo·syn·de·sis (spon"di·lo·sin·dee'sis) n. SPINAL FUSION.

spon·dy·lot·o·my (spon"di·lot'uh·mee) n. Section of a vertebra in correcting a deformity.

spon·dy·lus (spon'di·lus) n., pl. **spon·dy·li** (·lye) VERTEBRA. —**spondylous,** adj.

sponge (spunj) n. 1. A marine animal of the phylum Porifera. 2. The skeleton of the sponge, used as an absorbent. 3. GAUZE SPONGE.

sponge bath. A bath in which the body is sponged or washed one part at a time without being immersed.

sponge-gatherer's disease. A disease of divers due to a secretion of certain species of the sea anemone *Actinia,* found in waters where sponges grow. At the point of contact upon the body, the viscid excretion causes a swelling and intense itching, followed by a papule surrounded by a zone of redness which later becomes black and gangrenous and forms a deep ulcer.

sponge kidney. MEDULLARY SPONGE KIDNEY.

spongi-, spongio-. A combining form meaning *sponge, spongy.*

spon·gi·form (spun'ji·form) adj. Resembling a sponge.

spon·gio·blast (spon'jee·o·blast, spun'jee·o·) n. A nonnervous cell derived from the ectoderm of the embryonic neural tube, and later forming the neuroglia, the ependymal cells, the neurilemma sheath cells, the satellite cells of ganglions, and Müller's fibers of the retina.

spon·gio·blas·to·ma (spon"jee·o·blas·to'muh) n., pl. **spongioblastomas, spongioblastoma·ta** (·tuh) 1. SPONGIOBLASTOMA POLARE. 2. GLIOBLASTOMA MULTIFORME.

spongioblastoma mul·ti·for·me (mul-ti-for'mee). GLIOBLASTOMA MULTIFORME.

spongioblastoma po·la·re (po-lair'ee). A benign glial tumor composed of astrocytes with long polar cytoplasmic fibers.

spon·gio·cyte (spon'jee-o-site, spun') n. A cell, in the fasciculate zone of the adrenal cortex, which appears spongy because of the solution of lipids during preparation of the tissue for microscopical study.

spon·gio·cy·to·ma (spon''jee-o-sigh-to'muh) n. ASTROCYTOMA.

spon·gi·ose (spon'jee-oce) adj. Full of pores, like a sponge.

spon·gi·o·sis (spon''jee-o'sis, spun'') n. Accumulation of fluid in the intercellular spaces of the epidermis; an intercellular edema. **—spongi·ot·ic** (-ot'ick) adj.

spon·gi·o·si·tis (spon''jee-o-sigh'tis) n. Inflammation of the corpus spongiosum.

spon·gy (spun'jee) adj. Having the texture of sponge; very porous.

spongy bone. CANCELLOUS BONE.

spongy degeneration of infancy. A pathologic feature observed in the brains of infants and young children with a variety of conditions disturbing myelination of the brain including some of the aminoacidurias, characterized by the presence of rounded, empty spaces separated by strands of more or less intact neural tissue, resulting in the spongelike appearance. There may be edema, and demyelination may be extensive. Syn. *Canavan's disease, van Bogaert-Bertrand disease.*

spongy layer. The middle zone of the endometrium during the secretory phase of the menstrual cycle, characterized by the dilated portion of the glands and edematous connective tissue.

spon·ta·ne·ous (spon-tay'nee-us) adj. 1. Occurring naturally; not induced. 2. Occurring without external cause or influence. 3. Occurring without apparent cause. 4. Unpremeditated; not deliberate.

spontaneous abortion. Unexpected premature expulsion of the product of conception before the 20th completed week of gestation.

spontaneous amputation. 1. CONGENITAL AMPUTATION. 2. Amputation not caused by external trauma or injury, as in ainhum.

spontaneous fracture. A fracture occurring without apparent trauma; occurs in bone diseases.

spontaneous pneumothorax. Air in a pleural space and consequent lung collapse in the absence of trauma or deliberate introduction of air into the pleural space.

spontaneous subarachnoid hemorrhage. Bleeding confined to the subarachnoid space, due to rupture of a saccular (berry) aneurysm.

spoon, n. An instrument, usually made of metal, with a circular or oval bowl attached to a handle. A spoon is considered full when the contained liquid comes up to, but does not show a curve above, the upper edge or rim of the bowl. Teaspoons are popularly used to measure the dose of medicines on the assumption that they hold 5 ml.

spoon·er·ism (spoon'ur-iz-um) n. A psychic speech or writing defect characterized by the tendency to transpose sounds or syllables of two or more words.

spoon nail. KOILONYCHIA.

spor-, spori-, sporo- A combining form meaning *spore.*

spo·rad·ic (spo-rad'ick) adj. Scattered; occurring in an isolated manner.

spo·ran·gi·um (spo-ran'jee-um) n., pl. **sporan·gia** (-jee-ah) A specialized structure of a fungus; the enlarged end of a hypha within which spores develop.

spore, n. 1. *In bacteriology,* a refractile, resting body, highly resistant to heat, toxic chemicals, and dessication, found in the family Bacillaceae. 2. *In mycology and botany,* an asexual or sexual reproductive unit. 3. *In protozoology,* any of various reproductive cells, including the suborder of Eimeriidea; the sporoblasts resulting from nuclear division in the sporocyst.

spo·ri·cide (spo'ri-side) n. Any agent that destroys spores. **—spo·ri·ci·dal** (spo''ri-sigh'dul) adj.

spo·ro·cyst (spo'ro-sist) n. 1. The oocyst of certain protozoa, e.g., plasmodia and coccidia, in which sporozoites develop. 2. The larval stages of flukes in snails, from which cercariae develop.

spo·ro·cyte (spo'ro-site) n. A single binucleated cell formed in the life cycle of protozoa of the orders Myxosporidia and Actinomyxidia.

spo·ro·gen·e·sis (spo''ro-jen'e-sis) n. Production of spores. **—sporogen·ic** (-ick) adj.

spo·rog·e·nous (spo-roj'e-nus) adj. Spore-producing.

spo·rog·o·ny (spo-rog'uh-nee) n. Reproduction by spores; especially spore formation in Sporozoa following encystment of a zygote.

spo·ront (spo'ront) n. In Sporozoa, a cell that forms spores by encystment and subsequent division.

spo·ro·phyte (spo'ro-fite) n. The asexual, spore-producing phase in plants having alternation of generations.

spo·rot·ri·chin (spo-rot'ri-kin) n. An extract of cultures of *Sporotrichum schenckii,* used as a skin test antigen and in the agglutination test for sporotrichosis.

spo·ro·tri·cho·sis (spor''o-tri-ko'sis, -trye-ko'sis) n., pl. **sporotricho·ses** (-seez) A subacute or chronic granulomatous disease caused by the fungus *Sporotrichum.* The lesions are usually cutaneous and spread along lymph channels; occasionally the internal organs and bones may be involved. The disease is reported among farmers, florists, and others working in soil. Syn. *de Beurmann-Gougerot disease. Schenck's disease.*

Spo·rot·ri·chum (spo-rot'ri-kum) n. A genus of saprophytic or parasitic fungi.

Sporotrichum schenck·ii (shenk'ee-eye). A species of fungi that is the causative agent of sporotrichosis, growing at room temperature and on noncystine-containing media as a leathery, filamentous, brown-to-black colony, but in tissues and exudates of animals, rarely of man, as cigar-shaped, round, or fusiform budding yeast cells.

sporozoa. Plural of *sporozoon.*

spo·ro·zo·an (spo"ruh·zo'un) *adj.* & *n.* 1. Of or pertaining to the Sporozoa. 2. An organism of the class Sporozoa.

spo·ro·zo·ite (spo"ruh·zo'ite) *n.* The organism resulting from the schizogenesis or sporogony of the Sporozoa.

spo·ro·zo·on (spo"ruh·zo'on) *n.,* pl. **sporo·zoa** An organism of the class Sporozoa.

sport, *n.* An individual organism that differs from its parents to an unusual degree; a mutant.

spor·u·late (spor'yoo·late) *v.* To eject spores from a sporangium; to form spores.

spor·u·la·tion (spor"yoo·lay'shun) *n.* The formation of spores.

spot film. A small, highly collimated radiograph of an anatomic part, frequently obtained in conjunction with fluoroscopy.

spot test. Any test using small quantities of a reagent and substance tested, as on a plate or sheet of paper, for the determination of the presence of a substance.

spot·ting, *n.* Small amounts of bloody vaginal discharge, usually intermenstrual, and of significance in certain obstetric and gynecologic conditions.

sprain, *n.* A wrenching of a joint, producing a stretching or laceration of the ligaments.

sprain fracture. An injury in which a tendon or ligament, together with a shell of bone, is torn from its attachment; most commonly occurring at the ankle.

spray, *n.* 1. A stream of air and finely divided liquid produced with an atomizer, or other device. 2. A liquid pharmaceutical preparation intended for applying medication to the nose, throat, or other cavities by spraying from an atomizer; may be aqueous or oily in character.

spread·ing, *n.* Growth of bacteria beyond the line of inoculation.

Spreng·el's deformity (shpreng'el) Congenital elevation of the scapula; may be due to bony or muscular anomalies.

spring finger. A condition in which there is an obstruction to flexion and extension of one or more fingers; due to injuries or inflammation of the tendinous sheaths.

¹sprue (sproo) *n.* Generally a malabsorption syndrome characterized by impaired absorption of foods, minerals, and water by the small bowel; symptoms are due to nutritional deficiencies resulting from impaired absorption or due to altered intestinal activity.

²sprue, *n.* & *v.* 1. Wax, plastic, or metal that forms the pathway for molten metal in casting procedures; also the hardened metal that fills this pathway. 2. To form a sprue.

spud, *n.* A surgical instrument with a dull flattened blade, used for blunt dissection or removal of foreign bodies.

spur, *n.* 1. A sharp projection. Syn. *calcar.* 2. In biology, a pointed, spinelike outgrowth, either of the integument or of a projecting appendage.

spur·gall (spur'gawl) *n.* A calloused and hairless place on the side of a horse, caused by the use of a spur.

spu·ri·ous (spew'ree·us) *adj.* False; closely resembling a genuine instance functionally or in symptoms but not in pathological or morphological characteristics.

spu·tum (spew'tum) *n.,* pl. **spu·ta** (·tuh), **sputums** Material discharged from the surface of the air passages, throat, or mouth, and removed chiefly by spitting but in lesser degree by swallowing. It may consist of saliva, mucus, or pus, either alone or in any combination. It may also contain microorganisms, fibrin, blood or its decomposition products, or inhaled particulate foreign matter.

squa·lene (squay'leen) *n.* 2,6,10,15,19,23-Hexamethyl-2,6,10,14,18,22-tetracosahexaene, $C_{30}H_{50}$, an unsaturated hydrocarbon occurring in large proportion in shark-liver oil and in smaller proportion in various vegetable oils; an intermediate in the biosynthesis of cholesterol.

squa·ma (skway'muh) *n.,* pl. **squa·mae** (·mee) 1. A platelike mass, as the squama of the temporal bone. 2. A scale of the skin.

squame (skwame) *n.* SQUAMA.

squamo-. A combining form meaning *squamous.*

squa·mo·ba·sal (skway"mo·bay'sul) *adj.* Pertaining to the basal and squamous cells of a stratified squamous epithelium.

squa·mo·co·lum·nar (skway"mo·kol·um'nur) *adj.* Pertaining to squamous and columnar cells; usually refers to the junction of these two types of epithelium in the uterine cervix.

squa·mo·oc·cip·i·tal (skway"mo·ock·sip'i·tul) *adj.* Pertaining to the squamous portion of the occipital bone, or to the suture between the squamous part of the temporal bone and the occipital bone.

squa·mo·sa (skway·mo'suh) *n.,* pl. **squamo·sae** (·see) The squamous portion of the temporal bone.

squa·mo·sal (skway·mo'sul) *adj.* 1. SQUAMOUS. 2. Pertaining to the squamosa.

squa·mo·sphe·noid (skway"mo·sfee'noid) *adj.* Pertaining to the squamous portion of the temporal bone and to the sphenoid bone.

squa·mo·tym·pan·ic (skway"mo·tim·pan'ick) *adj.* Pertaining to the squamosal and tympanic parts of the temporal bone.

squa·mous (skway'mus) *adj.* 1. Thin and flat, like a fish's scale. 2. Consisting of or characterized by flat, scalelike cells, as squamous epithelium. 3. Pertaining to or constituting the thin anterior and superior portion of the temporal bone.

squamous cell carcinoma. A carcinoma whose parenchyma is composed of anaplastic squamous cells. Syn. *epidermoid carcinoma.*

squamous cell epithelioma. SQUAMOUS CELL CARCINOMA.

squill (skwil) *n.* The cut and dried fleshy inner scale of the bulb of the white variety of *Urginea maritima,* or of *U. indica.* Contains many glycosides, most of them cardioactive. Squill has been used as a diuretic and nauseant and more recently, as a cardiotonic drug, but the uncertainty of the absorption of its active principles has been a deterrent to the use of squill and its preparations and derivatives.

squint, *n.* STRABISMUS.

Sr Symbol for strontium.

sRNA Abbreviation for *soluble RNA.*

ss, ss Abbreviation for *semis,* one-half.

SS disease. Homozygous sickle cell disease: SICKLE CELL ANEMIA.

stab, *n. & v.* 1. A puncture wound. 2. The path formed by plunging an inoculation needle into nutrient media. 3. BAND CELL. 4. To puncture.

stab cell or **form** (stab, shtahp) BAND CELL.

sta·bile (stay'bil, stay'bile) *adj.* 1. Stationary; immobile; maintaining a fixed position. 2. Resistant to chemical change.

sta·bi·li·zer (stay'bi·lye''zur) *n.* 1. A retarding agent, or a substance that counteracts the effect of a vigorous accelerator and preserves a chemical equilibrium. 2. A substance added to a solution to render it more stable, as acetanilid to hydrogen peroxide solution.

stab·ker·ni·ge cell (shtahp'kerr''ni·guh) BAND CELL.

sta·ble, *adj.* 1. Steady, regular, not easily moved. 2. Secure; specifically, not subject to sudden alterations in mood. 3. Unlikely to break down or dissolve; in the case of a compound, likely to retain its composition under the application of physical or chemical forces.

stac·ca·to (sta·kah'to) *adj.* Designating an abrupt, jerky manner of speech with a noticeable interval between words.

stach·y·drine (stack'i·dreen) *n.* *N*-Methylproline methyl betaine, $C_7H_{13}NO_2$, an alkaloid occurring in *Stachys tuberifera* and other plants.

stach·y·ose (stack'ee·oce) *n.* A tetrasaccharide obtained from the tubers of *Stachys tuberifera* and some other plants. On complete hydrolysis, it yields one molecule each of fructose and glucose and two of galactose.

Stader's splint A metal bar with pins affixed at right angles. The pins are driven into the fragments of a fracture, and the bar maintains the alignment.

sta·di·um (stay'dee·um) *n.,* pl. **sta·dia** (·dee·uh) A stage or period in the course of a disease, especially a febrile disease.

stadium ac·mes (ack'meez). The height of a disease.

stadium an·ni·hi·la·ti·o·nis (a·nigh''i·lay·shee·o'nis). The convalescent stage of a disease.

stadium aug·men·ti (awg·men'tye). The period of increase in the intensity of disease.

stadium ca·lo·ris (ka·lo'ris). The period of disease during which there is fever.

stadium con·ta·gii (kon·tay'jee·eye). The prodromal stage of an infectious disease; the period of a disease during which it is contagious.

stadium con·va·les·cen·ti·ae (kon·va·le·sen'shee·ee). The period of recovery from disease.

stadium dec·re·men·ti (deck·re·men'tye). Defervescence of a febrile disease; the period of decrease in the severity of disease.

stadium de·crus·ta·ti·o·nis (dee''krus·tay·shee·o'nis). The stage of an exanthematous disease in which the lesions form crusts.

stadium des·qua·ma·ti·o·nis (des''kwa·may·shee·o'nis). The period of desquamation in an exanthematous disease.

stadium erup·ti·o·nis (e·rup·shee·o'nis). The period of an exanthematous disease in which the exanthem appears.

stadium flo·ri·ti·o·nis (flo·rish·ee·o'nis). The stage of an eruptive disease during which the exanthem is at its height.

stadium frig·o·ris (frig'o·ris). The cold or shivering stage of a febrile disease.

stadium in·cre·men·ti (ing·kre·men'tye). The stage of increase of a fever or disease.

stadium ma·ni·a·ca·le (ma·nigh·uh·kay'lee). The stage of greatest excitement and restlessness in a manic illness after which symptoms gradually subside.

stadium ner·vo·sum (nur·vo'sum). The paroxysmal stage of a disease.

stadium pro·dro·mo·rum (pro·dro·mo'rum). The stage immediately prior to the appearance of the signs and symptoms of disease.

stadium su·do·ris (sue·do'ris). The sweating stage of a febrile disease.

stadium sup·pu·ra·ti·o·nis (sup''yoo·ray·shee·o'nis). The period of suppuration in smallpox.

stadium ul·ti·mum (ul'ti·mum). The final stage of a febrile disease.

staff, *n.* 1. An instrument for passing through the urethra to the urinary bladder, used as a guide in operations on the bladder or for stricture. It is usually grooved. 2. The professional personnel, or a corps of specially trained persons, concerned with the care of patients in a hospital.

staff cell or **form.** BAND CELL.

stage, *n.* 1. A period or phase of disease characterized by certain symptoms; a condition in the course of a disease. 2. A period or step in a process, activity, or development; or of a surgical operation, or anesthesia. 3. The horizontal plate projecting from the pillar of a microscope for supporting the slide or object.

stages of general anesthesia. Divisions in the progressive sequence of clinical and physiological responses to general anesthetic agents: Stage 1. Period of repulsive responses to stimuli, loss of self-control, and altered sensibility (effects upon higher cortical centers); from initiation of the anesthesia to loss of consciousness. Stage 2. Period of reflex muscular activity and sometimes delirious excitement (effects upon basal ganglia and cerebellum); from the loss of consciousness to the onset of generalized muscular relaxation. Stage 3. Period of general muscular relaxation, complete anesthesia, abolished reflexes, and deep unconsciousness (effects upon the spinal cord, motor and sensory), which provides ideal conditions for many major surgical procedures; during this time vital functions are controlled by the automatic centers. Stage 4. Period of anesthetic overdosage (medullary paralysis), in which the vital centers are dangerously depressed, first the respiratory and then the cardiac centers. With present-day techniques, multiplicity of potent drugs, and balanced anesthesia, the stages described are not always clearly defined in practice.

stages of labor. Arbitrary divisions of the period of labor; the first begins with the onset of regular uterine contractions, and ends when dilatation of the ostium uteri is complete; the second ends with the expulsion of the child; the third (placental) ends with the expulsion of the placenta.

stag·gers, n. Any of various diseases manifested by lack of coordination in movement and a staggering gait, such as gid and sturdy of sheep, encephalomyelitis of horses, botulism, loco poisoning, and some cerebral affections of livestock.

stag·horn calculus. A large, irregularly branched calculus in the renal pelvis.

stag·na·tion (stag-nay'shun) n. 1. A cessation of motion. 2. In pathology, a cessation of motion in any fluid; stasis. **—stag·nate** (stag'nate) v.

stain, n. 1. A discoloration produced by absorption of, or contact with, foreign matter. 2. In microscopy, a pigment or dye used to render minute and transparent structures visible, to differentiate tissue elements, or to produce specific microchemical reactions.

staircase phenomenon. The stepwise increases in height of muscle contractions early in a series of responses to artificially applied stimuli of constant intensity. The mechanism of this phenomenon is not fully understood. Syn. TREPPE.

stal·ag·mom·e·ter (stal''ag-mom'e-tur) n. 1. An instrument for measuring the size of drops, or the number of drops in a given volume of liquid. 2. An instrument for measuring the surface tension of liquids.

stal·ing (stay'ling) n. Urination in farm animals.

stalk, n. Any lengthened supporting part, as of a plant or an organ.

sta·men (stay'mun) n., pl. **stamens, sta·mi·na** (stay'mi·nuh) The male organ of the flower, consisting of a stalk or filament and an anther containing pollen. **—stam·i·nate** (stam'i·nut) adj.

Stamey test A test of differential urinary excretion designed to detect unilateral renovascular disease.

stam·i·na (stam'i·nuh) n. Natural strength of constitution; vigor; inherent force; endurance.

stam·mer, n. & v. 1. Any of several irregularities of speech marked by involuntary halting, repetition of words or smaller segments, or transposition or mispronunciation of certain consonants, or by combinations of these defects. 2. To speak with such an irregularity. **—stammer·er,** n.

stammering bladder. Obsol. A condition in which there is interruption of the urinary stream; may be psychogenic or pathologic in origin.

stan·dard, n. & adj. 1. An established form of quality or quantity. 2. A substance of known strength used for determining the strength of an unknown by comparison. 3. Well established.

standard conditions. In measurements of gases, an atmospheric pressure of 760 mm and a temperature of 0°C. Syn. standard temperature and pressure.

standard deviation. The square root of the arithmetic average of the squares of the differences of each observation in a series from the mean of the series. The most commonly used measure of variation. Symbol, sigma (σ).

standard error. A measure of the variability any statistical constant would be expected to show in taking repeated random samples of a given size from the same universe of observations.

stan·dard·i·za·tion (stan''dur·di·zay'shun) n. The procedure whereby a preparation, a process, or a method is evaluated with respect to or brought into conformance with a standard.

standardized death rate. In biometry, the number of deaths per 1000 which would have occurred in some standard population with a known age-specific death rate. The rate may be standardized for race, sex, or other variables with known death rates.

stand·still, n. A state of quiescence dependent upon suspended action.

Stanford-Binet test. STANFORD REVISIONS OF BINET-SIMON TEST.

Stanford revisions of Binet-Simon test. Revisions of the Binet-Simon test to suit conditions in the United States. The last revision provides for more adequate sampling of intelligence at upper and lower levels by employing two new scales, by procedures for the administration and scoring of the test which have been defined more meticulously, and by standardization based upon larger and more representative samples of the population.

stan·nic (stan'ick) adj. Pertaining to tin; containing tin in the tetravalent state.

stan·nous (stan'us) adj. Containing tin as a bivalent element.

stan·num (stan'um) n. TIN.

sta·pe·dec·to·my (stay''pe·deck'tuh·mee) n. Surgical removal of the stapes and replacement with a prosthesis.

sta·pe·di·al (stay·pee'dee·ul) adj. Pertaining to, or located near, the stapes.

sta·pe·dio·te·not·o·my (sta·pee''dee·o·te·not'uh·mee) n. Cutting of the tendon of the stapedius muscle.

sta·pe·dio·ves·tib·u·lar (sta·pee''dee·o·ves·tib'yoo·lur) adj. Pertaining to the stapes and the vestibule.

sta·pe·di·us (stay·pee'dee·us) n., pl. **stape·dii** (·dee·eye). A muscle in the middle ear, inserted into the stapes.

sta·pes (stay'peez) n., pl. **stapes, sta·pe·des** (stay·pee'deez) The stirrup-shaped bone of the middle ear, articulating with the incus and the fenestra vestibuli. It is composed of the head, the crura or legs, and the footplate.

Staphcillin. A trademark for the sodium salt of methicillin, a semisynthetic penicillin antibiotic.

staphyl-, staphylo- A combining form meaning (a) grapelike (bunch or single); (b) pertaining to the uvula, velum palatinum, or the whole soft palate; (c) staphylococci, staphylococcal.

staph·y·lec·to·my (staf''i·leck'tuh·mee) n. Surgical removal of the uvula.

staph·yl·ede·ma, staph·yl·oe·de·ma (staf''il·e·

dee'muh) *n.* Edema of the uvula; any enlargement of the uvula.

staph·y·le·us (staf"i·lee'us) *L. adj.* Pertaining to the uvula.

staph·yl·he·ma·to·ma, staph·yl·hae·ma·to·ma (staf"il·hee"muh·to'muh, ·hem"uh·to'muh) *n.* An extravasation of blood into the uvula.

staph·y·line (staf'i·line, ·leen) *adj.* Pertaining to the uvula or to the entire palate.

staph·y·li·nus (staf"i·lye'nus) *adj.* Pertaining to the soft palate.

sta·phyl·i·on (sta·fil'ee·on) *n. In craniometry,* the point where the straight line that is drawn tangent to the two curved posterior borders of the horizontal plates of the palatine bones intersects the interpalatine suture.

staph·y·li·tis (staf"i·lye'tis) *n.* Inflammation of the uvula.

staph·y·lo·coc·cal (staf"i·lo·kock'ul) *adj.* Pertaining to or caused by staphylococci.

staph·y·lo·coc·ce·mia, staph·y·lo·coc·cae·mia (staf"i·lo·kock·see'mee·uh) *n.* The presence of staphylococci in the blood.

staph·y·lo·coc·cic (staf"i·lo·kock'sick) *adj.* Pertaining to, or caused by, staphylococci.

staph·y·lo·coc·cus (staf"i·lo·kock'us) *n.,* pl. **staphylococ·ci** (·sigh) A bacterium of the family Micrococcaceae, which is facultatively anaerobic, nonmotile, gram-positive, and tends to grow in irregular clusters.

Staphylococcus, *n.* A genus of cocci officially classified with *Micrococcus* by American bacteriologists.

Staphylococcus al·bus (al'bus). STAPHYLOCOCCUS EPIDERMIDIS.

staphylococcus antitoxin. An antitoxin prepared by immunizing horses with staphylococcus toxoid and/or staphylococcus toxin.

Staphylococcus au·re·us (aw'ree·us). A species of staphylococci, developing either yellow or white colonies, that is generally coagulase-positive and elaborates a number of soluble exotoxins and enzymes, and is responsible for a variety of clinical disturbances in man and animals, such as abscesses, endocarditis, pneumonia, osteomyelitis, and septicemia, but also may be normal inhabitants of the skin and mucous membranes without disease. Syn. *Staphylococcus pyogenes, Micrococcus aureus.*

Staphylococcus epi·der·mi·dis (ep"i·dur'mi·dis). A species of staphylococci, developing white colonies, that is coagulase-negative. It is rarely involved in human disease, such as endocarditis and infection of central nervous system shunts for hydrocephalus. Syn. *Staphylococcus albus, Micrococcus albus.*

Staphylococcus py·og·e·nes (pye·oj'e·neez). STAPHYLOCOCCUS AUREUS.

staphylococcus toxoid. Univalent or polyvalent, potently hemolytic and dermonecrotic toxins of *Staphylococcus aureus* altered by a formaldehyde-detoxifying process. Antigenicity is maintained, but toxicity is greatly diminished. Used in the prophylaxis and therapy of various staphylococcic pyodermas and localized pyogenic processes.

staph·y·lo·co·sis (staf"i·lo·ko'sis) *n.* Infection by staphylococci.

staph·y·lo·der·ma (staf"i·lo·dur'muh) *n.* A pyodermatous condition of the skin caused by staphylococci.

staph·y·lo·der·ma·ti·tis (staf"i·lo·dur"muh·tye' tis) *n.* Dermatitis due to staphylococci (*Staphylococcus aureus*).

staph·y·lo·di·al·y·sis (staf"i·lo·dye·al'i·sis) *n.* Relaxation of the uvula.

staph·y·lo·ma (staf"i·lo'muh) *n.* A bulging of the cornea or sclera of the eye. —**staph·y·lo·mat·ic** (·lo·mat'ick), **staphy·lom·a·tous** (·lom'uh·tus) *adj.*

staph·y·lon·cus (staf"i·lonk'us) *n.* Swelling of the uvula.

staph·y·lo·phar·yn·gor·rha·phy (staf"i·lo·far"in·gor'uh·fee) *n.* A plastic operation on the palate and pharynx, as for repair of a cleft palate.

staph·y·lo·plas·ty (staf"i·lo·plas'tee) *n.* A plastic operation on the soft palate or uvula.

staph·y·lop·to·sis (staf"i·lop·to'sis) *n.* Abnormal elongation of the uvula.

staph·y·lor·rha·phy (staf"i·lor'uh·fee) *n.* Repair of a cleft palate by plastic operation and suture.

staph·y·los·chi·sis (staf"i·los'ki·sis) *n.* 1. CLEFT UVULA. 2. A cleft soft palate. 3. See *cleft palate.*

staph·y·lot·o·my (staf"i·lot'uh·mee) *n.* 1. The operation of incising the uvula. 2. *In ophthalmology,* the operation of incising a staphyloma.

staph·y·lo·tox·in (staf"i·lo·tock'sin) *n.* One of several toxins which may be elaborated by various strains of *Staphylococcus aureus,* such as the alpha hemolysin possessing hemolytic, dermonecrotic, and acutely lethal activities; beta hemolysin with hot-cold activity against sheep erythrocytes; the delta and gamma hemolysins; enterotoxin; and leukocidin.

star·blind, *adj.* Half blind; blinking.

starch, *n.* 1. Any one of a group of carbohydrates or polysaccharides, of the general composition $(C_6H_{10}O_5)_n$, occurring as organized or structural granules of varying size and markings in many plant cells. It hydrolyzes to several forms of dextrin and glucose. Its chemical structure is not completely known, but the granules consist of concentric shells containing at least two fractions: an inner portion called amylose, and an outer portion called amylopectin. 2. CORNSTARCH.

starch-block electrophoresis. Electrophoresis in which a starch block is the supportive medium for the protein solution.

Star·ling's law of the heart. FRANK-STARLING LAW OF THE HEART.

Starr-Edwards valve prosthesis A prosthetic cardiac valve of the ball-in-cage type.

star·tle, *v.* To arouse unexpectedly and suddenly, causing a more or less involuntary response as of alarm, fear, or surprise.

startle response, reaction, reflex, or pattern. The complex psychophysiological response of an organism to a sudden unexpected stimulus such as a loud noise or blinding light; usually manifested by involuntary spasmodic movements of the limbs and often of the head and face so as to avoid or escape from the stimulus, but may include feelings of fear and a variety of visceral and autonomic changes; seen as the Moro reaction in infants.

star·va·tion, n. 1. Deprivation of food. 2. The state produced by deprivation of food. **—starve,** v.

stasi·basi·pho·bia (stas''i·bas''i·fo'bee·uh, stay''si·bay''si·) n. A pathologic fear of one's ability to walk or stand.

stasi·pho·bia (stas''i·fo'bee·uh, stay''si·) n. A pathologic fear of one's ability to stand upright.

sta·sis (stay'sis) n., pl. **sta·ses** (·seez) A cessation of flow in blood or other body fluids.

stasis dermatitis. Chronic inflammation of the skin of the legs, due to vascular stasis.

stasis ulcer. Ulceration, usually of the leg, due to chronic venous insufficiency or venous stasis. Syn. *varicose ulcer.*

stat. Abbreviation for *statim.*

stat, adv. Slang. Immediately.

-stat A combining form meaning (a) *a substance or device for checking or arresting;* (b) *a device, such as a servomechanism, for maintaining a process in a steady state;* (c) *a stand.*

state, n. 1. A condition; status. 2. The acme or crisis of a disease.

stat·ic (stat'ick) adj. 1. At rest; in equilibrium; nonfluctuating; unchanging. 2. Of or pertaining to static electricity. 3. Pertaining to the laws of statics. 4. CHRONIC.

stat·ics (stat'icks) n. The science that deals with bodies at rest or at equilibrium relative to some given state of reference.

static theory. A theory that every position of the head causes the endolymph of the semicircular canals to exert greatest pressure upon some part of the canals, thus in varying degree exciting the nerve endings of the ampullae.

static tremor. RESTING TREMOR.

stat·im (stat'im, stay'tim) adv. Immediately; at once. Abbreviated, stat.

sta·tion, n. 1. Standing position or attitude. 2. A place where first aid or treatment is given, as a dressing station, rest station.

statistical constant. A value such as the arithmetic mean, the standard error, or any other measure which characterizes a particular series of quantitative observations. Used as an estimate of the corresponding value for the universe from which the observations were chosen.

stato·acous·tic (stat''o·uh·koos'tick) adj. Of or pertaining to equilibrium and hearing.

statoacoustic nerve. VESTIBULOCOCHLEAR NERVE.

stato·co·nia (stat''o·ko'nee·uh) n., sing. **statoco·ni·um** (·nee·um) OTOCONIA.

stato·ki·net·ic (stat''o·ki·net'ick) adj. Pertaining to the balance and posture of the body or its parts during movement, as in walking.

sta·tom·e·ter (sta·tom'e·tur) n. An instrument for measuring the degree of exophthalmos.

stat·ure (statch'ur) n. The height of any animal when standing. In quadrupeds, it is measured at a point over the shoulders. In humans, it is the measured distance from the sole to the top of the head.

sta·tus (stay'tus, stat'us) n. A state or condition; often, a severe or intractable condition.

status an·gi·no·sus (an·ji·no'sus). A severe or protracted attack of angina pectoris.

status asth·mat·i·cus (az·mat'i·kus). Intractable asthma lasting from a few days to a week or longer.

status epi·lep·ti·cus (ep''i·lep'ti·kus). 1. A condition in which generalized convulsions occur at a frequency which does not allow consciousness to be regained in the interval between seizures. Syn. *grand mal status.* 2. Any of various other forms of prolonged seizures with variable degrees of impairment of consciousness, such as absence status, focal status, myoclonic status, or psychomotor status.

status mar·mo·ra·tus (mahr''mo·ray'tus, ·muh·). A cerebral lesion of obscure cause, affecting the thalamus, striatum, and border zones of the cerebral cortex, which are shrunken and have a whitish, marblelike appearance, representing foci of nerve cell loss and gliosis with peculiar condensations of myelinated fibers and even myelination of astroglial fibers (hypermyelination). This lesion does not develop after infancy, after the myelination glia have finished their developmental cycle. The usual clinical features are impairment of psychomotor development, defects in voluntary movement, choreoathetosis, and other extrapyramidal movement disorders. Syn. *état marbré, Vogt disease.*

status rap·tus (rap'tus). ECSTASY.

stat·u·to·ry rape (statch'oo·tor''ee). The violation of a female under the age of consent as fixed in the state or country in which the attack occurs. Syn. *rape of the second degree.*

sta·tu·vo·lence (sta·tew'vuh·lunce, stat''yoo·vo'lunce) n. 1. AUTOHYPNOTISM. 2. Voluntary somnambulism or clairvoyance. 3. A trance into which one voluntarily enters without aid from another. **—statuvo·lent** (·lunt) adj.

STD 1. Skin test dose, a standardized test dose of streptococcal erythrogenic toxin used in the Dick test. 2. Sexually transmitted disease (= VENEREAL DISEASE).

steal syndrome. Diversion of normal blood flow from a part, due to arterial narrowing or occlusion, which results in rerouting of the usual blood supply by reversal of flow in a large communicating arterial branch.

ste·ap·sin (stee·ap'sin) n. PANCREATIC LIPASE.

stea·rate (stee'uh·rate) n. An ester or salt of stearic acid, as stearin (glyceryl stearate) or sodium stearate.

stea·ric acid (stee·ar'ick, stee·ur'ick) A mixture of solid acids obtained from fats; consists chiefly of stearic acid, $CH_3(CH_2)_{16}COOH$, and palmitic acid, $CH_3(CH_2)_{14}COOH$. Used in the formulation of many dermatologic creams, in some enteric-coating compositions, and as a lubricant in compressing tablets.

stear·i·form (stee·ar'i·form) n. Having the appearance of, or resembling, fat.

stea·rin (stee'uh·rin) n. Tristearin, glyceryl tristearate, $C_3H_5O_3(C_{17}H_{35}CO)_3$, the glyceryl ester of stearic acid; occurs in many solid fats.

stea·rop·tene (stee''uh·rop'teen) n. The portion

of a volatile oil, usually consisting of oxygenated substances, which is solid at ordinary temperatures.

ste·a·ti·tis (stee″uh·tye′tis) *n.* Inflammation of adipose tissue.

ste·a·to·cryp·to·sis (stee″uh·to·krip·to′sis) *n.* Abnormal function of the sebaceous glands.

ste·a·to·cys·to·ma mul·ti·plex (stee″uh·to·sis·to′ muh mul′ti·plecks). A familial skin disorder inherited as a dominant trait, characterized by various-sized epidermal cysts on the trunk, back, arms, or thighs. Both men and women may be affected. Syn. *sebocystomatosis.*

ste·a·tog·e·nous (stee″uh·toj′e·nus) *adj.* 1. Producing steatosis or fat. 2. Causing sebaceous gland disease.

ste·a·tol·y·sis (stee″uh·tol′i·sis) *n.* The emulsifying process by which fats are prepared for absorption and assimilation. **—ste·a·to·lyt·ic** (stee″uh·to·lit′ick) *adj.*

ste·a·to·ma (stee″uh·to′muh) *n., pl.* **steatomas, steatoma·ta** (·tuh) 1. SEBACEOUS CYST. 2. LIPOMA.

ste·a·to·py·gia (stee″uh·to·pij′ee·uh, ·pye′jee·uh) *n.* Excessive accumulation of fat on the buttocks. Syn. *Hottentot bustle.* **—stea·top·y·gous** (·top′i·gus) *adj.*

ste·a·tor·rhea, ste·a·tor·rhoea (stee″uh·to·ree′ uh) *n.* 1. Fatty stools. 2. An increased flow of the secretion of the sebaceous follicles.

ste·a·to·sis (stee″uh·to′sis) *n., pl.* **steato·ses** (·seez) 1. FATTY DEGENERATION. 2. Disease of sebaceous glands.

stee·ple head or **skull.** OXYCEPHALY.

steer·horn stomach. A high, transversely located stomach. Syn. *cow-horn stomach.*

Stego·my·ia (steg″o·migh′ee·uh) *n.* A subgenus of the genus *Aëdes* of mosquitoes; includes a principal vector of yellow fever, *Aëdes aegypti.*

Stei·nach's method or **operation** (shtye′nahᵏh) Occlusion of the ductus deferens to promote production of testicular hormones and rejuvenation.

Stein-Leventhal syndrome A group of symptoms and findings characterized by amenorrhea or abnormal uterine bleeding or both, enlarged polycystic ovaries, hirsutism frequently, and occasionally retarded breast development and obesity.

Stein·mann pin or **nail** (shtine′mahn) A surgical nail inserted in distal portions of such bones as the femur or tibia for skeletal tractions.

Stelazine. Trademark for trifluoperazine, a tranquilizer used as the hydrochloride salt.

stel·late (stel′ate) *adj.* Star-shaped; with parts radiating from a center.

Stellwag's sign Infrequent blinking; seen in hyperthyroidism.

stem, *n.* 1. The pedicle or stalk of a tumor. 2. A supporting stalk, as of a leaf or plant.

stem bronchus. The continuation of the main bronchus which extends lengthwise in each lung, giving off anterior and posterior branches to the lobes.

stem cell leukemia. Leukemia in which the type of cell is so poorly differentiated that it is impossible to identify its series.

steno- A combining form meaning *narrow* or *constricted.*

steno·car·dia (sten″o·kahr′dee·uh) *n.* ANGINA PECTORIS.

steno·ce·pha·lia (sten″o·se·fay′lee·uh) *n.* STENOCEPHALY.

steno·ceph·a·ly (sten″o·sef′uh·lee) *n.* Unusual narrowness of the head. **—steno·ceph·a·lous** (·sef′uh·lus) *adj.*

steno·cho·ria (sten″o·ko′ree·uh) *n.* A narrowing; partial obstruction, particularly of a lacrimal duct.

steno·co·ri·a·sis (sten″o·ko·rye′uh·sis) *n.* Narrowing of the pupil.

sten·o·dont (sten′o·dont) *adj.* Provided with narrow teeth.

ste·nose (ste·noce′, ste·noze′, sten′oze) *v.* To constrict, narrow. **—ste·nosed** (ste·noazd′, ·noast′) *adj.;* **ste·nos·ing** (·no′zing, ·no′sing) *adj.*

ste·no·sis (ste·no′sis) *n., pl.* **steno·ses** (·seez) Constriction or narrowing, especially of a lumen or orifice; STRICTURE. **—steno·sal** (·sul), **ste·not·ic** (·not′ick) *adj.*

ste·nos·to·my (ste·nos′tuh·mee) *n.* Narrowing of any mouth or aperture.

steno·ther·mal (sten″o·thur′mul) *adj.* Capable of resisting a small range of temperature.

steno·tho·rax (sten″o·tho′racks) *n.* An unusually narrow chest.

stent, *n.* 1. A compound used for immobilizing some forms of skin graft. 2. A mold made of stent, used for immobilizing some forms of skin graft.

sten·to·roph·o·nous (sten″to·rof′o·nus) *adj.* Having a loud voice.

steph·a·no·fil·a·ri·a·sis (stef″uh·no·fil″uh·rye′uh· sis) *n.* A nematode dermatitis affecting cattle caused by any of several filarial worms in the genus *Stephanofilaria.*

steph·a·nu·ri·a·sis (stef″uh·new·rye′uh·sis) *n.* Infection of swine by the kidney worm *Stephanurus dentatus.*

step·page gait (step′ij). The high-stepping gait with exaggerated flexion at the hip and knee, the advancing foot hanging with the toes pointing toward the ground (foot drop). It is seen in various diseases that cause paralysis of the pretibial and peroneal muscles; may be unilateral or bilateral.

step sections. A series of histologic preparations made from a single block of tissue, succeeding sections being a significant distance apart from their predecessor.

sterco- A combining form meaning *feces, fecal.*

ster·co·bi·lin (stur″ko·bye′lin, ·bil′in) *n.* Urobilin as a constituent of the brown pigment found in feces; derived from bilirubin by reduction due to bacteria in the intestine.

ster·co·bi·lin·o·gen (stur″ko·bye·lin′o·jen) *n.* A reduction product of stercobilin which occurs in the feces; it is a colorless compound which becomes brown on oxidation, probably identical with urobilinogen.

ster·co·lith (stur′ko·lith) *n.* A calcified fecal concretion.

ster·co·ra·ceous (stur″ko·ray′shus) *adj.* FECAL; having the nature of or containing feces.

stercoraceous ulcer. An ulcer of the skin which is contaminated by feces.

stercoraceous vomiting. Ejection of fecal matter in vomit, usually due to intestinal obstruction. Syn. *fecal vomiting.*

ster·co·ral (stur'kuh·rul) *adj.* STERCORACEOUS.

ster·co·ro·ma (stur''kuh·ro'muh) *n.* FECALITH; a hard fecal mass usually in the rectum.

Ster·cu·lia (stur·kew'lee·uh) *n.* A large genus of tropical trees. *Sterculia urens* of India and *S. tragacantha* of Africa yield karaya gum; *S. acuminata* (*Cola nitida*) produces the kola nut.

ster·cus (stur'kus) *n.* FECES.

stere (steer, stair) *n.* A unit of volume equivalent to one cubic meter or one kiloliter.

stere-, stereo- A combining form meaning (a) *involving three dimensions;* (b) *involving depth perception, especially, stereoscopic;* (c) *firm, solid.*

ste·re·o·ag·no·sis (sterr''ee·o·ag·no'sis, steer''ee·o·) *n.* ASTEREOGNOSIS.

ste·re·o·an·es·the·sia, ste·re·o·an·aes·the·sia (sterr''ee·o·an''es·theezh'uh, steer''ee·o·) *n.* The failure to recognize the shape and form of objects due to interruption of traits transmitting postural and tactile sensation.

ste·re·o·ar·throl·y·sis (sterr''ee·o·ahr·throl'i·sis, steer''ee·o·) *n.* Loosening stiff joints by operation or manipulation in cases of ankylosis.

ste·re·o·blas·tu·la (sterr''ee·o·blas'tew·luh, steer''ee·o·) *n.* A solid blastula, not having a blastocoele, but having all its cells bounding the external surface.

ste·re·o·chem·is·try (sterr''ee·o·kem'is·tree, steer''ee·o·) *n.* A branch of science that deals with the spatial arrangement of atoms in a molecule. —**stereochem·i·cal** (·i·kul) *adj.*

ste·re·o·cil·ia (sterr''ee·o·sil'ee·uh, steer''ee·o·) *n.*, *sing.* **stereocil·i·um** (·ee·um) Irregular, nonmotile tufts of microvilli on the free surface of cells of the male reproductive tract, especially the epididymis, which are secretory in function.

ste·re·o·en·ceph·a·lo·tome (sterr''ee·o·en·sef'uh·lo·tome, steer''ee·o·) *n.* A device for localizing exactly any point within the brain, for the operation of stereoencephalotomy.

ste·re·o·en·ceph·a·lot·o·my (sterr''ee·o·en·sef''uh·lot'uh·mee, steer''ee·o·) *n.* Selective destruction, by cautery or electrolysis, of cerebral tracts or nuclei, using the pineal body or posterior commissure as the point of reference or zero point on the stereotaxic coordinates.

ste·re·og·no·sis (sterr''ee·og·no'sis, steer''ee·) *n.* The faculty of recognizing the size and shape of objects by palpation. —**stereog·nos·tic** (·nos'tick) *adj.*

ste·re·o·gram (sterr''ee·o·gram, steer''ee·o·) *n.* 1. A two-dimensional picture which represents an object with the impression of three dimensions, by means of contour lines or shading. 2. A stereoscopic picture.

ste·re·o·iso·mer (sterr''ee·o·eye'so·mur, steer''ee·o·) *n.* A compound that has the same number and kind of atoms as another compound, and is of similar structure, but with a different arrangement of the atoms in space.

ste·re·o·phoro·scope (sterr''ee·o·for'uh·skope,

steer''ee·o·) *n.* A stereoscopic stroboscope, an instrument for producing a series of images apparently in motion; used in tests of visual perception.

ste·re·op·sis (sterr''ee·op'sis, steer''ee·) *n.* STEREOSCOPIC VISION.

ste·re·op·ter (sterr''ee·op'tur, steer''ee·) *n.* An instrument to provide a rapid quantitative test for depth perception.

ste·re·o·scope (sterr''ee·o·skope, steer''ee·o·) *n.* An instrument by which two similar pictures of the same object are so mounted that the images are seen as one, thereby giving a three-dimensional impression. —**ste·re·os·co·py** (sterr''ee·os'kuh·pee, steer''ee·).

ste·re·o·scop·ic (sterr''ee·o·skop'ick, steer''ee·o·) *adj.* 1. Of or pertaining to the stereoscope. 2. Pertaining to or characterized by three-dimensional observation of objects.

stereoscopic vision. Disparity of retinal images resulting in depth perception.

ste·re·o·tac·tic (sterr''ee·o·tack'tick, steer''ee·o·) *adj.* Pertaining to or involving stereotaxis.

ste·re·o·tax·ic (sterr''ee·o·tack'sick, steer''ee·o·) *adj.* Pertaining to or characterized by precise spatial positioning.

ste·re·o·tax·is (sterr''ee·o·tack'sis, steer''ee·o·) *n.* 1. The accurate location of a definite circumscribed area within the brain by moving a probe or electrode along coordinates for measured distances from certain external points or landmarks of the skull. 2. STEREOTROPISM. —**stereo·tac·tic** (·tack'tick), **stereotac·ti·cal** (·ti·kul) *adj.*

ste·re·ot·ro·pism (sterr''ee·ot'ro·pizum, steer''ee·) *n.* Growth or movement toward a solid body (positive stereotropism) or away from a solid body (negative stereotropism). Syn. *thigmotropism.* —**ste·re·o·trop·ic** (sterr''ee·o·trop'ick, steer''ee·o·) *adj.*

ste·re·o·ty·py (sterr''ee·o·tye''pee, steer''ee·o·) *n.* Persistent repetition of an activity, as the repeatedly similar hallucinations heralding certain psychomotor convulsions, the mannerisms seen in retarded children or the morbidly selfsame movements or ideas encountered in certain psychoses, especially schizophrenia.

ste·ric (steer'ick, sterr'ick) *adj.* Pertaining to the arrangement of atoms in space.

ste·rid (steer''id, sterr') *n.* A proposed generic name for any substance that is either a sterol or a steroid.

ste·rig·ma (ste·rig'muh) *n.*, *pl.* **sterigma·ta** (·tuh), **sterigmas** In fungi, specialized cells involved in spore formation, such as those which arise from the vesicle of *Aspergillus.* —**ster·ig·mat·ic** (sterr''ig·mat'ick) *adj.*

ster·ile (sterr'il) *adj.* 1. Not fertile; not capable of reproducing. 2. Free from live microorganisms.

ste·ril·i·ty (ste·ril'i·tee) *n.* 1. Total inability to reproduce. 2. The condition of freedom from live microorganisms.

ster·il·ize (sterr'i·lize) *v.* 1. To render sterile or free from live microorganisms. 2. To render incapable of procreation. —**ster·il·iza·tion** (sterr''il·zay'shun) *n.*

ster·i·li·zer (sterr'i·lye"zur) *n.* An apparatus, such as an autoclave, used to sterilize equipment or other objects by destroying all contaminating microorganisms.

stern-, sterno- A combining form meaning (a) *sternum, sternal*; (b) *chest, breast.*

ster·nal (stur'nul) *adj.* Pertaining to, or involving, the sternum.

ster·nal·gia (stur·nal'jee·uh, ·juh) *n.* 1. Pain in the sternum. 2. ANGINA PECTORIS.

sternal puncture. Insertion of a hollow needle into the sternum to obtain bone marrow specimens.

Sternberg-Reed cell REED-STERNBERG CELL.

Stern·hei·mer-Mal·bin cells. Leukocytes with cytoplasm containing granules agitated by brownian movement, seen in urinary sediments of patients with urological disorders, as in pyelonephritis.

ster·no·cla·vic·u·lar (stur"no·kla·vick'yoo·lur) *adj.* Pertaining to the sternum and the clavicle.

ster·no·clei·do·mas·toid (stur"no·klye"do·mas'toid) *adj. & n.* 1. Pertaining to the sternum, the clavicle, and the mastoid process. 2. A muscle of the neck that flexes the head.

ster·no·cos·tal (stur"no·kos'tul) *adj.* Pertaining to the sternum and the ribs.

ster·no·dyn·ia (stur"no·din'ee·uh) *n.* Pain in the sternum.

ster·no·hy·oid (stur"no·high'oid) *adj. & n.* 1. Pertaining to the sternum and the hyoid bone. 2. A muscle arising from the manubrium of the sternum and inserted into the hyoid bone.

ster·no·mas·toid (stur"no·mas'toid) *n.* STERNO-CLEIDOMASTOID (2).

ster·nop·a·gus (stur·nop'uh·gus) *n.* Conjoined twins united at the sternum.

ster·nos·chi·sis (stur·nos'ki·sis) *n.* A congenital cleft or fissure of the sternum.

ster·no·thy·roid (stur"no·thigh'roid) *adj. & n.* 1. Pertaining to the sternum and thyroid cartilage. 2. A muscle arising from the manubrium of the sternum and inserted into the thyroid cartilage.

ster·not·o·my (stur·not'uh·mee) *n.* An operation cutting through the sternum.

ster·num (stur'num) *n.*, genit. **ster·ni** (·nye), pl. **sternums, ster·na** (·nuh) The flat, narrow bone in the median line in the front of the chest, composed of three portions—the manubrium, the body, and the xiphoid process.

ster·nu·ta·tion (stur"new·tay'shun) *n.* The act of sneezing.

ster·nu·ta·tor (stur'new·tay"tur) *n.* A substance capable of inducing sneezing, as certain war gases.

ste·roid (steer'oid, sterr'oid) *n. & adj.* 1. Generally any of the compounds having the cyclopentanoperhydrophenanthrene ring system of sterols but not including the latter. In common usage however, sterols are included. They include the primary sex hormones, androgen and estrogen, and the corticosteroids. 2. Pertaining to or characteristic of a steroid. —**steroid·al** (·ul) *adj.*

ste·rol (steer'ol, sterr'ol, ·ole) *n.* Any saturated or unsaturated alcohol derived from cyclopen-tanoperhydrophenanthrene; the alcohols occur both free and combined as esters or glycosides, and often are principal constituents of the nonsaponifiable fraction of fixed oils and fats.

ste·rone (steer'ohn, sterr'ohn) *n.* A steroid possessing one or more ketone groups.

ster·tor (sturt'ur) *n.* Sonorous breathing or snoring; the rasping, rattling sound produced when the larynx and the air passages are partially obstructed by mucus. —**stertor·ous** (·us) *adj.*

stertorous respiration. The sound produced by breathing through the nose and mouth at the same time, causing vibration of the soft palate between the two currents of air.

steth-, stetho- A combining form meaning *breast* or *chest.*

stetho·poly·scope (steth"o·pol'ee·skope) *n.* A stethoscope having several tubes for the simultaneous use of several listeners.

stetho·scope (steth'uh·skope) *n.* An instrument for mediate auscultation for the detection and study of sounds arising within the body. The sound is conveyed from the body surface to both ears of the examiner simultaneously.

Ste·vens-John·son syndrome A severe form of erythema multiforme, characterized by constitutional symptoms and marked involvement of the conjunctiva and oral mucosa.

Stewart-Morel-Morgagni syndrome Hyperostosis frontalis interna associated with obesity, headache, hypertension, and various endocrine or neurologic and psychologic symptoms.

Stewart-Treves syndrome. Postmastectomy lymphangiosarcoma.

sthe·nia (sthee'nee·uh) *n.* Normal force or vigor.

stib·amine glucoside (stib'uh·meen). A nitrogen glucoside of sodium *p*-aminophenylstibonate, a pentavalent antimony compound used in the treatment of kala azar.

stib·i·al·ism (stib'ee·ul·iz·um) *n.* Poisoning by antimony.

stib·i·um (stib'ee·um) *n.* ANTIMONY.

stib·o·phen (stib'o·fen) *n.* Pentasodium antimony III bis(pyrocatechol-2,4-disulfonate), $C_{12}H_4Na_5O_{16}S_4Sb$, a trivalent antimony compound used as an antischistosomal drug.

stiff-man syndrome A particularly malignant and progressive form of painful muscular spasms, of unknown cause but probably of central nervous system origin. Clinically, it resembles tetanus.

sti·fle, *v.* To choke; to kill by impeding respiration.

stig·ma (stig'muh) *n.*, pl. **stig·ma·ta** (stig·mah'tuh, stig'muh·tuh), **stigmas** 1. Any mark, blemish, spot, or scar on the skin. 2. Any one of the marks or features characteristic of a condition, as hysterical stigmas. 3. Specifically, any visible characteristic associated with or diagnostic of a medical disorder, such as café-au-lait spots in neurofibromatosis, the Kayser-Fleischer ring in hepatolenticular degeneration, or the physical appearance commonly seen in Down's syndrome (mongolism). 4. The part of a pistil that receives the pollen.

5. An opening between cells, especially one between the endothelial cells of a capillary, now considered an artifact. —**stig·mal** (·mul), **stig·mat·ic** (stig·mat'ick) adj.

stigma of the graafian follicle. The point of rupture through which the ovum escapes.

stig·mas·ter·ol (stig·mas'tur·ol) n. A sterol, $C_{29}H_{48}O$, obtained from the soybean.

stig·ma·tism (stig'muh·tiz·um) n. **1.** A condition of the refractive media of the eye in which rays of light from a point are accurately brought to a focus on the retina. **2.** The condition of having stigmas.

stig·ma·ti·za·tion (stig''muh·ti·zay'shun) n. The formation of stigmas.

stil·bes·trol, stil·boes·trol (stil·bes'trole, ·trol) n. DIETHYLSTILBESTROL.

sti·let, sti·lette (stye·let', sti·let') n. STYLET.

still·birth, n. **1.** The birth of a dead child. **2.** A child born dead.

still·born, adj. Born dead.

stil·lin·gia (sti·lin'jee·uh) n. The dried root of *Stillingia sylvatica*; preparations of the root have been used for the treatment of various afflictions.

Still's disease Juvenile rheumatoid arthritis in which visceral involvement is prominent. Syn. *Chauffard-Still disease*.

stim·u·lant (stim'yoo·lunt) n. & adj. **1.** An agent that stimulates. **2.** Producing a temporary increase in activity.

stim·u·late (stim'yoo·late) v. To quicken; to stir up; to excite; to increase functional activity. —**stimu·lat·ing** (·lay·ting) adj.

stim·u·la·tion (stim''yoo·lay'shun) n. **1.** The act of stimulating. **2.** The effect of a stimulant. **3.** EXCITATION.

stim·u·la·tor (stim'yoo·lay''tur) n. A person or thing that stimulates.

stim·u·lin (stim'yoo·lin) n. A substance supposed to stimulate the phagocytes to destroy germs.

stim·u·lus (stim'yoo·lus) n., pl. **stimu·li** (·lye) An excitant or irritant; an alteration in the environment of any living thing (cell, tissue, organism), capable of influencing its activity or of producing a response in or by it.

stimulus threshold. ABSOLUTE THRESHOLD.

sting, n. & v. **1.** The acute burning sensation caused by pricking, striking, or chemically stimulating the skin or a mucous membrane. **2.** The wound caused. **3.** The organ or part causing the injury, such as the sting of a bee. **4.** To prick or pierce with ensuing pain.

S-T interval. The period between the end of the QRS complex and the end of the T wave; the interval representing ventricular repolarization.

stip·ple cell. An erythrocyte with numerous fine blue or blue-black dots as seen in Romanovsky-stained preparations; occurs in lead poisoning, thalassemia, and other chronic anemias.

stippled epiphyses. CHONDRODYSTROPHIA CALCIFICANS CONGENITA.

stip·pling, n. **1.** A change of a surface whereby the presence of tiny nodules produces an appearance like that of a pebbled paper, as slight deposits of fibrin on a serous surface. **2.** BASO-

PHILIA (2). **3.** The pitted appearance of the surface of normal gingivae. **4.** An effect developed in the surface finishing of artificial dentures to simulate natural tissue. **5.** Multiple punctate opacities in radiographs, usually representing calcific deposits. **6.** The dotting with basophilic granules in Romanovsky-stained preparations.

stitch, n. **1.** A sudden, sharp, lancinating pain, often at a costal margin. **2.** SUTURE (2, 3).

stock·i·net (stock'i·net'') n. Cotton material or shirting, woven like a stocking, but of uniform caliber and used according to size to cover extremities or the body preparatory to the application of a fixed dressing, such as a plaster or splints.

stock·ing, n. A close-fitting covering for the leg and foot, sometimes designed and fitted for a special hygienic or therapeutic purpose; usually made of knitted or woven goods that sometimes contain an elastic thread.

stoi·chi·om·e·try (stoy''kee·om·e·tree) n. The branch of chemistry that deals with the numerical relationship between elements or compounds (atomic weights), the determination of the proportions in which the elements combine (formulas), and the weight relations in reactions (equations). —**stoichi·o·met·ric** (·o·met'rick) adj.

Stokes-Adams syndrome Syncope of cardiac origin occurring most frequently in patients with complete atrioventricular block and a pulse rate of 40 or less per minute; during an attack the electrocardiogram will show ventricular standstill, ventricular tachycardia or fibrillation, or slowing of the idioventricular impulses below a critical rate.

Stokes' expectorant EXPECTORANT MIXTURE.

sto·ma (sto'muh) n., pl. **stoma·ta** (·tuh), **stomas** **1.** A minute opening or pore in a surface. **2.** A surgically created opening.

sto·mac·a·ce (sto·mack'uh·see) n. ULCERATIVE STOMATITIS.

stom·ach (stum'uck) n. The most dilated part of the alimentary canal, in which food is stored immediately after swallowing and is partially digested by the gastric juice. It is situated below the diaphragm in the left hypochondriac, the epigastric, and part of the right hypochondriac regions. It is continuous at the cardiac end with the esophagus, at the pyloric end with the duodenum. Its wall consists of four coats: mucous, submucous, muscular, and serous.

sto·mach·ic (sto·mack'ick) n. A substance that may stimulate the secretory activity of the stomach.

stomat-, stomato- A combining form meaning *mouth*.

sto·ma·tal·gia (sto''muh·tal'jee·uh) n. Pain in the mouth.

sto·mat·ic (sto·mat'ick) adj. Pertaining to the mouth.

sto·ma·ti·tis (sto''muh·tye'tis) n., pl. **stoma·tit·i·des** (·tit'i·deez) Inflammation of the soft tissues of the mouth.

stomatitis med·i·ca·men·to·sa (med''i·kuh·men·to'suh). Inflammation of the mucus membranes of the mouth resulting from a systemic allergic reaction to a drug.

stomatitis ven·e·na·ta (ven-e-nay'tuh). STOMATITIS MEDICAMENTOSA.

sto·ma·toc·a·ce (sto''muh-tock'uh-see) *n.* ULCERATIVE STOMATITIS.

stoma·to·ca·thar·sis (sto''muh-to-ka-thahr'sis) *n.* The cleaning or disinfection of the mouth.

sto·ma·to·dyn·ia (sto''muh-to-din'ee-uh) *n.* Pain in the mouth.

sto·ma·to·dys·o·dia (sto''muh-to-di-so'dee-uh) *n.* Ill-smelling breath.

sto·ma·to·gas·tric (sto''muh-to-gas'trick) *adj.*
1. Pertaining to the mouth and the stomach.
2. Pertaining to the nerves that supply the anterior end of the digestive tract in various invertebrates.

sto·ma·to·gnath·ic (sto''muh-to-nath'ick) *adj.* Pertaining to the mouth, oral cavity, and jaws.

sto·ma·tol·o·gy (sto''muh-tol'uh-jee) *n.* The branch of medical science concerned with the anatomy, physiology, pathology, therapeutics, and hygiene of the oral cavity, the tongue, teeth, and adjacent structures and tissues, and of the relationship of that field to the entire body. —**stoma·to·log·ic** (·to-loj'ick) *adj.*

sto·ma·to·me·nia (sto''muh-to-mee'nee-uh) *n.* STOMENORRHAGIA.

sto·ma·to·mia (sto''muh-to'mee-uh, stom''uh·) *n.* A general term for the incision of a mouth, as of the uterus.

stomat·o·my (sto-mat'uh-mee) *n.* Incision of the ostium uteri.

sto·ma·to·my·co·sis (sto''muh-to-migh-ko'sis) *n.* THRUSH (1).

sto·ma·to·ne·cro·sis (sto''muh-to-ne-kro'sis) *n.* Noma of the mouth.

sto·ma·top·a·thy (sto''muh-top'uth-ee) *n.* Any disease of the mouth.

sto·ma·to·plas·ty (sto''muh-to-plas''tee) *n.* A plastic operation upon the mouth. —**sto·ma·to·plas·tic** (sto''muh-to-plas'tick) *adj.*

sto·ma·tor·rha·gia (sto''muh-to-ray'jee-uh) *n.* Copious hemorrhage from the mouth.

sto·ma·to·scope (sto''muh-to-skope) *n.* An instrument used for inspecting the cavity of the mouth.

sto·ma·to·sis (sto''muh-to'sis) *n.* Any disease of the mouth.

sto·men·or·rha·gia (sto-men''o-ray'jee-uh) *n.* Vicarious bleeding in the mouth, associated with abnormal menstruation.

sto·mo·de·um, sto·mo·dae·um (sto''mo-dee'um) *n.* The primitive oral cavity of the embryo; an ectodermal fossa formed by the growth of the facial processes about the buccopharyngeal membrane. —**stomode·al, stomodae·al** (·ul) *adj.*

sto·mos·chi·sis (sto-mos'ki-sis) *n.* A fissure of the mouth.

Sto·mox·ys (sto-mock'sis) *n.* A genus of bloodsucking flies of the family Muscidae. It is similar to the common housefly.

stone, *n.* 1. CALCULUS. 2. An English unit of weight equal to 14 lb.

stone·cut·ter's disease. Raynaud's phenomenon

related to the use of pneumatic or compressed-air tools.

stool, *n.* Material evacuated from the bowels; feces.

stop·page (stop'ij) *n.* Cessation of flow or action; closure or stenosis.

storage disease. Any metabolic disease, usually due to an inherited enzyme deficiency, characterized by excess deposition of exogenous or endogenous substances within the body. Syn. *thesaurosis.*

sto·rax (sto'racks) *n.* A balsam obtained from the wounded trunk of *Liquidambar orientalis,* or of *L. styraciflua;* occurs as a semiliquid, grayish to grayish-brown, sticky, opaque mass, or a semisolid, sometimes solid mass; consists largely of storesin, or storesin—both free and in the form of a cinnamic ester, and also cinnamic acid and its esters. Has been used as a stimulating expectorant, and externally as a parasiticide.

sto·ri·form (sto'ri-form) *adj.* Having the spiraled, whorled appearance of a nebula.

stra·bis·mus (stra-biz'mus) *n.* An abnormality of the eyes in which the visual axes do not meet at the desired objective point, in consequence of incoordinate action of the extrinsic ocular muscles. Syn. *squint, heterotropia.* —**strabis·mal** (·mul), **strabis·mic** (·mick) *adj.*

stra·bom·e·ter (stra-bom'e-tur) *n.* An instrument for the measurement of the deviation of the eyes in strabismus. Syn. *strabismometer.*

stra·bom·e·try (stra-bom'e-tree) *n.* The determination of the degree of ocular deviation in strabismus. Syn. *strabismometry.*

strabo·tome (strab'uh-tome) *n.* A knife used for strabotomy.

stra·bot·o·my (stra-bot'uh-mee) *n.* An operation for the correction of strabismus.

straight-leg-raising test. LASÈGUE'S SIGN.

straight sinus. A sinus of the dura mater running from the inferior sagittal sinus along the junction of the falx cerebri and tentorium to the transverse sinus.

¹**strain,** *n.* A group of organisms possessing a common characteristic which distinguishes them from other groups within the same species.

²**strain,** *v. & n.* 1. To injure by excessive stretching, overuse, or misuse. 2. To pass through a strainer or other device; to filter. 3. To exert great effort, as when retching or sometimes defecating. 4. Excessive stretching or overuse of a part, as of muscles or joints. 5. The condition produced in a part by overuse or wrong use, as eyestrain. 6. The condition or state of a system exposed to stress; the disturbance of normal and harmonious relationships of one part or person with other parts or persons as a result of such stress; mental tension.

strait, *n.* A narrow or constricted passage, as the inferior or superior pelvic strait.

strait·jack·et, *n.* A restraining apparatus, not always conforming to the jacket type, used to prevent violent, delirious, or otherwise physically uncontrollable persons from injuring themselves or others.

stra·mo·ni·um (stra-mo'nee·um) n. The dried leaves and flowering tops of *Datura stramonium* (including *D. tatula*); contains the alkaloids hyoscyamine and scopolamine. The actions of stramonium are similar to those of belladonna. Stramonium has been used in the treatment of asthma by smoking in cigarettes or by mixing with potassium nitrate and burning and inhaling the vapors, which contain atropine. Syn. *Jamestown weed, Jimson weed.*

stran·gle, v. 1. To choke or throttle by compression of the glottis or trachea. 2. To be choked, to suffocate from tracheal constriction or obstruction.

stran·gles, n. An infectious disease of solipeds caused by *Streptococcus equi*, involving the nasal passages and related structures; characterized by a purulent inflammation with involvement of the lymphatic system of the head and, in some instances, accompanied by difficult breathing. Syn. *equine distemper.*

stran·gu·lat·ed hernia (strang'gew·lay''tid). A hernia involving intestine in which circulation of the blood and the fecal current are blocked. If unrelieved, it leads to ileus and necrosis of the intestine.

stran·gu·la·tion (strang''gew·lay'shun) n. 1. Asphyxiation due to obstruction of the air passages, as by external pressure on the neck. 2. Constriction of a part producing arrest of the circulation, as strangulation of a hernia. —**stran·gu·lat·ed** (strang'gew·lay''tid) adj.

stran·gu·ria (strang·gew'ree·uh) n. STRANGURY.

stran·gu·ry (strang'gew·ree) n. Painful urination, the urine being voided drop by drop.

strap, n. & v. 1. A long band, as of adhesive plaster. 2. To compress or support a part by means of bands, especially bands of adhesive plaster.

strat·i·fi·ca·tion (strat''i·fi·kay'shun) n. Arrangement in layers or strata.

strat·i·fied (strat'i·fide) adj. Arranged in layers or strata.

strat·o·sphere (strat'uh·sfeer) n. The atmosphere above the tropopause, where temperature changes are small and winds essentially horizontal.

stra·tum (stray'tum, strah'tum) n., pl. **stra·ta** (·tuh) (tum).

stratum ba·sa·le (ba·say'lee). BASAL LAYER.

stratum cor·ne·um (kor'nee·um) [NA]. The layer of keratinized cells of the epidermis. Syn. *horny layer.*

stratum gra·nu·lo·sum (gran·yoo·lo'sum). A layer of minute cells containing many granules.

stratum lu·ci·dum (lew'si·dum) [NA]. A translucent layer of the epidermis consisting of irregular transparent cells with traces of nuclei.

stratum pa·pil·la·re (pap·i·lair'ee ko'ree·eye) [NA]. The zone of fine-fibered connective tissue within and immediately subjacent to the papillae of the corium. Syn. *papillary layer.*

stratum spon·gi·o·sum (spon·jee·o'sum). SPONGY LAYER.

stratum sub·mu·co·sum (sub·mew·ko'sum). The thin layer of smooth muscle of the myometrium adjacent to the endometrium.

stratum sub·se·ro·sum (sub·se·ro'sum). The thin layer of smooth muscle of the myometrium adjacent to the serous coat.

stratum su·pra·vas·cu·la·re (sue''pruh·vas·kew·lair'ee). The layer of muscle of the myometrium between the stratum vasculare and the stratum subserosum.

strawberry mark. A congenital hemangioma clinically characterized by its raised, bright-red, soft, often lobulated appearance. Syn. *nevus vasculosus.*

streak, n. 1. A furrow, line, or stripe. 2. *In bacteriology,* the process of distributing the inoculum over the surface of a solid culture medium. Cultures thus obtained are called streak cultures.

street rabies virus. The naturally occurring rabies virus, as contrasted with the fixed virus produced by intracerebral passage in rabbits.

Strep. An abbreviation for *Streptococcus.*

strepho·sym·bo·lia (stref''o·sim·bo'lee·uh) n. 1. MIRROR VISION. 2. Specifically, the tendency of many children first learning to read to reverse letters in a word or to fail to distinguish between similar letters, as *p* and *q,* or *n* and *u*; abnormal if persisting. 3. Reversal in direction of reading.

strept-, strepto- A combining form meaning (a) *twisted, curved;* (b) *streptococcal.*

strep·ti·dine (strep'ti·deen) n. 1,3-Diguanidino-2,4,5,6-tetrahydroxycyclohexane, $C_8H_{18}N_6O_4$, obtained when streptomycin undergoes acid hydrolysis; in the streptomycin molecule it is glycosidically linked to streptobiosamine.

strep·to·ba·cil·lary (strep''to·bas'i·lerr·ee) adj. Caused by a streptobacillus.

strep·to·ba·cil·lus (strep''to·ba·sil'us) n., pl. **streptobacil·li** (·eye) A bacillus that remains attached end to end, resulting in the formation of chains. It is a constant characteristic of some strains and appears atypically in others.

Streptobacillus, n. A genus of bacteria whose medical importance derives principally from *Streptobacillus moniliformis.*

Streptobacillus mo·nil·i·for·mis (mo·nil·i·for'mis). The species of *Streptobacillus* that is the etiologic agent of one type of rat-bite fever; namely, Haverhill fever.

strep·to·bi·o·sa·mine (strep''to·bye·o'suh·meen) n. A nitrogen-containing disaccharide, $C_{13}H_{23}NO_9$, obtained when streptomycin undergoes acid hydrolysis; in the streptomycin molecule it is glycosidically linked to streptidine.

strep·to·coc·cal (strep''to·kock'ul) adj. Pertaining to or due to streptococci.

Strep·to·coc·ce·ae (strep''to·kock'see·ee) n.pl. The tribe of gram-positive cocci occurring in pairs or in chains which includes the medically important genera *Diplococcus* and *Streptococcus.*

Strep·to·coc·cus (strep''to·kock'us) n. A genus of gram-positive, chain-forming bacteria of the tribe Streptococceae, family Lactobacteriaceae.

streptococcus. Singular of *streptococci*.

Streptococcus an·he·mo·lyt·i·cus (an-hee-mo-lit'i-kus). GAMMA STREPTOCOCCI.

Streptococcus fe·ca·lis (fee-kay'lis). Enterococci, characterized by group D polysaccharide, which are normal inhabitants of the intestinal contents of man and animals, and which are of importance as penicillin-resistant pathogens in endocarditis and in genitourinary and wound infections.

Streptococcus lac·tis (lack'tis). A group all the members of which produce Lancefield group N C-substance and are nonpathogenic for man. They readily coagulate milk and are important in the dairy industry.

Streptococcus pneu·mo·ni·ae (new-mo'nee-ee). A species of gram-positive, capsulated, nonmotile, facultatively aerobic streptococci which occur singly, in pairs, or in short chains in their natural habitat, the upper respiratory tract of man and other mammals. At least 84 serotypes are now known capable of causing such infectious diseases as pneumonia, meningitis, and otitis media. Formerly called *Diplococcus pneumoniae*. Syn. *pneumococcus*.

Streptococcus py·og·e·nes (pye-oj'e-neez). A species of beta-hemolytic streptococci, Lancefield group A, that causes a variety of suppurative diseases including acute pharyngitis, puerperal sepsis, cellulitis, impetigo, and erysipelas. Nonsuppurative diseases caused by this species include acute glomerulo-nephritis, rheumatic fever, and erythema nodosum.

strep·to·dor·nase (strep″to-dor'nace) n. An enzyme, occurring in filtrates of cultures of certain hemolytic streptococci, capable of hydrolyzing deoxyribonucleoproteins and deoxyribonucleic acid; used, along with streptokinase, for enzymic debridement of infected tissues. Abbreviated, SD. Syn. *streptococcal deoxyribonuclease*.

strep·to·ki·nase (strep″to-kigh'nace) n. A catalytic enzyme, a component of the fibrinolysin occurring in cultures of certain hemolytic streptococci. The enzyme activates the fibrinolytic system present in the euglobulin fraction of human blood. With streptodornase, it is used for enzymic debridement of infected tissues. Abbreviated, SK.

strep·to·ly·sin (strep″to-lye'sin, strep-tol'i-sin) n. A group of hemolysins produced by *Streptococcus pyogenes*. Streptolysin O is oxygen-labile and antigenic. Streptolysin S is an oxygen-stable hemolysin, probably not antigenic, and separable from the streptococcal cells by serum extraction.

Strep·to·my·ces (strep″to-migh'seez) n. A genus of aerobic nonacid-fast, nonfragmenting organisms with branching filaments 1 μm or less in diameter, occupying a position intermediate between the bacteria and the fungi, that are primarily saprophytic inhabitants of the soil. Some species (*Streptomyces somaliensis, S. madurae, S. pelletierii, S. paraguayensis*) are causes of localized mycetomas, and several

others (*S. aureofaciens, S. erythreus*) are sources of antibiotics.

Strep·to·my·ce·ta·ce·ae (strep″to-migh″se·tay′see·ee) n.pl. A family of principally soil-inhabiting organisms that form branching filaments not fragmenting into bacillary and coccoid forms, and which includes the genus *Streptomyces* from which many of the antibiotics have been derived.

strep·to·my·cin (strep″to-migh'sin) n. A water-soluble antibiotic, $C_{21}H_{39}N_7O_{12}$, obtained from *Streptomyces griseus*. It consists of a hydroxylated base, streptidine, glycosidally linked to the disaccharide-like molecule streptobiosamine. It is active against a variety of organisms, but its principal therapeutic use is in the treatment of tuberculosis. Resistant strains of organisms have appeared. The antibiotic may produce toxic effects, of which those involving the eighth cranial nerve are the most serious. It is administered, usually as the sulfate salt, by intramuscular injection; sometimes it is given intravenously or intrathecally.

strep·to·ni·grin (strep″to-nigh'grin) n. An antibiotic, $C_{25}H_{22}N_4O_8$, produced by *Streptomyces flocculus*, that has antineoplastic activity.

strep·to·sep·ti·ce·mia, strep·to·sep·ti·cae·mia (strep″to·sep″ti·see'mee·uh) n. Septicemia due to streptococci.

strep·to·so·mus (strep″to·so'mus) n. A nonhuman form of celosoma in which the spine is twisted so that the legs are displaced laterally.

strep·to·thri·cin (strep″to·thrye'sin, -thris'in) n. An antibiotic substance from *Streptomyces lavendulae*; active against various gram-negative and some gram-positive bacteria.

strep·to·thri·co·sis (strep″to·thri·ko'sis) n. Obsol. Any disease caused by microorganisms formerly included in the genus *Streptothrix*.

Strep·to·thrix (strep'to·thricks) n. A former genus including *Actinomyces, Streptomyces, Streptobacillus*, and other such microorganisms.

stress, n. 1. Force exerted by load, pull, pressure, or other mechanical means; also the exertion of such force. 2. *In medicine,* any stimulus or succession of stimuli of such magnitude as to tend to disrupt the homeostasis of the organism; when mechanisms of adjustment fail or become disproportionate or incoordinate, the stress may be considered an injury, resulting in disease, disability, or death. 3. *In dentistry,* the force exerted by the lower teeth against the upper during mastication.

stress incontinence. Involuntary loss of urine due to activity causing increased intrabdominal pressure.

stretch, v. & n. 1. To draw out to full length. 2. The act of stretching.

stretch·er, n. A litter, particularly one mounted on an easily maneuverable carriage with rubber-shod wheels, used in hospitals for transporting patients.

stretch marks. White or gray, shiny, slightly depressed lines on the anterior abdominal wall skin, or that of the breasts or thighs, following prolonged stretching from such causes as pregnancy, ascites, or obesity. Syn. *striae cutis distensae.*

stretch receptor. A receptor that responds to mechanical deformation wholly brought about by the stretching of the tissue in which the receptor is embedded, such as the stretch receptors stimulated by inflation of the lung which, via ascending vagal nerve fibers, reflexly inhibit the respiratory center.

stretch reflex. Contraction of a muscle in response to sudden brisk longitudinal stretching of the same muscle. Syn. *myotatic reflex.*

stria (strye'uh) *n.,* pl. **stri·ae** (·ee) 1. A streak, stripe, or narrow band. 2. FIBRINOID (2).

stria dis·ten·sa (dis·ten'suh). Singular of *striae (cutis) distensae;* STRETCH MARK.

striae. Plural of *stria.*

striae cu·tis dis·ten·sae (kew'tis dis·ten'see). STRETCH MARK.

stri·a·tal (strye·a'tul) *adj.* Pertaining to the corpus striatum.

striatal epilepsy. *Obsol.* Brief epileptic attacks consisting of tonic spasms of one or both limbs on one side, once attributed to a discharging focus in the corpus striatum.

stri·ate (strye'ate) *adj.* STRIATED.

stri·at·ed (strye'ay·tid) *adj.* Striped, as striated muscle.

striated muscle. Muscle characterized by the banding pattern of cross-striated muscle fibers, seen in skeletal and cardiac muscles.

stri·a·tion (strye·ay'shun) *n.* 1. The state of being striated. 2. STRIA (1).

stri·a·to·pal·li·dal (strye''uh·to·pal'i·dul, strye·ay'to·) *adj.* Of or pertaining to the corpus striatum and globus pallidus.

stri·a·tum (strye·ay'tum) *n.,* pl. **stri·a·ta** (·tuh). CORPUS STRIATUM.

stric·ture (strik'chur) *n.* A circumscribed narrowing of the lumen of a canal or hollow organ, as the esophagus, pylorus, ureter, or urethra, the result of inflammatory or other changes in its walls, and, occasionally, of external pressure. It may be temporary or permanent, depending upon the cause and the course of the disease producing it.

stri·dor (strye'dur) *n.* A high-pitched, harsh, vibrating rale.

stridor den·ti·um (den'shee·um). Grinding of the teeth.

strid·u·lous (strid'yoo·lus) *adj.* Characterized by stridor, as stridulous laryngismus.

strin·gent (strin'junt) *adj.* 1. Rigorous; strict. 2. ASTRINGENT (1). 3. Binding; constricting.

string·halt (string'hawlt) *n.* An involuntary, convulsive movement of the muscles in the hind legs of the horse; the leg is suddenly raised from the ground and lowered again with unnatural force. Syn. *springhalt.*

strio·cel·lu·lar (strye''o·sel'yoo·lur) *adj.* Composed of alternating bands of fibers and cells.

strio·cer·e·bel·lar (strye''o·serr''e·bel'ur) *adj.* Pertaining to the corpus striatum and the cerebellum.

strip, *v.* 1. To press with a milking movement so as to force out the contents of a canal or duct. 2. To remove lengths of varicose saphenous

veins, largely by blind subcutaneous tunneling dissection, using a vein stripper.

stripe, *n.* A streak; a discolored mark. **—striped,** *adj.*

strip·per, *n.* VEIN STRIPPER.

strip·ping, *n.* 1. Uncovering; unsheathing. 2. Removal, after ligation and division, of lengths of varicose saphenous veins from a lower extremity by blind, blunt dissection. 3. (pl.) The last and richest milk given at any one milking; so called because it is slowly removed by the milker, who strips the teats between the fingers.

strob·ic (strob'ick) *adj.* Resembling, or pertaining to, a top.

stro·bi·la (stro·bye'luh) *n.,* pl. **strobi·lae** (·lee) 1. The segmented body of the adult tapeworm. 2. The whole adult tapeworm including the scolex.

strob·i·lus (strob'i·lus) *n.,* pl. **strobi·li** (·lye). The adult tapeworm.

stro·bo·scope (stro'buh·skope, strob'o·) *n.* A device by which a moving object may appear to be at rest; a rapid motion may appear to be slowed, or motion can be depicted by a series of still pictures. The effect depends upon an accurately controlled, intermittent source of light or periodically interrupted vision. **—stro·bo·scop·ic** (·skop'ick) *adj.*

stroke, *n. Informal.* CEREBROVASCULAR ACCIDENT.

stro·ma (stro'muh) *n.,* pl. **stroma·ta** (·tuh) 1. [NA] The supporting framework of an organ, including its connective tissue, vessels, and nerves, as contrasted with the epithelial or other tissues performing the special function of the organ, the parenchyma. 2. The internal structure of erythrocytes after extraction of hemoglobin.

stromal endometriosis. STROMATOSIS.

stromal myosis. STROMATOSIS.

stro·ma·to·sis (stro''muh·to'sis) *n.* The presence throughout the myometrium of collections of tissue similar to the mesenchymal tissue which forms the bulk of the endometrial stroma. Syn. *stromal myosis, stromal endometriosis, endolymphatic stromal myosis.*

stro·muhr (stro'moor) *n.* An instrument for measuring the velocity of blood flow.

Stron·gy·loi·dea (stron''ji·loy'dee·uh) *n.pl.* A superfamily of roundworms, of the suborder Strongylinae, order Rhabditida. The genera *Ancylostoma* and *Necator* are included.

Stron·gy·loi·des (stron''ji·loy'deez) *n.* A genus of nematode worms.

Strongyloides ster·co·ra·lis (stur''ko·ray'lis). An intestinal parasite of man with the same distribution as hookworm. Other species are parasites of lower animals. Syn. *Strongyloides intestinalis.*

stron·gy·loi·di·a·sis (stron''ji·loy·dye'uh·sis) *n.* Infection of the intestines with a roundworm of the genus *Strongyloides.*

stron·ti·um (stron'chee·um, ·tee·um) *n.* Sr = 87.62. A silver-white to pale yellow, malleable, ductile metal; atomic number 38; decomposes in water and alcohol. Certain salts of strontium, notably the bromide and salicylate, have been used for the therapeutic effect of the anions; these have no advantage over the corresponding sodium salts.

stro·phan·thin (stro-fan'thin) n. A glycoside or a mixture of glycosides obtained from *Strophanthus kombé*; a cardioactive drug that has been used in the treatment of various heart ailments but, because of variation in potency, is no longer employed.

stro·phan·thus (stro-fanth'us) n. The dried ripe seeds of *Strophanthus kombé*, or of *S. hispidus*, deprived of the awns; formerly used like digitalis, as a cardiotonic drug.

stroph·u·lus (strof'yoo·lus) n., pl. **strophu·li** (·lye). A form of miliaria occurring in infants, and often unilateral.

struc·tur·al (struck'chur.ul) n. Pertaining to, characterized by, or affecting, a structure.

struc·ture (struck'chur) n. 1. The manner or method of the building up, arrangement, and formation of the different tissues and organs of the body or of a complete organism. 2. An organ, a part, or a complete organic body.

stru·ma (stroo'muh) n., pl. **stru·mae** (·mee) GOITER.

struma lym·pho·ma·to·sa (lim''fo·muh·to'suh). Diffuse thyroid enlargement of unknown origin characterized by retrogressive epithelial changes and lymphoid hyperplasia. Syn. *Hashimoto's struma, lymphadenoid goiter*.

struma ova·rii (o·vair'ee·eye). A rare teratoma of the ovary chiefly or entirely composed of thyroid tissue.

stru·mi·form (stroo'mi·form) adj. Having the appearance of struma; resembling scrofula or goiter.

stru·mi·pri·val (stroo''mi·priv'ul, ·prye'vul, stroo·mip'riv·ul) adj. THYROPRIVAL.

stru·mous (stroo'mus) adj. 1. GOITROUS. 2. SCROFULOUS.

strych·nine (strick'nin, ·nine, ·neen) n. An alkaloid, $C_{21}H_{22}N_2O_2$, obtained chiefly from nux vomica; formerly used for central nervous system stimulation in a variety of ailments but of little, if any, therapeutic merit. Various salts were employed.

strych·nin·iza·tion (strick''ni·ni·zay'shun) n. 1. The condition produced by large doses of strychnine or nux vomica. 2. Topical application of strychnine to areas of the central nervous system to increase nervous excitability and thus facilitate the study of neuron connections.

Strych·nos (strick'nos) n. A genus of the Loganiaceae, which includes *Strychnos nux-vomica*, the source of nux vomica.

S.T.S. Serologic test for syphilis.

S-T segment. The interval of the electrocardiogram between the end of the QRS complex and the beginning of the T wave; usually isoelectric. Syn. $R(S)$-T segment.

S.T.U. Skin test unit.

stump, n. The extremity, pedicle, or basis of the part left after surgical amputation, excision, or ablation.

stun, v. To render temporarily insensible, as by a blow.

stunt, v. To arrest the normal growth and development of an organism.

stu·pe·fa·cient (stew''pe·fay'shunt) n. & adj. NARCOTIC.

stu·pe·fac·tion (stew''pe·fack'shun) n. 1. STUPOR (1). 2. The process of succumbing to stupor. —**stu·pe·fy** (stew'pe·fye) v.

stu·pe·ma·nia (stew''pe·may'nee·uh) n. Mental stupor.

stu·por (stew'pur) n. 1. A state of depressed consciousness in which mental and physical activity are reduced to a minimum and from which one can be aroused only by vigorous and repeated stimuli, at which time response to spoken commands is either absent or slow and inadequate. 2. *In psychiatry*, a state in which impressions of the external environment are normally received but activity is suspended or marked by negativism, as in catatonic schizophrenia. —**stupor·ous** (·us) adj.

stur·dy (stur'dee) n. STAGGERS.

Sturge–Weber disease or **syndrome** A form of neurocutaneous dysplasia defined by the presence of a port-wine nevus of the upper part of the face or scalp and leptomeningeal angiomatosis. Rarely, both sides of the face and cortex may be involved and there may be cutaneous angiomatosis of other parts of the body, as well as buphthalmos, seizures, hemianopsia, hemiparesis, and mental retardation. Syn. *encephalofacial angiomatosis*.

stut·ter, n. & v. 1. Speech marked by the intermittent inability to enunciate a phonetic segment not more than one syllable in length without repeating it, straining unnaturally, or doing both. 2. To speak in such a manner. —**stutter·er** (·ur) n.

stutter spasm. Spasm of the lingual and palatal muscles, psychogenic in origin, resulting in stuttering speech.

sty, stye, n., pl. **sties, styes** HORDEOLUM.

styl-, stylo-. A combining form signifying *styloid process of the temporal bone*.

sty·let (stye'lit) n. 1. A wire inserted into a soft catheter or cannula to insure rigidity. 2. A fine wire inserted into a hollow hypodermic needle or other hollow needle to maintain patency.

sty·lo·glos·sus (stye''lo·glos'us) n. A muscle arising from the styloid process of the temporal bone, and inserted into the tongue. —**styloglos·sal** (·ul) adj.

sty·lo·hy·oid (stye''lo·high'oid) adj. Pertaining to the styloid process of the temporal bone and the hyoid bone.

sty·loid (stye'loid) adj. Having one end slender and pointed.

styloid process of the temporal bone. A sharp spine about an inch in length, descending downward, forward, and inward from the inferior surface of the petrous portion of the temporal bone.

sty·lo·man·dib·u·lar (stye''lo·man·dib'yoo·lur) adj. Pertaining to the styloid process of the temporal bone and the mandible.

sty·lo·mas·toid (stye''lo·mas'toid) adj. Pertaining to the styloid and the mastoid processes of the temporal bone.

sty·lo·pha·ryn·ge·us (stye″lo·fa·rin″jee·us) *n.* A muscle arising from the styloid process of the temporal bone, and inserted into the pharynx.

sty·ma·to·sis (stye″muh·to′sis) *n.* A violent erection of the penis attended with hemorrhage.

styp·tic (stip′tick) *adj. & n.* 1. Having the effect of checking hemorrhage. 2. An agent that checks hemorrhage by causing contraction of the blood vessels, as alum, tannic acid.

sub- A prefix meaning (a) *under, beneath;* (b) *less than, below;* (c) *just short of, immediately underlying;* (d) *partial, slight, mild;* (e) *subordinate, subsidiary;* (f) in chemistry, *basic;* (g) *containing less of a given radical than another compound of the same elements.*

sub·ab·dom·i·nal (sub″ab·dom′i·nul) *adj.* Beneath the abdomen.

sub·ac·e·tate (sub·as′e·tate) *n.* A basic acetate, as lead subacetate.

sub·acro·mi·al (sub″uh·kro′mee·ul) *adj.* Beneath the acromion.

sub·acute (sub″uh·kewt′) *adj.* 1. Somewhat less than acute in severity. 2. Of a disease, intermediate in character between acute and chronic.

subacute appendicitis. Mild acute appendicitis.

subacute bacterial endocarditis. BACTERIAL ENDOCARDITIS.

subacute combined degeneration of the spinal cord. Combined degeneration of posterior and lateral columns of the spinal cord due to deficiency of vitamin B_{12}; the neurological component of pernicious anemia.

subacute sclerosing panencephalitis. Diffuse inflammation of the brain affecting chiefly children and associated with inclusion bodies in neuronal nuclei or cytoplasm, pursuing an indolent course of months or years, with occasional partial remissions; personality changes, seizures, blindness, and progressive dementia terminate in a febrile, decerebrate state. Now linked etiologically to slow infection with measles virus.

subacute spongiform encephalopathy. A distinctive cerebral disease, in which a profound and rapidly progressive dementia is associated with ataxia and myoclonic jerks. The neuropathologic changes consist of widespread neuronal loss and gliosis accompanied by a striking vacuolation or spongy state in the cerebral and cerebellar cortices. Like kuru, subacute spongiform encephalopathy is due to a transmissible agent, possibly a virus.

sub·al·i·men·ta·tion (sub·al″i·men·tay′shun) *n.* Inadequate or deficient nourishment.

sub·aor·tic stenosis (sub·ay·or′tick). Narrowing of the left ventricular outflow tract immediately proximal to the orifice of the aortic valve; it may be localized or diffuse, membranous or muscular. Syn. *subvalvular aortic stenosis.*

sub·ap·i·cal (sub·ap′i·kul, ·ay′pi·kul) *adj.* Beneath an apex.

sub·ap·o·neu·rot·ic (sub·ap″o·new·rot′ick) *adj.* Beneath an aponeurosis.

sub·arach·noid (sub″uh·rack′noid) *adj.* Beneath the arachnoid.

subarachnoid block. A condition in which an obstruction in the subarachnoid space prevents the normal flow of cerebrospinal fluid.

subarachnoid hemorrhage. 1. Blood in the subarachnoid space from any cause. 2. SPONTANEOUS SUBARACHNOID HEMORRHAGE.

subarachnoid space. The space between the arachnoid and the pia mater, containing subarachnoid trabeculae and filled with cerebrospinal fluid.

sub·ar·cu·ate (sub·ahr′kew·ate) *adj.* Slightly arched or curved.

sub·are·o·lar (sub″a·ree′o·lur) *adj.* Situated, or occurring, beneath the mammary areola.

sub·atom·ic (sub″uh·tom′ick) *adj.* Pertaining to the structure or components of atoms.

sub·au·ric·u·lar (sub″aw·rick′yoo·lur) *adj.* Below the auricle or external ear.

sub·ax·il·lary (sub·ack′si·lerr″ee) *adj.* Under the armpit.

sub·cal·ca·rine (sub·kal′cuh·rine, ·reen) *adj.* Situated beneath the calcarine sulcus.

subcalcarine gyrus. A narrow convolution ventral to the cuneus and lying between the collateral and calcarine sulci.

sub·cal·lo·sal (sub″ka·lo′sul) *adj.* Below the corpus callosum.

sub·cap·su·lar (sub·kap′sue·lur) *adj.* Beneath a capsule.

sub·cer·vi·cal (sub″sur′vi·kul) *adj.* Beneath a neck.

sub·chlo·ride (sub·klo′ride) *n.* The chloride of a series which contains relatively the least chlorine.

sub·chon·dral (sub·kon′drul) *adj.* Situated beneath cartilage.

sub·cho·ri·on·ic (sub·ko″ree·on′ick) *adj.* Beneath the chorion.

sub·cho·roi·dal (sub″ko·roy′dul) *adj.* Beneath the choroid membrane of the eye.

sub·chron·ic (sub·kron′ick) *adj.* More nearly chronic than subacute.

sub·cla·vi·an (sub·klay′vee·un) *adj.* Lying under the clavicle, as the subclavian artery.

subclavian artery. See Table of Arteries in the Appendix.

subclavian steal syndrome. A vascular syndrome due to occlusion of the subclavian artery proximal to the origin of the vertebral artery, with reversal of the normal blood pressure gradient in the vertebral artery and decreased blood flow distal to the occlusion, manifested by pain in the mastoid and posterior head regions, episodes of flaccid paralysis of the arm, and diminished or absent radial pulse on the side involved.

sub·clin·i·cal (sub·klin′i·kul) *adj.* Pertaining to a disease in which manifestations are so slight as to be unnoticeable or even not demonstrable.

sub·cli·noid (sub·klye′noid) *adj.* Beneath a clinoid process.

sub·col·lat·er·al (sub″kuh·lat′ur·ul) *adj.* Ventral to the collateral sulcus of the brain.

sub·con·junc·ti·val (sub″kon·junk·tye′vul) *adj.* Situated beneath the conjunctiva.

sub·con·scious (sub·kon′shus) *n. & adj.* 1. In *psychiatry,* mental material outside the range of clear consciousness, including the preconscious which can be recalled with effort as well as the unconscious, which is nevertheless capable of determining conscious mental or physical reactions. 2. Of, pertaining, or belonging to such mental material.

sub·con·scious·ness (sub·kon′shus·nus) *n.* A state or condition in which mental processes take place without the mind being distinctly conscious of its own activity.

sub·cor·a·coid (sub·kor′uh·koid) *adj.* Situated below the coracoid process, as subcoracoid dislocation of the humerus.

sub·cor·ne·al (sub″kor′nee·ul) *adj.* Beneath the horny layer of the skin.

sub·cor·ti·cal (sub·kor′ti·kul) *adj.* 1. Beneath a cortex. 2. Beneath the cerebral cortex.

sub·cos·tal (sub·kos′tul) *adj.* Lying beneath a rib or the ribs.

sub·cos·tal·gia (sub″kos·tal′jee·uh) *n.* Pain beneath the ribs, or over a subcostal nerve.

sub·crep·i·tant (sub·krep′i·tunt) *adj.* Almost or faintly crepitant.

subcrepitant rale. A fine moist crackling sound similar to a crepitant rale, but coarser and lower pitched. Syn. *crackling rale.*

sub·crep·i·ta·tion (sub·krep″i·tay′shun) *n.* An indistinctly crepitant sound.

sub·cul·ture (sub′kul″chur) *n.* 1. *In microbiology,* the procedure of transferring organisms from one culture to fresh culture medium; also, the resulting culture. 2. *In anthropology and sociology,* the culture that is characteristic of a particular subgroup (community, class, ethnic group, age group, etc.) of a society.

sub·cu·ta·ne·ous (sub″kew·tay′nee·us) *adj.* Beneath the skin; HYPODERMIC.

subcutaneous emphysema. The accumulation of air or gas in the subcutaneous tissues.

subcutaneous inguinal ring. SUPERFICIAL INGUINAL RING.

subcutaneous tissue. The layer of loose connective tissue under the dermis.

sub·cu·tic·u·lar (sub″kew·tick′yoo·lur) *adj.* Beneath the epidermis.

sub·cu·tis (sub·kew′tis) *n.* The superficial fascia below the skin or cutis.

sub·de·lir·i·um (sub″de·lirr′ee·um) *n.* A slight or muttering delirium, with lucid intervals.

sub·del·toid (sub·del′toid) *adj.* Beneath the deltoid muscle.

sub·der·mal (sub·dur′mul) *adj.* HYPODERMIC (1, 2).

sub·di·a·phrag·mat·ic (sub″dye″uh·frag·mat′ick) *adj.* Under the diaphragm.

sub·di·vid·ed (sub″di·vye′did) *adj.* Redivided; making secondary or smaller divisions.

sub·duct (sub·dukt′) *v.* To draw downward.

sub·du·ral (sub·dew′rul) *adj.* Beneath the dura mater.

subdural hematoma. A collection of blood between the dura mater and the arachnoid, involving one or both hemispheres, usually due to head trauma, but also seen in blood dyscrasias and cachexia; classified as neonatal, acute, subacute, or chronic according to time of occurrence and the duration of the symptoms and signs, which vary with the age of the patient and extent of neurologic involvement, but which usually include depression of consciousness, seizures, and focal neurologic deficits such as hemiplegia.

subdural space. The space between the dura mater and the arachnoid which usually contains only a capillary layer of fluid.

sub·du·ro·peri·to·ne·al shunt (sub·dew″ro·perr″i·to·nee′ul). Surgical communication between the subdural space and the peritoneal cavity by means of a plastic or rubber tube for the relief of subdural effusion.

sub·en·do·car·di·al (sub″en″do·kahr′dee·ul) *adj.* Beneath the endocardium or between the endocardium and myocardium.

sub·en·do·the·li·al (sub″en″do·theel′ee·ul) *adj.* Underneath the endothelium.

sub·ep·en·dy·mal (sub″ep·en′di·mul) *adj.* Under the ependyma.

sub·ep·en·dy·mo·ma (sub″e·pen″di·mo′muh) *n.* A tumor usually found in the fourth ventricle of the brain, sometimes in relation to other ventricles, and often discovered accidentally at autopsy, due to proliferation of fibrillary subependymal astrocytes.

sub·epi·der·mal (sub″ep″i·dur′mul) *adj.* Beneath the epidermis.

sub·ep·i·the·li·al (sub″ep·i·theel′ee·ul) *adj.* Under the epithelium.

su·ber·o·sis (sue″bur·o′sis) *n.* A form of pneumoconiosis affecting cork workers, characterized by bronchial asthma or disordered gas exchange in the alveoli.

sub·gal·late (sub·gal′ate) *n.* A basic salt of gallic acid.

sub·gin·gi·val (sub·jin′ji·vul, ·jin·jye′vul) *adj.* Beneath the gingiva.

sub·gle·noid (sub·glee′noid, ·glen′oid) *adj.* Beneath the glenoid cavity of the scapula, as subglenoid dislocation of the humerus.

sub·glos·si·tis (sub″glos·eye′tis) *n.* Inflammation of the tissues under the tongue.

sub·gron·da·tion (sub″gron·day′shun) *n.* The intrusion of one fragment of a cranial bone beneath another part in a fracture.

sub·hy·a·loid (sub·high′uh·loid) *adj.* Beneath the hyaloid membrane.

sub·hy·oid (sub·high′oid) *adj.* Beneath the hyoid bone.

su·bic·u·lum (suh·bick′yoo·lum, sue·) *n.,* pl. **subic·u·la** (·luh) An underlying structure. —**subicu·lar** (·lur) *adj.*

sub·in·ci·sion (sub″in·sizh′un) *n.* Making a permanent opening into the urethra through the undersurface of the penis, a practice common in some primitive tribes, especially those of central Australia. It does not impair coitus or cause sterility.

sub·in·fec·tion (sub″in·feck′shun) *n.* Infection with slight or no overt clinical manifestations of disease.

sub·in·gui·nal (sub·ing′gwi·nul) *adj.* Distal to the inguinal region or groin.

sub·in·vo·lu·tion (sub″in·vo·lew′shun) *n.* Imperfect return to normal size after functional enlargement.

subinvolution of the uterus. The imperfect involution of the uterus after delivery.

sub·io·dide (sub·eye′o·dide) *n.* The iodide of a series containing the least iodine.

sub·ja·cent (sub-jay'sunt) *adj.* Lying beneath.

sub·jec·tive, *adj.* 1. Pertaining to or centered on the subject, or that which perceives or observes, as distinguished from the object or that which is observed. 2. Perceived or experienced by an individual himself but not directly observable by others, as sensations in general, or as a patient's symptoms in contrast to objective signs of disease. 3. Originating internally but mimicking to some extent sensations produced by external stimuli, as a ringing in the ears, dizziness, muscae volitantes, or hallucinations. 4. Conceived in terms of an individual's more immediate experiences and responses, with relatively little adjustment for perspective.

subjective sign. A sign or symptom recognized only by the patient.

sub·la·tion (sub-lay'shun) *n.* Removal; ABLATION.

sub·le·thal (sub-lee'thul) *adj.* Less than fatal, as a sublethal dose of poison.

sub·leu·ke·mic, sub·leu·kae·mic (sub''lew-kee'mick) *adj.* Less than leukemic; usually applied to states in which the peripheral blood manifestations of leukemia are temporarily suppressed.

¹sub·li·mate (sub'li·mate) *n.* A solid or condensed substance obtained by heating a material, which passes directly from the solid to the vapor phase and then back to the solid state.

²sub·li·mate (sub'li·mate) *v. In psychiatry,* to express or externalize instinctual impulses in a socially acceptable or conventional manner.

sub·li·ma·tion (sub''li·may'shun) *n.* 1. The transformation of a solid to the gaseous state, followed by condensation to the solid state; used to purify substances such as iodine and mercuric chloride. 2. *In psychiatry,* a defense mechanism, working unconsciously, whereby undesirable instinctual cravings and impulses gain outward expression by converting their energies into socially acceptable activities.

sub·lime (suh·blime') *v.* To successively volatilize and condense a solid. Noun *sublimation.*

sub·lim·i·nal (sub·lim'i·nul) *adj.* 1. Below the limit of conscious perception. 2. SUBTHRESHOLD.

sub·li·mis (sub·lye'mis) *adj.* Elevated; superficial, a qualification applied to certain muscles, as the flexor digitorum sublimis.

sub·lin·gual (sub·ling'gwul) *adj.* 1. Beneath the tongue. 2. Pertaining to the structures under the tongue.

sublingual gland. A complex of small salivary glands situated in the sublingual fold on each side of the oral floor. The anterior third to half of this complex on each side commonly is drained by a single duct, the major sublingual duct. The remaining glands are drained by the 5 to 15 or more minor sublingual ducts.

sub·lin·gui·tis (sub''ling-gwye'tis) *n.* Inflammation of sublingual gland.

sub·lob·u·lar (sub''lob'yoo·lur) *adj.* Situated beneath or at the base of a liver lobule or lobules.

sub·lux (sub·lucks') *v.* To cause subluxation.

sub·lux·a·tion (sub''luck·say'shun) *n.* IN-

COMPLETE DISLOCATION. —**sub·lux·at·ed** (sub·luck'say·tid) *adj.*

sub·mal·le·o·lar (sub''ma·lee'uh·lur) *adj.* Under the malleoli, as submalleolar amputation, removal of the foot at the ankle joint.

sub·mam·ma·ry (sub·mam'uh·ree) *adj.* Situated beneath a mammary gland.

sub·man·dib·u·lar (sub''man·dib'yoo·lur) *adj.* Below or beneath the mandible.

sub·max·il·lar·i·tis (sub''mack·sil''uh·rye'tis) *n.* Inflammation of a submandibular gland.

sub·max·il·lary (sub·mack'si·lerr''ee) *adj.* SUBMANDIBULAR.

sub·men·tal (sub·men'tul) *adj.* Situated under the chin.

sub·mi·cro·scop·ic (sub''migh·kruh·skop'ick) *adj.* Pertaining to a particle that is too small to be resolved by the optical microscope.

sub·mil·i·ary (sub·mil'ee·err·ee) *adj.* Smaller than the usual nodules that are described as miliary, or millet seed, in size.

sub·mor·phous (sub·mor'fus) *adj.* Having a structure intermediate between amorphous and true crystalline; often applied to the indefinite, partially crystalline structure of calculi.

sub·mu·co·sa (sub''mew·ko'suh) *n.* The layer of fibrous connective tissue that attaches a mucous membrane to its subjacent parts. —**sub·muco·sal** (·sul), **sub·mu·cous** (sub·mew'kus) *adj.*

submucous plexus. A visceral nerve network lying in the submucosa of the digestive tube. Syn. *Meissner's plexus.*

sub·nar·cot·ic (sub''nahr·kot'ick) *adj.* Moderately narcotic.

sub·ni·trate (sub·nigh'trate) *n.* A basic nitrate.

sub·nor·mal (sub·nor'mul) *adj.* Below normal. —**sub·nor·mal·ity** (sub''nor·mal'i·tee) *n.*

sub·nu·cle·us (sub·new'klee·us) *n.* Any one of the smaller groups of cells into which a large nerve nucleus is divided by the passage through it of nerve bundles.

sub·oc·cip·i·tal (sub''ock·sip'i·tul) *adj.* Situated beneath the occiput.

sub·or·bit·al (sub·or'bi·tul) *adj.* Situated beneath the orbit.

sub·or·di·na·tion, *n.* 1. The condition of being under subjection or control. 2. The condition of organs that depend upon or are controlled by other organs.

sub·pap·il·la·ry (sub·pap'i·lerr''ee) *adj.* Beneath the stratum papillare.

sub·par·a·lyt·ic (sub''păr''uh·lit'ick) *adj.* Not completely paralytic.

sub·pa·ri·e·tal (sub''puh·rye'e·tul) *adj.* Situated below the parietal lobe.

sub·pec·to·ral (sub·peck'tuh·rul) *adj.* Situated beneath the chest muscles.

sub·peri·car·di·al (sub''perr·i·kahr'dee·ul) *adj.* Situated beneath the pericardium.

sub·peri·os·te·al (sub''perr·ee·os'tee·ul) *adj.* Beneath the periosteum.

sub·peri·to·ne·al (sub''perr''i·to·nee'ul) *adj.* Beneath peritoneum.

sub·phren·ic (sub·fren'ick) *adj.* SUBDIAPHRAGMATIC.

sub·pla·cen·ta (sub''pluh·sen'tuh) *n.* DECIDUA PARIETALIS.

sub·pla·cen·tal (sub″pluh·sen′tul) *adj.* 1. Situated beneath the placenta. 2. Pertaining to the decidua parietalis.

sub·plan·ti·grade (sub·plan′ti·grade) *adj.* Incompletely plantigrade; walking with the heel slightly elevated.

sub·pleu·ral (sub·ploo′rul) *adj.* Situated beneath the pleura.

sub·pu·bic (sub·pew′bick) *adj.* Situated beneath the pubic arch or symphysis.

sub·sar·to·ri·al (sub″sahr·to′ree·ul) *adj.* Situated beneath the sartorius muscle.

sub·scap·u·lar (sub·skap′yoo·lur) *adj.* 1. Beneath the scapula. 2. Pertaining to the subscapularis muscle.

sub·scrip·tion, *n.* The part of a prescription containing the directions to the pharmacist, indicating how the ingredients are to be mixed and prepared.

sub·se·rous (sub·seer′us) *adj.* Beneath a serous membrane.

sub·sib·i·lant (sub·sib′i·lunt) *adj.* Having a sound like a muffled whistling.

sub·si·dence (sub·sigh′dunce, sub′si·dunce) *n.* Gradual cessation and disappearance, as of the manifestations of disease.

sub·sig·moid (sub·sig′moid) *adj.* Under the sigmoid flexure.

sub·spi·nous (sub·spye′nus) *adj.* 1. Beneath a spine. 2. Beneath the spinal column.

sub·stage, *n.* The parts beneath the stage of a microscope, including the diaphragm, condenser, mirror, and other accessories.

sub·stan·tia (sub·stan′shee·uh) *n.,* pl. & genit. sing. **substan·ti·ae** (·shee·ee) Substance; matter.

substantia al·ba (al′buh) [NA]. WHITE SUBSTANCE.

substantia alba me·dul·lae spi·na·lis (me·dul′ee spye·nay′lis) [NA]. The white matter of the spinal cord.

substantia com·pac·ta (kom·pack′tuh) [NA]. COMPACT BONE.

substantia ni·gra (nigh′gruh) [NA]. A broad, thick plate of large, pigmented nerve cells separating the basis pedunculi from the tegmentum and extending from the border of the pons through the mesencephalon into the hypothalamus.

substantia propria of the cornea. The central, transparent, lamellated layer of dense connective tissue in the cornea.

sub·ster·nal (sub″stur′nul) *adj.* Beneath the sternum, as substernal pain.

sub·sti·tu·tion, *n.* 1. The replacement of one thing by another to serve a similar function. 2. *In chemistry.* the replacing of one or more elements or radicals in a compound by other elements or radicals. 3. *In psychiatry,* a defense mechanism whereby alternative or substitutive gratifications are secured to reduce tension resulting from frustration. The substitutes are generally comparable to the pleasures and satisfactions which the individual was frustrated in obtaining.

substitution therapy. The use in treatment of substances the normal secretion of which is deficient or absent.

sub·strate (sub′strate) *n.* 1. An underlayer. 2. A substance upon which an enzyme acts.

sub·sul·to·ry (sub·sul′tuh·ree) *adj.* Leaping; twitching; convulsive.

sub·sul·tus (sub·sul′tus) *n.* A convulsive jerking or twitching.

subsultus ten·di·num (ten′di·num). *Obsol.* Involuntary twitching of the muscles, especially of the hands and feet, seen with some fevers.

sub·syn·ap·tic (sub″si·nap′tick) *adj.* POSTSYNAPTIC.

sub·ta·lar (sub·tay′lur) *adj.* Beneath the talus.

sub·tem·po·ral (sub·tem′puh·rul) *adj.* Situated beneath the temporal region of the skull.

subtemporal decompression. Cranial decompression by an approach in the temporal region.

sub·ten·to·ri·al (sub″ten·to′ree·ul) *adj.* Below or beneath the tentorium cerebelli.

sub·te·tan·ic (sub″te·tan′ick) *adj.* Not quite tetanic; applied to seizures which are tonic with brief periods of relaxation but not clonic.

sub·tha·lam·ic (sub″thuh·lam′ick) *adj.* Below the thalamus.

subthalamic nucleus. A biconvex nucleus between the internal capsule and the cerebral peduncle, having well-developed connections with the globus pallidus. Syn. *corpus Luysii.*

sub·thal·a·mus (sub·thal′uh·mus) *n.* SUBTHALAMIC REGION.

sub·thresh·old, *adj.* Pertaining to a stimulus of insufficient strength to produce a response.

sub·ti·lin (sub′ti·lin) *n.* An antibiotic substance obtained from *Bacillus subtilis,* active against gram-positive bacteria.

sub·to·tal (sub″to′tul) *adj.* Less than complete.

sub·tra·pe·zi·al (sub″tra·pee′zee·ul) *adj.* Located beneath the trapezius muscle.

sub·trig·o·nal (sub·trig′uh·nul, ·tri·go′nul) *adj.* Situated beneath the trigone.

sub·tro·chan·ter·ic (sub·tro″kan·terr′ick) *adj.* Below a trochanter.

sub·trop·i·cal (sub·trop′i·kul) *adj.* Almost tropical in climate.

sub·uber·es (sub·yoo′bur·eez) *n.pl.* Children at the breast; suckling children.

sub·um·bil·i·cal (sub″um·bil′i·kul) *adj.* Situated below the umbilicus.

sub·un·gual (sub″ung′gwul) *adj.* Beneath a nail.

sub·ure·thral (sub″yoo·ree′thrul) *adj.* Situated beneath the urethra.

sub·val·vu·lar (sub·val′vew·lur) *adj.* Beneath a valve, usually a cardiac semilunar valve.

sub·vir·ile (sub·virr′il) *adj.* Deficient in virility.

sub·vi·ta·min·o·sis (sub·vye″tuh·mi·no′sis) *n.* A state of vitamin deficiency.

sub·vo·lu·tion (sub″vo·lew′shun) *n.* A method of operating for pterygium, in which a flap is turned over so that an outer or cutaneous surface comes in contact with a raw, dissected surface. Adhesions are thus prevented.

sub·wak·ing (sub·way′king) *adj.* Pertaining to the state between sleeping and complete wakefulness.

Sucaryl. Trademark for the noncaloric sweeteners calcium cyclamate (Sucaryl Calcium) and sodium cyclamate (Sucaryl Sodium).

suc·ce·da·ne·ous (suck″se·day′nee·us)

1. Pertaining to, or acting as, a substitute.
2. Pertaining to that which follows after.

suc·cen·tu·ri·ate (suck″sen·tew′ree·ut) *adj.* ACCESSORY.

suc·cif·er·ous (suck·sif′ur·us) *adj.* Producing sap.

suc·ci·nate (suck′si·nate) *n.* A salt or ester of succinic acid.

suc·cin·ic acid (suck·sin′ick) Butanedioic acid, $HOOCCH_2CH_2COOH$, an intermediate in the tricarboxylic acid cycle. Formerly variously used for medicinal purposes. The sodium salt has been used as an analeptic in barbiturate poisoning.

suc·ci·nyl·sul·fa·thi·a·zole (suck″si·nil·sul′fuh·thigh′uh·zole) *n.* 4′-(2-Thiazolylsulfamoyl)-succinanilic acid, $C_{13}H_{13}N_3O_5S_2$, a poorly absorbed sulfonamide used as an intestinal antibacterial agent in preoperative preparation of patients for abdominal surgery; also postoperatively to maintain a low bacterial count.

suc·cor·rhea, suc·cor·rhoea (suck″o·ree′uh) *n.* An excessive flow of a secretion, as of saliva or gastric juice.

suc·cu·lent, *adj.* Juicy.

suc·cur·sal (suh·kur′sul) *adj.* Subsidiary.

suc·cus (suck′us) *n.,* pl. **suc·ci** (·sigh) 1. A vegetable juice. 2. An animal secretion.

succus en·ter·i·cus (en·ter′i·kus). The intestinal juice, secreted by the glands of the intestinal mucous membrane. It is thin, opalescent, alkaline, and has a specific gravity of 1.011.

succus gas·tri·cus (gas′tri·kus). GASTRIC JUICE.

succus pan·cre·a·ti·cus (pan·kree·at′i·kus). PANCREATIC JUICE.

suc·cus·sion (suh·kush′un) *n.* A shaking, especially of an individual, to determine the presence of free fluid and gas in a cavity or hollow organ of the body.

succussion sound or **splash.** The splashing sound heard on succussion when there is free fluid and gas in a body cavity or hollow organ.

suck, *v.* 1. To draw up a liquid or gel as by the partial vacuum created by a suction apparatus, or the motions of the mouth, tongue, and lips. 2. Specifically, to nurse at the breast or, in an animal, the udder.

suck·ing, *n.* Nursing; drawing with the mouth.

sucking reflex. Sucking movements of the lips, tongue, and jaw in response to contact of an object with the lips, seen normally in infants, but observed abnormally and often in exaggerated form in patients with bilateral frontal lobe lesions.

sucking wound. A wound in the chest wall through which air is taken in and expelled; seen in traumatopnea.

suck·le, *v.* To nurse at the breast.

suck·ling, *n.* A nursling; especially, a young child or animal that is not yet weaned.

su·crase (sue′krace) *n.* SACCHARASE.

su·crate (sue′krate) *n.* A salt of saccharic acid.

su·crose (sue′kroce, ·kroze) *n.* A sugar, $C_{12}H_{22}O_{11}$, obtained from the plants *Saccharum officinarum, Beta vulgaris,* and other sources; used as a carbohydrate food and as a sweetening agent. Syn. *saccharum, sugar.*

suc·tion, *n.* 1. The act of sucking. 2. The act or the force developed by reducing the atmospheric pressure over a surface or a substance.

suction abortion. SUCTION CURETTAGE.

suction curet. A small hollow tube with a cutting window to which suction may be applied; used for obtaining endometrial biopsy.

suction curettage. Abortion by means of a suction device inserted into the uterus; effective during the first trimester of pregnancy.

suction test. DALLDORF TEST.

sud-, sudo- A combining form meaning *perspiration. sweat.*

su·da·men (sue·day′mun) *n.,* pl. **su·dam·i·na** (·dam′i·nuh) A skin disease in which sweat accumulates under the superficial horny layers of the epidermis to form small, clear, transparent vesicles.

Su·dan dye or **stain** (soo·dan′). Any one of a number of related fat-soluble dyes used as biological stains. They are related by being oil-soluble and by being aromatic compounds, but fall into at least three chemical groups.

su·dano·phil·ia (soo·dan″o·fil′ee·uh) *n.* An affinity for or staining fat-soluble dyes in general, but especially Sudan dyes. **—sudanophil·ic** (·ick) *adj.*

sudanophilic leukodystrophy. An inherited disease of the nervous system, affecting only males and having its onset between four and sixteen years; characterized by atrophy of the adrenal cortex and widespread degeneration of myelin in the central nervous system associated, in recent lesions, with fat-laden (sudan-positive) macrophages; Originally included under the rubric of Schilder's disease but now considered to be an independent metabolic encephalopathy.

su·da·tion (sue·day′shun) *n.* Sweating.

su·da·to·ri·um (sue″duh·to′ree·um) *n.,* pl. **sudato·ria** (·ree·uh) 1. A hot-air bath. 2. A room for the administration of a hot-air bath.

sudden infant death syndrome. The syndrome of sudden, unexpected death of an apparently healthy infant, occurring almost always during a sleep period and most commonly between the ages of 1 and 4 months. Postmortem examination usually reveals only the results of a fatal apneic episode, and though the etiology remains essentially unknown and perhaps multiple, there is evidence that many such infant deaths are preceded by a period of chronic but subclinical hypoxia. Abbreviated, SIDS. Syn. *crib death, sleep apnea syndrome.*

Su·deck's atrophy, disease, or **dystrophy** (zoo′deck) Acute bone atrophy or aseptic necrosis of bone following injury. Syn. *traumatic osteoporosis.*

su·do·mo·tor (sue″do·mo′tur) *adj.* Pertaining to the efferent nerves that control the activity of sweat glands.

su·dor (sue′dur, ·dor) *n.* SWEAT. **—sudor·al** (·ul) *adj.*

su·do·re·sis (sue″duh·ree′sis) *n.* Excessive sweating.

su·do·rif·er·ous (sue″dur·if′ur·us) *adj.* Producing sweat.

su·do·rif·ic (sue″dur·if′ick) *adj. & n.* 1. Tending to induce sweating. 2. An agent that induces sweating.

su·do·rip·a·rous (sue″dur·ip′uh·rus) *adj.* Secreting sweat.

sudor noc·tur·nus (nock·tur′nus). NIGHT SWEAT.

suf·fo·cate (suf′uh·kate) *v.* ASPHYXIATE.

suf·fo·ca·tion (suf″uh·kay′shun) *n.* Interference with the entrance of air into the lungs and resultant asphyxiation.

suf·fu·sion (suh·few′zhun) *n.* 1. A spreading or flow of any fluid of the body into surrounding tissue; an extensive extravasation of blood. 2. The pouring of water upon a patient as a remedial measure. —**suf·fuse** (·fewz′) *v.*

sug·ar, *n.* 1. Any carbohydrate having a sweet taste and the general formula $C_nH_{2n}O_n$ or $C_nH_{2n-2}O_{n-1}$. 2. SUCROSE.

sugar-coated spleen. ICED SPLEEN.

sug·gest·ibil·i·ty (sug·jes″ti·bil′i·tee) *n.* The condition of being readily influenced by another; an abnormal state when the individual conforms with unusual readiness, as patients who too readily accept ideas of health or illness.

sug·gest·ible, *adj.* Amenable to suggestion.

sug·ges·tion, *n.* 1. *In psychiatry,* the influencing of an individual to accept uncritically a belief, attitude, or feeling put forward by the therapist. 2. The artificial production of a certain psychic state in which the individual experiences such sensations as are suggested to him or ceases to experience those which he is instructed not to feel. 3. The thing suggested.

sug·ges·tion·ist (sug·jes′chun·ist) *n.* A person who treats disease by means of suggestion or who employs hypnotherapy. —**suggestion·ize** (·ize) *v.*

suggestion therapy. Treating disordered states by means of suggestion.

sug·gil·la·tion (sug″ji·lay′shun, suj′i·) *n.* An ecchymosis or bruise.

sui·cide, *n.* 1. Self-murder; intentionally taking one's own life. 2. One who takes his own life. —**su·i·ci·dal** (sue″i·sigh′dul) *adj.*

su·i·ci·dol·o·gy (sue″i·si·dol′uh·jee) *n.* The study of the causes and prevention of suicide.

Sulamyd. A trademark for sulfacetamide.

sul·cal (sul′kul) *adj.* Pertaining to a sulcus.

sulci. Plural and genitive singular of sulcus.

sul·cus (sul′kus) *n.* pl. & genit. sing. **sul·ci** (·sigh) 1. A furrow or linear groove, as in a bone. When applied to linear depressions on the cerebral hemisphere, the term indicates a less deep depression than a fissure. Sulci in the brain separate the convolutions or gyri. 2. *In dentistry,* a longitudinal groove in the surface of a tooth the inclines of which meet at an angle; a developmental groove lies at the junction of the inclines.

sulcus terminalis lin·guae (ling′gwee) [NA]. TERMINAL LINGUAL SULCUS.

sul·fa·cet·a·mide (sul″fuh·set′uh·mide) *n.* N-Sulfanilylacetamide, $C_8H_{10}N_2O_3S$, used for the treatment of urinary tract infections; the sodium derivative is used for treatment of ophthalmic infections susceptible to sulfonamides.

sul·fa·di·a·zine (sul″fuh·dye′uh·zeen, ·zin, ·dye·az′een) *n.* N^1-2-Pyrimidinylsulfanilamide, $C_{10}H_{10}N_4O_2S$, an antibacterial sulfonamide used in the treatment of a variety of infections; frequently given in combination with sulfamerazine and sulfamethazine. Sodium sulfadiazine, which is freely soluble in water, is used when the drug is to be administered intravenously.

sul·fa drugs (sul′fuh). A family of drugs of the sulfonamide type which have marked bacteriostatic properties.

sul·fa·gua·ni·dine (sul″fuh·gwah′ni·deen, ·gwan′i·deen, ·din) *n.* N^1-Amidinosulfanilamide, $C_7H_{10}N_4O_2S$, an intestinal antibacterial sulfonamide proposed for treatment of dysentery and for sterilization of the colon prior to gastrointestinal tract surgery.

sul·fa·mer·a·zine (sul″fuh·merr′uh·zeen, ·zin) *n.* N^1-(4-Methyl-2-pyrimidinyl)sulfanilamide, $C_{11}H_{12}N_4O_2S$; used like sulfadiazine but generally employed in combination with it and with sulfamethazine.

sul·fa·meth·a·zine (sul″fuh·meth′uh·zeen, ·zin) *n.* N^1-(4,6-Dimethyl-2-pyrimidinyl)sulfanilamide, $C_{12}H_{14}N_4O_2S$; used like sulfadiazine but generally employed in combination with it and with sulfamerazine. Syn. *sulphadimidine, sulfamezathine.*

sul·fa·meth·i·zole (sul″fuh·meth′i·zole) *n.* N^1-(5-Methyl-1,3,4-thiadiazol-2-yl)sulfanilamide, $C_9H_{10}N_4O_2S_2$, a sulfonamide used for treatment of infections of the urinary tract.

sul·fa·meth·ox·a·zole (sul″fuh·meth·ock′suh·zole) *n.* 5-Methyl-3-sulfanilamidoisoxazole, $C_{10}H_{11}N_3O_3S$, an antibacterial sulfonamide.

sul·fa·me·thoxy·py·rid·a·zine (sul″fuh·me·thock″see·pi·rid′uh·zeen) *n.* N^1-(6-Methoxy-3-pyridazinyl)sulfanilamide, $C_{11}H_{12}N_4O_3S$, an antibacterial sulfonamide characterized by an exceptionally low rate of excretion.

Sulfamylon. Trademark for mafenide, an antibacterial sulfonamide.

sul·fa·nil·a·mide (sul″fuh·nil′uh·mide) *n.* p-Aminobenzenesulfonamide, $NH_2C_6H_4SO_2NH_2$, the predecessor of a large group of sulfonamides which, by virtue of being more effective and less toxic than sulfanilamide, have supplanted it.

sul·fa·nil·ic acid (sul″fuh·nil′ick). p-Aminobenzenesulfonic acid, $NH_2C_6H_4SO_3H$; used as a reagent.

sul·fa·pyr·i·dine (sul″fuh·pirr′i·deen, ·din) *n.* N^1-2-Pyridylsulfanilamide, $C_{11}H_{11}N_3O_2S$, a sulfonamide formerly used for the treatment of various infections but found to be too toxic for general use; now employed only as a suppressant for dermatitis herpetiformis.

sul·fa·tase (sul′fuh·tace, ·taze) *n.* Any enzyme that hydrolyzes an ethereal sulfate (ester sulfate).

sulfatase A deficiency. An enzyme deficiency state that may be responsible for metachromatic leukodystrophy.

Sulfathalidine. Trademark for phthalylsulfathiazole, a poorly absorbed sulfonamide used for suppressing growth of bacteria in the large intestine.

sul·fa·thi·a·zole (sul″fuh·thigh′uh·zole) *n.* N^1-2-Thiazolylsulfanilamide, $C_9H_9N_3O_2S_2$, formerly widely used in the treatment of pneumococcal, staphylococcal, and urinary tract infections; it has been replaced by less toxic sulfonamides.

sulfatide lipidosis. METACHROMATIC LEUKODYSTROPHY.

sul·fat·i·do·sis (sul·fat″i·do′sis) *n.* An excess of sulfatides, such as that occurring in the neural tissues in metachromatic leukodystrophy.

sulf·he·mo·glo·bin (sulf·hee″muh·glo′bin) *n.* A greenish substance derived from hemoglobin by the action of hydrogen sulfide. It may appear in the blood following the ingestion of sulfanilamide and other substances. Syn. *sulfmethemoglobin.*

sulf·he·mo·glo·bi·ne·mia (sulf·hee″muh·glo·bi·nee′mee·uh) *n.* A condition in which sulfhemoglobin is present in the blood; the symptoms are similar to those present in methemoglobinemia.

sulf·hy·drate (sulf·high′drate) *n.* A compound of a base with the univalent radical sulfhydryl, HS—.

sulf·hy·dryl (sulf·high′dril) *n.* The univalent radical HS—, usually attached to a carbon chain. The presence of active sulfhydryl groups is important for the activity of many enzymes. Syn. *SH group.*

sul·fide (sul′fide) *n.* A compound of sulfur with an element or basic radical.

sul·fi·sox·a·zole (sul″fi·sock′suh·zole, sulf″eye·) *n.* N¹-(3,4-Dimethyl-5-isoxazolyl)sulfanilamide, C₁₁H₁₃N₃O₃S, a sulfonamide of general therapeutic utility. For parenteral administration the soluble salt sulfisoxazole diethanolamine is used; for pediatric use the tasteless derivative acetyl sulfisoxazole is given. Syn. *sulphafurazole.*

sul·fite (sul′fite) *n.* A salt of sulfurous acid of the type M₂SO₃.

sulf·met·he·mo·glo·bin (sulf″met·hee″muh·glo′bin) *n.* SULFHEMOGLOBIN.

sulfo-. A combining form generally indicating *the presence of divalent sulfur* or *the sulfo- group,* —SO₃H.

sul·fo·bro·mo·phthal·ein sodium (sul″fo·bro″mo·thal′ee·in) *n.* Disodium 3,3′-(tetrabromophthalidylidene)bis (6-hydroxybenzenesulfonate), C₂₀H₈Br₄Na₂O₁₀S₂, a diagnostic aid used intravenously to determine the functional capacity of the liver.

sul·fon·amide (sul·fon′uh·mide, sul·fo′nuh·mide, ·mid) *n.* Any of a group of compounds derived from sulfanilamide, H₂NC₆H₄SO₂NH₂, and used in the treatment of various bacterial infections. Members of the group vary with respect to activity, degree and rate of absorption, metabolic alteration and excretion, and toxic manifestations produced. Prominent among their adverse effects is renal damage, particularly of the type caused by the crystallization of their N⁴-acetyl derivatives in the urinary tract; many other toxic effects have been noted, of which some can be attributed to sensitization.

sul·fo·nate (sul′fuh·nate) *v. & n.* 1. To treat an aromatic hydrocarbon with fuming sulfuric acid. 2. A sulfuric acid derivative. 3. The ester of a sulfonic acid.

sul·fo·na·tion (sul″fo·nay′shun) *n.* A chemical process resulting in the introduction in a compound of one or more sulfo- groups.

sul·fone (sul′fone) *n.* An oxidation product of thio- compounds containing the group SO₂ attached to a hydrocarbon group, such as RSO₂R.

sul·fon·eth·yl·meth·ane (sul″fone·eth″il·meth′ane) *n.* Diethylsulfonemethylethylmethane, CH₃C₂H₅C(SO₂C₂H₅)₂, formerly extensively used as a hypnotic. Syn. *methylsulfonal.*

sul·fon·meth·ane (sul″fone·meth′ane) *n.* Diethylsulfonedimethylmethane, (CH₃)₂C(SO₂C₂H₅)₂, formerly extensively used as a hypnotic.

sul·fo·sal·i·cyl·ic acid (sul″fo·sal″i·sil′ick). 3-Carboxy-4-hydroxybenzenesulfonic acid, C₇H₆O₆S; used as a reagent, mainly for protein in urine, and also for decalcification of bone for histologic study.

sulfosalicylic acid test. A test for urine protein, in which a sulfosalicylic acid solution produces cloudiness in the presence of protein.

sulf·ox·one sodium (sulf·ock′sone) *n.* Disodium [sulfonylbis(*p*-phenyleneimino)]di(methanesulfinate), C₁₄H₁₄N₂Na₂O₆S₃, a drug used in the treatment of lepromatous and tuberculoid leprosy, and as a suppressant for dermatitis herpetiformis.

sul·fur, sul·phur (sul′fur) *n.* S = 32.06. A solid, nonmetallic element, atomic number 16. Occurs as a yellow, brittle mass or in transparent monoclinic or rhombic crystals and exists in a number of modifications. Sometimes used as a laxative but mainly externally in the treatment of various parasitic and nonparasitic diseases of the skin.

sul·fu·rat·ed (sul′fuh·ray″tid, sul′few·) *n.* Combined with sulfur.

sul·fu·ra·tor (sul′few·ray″tur, sul′fuh·) *n.* An apparatus for applying sulfur dioxide fumes for purposes of disinfection.

sulfur dioxide. A gas, SO₂, with strong reducing action in water. Sometimes employed in preparation of medicinal dosage forms as an antioxidant; has been used as a space disinfectant.

sulfur granules. Yellow flecks composed of masses of densely packed, delicate, branching filaments characteristically exhibiting clublike structures at the periphery; found in tissues infected by *Actinomyces.*

sul·fu·ric acid (sul·few′rick). A solution containing about 96% H₂SO₄, the remainder being water; occurs as a colorless, odorless liquid of oily consistency. Used as a reagent, and in various syntheses, but not employed medicinally. Syn. *oil of vitriol.*

sul·fu·rous (sul′few·rus) *adj.* 1. Of the nature of sulfur. 2. Combined with sulfur; derived from sulfur dioxide.

sulfurous acid. H₂SO₃. A solution of sulfur dioxide in water; used as a decalcifying agent in histology. Formerly employed as a gastric antiseptic and for treatment of skin diseases.

Sul·ko·witch's test A test for calcium in the urine, in which equal parts of clear urine and Sulkowitch's reagent (oxalic acid, ammonium oxalate, glacial acetic acid, distilled water) are mixed. A fine white precipitate suggests normal serum calcium, no precipitate suggests reduced calcium, and a milky precipitate suggests increased serum calcium.

sul·lage (sul'ij) n. SEWAGE.

sum. Abbreviation for (a) *sume*, take; (b) *sumendus*, to be taken; used as a direction in prescriptions.

su·mac, su·mach (sue'mack, shoo'mack) n. A name applied to various species of *Rhus*, especially the nonpoisonous species.

sum·ma·tion (sum·ay'shun) n. The additory effect of individual events, especially of those of muscular, sensory, or mental stimuli. —**summation·al** (·ul) *adj.*

summation of stimuli. 1. SPATIAL SUMMATION. 2. TEMPORAL SUMMATION.

sum·mer diarrhea. An acute diarrhea, usually of children, especially during the summer, associated with an increased prevalence of enteropathogenic bacteria and viruses, as in poorly refrigerated food.

summer eruption. MILIARIA.

sump drain. An aspirating tubular drain of rubber, plastic, glass, etc., sometimes with lateral openings and fishtail ends, designed to provide continuous removal of accumulated secretions.

sun blindness. Blindness, either temporary or permanent, caused by retinal injury resulting from gazing at the sun without adequate protection. Syn. *photoretinitis*.

sun·burn, n. 1. Erythema, tenderness and vesiculobullous changes of the skin due to exposure to the sun. 2. Inflammation of the skin, due to the action of the sun's rays, which may be of the first or second degree. —**sun·burned, sun·burnt,** *adj.*

Sunday morning paralysis. DRUNKARD'S ARM PARALYSIS.

sun lamp. A lamp designed to give off radiations of wavelengths similar to those received from the sun.

sun·stroke, n. A form of heat stroke occurring on exposure to the sun, characterized by extreme pyrexia, prostration, convulsion, coma. Syn. *insolation, thermic fever.*

super- A prefix meaning (a) *above, upon;* (b) *extreme, in high degree;* (c) *excessive, over-;* (d) *ranking next above, superordinate to.*

su·per·ab·duc·tion (sue"pur·ab·duck'shun) n. HYPERABDUCTION.

su·per·acute (sue"pur·uh·kewt') *adj.* Extremely acute.

su·per·al·i·men·ta·tion (sue"pur·al"i·men·tay'shun) n. Overfeeding; the taking in or administration of food or nutritive substances in excess of ordinary metabolic requirements.

su·per·cer·e·bel·lar (sue"pur·serr"e·bel'ur) *adj.* Situated in the upper part of the cerebellum.

su·per·cil·i·um (sue"pur·sil'ee·um) n., pl. supercilia (·ee·uh) EYEBROW (1). —**supercili·ary** (·err"ee) *adj.*

su·per·duct (sue"pur·dukt') v. To elevate; to lead upward.

su·per·duc·tion (sue"pur·duck'shun) n. SURSUMDUCTION.

su·per·ego (sue"pur·ee'go) n. In psychoanalysis,

the subdivision of the psyche that acts as the conscience of the unconscious. Its components are derived from both the id and the ego, and are associated with standards of behavior, both personal and social, and self-criticism. It is formed in early life by identification with the individuals, primarily the parents or surrogates, who are esteemed and whose love is sought.

su·per·ex·ci·ta·tion (sue"pur·eck"si·ta'shun) n. Excessive excitement; overstimulation.

su·per·ex·ten·sion (sue"pur·eck·sten'shun) n. Excessive extension; HYPEREXTENSION.

su·per·fe·cun·da·tion (sue"pur·fee"kun·day'shun, ·feck"un·) n. The fertilization of two or more ova, ovulated more or less simultaneously, by two or more coital acts not necessarily involving the same male.

su·per·fe·cun·di·ty (sue"pur·fe·kun'di·tee) n. Superabundant fertility.

su·per·fe·ta·tion, su·per·foe·ta·tion (sue"pur·fee·tay'shun) n. The production or development of a second fetus after one is already present in the uterus.

su·per·fi·cial (sue"pur·fish'ul) *adj.* Confined to or pertaining to the surface.

superficial fascia. A sheet of subcutaneous tissue.

superficial inguinal ring. An obliquely placed triangular opening in the aponeurosis of the external oblique abdominal muscle forming the external opening of the inguinal canal. Syn. *external inguinal ring.*

superficial reflex. Any reflex occurring in response to superficial stimulation, as of the skin.

su·per·fi·ci·es (sue"pur·fish'ee·eez, ·fish'eez) n., pl. **superficies** The outer surface.

su·per·im·preg·na·tion (sue"pur·im"preg·nay'shun) n. 1. SUPERFETATION. 2. SUPERFECUNDATION.

su·per·in·duce (sue"pur·in·dewce') v. To add a new factor or a complication of a condition already existing.

su·per·in·fec·tion (sue"pur·in·feck'shun) n. A second or subsequent infection by the same microorganism, as seen in tuberculosis, or by a different organism, as seen following antibiotic therapy.

su·per·in·vo·lu·tion (sue"pur·in'vo·lew'shun) n. 1. HYPERINVOLUTION. 2. Excessive rolling up.

su·pe·ri·or (sue·peer'ee·ur) *adj.* In anatomy with reference to the human or animal body as poised for its usual manner of locomotion): upper; farther from the ground or surface of locomotion. —**superior·ly,** *adv.*

superior articular process. One of a pair of processes projecting upward from the side of the vertebral arch and articulating with an inferior articulating process of the vertebra above.

superior cerebellar peduncle. A large band of nerve fibers which arise in the dentate and emboliform nuclei of the cerebellum, form the dorsolateral part of the rostral portion of the fourth ventricle, decussate in the region of the inferior colliculi, and end in the red nucleus and ventrolateral thalamus. Syn. *brachium conjunctivum.*

superior colliculus. One of the posterior pair of rounded eminences arising from the dorsal portion of the mesencephalon. It contains primary visual centers especially for coordination of eye movement.

superior frontal gyrus. A convolution of the frontal lobe situated between the dorsal margin of the hemisphere and the superior frontal sulcus, immediately above the middle frontal gyrus.

su·pe·ri·or·i·ty complex (sue"peer"ee·or'i·tee). A general attitude or character trait, often pathologic and usually arising out of an underlying feeling of inferiority, which is characterized by the occurrence of some form of real or assumed ascendancy and by feelings of conceit, vanity, envy, jealousy, or revenge.

superior medullary velum. A thin layer of white substance which forms the anterior portion of the roof of the fourth ventricle.

superior orbital fissure. The elongated opening between the smaller and the greater wing of the sphenoid.

superior pelvic aperture or **strait.** The space within the brim of the pelvis; INLET OF THE PELVIS.

superior sagittal sinus. A sinus of the dura mater which runs along the upper edge of the falx cerebri, beginning in the front of the crista galli and terminating at the confluence of the sinuses.

superior strait of the pelvis. INLET OF THE PELVIS.

superior vena cava. A vein formed by the union of the brachiocephalic veins, and conveying the blood from the head, chest wall, and upper extremities to the right atrium of the heart.

superior vestibular nucleus. A nucleus dorsal and mostly rostral to the lateral vestibular nucleus in the angle formed by the floor and the lateral wall of the fourth ventricle.

su·per·lac·ta·tion (sue"pur·lack·tay'shun) *n.* 1. Excess of the secretion of milk. 2. Excessive continuance of lactation.

su·per·le·thal (sue"pur·lee'thul) *adj.* Highly lethal.

su·per·mo·ron (sue"pur·mo'ron) *n.* A person with dull normal or slightly below normal intelligence.

su·per·na·tant (sue"pur·nay'tant) *adj. & n.* 1. Floating on top. 2. The fluid that remains after the removal of suspended matter by centrifugation or other physical or chemical means. —**su·per·nate** (sue'pur·nate) *n.*

su·per·nor·mal (sue"pur·nor'mul) *adj.* 1. Characterizing a faculty or phenomenon that is beyond the level of ordinary experience. 2. Superior to, or greater than, the normal.

su·per·nu·mer·ary (sue"pur·new'mur·err"ee) *adj.* Existing in more than the usual number.

su·per·o·in·fe·ri·or (sue"pur·o·in·feer'ee·ur) *adj.* Pertaining to any dimension extending from above downward.

su·pe·ro·lat·er·al (sue"pur·o·lat'ur·ul) *adj.* Above and to the side.

su·pe·ro·me·di·al (sue"pur·o·mee'dee·ul) *adj.* Above and toward the middle.

Superoxol. Trademark for a 30% solution of hydrogen peroxide.

su·per·par·a·sit·ism (sue"pur·păr'uh·sigh·tiz·um) *n.* The infestation of parasites by other parasites.

su·per·sat·u·rate (sue"pur·satch'uh·rate) *v.* To saturate to excess; to add more of a substance than a liquid can normally and permanently dissolve.

su·per·scrip·tion (sue"pur·skrip'shun) *n.* The sign ℞ (abbreviation of Latin *recipe*, take) at the beginning of a prescription.

su·per·se·cre·tion (sue"pur·se·kree'shun) *n.* Excessive secretion.

su·per·sen·si·tive (sue"pur·sen'si·tiv) *adj.* Abnormally sensitive.

su·per·sen·si·ti·za·tion (sue"pur·sen"si·ti·zay'shun) *n.* Excessive susceptibility to the action of a protein following its injection.

su·per·son·ic (sue"pur·son'ick) *adj.* 1. A term, synonymous with ultrasonic but more commonly used than the latter in the physical sciences, describing or pertaining to soundlike waves with a frequency above that of audible sounds, that is, above 20,000 hertz. 2. Of or pertaining to speeds exceeding that of sound in air. —**su·per·sound** (sue'pur·saownd) *n.*

su·per·spi·na·tus (sue"pur·spye·nay'tus) *n. In veterinary medicine*, an extensor muscle of the humerus which has no exact homologue in man.

su·per·ten·sion (sue"pur·ten'shun) *n.* Extreme tension.

su·per·ve·nos·i·ty (sue"pur·ve·nos'i·tee) *n.* The condition in which the blood has become venous to a high degree.

su·per·ven·tion (sue"pur·ven'shun) *n.* That which is added; a new, extraneous, or unexpected condition added to another.

su·per·vi·sor, *n.* A supervising or head nurse.

su·per·volt·age, *adj.* Pertaining to x-rays produced by a very high-voltage current flow across an x-ray tube or very high-energy radiation produced by other devices, as telecobalt (radioactive cobalt used in telecobalt therapy) and linear accelerators.

supervoltage radiation. *In radiology,* roentgen radiation produced by voltages above 500,000 volts or equivalent gamma rays.

su·pi·na·tion (sue"pi·nay'shun) *n.* 1. Of the hand: the turning of the palm upward. 2. Of the foot: a turning of the sole inward so that the medial margin is elevated. 3. The condition of being supine; lying on the back. —**su·pi·nate** (sue'pi·nate) *v.*

su·pi·na·tor (sue'pi·nay"tur, sue'pi·nay'tor) *n.* A muscle of the forearm, which rotates the radius outward.

su·pine (suh·pine', sue'pine) *adj.* 1. Lying on the back face upward. 2. Of the hand: palm upward.

supine hypotensive syndrome. Severe hypotension in late pregnancy or during labor caused by compression of the abdominal aorta and vena cava by the gravid uterus when the mother assumes the supine position. The resulting reduction of uterine blood flow may produce fetal distress.

sup·pe·da·ne·ous (sup"e·day'nee·us) *adj.* Pertaining to the sole of the foot.

sup·pe·da·ne·um (sup″e·day′nee·um) *n.* An application to the sole of the foot.

sup·ple·men·tal (sup″le·men′tul) *adj.* Additional.

sup·ple·men·ta·ry (sup″le·men′tur·ee) *adj.* SUPPLEMENTAL.

sup·port, *v. & n.* 1. To sustain, prop, or hold in position. 2. Any appliance that supports a part or structure, as an arch support. 3. The providing for the needs of another person, particularly for a dependent, such as a child or invalid. 4. *In psychiatry,* the giving of approval, acceptance, sympathy, and encouragement to another person. Adj. *supportive.*

sup·port·er, *n.* An apparatus intended to hold in place a low-hanging or prolapsed organ, as the uterus, the scrotum and its contents, or the abdomen, or to limit the use of certain joints, as the knee or ankle.

sup·port·ive, *adj.* Characterizing or pertaining to any device, measure, person, or program which maintains, gives assistance to, sustains, or in any manner helps a patient.

supportive therapy. 1. Any form of treatment designed primarily to bolster and reinforce the patient's own defenses and to suppress disturbing influences or factors in such a way as to allow his own resources to help him back to health. 2. Specifically, a technique of psychotherapy in which the therapist, through encouragement, advice, reassurance, reeducation, and often even environmental manipulation, reinforces the patient's own psychic defenses and helps him suppress disturbing psychologic material; employed particularly in patients whose mental state is too fragile to achieve insight or whose symptoms are not sufficiently severe to justify intensive psychotherapy.

sup·pos·i·to·ry (suh·poz′i·tor″ee) *n.* A medicated solid body of varying weight and shape, intended for introduction into different orifices of the body, as the rectum, urethra, or vagina. Usually suppositories melt or are softened at body temperature, in some instances release of medication is effected through use of a hydrophilic vehicle. Typical vehicles or bases are theobroma oil (cocoa butter), glycerinated gelatin, sodium stearate, and propylene glycol monostearate.

sup·press, *v.* 1. To hold back, curtail, constrain, arrest; to prevent from functioning. 2. To exclude from overt manifestation or consciousness. —**suppres·sive,** *adj.*; **suppres·sant,** *adj. & n.*

sup·pres·sion, *n.* 1. A sudden cessation of secretion, as of the urine, or of a normal process, as the menses. 2. *In psychiatry,* the conscious effort to control and cover ideas, feelings, urges, and desires considered to be unacceptable, untenable, or unworthy.

sup·pu·rant (sup′yoo·runt) *adj. & n.* 1. Promoting suppuration. 2. Any agent that promotes suppuration.

sup·pu·ra·tion (sup″yoo·ray′shun) *n.* The formation of pus. —**sup·pu·rate** (sup′yoo·rate) *v.*

sup·pu·ra·tive (sup′yoo·ray″tiv) *adj. & n.* 1. Characterized by suppuration. 2. SUPPURANT (2).

suppurative parotitis. Suppurating inflammation of the parotid gland, usually due to *Staphylococcus aureus* and associated with chronic debilitating disease or blockage of the parotid gland by a calculus; characterized by local pain and swelling, often with fever and chills.

supra- A prefix meaning (a) *upon* or *above;* (b) *beyond, transcending, exceeding.*

su·pra·aor·tic (sue″pruh·ay·or′tick) *adj.* Above the level of the aortic valve, as supraaortic stenosis.

su·pra·cal·lo·sal (sue″pruh·ka·lo′sul) *adj.* Situated above the corpus callosum.

su·pra·cer·vi·cal (sue″pruh·sur′vi·kul) *adj.* Situated above the cervix of the uterus.

su·pra·cho·roid (sue″pruh·ko′roid) *adj.* Situated above or upon the choroid coat of the eye.

su·pra·cla·vic·u·lar (sue″pruh·kla·vick′yoo·lur) *adj.* Above the clavicle.

supraclavicular signal node. SIGNAL NODE.

su·pra·cli·noid (sue″pruh·klye′noid) *adj.* Above the clinoid processes.

su·pra·clu·sion (sue″pruh·klew′zhun) *n.* The position of a tooth that has overerupted in the plane of occlusion.

su·pra·con·dy·lar (sue″pruh·kon′di·lur) *adj.* Above a condyle.

su·pra·cris·tal (sue″pruh·kris′tul) *adj.* Above a ridge or crest.

su·pra·di·a·phrag·mat·ic (sue″pruh·dye″uh·frag·mat′ick) *adj.* Above the diaphragm.

su·pra·ge·nic·u·late (sue″pruh·je·nick′yoo·lut) *adj.* Situated above the medial geniculate body.

su·pra·gin·gi·val (sue″pruh·jin′ji·vul, jin·jye′vul) *adj.* Located above the gingiva.

supragingival calculus. A concretion deposited on the surface of a tooth above the level of the gingival margin. Syn. *extragingival calculus.*

su·pra·gle·noid (sue″pruh·glee′noid) *adj.* Above the glenoid cavity.

su·pra·glot·tic (sue″pruh·glot′ick) *adj.* Above the glottis.

su·pra·gran·u·lar (sue″pruh·gran′yoo·lur) *adj.* Situated above the external granular layer of the cerebrum.

su·pra·hy·oid (sue″pruh·high′oid) *adj.* Above the hyoid bone.

su·pra·in·gui·nal (sue″pruh·ing′gwi·nul) *adj.* Situated proximal to the inguinal region.

su·pra·le·thal (sue″pruh·lee′thul) *adj.* Above the lethal level.

su·pra·le·va·tor (sue″pruh·le·vay′tur) *adj.* Situated above a levator ani muscle.

su·pra·lim·i·nal (sue″pruh·lim′i·nul) *adj.* Above, or in excess of, a threshold; SUPRATHRESHOLD.

su·pra·mal·le·o·lar (sue″pruh·ma·lee′uh·lur) *adj.* Above a malleolus.

su·pra·ma·mil·lary (sue″pruh·mam′i·lerr·ee) *adj.* Situated above a mamillary body.

su·pra·man·dib·u·lar (sue″pruh·man·dib′yoo·lur) *adj.* Situated above the mandible.

su·pra·mar·gin·al (sue″pruh·mahr′jin·ul) *adj.* Above an edge or margin.

su·pra·mas·toid (sue″pruh·mas′toid) *adj.* Above the mastoid process of the temporal bone.

su·pra·max·il·lary (sue″pruh·mack′si·lerr·ee)

adj. Situated above a maxillary alveolar process.

su·pra·me·a·tal (sue"pruh·mee·ay'tul) *adj.* Situated above a meatus.

su·pra·nu·cle·ar (sue"pruh·new'klee·ur) *adj.* In the nervous system, central to a nucleus.

su·pra·oc·cip·i·tal (sue"pruh·ock·sip'i·tul) *adj.* Situated above the occipital bone.

su·pra·oc·clu·sion (use"pruh·o·kloo'zhun) *n.* The condition created by the abnormal elongation of teeth in their sockets.

su·pra·op·tic (sue"pruh·op'tick) *adj.* Situated above the optic tract.

supraoptic nucleus of the hypothalamus. A well-defined crescent-shaped nucleus that straddles the optic tract lateral to the chiasma. Its efferent fibers combine with those of the paraventricular nucleus to form the supraopticohypophyseal tract.

su·pra·op·ti·co·hy·poph·y·se·al (sue"pruh·op'ti·ko·high·pof''i·see'ul, ·high''po·fiz'ee·ul) *adj.* Pertaining to the supraoptic nucleus and the hypophysis.

su·pra·or·bit·al (sue"pruh·or'bi·tul) *adj.* Situated above the orbit.

supraorbital reflex. Contraction of the orbicularis oculi muscle in response to a tap of the outer region of the supraorbital ridge, resulting in closing the eye of the same side or even of both eyes; difficult to elicit normally, the response is exaggerated in lesions above the facial nucleus and absent in lesions of the facial nerve at or below the nucleus. Syn. *McCarthy's reflex, orbicularis oculi reflex.*

supraorbital ridge. The curved and prominent margin of the frontal bone that forms the upper boundary of the orbit.

su·pra·pa·tel·lar (sue"pruh·puh·tel'ur) *adj.* Above the patella.

su·pra·pel·vic (sue"pruh·pel'vick) *adj.* Above the pelvis.

su·pra·pleu·ral membrane (sue"pruh·ploo'rul). The extrapleural fascia attached to the inner margin of the first rib and covering the dome of the pleura. Syn. *Sibson's fascia.*

su·pra·pu·bic (sue"pruh·pew'bick) *adj.* Above the pubes.

suprapubic prostatectomy. Removal of the prostate through an incision into the urinary bladder through the abdominal (suprapubic) route in a one- or two-stage operation.

su·pra·re·nal (sue"pruh·ree'nul) *adj. & n.* 1. Located above or anterior to the kidneys; ADRENAL (1). 2. A tissue in suprarenal position, especially the adrenal gland.

su·pra·re·nal·ec·to·my (sue"pruh·ree''nul·eck'tuh·mee) *n.* ADRENALECTOMY.

suprarenal gland. ADRENAL GLAND.

Suprarenalin. A trademark for epinephrine.

su·pra·re·nal·ism (sue"pruh·ree'nul·iz·um) *n.* ADRENALISM.

su·pra·re·nal·op·a·thy (sue"pruh·ree''nul·op'uth·ee) *n.* A disordered condition resulting from disturbed function of the suprarenal glands.

Suprarenin. A trademark for epinephrine.

su·pra·scap·u·lar (sue"pruh·skap'yoo·lur) *adj.* Above or in the upper part of the scapula, as an artery or nerve.

su·pra·scle·ral (sue"pruh·skleer'ul) *adj.* Situated at or upon the outer surface of the sclera.

su·pra·sel·lar (sue"pruh·sel'ur) *adj.* Situated upon or above the sella turcica of the sphenoid bone.

suprasellar cyst. CRANIOPHARYNGIOMA.

su·pra·spi·nal (sue"pruh·spye'nul) *adj.* Situated above a spine or the spinal column.

su·pra·spi·na·tus (sue"pruh·spye·nay'tus) *n.* A muscle originating above the spine of the scapula and inserted on the greater tubercle of the humerus.

su·pra·spi·nous (sue"pruh·spye'nus) *adj.* Above the spinous process of the scapula or of a vertebra.

su·pra·sple·ni·al (sue"pruh·splee'nee·ul) *adj.* Situated above the splenium.

su·pra·ster·nal (sue"pruh·stur'nul) *adj.* Above the sternum.

suprasternal notch. JUGULAR NOTCH OF THE STERNUM.

su·pra·ste·rol (sue"pruh·sterr'ol, ·steer'ol) *n.* A type of sterol produced by the irradiation of ergosterol. Suprasterols are toxic.

su·pra·thresh·old (sue"pruh·thresh'hohld) *adj.* Above, or in excess of, a threshold.

su·pra·ton·sil·lar (sue"pruh·ton'si·lur) *adj.* Above a tonsil.

su·pra·troch·le·ar (sue"pruh·trock'lee·ur) *adj.* Above the trochlea of the superior oblique muscle.

su·pra·um·bil·i·cal (sue"pruh·um·bil'i·kul) *adj.* Above the navel; cranial to a transverse plane at the umbilicus.

su·pra·va·gi·nal (sue"pruh·vaj'i·nul, va·jye'nul) *adj.* Situated above or superior to the vagina.

su·pra·val·vu·lar (sue"pruh·val'vew·lur) *adj.* Above a valve, usually cardiac.

su·pra·ven·tric·u·lar (sue"pruh·ven·trick'yoo·lur) *adj.* Occurring or situated above a ventricle.

supraventricular tachycardia. A rapid regular tachycardia with the ectopic pacemaker originating above the ventricles, i.e., in the atria or atrioventricular node.

su·pra·ver·gence (sue"pruh·vur'junce) *n.* Divergence of the two eyes in a vertical plane, measured by a prism, of from 2 to 3°; the eye moving upwards is supraverging. Syn. *sursumvergence.* —**supra·verge** (·vurj') *v.*

su·pra·vi·tal (sue"pruh·vye'tul) *adj.* Pertaining to the staining of living cells after removal from a living animal or of still living cells within a recently killed animal. —**supravital·ly** (·lee) *adv.*

su·ra (sue'ruh) *n.* CALF. —**su·ral** (·rul) *adj.*

sur·al·i·men·ta·tion (sur"al''i·men·tay'shun) *n.* The method of forced feeding or overalimentation; SUPERALIMENTATION, HYPERALIMENTATION.

sur·di·tas (sur'di·tas) *n.* Deafness.

surd·i·ty (surd'i·tee) *n.* Deafness.

sur·do·car·di·ac (sur"do·kahr'dee·ack) *adj.* Characterized by deafness and cardiac abnormalities.

surdocardiac syndrome. CARDIOAUDITORY SYNDROME.

sur·face, *n.* 1. The exterior of a body. 2. The face

or faces of a body; a term frequently used in anatomy in the description of various structures.

surface-active, *adj.* Of a substance, such as a detergent; able to change, usually to lower, the interfacial tension between two phases.

surface tension. The force operating at surfaces (commonly at the interface of a liquid and a gas) which is due to the unequal molecular attraction on either side of the molecules at the surface. It is the contractile force in the surface of a liquid that causes the surface to shrink and assume the smallest area possible. The surface tension of a liquid is the force in dynes exerted on either side of an imaginary straight line 1 cm long lying on the surface of the liquid.

sur·fac·tant (sur·fack'tunt) *n.* 1. Any surface-active agent which reduces interfacial or surface tension. 2. The surface-active lipoprotein substance, secreted by great alveolar cells and lining the alveolar surface, which serves to maintain the stability of the alveolar mucosa.

surf·er's lumps. Skin nodules developing at points of contact between the bodies of surfboard riders and their boards, usually on the lower extremity.

sur·geon (sur'jun) *n.* A physician who is specially trained and qualified to perform operations and practice surgery.

surgeon general. The chief medical officer of an armed force or public health service unit.

surgeon's knot. DOUBLE KNOT.

sur·gery, *n.* 1. The branch of medicine dealing with trauma and diseases requiring operative procedure, including manipulation. 2. Any of the treatments and procedures developed and applied in surgery. 3. In British usage, any medical practitioner's place of consultation and treatment. —**sur·gi·cal,** *adj.*

surgical anesthesia. Stage 3 of general anesthesia where muscles are sufficiently relaxed to permit surgical procedures to be carried out readily.

surgical cleansing. Removal of devitalized tissue and foreign material from traumatic wounds with sterile cutting instruments.

surgical decompression. Any operative method to relieve excessive pressure, as in a body cavity, the gastrointestinal tract, or the cranium.

surgical diphtheria. Formation of a diphtheritic membrane on the surface of a wound. Syn. *wound diphtheria.*

surgical erysipelas. Erysipelas occurring in the site of a wound. Syn. *traumatic erysipelas.*

surgical neck. The constricted part of the humerus just below the tubercles.

surgical tetanus. Tetanus following infection of an operative site with *Clostridium tetani.*

surgical third space. THIRD SPACE.

Surital. Trademark for sodium thiamylal, an ultrashort-acting barbiturate used intravenously as an anesthetic.

sur·ra (soor'uh, surr'uh) *n.* A type of trypanosomiasis of domestic animals in southern Asia, caused by *Trypanosoma evansi* and transmitted by a number of bloodsucking flies.

sur·ro·gate (sur'uh·gut, ·gate) *n.* 1. Any medicine used as a substitute for a more expensive one, or for one to which there is a special objection in any particular case. 2. *In psychiatry,* an authority figure who takes the place of a parent (father or mother) in the emotional life of the patient.

sur·sum·duc·tion (sur''sum·duck'shun) *n.* 1. The power of the two eyes of fusing two images when one eye has a prism placed vertically before it. 2. SUPRAVERGENCE. 3. A movement of either eye alone upward.

sur·sum·ver·gence (sur''sum·vur'junce) *n.* SUPRAVERGENCE. —**sursumver·gent** (·junt) *adj.*

sur·sum·ver·sion (sur''sum·vur'zhun) *n.* The upward movement of both eyes.

sus·cep·ti·bil·i·ty (suh·sep''ti·bil'i·tee) *n.* The inherited or acquired disposition to develop a disease if exposed to the causative agent.

sus·cep·ti·ble (suh·sep'ti·bul) *adj.* 1. Sensitive to impression or influence. 2. Characterizing an individual who has neither natural nor acquired immunity to a disease and is liable to infection.

sus·ci·tate (sus'i·tate) *v.* To increase activity; to stimulate.

sus·pend·ed, *adj.* 1. Hanging; applied to any structure attached to or hanging from another structure, and attached by a pedicle or cord. 2. Interrupted.

sus·pen·sion, *n.* 1. Hanging or fixation in a higher position; a method of treatment, as suspension of the uterus. 2. *In chemistry and pharmacy,* a dispersion of solid particles in a continuous liquid medium.

sus·pen·soid (sus·pen'soid) *n.* An apparent solution which is seen, by the microscope, to consist of small particles of solid dispersed material in active Brownian movement.

sus·pen·so·ri·um (sus''pen·so'ree·um) *n.,* pl. **suspenso·ria** (·ree·uh) That upon which anything hangs for support.

sus·pen·so·ry (su·spen'suh·ree) *adj. & n.* 1. Serving for suspension or support. 2. SUPPORTER. 3. JOCKSTRAP.

suspensory bandage. A bandage for supporting the scrotum.

sus·pi·ra·tion (sus''pi·ray'shun) *n.* 1. SIGH. 2. The act of sighing.

sustentacular cell. One of the supporting cells of an epithelial membrane or tissue as contrasted with other cells with special function, as the nonnervous cells of the olfactory epithelium or the Sertoli cells of the seminiferous tubules. Syn. *Müller's fibers.*

sus·ten·tac·u·lum (sus''ten·tack'yoo·lum) *n.,* pl. **sustentacu·la** (·luh) A support. —**sustentacu·lar** (·lur) *adj.*

su·sur·ra·tion (sue''sur·ay'shun) *n.* Murmuring, susurrus.

su·sur·rus (suh·sur'us) *n.* A soft murmur.

Sut·ter blood group. An erythrocyte antigen defined by its reaction to anti-Js^a antibody, found in the blood of a Mr. Sutter, who had received transfusions. It occurs in about 20 percent of Negroes and is a Mendelian dominant trait.

su·tu·ra (sue·tew'ruh) *n.,* pl. & genit. sing. **sutu-**

rae (·ree), genit. pl. **su·tu·ra·rum** (sue·tew·rair' um) SUTURE.

su·tur·al (sue'chur·ul) *adj.* Pertaining to, or having the nature of, a suture.

sutural bone. Any supernumerary bone occurring in a cranial suture. Syn. *Wormian bone.*

su·ture (sue'chur) *n. & v.* 1. *In osteology,* a line of junction or closure between bones, as a cranial suture. 2. *In surgery,* a fine thread or cord-like absorbable or nonabsorbable material, such as catgut or silk, used to make a repair or close a wound. 3. The method used in suturing, such as interrupted or mattress suture. 4. To close a wound or effect a union of tissues by sewing.

Svedberg flotation unit A rate of flotation of a macromolecule, particularly a lipoprotein, in a medium of relatively greater density, of 10⁻¹³ cm per second under unit centrifugal force. Symbol, S_f.

Svedberg sedimentation unit A rate of sedimentation of a macromolecule, in a specified medium, of 10⁻¹³ cm per second under unit centrifugal force. Syn. *svedberg.*

swab (swahb) *n.* A small stick or clamp with cotton or gauze at the tip, used to clean wounds, clear mucous passageways, take cultures, apply drugs topically, etc.

swage, *n. & v.* 1. A counter-die used in shaping thin metal. 2. To conform a thin metal plate to the shape of a model, cast, or die with the aid of a counter-die, the swage. 3. To fuse a strand of suture thread onto the end of a suture needle.

swal·low, *v.* 1. To take into the stomach through the esophagus by means of a complex reflex (the swallowing reflex) initiated by voluntary muscles and resulting in esophageal peristalsis. 2. To go through the motions of swallowing something.

swallowing reflex. The chain of reflexes involved in the mechanism of swallowing which may be evoked by stimulation of the palate or pharynx.

swamp fever. LEPTOSPIROSIS.

swamp fever of horses. INFECTIOUS EQUINE ANEMIA.

swathe (swahth) *n. & v.* A broad band of cloth used to wrap or bind a part. 2. To wrap or bind in a swathe.

S wave of the electrocardiogram. The negative deflection of the ventricular depolarization complex, following R (positive) wave.

sway·back, *n.* In humans, increased lumbar lordosis with compensatory increased thoracic kyphosis; in horses, sinking of the back or lordosis.

sweat, *n. & v.* 1. The secretion of the sweat glands, consisting of a transparent, colorless, aqueous fluid, holding in solution neutral fats, volatile fatty acids, traces of albumin and urea, free lactic acid, sodium lactate, sodium chloride, potassium chloride, and traces of alkaline phosphates, sugar, and ascorbic acid. Its excretion, largely by the cooling effect of evaporation, helps regulate the temperature of the body. 2. To produce sweat.

sweat gland. One of the coiled tubular glands of the skin which secrete sweat.

sweat gland adenoma. A benign tumor whose parenchyma consists of one or more sweat gland components.

sweat gland carcinoma. A malignant tumor whose parenchymal cells form structures resembling eccrine glands.

sweat-retention syndrome. Inability to sweat because of plugging of sweat pores, followed by the classic clinical and histological signs of prickly heat, which may persist after heat rash has subsided. Syn. *thermogenic anhidrosis.*

sweaty-feet syndrome. ODOR-OF-SWEATY-FEET SYNDROME.

swee·ny (swee'nee, swin'ee) *n.* A wasting or atrophy of the scapular muscles of the horse, usually due to an injury of the nerve supply. Syn. *swinney.*

sweet clover disease. A hemorrhagic disease observed in animals after eating spoiled sweet clover; due to a toxic substance (dicoumarin) that lowers the prothrombin content of the blood plasma.

swell·ing, *n.* 1. Any morbid enlargement, inflation, or abnormal protuberance. 2. *In embryology,* a small eminence or ridge.

swim·mer's itch. SCHISTOSOME DERMATITIS.

swim·ming-pool conjunctivitis. INCLUSION CONJUNCTIVITIS.

swine erysipelas. An infectious disease of hogs, caused by *Erysipelothrix insidiosa,* in which skin involvement predominates.

swine influenza. Disease due to the swine influenza virus, a strain of influenza. A virus having the antigenic marker $H_{sw}1$, N1. The virus causes respiratory-tract inflammation in swine and rarely infects man. The virus is related antigenically to the virus believed to have caused the severe influenza pandemic of 1918-1919.

swine plague. 1. Hemorrhagic septicemia of swine caused by *Pasteurella suiseptica.* The disease is characterized by a pleuropneumonia with focal necrosis and occasionally by septicemia. 2. HOG CHOLERA.

swine pox. A frequent disease of hogs characterized by pox lesions on the body and inner surfaces of the legs. It is a benign infection and usually occurs in young pigs.

Swiss type agammaglobulinemia. The autosomal recessive form of severe combined immunodeficiency.

sy·co·ma (sigh·ko'muh) *n.* A condyloma or wart.

sy·co·sis (sigh·ko'sis) *n.* An inflammatory disease affecting the hair follicles, particularly of the beard, and characterized by papules, pustules, and tubercles, perforated by hairs, together with infiltration of the skin and crusting.

sy·co·sis bar·bae (sigh·ko'sis bahr'bee). Inflammation of the hair follicles of the beard.

sycosis cap·il·li·tii (kap''i·lish'ee·eye). KELOID ACNE.

sycosis par·a·sit·i·ca (păr''ih·sit'i·kuh). Barber's itch; a disease of the hair follicles, usually affecting the region covered by the beard and due to the presence of various trichophyta.

sycosis vul·ga·ris (vul·gair′is). A pustular, follicular lesion caused by staphylococci.

Syd·en·ham's chorea (sid′ᵉn·um) A disorder of childhood characterized by chorea, hypotonia, and hyporeflexia, and frequently by irritability and other psychic disturbances, often insidious in onset, and sometimes more manifest on one side of the body; related to streptococcal infection, with a high incidence of cardiac complications in later life unless prophylaxis against recurrent streptococcal infections is practiced. Syn. *Saint Vitus dance, acute chorea, dancing chorea, chorea minor.*

syl·lab·ic speech or **utterance** (si·lab′ick). SCANNING SPEECH.

syl·la·ble-stumbling. A form of dysphasia wherein each sound and syllable can be distinctly uttered, but the word as a whole is spoken with difficulty; seen in general paresis and other central nervous system disorders.

syl·la·bus (sil′uh·bus) *n.*, pl. **sylla·bi** (·bye), **syllabuses** 1. A compendium containing the headings of a discourse. 2. The main propositions of a course of lectures. 3. An abstract.

syl·lep·si·ol·o·gy (si·lep″see·ol′uh·jee) *n.* The physiologic study of conception and pregnancy.

syl·van yellow fever (sil′vun). Yellow fever transmitted to man from monkeys by forest mosquitoes.

syl·vat·ic plague (sil·vat′ick). Enzootic and epizootic plague occurring in some 50 rodent species, occurring in many western states of the United States and in many rural and sylvan areas of the world. Man may become infected accidentally by direct contact with these animals or by the bite of vectors, such as the flea.

Syl·vi·an (sil′vee·un) *adj.* 1. Described by or associated with Franciscus Sylvius (François de la Boë), Dutch physician, 1614–1672. 2. Described by or associated with Jacobus Sylvius (Jacques du Bois), French anatomist, 1478–1555.

Sylvian artery. The middle cerebral artery. See Table of Arteries in the Appendix.

Sylvian fissure LATERAL CEREBRAL SULCUS.

Sylvian triangle. In cerebral angiography, an area on the surface of the insula outlined by five to eight branches of the middle cerebral artery. The apex of the triangle is the Sylvian point; the inferior margin of the triangle is formed by the lower branches of the middle cerebral artery and the superior margin by the looping branches of this artery that are reversing their course.

sym·bal·lo·phone (sim·bal′o·fone) *n.* A stethoscope equipped with two chest pieces for simultaneous use as a special aid in localizing or in comparing sounds.

sym·bi·on (sim′bee·on, ·bye·on) *n.* SYMBIONT.

sym·bi·o·sis (sim″bee·o′sis, ·bye·o′sis) *n.* 1. A more or less intimate association between organisms of noncompeting species, such as parasitism, mutalism, or commensalism. 2. Specifically, an association or union between organisms of different species which is mutually beneficial or essential to the survival of both parties; MUTUALISM. 3. *In psychiatry,* the more or less mutually advantageous relationship between two or more mentally disturbed individuals who are emotionally dependent on one another. —**symbi·ot·ic** (·ot′ick) *adj.*

symbiotic psychosis. A mental disorder of early childhood characterized by severe developmental and social retardation and profound reactions to separation in a child who appears to be autistic, but whose relationships with his mother or surrogate are abnormally close.

sym·bleph·aron (sim·blef′uh·ron) *n.* Adhesion of the eyelids to the eyeball.

sym·bleph·a·ro·sis (sim·blef″uh·ro′sis) *n.* Adhesion of the eyelids to the eyeball or to each other.

sym·bo·lia (sim·bo′lee·uh) *n.* The ability to recognize an object by the sense of touch.

sym·bol·ic visual agnosia. Inability to recognize words or fractions of words (agnostic alexia), musical symbols, or numbers and other mathematical symbols, in spite of adequate vision, usually due to a lesion in the angular gyrus or connections thereof with other cortical regions such as Wernicke's and Broca's areas.

sym·bol·ism (sim′bul·iz·um) *n.* The delusional or hallucinational interpretation of all events or objects as having a mystic significance, common in certain forms of mental, particularly psychotic, disorders.

sym·bol·iza·tion (sim″bul·i·zay′shun) *n. In psychiatry,* an unconscious mental process by which a feeling, idea, or object is expressed by a substitute device, as in dreams, the meaning of which is not clear to the conscious mind. The symbol contains in disguised form the emotions vested in the initial idea or object.

sy·me·lia (si·mee′lee·uh) *n.* A coalescence of the lower extremities.

Syme's amputation Amputation above the ankle joint, the malleoli being sawed through, and a flap made with the skin of the heel.

sym·me·try (sim′e·tree) *n. In anatomy,* a harmonious correspondence of parts; also the relation of homologous parts at opposite sides or ends of the body. —**sym·met·ric** (si·met′rick), **symmet·ri·cal** (·ri·kul) *adj.*

sym·pa·thec·to·my (sim′puh·theck′tuh·mee) *n.* Excision of a portion of the autonomic or sympathetic nervous system.

sym·pa·thet·ic (sim″puh·thet′ick) *adj.* 1. Pertaining to or produced by sympathy. 2. Pertaining to the sympathetic nervous system.

sympathetic abscess. A secondary or metastatic abscess at a distance from the part in which the exciting cause has acted, as a bubo.

sympathetic irritation. Inflammation of an organ arising from inflammation of another related organ, as inflammation of an uninjured eye in association with inflammation of the other.

sympathetic meningitis. A form of aseptic meningitis with increased pressure, protein, and cell count in the cerebrospinal fluid in the absence of any infecting organism, due to a septic or necrotic focus in a structure contiguous to the leptomeninges.

sympathetic nervous system. 1. The thoraco-lumbar division of the autonomic nervous system; the ganglionated sympathetic trunk, sympathetic plexuses, and the associated preganglionic and postganglionic nerve fibers. 2. *Obsol.* AUTONOMIC NERVOUS SYSTEM.

sympathetic ophthalmia. A granulomatous inflammatory condition of the uveal tract which can occur in both eyes following ocular injury or intraocular surgery of one eye.

sym·path·ic (sim·path'ick) *adj.* SYMPATHETIC.

sym·path·i·co·blast (sim·path'i·ko·blast) *n.* SYMPATHOBLAST.

sym·path·i·co·blas·to·ma (sim·path"i·ko·blas·to'muh) *n.* NEUROBLASTOMA.

sym·path·i·co·go·ni·o·ma (sim·path"i·ko·go"nee·o'muh) *n.* NEUROBLASTOMA.

sym·path·i·co·neu·ri·tis (sim·path"i·ko·new·rye'tis) *n.* A neuropathy or neuritis involving ganglions and fibers of the sympathetic nervous system.

sym·path·i·cop·a·thy (sim·path"i·kop'uth·ee) *n.* A disordered condition resulting from disturbance of the sympathetic nervous system.

sym·path·i·co·to·nia (sim·path"i·ko·to'nee·uh) *n.* A condition produced by stimulation of the sympathetic nervous system, manifested by gooseflesh, increased blood pressure, or vascular spasm.

sym·path·i·co·trop·ic (sim·path"i·ko·trop'ick) *adj.* Possessing special affinity for the sympathetic nervous system.

sym·path·i·cus (sim·path'i·kus) *n. Obsol.* SYMPATHETIC NERVOUS SYSTEM.

sym·pa·thism (sim'puh·thiz·um) *n.* Susceptibility to hypnotic suggestion. **—sympa·thist** (·thist) *n.*

sym·pa·thi·zer (sim'puh·thigh"zur) *n.* SYMPATHIZING EYE.

sym·pa·thiz·ing eye (sim'puh·thigh"zing). The noninjured eye that becomes involved in sympathetic ophthalmia.

sym·pa·tho·blast (sim·path'o·blast, sim'puh·tho·) *n.* An embryonic sympathetic nerve cell which differentiates into the characteristic sympathetic ganglion cell. It is larger than the sympathogonia, with a less dense nucleus, more cytoplasm, and often a short cytoplasmic process.

sym·pa·tho·blas·to·ma (sim"puh·tho·blas·to'muh, sim·path"o·) *n.* NEUROBLASTOMA.

sym·pa·tho·go·nia (sim"puh·tho·go'nee·uh, sim·path"o·) *n.pl.* Primitive cells of the sympathetic nervous system derived from neuroblasts of the neural crest. They have dense nuclei, rich in chromatin, and only a thin rim of cytoplasm, and differentiate to form along one line ganglion cells and along another line chromaffin cells.

sym·pa·tho·go·ni·o·ma (sim"puh·tho·go"nee·o'muh, sim·path"o·) *n.* NEUROBLASTOMA.

sym·pa·tho·lyt·ic (sim"puh·tho·lit'ick, sim·path"o·) *adj.* Having or pertaining to an effect antagonistic to the activity produced by stimulation of the sympathetic nervous system.

sympatholytic agent. ADRENERGIC BLOCKING AGENT.

sym·pa·tho·mi·met·ic (sim"puh·tho·mi·met'ick,

sim·path"o·) *adj.* Having the power to cause physiologic changes similar to those produced by action of the sympathetic nervous system, usually with respect to a drug.

sym·pa·thy (sim'puth·ee) *n.* 1. The mutual relation between parts more or less distant, whereby a change in the one has an effect upon the other. 2. Feeling in response to similar feelings of another person; the close sharing of the experiences or feelings of and with another; close identification with another. 3. *Colloq.* The sharing of sad, painful, or unpleasant feelings; commiseration.

sym·pet·al·ous (sim·pet'ul·us) *adj. In botany,* having the petals united.

sym·phal·an·gism (sim·fal'un·jiz·um) *n.* An inherited condition of stiff fingers, or ankylosed finger joints.

sym·phys·i·al (sim·fiz'ee·eul) *adj.* Of or pertaining to a symphysis.

sym·phy·si·ec·to·my (sim"fi·zee·eck'tuh·mee) *n.* Excision of the symphysis pubis for the purpose of facilitating delivery.

sym·phy·si·or·rha·phy (sim"fi·zee·or'uh·fee) *n.* Suture of a divided symphysis.

sym·phy·si·ot·o·my (sim"fi·zee·ot'uh·mee) *n.* The dividing of the symphysis pubis to gain access to or to increase the diameters of the pelvic canal.

sym·phy·sis (sim'fi·sis) *n.,* pl. **symphy·ses** (·seez) A synchondrosis, especially one in the sagittal plane.

symphysis man·di·bu·lae (man·dib'yoo·lee). The midline osteochondral union of the halves of the mandible.

symphysis pu·bis (pew'bis). The fibrocartilaginous union (synchondrosis) of the pubic bones.

sym·plasm (sim'plaz·um) *n.* A protoplasmic mass resulting from the coalescence of originally separate cells.

sym·po·dia (sim·po'dee·uh) *n.* The condition of united lower extremities.

symp·tom (simp'tum) *n.* A phenomenon of physical or mental disorder or disturbance which leads to complaints on the part of the patient; usually a subjective state, such as headache or pain, in contrast to an objective sign such as papilledema.

symp·tom·at·ic (simp"tuh·mat'ick) *adj.* 1. Pertaining to, or of the nature of, a symptom. 2. Affecting symptoms, as symptomatic treatment. 3. Characteristic or indicative of a physical or mental disorder, as night sweating may be symptomatic of tuberculosis, or excessive alcoholic intake of emotional disturbance. 4. Pertaining to or having the characteristics of one disorder which reflects a known or diagnosable underlying pathologic cause, as epilepsy may be symptomatic of a brain injury or of a metabolic disorder, in contrast to idiopathic or essential epilepsy where the cause is not known.

symptomatic purpura. Purpura which may accompany acute infectious diseases or chronic diseases such as malignant tumors, nephritis, and blood dyscrasias, and following administration of certain drugs. Syn. *secondary purpura.*

symp·tom·atol·o·gy (simp″tuh-muh-tol′uh-jee) *n.* 1. The science of symptoms. 2. In common usage, the symptoms of disease taken together as a whole. —**symp·tom·ato·log·ic** (simp″tuh-mat″uh-loj′ick) *adj.*

symptom complex, group, or **grouping.** The ensemble of symptoms of a disease.

symp·to·sis (simp·to′sis) *n.* Wasting; emaciation; collapse.

sym·pus (sim′pus) *n.* A fetus characterized by greater or less fusion of the legs, rotation of the legs, and marked deficiencies of the pelvic region and genitalia. Syn. *cuspidate fetus, symelus, sirenoform fetus, mermaid fetus.*

syn-, sym- A prefix meaning (a) *with, together;* (b) (italicized) in chemistry, the stereoisomeric form of certain compounds, as aldoximes, in which substituent atoms or groups are in cis-relationship.

syn·ac·to·sis (sin″ack·to′sis) *n.* Malformations caused by the abnormal growing together of parts.

syn·apse (sin′aps, si·naps′) *n. & v.,* pl. **synap·ses** (·seez) 1. The region of communication between neurons; the point at which an impulse passes from an axon of one neuron to a dendrite or to the cell of another. A synapse is polarized, that is, nerve impulses are transmitted only in one direction, and is characterized by fatigability. 2. The union of the male and female chromosome pairs during meiosis, occurring either side-to-side or end-to-end without either univalent chromosome losing its identity. A bivalent chromosome results and is responsible for transmitting mixed characteristics from the parents to the offspring. 3. To make an interneuronal connection; a syncytium.

syn·ap·sis (sin·ap′sis) *n.,* pl. **synap·ses** (·seez) SYNAPSE.

syn·ap·tic (si·nap′tick) *adj.* Pertaining to or communicated by a synapse.

syn·ar·thro·phy·sis (sin·ahr″thro·figh′sis) *n.* Progressive ankylosis of the joints.

syn·ar·thro·sis (sin″ahr·thro′sis) *n.,* pl. **synarthro·ses** (·seez) A form of articulation in which the bones are immovably bound together without any intervening synovial cavity. The forms are sutura, in which processes are interlocked; schindylesis, in which a thin plate of one bone is inserted into a cleft of another; and gomphosis, in which a conical process is held by a socket. Adj. *synarthrodial.*

syn·can·thus (sin·kan′thus) *n.* Adhesions between the orbital tissues and the eyeball.

syn·chei·lia, syn·chi·lia (sin·kigh′lee·uh) *n.* Fusion of the lips.

syn·chon·dro·sis (sin·kon·dro′sis, sin·) *n.,* pl. **synchondro·ses** (·seez) A joint in which the surfaces are connected by a plate of cartilage. —**synchondro·sial** (·zee·ul, ·zhul) *adj.*

syn·chon·drot·o·my (sin″kon·drot′uh·mee) *n.* A division of the cartilage uniting bones, especially that of the symphysis pubis.

syn·chro·nism (sing′kruh·niz·um) *n.* SYNCHRONY.

syn·chro·nous (sing′kruh·nus) *adj.* Occurring at

the same time; concurrent. —**synchro·ny** (·nee) *n.*

synchysis scin·til·lans (sin′ti·lanz). The presence of bright, shining particles in the vitreous body of the eye.

syn·cli·tism (sing′kli·tiz·um, sin′) *n.* 1. A condition marked by parallelism or similarity of inclination. 2. Parallelism between the pelvic planes and those of the fetal head. —**syn·clit·ic** (sing·klit′ick, sin·) *adj.*

syn·clo·nus (sing′klo·nus, sin·) *n. Obsol.* 1. Tremor, or clonic spasm, of several muscles at the same time. 2. A disease thus characterized, as chorea.

syn·co·pe (sing′kuh·pee) *n.* A faint; an episodic pause in the stream of consciousness due to cerebral hypoxia, of abrupt onset and brief duration and from which recovery is usually complete. —**synco·pal** (·pul), **syn·cop·ic** (sing·kop′ick) *adj.*

Syncurine. Trademark for decamethonium bromide, a skeletal muscle relaxant.

syn·cy·tial (sin·sish′ul) *adj.* Pertaining to, or constituting, a syncytium.

syncytial endometritis or **deciduitis.** Excessive proliferation of the syncytiotrophoblastic cells near the site of the placenta with invasion of the endometrium, decidua, and adjacent myometrium by these cells.

syncytial knots. Protuberant masses of syncytiotrophoblast characteristic of the surface of mature placental villi.

syn·cy·tio·ly·sin (sin·sish″ee·o·lye′sin, sin·sit″ee·ol′i·sin) *n.* A cytolysin produced by injections of an emulsion made from placental tissue.

syn·cy·tio·tro·pho·blast (sin·sish″ee·o·tro′fo·blast, sin·sit″) *n.* An irregular sheet or net of deeply staining cytoplasm in which nuclei are irregularly scattered; it lies outside the cytotrophoblast from which it is derived by fusion of separate cells. Syn. *plasmoditrophoblast, syncytial trophoblast.*

syn·cy·tium (sin·sish′ee·um, sin·sit′ee·um) *n.,* pl. **syncy·tia** (·shee·uh, ·tee·uh) A mass of cytoplasm with numerous nuclei but with no division into separate cells.

syn·dac·tyl (sin·dack′til) *adj.* Having fingers or toes joined together.

syn·dac·ty·lism (sin·dack′ti·liz·um) *n.* SYNDACTYLY.

syn·dac·ty·lus (sin·dack′ti·lus) *n.* A person with webbed fingers or toes.

syn·dac·ty·ly (sin·dack′ti·lee) *n.* Adhesion of fingers or toes; webbed fingers or webbed toes. —**syndacty·lous** (·lus) *adj.*

syn·de·sis (sin·de′sis) *n.* The state of being bound together.

syn·des·mec·to·pia (sin·dez″meck·to′pee·uh) *n.* Displacement of a ligament.

syn·des·mi·tis (sin″dez·migh′tis) *n.* 1. Inflammation of a ligament. 2. CONJUNCTIVITIS.

syn·des·mo·di·as·ta·sis (sin·dez″mo·dye·as′tuh·sis) *n.* Separation of ligaments.

syn·des·mol·o·gy (sin″dez·mol′uh·jee) *n.* The study of ligaments.

syn·des·mo·pexy (sin·dez′mo·peck″see) *n.* The attachment of a ligament in a new position.

syn·des·mor·rha·phy (sin″dez·mor′uh·fee) n. Suture or repair of ligaments.

syn·des·mo·sis (sin″dez·mo′sis) n., pl. **syndesmoses** (·seez) A form of articulation in which the bones are connected by fibrous connective tissue.

syn·des·mot·omy (sin″dez·mot′uh·mee) n. The division of a ligament.

syn·drome (sin′drome, sin′dro·mee) n. A group of symptoms and signs, which, when considered together, are known or presumed to characterize a disease or lesion. —**syn·dro·mic** (sin·dro′mick, ·drom′ick) adj.

syn·dro·mol·o·gy (sin″dro·mol′uh·jee) n. The study of syndromes; the analysis of constellations of signs or symptoms with a view to determining which of them are significantly linked as probable results of the same underlying cause or causes.

syn·ech·ia (si·neck′ee·uh, si·nee′kee·uh) n., pl. **syn·echiae** (·ee·ee) An abnormal union of parts; especially adhesion of the iris to a neighboring part of the eye. —**synech·i·al** (·ee·ul) adj.

syn·ech·o·tome (si·neck′o·tome) n. An instrument for the division of adhesions, particularly of the tympanic membrane.

syn·ech·ot·o·my (sin″e·kot′uh·mee) n. The division of a synechia.

syn·en·ceph·a·lo·cele (sin″en·sef′uh·lo·seel) n. An encephalocele with adhesions.

syn·er·e·sis (sin·err′e·sis) n., pl. **synere·ses** (·seez) 1. Contraction of a clot, as blood, milk. 2. In colloid chemistry, the exudation of the liquid constituent of gels irrespective of the vapor pressure imposed upon the system. Lowered vapor pressure aids the process.

syn·er·get·ic (sin″er·jet′ick) adj. Exhibiting synergy; working together; synergic.

syn·er·gism (sin′ur·jiz·um) n. 1. SYNERGY. 2. The joint action of two types of microorganisms on a carbohydrate medium, leading to the production of gas that is not formed by either organism when grown separately. 3. POTENTIATION (2).

syn·er·gist (sin′ur·jist) n. 1. An agent that increases the action or effectiveness of another agent when combined with it. 2. SYNERGISTIC MUSCLE. —**syn·er·gis·tic** (sin″ur·jis′tick) adj.

synergistic muscle. A muscle which, though not directly concerned as a prime mover in a particular act, helps some other muscle to perform the movement more efficiently.

syn·er·gy (sin′ur·jee) n. 1. The combined action or effect of two or more organs or agents, often greater than the sum of their individual actions or effects. 2. Coordination of muscular or organ functions by the nervous system in such a way that specific movements and actions can be performed. —**syn·er·gic** (si·nur′jick) adj.

syn·es·the·sia, syn·aes·the·sia (sin″es·theezh′uh, ·theez′ee·uh) n. 1. A secondary sensation or subjective impression accompanying an actual perception of a different character, as a sensation of color or sound aroused by a sensation of taste. 2. A sensation experienced in one part of the body following stimulation of another part.

Syn·ga·mus (sing′guh·mus) n. A genus of nematode worms of the family Syngamidae, which inhabits the upper respiratory tract of fowl and mammals.

Syngamus la·ryn·ge·us (la·rin′jee·us). A species which is usually a parasite of ruminants; incidental infection of man has occurred.

Syngamus tra·che·a·lis (tray″kee·ay′lis). The nematode infesting the trachea of avians and causing the condition called gapes of chickens. Syn. gapeworm.

syn·ge·ne·ic (sin″je·nee′ick) adj. SYNGENESIOUS.

syngeneic graft. A transplant between individuals that have been inbred until their genetic similarity allows acceptance of grafts between strain members.

syn·ge·ne·sio·plas·ty (sin″je·nee′zee·o·plas″tee) n. Plastic surgery employing homografts taken from parents, siblings, or offspring. —**syn·ge·ne·sio·plas·tic** (·nee″zee·o·plas′tick) adj.

syn·ge·ne·sious (sin″je·nee′zhus, ·zee·us) adj. Of or derived from an individual of the same family or species, as of a tissue transplant.

syn·gig·no·scism (sin·jig′no·siz·um) n. HYPNOTISM.

syn·hi·dro·sis (sin″hi·dro′sis) n. Concurrent sweating; the association of perspiration with another condition.

syn·i·ze·sis (sin″i·zee′sis) n. SYNIZESIS PUPILLAE.

synizesis pu·pil·lae (pew·pil′ee). Closure of the pupil.

Synkamin. Trademark for 2-methyl-4-amino-1-naphthol hydrochloride, referred to as vitamin K_5, a water-soluble vitamin K compound.

Synkayvite. A trademark for menadiol sodium diphosphate, a water-soluble prothrombinogenic compound with the actions and uses of menadione.

syn·ki·ne·sia (sin″kigh·nee′zhuh) n. SYNKINESIS.

syn·ki·ne·sis (sin″kigh·nee′sis) n. Involuntary movement of muscles or limbs coincident with the deliberate or essential movements carried out by another part of the body, such as the swinging of the arms while walking. Syn. associated automatic movement, accessory movement. —**synki·net·ic** (·net′ick) adj.

syn·ne·ma·tin (si·nee′muh·tin, sin″e·may′tin) n. An antibiotic substance, produced by Cephalosporium salmosynnematum, found to be D-(4-amino-4-carboxybutyl) penicillin and now generally called penicillin N. Syn. cephalosporin N.

syn·odon·tia (sin″o·don′chee·uh) n. Production of one tooth, showing evidence of duplicity, by fusion of two tooth germs.

syn·oph·rys (sin·off′ris) n. Meeting of the eyebrows.

syn·or·chi·dism (sin·or′ki·diz·um) n. Partial or complete fusion of the two testes within the abdomen or scrotum.

syn·or·chism (sin·or′kiz·um) n. SYNORCHIDISM.

syn·os·che·os (sin·os′kee·os) n. A condition of adherence between the skin of the penis and that of the scrotum.

syn·os·teo·phyte (sin·os'tee·o·fite) n. A congenital bony ankylosis. Syn. *synostosis congenita.*

syn·os·to·sis (sin''os·to'sis) n., pl. **synosto·ses** (·seez) A union by osseous material of originally separate bones. **—synos·tot·ic** (·tot'ick) adj.

syn·o·tia (si·no'shee·uh) n. Approximation or union of the ears in the anterior cervical region in the absence, or marked reduction, of the lower jaw.

syn·o·vec·to·my (sin''o·veck'tuh·mee) n. Excision of synovial membrane.

syn·o·via (si·no'vee·uh) n. SYNOVIAL FLUID. **—syno·vi·al** (·vee·ul) adj.

synovial fluid. The clear fluid, resembling white of egg, found in various joints, bursas, and sheaths of tendons.

synovial joint. A freely movable articulation, in which contiguous bone surfaces are covered with collagenous fibrovascular tissue composed of flattened or cuboidal cells. For synovial joints listed by name, see Table of Synovial Joints and Ligaments in the Appendix.

synovial membrane. The sheet of flattened connective tissue cells that lines a synovial bursa, a synovial sheath, or the capsule of a synovial joint.

synovial sheath. A synovial membrane which lines the cavity through which a tendon glides.

syn·o·vio·en·do·the·lio·ma (si·no''vee·o·en''theel·ee·o'muh) n. A malignant synovioma.

syn·o·vi·o·ma (si·no''vee·o'muh) n. Any tumor, benign or malignant, whose parenchyma is composed of cells similar to those covering the synovial membranes.

syn·o·vi·tis (sin''o·vye'tis) n. Inflammation of a synovial membrane.

syn·tac·tic (sin·tack'tick) adj. Pertaining to syntax, or the system whereby linguistic units (especially, words) are combined to form larger units (phrases, sentences).

syn·tac·ti·cal (sin·tack'ti·kul) adj. SYNTACTIC.

syntactical or **syntactic aphasia.** A type of Wernicke's aphasia characterized by jargon and impaired comprehension, writing, and reading.

syn·ta·sis (sin'tuh·sis) n. A stretching, or tension.

syn·the·sis (sinthe'e·sis) n., pl. **synthe·ses** (·seez) 1. *In chemistry,* the processes and operations necessary to build up a compound. In general, a reaction, or series of reactions, in which a complex compound is obtained from elements or simple compounds. 2. The formation of a complex concept by the combination of separate ideas; the putting together of data to form a whole. 3. *In psychiatry,* the process in which the ego accepts unconscious ideas and feelings and amalgamates them within itself more or less consciously. **—syn·the·size** (sinth'e·size) v.

syn·thet·ic (sin·thet'ick) adj. Produced by artificial means.

syn·ton·ic (sin·ton'ick) adj. Characterizing a type of personality in which there is an appropriate harmony of thinking, feeling, and behavior, one in harmony with the environment.

syn·to·nin (sin'to·nin) n. 1. A metaprotein obtained by the action of dilute acid on more complex proteins. 2. The specific metaprotein thus obtained from the myosin of muscle.

syn·tro·pho·blast (sin·tro'fo·blast, ·trof'o·) n. SYNCYTIOTROPHOBLAST.

syn·tro·py (sin'truh·pee) n. *In psychobiology,* the state of felicitous and mutually satisfactory relationship with other individuals.

syph·i·le·mia (sif''i·lee'mee·uh) n. The presence of *Treponema pallidum* in the bloodstream.

syph·i·lid (sif'i·lid) n. Any skin eruption due to syphilis.

syph·i·lis (sif'i·lis) n. A prenatal or acquired systemic infection with *Treponema pallidum,* most often contracted in sexual intercourse. Lesions may occur in any tissue or vascular organ of the body, and the disease may produce various clinical pictures of its own, or give rise to symptoms characteristic of other diseases.

syphilis tech·ni·ca (teck'ni·kuh). Syphilis acquired in following one's occupation, as by physicians, midwives, nurses.

syph·i·lit·ic (sif''i·lit'ick) adj. & n. 1. Of, pertaining to, or affected with syphilis. 2. A person affected with syphilis.

syphilitic amyotrophy. A rare disease of questionable syphilitic etiology, characterized by progressive muscular atrophy of the upper limbs and shoulder girdles.

syphilitic cirrhosis. Hepatic fibrosis resulting from syphilitic destruction of liver parenchyma.

syphilitic meningomyelitis. A form of spinal syphilis, characterized pathologically by a chronic fibrosing meningitis with subpial loss of myelinated fibers and gliosis, and clinically by signs referable to disease of the lateral and posterior columns of the spinal cord.

syphilitic node. Localized swelling on bones due to syphilitic periostitis.

syph·i·li·za·tion (sif''i·li·zay'shun) n. 1. Inoculation with *Treponema pallidum.* 2. The occurrence and spread of syphilis in a community.

syph·i·lo·derm (sif'i·lo·durm) n. Any of the skin manifestations of syphilis. **—syph·i·lo·der·ma·tous** (sif''i·lo·dur'muh·tus) adj.

syph·i·lo·ma (sif''i·lo'muh) n., pl. **syphilomas, syphiloma·ta** (·tuh) 1. A syphilitic gumma. 2. A tumor due to syphilis. **—syph·i·lom·a·tous** (·lom'uh·tus) adj.

syph·i·lo·ma·nia (sif''i·lo·may'nee·uh) n. Extreme syphilophobia.

syph·i·lo·phobe (sif'i·lo·fobe) n. A person affected with syphilophobia.

syph·i·lo·pho·bia (sif''i·lo·fo'bee·uh) n. Abnormal fear of syphilis; the delusion of being infected with syphilis.

syr. Abbreviation for *syrupus.* syrup.

sy·rig·mo·pho·nia (si·rig''mo·fo'nee·uh) n. 1. A piping or whistling state of the voice. 2. A sibilant rale.

sy·rig·mus (si·rig'mus) n., pl. **syrig·mi** (·mye) Any subjective hissing, murmuring, or tinkling sound heard in the ear.

syr·ing·ad·e·no·ma (sirr''ing·gad''e·no'muh) n. SWEAT GLAND ADENOMA.

syr·ing·ad·e·no·sus (sirr''ing·gad''e·no'sus) adj. Pertaining to the sweat glands.

sy·ringe (suh·rinj', sirr'inj) *n.* 1. An apparatus commonly made of glass or plastic, fitted snugly onto a hollow metal needle, used to aspirate or inject fluids for diagnostic or therapeutic purposes. It consists essentially of a barrel, which may be calibrated, and a perfectly matched plunger. 2. A large glass barrel with a fitted rubber bulb at one end and a nozzle at the other, used primarily for irrigation purposes.

sy·rin·go·bul·bia (si·ring''go·bul'bee·uh) *n.* An extension of the cavity of syringomyelia into the brainstem, usually into the lateral tegmentum of the medulla and rarely into the pons.

sy·rin·go·car·ci·no·ma (si·ring''go·kahr''si·no'muh) *n.* 1. SWEAT GLAND ADENOMA. 2. SWEAT GLAND CARCINOMA.

sy·rin·go·cele, sy·rin·go·coele (si·ring'go·seel) *n.* The cavity or central canal of the spinal cord.

sy·rin·go·cyst·ad·e·no·ma (si·ring''go·sist''ad·e·no'muh) *n.* SYRINGOMA.

sy·rin·go·cys·to·ma (si·ring''go·sis·to'muh) *n.* SYRINGOMA.

sy·rin·goid (si·ring'goid) *adj.* Like a tube.

syr·in·go·ma (sir''ing·go'muh) *n.* A benign tumor of sweat glands, occurring most often in females and developing after puberty. Histologically, the dermis contains numerous small cystic ducts with comma-like tails of epithelium. Syn. *syringocystadenoma, syringocystoma.*

sy·rin·go·my·e·lia (si·ring''go·migh·ee'lee·uh) *n.* A chronic progressive degenerative disorder of the spinal cord, characterized clinically by brachial amyotrophy and segmental sensory loss of dissociated type, and pathologically by cavitation of the central parts of the cervical spinal cord and extending in some cases into the medulla oblongata or downward into the thoracic and lumbar segments.

sy·rin·go·my·e·lo·cele (si·ring''go·migh'e·lo·seel) *n.* Spina bifida with protrusion of a meningeal sac containing a portion of the spinal cord whose central canal is greatly distended with cerebrospinal fluid.

syr·inx (sirr'inks) *n.,* pl. **sy·rin·ges** (si·rin'jeez), **syrinxes** 1. A fistula or tube. 2. The posterior larynx of birds, found within the thorax at the tracheal bifurcation; the organ of voice in birds. 3. The glial-lined cavity in syringomyelia.

syr·up, sir·up (sur'up, sirr'up) *n.* 1. A concentrated solution of sugar in aqueous fluids, with the addition of medicating or flavoring ingredients. 2. Simple syrup: the U.S.P. preparation containing sucrose, 850 g and a sufficient quantity of purified water to make 1,000 ml.

Used in the preparation of other medicated or flavored syrups and preparations and in pharmaceutical operations where sucrose is in solution is required. Abbreviated, syr.

sys·sar·co·sis (sis''ahr·ko'sis) *n.,* pl. **syssarco·ses** (·seez) The failure of union of bones after fracture by the interposition of muscular tissue. —**syssar·cot·ic** (·kot'ick) *adj.*

sys·ta·sis (sis'tuh·sis) *n.* Consistency, density.

sys·tem, *n.* 1. A methodical arrangement. 2. A combination of parts into a whole, as the digestive system, the nervous system. 3. The body as a functional whole.

sys·tem·at·ic (sis''te·mat'ick) *adj.* 1. Pertaining to or constituting a system. 2. Methodical; orderly. 3. Of or pertaining to classification, as in taxonomy. 4. SYSTEMIC (1).

sys·tem·ic (sis·tem'ick) *adj.* 1. Of, pertaining to, or involving the body considered as a functional whole. 2. Of or pertaining to the systemic circulation.

systemic circulation. The general circulation, as distinct from the pulmonary circulation. Syn. *greater circulation.*

systemic lupus erythematosus. An often fatal disease of unknown cause, characterized clinically by fever, muscle and joint pains, anemia, leukopenia, and frequently by a skin eruption similar to chronic discoid lupus erythematosus. Pathologically it is characterized by alteration in the connective tissue, especially of the arterioles, and the presence of hematoxylin-staining bodies in areas of fibrinoid degeneration of involved tissues. Primarily involved are the kidney, spleen, skin, and endocardium.

sys·tem·oid (sis'te·moid) *adj.* Characterizing a tumor composed of a number of tissues resembling a system of organs.

sys·to·le (sis'tuh·lee) *n.* The contraction phase of the cardiac cycle.

sys·tol·ic (sis·tol'ick) *adj.* Pertaining to the systole; occurring during systole.

systolic blood pressure. The maximum systemic arterial blood pressure during ventricular systole.

systolic click. A single or multiple extra heart sound, occurring in mid- or late systole; usually related to an abnormality of the mitral valve but may occasionally be of extracardiac origin.

systolic thrill. A thrill felt during ventricular systole on palpation of the precordium, as in conditions such as ventricular septal defect and aortic or pulmonic stenosis.

sys·trem·ma (sis·trem'uh) *n.,* pl. **systremma·ta** (·tuh) A cramp in the muscles of the leg.

T

T 1. Abbreviation for *temperature.* 2. *In molecular biology,* symbol for thymine.

t½, t½ *In radiology,* symbol for half-life.

T 1824 EVANS BLUE.

Ta Symbol for tantalum.

tab·a·co·sis (tab″uh·ko′sis) *n.* A toxic state produced by the excessive use of tobacco, or by the inhalation of tobacco dust.

Ta·ban·i·dae (ta·ban′i·dee) *n.pl.* A family of the Diptera, which includes the horseflies, deerflies, and gadflies. They are medium to large in size, robust and worldwide in distribution. The females of the well-known species are bloodsuckers which attack man and warm-blooded animals generally. Certain species distribute diseases such as anthrax among cattle and sheep; others transmit the trypanosomes of animals, especially the *Trypanosoma evansi,* the cause of surra in horses and cattle. The important genera are *Chrysops, Haematopota, Tabanus,* and *Pangonia.*

ta·bar·dil·lo (tah″bahr·dee′yo) *n.* EPIDEMIC TYPHUS.

ta·bel·la (ta·bel′uh) *n.,* pl. **tabel·lae** (·ee) A medicinal troche or tablet.

ta·bes (tay′beez) *n.* 1. A wasting or consumption of a part of or the whole body. 2. TABES DORSALIS. Adj. *tabetic.*

tabes cox·a·ria (kock·sair′ree·uh). Wasting from hip disease.

tabes dor·sa·lis (dor·say′lis). A form of neurosyphilis which develops 15 to 20 years after the onset of infection. It is characterized clinically by lightning pains, ataxia, urinary incontinence, absent knee and ankle jerks, impaired vibratory and position sense in the feet and legs, and a Romberg posterior sign, and pathologically by a degeneration of the posterior roots and posterior columns of the spinal cord. Syn. *tabetic neurosyphilis, locomotor ataxia.*

tabes mes·en·ter·i·ca (mes″en·terr′i·kuh). Mesenteric lymphadenitis, usually due to infection with *Mycobacterium tuberculosis,* with paroxysmal abdominal symptoms resembling those of tabes dorsalis.

ta·bet·ic (ta·bet′ick) *adj.* 1. Affected with tabes; of or pertaining to tabes. 2. Pertaining to, or affected with, tabes dorsalis.

tabetic arthropathy. CHARCOT′S JOINT.

tabetic crisis. Paroxysmal pain occurring in the course of tabes dorsalis.

tabetic gait. The ataxic gait of tabes dorsalis.

ta·bet·i·form (ta·bet′i·form) *adj.* Resembling tabes.

ta·ble, *n.* 1. A flat-topped piece of furniture, as an operating table, examining table. 2. A flat plate, especially one of bone, as the inner or outer table (of compact bone) of a flat bone of the cranium. 3. An orderly presentation of numerical data in the form of rows and columns.

ta·ble·spoon, *n.* A large spoon, holding about 15 ml, or 4 fluidrams. Abbreviated, tbsp.

tab·let, *n.* A solid dosage form of a medicinal substance or substances, with or without suitable diluents, that may be prepared by compression or by molding.

ta·bo·pa·ral·y·sis (tay″bo·puh·ral′i·sis) *n.* TABOPARESIS.

tabo·pa·re·sis (tay″bo·puh·ree′sis, ·păr′e·sis) *n.* A form of neurosyphilis in which the symptoms and signs of tabes dorsalis are combined with those of general paresis.

tab·u·lar (tab′yoo·lur) *adj.* Having the form of a table.

tache (tash) *n.,* pl. **taches** (tash) A spot, macule, freckle; circumscribed discoloration on the skin or a mucous membrane.

tache cé·ré·brale (say·ray·bral′). A red streak, sometimes associated with petechiae, produced by drawing a fingernail over the skin, due to increased vasomotor irritability, occurring in certain neurologic disorders, especially in connection with meningeal irritation. Syn. *Trousseau′s sign.*

ta·chet·ic (ta·ket′ick) *adj.* Relating to the formation of reddish blue or purple patches (taches).

ta·chis·to·scope (ta·kis′tuh·skope) *n.* 1. An instrument used in physiologic psychology to observe the time rate and time conditions for apperception. 2. Any of several instruments using timed brief flashes of light for testing visual fields or in orthoptic correction procedures. —**ta·chis·to·scop·ic** (ta·kis''tuh·skop'ick) adj.

tacho- A combining form meaning speed.

tacho·gram (tack'o·gram) n. The record made in tachography.

ta·chog·ra·phy (ta·kog'ruh·fee) n. The estimation of the rate of flow of arterial blood by means of a flowmeter.

ta·chom·e·ter (ta·kom'e·tur) n. HEMOTACHOMETER. 2. A device for measuring frequency of rotation.

tachy- A combining form meaning rapid, quick, accelerated.

tachy·al·i·men·ta·tion (tack''ee·al'i·men·tay'shun) n. Eating more rapidly than normal.

tachy·ar·rhyth·mia (tack''ee·a·rith'mee·uh) n. Rapid heart action without control by the sinoatrial node.

tachy·aux·e·sis (tack''ee·awk·see'sis) n. Heterauxesis in which a part grows more rapidly than the whole organism.

tachy·car·dia (tack''i·kahr'dee·uh) n. Excessive rapidity of the heart's action.

tachy·car·di·ac (tack''i·kahr'dee·ack) adj. Pertaining to, or suffering from, tachycardia.

tachy·graph (tack'i·graf) n. A blood flowmeter.

ta·chyg·ra·phy (ta·kig'ruh·fee) n. The estimation of the rate of flow of arterial blood by means of a blood flowmeter.

tachy·lo·gia (tack''i·lo'jee·uh) n. Extreme rapidity or volubility of speech.

ta·chym·e·ter (ta·kim'e·tur) n. An instrument for measuring the speed of a moving object.

tachy·pha·gia (tack''i·fay'jee·uh) n. Rapid eating.

tachy·phy·lax·ia (tack''i·fi·lack'see·uh) n. TACHYPHYLAXIS.

tachy·phy·lax·is (tack''i·fi·lack'sis) n. 1. The rapid desensitization against toxic doses of organ extracts or serum by the previous inoculation of small, subtoxic doses of the same preparation. 2. Decreasing response to stimulation by such substances as hormones or drugs, as doses of the substance are repeatedly given.

tachy·pnea, tachy·pnoea (tack''i·nee'uh, tack''ip·) n. Abnormally rapid rate of breathing. —**tachy·pne·ic, tachy·pnoe·ic** (·nee'ick) adj.

tachy·rhyth·mia (tack''i·rith'mee·uh) n. TACHYCARDIA.

ta·chys·ter·ol (ta·kis'tur·ole, ·ol, tack''i·steer'ol) n. The precursor of calciferol in the irradiation of ergosterol; an isomer of ergosterol.

tachy·sys·to·le (tack''i·sis'tuh·lee) n. TACHYCARDIA.

tac·tile (tack'til) adj. 1. Pertaining to the sense of touch. 2. Capable of being felt.

tactile alexia. Inability to recognize language symbols by touch, as when a blind person loses the faculty of reading braille.

tactile fremitus. The vibratory sensation conveyed to the hand when applied to the chest of a person speaking.

ac·toid (tack'toid) n. A type of colloidal structure showing intense birefringence in which

elongated particles are oriented in a group and parallel to a central axis; a cigar-shaped colloidal particle.

tad·pole cells. Anaplastic squamous cells desquamated in cancer of the uterine cervix, appearing with one broad and one narrow end.

tae·di·um vi·tae (tee'dee·um vye'tee) Weariness of life, a symptom of depressive illness and sometimes a precursor of suicide.

Tae·nia (tee'nee·uh) n. A genus of parasitic worms of the class Cestoda; they are ribbonlike segmental flatworms. The adult is an intestinal parasite of vertebrates; the larvae parasitize both vertebrate and invertebrate tissues. The adult consists of a scolex, an undifferentiated germinal neck, and two or more hermaphroditic segments or proglottids that contain fertile ova when mature.

¹taenia, n., pl. **taenias.** 1. A member of the genus Taenia. 2. Any tapeworm.

²tae·nia (tee'nee·uh) n., pl. **tae·ni·ae** (·nee·ee) [NA]. Tenia (= BAND (3)).

tae·nia·cide, te·nia·cide (tee'nee·uh·side) n. Any agent that is destructive of tapeworms.

taeniae co·li (ko'lye) [BNA]. TENIAE COLI.

tae·nia·fuge, te·nia·fuge (tee'nee·uh·fewj) n. Any agent that brings about the expulsion of tapeworms.

Taenia sag·i·na·ta (saj·i·nay'tuh). A tapeworm that passes its larval stages in cattle, its adult stage in the intestine of man. The human infection is acquired by eating insufficiently cooked infected beef. Syn. beef tapeworm.

tae·ni·a·sis (tee·nye'uh·sis) n. The symptoms caused by infection with any of the species of Taenia.

Taenia so·li·um (so'lee·um). A tapeworm that passes the larval stages in hogs; the adult is found in the intestine of man. Ingestion of ova may result in larval infection in man; the larva is then called Cysticercus cellulosae. Infection is usually acquired by ingestion of viable larvae in pork. Syn. pork tapeworm.

tae·ni·form, te·ni·form (tee'ni·form) adj. Having a ribbonlike form; resembling a tapeworm.

tae·ni·oid, te·ni·oid (tee'nee·oid) adj. TAENIFORM.

tae·nio·pho·bia, te·nio·pho·bia (tee''nee·o·fo'bee·uh) n. An abnormal fear of becoming the host of a tapeworm.

tag, n. & v. 1. A flap or appendage. 2. LABEL. —**tagged,** adj.

tail, n. 1. The caudal extremity of an animal. 2. Anything resembling a tail.

tai·lor's ankle. An abnormal bursa over the lateral malleolus in tailors, due to pressure from sitting on the floor with crossed legs.

taint, n. 1. Hereditary predisposition to disease; affection by disease without unspoken manifestations. 2. Putrefaction or infestation, as in tainted meat. 3. Local discoloration, as a blemish.

Ta·ka·ta-Ara test A test for liver function in which a solution of mercuric chloride is used to determine an imbalance between albumin and globulin in blood plasma or cerebrospinal fluid.

Ta·ka·ya·su's disease or **syndrome** AORTIC ARCH SYNDROME.

take, *n.* 1. *In medicine,* a successful inoculation, as by a vaccine. 2. *In plastic surgery,* the survival of transplanted tissue in its new site, either temporarily or permanently.

tal-, talo-. A combining form meaning *talus, talar, ankle.*

ta·lal·gia (ta·lal'jee·uh) *n.* Pain in the ankle.

ta·lar (tay'lur) *adj.* Of or pertaining to the talus.

talc, *n.* A native hydrous magnesium silicate sometimes containing a little aluminum silicate. Used as a protective and lubricant dusting powder; also, in pharmacy, as a diluent and filter aid.

talc granuloma. TALCUM-POWDER GRANULOMA.

talc·o·sis (tal·ko'sis) *n.,* pl. **talco·ses** (·seez) Pneumoconiosis caused by talc dust.

tal·cum (tal'kum) *n.* TALC.

talcum-powder granuloma. A variety of siliceous granuloma produced by talcum powder. Syn. *surgical-glove talc granuloma, pseudosilicoticum.*

tal·i·pes (tal'i·peez) *n.* Any one of a variety of deformities of the human foot, especially those of congenital origin, such as clubfoot or equinovarus. Also embraces paralytic deformities and the numerous simple varieties of foot distortion, according to whether the forefoot is inverted or everted and whether the calcaneal tendon is shortened or lengthened. Combinations of the various types occur.

talipes cal·ca·neo·ca·vus (kal·kay''nee·o·kay'vus). A calcaneus deformity of the foot in which there is also a cavus; a dorsal rotation of the calcaneus with a relative plantar tilting of the foot.

talipes cal·ca·neo·val·gus (kal·kay''nee·o·val'gus). A calcaneus deformity of the foot with associated valgus deviation.

talipes cal·ca·ne·us (kal·kay'nee·us). Talipes in which the patient walks upon the heel alone.

talipes ca·vus (kay'vus). A foot having an abnormally high longitudinal arch, a depression of the metatarsal arch, and dorsal contractures of the toes. It exists in two forms: that in which the outstanding deformity is an exaggeration of the longitudinal arch, and that in which the exaggeration of the longitudinal arch is associated with contraction of the plantar fascia and limitation of dorsiflexion at the ankle. Syn. *hollow foot, contracted foot, nondeforming clubfoot, claw foot.*

talipes equi·no·ca·vus (e·kwye''no·kay'vus). A deformity of the foot characterized by fixed plantar flexion and a high longitudinal arch.

talipes equi·no·val·gus (e·kwye''no·val'gus, eck''wi·). Faulty development of the foot characterized by elevation and outward rotation of the heel.

talipes equi·no·va·rus (e·kwye''no·vair'us). A deformity of the foot characterized by fixed plantar flexion and a turning inward of the foot; CLUBFOOT.

talipes equi·nus (e·kwye'nus). Talipes in which the heel is elevated and the weight thrown upon the anterior portion of the foot.

talipes per·ca·vus (pur·kay'vus). Excessive plantar curvature.

talipes pla·nus (play'nus). FLATFOOT.

talipes spas·mod·i·ca (spaz·mod'i·kuh). Noncongenital talipes due to muscular spasm.

talipes val·gus (val'gus). Talipes in which the outer border of the foot is everted, with inward rotation of the tarsus and flattening of the plantar arch. Syn. *splayfoot.*

talipes va·rus (vair'us). A variety of talipes in which the foot is inverted, the weight falling on the outer border. If the inversion is extreme, with rotation of the forefoot, the condition is known as clubfoot.

tal·i·pom·a·nus (tal''i·pom'uh·nus, tal''i·po·man'us) *n.* CLUBHAND.

tal·low (tal'o) *n.* The fat extracted from suet, the solid fat of cattle, sheep, and other ruminants. It consists largely of stearin and palmitin.

ta·lo·cal·ca·ne·al (tay''lo·kal·kay'nee·ul) *adj.* Pertaining to the talus and the calcaneus.

talocalcaneal ligament. Any of the ligaments connecting the talus and the calcaneus in the subtalar articulation; the interosseous talocalcaneal ligament in the sinus tarsi, the lateral talocalcaneal ligament, connecting the lateral surfaces of the two bones, the medial talocalcaneal ligament, connecting the medial tubercle of the talus and the sustentaculum tali, the anterior talocalcaneal ligament, connecting the neck of the talus and the calcaneus just posterior to the interosseous talocalcaneal ligament, or the posterior talocalcaneal ligament, connecting the lateral tubercle of the talus and the superior and medial surfaces of the calcaneus.

ta·lo·cal·ca·neo·na·vic·u·lar (tay''lo·kal·kay''nee·o·na·vick'yoo·lur) *adj.* Pertaining to the talus, calcaneus, and navicular bones.

ta·lo·fib·u·lar (tay''lo·fib'yoo·lur) *adj.* Pertaining to the talus and the fibula.

talofibular ligament. Either of the ligaments connecting the talus and the fibula; the anterior talofibular ligament, which connects the anterior margins of the lateral malleolus of the fibula and the lateral articular facet of the talus, or the posterior talofibular ligament, a strong, almost horizontal ligament attached to the posterior medial surface of the lateral malleolus and the lateral tubercle on the posterior projection of the talus.

ta·lo·mal·le·o·lar (tay''lo·ma·lee'uh·lur) *adj.* Pertaining to the talus and a malleolus.

ta·lo·na·vic·u·lar (tay''lo·na·vick'yoo·lur) *adj.* Pertaining to the talus and navicular bones.

tal·ose (tal'oce, ·oze) *n.* A monosaccharide, $C_6H_{12}O_6$, isomeric with dextrose.

ta·lus (tay'lus) *n.,* pl. & genit. sing. **ta·li** (·lye) The bone of the ankle which articulates with the bones of the leg. Syn. *astragalus.*

Talwin. Trademark for the synthetic narcotic analgesic pentazocine.

Tamm–Hors·fall protein. A high-molecular-weight mucoprotein which is the major protein constituent of urinary casts.

tam·pan (tam'pan) *n.* An African name for *Ornithodorus moubata,* a parasitic tick infesting birds, small mammals, domestic animals, and occasionally man; an important vector of relapsing fever. Syn. *bibo, mabata.*

tam·pon (tam'pon) *n.* & *v.* 1. A plug of cotton

sponge, or other material inserted into the vagina, nose, or other cavity; a pack. 2. To plug with a tampon.

tam·pon·ade (tam′puh·nade′) *n.* 1. The act of plugging with a tampon. 2. Compression of a viscus, especially of the heart, by an external agent.

tam·pon·age (tam′puh·nij) *n.* TAMPONADE.

tam·pon·ing (tam′pon·ing) *n.* The act of inserting a pack or plug within a cavity, as for checking hemorrhage.

tan, *n. & v.* 1. The darker color produced by exposure of "white" skin to sun, wind, etc. 2. To make or become tan.

ta·na·pox (tah′nuh·pocks) *n.* A viral disease, observed in epidemics in Kenya, characterized by a short febrile illness with headache, malaise, and a single pocklike lesion on the upper part of the body, due to a pox virus which is not related to the vaccinia-variola group; probably a zoonosis, transmitted from monkey to man.

Tandearil. Trademark for oxyphenbutazone, an antiarthritic and anti-inflammatory drug.

tan·dem gait. A manner of walking in which the heel of the advancing foot is placed directly in front of the toes of the stationary foot; used to test a patient's equilibrium and coordination.

Tan·gier disease Greatly reduced serum alphalipoprotein (high-density lipoprotein) and deposition of cholesterol esters in the reticuloendothelial system, manifested clinically by markedly enlarged, strikingly yellow-gray tonsils, lymphadenopathy, splenomegaly, and in adult life by vascular and neurologic involvement.

tan·nase (tan′ace, ·aze) *n.* An enzyme found in cultures of *Penicillium* and *Aspergillus* which converts tannic acid to gallic acid.

tan·nic acid (tan′ick). A tannin usually obtained from nutgalls, the excrescences formed on the young twigs of *Quercus infectoria* and allied species. Used topically as a styptic and astringent, often in 20% solution in glycerin; has been used for treatment of burns but may be absorbed and cause serious systemic toxicity.

tan·nin (tan′in) *n.* 1. TANNIC ACID. 2. Any one of a group of astringent plant principles characterized by their ability to precipitate collagen and to produce dark-colored compounds with ferric salts. The source is frequently identified by a prefix, as gallotannin, quercitannin.

tan·ta·lum (tan′tuh·lum) *n.* Ta = 180.948. A lanthanide, atomic number 73; very hard, malleable, and ductile. It has been variously used in surgery because of its resistance to corrosion.

tan·trum (tan′trum) *n.* An expression of uncontrollable anger, sometimes accompanied by acts of violence.

tap, *n. & v.* 1. A sudden slight blow. 2. Withdrawal of fluid by the use of a trochar or hollow needle. 3. To withdraw fluid by the use of a trochar or hollow needle.

Tapazole. Trademark for the antithyroid drug methimazole.

tapetal reflex. The metallic luster reflected from the back of the eye of certain animals, as the shining green reflex seen in the eyes of cats at night.

ta·pe·to·ret·i·nal (ta·pee″to·ret′i·nul) *adj.* Pertaining to the tapetum and the retina.

ta·pe·tum (ta·pee′tum) *n.,* pl. **tape·ta** (·tuh) 1. [BNA] The layer forming the roof of the posterior horn of the lateral ventricle of the brain. It is composed of fibers from the corpus callosum. 2. A layer of tissue in the choroid of the eye, between its vascular and capillary layer, usually not present in man; it may be cellular as in carnivores or fibrous as in ruminants and contain crystals which reflect light strongly and which result in the metallic luster seen, as in the cat. In man, it is represented by a layer of fibers. —**tape·tal** (·tul) *adj.*

tape·worm, *n.* Any of the species of the class Cestoidea; segmented, ribbonlike flatworms which are parasites of man and other animals.

tapeworm anemia. A megaloblastic anemia, possibly identical with pernicious anemia, occurring in persons infected by the fish tapeworm, *Diphyllobothrium latum.*

taph·e·pho·bia, taph·i·pho·bia (taf″e·fo′bee·uh) *n.* An abnormal fear of being buried alive.

tap·i·no·ceph·a·ly (tap″i′no·sef′uh·lee, ta·pye″ no·) *n.* Flatness of the top of the cranium; flat top. —**tapino·ce·phal·ic** (·se·fal′ick) *adj.*

tap·i·o·ca (tap″ee·o′kuh) *n.* A variety of starch obtained from the cassava or manioc plant, *Jatropha manihot.* Used as food.

ta·pir mouth or **lip** (tay′pur). The peculiarly loose, thickened, protruding lips of the myopathic facies. The patient is unable to smile or whistle.

ta·pir·oid (tay′pur·oid) *adj.* Characterizing pertaining to an elongated cervix of the uterus, so called from its resemblance to a tapir's snout.

ta·pote·ment (ta·poht′munt, F. ta·po^ht·mahn^r) *n.* Percussion movements used in massage.

tar, *n.* A thick brown to black liquid consisting of a mixture of hydrocarbons and their derivatives obtained by the destructive distillation of many kinds of carbonaceous matter.

Taractan. Trademark for chlorprothixene, a tranquilizing drug with antiemetic activity.

tar·ant·ism (tār′un·tiz·um) *n.* A dancing mania, first described during the 15th to 17th centuries in Southern Europe and ascribed to the bite of a tarantula.

ta·ran·tu·la (tuh·ran′choo·luh) *n.,* pl. **tarantulas, taran·tu·lae** (·lee) 1. *Lycosa tarentula,* a large spider of southern Europe, whose bite, traditionally supposed to cause tarantism, is now considered innocuous. 2. Any of various very large, hairy New World spiders of the family Theraphosidae, not significantly poisonous to humans.

ta·rax·is (ta·rack′sis) *n.* CONJUNCTIVITIS.

tar cancer. Squamous cell carcinoma associated with prolonged exposure to tar.

Tar·dieu's ecchymoses (tar·dyceh′) Ecchymotic spots beneath the pleura after death from strangulation or suffocation.

tar·dive (tahr′div) *adj.* Tending to be late; tardy.

tar·get, *n.* 1. The anode in a roentgen-ray tube upon which the electrons are directed and from which the roentgen rays arise. 2. MIRE.

target cell. 1. An abnormal erythrocyte with a low mean corpuscular hemoglobin concentration (MHC) which, when stained, shows a central and peripheral zone of hemoglobin separated by an intermediate unstained area and thus resembles a bull's-eye target. Found after splenectomy and in several types of anemia. Syn. *Mexican hat cell.* 2. A cell bearing a specific surface membrane receptor or antigen which reacts with a given hormone, antibiotic, antibody, sensitized lymphocyte, or other agent and is therefore conceived of as the target of that agent.

target-cell anemia. THALASSEMIA.

target erythrocyte. TARGET CELL (1).

target gland. Any gland directly affected by the hormone of another gland.

target lesion. A vesicular skin lesion with a red rim, characteristic of such diseases as erythema multiforme.

ta·ro (tah'ro) *n.* The starchy root of *Colocasia antiquorum* or Indian kale; used as a food in certain Pacific islands.

tar·ry stools (tahr'ee). Stools having the color and consistency of tar, usually due to hemorrhage into the intestinal tract but also produced by iron, bismuth, or other medication.

tars-, tarso-. A combining form meaning *tarsus, tarsal.*

tars·ad·e·ni·tis (tahr"sad"e·nigh'tis) *n.* Inflammation of the tarsal glands and tarsal plate.

tar·sal (tahr'sul) *adj.* 1. Pertaining to the tarsus (1). 2. Pertaining to the tarsus (2), the dense connective tissue forming the support of an eyelid.

tar·sal·gia (tahr·sal'jee·uh) *n.* Pain, especially of neuralgic character, in the tarsus of the foot.

tarsal glands. Sebaceous glands in the tarsal plates of the eyelids. Syn. *Meibomian glands.* NA *glandulae tarsales.*

tarsal plate. Either of the thin, elongated plates, inferior or superior, which contribute to the form and support of the eyelids.

tarsal tenotomy. Division of the peroneal tendon in the horse for the relief of spavin.

tarsal tunnel syndrome. Pain and sensory loss involving the medial anterior foot and great toe due to compression of the medial plantar nerve by the flexor retinaculum and deep fascia.

tar·sec·to·my (tahr·seck'tuh·mee) *n.* Excision of a tarsal bone or bones.

tar·si·tis (tahr·sigh'tis) *n.* 1. Inflammation of the tarsus of the eyelid. 2. BLEPHARITIS. 3. Inflammation of the tarsus of the foot.

tar·so·chei·lo·plas·ty (tahr"so·kigh'lo·plas"tee) *n.* Plastic surgery of the edge of the eyelid.

tar·so·ma·la·cia (tahr"so·ma·lay'shee·uh, ·see·uh) *n.* Softening of the tarsus of the eyelid.

tar·so·meta·tar·sal (tahr"so·met"uh·tahr'sul) *adj.* Pertaining to the tarsus and the metatarsus.

tarsometatarsal ligament. Any of the ligaments between the tarsal and metatarsal bones, including the dorsal tarsometatarsal ligaments, the plantar tarsometatarsal ligaments, and the interosseous tarsometatarsal ligaments.

tar·so·phy·ma (tahr"so·figh'muh) *n.* Any morbid growth or tumor of the tarsus of the eyelid.

tar·so·plas·ty (tahr'so·plas"tee) *n.* Plastic surgery of the eyelid; BLEPHAROPLASTY.

tar·sop·to·sis (tahr"sop·to'sis) *n.,* pl. **tarsopto·ses** (·seez) Fallen arches; FLATFOOT.

tar·sor·rha·phy (tahr·sor'uh·fee) *n.* 1. The operation of sewing the eyelids together for a part or the whole of their extent. 2. Suture of a tarsal plate.

tar·sot·o·my (tahr·sot'uh·mee) *n.* 1. Operation upon the tarsus of the foot. 2. Operation upon a tarsal plate.

tar·sus (tahr'sus) *n.,* pl. & genit. sing. **tar·si** (·sigh) 1. The instep, or ankle, consisting of the calcaneus, talus, cuboid, navicular, medial, intermediate, and lateral cuneiform bones. 2. The dense connective tissue forming the support of an eyelid; TARSAL PLATE.

tar·tar (tahr'tur) *n.* 1. Crude potassium bitartrate, the principal component of argol, yielding cream of tartar when purified. 2. DENTAL CALCULUS.

tartar emetic. ANTIMONY POTASSIUM TARTRATE.

tart cell. A granulocyte which has ingested the nucleus of another cell, usually a lymphocyte; an important artifact in lupus erythematosus (L.E.) cell preparations.

Tarui's disease. An inborn error of glycogen metabolism, caused by a deficiency of the enzyme phosphofructokinase, with abnormal accumulation of glycogen in muscle.

taste, *n.* A sensation produced by stimulation of special sense organs in the tongue by sweet, sour, bitter, or salty substances.

taste blindness. Inability to recognize the acid, bitter, salty, or sweet flavor of substances, readily detected by others.

taste bud. The end organ of the sense of taste; one of the oval, flask-shaped bodies embedded, most commonly, in the epithelium of the tongue.

TAT Abbreviation for (a) *thematic apperception test;* (b) *toxin-antitoxin.*

tat·too·ing, ta·too·ing, *n.* The production of permanent colors in the skin by the introduction of foreign substances, vegetable or mineral, directly into the corium.

tau·rine (taw'reen, ·rin) *n.* 2-Aminoethanesulfonic acid, $NH_2CH_2CH_2SO_3H$; occurs in bile combined with cholic acids.

tau·ro·cho·lic acid (taw"ro·ko'lick, ·kol'ick). Cholyltaurine $C_{26}H_{45}NO_7S$, a bile acid resulting from conjugation of cholic acid and taurine.

Taus·sig-Bing complex or **malformation** A form of congenital incomplete transposition of the great arteries, in which the aorta arises from the right ventricle and is slightly posterior to the pulmonary trunk, which arises anteriorly from both ventricles.

Taussig-Blalock operation BLALOCK-TAUSSIG OPERATION.

tau·to·me·ni·al (taw"to·mee'nee·ul) *adj.* Pertaining to the same menstrual period.

tau·tom·er·al (taw·tom'ur·ul) *adj.* Pertaining to certain nerve fibers involved in the development of the spinal cord and derived from neurons from the same part of the spinal cord.

tau·tom·er·ism (taw·tom'ur·iz·um) *n.* The property of existing in a state of equilibrium between two isomeric forms and capable of reacting as either one.

Ta·wa·ra's node ATRIOVENTRICULAR NODE.

Ta wave. The electrocardiographic deflection due to repolarization of the atria; it is usually masked by the QRS complex but may be evident with prolongation of the P-R segment.

tax-, taxi-, taxo- A combining form meaning *arrangement.*

tax·is (tack'sis) *n.*, pl. **tax·es** (·seez) 1. A manipulation of an organ whereby it is brought into normal position; specifically, the reduction of a hernia by manual methods. 2. The involuntary response of an entire organism involving change of place toward (positive taxis) or away from (negative taxis) a stimulus.

-taxis A combining form meaning (a) *arrangement, order;* (b) *taxis* (2).

tax·on·o·my (tacks·on'uh·mee) *n. In biology,* the science of the classification of organisms. —**tax·o·nom·ic** (tack"suh·nom'ick) *adj.*

Tay-Sachs disease (sacks) A form of G_{M2} gangliosidosis which begins during the first 3 to 6 months of age and is characterized by an abnormal startle reaction, axial hypotonia leading to spasticity, and, in most cases, cherry-red spots in the retinas; death occurs at 3 to 5 years. The disease results from a deficiency of, or defect in, the enzyme hexosaminidase A.

TB Abbreviation for *tuberculosis.*

t.b. Abbreviation for *tubercle bacillus.*

T bandage. A bandage with three arms that form a letter T; especially used about the waist and the perineum to hold a dressing.

tbsp Abbreviation for *tablespoon.*

tea, *n.* 1. The leaves of *Camellia sinensis (Thea sinensis),* family Theaceae. Tea contains 1 to 5% caffeine, 5 to 15% tannin, and a fragrant volatile oil. An infusion is used as a stimulating beverage. 2. An infusion or decoction prepared from the leaves of *C. sinensis.* 3. Any vegetable infusion or decoction used as a beverage.

teaberry oil. The volatile oil from the leaves of *Gaultheria procumbens,* consisting essentially of methyl salicylate. Syn. *wintergreen oil.*

teach·er's node. SINGER'S NODE.

tear (teer) *n. & v.* 1. A drop of the secretion of the lacrimal glands. 2. A hardened drop or lump of any resinous or gummy drug. 3. To exude tears. 4. More generally, to exude drops or beads of liquid.

tear gas. Substances used to produce physical discomfort without injury by causing inflammation of the mucous membranes of the eyes and nose, followed by lacrimation.

tease, *v.* To tear or gently separate tissue into its component parts, by the use of needles.

tea·spoon, *n.* A spoon commonly assumed to hold about 5 ml. Abbreviated, tsp.

teat (teet) *n.* NIPPLE.

tech·ne·ti·um (teck·nee'shee·um) *n.* Tc = 98.9062. Element number 43, prepared in 1937 by electron or deuteron bombardment of molybdenum and later found among the fission products of uranium. Syn. *masurium.*

tech·ni·cian (teck·nish'un) *n.* A person trained and expert in the technical details of certain medical fields, as bacteriology, pathology, radiology.

tech·nique (teck·neek') *n.* The method of procedure in operations or manipulations of any kind.

tech·nol·o·gist (teck·nol'uh·jist) *n.* A specialist in the technology of a particular field.

tec·no·cyte, tek·no·cyte (teck'no·site) *n.* A young metamyelocyte.

tecta. Plural of *tectum.*

tec·tal (teck'tul) *adj.* Of or pertaining to a tectum; especially, to the tectum of the mesencephalon.

tec·ti·form (teck'ti·form) *adj.* Roof-shaped.

tec·to·ceph·a·ly (teck"to·sef'uh·lee) *n.* SCAPHOCEPHALY.

tec·to·ri·al (teck·to'ree·ul) *adj.* Serving as a roof or covering.

tec·to·spi·nal (teck"to·spye'nul) *adj.* Of or pertaining to the spinal cord and the corpora quadrigemina.

tec·tum (teck'tum) *n.*, pl. **tec·ta** (·tuh) A roof or covering.

tectum me·sen·ce·pha·li (mes·en·sef'uh·lye) [NA]. The dorsal portion of the mesencephalon, including the superior and inferior colliculi and adjacent areas.

te·di·ous (tee'dee·us) *adj.* Unduly protracted, as tedious labor.

teeth·ing (tee'thing) *n.* The eruption of the primary teeth; the process of dentition.

teg·men (teg'mun) *n.*, pl. **teg·mi·na** (·mi·nuh) A cover.

teg·men·tal (teg·men'tul) *adj.* Pertaining to a tegmentum, especially, the tegmentum of the midbrain.

teg·men·tum (teg·men'tum) *n.*, pl. **tegmen·ta** (·tuh) 1. A covering. 2. [NA] The dorsal portion of the midbrain, exclusive of the corpora quadrigemina and the central gray substance.

teg·u·ment (teg'yoo·munt) *n.* INTEGUMENT.

teg·u·men·ta·ry (teg"yoo·men'tur·ee) *adj.* Pertaining to an integument.

tei·chop·sia (tye·kop'see·uh) *n.* Temporary amblyopia, with subjective visual images.

tel-, tele-, teleo-, telo- A combining form meaning *distant, at a distance, remote.*

te·la (tee'luh) *n.*, pl. **te·lae** (·lee) A web or tissue.

tel·al·gia (tel·al'jee·uh) *n.* REFERRED PAIN.

tel·an·gi·ec·ta·sia (tel·an"jee·eck·tay'zhuh, ·zee·uh) *n.* TELANGIECTASIS.

tel·an·gi·ec·ta·sis (tel·an"jee·eck'tuh·sis) *n.* Dilatation of groups of capillaries. They form elevated, dark red, wartlike spots, varying in size from 1 to 7 mm. —**telangi·ec·tat·ic** (·eck·tat'ick) *adj.*

telangiectatic angioma. An angioma in which the component vessels are large.

telangiectatic carcinoma. Inflammatory carcinoma with prominent vascularity.

telangiectatic sarcoma. A variety of osteogenic sarcoma with a prominent vascular component.

tel·an·gi·o·ma (tel·an"jee·o'muh) *n.*, pl. **telangi·omas, telangioma·ta** (·tuh) A mass composed of dilated capillaries.

tel·an·gi·o·sis (te·lan"jee·o'sis) *n.* Any disease of minute blood vessels.

tel·an·gi·tis (tel"an·jye'tis) *n.* Inflammation of capillaries.

tele·car·dio·gram (tel′e-kahr′dee·o·gram) *n.* TEL-ELECTROCARDIOGRAM.

tele·cep·tor (tel′e·sep″tur) *n.* A sense organ that is activated by a distant stimulus, for example, the nose, eye, and cochlea. Syn. *teloreceptor.*

tele·co·balt therapy (tel″e·ko′bawlt). External radiation therapy with a radioactive cobalt source at some distance from the skin.

tele·di·as·tol·ic (te′dye″us·tol′ick) *adj.* Pertaining to the last phase of a diastole.

tele·flu·or·os·co·py (tel″e·floo″ur·os′kuh·pee) *n.* The procedure by which the usual distortion of a fluoroscopic picture by divergence of the roentgen rays is eliminated by placing the source of the rays 2 meters or more from the body part to be fluoroscoped.

tele·ki·ne·sis (tel″e·ki·nee′sis, ·kigh·nee′sis) *n.* The power claimed by some people of causing objects to move without touching them.

tel·elec·tro·car·dio·gram (tel″e·leck″tro·kahr′dee·o·gram) *n.* An electrocardiogram taken in a laboratory, the galvonometer being connected by a wire with the patient, who is elsewhere.

tel·elec·tro·ther·a·peu·tics (tel″e·leck″tro·therr″uh·pew′ticks) *n.* Treatment of hysterical paralysis by a series of electric discharges near the patient without actual contact.

te·lem·e·try (te·lem′e·tree) *n.* The measurement of a property, such as temperature or pressure, and the transmission of the result to a distant receiving station where it is indicated or recorded.

tel·en·ceph·a·lon (tel″en·sef′uh·lon) *n.* The anterior subdivision of the primary forebrain that develops into olfactory lobes, cerebral cortex, and corpora striata. —**telen·ce·phal·ic** (·se·fal′ick) *adj.*

te·le·ol·o·gy (teel″ee·ol′uh·jee, tel′ee·) *n.* The doctrine that explanations of phenomena are to be sought in terms of final causes, purpose, or design in nature. —**tele·o·log·ic** (·o·loj′ick) *adj.*

tele·op·sia (tel″ee·op′see·uh) *n.* A disorder in visual perception of space characterized by an excess of depth, or the illusion that close objects are far away.

tel·eo·roent·gen·o·gram (tel″ee·o·rent′gen·o·gram) *n.* A radiograph, usually of the heart, made at a distance of 6 or more feet, to minimize distortion.

te·leo·ther·a·peu·tics (teel″ee·o·therr″uh·pew′ticks, tel″ee·o·) *n.* SUGGESTION THERAPY.

te·lep·a·thy (te·lep′uh·ee) *n.* The direct awareness of what is taking place in another person′s mind. —**tele·path·ic** (tel″e·path′ick) *adj.*

tele·ra·di·og·ra·phy (tel″e·ray″dee·og′ruh·fee) *n.* Radiography with the tube about 6 feet from the body to avoid distortion and magnification.

tel·es·the·sia, tel·aes·the·sia (tel″es·theezh′uh, ·theez′ee·uh) *n.* 1. Perception of objects or sounds at a distance. 2. A perception of objects or conditions independently of the recognized channels of sense.

tele·sys·tol·ic (tel″e·sis·tol′ick) *adj.* Pertaining to the last phase of systole.

tele·ther·a·py (tel″e·therr′uh·pee) *n.* 1. SUGGES-

TION THERAPY. 2. Treatment with radiation from a distant source.

tel·lu·ri·um (te·lew′ree·um) *n.* Te = 127.60. A nonmetallic element, atomic number 52, of bluish-white color, obtained chiefly as a by-product in the refining of copper and lead.

tel·og·no·sis (tel″og·no′sis) *n.* Diagnosis by telephone-transmitted radiographs.

telo·lec·i·thal (tel″o·les′i·thul) *adj.* Pertaining to or characterizing an egg having a large mass of yolk that is concentrated at one pole or in one hemisphere.

telo·mere (tel′o·meer) *n.* An extremity or arm of a chromosome.

telo·phase (tel′o·faze) *n.* 1. The final stage of mitosis in which the chromosomes reorganize to form an interstage nucleus. 2. The final stage of the first (telophase I) or second (telophase II) meiotic division. 3. The final phase of any process.

Telo·spo·rid·ia (tel″o·spo·rid′ee·uh) *n.pl.* A class of Sporozoa, characterized by spore formation after the sporozoon has completed its growth. The subclasses included are Gregarinida, Coccidia, and Haemosporidia.

TEM Abbreviation for *triethylenemelamine.*

tem·per, *v. & n.* 1. To make metals hard and elastic by heating them and then suddenly cooling them. 2. The hardness or brittleness of a metal, as induced by heating and suddenly cooling. 3. Disposition, state of mind, temperament; a show of anger.

tem·per·a·ment (tem′pruh·munt) *n.* 1. The mixture of physical, intellectual, emotional, and moral qualities which make up a person′s personality, his attitudes, and his behavioral responses to varying life situations. 2. *In constitutional medicine,* the mixture of motivational drives in a personality. The level of personality just above physiologic function and just below acquired attitudes and beliefs. The quantitative patterning of viscerotonia, somatotonia, and cerebrotonia in a personality.

tem·per·ance, *n.* Moderation in satisfying desire, especially in the use of alcoholic beverages.

tem·per·ate, *adj.* Moderate; without excess.

tem·per·a·ture, *n.* The degree of intensity of heat of a body, especially as measured by the scale of a thermometer. Abbreviated, T.

tem·ple, *n.* The portion of the head anterior to the ear and above the zygomatic arch.

tem·po·ral (tem′puh·rul) *adj.* 1. Pertaining to, or in the direction of, the temple. 2. Pertaining to the temporal lobe. 3. Pertaining to time.

temporal fossa. The depression that lodges the temporal muscle.

tem·po·ra·lis (tem″po·ray′lis) *n.* A muscle of mastication, arising from the temporal fossa and inserted into the coronoid process of the mandible. Syn. *temporal muscle.*

temporal lobe. The part of the cerebral hemisphere below the lateral cerebral sulcus, continuous posteriorly with the occipital lobe.

temporal lobe epilepsy. Recurrent seizures originating in discharging lesions of the temporal lobe, characterized by hallucinations, illusions, feeling of increased reality or familiarity (déjà vu) or unfamiliarity (jamais vu) and a large variety of affective experiences (fear, anxiety and epigastric sensations). Syn. *partial complex seizures.*

temporal summation. The cumulative effect of successive subthreshold stimuli on excitable tissue, resulting in a response. Most phenomena formerly believed to be due to temporal summation can be explained by spatial summation.

tem·po·rary, *adj.* Not permanent.

temporary parasite. A parasite that is free-living during part of its life.

temporary teeth. 1. DECIDUOUS TEETH. 2. A provisional set of artificial teeth.

tem·po·rize (tem′puh·rize) *v.* To provide provisional or temporary treatment for a patient until a definitive diagnosis is established. —**tem·po·ri·za·tion** (tem″puh·roh·zay′shun) *n.*

tem·po·ro·fron·tal (tem″puh·roh·frun′tul) *adj.* Pertaining to the temporal and frontal bones or areas.

tem·po·ro·man·dib·u·lar (tem″puh·ro·man·dib′yoo·lur) *adj.* Pertaining to the temporal bone and the mandible.

tem·po·ro·oc·cip·i·tal (tem″puh·ro·ock·sip′i·tul) *adj.* Pertaining to the temporal and occipital bones, regions, or lobes.

tem·po·ro·pa·ri·e·tal (tem″puh·ro·pa·rye′e·tul) *adj.* Pertaining to the temporal and parietal bones, regions, or lobes.

tem·po·ro·pon·tine (tem″puh·ro·pon′tine, ·teen) *adj.* Pertaining to the temporal lobe and the pons.

te·na·cious (te·nay′shus) *adj.* Tough; cohesive, adhesive. —**te·nac·i·ty** (te·nas′i·tee) *n.*

te·nac·u·lum (te·nack′yoo·lum) *n.,* pl. **tenacu·la** (·luh), **tenaculums** A slender, hook-shaped instrument with a long handle for seizing and holding parts or approximating incised edges during surgical operations.

ten·der, *adj.* Painful to the touch or on palpation. —**tender·ness,** *n.*

ten·di·no·plas·ty (ten′di·no·plas″tee) *n.* Plastic surgery of tendons. —**ten·di·no·plas·tic** (ten′di·no·plas′tick) *adj.*

ten·di·nous (ten′di·nus) *adj.* Pertaining to, or having the nature of, a tendon.

tendinous cords. The tendons of the papillary muscles of the ventricles of the heart, attached to the atrioventricular valves.

ten·do (ten′do) *n.,* genit. **ten·di·nis** (ten′di·nis), pl. **tendi·nes** (·neez) TENDON.

ten·do·mu·cin (ten′do·mew′sin) *n.* A mucoid found in tendons.

ten·don (ten′dun) *n.* A band of dense fibrous tissue forming the termination of a muscle and attaching the latter to a bone.

ten·don·i·tis (ten′dun·eye′tis) *n.* Inflammation of a tendon, usually at the point of its attachment to bone.

tendon reflex. Contraction of a muscle in response to sudden stretching of the muscle by a brisk tap against its tendon.

tendon sheath. In particular, the synovial sheath surrounding a tendon crossing the wrist or ankle joints.

ten·do·plas·ty (ten·do·plas″tee) *n.* TENDINOPLAS-TY.

ten·do·vag·i·ni·tis (ten″do·vaj″i·nigh′tis) *n.* Inflammation of a tendon and its sheath; TENO-SYNOVITIS.

-tene A combining form designating *a chromosome filament in meiosis.*

te·neb·ric (te·neb′rick) *adj.* Dark, gloomy.

te·nec·to·my (te·neck′tuh·mee) *n.* 1. Excision of a lesion, as a ganglion or xanthoma, of a tendon or tendon sheath. 2. TENOPLASTY.

te·nes·mus (tuh·nez′mus) *n.* A straining, especially the painful straining to empty the bowels or bladder without the evacuation of feces or urine. —**tenes·mic** (·mick) *adj.*

¹**tenia.** ¹TAENIA.

²**te·nia.** (tee′nee·uh) *n.,* pl. **te·ni·ae** (·nee·ee) [NA]. BAND (3).

tenia cho·roi·dea (ko·roy′dee·uh) [NA]. The line of attachment of the lateral part of the choroid plexus to the medial side of the cerebral hemisphere in the lateral ventricle.

teniae. Plural of ²*tenia* (BAND (3)).

teniae co·li (ko′lye) [NA]. The three tapelike bands of the longitudinal layer of the tunica muscularis of the colon: the tenia libera, tenia mesocolica, and tenia omentalis.

teniafuge. TAENIAFUGE.

teniform. TAENIFORM.

tenioid. Taenioid (= TAENIFORM).

ten·nis elbow or **arm.** EPICONDYLITIS (2).

te·no·de·sis (te·nod′e·sis, ten″o·dee′sis) *n.,* pl. **te·node·ses** (·seez) Fixation of a tendon, as to a bone.

ten·o·dyn·ia (ten″o·din′ee·uh) *n.* Pain in a tendon.

teno·fi·bril (ten″o·figh′bril) *n.* A small, delicate fibril connecting one epithelial cell with another; TONOFIBRIL.

te·nol·y·sis (te·nol′i·sis) *n.* TENDOLYSIS.

te·nom·e·ter (te·nom′e·tur) *n.* A device for measuring intraocular tension.

teno·myo·plas·ty (ten″o·migh′o·plas″tee) *n.* TE-NONTOMYOPLASTY.

teno·my·ot·o·my (ten″o·migh·ot′uh·mee) *n.* In *ophthalmology,* a procedure for the treatment of squint, devised to enfeeble the action of one of the rectus muscles by incising portions of its tendon near the scleritic insertion.

ten·o·nec·to·my (ten″o·neck′tuh·mee) *n.* Excision of a portion of a tendon.

¹**ten·o·ni·tis** (ten″o·nigh′tis) *n.* TENDONITIS.

²**tenonitis,** *n.* Inflammation of the vagina bulbi (Tenon's capsule).

Te·non's capsule. (tuh·nohnⁿ′) VAGINA BULBI.

te·non·to·myo·plas·ty (te·non″to·migh′o·plas″tee) *n.* Reparative surgery involving both tendon and muscle; used particularly for hernia.

te·non·to·my·ot·o·my (te·non″to·migh·ot′uh·mee) *n.* Surgical division of tendons and muscles.

teno·phyte (ten′o·fite) *n.* A bony or cartilaginous growth on a tendon.

teno·plas·ty (ten′o·plas″tee) *n.* Reparative or plastic surgery of a tendon. —**teno·plas·tic** (ten″o·plas′tick) *adj.*

te·nor·rha·phy (te·nor′uh·fee) *n.* The uniting of a divided tendon by sutures.

ten·os·to·sis (ten″os·to′sis) *n.,* pl. **tenosto·ses** (·seez) Ossification of a tendon.

te·no·syn·o·vec·to·my (ten″o·sin″o·veck′tuh·mee) *n.* Excision of a tendon sheath.

teno·syn·o·vi·al (ten″o·sin·o·vee′ul) *adj.* Pertaining to a tendon and a synovial surface.

teno·syn·o·vi·tis (ten″o·sin″o·vye′tis) *n.* Inflammation of a tendon and its sheath.

teno·tome (ten′o·tome) *n.* A small, narrow-bladed knife mounted on a slender handle; a tenotomy knife.

te·not·o·mize (te·not′uh·mize) *v.* To perform tenotomy.

te·not·o·my (te·not′uh·mee) *n.* The operation of cutting a tendon.

teno·vag·i·ni·tis (ten″o·vaj″i·nigh′tis) *n.* Inflammation of the sheath of a tendon.

ten·sion, *n.* 1. The act of stretching; the state of being stretched or strained. 2. In electricity, the power of overcoming resistance; electric potential. 3. The partial pressure exerted by a component of a mixture of gases. 4. A state of mental or physical strain.

tension headache. MUSCLE-CONTRACTION HEADACHE.

tension pneumothorax. VALVULAR PNEUMOTHORAX.

ten·si·ty (ten′si·tee) *n.* Tenseness, the condition of being stretched.

ten·sive (ten′siv) *adj.* Giving the sensation of stretching or contraction.

ten·sor (ten′sor, ·sur) *n.* A muscle that serves to make a part tense.

tensor ve·li pa·la·ti·ni (vee′lye pal·uh·tye′nigh). A muscle of the soft palate arising from the cartilaginous medial end of the auditory tube and a nearby portion of the sphenoid bone and inserted into the palatal aponeurosis.

ten·sure (ten′shur) *n.* TENSION (1); a stretching or straining.

ten·ta·tive (ten′tuh·tiv) *adj.* Provisional; not final; offered or proposed for the time being.

ten·tig·i·nous (ten·tij′i·nus) *adj.* Characterized by insane lust.

ten·to·ri·um (ten·to′ree·um) *n.,* pl. **tento·ria** (·ree·uh) A partition of dura mater, roofing over the posterior cranial fossa, separating the cerebellum from the cerebral hemispheres. —**tentorial** (·ul) *adj.*

tentorium ce·re·bel·li (serr·e·bel′eye) [NA]. TENTORIUM.

ten·u·ate (ten′yoo·ate) *v.* To make thin.

ten·u·ous (ten′yoo·ous) *adj.* Thin; minute.

tep·id, *adj.* Moderately warm.

ter- A combining form meaning *three* or *threefold.*

te·ras (terr′us) *n.,* pl. **ter·a·ta** (terr′uh·tuh) MONSTER. —**ter·at·ic** (ter·at′ick) *adj.*

ter·a·tism (terr′uh·tiz·um) *n.* A congenital anomaly or monstrosity.

ter·a·to·blas·to·ma (terr″uh·to·blas·to′muh) *n.* TERATOMA.

ter·a·to·car·ci·no·ma (terr″uh·to·kahr″si·no′muh) *n.* A teratoma with carcinomatous elements.

ter·a·to·gen (terr′uh·to·jen, te·rat′o·jin) *n.* Any agent that brings about teratogenesis, such as a virus, medication, or radiation that can cause maldevelopment of the embryo in the first trimester of pregnancy. —**ter·a·to·gen·ic** (terr″uh·to·jen′ick) *adj.*

ter·a·to·gen·e·sis (terr″uh·to·jen′e·sis) *n.* Embryonic maldevelopment leading to teratism or serious congenital defects.

ter·a·tog·e·nous (terr″uh·toj′e·nus) *adj.* Arising from totipotential cells, such as those which produce a fetus under normal conditions.

ter·a·tog·e·ny (terr″uh·toj′e·nee) *n.* TERATOGENESIS.

ter·a·toid (terr′uh·toid) *adj.* Resembling a monster.

teratoid tumor. TERATOMA.

ter·a·tol·o·gy (terr″uh·tol′uh·jee) *n.* The science of malformations and monstrosities. —**tera·to·log·ic** (·to·loj′ick) *adj.;* —**tera·tol·o·gist** (·tol′uh·jist) *n.*

ter·a·to·ma (terr″uh·to′muh) *n.,* pl. **teratomas, teratoma·ta** (·tuh) A true neoplasm composed of bizarre and chaotically arranged tissues foreign embryologically as well as histologically to the area in which the tumor is found. —**tera·to·ma·tous** (·muh·tus) *adj.*

ter·a·to·pho·bia (terr″uh·to·fo′bee·uh) *n.* 1. Abnormal fear of monsters or of deformed people. 2. Abnormal dread, on the part of a pregnant woman, of giving birth to a deformed infant.

ter·a·to·sis (terr″uh·to′sis) *n.,* pl. **terato·ses** (·seez) A congenital deformity; TERATISM.

ter·a·to·sper·mia (terr″uh·to·spur′mee·uh) *n.* Abnormal sperm morphology.

ter·bi·um (tur′bee·um) *n.* Tb = 158.9254. A rare metallic element, atomic number 65.

ter·e·bin·thi·nate (terr″e·bin′thi·nate) *adj.* Containing or resembling turpentine.

ter·e·bra·che·sis (terr″e·bra·kee′sis) *n.* The operation of shortening the round ligament of the uterus.

te·res (teer′eez, terr′eez) *adj.* & *n.* pl. **ter·e·tes** (teer′e·teez, terr′) 1. CYLINDRICAL. 2. A muscle having a cylindrical shape.

term, *n.* 1. A limit; the time during which anything lasts. 2. The time of expected delivery. 3. A vocabulary item; especially, a word, phrase, or symbol used in specialized or technical language.

ter·mi·nal, *adj.* & *n.* 1. Pertaining to the end; placed at or forming the end. 2. The pole of a battery or other electric source, or the end of the conductors or wires connected thereto.

terminal anesthesia. The state of insensitivity produced by the deposition of the local anesthetic agent about the terminal arborizations of the afferent axon. These are designated as anoceptors. This anesthetic works best through very thin mucous membrane surfaces, such as conjunctiva, urethra, urinary bladder, larynx, peritoneum, and pleura.

terminal arborization. 1. The branched end of a sensory nerve fiber. 2. MOTOR END PLATE. 3. The terminal ramifications of the Purkinje system of the heart.

terminal artery. END ARTERY.

terminal hair. The longer, coarser hair which in humans grows on the scalp, eyebrows, and eyelashes and in the axillae and pubes of adults, and more sparsely and variably (especially in adult males of certain racial groups) on other parts of the body.

terminal lingual sulcus. The shallow, V-shaped

groove, with its apex directed backward, on the dorsum of the tongue; it separates the oral and pharyngeal parts of the organ.

ter·mi·nol·o·gy (tur″mi·nol′uh·jee) *n.* NOMENCLATURE; a system of technical terms.

ter·mi·nus (tur′mi·nus) *n.*, pl. **termi·ni** (·nigh) A term or expression.

terms, *n.pl.* MENSES.

ter·na·ry (tur′nuh·ree) *adj.* Pertaining to chemical compounds, made up of three elements or radicals.

ter·pene (tur′peen) *n.* Any hydrocarbon of the general formula $C_{10}H_{16}$, sometimes represented as a condensation of two isoprene (C_5H_8) units. By extension the term may include compounds representing any multiple of C_5H_8 units. Terpenes occur naturally in volatile oils and other plant sources; they are generally insoluble in water but soluble in alcohol and other organic liquids. Sesquiterpenes are hydrocarbons of the formula $C_{15}H_{24}$ or (C_5H_8)₃; diterpenes are hydrocarbons of the formula $C_{20}H_{32}$ or (C_5H_8)₄; triterpenes are hydrocarbons of the formula $C_{30}H_{48}$ or (C_5H_8)₆; polyterpenes are hydrocarbons of the formula (C_5H_8)ₙ. The term hemiterpene is sometimes applied to the hydrocarbon of the formula C_5H_8 (isoprene).

ter·pin·e·ol (tur·pin′ee·ol) *n.* A mixture of isomeric alcohols of the formula $C_{10}H_{17}OH$ occurring in many volatile oils; formerly used as an antiseptic.

ter·pin hydrate (tur′pin). *cis-p*-Menthane-1,8-diol hydrate, $C_{10}H_{20}O_2 \cdot H_2O$, used as an expectorant.

Ter-Po·gos·si·an camera (tur·puh·go′see·un) A direct-viewing radiation imaging apparatus consisting of a type of image amplifier tube designed for use with low gamma-ray photon energies.

Terramycin. Trademark for the antibiotic substance oxytetracycline and its hydrochloride salt.

ter·tian (tur′shun) *adj.* Recurring every other day, as tertian fever; the initial day is counted as the first, the recurrence taking place on the third.

tertian fever. VIVAX MALARIA.

tertian malaria. VIVAX MALARIA.

ter·ti·a·ry (tur′shee·err″ee) *adj.* Of the third order or stage.

tertiary syphilis. Late syphilis, including all the symptoms of disease occurring after the fourth year of infection.

ter·tip·a·ra (tur·tip′uh·ruh) *n.* A woman who has had three viable pregnancies.

ter·va·lence (tur·vay′lunce) *n.* TRIVALENCE.

test, *n.* 1. A trial or examination. 2. A procedure to identify a constituent, to detect changes of a function, or to establish the true nature of a condition. 3. The reagent for producing a special reaction.

tes·tal·gia (tes·tal′jee·uh) *n.* Testicular pain.

testes. Plural of *testis.*

tes·ti·cle (tes′ti·kul) *n.* A testis; especially, the scrotal testis of larger mammals.

tes·tic·u·lar (tes·tick′yoo·lur) *adj.* Pertaining to the testis.

tes·tis (tes′tis) *n.*, pl. **tes·tes** (·teez) One of a pair of male reproductive glands, after sexual maturity the source of the spermatozoa; a male gonad.

test meal. A specified quantity and type of food given to test the secretory function of the stomach.

tes·toid (tes′toid) *adj.* Pertaining to any substance, natural or synthetic, which is androgenic, i.e., capable of maintaining or stimulating development of secondary male-sex characters.

tes·tos·ter·one (tes·tos′tur·ohn) *n.* 17-Hydroxy-androst-4-en-3-one, $C_{19}H_{28}O_2$, a male sex hormone; the principal androgen secreted by human testes. May be synthesized from cholesterol and certain other sterols. Used for the treatment of deficiency or absence of testosterone in the male; also for palliation of advanced metastatic carcinoma of the female breast. Employed as the free alcohol and as the following esters: testosterone cypionate, testosterone enanthate, testosterone phenylacetate, and testosterone propionate.

test solution. A reagent solution. Abbreviated, T.S.

te·tan·ic (te·tan′ick) *adj.* 1. Of, pertaining to, or causing tetanus. 2. Of, pertaining to, or causing tetany.

tetanic contraction. 1. *In obstetrics,* a state of continued contraction of the uterine muscle; occurs in prolonged labors, usually in the second stage. Results from a pathologic retraction ring. 2. TETANUS (2).

te·tan·i·form (te·tan′i·form) *adj.* Resembling either tetanus or tetany.

tet·a·nig·e·nous (tet″uh·nij′e·nus) *adj.* Causing tetanus or tetanic spasms.

tet·a·nil·la (tet″uh·nil′uh) *n. Obsol.* 1. A mild form of tetanus. 2. MYOCLONUS.

tet·a·ni·za·tion (tet″uh·ni·zay′shun) *n.* Production of tetanus or tetanic spasms. —**tet·a·nize** (tet′uh·nize) *v.*

tet·a·node (tet′uh·node) *n.* The quiescent interval in tetanus, between the tonic spasms.

tet·a·noid (tet′uh·noid) *adj.* Resembling the muscular spasms of tetanus or tetany.

tet·a·nom·e·ter (tet″uh·nom′e·tur) *n.* An instrument for measuring tetanic spasms.

tet·a·no·pho·bia (tet″uh·no·fo′bee·uh) *n.* An abnormal fear of tetanus.

tet·a·no·spas·min (tet″uh·no·spaz′min) *n.* The potent exotoxin produced by the vegetative forms of *Clostridium tetani,* responsible for the principal manifestations of tetanus of man and animals.

tet·a·nus (tet′uh·nus) *n.* 1. An infectious disease characterized by extreme stiffness of the body, painful tonic spasms of the affected muscles including trismus and opisthotonus, exaggeration of reflex activity, and generalized spasms or convulsions without loss of consciousness; due to the exotoxin produced by *Clostridium tetani* which interferes with the function of the reflex arc by suppressing spinal and brainstem inhibitory neurons; results from contamination of a wound not exposed to oxygen. Syn. *lockjaw.* 2. Sustained muscular contraction artificially induced with repeated stimuli of such a frequency that individual contractions fuse.

tetanus antitoxin. Any serum containing specific antibodies that neutralize tetanus toxin; originally produced in horses, now generally produced in humans.

tetanus neo·na·to·rum (nee″o·na·to′rum) Tetanus of the newborn, usually due to infection of the umbilical stump.

tetanus toxoid. Inactivated tetanus toxin which is used to produce active immunity against the disease.

tet·a·ny (tet′uh·nee) n. A state of increased excitability and spontaneous activity of the central and peripheral nervous system, caused by alkalosis or a decrease of serum calcium, manifested by intermittent numbness and cramps or twitchings of the extremities, carpopedal spasm, laryngospasm, confusion, and such signs of neuromuscular hyperexcitability as the Chvostek, peroneal, Trousseau, and Erb signs. Associated with hypoparathyroidism, vitamin D deficiency, deficiencies in the absorption or utilization of calcium as in rickets or the celiac syndrome, and possibly magnesium deficiency.

te·tar·ta·no·pia (te·tahr″tuh·no′pee·uh) n. Loss of vision in a homonymous quadrant in each field of vision.

te·tar·to·cone (te·tahr′tuh·kone) n. The distolingual cone; the fourth or distolingual cusp of an upper molar tooth.

te·tar·to·co·nid (te·tahr″to·ko′nid, ·kon′id) n. The distolingual or fourth cusp of a lower molar tooth.

tetr-, tetra- A combining form meaning *four.*

tet·ra·ba·sic (tet″ruh·bay′sick) adj. With reference to acids, having four atoms of replaceable hydrogen.

tet·ra·caine (tet′ruh·kane) n. 2-(Dimethylamino)ethyl *p*-(butylamino)benzoate, $C_{15}H_{24}N_2O_2$, a potent local anesthetic with many uses; employed as the base and as the hydrochloride salt. Syn. *amethocaine.*

tet·ra·chlo·ro·eth·yl·ene (tet″ruh·klo″ro·eth′il·ene) n. Ethylene tetrachloride, $Cl_2C{=}CCl_2$, a nonflammable liquid; used as an anthelmintic, especially against the hookworm *Necator americanus.* Syn. *perchloroethylene.*

tet·ra·cy·cline (tet″ruh·sigh′kleen, ·klin) n. 1. Generic name for a group of biosynthetic antibiotic substances having in common the four-ring structure of chlortetracycline, the first tetracycline to be discovered, and found also in oxytetracycline, the second member of the group to be isolated. 2. The specific antibiotic having the composition $C_{22}H_{24}N_2O_8$; has a wide spectrum of activity.

tet·rad (tet′rad) n. 1. A group of four. 2. *In genetics,* a group of four chromatids which arises during meiosis from the pairing and splitting of maternal and paternal homologous chromosomes. 3. *In chemistry,* an element having a valence of four. 4. *Informal.* TETRALOGY OF FALLOT.

tetrad of Fallot. TETRALOGY OF FALLOT.

tet·ra·gen·ic (tet″ruh·jen′ick) adj. Pertaining to

genotypes of polysomic or polyploid organisms which contain four different alleles for any given locus.

tet·ra·hy·dric (tet″ruh·high′drick) adj. Containing four replaceable atoms of hydrogen.

tet·ra·hy·dro·can·nab·in·ol (tet″ruh·high″dro·ka·nab′i·nol) n. Any one of a group of isomeric substances, $C_{21}H_{30}O_2$, obtained from cannabis, that possess to a great degree the activity of that drug. Abbreviated, THC.

tet·ra·hy·dro·fo·lic acid (tet″ruh·high″dro·fo′lick). The reduced derivative, $C_{19}H_{23}N_7O_6$, of folic acid that serves as its active metabolite in various biochemical reactions, functioning as a carrier for groups having a single carbon, such as $-CH_3$, $-CH_2OH$, $-CHO$, and $-CH{=}NH$.

te·tral·o·gy (te·tral′uh·jee) n. The combination of four related symptoms or defects that are characteristic of a disease or syndrome.

tetralogy of Fal·lot (fah·lo′) A cyanotic congenital cardiac lesion consisting of pulmonary stenosis, ventricular septal defect, right ventricular hypertrophy, and overriding or dextroposition of the aorta. Syn. *tetrad of Fallot.*

tet·ra·mas·tia (tet″ruh·mas′tee·uh) n. The condition of having four breasts.

tet·ra·nop·sia (tet″ra·nop′see·uh) n. QUADRANTANOPIA.

tet·ra·nu·cle·o·tide (tet″ruh·new′klee·o·tide) n. 1. *Obsol.* Nucleic acid, which contains four constituent nucleotides. 2. Any molecule composed of four mononucleotides linked by phosphodiester bonds.

tet·ra·pa·re·sis (tet″ruh·pa·ree′sis, ·păr′e·sis) n. Weakness of all four extremities.

tet·ra·pho·co·me·lia (tet″ruh·fo″ko·mee′lee·uh) n. Phocomelia affecting all four extremities.

tet·ra·ple·gia (tet″ruh·plee′jee·uh) n. QUADRIPLEGIA.

tet·ra·ploid (tet′ruh·ploid) adj. Having four haploid sets of chromosomes.

tet·ras·ce·lus (te·tras′e·lus) adj. Having four legs.

tet·ra·sti·chi·a·sis (tet″ruh·sti·kigh′uh·sis) n. Arrangement of the eyelashes in four rows.

tet·ra·tom·ic (tet″ruh·tom′ick) adj. 1. Containing four atoms. 2. Having four hydroxyl radicals.

tet·ra·vac·cine (tet″ruh·vack′seen) n. A polyvalent vaccine containing four different cultures, as one containing typhoid, paratyphoid A and B, and cholera.

tet·ra·va·lent (tet″ruh·vay′lunt) adj. *In chemistry,* having a combining power equivalent to that of four hydrogen atoms. Syn. *quadrivalent.*

tet·relle (te·trel′, tet′rel) n. A device formerly used to enable a weak infant to obtain milk from its mother. It consists of a nipple shield and two tubes; the mother sucks one tube, and the milk flows to the infant's mouth through the other.

tet·rose (tet′roze) n. A monosaccharide whose molecule contains four atoms of carbon, as erythrose, $C_4H_8O_4$.

tet·ter (tet′ur) n. Any of various skin eruptions, particularly herpes, eczema, and psoriasis.

tex·ture (tecks′chur) n. 1. Any organized substance or tissue of which the body is composed. 2. The arrangement of the elementary parts of tissue. —**tex·tur·al** (·chur·ul) *adj.*

thalami. Plural of *thalamus.*

tha·lam·ic (tha·lam′ick) *adj.* Pertaining to or involving the thalamus.

thalamic pain. HYPERPATHIA.

thalamic syndrome. A symptom complex produced by a lesion, usually vascular, of the posterior portion of the lateral nuclear mass of the thalamus. It includes initially contralateral hemianesthesia and sometimes hemiparesis, followed by hypersensitivity to physical stimuli and severe paroxysmal pain over the contralateral half of the body, often aggravated by emotional stress and fatigue, as well as slight hemiataxia, and occasional hemichorea. Syn. *Dejerine-Roussy syndrome, thalamic apoplexy, thalamic hyperesthetic anesthesia.*

thal·a·mo·cor·ti·cal (thal″a·mo·kor′ti·kul) *adj.* Pertaining to the thalamus and the cortex of the brain.

thal·a·mo·len·tic·u·lar (thal″a·mo·len·tick′yoo·lur) *adj.* Pertaining to the thalamus and the lentiform nucleus.

thal·a·mo·ma·mil·lary (thal″a·mo·mam′i·lerr·ee) *adj.* Pertaining to the thalamus and the mamillary bodies.

thal·a·mo·pa·ri·e·tal (thal″mo·puh·ruh·rye′e·tul) *adj.* Pertaining to the thalamus and the parietal lobe.

thal·a·mo·teg·men·tal (thal″a·mo·teg·men′tul) *adj.* Pertaining to the thalamus and the tegmentum.

thal·a·mot·o·my (thal″a·mot′uh·mee) *n.* Surgical destruction of parts of the thalamus for the treatment of intractable pain, movement disorders; and rarely mental disorders.

thal·a·mus (thal′uh·mus) *n.,* pl. & genit. sing. **thal·a·mi** (·migh) Either one of two masses of gray matter situated one on either side of the third ventricle, and each forming part of the lateral wall of that cavity. The thalamus sends projection fibers to the primary sensory areas of the cortex, the tegmentum, and the optic tract. The internal medullary lamina divides each thalamic mass into groups of nuclei. The anterior thalamic nuclei lie between the diverging anterior sheets of the lamina. Medial to the lamina are the medial and midline thalamic nuclei. Lateral to the lamina are the lateral thalamic nuclei which are further divided into lateral or dorsal groups and ventral groups. The posterior thalamic nuclei include the pulvinar and medial and lateral geniculate bodies.

thal·as·se·mia, thal·as·sae·mia (thal″uh·see′mee·uh) *n.* A form of hemolytic anemia resulting from a group of hereditary defects in hemoglobin synthesis characterized in common by impaired synthesis of one of its polypeptide chains, resulting in hypochromic, microcytic erythrocytes. Thalassemia major is the homozygous state, with evident clinical disease from early life. Thalassemia minor, the heterozygous state, may or may not be accompanied by clinical illness. There are several variants of the disease, classified according to the globin chains involved.

tha·lid·o·mide (tha·lid′o·mide) *n.* N-(2,6-Dioxo-3-piperidyl)-phthalimide, $C_{13}H_{10}N_2O_4$, a sedative and hypnotic; its use has been discontinued because it may produce teratogenic effects when administered during pregnancy.

thalidomide embryopathy. A specific malformation syndrome related to maternal ingestion of thalidomide during the early development of the fetus. It consists of multiple congenital anomalies including one or more of the following: limb-reduction defects ranging from one or more missing digits to absence of all extremities, cardiac defects, deafness, gastrointestinal malformations and hemangiomas.

thal·li·um (thal′ee·um) *n.* Tl = 204.37 A bluish-white metallic element, atomic number 81, density 11.85. Salts of thallium are highly toxic.

Thal·loph·y·ta (tha·lof′i·tuh) *n.pl.* The phylum of plants having a thallus and no true roots, stems, and leaves; it includes the algae and the fungi.

thal·lo·phyte (thal′o·fite) *n.* A plant belonging to the phylum Thallophyta.

thal·lo·tox·i·co·sis (thal″o·tock″si·ko′sis) *n.* Poisoning by thallium or its derivatives.

THAM. Trademark for tromethamine, a systemic antacid used for the treatment of metabolic acidosis.

tha·mu·ria (tha·mew′ree·uh) *n.* Frequent urination.

thanat-, thanato- A combining form meaning *death.*

than·a·to·gno·mon·ic (than″uh·to·no·mon′ick, than″uh·tog″) *adj.* Indicative of death.

than·a·tog·ra·phy (than″uh·tog′ruh·fee) *n.* 1. A dissertation on death. 2. A description of symptoms and feelings experienced in the course of dying.

than·a·toid (than′uh·toid) *adj.* Resembling death.

than·a·tol·o·gy (than″uh·tol′uh·jee) *n.* The study of the phenomena of somatic death.

than·a·to·pho·bia (than″uh·to·fo′bee·uh) *n.* An abnormal fear of death.

than·a·tos (than′uh·tos) *n.* DEATH INSTINCT.

Thay·er-Mar·tin medium. A complex culture medium containing several antibiotics and used to isolate and grow gonococci. Used to screen patients for asymptomatic gonorrhea.

the·ba·ic (the·bay′ick) *adj.* Pertaining to, or derived from, opium.

the·ba·ine (theeb′uh·een, thi·bay′een, ·in) *n.* An alkaloid, $C_{19}H_{21}NO_3$, found in opium; it causes strychnine-like spasms. Syn. *paramorphine.*

thec-, theci-, theco-. A combining form meaning *theca, sheath.*

the·ca (thee′kuh) *n.,* pl. & genit. sing. **the·cae** (·kee, ·see) A sheath. —**the·cal** (·kul) *adj.*

theca ex·ter·na (ecks·tur′nuh). The outer fibrous layer of the theca folliculi.

theca fol·li·cu·li (fol·ick′yoo·lye) [NA]. The capsule of a growing or mature ovarian (graafian) follicle consisting of the theca interna and the theca externa.

the·ca in·ter·na (in·tur'nuh). The inner vascular, cellular layer of the theca folliculi.

theca lutein cyst. A cyst due to distention of the corpus luteum but with well-developed theca in the wall.

the·ci·tis (the·sigh'tis) n. Inflammation of the sheath of a tendon.

the·co·ma (the·ko'muh) n., L. pl. **thecoma·ta** (·tuh) A benign tumor of the ovary composed of cells derived from the ovarian stroma, in some instances resembling the thecal element of the follicle. Syn. *thelioma.*

the·e·lin (thee'e·lin, theel'in) n. ESTRONE.

the·e·lol (thee'e·lole, ·lol) n. ESTRIOL.

thel-, theli-, thelo- A combining form meaning *nipple.*

the·lal·gia (the·lal'jee·uh) n. Pain in a nipple.

the·lar·che (the·lahr'kee) n. The onset of female breast development.

the·las·is (the·las'is) n. The act of sucking.

the·le·plas·ty (theel'e·plas·tee) n. Plastic surgery of a nipple.

the·ler·e·thism (the·lerr'e·thiz·um) n. Erection of a nipple, caused by contraction of its smooth muscle.

the·li·tis (the·lye'tis) n. MAMILLITIS.

the·li·um (theel'ee·um) n. 1. NIPPLE. 2. PAPILLA.

the·lon·cus (the·lonk'us) n. Tumor of a nipple.

the·lo·phleb·o·stem·ma (theel''o·fleb''o·stem'uh) n. Venous circle around a nipple.

the·lor·rha·gia (theel''o·ray'juh, ·jee·uh) n. Hemorrhage from a nipple.

the·lo·thism (the'lo·thiz·um) n. THELERETHISM.

the·mat·ic apperception test (the·mat'ick). A projective psychological test using a set of pictures suggesting life situations from which the subject constructs a story, designed to reveal to the trained interpreter some of the dominant drives, emotions, sentiments, complexes, and conflicts of personality. Abbreviated, TAT

the·nar (theen'ahr) n. & adj. 1. The palm of the hand. 2. Of or pertaining to the palm. 3. [NA] The fleshy prominence of the palm corresponding to the base of the thumb.

The·o·bro·ma (thee''o·bro'muh) n. A genus of trees of the Sterculiaceae. The seeds of *Theobroma cacao* yield a fixed oil (cocoa butter) and contain the alkaloid theobromine. The seeds are used in the preparation of chocolate and cocoa.

the·o·bro·mine (thee''o·bro'meen, ·min) n. An alkaloid, 3,7-dimethylxanthine, $C_7H_8N_4O_2$, isomeric with theophylline, occurring in cacao beans and kola nuts; used as a diuretic and myocardial stimulant.

theo·ma·nia (thee''o·may'nee·uh) n. 1. A religious mania. 2. A mental disorder in which the individual believes himself to be a divine being. —**theoma·ni·ac** (·nee·ack) n.

theo·pho·bia (thee''o·fo'bee·uh) n. An abnormal fear of the deity or of divine punishment.

theo·phyl·line (thee''o·fil'een, thee·off'il·een, ·in) n. An alkaloid, 1,3-dimethylxanthine, $C_7H_8N_4O_2$, obtained from tea leaves and also prepared synthetically. It differs chemically

from theobromine only in the position of the methyl groups. Used as a diuretic and vasodilator; also to relax bronchial spasms.

theophylline meth·yl·glu·ca·mine (meth''il·gloo'kuh·meen, ·min). An equimolecular mixture of theophylline and *N*-methylglucosamine; has the action and uses of theophylline. Syn. *theophylline-meglumine.*

the·o·ry (thee'uh·ree) n. The abstract principles of science. Also, a reasonable supposition or assumption, generally better developed and more probable than a mere hypothesis.

ther·a·peu·sis (therr''uh·pew'sis) n. THERAPEUTICS.

ther·a·peu·tic (therr''uh·pew'tick) adj. 1. CURATIVE. 2. Pertaining to therapy or to therapeutics.

therapeutic abortion. 1. Broadly, any abortion induced in a woman for the sake of her physical or mental health or welfare. 2. More narrowly, any such abortion permitted by law.

therapeutic community. *In psychiatry,* the social organization of patients and personnel within a specially structured mental hospital setting which, through various techniques, promotes the patients' functioning within acceptable social bounds and helps the patients to overcome their dependency needs and to assume responsibility for their own rehabilitation and that of other patients.

therapeutic index. The ratio of the toxic dose of a substance to its therapeutic dose. It is intended to serve as an estimate of the safety of a drug.

therapeutic psychosis. *In psychoanalysis,* a temporary regression during therapy accompanied by primitive means of dealing with drives which provide the basis for the massive resynthesis of personality.

ther·a·peu·tics (therr''uh·pew'ticks) n. The branch of medical science dealing with the treatment of disease.

therapeutic test. A test in which the response to specific therapy is used to aid in the establishment of a diagnosis.

ther·a·pist (therr'uh·pist) n. A practitioner of some kind of therapy.

ther·a·py (therr'uh·pee) n. The means employed in effecting the cure or amelioration of disease or of diseased patients.

the·ri·od·ic (theer''ee·od'ick) adj. MALIGNANT.

the·ri·o·ma (theer''ee·o'muh) n., pl. **theriomas, therioma·ta** (·tuh) A malignant tumor.

therm-, thermo- A combining form meaning *heat* or *temperature.*

therm, n. A unit of heat to which many equivalents have been given, for example, a small calorie, a kilocalorie, 1,000 kilocalories.

ther·mal (thur'mul) adj. Pertaining to heat.

thermal capacity. HEAT CAPACITY.

thermal neutron. A neutron slowed down, following its release by fissioning, to a state of thermal equilibrium with its surrounding medium. Syn. *slow neutron.*

ther·ma·tol·o·gy (thur''muh·tol'uh·jee) n. The scientific use or understanding of heat or of the waters of thermal springs in the treatment of disease. —**therma·to·log·ic** (·to·loj'ick) adj.

therm·es·the·sia, therm·aes·the·sia (thurm″es-theezh′uh) n. 1. Temperature sensibility or ability to feel hot and cold or variations in temperature. 2. Sensitiveness to heat.

therm·es·the·si·om·e·ter, therm·aes·the·si·om·e·ter (thurm″es·theez″ee·om′e·tur) n. An instrument for measuring the sensitivity to heat of different regions of the skin.

therm·is·tor (thur′mis·tur, thur·mis′tur) n. A type of electrical resistance element made of material whose resistance value varies with temperature, allowing its use in temperature-measuring devices.

ther·mo·an·al·ge·sia (thur″mo·an″al·jee′zee·uh) n. Insensibility to heat or to contact with heated objects.

ther·mo·an·es·the·sia, ther·mo·an·aes·the·sia (thur″mo·an″es·theezh′uh) n. Loss of temperature sensation, the ability to recognize the difference between hot and cold, or to feel variations in temperature.

ther·mo·cau·tery (thur″mo·kaw′tur·ee) n. A cautery that depends for its action upon heat delivered to the metal end of the instrument, either by direct action of flame, aided by the passage of a current of hot air as in the Paquelin cautery, or by the passage of electric current.

ther·mo·chem·is·try (thur″mo·kem′is·tree) n. The branch of chemical science which treats of the mutual relations of heat and chemical changes.

ther·mo·chro·ism (thur″mo·kro′iz·um) n. The property of some substances of reflecting or transmitting some thermal radiations while absorbing or changing others.

ther·mo·co·ag·u·la·tion (thur″mo·ko·ag″yoo·lay′shun) n. 1. A method of destroying tissue by means of electrocautery or high-frequency current. 2. A method by which one or several layers of the cerebral cortex in a desired area can be destroyed without alteration of the surrounding tissue.

ther·mo·cou·ple (thur′mo·kup″ul) n. A device for measuring temperature in which plates or wires of two dissimilar metals form a junction that develops a thermoelectric current when heated and the electromotive force of which varies with the temperature at the junction.

ther·mo·dy·nam·ics (thur″mo·dye·nam′icks) n. The science that treats of the relations of heat and other forms of energy.

thermogenic anhidrosis. SWEAT-RETENTION SYNDROME.

ther·mo·gram (thur′mo·gram) n. A visual display of the surface temperatures of the body recorded from the spontaneous infrared emanations, as obtained by thermography.

ther·mog·ra·phy (thur·mog′ruh·fee) n. A diagnostic technique that records infrared radiations spontaneously emanating from the body's surface to provide a thermogram or mathematical recording of its temperature and local thermal differences.

ther·mo·hy·per·es·the·sia, ther·mo·hy·per·aes·the·sia (thur″mo·high″pur·es·theezh′uh) n. Increased sensibility to heat or cold, or to variations in temperature.

ther·mo·hyp·es·the·sia, ther·mo·hyp·aes·the·sia (thur″mo·hip″es·theezh′uh, high″pes·) n. Reduced perception of heat or cold, or reduced ability to recognize differences in temperatures.

ther·mo·in·hib·i·to·ry (thur″mo·in·hib′i·to·ree) adj. Inhibiting the production of heat.

ther·mo·la·bile (thur″mo·lay′bil, ·bile) adj. Sensitive to or destroyed or changed by heat.

ther·mo·mas·sage (thur″mo·muh·sahzh′) n. Massage with application of heat.

ther·mom·e·ter (thur·mom′e·tur) n. A device for measuring temperatures or thermal states, generally consisting of a substance capable of expanding and contracting with variation of temperature, and a graduated scale by means of which the expansion or contraction of the substance can be determined.

ther·mo·neu·ro·sis (thur″mo·new·ro′sis) n. In a conversion type of hysterical neurosis, fever of vasomotor origin.

ther·moph·a·gy (thur·mof′uh·jee) n. The habit of eating very hot food.

ther·mo·phile (thur′mo·file, ·fil) n. A microorganism for which the optimum temperature for growth is between 50 to 55°C; found in soil and water, especially hot springs.

ther·mo·phil·ic (thur″mo·fil′ick) adj. Pertaining to a microorganism that grows best at high temperatures.

ther·mo·pho·bia (thur″mo·fo′bee·uh) n. Abnormal dread of heat.

ther·mo·phy·lic (thur″mo·figh′lick) adj. THERMOSTABLE.

ther·mo·pile (thur′mo·pile) n. An instrument for measuring temperatures; it consists of a series of thermocouples combined to amplify the effect of each so as to permit measurement of minute temperature effects.

ther·mo·plas·tic (thur″mo·plas′tick) adj. Having the property of softening or melting when heated and becoming rigid again when cooled without appreciable chemical change.

ther·mo·ple·gia (thur″mo·plee′jee·uh, ·juh) n. SUNSTROKE.

ther·mo·reg·u·la·tion (thur″mo·reg″yoo·lay′shun) n. Regulation of temperature by regulation of heat production or heat loss, or both.

ther·mo·scope (thur′muh·skope) n. An instrument for detecting changes or differences in temperature by their effect on the volume of some material, as a gas.

ther·mo·sta·ble (thur″mo·stay′bul) adj. Exhibiting resistance to change in a defined, usually elevated, temperature range. —**thermo·sta·bil·i·ty** (·stuh·bil′i·tee) n.

ther·mo·stat (thur′mo·stat) n. A device for automatically regulating and maintaining a constant temperature.

ther·mo·ste·re·sis (thur″mo·ste·ree′sis) n. The removal or deprivation of heat.

ther·mo·ther·a·py (thur″mo·therr′uh·pee) n. Treatment of disease by heat of any kind.

ther·mo·to·nom·e·ter (thur″mo·to·nom′e·tur) n. An apparatus for determining the amount of muscular contraction induced by heat stimuli.

the·sau·ris·mo·sis (the·saw″riz·mo′sis) n. Thesaurosis (= STORAGE DISEASE).

the·sau·ro·sis (thee"saw·ro'sis, thes"aw·) n. STORAGE DISEASE.

theta rhythm. In electroencephalography, a succession of waves with a frequency of 4 to 7 hertz, best recorded from the temporal region.

thi-, thio- A combining form meaning sulfur.

thi·a·ben·da·zole (thigh"uh·ben'duh·zole) n. 2-(4-Thiazolyl)benzimidazole, $C_{10}H_7N_3S$, a veterinary anthelmintic that has been beneficial in humans in the treatment of creeping eruption due to larval forms of Ancylostoma braziliense and A. caninum.

thi·a·min (thigh'uh·min) n. THIAMINE.

thi·a·mine (thigh'uh·meen, ·min) n. 3-(4-Amino-2-methylpyrimidyl-5-methyl)-4-methyl-5-(β-hydroxyethyl)thiazolium chloride, $C_{12}H_{17}ClN_4OS$, a member of the vitamin B complex that occurs in many natural sources, frequently in the form of the pyrophosphate ester known as cocarboxylase. The commercial product is obtained by synthesis. A deficiency of this vitamin is evidenced chiefly in the nervous system, the circulation, and the alimentary tract. Among the symptoms are irritability, emotional disturbances, multiple neuritis, increased pulse rate, dyspnea, edema, loss of appetite, reduced intestinal motility. Syn. vitamin B_1.

thiamine hydrochloride. The salt, $C_{12}H_{17}ClN_4OS·HCl$, produced by neutralization of thiamine with hydrochloric acid; acid in reaction. The form in which thiamine is generally employed.

thiamine pyrophosphate. COCARBOXYLASE.

thi·am·y·lal sodium (thigh·am'i·lal). Sodium 5-allyl-5-(1-methylbutyl)-2-thiobarbiturate, $C_{12}H_{17}N_2NaO_2S$, an ultrashort-acting barbiturate used intravenously as an anesthetic.

thi·a·zide (thigh'uh·zide) n. A diuretic whose main function is to block sodium reabsorption in the first portion of the renal distal tubules, bringing about antihypertensive action.

thi·a·zine (thigh'uh·zeen, ·zin) n. Any of a group of heterocyclic compounds containing four carbon atoms, one nitrogen atom, and one sulfur atom in a ring.

thick-split graft. A split graft in which the grafted skin is relatively thick.

Thiersch graft (teersh) Extensive thin sheets or broad strips of skin, consisting largely of epidermis, sliced with a very sharp knife from healthy surfaces of the body, and transferred to cover large fresh or granulating wounds.

thigh, n. The part of the lower extremity from the pelvis to the knee.

thigh-bone, n. The long bone of the thigh; FEMUR.

thig·man·es·the·sia, thig·man·aes·the·sia (thig·man"es·theezh'uh) n. Loss of tactile sensibility.

thi·mero·sal (thigh·merr'o·sal, ·mur'o·) n. Sodium ethylmercurithiosalicylate, C_6H_4-(COONa)SHgC_2H_5, an organomercurial antiseptic used topically and also as a preservative of certain biological products.

thio·bac·te·ria (thigh"o·back·teer'ee·uh) n.pl. Bacteria that grow where decaying organic material releases hydrogen sulfide. Found in stagnant water and at the bottom of the sea. They are not pathogenic to man or animals.

thio·cy·a·nate (thigh"o·sigh'uh·nate) n. Any compound containing the monovalent radical —SCN. The sodium and potassium salts have been used in the control of hypertension, but are no longer employed because of their toxicity.

thio·gua·nine (thigh"o·gwah'neen) n. 2-Amino-purine-6-thiol, $C_5H_5N_5S$, an antineoplastic agent.

thi·on·ic (thigh·on'ick) adj. Pertaining to sulfur.

thio·pen·tal sodium (thigh"o·pen'tal, ·tol). Sodium 5-ethyl-5-(1-methylbutyl)-2-thiobarbiturate, $C_{11}H_{17}N_2NaO_2S$, an ultrashort-acting barbiturate used intravenously or by rectal instillation as an anesthetic.

thi·o·phene (thigh'o·feen) n. Thiofuran, C_4H_4S, a heterocyclic constituent of coal tar; used as a solvent and in the manufacture of medicinal agents.

thio·phile (thigh'o·file, ·fil) n. & adj. 1. A microorganism that requires sulfur compounds for metabolism. 2. THIOPHILIC.

thio·phil·ic (thigh"o·fil'ick) adj. 1. Pertaining to, or characteristic of, a thiophile. 2. Thriving in sulfur.

thio·sul·fate (thigh"o·sul'fate) n. Any salt or ester of thiosulfuric acid.

Thiosulfil. Trademark for sulfamethizole, a sulfonamide used for treatment of infections of the urinary tract.

thio·tepa (thigh"o·tep'uh) n. Tris(1-aziridinyl)-phosphine sulfide, $C_6H_{12}N_3PS$, an alkylating agent employed for palliation of certain malignant tumors.

thio·ura·cil (thigh"o·yoor'uh·sil) n. 2-Mercapto-4-hydroxypyrimidine, $C_4H_4N_2OS$, an antithyroid drug that interferes with synthesis of thyroxine but has adverse effects in many patients; certain of its derivatives are better tolerated.

thio·urea (thigh"o·yoo·ree'uh) n. Thiocarbamide, H_2NCSNH_2; has been used as an antithyroid drug in the treatment of hyperthyroidism.

third-degree burn. A burn that is more severe than a second-degree burn and that destroys the skin and its deeper underlying tissues.

third-degree heart block. A complete atrioventricular block.

third heart sound. The heart sound occurring at the end of rapid ventricular filling, related to the sudden deceleration of blood flow. Symbol, S_3 or SIII. Syn. ventricular filling sound.

third space. Any of the regions of the body, such as peritoneal cavity, mesentery, and gastrointestinal tract, viewed as a physiological unit, where excessive amounts of exudates may accumulate and be sequestered, especially in acute peritonitis. Syn. surgical third space.

third ventricle. The cavity of the diencephalon, a narrow cleft between the two thalami.

thirst, n. A sensation associated with the need of the body for water. The sensory nerve endings for thirst are principally in the mucous membrane of the pharynx, and less than normal content of water in this region supposedly produces thirst. Prolonged deprivation with dehydration of tissues produces severe unpleasant sensations probably of wide origin.

thix·ot·ro·py (thick·sot'ruh·pee) *n.* The property of some gels, when mechanically agitated, to undergo a reversible isothermal solution and reconversion to a gel when allowed to stand. The tobacco mosaic virus has this property of thixotropy. —**thixo·trop·ic** (thick"so·trop'ick) *adj.*

Thomas splint An appliance designed originally to provide support in the treatment of diseases of the hip or knee, now used chiefly to maintain traction or for emergency transportation in fractures of the femur or humerus. It is made in various sizes and forms, and consists essentially of a padded metal ring which fits around the thigh or upper arm, and long metal rods extending from the ring down each side of the extremity.

Thom·sen's disease MYOTONIA CONGENITA.

Thom·so·ni·an·ism (tom·so'nee·un·iz·um) *n.* An empirical system of medicine which insisted on the use of vegetable remedies only.

thorac-, thoraci-, thoracico-, thoraco- A combining form meaning *thorax, thoracic.*

tho·ra·cec·to·my (tho"ruh·seck'tuh·mee) *n.* Resection of a rib.

tho·ra·cen·te·sis (tho"ruh·sen·tee'sis) *n.,* pl. **tho·racente·ses** (·seez) Aspiration of the chest cavity for the removal of fluid, usually for hydrothorax or empyema.

tho·rac·ic (tho·ras'ick) *adj.* Pertaining to the thorax.

thoracic duct. The common lymph trunk beginning in the cisterna chyli, passing upward, and emptying into the left subclavian vein at its junction with the left internal jugular vein.

thoracic inlet. The superior opening of the thoracic cavity, bounded by the first thoracic vertebra, the first ribs, and the manubrium of the sternum.

thoracic-inlet tumors. Infiltrating tumors at the thoracic inlet which may produce the symptom complex commonly known as Pancoast syndrome.

thoracic kyphosis. A posterior angular deformity of the spine in the thoracic area.

thoracic nucleus. A prominent round or oval cell column in the medial part of the base of the dorsal gray horn of the spinal cord; contains cells of origin of the uncrossed dorsal spinocerebellar tract. Syn. *dorsal nucleus of Clarke.*

tho·rac·i·co·lum·bar (tho·ras'i·ko·lum'bur) *adj.* THORACOLUMBAR.

thoracic outlet syndrome. SCALENUS ANTERIOR SYNDROME.

thoracic respiration. Respiration caused by contraction of the intercostal and other thoracic muscles.

thoracic stomach. Congenital herniation of the stomach above the diaphragm due to imperfect development of the diaphragm.

thoracic surgery. Surgery limited to the thorax, particularly to the rib cage and structures within the thoracic cavity.

tho·ra·co·ab·dom·i·nal (tho"ruh·ko·ab·dom'i-nul) *adj.* Pertaining to the thorax and the abdomen.

tho·ra·co·acro·mi·al (tho"ruh·ko·a·kro'mee·ul) *adj.* Pertaining to the acromion and the chest, as the thoracoacromial artery.

thor·a·co·bi·lia (tho"ruh·ko·bye'lee·uh, ·bil'ee·uh) *n.* A syndrome characterized by bile expectoration, fever, and a large, tender liver; it results from a bronchobiliary fistula.

tho·ra·co·ce·li·ot·o·my, tho·ra·co·coe·li·ot·o·my (tho"ruh·ko·see"lee·ot'uh·mee) *n.* Surgical opening of the thoracic and abdominal cavities.

tho·ra·co·cen·te·sis (tho"ruh·ko·sen·tee'sis) *n.* THORACENTESIS.

tho·ra·co·cyl·lo·sis (tho"ruh·ko·sil·o'sis) *n.* Deformity of the thorax.

tho·ra·co·cyr·to·sis (tho"ruh·ko·sur·to'sis) *n.* Excessive curvature of the thorax.

tho·ra·co·dor·sal (tho"ruh·ko·dor'sul) *adj.* Pertaining to the thorax and the back, as: thoracodorsal artery.

tho·ra·co·gas·tros·chi·sis (thor"uh·ko·gas·tros'ki·sis) *n.* Congenital fissure of the thorax and abdomen. Syn. *thoracoceloschisis.*

tho·ra·co·lap·a·rot·o·my (tho"ruh·ko·lap"uh·rot'uh·mee) *n.* An operation in which both the thorax and the abdomen are opened.

tho·ra·co·lum·bar (tho"ruh·ko·lum'bur) *adj.* Pertaining to the thoracic and lumbar portions of the spine, or to thoracic and lumbar ganglions and fibers of the autonomic nervous system.

tho·ra·col·y·sis (tho"ruh·kol'i·sis) *n.* PNEUMONOLYSIS.

tho·ra·cop·a·gus (tho"ruh·kop'uh·gus) *n.,* pl. **tho·racopa·gi** (·jye, ·guy) Conjoined twins united by their thoraxes or epigastric regions. —**tho·racopagous,** *adj.*

tho·ra·co·plas·ty (tho'ruh·ko·plas"tee) *n.* The mobilization of the chest wall by the resection of any number of ribs, wholly or in part, in order to produce collapse of the chest wall and obliteration of the pleural cavity or reduction of the thoracic space. The operation is commonly extrapleural and may be partial or complete, the latter involving segments of the first to eleventh ribs. It is also referred to by location, as anterior, lateral, posterior, apical.

tho·ra·cos·chi·sis (tho"ruh·kos'ki·sis) *n.* Congenital fissure of the thorax.

tho·ra·co·scope (tho·ray'kuh·skope, tho·rack"o-) *n.* An electrically lighted, tubular instrument designed for insertion between ribs into a pneumothorax space. Used for visual examination of the pleural surfaces and for the severance of pleural adhesion bands by electrocautery.

tho·ra·cos·co·py (tho"ruh·kos'kuh·pee) *n.* Examination of the pleural cavity in the presence of a pneumothorax by means of a thoracoscope introduced through the thoracic wall. Syn. *pleuroscopy.*

tho·ra·cos·to·my (tho·ruh·kos'tuh·mee) *n.* Opening the chest; particularly, the removal of some ribs for drainage, or for access to the pleural cavity.

tho·ra·cot·o·my (tho"ruh·kot'uh·mee) *n.* Incision of the thoracic wall.

tho·rax (tho'racks) *n.*, genit. **tho·ra·cis** (tho·ray'sis), pl. **thoraxes, tho·ra·ces** (tho'ruh·seez, tho·ray'seez) The chest; the portion of the trunk above the diaphragm and below the neck; the framework of bones and soft tissues bounded by the diaphragm below, the ribs and sternum in front, the ribs and thoracic portion of the vertebral column behind, and above by the structures in the lower part of the neck, and containing the heart enclosed in the pericardium, the lungs invested by the pleura, and mediastinal structures.

Thorazine. Trademark for chlorpromazine, a tranquilizer and antiemetic drug used as the hydrochloride salt.

tho·ri·um (tho'ree·um) *n.* Th = 232.038. A radioactive, grayish-white, lustrous metal, atomic number 90, the parent of a series of radioactive elements.

Thorn test A test of adrenocortical reserve in which the eosinophil count in the fasting patient is compared with the eosinophil count four hours after the intramuscular injection of 25 units of lyophilized adrenocorticotropic hormone (ACTH); a decrease of 50 percent or more is seen in normal individuals, tending to exclude adrenal cortical insufficiency.

thor·ough·pin (thur'o·pin) *n.* A bursitis occurring over the tuber calcis of the hock joint of a horse.

Thor·son-Bioerck syndrome (tor'so^hn, byœrk). CARCINOID SYNDROME.

thread, *n.* 1. The spun and twisted fibers of cotton, linen, or silk. 2. *In surgery,* a fine suture. 3. Any fine filament or natural process resembling a thread.

thread reaction. The formation of long chains of bacillary forms of bacteria when grown in immune serum after agglutination.

thread-worm, *n.* ENTEROBIUS VERMICULARIS.

threat·ened abortion. The occurrence of signs and symptoms of impending loss of the embryo or fetus. It may be prevented by treatment or may go on to inevitable abortion.

three-day fever. PHLEBOTOMUS FEVER.

three-day measles. RUBELLA.

three-glass test. GLASS TEST.

thre·o·nine (three'o·neen, ·nin) *n.* α-Amino-β-hydroxybutyric acid, $CH_3CHOHCH-NH_2COOH$, an amino acid essential to human nutrition.

threp·sol·o·gy (threp·sol'uh·jee) *n.* The science of nutrition.

thresh·er's lung. FARMER'S LUNG.

thresh·old, *n.* 1. The lower limit of stimulus capable of producing an impression upon consciousness or of evoking a response in an irritable tissue. 2. The entrance of a canal.

threshold dose. *In therapeutics,* the minimum dose that will produce a detectable response of a specified kind.

threshold stimulus. The least intensity of a stimulus that produces response.

thrill, *n.* A fine vibration felt by the hand or fingertips, and associated in some instances with disease in underlying organs, such as the heart.

throat, *n.* The pharynx and the fauces.

throb, *n.* A pulsation or beating.

throm·bas·the·nia (throm''bas·theen'ee·uh) *n.* THROMBOASTHENIA.

throm·bec·to·my (throm·beck'tuh·mee) *n.* Excision of a thrombus.

thrombi. Plural of *thrombus.*

throm·bic (throm'bick) *adj.* Of or pertaining to a thrombus or thrombi.

throm·bin (throm'bin) *n.* An enzyme elaborated in shed blood from an inactive precursor, prothrombin. It induces clotting by converting fibrinogen to fibrin, possibly by proteolysis, and is used therapeutically as a topical hemostatic agent.

throm·bo·an·gi·itis (throm''bo·an''jee·eye'tis) *n.* Thrombosis associated with inflammation of the vessel wall.

throm·bo·as·the·nia (throm''bo·as·theen'ee·uh) *n.* A rare hereditary disorder in which about 25 percent of the blood platelets are large and poorly granular; it is associated with abnormal posttraumatic bleeding.

throm·bo·cav·er·no·si·tis (throm''bo·kav''ur·no·sigh'tis) *n.* Thrombosis combined with inflammation of the corpora cavernosa of the penis.

throm·bo·la·sis (throm·bock'luh·sis) *n.* Breaking up or destruction of a thrombus; thrombolysis. —**throm·bo·clas·tic** (throm''bo·klas'tick) *adj.*

throm·bo·cyte (throm'bo·site) *n.* BLOOD PLATELET. —**throm·bo·cyt·ic** (throm''bo·sit'ick) *adj.*

throm·bo·cy·the·mia, throm·bo·cy·thae·mia (throm''bo·sigh·theem'ee·uh) *n.* THROMBOCYTOSIS.

throm·bo·cy·to·crit (throm''bo·sigh'to·krit) *n.* A glass tube for counting blood platelets. Blood diluted with sodium oxalate is centrifuged in a special spherical sediment chamber so that the platelets are seen layered above the red cells. This volume can be measured. Normal is 0.35 to 0.67 percent.

throm·bo·cy·tol·y·sis (throm''bo·sigh·tol'i·sis) *n.* Destruction of blood platelets. —**thrombo·cy·to·lyt·ic** (·sigh''to·lit'ick) *adj.*

thrombocytolytic purpura. IDIOPATHIC THROMBOCYTOPENIC PURPURA.

throm·bo·cy·to·path·ia (throm''bo·sigh''to·path'ee·uh) *n.* A hemorrhagic state in which the blood platelets are functionally abnormal. —**thrombocytopath·ic** (·ick) *adj.*

thrombocytopathic purpura. Purpura associated with a normal number of qualitatively defective blood platelets.

throm·bo·cy·to·pe·nia (throm''bo·sigh''to·pee'nee·uh) *n.* A condition in which there is a decrease in the absolute number of platelets below normal. —**thrombocytope·nic** (·nick) *adj.*

thrombocytopenic purpura. Purpura associated with decreased numbers of blood platelets per unit volume of blood.

throm·bo·cy·to·pher·e·sis (throm''bo·sigh''to·ferr'e·sis) *n.* Selective removal of blood platelets from the circulation.

throm·bo·cy·to·sis (throm''bo·sigh·to'sis) *n.*, pl. **thrombocyto·ses** (·seez) A condition marked by an absolute increase in the number of blood platelets. Syn. *piastrinemia, thrombocytemia.*

throm·bo·em·bo·lec·to·my (throm''bo·em''bo-leck'tuh·mee) *n.* Surgical removal of an embolus representing a dislodged thrombus or part of a thrombus.

throm·bo·em·bo·lism (throm''bo·em'bo·liz·um) *n.* Embolism due to a dislodged thrombus, or part of a thrombus.

throm·bo·em·bo·li·za·tion (throm''bo·em''bo·li·zay'shun) *n.* The occlusion of a blood vessel by the lodgement of a portion of a thrombus.

throm·bo·em·bo·lus (throm''bo·em'bo·lus) *n.* An embolus composed of a thrombus.

throm·bo·en·do·car·di·tis (throm''bo·en''do·kahr·dye'tis) *n.* Bacterial or nonbacterial thrombotic vegetations on heart valves.

throm·bo·gen (throm'bo·jen) *n.* PROTHROMBIN.

throm·bo·gen·ic (throm''bo·jen'ick) *adj.* Producing thrombi.

throm·bo·ki·nase (throm''bo·kigh'nace, ·kin'ace) *n.* A proteolytic enzyme in blood plasma that, along with thromboplastin, calcium, and factor V, converts prothrombin to thrombin. May be identical with factor X.

throm·bol·y·sis (throm·bol'i·sis) *n.*, pl. **thrombolyses** (·seez) Destruction or dissolution of a thrombus; thromboclasis. —**throm·bo·lyt·ic** (throm''bo·lit'ick) *adj.*

throm·bop·a·thy (throm·bop'uth·ee) *n.* Disease characterized by disturbance of platelet function.

throm·bo·pe·nia (throm''bo·pee'nee·uh) *n.* THROMBOCYTOPENIA. —**thrombope·nic** (·nick) *adj.*

throm·bo·phil·ia (throm''bo·fil'ee·uh) *n.* A tendency to form thrombi.

throm·bo·phle·bi·tis (throm''bo·fle·bye'tis) *n.* Inflammation of a vein associated with thrombosis.

throm·bo·plas·tic (throm''bo·plas'tick) *adj.* 1. Causing or hastening the coagulation of the blood. 2. Of or pertaining to a thromboplastin.

throm·bo·plas·tin (throm''bo·plas'tin) *n.* Any of a group of substances that, along with procoagulants and calcium, accelerates the conversion of prothrombin to thrombin. Most such substances are complexes of lipids and proteins.

throm·bo·poi·e·sis (throm''bo·poy·e'sis) *n.* The production of blood platelets.

throm·bose (throm'boze) *v.* To form or become a thrombus.

throm·bosed (throm'boze'd) *adj.* 1. Affected with thrombosis. 2. Clotted.

throm·bo·sis (throm·bo'sis) *n.*, pl. **thrombo·ses** (·seez) The formation of a thrombus. —**throm·bot·ic** (·bot'ick) *adj.*

throm·bo·sta·sis (throm''bo·stay'sis, throm·bos'tuh·sis) *n.* Stasis of blood leading to formation of a thrombus.

thrombotic endocarditis. MARANTIC ENDOCARDITIS.

thrombotic thrombocytopenic purpura. Thrombi in the vascular channels associated with hyaline deposits in the walls and subendothelial areas of the vessels, and associated thrombocytopenia. Syn. *Moschcowitz's syndrome.*

throm·bus (throm'bus) *n.*, pl. **throm·bi** (·bye) A clot of blood formed during life within the heart or blood vessels.

throt·tle (throt'ul) *v. & n.* 1. To choke; to suffocate. 2. THROAT.

thrush, *n.* 1. A form of candidiasis due to infection by *Candida albicans.* It occurs most often in infants and children and is characterized by small, whitish spots on the tip and sides of the tongue and the buccal mucous membrane. Syn. *mycotic stomatitis, parasitic stomatitis.* 2. A diseased condition of the frog of the horse's foot, with a fetid discharge.

thryp·sis (thrip'sis) *n.* 1. A comminuted fracture. 2. The hypothetical softening and liquefaction of bone matrix preceding leaching out of bone salt in halisteresis.

thumb, *n.* The digit on the radial side of the hand, differing from the other digits in having but two phalanges, and in that its metacarpal bone is freely movable.

thumps, *n.* 1. A verminous pneumonia of swine caused by the larvae of *Ascaris lumbricoides* in the lungs. 2. An affection in the horse, similar to hiccup in man, due to spasmodic contraction of the diaphragm.

thyme (time) *n.* The dried leaves and flowering tops of *Thymus vulgaris* (family Lamiaceae); contains a volatile oil, thyme oil, of which one of the constituents is thymol. It has been used as a diaphoretic, carminative, and expectorant.

thy·mec·to·my (thigh·meck'tuh·mee) *n.* Excision of the thymus. —**thymecto·mize** (·mize) *v.*

thy·mer·ga·sia (thigh''mur·gay'zhuh, ·zee·uh) *n. In psychiatry,* Meyer's term for the affective illnesses. —**thymerga·sic** (·sick) *adj.*

-thymia A combining form designating *a condition involving mood or affect.*

¹**thy·mic** (tigh'mick) *adj.* Pertaining to, or derived from, thyme.

²**thy·mic** (thigh'mick) *adj.* Pertaining to the thymus.

thymic aplasia. Congenital absence of the thymus and of the parathyroids, and often cardiovascular malformations, with deficient cellular immunity; characterized clinically by frequent virus, fungus, or *Pneumocystis* infections, neonatal tetany, and early death. Syn. *Di George's syndrome, third and fourth (III-IV) branchial pouch syndrome.*

thymic corpuscle. A characteristic, rounded, acidophil body in the medulla of the thymus; composed of hyalinized epithelial cells concentrically arranged about a core which is occasionally calcified.

thy·mi·dine (thigh'mi·deen, ·din) *n.* Thymine-2-deoxyriboside, $C_{10}H_{14}N_2O_5$, a nucleoside obtained from deoxyribonucleic acid.

thy·mine (thigh'meen, ·min) *n.* 5-Methyluracil or 2,4-dihydroxy-5-methylpyrimidine, $C_5H_6N_2O_2$, one of the pyrimidine components of nucleic acids, first isolated from the thymus.

thy·mi·on (thigh'mee·on) *n.* WART; CONDYLOMA.

thy·mi·tis (thigh·mye'tis) *n.* Inflammation of the thymus.

thy·mo·cyte (thigh'mo·site) *n.* A lymphocyte formed in the thymus.

thy·mol (thigh'mol) n. 5-Methyl-2-isopropyl-phenol, $C_{10}H_{14}O$, present in thyme oil and other volatile oils and produced by synthesis; a bactericide and fungicide applied topically.

thymol flocculation test. A modification of the thymol turbidity test in which the mixture is allowed to stand overnight and the amount of flocculation is measured.

thymol turbidity test. A test for liver disease based on precipitation of altered serum proteins by a thymol solution.

thy·mo·ma (thigh·mo'muh) n., pl. **thymomas, thymoma·ta** (·tuh) A primary tumor of the thymus whose parenchyma is composed of mixtures of lymphocytic and epithelial cells, or of either element predominantly; its behavior is usually benign, and some forms are associated with myasthenia gravis or hypoplasia of erythrocyte precursors.

thy·mo·no·ic (thigh'mo·no'ick) adj. Pertaining to thoughts and ideas that are strongly influenced by deviations in mood.

thy·mop·a·thy (thigh·mop'uth·ee) n. Any disease of the thymus.

thy·mo·priv·ic (thigh'mo·priv'ick) adj. Related to, or caused by, removal of or premature involution of the thymus.

thy·mus (thy'mus) n., pl. **thymuses, thy·mi** (·migh) A lymphoepithelial organ developed from the third and fourth branchial pouches and normally situated in the anterior superior mediastinum. It is the site of differentiation of T lymphocytes and is a central lymphoid organ controlling many aspects of immunologic reactivity, particularly delayed hypersensitivity. It is well developed at birth but undergoes gradual involution after puberty. It is lobulated and contains primarily lymphocytes, densely packed in the cortex and more loosely packed in the medulla which also contains concentric arrangements of epithelial cells called thymic corpuscles.

thyr-, threreo-, thyro-. A combining form meaning thyroid.

thy·reo·apla·sia con·gen·i·ta (thigh''ree·o·uh·play'zhuh kon·jen'i·tuh). Anomalies found in congenital defects of the thyroid gland and in deficient thyroid secretion.

thy·reo·gen·ic (thigh''ree·o·jen'ick) adj. Of thyroid origin, as thyreogenic obesity.

thy·reo·priv·al (thigh''ree·o·prye'vul) adj. THYROPRIVAL.

thy·ro·ary·te·noid (thigh''ro·ăr'i·tee'noid) adj. Pertaining to the thyroid and arytenoid cartilages.

thy·ro·cal·ci·to·nin (thigh''ro·kal·si·to'nin) n. CALCITONIN.

thy·ro·car·di·ac (thigh''ro·kahr'dee·ack) adj. Pertaining to thyroid disease with cardiac symptoms predominating.

thy·ro·cele (thigh'ro·seel) n. A tumor affecting the thyroid gland; goiter.

thy·ro·cer·vi·cal (thigh''ro·sur'vi·kul) adj. Pertaining to the thyroid gland and the neck.

thy·ro·chon·drot·o·my (thigh''ro·kon·drot'uh·mee) n. THYROTOMY.

thy·ro·cri·cot·o·my (thigh''ro·krye·kot'uh·mee, ·kri·) n. Tracheotomy performed through the cricothyroid membrane.

thy·ro·epi·glot·tic (thigh''ro·ep''i·glot'ick) adj. Pertaining to the thyroid cartilage and the epiglottis.

thy·ro·gen·ic (thigh''ro·jen'ick) adj. THYREOGENIC.

thy·ro·glob·u·lin (thigh''ro·glob'yoo·lin) n. An iodinated protein found in the thyroid follicular lumen and epithelial cells which contains within its structure monoiodotyrosine, diiodotyrosine, triiodothyronine, and tetraiodothyronine. The storage form of the iodinated hormones.

thy·ro·glos·sal (thigh''ro·glos'ul) adj. Pertaining to the thyroid gland and the tongue.

thyroglossal cyst. Cystic distention of the remnants of the thyroglossal duct, filled with secretion of lining epithelial cells; most often presents over the thyrohyoid membrane in the midline.

thyroglossal fistula. A developmental abnormality, due to incomplete obliteration of the thyroglossal duct, resulting in a midline cervical fistula.

thy·ro·hy·al (thigh''ro·high'ul) n. The greater cornu of the hyoid bone.

thy·ro·hy·oid (thigh''ro·high'oid) adj. Pertaining to the thyroid cartilage and the hyoid bone.

¹thy·roid (thigh'roid) adj. & n. 1. Shield-shaped, as: thyroid cartilage. 2. Pertaining to the thyroid cartilage, as: thyroid gland. 3. Pertaining to the thyroid gland, its functions and secretions. 4. THYROID GLAND. 5. The cleaned, dried and powdered parenchymal tissue of the thyroid glands of domestic animals, containing about 0.2% iodine in thyroid combination, especially as thyroxine. Used in the treatment of thyroid-deficiency states.

²thyroid, adj. Comparable to a door or doorway, as: thyroid foramen (2).

thyroid cartilage The largest of the laryngeal cartilages, consisting of two laminas united at an angle in front called the laryngeal prominence.

thyroid crisis. THYROTOXIC CRISIS.

thyroid dwarfism. 1. CRETINISM. 2. Stunted growth resulting from hypothyroidism.

thy·roid·ec·to·mize (thigh''roy·deck'tuh·mize) v. To perform a thyroidectomy.

thy·roid·ec·to·my (thigh''roy·deck'tuh·mee) n. Partial or complete excision of the thyroid gland.

thyroid gland. One of the endocrine glands, lying in front of the trachea and consisting of two lateral lobes connected centrally by an isthmus. The organ is composed of follicles lined by epithelium, producing a colloid material.

thyroid heart. GOITER HEART.

thyroid heart disease. Heart disease or cardiac symptoms associated with alteration of thyroid function, either hyperthyroidism or myxedema.

thyroid hormone. Commonly, thyroxine (tetraiodothyronine) or liothyronine (triiodothyronine), or both.

thyroid infantilism. Physical and mental underdevelopment resulting from hypothyroidism.

thy·roid·i·tis (thigh''roid·eye'tis) n. Inflammation of the thyroid gland.

thy·roid·ot·o·my (thigh″roy·dot′uh·mee) *n.* Incision of the thyroid gland.

thy·roido·tox·in (thigh·roy″do·tock′sin) *n.* A substance specifically toxic for the cells of the thyroid gland.

thyroid-stimulating hormone. THYROTROPIC HORMONE. Abbreviated, TSH.

thyroid storm. THYROTOXIC CRISIS.

thy·ro·meg·a·ly (thigh″ro·meg′uh·lee) *n.* Enlargement of the thyroid gland.

thy·ro·mi·met·ic (thigh″ro·migh·met′ick, ·mi·) *adj.* Pertaining to or characterized by thyroid-like action, as of thyroid hormones.

thy·ro·para·thy·roid·ec·to·my (thigh″ro·păr″uh·thigh″roy·deck′tuh·mee) *n.* Excision of the thyroid and parathyroid glands.

thy·ro·pri·val (thigh″ro·prye′val) *adj.* Pertaining to the effects of loss of function, or removal, of the thyroid gland.

thyroprival tetany. Tetany following surgical removal of the thyroid gland when the parathyroids have inadvertently been removed also, or have been damaged.

thy·rop·to·sis (thigh″rop·to′sis) *n.* Displacement of a goitrous thyroid so that it is partially or completely concealed in the thorax.

thy·rot·o·my (thigh·rot′uh·mee) *n.* Incision or splitting of the thyroid cartilage.

thy·ro·tox·ic (thigh″ro·tock′sick) *adj.* 1. Pertaining to or affected with thyrotoxicosis. 2. Of or pertaining to thyrotoxin.

thyrotoxic crisis. Acute fulminating hyperthyroidism which may lead to extreme tachycardia, muscle weakness, coma, and death. Syn. *thyroid crisis.*

thyrotoxic heart. GOITER HEART.

thy·ro·tox·i·co·sis (thigh″ro·tock″si·ko′sis) *n.* HYPERTHYROIDISM.

thy·ro·tox·in (thigh″ro·tock′sin) *n.* Any substance that is toxic to the thyroid cells.

thy·ro·trop·ic (thigh″ro·trop′ick, ·tro′pick) *adj.* 1. Stimulating the thyroid gland. 2. Pertaining to thyrotropin (2).

thyrotropic hormone. A hormone of the adenohypophysis which controls the status of the thyroid. Syn. *thyroid-stimulating hormone.*

thy·ro·tro·pin (thigh″ro·tro′pin, thigh·rot′ro·pin) *n.* A thyroid-stimulating hormone produced by the adenohypophysis.

thy·ro·tro·pism (thigh″ro·tro′piz·um, thigh·rot′ro·piz·um) *n.* 1. An affinity for the thyroid. 2. Constitutional domination by thyroid influence.

thy·rox·ine (thigh·rock′seen, ·sin) *n.* L-3,3′,5,5′-Tetraiodothyronine, $C_{15}H_{11}I_4NO_4$, an active physiologic principle of the thyroid gland; used, in the form of the sodium salt (levothyroxine sodium), as replacement therapy where there is reduced or absent thyroid function.

tib·ia (tib′ee·uh) *n.,* L. pl. & genit. sing. **ti·bi·ae** (tib′ee·ee), E. pl. **tibias** The larger of the two bones of the leg, commonly called the shin-bone, articulating with the femur, fibula, and talus. **—tib·i·al** (·ee·ul) *adj.*

tibial collateral ligament. A broad, flat ligament on the medial side of the knee joint, connecting the medial condyle of the femur and the medial surface and surface of the shaft of the tibia, adhering also to the edge of the medial meniscus.

tib·i·al·gia (tib″ee·al′jee·uh) *n.* Pain in the tibia.

tib·i·a·lis (tib″ee·ay′lis) *n.* One of two muscles of the leg, tibialis anterior and tibialis posterior.

tibio–. A combining form meaning *tibia, tibial.*

tib·io·fem·o·ral (tib″ee·o·fem′o·rul) *adj.* Pertaining to the tibia and the femur.

tib·io·fib·u·lar (tib″ee·o·fib′yoo·lur) *adj.* Pertaining to the tibia and the fibula.

tibiofibular articulation. 1. Either of the articulations between the tibia and the fibula; the proximal or superior tibiofibular articulation, between the lateral condyle of the tibia and the head of the fibula, or the distal or inferior tibiofibular articulation, the tibiofibular syndesmosis, joining the distal ends of these two bones. 2. Specifically, the proximal tibiofibular articulation, as distinguished from the tibiofibular syndesmosis.

tibiofibular ligament. Either of the two ligaments joining the distal ends of the tibia and the fibula, in the tibiofibular syndesmosis; the anterior tibiofibular ligament, connecting the ends of the two bones at their anterior adjacent margins, or the posterior tibiofibular ligament, which passes between them on the posterior face of the syndesmosis.

tic, *n.* A habitual, irresistible, repetitious, stereotyped movement or complex of movements, of which the patient is aware but feels compelled to make in order to relieve tension. Syn. *habit spasm.*

tic dou·lou·reux (doo·loo·ruh′) TRIGEMINAL NEURALGIA.

tick, *n.* An arthropod of the order Acarina infesting vertebrate animals. They are important vectors and reservoirs of rickettsial diseases and also transmit many viral, bacterial, and protozoal diseases. Toxins produced by the female before oviposition produce tick paralysis. The important genera are *Amblyomma, Argas, Boophilus, Dermacentor, Haemaphysalis, Hyalomma, Ixodes, Ornithodorus,* and *Rhipicephalus.*

tick-bite paralysis. A flaccid type of paralysis occurring in animals, and occasionally in man, during the attachment of certain species of ticks. The paralysis will disappear a few hours after removal of the tick. The cause is thought to be a neurotoxin injected by the engorging tick. Syn. *tick paralysis.*

tick fever. ROCKY MOUNTAIN SPOTTED FEVER.

tick·ling, *n.* A rapid series of light, tactile stimulations of the skin or mucous membrane arousing a tingling sensation.

tick paralysis. TICK-BITE PARALYSIS.

t.i.d. Abbreviation for *ter in die,* three times a day.

tidal drainage. Drainage of a cavity, particularly a paralyzed urinary bladder, with an automatic irrigation apparatus which alternately fills and empties the cavity.

tidal volume. The amount of air moved by a single breath at any level of activity; normally, at rest, approximates 500 ml (resting tidal volume). Syn. *tidal air.*

Tie·tze's disease or **syndrome** (tee'tsuh) Painful nonsuppurative swelling of the rib cartilages.

ti·ger lily appearance. The speckled appearance of the myocardium observed in untreated pernicious anemia.

tigroid bodies. The Nissl bodies or chromophil granules of nerve cells.

ti·grol·y·sis (tye-grol'i·sis) *n.* Disintegration of the chromophil substance in a nerve cell.

tilt table. A table top on which a patient lies and which can be rotated to the vertical position, employed for a variety of therapeutic and investigative purposes.

tim·bre (tam'bur, tam'br) *n.* The peculiar quality of a tone, other than pitch and intensity, that makes it distinctive. It depends upon the overtones of the vibrating body.

tim·o·thy (tim'uth·ee) *n.* A common name for *Phleum pratense,* the most important meadow grass in America. It flowers during June and July, shedding quantities of pollen, one of the more common causes of the seasonal rhinitis of early summer.

tin, *n.* Sn = 118.69. A silver-white metallic element, atomic number 50; powdered tin was at one time used as a mechanical anthelmintic.

Tinactin. Trademark for tolnaftate, a topically applied antifungal drug.

tinc·to·ri·al (tink·to'ree·ul) *adj.* Pertaining to staining or dyeing.

tinc·ture (tink'chur) *n.* Alcoholic or hydroalcoholic solutions of medicinal substances, generally representing 10 or 20% (weight per volume) of drug and usually prepared by maceration or percolation of the drug with suitable menstruum. Abbreviated, tr.

tine, *n.* A fine pointed instrument, used in dentistry to explore fine crevices and cavities.

tin·ea (tin'ee·uh) *n.* The lesions of dermatophytosis; RINGWORM.

tinea bar·bae (bahr'bee). Ringworm of the bearded areas of the face and neck, caused by various species of *Trichophyton* and *Microsporum.* Syn. *tinea sycosis.*

tinea cap·i·tis (kap'i·tis). Fungus infection of the scalp and hair. Caused by several species of *Trichophyton* and *Microsporum.* Syn. *tinea tonsurans.*

tinea cir·ci·na·ta (sur''si·nay'tuh). TINEA CORPORIS.

tinea cor·po·ris (kor'po·ris). A fungus infection involving the glabrous skin. Caused by various species of *Trichophyton* and *Microsporum.* Syn. *tinea circinata.*

tinea cru·ris (kroo'ris). A fungus infection involving the skin of the groin, perineum, and perianal regions. Caused by *Epidermophyton floccosum* and several species of *Trichophyton.* Syn. *gum itch, jockey itch, laundryman's itch.*

tinea de·cal·vans (dee·kal'vanz). ALOPECIA AREATA.

tinea fa·ci·a·le (fay''shee·ay'lee). Fungous infection of the skin of the face, especially of the glabrous skin.

tinea gla·bro·sa (gla·bro'suh). Fungus infection of the nonhairy skin. Included under this heading are tinea corporis, tinea cruris, tinea versicolor, erythrasma, and dermatophytosis of the hands and feet.

tinea im·bri·ca·ta (im''bri·kay'tuh). A superficial fungus disease of the tropics characterized by the presence of concentric rings of pruritic papulosquamous patches scattered over the body. Caused by *Trichophyton concentricum.* Syn. *gogo, scaly ringworm, tropical tinea circinata, Malabar itch.*

tinea ni·gra (nye'gruh). A contagious cutaneous fungus infection caused by *Cladosporium mansonii* in the East and *Cladosporium werneckii* in the Americas, clinically characterized by its black or dark-brown coloration and its predominant occurrence on the trunk, neck, or palmar regions, though other sites may be involved. Syn. *pityriasis nigra, microsporosis nigra.*

tinea pedis. A fungus infection of the feet, especially the webs of the toes and the soles. Caused by *Epidermophyton floccosum,* various species of *Trichophyton,* and rarely by *Microsporum.*

tinea un·gui·um (ung'gwee·um). A chronic fungus infection involving the nails of the hands and feet. Caused by *Epidermophyton floccosum,* various species of *Trichophyton,* and *Candida albicans.*

tinea ver·si·co·lor (vur''si·ko'lor, vur'si·kul''ur). A chronic superficial fungus infection of the skin, usually of the trunk. It is caused by *Malassezia furfur.*

tin·gle, *n.* A pricking or stinging sensation; the feeling of a slight, sharp, and sudden thrill, as of pain; acanthesthesia.

tin·ni·tus (ti·nigh'tus) *n.* A ringing in one or both ears. Buzzing, hissing, humming, whistling, roaring, or clicking sounds are also reported. Syn. *tinnitus aurium.*

tire, *v.* To become weary; to become exhausted; used extensively by the medical profession and laymen in reference to muscular and mental fatigue, general bodily and mental exhaustion.

Ti·se·li·us apparatus (tee·se'y'lee·ōōs) An apparatus that permits the measurement of electrophoretic mobilities of proteins by use of moving-boundary electrophoresis. The cell is divided into compartments which permit isolation of the components separated by the electric current.

tis·sue (tish'oo) *n.* An aggregation of similar cells and their intercellular substance.

tissue dose. Radiant energy absorbed by a designated tissue at a point in question, measured in ergs per gram.

tissue protein. The part of the body protein present in the solid tissues as distinguished from the circulating protein of the blood.

tissue thromboplastin. Any of several lipid-rich clot accelerators prepared from tissues, particularly from brain or lung. Such preparations are effective in the absence of factors VIII, IX, XI, and XII, but require factors V, VII, and X for maximum acceleration of clotting.

tis·su·lar (tish'yoo·lur) *adj.* Pertaining to the tissues of living organisms.

ti·ta·ni·um (tye·tay'nee·um, ti·tay'nee·um) *n.* Ti = 47.90. A very hard, dark-gray, lustrous, metallic element, atomic number 22, density

4.51, used in certain alloys to impart toughness.

titanium dioxide. TiO₂; used as a protectant against sunburn.

ti·ter, ti·tre (tye'tur) *n.* 1. *In chemistry,* an expression of the strength of a volumetric solution. 2. The amount of one substance that corresponds to, reacts with, or is otherwise equivalent to a stated quantity of another substance.

tit·il·la·tion (tit''i-lay'shun) *n.* Tickling; the responses produced by tickling.

ti·tra·tion (tye-tray'shun) *n.* An operation involving the measurement of the concentration or volume of a standard solution required to react chemically or immunologically with a substance being analyzed or standardized. —**ti·trate** (ti'trate) *v.*

ti·trim·e·ter (tye-trim'e-tur) *n.* An apparatus or instrument for use in titrimetry.

tit·u·ba·tion (tit'yoo-bay'shun) *n.* Unsteadiness of posture, especially in diseases of the cerebellum and its connections; manifested as a rhythmic instability and swaying of the trunk or of the head on the trunk.

T loop. The vectorcardiographic representation of ventricular repolarization.

TNT Abbreviation for *trinitrotoluene.*

to-and-fro murmur. A pericardial murmur heard during both systole and diastole.

to·bac·co (tuh-back'o) *n.,* pl. **tobaccos, tobaccoes** A plant, *Nicotiana tabacum,* of the family Solanaceae, the dried leaves of which contain an alkaloid, nicotine. Formerly employed as an enema to overcome intestinal obstruction.

tobacco amblyopia. TOXIC AMBLYOPIA.

To·bey-Ay·er test A test for lateral sinus thrombosis, based on changes in the pressure of the spinal fluid during compression of one or both internal jugular veins.

toco-, toko- A combining form meaning (a) *childbirth, labor;* (b) *offspring.*

toco·dy·na·mom·e·ter, toko·dy·na·mom·e·ter (to''ko-dye''nuh-mom'e-tur, tock''o-) *n.* An instrument for measuring the amplitude, duration, and frequency of uterine muscular contraction, as during labor. Abbreviated, TKD

to·cog·ra·phy, to·kog·ra·phy (to-kog'ruh-fee) *n.* The making and interpreting of graphic recordings of the amplitude, duration, and frequency of uterine muscular contractions during labor. —**toco·graph·ic, toko·graph·ic** (to''ko-graf'ick) *adj.*

to·col·o·gy, to·kol·o·gy (to-kol'uh-jee) *n.* OBSTETRICS.

toco·ma·nia, toko·ma·nia (to''ko-may'nee-uh, tock''o-) *n.* PUERPERAL PSYCHOSIS.

to·com·e·try, to·kom·e·try (to-kom'e-tree) *n.* A study of the amplitude, duration, and frequency of the uterine muscular contractions, as during labor, with a tocodynamometer. —**tocome·ter, tokome·ter** (·tur)

to·coph·er·ol (to-kof'ur-ol) *n.* Any one of several related substances, occurring naturally in certain oils and also prepared by synthesis, that have vitamin E activity. The most potent of these, alpha tocopherol, is 2,5,7,8-tetramethyl-2-(4',8',12'-trimethyltridecyl)-6-chromanol,

C₂₉H₅₀O₂; the *d-* form is more active than the *l-* form.

toco·pho·bia, toko·pho·bia (to''ko-fo'bee-uh, tock''o-) *n.* Undue dread of childbirth.

to·cus, to·kus (to'kus) *n.* CHILDBIRTH.

toe, *n.* A digit of the foot.

toe-drop, *n.* DROPPED FOOT.

to·ga·vi·rus (to'guh-vye''rus) *n.* A spherical, encapsulated RNA virus that is categorized as either group A or group B. Group A viruses are larger and produce eastern and western equine encephalitis; group B viruses produce various illnesses including encephalitis, hemorrhagic diseases and severe systemic illnesses.

tol·bu·ta·mide (tol-bew'tuh-mide) *n.* 1-Butyl-3-(*p*-tolylsulfonyl)urea, C₁₂H₁₈N₂O₃S, an orally effective hypoglycemic drug.

tol·er·ance, *n.* 1. The ability of enduring or being less responsive to the influence of a drug or poison, particularly when acquired by continued use of the substance. 2. The allowable deviation from a standard, as the range of variation permitted for the content of a drug in one of its dosage forms. 3. IMMUNOLOGIC TOLERANCE.

tol·er·ant, *n.* TOLERANCE. —**tol·er·ate,** *v.*

tol·naf·tate (tol-naf'tate) *n.* O-2-Naphthyl *m,N*-dimethylthiocarbanilate, C₁₉H₁₇NOS, a topically applied antifungal drug.

tol·u·ene (tol'yoo-een) *n.* Methylbenzene, C₆H₅CH₃, a colorless liquid obtained chiefly from coal tar. Used as a solvent and reagent.

toluidine blue O. A basic dye of the thiazine series used in Albert's stain for the diphtheria organism, in the panchrome stain, and for many other purposes. Syn. *methylene blue O.*

tol·u·ol (tol'yoo-ol) *n.* TOLUENE.

tol·yl (tol'il) *n.* The univalent radical —C₆H₄CH₃.

-tome A combining form designating (a) *a part or a section;* (b) *an instrument for cutting.*

to·mo·gram (to'muh-gram) *n.* A radiograph obtained by sectional radiography.

to·mog·ra·phy (to-mog'ruh-fee) *n.* SECTIONAL RADIOGRAPHY. —**to·mo·graph·ic** (to''mo-graf'ick) *adj.*

to·mo·ma·nia (to''mo-may'nee-uh) *n.* 1. An abnormal desire to have a surgical procedure performed upon oneself. 2. An abnormal wish to perform surgical procedures.

to·mo·to·cia (to''mo-to'shee-uh, ·see-uh) *n.* CESAREAN SECTION.

-tomy A combining form meaning *cutting, incision, section.*

to·na·pha·sia (to''nuh-fay'zhuh, ·zee-uh, ton''uh-) *n.* AMUSIA.

tone, *n.* 1. A sound characterized by a definite pitch or harmonic combination of pitches. 2. The normal state of healthy tension and vigor in the body or in a part; specifically, TONUS. Adj. *tonal, tonic.*

tone deafness. Relative inability to distinguish between musical tones of different pitch; due to abnormalities of the end organ, as opposed to amusia, which is due to lesion of the cerebral cortex.

tongue, *n.* The movable muscular organ attached to the floor of the mouth, and concerned in tasting, masticating, swallowing, and speaking. It consists of a number of muscles, and is covered by mucous membrane from which project numerous papillae, and in which are placed the terminal organs of taste.

tongue-tie, n. A congenital abnormality of the frenulum of the tongue, interfering with its mobility.

tongue worm. PENTASTOME.

-tonia. A combining form designating a condition or degree of tonus.

ton·ic (ton′ick) adj. & n. 1. Pertaining to tone; producing normal tone or tension. 2. Pertaining to or characterized by continuous tension or contraction. 3. An agent or drug given to improve the normal tone of an organ or of the patient generally.

tonic-clonic, adj. Pertaining to muscular spasms, especially as seen in generalized seizures, in which there is a tonic and a clonic phase.

tonic-clonic convulsion or **seizure.** Any convulsive seizure with a phase of tonic contraction and one of clonic contraction; almost always a generalized seizure.

tonic contraction. TONIC SPASM.

to·nic·i·ty (to-nis′i-tee) n. 1. The condition of normal tone or tension of an organ. 2. The condition of a solution with respect to its being hypertonic, isotonic, or hypotonic.

tonic postural epilepsy. Epilepsy characterized by tonic seizures.

tonic seizure. A major generalized seizure in which the motor manifestations are limited to a tonic spasm of the entire musculature; characterized by a forceful closure of the jaws, often with biting of the tongue, and a piercing cry, as air is forced through closed vocal cords.

tonic spasm. A spasm that persists without relaxation for some time.

To·ni-Fan·co·ni syndrome (toh′nee, fah′ng·ko′nee) FANCONI SYNDROME.

ton·i·tro·pho·bia (ton′i·tro·fo′bee·uh) n. Abnormal fear of thunder.

tono– A combining form meaning (a) tone; (b) pressure.

tono·clon·ic (ton′′o·klon′ick) adj. TONIC-CLONIC.

tono·fi·brils (to′′no·figh′brilz) n.pl. Delicate fibrils, found particularly in epithelial cells, which converge on desmosomes.

tono·gram (to′nuh·gram, ton′o·) n. A record made by a tonograph.

tono·graph (to′nuh·graf, ton′o·) n. A device for determining or recording pressure.

to·nog·ra·phy (to·nog′ruh·fee) n. Continuous recording of pressure with an electric tonometer; used especially in measuring intraocular pressure.

to·nom·e·ter (to·nom′e·tur) n. 1. An instrument to measure tension, as that of the eyeball. 2. An instrument used to equilibrate samples of fluid, as blood, with gases at known concentrations.

to·nom·e·try (to·nom′e·tree) n. The measurement of pressure or tension with a tonometer.

ton·os·cil·log·ra·phy (to·nos′′si·log′ruh·fee) n. A

method of automatically recording blood pressure in the extremities.

tono·scope (to′nuh·skope) n. An instrument for examination of the interior of the cranium by means of sound.

ton·sil (ton′sil) n. 1. Aggregated lymph nodules and associated lymph vessels surrounding crypts or depressions of the pharyngeal mucosa; specifically, the palatine tonsil. 2. The tonsilla of the cerebellum; TONSILLA (1). —**ton·sil·lar** (·ur) adj.

tonsill-, tonsillo-. A combining form meaning tonsil.

ton·sil·la (ton·sil′uh) n., pl. **tonsil·lae** (·ee) 1. (of the cerebellum:) A small lobe of the cerebellar hemisphere, on its inferior medial aspect. 2. TONSIL (1).

tonsillar herniation. Informal. CEREBELLAR PRESSURE CONE.

ton·sil·lec·to·my (ton′′si·leck′tuh·mee) n. Removal of the palatine tonsils.

ton·sil·li·tis (ton′′si·lye′tis) n. Inflammation of the tonsils. —**ton·sil·lit·ic** (ton′′si·lit′ick) adj.

ton·sil·lo·lith (ton·sil′o·lith) n. A concretion within a tonsil.

ton·sil·lo·phar·yn·gi·tis (ton′′si·lo·far′′in·jye′tis) n. Inflammation of the tonsils and pharynx.

ton·sil·lo·tome (ton·sil′uh·tome) n. An instrument for removing a tonsil.

ton·sil·lot·o·my (ton′′si·lot′uh·mee) n. The operation of cutting into or removing part of a tonsil.

ton·sil·sec·tor (ton′′sil·seck′tur) n. A tonsillotome consisting of a pair of circular or oval scissor blades moving inside a guarding ring.

ton·sure (ton′shur) n. The shaving or removal of the hair from the crown of the head.

to·nus (to′nus) n. The sustained partial contraction present in relaxed skeletal muscles; the slight resistance that normal, relaxed muscle offers to passive movement.

tooth, n., pl. **teeth.** One of the calcified organs supported by the alveolar processes and gingivae of both jaws, serving to masticate food, aid speech, and influence facial contour. Each tooth consists of an enamel-covered crown, a single, bifid, or trifid cementum-covered root, and a neck (the conjunction of crown and root), and a pulp chamber which contains the dental pulp with its nerves and vessels and is surrounded by a mass of dentin.

tooth·ache, n. Any pain in or about a tooth. Syn. odontalgia.

toothed, adj. Having teeth or indentations.

Tooth's muscular atrophy PERONEAL MUSCULAR ATROPHY.

top-, topo- A combining form meaning (a) place, part; (b) local.

top·ag·no·sis (top′′ag·no′sis) n. TOPAGNOSIA.

to·pal·gia (to·pal′jee·uh) n. Localized pain, without evident organic basis, common in certain mental disorders, as in the conversion type of hysterical neurosis.

to·pec·to·my (to·peck′tuh·mee) n. A form of psychosurgery with excision of a limited portion of the cerebral cortex, usually in the frontal area, as applied in the treatment of certain mental disorders or intractable pain.

top·es·the·sia (top''es·theezh'uh) *n.* Ability to localize a tactile sensation.

Töp·fer's reagent (tœp'fur) A 0.5% solution of dimethylaminoazobenzene in 95% alcohol; most commonly used as an indicator to titrate free hydrochloric acid in the gastric contents.

Töpfer's test A test for free hydrochloric acid in gastric contents in which a few drops of Töpfer's reagent gives a cherry-red color to a fluid containing free hydrochloric acid.

to·pha·ceous (to·fay'shus) *adj.* Of the nature of tophi; sandy or gritty.

tophaceous gout. Prominent deposits of sodium urate (tophi) in the subcutaneous and periarticular tissues in gout.

to·phus (to'fus) *n.,* pl. **to·phi** (·fye) 1. A sodium urate deposit in the skin about a joint, in the ear, or in bone, in gout. 2. A mineral concretion in the body, especially about the joints.

top·i·cal (top'i·kul) *adj.* LOCAL.

topical anesthesia. Application of an anesthetic to one of the body surfaces, as with a swab.

top·og·nos·tic (top''og·nos'tick) *adj.* Pertaining to the recognition of changes, positions, or symptoms of parts of the body, as topognostic sensibility.

to·po·graph·ic (top''o·graf'ick, to''po·) *adj.* Of or pertaining to topography.

to·po·graph·i·cal (top''o·graf'i·kul, to''po·) *adj.* TOPOGRAPHIC.

topographic anatomy. Anatomy of a part in its relation to other parts.

to·pog·ra·phy (to·pog'ruh·fee) *n.* A study of the regions of the body or its parts, as cerebral topography.

to·pol·o·gy (to·pol'uh·jee) *n.* 1. TOPOGRAPHIC ANATOMY. 2. The relation of the presenting part of a fetus to the pelvic canal.

topo·nar·co·sis (top''o·nahr·ko'sis) *n.* Local insensibility or anesthesia.

topo·neu·ro·sis (top''o·new·ro'sis) *n.* A localized neurosis.

topo·pho·bia (top''o·fo'bee·uh) *n.* An abnormal dread of certain places.

torch syndrome A group of clinical manifestations that are similar in perinatal infection by the diverse agents *Toxoplasma gondii,* rubella virus, cytomegalovirus, and herpes simplex virus.

Torek's operation 1. An operation for undescended testis. 2. A resection of the thoracic esophagus for cancer.

tori. Plural of *torus.*

Tor·kild·sen procedure Surgical establishment of a communication between a lateral ventricle and the cisterna magna.

Torn·waldt's abscess (torn'vah\ᵇlt) An abscess located in the pharyngeal tonsil or surrounding structures and caused by an infection of the pharyngeal bursa.

Tornwaldt's bursitis or **disease** PHARYNGEAL BURSITIS.

tor·pid (tor'pid) *adj.* Affected with or exhibiting torpor.

tor·pid·i·ty (tor·pid'i·tee) *n.* TORPOR.

tor·por (tor'pur) *n.* Sluggishness; inactivity.

torque, *n.* The measure of the effectiveness of a force in producing rotation or torsion of a body about an axis; the moment of force, i.e., the magnitude of the force times the perpendicular distance from the axis to the line of action of the force.

tor·si·oc·clu·sion (tor''see·uh·kloo'zhun) *n.* Occlusion of a tooth that is in torsiversion.

tor·si·om·e·ter (tor''see·om'e·tur) *n.* An instrument for measuring ocular torsion.

tor·sion (tor'shun) *n.* 1. A twisting; also, the rotation of the eye about the visual axis. 2. The tilting of the vertical meridian of the eye.

tor·sive (tor'siv) *adj.* Twisted; twisting.

tor·si·ver·sion (tor''si·vur'zhun) *n.* Rotated position of a tooth in its alveolus.

tor·so (tor'so) *n.,* pl. **torsos, tor·si** (·see), **torsoes** The trunk; the body without head or limbs.

tort, *v.* To tilt the vertical meridian of the eye.

tor·ti·col·lis (tor''ti·kol'is, ·kol'ee) *n.* Deformity of the neck due to contraction of cervical muscles or fascia, but most prominently involving the sternocleidomastoid muscle unilaterally, resulting in abnormal position and limitation of movements of the head. Syn. *wryneck.*

tor·tu·ous (tor'choo·us) *adj.* Twisted, sinuous. —**tor·tu·os·i·ty** (tor''choo·os'i·tee) *n.*

Tor·u·la (tor'yoo·luh) *n.* CRYPTOCOCCUS. —**torular** (·lur) *adj.*

tor·u·lo·ma (tor''yoo·lo'muh) *n.* A tumorlike nodule resulting from cryptococcal (torular) infection.

tor·u·lo·sis (tor''yoo·lo'sis) *n.* CRYPTOCOCCOSIS.

tor·u·lus (tor'yoo·lus) *n.,* pl. **tor·u·li** (·lye) A minute elevation.

to·rus (to'rus) *n.,* pl. **to·ri** (·rye) 1. A surface having a regular curvature with two principal meridians of dissimilar curvature at right angles to each other. 2. An elevation or prominence.

torus pa·la·ti·nus (pal·uh·tye'nus) [NA] A nodular elevation along the median suture of the hard palate; due to an exostosis.

total color blindness. The complete inability to distinguish different hues and saturation. Syn. *monochromatism.*

total hyperopia. The entire amount of hyperopia, both latent and manifest, detected after accommodation has been paralyzed by a mydriatic or during complete relaxation of the ciliary muscle. Symbol, Ht.

to·tip·o·tence (to·tip'o·tunce) *n.* The capacity of a precursor stage of a cell or organism to give rise to a full range of types, or a complete organism, at a later stage. —**totipo·tent** (·tunt), **to·ti·po·ten·tial** (to''ti·po·ten'chul) *adj.*

touch, *n.* 1. The tactile sense. 2. PALPATION.

Tou·louse–Lau·trec disease (too·looz' lo·treck') PYKNODYSOSTOSIS.

tour·ni·quet (toor'ni·kut, tur') *n.* Any apparatus for controlling hemorrhage from, or circulation in, a limb or part of the body, where pressure can be brought upon the blood vessels by means of straps, cords, rubber tubes, or pads. Tourniquets are made in a multiplicity of forms, from the simplest emergency adaptation to elaborate instruments.

tourniquet paralysis. Pressure paralysis caused by too long application of a tourniquet to a limb while checking hemorrhage. It is most common in the nerves of the arm.

tourniquet test. A test for capillary resistance in which a blood pressure cuff about the upper arm is used to occlude the vein effectively for a measured time, after which the skin of the forearm and hand is examined for petechiae.

Tou·ton cells Multinucleated giant cells having foamy, fat-containing cytoplasm which forms a distinct rim outside a wavy row of nuclei; they are associated with disease that destroys adipose tissue.

tox-, toxi-, toxo-. A combining form meaning *toxic, poisonous, toxin, poison.*

tox·al·bu·min (tock″sal·bew′min) *n.* A poisonous protein, obtained from cultures of bacteria and from certain plants.

tox·ae·mia, tox·ae·mia (tock·see′mee·uh) *n.* A condition in which the blood contains poisonous products, either those produced by the body cells or those resulting from microorganisms.

toxemia of pregnancy. A pathologic condition sometimes occurring in the latter half of pregnancy, manifested by symptoms of eclampsia or preeclampsia.

tox·emic, tox·ae·mic (tock·see′mick) *adj.* Pertaining to, affected with, or caused by toxemia.

toxic-, toxico-. A combining form meaning *poison, toxic.*

tox·ic (tock′sick) *adj.* POISONOUS.

toxic amblyopia. A relative or absolute loss of a portion or all of the visual field caused by a chronic or by an acute toxemia, which may be endogenous, such as uremia, diabetes, or beri beri; or exogenous, such as quinine, lead, tobacco, or methyl alcohol.

tox·i·cant (tock′si·kunt) *adj. & n.* 1. Poisonous or toxic. 2. A poison or toxin.

toxic cirrhosis. POSTNECROTIC CIRRHOSIS.

toxic convulsion or **seizure.** A seizure due to the action of some toxic agent upon the nervous system. The responsible substance may be inorganic (for example, carbon monoxide), organic (for example, alcohol), metallic (for example, lead, arsenic), a foreign protein, or a convulsant substance such as strychnine; or the seizure may be associated with toxemia of pregnancy or uremia.

toxic encephalopathy. 1. Any brain disorder due to toxic factors. 2. A severe, not uncommon, neurologic disorder of infants and children of unknown cause, characterized clinically by rapid onset of fever, depression of consciousness or coma, seizures, and often a fulminant fatal course, and pathologically by acute cerebral edema without other significant histopathological changes.

toxic epidermal necrolysis. A condition characterized by sudden development of high fever and large, flaccid bullae on the skin generally, and in or about the mucous membranes; in some cases thought to be caused by drugs; in others, due to an exfoliative toxin produced by some strains of *Staphylococcus aureus.* Syn. *scalded skin syndrome, Lyell's syndrome.*

toxic hepatitis. Inflammation of the liver resulting from the action of toxic compounds. Examples of hepatotoxins include such diverse compounds as the chlorinated hydrocarbons, phosphorus, and certain alkaloids.

tox·i·cide (tock′si·side) *n.* A remedy or principle that destroys toxic agents.

tox·ic·i·ty (tock·sis′i·tee) *n.* 1. The quality of being toxic. 2. The kind and amount of poison or toxin produced by a microorganism, or possessed by a chemical substance not of biologic origin.

tox·i·co·den·drol (tock″si·ko·den′drol) *n.* A toxic nonvolatile oil from poison ivy and poison oak.

Tox·i·co·den·dron (tock″si·ko·den′drun) *n.* A genus of plants and shrubs, formerly classified as *Rhus,* including poison ivy, *Toxicodendron radicans;* poison oak, *T. quercifolium;* poison sumac, *T. vernix;* and other species.

tox·i·co·der·ma (tock″si·ko·dur′muh) *n.* Disease of the skin due to poison.

tox·i·co·gen·ic (tock″si·ko·jen′ick) *adj.* Producing poisons.

tox·i·coid (tock′si·koid) *adj.* Resembling a poison or a toxin.

tox·i·col·o·gist (tock″si·kol′uh·jist) *n.* A person versed in toxicology.

tox·i·col·o·gy (tock″si·kol′uh·jee) *n.* The science of the nature and effects of poisons, their detection, and treatment of their effects. —**toxi·co·log·ic** (·ko·loj′ick), **toxicolog·i·cal** (·i·kul) *adj.*

tox·i·co·ma·nia (tock″si·ko·may′nee·uh) *n.* An abnormal desire to consume poison. —**toxico·ma·ni·ac** (·nee·ack) *n.*

tox·i·co·path·ic (tock″si·ko·path′ick) *adj.* Pertaining to any abnormal condition due to the action of a poison.

tox·i·co·pho·bia (tock″si·ko·fo′bee·uh) *n.* An abnormal fear of being poisoned.

tox·i·co·sis (tock″si·ko′sis) *n.,* pl. **toxico·ses** (·seez) A state of poisoning.

toxic psychosis. Any acute confusional or delirious state supposedly due to a toxin and associated with medical or surgical diseases, postoperative or posttraumatic states, exogenous intoxications, withdrawal of alcohol or barbiturates, congestive heart failure, or metabolic disorders.

toxic purpura. Purpura caused by various poisons such as arsenic, phosphorus, phenolphthalein, heparin.

toxic unit. Any arbitrarily established unit of activity, often expressed in terms of an accepted official reference standard. In the case of diphtheria toxin, the unit is defined as the least amount that will, on the average, kill a 250g guinea pig within 96 hours after subcutaneous injection.

tox·if·er·ous (tock·sif′ur·us) *adj.* Producing or conveying poison.

tox·i·ge·nic·i·ty (tock″see·je·nis′i·tee) *n.* The degree of ability of an organism to produce toxicity or disease.

tox·in (tock′sin) *n.* Any poisonous substance formed by plant or animal cells. Some bacterial toxins, such as diphtheria and tetanus toxins, are readily separable from the cells (exotoxin); others are intimately bound to the cells (endotoxin). Phytotoxins include ricin and abrin. Zootoxins include the venoms of snakes, spiders, scorpions, toads, or sting rays. Many toxins are proteins capable of stimulating the production in man or animals of neutralizing antibodies or antitoxins.

toxin–antitoxin, *n.* A combination of a toxin and an antitoxin for therapeutic use. Abbreviated, T.A., T.A.T.

tox·is·ter·ol (tock·sis′tur-ol) *n.* A product of the excessive irradiation of ergosterol. Although isomeric with calciferol, it has little antirachitic action and is highly toxic.

Tox·o·cara (tock″so-kār′uh) *n.* A genus of ascarid worms; the larvae of a few species are important causes of human visceral larva migrans.

Toxocara can·is (kan′is, kay′nis). The common ascarid of dogs.

Toxocara cati (kat′eye). The common ascarid of cats.

tox·oid (tock′soid) *n.* A toxin detoxified by moderate heat or chemical treatment (formaldehyde) but with antigenic properties intact. The toxoids of diphtheria and tetanus are used frequently for immunization.

toxo·no·sis (tock″suh-no′sis) *n.* An affection resulting from a poison.

toxo·phil (tock′so-fil) *adj.* Having an affinity for toxins or poisons.

Toxo·plas·ma (tock″so-plaz′muh) *n.* A genus of parasitic protozoans.

Toxoplasma dye test. DYE TEST.

Toxoplasma gon·dii (gon′dee-eye). The causative agent of toxoplasmosis.

tox·o·plas·min (tock″so-plaz′min) *n.* The *Toxoplasma* antigen, prepared either from infected mouse peritoneal fluid or in embryonated eggs, used in a skin test to demonstrate delayed hypersensitivity to toxoplasmosis.

tox·o·plas·mo·sis (tock″so-plaz-mo′sis) *n.*, pl. **toxoplasmo·ses** (·seez) Infection by the protozoon *Toxoplasma gondii* widely distributed in nature, and causing in man congenital and acquired, often inapparent, illness. The protean clinical manifestations of the congenital form include jaundice, hepatomegaly, and splenomegaly; chorioretinitis, convulsions, hydrocephaly or microcephaly; cerebral calcifications and psychomotor retardation evident at birth or later in life; in acquired form, febrile illness with rash resembling Rocky Mountain spotted fever, lymphadenopathy, hepatosplenomegaly, encephalomyelitis, myocarditis, and granulomatous uveitis may occur.

TPI *TREPONEMA PALLIDUM* IMMOBILIZATION TEST.

TPI test. Abbreviation for *Treponema pallidum immobilization test.*

TPN Abbreviation for *triphosphopyridine nucleotide* (= NICOTINAMIDE ADENINE DINUCLEOTIDE PHOSPHATE).

TPNH Symbol for the reduced form of triphosphopyridine nucleotide, now more often described as the reduced form of nicotinamide-adenine dinucleotide phosphate and symbolized NADPH.

T.P.R. 1. Total peripheral resistance. 2. Total pulmonary resistance. 3. Temperature, pulse, respiration; also given without periods.

T–P segment. The interval between the end of the T wave and the beginning of the subsequent P wave.

tr. Abbreviation for *tinctura*, tincture.

tra·bec·u·la (tra-beck′yoo-luh) *n.*, pl. **trabecu·lae** (·lee) 1. Any one of the fibrous bands extending from the capsule into the interior of an organ. 2. One of the variously shaped spicules of bone in cancellous bone.

trabeculae car·ne·ae (kahr′nee-ee) [NA]. The interlacing muscular columns projecting from the inner surface of the ventricles of the heart.

tra·bec·u·lar (tra-beck′yoo-lur) *adj.* Pertaining to, constituting, or consisting of a trabecula or trabeculae.

trace, *n.* A slight amount, degree, or indication, often barely detectable and often treated as quantitatively indeterminate.

trac·er, *n.* An isotope which, because of its unique physical properties, can be detected in extremely minute quantity, and hence is used to trace the chemical behavior of the natural element. As isotopes of the same element differ in physical properties only, but have identical chemical properties (with a few exceptions), an isotope detectable by physical properties may be used to trace the pattern of biochemical reactions. Such use of isotopes is referred to as a tracer study. The isotope itself is a tracer. Stable (by measurement of isotopic ratios) or unstable (by detection of their ionizing radiation) isotopes may be used.

trache-, tracheo-. A combining form meaning *trachea, tracheal.*

tra·chea (tray′kee-uh) *n.*, L. pl. & genit. sing. **tra·che·ae** (·kee-ee), E. pl. **tracheas** The cartilaginous and membranous tube extending from the lower end of the larynx to its division into the two principal bronchi; the windpipe. —**tra·che·al** (·kee-ul) *adj.*

tra·che·ec·ta·sy (tray″kee-uh-eck′tuh-see) *n.* Dilatation of the trachea.

tra·che·al·gia (tray″kee-al′jee-uh) *n.* Pain in the trachea.

tracheal tug. The downward tugging movement of the larynx, sometimes observed in aneurysm of the aortic arch.

tra·che·i·tis (tray″kee-eye′tis) *n.* Inflammation of the trachea.

trachel-, trachelo- A combining form meaning *neck, cervix, cervical.*

trach·e·lec·to·my (track″e-leck′tuh-mee) *n.* Excision of the neck of the uterus.

trach·e·lis·mus (track″e-liz′mus) *n.* Spasmodic contraction of the muscles of the neck, with marked retraction of the head, as seen in the tonic phase of a seizure.

trach·e·li·tis (track″e-lye′tis) *n.* Inflammation of the neck of the uterus.

trach·e·lo·cyl·lo·sis (track″e-lo-si-lo′sis) *n. Obsol.* TORTICOLLIS.

trach·e·lo·dyn·ia (track″e-lo-din′ee-uh) *n.* Pain in the neck.

trach·e·lo·ky·pho·sis (track"e·lo·kigh·fo'sis) *n.* An abnormal anterior curvature of the cervical portion of the spinal column.

trach·e·lo·par·a·si·tus (track"e·lo·păr"uh·sigh'tus) *n.* Any parasitic growth upon the neck or jaws.

trach·e·lo·pex·ia (track"e·lo·peck'see·uh) *n.* Surgical fixation of the neck of the uterus.

trach·e·lo·plas·ty (track"e·lo·plas'tee) *n.* Plastic operation on the neck of the uterus.

trach·e·lor·rha·phy (track"e·lor'uh·fee) *n.* Repair of a laceration of the cervix of the uterus.

trach·e·lor·rhec·tes (track"e·lo·reck'teez) *n.* An instrument for crushing the cervical vertebrae; used in embryotomy.

trach·e·los·chi·sis (track"e·los'ki·sis) *n.* CERVICAL FISSURE.

trach·e·lo·syr·in·gor·rha·phy (track"e·lo·sirr"ing·gor'uh·fee) *n.* An operation for vaginal fistula with stitching of the cervix of the uterus.

trach·e·lot·o·my (track"e·lot'uh·mee) *n.* Incision into the cervix of the uterus.

tra·cheo·blen·nor·rhea, tra·cheo·blen·nor·rhoea (tray"kee·o·blen"o·ree'uh) *n.* A profuse discharge of mucus from the trachea.

tra·cheo·bron·chi·al (tray"kee·o·bronk'ee·ul) *adj.* Pertaining to the trachea and a bronchus or the bronchi.

tra·cheo·bron·chi·tis (tray"kee·o·brong·kigh'tis) *n.* Inflammation of the trachea and bronchi.

tra·cheo·bron·chos·co·py (tray"kee·o·brong·kos'kuh·pee) *n.* Inspection of the interior of the trachea and bronchi.

tra·cheo·esoph·a·ge·al, tra·cheo·oe·soph·a·ge·al (tray"kee·o·e·sof"uh·jee'ul, ·ee"so·faj'ee·ul) *adj.* Pertaining to the trachea and the esophagus; usually refers to a congenital fistulous tract between the two structures.

tra·cheo·fis·sure (tray"kee·o·fish'ur) *n.* Congenital longitudinal cleft of the trachea.

tra·cheo·gram (tray"kee·o·gram) *n.* A radiographic depiction of the trachea following the instillation of a contrast medium.

tra·che·og·ra·phy (tray"kee·og'ruh·fee) *n.* The process of making a tracheogram.

tra·cheo·la·ryn·ge·al (tray"kee·o·la·rin'jee·ul) *adj.* Pertaining to the trachea and the larynx.

tra·cheo·lar·yn·got·o·my (tray"kee·o·lar"in·got'uh·mee) *n.* Incision into the larynx and trachea; combined tracheotomy and laryngotomy.

tra·cheo·ma·la·cia (tray"kee·o·ma·lay'shee·uh) *n.* Softening and destruction of the tracheal wall, especially the cartilaginous rings.

tra·cheo·path·ia os·teo·plas·ti·ca (tray"kee·o·path'ee·uh os·tee·o·plas'ti·kuh) A deposit of cartilage and bone in the mucosa of the trachea.

tra·che·oph·o·ny (tray"kee·off'uh·nee) *n.* The sound heard over the trachea on auscultation.

tra·cheo·py·o·sis (tray"kee·o·pye·o'sis) *n.* Purulent tracheitis.

tra·che·or·rha·gia (tray"kee·o·ray'jee·uh) *n.* Hemorrhage from the trachea.

tra·che·or·rha·phy (tray"kee·or'uh·fee) *n.* Suturing of the trachea.

tra·che·os·chi·sis (tray"kee·os'ki·sis) *n.* Congenital fissure of the trachea.

tra·che·os·co·py (tray"kee·os'kuh·pee) *n.* Inspection of the interior of the trachea by means of a laryngoscopic mirror and reflected light, or through a bronchoscope. —**trache·o·scop·ic** (·o·skop'ick) *adj.*

tra·cheo·ste·no·sis (tray"kee·o·ste·no'sis) *n.* Abnormal constriction or narrowing of the trachea.

tra·che·os·to·my (tray"kee·os'tuh·mee) *n.* The formation of an opening into the trachea, and suturing the edges of the opening to an opening in the skin of the neck, as in laryngectomy.

tra·che·ot·o·mize (tray"kee·ot'uh·mize) *v.* To perform tracheotomy upon a living subject.

tra·chi·el·co·sis (tray"kee·el·ko'sis) *n.* Ulceration of the trachea.

tra·chi·el·cus (tray"kee·el'kus) *n.* A tracheal ulcer.

tra·cho·ma (tra·ko'muh) *n.* An infectious disease of the conjunctiva and cornea, producing photophobia, pain, excessive lacrimation, and sometimes blindness, caused by *Chlamydia trachomatis*. The lesion is characterized initially by inflammation and later by pannus and follicular and papillary hypertrophy of the conjunctiva. Syn. *Egyptian conjunctivitis, Egyptian ophthalmia, conjunctivitis granulosa, granular lids.* —**trachoma·tous** (·tus) *adj.*

trachoma bodies. PROWAZEK-HALBERSTAEDTER BODIES.

tra·chy·chro·mat·ic (tray"kee·kro·mat'ick, track"i·) *adj.* Deeply staining.

tra·chy·onych·ia (tray"kee·o·nick'ee·uh, track"ee·) *n.* Inflammation of the proximal portion of the nail matrix causing the nail to become covered with an opaque, corrugated, lamellated, grayish superficial layer.

tra·chy·pho·nia (tray"kee·fo'nee·uh, track"i·) *n.* Rough or hoarse voice.

trac·ing, *n.* A recording or marking out of a movement, design, or action.

tract, *n.* 1. A pathway or course. 2. A bundle or collection of nerve fibers. 3. Any one of the nervous pathways of the spinal cord or brain as an anatomic and functional entity. 4. A group of parts or organs serving some special purpose.

trac·tion, *n.* The act of drawing or pulling.

traction diverticulum. A circumscribed sacculation, usually of the esophagus, with bulging of the full thickness of the wall; due to the pull of adhesions arising from adjacent organs.

traction splint. A splint so devised that traction can be exerted on the distal fragment of a fracture to overcome muscle pull and maintain proper alignment of the fractured bone, such as a banjo splint, Thomas splint, or caliper splint.

trac·tor (track'tur) *n.* An instrument or apparatus for making traction.

trac·tot·o·my (track·tot'uh·mee) *n.* The surgical resection of a nerve-fiber tract of the central nervous system, usually for relief of pain.

trac·tus (track'tus) *n.,* pl. & genit. sing. **trac·tus** (track'toos, track'tus) TRACT.

trade·mark, *n.* A name or mark applied to a substance or product whereby its origin as of a particular producer is indicated; such a name or mark, which may or may not be officially registered, is the property of the producer. A name in this category is frequently called a trademarked name.

trade name. A name, commonly not descriptive or invested with ownership rights, by which a substance or product is known in commerce and industry. If it is intended to indicate the origin of the substance or product as of a particular producer, it is preferably called a trademark or trademarked name.

trag·a·canth (trag'uh·kanth) n. A gummy exudation from various Asiatic species of *Astragalus*, of the family Leguminosae. Almost white ribbons or powder; swells with 50 parts of water to make a stiff opalescent mucilage. A soluble portion is said to consist chiefly of uronic acid and arabinose; the insoluble portion that swells in water is largely bassorin, $(C_{11}H_{20}O_{10})_n$. Used as a suspending agent.

tra·gus (tray'gus) n., pl. **tra·gi** (·jye) 1. [NA] The small prominence of skin-covered cartilage projecting over the meatus of the external ear. 2. One of the coarse hairs at the external auditory meatus.

trait, n. Any characteristic, quality, or property of an individual or a genotype.

trance, n. 1. The state of hypnosis resembling sleep. 2. The state of being mentally out of touch with the environment. 3. A state of altered consciousness characterized by a prolonged condition of abnormal sleep, in which the vital functions are depressed and from which the patient ordinarily cannot be aroused; breathing is almost imperceptible and sensation abolished; onset and awakening may be sudden.

tran·quil·iz·er, tran·quil·liz·er (tran'kwi·lye''zur, trang') n. 1. In popular usage, any agent that brings about a state of peace of mind or relief from anxiety; an ataraxic. 2. Any agent that produces a calming or sedative effect without inducing sleep. 3. Any drug such as chlorpromazine, used primarily for its calming and antipsychotic effects, or meprobamate, used for symptomatic treatment of common psychoneuroses and as an adjunct in somatic disorders complicated by anxiety and tension. —**tranquil·ize, tranquil·lize** (·lize) v.

trans- A combining form meaning (a) *through* or *across;* (b) (italicized) in chemistry, a prefix indicating that *certain atoms or groups are on opposite sides of a molecule;* usually restricted to cyclic compounds with two stereogenic atoms.

trans·ab·dom·i·nal (trans''ab·dom'i·nul) adj. Through or across the abdomen or abdominal wall.

trans·am·i·nase (trans·am'i·nace, ·naze) n. One of a group of enzymes that catalyze the transfer of the amino group of an amino acid to a keto acid, to form another amino acid.

trans·am·i·na·tion (trans·am''i·nay'shun) n. 1. The transfer of one or more amino groups from one compound to another. 2. The transposition of an amino group within a single compound.

trans·an·i·ma·tion (trans·an''i·may'shun) n. MOUTH-TO-MOUTH BREATHING.

trans·aor·tic (trans''ay·or'tick) adj. Through or across the aorta.

trans·atri·al (trans·ay'tree·ul) adj. Through or across an atrium.

trans·au·di·ent (trans·aw'dee·unt) adj. Allowing the transmission of sound.

trans·cav·i·tary (trans·kav'i·terr''ee) adj. Through or across a cavity; usually referring to metastasis of tumor cells, most often in the peritoneal cavity.

trans·con·dy·lar (trans·kon'di·lur) adj. Across or through condyles.

trans·cor·ti·cal (trans·kor'ti·kul) adj. 1. Pertaining to connections between different parts of the cerebral cortex. 2. Through or across the cortex of an organ.

tran·scrip·tion (tran·skrip'shun) n. The deoxyribonucleic acid-directed synthesis of messenger ribonucleic acid.

trans·cu·ta·ne·ous (trans''kew·tay'nee·us) adj. PERCUTANEOUS.

trans·duc·tion (tranz·duck'shun) n. 1. The process of transferring energy from one system to another; the transferred energy may be of the same or of a different form, for example, a steam engine converting thermal energy to mechanical energy. 2. The transfer from bacterium to bacterium of genetic material carried by a bacterial virus. —**trans·duc·er** (·dew'sur) n.

trans·du·o·de·nal (trans''dew·od'e·nul, ·dew·o·dee'nul) adj. Through or across the duodenum.

tran·sect (tran·sekt') v. To cut across.

tran·sec·tion (tran·seck'shun) n. A section made across the long axis of a part, as transection of the spinal cord.

trans·fer, n. In prosthodontics, a nonanatomic cover for a tooth, which may be removed in an impression and used as a receptacle for dies to assure their correct relationship in the poured working cast; usually made of resin, low-fusing metal, or cast gold alloy.

trans·fer·ase (trans'fur·ace, ·aze) n. Any of many types of enzymes that catalyze transfer of a chemical group from one molecule to another; among groups that may be transferred are phosphate, methyl, amine, keto.

trans·fer·ence (trans·fur'unce, trans'fur·unce) n. In psychiatry, the unconscious transfer of the patient's feelings and reactions originally associated with important persons in the patient's life, usually father, mother, or siblings, toward others and in the analytic situation, toward the therapist. Transference may be positive, when the feelings and reactions are affectionate, friendly, or loving; it may be negative, when these feelings and reactions are hostile.

trans·fer·rin (trans·ferr'in) n. A beta-l globulin of blood serum concerned with binding and transportation of iron. Syn. *siderophilin, siderophyllin.*

transfer RNA. A type of ribonucleic acid that combines with specific amino acids and then with messenger RNA to allow amino acid residues to combine in a certain sequence during protein synthesis. It constitutes 10 to 20 percent of total cellular ribonucleic acid, and its structure is complementary to messenger RNA. Abbreviated, tRNA

trans·fix·ion (trans-fick'shun) n. 1. The act of piercing through and through. 2. A method of amputation in which the knife is passed directly through the soft parts, the cutting being done from within outward. —**trans·fix** (·ficks') v.

trans·fo·ra·tion (trans"fo·ray'shun) n. The act of perforating the fetal skull. —**trans·fo·rate** (trans'fo·rate) v.

trans·for·ma·tion (trans"for·may'shun) n. 1. A marked change in form, structure, or function. 2. *In bacterial genetics,* the acquisition of genetic properties by the uptake and expression of free DNA. 3. *In cell biology and oncology,* the conversion of a normal cell into one which is capable of malignant growth or, by extension, into one exhibiting properties in culture which are those characterizing cultured malignant cells. These may include loss of density-dependent inhibition of growth, ability to form colonies in soft agar; may be spontaneous or induced by viruses of certain chemicals.

trans·form·er (trans·for'mur) n. An electrical apparatus for the transformation of lower potentials to higher potentials, or vice versa. It consists of a laminated iron core on which are wound two coils, a primary and a secondary coil, properly insulated from each other. The primary coil is energized by an alternating current at a given voltage, which induces in the secondary coil a voltage related to that in the primary by the ratio of the number of turns of wire in the two coils.

trans·fuse (trans·fewz') v. To perform a transfusion of or on.

trans·fu·sion (trans·few'zhun) n. The introduction into a blood vessel of blood, saline solution, or other liquid.

transfusion jaundice. SERUM HEPATITIS.

tran·sient (tran'shunt, ·zee·unt) adj. Present for only a short period of time; impermanent; temporary; transitory.

transient flora. *In surgery,* the loosely attached, easily removed or destroyed portion of the cutaneous bacterial flora, which is acquired largely by contact with germ-laden objects. It is subject to great variations, both quantitative and qualitative.

transient hypogammaglobulinemia. The temporary deficiency of gamma globulins sometimes seen in infants due to a delay in the onset of gamma-globulin synthesis and occasionally accompanied by increased susceptibility to bacterial infection.

transient ischemic attack. An episode of transient cerebral symptoms, varying from patient to patient but consisting most often of dim vision, hemiparesis, numbness on one side of the body, dizziness and thick speech, that usually lasts 10 minutes or less, but may last as long as 24 hours in some cases. These attacks are usually related to atherosclerotic throm-

botic disease; the longer-lasting attacks are probably due to cerebral embolism.

trans·il·i·ac (tran-zil'ee·ack) adj. Passing across from one ilium to the other, as the transiliac diameter.

trans·il·lu·mi·na·ble (trans"i·lew'mi·nuh·bul) adj. Capable of being transilluminated.

trans·il·lu·mi·na·tion (trans"i·lew'mi·nay'shun) n. 1. Illumination of an object by transmitted light. 2. Illumination of the paranasal sinuses by means of a light placed in the patient's mouth. 3. Illumination of an infant's skull, positive in hydrocephaly, porencephaly, and other brain defects or where there is fluid over the brain.

tran·sis·tor (tran-zis'tur) n. A solid-state device, considerably smaller than a vacuum tube used similarly, for amplifying electric currents through utilization of a semiconductor such as germanium or silicon.

tran·si·tion·al (tran-zish'un·ul) adj. & n. 1. Of, pertaining to, or characterized by change. 2. According to Ehrlich, a monocyte having a U-shaped nucleus, which he regarded, incorrectly, as a transitional form in the development of a polymorphonuclear granulocyte; now considered to be an older form of monocyte.

transitional cell. 1. A cell having characteristics of two or more other cell types. 2. An epithelial cell of the urinary collecting system and bladder which assumes different forms under different conditions of distention. 3. MONOCYTE. 4. A large plasma cell, considered transitional between a blast cell and a definitive small plasma cell.

transitional-cell carcinoma. A malignant tumor whose parenchyma is composed of anaplastic transitional epithelial cells.

transitional denture. A removable partial denture to which artificial teeth can be added as natural teeth are lost.

transitional epithelium. The stratified epithelium of the urinary tract. The cells of this form vary in shape between squamous, when the epithelium is stretched, and columnar or cuboidal when not stretched.

tran·si·to·ry (tran'si·to·ree) adj. TRANSIENT.

trans·la·tion (tranz·lay'shun) n. The ribonucleic acid–directed synthesis of protein.

trans·lo·ca·tion (tranz"lo·kay'shun) n. The displacement of part or all of one chromosome to another.

trans·lu·cent (tranz·lew'sunt) adj. Permitting a partial transmission of light; somewhat transparent.

trans·lu·mi·nal (trans·lew'mi·nul) adj. Across or through a lumen.

transluminal angioplasty. The removal of thrombi or emboli from blood vessels, especially arteries, by catheters inserted through their lumens.

trans·mi·gra·tion (tranz"migh·gray'shun) n. Movement from one place to another which may involve crossing a membrane or other barrier, such as the passage of leukocytes or erythrocytes through the capillary walls (diapedesis).

trans·mis·si·bil·i·ty (tranz·mis″i·bil′i·tee) *n.* The capability of being transmitted or communicated from one person to another. —**trans·mis·si·ble** (·mis′i·bul) *adj.*

trans·mis·sion (tranz·mish′un) *n.* The communication or transfer of anything, especially infectious or heritable disease, from one person or place to another.

trans·mit·tance (tranz·mit′unce) *n.* In applied spectroscopy, the ratio of the radiant power transmitted by a sample to the radiant power incident on the sample, both measurements being made at the same spectral position and with the same slit width. Symbol, *T*.

trans·mu·ral (trans·mew′rul) *adj.* Across a wall, used to describe myocardial infarction involving the full thickness of the myocardium in a given location.

trans·mu·ta·tion (tranz″mew·tay′shun) *n. In physics,* any process by which an atomic nucleus is converted into another of different atomic number.

trans·oc·u·lar (tranz·ock′yoo·lur) *adj.* Extending across the eye.

trans·o·nance (trans·uh·nunce) *n.* Transmission of sounds originating in one organ through another organ.

trans·or·bit·al (tranz·or′bit·ul) *adj.* Passing through the eye socket.

trans·par·ent (trans·pār′unt) *adj.* Permitting the passage of light rays without material obstruction, so that objects beyond the transparent body can be seen.

trans·peri·to·ne·al (trans·perr″i·to·nee′ul) *adj.* Passing through or across the peritoneum.

tran·spir·able (trans·pye′ruh·bul) *adj.* Capable of passing in a gaseous state through the respiratory epithelium or the skin.

tran·spi·ra·tion (tran″spi·ray′shun) *n.* 1. Exhalation of fluid through the skin. 2. PERSPIRATION.

trans·pla·cen·tal (trans″pluh·sen′tul) *adj.* Across the placenta.

trans·plant (trans′plant) *n.* Tissue removed from any portion of the body and placed in a different site. —**trans·plant** (trans·plant′) *v.*

trans·plan·ta·tion (trans″plan·tay′shun) *n.* The operation of transplanting or of applying to a part of the body tissues taken from another body or from another part of the same body.

trans·pleu·ral (trans·ploor′ul) *adj.* Through the pleura.

trans·pose (trans·poze′) *v.* To displace; to change about, as tissue from one location to another by operation.

trans·po·si·tion (trans″puh·zish′un) *n.* A change of position; a change from the usual order.

transposition of the great arteries or **vessels.** A congenital anomaly in which the aorta arises from the right ventricle and the pulmonary trunk from the left ventricle; this exchange of position may be complete or incomplete.

transposition of the heart. A reversal in the position of the heart.

transposition of the pulmonary veins. Drainage of the pulmonary veins into the right rather than left atrium; may be complete or incomplete. Syn. *anomalous pulmonary venous drainage.*

transposition of the viscera. A change in the position of the viscera to the side opposite to that normally occupied; situs inversus viscerum.

trans·sex·u·al (trans·seck′shoo·ul) *n.* An individual whose chromosomes, gonads, and body habitus mark him or her as a member of one sex, but who identifies psychically with the other sex, with an overwhelming desire for sex reassignment through surgical and hormonal intervention. Such an individual may dress and live routinely as a member of the opposite sex.

trans·sex·u·a·lism (trans·seck′shoo·uh·liz·um) *n.* The condition of being a transsexual.

trans·sub·stan·ti·a·tion (trans″sub·stan″shee·ay′shun) *n.* The replacement of tissue of one kind by another.

trans·ten·to·ri·al (trans″ten·to′ree·ul) *adj.* Into the incisure of or across the tentorium.

trans·tho·rac·ic (trans″tho·ra′sick) *adj.* Across or through the thorax.

tran·su·date (tran′sue·date) *n.* A liquid or other substance produced by transudation.

tran·su·da·tion (tran″sue·day′shun) *n.* The passing of fluid or a solute through a membrane by means of a hydrostatic or osmotic pressure gradient, especially passage of blood serum through the vessel walls. —**tran·su·da·tory** (tran·sue′duh·tor″ee) *adj.*; **tran·sude** (tran·sue′d′) *v.*

trans·ure·thral (trans″yoo·ree′thrul) *adj.* Via the urethra.

transurethral prostatectomy. Removal of the prostate by means of an operating cystoscope or resectoscope inserted through the urethra.

transurethral resection. Resection of the prostate or a portion of the lower urinary tract by means of a resectoscope passed through the urethra. Abbreviated, TUR

trans·va·gi·nal (trans·vuh·jye′nul, vaj′i·nul) *adj.* Across or through the vagina.

trans·ver·sa·lis (trans″vur·say′lis) *adj.* TRANSVERSE.

transversalis fascia. The thin membrane lying between the transversus abdominis muscle and the peritoneum.

trans·verse (trans·vurce′) *adj.* Crosswise; at right angles to the longitudinal axis of the body or of a part.

transverse acetabular ligament. The fibrous continuation of the acetabular lip which crosses the acetabular notch, completing the ring formed by the lip and converting the notch into a foramen.

transverse arch of the foot. The transverse hollow on the inner part of the sole of the foot in the line of the tarsometatarsal articulations.

transverse colon. The portion of the colon between the hepatic flexure and the splenic flexure.

trans·ver·sec·to·my (trans″vur·seck′tuh·mee) *n.* Excision of a transverse process of a vertebra; specifically, in orthopedics, removal of the transverse process of the fifth lumbar vertebra for pain due to irritation of the lower spinal nerve roots.

transverse diameter of the pelvic inlet. The

distance between the two most widely separated points of the pelvic inlet.

transverse diameter of the pelvic outlet. The distance between the two ischial tuberosities.

transverse facial cleft. An embryonic fissure at the angle of the mouth, causing macrostomia.

transverse fissure of the liver. A fissure crossing transversely the lower surface of the right lobe of the liver. It transmits the portal vein, hepatic artery and nerves, and hepatic duct.

transverse mesocolon. The transverse portion of the mesentery connecting the transverse colon with the posterior abdominal wall.

transverse myelitis or **myelopathy.** 1.Paraplegia or quadriplegia due to a sudden total or near-total transection of the spinal cord, occurring most often as a result of trauma, but also as a result of infarction or hemorrhage or rapidly advancing necrotizing, demyelinative or compressive inflammatory or neoplastic lesions. 2. More specifically, the sudden transverse spinal cord lesion of demyelinative disease.

transverse process. A process projecting outward from the side of a vertebra, at the junction of the pedicle and the lamina.

transverse rectal folds. Large, semilunar folds projecting into the lumen of the rectum.

trans·ver·sus (trans-vur'sus) *adj.* TRANSVERSE.

trans·ves·tism (trans-ves'tiz-um) *n.* Dressing or masquerading in the clothing of the opposite sex; usually due to an unconscious wish to appear and be accepted as a member of the opposite sex.

trans·ves·tite (trans-ves'tīte) *n.* An individual who dresses in the clothes of the opposite sex; usually applied only when this is done rather habitually, as by a homosexual or a transsexual.

tran·yl·cy·pro·mine (tran''il-sigh'pro-meen) *n.* *trans-dl*-2-Phenylcyclopropylamine, $C_9H_{11}N$, a nonhydrazine monoamine oxidase inhibitor used, as the sulfate salt, for the treatment of severe mental depression.

tra·pe·zio·meta·car·pal (tra-pee''zee-o-met''uh-kahr'pul) *adj.* Pertaining to the trapezium and metacarpals.

tra·pe·zi·um (tra-pee'zee-um) *n.*, pl. **trape·zia** (-zee-uh) The first bone of the second row of the carpal bones.

tra·pe·zi·us (tra-pee'zee-us) *n.* A muscle arising from the occipital bone, the nuchal ligament, and the spines of the thoracic vertebrae, and inserted into the clavicle, acromion, and spine of the scapula.

trap·e·zoid (trap'e-zoid) *n.* 1. A geometric, four-sided figure having two parallel and two diverging sides. 2. The second bone of the second row of the carpus.

Traube's semilunar space An area of the lower left lateral and anterior chest wall which is tympanitic to percussion because of gas in the underlying stomach.

trau·ma (traw'muh, trɔw'muh) *n.*, pl. **trauma·ta** (-tuh), **traumas** 1. An injury caused by a mechanical or physical agent. 2. A severe psychic injury.

trau·mat·ic (traw-mat'ick) *adj.* Pertaining to or caused by a wound or injury.

traumatic neurosis. Any neurotic reaction in which an injury is the precipitating cause; encompasses combat, compensation, and occupational neuroses. The traumatic event usually has specific symbolic significance for the patient, which may be further enforced by secondary gain.

trau·ma·tism (traw'muh-tiz-um, trɔw') *n.* The general or local condition produced by a wound or injury. —**trauma·tize** (-tize) *v.*

trau·ma·tol·o·gy (traw''muh-tol'uh-jee, trɔw'') *n.* The science or description of wounds and injuries, especially as they occur as disability in industry.

trau·ma·top·a·thy (traw''muh-top'uth-ee, trɔw'') *n.* Pathologic condition due to wounds or other violence.

trau·ma·top·nea, trau·ma·top·noea (traw''muh-top-nee'uh, trɔw'') *n.* The passage of respiratory air through a wound in the chest wall.

tra·vail (trav'ail, truh-vail') *n.* Labor of parturition.

trav·el·er's diarrhea. Transitory diarrhea and abdominal cramping often encountered by travelers to foreign countries. Enterotoxin-producing strains of *Escherichia coli* are thought to be etiologically important in many cases.

tray, *n.* A flat, shallow vessel of glass, hard rubber, or metal, for holding instruments during a surgical operation.

tread, *n. In veterinary medicine.* injury to the coronet of a horse's hoof, due to striking with the shoe of the opposite side.

treat, *v.* To combat disease by the application of remedies; to care for medically or surgically.

treat·ment, *n.* 1. Application of therapeutic measures; therapy. 2. Application of a chemical agent or a physical process to a substance or object to render it fit for use or disposal.

Trem·a·to·da (trem''uh-to'duh) *n.pl.* The flukes; a class of flat worms of which the digenetic species are endoparasites of man. The life cycle is complex, involving sexual and asexual reproduction; two intermediate hosts are required. Some of the genera seen most often are *Clonorchis, Fasciola, Fasciolopsis, Opisthorchis, Paragonimus, Schistosoma,* and *Troglotrema.* —**trem·a·tode** (-uh-tode) *adj. & n.*

trem·a·to·di·a·sis (trem''uh-to-dye'uh-sis) *n.*, pl. **trematodia·ses** (-seez) Infection with a trematode.

trem·bles, *n.pl.* 1. A disease of cattle and sheep, manifest by weakness and falling, presumed due to ingestion of white snakeroot, *Eupatorium urticaefolium,* or the rayless goldenrod, *Aplopappus heterophyllus.* 2. MILK SICKNESS. 3. A congenital disease of neonatal pigs of unknown etiology, characterized by severe trembling, difficulty in nursing, and occasionally death.

trembling ill. LOUPING ILL.

tremo·graph (trem'o-graf, tree'mo-) *n.* A device for recording tremor.

trem·o·lo (trem'uh-lo) *n.* An irregular, exaggerated vibrato; a voice tremor, symptomatic of psychogenic disturbance, old age, or diseases affecting the organs of respiration and phonation or their nervous control.

tremo·pho·bia (trem″o·fo′bee·uh, tree″mo·) n. An abnormal fear of trembling.

trem·or (trem′ur) n. A more or less regular, rhythmic oscillation of a part of the body around a fixed point involving alternate contraction of agonist and antagonist muscles.

tremor ar·tu·um (ahr′tew·um). PARKINSONISM.

tremo·sta·ble (trem″o·stay′bul, tree′mo·) adj. Not easily inactivated or destroyed by agitation.

trem·u·lous (trem′yoo·lus) adj. Trembling, quivering, as tremulous iris; affected by tremor.

trench back. Dorsolumbar pain and rigidity experienced by troops engaged in trench warfare.

trench fever. A louse-borne infection caused by *Rochalimaea quintana*, epidemic during World Wars I and II but rare now; characterized by headache, chills, rash, pain in the legs and back, and frequently by a relapsing fever.

trench foot. A condition of the feet, somewhat like immersion foot, due to exposure to cold and dampness.

trench mouth. NECROTIZING ULCERATIVE GINGIVITIS.

Tren·de·len·burg's position (tren′de·len·boork′) The posture of a patient lying supine on a table which is tilted head downward 45° or less.

Trendelenburg's test 1. A test of competence of the saphenous vein valves; the legs are raised to empty the veins and quickly lowered; the veins become immediately distended if the valves are incompetent. 2. A test for abnormality of the pelvis seen in congenital hip dislocation, poliomyelitis, etc.; when the patient stands on the involved foot, the opposite (normal) gluteal fold falls rather than rises.

tre·pan (tre·pan′) n. TREPHINE.

trep·a·na·tion (trep′uh·nay′shun) n. The operation of trephining.

tre·pan·ning (tre·pan′ing) n. Boring; using the trephine.

tre·phine (tre·fine′, tre·feen′) n. & v. 1. A circular instrument with a sawlike edge for cutting out a disk of bone, usually from the skull. 2. To cut with a trephine.

trep·i·da·tion (trep′i·day′shun) n. 1. Trembling. 2. A state of fear, alarm, or anxiety.

Trep·o·ne·ma (trep″o·nee′muh) n. A genus of spirochetes of the family Treponemataceae.

Treponema cu·nic·u·li (kew·nick′yoo·lye). The organism that causes pallidoidosis, a venereal disease of rabbits.

Treponema pal·li·dum (pal′i·dum). The organism that causes syphilis.

Treponema pallidum immobilization test. A specific serologic test for syphilis involving antibodies differing from the Wassermann antibody, in which suspensions of *Treponema pallidum* are immobilized in the presence of the syphilitic serum and complement. Abbreviated, TPI test.

Treponema per·ten·ue (pur·ten′yoo·ee). The organism that causes yaws.

Trep·o·ne·ma·ta·ce·ae (trep″o·nee″muh·tay′see·ee) n.pl. The family of spiral microorganisms which includes the genera *Borrelia*, *Leptospira*, and *Treponema*.

trep·o·ne·ma·to·sis (trep″o·nee″muh·to′sis) n., pl. **treponemato·ses** (·seez) Infection caused by a spirochete of the genus *Treponema*.

trep·o·ne·mi·a·sis (trep″o·ne·migh′uh·sis) n., pl. **treponemia·ses** (·seez) Infection caused by a spirochete of the genus *Treponema*.

trep·o·ne·mi·ci·dal (trep″o·nee″mi·sigh′dul) adj. 1. Destructive to any organism of the genus *Treponema*. 2. ANTISYPHILITIC.

tre·pop·nea, tre·pop·noea (tre·pop′nee·uh) n. A respiratory distress present in one posture and absent in another. Syn. *selective orthopnea*.

-tresia A combining form meaning *perforation*.

tri- A combining form meaning *three*.

tri·ac·yl·glyc·er·ol (trye·as″il·glis′ur·ole) n. An ester of glycerin in which all three hydroxyl groups of the latter are esterified with an acid; animal and vegetable fixed oils are composed chiefly of triacylglycerols of fatty acids. Syn. *triglyceride*.

tri·ad (trye′ad) n. 1. A set of three related elements, objects, or symptoms. 2. *In chemistry*, a trivalent element, atom, or radical.

tri·age (tree·ahzh′) n. 1. *In military medicine*, the process of sorting sick and wounded on the basis of urgency and type of condition presented, so that they may be properly routed to medical installations appropriately situated and equipped; with large numbers of wounded, it may become a process of concentrating limited resources on those who have a reasonable chance of survival. 2. More broadly, any of various comparable processes of screening patients in civilian institutions such as hospitals or community health clinics.

tri·al (trye′ul) n. The act of trying or testing.

tri·am·cin·o·lone (trye″am·sin′o·lone) n. 9α-Fluoro-16α-hydroxyprednisolone, $C_{21}H_{27}FO_6$, a potent glucocorticoid with anti-inflammatory, hormonal, and metabolic effects similar to those of prednisolone. Administered orally as the free alcohol or its diacetate ester; topically or by intraarticular, intrasynovial, or intrabursal injection as the acetonide derivative.

tri·an·gle (trye′ang·gul) n. 1. A geometrical figure having three sides and three angles. 2. A three-sided area or region having natural or arbitrary boundaries. —**tri·an·gu·lar** (trye·ang′gew·lur) adj.

Tri·at·o·ma (trye·at′o·muh) n. A genus of bloodsucking Hemiptera, commonly called conenose bugs. The most important species is *Triatoma megista*, the chief carrier of *Trypanosoma cruzi*. Other species are *Triatoma sordida*, *T. dimidiata*, and *T. infestans*.

Tri·a·tom·i·dae (trye″uh·tom′i·dee) n.pl. REDUVIIDAE. —**tri·at·o·mid** (trye·at′o·mid) adj. & n.

tri·atri·al (trye·ay′tree·ul) adj. The anomalous condition of having three atria.

tri·ax·i·al reference system (trye·ack′see·ul). Superimposition of the lead axes of electrocardiographic leads I, II, and III so that their midpoints coincide. A reference frame for frontal plane vectors.

trib·ade (trib'ud, tri·bahd') *n.* A woman who plays the role of the male in lesbian practices. —**trib·a·dism** (trib'uh·diz·um) *n.*

tri·ba·sic (trye·bay'sick) *adj.* Having three hydrogen atoms replaceable by bases.

tribe, *n.* A taxonomic category intermediate in the hierarchy between a genus and a family.

-tribe A combining form designating *an instrument for crushing or compressing.*

tribo·lu·mi·nes·cence (trye"bo·lew"mi·nes'unce, trib"o·) *n.* Luminosity induced by friction, as by grinding and pulverizing of solids.

tri·bro·mo·eth·a·nol (trye·bro"mo·eth'uh·nol) *n.* 2,2,2-Tribromoethanol, Br_3CCH_2OH; used as a basal anesthetic when dissolved in amylene hydrate.

tri·car·box·yl·ic acid (trye·kahr"bock·sil'ick). An organic compound with three —COOH groups.

tri·ceph·a·lus (trye·sef'uh·lus) *n.,* pl. **tricepha·li** (·lye) An individual with three heads.

tri·ceps (trye'seps) *adj. & n.* 1. Three-headed. 2. A muscle having three heads, as the triceps brachii muscle.

trich-, tricho- A combining form meaning (a) *hair;* (b) *filament.*

trich·an·gi·ec·ta·sia (trick·an"jee·eck·tay'zhuh, ·zee·uh) *n.* Dilatation of the capillaries.

trich·atro·phia (trick"a·tro'fee·uh) *n.* A brittle state of the hair from atrophy of the hair bulbs.

trich·es·the·sia, trich·aes·the·sia (trick"es·theezh'uh, ·theez'ee·uh) *n.* 1. A particular form of tactile sensibility in regions covered with hairs. 2. TRICHOESTHESIA.

tri·chi·a·sis (tri·kigh'uh·sis) *n.* 1. An abnormal position of the eyelashes which produces irritation by friction upon the globe. The acquired type usually follows an inflammatory condition that produces distortion. 2. The presence of minute hairlike filaments in the urine.

Trich·i·nel·la (trick"i·nel'uh) *n.* A genus of nematode worms that are parasites of man, hogs, rats, dogs, cats, and many other mammals.

Trichinella spi·ra·lis (spye·ray'lis). The species of nematode responsible for trichinosis in man.

trich·i·ni·a·sis (trick"i·nigh'uh·sis) *n.* TRICHINOSIS.

trich·i·no·pho·bia (trick"i·no·fo'bee·uh) *n.* An abnormal fear of trichinosis.

trich·i·no·sis (trick"i·no'sis) *n.,* pl. **trichino·ses** (·seez) A disease produced by the ingestion of uncooked or insufficiently cooked pork containing *Trichinella spiralis.* It is characterized by eosinophilia, nausea, fever, diarrhea, stiffness and painful swelling of muscles, and edema of the face. The intestinal symptoms are due to the development of the adult stage of the organisms; the muscular and systemic symptoms are due to the larval migration of the organisms through the tissues.

tri·chlo·ro·ace·tic acid (trye·klor"o·uh·see'tick). $Cl_3CCOOH.$ A crystalline, deliquescent acid, very corrosive; used topically as a caustic and astringent, and also as a protein precipitant.

tri·chlo·ro·eth·yl·ene (trye·klo"ro·eth'il·een) *n.* $CHCl=CCl_2.$ A liquid anesthetic and analgesic often self-administered by inhalation to relieve facial neuralgias.

tricho·an·es·the·sia, tricho·an·aes·the·sia (trick"o·an"es·theezh'uh, ·theez'ee·uh) *n.* Lack of sensation when the hair is stimulated or moved.

tricho·be·zoar (trick"o·bee'zo·ur) *n.* A hair ball or concretion in the stomach or intestine.

tricho·ceph·a·li·a·sis (trick"o·sef"uh·lye'uh·sis) *n.* TRICHURIASIS.

tri·choc·la·sis (tri·kock'luh·sis) *n.* TRICHORRHEXIS NODOSA.

tricho·clas·ma·nia (trick"o·klaz·may'nee·uh) *n.* An abnormal desire to pull out the hair, usually of the scalp.

tricho·cryp·to·sis (trick"o·krip·to'sis) *n.* Any disease of the hair follicles.

tricho·epi·the·li·o·ma (trick"o·ep"i·theel"ee·o'muh) *n.* A benign tumor characterized by many pin-headed to pea-sized, round, yellow, or skin-colored papules chiefly on the central face. It may be associated with syringoma or cylindroma.

tricho·es·the·sia, tricho·aes·the·sia (trick"o·es·theezh'uh, ·theez'ee·uh) *n.* 1. The sensation received when a hair is touched. 2. A type of paresthesia wherein there is a sensation as of uticaria on the skin, on the oral mucosa, or on the conjunctiva.

tricho·glos·sia (trick"o·glos'ee·uh) *n.* Hairy tongue, a lengthening of the filiform papillae, producing an appearance as if the tongue were covered with hair.

trich·oid (trick'oid) *adj.* Resembling hair.

tricho·lith (trick'o·lith) *n.* A calcified hair ball within the stomach or intestines.

tricho·lo·gia (trick"o·lo'jee·uh) *n.* 1. CARPHOLOGY. 2. The plucking out of one's hair.

tri·cho·ma (tri·ko'muh) *n.* 1. TRICHOMATOSIS. 2. TRICHIASIS.

tricho·ma·de·sis (trick"o·ma·dee'sis) *n.* The falling out of hair which may lead to alopecia.

tri·cho·ma·tose (tri·ko'muh·toze) *adj.* Matted together.

tricho·ma·to·sis (trick"o·muh·to'sis, tri·ko") *n.* An affection of the hair characterized by a matted condition, a result of neglect, filth, and the invasion of parasites.

trich·o·mo·na·ci·dal (trick"o·mo"nuh·sigh'dul) *adj.* Lethal for trichomonads.

trich·o·mo·na·cide (trick"o·mo'nuh·side) *n.* Any drug that destroys *Trichomonas* parasites.

trich·o·mo·nad (trick"o·mo'nad, ·mon'ad) *n. & adj.* A flagellate belonging to the genus *Trichomonas.* 2. Belonging or pertaining to the genus *Trichomonas.*

Trich·o·mo·nas (trick"o·mo'nas) *n.* A genus of flagellate protozoa, belonging to the subphylum Mastigophora. Three to five flagella, a thick rodlike axostyle extending throughout the pear-shaped body, and an undulating membrane characterize members of the genus.

Trichomonas hom·i·nis (hom'i·nis). The species found in the human intestine; it is not pathogenic.

Trichomonas vag·i·na·lis (vaj·i·nay'lis). The species of flagellate protozoa that has been implicated in vaginitis.

trich·o·mo·ni·a·sis (trick"o·mo·nigh'uh·sis) *n.*, pl. **trichomonia·ses** (·seez) Infection with *Trichomonas.*

tricho·my·co·sis (trick"o·migh·ko'sis) *n.* A disease of the hair produced by fungi.

trichomycosis ax·il·la·ris (ack"si·lair'is) Nodules formed on the axillary hairs by the saprophytic growth of species of *Nocardia* and bacteria. Syn. *trichonocardiosis axillaris, chromotrichomycosis.*

trichomycosis no·do·sa (no·do'suh). The growth of masses of fungous and bacterial material along the axillary and scrotal hair to form nodules; lepothrix.

tri·chon (trye'kon) *n.* A substance produced by autolysis of fungi of the genus *Trichophyton.*

tricho·no·car·di·o·sis (trick"o·no·kahr"dee·o'sis) *n.* Nodular appearance of the hair due to a species of *Nocardia*; axillary hair is most often affected.

tricho·no·do·sis (trick"o·no·do'sis) *n.* Fraying of the hair, with formation of true and false knots, associated with thinning and breaking of the hair shaft. Syn. *knotting hair.*

tricho·patho·pho·bia (trick"o·path"o·fo'bee·uh) *n.* Undue anxiety and fear regarding the hair, its growth, color, or diseases.

tri·chop·a·thy (tri·kop'uh·tee) *n.* Any disease of the hair. —**tricho·path·ic** (tricho"o·path'ick) *adj.*

trich·oph·a·gy (trick·off'uh·jee) *n.* The eating of hair.

tricho·pho·bia (trick"o·fo'bee·uh) *n.* 1. An abnormal fear of hair. 2. TRICHOPATHOPHOBIA.

tricho·phy·tin (trick"o·figh'tin, tri·kof'i·tin) *n.* A group antigen generally derived from filtrates of *Trichophyton mentagrophytes*, used in a skin test to determine past or present infection with the dermatophytes. Immediate and delayed hypersensitivity reactions occur; the test is of limited value diagnostically but is useful in confirming or disproving the diagnosis of a dermatophytid reaction.

tricho·phy·to·be·zoar (trick"o·figh"to·bee'zo·ur) *n.* A ball or concretion in the stomach or intestine, made of hair and fibers of vegetable matter and food detritus.

Trich·o·phy·ton (trick"o·figh'ton, tri·kof'i·ton) *n.* A principal genus of keratophilic fungi, attacking the hair, skin, and nails, causing dermatophytosis of man and animals. The genus has distinctive macroconidia, and the many species are distinguished by cultural and nutritional characteristics. When involving the hair, some species are called ectothrix, in which a prominent sheath of spore forms outside the hair shaft in addition to the invasion of the interior of the hair (e.g. *Trichophyton mentagrophytes, T. rubrum, T. verrucosum*); others are called endothrix, in which invasion of the hair shaft is not accompanied by the formation of the outside sheath of spores (e.g., *T. schoenleinii, T. tonsurans*).

trich·o·phy·to·sis (trick"o·figh·to'sis) *n.* A contagious disease of skin and hair, occurring mostly in children, and due to skin invasion by the *Trichophyton* fungus. It is characterized

by circular scaly patches and partial loss of hair.

tricho·pti·lo·sis (trick"o·ti·lo'sis, tri·kop"ti·lo'sis) *n.* TRICHORRHEXIS NODOSA.

trich·or·rhex·is (trick"o·reck'sis) *n.* Brittleness of the hair.

trichorrhexis no·do·sa (no·do'suh). An atrophic condition of the hair, affecting more often the male beard, and characterized by irregular thickenings resembling nodes on the hair shaft that are really partial fractures of the hair. The hairs often break, leaving a brush-like end; a certain amount of alopecia is thus produced.

trich·or·rhexo·ma·nia (trick"o·reck"so·may'nee·uh) *n.* A compulsion to break off hairs of the scalp or beard with the fingernails.

tri·cho·sis (tri·ko'sis) *n.* Any morbid affection of the hair.

Trich·o·spo·ron (trick"o·spor'on, trick·os'po·ron) *n.* A genus of fungi which grow on hair shafts. A causative agent of piedra. *Trichosporon beigelii* (*T. giganteum*) is the principal cause of white piedra.

trich·o·spo·ro·sis (trich"o·spo·ro'sis) *n.* A fungous infection of the hair shaft.

trich·o·stron·gy·li·a·sis (trick"o·stron"ji·lye'uh·sis) *n.* Infection with *Trichostrongylus.*

Trich·o·stron·gy·lus (trick"o·stron'ji·lus) *n.* A genus of nematode worms which usually are parasites of ruminants. Man is infected by consuming raw plants grown in contaminated soil. The species identified from human cases are *Trichostrongylus colubriformis, T. orientalis, T. probolurus, T. vitrinus.*

tricho·til·lo·ma·nia (trick"o·til"o·may'nee·uh) *n.* An uncontrollable impulse to pull out one's hair.

tri·chro·ma·top·sia (trye"kro·muh·top'see·uh) *n.* Normal color vision; ability to see the three primary colors.

tri·chrome (trye'krome) *adj.* Three-colored.

tri·chro·mic (trye·kro'mick) *adj.* 1. Able to distinguish the three colors red, blue, and green. 2. Having three colors, as in a histologic stain.

trich·u·ri·a·sis (trick"yoo·rye'uh·sis) *n.*, pl. **trichuria·ses** (·seez) Infection by *Trichuris trichiura.*

Trich·u·ris (trick·yoo'ris) *n.* A genus of nematodes of the superfamily Trichuroidea, parasitic in the digestive tracts of mammals.

Trichuris trich·i·u·ra (trick"ee·yoo'ruh). The species infecting man. Transmission is from man to man by ingestion of mature ova. Syn. *Trichocephalus dispar, Trichocephalus trichiurus, whipworm.*

tri·cip·i·tal (trye·sip'i·tul) *adj.* 1. Having three heads. 2. Pertaining to a triceps muscle.

tri·cre·sol (trye·kree'sole, ·sol) *n.* CRESOL, a mixture of three isomeric compounds of the composition $HOC_6H_4CH_3$.

tricrotic pulse. A pulse in which the three waves are palpated during each cardiac cycle.

tri·cro·tism (trye'kro·tiz·um) *n.* The condition of having three waves corresponding to one pulse beat. —**tri·crot·ic** (trye·krot'ick) *adj.*

tri·cus·pid (trye·kus'pid) *adj.* 1. Having three cusps. 2. Pertaining to or affecting the tricuspid valve.

tricuspid atresia. A complex cogenital cardiac

anomaly with failure of development of the tricuspid valve, underdevelopment of the right ventricle, an atrial septal defect, and a large but normal mitral valve and left ventricle; there is usually also a ventricular septal defect and pulmonary artery hypoplasia.

tricuspid insufficiency. TRICUSPID REGURGITATION.

tricuspid regurgitation. Reflux of blood into the right atrium during ventricular systole, due to incomplete or inadequate closure of the tricuspid valve.

tricuspid stenosis. Narrowing of the tricuspid valve, with resultant elevation of right atrial and venous pressure.

tricuspid valve. The three-cusped valve situated between the right atrium and right ventricle. Syn. *right atrioventricular valve, valva atrioventricularis dextra.*

tri·dac·tyl (trye-dack′til) *adj.* Having three digits.

trid·y·mus (trid′i·mus) *n.* A triplet.

tri·eth·a·nol·am·ine (trye-eth″uh-nol′uh-meen, -min) *n.* Trihydroxytriethylamine, $N(CH_2CH_2OH)_3$, a strongly basic, hygroscopic liquid; used as a solvent, emulsifying agent, and intermediate in many syntheses. Syn. *trolamine.*

tri·eth·yl·ene·mel·a·mine (trye-eth″il·een·mel′uh·meen, -min) *n.* 2,4,6-Tris(1-aziridinyl)-s-triazine, $C_9H_{12}N_6$, an antineoplastic drug that forms ethyleneammonium ion in the body, as does nitrogen mustard, and is effective for palliative treatment of certain cancers. Abbreviated, TEM

tri·fa·cial nerve (trye-fay′shul). The fifth cranial or trigeminal nerve, so called because it divides into three main branches that supply the face.

tri·fid (trye′fid) *adj.* Three-cleft, tripartite.

tri·flu·o·per·a·zine (trye-floo″o·perr′uh·zeen) *n.* 10-[3-(4-Methyl-1-piperazinyl)propyl]-2-trifluoromethylphenothiazine, $C_{21}H_{24}F_3N_3S$, a tranquilizer used as the hydrochloride salt principally to control acute and chronic psychoses marked by psychomotor activity.

tri·fo·cal glasses or **spectacles** (trye-fo′kul). Glasses or spectacles having three refractive powers to correct for distant, intermediate, and near vision.

tri·fo·li·o·sis (trye-fo″lee·o′sis, tri·) *n., pl.* **trifolioses** (·seez) *In veterinary medicine,* a superficial necrosis of the white markings, caused by exposure to the sun after the animals have been sensitized to light by eating certain substances, chiefly the legumes.

tri·fur·ca·tion (trye″fur·kay′shun) *n.* Division into three prongs. —**tri·fur·cate** (trye′fur·kate) *adj. & v.*

tri·gas·tric (trye·gas′trick) *adj.* Having three fleshy bellies, as certain muscles.

tri·gem·i·nal (trye·jem′i·nul) *adj.* Triple; dividing into three parts.

trigeminal ganglion. The large ganglion of the sensory portion of the trigeminal nerve; the ophthalmic, maxillary, and mandibular divisions of the fifth nerve are attached to it.

trigeminal nerve. The fifth cranial nerve with central attachment at the lateral aspect of the pons. At the trigeminal (semilunar or Gasserian) ganglion it divides into three divisions: mandibular, maxillary, and ophthalmic. Syn. *nervus trigeminus.* See also *mandibular nerve, maxillary nerve, ophthalmic nerve.*

trigeminal neuralgia. Sudden, severe, lancinating pains in the distribution of one or more divisions of the trigeminal nerve, generally of unknown cause, but triggered by irritation of a fairly constant zone, such as the angle of the mouth or the side of the nose.

trigeminal pulse. A pulse in which a pause occurs after every third beat.

tri·gem·i·nus (trye·jem′i·nus) *n.* TRIGEMINAL NERVE.

tri·gem·i·ny (trye·jem′i·nee) *n.* 1. Any grouping in threes. 2. Grouping of arterial pulse beats in groups of three.

trig·ger action. A sudden stimulus that initiates a physiologic or pathologic process that may have nothing in common with the action that started it.

trigger finger. A condition in which flexion or extension of a finger is at first obstructed, but finally accomplished with a jerk or sweep. It is due to chronic tenosynovitis.

trigger zone. Any area of hyperexcitability, stimulation of which will precipitate a specific response such as the lancinating pain of trigeminal neuralgia.

tri·glyc·er·ide (trye·glis′ur·ide) *n.* An ester of glycerin in which all three hydroxyl groups of the latter are esterified with an acid; animal and vegetable fixed oils are composed chiefly of triglycerides of fatty acids; TRIACYLGLYCEROL.

tri·gone (trye′gohn) *n.* 1. Any of various triangular anatomic areas or structures. 2. The smooth triangular area on the inner surface of the urinary bladder between the openings of the two ureters and the internal urethral opening. —**trig·o·nal** (trig′uh·nul) *adj.*

Trig·o·nel·la (trig″o·nel′uh) *n.* A genus of the Leguminosae, certain species of which have been used medicinally.

tri·go·nid (trye·go·nid, trye·gon′id, trig′o·) *n.* The first three cusps (viewed as one) of a lower molar tooth.

tri·go·ni·tis (trye″go·nigh′tis) *n.* Inflammation of the trigone of the urinary bladder.

trig·o·no·ceph·a·ly (trig″uh·no·sef′uh·lee, tri·go″no·) *n.* Triangular or egg-shaped head, due to early synostosis of the metopic suture.

tri·go·num (trye·go′num) *n., pl.* **trigo·na** (·nuh) TRIGONE.

tri·i·do·thy·ro·nine (trye·eye″o·do·thigh′ro·neen, ·nin) *n.* Either of two isomeric hormones present in thyroid, specifically identified as L-3,3′,5-triiodothyronine and L-3,3′,5′-triiodothyronine. The former, now called liothyronine, is more active than thyroxine and also more rapid in action, and is used for the treatment of hypothyroid states in the form of its sodium salt.

Trilafon. Trademark for the tranquilizer and antiemetic drug perphenazine.

tri·lam·i·nar (trye·lam′i·nur) *adj.* Three-layered.

Trilene. A trademark for trichloroethylene, a liquid anesthetic and analgesic.

tri·lo·bate (trye·lo'bate) *adj.* Three-lobed.

tri·loc·u·lar (trye·lock'yoo·lur) *adj. In biology,* having three chambers or cells.

trilocular heart. A three-chambered heart; in humans, a congenital anomaly in which there is either a single atrium or single ventricle. Syn. *cor triloculare.*

tri·man·u·al (trye·man'yoo·ul) *adj.* Accomplished by the aid of three hands.

tri·men·su·al (trye·men'syoo·ul, shoo·ul) *adj.* Occurring at periods of 3 months.

tri·mes·ter (trye·mes'tur) *n.* A stage or period of 3 months.

tri·meth·a·di·one (trye″meth·uh·dye'ohn) *n.* 3,5,-5-Trimethyl-2,4-oxazolidinedione, $C_6H_9NO_3$, an anticonvulsant drug used for the treatment of petit mal and akinetic epilepsy.

tri·meth·a·phan cam·syl·ate (trye·meth'uh·fan kam'zil·ate). (+)-1,3-Dibenzyldecahydro-2-oxoimidazo[4,5-*c*]thieno[1,2-*a*]thiolium 2-oxo-10-bornanesulfonate, $C_{32}H_{40}N_2O_5S_2$, a ganglionic blocking agent used as an antihypertensive drug.

tri·meth·yl·xan·thine (trye·meth″il·zan'theen, ·thin) *n.* CAFFEINE.

tri·ni·tro·glyc·er·in (trye·nigh″tro·glis'ur·in) *n.* Glyceryl trinitrate; NITROGLYCERIN.

tri·ni·tro·phe·nol (trye·nigh″tro·fee'nol) *n.* 2,4,6-Trinitrophenol, $C_6H_2(NO_2)_3OH$, a yellow, crystalline solid; has been used topically as an antiseptic, astringent, and epithelization stimulant. Syn. *picric acid.*

tri·ni·tro·tol·u·ene (trye·nigh″tro·tol'yoo·een) *n.* $(NO_2)_3C_6H_2CH_3$; any of six isomers of this formula, but especially 1-methyl-2,4,6-trinitrobenzene, occurring as pale-yellow crystals; used in explosives. Abbreviated, TNT.

tri·nu·cle·ate (trye·new'klee·ut) *adj.* Having three nuclei.

tri·or·chid (trye·or'kid) *adj. & n.* 1. Having three testes. 2. An individual having three testes. —**trior·chidy** (·ki·dee) *n.*

tri·or·tho·cres·yl phosphate (trye·or″tho·kres'il). A mixture of esters of the composition $(CH_3C_6H_4)_3PO_4$; a colorless or pale-yellow liquid used in industry as a plasticizer and solvent and for other purposes. It is neurotoxic.

triorthocresyl phosphate neuropathy. A polyneuropathy resulting from the ingestion of grain, cooking oil, or ginger extract contaminated with triorthocresyl phosphate. The neural effects are mainly those of a motor polyneuropathy, but the spinal cord, particularly the corticospinal tracts, is also affected. The effects on the latter are usually permanent. Syn. *Jamaica ginger paralysis, jake palsy.*

tri·o·tus (trye·o'tus) *n.* Having three ears.

tri·oxy·pu·rine (trye·ock″see·pew'reen, ·rin) *n.* URIC ACID.

trip·a·ra (trip'uh·ruh) *n.* A woman who has had three viable pregnancies.

tri·pel·en·na·mine (trye″pel·en'uh·meen, ·min) *n.* 2-{Benzyl[2-(dimethylamino)ethyl]amino}-pyridine, $C_{16}H_{21}N_3$, an antihistaminic drug used as the citrate and hydrochloride salts.

tri·pep·tide (trye·pep'tide) *n.* A protein hydrolysis product representing condensation of three molecules of amino acids, or a natural or synthetic peptide containing three amino acids.

tri·pha·lan·gism (trye″fa·lan'jiz·um) *n.* The presence of three phalanges in the thumb or great toe.

tri·pha·sic (trye·fay'zick) *adj.* Having three phases or variations.

tri·phos·pho·pyr·i·dine nucleotide (trye·fos″fo·pirr'i·deen). NICOTINAMIDE ADENINE DINUCLEOTIDE PHOSPHATE. Abbreviated, TPN

tri·ple·gia (trye·plee'jee·uh) *n.* Hemiplegia with the additional paralysis of one limb on the opposite side.

triple phosphate crystals. Coffin-lid shaped or feathery crystals of ammonium magnesium phosphate occurring in alkaline urine.

triple response. The three stages of normal vasomotor reaction resulting when a pointed instrument is drawn heavily across the skin. They are: reddening of the area stimulated, wide spreading of flush to adjacent skin, and development of wheals. The response is said to be due to a histamine-like substance liberated from injured tissue by a noxious stimulus.

triple rhythm. A cardiac cadence in which three sounds recur in successive cycles; it may be normal or abnormal.

trip·let *n.* 1. One of three children born at one birth. 2. *In optics,* a system consisting of three lenses.

triple-X syndrome. A human chromosomal abnormality in which somatic cells contain 47 chromosomes, with X-trisomy; subjects are phenotypic females, often mentally retarded.

tri·plo·pia (trip·lo'pee·uh) *n.* A disturbance of vision in which three images of a single object are seen.

trip·sis (trip'sis) *n.* 1. TRITURATION. 2. MASSAGE.

tri·que·trum (trye·kwee'trum, trye·kwet'rum) *n.,* pl. **trique·tra** (·truh) 1. The third carpal bone from the radial side in the proximal row. 2. Any of the Wormian bones.

tri·sac·cha·ride (trye·sack'uh·ride, ·rid) *n.* A carbohydrate which, on hydrolysis, yields three molecules of monosaccharides.

tri·sect (trye'sekt) *v.* To cut into three parts.

tris·mus (triz'mus) *n.* Tonic spasms of the muscles of the jaw; a frequent and sensitive sign of tetanus.

tri·so·mic (trye·so'mick) *adj. & n.* 1. Having three chromosomes of a given kind, but otherwise only two of each of the other chromosomes of a haploid set. 2. A trisomic individual, having three chromosomes of a given kind in an otherwise diploid set.

tri·so·my (trye'so·mee) *n.* The occurrence of three of a given chromosome rather than the normal diploid number of two; often followed by a specification of the aberrant chromosome or chromosome group, as trisomy 13 (Patau's) syndrome, trisomy 18 (Edwards') syndrome, and trisomy 21 syndrome.

trisomy 13 syndrome. A congenital disorder due to trisomy of the number 13 chromosome (D trisomy) and rarely of an unbalanced translocation (D/D), characterized by the infant's failure to thrive, severe mental retardation, seizures, arhinencephalia, sloping forehead, deformities of the eyes, low-set ears, cleft lip and palate, rocker-bottom shaped feet, congenital heart defects, and multiple other anomalies. Syn. *Patau's syndrome*.

trisomy 18 syndrome. A congenital disorder due to trisomy for all, or a large part of, the 18 chromosome, characterized by severe mental deficiency, hypertonicity with clenched hands, anomalies of the hands, sternum, and pelvis, abnormal facies with low-set malformed ears and prominent occiput, ventricular septal defect with or without patent ductus arteriosus, and renal anomalies; the majority of infants are female, and most infants fail to thrive. Syn. *Edwards' syndrome*.

trisomy 21 syndrome. DOWN'S SYNDROME.

tris·ti·chi·a·sis (tris″ti·kigh′uh·sis) *n.* The arrangement of the cilia (eyelashes) in three rows.

tris·tis (tris′tis) *adj.* 1. Sad; gloomy. 2. Dull in color.

trit·an·o·pia (trit″an·o′pee·uh, trye″tan·) *n.* A defect in a third constituent essential for color vision, as in violet blindness.

trit·i·um (trit′ee·um, trish′ee·um) *n.* The radioactive isotope of hydrogen of mass 3; used as a tracer. Symbol, ^{3}H.

tri·ton (trye′ton) *n.* The nucleus of the tritium atom. It contains two neutrons and one proton, and thus bears unit positive charge.

trit·o·pine (trit′o·peen, ·pin, trye·to′pin) *n.* An alkaloid, $C_{20}H_{25}NO_4$, of opium. Syn. *laudanine*.

trit·u·rate (trit′yoo·rate) *v. & n.* 1. To reduce to a fine powder. 2. To mix powdered substances in a mortar with the aid of a pestle. 3. A finely divided powder. 4. TRITURATION (2).

trit·u·ra·tion (trit″yoo·ray′shun) *n.* 1. The process of reducing a solid substance to a powder by rubbing. 2. The product obtained by triturating a potent medicinal substance with powdered lactose or other diluent. 3. The process of amalgamation.

tri·va·lence (trye·vay′lunce, triv′uh·) *n.* The quality of having a valence of three. —**trivalent** (·lunt) *adj.*

tri·val·vu·lar (trye·val′vyoo·lur) *adj.* Having three valves.

tRNA Abbreviation for *transfer RNA*.

tro·car (tro′kahr) *n.* A sharp-pointed surgical instrument, fitted with a hollow cannula, used to puncture a body cavity for withdrawal of fluid. When the instrument is withdrawn the cannula is left in place to act as a drainage outlet.

tro·char (tro′kahr) *n.* TROCAR.

tro·che (tro′kee) *n.* LOZENGE.

troch-, trocho- A combining form meaning (a) *round, resembling a wheel*; (b) *rotation*; (c) *trochoid*.

tro·chan·ter (tro·kan′tur) *n.* One of two processes on the upper extremity of the femur below the neck, the greater trochanter and the lesser trochanter. —**tro·chan·ter·ic** (tro″kan·terr′ick). *adj.*

troch·lea (trock′lee·uh) *n.,* pl. & genit. sing. **troch·le·ae** (·lee·ee) A part or process having the nature of a pulley.

troch·le·ar (trock′lee·ur) *adj.* 1. Of or pertaining to a trochlea. 2. Of or pertaining to the trochlear nerve.

trochlear nerve. The fourth cranial nerve, whose fibers emerge from the brainstem on the dorsal surface just caudal to the inferior colliculus and go to supply the superior oblique muscle of the eye.

trocho·car·dia (trock″o·kahr′dee·uh, tro″ko·) *n.* Displacement of the heart by rotation on its long axis.

trocho·ceph·a·lus (trock″o·sef′uh·lus) *n.* A rounded appearance of the head, due to early partial synostosis of the frontal and parietal bones.

tro·choid (tro′koid) *adj.* Serving as a pulley or pivot; involving a pivotal action.

troch·o·ri·zo·car·dia (trock″o·rye″zo·kahr′dee·uh) *n.* A form of displacement of the heart characterized by trochocardia and change to horizontal position.

Troi·sier's sign (trwah‾z·yey′) Enlargement of the supraclavicular lymph nodes; a sign of advanced abdominal or thoracic neoplasm.

tro·le·an·do·my·cin (tro″lee·an″do·migh′sin) *n.* Triacetyloleandomycin, $C_{41}H_{67}NO_{15}$, the triacetyl ester of the antibiotic substance oleandomycin.

trol·ni·trate (trol·nigh′trate) *n.* Triethanolamine trinitrate, $N(CH_2CH_2ONO_2)_3$, a vasodilator used as the phosphate salt to reduce the frequency and severity of attacks of angina pectoris.

Trom·bic·u·la (trom·bick′yoo·luh) *n.* A genus of mites; the larvae are blood suckers and cause a severe dermatitis.

Trombicula alfreddugesi. EUTROMBICULA ALFREDDUGESI.

Trombicula ir·ri·tans (irr′i·tanz). EUTROMBICULA ALFREDDUGESI.

trom·bic·u·lo·sis (trom·bick″yoo·lo′sis) *n.* Infestation with *Trombicula*.

tro·meth·a·mine (tro·meth′uh·meen) *n.* Tris(hydroxymethyl)aminomethane, $C_4H_{11}NO_3$, a systemic antacid.

tromo·ma·nia (trom″o·may′nee·uh) *n. Obsol.* DELIRIUM TREMENS.

-tron A suffix designating *an electronic or atomic apparatus.*

trop-, tropo- A combining form meaning (a) *turn, turning, change;* (b) *tendency, affinity.*

tro·pa·co·caine (tro″puh·ko·kain′, ·ko′kain) *n.* Benzoylpseudotropine, $C_{15}H_{19}NO_2$, an alkaloid in Java coca leaves; the hydrochloride salt has been used as a local anesthetic.

troph-, tropho- A combining form meaning *nutrition, nutritive, nourishment.*

troph·ede·ma, troph·oe·de·ma (tro″fe·dee′muh, trof″e·) *n. Obsol.* Localized chronic edema of the feet or legs due to damaged nourishment or nerve supply.

troph·e·sy (trof′e·see) *n. Obsol.* TROPHONEUROSIS. —**tro·phe·si·al** (tro·fee′zee·ul), **trophe·sic** (·sick) *adj.*

troph·ic (trof′ick) *adj.* Pertaining to the functions concerned in nutrition, digestion, assimilation, and growth.

-trophic A combining form designating (a) *a specified type of nutrition;* (b) *a specified nutritional requirement.*

trophic center. Any part of the central nervous system whose proper functioning is thought to be necessary for the nutrition, growth, or maintenance of a peripheral part of the body, as the parietal lobe for the development of the muscles of an extremity.

tro·phic·i·ty (tro-fis′i-tee) *n.* A trophic influence or state.

trophic keratitis. Keratitis due to chronic or repeated infections of the cornea by herpesvirus.

trophic ulcer. NEUROTROPHIC ULCER.

troph·ism (trof′iz-um) *n.* 1. NUTRITION. 2. TROPHICITY.

tro·pho·blast (trof′o-blast, tro′fo-) *n.* The outer, ectodermal epithelium of the mammalian blastocyst or chorion and chorionic villi. —**tro·pho·blas·tic** (trof″o-blas′tick, tro″fo-) *adj.*

tro·pho·dy·nam·ics (trof″o-dye-nam′icks, tro″fo-) *n.* The branch of medical science dealing with the forces governing nutrition.

tro·pho·neu·ro·sis (trof″o-new-ro′sis, tro″fo-) *n.,* pl. **trophoneu·ro·ses** (-seez) Any disease of a part due to disturbance of the nerves or nerve centers with which it is connected. —**tropho·neu·rot·ic** (-rot′ick) *adj.*

tro·pho·ther·a·py (trof″o-therr′uh-pee, tro″fo-) *n.* Dietary therapy.

tro·pho·zo·ite (trof″o-zo′ite, tro″fo-) *n.* The active, motile, feeding stage of a protozoon. In ameba, the motile feeding stage forms in contrast to the nonmotile cysts; in the plasmodia of malaria, the motile stage between the signet rings and the schizonts during development in the red blood cells of the vertebrate host.

-trophy A combining form meaning *nutrition, nourishment, growth.*

tro·pia (tro′pee-uh) *n.* 1. A deviation of an eye from the normal position when both eyes are uncovered and open. 2. STRABISMUS.

-tropia A combining form designating *a (specified) deviation in the line of vision.*

-tropic A combining form meaning *turning toward, having an affinity for.*

trop·i·cal (trop′i-kul) *adj.* Pertaining to the zone of the earth lying between the Tropic of Cancer and the Tropic of Capricorn.

tropical abscess. AMEBIC ABSCESS.

tropical anhidrotic asthenia. Heat exhaustion due to inability to sweat.

tropical eosinophilia. A condition of unknown cause, described in India and the South Pacific area, which is similar to Loeffler's syndrome; characterized clinically by cough, asthmatic attacks, a pulmonary infiltrate on x-ray, splenomegaly, and eosinophilia.

tropical medicine. The branch of medical science concerned chiefly with problems of health and disease found commonly or exclusively in the tropical or subtropical regions.

tropical sore. CUTANEOUS LEISHMANIASIS.

tropical ulcer. A chronic, often progressive, sloughing ulcer, usually on the lower extrem-

ities and occasionally extending deeply with destruction of underlying muscles, tendons, and bones. Etiology is uncertain but spirochetes, fusiform bacilli and other bacteria are generally present in the lesions.

tro·pin (tro′pin) *n.* Any one of the substances in the blood serum which make bacteria susceptible to phagocytosis.

tro·pism (tro′piz-um) *n.* The involuntary bending, turning, or orientation of an organism or a part toward (positive tropism), or away from (negative tropism), a stimulus. Various types, depending upon the directing influence, include chemotropism, galvanotropism, geotropism, phototropism, rheotropism, stereotropism, thermotropism.

-tropism A combining form meaning (a) *a tendency to turn;* (b) *an affinity for.*

tro·po·col·la·gen (tro″po·kol′uh-jin, trop″o-) *n.* The fundamental unit of collagen fibrils, obtained by prolonged extraction of insoluble collagen with dilute acid.

tro·pom·e·ter (tro-pom′e·tur) *n.* 1. An instrument for measuring the various rotations of the eyeball. 2. An instrument for estimating the amount of torsion in long bones.

tro·po·sphere (tro′po·sfeer, trop′o-) *n.* The atmosphere that lies between the stratosphere and the earth's surface, a zone of marked changes in temperature, with ascending and descending air currents and cloud formations.

Trous·seau's disease (troo-so′) HEMOCHROMATOSIS.

Trousseau's sign or **phenomenon** 1. A sign of tetany in which carpal spasm can be elicited by compressing the upper arm. 2. TACHE CÉRÉBRALE.

troy weight. A system of weights in which a pound is twelve ounces or 5,760 grains.

true, *adj.* 1. Real; not false. 2. Typical, as true vipers.

true aneurysm. An aneurysm in which the sac is formed of one, two, or all of the arterial coats.

true hernia. A hernia having a sac, usually of peritoneum, covering the hernial contents.

true knot. A knot of the umbilical cord formed by the fetus slipping through a loop in the cord.

true pelvis. The part of the pelvic cavity situated below the iliopectineal line.

true ribs. The seven upper ribs on each side that are attached to the sternum.

True·ta's shunt (Sp. trweʰ′taʰ). A part of the renal circulation in which blood passes through the juxtamedullary glomeruli into the capillary beds of the medulla, bypassing the cortex. It results in greatly decreased production of urine and may be of special significance under certain abnormal circulatory conditions, as hemorrhage and shock. Syn. *Oxford shunt, renal shunt.*

trun·cal (trunk′ul) *adj.* Pertaining to the trunk.

trun·cat·ed (trunk′ay·tid) *adj.* 1. With the top cut off; shortened in height. 2. Deprived of limbs or accessory parts.

trun·cus (trunk′us) *n.,* pl. & genit. sing. **trun·ci** (·sigh) TRUNK.

trunk, *n.* 1. The torso; the body without head or

limbs.   2. The main stem of a blood vessel, lymphatic, or nerve.

trunk-thigh sign of Babinski The patient, lying flat on his back and with legs abducted, tries to rise to the sitting position while keeping his arms crossed in front of his chest. Normally, the legs stay motionless and the heels are pressed down. In the patient with hemiplegia, there is flexion of the thigh in association with flexion of the trunk, resulting in an involuntary elevation of the paretic limb; the normal limb is either not raised or only slightly. In paraplegia, both legs are raised. In hysterical hemiplegia, the normal leg may be elevated, while in hysterical paraplegia neither leg is raised. The sign may also be elicited by having the patient attempt to sit up from the recumbent position with his legs hanging over the edge of the bed, at which time the thigh is flexed and the lower leg extended on the paretic side.

truss, *n.* Any mechanical apparatus for preventing the recurrence of a hernial protrusion which has been reduced. The term includes simple devices such as a yarn truss for the control of infantile hernia, as well as complicated pieces of apparatus with pressure pads designed to hold large inguinal or abdominal hernias.

truth serum. An intravenous solution of a barbiturate used in narcoanalysis; sodium amytal or thiopental are the most common ones.

T.S. Abbreviation for *test solution.*

tryp·an blue (trip'an, trye'pan). An acid diazo dye of the benzopurpurin series used in vital staining, and also as a trypanocide.

try·pa·no·cide (tri·pan'o·side, trip'uh·no·side) *n.* An agent that destroys trypanosomes. —**try·pano·ci·dal** (tri·pan''o·sigh'dul) *adj.*

Try·pa·no·so·ma (tri·pan''o·so''muh, trip''uh·no·) *n.* A genus of protozoa belonging to the subphylum Mastigophora, which are slender, elongate organisms with a central nucleus, posterior blepharoplast, and an undulatory membrane, from which flagellum projects forward; transmitted by insect vectors, and responsible for such infections as trypanosomiasis and Chagas' disease in man and dourine, nagana, and surra in animals.

Trypanosoma cru·zi (kroo'zye). The causative agent of Chagas' disease.

try·pa·no·some (tri·pan'o·sohm, trip'uh·no·) *n.* One of any species of *Trypanosoma,* a flagellated protozoan living in the blood and tissues of its host. —**trypano·som·ic** (·so'mick) *adj.*

try·pa·no·so·mi·a·sis (tri·pan''o·so·migh'uh·sis, trip''uh·no·) *n.,* pl. **trypanosomia·ses** (·seez) Any of many diseases of man and animals caused by infection with species of *Trypanosoma* and transmitted by tsetse flies or other insects.

tryp·sin (trip'sin) *n.* The proteolytic enzyme resulting from the action of the enterokinase of intestinal juice upon the trypsinogen secreted in the pancreatic juice. It catalyzes the hydrolysis of peptide linkages in proteins and partially hydrolyzed proteins, more readily on the latter. Syn. *tryptase.* —**tryp·tic** (·tick) *adj.*

tryp·sin·o·gen (trip·sin'uh·jen) *n.* The zymogen

of trypsin, occurring in the pancreatic juice and converted to trypsin by enterokinase in the small intestine. Syn. *protrypsin.*

tryp·ta·mine (trip'tuh·meen, ·min) *n.* 3-(2-Aminoethyl)indole, $C_{10}H_{12}N_2$, the decarboxylation product of tryptophan; an intermediate substance in certain metabolic processes in plants and animals.

tryp·tase (trip'tace) *n.* TRYPSIN.

tryp·to·lyt·ic (trip''to·lit'ick) *adj.* Of or pertaining to the hydrolysis of proteins caused by trypsin.

tryp·to·phan (trip'to·fan) *n. l-α-*Aminoindole-3-propionic acid, $C_{11}H_{12}N_2O_2$, an amino acid component of casein and other proteins that is essential in human nutrition but is not synthesized by the human body.

tryp·to·pha·nase (trip'to·fa·nace, trip·tof'uh·) *n.* A bacterial enzyme that catalyzes degradation of tryptophan to indole, pyruvic acid, and ammonia.

tryp·to·phan·uria (trip''to·fan·yoo'ree·uh) *n.* 1. The presence of tryptophan in the urine. 2. A rare inborn error of metabolism characterized by an increase in urinary tryptophan and delayed clearing of tryptophan from the plasma following an oral load. Clinical manifestations include mental retardation, dwarfism, photosensitivity, ataxia, telangiectasia, and hyperpigmentation. The nature of the basic defect is unknown.

T.S. Abbreviation for *test solution.*

tset·se fly (tset'see, tsee'tsee) *n.* Any dipterous insect of the genus *Glossina,* almost wholly restricted to Africa. *Glossina* flies carry the flagellate trypanosomes, the causative agents of nagana in cattle and of trypanosomiasis in man.

TSH Abbreviation for *thyroid-stimulating hormone.*

tsp Abbreviation for *teaspoon.*

T splint. A splint used to hold back the shoulders, and adapted by bandaging to hold the fragments in apposition in fractures of the clavicle.

TSTA Tumor-specific transplantation antigens; antigens on the surfaces of tumor cells capable of intiating a rejection phenomenon.

tsu·tsu·ga·mu·shi disease or **fever** (tsoo''tsuh·ga·moo'shee) A disease characterized by headache, high fever, and a rash, occurring in Japan, Formosa, and islands of the South Pacific; caused by *Rickettsia tsutsugamushi* and transmitted to man by the bite of the larval forms of mites of the genus *Trombicula.*

T tube. A rubber or glass tube in the form of the letter T.

tu·bage (tew'bij) *n.* The introduction of a tube or catheter.

tub·al (tew'bul) *adj.* Pertaining to a tube, especially the uterine or the auditory.

tubal pregnancy. Gestation within an oviduct.

tube, *n.* A hollow, cylindrical structure, especially a uterine tube or an auditory tube.

tu·bec·to·my (tew·beck'tuh·mee) *n.* SALPINGECTOMY; excision of a tube, specifically a uterine tube.

tu·ber (tew'bur) *n.,* pl. **tubers, tu·be·ra** (·be·ruh)

1. A thickened portion of an underground stem. 2. Any rounded swelling. —**tu·ber·al** (·ul) *adj.*

tuberal nuclei. Circular cell groups, in the lateral part of the tuber cinereum, which often produce small eminences on the basal surface of the hypothalamus.

tu·ber·cle (tew′bur·kul) *n.* 1. A small nodule. 2. A rounded prominence on a bone. 3. The specific lesion produced by the tubercle bacillus, consisting of a collection of lymphocytes and epithelioid cells, at times with giant cells.

tubercle bacillus. *MYCOBACTERIUM TUBERCULO-SIS.* Abbreviated, t.b.

tubercul-, tuberculo-. A combining form meaning *tuberculous, tuberculosis, tubercle bacillus.*

tu·ber·cu·lar (tew·bur′kew·lur) *adj.* 1. Characterized by the presence of small nodules or tubercles. 2. Of or pertaining to a tubercle. 3. *Erron.* TUBERCULOUS.

tu·ber·cu·lat·ed (tew·bur′kew·lay″tid) *adj.* Having tubercles; TUBERCULAR.

tu·ber·cu·la·tion (tew·bur″kew·lay′shun) *n.* 1. The formation, development, or arrangement of tubercles. 2. The process of affecting a part with tubercles.

tu·ber·cu·lid (tew·bur′kew·lid) *n.* Any of a group of varied skin manifestations, always free of tubercle bacilli, presumed to be reactions of hypersensitivity to a focus of tuberculous infection elsewhere in the body. Included are papular and papulonecrotic skin lesions, lichen scrofulosus, and erythema induratum.

tu·ber·cu·lin (tew·bur′kew·lin) *n.* A preparation containing tuberculoproteins derived from *Mycobacterium tuberculosis* which elicit reactions of delayed hypersensitivity, namely erythema, induration, and even necrosis in human or animal hosts with past or present sensitization to tubercle bacilli. Similar preparations may be derived from mycobacteria other than *M. tuberculosis.*

tuberculin reaction. The prototype of delayed hypersensitivity upon the introduction of tuberculin in an individual with prior or present sensitization with *Mycobacterium tuberculosis.* Locally, induration and erythema, with or without necrosis, reaches its height in 48 to 72 hours. Focal reactions at the site of tuberculous lesions, and constitutional reactions, including fever and malaise, may also occur.

tuberculin test. A test for past or present infection with tubercle bacilli, based on a delayed hypersensitivity reaction of edema, erythema, or necrosis at the site, reaching its height in 48 to 72 hours. It is elicited by such products as old tuberculin or purified protein derivative, usually introduced into the skin.

tuberculin-type allergy. DELAYED HYPERSENSITIVITY.

tuberculin-type sensitivity. TUBERCULIN REACTION.

tu·ber·cu·lo·der·ma (tew·bur″kew·lo·dur′muh) *n.* TUBERCULID.

tu·ber·cu·lo·fi·broid (tew·bur″kew·lo·figh′broid) *adj.* Pertaining to a tubercle (3) that has undergone dense fibrosis.

tu·ber·cu·loid (tew·bur′kew·loid) *adj.* Resembling tuberculosis or a tubercle.

tuberculoid leprosy. A principal form of leprosy, characterized by a paucity or absence of *Mycobacterium leprae* in the tissues, a positive lepromin reaction, and principally by asymmetric maculoanesthetic skin lesions, with involvement of peripheral nerve trunks leading to sensorimotor deficit in the distribution of the involved nerve in addition to the patch of cutaneous anesthesia.

tu·ber·cu·lo·ma (tew·bur″kew·lo′muh) *n.*, pl. **tu·berculomas, tuberculo·ma·ta** (·tuh) A conglomerate caseous tubercle, usually solitary, whose size and sharp circumscription resemble that of a neoplasm.

tuberculoma en plaque. A rare type of chronic tuberculous meningoencephalitis, characterized by a flat plaque of a granulomatous reaction in the meninges.

tu·ber·cu·lo·ma·nia (tew·bur″kew·lo·may′nee·uh) *n.* An unalterable and unfounded conviction that one is suffering from tuberculosis.

tu·ber·cu·lo·pho·bia (tew·bur″kew·lo·fo′bee·uh) *n.* An abnormal fear of tuberculosis.

tu·ber·cu·lo·pro·tein (tew·bur″kew·lo·pro′teen, ·tee·in) *n.* A variety of protein not exerting appreciable toxic effect upon the normal body but highly toxic for the tuberculous, hypersensitive individual, leading to necrosis, fever, and severe constitutional symptoms. Smaller, standardized doses elicit the tuberculin reaction of delayed hypersensitivity.

tu·ber·cu·lose (tew·bur′kew·loce) *adj.* TUBERCULATED.

tu·ber·cu·sil·i·co·sis (tew·bur″kew·lo·sil″i·ko′sis) *n.* SILICOTUBERCULOSIS.

tu·ber·cu·lo·sis (tew·bur″kew·lo′sis) *n.* A chronic infectious disease with protean manifestations, primarily involving the lungs but capable of attacking most organs of the body, caused by *Mycobacterium tuberculosis.* Usually the primary infection becomes arrested, but widespread tuberculous disease occasionally occurs. Severe clinical manifestations may include fever, weight loss, cough, chest pain, sputum, and hemoptysis. The pathological response may include tubercle formation, exudation, necrosis, and fibrosis, depending on local biochemical factors, the hypersensitive state, the number and virulence of the organisms, and the resistance of the host. Abbreviated, TB. Syn. *phthisis, consumption.*

tuberculosis li·chen·oi·des (lye″ke·noy′deez). A skin eruption consisting of groups of papules, usually on the trunk, seen especially in subjects suffering from tuberculosis of the lymph nodes and bone. Syn. *lichen scrofulosus.*

tuberculosis ver·ru·co·sa (verr″oo·ko′suh). A type of warty skin eruption, usually on the hands and arms, due to inoculation with the tubercle bacillus from handling meat of infected cattle or infected human material. Syn. *anatomic tubercle, dissection tubercle, verruca necrogenica.*

tu·ber·cu·lo·stat·ic (tew·bur″kew·lo·stat′ick) *adj.* Inhibiting the growth of tubercle bacilli.

tu·ber·cu·lous (tew·bur'kew·lus) *adj.* Affected with, or caused by, tuberculosis.

tu·ber·cu·lum (tew·bur'kew·lum) *n.*, pl. **tubercu·la** (·luh) TUBERCLE.

tuberculum sel·lae tur·ci·cae (sel'ee tur'si·see) [NA]. The anterior boundary of the sella turcica.

tu·be·ro·si·tas (tew·bur·os'i·tas) *n.*, pl. **tube·ro·si·ta·tes** (·os·i·tay'teez) TUBEROSITY.

tu·ber·os·i·ty (tew'bur·os'i·tee) *n.* A protuberance on a bone.

tuberosity of the ischium. ISCHIAL TUBER or TUBEROSITY.

tuberosity of the tibia. An oblong elevation on the anterior surface of the upper extremity of the tibia, to which the patellar ligament is attached.

tu·ber·ous (tew'bur·us) *adj.* 1. Resembling a tuber. 2. Having, or characterized by the presence of, tubers or tuberosities.

tuberous mole. BREUS' MOLE.

tuberous sclerosis. A familial neurocutaneous syndrome characterized in its complete form by epilepsy, adenoma sebaceum, and mental deficiency and pathologically by nodular sclerosis of the cerebral cortex. Retinal phacoma, other skin lesions such as areas of depigmentation, hyperpigmentation and shagreen patches, intracranial calcification, and hamartomas of different viscera are frequently present.

tuber ver·mis (vur'mis) [NA]. A portion of the inferior vermis just caudal to the horizontal fissure of the cerebellum.

tubo-. A combining form meaning *tube.*

tu·bo·ab·dom·i·nal (tew''bo·ab·dom'i·nul) *adj.* Pertaining to a uterine tube and to the abdomen.

tu·bo·cu·ra·re (tew''bo·kew·rah'ree) *n.* Curare so named because of its tube shape, the result of being packed in hollow bamboo canes.

***d*-tu·bo·cu·ra·rine** (tew''bo·kew·rah'reen, ·rin) *n.* TUBOCURARINE CHLORIDE.

tubocurarine chloride. The chloride of a quaternary base obtained from the bark and stems of plants of the genus *Chondodendron,* $C_{38}H_{44}Cl_2N_2O_6$; a skeletal muscle relaxant used as an adjunct in surgical anesthesia to soften convulsions in electroshock therapy, to reduce muscle spasm in fractures, and for diagnosis of myasthenia gravis. Syn. *d-tubocurarine.*

tu·bo·lig·a·men·ta·ry pregnancy (tew''bo·lig''uh·men'tuh·ree) Gestation arising in a uterine tube with extension into the broad ligament.

tu·bo·lig·a·men·tous (tew''bo·lig''uh·men'tus) *adj.* Pertaining to the uterine tube and the broad ligament.

tu·bo·ovar·i·an (tew''bo·o·vār''ee·un) *adj.* Pertaining to the uterine tube and the ovary.

tuboovarian pregnancy. Gestation arising in a uterine tube and extending into the ovary.

tu·bo·ovar·i·ot·o·my (tew''bo·o·vār''ee·ot'uh·mee) *n.* Excision of a uterine tube and ovary.

tu·bo·peri·to·ne·al (tew''bo·perr''i·to·nee'ul) *adj.* Pertaining to the uterine tubes and the peritoneum.

tu·bo·plas·ty (tew'bo·plas''tee) *n.* Plastic repair of a uterine tube.

tu·bo·tym·pan·ic (tew''bo·tim·pan'ick) *adj.* Pertaining to the auditory tube and the tympanic cavity.

tu·bo·uter·ine (tew''bo·yoo'tur·in, ·ine) *adj.* Pertaining to the uterine tube and the uterus.

tu·bo·va·gi·nal (tew''bo·vuh·jye'nul, ·vaj'i·nul) *adj.* Pertaining to a uterine tube and the vagina.

tu·bu·lar (tew'bew·lur) *adj.* 1. Shaped like a tube. 2. Pertaining to or affecting tubules, as tubular nephritis. 3. Produced in a tube, as tubular breathing.

tubular acidosis. RENAL TUBULAR ACIDOSIS.

tubular adenoma. An adenoma in which the parenchymal cells form tubules.

tubular vision. A hysterical phenomenon in which the constricted visual field defies the laws of physical projection and maintains a uniform small size, despite a change in distance of the patient from the tangent screen or the size of the test object. Syn. *gun-barrel vision, tunnel vision.*

tu·bule (tew'bewl) *n.* 1. A small tube. 2. *In anatomy,* any minute, tube-shaped structure.

tubuli. Plural and genitive singular of *tubulus.*

tu·bu·lin (tew'bew·lin) *n.* A globular protein containing two protomers; 10 to 14 tubulin molecules are arranged in a helix to form the microtubuls of cells.

tu·bu·li·za·tion (tew''bew·li·zay'shun) *n.* Protection of the ends of nerves, after neurorrhaphy, by an absorbable cylinder.

tu·bu·lo·ac·i·nous (tew''bew·lo·as'i·nus) *adj.* TUBULOALVEOLAR.

tu·bu·lo·al·ve·o·lar (tew''bew·lo·al·vee'o·lur) *adj.* Consisting of a system of branching tubules that terminate in alveoli, as in the salivary glands.

tu·bu·lo·cyst (tew'bew·lo·sist'') *n.* A cystic dilatation in an occluded canal or duct.

tu·bu·lo·rac·e·mose (tew''bew·lo·ras'e·moce) *adj.* Characterizing a gland that is both tubular and racemose.

tu·bu·lus (tew'bew·lus) *n.*, pl. & genit. sing. **tubu·li** (·lye) TUBULE.

tu·bus (tew'bus) *n.*, pl. & genit. sing. **tu·bi** (·bye) TUBE, CANAL.

tu·la·re·mia (tew''luh·ree'mee·uh) *n.* An infectious disease caused by *Francisella tularensis* (*Pasteurella tularensis*) widely prevalent in wild animals, birds, and ancillary hosts, primarily transmitted to man by contact with infected tissues or fluids (for example, skinning rabbits), or by insect bites, but also by ingestion and inhalation. Depending on the host response and point of entry, a variety of forms are recognized, such as ulceroglandular, oculoglandular, typhoidal, pneumonic, or gastrointestinal. Syn. *deer-fly fever, rabbit fever.*

tu·me·fa·cient (tew''me·fay'shunt) *adj.* Tending to cause swelling.

tu·me·fac·tion (tew''me·fack'shun) *n.* 1. A swelling. 2. The act or process of swelling.

tu·me·fy (tew′me·fye) v. To swell or cause to swell.

tu·mes·cence (tew·mes′unce) n. 1. The condition of growing tumid. 2. A swelling. 3. The vascular congestion of the sex organs, as the swelling of the penis, associated with heightened emotional and physical excitement, characteristic of the readiness to engage in copulation. —**tumes·cent** (·unt) adj.

tu·mid (tew′mid) adj. Swollen.

tu·mor, tu·mour (tew′mur) n. 1. Any abnormal mass resulting from the excessive multiplication of cells. 2. A swelling. —**tumor·al** (·ul) adj.

tumor blush. TUMOR STAIN.

tu·mori·gen·ic (tew″mur·i·jen′ick) adj. Tumorforming.

tu·mor·let (tew′mur·lit) n. 1. A tumorlike proliferation of cells in scarred lung tissue; thought to be of bronchial epithelial origin. 2. A small tumor.

tu·mor·ous (tew′mur·ous) adj. Of the nature of a neoplasm or tumor.

tumor stain. An angiographic appearance of contrast media in very small vessels and vascular spaces of a highly vascular tumor, usually resulting in diffuse, prolonged opacification. Syn. tumor blush.

tumour. TUMOR.

Tun·ga (tung′guh) n. A genus of fleas that burrow beneath the skin to lay their eggs; serious local inflammation results.

Tunga pen·e·trans (pen′e·tranz). A flea prevalent in the tropical regions of Africa and America; often attacks between the toes or on the foot; a chigoe or a jigger.

tun·gi·a·sis (tung·guy′uh·sis, tun·jye′) n. The cutaneous pustular inflammation caused by the gravid female sandflea, Tunga penetrans.

tung·sten (tung′stun) n. W = 183.85. A heavy metallic element, atomic number 74, density 19.3. Used in steel to increase hardness and tensile strength, in the manufacture of filaments for electric lamps, in contact points, and other products where hardness and toughness are demanded. Syn. wolfram.

tu·nic (tew′nick) n. A coat, layer, membrane, or sheath.

tu·ni·ca (tew′ni·kuh) n., pl. & genit. sing. **tuni·cae** (·see). A coat, layer, membrane, or sheath.

tunica ad·ven·ti·tia (ad·ven·tish′ee·uh) [NA]. The outer connective tissue coat of an organ where it is not covered by a serous membrane.

tunica al·bu·gi·nea (al·bew·jin′ee·uh) [NA]. A general term for a dense connective-tissue covering layer.

tunica elas·ti·ca (e·las′ti·kuh). TUNICA INTIMA.

tunica ex·ter·na (ecks·tur′nuh) [NA]. The outermost coat of a blood or lymph vessel.

tunica in·ti·ma (in′ti·muh) [NA]. The inner coat of a blood or lymph vessel.

tunica me·dia (mee′dee·uh) [NA]. The middle coat of a blood or lymph vessel, composed of varying amounts of smooth muscle and elastic tissue.

tunica mu·co·sa (mew·ko′suh) [NA]. MUCOUS MEMBRANE.

tunica mus·cu·la·ris (mus·kew·lair′ris) [NA]. The muscular coat of certain hollow organs, for example, the bronchi.

tunica vaginalis tes·tis (tes′tis) [NA]. The serous membrane covering the testis and epididymis and lining the serous cavity of the scrotum.

tun·ing fork. A two-tined metallic fork capable of vibrating at a rate which will produce a pure tone of a specific frequency.

tuning-fork test. The testing of hearing acuity or loss by use of a tuning fork.

tunnel graft. A skin graft with the epithelial side inward, introduced into tissues under a contracted scar, etc. The tunnel is split later, and the epithelial surface becomes superficial or is left in place to replace a part, such as the urethra.

tunnel of Cor·ti (kor′tee) The triangular canal formed by the pillar cells of the spiral organ (of Corti) and the lamina basilaris. It extends over the entire length of the lamina basilaris. Syn. canal of Corti, tunnel space.

tunnel vision. TUBULAR VISION.

TUR Abbreviation for transurethral resection.

tur·ban tumor (tur′bun). CYLINDROMA.

tur·bid (tur′bid) adj. Cloudy. —**tur·bid·i·ty** (tur·bid′i·tee) n.

tur·bi·dim·e·ter (tur″bi·dim′e·tur) n. An instrument for measuring the degree of turbidity of a liquid. —**turbi·di·met·ric** (·di·met′rick) adj.; **turbi·dim·e·try** (·dim′e·tree) n.

tur·bid·i·ty (tur·bid′i·tee) n. The characteristic of being turbid.

tur·bi·nal (tur′bi·nul) adj. TURBINATE.

tur·bi·nate (tur′bin·ut, ·ate) adj. & n. 1. Shaped like a top. 2. NASAL CONCHA. 3. Pertaining to a concha.

tur·bi·nat·ed (tur′bi·nay″tid) adj. Top-shaped; scroll-shaped.

tur·bi·nec·to·my (tur″bi·neck′tuh·mee) n. Excision of a nasal concha.

tur·bi·no·tome (tur′bi·no·tome) n. An instrument used in turbinotomy.

tur·bi·not·o·my (tur″bi·not′uh·mee) n. Cutting of a turbinated bone.

tur·ges·cense (tur·jes′unce) n. Swelling.

tur·ges·cent (tur·jes′unt) adj. Becoming or being swollen, tumid.

tur·gid (tur′jid) adj. 1. Swollen. 2. CONGESTED.

tur·gor (tur′gur) n. Active hyperemia; turgescence.

turgor vi·ta·lis (vye·tay′lis). The normal fullness of the capillaries.

Türk cell (tü͡erk) An abnormal cell of the peripheral blood closely resembling a plasma cell in nuclear placement and cytoplasmic staining, but having a chromatin pattern roughly intermediate between a lymphocyte and plasma cell.

Türk's irritation cell or **leukocyte** TÜRK CELL.

tur·mer·ic (tur′mur·ick) n. CURCUMA.

turn, v. 1. To cause to revolve about an axis. 2. To change the position of the fetus so as to facilitate delivery.

Tur·ner's sign Local discoloration of the abdominal wall in the flanks as a sign of acute pancreatitis.

Turner's syndrome GONADAL DYSGENESIS.

Turner's tooth. Hypoplasia, usually of a single

tooth, most commonly involving the permanent maxillary incisor or a premolar.

TURP Transurethral resection of the prostate.

tur·pen·tine (tur'pun·tine) *n.* 1. A concrete or liquid oleoresin obtained from coniferous trees. 2. The concrete oleoresin from *Pinus palustris* and other species of *Pinus*. Yellow-orange, opaque masses of characteristic odor and taste; contains a volatile oil. Has been used for local irritant effect. Syn. *gum thus. gum turpentine.*

tur·ri·ceph·a·ly (tur''i·sef'uh·lee) *n.* OXYCEPHALY.

tusk, *n.* A large, projecting tooth; in man, usually an upper canine tooth; in animals, a tooth that projects outside the mouth, as in the elephant, walrus, or boar.

tus·sic·u·la·tion (tuh·sick''yoo·lay'shun) *n.* A hacking cough.

tus·sis (tus'is) *n.* COUGH.

tus·sive (tus'iv) *adj.* Pertaining to, or caused by, a cough.

tussive fremitus. A thrill felt by the hand when applied to the chest of a person coughing.

tussive syndrome or **syncope.** COUGH SYNCOPE.

T wave of the electrocardiogram. The electrocardiographic deflection due to repolarization of the ventricles; it may be positive, negative, or both in succession. Syn. *ventricular repolarization complex.*

Tween. Trademark for any of several polysorbate fatty acid esters individually identified by appending a number to the trademark; the substances are surfactants.

Tween 80. Trademark for polysorbate 80, a surfactant.

tweez·ers, *n.pl.* Delicate surgical forceps that are capable of seizing without crushing easily damaged structures, as nerves; they are also used for removing eyelashes or hairs.

twelfth (XIIth) cranial nerve. HYPOGLOSSAL NERVE.

twelve-year molars. The second permanent molars.

twi·light sleep. *In obstetrics,* an injection of scopolamine and morphine to produce amnesia and analgesia.

twin, *n.* One of two born at the same birth.

twinge, *n.* A sudden short, sharp pain.

twin·ning, *n.* 1. Production of like structures by division. 2. The occurrence of twin pregnancies.

twitch, *n.* 1. A brief phasic contraction of a muscle fiber or the short, sudden, visible contractile response of a small muscular unit to a single maximal stimulus. 2. A spasmodic jerk of a muscle or group of muscles.

two-glass test. GLASS TEST.

two-point discrimination or **sensibility.** The ability to discriminate between two punctate stimuli applied simultaneously to the skin. The minimal separation at which discrimination is possible is proportional to the distance between the points, and varies in different skin areas.

two-step test. Repeated ascents over two 9-inch steps as a simple exercise test of cardiovascular function.

ty·lec·to·my (tye·leck'tuh·mee) *n.* Excision of a lump of tissue.

ty·lo·ma (tye·lo'muh) *n.* CALLOSITY.

ty·lo·sis (tye·lo'sis) *n.,* pl. **tylo·ses** (·seez) 1. A localized patch of hyperkeratotic skin due to chronic pressure and friction. 2. A form of blepharitis with thickening and hardening of the edge of the lid. **—ty·lot·ic** (·lot'ick) *adj.*

tympan-, tympano-. A combining form meaning (a) *tympanum, tympanic;* (b) *tympanites, tympanitic.*

tym·pa·nal (tim'puh·nul) *adj.* TYMPANIC.

tym·pa·nec·to·my (tim''puh·neck'tuh·mee) *n.* Excision of the tympanic membrane.

tym·pan·ic (tim·pan'ick) *adj.* 1. Of, pertaining to, or associated with the tympanum. 2. RESONANT.

tympanic antrum. MASTOID ANTRUM.

tympanic cavity. The cavity of the middle ear; an irregular, air-containing, mucous membrane-lined space in the temporal bone. The chain of auditory ossicles extends from its lateral wall, the tympanic membrane, to its medial wall, the bony labyrinth. It communicates anteriorly with the nasopharynx through the auditory tube and posterosuperiorly with the mastoid cells through the mastoid antrum.

tympanic membrane. The membrane separating the external from the middle ear. It consists of three layers: an outer or skin layer, a fibrous layer, and an inner mucous layer. Syn. *eardrum.*

tym·pa·nism (tim'puh·niz·um) *n.* Distention with gas; TYMPANITES.

tym·pa·ni·tes (tim'puh·nigh'teez) *n.* A distention of the abdomen from accumulation of gas in the intestine or peritoneal cavity.

tym·pa·nit·ic (tim'puh·nit'ick) *adj.* 1. Caused by, or of the nature of, tympanites. 2. Tympanic or resonant to percussion.

tympanitic resonance. 1. The prolonged musical sound heard on percussion over an air-containing cavity with flexible walls. Its sounds vary widely in pitch. 2. A percussion note which exhibits in varying proportion the characteristics of both resonance and tympany. Syn. *bandbox resonance. Skoda's resonance.*

tym·pa·ni·tis (tim''puh·nigh'tis) *n.* Inflammation of the tympanum; OTITIS MEDIA.

tym·pa·no·mas·toid (tim''puh·no·mas'toid) *adj.* Pertaining to the tympanum and the mastoid process or the mastoid cells.

tym·pa·no·mas·toid·itis (tim''puh·no·mas''toy·dye'tis) *n.* Inflammation of the tympanum and mastoid cells.

tym·pa·no·plas·ty (tim'puh·no·plas''tee) *n.* 1. Surgical repair of the eardrum. 2. Surgical repair of the eardrum and reconstruction of the bony pathway of the middle ear.

tym·pa·no·scle·ro·sis (tim''puh·no·skle·ro'sis) *n.* Fibrosis and sclerosis of the mucous membrane of the middle ear secondary to infection.

tym·pa·no·squa·mous (tim''puh·no·skway'mus) *adj.* Pertaining to the tympanic and squamous parts of the temporal bone.

tym·pa·no·sta·pe·di·al (tim''puh·no·stay·pee'

dee·ul) *adj.* Pertaining to the tympanum and stapes.

tym·pa·not·o·my (tim″puh·not′uh·mee) *n.* MYRINGOTOMY.

tym·pa·nous (tim′puh·nus) *adj.* Distended with gas; pertaining to tympanism.

tym·pa·num (tim′puh·num) *n.*, *genit.* **tympa·ni** (·nye), *pl.* **tympa·na** (·nuh) MIDDLE EAR.

tym·pa·ny (tim′puh·nee) *n.* 1. TYMPANITES. 2. A tympanitic percussion note. 3. BLOAT (2).

typ-, typo- A combining form meaning *image, model.*

type, *n. & v.* 1. A category or subcategory based on specified characteristics. 2. An example of such a category taken as a standard. 3. *In pathology,* the grouping of the distinguishing features of a fever, disease, etc., whereby it is referred to its proper class. 4. *In bacteriology,* members of a species having some further characteristic in common. 5. To identify or classify, as a blood group or a bacterial culture.

type A encephalitis. *Obsol.* ENCEPHALITIS LETHARGICA.

type B encephalitis. *Obsol.* JAPANESE B ENCEPHALITIS.

type C encephalitis. *Obsol.* ST. LOUIS ENCEPHALITIS.

type I of Cori VON GIERKE'S DISEASE.

type II of Cori POMPE'S DISEASE.

type III of Cori LIMIT DEXTRINOSIS.

type IV of Cori AMYLOPECTINOSIS.

type V of Cori McARDLE'S DISEASE.

type VI of Cori HERS' DISEASE.

typh-, typho- A combining form meaning (a) *typhus;* (b) *typhoid.*

typhl-, typhlo- A combining form meaning (a) *blind, blindness;* (b) *cecum.*

typh·lat·o·ny (tif·lat′uh·nee) *n.* An atonic condition of the wall of the cecum.

typh·lec·ta·sia (tif″leck·tay′zhuh, ·zee·uh) *n.* Dilatation of the cecum.

typh·lec·to·my (tif·leck′tuh·mee) *n.* Excision of the cecum.

typh·li·tis (tif·lye′tis) *n.* CECITIS.

typh·lo·dic·li·di·tis (tif″lo·dick″li·dye′tis, ·dye″kli-) *n.* Inflammation of the ileocecal valve.

typh·lo·em·py·e·ma (tif″lo·em″pye·ee′muh) *n.* Abscess attending cecitis or appendicitis.

typh·loid (tif′loid) *adj.* Having defective vision.

typh·lo·li·thi·a·sis (tif″lo·li·thigh′uh·sis) *n.* The formation of calculi in the cecum.

typh·lo·meg·a·ly (tif″lo·meg′uh·lee) *n.* Enlargement or hypertrophy of the cecum.

typh·lo·pto·sis (tif″lo·to′sis, tif″lo·pto′sis) *n.* Downward displacement or prolapse of the cecum.

typh·lo·sis (tif·lo′sis) *n.* BLINDNESS.

typh·lo·spasm (tif′lo·spaz·um) *n.* Spasm of the cecum.

typh·lo·ste·no·sis (tif″lo·ste·no′sis) *n.* Stenosis of the cecum.

typh·los·to·my (tif·los′tuh·mee) *n.* A cecal colostomy.

ty·pho·bac·ter·in (tye″fo·back′tur·in) *n.* A vaccine prepared from the typhoid bacillus.

ty·phoid (tye′foid) *adj. & n.* 1. Resembling typhus fever, as: typhoid fever. 2. TYPHOID FE-

VER. 3. Of or pertaining to typhoid fever; typhoidal.

ty·phoid·al (tye·foy′dul) *adj.* Of or pertaining to typhoid fever.

typhoid bacillus. SALMONELLA TYPHOSA.

typhoid fever. An acute systemic infection caused by *Salmonella typhosa:* characterized clinically by fever, headache, cough, toxemia, abnormal pulse, rose spots on the skin, leukopenia, and bacteremia and pathologically by hyperplasia and ulceration of intestinal lymph follicles, mesenteric lymphadenopathy, and splenomegaly.

typhoid nodules. Characteristic lesions found in the liver after fatal typhoid.

typhoid-paratyphoid A and B vaccine. A vaccine containing organisms of typhoid, and paratyphoid A and B strains, for simultaneous immunization against all three diseases. Abbreviated, T.A.B. vaccine.

typhoid spots. ROSE SPOTS.

typhoid state. A condition of stupor and hebetude, with dry, brown tongue, sordes on the teeth, rapid, feeble pulse, incontinence of feces and urine, and rapid wasting; seen in typhoid fever and other continued fevers.

typhoid vaccine. A sterile suspension of killed typhoid bacilli (*Salmonella typhosa*) of a strain selected for high antigenic efficiency. The vaccine contains not less than 1 billion typhoid organisms in each milliliter. An active immunizing agent against typhoid fever.

ty·pho·pneu·mo·nia (tye″fo·new·mo′nyuh) *n.* PNEUMOTYPHUS.

ty·phus (tye′fus) *n.* TYPHUS FEVER.

typhus ex·an·thé·ma·tique (eg·zahn·tay·ma·teek′). EPIDEMIC TYPHUS.

typhus fever. An acute infectious disease caused by a rickettsia and characterized by severe headache, sustained high fever, generalized macular or maculopapular rash, and termination by lysis in about 2 weeks.

typ·i·cal (tip′i·kul) *adj.* 1. Constituting a characteristic type or form for comparison. 2. Illustrative. 3. Complete.

tyr-, tyro- A combining form meaning *cheese* or *cheeselike substance.*

ty·ra·mine (tye′ruh·meen) *n.* 4-Hydroxyphenethylamine, $HOC_6H_4CH_2NH_2$, a decarboxylation product of tyrosine; occurs in putrefied animal tissue, ripe cheese, and ergot. Has been used as a sympathomimetic agent. Syn. *tyrosamine.*

ty·ro·ci·dine, ty·ro·ci·din (tye″ro·sigh′din) *n.* An antibiotic substance that is a major component of tyrothricin.

Ty·rode solution A solution containing sodium chloride, calcium chloride, potassium chloride, sodium bicarbonate, glucose, magnesium chloride, and sodium diphosphate; used in certain pharmacological experiments.

ty·ro·sin·ase (tye′ro·sin·ace, ·aze, tirr′o·) *n.* A copper-containing enzyme found in plants, molds, crustaceans, mollusks, and some bacteria. In the presence of oxygen, it causes the oxidation of monophenols and polyphenols with the introduction of —OH groups and/or formation of quinones.

ty·ro·sine (tye'ro·seen, ·sin) *n.* β-*p*-Hydroxyphe-nylalanine, $C_9H_{11}NO_3$, an amino acid widely distributed in proteins; a precursor of epi-nephrine, thyroxine, and melanin.

tyro·sin·emia, tyro·si·nae·mia (tye"ro·si·nee'mee·uh) *n.* An inborn error of metabolism in which there is a deficiency of *p*-hydroxyphen-ylpyruvic acid oxidase with abnormally high blood levels of tyrosine and sometimes me-thionine, increased urinary excretion of *p*-hydroxyphenylpyruvic, acetic, and lactic acids and sometimes methionine; manifested clinically by hepatic cirrhosis, mild general-ized aminoaciduria, renal glycosuria, and re-nal rickets.

ty·ro·sin·osis (tye"ro·si·no'sis) *n.* 1. Excretion in the urine of unusual amounts of tyrosine and of its first oxidation products. 2. A transient deficiency of the enzyme *p*-hydroxyphenylpy-ruvic oxidase in early life, resulting in tyrosi-nuria as a part of a generalized aminoaciduria;

clinically similar to phenylketonuria; the in-fant may exhibit seizures, gastrointestinal dis-turbances, failure to thrive, and unless treated by diet, mental retardation.

tyro·sin·uria (tye"ro·sin·yoo'ree·uh) *n.* The pres-ence of tyrosine in the urine.

ty·ro·thri·cin (tye"ro·thrigh'sin) *n.* A polypeptide mixture produced by the growth of *Bacillus brevis* and consisting of the antibiotic sub-stances gramicidin and tyrocidine; used as an antibacterial applied locally in infections due to gram-positive organisms.

Tyz·zer's disease A fatal infection of animals due to *Actinobacillus piliformis* (*Bacillus pilifor-mis*) originally described in Japanese waltzing mice.

Tzanck test (tsaᵇn'k) The demonstration of de-generative changes in epidermal cells in bul-lae of pemphigus by microscopic examination of a smear made from the base of an early intact bulla and stained with Giemsa stain.

U

U 1. Symbol for uranium. 2. *In molecular biology*, a symbol for uracil.

U. Abbreviation for *unit*.

uber·ty (yoo'bur·tee) *n.* Fertility; productiveness. —**uber·ous** (·us) *adj.*

ubi·qui·none (yoo-bick'wi·nohn, yoo''bi·kwi·nohn') *n.* Any of a group of lipid-soluble compounds that have a 2,3-dimethoxy-5-methylbenzoquinone nucleus with a variable substituent containing 1 to 10 terpene-like units, and that function as electron carriers in the mitochondrial electron transport system. Syn. *coenzyme Q, mitoquinone.*

ud·der, *n.* The mammary gland of the cow and other animals.

Uhl's anomaly [H.S.M. *Uhl,* U.S. internist, b. 1921]. Marked congenital hypoplasia of the right atrial and ventricular myocardium. Syn. *parchment heart.*

¹ul-, ule-, ulo- A combining form meaning *scar.*

²ul-, ule-, ulo- A combining form meaning *gums, gingival.*

ula (yoo'luh) *n.pl.* GINGIVA.

ul·cer (ul'sur) *n.* An interruption of continuity of an epithelial surface, with an inflamed base.

ul·cer·ate (ul'sur·ate) *v.* To become converted into, or affected with, an ulcer.

ul·cer·a·tion (ul''sur·ay'shun) *n.* The process of formation of an ulcer.

ul·cer·a·tive (ul'sur·uh·tiv) *adj.* Pertaining to, or characterized by, ulceration.

ulcerative colitis. An inflammatory disease of unknown etiology involving primarily the mucosa and submucosa of the colon. It is peculiar to man and not contagious; manifested clinically by abdominal pain, diarrhea, and rectal bleeding.

ulcerative stomatitis. Stomatitis characterized by the formation of ulcers and necrosis of oral tissues.

ul·cero·gen·ic (ul''sur·o·jen'ick) *adj.* Tending to produce ulcers.

ul·cero·glan·du·lar (ul''sur·o·glan'dew·lur) *adj.* Tending to produce ulcers and involve lymph nodes; said of one form of tularemia.

ul·cero·mem·bra·nous (ul''sur·o·mem'bruh·nus) *adj.* Pertaining to, or characterized by, ulceration, and accompanied by fibrinous inflammation with accompanying formation of a false membrane.

ul·cer·ous (ul'sur·us) *adj.* Characterized by or pertaining to ulcers.

ul·cus (ul'kus) *n.,* pl. **ul·cera** (·sur·uh) ULCER.

ule·gy·ria (yoo''le·jye'ree·uh) *n.* Shrinkage and sclerosis of individual gyri or groups of gyri, with preservation of the general convolutional pattern of the cerebral cortex. Characteristically, there is destruction of the lower parts of the walls of the convolution, with relative sparing of the crown.

uler·y·the·ma (yoo·lerr''i·theem'uh) *n.* An erythematous skin disease marked by the formation of cicatrices.

ulet·ic (yoo·let'ick) *adj.* Pertaining to the gums.

uli·tis (yoo·lye'tis) *n.* A generalized inflammation of the gums.

Ull·rich-Turner syndrome (ōōl'ri^k^h) Webbing of the neck, short stature, cubitus valgus, and hypogonadism in the male. Syn. *male Turner's syndrome.*

ul·na (ul'nuh) *n.,* L. pl. & genit. sing. **ul·nae** (·nee) The bone on the inner side of the forearm, articulating with the humerus and the head of the radius above and with the radius below. —**ul·nar** (ul'nur) *adj.*

ulnar collateral ligament. 1. (of the elbow:) A triangular ligament on the medial side of the elbow joint attached to the medial epicondyle of the humerus, with an anterior band of fibers passing to the coronoid process of the ulna, a posterior band to the olecranon, and a transverse band connecting the olecranon and the coronoid process. 2. (of the wrist:) A ligament passing from the styloid process of the ulna to the pisiform and triquetral bones.

uloc·a·ce (yoo-lock'uh·see) *n.* Ulcerative inflammation of the gums.

ulo·der·ma·ti·tis (yoo''lo·dur'muh·tye'tis) *n.* Inflammation of the skin with formation of cicatrices.

uloid (yoo'loid) *adj.* Scarlike.

ulor·rha·gia (yoo'lo·ray'jee·uh) *n.* Bleeding from the gums.

ulot·ic (yoo·lot'ick) *adj.* Pertaining to, or tending toward, cicatrization.

ulot·o·my (yoo·lot'uh·mee) *n.* Incision into the gum.

ul·ti·mate (ul'ti·mut) *adj.* 1. Final, farthest, extreme. 2. Elemental, basic.

ul·ti·mo·bran·chi·al (ul''ti·mo·brank'ee·ul) *adj.* Pertaining to the caudal pharyngeal or branchial pouch derivatives.

ultimobranchial bodies. Bodies considered by some to be rudimentary fifth pharyngeal pouches, by others, to be lateral thyroid primordia and fourth pouch derivatives. They are the source of the cells in the thyroid gland which produce calcitonin. Syn. *postbranchial bodies, lateral thyroids.*

ul·ti·mo·gen·i·ture (ul''ti·mo·jen'i·chur) *n.* The state of being the last born. —**ultimogeni·tary** (·terr·ee) *adj.*

ultra- A prefix meaning *beyond, excess.*

ul·tra·cen·tri·fuge (ul''truh·sen'tri·fewj) *n.* A high-speed centrifuge that will produce centrifugal fields up to several hundred thousand times the force of gravity; used for the determination of particle sizes, as in proteins or viruses, and for the analysis of such materials in complex fluids as blood plasma; may be equipped with instrumentation to permit optical observation of the sedimentation of substances in solution. —**ultra·cen·trif·u·gal** (·sen·trif'yoo·gul) *adj.*

ul·tra·fil·tra·tion (ul''truh·fil·tray'shun) *n.* 1. The removal of all but the smallest particles, such as viruses, by filtration. 2. A method for the separation of colloids from their dispersion mediums and dissolved crystalloids by the use of ultrafilters.

ul·tra·mi·cro·scope (ul''truh·migh'kruh·skope) *n.* A light microscope that is equipped to detect or resolve objects not detectable with the conventional light microscopy, generally by means of dark-field microscopy. —**ultra·mi·cro·scop·i·cal** (·migh''kruh·skop'i·kul) *adj.;* **ultra·mi·cros·co·py** (·migh·kros'kuh·pee) *n.*

ul·tra·son·ic (ul''truh·son'ick) *adj.* A term, synonymous with supersonic but more commonly used than the latter in the health and life sciences, describing or pertaining to soundwave waves with a frequency above that of audible sounds, that is, above 20,000 Hz.

ul·tra·sono·gram (ul''truh·son'o·gram) *n.* ECHOGRAM.

ul·tra·so·nog·ra·phy (ul''truh·so·nog'ruh·fee) *n.* PULSE-ECHO DIAGNOSIS.

ul·tra·sono·scope (ul''truh·son'o·skope) *n.* An instrument used to detect and locate the position of regions of varying density in a medium by recording the echoes of ultrasonic waves reflected from these regions. The ultrasonic waves, modulated by pulsations, are introduced into the medium usually by means of a piezoelectric transducer.

ul·tra·sound (ul'truh·sæownd'') *n.* The energy produced by pulsing a lead zirconate, quartz, or barium titanate crystal; utilized in medicine in three ways, depending on the power levels generated: power levels below 0.1 watt per sq cm are employed for diagnostic purposes using echo reflection techniques (echogram); power levels between 1 and 3 watts per sq cm are used in the physiotherapy of various joint and muscle disorders; power levels above 5 watts per sq cm are used to destroy tissue as in treatment of cancer.

ul·tra·struc·ture (ul'truh·struck''chur) *n.* Ultramicroscopic structure; the arrangement of ultramicroscopic particles.

ul·tra·vi·o·let (ul''truh·vye'uh·lit) *adj.* Of or pertaining to electromagnetic radiation having a wavelength shorter than that at the violet end of the visible spectrum and longer than that of any x-ray. Abbreviated, UV.

um·bi·lec·to·my (um''bi·leck'tuh·mee) *n.* 1. Excision of the umbilicus. 2. An operation for the relief of umbilical hernia.

um·bil·i·cal (um·bil'i·kul) *adj.* Of or pertaining to the umbilicus.

umbilical cord. The long, cylindrical structure, invested by the amnion, containing the umbilical arteries and vein, and connecting the fetus with the placenta.

umbilical hernia. A hernia occurring through the umbilical ring, either early in life (infantile) from imperfect closure, or later (acquired) from diastasis of the rectus abdominis muscles, obesity, or muscular weakness. Syn. *annular hernia.*

umbilical region. The middle of the three median abdominal regions, below the epigastric region and above the pubic region.

umbilical ring. A dense fibrous ring surrounding the umbilicus at birth; normally the ring is obliterated by the formation of a mass of dense fibrous tissue.

umbilical souffle. FUNICULAR SOUFFLE.

um·bil·i·cate (um·bil'i·kut) *adj.* Having a depression like that of the navel.

um·bil·i·cat·ed (um·bil'i·kay·tid) *adj.* UMBILICATE.

um·bil·i·ca·tion (um·bil''i·kay'shun) *n.* 1. A depression like the navel. 2. The state of being umbilicated.

um·bil·i·cus (um·bil'i·kus, um''bi·lye'kus) *n.,* L. pl. & genit. sing. **umbili·ci** (·kigh, ·sigh) The navel; the round, depressed cicatrix in the median line of the abdomen, marking the site of the aperture that in fetal life gave passage to the umbilical vessels.

um·bo (um'bo) *n.,* pl. **um·bo·nes** (um·bo'neez), **umbos** 1. A boss or bosselation. 2. Any central convex structure.

umbo of the tympanic membrane. The projection in the center of the lateral surface of the tympanic membrane.

um·brel·la bella (um·brel'uh). IRIS BOMBÉ.

un·bal·anced, *adj.* 1. Not in equilibrium. 2. EMOTIONALLY DISTURBED.

un·cal (unk'ul) *adj.* Pertaining to the uncus (2).

un·cia (un'see·uh) *n.,* pl. **un·ci·ae** (·see·ee) OUNCE.

Un·ci·nar·ia (un''si·nair'ee·uh) *n.* A generic name formerly applied to hookworms.

un·ci·na·ri·a·sis (un''si·na·rye'uh·sis) *n.* ANCYLOSTOMIASIS.

un·ci·nate (un'si·nate) *adj.* 1. Hooked. 2. Pertaining to the uncus (2).

uncinate epilepsy. A form of epilepsy characterized by recurrent uncinate fits.

uncinate fit or **seizure.** A form of psychomotor or temporal lobe seizure announced by an aura of olfactory hallucinations that are often disagreeable, such as of something burning, and frequently followed by disturbances of consciousness and automatisms, such as smacking of the lips; usually associated with irritative lesions of the uncus and hippocampus.

un·con·di·tioned (un''kun·dish'und) *adj.* Not dependent on learning or conditioning.

un·con·ju·gat·ed bile acid (un·kon'joo·gay·tid). The residual cholic acid remaining when glycine or taurine is removed from the bile acid.

unconjugated bilirubin. Bilirubin in a form that is not combined as a glucuronate or sulfate.

un·con·scious (un·kon'shus) *adj. & n.* 1. *In psychiatry,* pertaining to behavior or experiences not controlled by the conscious ego. 2. Insensible; in a state lacking conscious awareness and with reflexes abolished. 3. The part of the mind, mental functioning, or personality not in the immediate field of awareness; the repository for data that may never have entered consciousness or which the individual may have become conscious of for a short time and then repressed. —**unconscious·ness** (·nus) *n.*

unc·tion (unk'shun) *n.* 1. The act or process of anointing. 2. OINTMENT.

unc·tu·ous (unk'choo·us) *adj.* Greasy; oily.

un·cus (unk'us) *n.,* pl. & genit. sing. **un·ci** (un'sigh) 1. HOOK. 2. The rostromedial protrusion of the gyrus parahippocampalis.

un·dec·y·len·ic acid (un·des''i·len'ick, ·lee'nick). 10-Undecenoic acid, $CH_2=CH-(CH_2)_8COOH$, an unsaturated acid present in human sweat. It has fungistatic action and is used for the treatment of fungous infections.

un·der·achiev·er (un''dur·uh·chee'vur) *n.* 1. A person who performs less well in specific areas than would be expected from certain known characteristics or a previous record. 2. Specifically, a student whose scholastic achievement falls below his measured aptitude or intelligence. —**under·achieve** (·a·cheev') *v.;* **underachieve·ment** (·munt) *n.*

un·der·weight (un''dur·wate', un'dur·wate'') *adj.* Below the normal weight range for age and height.

undescended testis. The condition in which a testis is either in the abdomen or in the inguinal canal.

un·dif·fer·en·ti·at·ed (un''dif''ur·en·shee·ay·tid) *adj.* Not differentiated.

undifferentiated–cell leukemia. STEM CELL LEUKEMIA.

undifferentiated type of schizophrenia. A form of schizophrenia with mixed symptomatology, unclassifiable as one of the more distinct types. It includes all early, as yet undifferentiated, forms at the first attack, and may be acute, appearing suddenly and disappearing within a brief period though often recurring; or chronic, not classifiable as of another type.

un·dine (un·deen', un'dine) *n.* A glass container for irrigating the eye.

un·din·ism (un'di·niz·um) *n.* Sexual excitation aroused by running water, urine, or micturition.

un·du·lant (un'dew·lunt) *adj.* Fluctuating; rising and falling like waves.

undulant fever. BRUCELLOSIS.

un·du·la·tion (un''dew·lay'shun) *n.* A wavelike motion.

un·du·la·to·ry (un'dew·luh·to''ree) *adj.* Moving like waves.

un·equal (un·ee'kwul) *adj.* Differing in size, amount, or degree.

ung. Abbreviation for *unguentum,* ointment.

un·gual (ung'gwul) *adj.* Pertaining to the nails.

un·guen·tum (ung·gwen'tum) *n.* OINTMENT. Abbreviated, **ung.**

un·guis (ung'gwis) *n.,* pl. **un·gues** (·gweez) A fingernail or toenail.

un·gu·la (ung'gew·luh) *n.,* pl. **un·gu·lae** (·lee) 1. An instrument for extracting a dead fetus. 2. A hoof; a claw.

un·gu·late (ung'gew·lut, ·late) *n. & adj.* 1. A hoofed mammal. 2. Hooved.

un·health·ful, *adj.* Injurious to health.

un·healthy (un·helth'ee) *adj.* 1. Lacking health; sickly. 2. *Colloq.* UNHEALTHFUL.

uni- A combining form meaning *one.*

uni·ar·tic·u·lar (yoo''nee·ar·tick'yoo·lur) *adj.* Pertaining to a single joint.

uni·ax·i·al (yoo''nee·ack'see·ul) *adj.* Pertaining to, on, or having one axis, as the uniaxial movement of a pivot joint.

uni·cam·er·al (yoo''ni·kam'ur·ul) *adj.* Having only one cavity or chamber.

UNICEF (yoo'ni·sef). An acronym for *United Nations International Children's Emergency Fund.*

uni·cel·lu·lar (yoo''ni·sel'yoo·lur) *adj.* Composed of one cell.

uni·cen·tric (yoo''ni·sen'trick) *adj.* Having a single center.

uni·cor·nous (yoo''ni·kor'nus) *adj.* Having one horn.

uni·cus·pid (yoo''ni·kus'pid) *adj.* Having one cusp.

uni·fa·mil·ial (yoo''ni·fuh·mil'ee·ul) *adj.* Pertaining to a single family.

uni·grav·i·da (yoo''ni·grav'i·duh) *n.* A woman who is pregnant for the first time. Syn. *primigravida.*

uni·lat·er·al (yoo''ni·lat'ur·ul) *adj.* Pertaining to, or affecting, but one side.

unilateral hermaphroditism. The form of human hermaphroditism in which the following combinations are known: an ovary on one side and a testis, testis and ovary, or two ovotestes on the other; a testis on one side and an ovotestis on the other; no gonads on one side, with an ovary and a testis on the other.

uni·lo·bar (yoo''ni·lo'bur) *adj.* Having one lobe.

uni·loc·u·lar (yoo''ni·lock'yoo·lur) *adj.* Having but one loculus or cavity.

un·in·cised (un''in·size'd') *adj.* Uncut; unopened; undrained.

u·ni·nu·cle·ar (yoo″ni·new′klee·ur) *adj.* Having a single nucleus.

u·ni·oc·u·lar (yoo″nee·ock′yoo·lur) *adj.* MONOCULAR.

un·ion (yoon′yun) *n.* 1. A joining. 2. A coming or growing together into one; specifically, the consolidation of bone fractures or the healing of a wound.

u·ni·ov·u·lar (yoo″nee·ov′yoo·lur) *adj.* Pertaining to or derived from one egg.

uniovular twins. Twins arising from a single ovum.

u·nip·a·ra (yoo·nip′uh·ruh) *n.* A woman who has borne but one child.

u·nip·a·rous (yoo·nip′uh·rus) *adj.* Bearing one offspring, or producing one ovum, at a time.

u·ni·po·lar (yoo″ni·po′lur) *adj.* 1. Having but one pole or process. 2. Pertaining to one pole.

unipolar lead. An electrocardiographic lead with the negative, or indifferent, electrode at zero potential and the voltage determined by the positive, or exploring, electrode.

u·nip·o·tent (yoo·nip′o·tunt) *adj.* Giving rise to only one cell or tissue type; said of embryonic or multiplying cells. —**u·ni·po·ten·cy** (yoo″ni·po′ten·see) *n.*; **u·ni·po·ten·tial** (·po·ten′chul) *adj.*

unit, *n.* 1. A single thing or person or a group considered as a whole. 2. A standard weight or measurement. Abbreviated, U. 3. A molecule or distinctive portion of a larger molecule.

u·ni·tar·i·an (yoo″ni·tār′ee·un) *adj.* UNITARY (1).

unitarian theory. A theory of blood-cell formation which supposes that all blood cells come from a single parental blood cell, the hemocytoblast or hematopoietic stem cell. Syn. *monophyletic theory of hemopoiesis.*

u·ni·tary (yoo′ni·terr″ee) *adj.* 1. Pertaining to, or having the qualities of, a unit. 2. Pertaining to monsters having the organs of a single individual.

United Nations International Children's Emergency Fund. An organization, often identified by the acronym UNICEF and created by and dependent on the General Assembly of the United Nations, which deals with rehabilitation of children in war-ravaged countries, with maternal and child welfare, and, where necessary, with development of a technical and health program particularly as applied to children.

United States Pharmacopeia. The pharmacopeia of the United States of America, officially recognized by the Federal Food, Drug, and Cosmetics Act. Abbreviated, U.S.P.

United States Public Health Service. The agency concerned with the development of a public-health program and the handling of health problems within the jurisdiction of the federal government. Abbreviated, USPHS.

u·ni·va·lent (yoo″ni·vay′lunt) *adj.* 1. Having a valence of one. 2. Of vaccines: effective against one specific pathogenic agent.

universal calcinosis. CALCINOSIS UNIVERSALIS.

universal donor. A blood donor of group O.

universal recipient. An individual of AB blood group.

un·my·e·li·nat·ed (un·migh′e·li·nay·tid) *adj.* Lacking a myelin sheath; especially, never having formed one.

Un·na bodies or **cells** (ōōn′ah) RUSSELL BODIES.

Unna's paste boot A sheath or casing for the leg used in treating varicose ulcers and veins by relieving venous hydrostatic pressure. A paste of zinc oxide (Unna's), gelatin, and glycerin is applied to the leg, and a bandage is placed over the paste.

un·of·fi·cial, *adj.* Describing a drug or remedy that is not included in the United States Pharmacopeia or National Formulary.

un·or·ga·nized, *adj.* 1. Without organs. 2. Not arranged in the form of an organ or organs.

un·re·al·i·ty, *n. In psychiatry,* the distorted picture that a patient may have of a situation or event of life. What he sees is not in keeping with an interpretation of the same facts by an independent observer, but has been altered by his feelings or preconceptions.

un·re·solved pneumonia. ORGANIZING PNEUMONIA.

un·rest, *n.* A state of uneasiness characterized by general body and mental tension, and sometimes excessive muscular activity.

un·sat·u·rat·ed (un·satch′uh·ray″tid) *adj.* 1. Not saturated. 2. Characterizing an organic compound having double or triple bonds.

un·sex, *v.* To remove the testes in male, or the ovaries in female, animals.

un·sound, *adj.* Unhealthy, diseased, or not properly functioning. —**un·sound·ness,** *n.*

un·spec·i·fied, *adj.* Not specific.

un·sta·ble (un·stay′bul) *adj.* 1. Movable, not fixed in position, irregular, unsteady, vacillating. 2. Insecure; changeable; specifically, characterized by emotional lability, alterations of mood, or a volatile temperament. 3. Readily decomposing, said of chemical compounds.

un·stri·at·ed (un·strye′ay·tid) *adj.* Not striated.

un·thrift·y, *adj.* Of a domestic animal: not thriving; low in body weight for its age. —**unthrift·i·ness,** *n.*

un·unit·ed (un″yoo·nigh′tid) *adj.* Not joined.

Un·ver·richt-Lund·borg disease (ōōn′feh·rikht, lu^end′bor^y) PROGRESSIVE FAMILIAL MYOCLONIC EPILEPSY.

un·well, *n.* 1. Ill; sick. 2. *Obsol. colloq.* Menstruating.

unwinding protein. A protein involved in the replication of DNA which acts by attaching to the double helix and helping to separate the strands, thus permitting duplication.

upper brachial plexus paralysis. Paralysis due to a lesion of the fifth and sixth cervical nerve roots, commonly from birth injury, and affecting chiefly the functions of the biceps, deltoid, brachialis, and brachioradialis muscles, with loss of abduction and external rotation of the arm and weak forearm flexion and supination. Sensation over the deltoid and radial surfaces of the arm and forearm may be impaired. The paralysis may be transient or permanent, depending on the degree of injury. Syn. *Erb-Duchenne paralysis.*

upper motor neuron. Any efferent neuron having its cell body in the motor cortex and connecting with the motor nuclei of the brain-stem and anterior horns of the spinal cord.

upper motor neuron lesion. An injury to the cell body or axon of an upper motor neuron, resulting in spastic paralysis of the muscle involved, hyperactive deep reflexes but diminished or absent superficial reflexes, little or no muscle atrophy, absence of reaction of degeneration, and the presence of pathological reflexes and signs. Lesions may be located in the cerebral cortex, internal capsule, cerebral peduncles, brainstem, or spinal cord, and may be due to various causes.

upper urinary tract. The kidneys and the ureters; the urinary system above the ureteral insertion into the bladder.

upper uterine segment. The upper and major portion of the uterine musculature, which actively contracts and thickens during labor.

up·right·ing. *n.* An orthodontic tipping movement to place teeth in a more vertical axial inclination.

¹ur-, uro-. A combining form meaning *urine, urinary.*

ura·chus (yoor'uh·kus) *n.* An epithelial tube or cord connecting the apex of the urinary bladder with the allantois, regarded as the stalk of the allantois or as the degenerate apex of the primitive bladder. Its connective tissue forms the median umbilical ligament. **—ura·chal** (·kul) *adj.*

ura·cil (yoor'uh·sil) *n.* 2,4(1*H*,3*H*)-Pyrimidinedione, C₄H₄N₂O₂, a pyrimidine base important mainly as a component of ribonucleic acid. Symbol, U

uracil mustard. 5-[Bis(2-chloroethyl)amino]uracil, C₈H₁₁Cl₂N₃O₂, a compound similar to nitrogen mustard (mechlorethamine hydrochloride); useful for palliative treatment of certain neoplastic diseases.

ura·cra·sia (yoor'uh·kray'see·uh, ·zee·uh) *n.* Incontinence of urine; enuresis.

ura·gogue (yoor'uh·gog) *n.* A diuretic. **—ura·gog·ic** (yoor'uh·goj'ick) *adj.*

ura·nis·cus (yoor'uh·nis'kus) *n.* PALATE.

ura·nism (yoor'uh·niz·um) *n.* HOMOSEXUALITY.

ura·ni·um (yoo·ray'nee·um) *n.* U = 238.03. A heavy metallic element, atomic weight 92, density 19.05, of the radium group; occurs as silver-white, lustrous, radioactive crystals or powder. As concentrated from its ores uranium contains 99.3% of the isotope weighing 238, 0.7% of the 235 isotope, and a negligible amount of the 234 isotope. Uranium 235 may be made to undergo fission with the release of a large amount of energy. Uranium 238 can absorb a neutron to produce uranium 239; this spontaneously loses a beta particle to form neptunium, which, in turn, loses another beta particle to form plutonium, the last also being fissionable.

ura·no·col·o·bo·ma (yoor'uh·no·kol'uh·bo' muh) *n.* Cleft hard palate, not involving the alveolar process.

ura·no·plas·ty (yoor'uh·no·plas'tee) *n.* A plastic operation for the repair of cleft palate. **—ura·no·plas·tic** (yoor'uh·no·plas'tick) *adj.*

ura·no·ple·gia (yoor'uh·no·plee'jee·uh) *n.* Paralysis of the muscles of the soft palate.

ura·nos·chi·sis (yoor'uh·nos'ki·sis) *n.* 1. Cleft hard palate. See *cleft palate.* 2. Cleft hard palate and alveolar process. Syn. *gnathopalatoschisis.*

ura·no·staph·y·lor·rha·phy (yoor'uh·no·staf'i·lor'uh·fee) *n.* Repair of a cleft in both the hard and soft palates.

ura·nyl (yoo'ruh·nil) *n.* The bivalent uranium radical UO₂²⁺, which forms salts with many acids, as, for example uranyl acetate, UO₂(C₂H₃O₂)₂.2H₂O.

ura·ro·ma (yoor'uh·ro'muh) *n.* Aromatic odor of urine.

urate (yoor'ate) *n.* A salt of uric acid. **—urat·ic** (yoo·rat'ick) *adj.*

ura·te·mia, ura·tae·mia (yoor'uh·tee'mee·uh) *n.* The presence of urates in the blood.

ura·tu·ria (yoor'uh·tew'ree·uh) *n.* The presence of urates in the urine.

urban typhus. MURINE TYPHUS.

urban yellow fever. Yellow fever transmitted from man to man by the bite of the mosquito *Aëdes aegypti.*

urea (yoo·ree'uh) *n.* Carbamide, CO(NH₂)₂, a product of protein metabolism; formerly used externally to treat infected wounds but now used mainly as a diuretic, administered orally or intravenously. **—ure·al** (·ul) *adj.*

urea clearance test. A test for kidney function in which the excretory efficiency of the kidneys is tested by the amount of blood cleared of urea in 1 minute as determined by the ratio of the blood urea to the amount of urea excreted in urine during a fixed time.

urea nitrogen. The nitrogen of urea, as distinguished from the nitrogen in the form of protein or other nitrogenous substances.

ure·ase (yoor'ee·ace, ·aze) *n.* An enzyme, obtained from jack bean, that catalyzes hydrolysis of urea to ammonia and carbon dioxide and is used in the estimation of urea.

urec·chy·sis (yoo·reck'i·sis) *n.* Extravasation of urine into the tissues.

Urecholine Chloride. Trademark for bethanechol chloride, a cholinergic drug.

ure·de·ma, uroe·de·ma (yoor'e·dee'muh) *n.* Swelling of tissues from extravasation of urine.

ure·ide (yoor'ee·ide) *n.* A compound of urea and an acid radical.

ure·mia, urae·mia (yoo·ree'mee·uh) *n.* A complex biochemical abnormality occurring in kidney failure; characterized by azotemia, chronic acidosis, anemia, and a variety of systemic and neurologic symptoms and signs. **—ure·mic, urae·mic** (·mick) *adj.*

uremic acidosis. Metabolic acidosis due to decreased renal ability to excrete acids; seen in chronic kidney disease.

uremic frost. A whitish appearance of the skin due to dried urea aggregates; seen in advanced renal failure.

ure·si·es·the·sia, ure·si·aes·the·sia (yoo·ree'see·es·theezh'uh, ·theez'ee·uh) *n.* The feeling of a need to urinate.

ure·sis (yoo·ree'sis) *n.* URINATION.

ure·ter (yoo·ree′tur, yoor′e·tur) *n.* Either of the long, narrow tubes conveying the urine from the pelvis of each kidney to the urinary bladder. —**ure·ter·al** (yoo·ree′tur·ul), **ure·ter·ic** (yoor″e·terr′ick) *adj.*

ure·ter·ec·ta·sis (yoo·ree″tur·eck′tuh·sis, yoor″e·tur·) *n.* Dilatation of a ureter.

ure·ter·ec·to·my (yoo·ree″tur·eck′tuh·mee, yoor″e·tur·) *n.* Excision of a ureter.

ureteric bud. A dorsomedial outgrowth of a mesonephric duct; the anlage of a ureter, a renal pelvis and its calyxes, and the collecting tubules of a kidney.

ure·ter·itis (yoo·ree″tur·eye′tis, yoor″e·tur·) *n.* Inflammation of a ureter.

ureteritis cys·ti·ca (sis′ti·kuh). A form of chronic ureteral inflammation in which minute cysts are formed in the epithelium.

uretero-. A combining form meaning *ureter, ureteral.*

ure·tero·cele (yoo·ree′tur·o·seel) *n.* A cyst-like dilatation at the termination of a ureter; of congenital origin or due to a narrowing of the terminal orifice.

ure·tero·ce·lec·to·my (yoo·ree″tur·o·se·leck′tuh·mee) *n.* Surgical removal of a ureterocele.

ure·tero·co·los·to·my (yoo·ree″tur·o·ko·los′tuh·mee) *n.* Implantation of a ureter, severed from the urinary bladder, into the colon.

ure·tero·cys·tic (yoo·ree″tur·o·sis′tick) *adj.* Pertaining to a ureter and the urinary bladder.

ure·tero·cys·tos·to·my (yoo·ree″tur·o·sis·tos′tuh·mee) *n.* The surgical formation of a communication between a ureter and the urinary bladder.

ure·tero·en·ter·ic (yoo·ree″tur·o·en·terr′ick) *adj.* Pertaining to, or connected with, a ureter and adjacent bowel.

ure·tero·en·ter·os·to·my (yoo·ree″tur·o·en″tur·os′tuh·mee) *adj.* Surgical formation of a passage from a ureter to some portion of the intestine.

ure·ter·og·ra·phy (yoo·ree″tur·og′ruh·fee) *n.* Radiography of the ureters after the injection of a radiopaque substance, usually through a ureteral catheter.

ure·tero·hemi·ne·phrec·to·my (yoo·ree″tur·o·hem″ee·ne·freck′tuh·mee) *n.* Surgical removal of a portion of a kidney and its ureter in cases of reduplication of ureter, pelvis, or the entire upper urinary tract.

ure·tero·hy·dro·ne·phro·sis (yoo·ree″tur·o·high″dro·ne·fro′sis) *n.* Distention of a ureter and the pelvis of its kidney, due to distal obstruction to outflow of urine.

ure·tero·il·e·al (yoo·ree″tur·o·il′ee·ul) *adj.* Pertaining to a ureter and the ileum.

ure·tero·in·tes·ti·nal (yoo·ree″tur·o·in·tes′ti·nul) *adj.* Pertaining to the ureter and the intestine.

ure·tero·lith (yoo·ree′tur·o·lith) *n.* A calculus in a ureter.

ure·ter·o·li·thi·a·sis (yoo·ree″tur·o·li·thigh′uh·sis) *n.* The presence or formation of a calculus in a ureter.

ure·tero·li·thot·o·my (yoo·ree″tur·o·li·thot′uh·mee) *n.* Incision of a ureter for removal of a calculus.

ure·ter·ol·y·sis (yoo·ree″tur·ol′i·sis) *n.* Surgical mobilization of a ureter to relieve obstruction due to kinking or external compression.

ure·tero·meg·a·ly (yoo·ree″tur·o·meg′uh·lee) *n.* Abnormal enlargement, chiefly circumferential, of the ureter.

ure·tero·neo·cys·tos·to·my (yoo·ree″tur·o·nee″o·sis·tos′tuh·mee) *n.* Surgical reimplantation of the upper end of a divided ureter into the urinary bladder.

ure·tero·neo·py·elos·to·my (yoo·ree″tur·o·nee″o·pye″e·los′tuh·mee) *n.* Suturing the distal end of a severed ureter into a new opening in the pelvis of the kidney.

ure·tero·ne·phrec·to·my (yoo·ree″tur·o·ne·freck′tuh·mee) *n.* Surgical removal of a kidney and its ureter.

ure·tero·pel·vic (yoo·ree″tur·o·pel′vick) *adj.* Pertaining to a ureter and renal pelvis.

ure·tero·pel·vio·plas·ty (yoo·ree″tur·o·pel′vee·o·plas·tee) *n.* A surgical procedure aimed at the correction of abnormalities of a ureter and renal pelvis.

ure·tero·plas·ty (yoo·ree″tur·o·plas′tee) *n.* A plastic operation on a ureter.

ure·tero·py·eli·tis (yoo·ree″tur·o·pye″e·lye′tis) *n.* Inflammation of a ureter and the pelvis of a kidney.

ure·tero·py·elog·ra·phy (yoo·ree″tur·o·pye″e·log′ruh·fee) *n.* Radiographic visualization of the upper urinary tract by the injection of a contrast medium, usually through a ureteral catheter.

ure·tero·py·elo·ne·os·to·my (yoo·ree″tur·o·pye″e·lo·nee·os′tuh·mee) *n.* Surgical formation of a new passageway from the pelvis of a kidney to its ureter.

ure·tero·py·elo·ne·phri·tis (yoo·ree″tur·o·pye″e·lo·ne·frye′tis) *n.* Inflammation of a ureter and its kidney and pelvis.

ure·tero·py·elo·ne·phros·to·my (yoo·ree″tur·o·pye″e·lo·ne·fros′tuh·mee) *n.* Surgical anastomosis of the ureter with the pelvis of its kidney.

ure·tero·py·elo·plas·ty (yoo·ree″tur·o·pye″e·lo·plas·tee) *n.* Any plastic operation involving the upper portion of a ureter and the adjacent pelvis of the kidney.

ure·tero·py·elos·to·my (yoo·ree″tur·o·pye″e·los′tuh·mee) *n.* Surgical excision of part of a ureter and implantation of the remaining part into a new aperture made into the pelvis of the kidney.

ure·ter·or·rha·gia (yoo·ree″tur·o·ray′jee·uh) *n.* Hemorrhage from a ureter.

ure·ter·or·rha·phy (yoo·ree″tur·or′uh·fee) *n.* Surgical suture of a ureter.

ure·tero·sig·moid·os·to·my (yoo·ree″tur·o·sig″moy·dos′tuh·mee) *n.* Surgical implantation of a ureter, severed from the urinary bladder, into the sigmoid colon.

ure·ter·os·to·my (yoo·ree″tur·os′tuh·mee) *n.* Transplantation of a ureter to the skin; the formation of an external ureteral fistula.

ure·ter·ot·o·my (yoo·ree″tur·ot′uh·mee) *n.* Surgical incision of a ureter.

ure·tero·ure·ter·al (yoo·ree″tur·o·yoo·ree′tur·al) *adj.* Pertaining to both ureters, or to two parts of one ureter, as ureteroureteral anastomosis.

ure·tero·ure·ter·os·to·my (yoo·ree″tur·o·yoo·ree″tur·os′tuh·mee) n. Surgical formation of a passage between the ureters or between different parts of the same ureter.

ure·tero·uter·ine (yoo·ree″tur·o·yoo′tur·ine) adj. Pertaining to the ureters and the uterus.

ure·tero·va·gi·nal (yoo·ree″tur·o·vaj′i·nul, ·va·jye′nul) adj. Pertaining to the ureters and the vagina.

ure·tero·ves·i·cal (yoo·ree″tur·o·ves′i·kul) adj. Pertaining to the ureters and the urinary bladder.

ure·tero·ves·i·co·pexy (yoo·ree″tur·o·ves′i·ko·peck″see) n. Fixation of the distal ureter along and outside the posterior wall of the urinary bladder, for correction of vesicoureteral reflux in children.

ure·than (yoor′e·than) n. 1. Ethyl carbamate, $NH_2COOC_2H_5$; has been used as a hypnotic and as a neoplastic suppressant drug. 2. Any ester of carbamic acid.

ure·thane (yoor′e·thane) n. URETHAN.

ure·thra (yoo·ree′thruh) n., L. pl. & genit. sing. **ure·thrae** (·three) The canal through which the urine is discharged, extending from the neck of the urinary bladder to the external urethral orifice, divided in the male into the prostatic portion, the membranous portion, and the spongy or penile portion, and 8 to 9 inches long. (See Plate 25.) In the female, it is about 1½ inches in length. (See Plates 23, 24.) —**ure·thral** (·thrul) adj.

urethral caruncle. A small, red, benign, inflammatory, tender mass on the posterior wall of the female urethral meatus.

urethral glands. Small, branched, tubular mucous glands in the mucous membrane of the urethra. Syn. Littré's glands.

ure·threc·to·my (yoor″e·threck′tuh·mee) n. Surgical excision of the urethra or portion of it.

ure·thri·tis (yoor″e·thrye′tis) n., pl. **ure·thrit·i·des** (·thrit′i·deez) Inflammation of the urethra.

urethritis cys·ti·ca (sis′ti·kuh). Urethral inflammation characterized by submucosal cyst formation.

ure·thro·bul·bar (yoo·ree″thro·bul′bur) adj. Pertaining to the urethra and the bulb of the corpus spongiosum penis.

ure·thro·cele (yoo·ree′thro·seel) n. A urethral protrusion or diverticulum occurring, usually, in the female urethra.

ure·thro·cu·ta·ne·ous (yoo·ree″thro·kew·tay′ne·us) adj. Pertaining to the urethra and the skin.

ure·thro·cys·ti·tis (yoo·ree″thro·sis·tye′tis) n. Inflammation of the urethra and urinary bladder.

ure·thro·cys·to·cele (yoo·ree″thro·sis′to·seel) n. A herniation of the urethra and urinary bladder into the vagina.

ure·thro·gram (yoo·ree′thro·gram) n. A radiographic visualization of the urethra by the use of a contrast medium.

ure·thro·graph (yoo·ree′thro·graf) n. A recording urethrometer.

ure·throg·ra·phy (yoor″e·throg′ruh·fee) n. Radiography of the urethra employing an opaque contrast substance.

ure·throm·e·ter (yoor″e·throm′e·tur) n. An instrument for determining the caliber of the urethra or for measuring the lumen of a urethral stricture.

ure·thro·per·i·ne·al (yoo·ree″thro·perr″i·nee′ul) adj. Pertaining to, or involving, both the perineum and the urethra.

ure·thro·plas·ty (yoo·ree′thro·plas″tee) n. A plastic operation upon the urethra; surgical repair of the urethra.

ure·thro·pros·tat·ic (yoo·ree″thro·pros·tat′ick) adj. Relating to the urethra and the prostate.

ure·thro·rec·tal (yoo·ree″thro·reck′tul) adj. Involving both the urethra and the rectum.

ure·thror·rha·phy (yoo″e·thror′uh·fee) n. Surgical restoration of the continuity of the urethra.

ure·thror·rhea, ure·thror·rhoea (yoo·ree″thro·ree′uh) n. A discharge from the urethra.

ure·thro·scope (yoo·ree′thruh·skope) n. An instrument for inspecting the interior of the urethra. —**ure·thro·scop·ic** (yoo·ree″thruh·skop′ick) adj.

ure·thros·co·py (yoor″e·thros′kuh·pee) n. Inspection of the urethra with the aid of the urethroscope.

ure·thro·spasm (yoo·ree′thro·spaz·um) n. Spasmodic contraction of the urethral sphincter.

ure·thro·ste·no·sis (yoo·ree″thro·ste·no′sis) n. Stricture of the urethra.

ure·thros·to·my (yoor″e·thros′tuh·mee) n. A fistula created between the penile or perineal skin with some portion of the anterior urethra.

ure·thro·tome (yoo·ree′thruh·tome) n. An instrument used for performing an internal urethrotomy.

ure·throt·o·my (yoor″e·throt′uh·mee) n. The operation of cutting a stricture of the urethra.

ure·thro·tri·go·ni·tis (yoo·ree″thro·trye″go·nigh′tis) n. Inflammation of the trigone of the urinary bladder, usually the anterior segment, and the adjacent urethra.

ure·thro·va·gi·nal (yoo·ree″thro·vaj′i·nul, ·va·jye′nul) adj. Pertaining to the urethra and the vagina.

ure·thro·ves·i·cal (yoo·ree″thro·ves′i·kul) adj. Pertaining to the urethra and the urinary bladder.

ure·thro·ves·i·co·va·gi·nal (yoo·ree″thro·ves″i·ko·va·jye′nul, ·vaj′i·nul) adj. Pertaining to the urethra, urinary bladder, and vagina.

ur·gen·cy (ur′jun·see) n. Urgent desire to empty the urinary bladder.

ur·hi·dro·sis (yoor″hi·dro′sis) n. Excretion in the sweat of some of the constituents of the urine, chiefly urea, in excess of normal, as in uremia.

-uria A combining form designating (a) a (specified) condition of urine; (b) the presence of a (specified) substance in urine.

uric (yoor′ick) adj. Pertaining to the urine.

uric acid. 2,6,8-Trioxypurine, $C_5H_4N_4O_3$, a product of protein metabolism; present in blood and urine.

uric·ac·i·de·mia, uric·ac·i·dae·mia (yoor″ick·as″i·dee′mee·uh) n. HYPERURICEMIA.

uric·ac·i·du·ria (yoor″ick·as″i·dew′ree·uh) n. The presence of excessive amounts of uric acid in the urine.

uri·can·i·case (yoor″i·kan′i·kace, ·kaze) n. An

enzyme in the liver that catalyzes conversion of urocanic acid to *l*-glutamic acid.

uri·ce·mia, uri·cae·mia (yoor″i·see′mee·uh) *n.* HYPERURICEMIA.

uri·col·y·sis (yoor″i·kol′i·sis) *n.* The disintegration of uric acid.

uri·co·su·ria (yoor″i·ko·sue′ree·uh) *n.* Urinary excretion of uric acid.

uri·co·su·ric (yoo″ri·ko·sue′rick) *adj. & n.* 1. Promoting or relating to uricosuria. 2. A drug or substance that promotes uricosuria.

uri·dine (yoor′i·deen, ·din) *n.* Uracil riboside, $C_9H_{12}N_2O_6$, a nucleoside composed of one molecule each of uracil and D-ribose. One of the four main riboside components of ribonucleic acid.

urin-, urino-. A combining form meaning *urine.*

uri·nal (yoor′i·nul) *n.* A vessel for receiving urine.

uri·nal·y·sis (yoor″i·nal′i·sis) *n.* Analysis of the urine; in routine examination, this involves chemical, physical, and microscopical tests.

uri·nary (yoor′i·nerr·ee) *adj.* 1. Of or pertaining to urine. 2. Pertaining to, part of, in, or associated with the urinary system.

urinary abscess. An abscess resulting from extravasation of urine.

urinary infiltration. Passage of urine into tissue spaces, as into tissues of the perineum following rupture of the urethra or the urinary bladder.

urinary reflex. VESICAL REFLEX.

urinary sediment. Sediment consisting of the formed elements in urine, including casts, epithelial cells, erythrocytes, leukocytes, mucous threads, and spermatozoa.

urinary stammering. *Obsol.* STAMMERING BLADDER.

urinary stuttering. *Obsol.* STAMMERING BLADDER.

urinary system. The system made up of the kidneys, ureters, urinary bladder, and urethra, whose function is the elaboration and excretion of urine.

uri·nate (yoor′i·nate) *v.* To discharge urine from the bladder. —**uri·na·tion** (yoor″i·nay′shun) *n.*

uri·na·tive (yoor′i·nay″tiv) *n.* A drug that stimulates the flow of urine; a diuretic.

urine (yoor′in) *n.* The fluid excreted by the kidneys. In health, urine has an amber color, a slightly acid reaction, a faint odor, a saline taste, and a specific gravity of 1.005 to 1.030. The quantity excreted in 24 hours varies with the amount of fluids consumed but averages between 1,000 and 1,500 ml. The amount of solids in the urine varies with the diet, more being excreted on a high-protein, high-salt diet. Normally between 40 to 75 g of solids are present in the 24-hour urine, of which approximately 25% is urea, 25% chlorides, 25% sulfates and phosphates, and the remainder organic substances including organic acids, pigments, neutral sulfur, hormones. The most important abnormal constituents present in disease are protein, sugar, blood, pus, acetone, diacetic acid, fat, chyle, tube casts, various cells, and bacteria.

uri·nif·er·ous (yoor″i·nif′ur·us) *adj.* Carrying or conveying urine.

uriniferous tubule. One of the numerous winding tubules of the kidney.

uri·nif·ic (yoor″i·nif′ick) *adj.* Excreting or producing urine.

uri·nip·a·rous (yoor″i·nip′uh·rus) *adj.* Producing urine.

uri·no·ma (yoor″i·no′muh) *n.,* pl. **urinomas, uri·no·ma·ta** (·tuh) A cyst containing urine.

uri·nom·e·ter (yoor″i·nom′e·tur) *n.* A hydrometer for measuring the specific gravity of urine.

uri·nom·e·try (yoor″i·nom′e·tree) *n.* The determination of the specific gravity of urine.

uri·nous (yoor′i·nus) *adj.* Having the characteristics of urine.

uri·po·sia (yoor″i·po′see·uh) *n.* The drinking of urine.

uri·sol·vent (yoor″i·sol′vunt) *adj.* Dissolving uric acid.

ur·ning (oor′ning) *n.* A male homosexual.

uro·bi·lin (yoor″o·bye′lin, ·bil′in) *n.* A bile pigment produced by reduction of bilirubin by intestinal bacteria, with intermediate formation of urobilinogen, and excreted by the kidneys or removed by the liver.

uro·bi·lin·emia, uro·bi·lin·aemia (yoor″o·bye″li·nee′mee·uh, ·bil′i·) *n.* The presence of urobilin in the blood.

uro·bi·lino·gen (yoor″o·bye·lin′o·jen) *n.* A chromogen, formed in feces and present in urine, from which urobilin is formed by oxidation.

uro·bi·lino·gen·uria (yoor″o·bye·lin″o·je·new′ree·uh) *n.* 1. An excess of urobilinogen in the urine. 2. Urobilinogen in the urine.

uro·bi·lin·oi·din (yoor″o·bye″li·noy′din) *n.* A form of urinary pigment derived from hematin and resembling urobilin though not identical with it.

uro·bi·lin·uria (yoor″o·bye″li·new′ree·uh, ·bil′i·) *n.* The presence of an excess of urobilin in urine.

uro·che·sia (yoor″o·kee′zhuh, ·zee·uh) *n.* Discharge of urine through the anus.

uro·chrome (yoor′o·krome) *n.* A yellow pigment in urine.

uro·chro·mo·gen (yoor″o·kro′muh·jen) *n.* A substance occurring in tissues, which is oxidized to urochrome.

uro·clep·sia (yoor″o·klep′see·uh) *n.* Involuntary or unconscious urination.

uro·cris·ia (yoor″o·kriz′ee·uh, ·kris′ee·uh) *n.* Diagnosis by means of urinary examination and analysis.

uro·cri·sis (yoo″ro·krye′sis) *n.* 1. Painful spasms of the urinary tract in tabes dorsalis. 2. The critical stage of a disease distinguished by the excretion of a large volume of urine.

uro·cy·an·o·gen (yoor″o·sigh·an′o·jin) *n.* A blue pigment found in urine.

uro·cy·a·no·sis (yoor″o·sigh″uh·no′sis) *n.* Blue discoloration of the urine, usually from the presence of excess amounts of indican oxidized to indigo blue; also from drugs such as methylene blue.

uro·dy·nam·ics (yoor″o·dye·nam′icks) *n.* The study of the forces responsible for moving urine along the urinary tract; urinary tract hydrodynamics.

uro·er·y·thrin (yoor″o·err′i·thrin) *n.* A red pigment found in urine.

uro·fla·vin (yoor″o·flay′vin) *n.* A fluorescent compound of unknown structure, with properties similar to riboflavin, excreted in the urine along with the vitamin, following ingestion of riboflavin.

uro·fus·cin (yoor″o·fus′in) *n.* A pigment found occasionally in urine in cases of porphyrinuria.

uro·fus·co·hem·a·tin, uro·fus·co·haem·a·tin (yoor″o·fus′ko·hem′uh·tin) *n.* A red pigment derived from hematin, occurring in the urine.

uro·gas·trone (yoor′o·gas′trone) *n.* A substance extracted from urine which inhibits gastric secretion.

uro·gen·i·tal (yoor″o·jen′i·tul) *adj.* Pertaining to the urinary and genital organs.

urogenital diaphragm. The sheet of tissue stretching across the pubic arch, formed by the deep transverse perineal and the sphincter urethrae muscles. Syn. *triangular ligament, trigonium urogenitale.*

urogenital duct. 1. The male urethra from the orifices of the ejaculatory ducts to the fossa navicularis. 2. In certain vertebrates, the mesonephric duct.

urogenital system. The combined urinary and genital systems, which are intimately related embryologically and anatomically.

urog·e·nous (yoo·roj′e·nus) *adj.* Producing urine; derived from urine.

uro·glau·cin (yoor″o·glaw′sin) *n.* A blue pigment sometimes occurring in urine.

uro·gram (yoor′o·gram) *n.* A radiograph or radiographic visualization of the urinary tract made after intravenous or retrograde injection of an opaque contrast medium.

urog·ra·phy (yoo·rog′ruh·fee) *n.* Radiographic visualization of the urinary tract by the use of a contrast medium.

uro·hem·a·tin, uro·haem·a·tin (yoor″o·hem′uh·tin, ·hee′muh·tin) *n.* Hematin in the urine.

uro·hem·a·to·ne·phro·sis, uro·haem·a·to·ne·phro·sis (yoor″o·hem″uh·to·ne·fro′sis, ·hee″muh·to·) *n.* Distention of the pelvis of a kidney with blood and urine.

uro·hem·a·to·por·phy·rin, uro·haem·a·to·por·phy·rin (yoor″o·hem″uh·to·por′fi·rin, ·hee″muh·to·) *n.* Hematoporphyrin, occasionally occurring in urine in certain pathologic states.

uro·ki·nase (yoor″o·kigh′nace, ·kin′aze) *n.* An enzyme, present in human urine, that catalyzes conversion of the active proteolytic enzyme plasmin. It produces lysis of blood clots and has therapeutic utility as a thrombolytic (fibrinolytic) agent.

uro·ki·net·ic (yoor″o·ki·net′ick, ·kigh·net′ick) *adj.* Caused by a reflex from the urinary system; generally denotes indigestion secondary to irritation or disease of the urinary tract.

uro·leu·kin·ic acid (yoor″o·lew·kin′ick). An acid found in the urine in alkaptonuria.

uro·lith (yoor′o·lith) *n.* A calculus occurring in urine. —**uro·lith·ic** (yoor″o·lith′ick) *adj.*

uro·li·thi·a·sis (yoor″o·li·thigh′uh·sis) *n.* 1. The presence of, or a condition associated with, urinary calculi. 2. The formation of urinary calculi.

uro·li·thot·o·my (yoor″o·li·thot′uh·mee) *n.* Removal of a calculus from anywhere in the urinary tract.

urol·o·gist (yoo·rol′uh·jist) *n.* A person skilled in urology; a specialist in the diagnosis and treatment of diseases of the urogenital tract in the male and the urinary tract in the female. Syn. *genitourinary surgeon.*

urol·o·gy (yoo·rol′uh·jee) *n.* 1. The branch of medical science embracing the study and treatment of the diseases and the abnormalities of the urogenital tract in the male and the urinary tract in the female. 2. The scientific study of the urine. —**uro·log·ic** (yoor″o·loj′ick) *adj.*

uro·lu·te·in (yoor″o·lew′tee·in) *n.* A yellow pigment sometimes found in urine.

uro·mel·a·nin (yoo″ro·mel′uh·nin) *n.* A black pigment that sometimes appears in urine as a decomposition product of urochrome.

urom·e·ter (yoo·rom′e·tur) *n.* URINOMETER.

uron-, urono- A combining form meaning *urine, urinary.*

uron·on·com·e·try (yoor″on·ong·kom′e·tree) *n.* Measurement of the quantity of urine passed or excreted in a definite period, as 24 hours.

uro·nos·co·py (yoor″o·nos′kuh·pee) *n.* Examination of urine by inspection and use of the microscope.

urop·a·thy (yoo·rop′uth·ee) *n.* Any disease involving the urinary tract.

uro·pep·sin (yoor″o·pep′sin) *n.* The urinary end product of the secretion of pepsinogen into the bloodstream by gastric cells, followed by transport to the kidneys and excretion in urine.

uro·phe·in (yoor″o·fee′in) *n.* A gray pigment found in urine.

uro·pla·nia (yoor″o·play′nee·uh) *n.* The presence of urine elsewhere than in the urinary organs; discharge of urine from an orifice other than the urethra.

uro·poi·e·sis (yoor″o·poy·e′sis) *n.* The production of urine.

uro·por·phy·rin (yoor″o·por′fi·rin) *n.* Any of several isomeric, metal-free porphyrins, occurring in small amounts in normal urine and feces, characterized by having as substituents four acetic acid ($-CH_2COOH$) and four propionic acid ($-CH_2CH_2COOH$) groups.

uro·rec·tal (yoor″o·reck′tul) *adj.* Pertaining to the urinary organs and the rectum.

uro·ro·se·in (yoor″o·ro′zee·in) *n.* A urinary pigment that does not occur preformed in the urine, but is present in the form of a chromogen, indoleacetic acid, which is transformed into the pigment upon treatment with a mineral acid. It is said to be identical with urorrhodin.

uror·rha·gia (yoor″o·ray′jee·uh) *n.* Excessive discharge of urine, as in diabetes insipidus.

uror·rho·din, uror·rho·din (yoor″o·ro′din) *n.* A red pigment found in urine and derived from uroxanthin.

uror·rho·dino·gen (yoor″o·ro·din′uh·jen) *n.* The

chromogen which by decomposition produces urorrhodin.

uro·ru·bin (yoor''o·roo'bin) *n.* A red pigment found in urine, seen only in disease.

uros·che·sis (yoo·ros'ke·sis) *n.* Urinary retention.

uros·co·py (yoo·ros'kuh·pee) *n.* Examination of urine; URONOSCOPY. —**uro·scop·ic** (yoor''o·skop'ick) *adj.*

uro·se·mi·ol·o·gy (yoor''o·sem''ee·ol'uh·jee) *n.* Examination of the urine as an aid to diagnosis.

uro·sep·sis (yoor''o·sep'sis) *n.* Systemic toxicity from extravasated urine.

uro·spec·trin (yoor''o·speck'trin) *n.* A pigment of normal urine.

uro·ste·a·lith (yoor''o·stee'uh·lith) *n.* A fatlike substance occurring in some urinary calculi.

uro·the·li·um (yoor''o·theel'ee·um) *n.* The epithelium of the urinary tract. —**urotheli·al** (·ul) *adj.*

uro·tox·ic (yoor''o·tock'sick) *adj.* 1. Pertaining to poisonous substances eliminated in urine. 2. Pertaining to poisoning by urine or some of its constituents.

uro·tox·ic·i·ty (yoor''o·tock·sis'i·tee) *n.* The toxic properties of urine.

uro·xan·thin (yoor''o·zan'thin) *n.* A yellow pigment in human urine which yields indigo blue on oxidation.

ur·ti·cant (ur'ti·kunt) *n.* Something that produces urticaria.

ur·ti·car·i·a (ur''ti·kār'ee·uh) *n.* Hives or nettle rash. A skin condition characterized by the appearance of intensely itching wheals or welts with elevated, usually white, centers and a surrounding area of erythema. They appear in crops, widely distributed over the body surface, tend to disappear in a day or two, and usually are unattended by constitutional symptoms. —**urticar·i·al** (·ee·ul) *adj.*

urticaria bul·lo·sa (buh·lo'suh, bŏŏl·o'suh). Urticaria with the formation of fluid-filled vesicles or bullae on the surface of the wheals.

urticaria med·i·ca·men·to·sa (med''i·kuh·men·to'suh). Urticaria due to the ingestion of a drug to which the individual is allergic.

urticaria pap·u·lo·sa (pap''yoo·lo'suh). An intensely pruritic skin eruption seen in children, characterized by recurrent crops of erythematous patches and papules on the extensor surfaces of the extremities; it is related to insect bites. Syn. *lichen urticatus, prurigo simplex.*

urticaria pig·men·to·sa (pig''men·to'suh). A disease involving mast cells and occurring in several different forms. There are cutaneous manifestations of urticaria in a form affecting children and one affecting adults, and there is a systemic form usually without skin lesions. The skin manifestations have a variety of appearances, ranging from innumerable brown macules to solitary red-brown nodules; urtication occurs on stroking the lesions.

urticaria so·la·ris (so·lair'is). Urticaria occurring in certain individuals due to exposure to sunlight.

ur·ti·car·i·o·gen·ic (ur''ti·kār''ee·o·jen'ick) *adj.* Producing urticaria.

ur·ti·cate (ur'ti·kate, ·kut) *adj. & v.* 1. Characterized by the presence of wheals. 2. To produce urticaria or urtication (1).

ur·ti·ca·tion (ur''ti·kay'shun) *n.* 1. A sensation as if one had been stung by nettles. 2. Production of wheals.

uru·shi·ol (uh·roo'shee·ol) *n.* The irritant fraction of poison ivy and poison oak, consisting of derivatives of catechol with an unsaturated 15-carbon side chain.

U.S.P. Abbreviation for *United States Pharmacopeia.*

USPHS Abbreviation for *United States Public Health Service.*

us·ti·lag·i·nism (us''ti·laj'i·niz·um) *n.* A condition resembling ergot poisoning; caused by eating corn containing the fungus *Ustilago maydis.*

Us·ti·la·go (us''ti·lay'go) *n.* A genus of parasitic fungi; the smuts.

us·tion (us'chun) *n. In surgery,* CAUTERIZATION.

uta (oo'tah) *n.* A form of American mucocutaneous leishmaniasis, consisting of single or multiple skin ulcers of the nose and lips. It occurs in cool climates and at altitudes over 600 m. The etiologic agent is *Leishmania brasiliensis.*

uter-, utero-. A combining form meaning *uterus. uterine.*

uter·al·gia (yoo''tur·al'jee·uh) *n.* Pain in the uterus.

uter·ine (yoo'tur·in, yoo'tuh·rine) *adj.* Pertaining to the uterus.

uterine apoplexy. Massive infiltration of blood into the myometrium of the pregnant uterus, subsequent to premature separation of the placenta.

uterine inertia. *In obstetrics,* the diminution or cessation of uterine contractions during labor.

uterine souffle. A soft, blowing sound, synchronous with the maternal heart, heard over the abdomen at the sides of the uterus. The sound is due to the circulation of the blood in the large uterine arteries and veins. Its value as a diagnostic sign of pregnancy is doubtful.

uterine tube. The oviduct in mammals. Syn. *fallopian tube.*

uter·is·mus (yoo''tur·iz'mus) *n.* Uterine contraction of a spasmodic and painful character.

uter·i·tis (yoo''tur·eye'tis) *n.* Inflammation of the uterus; METRITIS.

utero·ab·dom·i·nal (yoo''tur·o·ab·dom'i·nul) *adj.* Pertaining to the uterus and the abdomen.

uteroabdominal pregnancy. Gestation with one fetus in the uterus and another within the peritoneal cavity.

utero·ad·nex·al (yoo''tur·o·ad·neck'sul) *adj.* Pertaining to the uterus and its tubes and ovaries.

utero·cer·vi·cal (yoo''tur·o·sur'vi·kul) *adj.* Pertaining to the uterus and the cervix of the uterus.

utero·co·lic (yoo''tur·o·ko'lick, ·kol'ick) *adj.* Pertaining to the uterus and the colon.

utero·en·ter·ic (yoo''tur·o·en·terr'ick) *adj.* UTEROINTESTINAL.

utero·ges·ta·tion (yoo''tur·o·jes·tay'shun) *n.* Gestation within the cavity of the uterus; normal pregnancy.

uter·og·ra·phy (yoo''tur·og'ruh·fee) *n.* Radiographic visualization of the uterine cavity by means of contrast medium injected therein through the cervical canal; metrography, hysterography.

utero·in·tes·ti·nal (yoo″tur-o-in-tes′ti-nul) *adj.* Pertaining to the uterus and the intestine.

uter·om·e·ter (yoo″tur-om′e-tur) *n.* An instrument used to measure the uterus.

utero·ovar·i·an (yoo″tur-o-o-vār′ee-un) *adj.* Pertaining to the uterus and the ovaries.

utero-ovarian pregnancy. Gestation with one fetus in the uterus and another in the ovary.

utero-ovarian varicocele. A varicose condition of the veins of the pampiniform plexus in the broad ligament.

utero·pa·ri·e·tal (yoo″tur-o-puh-rye′e-tul) *adj.* Pertaining to the uterus and the abdominal wall.

utero·pel·vic (yoo″tur-o-pel′vick) *adj.* Pertaining to the uterus and the pelvic ligaments.

utero·pexy (yoo′tur-o-peck″see) *n.* HYSTEROPEXY.

utero·pla·cen·tal (yoo″tur-o-pluh-sen′tul) *adj.* Pertaining to the uterus and the placenta.

uteroplacental apoplexy. COUVELAIRE UTERUS.

utero·plas·ty (yoo′tur-o-plas″tee) *n.* A plastic operation on the uterus.

utero·rec·tal (yoo″tur-o-reck′tul) *adj.* Pertaining to the uterus and the rectum.

utero·sa·cral (yoo″tur-o-say′krul) *adj.* Pertaining to the uterus and the sacrum.

utero·sal·pin·gog·ra·phy (yoo″tur-o-sal″pin-gog′ruh-fee) *n.* HYSTEROSALPINGOGRAPHY.

utero·scope (yoo′tur-o-skope) *n.* A uterine speculum.

uter·ot·o·my (yoo″tur-ot′uh-mee) *n.* HYSTEROTOMY.

utero·ton·ic (yoo″tur-o-ton′ick) *adj.* Increasing muscular tone of the uterus.

utero·trac·tor (yoo″tur-o-track′tur) *n.* 1. A uterine tenaculum or volsella forceps. 2. A wide, heavy, sharp-toothed retractor used to make continuous traction on the anterior portion of the cervix of the uterus during surgery.

utero·tu·bal (yoo″tur-o-tew′bul) *adj.* Pertaining to the uterus and the oviducts.

uterotubal pregnancy. Gestation with one fetus in the uterus and another in an oviduct.

utero·va·gi·nal (yoo″tur-o-va-jye′nul, -vaj′i-nul) *adj.* Pertaining to the uterus and vagina.

utero·ven·tral (yoo″tur-o-ven′trul) *adj.* Pertaining to the uterus and the abdomen.

utero·ves·i·cal (yoo″tur-o-ves′i-kul) *adj.* Pertaining to the uterus and the urinary bladder.

uter·us (yoo′tur-us) *n.*, pl. & genit. sing. **uteri** (yoo′tur-eye) The womb; the organ of gestation which receives and holds the fertilized ovum during the development of the fetus, and becomes the principal agent in its expulsion during parturition.

uterus acol·lis (a-kol′is). A uterus in which the vaginal part of the cervix is abnormally small or absent.

uterus ar·cu·a·tus (ahr-kew-ay′tus). A subvariety of uterus bicornis in which there is merely a vertical depression in the middle of the fundus uteri.

uterus bi·cor·nis (bye-kor′nis). 1. A human

uterus divided into two horns or compartments due to an arrest of development. 2. The normal uterus in many mammals, as carnivores.

uterus bi·loc·u·la·ris (bye-lock″yoo-lair′is). UTERUS SEPTUS.

uterus di·del·phys (dye-del′fis). UTERUS DUPLEX.

uterus du·plex (dew′plecks). A uterus that is double from failure of the paramesonephric ducts to unite.

uterus mas·cu·li·nus (mas-kew-lye′nus). UTRICLE (2).

uterus par·vi·col·lis (pahr-vi-kol′is). A malformation in which the vaginal portion of the uterus is small but the body is normal.

uterus sep·tus (sep′tus). A uterus in which a median septum more or less completely divides the lumen into halves.

uterus uni·cor·nis (yoo-ni-kor′nis). A uterus having but a single lateral half with usually only one uterine tube; it is the result of faulty development.

utri·cle (yoo′tri-kul) *n.* 1. A delicate membranous sac communicating with the semicircular canals of the ear. 2. The uterus masculinus, or prostatic utricle; a vestigial blind pouch in the colliculus seminalis opening into the prostatic urethra. The homolog of a part of the female vagina; derived from the fused distal ends of the paramesonephric ducts. Syn. *utriculus masculinus, sinus pocularis.* —**utric·u·lar** (yoo-trick′yoo-lur) *adj.*

utric·u·li·tis (yoo-trick″yoo-lye′tis) *n.* 1. Inflammation of the prostatic utricle. 2. Inflammation of the utricle of the ear.

utric·u·lo·sac·cu·lar (yoo-trick″yoo-lo-sack′yoo-lur) *adj.* Pertaining to the utricle and saccule of the ear.

utri·cu·lus (yoo-trick′yoo-lus) *n.*, pl. **utricu·li** (·lye) UTRICLE.

UV Abbreviation for *ultraviolet.*

uvea (yoo′vee-uh) *n.* The pigmented, vascular layer of the eye, the iris, ciliary body, and choroid. —**uve·al** (·ul) *adj.*

uveal tract. The iris, ciliary body, and choroid.

uve·itis (yoo″vee-eye′tis) *n.* Inflammation of the uvea. —**uve·it·ic** (·it′ick) *adj.*

uveo·me·nin·go·en·ceph·a·li·tis (yoo″vee-o-me-nin″go-en-sef″uh-lye′tis) *n.* A syndrome of unknown cause, characterized by severe bilateral nontraumatic uveitis, meningoencephalitis of varying severity with increased cells and protein in the cerebrospinal fluid, poliosis and patchy vitiligo most often distributed symmetrically, and dysacousia in a high percentage of patients; usually observed in young adults. Syn. *Vogt-Koyanagi-Harada syndrome.*

uveo·par·otid (yoo″vee-o-puh-rot′id) *adj.* Pertaining to the uvea and the parotid gland.

uveoparotid fever. A manifestation of sarcoidosis consisting of uveitis, parotitis, and fever. Syn. *Heerfordt's disease, uveoparotitis.*

uveo·par·o·ti·tis (yoo″vee-o-păr″o-tye′tis) *n.* UVEOPAROTID FEVER.

uvu·la (yoo′vew-luh) *n.*, genit. **uvu·lae** (·lee) The conical appendix hanging from the free edge of the soft palate, containing the uvular muscle covered by mucous membrane. **—uvu·lar** (·lur) *adj.*

uvu·lec·to·my (yoo″vew·leck′tuh·mee) *n.* Surgical resection of the uvula.

uvu·li·tis (yoo″vew·lye′tis) *n.* Inflammation of the uvula.

uvu·lo·nod·u·lar (yoo″vew·lo·nod′yoo·lur) *adj.* Pertaining to the uvula and the nodulus of the cerebellum.

uvu·lop·to·sis (yoo″vew·lop·to′sis, ·lop′tuh·sis) *n.* A relaxed and pendulous condition of the uvula.

uvu·lo·tome, uvu·la·tome (yoo′vew·luh·tome) *n.* An instrument used in uvulotomy.

uvu·lot·o·my (yoo″vew·lot′uh·mee) *n.* UVULEC-TOMY.

U wave of the electrocardiogram. A deflection, usually of low amplitude, following the T wave. It is often absent normally; its cause and significance are not certain.

V

V Symbol for vanadium.

v Abbreviation for *volt*.

vac·ci·na·ble (vack'si·nuh·bul) *adj.* Susceptible of successful vaccination.

vac·ci·nal (vack'si·nul) *adj.* Pertaining to vaccination or to vaccine.

vac·ci·nate (vack'si·nate) *v.* 1. To administer vaccine to produce immunity. 2. To inoculate to produce immunity to smallpox.

vac·ci·na·tion (vack''si·nay'shun) *n.* 1. Inoculation with the virus of vaccinia in order to protect against smallpox. 2. The inoculation or ingestion of organisms or antigens to produce immunity in the recipient.

vac·cine (vack'seen, vack·seen') *n.* 1. Originally, a suspension of cowpox virus used to produce immunity against smallpox. 2. A preparation administered to induce immunity in the recipient; may be a suspension of living or dead organisms or a solution of either pollens or viral or bacterial antigens.

vaccine lymph. The virus of vaccinia as obtained from the calf.

vac·cin·ia (vack·sin'ee·uh) *n.* An acute infectious disease caused by smallpox vaccination or by accidental contact of abraded skin with vaccinia virus. It is characterized by the development of a localized lesion that progresses from papule to vesicle to pustule to crust. The infection stimulates the production of antibodies that are protective against smallpox.

vac·cin·i·al (vack·sin'ee·ul) *adj.* 1. Pertaining to or characteristic of vaccinia. 2. Resembling vaccinia.

vac·cin·i·form (vack·sin'i·form) *adj.* Resembling vaccinia.

vac·ci·no·pho·bia (vack''si·no·fo'bee·uh) *n.* Abnormal fear of vaccination.

vac·ci·no·ther·a·py (vack''si·no·therr'uh·pee) *n.* The therapeutic use of vaccine.

vac·u·o·late (vack'yoo·o·late) *adj.* Having, or pertaining to, vacuoles.

vac·u·o·lat·ed (vack'yoo·o·lay'tid) *adj.* Containing one or more vacuoles; said of a cell or cytoplasm.

vac·u·o·la·tion (vack''yoo·o·lay'shun) *n.* The formation of vacuoles; the state of being vacuolated.

vac·u·ole (vack'yoo·ole) *n.* 1. A clear space in a cell. 2. A cavity bound by a single membrane; usually a storage area for fat, glycogen, secretion precursors, liquid, or debris, in contradistinction to the artifacts induced by technical manipulation.

vac·u·ol·iza·tion (vack''yoo·o·li·zay'shun) *n.* VACUOLATION.

vac·u·um (vack'yoo·um) *n.,* pl. **vacuums, vac·ua** (·yoo·uh) A space from which most of the air has been exhausted.

vacuum extractor. An obstetrical instrument employing suction rather than forceps in the second stage of labor.

vag-, vago-. A combining form meaning *vagus, vagal.*

vag·a·bond·age (vag'uh·bon·dij) *n.* Uncontrollable desire to wander from home.

vagabond's disease. Pigmentation and lichenification of the skin due to chronic scratching associated with long-standing cases of pediculosis corporis.

va·gal (vay'gul) *adj.* Pertaining to the vagus nerve.

vagi. Plural and genitive singular of *vagus.*

vagin-, vagino-. A combining form meaning *vagina, vaginal.*

va·gi·na (va·jye'nuh) *n.,* L. pl. & genit. sing. **vaginae** (·nee), E. pl. **vaginas** 1. SHEATH (2). 2. [NA] The musculomembranous canal from the vulvar opening to the cervix of the uterus.

va·gi·nal (va·jye'nul, vaj'i·nul) *adj.* 1. Pertaining to or resembling a vagina or sheath. 2. Pertaining to or affecting the vagina.

vaginal ballottement. The rebound of the fetus against a finger inserted into the vagina. Syn. *internal ballottement.*

vag·i·na·lec·to·my (vaj''i·nuh·leck'tuh·mee) *n.* VAGINECTOMY (2).

vaginal gland. One of the mucous glands found exceptionally in the mucous membrane of the fornices of the vagina.

vaginal hernia. A perineal hernia that follows the course of the vagina after leaving the abdomen, and which may enter the labium majus; resembles a labial inguinal hernia.

vag·i·nal hysterectomy. Hysterectomy in which the removal is effected through the vagina.

vaginal process of the peritoneum. A tube of peritoneum which evaginates through the inguinal canal into the scrotum (or labium majus) during embryonic life. In the male, the distal portion persists as the tunica vaginalis testis. In the female, a portion occasionally persists, forming the canal of Nuck.

va·gi·na·pexy (va·jye′nuh·peck″see) n. COLPOPEXY.

vag·i·nec·to·my (vaj′i·neck′tuh·mee) n. 1. Excision of the vagina or a portion of it. 2. Excision of the tunica vaginalis.

vag·i·nic·o·line (vaj′i·nick′uh·line) adj. Of, or pertaining to, microorganisms that inhabit the vagina.

vag·i·nif·er·ous (vaj′i·nif′ur·us) adj. Producing, or bearing, a sheath.

vag·i·nis·mus (vaj′i·niz′mus) n. Painful spasm of the vagina.

vag·i·ni·tis (vaj′i·nigh′tis) n. 1. Inflammation of the vagina. 2. Inflammation of a sheath.

vag·i·no·cele (vaj′i·no·seel) n. COLPOCELE.

vag·i·no·dyn·ia (vaj′i·no·din′ee·uh) n. Neuralgic pain of the vagina.

vag·i·no·fix·a·tion (vaj′i·no·fick·say′shun) n. Fixation of the uterus to the vagina.

vag·i·no·my·co·sis (vaj′i·no·migh·ko′sis) n. A fungous infection of the vagina, usually by Candida albicans.

vag·i·no·plas·ty (vaj′i·no·plas″tee) n. A plastic operation on the vagina.

vag·i·no·scope (vaj′i·nuh·scope) n. A vaginal speculum.

vag·i·nos·co·py (vaj′i·nos′kuh·pee) n. Inspection of the vagina.

vag·i·not·o·my (vaj′i·not′uh·mee) n. 1. Incision of the vagina; COLPOTOMY. 2. Incision of a tendon sheath.

va·gi·tus (va·jye′tus) n. The cry of an infant.

vagitus ute·ri·nus (yoo·te·rye′nus). The cry of a child while still in the uterus.

vagitus va·gi·na·lis (vaj·i·nay′lis). The cry of a child while the head is still in the vagina.

va·go·ac·ces·so·ry (vay″go·ack·ses′uh·ree) adj. Pertaining to the vagus and spinal accessory nerves.

va·go·gram (vay′go·gram) n. ELECTROVAGOGRAM.

va·got·o·mized (vay·got′uh·mize′d) adj. Pertaining to a person or animal whose vagus nerves have been severed for therapeutic or experimental purposes.

va·got·o·my (vay·got′uh·mee) n. 1. Surgical division of vagus nerves. 2. Specifically, section of thoracic and abdominal vagal branches, usually for treatment of peptic ulcer; described as selective when only gastric branches are divided and as highly selective or superselective when only the gastric fundus and corpus are denervated, leaving the antrum and pylorus unaffected.

va·go·to·nia (vay″go·to′nee·uh) n. A condition due to overaction of the vagus nerves and

modification of functions in organs innervated by them. —**vago·ton·ic** (·ton′ick) adj.

va·got·o·nin (vay·got′uh·nin, vay″go·to′nin) n. A substance derived from the pancreas that stimulates the parasympathetic system.

va·go·tro·pic (vay″go·tro′pick) adj. Having an effect upon, or influencing, the vagus nerve.

va·go·va·gal (vay″go·vay′gul) adj. Due to both the afferent and efferent impulses of the vagus nerve.

vagovagal syncope. Syncope of reflex origin in which the entire reflex arc is within the vagal system. Syncope is due to reflex cardiac asystole and is associated with distention of the esophagus, bronchus, etc.; it can be inhibited by anticholinergic agents such as atropine.

va·grant (vay′grunt) adj. Wandering, as a vagrant cell.

va·gus (vay′gus) n., pl. & genit. sing. **va·gi** (·guy, ·jye) The tenth cranial nerve; a mixed nerve whose voluntary motor fibers arise in the nucleus ambiguus and are distributed to the muscles of larynx and pharynx; parasympathetic fibers from the dorsal motor nucleus of the vagus are widely distributed to autonomic ganglia to function in the regulation of motor and secretory activities of the abdominal and thoracic viscera. Somatic sensory fibers go to the skin of the external auditory meatus and the meninges, and visceral sensory fibers reach the pharynx, larynx, and thoracic and abdominal viscera. Syn. pneumogastric nerve.

va·lence (vay′lunce) n. 1. The capacity of an atom to combine with other atoms in definite proportions. 2. By analogy, also applied to radicals and atomic groups. Valence is measured with the combining capacity of a hydrogen atom taken as unity. —**va·lent** (·lunt) adj.

va·len·cy (vay′lun·see) n. VALENCE.

valer-, valero-. A combining form meaning valeric.

val·er·ate (val′ur·ate) n. A salt of valeric acid.

va·le·ric acid (va·lerr′ick, va·leer′ick). $C_5H_{10}O_2$. Four isomeric modifications of this acid are known: Normal valeric or propylacetic acid, $CH_3(CH_2)_3COOH$; isovaleric or isopropyl-acetic acid, $(CH_3)_2CHCH_2COOH$, the valeric acid of commerce; methylethylacetic acid, $CH_3(C_2H_5)CHCOOH$; and trimethylacetic acid, $(CH_3)_3CCOOH$.

val·e·tu·di·nar·i·an (val″e·tew″di·nerr′ee·un) adj. INVALID.

val·e·tu·di·nar·i·an·ism (val″e·tew″di·nerr′ee·an·iz·um) n. Feeble or infirm state due to invalidism.

val·gus (val′gus) adj. Usually, indicating an abnormal turning away from the midline of the body, as in talipes valgus.

val·ine (val′een, ·in, vay′leen, ·lin) n. α-Amino-isovaleric acid, $C_5H_{11}NO_2$, an amino acid constituent of many proteins. It is considered essential to man, as well as to certain animals.

Valium. Trademark for diazepam, a tranquilizer.

val·late (val′ate) adj. Surrounded by a walled depression; cupped.

vallate papilla. One of the large, flat papillae, each surrounded by a trench, in a group anterior to the sulcus terminalis of the tongue. Syn. *circumvallate papilla.*

val·lec·u·la (va·leck'yoo·luh) *n.*, pl. **vallecu·lae** (·lee) A shallow groove or depression.

Vallestril. Trademark for methallenestril, an orally effective, nonsteroid estrogen.

val·ley fever. COCCIDIOIDOMYCOSIS.

Val·sal·va maneuver (vahl·sahl'vah) Forcible exhalation against the closed glottis, increasing intrathoracic pressure and impeding venous return to the heart.

Valsalva's test A maneuver to test the patency of the auditory tubes. While the nose and mouth are kept closed, forcible expiratory efforts are made; if the auditory tubes are patent, air should pass into the tympanic cavities.

val·va (val'vuh) *n.*, pl. & genit. sing. **val·vae** (·vee) VALVE.

valve, *n.* A device in a vessel or passage which prevents reflux of its contents.

val·vot·o·my (val·vot'uh·mee) *n.* Surgical incision into a valve. Syn. *diclidotomy.*

valvul-, valvulo-. A combining form meaning *valve, valvular.*

val·vu·la (val'vew·luh) *n.*, pl. & genit. sing. **val·vu·lae** (·lee) VALVE.

val·vu·lar (val'vew·lur) *adj.* 1. Pertaining to a valve. 2. Resembling a valve.

valvular pneumothorax. A type of open pneumothorax in which a margin of the wound acts as a valve. Air enters the pleural space with an inhalation, and is prevented by the valve from escaping during exhalation. Therefore, the air remains in the pleural space increases. Syn. *tension pneumothorax.*

val·vu·lec·to·my (val'vew·leck'tuh·mee) *n.* Surgical excision of a valve, usually a heart valve.

val·vu·li·tis (val'vew·lye'tis) *n.* Inflammation of a valve, especially of a cardiac valve.

val·vu·lo·plas·ty (val'vew·lo·plas''tee) *n.* Plastic surgical repair of a valve, usually a heart valve.

val·vu·lo·tome (val'vew·lo·tome) *n.* An instrument designed especially for incising the valves of the heart.

val·vu·lot·o·my (val'vew·lot'uh·mee) *n.* The surgical incision of a valve of the heart, as in mitral stenosis.

vam·pire, *n.* 1. In worldwide folk belief, a living corpse that rises from its grave at night and sucks the blood of the living. 2. A bloodsucking bat, belonging to the family Phyllostomidae, found in South and Central America and along the southern border of the United States.

vam·pir·ism (vam'pi·riz·um) *n.* 1. Belief in vampires (1). 2. The acts or practice of vampires; blood sucking. 3. NECROPHILISM.

·a·na·di·um (vuh·nay'dee·um) *n.* V = 50.9415. A rare metallic element, atomic number 23, density 6.11.

·a·na·di·um·ism (vuh·nay'dee·um·iz·um) *n.* A chronic form of intoxication due to the absorption of vanadium; occurs in workers using the metal or its compounds.

an·co·my·cin (van''ko·migh'sin) *n.* A complex antibiotic substance produced by *Streptomyces*

orientalis; useful for treatment of severe staphylococcic infections.

van den Bergh's method (vahn d**e**n berr**g**h', d**e** berr'u**g**h) The indirect form of van den Bergh's test.

van den Bergh's test or **reaction** Either of the two tests for serum bilirubin. In the direct test, diluted serum is added to diazo reagent. A bluish-violet color becoming maximal in 10 to 30 seconds is an immediate direct reaction supposedly indicating conjugated bilirubin and therefore the presence of obstructive jaundice. A red color beginning after 1 to 15 minutes and gradually turning to violet is a delayed direct reaction, indicating impaired liver function. A red color appearing at once and changing to violet is a biphasic direct reaction. In the indirect test, alcohol is added to serum which is then centrifuged. The diazo reagent is added to the supernatant fluid. An immediate violet-red color supposedly indicates nonconjugated bilirubin and signifies a hemolytic jaundice. The tests are now used as a modification in which diazotized serum and plasma is compared with a standard solution of diazotized bilirubin.

va·nil·la (vuh·nil'uh) *n.* The cured, full-grown, unripe fruit of *Vanilla planifolia,* or *V. tahitensis.* The fresh fruit possesses none of the pleasant odor commonly associated with the fruit. Two enzymes, under the influence of gentle heat and moisture, produce vanillin from two of three glycosides, and perhaps another aromatic substance from a third glycoside. Vanilla is used solely as a flavoring agent. Syn. *vanilla bean.*

vanilla-worker's itch. Acarodermatitis urticarioides caused by *Tyroglyphus siro.*

va·nil·lic acid (vuh·nil'ick). 3-Methoxy-4-hydroxybenzoic acid, $C_8H_8O_4$, the crystalline solid resulting from oxidation of vanillin.

va·nil·lin (va·nil'in, van'i·lin) *n.* 3-Methoxy-4-hydroxybenzaldehyde, $C_8H_8O_3$; used as a flavoring agent in place of vanilla.

va·nil·lyl·man·del·ic acid (van''i·lil·man·del'ick, va·nil''il·). 3-Methoxy-4-hydroxymandelic acid, $C_9H_{10}O_5$, a major degradation product of adrenal medullary catecholamines excreted in the urine, where its measurement is used as a test for pheochromocytoma. Abbreviated, VMA

van·ish·ing lungs. Thin-walled abnormal air spaces, which develop under the effect of chemotherapy when the disease process in the lungs resolves.

va·po·cau·ter·i·za·tion (vay''po·kaw''tur·i·zay' shun) *n.* Cauterization by live steam.

va·por (vay'pur) *n.* A gas, especially the gaseous form of a substance which at ordinary temperatures is liquid or solid.

vapor bath. A bath in which the bather is exposed to moist vapors.

va·po·ri·za·tion (vay''por·i·zay'shun) *n.* The conversion of a solid or liquid into a vapor. —**va·por·ize** (vay'pur·ize) *v.*

va·por·iz·er (vay'pur·eye''zur) *n.* 1. ATOMIZER. 2. A device for converting a substance, usually a liquid, into vapor.

va·po·ther·a·py (vay"po·therr'uh·pee) *n.* The therapeutic employment, as in respiratory diseases, of medicated or nonmedicated vapor, steam, or spray.

Va·quez's disease (vah·kez') POLYCYTHEMIA VERA.

vari·abil·i·ty, *n.* Differences among members of a species resulting from genetic or environmental causes.

vari·able, *adj & n.* 1. Inconstant; subject to variation. 2. A quantity or magnitude which may vary in value under differing conditions.

vari·ance (vár'ee·unce) *n.* The square of the standard deviation. The second moment when deviations are taken from the mean.

vari·ant (vár'ee·unt) *n. & adj.* 1. *In bacteriology,* a colony which differs in appearance from the parent colony grown on the same medium; MUTANT. 2. Exhibiting or constituting variation.

vari·a·tion (vár"ee·ay'shun) *n.* 1. Deviation from a given type as the result of environment, natural selection, or cultivation and domestication. 2. Diversity in characteristics among related objects.

varic-, varico-. A combining form meaning *varix, varicose.*

vari·ca·tion (vár"i·kay'shun) *n.* 1. The formation of a varix. 2. A system of varices.

vari·ce·al (vár"i·see'ul, va·ris'ee·ul) *adj.* Of or pertaining to a varix or varices.

vari·cec·to·my (vár"i·seck'tuh·mee) *n.* Excision of a varix or varicose vein, as distinguished from avulsion of a vein.

vari·cel·la (vár"i·sel'uh) *n.* CHICKENPOX.

vari·cel·la·tion (vár"i·se·lay'shun) *n.* Preventive inoculation with the virus of chickenpox (varicella).

varicella-zoster virus. A virus of the herpesvirus group causing chickenpox and herpes zoster infections in man; the viruses for these diseases have been considered identical as they are physically and immunologically indistinguishable.

vari·cel·li·form (vár"i·sel'i·form) *adj.* Characterized by vesicles resembling those of chickenpox (varicella).

varices. Plural of *varix.*

vari·ci·form (va·ris'i·form, vár'i·si·) *n.* Having the form of a varix; VARICOSE.

vari·co·bleph·a·ron (vár"i·ko·blef'uh·ron) *n.* Varicose veins of an eyelid.

vari·co·cele (vár'i·ko·seel) *n.* Dilatation of the veins of the pampiniform plexus of the spermatic cord, forming a soft, elastic, often uncomfortable swelling.

vari·co·ce·lec·to·my (vár"i·ko·se·leck'tuh·mee) *n.* Surgical excision of dilated spermatic veins for relief of varicocele.

vari·cog·ra·phy (vár"i·kog'ruh·fee) *n.* Radiographic visualization of the course and extent of a collection of varicose veins.

vari·coid (vár'i·koid) *adj.* Resembling a varix.

vari·com·pha·lus (vár"i·kom'fuh·lus) *n.* A varicosity at the navel.

vari·co·phle·bi·tis (vár"i·ko·fle·bye'tis) *n.* Inflammation of a varicose vein or veins.

vari·cose (vár'i·koce, ·koze) *adj.* 1. Characterizing blood vessels that are dilated, knotted, and tortuous. 2. Due to varicose veins.

varicose ulcer. STASIS ULCER.

varicose veins. Veins that have become abnormally dilated and tortuous, because of interference with venous drainage or weakness of their walls.

vari·co·sis (vár"i·ko'sis) *n.,* pl. **varico·ses** (·seez') An abnormal dilatation of the veins.

vari·cos·i·ty (vár"i·kos'i·tee) *n.* 1. The state of exhibiting varices or being varicose. 2. VARICOSE VEIN.

vari·cot·o·my (vár"i·kot'uh·mee) *n.* Surgical excision of a varicose vein.

va·ric·u·la (va·rick'yoo·luh) *n.,* pl. **varicu·lae** (·lee) A varix of the conjunctiva.

Varidase. Trademark for a purified mixture of streptokinase and streptodornase, enzymes elaborated by hemolytic streptococci. The mixed enzymes cause liquefaction and removal of necrotic tissue and thickened or clotted exudates resulting from wounds or inflammatory processes, thereby promoting normal repair of tissue.

va·ri·ety, *n.* A subdivision of a species; a stock, strain, breed.

vari·form (vár'i·form) *adj.* Having diversity of form.

va·ri·o·la (va·rye'o·luh) *n.* SMALLPOX.

variola minor. A mild form of smallpox due to a less virulent strain. Syn. *alastrim.*

va·ri·o·lar (va·rye'o·lur) *adj.* Pertaining to or characterized by smallpox.

va·ri·o·late (vár'ee·o·late) *v.* To inoculate with smallpox virus. —**va·ri·o·la·tion** (vár"ee·o·lay'shun) *n.*

va·ri·ol·i·form (vár"ee·o'li·form, ·ol'i·form) *adj.* Resembling smallpox.

va·ri·o·li·za·tion (vár"ee·uh·li·zay'shun) *n.* VARIOLATION.

va·ri·o·loid (vár'ee·o·loid) *adj. & n.* 1. Resembling smallpox. 2. A mild form of smallpox in persons who have been successfully vaccinated or who had previously had the disease.

va·ri·o·lous (va·rye'o·lus) *adj.* VARIOLAR.

var·ix (vár'icks) *n.,* pl. **var·i·ces** (·i·seez) 1. A dilated and tortuous vein. 2. A tortuous, enlarged artery or lymphatic vessel.

va·rus (vair'us) *adj.* Usually, denoting an abnormal turning inward toward the midline of the body, as in talipes varus and coxa vara; occasionally, as in genu varus (bowleg), denoting an abnormal turning outward.

vas (vas) *n.,* pl. **va·sa** (vay'suh, ·zuh), genit. pl. **va·so·rum** (vay·so'rum) VESSEL.

vas-, vasi-, vaso-. A combining form meaning (a) *vessel, vascular;* (b) *ductus deferens;* (c) *vasomotor.*

vasa prae·via (pree'vee·uh). Presentation of the velamentous vessels across the lower uterine segment, seen with a low implantation of the placenta.

vasa va·so·rum (vay·so'rum) [NA]. The blood vessels supplying the walls of arteries and veins having a caliber greater than 1 mm.

vascul-, vasculo-. A combining form meaning *vascular.*

vas·cu·lar (vas'kew·lur) *adj.* Consisting of, pertaining to, or provided with, vessels.

vascular bed. The total blood supply—arteries, capillaries, and veins—of an organ or region.

vascular flap. A pedicle flap that includes an artery and vein in its base.

vascular headache. A throbbing headache due to painful dilatation and distention of branches of the external carotid artery.

vascular hemophilia. A bleeding disorder associated with increased bleeding time and low factor VIII activity.

vas·cu·lar·i·ty (vas'kew·lăr'i·tee) *n.* The quality of being vascular.

vas·cu·lar·i·za·tion (vas'kew·lur·i·zay'shun) *n.* 1. The process of tissues becoming vascular. 2. The formation and extension of vascular capillaries within and into tissues. —**vas·cu·lar·ize** (vas'kew·lur·ize) *v.*

vascular retinopathy. Retinal manifestations of such diseases as arterial hypertension, chronic nephritis, eclampsia, and advanced arteriosclerosis, characterized by various combinations and degrees of hemorrhages, exudates, vascular sclerosis, and sometimes by papilledema (malignant hypertension).

vas·cu·la·ture (vas'kew·luh·chur) *n.* The distribution or arrangement of blood vessels in an organ or part.

vas·cu·li·tis (vas'kew·lye'tis) *n.*, pl. **vascu·lit·i·des** (·lit'i·deez) Inflammation of a vessel; ANGIITIS.

vas·cu·lo·gen·e·sis (vas'kew·lo·jen'e·sis) *n.* The formation of the vascular system.

vas·ec·to·my (vas·eck'tuh·mee) *n.* Surgical division or resection of the ductus deferens; used to produce male sterility for birth control.

vas·i·fac·tion (vas'i·fack'shun) *n.* VASOFORMATION.

vas·i·for·ma·tion (vas'i·for·may'shun) *n.* The process by which a structure assumes the appearance of a vessel or duct.

vas·i·tis (vas·eye'tis) *n.* Inflammation of the ductus deferens.

vaso-. See **vas-.**

vaso·con·stric·tion (vay'zo·kun·strick'shun, vas'o·) *n.* The constriction of blood vessels; particularly, functional narrowing of the arteriolar lumen.

vaso·con·stric·tive (vay'zo·kun·strick'tiv, vas'o·) *adj.* Promoting, stimulating, or characterized by constriction of blood vessels.

vaso·con·stric·tor (vay'zo·kun·strick'tur, vas'o·) *n. & adj.* 1. A nerve or an agent that causes constriction of blood vessels. 2. Causing vasoconstriction.

vaso·de·pres·sor (vay'zo·de·pres'ur, vas'o·) *n. & adj.* 1. An agent that produces vasomotor depression. 2. Lowering blood pressure or causing vasomotor depression.

vaso·dil·a·ta·tion (vay''zo·dil''uh·tay'shun, dye''luh·tay'shun, vas'o·) *n.* Dilatation of the blood vessels, particularly functional increase of the arteriolar lumen.

vaso·di·la·tion (vay''zo·dye·lay'shun, vas'o·) *n.* VASODILATATION.

vaso·di·la·tor (vay''zo·dye·lay'tur, vas'o·) *n. & adj.* 1. A nerve or agent that causes dilatation of blood vessels. 2. Pertaining to the relaxation of the smooth muscle of the vascular system. 3. Producing dilatation of blood vessels.

vaso·epi·did·y·mos·to·my (vaz''o·ep''i·did''i·mos'tuh·mee, vas''o·) *n.* Anastomosis of a ductus deferens with its epididymal duct.

vaso·for·ma·tion (vay'zo·for·may'shun, vas'o·) *n.* The process in which blood vessels are produced or formed.

vaso·for·ma·tive (vay'zo·for'muh·tiv, vas'o·) *adj.* Forming or producing vessels.

vaso·gen·ic (vay'zo·jen'ick, vas'o·) *adj.* 1. Pertaining to the development of blood or lymph vessels. 2. Vascular in origin.

vasogenic shock. Peripheral circulatory failure due to arteriolar and capillary vasodilatation.

va·sog·ra·phy (vay·zog'ruh·fee, vas·og') *n.* Radiography of blood vessels.

vaso·hy·per·ton·ic (vay''zo·high''pur·ton'ick, vas''o·) *adj.* VASOCONSTRICTOR (2).

vaso·hy·po·ton·ic (vay''zo·high''po·ton'ick, vas'o·) *adj.* VASODILATOR (2, 3).

vaso·in·hib·i·tor (vay''zo·in·hib'i·tur, vas''o·) *n.* A drug or agent tending to inhibit the action of the vasomotor nerves. —**vasoinhibi·to·ry** (·to·ree) *adj.*

vaso·li·ga·tion (vay''zo·lye·gay'shun, vas'o·) *n.* Surgical ligation of a ductus deferens.

vaso·mo·tion (vay''zo·mo'shun, vas'o·) *n.* The rhythmic increase or decrease of the caliber of a blood vessel, especially precapillary sphincters.

vaso·mo·tor (vay''zo·mo'tur, vas'o·) *adj.* 1. Pertaining to or regulating the contraction (vasoconstriction) and expansion (vasodilatation) of blood vessels. 2. VASOCONSTRICTOR (2).

vasomotor center. A large, diffuse area in the reticular formation of the lower brainstem, extending from just below the obex to the region of the vestibular nuclei, and from the floor of the fourth ventricle almost to the pyramids; stimulation of the rostral and lateral portions of this center (pressor area) causes a rise in blood pressure and tachycardia, and stimulation of a smaller portion around the obex (depressor area) results in a fall in blood pressure and bradycardia. It is now thought that variations in the interaction between the two areas, with excitatory fibers from the pressor area and inhibitory fibers from the depressor area converging on vasoconstrictor nerves, control vasomotor activity.

vasomotor headache. CLUSTER HEADACHE.

vasomotor neurosis. ANGIONEUROSIS.

vasomotor paralysis. Paralysis of the vasomotor mechanism with resultant atony and dilatation of the blood vessels.

vasomotor reflex. Constriction or dilatation of a blood vessel in response to stimulation. Syn. *vascular reflex.*

vasomotor rhinitis or **catarrh.** ALLERGIC RHINITIS.

vasomotor syncope. VASOVAGAL SYNCOPE.

vaso·neu·ro·sis (vay''zo·new·ro'sis, vas'o·) *n.* ANGIONEUROSIS.

vaso·or·chid·os·to·my (vas'o·or''kid·os'tuh·mee,

vay"zo·) n. Surgical anastomosis of a ductus deferens with any portion of its testis.

vaso·pa·ral·y·sis (vay"zo·puh·ral'i·sis, vas"o·) n. VASOMOTOR PARALYSIS.

vaso·pa·re·sis (vay"zo·puh·ree'sis, ·păr'e·sis, vas"o·) n. A partial vasomotor paralysis.

vaso·pres·sin (vay"zo·pres'in, vas"o·) n. ANTIDIURETIC HORMONE.

vaso·pres·sor (vay"zo·pres'ur, vas"o·) n. Any substance that causes contraction of the smooth muscle of vessels.

vaso·punc·ture (vay"zo·punk'chur, vas"o·) n. Surgical puncture of a ductus deferens.

vaso·re·lax·a·tion (vay"zo·re·lack·say'shun, vas' o·) n. Diminution of vascular tension.

vas·or·rha·phy (vaz·or'uh·fee) n. End-to-end or end-to-side suture of a ductus deferens or of a blood vessel.

vaso·sec·tion (vay"zo·seck'shun, vaz"o·) n. Severing of a ductus deferens.

vaso·spasm (vay'zo·spaz·um, vaz"o·) n. VASOCONSTRICTION; ANGIOSPASM.

vaso·spas·tic (vay"zo·spas'tick, vaz"o·) adj. ANGIOSPASTIC.

vasospastic syndrome. RAYNAUD'S PHENOMENON.

vaso·stim·u·lant (vay"zo·stim'yoo·lunt, vaz"o·) adj. & n. 1. Inducing or exciting vasomotor action. 2. Any agent that promotes vasomotor action.

vas·os·to·my (va·zos'tuh·mee) n. The surgical establishment of an artificial opening into a ductus deferens.

vas·ot·o·my (va·zot'uh·mee) n. Surgical incision of a ductus deferens.

vaso·ton·ic (vay"zo·ton'ick, vas"o·) adj. & n. 1. Pertaining to the tone or degree of vasoconstriction of the blood vessels. 2. VASOSTIMULANT (2).

vaso·to·nin (vay"zo·to'nin, vas"o·) n. A vasoconstrictor substance present in the blood.

vaso·troph·ic (vay"zo·trof'ick, vas"o·) adj. Concerned in the nutrition of blood vessels.

vaso·va·gal (vay"zo·vay'gul, vas"o·) adj. Pertaining to the blood vessels and vagus nerve.

vasovagal attack (of Gowers) Anxiety, pallor, bradycardia, hypotension, sweating, nausea, precordial and respiratory distress, often culminating in syncope; due to excessive vagal effect on the vascular system.

vasovagal syncope. The common faint, occurring as a response to sudden emotional stress, pain, or injury; characterized by hypotension, pallor, sweating, hyperventilation, bradycardia, and loss of consciousness from excessive vagal effect on the vascular system. Syn. *vasodepressor syncope.*

vaso·vas·os·to·my (vay"zo·va·zos'tuh·mee, vas" o·) n. Surgical anastomosis of one portion of a ductus deferens to another.

vaso·ve·sic·u·lec·to·my (vay"zo·ve·sick"yoo·leck'tuh·mee, vas"o·) n. Surgical excision of a ductus deferens and seminal vesicle.

Vater's ampulla The hepatopancreatic ampulla, where the common bile duct and main pancreatic duct empty.

vault, n. 1. An arched structure, as a dome.

2. Specifically, the vault of the skull; CALVARIA.

V.C.G. Abbreviation for *vectorcardiogram.*

VD Abbreviation for *venereal disease.*

V.D.H. Valvular disease of the heart.

vec·tion (veck'shun) n. The conveyance of disease germs from sick to well persons.

vec·tis (veck'tis) n. An instrument similar to the single blade of a forceps, used in hastening the delivery of the fetal head in labor.

vec·tor (veck'tur) n. 1. An arthropod or other agent that carries microorganisms from an infected person to some other person. 2. A quantity involving both magnitude and direction, as velocity, force, momentum, which may be represented by a straight line of suitable length and direction. —**vec·to·ri·al** (veck to'ree·ul) adj.

vec·tor·car·di·o·gram (veck"tur·kahr'dee·o·gram) n. The part of the pathway of instantaneous vectors during one cardiac cycle, consisting o P, QRS, and T loops. Abbreviated, V.C.G Syn. *monocardiogram.*

vec·tor·car·di·o·graph (veck"tur·kahr'dee·o·graf n. An apparatus for recording a vectorcardio gram.

vec·tor·car·di·og·ra·phy (veck"tur·kahr"dee·og ruh·fee) n. A method of recording the direc tion and magnitude of the instantaneous car diac vectors. Continuous loops are recorded in the frontal, horizontal, and sagittal planes

veg·e·ta·ble, adj. Of or pertaining to plants.

vegetable casein. A protein of plant origin re sembling the casein of milk, as legumin cor glutin. Syn. *gluten casein.*

veg·e·tal (vej'e·tal) adj. 1. VEGETABLE. 2. Pertain ing to the basic functions shared by bot plants and animals such as metabolism, resp ration, reproduction, and growth.

veg·e·ta·tion, n. 1. An excrescence on a cardia valve or other portion of the heart, compose of platelets, fibrin, and often bacteria, an resembling a plant in general shape; seen i bacterial endocarditis and other disease 2. Any plant-shaped abnormal structure.

veg·e·ta·tive (vej'e·tay"tiv) adj. 1. Involved i or pertaining to, growth and nutrition rath than reproduction. 2. Functioning involunta ily or unconsciously; pertaining to the aut nomic nervous system. 3. Pertaining to veg tation, or a pathologic growth.

ve·hi·cle (vee'i·kul) n. A liquid or solid su stance, generally inactive therapeutically, en ployed as a medium or carrier for the acti component of a medicine.

Veil·lo·nel·la (vay"o·nel'uh) n. A genus of m croorganisms belonging to the family Neisse iaceae; they are small, gram-negative, anaer bic cocci.

vein, n. A blood vessel carrying blood from t tissues toward the heart. Veins, like arterie have three coats, but the media is less w developed; many also possess valves.

vein stripper. A long-handled surgical instr ment, used to remove varicose veins, usua introduced intraluminally throughout the volved length of vein.

ve·la·men (ve·lay'mun) *n.*, pl. **ve·lam·i·na** (·lam'i·nuh) A veil or covering membrane.

velamentous insertion. The insertion of the umbilical cord, which first attaches to fetal membranes and then passes on to the placenta.

velamentous placenta. A placenta with the umbilical cord arising from the outer border.

vel·a·men·tum (vel''uh·men'tum, vee''luh·) *n.*, pl. **velamen·ta** (·tuh) A veil, or covering membrane. —**velamen·tous** (·tus) *adj.*

ve·lar (vee'lur) *adj.* 1. Of or pertaining to a velum, especially the velum palatinum. 2. Of consonant sounds: formed with the back of the tongue touching or almost touching the soft palate or the back part of the hard palate, as *g* in gut, *k* in talk, or *ch* in Bach.

Velban. Trademark for vinblastine, an antineoplastic drug used as the sulfate salt.

veldt or **veld sore** (velt). Chronic shallow ulcers of exposed parts of the body, noted particularly in subtropical hot desert regions of Australia, Africa, and the Middle East; of uncertain, but possibly diphtheritic, etiology.

vel·li·cate (vel'i·kate) *v.* To twitch spasmodically.

vel·li·ca·tion (vel''i·kay'shun) *n.* Spasmodic twitching of muscular fibers.

vel·lus (vel'us) *n.* The fine, downy hair that appears on all parts of the human body except the palms and soles and those parts, such as the scalp, where terminal hair grows.

ve·loc·i·ty (ve·los'i·tee) *n.* RATE; change per unit of time.

Vel·peau's bandage (vel·po') A bandage that fixes the arm against the side, with the forearm flexed at an angle of 135°, the palm resting upon the midclavicular region opposite. By successive turns about the body, the bandage envelops the shoulder, arm, forearm, and hand.

ve·lum (vee'lum) *n.*, genit. **ve·li** (·lye), pl. **ve·la** (·luh) 1. A veil or veil-like structure. 2. A band of cilia in front of the mouth, seen in certain larval stages of various mollusks.

velum pa·la·ti·num (pal''uh·tye'num) [NA]. The posterior portion of the soft palate.

ve·na (vee'nuh) *n.*, pl. & genit. sing. **ve·nae** (·nee) genit. pl. **ve·na·rum** (vee·nair'um) VEIN.

vena ca·va (kay'vuh, kav'uh), pl. **ve·nae ca·vae** (vee'nee kay'vee). Either of the two veins which empty into the right atrium; the vena cava inferior or the vena cava superior.

vena cava inferior [NA]. INFERIOR VENA CAVA.

vena cava superior [NA]. SUPERIOR VENA CAVA.

venae. Plural and genitive singular of *vena.*

venae comitantes. Plural of *vena comitans.*

venae em·is·sa·ri·ae (em·i·sair'ee·ee) [NA]. EMISSARY VEINS.

ve·na·tion (vee·nay'shun) *n.* 1. Distribution of venous circulation of a part or organ. 2. *In botany,* the pattern of the veins of leaves.

ve·nec·to·my (ve·neck'tuh·mee) *n.* Surgical excision of a vein or a portion of one.

ve·nene (ve·neen') *n.* VENIN.

ve·nen·if·er·ous (ven''e·nif'ur·us) *adj.* Conveying poison.

venepuncture. VENIPUNCTURE.

ve·ne·re·al (ve·neer'ee·ul) *adj.* Pertaining to, or produced by, sexual intercourse.

venereal disease. A contagious disease generally acquired during sexual intercourse, including gonorrhea, syphilis, chancroid, granuloma inguinale, and lymphogranuloma venereum. Abbreviated, VD.

venereal sore. CHANCRE (1).

venereal ulcer. CHANCROID.

venereal verruca. CONDYLOMA ACUMINATUM.

venereal wart. CONDYLOMA ACUMINATUM.

ve·ne·re·ol·o·gist (ve·neer''ee·ol'uh·jist) *n.* An expert in venereal diseases.

ve·ne·re·ol·o·gy (ve·neer''ee·ol'uh·jee) *n.* The study of venereal diseases.

ve·ne·re·o·pho·bia (ve·neer''ee·o·fo'bee·uh) *n.* Abnormal fear of getting a venereal disease.

ven·ery (ven'ur·ee) *n.* Indulgence in sexual activities.

vene·sec·tion, veni·sec·tion (ven''i·seck'shun, vee''ni·) *n.* PHLEBOTOMY.

vene·su·ture, veni·su·ture (ven''i·sue'chur) *n.* The suturing of a vein.

Ven·e·zue·lan equine encephalitis. Equine encephalomyelitis due to Venezuelan virus.

Venezuelan virus. An immunologically distinct type of arbovirus originally recovered from the brains of Venezuelan horses affected with equine encephalomyelitis. Infection of man is generally less serious with this strain.

ven·in (ven'in) *n.* A mixture of the venom of various poisonous snakes; once used in neurasthenia, hysteria, chorea.

veni·punc·ture (ven'i·punk''chur) *n.* The surgical puncture of a vein.

venisection. Venesection (= PHLEBOTOMY).

ve·noc·ly·sis (ve·nock'li·sis) *n.*, pl. **venocly·ses** (·seez) Injection of a nutritive solution or of drugs into a vein.

ve·no·fi·bro·sis (vee''no·figh·bro'sis) *n.* An increase in fibrous connective tissue in a vein wall, usually at the expense of muscular and elastic elements.

ve·no·gram (vee'no·gram) *n.* A radiograph of veins following the injection of a contrast medium. Syn. *phlebogram.*

ve·nog·ra·phy (ve·nog'ruh·fee) *n.* Radiographic examination of veins following injection of a contrast medium.

ven·om (ven'um) *n.* Poison, especially a poison secreted by certain reptiles and arthropods.

ve·no·mo·tor (vee''no·mo'tur) *adj.* Causing veins to contract.

ven·om·ous (ven'uh·mus) *adj.* POISONOUS.

ve·no·peri·to·ne·os·to·my (vee''no·perr''i·to·nee·os'tuh·mee) *n.* Surgical implantation of a divided greater saphenous vein into the peritoneal cavity for drainage of ascites. Syn. *Ruotte's operation.*

ve·no·pres·sor (vee''no·pres'ur) *adj.* Tending to raise the blood pressure in the veins.

ve·no·scle·ro·sis (vee''no·skle·ro'sis) *n.* Induration of veins; PHLEBOSCLEROSIS.

ve·nos·i·ty (ve·nos'i·tee) *n.* 1. A condition in which arterial blood shows characteristics of venous blood. 2. An excess of blood in the venous system. 3. A large number of blood vessels in a part.

ve·nos·ta·sis (ve·nos'tuh·sis, vee''no·stay'sis) *n.* Retardation or prevention of the return flow of the blood to the heart, as by compression of veins, obstruction, or varicosities.

ve·no·throm·bot·ic (vee''no·throm·bot'ick) *adj.* Having the property of producing venous thrombosis.

ve·not·o·my (ve·not'uh·mee) *n.* PHLEBOTOMY; surgical incision of a vein.

ve·nous (vee'nus) *adj.* Pertaining to the veins.

venous blood. The blood in the vascular system from the point of origin of the small venules in tissues to the capillary beds in the lungs where free carbon dioxide is released into the alveoli and oxygen taken up; includes the blood in the pulmonary arteries.

venous capillary. The terminal part of a capillary network, opening into a venule. Syn. *postcapillary.*

venous claudication. Lameness due to venous stasis. Syn. *angiosclerotic paroxysmal myasthenia.*

venous hum. A continuous blowing or singing murmur heard on auscultation in the neck veins, normally in children and also in states of high cardiac output. Syn. *humming-top murmur, bruit de diable.*

ve·no·ve·nos·to·my (vee''no·ve·nos'tuh·mee) *n.* The anastomosing of two veins.

vent, *n. & v.* 1. Any aperture or outlet. 2. VENTILATE (v).

ven·ter (ven'tur) *n.* 1. BELLY; ABDOMEN. 2. BELLY OF A MUSCLE. 3. The cavity of the abdomen.

ven·ti·late, *v.* 1. To renew the air in a place. 2. To oxygenate the blood in the capillaries of the lungs. 3. To air or discuss (one's feelings and emotional problems).

ven·ti·la·tion, *n.* 1. The act or process of supplying fresh air, i.e., air whose partial pressure of oxygen is higher and of carbon dioxide lower than in the air being replaced. 2. The act or process of purifying the air of a place. 3. *In psychiatry,* the ready verbal expression of an individual's emotional problems, whether in a psychotherapeutic setting or in a conversation with another person in whom the person confides.

ven·trad (ven'trad) *adv.* In a dorsal-to-ventral direction.

ven·tral (ven'trul) *adj.* Situated on or relatively near the "belly side" of the trunk or of the body as a whole; in human anatomy: ANTERIOR.

ventral hernia. A hernia of any part of the abdominal wall not involving the inguinal, femoral, or umbilical openings. Three varieties occur: median, lateral, and postincision. Syn. *abdominal hernia.*

ventral nucleus of the thalamus. A nucleus of the thalamus which may be subdivided into three separate nuclei: the ventral posterior nucleus, which relays specific sensory impulses to cortical regions, and the ventral anterior and ventral lateral nuclei, which relay impulses from the basal ganglia and cerebellum.

ventri-, ventro- A combining form meaning (a) *abdomen;* (b) *ventral.*

ven·tri·cle (ven'tri·kul) *n.* A small cavity or pouch.

ventricles of the brain. Cavities in the interior of the brain, comprising the two lateral ventricles and the third and fourth ventricles.

ven·tric·u·lar (ven·trick'yoo·lur) *adj.* Of or pertaining to a ventricle.

ventricular block. Block of one or both of the interventricular foramens, the cerebral aqueduct, or the lateral and medial apertures of the fourth ventricle; interfering with the flow of cerebrospinal fluid from the brain ventricles and causing obstructive hydrocephalus.

ventricular complex. The QRS complex (ventricular depolarization complex) and T wave (ventricular repolarization complex) of the electrocardiogram.

ventricular depolarization complex. QRS COMPLEX OF THE ELECTROCARDIOGRAM.

ventricular escape. Temporary assumption of pacemaker function by the ventricular myocardium, due to absence or abnormal slowing of impulses from the sinoauricular and atrioventricular nodes.

ventricular fibrillation. A cardiac arrhythmia characterized by rapid, irregular, uncoordinated ventricular excitation without effective ventricular contraction and cardiac output; direct-current defibrillation is the emergency treatment of choice.

ventricular gradient. *In electrocardiography,* the vectorial sum of the mean QRS (Â QRS) and T (Â T) vectors; this relationship between the electrical sequence of depolarization and repolarization provides a means of differentiating primary from secondary T wave changes. Symbol, G, Ĝ, ḡ.

ventricular puncture. The introduction of a hollow needle into one of the ventricles of the brain, almost always one of the lateral ones, for diagnostic or therapeutic purposes.

ventricular septal defect. A defect, usually congenital, of the septum between the ventricles of the heart. Syn. *maladie de Roger.*

ventricular septum. INTERVENTRICULAR SEPTUM.

ventricular strain. A nonspecific electrocardiographic term describing QRS and T changes presumed related to right and left ventricular hypertrophy, respectively; at present there is disagreement as to the electrocardiogram patterns and their significance.

ventricular tachycardia. A serious cardiac arrhythmia characterized by rapid regular, or only slightly irregular beats, originating in the ventricle at the rate of 150 to 200 per minute; the QRS complex of the electrocardiogram is widened and slurred and is completely unrelated to the normal atrial complex (P wave).

ven·tric·u·li·tis (ven·trick''yoo·lye'tis) *n.* Inflammation of the ependymal lining of the ventricles of the brain.

ven·tric·u·lo·a·tri·al (ven·trick''yoo·lo·ay'tree·ul) *adj.* Concerning a cerebral ventricle and cardiac atrium; usually refers to shunting cerebrospinal fluid to the heart through ventriculoatriostomy.

ven·tric·u·lo·cor·dec·to·my (ven·trick''yoo·lo·kor·deck'tuh·mee) *n.* Surgical excision of the wall of the laryngeal ventricle and part of the vocal folds, for the relief of laryngeal stenosis, as from bilateral abductor paralysis of the vocal folds. Syn. *Chevalier Jackson's operation.*

ven·tric·u·lo·gram (ven-trick′yoo·lo·gram) n. A radiograph of the brain after the direct introduction of gas or an opaque medium into the cerebral ventricles.

ven·tric·u·log·ra·phy (ven-trick″yoo·log′ruh·fee) n. A method of demonstrating the ventricles of the brain by radiography after the ventricular fluid has been replaced by gas or by an opaque medium injected directly into the ventricular system.

ven·tric·u·lo·jug·u·lar (ven-trick″yoo·lo·jug′yoo·lur) adj. Of or pertaining to a cerebral ventricle and a jugular vein.

ven·tric·u·lom·e·try (ven-trick″yoo·lom′e·tree) n. Measurement of the intraventricular (intracranial) pressure.

ven·tric·u·lo·peri·to·ne·al (ven-trick″yoo·lo·perr″i·to·nee′ul) adj. Pertaining to a cerebral ventricle and the peritoneal cavity.

ventriculoperitoneal shunt. Surgical communication between a lateral cerebral ventricle and the peritoneal cavity by means of a plastic or rubber tube, for the relief of hydrocephalus.

ven·tric·u·lo·pleur·al (ven-trick″yoo·lo·ploor′ul) adj. Pertaining to a cerebral ventricle and the pleural cavity.

ven·tric·u·lo·punc·ture (ven-trick″yoo·lo·punk′chur) n. VENTRICULAR PUNCTURE.

ven·tric·u·lo·scope (ven-trick′yoo·lo·skope) n. An instrument for inspecting the interior of the cerebral ventricles and for electrocoagulation of the choroid plexus.

ven·tric·u·los·co·py (ven-trick″yoo·los′kuh·pee) n. Examination of the ventricles of the brain by means of an endoscope.

ven·tric·u·los·to·my (ven-trick″yoo·los′tuh·mee) n. The surgical establishment of drainage of cerebrospinal fluid from the ventricles of the brain.

ven·tric·u·lo·sub·arach·noid (ven-trick″yoo·lo·sub″uh·rack′noid) adj. Of or pertaining to the subarachnoid space and the ventricles of the brain.

ven·tric·u·lo·ve·nous (ven-trick″yoo·lo·vee′nus) adj. Pertaining to a cerebral ventricle and the venous system.

ven·tric·u·lus (ven-trick′yoo·lus) n., pl. & genit. sing. **ventric·u·li** (·lye) 1. GIZZARD. 2. VENTRICLE. 3. [NA] STOMACH.

ven·tri·cum·bent (ven″tri·kum′bunt) adj. PRONE.

ven·tri·duc·tion (ven″tri·duck′shun) n. Drawing a part toward the abdomen.

ven·tri·lat·er·al (ven″tri·lat′ur·ul) adj. At the side of the ventral surface.

ven·tri·me·sal (ven″tri·mee′sul) adj. In the middle in front.

ven·tro·cys·tor·rha·phy (ven″tro·sis·tor′uh·fee) n. The suturing of an incised cyst, or bladder, to an opening in the abdominal wall.

ven·tro·fix·a·tion (ven″tro·fick·say′shun) n. The stitching of a displaced viscus to the abdominal wall; specifically, the operative attachment of the uterus to the anterior abdominal wall for prolapse or displacement.

ven·tro·hys·tero·pexy (ven″tro·his′tur·o·peck″ see) n. Ventrofixation of the uterus.

ven·tro·lat·er·al (ven″tro·lat′ur·ul) adj. Pertaining to or directed toward the ventral and lateral aspects of the body or a part.

ven·tro·me·di·al (ven″tro·mee′dee·ul) adj. Pertaining to or directed toward the anterior aspect and toward the midline.

ventromedial hypothalamic nucleus. The larger of two cell groups of the medial hypothalamic area.

ven·tro·me·di·an (ven″tro·mee′dee·un) adj. At the middle of the ventral surface.

ven·tros·co·py (ven·tros′kuh·pee) n. PERITONEOSCOPY.

ven·trose (ven′troce) adj. Having a belly, or a swelling like a belly (potbelly).

ven·tros·i·ty (ven·tros′i·tee) n. OBESITY.

ven·tro·sus·pen·sion (ven″tro·sus·pen′shun) n. The operation of correcting a displacement of the uterus by shortening the round ligaments or attaching them to the anterior abdominal wall.

ven·tro·ves·i·co·fix·a·tion (ven″tro·ves″i·ko·fick·say′shun) n. Suturing of the uterus to the urinary bladder and abdominal wall.

ve·nu·la (ven′yoo·luh) n., pl. **venu·lae** (·lee) VENULE.

ven·ule (ven′yool) n. A small vein. —**ven·u·lar** (·yoo·lur) adj.

ve·nus (vee′nus) n. 1. Sexual intercourse. 2. Alchemic name for copper.

ver·a·trine (verr′uh·treen, ·trin) n. 1. CEVADINE. 2. A mixture of alkaloids from veratrum viride.

veratrum vir·i·de (virr′i·dee). The dried rhizome and roots of green hellebore (*Veratrum viride*); contains a number of hypotensive alkaloids, including protoveratrine A and protoveratrine B. Certain of its alkaloids and alkaloidal extracts are used in the treatment of acute hypertensive states. Syn. *green hellebore, American hellebore.*

ver·bal (vur′bul) adj. 1. Pertaining to words. 2. Pertaining to speech or discourse.

verbal agraphia. Inability to write words, although single letters can be written.

ver·big·er·a·tion (vur·bij″ur·ay′shun) n. The frequent and obsessional repetition of the same word, phrase, or even sound without reference to its meaning.

verd-, verdo- A combining form meaning *green-colored.*

ver·di·gris (vur′di·gree, ·gris) n. 1. A mixture of basic copper acetates. 2. A deposit upon copper, from the formation of cupric salts.

ver·do·he·min (vur″do·hee′min) n. A green-colored bile pigment; a derivative of hemin in which the porphyrin ring has opened, rendering the iron labile.

ver·do·nych·ia (vur″do·nick′ee·uh) n. Green discoloration of the nails.

ver·gence (vur′junce) n. In ophthalmology, a disjunctive reciprocal movement of the eyes, as convergence, divergence.

ver·gens (vur′jenz) adj. Inclining.

Veriloid. Trademark for the fraction of veratrum

viride alkaloids known by the generic name alkavervir.

vermi- A combining form meaning *worm*.

ver·mi·ci·dal (vur″mi·sigh′dul) *adj.* Destructive of worms.

ver·mi·cide (vur′mi·side) *n.* An agent that destroys worms.

ver·mic·u·lar (vur·mick′yoo·lur) *adj.* Wormlike.

ver·mic·u·late (vur·mick′yoo·lut, ·late) *adj.* Resembling or shaped like a worm.

ver·mic·u·la·tion (vur·mick″yoo·lay′shun) *n.* A wormlike motion; peristaltic motion.

ver·mic·u·lus (vur·mick′yoo·lus) *n.* A little worm or grub.

ver·mi·form (vur′mi·form) *adj.* Worm-shaped.

vermiform appendix. The small, blind gut projecting from the cecum.

vermiform process. VERMIFORM APPENDIX.

ver·mi·fuge (vur′mi·fewj) *n.* Any agent that kills or expels intestinal worms. — **ver·mif·u·gal** (vur·mif′yoo·gul, vur″mi·few′gul) *adj.*

ver·mi·lin·gual (vur″mi·ling′gwul) *adj.* Having a worm-shaped tongue.

ver·mil·ion border (vur·mil′yun). The mucocutaneous junction of the lips.

ver·mil·ion·ec·to·my, ver·mil·lion·ec·to·my (vur·mil″yun·eck′tuh·mee) *n.* Surgical removal of the vermilion border of the lips.

ver·min (vur′min) *n.* Animals that are obnoxious or harmful to man, especially those infesting his person, domesticated animals, or buildings, as flies, lice, rats, or mice.

ver·min·ous (vur′min·us) *adj.* Infested with, or pertaining to, vermin.

ver·mi·pho·bia (vur″mi·fo′bee·uh) *n.* Abnormal fear of worms or of infection by worms.

ver·mis (vur′mis) *n.*, *pl.* **ver·mes** (·meez) 1. WORM. 2. [NA] The median lobe of the cerebellum, between the hemispheres, or lateral lobes.

vermis syndrome. Cerebellar dysfunction marked chiefly by disturbances in gait and the tendency to lose balance while sitting or standing, due to disease involving the vermis.

ver·nal (vur′nul) *adj.* 1. Occurring in the spring. 2. Pertaining to the spring.

vernal conjunctivitis. A form of conjunctivitis, allergic in origin, recurring each spring or summer and usually disappearing with frost. Syn. *conjunctivitis catarrhalis aestiva, spring catarrh, spring conjunctivitis.*

ver·nix ca·se·o·sa (vur′nicks kay″see·o′suh) A cheesy deposit on the surface of the fetus derived from the stratum corneum, sebaceous secretion, and remnants of the epitrichium.

Ve·ro·cay bodies (beʰ·ro·kigh′) Small whorls of fibrils, surrounded by radially arranged elongated cells, seen in neurofibromas.

Veronal. Trademark for barbital, a barbiturate sedative and hypnotic.

ver·ru·ca (ve·roo′kuh) *n.* WART.

verruca acu·mi·na·ta (a·kew″mi·nay′tuh). CONDYLOMA ACUMINATUM.

verruca dig·i·ta·ta (dij″i·tay′tuh). A soft, warty papule usually seen on the scalp or in the beard with fingerlike projections and a horny cap.

verruca fi·li·for·mis (fye″li·for′mis). A soft, slender, soft-pointed, threadlike warty papule usually seen on the face and neck.

verruca pe·ru·a·na (pe·roo·ah′nuh) VERRUGA PERUANA.

verruca pe·ru·vi·a·na (pe·roo·vee·ay′nuh) VERRUGA PERUANA.

verruca pla·na ju·ve·ni·lis (play′nuh joo″ve·nigh′lis). A smooth, flat, small type of wart seen most often in children on the back of the hands and face, often arranged in lines.

verruca plan·ta·ris (plan·tair′is). Verruca vulgaris occurring on the sole of the foot as a painful, callus-covered papule. Syn. *plantar wart.*

verruca se·ni·lis (se·nigh′lis). SEBORRHEIC KERATOSIS.

verruca vul·ga·ris (vul·gair′is). The common wart, a viral disease producing hard hyperkeratotic papules, most commonly on the fingers.

ver·ru·ci·form (ve·roo′si·form) *adj.* Wartlike.

ver·ru·coid (verr′uh·koid) *adj.* Resembling a wart.

ver·ru·cose (verr′uh·koce, ve·roo′) *adj.* Warty; covered with or having warts.

ver·ru·cous (ve·roo′kus) *adj.* VERRUCOSE.

verrucous carcinoma. A low-grade malignant tumor of squamous epithelial cells presenting a grossly warty appearance.

verrucous endocarditis. Small thrombotic nonbacterial wart-like lesions on the heart valves and endocardium. Occurs frequently in systemic lupus erythematosus; may occur terminally, with or without clinical symptoms, in a variety of illnesses.

verrucous nevus. NEVUS VERRUCOSUS.

ver·ru·ga (ve·roo′guh) *n.* Verruca (= WART).

ver·si·col·or (vur′si·kul″ur) *adj.* 1. Many-colored, variegated. 2. Iridescent, changing in color.

ver·sion (vur′zhun) *n.* 1. Turning; manipulation during delivery to alter the presentation of the fetus. 2. Movement of both eyes in conjugate gaze. 3. The condition of an organ or part being turned or placed away from its normal position.

vertebr-, vertebro-. A combining form meaning *vertebrae, vertebral.*

ver·te·bra (vur′te·bruh) *n.*, L. *pl. & genit. sing.* **ver·te·brae** (·bree), *genit. pl.* **ver·te·bra·rum** (vur′te·brair′um) One of 33 bones forming the spinal or vertebral column. A typical vertebra consists of a body and an arch, the latter being formed by two pedicles and two laminas. The arch supports seven processes—four articular, two transverse, and one spinous.

ver·te·bral (vur′te·brul) *adj.* Of or pertaining to vertebra or vertebrae.

vertebral arch. An arch formed by the paired pedicles and laminas of a vertebra; the posterior part of a vertebra which together with the anterior part, the body, encloses the vertebral foramen in which the spinal cord is lodged.

vertebral body. A short column of bone forming the anterior, weight-bearing segment of a vertebra.

vertebral canal. A canal formed by the foramens of the vertebrae; it contains the spinal cord and its meninges.

vertebral column. The flexible supporting column of the body made up of vertebrae separated by intervertebral disks and bound together by ligaments. Syn. *spinal column.*

vertebral foramen. The space included between the body and arch of a vertebra, passage to the spinal cord and its appendages.

vertebral venous system. A group of venous anastomoses that pass through the intervertebral foramens to connect the veins of the pelvic cavity, the pelvic girdle, the shoulder girdle, and the body wall with the vertebral veins and thus with the sinuses of the dura mater. Syn. *system of Batson.*

Ver·te·bra·ta (vur″te·brah′tuh, ·bray′tuh) *n.pl.* A major group in the animal kingdom, commonly classified as a subphylum of the Chordata, and comprising the mammals, birds, reptiles, amphibians, and fishes. They are characterized by a spinal column, which develops in embryonic life about a notochord, composed of bony or, in certain fishes, cartilaginous vertebrae, and which contains the spinal cord that connects with a brain enclosed in a skull.

ver·te·brate (vur·te·brut) *adj. & n.* 1. Having a vertebral column; belonging to the Vertebrata. 2. Resembling a vertebral column in flexibility, as a vertebrate catheter. 3. A member of the Vertebrata.

ver·te·brec·to·my (vur″te·breck′tuh·mee) *n.* Surgical excision of a portion of a vertebra.

vertebro-. See *vertebr-.*

ver·te·bro·chon·dral (vur″te·bro·kon′drul) *adj.* Pertaining to, or involving, a vertebra and a costal cartilage.

ver·te·bro·cos·tal (vur″te·bro·kos′tul) *adj.* Pertaining to or involving a vertebra and a rib.

ver·tex (vur′tecks) *n.,* L. pl. **ver·ti·ces** (vur′ti·seez) 1. *In craniometry,* the highest point, in the sagittal plane, on the outer surface of a skull oriented on the Frankfort horizontal plane. 2. [NA] The crown of the head. 3. The center of a lens surface; the point on either lens surface which lies on the principal axis.

vertex presentation. *In obstetrics,* the most usual type of presentation, with the occiput the presenting part.

ver·ti·cal (vur′ti·kul) *adj.* 1. Pertaining to the vertex. 2. Pertaining to the position of the long axis of the human body in the erect posture.

vertical strabismus. Squint in the vertical direction, called sursumversion when involving both eyes upward, deorsumduction when downward, and right or left hypertropia according to the higher eye.

ver·ti·cil (vur′ti·sil) *n.* A whorl; a circle of leaves, tentacles, hairs, organs, or processes radiating from an axis on the same horizontal plane. **—ver·ti·cil·late** (vur″ti·sil′ate) *adj.*

ver·tig·i·nous (vur·tij′i·nus) *adj.* Resembling or affected with vertigo.

ver·ti·go (vur′ti·go) *n.,* pl. **vertigoes, ver·tig·i·nes** (vur·tij′i·neez) 1. The sensation that the outer world is revolving about oneself (objective vertigo) or that one is moving in space (subjective vertigo). 2. Any subjective or objective illusion of motion or position.

ver·u·mon·ta·ni·tis (verr″yoo·mon″tuh·nigh′tis) *n.* Inflammation of the colliculus seminalis.

ve·si·ca (ve·sigh′kuh, ves′i·kuh) *n.,* pl. & genit. sing. **vesi·cae** (·see, ·kee) BLADDER.

ves·i·cal (ves′i·kul) *adj.* Of or pertaining to a bladder, especially the urinary bladder.

vesical crisis. Paroxysmal attack of bladder pain, with difficulty in urination, seen in tabes dorsalis.

vesical reflex. The reflex or automatic response of the urinary bladder to empty itself, induced by distention of the organ to a certain capacity or degree, normally controlled by voluntary inhibition and release. Syn. *urinary reflex, vesicourethral reflex.*

ves·i·cant (ves′i·kunt) *n.* 1. A blistering agent. 2. *In military medicine,* BLISTER GAS.

ves·i·ca·tion (ves″i·kay′shun) *n.* The formation of a blister; a blister. **—ves·i·cate** (ves′i·kate) *v.*

ves·i·ca·to·ry (ves′i·kuh·tor·ee) *adj. & n.* 1. Blistering; causing blisters. 2. A blistering agent.

ves·i·cle (ves′i·kul) *n.* 1. A small bladder; especially a small sac containing fluid. 2. A small bulla, as seen in herpes simplex or chickenpox.

vesico- A combining form meaning (a) *bladder;* (b) *vesicle or blister.*

ves·i·co·ab·dom·i·nal (ves″i·ko·ab·dom′i·nul) *adj.* Pertaining to the urinary bladder and the abdomen.

ves·i·co·bul·lous (ves″i·ko·bul′us) *adj.* VESICULOBULLOUS.

ves·i·co·cele (ves′i·ko·seel) *n.* CYSTOCELE.

ves·i·co·cer·vi·cal (ves″i·ko·sur′vi·kul) *adj.* Pertaining to the urinary bladder and the uterine cervix.

ves·i·co·en·ter·ic (ves″i·ko·en·terr′ick) *adj.* VESICOINTESTINAL.

ves·i·co·fix·a·tion (ves″i·ko·fick·say′shun) *n.* CYSTOPEXY.

ves·i·co·in·tes·ti·nal (ves″i·ko·in·tes′ti·nul) *adj.* Pertaining to the urinary bladder and the intestinal tract.

ves·i·co·pros·tat·ic (ves″i·ko·pros·tat′ick) *adj.* Pertaining to the prostate gland and the urinary bladder.

ves·i·co·pu·den·dal (ves″i·ko·pew·den′dul) *adj.* Of or pertaining to both the urinary bladder and the pudendum.

ves·i·co·pus·tule (ves″i·ko·pus′tewl) *n.* A vesicle which is developing into a pustule. **—vesico·pus·tu·lar** (·tew·lur) *adj.*

ves·i·co·rec·tal (ves″i·ko·reck′tul) *adj.* Pertaining to the urinary bladder and the rectum.

ves·i·co·rec·to·va·gi·nal (ves″i·ko·reck″to·va·jye′nul, ·vaj′i·nul) *adj.* Pertaining to the urinary bladder, rectum, and vagina.

ves·i·co·sig·moid (ves″i·ko·sig′moid) *adj.* Pertaining to the urinary bladder and the sigmoid colon.

ves·i·cos·to·my (ves″i·kos′tuh·mee) *n.* CYSTOSTOMY.

ves·i·cot·o·my (ves″i·kot′uh·mee) *n.* Surgical incision of the urinary bladder; CYSTOTOMY (1).

ves·i·co·um·bil·i·cal (ves″i·ko·um·bil′i·kul) *adj.* Pertaining to the urinary bladder and the umbilicus.

ves·i·co·ure·ter·al (ves″i·ko·yoo·ree′tur·ul) *adj.*

Pertaining to the urinary bladder and to a ureter or to the ureters.

ves·i·co·ure·thral (ves"i·ko·yoo·ree'thrul) *adj.* Pertaining to the urinary bladder and the urethra.

ves·i·co·ure·thro·va·gi·nal (ves"i·ko·yoo·ree"thro·va·jye'nul, ·vaj'i·nul) *adj.* Pertaining to the urinary bladder, urethra, and vagina.

ves·i·co·uter·ine (ves"i·ko·yoo'tur·in, ·yoo'tuh·rine) *adj.* Pertaining to the urinary bladder and the uterus.

ves·i·co·utero·va·gi·nal (ves"i·ko·yoo"tur·o·va·jye'nul, ·vaj'i·nul) *adj.* Pertaining to the urinary bladder, uterus, and vagina.

ves·i·co·va·gi·nal (ves"i·ko·va·jye'nul, ·vaj'i·nul) *adj.* Pertaining to the urinary bladder and the vagina.

vesicul-, vesiculo-. A combining form meaning *vesicle, vesicular.*

ve·sic·u·la (ve·sick'yoo·luh) *n.,* pl. **vesicu·lae** (·lee) VESICLE.

ve·sic·u·lar (ve·sick'yoo·lur) *adj.* 1. Pertaining to, or composed of, vesicles. 2. Produced in air vesicles. 3. *In cytology,* pertaining to nuclei whose chromatin is widely dispersed, with or without a thin nuclear membrane.

vesicular emphysema. Emphysema characterized pathologically by enlarged, deformed air spaces involving the alveoli, alveolar ducts, and respiratory bronchioles.

ve·sic·u·late (ve·sick'yoo·late, ·lut) *adj. & v.* 1. Like a vesicle. 2. Covered with or composed of vesicles. 3. To produce, or be transformed into, vesicles.

ve·sic·u·la·tion (ve·sick"yoo·lay'shun) *n.* The formation of vesicles; the state of becoming vesiculated.

ve·sic·u·lec·to·my (ve·sick"yoo·leck'tuh·mee) *n.* Surgical resection, complete or partial, of the seminal vesicles.

ve·sic·u·li·tis (ve·sick"yoo·lye'tis) *n.* Inflammation of the seminal vesicles.

ve·sic·u·lo·bron·chi·al (ve·sick"yoo·lo·bronk'ee·ul) *adj.* Having vesicular and bronchial characteristics.

ve·sic·u·lo·bul·lous (ve·sick"yoo·lo·bul'us) *adj.* Characterized by both vesicles and bullae at the same time.

ve·sic·u·lo·cav·ern·ous (ve·sick"yoo·lo·kav'ur·nus) *adj.* Having vesicular and cavernous characteristics.

ve·sic·u·lo·gram (ve·sick"yoo·lo·gram) *n.* A radiograph of the seminal vesicles, following injection of a radiopaque medium by way of the ejaculatory ducts or the ductus deferens.

ve·sic·u·log·ra·phy (ve·sick"yoo·log'ruh·fee) *n.* Radiography of the seminal vesicles with the injection of a contrast medium. Syn. *seminal vesiculography.*

ve·sic·u·lo·pap·u·lar (ve·sick"yoo·lo·pap'yoo·lur) *adj.* 1. Consisting of vesicles and papules. 2. Having characteristics of both vesicles and papules.

ve·sic·u·lo·pus·tu·lar (ve·sick"yoo·lo·pus'tew·lur) *adj.* 1. Consisting of vesicles and pustules. 2. Having characteristics of both vesicles and pustules.

ve·sic·u·lot·o·my (ve·sick"yoo·lot'uh·mee) *n.* Surgical incision of a seminal vesicle.

ves·sel (ves'ul) *n.* A receptacle for fluids, especially a tube or canal for conveying blood or lymph. Comb. form *vasculo(o)-.*

ves·tib·u·lar (ves·tib'yoo·lur) *adj.* 1. Pertaining to a vestibule. 2. Particularly, pertaining to the vestibular part of the eighth cranial nerve, concerned with equilibration.

vestibular apparatus. The anatomical parts concerned with the vestibular portion of the eighth cranial nerve, including the saccule, utricle, semicircular canals, vestibular nerve, and vestibular nuclei. Syn. *vestibulolabyrinthine apparatus.*

vestibular fossa of the vagina. The part of the vestibule of the vagina which lies posterior to the vaginal orifice.

vestibular glands. Glands of the vestibule of the vagina, comprising the compound tubuloalveolar major vestibular glands (of Bartholin), one in each lateral wall, and the minor vestibular glands, which are several small branched tubular mucous glands around the urethral orifice.

vestibular nerve. The portion of the vestibulocochlear nerve concerned with the sense of equilibrium.

vestibular nuclei. Lateral vestibular nucleus, medial vestibular nucleus, spinal vestibular nucleus, and superior vestibular nucleus.

vestibular paralysis. Loss of vestibular function, as may be caused by certain antibiotics, manifested by vertigo, tinnitus, nausea, and vomiting, followed by disturbances of gait, posture, and impaired response to the caloric stimulation of the tympanic membranes.

vestibular window. An oval opening in the medial wall of the middle ear, closed by the foot plate of the stapes. Syn. *oval window.*

ves·ti·bule (ves'ti·bewl) *n.* An approach; an antechamber.

vestibule of the ear. The oval cavity of the internal ear, which forms the entrance to the cochlea.

vestibule of the mouth. The space bounded internally by the teeth and gums, externally by the lips and cheeks.

vestibule of the nose. The skin-lined portion of each nasal cavity, between the naris and the limen nasi.

vestibule of the vagina. The portion of the vulva bounded by the minor lips.

ves·tib·u·lo·cer·e·bel·lar (ves·tib"yoo·lo·serr"e·bel'ur) *adj.* Pertaining to vestibular fibers and the cerebellum.

ves·tib·u·lo·coch·le·ar (ves·tib"yoo·lo·kock'lee·ur) *adj.* 1. Pertaining to the vestibule and the cochlea of the internal ear. 2. Pertaining to or comprising the vestibular and cochlear nerves.

vestibulocochlear nerve. The common trunk of the vestibular and cochlear nerves. Syn. *acoustic nerve, eighth cranial nerve.*

ves·tib·u·lo·oc·u·lar (ves·tib"yoo·lo·ock'yoo·lur) *adj.* Pertaining to the vestibular and the ocular nerves.

ves·tib·u·lo·spi·nal (ves·tib"yoo·lo·spye'nul) *adj.* Pertaining to vestibular and spinal regions of the central nervous system.

ves·tib·u·lot·o·my (ves·tib"yoo·lot'uh·mee) *n.* A

surgical opening into the vestibule of the laby-rinth.

ves·ti·bu·lum (ves·tib'yoo·lum) *n.*, genit. **vestibu·li** (·lye), pl. **vestibu·la** (·luh) VESTIBULE.

ves·tige (ves'tij) *n.* A trace or remnant of some-thing formerly present or more fully devel-oped; a vestigium. **—ves·tig·ial** (ves·tij'ee·ul) *adj.*

ves·tig·i·um (ves·tij'ee·um) *n.*, pl. **vestig·ia** (·ee·uh) An anatomic relic of fetal or embryonic life.

vet·er·i·nar·i·an (vet''ur·i·nerr'ee·un) *n.* A person who practices veterinary medicine.

vet·er·i·nary (vet'ur·i·nerr''ee) *adj. & n.* 1. Per-taining to the practice of medicine with ani-mals, especially domesticated animals. 2. VET-ERINARIAN.

vi·a·ble (vye'uh·bul) *adj.* Capable of living; likely to live. **—vi·a·bil·i·ty** (vye''uh·bil'i·tee) *n.*

Viadril. Trademark for sodium hydroxydione succinate, a steroid with hypnotic, mild anal-gesic, and, possibly, some amnesic action.

vi·al (vye'ul) *n.* A small glass bottle.

Vi antigen (vee eye) *n.* One of the sheath or envelope antigens of enterobacteria, such as the *Salmonella*, which inhibit the agglutina-tion of the organisms in O (somatic) antise-rums.

vi·bex (vye'becks) *n.*, pl. **vi·bi·ces** (·bi·seez) A linear hemorrhage giving the appearance that it was caused by a whiplash.

vi·bra·tile (vye'bruh·til, ·tile) *adj.* Characterized by an oscillating movement; vibratory.

vi·bra·tion (vye·bray'shun) *n.* Oscillation; a rapid fluctuation; a periodic movement in alternately opposite directions from a position of equilibrium. **—vi·brate** (vye'brate) *v.*; **vi·brat·ing** (vye'bray·ting) *adj.*

vi·bra·tor (vye'bray·tur) *n.* A device for convey-ing mechanical vibration to a part.

vi·bra·to·ry (vye'bruh·tor·ee) *adj.* Characterized by vibrations.

Vib·rio (vib'ree·o) *n.* A genus of bacteria of the family Spirillaceae; being typically short, bent, motile rods, single or united end to end in spirals. Many species liquefy gelatin.

vibrio, *n.* 1. Any bacterium of the genus *Vibrio.* 2. Any curved, motile microorganism.

Vibrio chol·e·rae (kol'e·ree). The causative orga-nism of cholera.

Vibrio com·ma (kom'uh). VIBRIO CHOLERAE.

Vibrio fe·tus (fee'tus). The species of bacteria that causes vibriosis.

vi·bri·o·sis (vib''ree·o'sis) *n.*, pl. **vibrio·ses** (·seez) An infectious disease, primarily of cattle, sheep, and goats, caused by *Vibrio fetus* and characterized by abortion, retained placenta, and metritis; occasionally a disease in hu-mans, primarily infants, including enteritis and bacteremia.

vi·bris·sa (vye·bris'uh, vi·) *n.*, pl. **vibris·sae** (·ee) 1. One of the hairs in the vestibule of the nose. 2. One of the long, coarse hairs on the face of certain animals, such as the whiskers of a cat.

Vi·bur·num opu·lus (vye·bur'num op'yoo·lus). The dried bark of *Viburnum opulus,* prepara-tions of which have been used empirically in various menstrual disorders. Syn. *high-bush cranberry bark, true cramp bark.*

vi·car·i·ous (vye·kăr'ee·us) *adj.* Taking the place of something else; said of a habitual discharge occurring in an abnormal situation.

vicarious menstruation. The discharge of blood at the time of menstruation from some place other than the vagina, as in endometriosis.

vice, *n.* 1. A physical defect. 2. Depravity. 3. Im-morality. **—vi·cious** (vish'us) *adj.*

Vi·chy water (vish'ee, F. vee·shee'). A mildly laxative and antacid mineral water obtained from Vichy, France.

vi·ci·a·nose (vis'ee·uh·noce) *n.* A disaccharide, $C_{11}H_{20}O_{10}$, which, on hydrolysis, yields *l*-arabinose and dextrose.

vi·cious (vish'us) *adj.* Faulty, defective, badly formed.

vid·e·og·no·sis (vid''ee·og·no'sis) *n.* Television transmission of x-ray pictures; makes possible long-distance consultation and diagnosis.

vig·il (vij'il) *n.* Watchful wakefulness; a period of sleeplessness.

vig·i·lance (vij'i·lunce) *n.* The state of being awake, alert.

villi. Plural of *villus.*

vil·li·ki·nin (vi·lick'i·nin) *n.* A substance, present in acid extracts of intestinal mucosa, that produces strong movements of the intestinal villi.

vil·li·tis (vi·lye'tis) *n.* Inflammation of the lami-nas of the corium of a horse's hoof.

vil·lo·si·tis (vil''o·sigh'tis) *n.* Inflammation of the villous surface of the placenta.

vil·lous (vil'us) *adj.* Pertaining to a villus; cov-ered with villi; characterized by villus-like projections.

villous adenoma. A slow-growing potentially malignant neoplasm of the intestinal, usually colonic, mucosa; may be clinically manifested by bleeding and large volumes of mucoid diarrhea with high potassium content.

villous carcinoma. A type of papillary carci-noma in which the papillae are exceptionally long and grossly of velvety appearance.

villous synovitis. A type of synovitis in which villous growths develop within the articular cavity.

villous tenosynovitis. A chronic inflammatory reaction of a tendon sheath producing thick-ening of the lining with the formation of re-dundant folds and villi.

vil·lus (vil'us) *n.*, pl. **vil·li** (·eye) A minute, elon-gated projection from the surface of a mucous membrane or other membrane.

vil·lus·ec·to·my (vil''us·eck'tuh·mee) *n.* Synovec-tomy; surgical excision of a hypertrophied fold of the synovial membrane of a joint.

vin·bar·bi·tal (vin·bahr'bi·tol, ·tal) *n.* 5-Ethyl-5-(1-methyl-1-butenyl)barbituric acid, $C_{11}H_{16}N_2O_3$, a barbiturate with intermediate duration of action; used also as the sodium derivative.

vin·blas·tine (vin·blas'teen) *n.* An alkaloid, $C_{46}H_{58}N_4O_9$, from the periwinkle plant, *Vinca rosea;* an antineoplastic drug, used as the sulfate salt. Syn. *vincaleukoblastine.*

Vin·cent's angina (væn·sahn'', angl. vin'sunt)

1. VINCENT'S INFECTION, involving the pharyngeal and tonsillar tissues. 2. VINCENT'S INFECTION, in general.

Vincent's infection or **disease** A noncontagious infection principally of the oral mucosa, characterized by ulceration and formation of a gray pseudomembrane. Fusiform bacteria *(Fusobacterium fusiforme)* and spirochetes (principally *Borrelia vincenti)* always in association with other microorganisms, are present in abundance but are not known to be causally involved.

vin·cris·tine (vin·kris′teen) *n.* An alkaloid, $C_{46}H_{56}N_4O_{10}$, from the periwinkle plant, *Vinca rosea;* an antineoplastic drug, differing from vinblastine in its spectrum of activity, used as the sulfate salt. Syn. *leurocristine.*

vin·cu·lum (vink′yoo·lum) *n.,* pl. **vincu·la** (·luh) A ligament or frenum.

Vine·berg operation or **procedure** Implantation of the internal thoracic artery and vein into the ventricular myocardium; a procedure for myocardial revascularization in severe coronary atherosclerotic heart disease.

vin·e·gar, *n.* 1. A weak (approximately 6%) solution of acetic acid containing coloring matter and other substances (esters, mineral matter, etc.) formed by fermentation of alcoholic liquids or other sugar-containing liquids that have first undergone alcoholic fermentation. The process involves the oxidation of ethyl alcohol, forming acetic acid as the final product. 2. A pharmaceutical preparation obtained by macerating a drug with diluted acetic acid and filtering.

vinyl ether. Divinyl ether, $(CH_2{=}CH{-})_2O$, a volatile liquid used as a general anesthetic for short operative procedures and as an adjunct to other anesthetics when the operation is of longer duration.

Vioform. Trademark for iodochlorhydroxyquin, a local anti-infective agent.

vi·o·la·ceous (vye′o·lay′shus) *adj.* Violet; said of a discoloration, usually of the skin.

vi·o·la·tion (vye′uh·lay′shun) *n.* 1. RAPE; the act of violating or ravishing. 2. *In legal medicine,* the act of coitus without violence or force but by means of deception, by the influence of alcohol or drugs, or by intimidation.

vi·o·my·cin (vye′o·migh′sin) *n.* A polypeptide antibiotic substance or a mixture of substances produced by strains of *Streptomyces griseus* var. *purpureus* (more commonly called *Streptomyces puniceus);* used as the sulfate salt, intramuscularly administered, for treatment of tuberculosis resistant to other therapy.

vi·os·ter·ol (vye·os′tur·ole, ·ol) *n.* Vitamin D_2 or CALCIFEROL; now officially designated ergocalciferol.

vi·per (vye′pur) *n.* Any of various poisonous snakes of the family Viperidae.

Vi·pera (vye′pur·uh) *n.* A genus of the family Viperidae or true vipers.

Vi·per·i·dae (vye·perr′i·dee) *n. pl.* A family of venomous snakes possessing long, curved, movable front fangs which can be erected when striking. Some Viperidae are: *Vipera*

berus, the European viper; *V. russellii,* Russell's viper; *Bitis gabonica,* Gaboon viper; *B. lachesis,* puff adder; *B. nasicornis,* rhinoceros viper; *Echis carinatus,* saw-scaled viper; night adders of the genus *Causus; Aspis cornutus,* horned viper.

vi·ral (vye′rul) *adj.* Belonging to, caused by, or involving a virus.

viral gastroenteritis or **enteritis.** An acute sporadic epidemic self-limited infectious gastroenteritis with negative bacteriologic studies, characterized by diarrhea, nausea, vomiting, and variable systemic symptoms. Various viruses have been implicated, including echoviruses and parvoviruses.

Virchow's node SIGNAL NODE.

vi·re·mia, vi·rae·mia (vye·ree′mee·uh) *n.* The presence of a virus in the bloodstream.

vir·gin (vur′jin) *n.* 1. A female who has never experienced sexual intercourse as normally understood; medicolegally, perforation of the hymen need not have occurred for loss of virginity. 2. A person of either sex who has not experienced sexual intercourse. —**virgin·al** (·ul) *adj.* —**vir·gin·i·ty** (vur·jin′i·tee) *n.*

vir·i·dans streptococci (virr′i·danz) A group of streptococci including strains not causing beta hemolysis, although many members cause alpha hemolysis; they do not elaborate a C substance and therefore cannot be classified by the Lancefield method. Both pathogenic and saprophytic organisms are involved, the former often being isolated in conditions such as subacute bacterial endocarditis, bronchopneumonia, urinary-tract infections, and focal inflammations.

vir·ile (virr′il) *adj.* Pertaining to, or characteristic of, the male.

virile reflex. 1. PENILE REFLEX. 2. A sudden downward movement of the penis when the prepuce or glans of the relaxed organ is pulled upward.

vir·i·les·cence (virr′i·les′unce) *n.* The acquiring of characters more or less like those of the male.

vir·i·lism (virr′i·liz·um) *n.* 1. Masculinity; the development of male traits or characteristic in the female. 2. FEMALE PSEUDOHERMAPHRODITISM.

vi·ril·i·ty (vi·ril′i·tee) *n.* 1. The condition of being virile. 2. Sexual potency.

vir·il·iza·tion (virr′i·li·zay′shun) *n.* The assumption or appearance of male secondary sexual characters.

vir·il·iz·ing (virr″i·lye′zing) *adj.* 1. Producing male secondary sex characters. 2. Producing virility.

vi·ri·on (vye′ree·on) *n.* The complete, mature virus particle, identical to the infectious unit.

vi·rip·o·tent (vi·rip′o·tunt, vye·) *adj.* Of the human male, sexually mature.

vi·ro·cyte (vye′ro·site) *n. Obsol.* An atypical lymphocyte resembling those seen in infectious mononucleosis, present in some cases of viral diseases, such as influenza, infectious hepatitis, and acute respiratory disease.

vi·rol·o·gist (vi·rol′o·jist, vye·) *n.* A person who studies viruses and virus diseases.

vi·rol·o·gy (vi·rol'o·jee, vye-) *n.* The study of viruses and virus diseases.

vi·ro·pex·is (vye'ro·peck'sis) *n.* The mechanism by which animal viruses enter the host cell intact, thought to be through phagocytosis into vacuoles.

vir·tu·al (vur'choo·ul) *adj.* 1. Being a specified kind of thing in effect, or by way of function, but not in fact, as a virtual focus. 2. Formed of virtual foci, as a virtual image.

vi·ru·ci·din (vye'ruh·sigh'din, virr'yoo·) *n.* An agent capable of destroying a virus.

vir·u·lence (virr'yoo·unce) *n.* Malignancy; noxiousness; infectiousness. The disease-producing power of a microorganism. **—viru·lent** (·lunt) *adj.*

vi·rus (vye'rus) *n.* Any of a vast group of minute structures, in the range of 250 to 10 nm, composed of a sheath of protein encasing a core of nucleic acids (deoxyribonucleic or ribonucleic acids), capable of infecting almost all members of the animal and plant kingdoms, including bacteria (bacteriophage), characterized by a total dependence on living cells for reproduction, and lacking independent metabolism. Heterogeneous in form and function, viruses may be considered as either living objects or inert chemicals, and a growing number have been crystallized.

virus meningitis. Aseptic meningitis caused by a virus, such as nonparalytic poliomyelitis, Coxsackie, echo, and mumps viruses.

virus pneumonia. Pneumonia caused by one of a number of viruses, such as influenza viruses, adenovirus, and respiratory syncytial virus.

vis (vis) *n.*, pl. **vi·res** (vye'reez) Force; energy; power.

vis a fron·te (a fron'tee) 1. A force that attracts or a force pulling from the front. 2. The factors promoting return of blood to the right side of the heart.

vis·am·min (vis·am'in) *n.* KHELLIN.

vis a ter·go (a tur'go) 1. A force that pushes something before it, or a force that pushes from behind. 2. The function of the left ventricular pump in returning blood to the right side of the heart.

vis·cera. Plural of *viscus.*

vis·cer·al (vis'ur·ul) *adj.* Pertaining to a viscus or to the viscera.

visceral arch. 1. One of the series of mesodermal ridges covered by epithelium bounding the lateral wall of the oral and pharyngeal region of vertebrates; embryonic in higher forms, they contribute to the formation of the face and neck. 2. The skeleton of a visceral arch. 3. In gill-bearing vertebrates, one of the first two arches as opposed to the remaining or branchial arches.

visceral cleft. An embryonic fissure between the visceral arches, produced by rupture of the closing plate between a pharyngeal pouch and its corresponding external visceral groove.

visceral cranium. The portion of the skull which forms the face and jaws.

visceral crisis. Lightning pains referable to a viscus, seen in tabes dorsalis.

visceral ectopia. A congenital hernia into the umbilical cord.

vis·cer·al·gia (vis'ur·al'jee·uh) *n.* Pain in a viscus.

visceral leishmaniasis. KALA AZAR.

visceral lymphomatosis. A form of the avian leukosis complex affecting primarily the liver and kidney and to a lesser extent all organs of the body.

viscero-. A combining form meaning *viscus, viscera, visceral.*

vis·cero·car·di·ac (vis'ur·o·kahr'dee·ack) *adj.* Pertaining to the viscera and the heart.

vis·cero·cep·tor (vis'ur·o·sep'tur) *n.* INTEROCEPTOR.

vis·cero·in·hib·i·to·ry (vis'ur·o·in·hib'i·tor·ee) *adj.* Inhibiting the movements of viscera.

vis·cero·meg·a·ly (vis'ur·o·meg'uh·lee) *n.* SPLANCHNOMEGALY.

vis·cer·op·to·sis (vis'ur·op·to'sis) *n.* Prolapse of a viscus, especially of the intestine; downward displacement of the intestine in the abdominal cavity; once considered clinically significant.

vis·cero·sen·so·ry (vis'ur·o·sen'suh·ree) *adj.* Pertaining to sensation in the viscera.

vis·cero·tome (vis'ur·o·tome) *n.* 1. An instrument used only in postmortem examinations to secure specimens of the liver or other internal organ. 2. The areas of the viscera supplied with sensory fibers from a single spinal nerve.

vis·cer·ot·o·my (vis'ur·ot'uh·mee) *n.* The process of cutting out a piece of liver or other internal organ with the viscerotome.

vis·cero·to·nia (vis'ur·o·to'nee·uh) *n.* The behavioral counterpart of component I (endomorphy) of the somatotype, manifested predominantly by a desire for assimilation and the conservation of energy through sociability, relaxation, and love of food. **—viscero·ton·ic** (·ton'ick) *adj.*

vis·cero·tro·pic (vis'ur·o·tro'pick, ·trop'ick) *adj.* Attracted to or seeking the viscera.

vis·cid (vis'id) *adj.* Adhesive; glutinous.

vis·cid·i·ty (vi·sid'i·tee) *n.* The quality or state of being viscid.

vis·co·liz·er (vis'ko·lye''zur) *n.* A machine used in reduction of size of fat particles, or in homogenization of a mixture or tissue.

vis·co·sim·e·ter (vis'ko·sim'e·tur) *n.* An apparatus for determining the degree of viscosity of a fluid.

vis·cos·i·ty (vis·kos'i·tee) *n.* The resistance that a liquid exhibits to the flow of one layer over another. The property of offering resistance to a change of form, arising from the molecular attraction between the molecules of a liquid.

vis·cous (vis'kus) *adj.* Glutinous; sticky; semifluid; having high viscosity.

vis·cus (vis'kus) *n.*, pl. **vis·cera** (vis'ur·uh) Any one of the organs enclosed within one of the four great cavities, the cranium, thorax, abdomen, or pelvis; especially an organ within the abdominal cavity.

vis in·er·ti·ae (i·nur'shee·ee) The force by virtue of which a body at rest tends to remain at rest.

vi·sion (vizh'un) *n.* 1. The act of seeing; sight. 2. The capacity or ability to see. 3. Loosely, visual acuity. 4. A mental image. 5. *In psychi-*

atry, a hallucinatory phenomenon in which the patient sees something not actually present. 6. A dream.

vis me·di·ca·trix na·tu·rae (med·i·kay'tricks na·tew'ree). The healing power of nature apart from medicinal treatment.

vis·na (vis'nuh) *n.* A chronic disease of the central nervous system of sheep, observed in Iceland and caused by a conventional RNA virus with a long incubation period, during which the animal appears well. It was in relation to this disease that Sigurdsson first used the term "slow infection."

vi·su·al (vizh'yoo·ul) *adj.* 1. Pertaining to sight. 2. Producing mental images.

visual acuity. The measured central vision, dependent upon the clarity of the retinal focus, integrity of the nervous elements, and cerebral interpretation of a given stimulus at a given distance as tested with a Snellen or similar chart; the result is usually expressed as a fraction with the numerator the distance at which the test was performed and the denominator the distance at which the symbol (letter, picture, E) should be seen by a normal eye. In the U.S.A. using Snellen's letter chart at 20 feet, normal visual acuity is 20/20.

visual agnosia. A condition characterized by inability to name a seen object or to indicate its use by gesture, despite intactness of vision, clarity of mind, and absence of aphasia.

visual allesthesia. Displacement of an image to the opposite half of the visual field; seen in patients with gross unilateral field defects and diffuse brain disease, but also in severe psychotic states and in migraine.

visual aura. The initial event of a seizure which consists either of unformed visual images, such as flashes or balls of light, suggesting an occipital lobe origin, or of formed visual images, such as persons, suggesting a temporal lobe origin.

visual field. FIELD OF VISION.

vi·su·al·iza·tion (vizh''yoo·ul·i·zay'shun) *n.* 1. Perceiving images in the mind with such distinctness that they seem to be seen by the eyes. 2. The act of making visible or of becoming visible, as by means of a microscope, x-ray photograph, otoscope, or other indirect means.

visual object agnosia. The inability to recognize objects by sight in spite of adequate vision; may be total or may pertain only to inanimate objects, to all animate objects, to a person's body or any part or side of it, or to the attributes, such as form, color, or dimensions of objects; lesions in the visuopsychic area are considered to be responsible. Syn. *nonsymbolic visual agnosia.*

visual projection area. The cortical receptive center for visual impulses, located in the walls and margins of the calcarine sulcus of the occipital lobe, characterized by the stripe (stria) of Gennari. Syn. *Brodmann's area 17, striate area.*

visual purple. RHODOPSIN.

visual seizure. VISUAL AURA.

visual verbal agnosia. The inability to recognize

words or fractions of words (agnostic alexia), musical symbols, or numbers and other mathematical symbols, in spite of adequate vision, usually due to a lesion in the angular gyrus or connections thereof with other cortical regions such as Wernicke's and Broca's areas. Syn. *symbolic visual agnosia.*

visual violet. IODOPSIN.

visual white. LEUKOPSIN.

visual yellow. An intermediary substance formed in the retina from rhodopsin after exposure to light first results in a transient orange, which then is converted into an indicator yellow before finally breaking up into retinene (vitamin A aldehyde) and vitamin A.

vi·suo·au·di·to·ry (vizh''yoo·o·aw'di·tor·ee) *adj.* Pertaining to hearing and seeing, as visuoauditory nerve fibers, which connect the visual and auditory centers.

vi·su·og·no·sis (vizh''yoo·og·no'sis) *n.* Appreciation and recognition of visual impressions.

vi·suo·mo·tor (vizh''yoo·o·mo'tur) *adj.* 1. Pertaining to seeing and the performance of skilled voluntary movements, as in the ability to copy a simple design or writing. 2. Of or pertaining to the connections between the visual and the motor cortex.

vi·suo·psy·chic (vizh''yoo·o·sigh'kick) *adj.* Pertaining to the visuopsychic area.

visuopsychic area or **cortex.** The visual association areas of the occipital cortex surrounding the visual projection area; the parastriate area and the peristriate area, collectively.

vi·suo·sen·so·ry (vizh''yoo·o·sen'sur·ee) *adj.* Pertaining to the visual projection area of the occipital cortex, Brodmann's area 17.

vi·sus (vye'sus) *n.* VISION.

vi·tal (vye'tul) *adj.* Pertaining to life.

vital capacity. The volume of air that can be expelled from the lungs by the most forcible expiration after the deepest inspiration. It is the maximum stroke volume of the thoracic pump and is affected by any factor restricting either the amount of filling or emptying of the lungs. A timed vital capacity is a measure of rate of emptying of the lungs and aids greatly in determining the maximum ventilatory capacity. A normal individual can exhale three fourths or more of his vital capacity in one second.

vital dye. A dye suitable for staining living tissues within the whole living body.

vi·tal·ism (vye'tul·iz·um) *n.* The theory that the activities of a living organism are under the guidance of a special form of energy, force, or agency which has none of the attributes of matter or energy. —**vital·ist** (·ist) *n.*, **vital·is·tic** (·ist'ick) *adj.*

vi·tal·i·ty (vye·tal'i·tee) *n.* The power to grow, develop, perform living functions; vigor.

vi·tal·ize (vye'tul·ize) *v.* To endow with the capacity to grow or develop as a living thing.

Vitallium. Trademark for an alloy of cobalt, chromium, and molybdenum used in certain surgical appliances and procedures.

vi·tals (vye'tulz) *n. pl.* The organs essential to life.

vital stain. INTRAVITAL STAIN.

vital statistics. The data concerning births, marriages, and deaths; a branch of biostatistics.

vi·ta·mer (vye'tuh·mur) *n.* Any of a group of chemically related substances that possess a specific vitamin activity, as the D vitamers, or the K vitamers.

vi·ta·min, vi·ta·mine (vye'tuh·min) *n.* Any of a group of organic compounds present in variable, minute quantities in natural foodstuffs, required for the normal growth and maintenance of the life of animals, including man, who, as a rule, are unable to synthesize these compounds. They are effective in small amounts and do not furnish energy, but are essential for transformation of energy and for the regulation of the metabolism in the organism.

vitamin A. 3,7-Dimethyl-9-(2,6,6-trimethyl-1-cyclohexen-1-yl)-2,4,6,8-nonatetraen-1-ol, $C_{20}H_{29}OH$, a component of liver oils that may be obtained also from certain carotenoids and produced by synthesis. It is a component of pigments concerned with visual accommodation to light and color vision; is essential for development, maturation, and metabolism of epithelial cells; and may have a role in promotion of growth and in synthesis of glucocorticoids. Used medicinally in the form of the alcohol or one of its esters with edible fatty acids. One unit of vitamin A is the biological activity of 0.30 microgram of the alcohol form of vitamin A. Syn. *retinol, vitamin A₁, vitamin A alcohol, anti-infective vitamin, antixerophthalmic vitamin.*

vitamin A acid. RETINOIC ACID.

vitamin B₁. Thiamine, occurring naturally as the hydrochloride and pyrophosphate, and used medicinally principally as the hydrochloride and nitrate salts.

vitamin B₂. RIBOFLAVIN.

vitamin B₆. 1. PYRIDOXINE. 2. A group name for pyridoxal, pyridoxamine, and pyridoxine, or any member of the group.

vitamin B₁₂. The anti-pernicious-anemia factor, present in liver, essential for normal hemopoiesis; identical with cyanocobalamin. Syn. *extrinsic factor.*

vitamin B₁₇. A misnomer for Laetrile.

vitamin B_c. FOLIC ACID.

vitamin B complex. A group of water-soluble vitamins, occurring in various foods, that include thiamine (vitamin B₁), riboflavin (vitamin B₂), niacin (nicotinic acid), pyridoxine (vitamin B₆), pantothenic acid, inositol, *p*-aminobenzoic acid, biotin, folic acid, and vitamin B₁₂.

vitamin C. ASCORBIC ACID.

vitamin D. Any one of several sterols having antirachitic activity, as ergocalciferol (vitamin D₂, calciferol) and cholecalciferol (vitamin D₃). Vitamin D occurs in fish liver oils (principally D₃) and is also obtained by irradiating ergosterol (D₂). It is essential for normal deposition of calcium and phosphorus in bones and teeth. Deficiency leads to rickets in children, osteomalacia in adults. Syn. *antirachitic vitamin.*

vitamin D–refractory rickets. Rickets that develops despite nutritional doses of vitamin D and that fails to respond to therapeutic amounts.

vitamin E. 5,7,8-Trimethyltocol, $C_{29}H_{50}O_2$, commonly known as α-tocopherol (alpha tocopherol), biologically the most active of a series of related compounds called tocopherols. Vitamin E occurs in wheat germ and other oils, and is also produced by synthesis. Its deficiency in rats may produce reproductive sterility, muscular dystrophy, and degeneration. It is believed to be needed in human physiological processes, but its role is not understood. One international unit is equivalent to 1 mg of *dl-α-tocopheryl acetate.*

vitamin F. A term formerly used for essential fatty acids, as linoleic acid ($C_{18}H_{32}O_2$), linolenic acid ($C_{18}H_{30}O_2$), and arachidonic acid ($C_{20}H_{32}O_2$).

vitamin G. Vitamin B₂; RIBOFLAVIN.

vitamin H. A water-soluble component of the vitamin B complex identical with biotin (coenzyme R).

vitamin K. Any one of at least three naphthoquinone derivatives, vitamin K₁, vitamin K₂, and vitamin K₃. Vitamin K is essential for formation of prothrombin. In vitamin-K deficiency, the blood clotting time is markedly prolonged and hemorrhages result. Syn. *antihemorrhagic vitamin, prothrombin factor.*

vitamin K₁. PHYTONADIONE.

vitamin K₃. MENADIONE.

vitamin K₅. 2-Methyl-4-amino-1-naphthol, $C_{11}H_{11}NO$, a vitamin K compound used as the water-soluble hydrochloride.

Vitamin K Analogue. A trademark for menadiol sodium diphosphate, a water-soluble prothrombinogenic compound with the actions and uses of menadione.

vitamin-K test. A liver-function test in which 2 mg of menadione is administered intramuscularly. If the prothrombin level rises more than 20 percent in 24 hours, liver function is normal.

vitamin M. *Obsol.* FOLIC ACID.

vitamin P. A collective term for substances, such as citrin or one or more of its components, believed to be concerned with maintenance of the normal state of the walls of small blood vessels, and that have been used for the treatment of conditions characterized by increased capillary permeability and fragility.

vitamin P-P. NIACIN.

vi·tel·lin (vi·tel'in, vye·) *n.* A phosphoprotein in egg yolk.

vi·tel·line (vi·tel'in, ·een, ·ine) *adj.* Pertaining to the vitellus or yolk.

vi·tel·lo·lu·te·in (vi·tel"o·lew'tee·in) *n.* A yellow pigment of yolk.

vi·tel·lo·ru·bin (vi·tel"o·roo'bin) *n.* A reddish pigment obtained from the yolk of egg.

vi·tel·lus (vi·tel'us, vye·tel'us) *n.* YOLK.

vi·ti·a·tion (vish"ee·ay'shun) *n.* A change that lessens utility or efficiency or neutralizes an action.

vit·i·lig·i·nes (vit"i·lij'i·neez) *n.pl.* Depigmented areas in the skin, as the lineae albicantes and the variously shaped foci of vitiligo.

vit·i·li·go (vit"i·lye'go) *n.* A skin disease characterized by an acquired achromia in areas of various sizes and shapes. There is an almost complete lack of pigment with hyperpigmented borders. Lesions are more marked in areas exposed to sun. —**viti·lig·i·nous** (·lij'i·nus) *adj.*

vit·re·ous (vit'ree·us) *adj. & n.* 1. Glassy; hyaline. 2. VITREOUS BODY.

vitreous body. The transparent, gelatin-like substance filling the greater part of the eyeball.

vitreous chamber. The portion of the eyeball posterior to the crystalline lens and anterior to the retina, which is filled by the vitreous humor.

vitreous humor. 1. VITREOUS BODY. 2. The more fluid portion of the vitreous body enmeshed in the more fibrous portion.

vitreous stroma. The more fibrous portion of the vitreous body.

vi·tres·cence (vi·tres'unce) *n.* The condition of becoming hard and transparent like glass.

vi·tri·na (vi·trye'nuh) *n.* VITREOUS HUMOR.

vit·ri·ol (vit'ree·ul) *n.* 1. Any substance having a glassy fracture or appearance. 2. SULFURIC ACID. 3. Any crystalline salt of sulfuric acid. —**vit·ri·o·lat·ed** (vit'ree·o·lay''tid), **vit·ri·ol·ic** (vit''ree·ol'ick) *adj.*

vitriolic acid. SULFURIC ACID.

vit·ro·pres·sion (vit''ro·presh'un) *n.* Pressure with a glass slide on the skin to aid in study and diagnosis of skin lesions.

vi·var·i·um (vye·vâr'ee·um) *n.*, pl. **vivar·ia** (·ee-uh), **vivariums** A place where live animals are kept.

vi·vax malaria (vye'vacks). Malaria caused by *Plasmodium vivax*, characterized by typical paroxysms occurring every two or three days, typically every second day. Syn. *benign tertian malaria, tertian malaria.*

vivi- A combining form meaning *alive, living.*

viv·i·fi·ca·tion (viv''i·fi·kay'shun) *n.* The act of making alive or of converting into living tissue.

vi·vip·a·rous (vye·vip'uh·rus, vi·) *adj.* Bringing forth the young alive. —**vivi·par·i·ty** (vye''vi·pâr'i·tee) *n.*

vivi·sec·tion (viv''i·seck'shun) *n.* The cutting of a living individual; especially, a surgical procedure upon an anesthetized animal for research purposes. —**vivi·sect** (viv'i·sekt) *v.*

VMA Abbreviation for *vanillylmandelic acid.*

vo·cal (vo'kul) *adj.* Pertaining to the voice or the organs of speech.

vocal asynergy. Faulty coordination of the muscles of the larynx, as in chorea.

vocal fold. In the larynx, either the right or left fold bounding the rima glottidis. Each is covered by mucous membrane which is supported anteriorly by a vocal ligament, posteriorly by the vocal process of an arytenoid cartilage.

vocal fremitus. The sounds of the voice transmitted to the ear when it is applied to the chest of a person speaking.

vocal lip. Either of the shelflike projections into the cavity of the larynx whose edges constitute the vocal cords or folds.

vocal node or **nodule.** SINGER'S NODE.

vocal resonance. The sound of the spoken voice transmitted through the lungs and the chest wall and heard on auscultation. Abbreviated, V.R.

voice, *n.* The sounds produced by the vibration of the vocal folds and modified by the resonance organs, especially as used in speaking or singing.

void, *v.* To evacuate, emit, discharge (especially excrement).

vol. %. Abbreviation for *volume percent.*

vo·la (vo'luh) *n.* The palm of the hand or the sole of the foot. —**vo·lar** (·lur) *adj.*

vol·a·tile (vol'uh·til) *adj.* Readily vaporizing; evaporating. —**vol·a·til·iza·tion** (vol''uh·til·i·zay'shun) *n.;* **vol·a·til·ize** (vol'uh·til·ize) *v.*

volatile oil. Oil characterized by volatility, variously obtained from tissues of certain plants, particularly odoriferous ones. The oil may exist as such in the plant or may be formed during the process of obtaining it, as by hydrolytic or pyrolytic action. Volatile oils may contain a variety of chemical compounds, for example hydrocarbons, alcohols, ethers, aldehydes, ketones, acids, phenols, esters, and sulfur and nitrogen compounds. Syn. *essential oil.*

vo·le·mic (vo·lee'mick) *adj.* Pertaining to volume of blood or plasma.

vo·li·tion (vo·li'shun) *n.* The conscious will or determination to act. —**volition·al** (·ul) *adj.*

Volk·mann's canals (fohlk'mah^hn) In compact bone, the vascular channels that lack the concentric lamellae of haversian systems. The term is commonly erroneously applied to nutrient canals in compact bone, whether haversian or Volkmann's.

Volkmann's contracture Ischemic muscular contracture of the arm and hand resulting from pressure injury or a tight cast; often accompanied by muscle degeneration and ultimate extensive fibrosis and claw hand.

Volkmann's paralysis The paralysis that accompanies Volkmann's contracture.

vol·ley, *n.* Approximately simultaneous discharges, as nerve impulses that travel simultaneously in different axons of a nerve or that are discharged simultaneously from groups of central neurons.

Vollmer patch test A tuberculin test in which gauze saturated with tuberculin is applied to an intact skin surface under adhesive plaster.

vol·sel·la (vol·sel'uh) *n.* A forceps having one or more hooks at the end of each blade.

volt, *n.* The unit of electromotive force and electric potential; the electromotive force that, steadily applied to a conductor whose resistance is one ohm, will produce a current of one ampere. Abbreviated, v

volt·age, *n.* Electromotive force measured in volts.

volt-ammeter, *n.* An instrument for measuring both voltage, or potential, and amperage, or amount of current.

volt-ampere, *n.* The power developed in an electric circuit when the current is one ampere and the potential one volt; equivalent in a direct current to a watt.

volt·me·ter (vohlt′mee″tur) *n*. An instrument for measuring voltage, or electromotive force.

volume dose. *In radiation therapy*, the total energy absorbed by an entire irradiated volume of tissue.

volume index. The relation of the volume of the red corpuscles to their number.

volume percent. The number of milliliters of a substance contained in 100 ml of medium. Usually refers to gas (O_2 or CO_2) contained in blood. Symbol, vol. %.

vol·u·met·ric (vol″yoo·met′rick) *adj*. Pertaining to measurement by volume.

vol·un·tary, *adj*. Under control of the will; performed by an exercise of the will.

vol·u·tin granules (vol′yoo·tin) Granules found in the cytoplasm of many bacterial and yeast cells, composed chiefly of complex salts of metaphosphoric acid polymers and staining red with methylene blue or toluidine blue. Syn. *metachromatic granules*.

vol·vu·lo·sis (vol·vew·lo′sis) *n*. ONCHOCERCIASIS.

vol·vu·lus (vol′vew·lus) *n*. A twisting of the bowel upon itself so as to occlude the lumen and, in severe cases, compromise its circulation. It occurs most frequently in the sigmoid flexure.

vo·mer (vo′mur) *n*. The thin plate of bone which is situated vertically between the nasal cavities, and which forms the posterior portion of the septum of the nose.

vom·ero·na·sal (vom″ur·o·nay′zul, vo″mur·o·) *adj*. Pertaining to the vomer and the nasal cavity.

vom·it, *v. & n*. 1. To expel from the stomach by vomiting. 2. Matter expelled from the stomach by vomiting.

vom·it·ing, *n*. The forcible ejection of the contents of the stomach through the mouth.

vomiting gas. A chemical agent that causes coughing, sneezing, pain in nose and throat, nasal discharge, sometimes tears, often followed by headache and vomiting; as, for example, adamsite. Syn. *irritant smoke* (obsol.).

vom·i·tive (vom′i·tiv) *adj*. EMETIC.

vom·i·to·ry (vom′i·to·ree) *n*. 1. Any agent that induces emesis. 2. A vessel used to receive vomited material.

vom·i·tu·ri·tion (vom″i·tew·rish′un) *n*. RETCHING.

vom·i·tus (vom′i·tus) *n*. VOMIT (2).

vomitus cru·en·tes (kroo·en′teez) Bloody vomit.

vomitus ma·ri·nus (ma·rye′nus). SEASICKNESS.

vomitus ma·tu·ti·nus (ma·tew·tye′nus). MORNING SICKNESS.

von Eco·no·mo's disease (fohn eʸ·ko·no′mo) ENCEPHALITIS LETHARGICA.

Vonedrine. Trademark for phenylpropylmethylamine, a vasoconstrictor applied topically, as the hydrochloride salt, to relieve nasal congestion.

von Gier·ke's disease (fohn geer′keʰ) A form of glycogenosis characterized by marked diminution in, or absence of, hepatic glucose 6-phosphatase resulting in hepatic glycogenosis, hypoglycemia, and acidosis. Syn. *glycogen storage disease, hepatic glycogenosis, type I of Cori, van Creveld-von Gierke's disease.*

von Graefe's sign Lid lag in hyperthyroidism.

von Jaksch's anemia or **disease** (fohn yaʰksh′) A nonspecific symptom complex of childhood consisting of severe anemia, extreme leukocytosis with lymphocytosis, lymphadenopathy, and hepatosplenomegaly in response to rickets, congenital syphilis, malnutrition, gastrointestinal disturbances, and a wide variety of other conditions and infections.

von Pir·quet test (fohn peer·keʰ) A tuberculin test in which the substance is applied to a superficial abrasion of the skin.

von Reck·ling·hausen's disease (fohn rek·ling·haʊw′zᵉn) 1. NEUROFIBROMATOSIS. 2. HEMOCHROMATOSIS. 3. Generalized osteitis fibrosa cystica.

von Wil·le·brand's disease (fohn vil′eʰ·braʰnt) VASCULAR HEMOPHILIA.

vo·ra·cious (vo·ray′shus) *adj*. Having an insatiable appetite or desire for food.

vor·tex (vor′tecks) *n*., pl. **vor·ti·ces** (·ti·seez) A structure having the appearance of being produced by a rotary motion about an axis.

vortices. Plural of *vortex*.

vor·ti·cose (vor′ti·koce) *adj*. Whirling; having a whorled appearance.

vox (vocks) *n*. VOICE.

vo·yeur (vwah·yur′) *n*. A person, usually a male, who obtains sexual gratification from witnessing the sexual acts of others or from viewing persons in the nude. —**voyeur·ism** (·iz·um) *n*.

VPB Abbreviation for *ventricular premature beat*.

vu·e·rom·e·ter (vew′ur·om′e·tur) *n*. An apparatus for determining the interpupillary distance.

vul·can·ize (vul′kuh·nize) *v*. To subject rubber to a process wherein it is treated with sulfur at a high temperature, and thereby rendered either flexible or very hard.

vul·ner·a·ble (vul′nur·uh·bul) *adj*. Susceptible to injury of any kind.

vul·nus (vul′nus) *n*. WOUND.

vulv-, vulvo-. A combining form meaning *vulva, vulvar*.

vul·va (vul′vuh) *n*., genit. **vul·vae** (·vee) The external genital organs in woman. —**vul·var** (·vur), **vul·val** (·vul) *adj*.

vulva con·ni·vens (ko·nye′venz). A form of vulva in which the labia majora are in close apposition.

vulva hi·ans (high′anz) The form of vulva in which the labia majora are gaping.

vulvar anus. An anomalous condition in whic' the anus is imperforate, the rectum opening into the vulva.

vul·vec·to·my (vul·veck′tuh·mee) *n*. Surgical excision of the vulva.

vul·vis·mus (vul·viz′mus) *n*. VAGINISMUS.

vul·vi·tis (vul·vye′tis) *n*. Inflammation of the vulva.

vul·vo·va·gi·nal (vul″vo·va·jye′nul, ·vaj′i·nul) *adj*. Of or pertaining to both the vulva and vagina.

vul·vo·vag·i·ni·tis (vul″vo·vaj″i·nigh′tis) *n*. Inflammation of the vulva and of the vagina existing at the same time.

v wave. 1. The positive-pressure wave in the

atrial or venous pulse due to caval and atrial filling during ventricular systole. 2. The giant positive-pressure wave in the atrial or venous pulse, produced by fusion of the regurgitant wave with the c and v waves, obliterating the negative x wave and producing a venous pulse wave similar to that found in the ventricles.

V-Z virus. VARICELLA-ZOSTER VIRUS.

W

W 1. Symbol for wolfram (= TUNGSTEN). 2. Abbreviation for *watt*.

wad·ding, *n.* 1. Carded cotton or wool, used for surgical dressings, generally not of the first quality. 2. Cotton batting, sometimes glazed to render it nonabsorbent.

wa·fer, *n.* A thin sheet made by heating moistened flour and formerly used to enclose powders that are taken internally. Syn. *cachet.*

waist, *n.* The narrowest portion of the trunk between the hips and the ribs.

waist·line, *n.* The circumference of the waist.

wake·ful·ness, *n.* 1. A physiologic state in which the organism is alert and aware or conscious of itself and its responses to internal and external stimuli. 2. INSOMNIA.

Waldeyer's tonsillar ring A ring of lymphatic tissue formed by the two palatine tonsils, the pharyngeal tonsil, and smaller groups of lymphatic follicles at the base of the tongue and behind the posterior pillars of the fauces.

walking iron or **splint.** A metal support attached to a splint, shoe, or plaster cast designed to permit walking without the sole of the foot coming in contact with the ground, used in ambulatory treatment of fractures of the lower leg.

wall, *n.* The bounding side or inside surface of a natural or artificial cavity or vessel.

wal·le·ri·an degeneration (wah·lirr'ee·un) A basic pathologic process affecting peripheral nerves, in which there is degeneration of the axis cylinder and myelin distal to the site of axonal interruption, associated with central chromatolysis.

wall·eye (wawl'eye) *n.* 1. LEUKOMA (1). 2. EXOTROPIA. —**wall-eyed** (·ide) *adj.*

Wal·thard's inclusions, islets, or **rests** (vahʰl'tart) Groups of epithelial cells found in the superficial part of the ovaries, uterine tubes, and ligaments.

wan·der·ing, *adj.* 1. Moving about. 2. Abnormally movable.

wandering abscess. An abscess in which the pus has traveled along the connective-tissue planes and points at some locality distant from its origin. Syn. *abscessus per decubitum.*

wandering atrial pacemaker. WANDERING SUPRAVENTRICULAR PACEMAKER.

wandering erysipelas. A form of erysipelas in which the erysipelatous process successively disappears from one part of the body to appear subsequently in another part.

wandering supraventricular pacemaker. Shifting of the cardiac impulse formation from the sinus node to the atrium or atrioventricular node; recognizable on the electrocardiogram.

Wang·en·steen's apparatus A suction apparatus connected with a Wangensteen or Miller-Abbott tube, which provides and maintains constant gentle aspiration, used for relief of gastric and intestinal distention, and in the treatment of obstruction.

Wangensteen tube A long slender catheter, passed through the nose into the stomach or duodenum to provide continuous drainage.

war·ble fly (wor'bul). A fly of the family Oestridae, the cause of warbles.

war·bles, *n.* The disease produced by infestation of domestic animals and man with the larva of the warble fly or botfly.

ward, *n.* A division or large room of a hospital.

war·fa·rin sodium (wahr'fuh·rin) 3-(α-Acetonylbenzyl)-4-hydroxycoumarin sodium. $C_{19}H_{15}NaO_4$, an anticoagulant drug.

war fever. EPIDEMIC TYPHUS.

warm-blooded, *adj.* Having a relatively high and constant body temperature, as birds and mammals; HOMEOTHERMIC. Syn. *hematothermal.*

war neurosis. A gross stress reaction to combat, and sometimes to the war situation in general, resulting in a transient situational personality disturbance usually accompanied by somatic complaints and conversion symptoms.

wart (wort) *n.* 1. VERRUCA VULGARIS. 2. Any rough-surfaced skin papule.

War·thin-Fin·kel·dey giant cells Multinucleated giant cells found in lymphoid tissue in patients with measles. They contain many small moderately vesicular nuclei closely clumped together and relatively scanty cytoplasm. The nuclei may number 100 in a cell and give the so-called mulberry outline.

Warthin's tumor A benign salivary gland tumor, usually of the parotid gland, composed of lymphoid interstitial tissue arranged in papillary processes and covered by a layer of epithelium. Syn. *adenocystoma lymphomatosum.*

wash, *n.* Any of a class of liquid medicinal preparations, usually solutions but sometimes suspensions, for local application without friction or rubbing.

wash·er·wom·an's itch. Dermatitis of the hands, a general term for various eruptions, usually a fungus infection or contact dermatitis; seen in those who wash their hands frequently in water.

washing soda. A hydrous form of sodium carbonate, $Na_2CO_3.10H_2O$.

wasp waist. A very slender waist caused by atrophy of the trunk muscles, as seen in muscular dystrophy.

Wassermann's test A complement-fixation test for syphilis currently utilizing sensitized lipid extracts of beef heart as antigen in order to detect reagin.

waste, *n. & v.* 1. Useless matter. 2. Material of no metabolic utility. 3. EXCREMENT. 4. To become thin; to pine away. —**wast·ing,** *adj.*

wast·er (way'stur) *n.* 1. A child suffering from marasmus. 2. An animal affected with tuberculosis, usually bovine types.

wa·ter, *n.* 1. The liquid consisting of molecules of the composition H_2O, or aggregates thereof. 2. *In pharmacy,* any saturated aqueous solution of a volatile oil or other aromatic or volatile substance. Syn. *aromatic water.*

water brash. PYROSIS.

water-drinking test or **tonography.** A provocative test for open-angle glaucoma in which the patient drinks water. Increase in ocular pressure of more than 6 mmHg when the initial tension is 30 mm, or of more than 9 mmHg when initial tension is less than 30 mm, is indicative of a positive reaction. Osmotic changes in blood serum are responsible for the change in ocular tension.

water-hammer pulse. A pulse characterized by a rapid forceful ascent or upstroke.

Wa·ter·house-Fri·de·rich·sen syndrome The association of bacteremia, particularly acute meningococcemia, massive skin hemorrhage, shock, and acute adrenal hemorrhage and insufficiency.

water intoxication. Cramps, dizziness, headache, vomiting, convulsions, and coma, produced by excessive administration of water or hypotonic solutions, or from water retention, resulting in hemodilution; may occur after administration of tap water enemas, especially to small children, or after head trauma, encephalitis, or from hypothalamic tumors or administration of drugs or anesthetics which result in inappropriate secretion of antidiuretic hormone.

water itch. 1. SCHISTOSOME DERMATITIS. 2. ANCYLOSTOMIASIS.

water mattress. A large, mattress-shaped, leak-proof bag which, when filled with water, conforms to the patient's body with uniform pressure, and supports his weight without excessive pressure on tissues overlying bony prominences.

water of crystallization. Water that is coordinated, bound, or held in a lattice position in a crystal in definite molecular proportion and is essential for the characteristic form of the crystal. It may often be removed by heating, with resultant physical disruption of the crystal.

water of hydration. Water that may be variously combined in a substance in definite molecular proportion and that may be expelled by heating without essentially altering the physical form of the substance or changing its chemical identity.

water-pitressin test. A combination of water intoxication induced by forced liquid intake, with administration of pitressin to detect the existence of epilepsy in a patient. A seizure will be produced in about 50% of all persons predisposed to convulsions. Since the test is positive in a high percentage of normal individuals, and does not rule out epilepsy if negative, it is no longer used, although it was extensively employed around World War I.

wa·ter·shed, *n. In neurology,* the territory at the distal extent of any major arterial supply, and particularly the region at the junction between the terminal branches of two major cerebral arteries, such as the anterior and middle cerebral.

water test. A test for Addison's disease based on the fact that patients with this disease do not have a normal diuresis following the rapid intake of a large quantity of water. After a water load any hourly urine volume will not exceed the total night urine volume in a patient with Addison's disease.

Watson-Schwartz test A test for porphobilinogen in the urine; used to diagnose acute porphyria.

watt, *n.* A unit of power, in the meter-kilogram-second system, that produces energy at the rate of one joule per second. It is the power required to cause an unvarying current of one ampere to flow between points differing in potential by one volt. Abbreviated, W.

watt·age (wot'ij) *n.* Consumption or output of an electric device in watts.

watt·me·ter (wot'mee''tur) *n.* An instrument for measuring electric power or activity in watts.

wave, *n.* 1. A uniform movement in a body which is propagated with a continuous motion, each part of the body vibrating through a fixed path. 2. The course traced by a lever or a beam of light on a surface moving at right angles to the direction of lever or beam. 3. A curve or undulation traced by a recording device, as an electrocardiograph or electroencephalograph, and reflecting alterations in electrical activity or in pressure of a part.

wave-and-spike. SHARP AND SLOW WAVE COMPLEX.

wave·length, *n.* The distance in the line of advancement between two points of a sine wave such that the two points are in the identical phase of the wave cycle. Differences in wavelength distinguish visible light, roentgen rays, and gamma rays from one another. Frequency and wavelength are related by the equation, $C = f\lambda$, where C is the velocity of wave propagation, f is the frequency of the waves, and λ is their wavelength. Abbreviated, wl. Symbol, λ.

wave number. The number of waves or cycles of light flux or radiant energy. measured through a distance of 1 cm.

wax, *n.* Any substance, of plant, animal, or mineral origin, consisting of a mixture of one or more of the following constituents: high molecular weight fatty acids, high molecular weight monohydric alcohols, esters of the fatty acids and alcohols, and solid hydrocarbons. Waxes are usually hard, brittle solids that become pliable on warming and melt on further heating.

waxy, *adj.* 1. Resembling or covered with wax. 2. Affected with amyloid degeneration or amyloidosis.

waxy cast. A tubal renal cast composed of translucent, usually amyloid, material.

waxy degeneration. 1. AMYLOID DEGENERATION. 2. ZENKER'S DEGENERATION.

waxy flexibility. *In psychiatry,* a form of stereotypy in which the patient maintains a posture in which he was placed with waxlike rigidity for a much longer period than is normally tolerable; typical of the catatonic type of schizophrenia.

WBC Abbreviation for (a) *white blood cell;* (b) *white blood count.*

wean, *v.* To cease to suckle or nurse offspring at a period when the latter is capable of taking substantial food from sources other than the breast. —**wean·ing,** *n.*

wean·ling, *n.* A child or an animal that has been newly weaned.

wear-and-tear pigments. Pigments such as hemofuscin, hemosiderin, and lipochrome, observed in increased amounts in tissues of older individuals.

weav·er's bottom. LIGHTERMAN'S BOTTOM.

web, *n.* A membranelike structure; especially, the skin and underlying tissue between the bases of fingers or toes. —**webbed,** *adj.*

webbed neck. A condition in which a thick triangular fold of loose skin extends from each lateral side of the neck across the upper aspect of the shoulder, as seen in gonadal dysgenesis. Syn. *pterygium colli.*

Weber-Christian disease Febrile, relapsing, nodular nonsuppurative panniculitis.

Weber's test A hearing test in which the vibrations from a tuning fork placed on the forehead of a normal patient are referred to the midline and heard equally in both ears; in unilateral middle-ear deafness, the sound is heard in the diseased ear; in deafness due to disease of the auditory nerve on one side, it is heard better in the normal ear.

Wechs·ler-Belle·vue intelligence scale A verbal and performance test for persons aged 16 to 64 years, comprising 11 subtests: information,

comprehension, arithmetical reasoning, digit memory, similarities, vocabulary, picture arrangement, picture completion, block design, object assembly, and digit symbol.

wedge pressure. Pulmonary capillary pressure, measured at cardiac catheterization by wedging the cardiac catheter in the most distal pulmonary artery branch; it reflects mean left atrial pressure. Syn. *pulmonary artery wedge pressure.*

weep·ing, *adj. & n.* 1. Exuding, as a raw or excoriated surface bathed with a moist discharge. 2. LACRIMATION. 3. Exudation or leakage of a fluid.

We·ge·ner's granulomatosis (ve⁷guh-nur) A rare disease of unknown causation characterized by necrotizing granulomas in the air passages, necrotizing vasculitis, and glomerulitis.

weight, *n.* The force with which a body is attracted by the earth. For weights listed by name, see Tables of Weights and Measures in the Appendix.

Weil-Fe·lix reaction (vile, fee'licks) The agglutination of certain strains of *Proteus vulgaris* (OX 19, OX 2, OX K) by the serums of patients with certain rickettsial infections, probably due to the presence of similar antigens in both *Proteus* and *Rickettsia.*

Weil-Felix test. An agglutination test based on the Weil-Felix reaction; used in the diagnosis of certain rickettsial diseases.

Weill-Mar·che·sa·ni syndrome (veʰl, mar"keʹzahʹnee) A heritable disorder of connective tissue manifested by short stature, brachydactylia, and spherophakia with associated myopia and glaucoma. Syn. *Marchesani syndrome.*

Weil's disease A severe form of leptospirosis, characterized by jaundice, oliguria, circulatory collapse, and hemorrhagic tendencies. Syn. *icterohemorrhagic fever. leptospirosis icterohemorrhagica. spirochetal jaundice.*

Welch bacillus CLOSTRIDIUM PERFRINGENS.

wen, *n.* A sebaceous cyst. The term is commonly used when the lesion occurs on the scalp.

Wenck·e·bach phenomenon (venk'eʰ.baᵏh) A form of second-degree atrioventricular block with progressive prolongation of the P-R interval, resulting finally in a nonconducted P wave; at this point the P-R interval shortens and the sequence recurs.

Werd·nig-Hoff·mann atrophy, disease, paral· sis, or **syndrome** (veʰrtʹnik, hoʰfʹmahn) I. FANTILE SPINAL MUSCULAR ATROPHY.

Werl·hof's disease (veʰrlʹhofe) IDIOPATHIC THROMBOCYTOPENIC PURPURA.

Werner's syndrome A multisystem disorder, probably of autosomal recessive inheritance, characterized by premature senescence, diminished body growth (dwarfism), cataracts, scleroderma-like skin changes, osteoporosis, and multiglandular dysfunction, particularly hypogonadism.

Wernicke's area The posterior portion of the left superior temporal gyrus, Brodmann's areas 41 and 42, destruction of which gives rise to a loss of comprehension of spoken language.

Wernicke's encephalopathy A disease of acute onset, characterized clinically by nystagmus, abducens and conjugate gaze palsies, ataxia of gait, mental confusion, and, in patients who recover, by an amnesic (Korsakoff's) psychosis; pathologically there are symmetrical areas of necrosis in the paraventricular regions of the thalamus and hypothalamus, the mamillary bodies, the periaqueductal region of the midbrain, floor of the fourth ventricle, and the superior vermis. The disease is usually observed in alcoholics and is due to nutritional deficiency, more specifically a deficiency of thiamine.

Wertheim's operation A radical total hysterectomy for carcinoma of the uterine cervix.

Wes·ter·gren method (ves'tur·grē'n″) A method to determine the blood sedimentation rate in which normal for men is 0 to 15 and for women is 0 to 20 mm in 1 hour.

West Nile fever. An acute febrile disease clinically resembling dengue fever and occurring principally in the Near East, caused by the West Nile virus. Syn. *Mediterranean dengue.*

West Nile virus A group B arbovirus, widespread in Africa and southern Asia, producing a very mild encephalitis similar to the St. Louis and Japanese B encephalitides. In the Near East it causes West Nile fever.

wet brain. Edema of the brain.

wet gangrene. MOIST GANGRENE.

wet nurse. A woman who furnishes breast feeding to an infant not her own.

wetting agent. A substance, commonly a synthetic organic compound, that causes a liquid to spread more readily upon a solid surface, chiefly through reduction of surface tension. Wetting agents are either ionic or nonionic, the former being further classified as cationic or anionic, depending on whether the characteristic activity is inherent in the cation or anion.

Wet·zel's grid A precision control chart for measuring and guiding growth and development of children from 5 to 18 years. Body build, maturation, nutritional grade, metabolic rate, and caloric intake are all determined by this graphic method.

W factor. BIOTIN.

Wharton's jelly The mucoid connective tissue that constitutes the matrix of the umbilical cord.

heal, *n.* A primary lesion of the skin that is a pruritic, circumscribed, edematous, usually transitory elevation that varies in size from a pin-head to that of the palm or larger, occurring classically in urticaria but also after insect bites, animal bites, trauma, or even as an effect of such physical agents as heat, cold, or sunlight. Syn. *pomphus, urtica.*

wheeze, *n.* A whistling or sighing noise produced in the act of breathing, often audible only on stethoscopic examination.

whey (whay) *n.* The liquid part of milk separating from the curd.

whip·lash injury. A syndrome, including headache, pain and tenderness of the occipitonuchal muscles and other supporting structures of the head and neck, related to the sudden extension or flexion of the neck which may occur in automobile occupants when their car is struck from behind or from the front.

Whip·ple operation Radical pancreaticoduodenectomy for carcinoma of the ampullary area and pancreatic head.

Whip·ple's disease A generalized disease associated with an intracellular bacterium and characterized by infiltration of the intestinal wall and lymphatics by glycoprotein-filled macrophages; there is steatorrhea, lymphadenopathy, arthritis, polyserositis, emaciation, and lipophagic intestinal granulomatosis. Syn. *intestinal lipodystrophy.*

Whipple's triad The three conditions which together are diagnostic of hyperinsulinism: attacks invariably occur while fasting; fasting blood sugar is below 50 mg/dl; immediate recovery from an acute attack occurs upon administration of glucose.

whip·worm, *n.* TRICHURIS TRICHIURA.

whirl·pool bath. A bath in which an arm, or a leg, or the greater part of the body is immersed in hot water which is agitated by a whirling or churning current of equally hot water mixed with air.

whis·key nose. RHINOPHYMA.

whis·per, *n.* A low, sibilant sound produced by the passage of the breath through the glottis without vibrating the vocal folds.

whispered pectoriloquy. The transmission of whispered voice sounds through the chest wall, heard stethoscopically; indicates consolidation near a large air passage.

white, *adj.* Having a color produced by reflection of all the rays of the spectrum; opposed to black.

white blood cell. LEUKOCYTE. Abbreviated, WBC.

white blood count. The calculation of the number of white blood cells per volume of blood or the determination of the percentages of each type of leukocyte. Abbreviated, WBC.

white comb. COMB DISEASE.

white commissure. 1. A band of myelinated nerve fibers in the spinal cord separating the anterior gray commissure from the bottom of the anterior median fissure. Syn. *anterior white commissure.* 2. See *white commissure* (1) (= anterior white commissure), *posterior white commissure.*

white fat. Ordinary adipose tissue as distinguished from brown fat; characterized by unilocular cells and white or yellow color.

white-grained mycetoma. A form of mycetoma, caused by any of eleven different etiological agents, in which the grains discharged in the exudate or on unstained tissue sections are white.

white infarct. An infarct in which the hemorrhage is slight, or the blood and blood pigments have been removed so that the infarct has become decolorized.

white matter. WHITE SUBSTANCE.

white-muscle disease. A degenerative process of skeletal or cardiac muscle affecting cattle and chickens and thought to result from at least three causes: vitamin E deficiency, selenium deficiency, and the toxic effect of certain poisonous plants.

white noise. WHITE SOUND.

white pulp. The lymphocytic portion of the spleen consisting of B and T lymphocyte zones and associated arterial vasculature and lymphatics; the site of antibody formation in the spleen.

whites, *n.* LEUKORRHEA.

white sound. 1. A noise made up of pure tones, harmonics, and discordants throughout the range of human hearing in equal parts and at equal intensities. It is used as a background noise in speech intelligibility tests. 2. The noise component in audio analgesia.

white substance or **matter.** The part of the central nervous system composed of myelinated nerve fibers.

Whit·field's ointment An ointment used in treatment of superficial fungous infections of the skin. It contains 6% benzoic acid, and 3% salicylic acid in a petrolatum or polyethylene glycol ointment base.

whit·low (whit'lo) *n.* Suppurative inflammation of the end of a finger or toe.

WHO Abbreviation for *World Health Organization.*

whole-body counter. A device, with heavy shielding to keep out background radiation and with ultrasensitive scintillation detectors and electronic equipment, used to identify and measure the radiation in the body of humans and animals.

whoop (hoop, whoop) *n.* The inspiratory crowing sound that precedes or occurs during a coughing paroxysm.

whoop·ing cough (hoop'ing). PERTUSSIS.

Wick·ham's striae A network of delicate bluishwhite lines associated with the characteristic lesions of lichen planus.

wick·ing, *n.* Loosely twisted unspun cotton or gauze, employed in packing cavities; a gauze wick.

Widal test A microscopic or macroscopic agglutination test for the diagnosis of typhoid fever and other Salmonella infections. Living cultures may be used specially prepared to preserve the Vi antigen; killed bacterial suspensions may be prepared with formalin to preserve the flagellar (H) antigen or with alcohol to preserve the somatic (O) antigen.

will, *n. In psychology,* the faculty by which the mind chooses its ends and directs action in carrying out its purpose.

Willis's glands CORPORA ALBICANTIA.

Wilms's or **Wilms' tumor** (vilms) A malignant mixed mesodermal tumor of the kidney, usually affecting infants and children.

Wilson-Mikity syndrome Progressive pulmonary insufficiency with dyspnea, tachypnea, rib retraction, and cyanosis, coming on at or soon after birth in very premature infants, whose chest radiographs characteristically show numerous small radiolucent cystlike lesions of the lungs.

Wilson's disease HEPATOLENTICULAR DEGENERATION.

wind·age (win'dij) *n.* Compression of air by the passage of a missile, shell, etc., near the body, causing blast injury.

wind-broken, *adj.* Affected with expiratory dyspnea; said especially of horses.

wind-gall (wind'gawl) *n.* A soft tumor or synovial swelling in the region of the fetlock joint of the horse.

wind·kes·sel (wind'kes·ul, vint') *n.* Compression chamberlike action of the aorta and its immediate branches in buffering pressure and flow changes during the cardiac cycle. This function of the large capacity and elastic walls of the vessels converts pulsatile flow to nearly continuous flow.

win·dow, *n. In anatomy,* a small aperture in a bone or other unyielding tissue.

wind·pipe, *n.* TRACHEA.

wind-puff, *n.* WINDGALL.

wind-stroke, *n.* Acute spinal paralysis of a horse.

wine-glass, *n.* A measure of nearly two fluidounces, or 60 ml.

wine spot. PORT-WINE NEVUS.

winged scapula. Projection of the scapula posteriorly, particularly noticeable when the arm is extended and pressed against a fixed object in front of the patient, due to weakness or paralysis of the serratus anterior muscle.

wink, *v.* 1. To close and open one eye voluntarily. 2. To blink.

winking spasm. Spasmodic twitching or blinking of the eyelids. May be a habit tic or be associated with irritative conditions of the eye or of the trigeminal or facial nerve. Syn. *spasmus nictitans.*

win·ter cough. Chronic bronchitis recurring every winter.

wintergreen oil. TEABERRY OIL.

Win·trobe-Lands·berg method A blood sedimentation rate technique in which a single tube is used for sedimentation rate and hematocrit determination.

wir·ing, *n.* Securing in position, by means of wire, fragments of a broken bone.

wiry, *adj.* Resembling wire; tough and flexible.

wis·dom tooth. The third molar tooth in man.

wish fulfilment. The discharge of psychologic or emotional tension by imagining a satisfactory solution or satisfying situation which reduces anxiety; a central theme in psychoanalytic theory, serving to explain the manifestation of repressed wishes in the form of neurotic symptoms, common errors, and (normally) dreams; a partial substitute for the forbidden or unattainable satisfaction.

Wis·kott-Al·drich syndrome A familial, sexlinked recessive disease, characterized by thrombocytopenia, bleeding diathesis, chronic eczema, recurrent infections (especially of ears), leukopenia with decreased lymphocytes in lymph nodes and spleen but not in the bone marrow, decreased gamma-A and gamma-M globulins, and deficient thymic maturation. Incomplete forms may exist.

witch's milk. Milk sometimes secreted from the breasts of a newborn infant.

Wi·teb·sky's substances. GROUP-SPECIFIC SUBSTANCES.

with·draw·al, *n.* 1. The taking away or removal of anything. 2. The discontinuance of a drug or medication. 3. COITUS INTERRUPTUS. 4. *In psychiatry,* a pattern of behavior in which an individual removes himself from conflicts by retreating from people and the world of reality; seen in its most pathologic form in schizophrenics.

withdrawal syndrome or symptoms. The complex of physical and psychological disturbances observed in addicts upon withdrawal of the addicting agent. Severity of the autonomic and psychomotor disturbances varies with the agent, length of addiction, and size of dosage.

with·ers (with'urz) *n.pl.* The ridge above the shoulders of the horse, formed by the spinous processes of the first eight or ten thoracic vertebrae.

wit·zel·sucht (vit'sul-zo͞okht) *n.* A mental condition characterized by silly behavior, shallow facetiousness, and unstable mood; regarded as a symptom of frontal lobe disease such as brain tumor.

wl Abbreviation for *wavelength.*

Wohl·fahr·tia (vohl·fahr'tee·uh) *n.* A genus of flesh flies.

Wohlfahrtia mag·nif·i·ca (mag·nif'i·kuh). The Old World flesh fly; the larvae are deposited in cutaneous lesions or in one of the body openings.

Wohlfahrtia mei·geni (migh'ge·nigh). A North American flesh fly.

Wohlfahrtia vig·il (vij'il). A North American flesh fly.

Wolff·ian (wŏol'fee·un, vol') *adj.* Described by or named after K. F. Wolff, German anatomist, 1733–1794.

Wolffian adenoma. ADRENOCORTICOID ADENOMA OF THE OVARY.

Wolffian body. MESONEPHROS.

Wolffian cyst. A cyst of mesonephric origin, usually near the ovary or uterine tube.

Wolffian duct. MESONEPHRIC DUCT.

Wolffian rests. MESONEPHRIC RESTS.

Wolff-Parkinson-White syndrome A disorder of activation of the heart due to accelerated conduction between the atria and ventricles and an abnormal excitation of the ventricles; characterized electrocardiographically by a short PR interval and a wide abnormal QRS complex, and clinically often by paroxysmal supraventricular tachycardia. Abbreviated, W-P-W syndrome. Syn. *pre-excitation syndrome.*

wolf-jaw, *n.* Bilateral cleft of the lip, jaw, and palate.

wolf-ram (wŏol'frum) *n.* TUNGSTEN.

wolfs·bane (wŏolfs'bane) *n.* 1. ACONITE. 2. Any plant of the genus *Aconitum,* especially *A. lycoctonum.*

Wol·man's disease A rare, autosomal recessive, inborn error of lipid metabolism in which large amounts of cholesteryl esters and triglycerides accumulate in the liver and other organs.

womb (woom) *n.* UTERUS.

wood alcohol. METHYL ALCOHOL.

wood charcoal. Charcoal prepared by incomplete combustion of wood.

wooden tongue. A disease of the tongue of cattle caused by a gram-negative rod, *Actinobacillus lignieresi;* formerly confused with actinomycosis.

Wood's light, filter, or lamp A light filter, made of glass containing nickel oxide, which transmits only ultraviolet rays; has been used in the diagnosis of infections by fungi, such as tinea capitis, which fluoresce when radiated with ultraviolet light.

wood spirit. METHYL ALCOHOL.

wood sugar. XYLOSE.

wood tick. DERMACENTOR ANDERSONI.

wood vinegar. Vinegar obtained by the dry distillation of wood.

woody thyroiditis. RIEDEL'S DISEASE.

wool fat. The purified, anhydrous, fatlike substance from the wool of sheep, *Ovis aries;* chiefly composed of esters of high molecular weight alcohols, as cholesterol and lanosterol, with fatty acids. Used as an ointment base. Syn. *anhydrous lanolin.*

wool-sort·er's disease. Anthrax brought on by inhalation of anthrax bacilli found in woolen particles.

word blindness. ALEXIA.

word deafness. AUDITORY VERBAL AGNOSIA.

word sal·ad. Meaningless words or neologisms emitted by psychotic patients, particularly with schizophrenia. Syn. *schizophasia.*

work-up, *n.* The results of investigation of a patient's illness, including history, physical examination, and laboratory and x-ray studies.

work up, *v.* To investigate a patient's illness by a variety of means.

World Health Organization. A specialized agency of the United Nations Organization whose broad purposes in the international health field are primarily to assist governments upon request in the field of health; to promote standards, provide information, and foster research in the field of health; to promote cooperation among scientific and professional groups; to promote and foster activities in the field of maternal and child health and of mental health; and to study and report on administrative and social techniques as relating to preventive medicine. It has authority to make sanitary and quarantine regulations, to regulate morbidity and mortality nomenclature, and to set standards for purity and potency of biological and pharmaceutical products. Abbreviated, WHO.

worm, *n.* A member of the phyla Annelida, Nemathelminthes, or Platyhelminthes. The medically important forms belong to the last two phyla.

Wor·mi·an bone (wur'mee·un) SUTURAL BONE.

wound (woond) *n.* The disruption of normal anatomical relationships, or loss of tissue, resulting from surgery or physical injury.

wound diphtheria. SURGICAL DIPHTHERIA.

wound shock. HYPOVOLEMIC SHOCK.

W-P-W syndrome. Abbreviation for *Wolff-Parkinson-White syndrome.*

Wright's stain A specially prepared polychrome methylene blue stain used to color the formed elements of blood in smears.

wrin·kles, *n.pl.* Minute crevices or furrows in the skin sometimes caused by habitual frowning, but particularly by old age, due to dehydration and atrophy of the corium.

wrist, *n.* 1. The part of the upper limb at which the hand joins the forearm. 2. WRIST JOINT.

wrist drop, wrist-drop. Inability to extend the hand at the wrist due to paralysis of the extensor muscles of the forearm and hand.

wrist flexion reflex. Flexion of the fingers induced by percussion of the flexor tendons of the wrist on the palmar surface of the forearm when the hand is in supination and the fingers are slightly flexed.

wrist joint. The joint in which the proximal row of carpal bones articulates with the radius and the articular disk of the distal radioulnar joint.

writer's cramp or **paralysis.** An occupational spasm affecting a hand.

writing hand. A peculiar position assumed by the hand in parkinsonism, with an exaggerated flexion of the metacarpophalangeal joints and an extension of the fingers.

wry-head, *n.* PLAGIOCEPHALY.

w.s. Abbreviation for *water soluble.*

Wuch·er·er·ia (voo″kur·err′ee·uh, wooch·ur·eer′ ee·uh) *n.* A genus of filarial worms found in all the warm regions of the world. The larva or microfilaria must be ingested by a mosquito for metamorphosis to take place.

Wuchereria ban·crof·ti (ban·krof′tye). A species of filaria of worldwide distribution. Man is the only known definitive host.

Wuchereria ma·layi (may·lay′eye). BRUGIA MA-LAYI.

wuch·er·e·ri·a·sis (wooch″ur·e·rye′uh·sis, vook″ ur·) *n.* Infection with worms of the genus *Wuchereria.*

w/v Weight in volume; indicating that a weighed quantity of a solid substance is contained in solution in a measured volume of liquid.

X

X. Symbol for the decimal scale of potency or dilution; used by homeopaths.

xanth-, xantho- A combining form meaning *yellow.*

xan·the·las·ma (zanth″e·laz′muh) *n.* Yellowish raised plaques occurring around the eyelids, resulting from lipid-filled cells in the dermis.

xan·thene (zan′theen) *n.* 1. Dibenzopyran, $C_{13}H_{10}O$, a three-ring heterocyclic compound resulting from the joining of two benzene rings by a methylene (CH_2) and also an oxygen bridge. Certain derivatives are medicinally important. 2. Any of several derivatives of xanthene (1).

xan·thine (zan′theen, ·thin) *n.* 2,6($1H,3H$)-Purinedione, or 2,6-dioxopurine, $C_5H_4N_4O_2$, found in plant and animal tissues; an intermediate product in the transformation of adenine and guanine into uric acid.

xanthine oxidase. A flavoprotein enzyme catalyzing the oxidation of certain purines.

xan·thi·nu·ria (zan″thi·new′ree·uh) *n.* The presence of xanthine in urine.

xan·tho·chro·mat·ic (zan″tho·kro·mat′ick) *adj.* Yellow-colored.

xan·tho·chro·mia (zan″tho·kro′mee·uh) *n.* 1. A yellow discoloration of the skin. 2. The yellow discoloration of the cerebrospinal fluid, diagnostic of hemorrhage in the spinal cord, brain, or subarachnoid or subdural space. —**xan·thochro·mic** (·mick) *adj.*

xan·tho·cy·a·no·pia (zan″tho·sigh″uh·no′pee·uh) *n.* A defect of color vision in which yellow and blue are perceived, while red and green are not.

xan·tho·cy·a·nop·sia (zan″tho·sigh″uh·nop′see·uh) *n.* XANTHOCYANOPIA.

xan·tho·der·ma (zan″tho·dur′muh) *n.* A yellow discoloration of the skin.

xan·tho·gran·u·lo·ma (zan″tho·gran′yoo·lo′muh) *n.* JUVENILE XANTHOGRANULOMA. —**xanthogranu·lom·a·tous** (·lom′uh·tus) *adj.*

xan·tho·gran·u·lo·ma·to·sis (zan″tho·gran″yoo·lo′muh·to′sis) *n.* HAND-SCHÜLLER-CHRISTIAN SYNDROME.

xan·tho·ma (zan·tho′muh) *n.,* pl. **xanthomas, xanthoma·ta** (·tuh) A collection of lipid-filled histiocytes, appearing grossly as a yellow mass, and usually found in the subcutaneous tissue, often around tendons.

xanthoma dis·sem·i·na·tum (di·sem″i·nay′tum). Xanthomas appearing as papules or plaques diffusely distributed chiefly over the face, flexor surfaces, and often the mucous membranes.

xan·tho·ma·to·sis (zan·tho″muh·to′sis) *n.* A condition marked by the deposit of a yellow or orange lipid material in the reticuloendothelial cells, the skin, and the internal organs.

xan·tho·ma·tous (zan·tho″muh·tus, ·thom′uh·) *adj.* Of the nature of, or affected with, xanthoma.

xanthomatous cirrhosis. Intrahepatic biliary cirrhosis complicated by high blood lipid levels and xanthomatous deposits in various tissues and organs.

xanthomatous giant-cell tumor of the tendon sheath. A benign, usually well-defined tumor composed of vacuolated macrophages and multinucleated giant cells set in a collagenic stroma, which varies greatly in amounts.

xanthoma tu·ber·o·sum (tew″bur·o′sum). Xanthomas appearing as papules, nodules, plaques, or linear lesions on the extensor surfaces, usually grouped together and often found about the joints. Tendon sheaths or other internal structures may be involved, giving various and bizarre symptoms.

xan·tho·phyll (zan′tho·fil) *n.* A dihydroxy-α-carotene, $C_{40}H_{56}O_2$, a yellow pigment widely distributed in nature. Syn. *lutein.*

xanthoproteic reaction or **test.** A test for proteins based on treatment with concentrated nitric acid. The yellow color that develops changes to deep orange on alkalization with ammonia.

xan·tho·pro·tein (zanth″o·pro′tee·in, ·teen) *n.* A yellowish derivative formed by the action of concentrated nitric acid on proteins. —**xan·tho·pro·te·ic** (·pro·tee′ick) *adj.*

xan·thop·sia (zan-thop'see·uh) *n.* Yellow vision; the condition in which objects look yellow; sometimes occurring in jaundice.

xan·thop·sin (zan-thop'sin) *n.* Visual yellow, produced by the action of light on rhodopsin.

xan·thop·ter·in (zan-thop'tur·in) *n.* 2-Amino-4,6-dihydroxypteridine, $C_6H_5N_5O_2$, a yellow pigment, widely distributed in animal organisms and representing an element of the structure of folic acid; it may have a role in hemopoiesis.

xan·thor·rhea, xan·thor·rhoea (zan''tho·ree'uh) *n.* An acrid, purulent, yellow discharge from the vagina.

xan·tho·sine (zanth'o·seen, ·sin) *n.* A nucleoside made up of xanthine and ribose.

xan·tho·sis (zan·tho'sis) *n.* A reversible discoloration of the skin due to a deposit of carotenoid pigment; occurs from eating quantities of carrots, squash, sweet potatoes, etc. A similar dicoloration results from taking quinacrine over a period of time.

xan·thu·re·nic acid (zan''thew·ree'nick). 4,8-Dihydroxyquinaldic acid, $C_{10}H_7NO_4$, excreted in the urine of pyridoxine-deficient animals following ingestion of tryptophan.

xan·thyl·ic (zan-thil'ick) *adj.* Pertaining to xanthine.

X chromosome. A sex-determining factor in ovum and approximately one-half of sperm. Ova fertilized by spermatozoa having the X chromosome give rise to female offspring.

Xe Symbol for xenon.

xen-, xeno- A combining form meaning (a) *different, foreign*; (b) *alien, intrusive*; (c) *host*, as in relation to parasites.

xe·no·di·ag·no·sis (zen''o·dye''ug·no'sis, zee''no·) *n.* The procedure of using a suitable arthropod to transfer an infectious agent from a patient to a susceptible laboratory animal.

xe·no·graft (zen'o·graft, zee''no·) *n.* A transplant from one species to another, especially one involving a wider genetic or species disparity than a heterograft.

xe·no·me·nia (zen''o·mee'nee·uh, zee''no·) *n.* VICARIOUS MENSTRUATION.

xe·non (zee'non, zen'on) *n.* Xe = 131.30. An inert gaseous element, atomic number 54, found in the atmosphere.

xe·no·pho·bia (zen''o·fo'bee·uh, zée''no·) *n.* An abnormal fear of strangers.

Xen·op·syl·la (zen''op·sil'uh, zen''o·) *n.* A genus of fleas of the family Pulicidae.

Xenopsylla che·o·pis (kee·o'pis). The tropical rat flea; found chiefly in tropical and subtropical regions. A vector for bubonic plague and *Hymenolepis diminuta*, a tapeworm. This flea attacks man and other mammals, in addition to the rat, its natural host. It transmits the organism of murine typhus, *Rickettsia mooseri*, from rat to man and from rat to rat.

Xen·o·pus (zen'o·pus) *n.* A genus of African toad belonging to the Pipidae, used in laboratory tests for pregnancy.

xer-, xero- A combining form meaning *dry*.

xe·ran·tic (ze·ran'tick) *adj.* Having desiccative properties; drying. —**xeran·sis** (·sis) *n.*

xe·ro·der·ma (zeer''o·dur'muh) *n.* A condition of excessively dry skin.

xeroderma pig·men·to·sum (pig·men·to'sum). A genodermatosis characterized by premature degenerative changes in the form of keratoses, malignant epitheliomatosis, and hyper- and hypopigmentation.

xe·ro·mam·mo·gram (zeer''o·mam'o·gram) *n.* A xeroradiographic depiction of the breast.

xe·ro·mam·mog·ra·phy (zeer''o·ma·mog'ruh·fee) *n.* Xeroradiography of the breast.

xe·ro·me·nia (zeer''o·mee'nee·uh) *n.* The presence of the usual constitutional disturbances at the menstrual period but without the menstrual flow of blood.

xe·ro·myc·te·ria (zeer''o·mick·teer'ee·uh) *n.* Lack of moisture in the nasal passages.

xe·ro·pha·gia (zeer''o·fay'jee·uh) *n.* The habitual eating of dry or desiccated food.

xe·roph·thal·mia (zeer''off·thal'mee·uh) *n.* A dry and thickened condition of the conjunctiva, sometimes following chronic conjunctivitis, disease of the lacrimal apparatus, or vitamin-A deficiency.

xe·ro·ra·di·og·ra·phy (zeer''o·ray''dee·og'ruh·fee) *n.* A rapid method of recording a roentgen image by a dry process. A powdered surface of an electrically charged selenium plate records the roentgen image. —**xeroradi·o·graph·ic** (·o·graf'ick) *adj.*

xe·ro·sis (ze·ro'sis) *n.*, pl. **xero·ses** (·seez) Abnormal dryness of a tissue, as of the skin, eye, or mucous membranes.

xerosis con·junc·ti·vae (kon·junk·tye'vee). A condition marked by silver-gray, shiny, triangular spots on both sides of the cornea, within the region of the palpebral aperture, consisting of dried epithelium, flaky masses, and microorganisms. The spots are observed in some cases of hemeralopia.

xerosis in·fan·ti·lis (in·fan'ti·lis). Xerophthalmia marked by a lusterless, grayish white, foamy, greasy, very persistent deposit on the conjunctiva. Syn. *keratitis sicca*.

xe·ro·sto·mia (zeer''o·sto'mee·uh) *n.* Dry mouth, caused by insufficient secretion of saliva.

xe·ro·tes (zeer'o·teez) *n.* Dryness of the body.

xe·ro·to·cia (zeer''o·to'shee·uh) *n.* DRY LABOR.

xiph-, xiphi-, xipho- A combining form meaning *xiphoid*.

xiphi·ster·nal (zif''i·stur'nul) *adj.* Pertaining to the body and xiphoid process of the sternum.

xiphi·ster·num (zif''i·stur'num) *n.* XIPHOID PROCESS.

xipho·cos·tal (zif''o·kos'tul) *adj.* Pertaining to the xiphoid process and to the ribs.

xiph·o·dyn·ia (zif''o·din'ee·uh) *n.* Pain in the xiphoid process.

xiph·oid (zif'oid, zye'foid) *adj. & n.* 1. Sword-shaped; ensiform. 2. Pertaining to the xiphoid process. 3. XIPHOID PROCESS.

xiphoid appendix or **cartilage.** XIPHOID PROCESS.

xiph·oid·itis (zif''oid·eye'tis) *n.* Inflammation of the xiphoid process.

xiphoid process. The elongated process projecting caudad from the lower end of the sternum between the cartilages of the seventh ribs.

XYZ

Cartilaginous in early life, it usually becomes osseous after the age of 50. Syn. *ensiform process*.

X-linkage. The usual case of sex-linkage in which a gene is physically located on the X chromosome. An X-linked recessive trait will be expressed in all males but only in homozygous females.

X-linked. Of a genetically determined trait: caused or controlled by a gene on the X chromosome.

x-ray, X-ray, *n.* 1. Any electromagnetic radiation having a wavelength in the approximate range of 0.1 to 100 angstroms, usually produced by bombarding a metal target with fast electrons in a highly evacuated tube and that has a spectrum characteristic of the target metal. X-rays penetrate various thicknesses of solids, strongly ionize tissues, affect photographic plates, and cause certain substances to fluoresce. Syn. *roentgen ray.* 2. Any photograph taken with x-rays.

x-ray photography. RADIOGRAPHY.

x-ray unit. Any assemblage of equipment primarily for diagnostic or therapeutic use of x-rays.

xyl-, xylo- A combining form meaning *wood*.

xy·lene (zye'leen) *n.* Dimethylbenzene, $C_6H_4(CH_3)_2$, a colorless, mobile, flammable liquid. The xylene of commerce is a mixture of the three isomerides: *ortho-, meta-,* and *para-*xylenes. Has many industrial uses, and is used as a solvent and clearing agent in microscopy. Syn. *xylol.*

xy·lo·pho·bia (zye''lo·fo'bee·uh) *n.* An abnormal fear of trees, wooded plants, or forests.

xy·lose (zye'loce) *n.* Wood sugar, $C_5H_{10}O_5$, obtained from vegetable fibers; used medicinally as a diabetic food.

XYY male. An aneuploid state in which affected males with an extra Y chromosome are taller than usual and are regarded by some as having a tendency to sociopathic behavior.

Y

Y Symbol for yttrium.

yawn·ing, *n.* The often involuntary act of opening the mouth widely, accompanied by deep inspiration, and frequently stretching of the arms, shoulders, and chest to assist in the inspiratory act followed by relaxation of the muscles involved, usually performed when sleepy or bored.

yaws (yawz) *n.* An infectious tropical disease caused by *Treponema pertenue;* manifested by a primary cutaneous lesion followed by a granulomatous skin eruption, and occasionally late destructive lesions of the skin and bones.

Yb Symbol for ytterbium.

Y chromosome. A sex-determining factor in the spermatozoon giving rise to male offspring.

yeast, *n.* The name applied to cells of various species of *Saccharomyces.* Certain of these, in dried form, are employed nutritionally as a source of protein and members of the B-complex group of vitamins.

yellow fat. Ordinary adipose tissue as distinguished from brown fat; characterized by unilocular cells and white or yellow color.

yellow fever. An acute viral disease transmitted to man by mosquitoes and characterized by fever, icterus, bradycardia, proteinuria, and a bleeding tendency.

yel·low·root, *n.* HYDRASTIS.

yellow wax. The purified wax from the honeycomb of the bee, *Apis mellifera.* It consists chiefly of myricin (myricyl palmitate); also contains cerotic acid (cerin), melissic acid, and about 6% hydrocarbons of the paraffin series. Used in the formulation of ointments, cerates, plasters, suppositories, and surgical dressings in which it acts mechanically, either giving stiffness or serving to repel water. Syn. *beeswax.*

Y factor. PYRIDOXINE.

Y-linkage. A special case of sex linkage in which a gene is physically located on the Y chromosome. Y-linked traits can only be expressed in males.

yo·him·bé, yo·him·bi (yo·him′bee) *n.* The rubiaceous tree *Corynanthe yohimbi (Pausinystalia yohimbe)* growing in the southern Cameroons district in Africa. The bark contains several alkaloids of which the most important is yohimbine; both bark and yohimbine have been employed for reputed aphrodisiac effect.

yo·him·bine (yo·him′been) *n.* The principal alkaloid, $C_{21}H_{26}N_2O_3$, of yohimbé, identical with quebrachine. Has been used as an aphrodisiac and also in treating angina pectoris and arteriosclerosis.

yolk, *n.* The nutritive part of an ovum.

yolk sac. An extraembryonic membrane composed of endoderm and splanchnic mesoderm. It encloses the yolk mass in reptiles, birds, and monotremes, or a cavity in higher mammals. It is also the site of the formation of the primitive blood cells.

youth, *n.* The period between childhood and maturity.

yper·ite (ee′pur·ite) *n.* Bis(2-chloroethyl)sulfide, $(C_2H_4Cl)_2S$, so-called mustard gas, a vesicant liquid that has been used in chemical warfare.

Yt Alternate symbol for yttrium.

yt·tri·um (it′ree·um) *n.* $Y = 88.9059$. A rare metallic element, atomic number 39, density 4.34.

Z

Zen·ker's degeneration (tsenk'ur) Necrosis and hyaline degeneration in striated muscle, seen especially in infectious disease.

Zenker's diverticulum or **pouch** A pulsion diverticulum of the esophagus.

Zenker's fixative or **fixing fluid** A mixture of potassium bichromate, mercuric chloride, distilled water, and glacial acetic acid; used in numerous fixing techniques.

ze·o·lite (zee'o·lite) *n.* Any one of a group of hydrated aluminum and calcium or sodium silicates, of the type $Na_2O.2Al_2O_3.5SiO_2$ or $CaO.2Al_2O_3.5SiO_2$, certain of which may be used for water softening by an ion-exchange process.

Zephiran Chloride. A trademark for benzalkonium chloride, a quaternary antiseptic for topical application.

ze·ro, *n.,* pl. **xeros, xeroes** 1. Any character denoting absence of quantity. 2. The point on thermometers from which temperatures are counted.

zinc, *n.* $Zn = 65.37$. A bluish-white, lustrous, metallic element, atomic number 30, density 7.14. Salts of zinc are used as astringents and antiseptics.

zinc acetate. $Zn(C_2H_3O_2)_2.2H_2O$. White crystals or granules, freely soluble in water. Variously used as a topical astringent.

zinc chloride. $ZnCl_2$. White crystalline powder or granules, very soluble in water. Used topically as an astringent and desensitizer for dentin.

zinc oxide. ZnO. Very fine, amorphous, white or yellowish-white powder, insoluble in water. Variously used in lotions, ointments, and pastes, as a topical astringent and protectant.

zinc phenolsulfonate. $Zn(HOC_6H_4SO_3)_2.8H_2O$. Colorless, transparent crystals, freely soluble in water. Has been used topically as an antiseptic and astringent, and internally as an intestinal antiseptic. Syn. *zinc sulfocarbolate.*

zinc stearate. A compound of zinc with variable proportions of stearic and palmitic acids; a fine, white, bulky powder; insoluble in water and alcohol. Used in eczema and other cutaneous diseases, in the form of powder or made into an ointment.

zinc sulfate. $ZnSO_4.7H_2O$. Colorless, transparent prisms or needles, or granular, crystalline powder, very soluble in water. Used topically as an astringent, and internally as an emetic in poisoning.

zinc sulfocarbolate. ZINC PHENOLSULFONATE.

zinc·um (zink'um) *n.* ZINC.

zir·co·ni·um (zur·ko'nee·um) *n.* $Zr = 91.22$. A metallic element, atomic number 40, density 6.53; resembles titanium and silicon.

Zn Symbol for zinc.

zo-, zoo- A combining form meaning *animal.*

zo·an·thro·py (zo·an'thruh·pee) *n.* A delusional state in which the person imagines himself transformed into or inhabited by an animal.

Zollinger-Ellison syndrome Gastric hypersecretion and hyperacidity, fulminating intractable atypical peptic ulceration, and hyperplasia of the islet cells of the pancreas.

zo·na (zo'nuh) *n.,* pl. & genit. sing. **zo·nae** (·nee) 1. ZONE; belt, or girdle. 2. HERPES ZOSTER.

zona glo·me·ru·lo·sa (glo·merr·yoo·lo'suh). The outer zone of the adrenal cortex in which the cells are grouped in rounded masses.

zona pel·lu·ci·da (pe·lew'si·duh). The thick, solid, elastic envelope of the ovum. Syn. *oolemma.*

zone, *n.* A delimited area or region. —**zon·al** (zo'nul) *adj.*

zone of antigen excess. The zone in which the antigen-antibody complexes are soluble.

zone of inhibition. ZONE OF ANTIGEN EXCESS.

zon·es·the·sia, zon·aes·the·sia (zo''nes·theezh'uh, ·theez'ee·uh) *n.* GIRDLE PAIN.

zo·nif·u·gal (zo·nif'yoo·gul) *adj.* Pertaining to the tendency to pass out of, or away from, a zone.

zo·nip·e·tal (zo·nip'e·tul) *adj.* Pertaining to the tendency to pass into a zone from without.

zo·nu·la (zo'new·luh) *n.,* pl. **zonu·lae** (·lee). ZONULE.

zo·nu·lar (zo'new·lur) *adj.* Pertaining to a zonule.

zonular cataract. A partial, stationary cataract, which is bilateral and may be congenital or form in infancy, due to a disturbance of calcium metabolism; characterized by a grayish central disk surrounded by a clear lens substance. Syn. *lamellar cataract.*

zo·nule (zo'newl, zon'yool) *n.* A small band.

zo·nu·li·tis (zo'new·lye'tis, zon'yoo·) *n.* Inflammation of the ciliary zonule.

zo·nu·lot·o·my (zo'new·lot'uh·mee, zon'yoo·) *n.* The severing of the ciliary zonular fibers.

zo·nu·ly·sis (zo'new·lye'sis, zon'yoo·) *n.* Enzymatic dissolution of the ciliary zonular fibers of the eye.

zoo·der·mic (zo'o·dur'mick) *adj.* Pertaining to, or taken from, the skin of some animal other than man; applied to a form of skin grafting.

zoo·eras·tia (zo'o·e·ras'tee·uh) *n.* Sexual intercourse with an animal.

zoo·ge·og·ra·phy (zo'o·jee·og'ruh·fee) *n.* The geography of animal life.

zoo·graft (zo'o·graft) *n.* A graft of tissue taken from an animal and transplanted to a human.

zoo·lag·nia (zo'o·lag'nee·uh) *n.* Sexual attraction toward animals.

-zoon A combining form meaning *living being, animal.*

zoo·no·sis (zo'o·no'sis, zo·on'o·sis) *n.,* pl. **zoono·ses** (·seez) A disease of lower animals transmissible to other vertebrate animals and man. **—zoo·not·ic** (·not'ick) *adj.*

zo·o·par·a·site (zo'o·păr'uh·site) *n.* An animal parasite. **—zoo·par·a·sit·ic** (·păr''uh·sit'ick) *adj.*

zooparasitic cirrhosis. Cirrhosis resulting from the invasion of animal parasites or their ova, such as *Schistosoma.*

zo·oph·a·gous (zo·off'uh·gus) *adj.* Subsisting on animal food.

zo·oph·i·lism (zo·off'i·liz·um) *n.* 1. The love of animals; it is usually immoderate, and toward certain animals. 2. *In psychiatry,* sexual pleasure from stroking or fondling animals.

zoo·pho·bia (zo'o·fo'bee·uh) *n.* Abnormal fear of animals.

zoo·plasty (zo'o·plas'tee) *n.* The surgical transfer of zoografts; the transplantation of tissue from any of the lower animals to man. **—zoo·plas·tic** (zo'o·plas'tick) *adj.*

zo·op·sia (zo·op'see·uh) *n.* The seeing of animals, as an illusion or as a hallucination or in a dream; occurs commonly in delirium tremens.

zoo·tox·in (zo'o·tock'sin) *n.* Any toxin or poison of animal origin.

zos·ter (zos'tur) *n.* HERPES ZOSTER.

zoster fa·ci·a·lis (fay·shee·ay'lis). Herpes zoster involving the sensory fibers of the trigeminal nerve distributed over the face. Any or all of the three branches may be involved.

zos·ter·i·form (zos·terr'i·form) *adj.* Resembling herpes zoster.

zos·ter·oid (zos'tur·oid) *adj.* ZOSTERIFORM.

zoster oph·thal·mi·cus (off·thal'mi·kus). A herpes zoster eruption in the course of the ophthalmic division of the fifth nerve.

Z-plastic relaxing operation. An operation for the relaxation of scar contractures, effected by a Z-shaped incision, with transposition of the flaps.

Z-plas·ty (zee'plas·tee) *n.* Z-PLASTIC RELAXING OPERATION.

Zr Symbol for zirconium.

zuck·er·guss (tsook'ur·goos) *adj.* Sugar-coated; applied especially to hyaline thickening of the splenic capsule, but also to hyaline thickening of other mesothelial coverings.

Zuck·er·kan·dl's bodies (tsook'ur·kahn''d'l) PARAAORTIC BODIES.

zuck·ung (tsook'oong) *n.* CONTRACTION; a term used in electrotherapeutics. Abbreviated, Z.

zwit·ter·ion (tsvit'ur·eye''un) *n.* An ion that contains both a positive and a negative charge, but is neutral as a whole; a dipolar ion. Amino acids may form such ions by migration of a hydrogen ion from the carboxyl group to the basic nitrogen atom as, for example, when RNH_2COOH is thus converted to $RNH_3{}^+COO^-$.

zyg-, zygo- A combining form meaning (a) *yoke, joining;* (b) *union, fusion;* (c) *pair.*

zyg·apoph·y·sis (zig''uh·pof'i·sis, zye''guh·) *n.,* pl. **zygapophy·ses** (·seez) An articular process of a vertebra. **—zyg·apoph·y·se·al** (·uh·pof''i·see'ul, ·uh·po·fiz'ee·ul) *adj.*

zy·go·dac·ty·ly (zye''go·dack'ti·lee) *n.* SYNDACTYLY.

zy·go·ma (zye·go'muh, zi·go'muh) *n.,* pl. **zygo·ma·ta** (·tuh), **zygomas** ZYGOMATIC BONE.

zy·go·mat·ic (zye''go·mat'ick) *adj. & n.* 1. Of or pertaining to the zygomatic bone. 2. Either of two small subcutaneous muscles arising from, or in relation with, the zygomatic bone. 3. A somatic sensory nerve, a branch of the maxillary nerve which innervates the skin in the region of the zygomatic bone and temple.

zygomatic arch. The arch formed by the zygomatic process of the temporal bone, the zygomatic bone, and the temporal process of the zygomatic bone.

zygomatic bone. The bone that forms the prominence of the cheek. Syn. *cheekbone.*

zy·go·mat·i·co·fa·cial (zye''go·mat''i·ko·fay'shul) *adj.* Pertaining to the zygomatic bone and the face.

zy·go·mat·i·co·max·il·lary (zye''go·mat''i·ko·mack'si·lerr·ee) *adj.* Pertaining to the zygomatic bone and the maxilla.

zy·go·mat·i·co·or·bit·al (zye''go·mat''i·ko·or'bi·tul) *adj.* Pertaining to the zygomatic bone and the orbit.

zy·go·mat·i·co·tem·po·ral (zye''go·mat''i·ko·tem'po·rul) *adj.* Pertaining to the zygomatic bone and the temporal bone or fossa.

zy·go·mat·i·cus (zye''go·mat'i·kus) *n.* A muscle of facial expression associated with the zygoma; ZYGOMATIC (2).

Zy·go·my·ce·tes (zye''go·migh·see'teez) *n. pl.* A group of fungi characterized by sexual reproduction through the union of two similar gametes.

zy·gos·ity (zye·gos'i·tee) *n.* The genetic state of the zygote, particularly with reference to identity (homozygosity) or nonidentity (heterozygosity) for one or more genes.

zy·go·spore (zye′go·spore) *n.* The spore resulting from the fusion of two similar gametes, as in certain algae and fungi.

zy·gote (zye′gote) *n.* 1. An organism produced by the union of two gametes. 2. The fertilized ovum before cleavage. —**zy·got·ic** (zye·got′ick) *adj.*

zy·go·tene (zye′go·teen) *n.* The stage in the first meiotic prophase in which pairing of homologous chromosomes occurs.

Zyloprim. Trademark for allopurinol, a suppressant for gout.

zy·mo·gen (zye′mo·jen) *n.* The inactive precursor of an enzyme which, on reaction with an appropriate kinase or other chemical agent, liberates the enzyme in active form.

zymogen granules. Secretion antecedent granules in gland cells, particularly those of the pancreatic acini and of the chief cells of the stomach, which are precursors of the enzyme secretion.

zy·mo·gen·ic (zye″mo·jen′ick) *adj.* 1. Causing fermentation. 2. Pertaining to, or producing, a zymogen.

zy·mo·hy·drol·y·sis (zye″mo·high·drol′i·sis) *n.* Hydrolysis produced by the action of an enzyme. Syn. *enzymatic hydrolysis.*

zy·mol·o·gy (zye·mol′uh·jee) *n.* The science of fermentation. —**zy·mo·log·ic** (zye″mo·loj′ick) *adj.*

zy·mol·y·sis (zye·mol′i·sis) *n.* FERMENTATION. —**zy·mo·lyt·ic** (zye″mo·lit′ick) *adj.*

zy·mom·e·ter (zye·mom′e·tur) *n.* An instrument for measuring fermentation.

zy·mo·phore (zye′mo·fore) *n.* The active part or moiety of an enzyme which possesses its characteristic activity. —**zy·mo·pho·ric** (zye″mo·fo′rick) *adj.*

zy·mo·pro·tein (zye″mo·pro′tee·in, ·teen) *n.* Any one of a class of proteins possessing catalytic powers.

zy·mo·sis (zye·mo′sis) *n.,* pl. **zymo·ses** (·seez) 1. FERMENTATION. 2. Any infectious or contagious disease. 3. The development or spread of an infectious disease. —**zy·mot·ic** (zye·mot′ick) *adj.*

zy·mos·ter·ol (zye·mos′tur·ole, ·ol) *n.* A sterol from yeast.

zy·mur·gy (zye′mur·jee) *n.* The branch of chemical technology dealing with the application of fermentation or enzymic action to any industrial process, as the curing of cheese, processing of leather, production of organic solvents.

Appendix

Name	Origin	Branches	Distribution
Accompanying median nerve	See *Median*		
Accompanying phrenic nerve	See *Pericardiacophrenic*		
Accompanying sciatic nerve	See *Sciatic*		
Acromiothoracic	See *Thoracoacromial*		
Alveolar, anterior superior (arteriae alveolares superiores anteriores [NA])	Infraorbital	Dental branches	Upper incisor and canine teeth; mucous membrane of maxillary sinus
Alveolar, inferior (arteria alveolaris inferior [NA])	Maxillary	Mental artery; dental and mylohyoid branches	Lower teeth; mandible and gums; mylohyoid muscle; buccal mucous membrane
Alveolar, posterior superior (arteria alveolaris superior posterior [NA])	Maxillary	Dental branches	Upper molar and premolar teeth and gums; mucous membrane of maxillary sinus; buccinator muscle
Angular (arteria angularis [NA])	Facial		Orbicularis oculi, nasalis, levator labii superioris, and procerus muscles; lacrimal sac; anastomoses with dorsal nasal branch of ophthalmic artery
Aorta, abdominal (aorta abdominalis [NA])	Continuation of descending aorta from level of lower border of twelfth thoracic vertebra	(1) Visceral celiac trunk superior mesenteric inferior mesenteric middle suprarenal renal testicular or ovarian (2) Parietal inferior phrenic lumbar (4 pairs) median sacral (3) Terminal common iliac	Diaphragm; body wall; abdominal and pelvic viscera; lower extremities
Aorta, abdominal (aorta abdominalis [NA])	Continuation of ascending aorta from upper border of right second costal cartilage to lower border of fourth thoracic vertebra	Brachiocephalic, left common carotid, left subclavian, lowest thyroid (occasionally)	
Aorta, ascending (aorta ascendens [NA])	Left ventricle	Left and right coronary	

Name	Origin	Branches	Distribution
Aorta, descending (aorta descendens [NA])	Continuation of arch of aorta. See *Aorta, abdominal; Aorta, thoracic*		
Aorta, thoracic (aorta thoracica [NA])	Portion of descending aorta in posterior mediastinum	Superior phrenic, posterior intercostal, subcostal arteries; bronchial, esophageal, mediastinal, and pericardial branches	Body wall; thoracic viscera; diaphragm
Appendicular (arteria appendicularis [NA])	Ileocolic		Vermiform appendix
Arch, deep palmar	See *Palmar arch, deep*		
Arch, plantar	See *Plantar arch*		
Arch, superficial palmar	See *Palmar arch, superficial*		
Arcuate of foot (arteria arcuata pedis [NA])	Dorsal pedal	Dorsal metatarsal, dorsal digital	Dorsal metatarsal portion of foot
Arcuate of kidney (arteriae arcuatae renis [NA])	Interlobar	Interlobular	Renal parenchyma
Auditory, internal	See *Labyrinthine*		
Auricular, deep (arteria auricularis profunda [NA])	Maxillary		Skin of external acoustic meatus; external surface of tympanic membrane
Auricular, posterior (arteria auricularis posterior [NA])	External carotid	Stylomastoid and posterior tympanic arteries; auricular, occipital, and stapedial branches	Digastric, stylohyoid, sternocleidomastoid, posterior auricular, occipitalis, and stapedius muscles; tympanic membrane and cavity; mastoid antrum; mastoid cells; semicircular canals; auricle; scalp; parotid gland
Axillary (arteria axillaris [NA])	Continuation of subclavian	Continues as brachial; highest thoracic, thoracoacromial, lateral thoracic, subscapular, anterior and posterior humeral circumflex	Muscles of upper arm, chest, and shoulder; mammary gland; shoulder joint; skin of pectoral region and shoulder; rete acromiale; head of humerus

Name	Origin	Branches	Distribution
Basilar (arteria basilaris [NA])	Formed by junction of two vertebral	Anterior inferior and superior cerebellar, labyrinthine, and posterior cerebral arteries; pontine branches	Pons; internal ear; cerebellum; pineal body; superior medullary velum; tela choroidea of third ventricle; temporal and occipital lobes of cerebrum
Brachial (arteria brachialis [NA])	Continuation of axillary	Deep brachial, inferior and superior ulnar collateral; terminates in radial and ulnar	Upper arm; elbow; forearm; hand
Brachial, deep (arteria profunda brachii [NA])	Brachial	Medial and radial collateral arteries; deltoid branch	Humerus; muscles of upper arm; radial nerve; rete olecrani
Brachiocephalic trunk (truncus brachiocephalicus [NA])	Arch of aorta	Right common carotid and right subclavian arteries; occasionally lowest thyroid artery, thymic and bronchial branches	Right side of neck and head; right shoulder girdle and arm; occasionally thymus gland, bronchus, inferior portion of thyroid gland
Buccal (arteria buccalis [NA])	Maxillary		Buccinator muscle; skin and mucous membrane of cheek; upper gums
Bulb of penis (arteria bulbi penis [NA])	Internal pudendal		Bulb of the penis; bulbourethral gland
Bulb of vestibule (of vagina) (arteria bulbi vestibuli [NA])	Internal pudendal		Bulb of the vestibule; major vestibular glands
Carotid, common (arteria carotis communis [NA])	Right from brachiocephalic, left from arch of aorta	External and internal carotid (terminal)	Region of neck and head
Carotid, external (arteria carotis externa [NA])	Common carotid	Superior thyroid, ascending pharyngeal, lingual, facial (linguofacial trunk), occipital, posterior auricular, superficial temporal, maxillary	Anterior portion of neck; face; scalp; side of head; ear; dura mater
Carotid, internal (arteria carotis interna [NA])	Common carotid	Ophthalmic, posterior communicating, anterior cerebral, middle cerebral arteries; caroticotympanic and anterior choroid branches	Anterior portion of cerebrum; eye; forehead; nose; internal ear; trigeminal nerve; dura mater; hypophysis
Celiac (trunk) (truncus celiacus [NA])	Abdominal aorta	Left gastric, common hepatic, lienal, dorsal pancreatic	Esophagus; cardia and lesser curvature of stomach; liver; gallbladder; pylorus; duodenum; pancreas; greater omentum; spleen

Name	Origin	Branches	Distribution
Central of retina (arteria centralis retinae [NA])	Ophthalmic		Retina
Cerebellar, anterior inferior (arteria cerebelli inferior anterior [NA])	Basilar	Labyrinthine	Anterior portion of inferior surface of cerebellum
Cerebellar, posterior inferior (arteria cerebelli inferior posterior [NA])	Vertebral		Medulla; choroidplexus of fourth ventricle; inferior portion of cerebellum
Cerebellar, superior (arteria cerebelli superior [NA])	Basilar		Vermis and superior surface of cerebellum; pineal body; superior medullary velum; tela choroidea of third ventricle
Cerebral, anterior (arteria cerebri anterior [NA])	Internal carotid	Anterior communicating artery; cortical, central, orbital, frontal, and parietal branches	Cortex of frontal and parietal lobes; portion of basal ganglia
Cerebral, middle (arteria cerebri media [NA])	Internal carotid	Cortical, central, orbital, frontal, parietal, temporal, and striate branches	Corpus striatum; cortex of orbital, frontal, parietal, and temporal lobes
Cerebral, posterior (arteria cerebri posterior [NA])	Basilar	Cortical, temporal, occipital, parietooccipital, central, and posterior choroid branches	Thalamus; tela choroidea and choroid plexus of third ventricle, cortex of temporal and occipital bones
Cervical, ascending (arteria cervicalis ascendens [NA])	Inferior thyroid	Spinal branches	Muscles of neck; spinal cord and its membranes; vertebrae
Cervical, deep (arteria cervicalis profunda [NA])	Costocervical trunk		Deep neck muscles; spinal cord
Cervical, superficial (arteria cervicalis superficialis [NA])	Transverse cervical		Trapezius, levator scapulae, splenius cervicis, and splenius capitis muscles; posterior chain of lymph nodes
Cervical, transverse (arteria transversa colli [NA])	Thyrocervical trunk	Superficial cervical, descending scapular	Trapezius, levator scapulae, splenius, rhomboid, and latissimus dorsi muscles; posterior chain of lymph nodes

Name	Origin	Branches	Distribution
Choroid, anterior (arteria choroidea anterior [NA])	Internal carotid		Optic tract; cerebral peduncle; base of cerebrum; lateral geniculate body; tail of caudate nucleus; globus pallidus; internal capsule; choroid plexus of inferior horn of lateral ventricle.
Choroid, posterior (ramus choroideus arteriae cerebri posterioris [NA])	Posterior cerebral		Tela choroidea and choroid plexus of third ventricle
Ciliary, anterior (arteriae ciliares anteriores [NA])	Ophthalmic		Iris and conjunctiva
Ciliary, long posterior (arteriae ciliares posteriores longae [NA])	Ophthalmic		Ciliary muscle and iris
Ciliary, short posterior (arteriae ciliares posteriores breves [NA])	Ophthalmic		Choroid and ciliary processes
Circumflex, anterior humeral (arteria circumflexa humeri anterior [NA])	Axillary		Coracobrachialis, biceps brachii, and deltoid muscles; shoulder joint; head of humerus
Circumflex, deep iliac (arteria circumflexa ilium profunda [NA])	External iliac	Ascending branch	Abdominal muscles; psoas, iliacus, sartorius, and tensor fasciae latae muscles; skin over course of vessel
Circumflex, lateral femoral (arteria circumflexa femoris lateralis [NA])	Deep femoral	Ascending, descending, and transverse branches	Muscles of thigh
Circumflex, medial femoral (arteria circumflexa femoris medialis [NA])	Deep femoral	Deep, ascending, transverse, and acetabular branches	Muscles of thigh; hip joint
Circumflex, posterior humeral (arteria circumflexa humeri posterior [NA])	Axillary		Deltoid, teres minor, and triceps brachii muscles; posterior portion of shoulder joint; rete acromiale
Circumflex, scapular (arteria circumflexa scapulae [NA])	Subscapular		Subscapularis, infraspinatus, teres, deltoid, and triceps brachii muscles; scapula; shoulder joint
Circumflex, superficial iliac (arteria circumflexa ilium superficialis [NA])	Femoral		Sartorius, iliacus, and tensor fasciae latae muscles; inguinal lymph nodes; skin over course of vessel

Name	Origin	Branches	Distribution
Clitoris, deep of (arteria profunda clitoridis [NA])	Internal pudendal		Corpus cavernosum of the clitoris
Clitoris, dorsal of (arteria dorsalis clitoridis [NA])	Internal pudendal		Clitoris
Colic, left (arteria colica sinistra [NA])	Inferior mesenteric	Ascending and descending branches	Left portion of transverse colon; upper portion of descending colon; splenic flexure
Colic, middle (arteria colica media [NA])	Superior mesenteric	Left and right branches	Upper portion of ascending colon; hepatic flexure; right portion of transverse colon
Colic, right (arteria colica dextra [NA])	Superior mesenteric	Ascending and descending branches	Ascending colon
Collateral, inferior ulnar (arteria collateralis ulnaris inferior [NA])	Brachial		Triceps brachii, brachialis, and pronator teres muscles; rete olecrani
Collateral, middle or medial (arteria collateralis media [NA])	Deep brachial		Triceps brachii muscle; rete olecrani
Collateral, radial (arteria collateralis radialis [NA])	Deep brachial		Triceps brachii and brachioradialis muscle; rete olecrani
Collateral, superior ulnar (arteria collateralis ulnaris superior [NA])	Brachial		Triceps brachii muscle; elbow joint and rete olecrani
Communicating, anterior (arteria communicans anterior cerebri [NA])	Anterior cerebral		Anterior perforated substance
Communicating, posterior (arteria communicans posterior cerebri [NA])	Internal carotid		Optic chiasm; optic tract; tuber cinereum; mamillary body; hippocampal gyrus; internal capsule; cerebral peduncle; interpeduncular region; thalamus
Companion of sciatic nerve (arteria comitans nervi ischiadici [NA])	See *Sciatic*		
Conjunctival, anterior (arteriae conjunctivales anteriores [NA])	Ophthalmic		Conjunctiva
Conjunctival, posterior (arteriae conjunctivales posteriores [NA])	Ophthalmic		Conjunctiva

Name	Origin	Branches	Distribution
Coronary, left (arteria coronaria sinistra [NA])	Left posterior aortic sinus	Anterior interventricular, and circumflex branches	Left atrium; root of aorta and pulmonary artery; myocardium of both ventricles; interventricular septum
Coronary, right (arteria coronaria dextra [NA])	Anterior aortic sinus	Posterior interventricular branches	Right atrium; root of aorta and pulmonary artery; anterior wall of right ventricle; septal myocardium; left ventricle adjoining posterior interventricular sulcus
Costocervical trunk (truncus costocervicalis [NA])	Subclavian	Deep cervical, highest intercostal	First and second intercostal spaces; muscles of neck; spinal cord and its membranes
Cremasteric (arteria cremasterica [NA])	Inferior epigastric		Spermatic cord and cremaster muscle in the male (corresponds to artery of the round ligament of the uterus in the female)
Cystic (arteria cystica [NA])	Right hepatic branch of hepatic proper		Surface of gallbladder
Deferential (arteria ductus deferentis [NA])	Internal iliac	Ureteric branches	Seminal vesical; ductus deferens; epididymis
Dental	See *Alveolar*		
Digital, common palmar (arteriae digitales palmares communes [NA])	Superficial palmar arch	Proper palmar digital	Fingers
Digital, common plantar (arteriae digitales plantares communes [NA])	Plantar metatarsal	Proper plantar digital	Toes
Digital, dorsal (of foot) (arteriae digitales dorsales pedis [NA])	Arcuate		Dorsal areas of toes
Digital, dorsal (of hand) (arteriae digitales dorsales manus [NA])	Dorsal metacarpal		Dorsal areas of fingers
Digital, palmar proper (arteriae digitales palmares propriae [NA])	Common palmar digital		Fingers
Digital, plantar proper (arteriae digitales plantares propriae [NA])	Common plantar digital		Toes
Dorsal pedal (arteria dorsalis pedis [NA])	Anterior tibial	Lateral tarsal, medial tarsal, and arcuate arteries; deep plantar branch	Dorsal portion of foot and toes

Name	Origin	Branches	Distribution
Epigastric, deep	See *Epigastric, inferior*		
Epigastric, inferior (arteria epigastrica inferior [NA])	External iliac	Cremasteric or artery of round ligament of uterus; pubic and obturator branches	Skin and muscles of anterior abdominal wall; round ligament of uterus in the female, cremaster muscle and spermatic cord in the male; peritoneum
Epigastric, superficial (arteria epigastrica superficialis [NA])	Femoral		Skin of abdominal wall below umbilicus; superficial fascia; inguinal lymph nodes
Epigastric, superior (arteria epigastrica superior [NA])	Internal thoracic		Skin, fascia, muscles, and peritoneum of upper abdominal wall; diaphragm; falciform ligament of the liver
Episcleral (arteriae episclerales [NA])	Ophthalmic		Iris; ciliary processes; conjunctiva
Ethmoid, anterior (arteria ethmoidalis anterior [NA])	Ophthalmic	Anterior meningeal	Anterior and middle ethmoidal cells; dura mater of anterior cranial fossa; mucoperiosteum of middle nasal meatus; lateral wall and septum of nose; frontal air sinus; skin of dorsum of nose
Ethmoid, posterior (arteria ethmoidalis posterior [NA])	Ophthalmic		Posterior ethmoid cells; dura mater around cribriform plate; superior nasal meatus; superior nasal concha
Facial (arteria facialis [NA])	External carotid	Ascending palatine, submental, inferior and superior labial, angular arteries; tonsillar and glandular branches	Face; tonsil; auditory tube; root of tongue; submandibular gland
Facial, transverse (arteria transversa faciei [NA])	Superficial temporal		Masseter muscle; parotid gland; skin of face
Femoral (arteria femoralis [NA])	Continuation of external iliac	Continues as popliteal; superficial epigastric, superficial circumflex iliac, external pudendal, deep femoral, descending genicular	Skin of lower part of abdomen and groin; external genitalia; inguinal lymph nodes; muscles of medial, lateral, and anterior aspects of thigh; femur; knee joint

Name	Origin	Branches	Distribution
Femoral, deep (arteria profunda femoris [NA])	Femoral	Lateral and medial femoral circumflex, perforating	Muscles of thigh; hip joint; head and shaft of femur
Fibular (arteria fibularis [NA alternative])	See *Peroneal*		
Frontal	See *Supraorbital*		
Gastric, left (arteria gastrica sinistra [NA])	Celiac trunk	Esophageal branches	Lesser curvature and cardia of stomach; lower end of esophagus; occasionally left lobe of liver
Gastric, right (arteria gastrica dextra [NA])	Common hepatic		Pyloric portion of stomach
Gastric, short (arteriae gastricae breves [NA])	Lienal		Greater curvature of stomach
Gastroduodenal (arteria gastroduodenalis [NA])	Common hepatic	Superior, pancreaticoduodenal, right gastroepiploic	Pylorus; duodenum; pancreas; greater omentum; common bile duct
Gastroepiploic, left (arteria gastroepiploica sinistra [NA])	Lienal	Epiploic branches	Greater curvature of the stomach; greater omentum
Gastroepiploic, right (arteria gastroepiploica dextra [NA])	Gastroduodenal	Epiploic branches	Greater curvature of the stomach; greater omentum
Genicular, descending (arteria genus descendens [NA])	Femoral	Saphenous and articular branches	Knee joint; skin of medial distal portion of thigh; arterial retina on medial and lateral sides of knee; thigh muscles
Genicular, highest	See *Genicular, descending*		
Genicular, lateral inferior (arteria genus inferior lateralis [NA])	Popliteal		Knee joint
Genicular, lateral superior (arteria genus superior lateralis [NA])	Popliteal		Knee joint; thigh muscles
Genicular, medial inferior (arteria genus inferior medialis [NA])	Popliteal		Knee joint; proximal end of tibia; popliteus muscle
Genicular, medial superior (arteria genus superior medialis [NA])	Popliteal		Knee joint; patella; femur; vastus medialis muscle
Genicular, middle (arteria genus media [NA])	Popliteal		Knee joint; cruciate ligaments; patellar synovial and alar folds

Name	Origin	Branches	Distribution
Gluteal, inferior (arteria glutea inferior [NA])	Internal iliac	Sciatic	Buttock; hip joint; skin and muscles of back of upper thigh
Gluteal, superior (arteria glutea superior [NA])	Internal iliac	Superficial and deep branches	Buttock
Hemorrhoidal	See *Rectal*		
Hepatic, common (arteria hepatica communis [NA])	Celiac trunk	Right gastric, gastroduodenal, hepatic proper	Lesser and greater curvatures of stomach; pylorus; pancreas; greater omentum; gallbladder; liver
Hepatic, proper (arteria hepatica propria [NA])	Common hepatic	Cystic artery; right and left branches	Liver; gallbladder
Hypogastric	See *Iliac, internal*		
Ileal (arteriae ilei [NA])	Superior mesenteric		Ileum
Ileocolic (arteria ileocolica [NA])	Superior mesenteric	Appendicular artery; cecal branches	Ascending colon; cecum; vermiform process; lower part of ileum
Iliac, common (arteria iliaca communis [NA])	Abdominal aorta	Internal and external iliac	Psoas major muscle; peritoneum; fascia; pelvic viscera; external genitalia; gluteal region; lower limb
Iliac, external (arteria iliaca externa [NA])	Common iliac	Continues as femoral; inferior epigastric, deep circumflex iliac	Psoas major, iliacus, sartorius, tensor fasciae latae, cremaster, and abdominal wall muscles; external iliac lymph nodes; peritoneum; skin of lower abdominal wall; spermatic cord or round ligament of the uterus; lower limb
Iliac, internal (arteria iliaca interna [NA])	Common iliac	Iliolumbar, obturator, superior and inferior gluteal, inferior vesical, middle rectal, internal pudendal, umbilical (fetal), uterine or deferential	Pelvic wall and contents; gluteal region; medial portion of thigh; external genitalia; anal region
Iliolumbar (arteria iliolumbalis [NA])	Internal iliac	Lateral sacral arteries; lumbar, iliac, and spinal branches	Muscles and bones of pelvis; cauda equina

Name	Origin	Branches	Distribution
Infraorbital (arteria infraorbitalis [NA])	Maxillary	Anterior superior alveolar	Inferior rectus and inferior oblique muscles of the eye; orbicularis oculi muscle; lacrimal gland and sac; upper lip; anterior upper teeth; mucosa of maxillary sinuses
Innominate	See *Brachiocephalic*		
Intercostal, highest (arteria intercostalis suprema [NA])	Costocervical trunk	Posterior intercostal (I, II)	Posterior vertebral muscles; contents of first and second intercostal spaces; contents of vertebral canal
Intercostal, posterior (I, II) (arteriae intercostales posteriores I, II [NA])	Highest intercostal	Dorsal and spinal branches	First and second intercostal spaces
Intercostal, posterior (III–XI) (arteriae intercostales posteriores III–XI [NA])	Thoracic aorta	Dorsal, spinal, cutaneous, collateral, and mammary branches	Intercostal, pectoral, serratus anterior, iliocostalis, longissimus dorsi, multifidus spinae, and semispinalis dorsi muscles; abdominal wall; vertebrae; ribs; mammary gland; skin of body wall and back; contents of vertebral canal
Interlobar of kidney (arteriae interlobares renis [NA])	Renal	Arcuate of kidney	Renal lobes
Interlobular of kidney (arteriae interlobulares renis [NA])	Arcuate of kidney		Glomeruli of kidney
Interlobular of liver (arteriae interlobulares hepatis [NA])	Proper hepatic (right or left branch)		Lobules of liver
Interosseous, anterior (arteria interossea anterior [NA])	Common interosseous	Median artery	Deep anterior forearm
Interosseous, common (arteria interossea communis [NA])	Ulnar	Anterior and posterior interosseous	Forearm; rete olecrani
Interosseous, posterior (arteria interossea posterior [NA])	Common interosseous	Recurrent interosseous	Muscles and skin of posterior forearm; rete olecrani
Interosseous, recurrent (arteria interossea recurrens [NA])	Posterior interosseous		Supinator and anconeus muscles; rete olecrani
Interosseous, volar	See *Interosseous, anterior*		
Intestinal	See *Ileal; Jejunal*		

Name	Origin	Branches	Distribution
Jejunal (arteriae jejunales [NA])	Superior mesenteric		Jejunum
Labial, inferior (arteria labialis inferior [NA])	Facial		Mucous membrane, skin, muscles, and glands of lower lip
Labial, superior (arteria labialis superior [NA])	Facial		Mucous membrane, skin, muscles, and glands of upper lip; nasal septum; ala of nose
Labyrinthine (arteria labyrinthi [NA])	Basilar or anterior inferior cerebellar		Internal ear
Lacrimal (arteria lacrimalis [NA])	Ophthalmic		Lacrimal gland; superior and lateral rectus muscles; eyelids; conjunctiva; sclera; iris; ciliary processes; temporal fossa
Laryngeal, inferior (arteria laryngea inferior [NA])	Inferior thyroid		Constrictor pharyngis inferior muscle; mucous membrane of lower part of larynx
Laryngeal, superior (arteria laryngea superior [NA])	Superior thyroid		Muscles, mucous membrane, and glands of larynx
Lienal (arteria lienalis [NA])	Celiac trunk	Left gastroepiploic, short gastric, great pancreatic, dorsal pancreatic arteries; pancreatic and lienal branches	Pancreas; pancreatic duct; fundus and greater curvature of stomach; both surfaces of greater omentum; body of spleen
Lingual (arteria lingualis [NA])	External carotid	Sublingual and deep lingual arteries; suprahyoid and dorsal thyroid branches	Intrinsic and extrinsic muscles of tongue; mucous membrane of tongue and mouth; gums; sublingual gland; glossopalatine arch; tonsil; soft palate; epiglottis; frenulum of the tongue
Lingual, deep (arteria profunda lingualis [NA])	Lingual		Genioglossus muscle; intrinsic muscles of the tongue; mucous membrane of inferior surface of tongue
Linguofacial trunk	Combined facial and lingual arteries		
Lumbar (arteriae lumbales [NA])	Abdominal aorta	Dorsal and spinal branches	Muscles of back; lumbar vertebrae; fibrous capsule of the kidney

Name	Origin	Branches	Distribution
Lumbar, lowest (arteria lumbalis ima [NA])	Median sacral		Iliacus and gluteus maximus muscles; sacrum
Malleolar, anterior lateral (arteria malleolaris anterior lateralis [NA])	Anterior tibial		Lateral side of ankle
Malleolar, anterior medial (arteria malleolaris anterior medialis [NA])	Anterior tibial		Medial side of ankle
Mammary, external	See *Thoracic, lateral*		
Mammary, internal	See *Thoracic, internal*		
Masseteric (arteria masseterica [NA])	Maxillary		Masseter muscle
Maxillary (arteria maxillaris [NA])	External carotid	Deep auricular, anterior tympanic, inferior alveolar, middle meningeal, masseteric, buccal, deep temporal, posterior superior alveolar, infraorbital, artery of pterygoid canal, descending palatine, sphenopalatine, nasal	Jaws, teeth, and other deep structures of face; ear
Maxillary, external	See *Facial*		
Maxillary, internal	See *Maxillary*		
Median (arteria mediana [NA])	Anterior interosseous		Median nerve
Meningeal, anterior (arteria meningea anterior [NA])	Anterior ethmoid		Dura mater of anterior cranial fossa
Meningeal, middle (arteria meningea media [NA])	Maxillary	Accessory, meningeal, and petrous branches	Tensor, tympani muscle; semilunar ganglion; trigeminal nerve; dura mater of anterior and middle cranial fossae; skull; tympanic cavity; orbit; infratemporal fossa
Meningeal, posterior (arteria meningea posterior [NA])	Ascending pharyngeal		Dura mater of posterior and middle cranial fossae
Mental (arteria mentalis [NA])	Inferior alveolar		Lower lip and chin
Mesenteric, inferior (arteria mesenterica inferior [NA])	Abdominal aorta	Left colic, sigmoid, superior rectal	Transverse colon; splenic flexure; descending colon; sigmoid flexure; proximal portion of rectum

Name	Origin	Branches	Distribution
Mesenteric, superior (arteria mesenterica superior [NA])	Abdominal aorta	Inferior pancreatico-duodenal, jejunal, ileal, ileocolic, right colic, middle colic	Pancreas; duodenum; jejunum; ileum; mesentery; mesenteric lymph nodes; cecum; vermiform appendix; ascending colon; hepatic flexure
Metacarpal, dorsal (arteriae metacarpeae dorsales [NA])	Radial (dorsal carpal rete)	Dorsal digital	Dorsal areas of fingers
Metacarpal, palmar (arteriae metacarpeae palmares [NA])	Deep palmar arch		Interosseus and second, third, and fourth lumbrical muscles; metacarpal bones
Metacarpal, volar	See *Metacarpal, palmar*		
Metatarsal, dorsal (arteriae metatarseae dorsales [NA])	Arcuate of foot		Adjacent sides of toes
Metatarsal, plantar (arteriae metatarseae plantares [NA])	Plantar arch	Common digital arteries; perforating branches	Toes
Musculophrenic (arteria musculophrenica [NA])	Internal thoracic		Muscles of abdominal wall; diaphragm; lower six intercostal spaces
Nasal, dorsal (arteria dorsalis nasi [NA])	Ophthalmic		Dorsum of nose
Nasal, lateral posterior and septal posterior (arteriae nasales posteriores, laterales et septi [NA])	Maxillary		Nasal conchae, cavity, and septum
Nasopalatine	See *Sphenopalatine*		
Nutrient	A branch of any artery that supplies a bone. There may be a number of nutrient branches from any nearby artery		
Obturator (arteria obturatoria [NA])	Internal iliac	Pubic, acetabular, anterior, and posterior branches	Pelvic and thigh muscles (including obturators); pubis; hip joint; head of femur; bladder; ilium
Occipital (arteria occipitalis [NA])	External carotid	Mastoid, auricular, occipital, sternocleidomastoid, descending, and meningeal branches	Muscles of neck; posterior surface of auricle; mastoid cells; pericranium and scalp of posterolateral surface of the head

Name	Origin	Branches	Distribution
Ophthalmic (arteria ophthalmica [NA])	Internal carotid	Central retinal lacrimal, palpebral, ciliary, conjunctival, episcleral, supraorbital, ethmoid, meningeal, supratrochlear, dorsal nasal	Contents of orbit; diploë of frontal bone; mucous membrane of frontal sinus and ethmoidal cells; dura mater of anterior fossa of skull; superior nasal concha and meatus; lacrimal sac; skin of dorsum of nose
Ovarian (arteria ovarica [NA])	Abdominal aorta	Ureteric branches	Ovary; ureter; suspensory ligament of the ovary; broad ligament of the uterus; uterine tube; round ligament of the uterus; skin of labium majus and groin
Palatine, ascending (arteria palatina ascendens [NA])	Facial	Tonsillar branch	Styloglossus, stylopharyngeus, superior constrictor of pharynx, and levator veli palatini muscles; auditory tube; lateral wall of upper part of pharynx; soft palate; palatine tonsil
Palatine, descending (arteria palatina descendens [NA])	Maxillary	Greater and lesser palatine	Soft palate; palatine tonsil; mucous membrane of roof of mouth; gums; palatine glands; palatine bone; maxilla
Palatine, greater (arteria palatina major [NA])	Descending palatine		Mucous membrane of hard palate; gums; palatine glands; palatine bone; maxilla
Palatine, lesser (arteriae palatinae minores [NA])	Descending palatine		Soft palate; palatine tonsil
Palmar arch, deep (arcus palmaris profundus [NA])	Radial	Palmar metacarpal	Interossei and second, third, and fourth lumbrical muscles; metacarpals; joints of fingers
Palmar arch, superficial (arcus palmaris superficialis [NA])	Ulnar	Common palmar digital	Flexor tendons and tendon sheaths; joints and bones of fingers; skin of palm and fingers
Palpebral, lateral (arteriae palpebrales laterales [NA])	Ophthalmic	Superior palpebral arch, inferior palpebral arch	Upper and lower eyelids; conjunctiva

TABLE OF ARTERIES (Continued)

Name	Origin	Branches	Distribution
Palpebral, medial (arteriae palpebrales mediales [NA])	Ophthalmic	Superior palpebral arch, inferior palpebral arch	Upper and lower eyelids; conjunctiva; lacrimal caruncle; lacrimal sac
Pancreatic, dorsal (arteria pancreatica dorsalis [NA])	Lienal or celiac	Inferior pancreatic	Head and body of pancreas
Pancreatic, great (variable) (arteria pancreatica magna [NA])	Lienal		Posterior surface of pancreas, following course of pancreatic duct
Pancreatic, inferior (arteria pancreatica inferior [NA])	Dorsal pancreatic		Body and tail of pancreas
Pancreaticoduodenal, inferior (arteriae pancreaticoduodenales inferiores [NA])	Superior mesenteric		Head of pancreas; descending and inferior parts of duodenum
Pancreaticoduodenal, superior	Gastroduodenal	Pancreatic and duodenal branches	Second part of duodenum; common bile duct; pancreas
Pedal, dorsal	See *Dorsal pedal*		
Penis, deep (arteria profunda penis [NA])	Internal pudendal		Corpus cavernosum of the penis
Penis, dorsal (arteria dorsalis penis [NA])	Internal pudendal		Dorsum of penis; prepuce; glans; corpus cavernosum and its fibrous sheath
Perforating (arteriae perforantes [NA])	Deep femoral		Gluteus maximus, pectineus, adductor, biceps femoris, and posterior femoral muscles; shaft of femur
Pericardiacophrenic (arteria pericardiacophrenica [NA])	Internal thoracic		Phrenic nerve; pleura; pericardium; diaphragm
Perineal (arteria perinealis [NA])	Internal pudendal	Scrotal or labial branches	Perineum; posterior portion of scrotum or labium majus; subcutaneous structures in urogenital triangle
Peroneal (arteria peronea [NA])	Posterior tibial	Perforating, communicating, malleolar, and calcaneal branches	Soleus, tibialis posterior, flexor hallucis longus, peroneus, and extensor digitorum longus muscles; shaft of fibula; tibiofibular syndesmosis; ankle joint; dorsum of foot

Name	Origin	Branches	Distribution
Pharyngeal, ascending (arteria pharyngea ascendens [NA])	External carotid	Posterior meningeal and inferior tympanic arteries; pharyngeal branches	Pharynx; soft palate; palatine tonsil; auditory tube; cervical lymph nodes; tympanic cavity; dura mater of middle and posterior cranial fossae
Phrenic, inferior (arteriae phrenicae inferiores [NA])	Abdominal aorta	Superior suprarenal	Inferior surface of diaphragm; suprarenal gland; vena cava inferior; liver; esophagus; pericardium (from the right artery); spleen (from the left)
Phrenic, superior (arteriae phrenicae superiores [NA])	Thoracic aorta		Posterior surface of diaphragm
Plantar arch (arcus plantaris [NA])	Lateral plantar	Plantar metatarsal	Interosseous muscles; toes
Plantar, lateral (arteria plantaris lateralis [NA])	Posterior tibial	Plantar arch	Toes and related muscles; heel; skin on lateral side of foot
Plantar, medial (arteria plantaris medialis [NA])	Posterior tibial	Deep and superficial branches	Abductor hallucis and flexor digitorum brevis muscles; skin on medial surface of sole of foot
Popliteal (arteria poplitea [NA])	Continuation of femoral	Genicular, sural; anterior and posterior tibial	Knee and calf; muscles of thigh
Popliteal, lateral	See *Peroneal*		
Popliteal, medial	See *Tibial*		
Principal of thumb (arteria princeps pollicis [NA])	Radial	Radial index	Sides and palmar surface of thumb
Profunda brachii	See *Brachial, deep*		
Profunda femoris	See *Femoral, deep*		
Pterygoid canal, artery of (arteria canalis pterygoidei [NA])	Maxillary		Upper portion of pharynx; levator and tensor veli palatini muscles; auditory tube; tympanic cavity
Pudendal, external (arteriae pudendae externae [NA])	Femoral	Inguinal and anterior scrotal or labial branches	Scrotum or labium majus; skin of lower abdomen, of penis or clitoris, of scrotum or labium majus, and of perineum

TABLE OF ARTERIES (Continued)

Name	Origin	Branches	Distribution
Pudendal, internal (arteria pudenda interna [NA])	Internal iliac	Inferior rectal, perineal, urethral, artery of bulb of penis or of vestibule, dorsal and deep penile or clitoridal arteries; posterior scrotal or labial branches	External genitalia; perineum; anus and rectum
Pulmonary, left (arteria pulmonis sinistra [NA])	Pulmonary trunk	Branches to lobes and segments of left lung	Left lung
Pulmonary, right (arteria pulmonis dextra [NA])	Pulmonary trunk	Branches to lobes and segments of right lung	Right lung
Pulmonary trunk (truncus pulmonalis [NA])	Right ventricle	Left and right pulmonary	Lungs
Radial (arteria radialis [NA])	Brachial	Radial recurrent artery, principal artery of thumb, and deep palmar arch; dorsal and palmar carpal and superficial palmar branches	Muscles of forearm; radius; elbow, wrist, and carpal joints; skin of dorsum of hand and fingers; skin of palmar surface of thumb and lateral side of index finger
Radial of index finger (arteria radialis indicis [NA])	Principal artery of thumb		Lateral palmar aspect of index finger
Radial recurrent (arteria recurrens radialis [NA])	Radial		Supinator, brachialis, brachioradialis, and extensor carpi radialis brevis and longus muscles; elbow joints; rete olecrani
Ranine	See *Lingual, deep*		
Rectal, inferior (arteria rectalis inferior [NA])	Internal pudendal		Anal canal; levator ani and sphincter ani externus muscles; skin around anus and lower region of buttock
Rectal, middle (arteria rectalis media [NA])	Internal iliac		Rectum; ductus deferens; seminal vesicle; prostate gland
Rectal, superior (arteria rectalis superior [NA])	Inferior mesenteric		Muscular and mucous coats of the pelvic colon and proximal portion of the rectum; mucous coat of distal portion of rectum
Renal (arteria renalis [NA])	Abdominal aorta	Inferior suprarenal and interlobar arteries; ureteric branches	Suprarenal gland; upper end of ureter; kidney

Name	Origin	Branches	Distribution
Round ligament of the uterus, artery of (arteria ligamenti teretis uteri [NA])	Inferior epigastric		Round ligament of the uterus (corresponds to cremasteric artery in the male)
Sacral, lateral (arteriae sacrales laterales [NA])	Iliolumbar		Sacrum
Sacral, median (arteria sacralis mediana [NA])	Abdominal aorta	Lowest lumbar	Sacrum; rectum; coccyx
Scapular, circumflex	Subscapular		
Scapular, descending (arteria scapularis descendens [NA])	Transverse cervical		Muscles in the region of the medial border of the scapula
Scapular, transverse	See *Suprascapular*		
Sciatic (arteria comitans nervi ischiadici [NA])	Inferior gluteal		Sciatic nerve
Sigmoid (arteriae sigmoideae [NA])	Inferior mesenteric		Sigmoid colon and lower part of descending colon
Spermatic, external	See *Cremasteric*		
Spermatic, internal	See *Ovarian; Testicular*		
Sphenopalatine (arteria sphenopalatina [NA])	Maxillary		Nasal conchae and meati; mucous membrane of frontal, maxillary, sphenoidal, and ethmoidal air sinuses; posterior portion of nasal septum
Spinal, anterior (arteria spinalis anterior [NA])	Spinal branches of vertebral		Spinal cord and its coverings
Spinal, posterior (arteria spinalis posterior [NA])	Spinal branches of vertebral		Spinal cord and its coverings
Splenic	See *Lienal*		
Stylomastoid (arteria stylomastoidea [NA])	Posterior auricular		Mastoid cells; stapes; stepedius muscle and tendon; posterior portion of tympanic membrane

Name	Origin	Branches	Distribution
Subclavian (arteria subclavia [NA])	Left—arch of aorta Right—brachiocephalic	Continues as axillary; vertebral and internal thoracic arteries; thyrocervical and costocervical trunks	Muscles of neck and upper extremity; cervical vertebrae and canal; skull, brain, and meninges; pericardium; pleura; mediastinum; bronchi; sternum; skin over shoulder and anterior body wall; mammary gland; peritoneum
Subcostal (arteria subcostalis [NA])	Thoracic aorta	Dorsal and spinal branches	Quadratus lumborum, transversus abdominis, and obliquus abdominis internus muscles; lumbar vertebrae and contents of canal; skin of back
Sublingual (arteria sublingualis [NA])	Lingual		Mylohyoid,, geniohyoid, and genioglossus muscles; sublingual gland; frenulum of the tongue
Submental (arteria submentalis [NA])	Facial	Glandular branches	Mylohyoid, digastric, platysma, and depressor labii inferioris muscles; submandibular and sublingual glands
Subscapular (arteria subscapularis [NA])	Axillary	Thoracodorsal, scapular circumflex	Muscles of scapular and shoulder region; scapula; shoulder joint; axillary lymph nodes
Supraorbital (arteria supraorbitalis [NA])	Ophthalmic		Rectus superior and levator palpebrae superioris muscles; periosteum of root of orbit; diploë of frontal bone; mucous membrane of frontal sinus; trochlea of obliquus superior muscle; upper eyelid
Suprarenal, inferior (arteria suprarenalis inferior [NA])	Renal		Suprarenal gland
Suprarenal, middle (arteria suprarenalis media [NA])	Abdominal aorta		Suprarenal gland
Suprarenal, superior (arteria suprarenalis superior [NA])	Inferior phrenic		Suprarenal gland

Name	Origin	Branches	Distribution
Suprascapular (arteria suprascapularis [NA])	Thyrocervical trunk	Acromial branch	Clavicle; scapula; acromioclavicular and shoulder joints; muscles of these areas
Supratrochlear (arteria supratrochlearis [NA])	Ophthalmic		Anterior scalp
Sural (arteriae surales [NA])	Popliteal		Gastrocnemius, soleus, and plantaris muscles; skin and fascia of calf
Tarsal, lateral (arteria tarsea lateralis [NA])	Dorsal pedal		Extensor digitorum brevis muscle; navicular and cuboid bones and joint between them
Tarsal, lateral (arteria tarsea lateralis [NA])	Dorsal pedal		Skin of medial surface of foot; tarsal joints
Temporal, deep (arteriae temporales profundae [NA])	Maxillary		Temporal muscle; orbit; pericranium; skull
Temporal, middle (arteria temporalis media [NA])	Superficial temporal		Temporal muscle; temporal fascia
Temporal, superficial (arteria temporalis superficialis [NA])	External carotid	Transverse facial, middle temporal, zygomaticoorbital arteries; parotid, anterior auricular, frontal, and parietal branches	Temporal, masseter, frontalis, and orbicularis oculi muscles; parotid gland and duct; skin of face; external ear; external acoustic meatus; scalp
Testicular (arteria testicularis [NA])	Abdominal aorta	Ureteric branches	Testicle; ureter; epididymis
Thoracic, highest (arteria thoracica suprema [NA])	Axillary		Pectoral, intercostal, and serratus anterior muscles; thoracic wall
Thoracic, internal (arteria thoracica interna [NA])	Subclavian	Pericardiacophrenic, musculophrenic, and superior epigastric arteries; mediastinal, thymic, bronchial, sternal, perforating, mammary, and intercostal branches	Mediastinum and anterior thoracic wall
Thoracic, lateral (arteria thoracica lateralis [NA])	Axillary	Mammary branches	Pectoral, serratus anterior, and subscapularis muscles; axillary lymph nodes; mammary gland
Thoracic, twelfth	See *Subcostal*		

Name	Origin	Branches	Distribution
Thoracoacromial (arteria thoraco-acromialis [NA])	Axillary	Acromial, clavicular, deltoid, and pectoral branches	Pectoral, deltoid, and subclavius muscles; mammary gland; sternoclavicular joint
Thoracodorsal (arteria thoraco-dorsalis [NA])	Subscapular		Latissimus dorsi, teres major, and serratus anterior muscles
Thyrocervical trunk (truncus thyrocervicalis [NA])	Subclavian	Inferior thyroid, suprascapular, transverse cervical	Muscles of neck, scapular region, and upper back; cervical spinal cord and vertebrae; larynx; trachea; esophagus; thyroid gland; pharynx
Thyroid, inferior (arteria thyroidea inferior [NA])	Thyrocervical trunk	Inferior laryngeal, and ascending cervical arteries; pharyngeal, esophageal, and tracheal branches	Esophagus; pharynx; larynx; trachea; posterior surface of thyroid gland; vertebrae; contents of vertebral canal; related muscles
Thyroid, lowest (inconsistent) (arteria thyroidea ima [NA])	Arch of aorta, brachiocephalic trunk or elsewhere		Lower part of thyroid gland
Thyroid, superior (arteria thyroidea superior [NA])	External carotid	Superior laryngeal artery; muscular, anterior, and posterior branches	Thyroid gland; esophagus; intrinsic muscles and mucous membrane of larynx; related muscles
Tibial anterior (arteria tibialis anterior [NA])	Popliteal	Tibial recurrent and malleolar arteries; malleolar branches	Knee, proximal tibiofibular, and ankle joints; muscles of lower leg; fascia and skin on front of leg
Tibial, anterior-recurrent (arteria recurrens tibialis anterior [NA])	Anterior tibial		Knee joint and overlying fascia and skin; tibialis anterior and extensor digitorum longus muscles
Tibial, posterior (arteria tibialis posterior [NA])	Popliteal	Plantar arteries; circumflex fibular branch	Shaft of tibia; shaft of fibula; sole of foot; muscles of lower leg; skin of medial and posterior part of leg and tarsus

Name	Origin	Branches	Distribution
Tibial, posterior recurrent (arteria recurrens tibialis posterior [NA])	Anterior tibial		Soleus, tibialis, posterior, flexor hallucis longus, flexor digitorum longus, and peroneus muscles; ankle joint; skin of medial and posterior part of leg and foot; sole of foot; shaft of tibia; shaft of fibula
Transverse facial	See *Facial, transverse*		
Tympanic, anterior (arteria tympanica anterior [NA])	Maxillary		Mucous membrane of tympanic cavity
Tympanic, inferior (arteria tympanica inferior [NA])	Ascending pharyngeal		Lining of medial wall of tympanic cavity
Tympanic, posterior (arteria tympanica posterior [NA])	Posterior auricular	Mastoid and stapedial branches	Tympanic membrane
Tympanic, superior (arteria tympanica superior [NA])	Middle meningeal	Frontal, parietal, and anastomotic branches	Tensor tympani muscle; lining of wall of tympanic cavity
Ulnar (arteria ulnaris [NA])	Brachial	Recurrent ulnar and common interosseous arteries; superficial palmar arch; dorsal carpal, deep palmar, and palmar carpal branches	Muscles of forearm; shafts of radius and ulna; median nerve; ulnar half of hand; carpal joints; skin over course of vessels
Ulnar, recurrent (arteria recurrens ulnaris [NA])	Ulnar	Anterior and posterior branches	Brachialis, pronator teres, flexor digitorum profundus, flexor digitorum sublimis, and flexor carpi ulnaris muscles; skin over medial cubital region; elbow joint; ulnar nerve
Umbilical (fetal) (arteria umbilicalis [NA])	Internal iliac		Ductus deferens; seminal vesicles; epididymis; ureter; bladder
Urethral (arteria urethralis [NA])	Internal pudendal		Urethra
Uterine (arteria uterina [NA])	Internal iliac	Vaginal artery; ovarian and tubal branches	Uterus; broad ligament of uterus; round ligament of uterus; uterine tube; portion of vagina
Vaginal (arteria vaginalis [NA])	Uterine		Vagina; fundus of bladder; rectum; vestibular bulb

Name	Origin	Branches	Distribution
Vertebral (arteria vertebralis [NA])	Subclavian	Basilar, anterior spinal, posterior spinal, and posterior inferior cerebellar arteries; meningeal branch	Muscles of neck; cervical vertebrae; cervical spinal cord and its membranes; intervertebral disks; bone and dura mater of posterior fossa of skull; falx cerebelli; cerebellum; medulla oblongata
Vesical, inferior (arteria vesicalis inferior [NA])	Internal iliac		Fundus of bladder; prostate gland; ductus deferens; seminal vesicle; lower part of ureter
Vesical, superior (arteriae vesicales superiores [NA])	Internal iliac (umbilical)		Lower part of ureter; upper part of bladder; ductus deferens; medial umbilical ligament
Vidian	See *Pterygoid canal, artery of*		
Volar arch	See *Palmar arch*		
Zygomaticoorbital (arteria zygomaticoorbitalis [NA])	Superficial temporal		Orbicularis oculi muscle; lateral portion of orbit

Name	Principal features	Bones with which articulation occurs and type of joint
Anvil	See *Incus*	
Astragalus	See *Talus*	
Atlas [NA]	First cervical vertebra; ringlike; lateral masses; anterior and posterior arches and tubercles; articular surfaces; vertebral and transverse foramens; sulcus for vertebral artery; ossifies in cartilage	Occipital bone, *bilateral gliding* Axis, 3 joints, *bilateral gliding* and *pivot* with dens
Axis [NA]	Second cervical vertebra; body; dens (odontoid process); laminae, pedicles; transverse processes and foramens; articular surfaces; thick spine; vertebral foramen; ossifies in cartilage	Atlas, 3 joints, *bilateral gliding* and *pivot* with dens Third cervical vertebra, *cartilaginous*
Calcaneum	See *Calcaneus*	
Calcaneus [NA]	Heel bone; largest tarsal bone; irregularly cuboid; tuber with medial and lateral processes; sustentaculum tali; trochlea; sinus tarsi; grooves for tendons of flexor hallucis longus and peroneal muscles; articular surfaces; ossifies in cartilage	Talus (3 facets) ⎫ Cuboid ⎭ *gliding*
Calvaria [NA]	Skullcap or upper part of skull	
Calvarium	See *Calvaria*	
Capitate (os capitatum [NA])	Usually largest carpal bone; in distal row of carpal bones; occupies center of wrist; head; neck; body; ossifies in cartilage	Scaphoid ⎫ Lunate ⎪ Trapezoid ⎪ Hamate ⎬ *gliding* Second ⎫ ⎪ Third ⎬ metacarpal ⎪ Fourth ⎭ ⎭
Carpus (ossa carpi [NA])	Consists of 8 short bones arranged in a proximal row (scaphoid; lunate; triquetrum; pisiform) and a distal row (trapezium; trapezoid; capitate; hamate)	
Central (os centrale [NA])	Occasional accessory bone of carpus; usually in man fuses with scaphoid but remains separate in many mammals	
Clavicle (clavicula [NA])	Collarbone; resembles the italic "*f*"; body; sternal and acromial extremities; conoid tubercle; trapezoid line; coracoid tuberosity; costal tuberosity; subclavian groove; first bone to ossify; ossifies partly in cartilage and partly in membrane	Sternum ⎫ Scapula ⎬ *gliding* Cartilage of first rib ⎭
Coccyx (os coccygis [NA])	Last bone of vertebral column; usually composed of 4 small incomplete vertebrae fused together; base; apex; cornua; transverse processes; ossifies in cartilage	Sacrum, *cartilaginous*

Name	Principal features	Bones with which articulation occurs and type of joint
Concha, inferior nasal (concha nasalis inferior [NA])	Irregular scroll-shaped bone situated on lateral wall of nasal cavity; lacrimal, ethmoid, and maxillary processes; ossifies in cartilage	Ethmoid, Maxilla, Lacrimal, Palatine } *sutures*
Costal	See *Ribs*	
Coxal	See *Hipbone*	
Cranium [NA]	Braincase; composed of occipital, parietal (2), frontal, temporal (2), sphenoid, and ethmoid. Sometimes cranium is used to designate entire skull without mandible	
Cuboid (os cuboideum [NA])	Roughly cubical bone in lateral part of tarsus; tuberosity; groove for tendon of peroneus longus	Calcaneus, Lateral cuneiform, Fourth and fifth metatarsals, Navicular } *gliding*
Cuneiform, inner	See *Cuneiform, medial*	
Cuneiform, intermediate (second cuneiform) (os cuneiforme intermedium [NA])	Wedge-shaped; smallest of the 3; articular surfaces; ossifies in cartilage	Navicular, Medial cuneiform, Lateral cuneiform, Second metatarsal } *gliding*
Cuneiform, lateral (third cuneiform) (os cuneiforme laterale [NA])	Wedge-shaped; articular surfaces; ossifies in cartilage	Navicular, Intermediate cuneiform, Cuboid, Second, Third, Fourth } metatarsal } *gliding*
Cuneiform, medial (first cuneiform) (os cuneiforme mediale [NA])	Irregularly wedge-shaped; articular surfaces; largest of the 3; ossifies in cartilage	Navicular, Intermediate cuneiform, First and second metatarsals } *gliding*
Cuneiform, middle	See *Cuneiform, medial*	
Cuneiform, outer	See *Cuneiform, lateral*	
Epistropheus	See *Axis*	
Ethmoid (os ethmoidale [NA])	Irregular shape; situated in anterior part of base of skull and forming medial wall of each orbit and portion of roof and lateral wall of each nasal cavity; cribriform or horizontal plates; nasal slit; perpendicular plate; crista galli; alar processes; labyrinth with air cells; superior and middle nasal conchae, uncinate process; bulla; orbital plate; semilunar hiatus; ethmoid foramens; ossifies in cartilage	Sphenoid, Frontal, Nasal (2), Maxilla (2), Lacrimal (2), Palatine (2), Inferior nasal concha (2), Vomer } *sutures*

Name	Principal features	Bones with which articulation occurs and type of joint
Facial (ossa faciei [NA])	Bones of nose and jaws; maxilla, zygoma, nasal, lacrimal, palatine, inferior nasal concha, vomer, mandible, and parts of ethmoid and sphenoid	
Femur [NA]	Thighbone; largest, longest, and heaviest bone in the body; head; neck; greater and lesser trochanters; trochanteric fossa; quadrate tubercle; intertrochanteric line and crest; shaft; linea aspera and pectineal line; gluteal tuberosity; intercondylar line and fossa; medial and lateral condyles and epicondyles; adductor tubercle; articular surfaces; ossifies in cartilage	Hipbone, *ball-and-socket* Patella, *gliding* Tibia, combined *hinge* and *gliding*
Fibula [NA]	Splint bone; lateral bone of leg; head; body; medial crest; lateral malleolus; lateral malleolar fossa; articular surfaces; ossifies in cartilage	Tibia, *gliding* Talus with tibia and fibula, *hinge*
Flabella	Inconstant sesamoid bone occurring in lateral head of gastrocnemius muscle	
Foot	Composed of tarsus, metatarsus, and phalanges of foot	
Frontal (os frontale [NA])	Forehead bone; flat bone; frontal (squamous) part with eminences, glabella; superciliary arch, supraorbital margin and notch (foramen), zygomatic processes, temporal line, sagittal sulcus; orbital part forming upper portion of each orbit, anterior and posterior ethmoid foramens, spine or fovea for trochlea, fossa for lacrimal gland, frontal sinus; nasal part with spine; ossifies in membrane	Parietal (2) Sphenoid Ethmoid Nasal (2) Maxilla (2) *sutures* Lacrimal (2) Zygoma (2)
Greater multangular	See *Trapezium*	
Hamate (os hamatum [NA])	Wedge-shaped; in distal row of carpal bones; hook-like process (hamulus); articular surfaces; ossifies in cartilage	Lunate Fourth and fifth metacarpals Triquetrum *gliding* Capitate
Hammer	See *Malleus*	
Hand	Composed of carpus, metacarpus, and phalanges of hand	
Hipbone (os coxae [NA])	Large broad bone consisting of 3 parts; the ilium, ischium, and pubis; with its fellow pelvic girdle; with its fellow, sacrum and coccyx forms bony pelvis; acetabulum; obturator foramen; pubic arch; greater and lesser sciatic notches; articular surfaces; ossifies in cartilage	With its fellow of opposite side (symphysis pubis), *cartilaginous* Sacrum, *gliding*, very little movement Femur, *ball-and-socket*

Name	Principal features	Bones with which articulation occurs and type of joint
Humerus [NA]	Largest bone of upper limb; head; anatomic neck; greater and lesser tubercles; surgical neck; intertubercular sulcus; body; deltoid tuberosity; radial sulcus; condyle; capitulum; olecranon, coronoid, and radial fossae; trochlea; medial and lateral epicondyles; sulcus for ulnar nerve; articular surfaces; ossifies in cartilage	Scapula (glenoid cavity), *ball-and-socket* Ulna, *hinge* Radius, *gliding*
Hyoid (os hyoideum [NA])	U-shaped bone in front of neck; body; greater and lesser cornua; ossifies in cartilage	None
Ilium (os ilium [NA])	Broad expanded upper portion, the ala; body; crest; spines; gluteal lines; fossa; tuberosity; auricular surface; two-fifths (about) of acetabulum. See also *Hipbone*	
Incarial	See *Sutural*	
Incus [NA]	Resembles a premolar tooth with 2 roots; middle bone of auditory ossicles; body; long and short processes or crura; lenticular process; ossifies in cartilage	Malleus } *gliding* Stapes }
Inferior maxilla	See *Mandible*	
Inferior concha	See *Concha, inferior nasal*	
Inferior turbinate	See *Concha, inferior nasal*	
Innominate	See *Hipbone*	
Intermediate cuneiform	See *Cuneiform, intermediate*	
Ischium (os ischii [NA])	Heavy, posterior lower portion; body; tuber; ramus; spine; notches; lower boundary of obturator foramen; two-fifths (about) of acetabulum. See also *Hipbone*	
Lacrimal (os lacrimale [NA])	Small scale of bone resembling a fingernail; situated in the anterior medial wall of orbit; crest; descending process; hamulus; groove; ossifies in membrane	Frontal } Ethmoid } *sutures* Maxilla } Inferior nasal concha }
Lateral cuneiform	See *Cuneiform, lateral*	
Lesser multangular	See *Trapezoid*	
Lunate (os lunatum [NA])	One of proximal row of carpal bones; named from crescent-shaped articular facet; articular surfaces; ossifies in cartilage	Radius, *biaxial* Capitate } Hamate } Triquetrum } *gliding* Scaphoid }

Name	Principal features	Bones with which articulation occurs and type of joint
Magnum	See *Capitate*	
Malar	See *Zygoma*	
Malleus [NA]	Resembles a small hammer; head; neck; spur; crest; handle; anterior and lateral processes; ossifies in cartilage	Incus, *gliding*
Mandible (mandibula [NA])	Lower jaw; body, 2 rami; angle; coronoid and condyloid processes; symphysis; alveolar part; mental protuberance and tubercle; mylohyoid line and groove; mandibular and mental foramens; lingula; canal; articular surfaces; ossifies partly in membrane and partly in cartilage	Each temporal bone, combined *gliding* and *hinge*
Maxilla [NA]	Upper jaw; body with infraorbital foramen, sulcus, and canal, maxillary sinus, lacrimal groove, greater palatine sulcus, and foramen; zygomatic process; frontal process; ethmoid crest; alveolar process; maxillary tuber; palatine process; incisive crest, spine, and canal; nasal crest; maxillary hiatus; ossifies in membrane	Frontal Ethmoid Nasal Zygoma Lacrimal *sutures* Inferior nasal concha Palatine Vomer Other maxilla
Medial cuneiform	See *Cuneiform, medial*	
Metacarpus (ossa metacarpalia I–V [NA])	Five bones of the hand proper; each with head, shaft, and base; numbered from 1 to 5 beginning on the thumb side; styloid process on lateral side of base of third; articular surfaces; each ossified in cartilage	Base of first with trapezium Base of others with each other and with distal row of carpal bones *gliding* Heads with corresponding phalanges, *ball-and-socket*
Metatarsus (ossa metatarsalia I–V [NA])	Five bones of foot proper; each with head, shaft, and base; numbered from 1 to 5 beginning on the great toe side; tuberosity on 1 and 5; articular surfaces; each ossifies in cartilage	Distal tarsal bones Bases with each other *gliding* Heads with corresponding phalanges, *ball-and-socket*
Middle turbinate	See *Ethmoid*, middle nasal concha (not a separate bone)	
Multangulum majus	See *Trapezium*	
Multangulum minus	See *Trapezoid*	
Nasal (os nasale [NA])	Rectangular plate; 2 form bridge of nose; ethmoid sulcus and crest; ossifies in membrane	Frontal Ethmoid *sutures* Maxilla Other nasal
Navicular (os naviculare [NA])	Boat-shaped; proximal articular facet markedly concave; tuberosity; articular surfaces; ossifies in cartilage	Talus Three cuneiforms *gliding* Cuboid

Name	Principal features	Bones with which articulation occurs and type of joint
Navicular of hand	See *Scaphoid*	
Occipital (os occipitale [NA])	Posterior part and base of cranium; saucer-shaped; squamous part with internal and external protuberances, highest, superior, and inferior nuchal lines; sagittal and transverse sulci; lateral part with condyles, canal for hypoglossal nerve, condyloid canal, jugular notch, process and tubercle; basal part with pharyngeal tubercle and foramen magnum; squamous part ossifies in membrane, the rest in cartilage	Parietal (2) ⎫ Temporal (2) ⎬ *sutures* Sphenoid ⎭ Atlas, *bilateral gliding*
Os calcis [NA alternative]	See *Calcaneus*	
Os intercuneiforme	A very rare accessory ossicle of the foot situated between the medial and intermediate cuneiforms	
Os intermetatarseum	A very rare accessory ossicle of the foot situated between the bases of the first and second metatarsal bones	
Os magnum	See *Capitate*	
Os paracuneiforme	A very rare accessory ossicle of the foot situated between the navicular and medial cuneiform bones	
Ossa cranii [NA]	See *Cranium*	
Os vesalianum	See *Vesalian bone*, 1 and 2	
Ossicula auditus [NA]	See *Tympanic*	
Palatine (os palatinum [NA])	Forms portions of hard palate, orbits, and nasal cavities; irregularly L-shaped; horizontal part with nasal and palatine aspects, nasal and palatine crests, posterior nasal spine, lesser palatine foramens; perpendicular part with nasal and maxillary aspects, pyramidal, orbital, and sphenoid processes, conchal and ethmoid crests, greater palatine sulcus, and sphenopalatine notch; ossifies in membrane	Sphenoid ⎫ Ethmoid ⎪ Maxilla ⎪ Inferior nasal concha ⎬ *sutures* Palatine (opposite) ⎪ Vomer ⎭
Parietal (os parietale [NA])	Forms side and roof of cranium; quadrilateral plate of bone; superior and inferior temporal lines; parietal foramen; tubers; sulcus for superior sagittal sinus; sulcus for sigmoid sinus; ossifies in membrane	Parietal (opposite) ⎫ Occipital ⎪ Frontal ⎬ *sutures* Temporal ⎪ Sphenoid ⎭
Patella [NA]	Kneecap; triangular; largest sesamoid; ossifies in cartilage	Condyles of femur, *gliding*

Name	Principal features	Bones with which articulation occurs and type of joint
Pelvis [NA]	Bony pelvis composed of 2 hipbones, sacrum, and coccyx	
Phalanges (of foot) (ossa digitorum pedis [NA])	Two for great toe, 3 for each of others, 14 in all, usually fifth toe has only 2; each phalanx is a miniature long bone with head, shaft, and base; articular surfaces; tuberosity on distal phalanx; each ossifies in cartilage	Proximal row with corresponding metatarsal bones, *ball-and-socket* Interphalangeal joints, *hinge*
Phalanges (of hand) (ossa digitorum manus [NA])	Two for thumb, 3 for each finger, 14 in all; each phalanx is a miniature long bone with head, shaft, and base; articular surfaces; tuberosity on distal phalanx; each ossifies in cartilage	Proximal row with corresponding metacarpal bones, *ball-and-socket* Interphalangeal joints, *hinge*
Pisiform (os pisiforme [NA])	Most medial of proximal row of carpus; smallest carpal; resembles half a pea; articular surface; ossifies in cartilage	Triquetrum, *gliding*
Pubis (os pubis [NA])	Anterior lower portion; body; superior and inferior rami; tubercle; crest; pecten; upper boundary of obturator foramen, obturator crest and groove; one-fifth (about) of acetabulum. See also *Hipbone*	
Pyramidal	See *Triquetrum*	
Radius [NA]	Lateral bone of forearm; head; shaft; neck; tuberosity; styloid process; interosseous margin; ulnar notch; articular surfaces; ossifies in cartilage	Humerus, *gliding* Ulna, proximal, *pivot* Ulna, distal, *gliding* Lunate ⎫ Scaphoid ⎬ *biaxial* Triquetrum ⎭
Ribs (costae [NA])	Twelve on each side; head; neck; body; tubercle; angle; costal groove; first is relatively broad and flat; second has tubercle; 11 and 12 are floating; each ossifies in cartilage	Head with vertebral bodies ⎫ Tubercle with transverse ⎬ *gliding* processes ⎭ Sternum with first rib ⎫ Sternum with others ⎬ *cartilaginous*
Sacrum (os sacrum [NA])	Large triangular bone composed of 5 fused vertebrae; base; apex; intervertebral, pelvic, and dorsal foramens; articular processes; promontory; sacral crests; cornua; canal; hiatus; auricular facet; articular surfaces; ossifies in cartilage	Last lumbar vertebra ⎫ *cartilaginous* Coccyx ⎬ Hipbones, *gliding* (very little movement)
Scaphoid of foot	See *Navicular*	
Scaphoid (os scaphoideum [NA])	Largest bone of proximal row of carpal bones; comma-shaped; tubercle; articular surfaces; ossifies in cartilage	Trapezium ⎫ Trapezoid ⎬ *gliding* Capitate ⎪ Lunate ⎭ Radius, *biaxial*

Name	Principal features	Bones with which articulation occurs and type of joint
Scapula [NA]	Shoulder blade; flat, triangular bone of posterior part of shoulder; neck; spine; acromion; coracoid process; glenoid cavity; infraglenoid and supraglenoid tubercles; notch; subscapular, infraspinatus, and supraspinatus fossae; costal and dorsal aspects; medial, lateral, and superior margins; inferior, lateral, and superior angles; ossifies in cartilage	Humerus, *ball-and-socket* Clavicle, *gliding*
Semilunar	See *Lunate*	
Sesamoids (ossa sesamoidea [NA])	Small seed-like nodules of bone which develop in muscular tendons where they play against bone; patella, one in each tendon of insertion of flexor hallucis brevis muscle, and one in tendon of insertion of flexor pollicis brevis and of adductor pollicis are constant; others are variable; each develops in cartilage	
Skull	See *Cranium.* Sometimes used to include mandible as well	
Sphenoid (os sphenoidale [NA])	Forms anterior part of base of skull and portions of cranial, orbital, and nasal cavities; in shape resembles a butterfly with extended wings; body with air sinuses, sella turcica, hypophyseal fossa, dorsum sellae, posterior clinoid processes, clivus, chiasmatic groove, spine, carotid groove, crest, pterygoid fossa, rostrum; small wings each with optic canal, anterior clinoid process, superior orbital fissure; great wings each with foramen rotundum, foramen ovale, foramen spinosum, pterygoid processes, medial and lateral pterygoid plates, hamulus, scaphoid fossa, pterygoid canal; ossifies partly in membrane and partly in cartilage	Frontal Parietal (2) Occipital Temporal (2) Ethmoid Palatine (2) Zygoma (2) Vomer } *sutures*
Stapes [NA]	Resembles a stirrup; smallest of auditory ossicles; head; base; anterior and posterior crura; ossifies in cartilage	Incus Oval window } *gliding*
Sternum [NA]	Breastbone; dagger-shaped; manubrium; angle; body; xiphoid process; ossifies in cartilage	Clavicle (2), *gliding* First rib (2), *cartilaginous* Costal cartilages of ribs 2 to 7, *cartilaginous*
Stirrup	See *Stapes*	
Superior maxilla	See *Maxilla*	
Superior turbinate	See *Ethmoid,* superior nasal concha (not a separate bone)	

Name	Principal features	Bones with which articulation occurs and type of joint
Sutural (ossa suturarum [NA])	Irregular variable bones occasionally found along cranial sutures; most frequent in lambdoid suture	
Talus [NA]	Second largest bone of tarsus; head; neck; body; trochlea; lateral and posterior processes; medial and lateral tubercles; sulcus; articular surfaces; ossifies in cartilage	Tibia, Fibula } *hinge* Calcaneus (3 facets), Navicular } *gliding*
Tarsus (ossa tarsi [NA])	Posterior portion of foot; consists of 7 bones: calcaneus, talus, cuboid, navicular, and 3 cuneiforms	
Temporal (os temporale [NA])	Forms a portion of lateral aspect of skull and part of base of cranium; squamous part with zygomatic process, mandibular fossa, articular tubercle; tympanic part with external acoustic meatus, tympanic spine, styloid process and sheath, stylomastoid foramen, tympanic sulcus; mastoid part with air cells, notch, foramen, sigmoid sulcus; petrous part with apex, caroticotympanic and musculotubarial canals, jugular fossa, internal ear, carotid canal, internal acoustic meatus; articular surfaces; ossifies partly in membrane and partly in cartilage	Occipital, Parietal, Sphenoid, Zygoma } *sutures* Mandible, combined *gliding* and *hinge*
Tibia [NA]	Shinbone; large medial bone of leg; medial and lateral condyles; intercondylar eminence and intercondylar tubercles; tuberosity; body; soleal line; medial malleolus; articular surfaces; ossifies in cartilage	Femur, combined *hinge* and *gliding* Fibula, superior, Fibula, inferior } *gliding* Talus with fibula, *hinge*
Trapezium (os trapezium [NA])	In distal row of carpal bones; irregular bone with 6 surfaces; tubercle; articular surfaces; ossifies in cartilage	Scaphoid, Trapezoid, Second metacarpal } *gliding* First metacarpal, *saddle*
Trapezoid (os trapezoideum [NA])	Smallest bone in distal row of carpal bones; irregular bone with 6 surfaces; articular surfaces; ossifies in cartilage	Scaphoid, Second metacarpal, Trapezium, Capitate } *gliding*
Trigonal (os trigonum [NA])	Occasional extra tarsal bone; due to failure of center of ossification in lateral tubercle of talus to fuse with main center	
Triquetrum (os triquetrum [NA])	One of proximal row of carpal bones; wedge-shaped; articular surfaces; ossifies in cartilage	Lunate, Pisiform, Hamate } *gliding* Radius, *biaxial*
Turbinate, inferior	See *Concha, inferior nasal*	

Name	Principal features	Bones with which articulation occurs and type of joint
Turbinate, middle	See *Ethmoid*, middle nasal concha (not a separate bone)	
Turbinate, superior	See *Ethmoid*, superior nasal concha (not a separate bone)	
Tympanic (ossicula auditus [NA])	Includes 3 auditory ossicles. See *Incus; Malleus; Stapes*	
Ulna [NA]	Medial bone of forearm; olecranon; coronoid process; radial and trochlear notches; tuberosity; body; head; styloid process; interosseous margin; supinator crest; articular surfaces; ossifies in cartilage	Humerus, *hinge* Radius, proximal, *pivot* Radius, distal, *gliding*
Unciform	See *Hamate*	
Vertebrae [NA]	Bones of vertebral column, 33 in all: cervical 7, thoracic 12, lumbar 5, sacrum 5 (fused), coccyx 4 (fused); each has body; arch; articular processes; transverse processes; spinous process; foramens; each vertebra ossifies in cartilage. See also *Atlas, Axis, Coccyx, Sacrum*	Between vertebral bodies, *cartilaginous* Between articular processes, *gliding*
Vesalian	(1) Occasional extra ossicle in carpus (2) Occasional extra ossicle at base of fifth metatarsal due to failure of separate center of ossification to fuse with main center	
Vomer [NA]	Forms posterior part of nasal septum; ala; ossifies in membrane	Sphenoid Ethmoid *sutures* Maxilla (2) Palatine (2)
Wormian	See *Sutural*	
Wrist	See *Carpus*	
Zygoma (os zygomaticum [NA])	Cheekbone; forms cheek and lateral aspect of orbit; tubercle; temporal process; frontal process; foramens; ossifies in membrane	Frontal Sphenoid *sutures* Temporal Maxillary

Name	Origin	Insertion	Innervation	Function
Abductor accessorius digiti quinti	Rare variant of opponens digiti minimi of foot	Base of proximal phalanx of little toe	Lateral plantar	
Abductor digiti minimi of foot (musculus abductor digiti minimi [NA])	Medial and lateral tubercles of calcaneus and plantar fascia	Lateral surface of base of proximal phalanx of little toe	Lateral plantar	Supports lateral longitudinal arch and abducts little toe
Abductor digiti minimi of hand (musculus abductor digiti minimi [NA])	Pisiform and tendon of flexor carpi ulnaris	Medial surface of base of proximal phalanx of little finger	Ulnar	Abducts little finger
Abductor digiti quinti	See *Abductor digiti minimi of foot* or *of hand*			
Abductor hallucis (musculus abductor hallucis [NA])	Medial tubercle of calcaneus and plantar fascia	Medial surface of base of proximal phalanx of great toe	Medial plantar	Supports medial longitudinal arch; flexes great toe
Abductor indicis	See *Interossei, dorsal*			
Abductor ossis metatarsid quinti	Small variable portion of abductor digiti minimi of foot	Lateral side of base of fifth metatarsal	Lateral plantar	
Abductor pollicis brevis (musculus abductor pollicis brevis [NA])	Scaphoid, ridge of trapezium and flexor retinaculum	Lateral surface of base of proximal phalanx of thumb	Median	Abducts and flexes thumb
Abductor pollicis longus (musculus abductor pollicis longus [NA])	Posterior aspect of ulna, radius, and interosseous membrane	Lateral aspect of base of first metacarpal and trapezium	Dorsal interosseous of radial	Abducts and extends thumb
Accelerator urinae	See *Bulbospongiosus, male*			
Accessorius	See *Quadratus plantae; Iliocostalis thoracis*			
Accessorius ad flexorem carpi radialem	Variable additional slip of flexor carpi radialis			
Accessorius ad flexorem digitorum profundum	Variable additional slip of flexor digitorum profundus arising from coronoid process of ulna	Usually associated with tendons to middle and index fingers		
Accessorius ad flexorem pollicis longum	Variable extra part of flexor pollicis longus			

Name	Origin	Insertion	Innervation	Function
Accessorius of gluteus minimus	Occasional extra slip	Capsule of hip joint		
Accessory peroneal	Occasional variable extra slip of peroneus longus or brevis	Variable along lateral side of foot		
Accessory pterygoid	Occasional extra slip from body of sphenoid	Lateral pterygoid plate		
Adductor brevis (musculus adductor brevis [NA])	Pubis	Proximal part of linea aspera of femur and femur proximal to that line	Obturator	Adducts thigh
Adductor digiti secundi	Occasional extra part of oblique head of adductor of great toe			
Adductor hallucis (musculus adductor hallucis [NA])		Lateral aspect of base of proximal phalanx of great toe	Lateral plantar	Adducts great toe
(1) Oblique head (caput obliquum musculi adductoris hallucis [NA])	Plantar fascia and bases of second, third, and fourth metatarsals			
(2) Transverse head (caput transversum musculi adductoris hallucis [NA])	Transverse metatarsal ligament, and capsules of 4 lateral metatarsophalangeal joints			
Adductor hallucis transversus	See *Adductor hallucis, transverse head*			
Adductor longus (musculus adductor longus [NA])	Pubis	Linea aspera of femur	Obturator	Adducts thigh
Adductor magnus (musculus adductor magnus [NA])	(1) Inferior ramus of pubis and ramus of ischium	Linea aspera of femur	Obturator	Adducts thigh
	(2) Ischial tuber	Adductor tubercle of femur	Tibial	Extends thigh
Adductor minimus (musculus adductor minimus)	When present is a separate proximal portion of adductor magnus			

Name	Origin	Insertion	Innervation	Function
Adductor pollicis (musculus adductor pollicis [NA])		Medial aspect of base of proximal phalanx of thumb	Ulnar	Adducts and opposes thumb
(1) Oblique head (caput obliquum musculi adductoris pollicis [NA])	Trapezium, trapezoid, capitate, and bases of second, third, and fourth metacarpals			
(2) Transverse head (caput transversum musculi adductoris pollicis [NA])	Third metacarpal			
Adductor pollicis obliquus	See *Adductor pollicis, oblique head*			
Adductor pollicis transversus	See *Adductor pollicis, transverse head*			
Agitator caudae (variable)	Variable portion of gluteus maximus; sometimes arises separately from coccyx			
Amygdaloglossus (variable)	Scattered fibers of palatoglossus to tonsil			
Anconeus (musculus anconeus [NA])	Dorsal surface of lateral epicondyle of humerus	Olecranon of ulna	Radial	Extends elbow joint
Anconeus internus (variable)	See *Epitrochleo-olecranonis*			
Anconeus lateralis	See *Triceps brachii, lateral head*			
Anconeus longus	See *Triceps brachii, long head*			
Anconeus medialis	See *Triceps brachii, medial head*			
Antitragicus (vestigial) (musculus antitragicus [NA])	Lateral surface of antitragus	Anthelix and cauda helicis	Facial	
Arrectores pilorum (smooth) (musculi arrectores pilorum [NA])	Found in corium	Hair follicles	Sympathetic	Elevate hairs of skin

Name	Origin	Insertion	Innervation	Function
Articularis cubiti (musculus articularis cubiti [NA])	Posterior distal surface of humerus	Posterior aspect of elbow joint	Radial	Pulls capsule upward in extension of elbow joint
Articularis genus (musculus articularis genus [NA])	Distal fourth of anterior surface of femur	Synovial membrane of knee joint	Femoral	Draws synovial membrane proximally in extension of knee joint
Aryepiglotticus (inconstant) (musculus aryepiglotticus [NA])	Apex of arytenoid cartilage	Lateral margin of epiglottis	Recurrent laryngeal	Closes inlet of larynx
Arymembranous (inconstant)	Apex of arytenoid cartilage	Lateral margin of membranous part of aryepiglottic fold	Recurrent laryngeal	Closes inlet of larynx
Arytenoid				
(1) Oblique (musculus arytenoideus obliquus [NA])	Dorsal aspect of muscular process of arytenoid cartilage	Apex of opposite arytenoid cartilage	Recurrent laryngeal	Closes inlet of larynx
(2) Transverse (musculus arytenoideus transversus [NA])		Becomes continuous with thyroarytenoid		Approximates arytenoid cartilages
Aryvocalis (variable)	Variable slip of vocalis			
Atlantobasilaris internus (variable)	Occasional slip of longus capitis			
Attollens aurem (vestigial)	See *Auricular, superior*			
Attrahens aurem (vestigial)	See *Auricular, anterior*			
Auricular (vestigial)		Helix	Facial	Move auricle
(1) Anterior (musculus auricularis anterior [NA])	Galea aponeurotica			
(2) Inferior	Scattered fibers			
(3) Oblique (musculus obliquus auriculae [NA])	Scattered fibers over transverse sulcus of anthelix			
(4) Posterior (musculus auricularis posterior [NA])	Mastoid process			

Name	Origin	Insertion	Innervation	Function
Auricular (vestigial) (Continued)				
(5) Superior (musculus auricularis superior [NA])	Galea aponeurotica			
(6) Transverse (musculus transversus auriculae [NA])	Scattered fibers from concha to scapha			
Auriculofrontalis	Occasional slip of auricular anterior			
Axillary arches	Occasional slips of muscle in axillary fascia with various names			
Azygos uvulae	See *Uvulae*			
Biceps brachii (musculus biceps brachii [NA])		Tuberosity of radius and deep fascia of forearm	Musculocutaneous	Supinates and flexes forearm
(1) Long head (caput longum musculi bicipitis brachii [NA])	Supraglenoid tubercle of scapula			
(2) Short head (caput breve musculi bicipitis brachii [NA])	Tip of coracoid process of scapula			
Biceps femoris (musculus biceps femoris [NA])		Head of fibula, lateral condyle of tibia, and deep fascia on lateral aspect of knee		
(1) Long head (caput longum musculi bicipitis femoris [NA])	Ischial tuber		Tibial	Flexes knee joint and extends hip joint
(2) Short head (caput breve musculi bicipitis femoris [NA])	Linea aspera of femur		Peroneal	Flexes knee joint
Biceps flexor cruris	See *Biceps femoris*			
Biventer cervicis	See *Spinalis capitis*			
Biventer mandibulae	See *Digastric*			
Brachialis (musculus brachialis [NA])	Anterior aspect of humerus	Coronoid process of ulna	Musculocutaneous	Flexes elbow joint

Name	Origin	Insertion	Innervation	Function
Brachioradialis (musculus brachioradialis [NA])	Lateral supracondylar ridge of humerus	Lower end of radius	Radial	Flexes elbow joint
Bronchoesophageal (smooth) (musculus bronchoesophageus [NA])	Fibers from left bronchus to esophagus		Autonomic	
Buccinator (musculus buccinator [NA])	Alveolar process of maxilla and of mandible and pterygomandibular raphe	Blends about mouth with orbicularis oris	Facial	Compresses cheek and retracts angle of mouth
Buccopharyngeus (pars buccopharyngea musculi constrictoris pharyngis superioris [NA])	Portion of superior constrictor of pharynx			
Bulbocavernosus	See *Bulbospongiosus*			
Bulbospongiosus, male and female (musculus bulbospongiosus [NA])	Central part of perineum and median raphe of bulb in male	Fascia of perineum and of penis (clitoris)	Perineal	In male compresses urethra; in female contracts vaginal orifice and compresses bulb of vestibule
Caninus	See *Levator anguli oris*			
Cephalopharyngeus	Portion of superior constrictor of pharynx			
Ceratocricoid (musculus ceratocricoideus [NA])	Variable slip of posterior cricoarytenoid			
Ceratopharyngeus (pars ceratopharyngea musculi constrictoris pharyngis medii [NA])	Part of middle constrictor of pharynx			
Cervicalis ascendens	See *Iliocostalis cervicis*			
Chondroepitrochlearis (variable)	Occasional slip of muscle in axillary fascia			
Chondroglossus (variable portion of hyoglossus) (musculus chondroglossus [NA])	Lesser cornu of hyoid	Side of tongue	Hypoglossal	Depresses tongue

Name	Origin	Insertion	Innervation	Function
Chondrohumeralis	Occasional slip of muscle in axillary fascia			
Chondropharyngeus (pars chondropharyngea musculi constrictoris pharyngis medii [NA])	Portion of middle constrictor of pharynx			
Ciliary (smooth) (musculus ciliaris [NA])		Ciliary processes	Oculomotor; parasympathetic	Visual accommodation
(1) Meridional portion (fibrae meridionales musculi ciliaris [NA])	Scleral spur			
(2) Circular portion (fibrae circulares musculi ciliaris [NA])	Sphincter of ciliary body			
Ciliary (striate)	Portion of orbicularis oculi near lid margins		Facial	
Circumflexus palati	See *Tensor veli palatini*			
Cleidomastoid	Portion of sternocleidomastoid			
Cleidooccipital	Portion of sternocleidomastoid			
Coccygeofemoralis (variable)	Occasional slip of the gluteus maximus arising separately from coccyx			
Coccygeus (musculus coccygeus [NA])	Ischial spine and sacrospinous ligament	Lateral border of lower sacrum and upper coccyx	Sacral	Helps to form pelvic diaphragm
Complexus	See *Semispinalis capitis*			
Complexus minor	See *Longissimus capitis*			
Compressor bulbi proprius	Portion of bulbospongiosus, male			
Compressor hemispherium bulbi	Portion of bulbospongiosus, male			

Name	Origin	Insertion	Innervation	Function
Compressor labii	Portion of orbicularis oris			
Compressor naris	See *Nasalis, transverse part*			
Compressor nasi	See *Nasalis, transverse part*			
Compressor urethrae	See *Sphincter urethrae*			
Compressor vaginae	See *Bulbospongiosus, female*			
Compressor venae dorsalis (variable)	Portion of bulbospongiosus, male			
Constrictor of pharynx, inferior (musculus constrictor pharyngis inferior [NA])	Oblique line of thyroid cartilage, side of cricoid cartilage	Median raphe of posterior wall of pharynx	Pharyngeal plexus	Constricts pharynx
Constrictor of pharynx, middle (musculus constrictor pharyngis medius [NA])	Stylohyoid ligament and both cornua of hyoid	Median raphe of pharynx	Pharyngeal plexus	Constricts pharynx
Constrictor of pharynx, superior (musculus constrictor pharyngis superior [NA])	Medial pterygoid plate, pterygomandibular ligament, and mylohyoid line of mandible	Median raphe of pharynx	Pharyngeal plexus	Constricts pharynx
Constrictor radicis penis	Portion of bulbospongiosus, male			
Constrictor vaginae	See *Bulbospongiosus, female*			
Coracobrachialis (musculus coracobrachialis [NA])	Coracoid process of scapula	Medial aspect of shaft of humerus	Musculocutaneous	Flexes and adducts humerus
Coracobrachialis superior or brevis	Occasional proximal slip of coracobrachialis			
Corrugator cutis ani (smooth)	Found in skin about anus		Sympathetic	
Corrugator supercilii (musculus corrugator supercilii [NA])	Superciliary arch of frontal bone	Skin of forehead	Facial	Muscle of facial expression

Name	Origin	Insertion	Innervation	Function
Costalis	See *Iliocostalis thoracis*			
Costocervicalis	See *Iliocostalis cervicis*			
Costocoracoid (variable)	Occasional slip of muscle in axillary fascia			
Cremaster (musculus cremaster [NA])	Inferior margin of internal oblique abdominal muscle	Pubic tubercle	Genitofemoral	Elevates testis
Cricoarytenoid, lateral (musculus cricoarytenoideus lateralis [NA])	Lateral surface of cricoid cartilage	Muscular process of arytenoid cartilage	Recurrent laryngeal	Approximates vocal folds
Cricoarytenoid, posterior (musculus cricoarytenoideus posterior [NA])	Dorsal surface of cricoid cartilage	Muscular process of arytenoid cartilage	Recurrent laryngeal	Separates vocal folds
Cricopharyngeus (pars cricopharyngea musculi constrictoris pharyngis inferioris [NA])	Part of inferior constrictor of pharynx			
Cricothyroid (musculus cricothyroideus [NA])	Arch of cricoid cartilage	Lamina of thyroid cartilage	External branch of superior laryngeal	Tenses vocal folds
Crureus	See *Vastus intermedius*			
Cucullarius	See *Trapezius*			
Dartos (smooth) (tunica dartos [NA])	Found in skin and superficial fascia of scrotum		Sympathetic	Corrugates skin of scrotum
Deep transverse perineal (musculus transversus perinei profundus [NA])	Ramus of ischium	Central point of perineum	Perineal	Supports perineum
Deltoid (musculus deltoideus [NA])	Clavicle, acromion, and spine of scapula	Deltoid tuberosity of humerus	Axillary	Abducts humerus; anterior fibers flex and medially rotate humerus, posterior fibers extend and laterally rotate humerus
Depressor alae nasi	See *Nasalis, alar part*			

Name	Origin	Insertion	Innervation	Function
Depressor anguli oris (musculus depressor anguli oris [NA])	Mandible	Skin of angle of mouth	Facial	Muscle of facial expression
Depressor epiglottidis	Some fibers of thyro-epiglottic			
Depressor labii inferioris (musculus depressor labii inferioris [NA])	Mandible	Skin of lower lip	Facial	Muscle of facial expression
Depressor septi nasi (musculus depressor septi [NA])	Maxilla	Septum of nose	Facial	Muscle of facial expression
Depressor supercilii (musculus depressor supercilii [NA])	A few fibers of orbicularis oculi	Eyebrow	Facial	Muscle of facial expression
Detrusor urinae	See Detrusor vesicae			
Detrusor vesicae (smooth)	In wall of urinary bladder		Autonomic	Empties urinary bladder
Diaphragm (diaphragma [NA])	Xiphoid cartilage, costal cartilages of ribs 5 to 9, lower ribs, and lumbar vertebrae	Central tendon	Phrenic	Acts as main muscle of inhalation; aids in expulsive actions such as sneezing and parturition
Digastric (musculus digastricus [NA])		Lesser cornu of hyoid via fascial sling		Elevates and fixes hyoid bone
(1) Anterior belly (venter anterior musculi digastrici [NA])	Inner surface of mandible near symphysis		Mylohyoid	
(2) Posterior belly (venter posterior musculi digastrici [NA])	Mastoid notch		Facial	
Dilator naris	See Nasalis, alar part			
Dilator pupillae (smooth) (musculus dilator pupillae [NA])	Circumference of iris	Margin of pupil	Sympathetic	Dilates pupil
Dilator tubae	See Tensor veli palatini			
Dorsoepitrochlearis (variable)	Occasional slip of muscle in axillary fascia			

Name	Origin	Insertion	Innervation	Function
Ejaculator urinae	See *Bulbospongiosus, male*			
Epicraniotemporalis	See *Auricular, anterior*			
Epicranius (musculus epicranius [NA])	See *Occipitofrontalis; Temporoparietalis*			
Epitrochlearis	See *Chondrohumeralis*			
Epitrochleo-olecranonis (variable)	Medial epicondyle of humerus	Olecranon	Radial	
Erector clitoridis	See *Ischiocavernosus*			
Erector penis	See *Ischiocavernosus*			
Erector pili	See *Arrectores pilorum*			
Erector spinae (musculus erector spinae [NA])	Composed of iliocostalis, longissimus, and spinalis			
Extensor carpi radialis accessorius (variable part of extensor carpi radialis brevis)				
Extensor carpi radialis brevior	See *Extensor carpi radialis brevis*			
Extensor carpi radialis brevis (musculus extensor carpi radialis brevis [NA])	Lateral epicondyle of humerus	Base of second and third metacarpals		Extends wrist
Extensor carpi radialis intermedius (variable part of extensor carpi radialis brevis)				
Extensor carpi radialis longior	See *Extensor carpi radialis longus*			
Extensor carpi radialis longus (musculus extensor carpi radialis longus [NA])	Lateral epicondyle of humerus	Base of second metacarpal	Radial	Extends wrist

Name	Origin	Insertion	Innervation	Function
Extensor carpi ulnaris (musculus extensor carpi ulnaris [NA])	Lateral epicondyle of humerus and dorsal margin of ulna	Base of fifth metacarpal	Radial	Extends wrist
Extensor coccygeus (vestigial)	See *Sacrococcygeus dorsalis*			
Extensor communis pollicis et indicis (variable)	Occasional extra slip of extensor pollicis longus			
Extensor digiti annularis (variable)	Occasional extra slip of muscle to ring finger			
Extensor digiti minimi (musculus extensor digiti minimi [NA])	Lateral epicondyle of humerus	Dorsum of proximal phalanx of little finger	Radial	Extends metacarpophalangeal joint of little finger
Extensor digitorum (musculus extensor digitorum [NA])	Lateral epicondyle of humerus	Tendon to dorsal aspect of each finger	Radial	Extends fingers at metacarpophalangeal joints
Extensor digitorum brevis (musculus extensor digitorum brevis [NA])	Dorsal surface of calcaneus	Extensor tendons of 4 medial toes	Deep peroneal	Dorsiflexes toes at metatarsophalangeal joints
Extensor digitorum brevis of hand (variable)	Carpal bones	Extensor tendons of metacarpals	Radial	Aids common extensor (extensor digitorum)
Extensor digitorum communis	See *Extensor digitorum*			
Extensor digitorum longus (musculus extensor digitorum longus [NA])	Anterior aspect of fibula, lateral aspect of lateral malleolus, and interosseous membrane	Common extensor tendons of 4 lateral toes	Deep peroneal	Dorsiflexes at metatarsophalangeal joints
Extensor hallucis brevis (most medial portion of extensor digitorum brevis) (musculus extensor hallucis brevis [NA])	Dorsal surface of calcaneus	Base of proximal phalanx of great toe	Deep peroneal	Dorsiflexes great toe at metatarsophalangeal joint
Extensor hallucis longus (musculus extensor hallucis longus [NA])	Medial surface of fibula and interosseous membrane	Base of proximal phalanx of great toe	Deep peroneal	Dorsiflexes ankle joint and great toe

Name	Origin	Insertion	Innervation	Function
Extensor indicis (musculus extensor indicis [NA])	Dorsal surface of ulna	Common extensor tendon of index finger	Dorsal interosseous	Extends metacarpophalangeal joint of index finger
Extensor medii digiti (variable)	Occasional extra slip of muscle to middle finger			
Extensor ossis metacarpi pollicis	See *Abductor pollicis longus*			
Extensor ossis metatarsi hallucis	Occasional separate slip of insertion of extensor hallucis longus into first metatarsal			
Extensor pollicis brevis (musculus extensor pollicis brevis [NA])	Dorsal surface of radius and interosseous membrane	Dorsal surface of proximal phalanx of thumb	Dorsal interosseous	Extends metacarpophalangeal joint of thumb
Extensor pollicis longus (musculus extensor pollicis longus [NA])	Dorsal surface of radius and interosseous membrane	Dorsal surface of proximal phalanx of thumb	Dorsal interosseous	Extends metacarpophalangeal joint of thumb
Extensor primi internodii longus hallucis	Occasional extra slip of insertion of extensor hallucis longus into proximal phalanx of great toe			
Extensor primi internodii pollicis	See *Extensor pollicis brevis*			
Extensor secundi internodii pollicis	See *Extensor pollicis longus*			
External oblique of abdomen	See *Oblique, external abdominal*			
External thyroarytenoid (lateral part of thyroarytenoid)				
Fibularis brevis (musculus fibularis brevis [NA alternative])	See *Peroneus brevis*			
Fibularis longus (musculus fibularis longus [NA alternative])	See *Peroneus longus*			

TABLE OF MUSCLES (Continued)

Name	Origin	Insertion	Innervation	Function
Fibularis tertius (musculus fibularis tertius [NA alternative])	See *Peroneus tertius*			
Fibulocalcaneus (variable)	Occasional extra slip of quadratus plantae or of flexor digitorum longus			
Fibulotibialis (variable)	Occasional extra slip of popliteus			
Flexor accessorius (musculus flexor accessorius [NA alternative])	See *Quadratus plantae*			
Flexor carpi radialis (musculus flexor carpi radialis [NA])	Medial epicondyle of humerus	Base of second metacarpal	Median	Flexes wrist joint
Flexor carpi radialis brevis (variable)	Lateral surface of distal half of radius	Variable into carpus or index finger	Median	Flexes wrist joint
Flexor carpi ulnaris (musculus flexor carpi ulnaris [NA])	Medial epicondyle of humerus	Pisiform, hamulus of hamate, and proximal end of fifth metacarpal	Ulnar	Flexes wrist joint
Flexor carpi ulnaris brevis (variable)	Distal one-fourth of palmar surface of ulna	Pisiform, hamulus of hamate, and proximal end of fifth metacarpal	Ulnar	Flexes wrist joint
Flexor digiti minimi brevis of foot (musculus flexor digiti minimi brevis [NA])	Base of fifth metatarsal and plantar fascia	Lateral side of proximal phalanx of little toe	Lateral plantar	Flexes little toe at metatarsophalangeal joint
Flexor digiti minimi brevis of hand (musculus flexor digiti minimi brevis [NA])	Hamulus of hamate and flexor retinaculum	Medial side of proximal phalanx of little finger	Ulnar	Flexes metacarpophalangeal joint of little finger
Flexor digitorum accessorius (musculus flexor accessorius [NA alternative])	See *Quadratus plantae*			
Flexor digitorum brevis (musculus flexor digitorum brevis [NA])	Medial tubercle of calcaneus and plantar aponeurosis	Four tendons, one to middle phalanx of each of 4 lateral toes	Medial plantar	Flexes toes at metatarsophalangeal and proximal interphalangeal joints

Name	Origin	Insertion	Innervation	Function
Flexor digitorum longus (musculus flexor digitorum longus [NA])	Posterior aspect of tibia	Four tendons, one to base of distal phalanx of each of 4 lateral toes	Tibial	Flexes toes at metatarsophalangeal and interphalangeal joints
Flexor digitorum profundus (musculus flexor digitorum profundus [NA])	Medial and anterior aspects of ulna and interosseous membrane	Four tendons, one to base of distal phalanx of each finger	Ulnar to medial portion, median to lateral portion	Flexes fingers primarily at distal interphalangeal joints; aids in flexing at wrist and other joints of fingers
Flexor digitorum sublimis	See *Flexor digitorum superficialis*			
Flexor digitorum superficialis (musculus flexor digitorum superficialis [NA])	Medial epicondyle of humerus, coronoid process of ulna, and anterior process of radius	Four tendons, one to base of middle phalanx of each finger	Median	Flexes fingers primarily at proximal interphalangeal joints; aids in flexing wrist and metacarpophalangeal joints
Flexor hallucis brevis (musculus flexor hallucis brevis [NA])	Plantar aspect of cuboid and plantar fascia	Base of proximal phalanx of great toe	Medial plantar	Flexes metatarsophalangeal joint of great toe
Flexor hallucis longus (musculus flexor hallucis longus [NA])	Posterior aspect of fibula	Base of distal phalanx of great toe	Tibial	Flexes great toe; plantar flexes foot; supports arches of foot
Flexor ossis metacarpi pollicis	See *Opponens pollicis*			
Flexor pollicis brevis (musculus flexor pollicis brevis [NA])	Flexor retinaculum and ridge of trapezium	Base of proximal phalanx of thumb	Median	Flexes metacarpophalangeal joint of thumb
Flexor pollicis longus (musculus flexor pollicis longus [NA])	Anterior aspect of radius and interosseous membrane	Base of distal phalanx of thumb	Median	Flexes thumb
Frontalis	See *Occipitofrontalis*			
Gastrocnemius (musculus gastrocnemius [NA])		Posterior surface of calceneus via calcaneal tendon	Tibial	Plantar flexes ankle joint; flexes knee joint
(1) Lateral head (caput laterale musculi gastrocnemii [NA])	Lateral condyle of femur			
(2) Medial head (caput mediale musculi gastrocnemii [NA])	Medial condyle of femur			

Name	Origin	Insertion	Innervation	Function
Gemellus, inferior (musculus gemellus inferior [NA])	Tuber of ischium	Greater trochanter of femur	Nerve to quadratus femoris	Rotates femur laterally
Gemellus, superior (musculus gemellus superior [NA])	Spine of ischium	Greater trochanter of femur	Nerve to obturator internus	Rotates femur laterally
Genioglossus (musculus genioglossus [NA])	Upper mental tubercle of mandible	Hyoid and lateral side of tongue	Hypoglossal	Protrudes and depresses tongue
Geniohyoglossus	See *Genioglossus*			
Geniohyoid (musculus geniohyoideus [NA])	Lower mental tubercle of mandible	Body of hyoid	Superior ramus of ansa cervicalis	Elevates and draws hyoid forward
Geniopharyngeus (variable)	Occasional slip of genioglossus to superior constrictor of pharynx			
Glossopalatinus	See *Palatoglossus*			
Glossopharyngeus (pars glossopharyngea musculi constrictoris pharyngis superioris [NA])	Part of superior constrictor of pharynx			
Gluteus maximus (musculus gluteus maximus [NA])	Lateral surface of ilium, posterior surface of ischium and coccyx, and sacrotuberous ligament	Gluteal tuberosity and iliotibial tract	Inferior gluteal	Extends hip joint; extends trunk on legs when raising body from a seated position
Gluteus medius (musculus gluteus medius [NA])	Lateral surface of ilium	Greater trochanter	Superior gluteal	Abducts femur
Gluteus minimus (musculus gluteus minimus [NA])	Lateral surface of ilium	Greater trochanter	Superior gluteal	Abducts and medially rotates femur
Gluteal, small anterior (variable) (gluteal, fourth)	Occasional accessory slip of gluteus minimus			
Gracilis (musculus gracilis [NA])	Pubis	Medial surface of tibia	Obturator	Adducts femur; flexes knee joint
Hamstrings	Semimembranosus, semitendinosus, and biceps femoris as a group			

Name	Origin	Insertion	Innervation	Function
Helicis major (vestigial) (musculus helicis major [NA])	Spina helicis	Ascending part of helix	Facial	
Helicis minor (vestigial) (musculus helicis minor [NA])	Spina helicis	Crux of helix	Facial	
Hyoglossus (musculus hyoglossus [NA])	Body and greater cornu of hyoid	Side of tongue	Hypoglossal	Depresses tongue
Hyopharyngeus	See *Constrictor of pharynx, middle*			
Iliacus (musculus iliacus [NA])	Iliac fossa and sacrum	Lesser trochanter	Femoral	Flexes hip joint and trunk on lower extremity
Iliacus minor (variable) (musculus psoas minor [NA])	Occasional separate lateral part of iliacus			
Iliocapsulotrochantericus (variable)	Occasional separate slip of iliacus			
Iliococcygeus (musculus iliococcygeus [NA])	Part of levator ani			
Iliocostalis (lateral part of erector spinae) (musculus iliocostalis [NA])			Posterior rami of spinal	Extends vertebral column and assists in lateral movements of trunk
(1) Cervicis (musculus iliocostalis cervicis [NA])	Upper 6 ribs	Posterior tubercles of transverse processes of fourth, fifth, and sixth cervical vertebrae		
(2) Lumborum (musculus iliocostalis lumborum [NA])	Iliac crest, lumbar vertebrae, sacrum, and lumbodorsal fascia	Lower 6 ribs		
(3) Thoracis (musculus iliocostalis thoracis [NA])	Lower 6 ribs	Upper 6 ribs		
Iliocostalis dorsi	See *Iliocostalis thoracis*			
Iliocostocervicalis	See *Iliocostalis cervicis; Iliocostalis thoracis*			

Name	Origin	Insertion	Innervation	Function
Iliopsoas (musculus iliopsoas [NA])	Combined iliacus and psoas			
Incisive, of lower lip (musculi incisivi labii inferioris)	Portion of orbicularis oris			
Incisive, of upper lip (musculi incisivi labii superioris)	Portion of orbicularis oris			
Inferior constrictor of pharynx	See *Constrictor of pharynx, inferior*			
Inferior lingual	See *Longitudinalis of tongue*			
Inferior oblique	See *Oblique, inferior*			
Inferior rectus	See *Rectus inferior bulbi*			
Inferior tarsal	See *Tarsal*			
Infraclavicularis (variable)	Occasional slip of pectoralis major passing over clavicle			
Infracostals	See *Subcostals*			
Infraspinatus (musculus infraspinatus [NA])	Infraspinous fossa of scapula	Greater tubercle of humerus	Suprascapular	Rotates humerus laterally
Interarytenoideus	See *Arytenoid*			
Intercostal, external (musculi intercostales externi [NA])	Lower border of rib above	Superior border of rib below	Anterior rami of thoracic	Accessory muscles of respiration (inhalation)
Intercostal, innermost (musculi intercostales intimi [NA])	Lower border of rib above	Superior border of rib below	Anterior rami of thoracic	Accessory muscles of respiration (exhalation)
Intercostal, internal (musculi intercostales interni [NA])	Lower border of rib above	Superior border of rib below	Anterior rami of thoracic	Accessory muscles of respiration (exhalation)
Internal oblique of abdomen	See *Oblique, internal abdominal*			
Interossei, dorsal (of foot) (4) (musculi interossei dorsales [NA])	Each by 2 heads from sides of adjacent metatarsals	Extensor tendon of each of 4 lateral toes	Lateral plantar	Abduct toes; aid in flexion at metatarsophalangeal joints and in extension at interphalangeal joints

Name	Origin	Insertion	Innervation	Function
Interossei, dorsal (of hand) (4) (musculi interossei dorsales [NA])	Each by 2 heads from sides of adjacent metacarpals	Extensor tendons of second, third, and fourth fingers	Ulnar	Abduct fingers; aid in flexion at metacarpophalangeal joints and in extension at interphalangeal joints
Interossei, palmar (3) (musculi interossei palmares [NA])	Medial side of second and lateral side of fourth and fifth metacarpals, respectively	Extensor tendons of second, third, and fourth fingers	Ulnar	Adduct second, fourth, and fifth fingers and assist dorsal interossei
Interossei, plantar (3) (musculi interossei plantares [NA])	Medial side of third, fourth, and fifth metatarsals, respectively	Extensor tendons of third, fourth, and fifth toes	Lateral plantar	Adduct toes and assist dorsal interossei
Interossei, volar	See *Interossei, palmar*			
Interspinales (musculi interspinales [NA])			Dorsal rami of spinal	Rotate and extend the vertebral column
(1) Cervicis (musculi interspinales cervicis [NA])	Spine of vertebra below	Spine of vertebra above		
(2) Lumborum (musculi interspinales lumborum [NA])	Spine of vertebra below	Spine of vertebra		
(3) Thoracis (musculi interspinales thoracis [NA])	Spine of vertebra below	Spine of vertebra above		
Intertransversales	See *Intertransverse*			
Intertransverse (musculi intertransversarii [NA])			Anterior rami of spinal for lateral portions; posterior rami of spinal for medial portions	Lateral movements of vertebral column
(1) Cervical (a) Anterior (musculi intertransversarii anteriores cervicis [NA])	Transverse process of cervical vertebra	Transverse process of contiguous cervical vertebra		
(b) Posterior (musculi intertransversarii posteriores cervicis [NA])				

Name	Origin	Insertion	Innervation	Function
Intertransverse (musculi intertransversarii [NA]) (Continued)				
(2) Lumbar (a) Lateral(musculi intertransversarii laterales lumborum [NA])	Transverse process of lumbar vertebra	Transverse process of contiguous lumbar vertebra		
(b) Medial(musculi intertransversarii mediales lumborum [NA])				
(3) Thoracic (variable) (musculi intertransversarii thoracis [NA])	Transverse process of thoracic vertebra	Transverse process of contiguous thoracic vertebra		
Invertor femoris (variable)	Occasional extra slip of gluteus minimus			
Ischiobulbosus (variable)	Ischium	Perineal raphe	Perineal	Assists bulbospongiosus
Ischiocavernosus (musculus ischiocavernosus [NA])	Ischium	Crus of penis (clitoris)	Perineal	Assists in erection
Ischiococcygeus	See *Coccygeus*			
Ischiofemoralis (variable)	Occasional extra slip of gluteus maximus arising from ischial tuber			
Ischiopubicus (variable)	Portion of sphincter of urethra			
Laryngopharyngeus	See *Constrictor of pharynx, inferior*			
Lateral cricoarytenoid	See *Cricoarytenoid, lateral*			
Lateral rectus	See *Rectus lateralis*			
Latissimocondyloid (variable)	Occasional slip of latissimus dorsi to olecranon			
Latissimus colli	See *Platysma*			

Name	Origin	Insertion	Innervation	Function
Latissimus dorsi (musculus latissimus dorsi [NA])	Spines of lower 6 thoracic vertebrae, spines of lumbar vertebrae, lumbodorsal fascia, crest of ilium, lower ribs, and inferior angle of scapula	Intertubercular sulcus of humerus	Thoracodorsal	Adducts and extends humerus; used to pull body upward in climbing; accessory muscle of respiration
Latissimus thoracis	See *Latissimus dorsi*			
Levator anguli oris (musculus levator anguli oris [NA])	Maxilla	Skin of angle of mouth	Facial	Muscle of facial expression
Levator anguli scapulae	See *Levator scapulae*			
Levator ani (musculus levator ani [NA])			Anterior rami of third and fourth sacral, and perineal	Supports pelvic viscera
(1) Iliococcygeus (musculus iliococcygeus [NA])	Pelvic surface of ischial spine and pelvic fascia	Central point of perineum, anococcygeal raphe, and coccyx		
(2) Levator prostatae (musculus levator prostatae [NA])		Some fibers inserted into the prostate		
(3) Pubococcygeus (musculus pubococcygeus [NA])	Pubis and pelvic fascia			
(4) Puborectalis (musculus puborectalis [NA])	Pubis	Some fibers that form a sling around the lower part of the rectum		
Levator claviculae (variable)	Occasional slip of levator scapulae inserted into clavicle			
Levator epiglottiidis (variable)	Occasional slip of genioglossus to epiglottis			
Levator glandulae thyroideae (variable) (musculus levator glandulae thyroideae [NA])	Hyoid	Isthmus of thyroid gland		
Levator labii superioris (musculus levator labii superioris [NA])	Maxilla	Skin of upper lip	Facial	Muscle of facial expression

Name	Origin	Insertion	Innervation	Function
Levator labii superioris alaeque nasi (musculus levator labii superioris alaeque nasi [NA])	Maxilla	Skin of upper lip and ala of nose	Facial	Muscle of facial expression
Levator menti	See *Mentalis*			
Levator palati	See *Levator veli palatini*			
Levator palpebrae superioris (musculus levator palpebrae superioris [NA])	Roof of orbit	Skin of upper eyelid and superior tarsus	Oculomotor	Raises upper eyelid
Levator prostatae	See *Levator ani*			
Levator scapulae (musculus levator scapulae [NA])	Transverse process of upper cervical vertebrae	Medial margin and superior angle of scapula	Dorsal scapular and anterior rami of third and fourth cervical	Elevates shoulder; rotates inferior angle of scapula medially
Levator veli palatini (musculus levator veli palatini [NA])	Apex of petrous part of temporal bone and cartilaginous part of auditory tube	Aponeurosis of soft palate	Pharyngeal plexus	Raises soft palate
Levatores costarum (12 pairs) (musculi levatores costarum [NA])	Transverse process of vertebra (seventh cervical to eleventh thoracic)	Angle of rib below	Anterior rami of thoracic	Aid in raising ribs
(1) Breves (musculi levatores costarum breves [NA])				
(2) Longi (musculi levatores costarum longi [NA])				
Longissimus (middle part of erector spinae) (musculus longissimus [NA])			Posterior rami of spinal	Extends vertebral column and assists in rotation and lateral movements of trunk
(1) Capitis (musculus longissimus capitis [NA])	Transverse processes of upper 6 thoracic vertebrae and articular processes of lower 4 cervical vertebrae	Mastoid process of temporal bone		
(2) Cervicis (musculus longissimus cervicis [NA])	Transverse processes of upper 6 thoracic vertebrae	Transverse processes of second to sixth cervical vertebrae		

Name	Origin	Insertion	Innervation	Function
Longissimus (middle part of erector spinae) (musculus longissimus [NA]) (Continued)				
(3) Thoracis (musculus longissimus thoracis [NA])	Iliac crest, sacroiliac ligament, spines of lumbar and sacral vertebrae	Ribs and transverse processes of thoracic and upper lumbar vertebrae		
Longissimus dorsi	See *Longissimus thoracis*			
Longitudinalis of tongue	Base of tongue	Tip of tongue	Hypoglossal	Alters shape of tongue
(1) Inferior (musculus longitudinalis inferior [NA])				
(2) Superior (musculus longitudinalis superior [NA])				
Longus capitis (musculus longus capitis [NA])	Transverse processes of third and sixth cervical vertebrae	Basal portion of occipital bone	Anterior rami of upper 4 cervical	Flexes head
Longus cervicis	See *Longus colli*			
Longus colli (musculus longus colli [NA])			Anterior rami of cervical	Flexes vertebral column
(1) Inferior oblique portion	Bodies of first 3 thoracic vertebrae	Anterior tubercles of fifth and sixth cervical vertebrae		
(2) Superior oblique portion	Transverse processes of third to fifth thoracic vertebrae	Anterior tubercle of atlas		
(3) Vertical portion	Bodies of last 3 cervical and first 3 thoracic vertebrae	Bodies of second to fourth cervical vertebrae		
Lumbricals of fingers (4) (musculi lumbricales [NA])	Tendons of flexor digitorum profundus muscle	One to extensor tendon of each finger	Two lateral by median and 2 medial by ulnar	Flex at metacarpophalangeal joints and extend at interphalangeal joints
Lumbricals of toes (4) (musculi lumbricales [NA])	Tendons of flexor digitorum longus	One to extensor tendon of each of 4 lateral toes	Medial one by medial plantar, others by lateral plantar	Flex at metatarsophalangeal joints and extend at interphalangeal joints
Masseter (musculus masseter [NA])	Arch of zygoma	Ramus and angle of mandible	Mandibular	Muscle of mastication; closes mouth and clenches teeth

Name	Origin	Insertion	Innervation	Function
Mentalis (musculus mentalis [NA])	Incisor fossa of mandible	Skin of chin	Facial	Muscle of facial expression
Middle constrictor of pharynx	See *Constrictor of pharynx, middle*			
Multifidus (part of transverse spinal) (musculi multifidi [NA])	Sacrum, sacroiliac ligament, mammillary processes of lumbar vertebrae, transverse processes of thoracic vertebrae, articular processes of lower 4 cervical vertebrae	Spines of vertebrae	Posterior rami of spinal	Extends and rotates vertebral column
Mylohyoid (musculus mylohyoideus [NA])	Mylohyoid line of mandible	Hyoid	Nerve to mylohyoid	Elevates hyoid and supports floor of mouth
Mylopharyngeal (pars mylopharyngea musculi constrictoris pharyngis superioris [NA])	Portion of superior constrictor of pharynx			
Nasalis (musculus nasalis [NA])			Facial	
(1) Alar part (pars alaris musculi nasalis [NA])	Maxilla	Ala of nose		Widens nasal opening
(2) Transverse part (pars transversa musculi nasalis [NA])	Maxilla	Bridge of nose		Depresses nasal cartilage
Oblique arytenoid	See *Arytenoid, oblique*			
Oblique, auricular	See *Auricular, oblique*			
Oblique, external abdominal (musculus obliquus externus abdominis [NA])	Lower 8 ribs	Xiphoid, linea alba, crest of ilium, pubis	Lower 6 thoracic	Supports abdominal viscera; flexes vertebral column
Oblique, inferior of eye (musculus obliquus inferior bulbi [NA])	Medial aspect of floor of orbit	Sclera	Oculomotor	Rotates eyeball upward and outward
Oblique, inferior of head (musculus obliquus capitis inferior [NA])	Spine of axis	Transverse process of atlas	Posterior ramus of first cervical	Aids in extension and lateral movements of head

Name	Origin	Insertion	Innervation	Function
Oblique, internal abdominal (musculus obliquus internus abdominis [NA])	Lumbodorsal fascia, iliac crest, inguinal ligament	Lower 3 ribs, linea alba, xiphoid, pubis	Lower 6 thoracic and iliohypogastric	Supports abdominal viscera; flexes vertebral column
Oblique, superior of eye (musculus obliquus superior [NA])	Margin of optic canal	Sclera	Trochlear	Rotates eyeball downward and outward
Oblique, superior of head (musculus obliquus capitis superior [NA])	Transverse process of atlas	Occipital bone	Posterior ramus of first cervical	Aids in extension and lateral movements of head
Obturator externus (musculus obturatorius externus [NA])	Pubis, ischium, and superficial surface of obturator membrane	Trochanteric fossa of femur	Obturator	Rotates femur laterally
Obturator internus (musculus obturatorius internus [NA])	Pubis, ischium, and deep surface of obturator membrane	Greater trochanter of femur	Nerve to obturator internus	Rotates femur laterally
Occipitalis	See *Occipitofrontalis*			
Occipitalis minor (variable)	See *Transverse nuchal*			
Occipitofrontalis (musculus occipitofrontalis [NA])			Facial	
(1) Frontal part (venter frontalis musculi occipitofrontalis [NA])	Galea aponeurotica	Skin of forehead		Elevates eyebrows and draws scalp forward
(2) Occipital part (venter occipitalis musculi occipitofrontalis [NA])	Superior nuchal line of occipital bone	Galea aponeurotica		Draws scalp backward
Occipitoscapular (variable)	Occasional extra slip of rhomboideus major			
of Aeby	See *Depressor labii inferioris*			
of Albinus	See *Risorius; Scalene, least*			
of Bell	Smooth muscle of urinary bladder running forward from each ureteric orifice			

Name	Origin	Insertion	Innervation	Function
of Bochdalak	See *Triticeoglossus*			
of Bowman	See *Ciliary*			
of Boyden	See *Sphincter of common bile duct*			
of Brücke	See *Ciliary, meridional portion*			
of Chassaignac	One of the axillary arch muscles			
of Gantzer	See *Accessorius ad flexorem digitorum profundum; Accessorius ad flexorem carpi radialem; Accessorius ad flexorem pollicis longum*			
of Gegenbauer	See *Auriculofrontalis*			
of Gruber	See *Peroneocalcaneus externus*			
of Guthrie	See *Sphincter urethrae*			
of Hall	See *Ischiobulbosus*			
of Henle	See *Auricular, anterior*			
of Hilton	See *Aryepiglotticus*			
of Horner	See *Orbicularis oculi, lacrimal part*			
of Houston	See *Compressor venae dorsalis*			
of incisure of helix (variable)	Bridges incisure of helix			
of Jung	See *Pyramidal of ear*			
of Klein	See *Compressor labii*			
of Langer	One of axillary arch muscles			
of Landström	Smooth fibers in orbital fascia			
of Ludwig	See *Aryvocalis*			
of Macallister	See *Fibulocalcaneus*			

Name	Origin	Insertion	Innervation	Function
of Merkel	See *Ceratocricoid*			
of Müller	See *Orbital; Tarsal; Ciliary, circular portion*			
of Oddi	See *Sphincter of hepatopancreatic ampulla*			
of Raux	See *Rectourethralis*			
of Riolan	See *Orbicularis oculi, ciliary part*			
of Rouget	See *Ciliary, circular portion*			
of Santorini	See *Risorius*			
of Treitz	See *Rectococcygeus; Suspensory of duodenum*			
of Wilson	See *Sphincter urethrae*			
of Wood	See *Extensor carpi radialis intermedius*			
Omohyoid(musculus omohyoideus [NA])			Ansa cervicalis	Depresses hyoid
(1) Inferior belly (venter inferior musculi omohyoidei [NA])	Superior margin of scapula	Intermediate tendon		
(2) Superior belly (venter superior musculi omohyoidei [NA])	Intermediate tendon	Hyoid		
Opponens digiti minimi of foot	See *Opponens digiti quinti of foot*			
Opponens digiti minimi of hand (musculus opponens digiti minimi [NA])	Flexor retinaculum and hamulus of hamate	Medial aspect of fifth metacarpal	Ulnar	Deepens palm
Opponens digiti quinti of foot (variable) (musculus opponens digiti quinti)	Occasional insertion of part of flexor digiti minimi brevis into fifth metatarsal			

Name	Origin	Insertion	Innervation	Function
Opponens digiti quinti of hand	See *Opponens digiti minimi of hand*			
Opponens hallucis (variable)	Occasional insertion of some fibers of flexor hallucis brevis into shaft of first metatarsal			
Opponens pollicis (musculus opponens pollicis [NA])	Ridge of trapezium and flexor retinaculum	First metacarpal	Median	Opposes thumb
Orbicularis oculi (musculus orbicularis oculi [NA])	Medial aspect of orbit	Skin about eyelids	Facial	Closes lids; muscle of facial expression
(1) Ciliary part				
(2) Lacrimal part (pars lacrimalis musculi orbicularis oculi [NA])				
(3) Orbital part (pars orbitalis musculi orbicularis oculi [NA])				
(4) Palpebral part (pars palpebralis musculi orbicularis oculi [NA])				
Orbicularis oris (musculus orbicularis oris [NA])	Lies in skin about mouth		Facial	Closes lips; muscle of facial expression
(1) Labial part (pars labialis musculi orbicularis oris [NA])				
(2) Marginal part (pars marginalis musculi orbicularis oris [NA])				
Orbicularis palpebrarum	See *Orbicularis oculi*			
Orbital (smooth) (musculus orbitalis [NA])	Bridges inferior orbital fissure		Sympathetic	
Palatoglossus (musculus palatoglossus [NA])	Inferior surface of soft palate	Side of tongue	Accessory	Elevates tongue and constricts fauces

Name	Origin	Insertion	Innervation	Function
Palatopharyngeus (musculus palatopharyngeus [NA])	Soft palate and auditory tube	Aponeurosis of pharynx	Accessory	Aids in swallowing
Palmaris brevis (musculus palmaris brevis [NA])	Palmar aponeurosis	Skin of medial border of hand	Ulnar	Deepens palm
Palmaris longus (variable) (musculus palmaris longus [NA])	Medial epicondyle of humerus	Flexor retinaculum and palmar aponeurosis	Median	Flexes wrist joint
Papillary (cardiac) (musculi papillares [NA])	Ventricles of heart		Autonomic	Contract in systole of heart
(1) Anterior of left ventricle (musculus papillaris anterior ventriculi sinistri [NA])				
(2) Anterior of right ventricle (musculus papillaris anterior ventriculi dextri [NA])				
(3) Posterior of left ventricle (musculus papillaris posterior ventriculi sinistri [NA])				
(4) Posterior of right ventricle (musculus papillaris posterior ventriculi dextri [NA])				
(5) Septal of right ventricle (musculi papillares septales [NA])				
Pectinate (cardiac) (musculi pectinati [NA])	Auricles of heart		Autonomic	Contract in systole of heart
Pectineus (musculus pectineus [NA])	Pubis	Femur distal to lesser trochanter	Femoral (occasionally obturator)	Adducts femur and flexes hip joint
Pectoralis major (musculus pectoralis major [NA])	Clavicle, sternum, first 6 ribs, aponeurosis of external oblique abdominal muscle	Intertubercular sulcus of humerus, lateral side	Medial and lateral anterior thoracic	Adducts and medially rotates humerus; flexes shoulder joint; depresses shoulder girdle

Name	Origin	Insertion	Innervation	Function
Pectoralis minor (musculus pectoralis minor [NA])	Third to fifth ribs	Coracoid process of scapula	Medial and lateral anterior thoracic	Draws shoulder forward
Pectorodorsalis (variable)	Occasional slip of muscle in axillary fascia			
Peroneocalcaneus externus (variable)	Occasional slip of insertion of peroneus brevis or longus into calcaneus			
Peroneocalcaneus internus (variable)	Occasional extra slip of tibialis posterior			
Peroneocuboideus (variable)	Occasional slip of insertion of peroneus brevis or longus into cuboid			
Peroneotibialis (variable)	Occasional extra slip of popliteus			
Peroneus accessorius (variable)	Occasional extra slip of peroneus brevis or longus			
Peroneus brevis (musculus peroneus brevis [NA])	Lateral surface of fibula	Base of fifth metatarsal	Superficial peroneal	Everts and plantar flexes foot
Peroneus longus (musculus peroneus longus [NA])	Lateral condyle of tibia and lateral surface of fibula	First cuneiform and first metatarsal	Superficial peroneal	Everts and plantar flexes foot; supports arches
Peroneus tertius (musculus peroneus tertius [NA])	Medial surface of fibula	Fifth metatarsal	Deep peroneal	Everts and dorsiflexes foot
Petropharyngeus (variable)	Occasional slip from petrous part of temporal bone to pharynx			
Petrosalpingostaphylinus	See *Levator veli palatini*			
Petrostaphylinus	See *Levator veli palatini*			
Pharyngopalatinus (musculus pharyngopalatinus)	See *Palatopharyngeus*			

Name	Origin	Insertion	Innervation	Function
Piriformis (musculus piriformis [NA])	Second to fifth sacral vertebrae, ilium, and sacrotuberous ligament	Greater trochanter of femur	Anterior rami of first and second sacral	Rotates femur laterally
Plantaris (variable) (musculus plantaris [NA])	Lateral condyle of femur	Calcaneus	Tibial	Flexes knee joint; plantar flexes foot
Platysma (platysma [NA])	Fascia of neck	Mandible and skin about mouth	Facial	Muscle of facial expression
Platysma myoides	See *Platysma*			
Pleuroesophageal (smooth) (musculus pleuroesophageus [NA])	Fibers from left mediastinal pleura to esophagus		Autonomic	
Popliteus (musculus popliteus [NA])	Lateral condyle of femur	Back of tibia	Tibial	Rotates tibia medially; flexes knee joint
Popliteus minor	Part of popliteus inserted into back of capsule of knee joint			
Posterior cricoarytenoid	See *Cricoarytenoid, posterior*			
Procerus (musculus procerus [NA])	Skin over nose	Skin of forehead	Facial	Muscle of facial expression
Pronator pedis	See *Quadratus plantae*			
Pronator quadratus (musculus pronator quadratus [NA])	Anterior surface of ulna	Anterior surface of radius	Palmar interosseous	Pronates forearm
Pronator radii teres	See *Pronator teres*			
Pronator teres (musculus pronator teres [NA])	(1) Medial epicondyle of humerus (2) Coronoid of ulna	Lateral aspect of radius	Median	Pronates forearm
Psoas magnus	See *Psoas major*			
Psoas major (part of iliopsoas) (musculus psoas major [NA])	Lumbar vertebrae and fascia	Lesser trochanter of femur	Anterior rami of second and third lumbar	Flexes hip joint and trunk on lower extremity
Psoas minor (variable) (musculus psoas minor [NA])	Last thoracic and first lumbar vertebrae	Iliopectineal eminence	Anterior ramus of first lumbar	Flexes trunk on pelvis

TABLE OF MUSCLES (Continued)

Name	Origin	Insertion	Innervation	Function
Psoas parvus	See *Psoas minor*			
Pterygoid, external	See *Pterygoid, lateral*			
Pterygoid, internal	See *Pterygoid, medial*			
Pterygoid, lateral (musculus pterygoideus lateralis [NA])	(1) Sphenoid (2) Lateral pterygoid plate	Neck of mandible and capsule of temporomandibular joint	Mandibular	Muscle of mastication; protrudes mandible
Pterygoid, medial (musculus pterygoideus medialis [NA])	(1) Lateral pterygoid plate (2) Tubercle of maxilla	Medial surface of angle of mandible	Mandibular	Muscle of mastication; clenches teeth
Pterygopharyngeus (pars pterygopharyngea musculi constrictoris pharyngis superioris [NA])	Portion of superior constrictor of pharynx			
Pterygospinous (variable)	Occasional slip from spine of sphenoid to medial pterygoid plate			
Pubocavernosus (variable)	Occasional slip of ischiocavernosus arising from pubis			
Pubococcygeus (musculus pubococcygeus [NA])	Portion of levator ani			
Puboprostatic (smooth) (musculus puboprostaticus [NA])	Fibers in pelvic fascia between pubis and prostate		Autonomic	
Puborectalis (musculus puborectalis [NA])	Part of levator ani			
Pubovaginalis (musculus pubovaginalis [NA alternative])	Part of levator ani; in female corresponds to levator prostatae in male			
Pubovesicalis (smooth) (musculus pubovesicalis [NA])	Fibers in pelvic fascia between pubis and urinary bladder		Autonomic	
Pyramidal, abdominal (variable) (musculus pyramidalis [NA])	Pubis	Linea alba	Anterior ramus of twelfth thoracic	Supports abdominal viscera

Name	Origin	Insertion	Innervation	Function
Pyramidal of ear (vestigial) (musculus pyramidalis auriculae [NA])	Part of tragicus			
Pyramidalis nasi	See *Procerus*			
Quadratus femoris (musculus quadratus femoris [NA])	Ischial tuber	Quadrate tubercle of femur	Nerve to quadratus femoris	Adducts and laterally rotates femur
Quadratus labii inferiores	See *Depressor labii inferioris*			
Quadratus labii superioris	See *Levator labii superioris*			
Quadratus lumborum (musculus quadratus lumborum [NA])	Iliac crest, lumbodorsal fascia, and lumbar vertebrae	Last rib	Anterior rami of first 3 lumbar	Assists in lateral movements of vertebral column
Quadratus menti	See *Depressor labii inferioris*			
Quadratus plantae (musculus quadratus plantae [NA])	Calcaneus and plantar fascia	Tendons of flexor digitorum longus	Lateral plantar	Assists in flexion of toes
Quadriceps extensor	See *Quadriceps femoris*			
Quadriceps femoris (musculus quadriceps femoris [NA])	Combined rectus femoris and vastus muscles			
Radialis externus brevis	See *Extensor carpi radialis brevis*			
Radialis externus longus	See *Extensor carpi radialis longus*			
Radialis internus	See *Flexor carpi radialis*			
Radiocarpeus (variable)	See *Flexor carpi radialis brevis*			
Rectococcygeus (smooth) (musculus rectococcygeus [NA])	Fibers in pelvic fascia between coccyx and rectum		Autonomic	
Rectourethralis (smooth) (musculus rectourethralis [NA])	Fibers in pelvic fascia between rectum and membranous urethra of male		Autonomic	

Name	Origin	Insertion	Innervation	Function
Rectouterine (smooth) (musculus rectouterinus [NA])	Fibers in pelvic fascia between rectum and cervix of uterus		Autonomic	
Rectovesical (smooth) (musculus rectovesicalis [NA])	Fibers in pelvic fascia between rectum and urinary bladder		Autonomic	
Rectus abdominis (musculus rectus abdominis [NA])	Pubis	Xiphoid, fifth to seventh costal cartilages	Anterior rami of lower 6 thoracic	Supports abdominal viscera; flexes vertebral column
Rectus capitis anterior (musculus rectus capitis anterior [NA])	Lateral portion of atlas	Occipital bone	Anterior rami of first and second cervical	Flexes head
Rectus capitis anticus major	See *Longus capitis*			
Rectus capitis anticus minor	See *Rectus capitis anterior*			
Rectus capitis lateralis (musculus rectus capitis lateralis [NA])	Transverse process of atlas	Occipital bone	Anterior ramus of first cervical	Assists in lateral movements of head
Rectus capitis posterior major (musculus rectus capitis posterior major [NA])	Spine of axis	Occipital bone	Posterior ramus of first cervical	Extends head
Rectus capitis posterior minor (musculus rectus capitis posterior minor [NA])	Posterior tubercle of atlas	Occipital bone	Posterior ramus of first cervical	Extends head
Rectus capitis posticus major	See *Rectus capitis posterior major*			
Rectus capitis posticus minor	See *Rectus capitis posterior minor*			
Rectus externus oculi	See *Rectus lateralis bulbi*			
Rectus femoris (musculus rectus femoris [NA])		Patella and ultimately into tubercle of tibia	Femoral	
(1) Reflected head	Dorsum ilii			Flexes hip joint
(2) Straight head	Anterior inferior spine of ilium			Extends knee joint

Name	Origin	Insertion	Innervation	Function
Rectus inferior bulbi (musculus rectus inferior bulbi [NA])	Lower border of optic canal	Sclera	Oculomotor	Rotates eyeball downward and somewhat inward
Rectus inferior oculi	See *Rectus inferior bulbi*			
Rectus internus oculi	See *Rectus medialis bulbi*			
Rectus lateralis bulbi (musculus rectus lateralis bulbi [NA])	Lateral border of optic canal	Sclera	Abducent	Rotates eyeball laterally
Rectus lateralis oculi	See *Rectus lateralis bulbi*			
Rectus medialis bulbi (musculus rectus medialis bulbi [NA])	Medial border of optic canal	Sclera	Oculomotor	Rotates eyeball medially
Rectus medialis oculi	See *Rectus medialis bulbi*			
Rectus superior bulbi (musculus rectus superior bulbi [NA])	Upper border of optic canal	Sclera	Oculomotor	Rotates eyeball upward and somewhat inward
Rectus superior oculi	See *Rectus superior bulbi*			
Rectus thoracis (variable)	Occasional separate slip associated with sternalis			
Retrahens aurem (vestigial)	See *Auricular, posterior*			
Rhomboideus major (musculus rhomboideus major [NA])	Spines of second to fifth thoracic vertebrae	Medial margin of scapula	Dorsal scapular	Draws scapula backward and aids in rotating inferior angle medially
Rhomboideus minor (musculus rhomboideus minor [NA])	Spines of seventh cervical and first thoracic vertebrae	Medial margin of scapula	Dorsal scapular	Same as rhomboideus major
Rhomboatloideus (variable)	Occasional extra slip of rhomboideus major to atlas			
Rhombooccipitalis	Occipitoscapular			
Risorius (musculus risorius [NA])	Fascia over masseter	Skin at angle of mouth	Facial	Muscle of facial expression

Name	Origin	Insertion	Innervation	Function
Rotatores (part of transversospinalis) (musculi rotatores [NA])			Posterior rami of spinal	Extend and rotate vertebral column
(1) Cervicis (musculi rotatores cervicis [NA])	Transverse processes of cervical vertebrae	Laminae of vertebrae above		
(2) Lumborum (musculi rotatores lumborum [NA])	Transverse processes of lumbar vertebrae	Laminae of vertebrae above		
(3) Thoracis (musculi rotatores thoracis [NA])	Transverse processes of thoracic vertebrae	Laminae of vertebrae above		
Rotatores breves (musculi rotatores breves)	Transverse process of vertebrae below	Laminae of vertebrae above	Posterior rami of spinal	Extend and rotate vertebral column
Rotatores longi (musculi rotatores longi)	Transverse processes of vertebrae	Laminae of vertebrae second above	Posterior rami of spinal	Extend and rotate vertebral column
Sacrococcygeus anterior (musculus sacrococcygeus anterior)	See *Sacrococcygeus ventralis*			
Sacrococcygeus dorsalis (vestigial) (musculus sacrococcygeus dorsalis [NA])	Dorsal aspect of sacrum	Coccyx	Posterior rami of sacral	
Sacrococcygeus posterior	See *Sacrococcygeus dorsalis*			
Sacrococcygeus ventralis (vestigial) (musculus sacrococcygeus ventralis [NA])	Ventral aspect of sacrum	Coccyx	Anterior rami of sacral	
Sacrolumbalis	See *Iliocostalis lumborum*			
Sacrospinalis (musculus sacrospinalis)	See *Erector spinae*			
Salpingopharyngeus (musculus salpingopharyngeus [NA])	Portion of palatopharyngeus arising from auditory tube			
Sartorius (musculus sartorius [NA])	Anterior superior iliac spine	Tibia	Femoral	Flexes hip and knee joints; rotates femur laterally

Name	Origin	Insertion	Innervation	Function
Scalene, anterior (musculus scalenus anterior [NA])	Transverse processes of third to sixth cervical vertebra	Tubercle of first rib	Anterior rami of third and fourth cervical	Flexes vertebral column laterally; accessory muscle of respiration (inhalation)
Scalene, least (variable) (musculus scalenus minimus [NA])	Occasional extra slip of posterior scalene			
Scalene, middle (musculus scalenus medius [NA])	Transverse processes of second to sixth cervical vertebrae	First rib	Anterior rami of third and fourth cervical	Flexes vertebral column laterally; accessory muscle of respiration (inhalation)
Scalene, posterior (musculus scalenus posterior [NA])	Tubercles of fourth to sixth cervical vertebrae	Second rib	Anterior rami of third and fourth cervical	Flexes vertebral column laterally; accessory muscle of respiration (inhalation)
Scalenus anticus	See *Scalene, anterior*			
Scalenus minimus	See *Scalene, least*			
Scalenus posticus	See *Scalene, posterior*			
Scansorius (variable)	Occasional extra slip of gluteus minimus			
Semimembranosus (musculus semimembranosus [NA])	Ischial tuber	Medial condyle of tibia	Tibial	Flexes knee joint and extends hip joint
Semispinalis (part of transversospinalis) (musculus semispinalis [NA])			Posterior rami of spinal	
(1) Capitis (musculus semispinalis capitis [NA])	Transverse processes of upper 6 thoracic and articular processes of lower 4 cervical vertebrae	Occipital bone		Extends head
(2) Cervicis (musculus semispinalis cervicis [NA])	Transverse processes of upper 6 thoracic and lower 4 cervical vertebrae	Spines of second to fifth cervical vertebrae		Extends and rotates vertebral column
(3) Thoracis (musculus semispinalis thoracis [NA])	Transverse processes of lower 6 thoracic vertebrae	Spines of last 2 cervical and first 4 thoracic vertebrae		
Semispinalis colli	See *Semispinalis cervicis*			

Name	Origin	Insertion	Innervation	Function
Semispinalis dorsi	See *Semispinalis thoracis*			
Semitendinosus (musculus semitendinosus [NA])	Ischial tuber	Medial aspect of proximal portion of tibia	Tibial	Flexes knee joint and extends hip joint
Serratus anterior (musculus serratus anterior [NA])	Upper 8 or 9 ribs	Medial border of scapula	Long thoracic	Draws scapula forward; draws inferior angle laterally
Serratus anticus	See *Serratus anterior*			
Serratus magnus	See *Serratus anterior*			
Serratus posterior inferior (musculus serratus posterior inferior [NA])	Lumbodorsal fascia, spines of lowest thoracic and upper lumbar vertebrae	Last 4 ribs	Lower thoracic	Accessory muscle of respiration
Serratus posterior superior (musculus serratus posterior superior [NA])	Ligamentum nuchae, spines of seventh cervical and upper thoracic vertebrae	Second to fifth ribs	Second and third thoracic	Accessory muscle of respiration
Serratus posticus inferior	See *Serratus posterior inferior*			
Serratus posticus superior	See *Serratus posterior superior*			
Soleus (musculus soleus [NA])	Fibula, popliteal fascia, and tibia	Calcaneus	Tibial	Plantar flexes foot
Sphenosalpingostaphylinus	See *Tensor veli palatini*			
Sphincter ani externus (divided into subcutaneous, superficial, and deep portions) (musculus sphincter ani externus [NA])	Tip of coccyx	Surrounds anus	Pudendal	Closes anus
Sphincter ani internus (smooth) (musculus sphincter ani internus [NA])			Autonomic	
Sphincter of Boyden	See *Sphincter of common bile duct*			
Sphincter of common bile duct (smooth) (musculus sphincter ductus choledochi [NA])	Sphincter in distal part of common duct		Autonomic	

Name	Origin	Insertion	Innervation	Function
Sphincter of hepato-pancreatic ampulla (smooth) (musculus sphincter ampullae hepatopancreaticae [NA])	Sphincter of major duodenal papilla		Autonomic	
Sphincter of Oddi	See *Sphincter of hepatopancreatic ampulla*			
Sphincter pupillae (smooth) (musculus sphincter pupillae [NA])	Circular fibers of iris		Parasympathetic (oculomotor)	
Sphincter of pylorus (smooth) (musculus sphincter pylori [NA])	Sphincter of pylorus of stomach		Autonomic	
Sphincter of urinary bladder (smooth) (musculus sphincter vesicae [NA])	Outlet of urinary bladder		Autonomic	
Sphincter oris	See *Orbicularis oris*			
Sphincter urethrae (musculus sphincter urethrae [NA])	Ramus of pubis	Median raphe	Perineal	Compresses urethra
Sphincter vaginae	See *Bulbospongiosus, female*			
Spinalis (medial part of erector spinae) (musculus spinalis [NA])			Posterior rami of spinal	
(1) Capitis (variable) (musculus spinalis capitis [NA])	Spines of upper thoracic and lowest cervical vertebrae	Occipital bone		Extends head
(2) Cervicis (variable) (musculus spinalis cervicis [NA])	Spines of lower cervical and upper thoracic vertebrae	Spines of second to fourth cervical vertebrae		Extends and assists in rotation and lateral movements of trunk
(3) Thoracis (musculus spinalis thoracis [NA])	Spines of lower 2 thoracic and upper 2 lumbar vertebrae	Spines of fourth to eighth thoracic vertebrae		
Spinalis colli	See *Spinalis cervicis*			
Spinalis dorsi	See *Spinalis thoracis*			

Name	Origin	Insertion	Innervation	Function
Splenius capitis (musculus splenius capitis [NA])	Ligamentum nuchae, spines of last cervical and upper thoracic vertebrae	Mastoid process	Posterior rami of spinal	Extends head
Splenius cervicis (musculus splenius cervicis [NA])	Ligamentum nuchae, spines of last cervical and upper thoracic vertebrae	Transverse processes of upper cervical vertebrae	Posterior rami of spinal	Extends vertebral column
Splenius colli	See *Splenius cervicis*			
Stapedius (musculus stapedius [NA])	Pyramidal process	Neck of stapes	Facial	Draws base of stapes toward tympanic cavity
Staphylinus externus	See *Tensor veli palatini*			
Staphylinus internus	See *Levator veli palatini*			
Staphylinus medius	See *Uvulae*			
Sternalis (variable) (musculus sternalis [NA])	Fascia of chest wall		Anterior thoracic	
Sternochondroscapular (variable)	Occasional slip of muscle in axillary fascia			
Sternoclavicularis (variable)	Small extra slip of subclavius occasionally arising from sternum			
Sternocleidomastoid (musculus sternocleidomastoideus [NA])	Manubrium of sternum and clavicle	Mastoid process	Accessory	Flexes head
Sternocostalis	See *Transverse thoracic*			
Sternofascialis (variable)	Occasional slip from manubrium of sternum to fascia of neck			
Sternohyoid (musculus sternohyoideus [NA])	Manubrium of sternum	Hyoid	Ansa cervicalis	Depresses hyoid
Sternothyroid (musculus sternothyroideus [NA])	Manubrium of sternum	Thyroid cartilage	Ansa cervicalis	Depresses larynx

Name	Origin	Insertion	Innervation	Function
Styloauricularis (variable)	Occasional slip from styloid process to cartilage of external ear			
Styloglossus (musculus styloglossus [NA])	Styloid process	Side of tongue	Hypoglossal	Elevates tongue
Stylohyoid (musculus stylohyoideus [NA])	Styloid process	Hyoid	Facial	Elevates hyoid
Stylopharyngeus (musculus stylopharyngeus [NA])	Styloid process	Lateral wall of pharynx	Glossopharyngeal	Pulls up pharynx
Subanconeus	See *Articularis cubiti*			
Subclavius (musculus subclavius [NA])	First costal cartilage and first rib	Clavicle	Nerve to subclavius	Depresses lateral end of clavicle
Subcostals (variable) (musculi subcostales [NA])	Lower ribs	Chest wall	Thoracic	Muscles of respiration
Subcrureus	See *Articularis genus*			
Subcutaneous colli	See *Platysma*			
Subscapular (musculus subscapularis [NA])	Subscapular fossa	Lesser tubercle of humerus	Subscapular	Rotates humerus medially
Superficial transverse of perineum (musculus transversus perinei superficialis [NA])	Tuber of ischium	Central point of perineum	Perineal	Supports perineum
Superior lingual	See *Longitudinalis of tongue*			
Superior oblique	See *Oblique, superior*			
Supinator (musculus supinator [NA])	Lateral epicondyle of humerus, fascia about elbow joint, and shaft of ulna	Radius	Dorsal interosseous of forearm	Supinates forearm
Supinator longus	See *Brachioradialis*			
Supinator radii brevis	See *Supinator*			

Name	Origin	Insertion	Innervation	Function
Supraclavicularis (variable)	Occasional slip from manubrium to clavicle			
Supraspinalis (variable)	Occasional slips between tips of spines of cervical vertebrae			
Supraspinatus (musculus supraspinatus [NA])	Supraspinous fossa	Greater tubercle of humerus	Suprascapular	Abducts humerus
Suspensory of duodenum (smooth) (musculus suspensorius duodeni [NA])	Scattered fibers in suspensory ligament of duodenum		Autonomic	
Tarsal (smooth) (musculus tarsalis inferior et superior [NA])	Smooth muscle in eyelids		Sympathetic	
Temporal	See *Temporalis*			
Temporalis (musculus temporalis [NA])	Temporal fossa	Coronoid process of mandible	Mandibular	Closes mouth; clenches teeth; retracts lower jaw
Temporoparietalis (musculus temporoparietalis [NA])	Part of epicranius			
Tensor fasciae latae (musculus tensor fasciae latae [NA])	Iliac crest	Iliotibial tract and ultimately into tibia	Superior gluteal	Abducts lower extremity; flexes hip joint; extends knee joint
Tensor fasciae suralis (variable)	Occasional slip of biceps femoris into fascia of calf			
Tensor palati	See *Tensor veli palatini*			
Tensor tarsi	Part of orbicularis oculi			
Tensor tympani (musculus tensor tympani [NA])	Cartilaginous portion of auditory tube	Manubrium of malleus	Mandibular	Tenses tympanic membrane
Tensor vaginae femoris	See *Tensor fasciae latae*			
Tensor veli palatini (musculus tensor veli palatini [NA])	Scaphoid fossa of sphenoid and wall of auditory tube	Aponeurosis of soft palate	Mandibular	Tenses soft palate and opens auditory tube

Name	Origin	Insertion	Innervation	Function
Teres major (musculus teres major [NA])	Lateral margin of scapula	Intertubercular sulcus of humerus	Subscapular	Adducts and medially rotates humerus
Teres minor (musculus teres minor [NA])	Lateral margin of scapula	Greater tubercle of humerus	Axillary	Laterally rotates humerus
Thyroarytenoid (musculus thyroarytenoideus [NA])	Lamina of thyroid cartilage	Muscular process of arytenoid cartilage	Recurrent laryngeal	Relaxes vocal folds; closes vestibule of larynx
Thyroarytenoid, external	See *Thyroarytenoid*			
Thyroarytenoid, internal	See *Vocalis*			
Thyroarytenoid, superior (variable)	See *Ventricular*			
Thyroepiglottic (musculus thyroepiglotticus [NA])	Lamina of thyroid cartilage	Epiglottis	Recurrent laryngeal	Closes inlet of larynx
Thyrohyoid (musculus thyrohyoideus [NA])	Thyroid cartilage	Hyoid	Ansa cervicalis	Draws hyoid and thyroid cartilages toward each other
Thyropharyngeus (pars thyropharyngea musculi constrictoris pharyngis inferioris [NA])	Portion of inferior constrictor of pharynx			
Tibialis anterior (musculus tibialis anterior [NA])	Tibia and interosseous membrane	First cuneiform and first metatarsal	Deep peroneal	Dorsiflexes and inverts foot
Tibialis anticus	See *Tibialis anterior*			
Tibialis gracilis	See *Plantaris*			
Tibialis posterior (musculus tibialis posterior [NA])	Fibula, tibia, and interosseous membrane	Bases of metatarsals and all tarsal bones except talus	Tibial	Plantar flexes and inverts foot; supports arches of foot
Tibialis posticus	See *Tibialis posterior*			
Tibialis secundus (variable)	Back of tibia	Capsule of ankle joint		
Tibioaccessorius	See *Quadratus plantae*			

Name	Origin	Insertion	Innervation	Function
Tibiofascialis (variable)	Occasional extra slip of tibialis anterior inserted into fascia of dorsum of foot			
Trachealis (smooth) (musculus trachealis [NA])	Transverse fibers in dorsal wall of trachea	Tracheal cartilages	Autonomic	Lessens caliber of trachea
Trachelomastoid	See *Longissimus capitis*			
Tragicus (vestigial) (musculus tragicus [NA])	Crosses tragus		Facial	
Transversalis abdominis	See *Transverse abdominal*			
Transversalis colli	See *Longissimus cervicis*			
Transverse abdominal (musculus transversus abdominis [NA])	Costal cartilages of lower 6 ribs, lumbodorsal fascia, iliac crest, and inguinal ligament	Xiphoid, linea alba, inguinal ligament, and pubis	Anterior rami of lower 6 thoracic and iliohypogastric	Supports abdominal viscera and flexes vertebral column
Transverse arytenoid	See *Arytenoid*			
Transverse auricular (vestigial)	See *Auricular*			
Transverse of neck	See *Longissimus cervicis*			
Transverse lingual (musculus transversus linguae [NA])	Median septum of tongue	Dorsum and sides of tongue	Hypoglossal	Alters shape of tongue
Transverse mental (musculus transversus menti [NA])	Part of depressor anguli oris			
Transverse nuchal (variable) (musculus transversus nuchae [NA])	Occasional extra slip of occipitofrontalis			
Transverse of foot	See *Adductor hallucis*			
Transverse pedis	See *Adductor hallucis, transverse head*			
Transverse, deep of perineum	See *Deep transverse perineal*			

Name	Origin	Insertion	Innervation	Function
Transverse, superficial perineal	See *Superficial transverse of perineum*			
Transverse spinal	Multifidus, rotatores, and semispinales as a group			
Transverse thoracic (musculus transversus thoracis [NA])	Mediastinal surface of xiphoid and body of sternum	Second to sixth costal cartilages	Anterior rami of thoracic	
Transverse urethral	Part of sphincter urethrae			
Transverse vaginal	Part of sphincter of urethra of female			
Transversospinalis (musculus transversospinalis [NA])	Composed of multifidus, rotatores, and semispinales			
Transversus colli	See *Longissimus cervicis*			
Trapezius (musculus trapezius [NA])	Occipital bone, ligamentum nuchae, spines of seventh cervical and all thoracic vertebrae	Clavicle, acromion, and spine of scapula	Accessory	Rotates inferior angle of scapula laterally; raises shoulder; draws scapula backward
Triangularis	See *Depressor anguli oris*			
Triangularis labii inferioris	See *Depressor anguli oris*			
Triangularis labii superioris	See *Levator anguli oris*			
Triangularis sterni	See *Transverse thoracic*			
Triceps brachii (musculus triceps brachii [NA])		Olecranon of ulna	Radial	Extends elbow joint; long head also aids in adducting humerus
(1) Long head (caput longum musculi tricipitis brachii [NA])	Infraglenoid tubercle			
(2) Lateral head (caput laterale musculi tricipitis brachii [NA])	Shaft of humerus			

Name	Origin	Insertion	Innervation	Function
Triceps brachii (musculus triceps brachii [NA]) (Continued)				
(3) Medial head (caput mediale musculi tricipitis brachii [NA])	Shaft of humerus			
Triceps surae (musculus triceps surae [NA])	Combined gastrocnemius and soleus			
Triticeoglossus (variable)	Occasional slip from base of tongue to triticeous cartilage			
Trochlear	See *Oblique, superior of eye*			
Ulnaris externus	See *Extensor carpi ulnaris*			
Ulnaris internus	See *Flexor carpi ulnaris*			
Uvulae (musculus uvulae [NA])	Posterior nasal spine	Aponeurosis of soft palate	Accessory	
Vastus crureus	See *Vastus intermedius*			
Vastus externus	See *Vastus lateralis*			
Vastus intermedius (musculus vastus intermedius [NA])	Anterior and lateral aspect of femur	Patella and ultimately into tubercle of tibia	Femoral	Extends knee joint
Vastus internus	See *Vastus medialis*			
Vastus lateralis (musculus vastus lateralis [NA])	Capsule of hip joint and lateral aspect of femur	Patella and ultimately into tubercle of tibia	Femoral	Extends knee joint
Vastus medialis (musculus vastus medialis [NA])	Medial aspect of femur	Patella and ultimately into tubercle of tibia	Femoral	Extends knee joint
Ventricular (musculus ventricularis)	Lateral fibers of thyroarytenoid		Vagus	
Vertical lingual (musculus verticalis linguae [NA])	Dorsal aspect of tongue	Sides and base of tongue	Hypoglossal	Alters shape of tongue

Name	Origin	Insertion	Innervation	Function
Vocalis (musculus vocalis [NA])	Medial fibers of thyroarytenoid, internal		Vagus	
Zygomatic	See *Zygomatic, major*			
Zygomatic, major (musculus zygomaticus major [NA])	Zygoma	Skin about mouth	Facial	Muscle of facial expression
Zygomatic, minor (musculus zygomaticus minor [NA])	Zygoma	Skin about mouth	Facial	Muscle of facial expression

Name	Central attachment	Components*	Branches	Distribution
Abducens (sixth cranial) (nervus abducens [NA])	Brainstem at inferior border of pons	Motor	Muscular filaments	Lateral rectus muscle of eyeball
Accessory (eleventh cranial) (nervus accessorius [NA])				
(1) Bulbar part (cranial) (radices craniales [NA])	Lateral aspect of medulla oblongata	Motor	Internal ramus to vagus	Striate muscles of larynx and pharynx
(2) Spinal part (radices spinales [NA])	Upper 5 or 6 cervical segments of cord	Motor	External ramus to cervical plexus	Trapezius and sternocleidomastoid muscles
Accessory obturator	See *Obturator, accessory*			
Accessory phrenic (nervi phrenici accessorii [NA])	Occasional branch from fifth cervical which arises with the subclavian		Joins phrenic	Diaphragm
Acoustic	See *Vestibulocochlear*			
Alveolar, anterior superior (rami alveolares superiores anteriores nervi infraorbitalis [NA])	Infraorbital	Somatic sensory	Filaments	Upper incisor and cuspid teeth, mucosa of nasal floor
Alveolar, inferior (nervus alveolaris inferior [NA])	Mandibular	Somatic sensory	Mental and filaments	Lower teeth, skin of lower lip and chin
		Motor	Mylohyoid	Mylohyoid and anterior belly of digastric muscles
Alveolar, middle superior (ramus alveolaris superior medius nervi infraorbitalis [NA])	Maxillary	Somatic sensory	Filaments	Upper premolar teeth
Alveolar, posterior superior (rami alveolares superiores posteriores nervi infraorbitalis [NA])	Maxillary	Somatic sensory	Filaments	Upper molar teeth and mucosa of maxillary sinus
Alveolar, superior (nervi alveolares superiores [NA])	See *Alveolar, anterior superior, middle superior,* and *posterior superior*			

*Nerves to muscles contain proprioceptive sensory fibers in addition to motor fibers; muscular branches of third, fourth, sixth, and twelfth cranial nerves may be exceptions.

Name	Central attachment	Components*	Branches	Distribution
Ampullary, anterior (nervus ampullaris anterior [NA])	Vestibular	Sensory (movement of head in space—dynamic)	Filaments	Ampulla of anterior semicircular duct
Ampullary, inferior	See *Ampullary, posterior*			
Ampullary, lateral (nervus ampullaris lateralis [NA])	Vestibular	Sensory (movement of head in space—dynamic)	Filaments	Ampulla of lateral semicircular duct
Ampullary, posterior (nervus ampullaris posterior [NA])	Vestibular	Sensory (movement of head in space—dynamic)	Filaments	Ampulla of posterior semicircular duct
Anastomotic, peroneal	See *Peroneal, anastomotic*			
Anococcygeal (nervi anococcygei [NA])	Fourth and fifth sacral and coccygeal segments of cord	Somatic sensory	Filaments	Skin in vicinity of coccyx
Ansa cervicalis (ansa cervicalis [NA])	By a superior and an inferior ramus from first, second, and third cervical segments of spinal cord	Motor	Filaments	Omohyoid, sternohyoid, and sternothyroid muscles
Auditory	See *Vestibulocochlear*			
Auricular (ramus auricularis nervi vagi [NA])	Vagus	Somatic sensory	Filaments	Skin of auricle and external acoustic meatus
Auricular, anterior (nervi auriculares anteriores [NA])	Mandibular	Somatic sensory	Filaments	Skin anterior to external ear
Auricular, great (nervus auricularis magnus [NA])	Second and third cervical segments (cervical plexus)	Somatic sensory	Auricular, facial, and mastoid branches	Skin about ear
Auricular, posterior (nervus auricularis posterior [NA])	Facial	Motor	Filaments	Occipital and intrinsic muscles of auricle, stylohyoid and posterior belly of digastric muscles
Auriculotemporal (nervus auriculotemporalis [NA])	Mandibular	Somatic sensory	Filaments	Skin of scalp and temple, temporomandibular joint
Axillary (nervus axillaris [NA])	Fifth and sixth cervical segments of cord (brachial plexus)	Motor	Muscular, articular, and cutaneous branches	Deltoid and teres minor muscles
		Somatic sensory	Lateral cutaneous of arm	Skin of lateral aspect of shoulder and arm

Name	Central attachment	Components*	Branches	Distribution
Bigeminus	Old name for third sacral nerve			
Buccal (nervus buccalis [NA])	Mandibular	Somatic sensory	Filaments	Skin and mucosa of cheek
Buccinator	See *Buccal*			
Calcaneal (rami calcanei laterales nervi suralis [NA])	Sural	Somatic sensory	Filaments	Skin of heel
Cardiac, inferior cervical (nervus cardiacus cervicalis inferior [NA])	Inferior cervical ganglion	Sympathetic. Visceral sensory	To cardiac plexuses	Heart
Cardiac, inferior or thoracic (nervus cardiacus inferior)	Vagus	Parasympathetic. Visceral sensory	To cardiac plexuses	Heart
Cardiac, middle (nervus cardiacus medius)	Vagus	Parasympathetic. Visceral sensory	To cardiac plexuses	Heart
Cardiac, middle cervical (nervus cardiacus cervicalis medius [NA])	Middle cervical ganglion	Sympathetic. Visceral sensory	To cardiac plexuses	Heart
Cardiac, superior (nervus cardiacus superior)	Vagus	Parasympathetic. Visceral sensory	To cardiac plexuses	Heart
Cardiac, superior cervical (nervus cardiacus cervicalis superior [NA])	Superior cervical ganglion	Sympathetic. Visceral sensory	To cardiac plexuses	Heart
Cardiac, thoracic (nervi cardiaci thoracici [NA])	Second to fifth thoracic ganglia	Sympathetic. Visceral sensory	To cardiac plexuses	Heart
Caroticotympanic (nervi caroticotympanici [NA]) (1) Inferior (2) Superior	Branches between tympanic plexus and internal carotid plexus			
Carotid, external (nervi carotici externi [NA])	Superior cervical ganglion	Sympathetic	Plexuses on external carotid artery and its branches	Filaments to smooth muscle and glands of head
Carotid, internal (nervus caroticus internus [NA])	Superior cervical ganglion	Sympathetic	Plexus on internal carotid artery and its branches	Filaments to smooth muscle and glands of head

Name	Central attachment	Components*	Branches	Distribution
Cavernous of penis or clitoris (nervi cavernosi penis, nervi cavernosi clitoridis [NA])	Pelvic plexus	Autonomic	Filaments	Corpora cavernosa of penis or clitoris
Cervical, first (dorsal ramus)	First cervical segment of cord	Motor	Muscular	Deep muscles of back of neck
Cervical, first (ventral ramus)	First cervical segment of cord	Motor	To cervical plexus	Neck muscles
Cervical, second (dorsal ramus)	Second cervical segment of cord	Motor. Somatic sensory	Greater occipital	Deep muscles of back of neck and skin of back of neck
Cervical, second (ventral ramus)	Second cervical segment of cord	Motor. Somatic sensory	To cervical plexus	Neck muscles and skin
Cervical, third (dorsal ramus)	Third cervical segment of cord	Motor. Somatic sensory	Third occipital	Neck muscles and skin
Cervical, third (ventral ramus)	Third cervical segment of cord	Motor. Somatic sensory	To cervical plexus	Neck muscles and skin
Cervical, fourth to eighth (dorsal rami)	Fourth to eighth cervical segments of cord	Motor. Somatic sensory	Muscular and cutaneous	Deep muscles of neck and upper portion of back, skin of upper back
Cervical, fourth (ventral ramus)	Fourth cervical segment of cord	Motor. Somatic sensory	To cervical plexus	Neck muscles, diaphragm
Cervical, fifth to eighth (ventral rami)	Fifth to eighth cervical segments of cord	Motor. Somatic sensory	To brachial plexus	Muscles and skin of upper extremity
Cervical, descending	See *Ansa cervicalis, inferior ramus*			
Cervical, superficial	See *Transverse of neck*			
Chorda tympani [NA]	Intermedius	Parasympathetic	Filaments via lingual	Submandibular and sublingual salivary glands
		Sensory (taste)	Filaments via lingual	Taste buds of anterior two-thirds of tongue
Ciliary, long (nervi ciliares longi [NA])	Nasociliary	Somatic sensory	Filaments	Eyeball
Ciliary, short (nervi ciliares breves [NA])	Ciliary ganglion	Parasympathetic	Filaments	Ciliary muscle and constrictor fibers of iris
	Nasociliary	Somatic sensory	Filaments	Eyeball
Circumflex	See *Axillary*			
Cluneal, inferior (nervi clunium inferiores [NA])	Posterior cutaneous nerve of thigh	Somatic sensory	Filaments	Skin of lower gluteal region

Name	Central attachment	Components*	Branches	Distribution
Cluneal, medial (nervi clunium medii [NA])	First, second, and third sacral (dorsal rami)	Somatic sensory	Filaments	Skin of medial gluteal region
Cluneal, superior (nervi clunium superiores [NA])	First, second, and third sacral (dorsal rami)	Somatic sensory	Filaments	Skin of upper gluteal region
Clunial	See *Cluneal*			
Coccygeal (nervus coccygeus [NA])	Coccygeal segment of cord	Somatic sensory	Filaments	Skin over coccyx
Cochlear (cochlear part of eighth cranial—vestibulocochlear) (pars cochlearis nervi octavi [NA])	Brainstem at lower border of pons	Somatic sensory	Filaments	Spiral organ (of Corti) of internal ear
Common peroneal	See *Peroneal, common*			
Crural, anterior	See *Femoral*			
Cutaneous, abdominal anterior	Iliohypogastric	Somatic sensory	Filaments	Skin over lower anterior abdomen
Cutaneous, antebrachial, lateral (nervus cutaneus antebrachii lateralis [NA])	Musculocutaneous	Somatic sensory	Filaments	Skin of lateral aspect of forearm
Cutaneous, antebrachial, medial (nervus cutaneus antebrachii medialis [NA])	Brachial plexus	Somatic sensory	Filaments	Skin of medial aspect of forearm
Cutaneous, antebrachial, posterior (nervus cutaneus antebrachii posterior [NA])	Radial	Somatic sensory	Filaments	Skin of posterior aspect of forearm
Cutaneous, antibrachial	See *Cutaneous, antebrachial*			
Cutaneous, brachial, lateral inferior (nervus cutaneus brachii lateralis inferior [NA])	Radial	Somatic sensory	Filaments	Skin of lower lateral aspect of arm
Cutaneous, brachial, lateral superior (nervus cutaneus brachii lateralis superior [NA])	Axillary	Somatic sensory	Filaments	Skin of lateral aspect of arm

Name	Central attachment	Components*	Branches	Distribution
Cutaneous, brachial, medial (nervus cutaneus brachii medialis [NA])	Brachial plexus	Somatic sensory	Filaments	Skin of medial aspect of arm
Cutaneous, brachial, posterior (nervus cutaneus brachii posterior [NA])	Radial	Somatic sensory	Filaments	Skin of posterior aspect of arm
Cutaneous colli	See *Transverse of neck*			
Cutaneous, femoral, medial (anterior internal of thigh)	Femoral	Somatic sensory	Filaments	Skin of medial aspect of thigh
Cutaneous, femoral, middle (anterior middle of thigh)	Femoral	Somatic sensory	Filaments	Skin of anterior middle aspect of thigh
Cutaneous, femoral, lateral (nervus cutaneus femoris lateralis [NA])	Lumbar plexus	Somatic sensory	Filaments	Skin of lateral aspect of thigh
Cutaneous, femoral, posterior (nervus cutaneus femoris posterior [NA])	Sacral plexus	Somatic sensory	Filaments	Skin of posterior aspect of thigh
Cutaneous of arm	See *Cutaneous, brachial*			
Cutaneous of calf	See *Cutaneous, sural*			
Cutaneous of foot				
(1) Cutaneous, dorsal intermediate (nervus cutaneus dorsalis intermedius [NA])	Superficial peroneal	Somatic sensory	Filaments	Skin of dorsum of foot
(2) Cutaneous, dorsal lateral (nervus cutaneus dorsalis lateralis [NA])	Sural	Somatic sensory	Filaments	Skin of dorsolateral part of foot
(3) Cutaneous, dorsal medial (nervus cutaneus dorsalis medialis [NA])	Superficial peroneal	Somatic sensory	Filaments	Skin of dorsomedial part of foot
Cutaneous of forearm	See *Cutaneous, antebrachial*			

Name	Central attachment	Components*	Branches	Distribution
Cutaneous of hand				
(1) Cutaneous, dorsal (ramus dorsalis nervi ulnaris [NA])	Ulnar	Somatic sensory	Filaments	Skin of medial dorsal part of hand
(2) Cutaneous, palmar, lateral (ramus palmaris nervi mediani [NA])	Median	Somatic sensory	Filaments	Skin of lateral part of palm
(3) Cutaneous, palmar, medial (ramus palmaris nervi ulnaris [NA])	Ulnar	Somatic sensory	Filaments	Skin of medial part of palm
Cutaneous of leg	See *Cutaneous, sural*			
Cutaneous of neck	See *Transverse of neck*			
Cutaneous of thigh	See *Cutaneous, femoral*			
Cutaneous, sural, lateral (nervus cutaneus surae lateralis [NA])	Common peroneal	Somatic sensory	Filaments	Skin of lateral part of calf
Cutaneous, sural, medial (nervus cutaneus surae medialis [NA])	Tibial	Somatic sensory	Filaments	Skin of medial part of calf
Cutaneous, perforating (variable)	Pudendal plexus	Somatic sensory	Filaments	Skin of posterior aspect of buttocks
Deep peroneal	See *Peroneal, deep*			
Deep temporal	See *Temporal, deep*			
Dental	See *Alveolar*			
Descendens cervicis	See *Ansa cervicalis, inferior ramus*			
Descendens hypoglossi	See *Ansa cervicalis, superior ramus*			
Digital of fingers				
(1) Dorsal radial (nervi digitales dorsales nervi radialis [NA])	Radial	Somatic sensory	Filaments	Skin of dorsum of lateral fingers
(2) Dorsal ulnar (nervi digitales dorsales nervi ulnaris [NA])	Ulnar	Somatic sensory	Filaments	Skin of dorsum of medial fingers and tips of fingers
(3) Palmar common median (nervi digitales palmares communes nervi mediani [NA])	Median	Somatic sensory	Proper palmar	

Name	Central attachment	Components*	Branches	Distribution
Digital of fingers (Continued)				
(4) Palmar common ulnar (nervi digitales palmares communes nervi ulnaris [NA])	Ulnar	Somatic sensory	Proper palmar	
(5) Palmar proper median (nervi digitales palmares proprii nervi mediani [NA])	Common palmar median	Somatic sensory	Filaments	Palmar surface of lateral fingers
(6) Palmar proper ulnar (nervi digitales palmares proprii nervi ulnaris [NA])	Common palmar ulnar	Somatic sensory	Filaments	Palmar surface of medial fingers
Digital of toes				
(1) Dorsal (nervus cutaneus dorsalis intermedius [NA])	Intermediate dorsal cutaneous of foot	Somatic sensory	Filaments	Dorsal aspect of toes
(2) Dorsal of lateral side of great toe and medial side of second toe (nervi digitales dorsales hallucis lateralis et digiti secundi medialis [NA])	Deep peroneal	Somatic sensory	Filaments	Adjacent sides of great and second toes
(3) Plantar common lateral (nervi digitales plantares communes nervi plantaris lateralis [NA])	Lateral plantar	Somatic sensory	Proper plantar	
(4) Plantar common medial (nervi digitales plantares communes nervi plantaris medialis [NA])	Medial plantar	Somatic sensory	Proper plantar	
(5) Plantar proper lateral (nervi digitales plantares proprii nervi plantaris lateralis [NA])	Common lateral plantar	Somatic sensory	Filaments	Plantar aspect of lateral toes
(6) Plantar proper medial (nervi digitales plantares proprii nervi plantaris medialis [NA])	Common medial plantar	Somatic sensory	Filaments	Plantar aspect of medial toes
Dorsal of penis or clitoris (nervus dorsalis penis, nervus dorsalis clitoridis [NA])	Pudendal	Somatic sensory	Filaments	Penis (clitoris)

Name	Central attachment	Components*	Branches	Distribution
Dorsal scapular (nervus dorsalis scapulae [NA])	Brachial plexus	Motor	Filaments	Major and minor rhomboids, levator scapulae
Erigent (nervi erigentes [NA alternative])	See *Splanchnic, pelvic*			
Ethmoid, anterior (nervus ethmoidalis anterior [NA])	Nasociliary	Somatic sensory	Filaments, external nasal	Mucosa of nasal cavity and anterior ethmoid air cells
Ethmoid, posterior (nervus ethmoidalis posterior [NA])	Nasociliary	Somatic sensory	Filaments	Mucosa of sphenoid and posterior ethmoid air cells
Facial (seventh cranial) (nervus facialis [NA])	Brainstem at level of inferior border of pons	Motor Parasympathetic. Sensory (taste) See *Intermedius*	Stapedial, auricular, temporal, zygomatic, buccal, mandibular, and cervical branches	Stapedius, stylohyoid, posterior belly of digastric, and muscles of facial expression
Femoral (nervus femoralis [NA])	Lumbar plexus	Motor. Somatic sensory	Muscular, articular, saphenous, and cutaneous of thigh	Pectineus, quadriceps femoris, sartorius, iliacus, and skin
Fibular (nervus fibularis communis [NA alternative])	See *Peroneal*			
Fibular, communicating	See *Peroneal, anastomotic*			
Frontal (nervus frontalis [NA])	Ophthalmic	Somatic sensory	Supraorbital, supratrochlear	Skin of upper eyelid, forehead, and scalp
Furcal (nervus furcalis)	Old term for fourth lumbar nerve, ventral ramus			
Genitocrural	See *Genitofemoral*			
Genitofemoral (nervus genitofemoralis [NA])	Lumbar plexus	Somatic sensory	Genital and femoral	Skin of thigh and scrotum (labium majus)
Glossopalatine	See *Intermedius*			

Name	Central attachment	Components*	Branches	Distribution
Glossopharyngeal (ninth cranial) (nervus glossopharyngeus [NA])	Lateral aspect of medulla oblongata	Motor	Muscular, pharyngeal, tonsillar, lingual, tympanic	Stylopharyngeus, and muscles of soft palate and pharynx via pharyngeal plexus
		Visceral sensory		Mucosa of posterior one-third of tongue, pharynx, middle ear and mastoid air cells
		Sensory (taste)		Taste buds of posterior one-third of tongue
		Parasympathetic		Parotid gland via otic ganglion
Gluteal (cutaneous)	See *Cluneal*			
Gluteal, inferior (nervus gluteus inferior [NA])	Sacral plexus	Motor		Gluteus maximus muscle
Gluteal, superior (nervus gluteus superior [NA])	Sacral plexus	Motor		Gluteus medius and minimus and tensor fasciae latae muscles
Hamstrings, nerve to (part of sciatic)	Sacral plexus	Motor		Biceps femoris, semitendinosus, semimembranosus, and part of adductor magnus muscles
Hemorrhoidal, inferior	See *Rectal, inferior*			
Hemorrhoidal, middle	Pudendal plexus	Sympathetic. Visceral sensory	Filaments	Rectum
Hemorrhoidal, superior	Hypogastric plexus	Sympathetic. Visceral sensory	Filaments	Rectum
Hypogastric (nervus hypogastricus [NA])	Superior hypogastric plexus (presacral)	Sympathetic. Visceral sensory	Inferior hypogastric or pelvic plexus	
Hypoglossal (twelfth cranial) (nervus hypoglossus [NA])	Medulla oblongata	Motor	Filaments	Intrinsic and extrinsic muscles of tongue
Iliohypogastric (nervus iliohypogastricus [NA])	Lumbar plexus	Motor. Somatic sensory	Filaments	Muscles and skin of anterior abdominal wall
Ilioinguinal (nervus ilioinguinalis [NA])	Lumbar plexus	Motor. Somatic sensory	Anterior scrotal (labial)	
Infraorbital (nervus infraorbitalis [NA])	Maxillary	Somatic sensory	Alveolar, palpebral, nasal, labial	Upper teeth, mucosa of nasal floor, skin of face

Name	Central attachment	Components*	Branches	Distribution
Infratrochlear (nervus infratrochlearis [NA])	Nasociliary	Somatic sensory	Filaments	Skin of eyelids and root of nose
Intercostobrachial (nervi intercostobrachiales [NA])	Second thoracic segment ventral ramus	Somatic sensory	Filaments	Skin of axilla and medial aspect of arm
Intermedius (part of seventh cranial) (nervus intermedius [NA])	Brainstem at inferior border of pons	Parasympathetic	Greater petrosal, chorda tympani	Glands of soft palate and nose via pterygopalatine ganglion submandibular and sublingual glands via submandibular ganglion
		Sensory (taste)		Taste buds of anterior two-thirds of tongue
Interosseous, anterior of forearm (nervus interosseus anterior [NA])	Median	Motor. Somatic sensory	Muscular and articular	Deep flexor muscles of forearm, articular
Interosseous, dorsal of forearm	See *Interosseous, posterior of forearm*			
Interosseous, posterior of forearm (nervus interosseus posterior [NA])	Radial	Motor. Somatic sensory	Muscular and articular	Deep extensor muscles of forearm, articular
Interosseous, crural (nervus interosseus cruris [NA])	Tibial	Somatic sensory	Filaments	Ankle joint
Interosseous, volar	See *Interosseous, anterior of forearm*			
Ischiatic (nervus ischiadicus [NA])	See *Sciatic*			
Jugular (nervus jugularis [NA])	Superior cervical ganglion	Sympathetic	Filaments	To glossopharyngeal and vagus nerves
Labial, anterior (nervi labiales anteriores [NA])	Ilioinguinal	Somatic sensory	Filaments	Labia majora and minora
Labial, inferior (rami labiales inferiores [NA])	Inferior alveolar	Somatic sensory	Filaments	Skin of lower lip
Labial, posterior (nervi labiales superiores [NA])	Pudendal	Somatic sensory	Filaments	Labia majora and minora
Labial, superior (rami labiales superiores [NA])	Superior alveolar	Somatic sensory	Filaments	Skin of upper lip

Name	Central attachment	Components*	Branches	Distribution
Lacrimal (nervus lacrimalis [NA])	Ophthalmic	Somatic sensory	Filaments	Lacrimal gland and skin about lateral commissure of eye
Laryngeal, external (ramus externus nervi laryngei superioris [NA])	Superior laryngeal	Motor	Filaments	Cricothyroid muscle
Laryngeal, inferior (nervus laryngeus inferior [NA])	Recurrent laryngeal	Motor	Filaments	Intrinsic muscles of larynx
Laryngeal, internal (ramus internus nervi laryngei superioris [NA])	Superior laryngeal	Visceral sensory	Filaments	Mucosa of larynx
Laryngeal, recurrent (nervus laryngeus recurrens [NA])	Vagus	Motor. Parasympathetic	Inferior laryngeal, cardiac	Heart
Laryngeal, superior (nervus laryngeus superior [NA])	Vagus	Motor. Visceral sensory	Internal and external laryngeal	
Lingual (nervus lingualis [NA])	Mandibular	Somatic sensory	Filaments, sublingual	Mucosa of floor of mouth and anterior two-thirds of tongue
Long thoracic	See *Thoracic, long*			
Lumbar (5 pairs) (nervi lumbales [NA])	Lumbar segments of cord	Motor. Somatic sensory. Visceral sensory. Sympathetic (upper segments only)	Ventral and dorsal rami	Dorsal rami to skin and deep muscles of lower back, ventral rami to lumbar plexus
Lumboinguinal	See *Genitofemoral*			
Malar	See *Zygomaticofacial*			
Mandibular (nervus mandibularis [NA])	Trigeminal	Motor (masticator nerve). Somatic sensory	Masseteric, temporal, pterygoid, buccal, auriculotemporal, inferior alveolar, mylohyoid, meningeal, lingual	Tensor tympani, tensor veli palatini, mylohyoid, anterior belly of digastric and muscles of mastication; lower teeth and adjacent mucosa, anterior two-thirds of tongue, cheek, lower face, meninges
Masseteric (nervus massetericus [NA])	Mandibular	Motor	Filaments	Masseter muscle
Masticator	Motor part of mandibular			

Name	Central attachment	Components*	Branches	Distribution
Maxillary (nervus maxillaris [NA])	Trigeminal	Somatic sensory	Middle meningeal, pterygopalatine, zygomatic, infraorbital, superior alveolar	Skin of upper part of face, upper teeth, mucosa of nose and palate, meninges
Meatal, external acoustic (nervus meatus acustici externi [NA])	Auriculotemporal	Somatic sensory	Filaments	External acoustic meatus
Median (nervus medianus [NA])	Brachial plexus	Motor. Somatic sensory	Articular, muscular, anterior interosseous, digital	Flexor muscles of forearm, small muscles of thumb, two lateral lumbricals, skin of hand, hand joints
Meningeal	Vagus	Somatic sensory	Filaments	Meninges
Meningeal, middle (ramus meningeus medius nervi maxillaris [NA])	Maxillary	Somatic sensory	Filaments	Meninges
Mental (nervus mentalis [NA])	Inferior alveolar	Somatic sensory	Filaments	Skin of lower lip and chin
Musculocutaneous (of lower extremity)	See *Peroneal, superficial*			
Musculocutaneous (of upper extremity) (nervus musculocutaneous[NA])	Brachial plexus	Motor. Somatic sensory	Muscular, lateral cutaneous of forearm	Coracobrachialis, brachialis and biceps brachii muscles, skin of lateral aspect of forearm
Musculospiral	See *Radial*			
Mylohyoid (nervus mylohyoideus [NA])	Inferior alveolar	Motor	Filaments	Mylohyoid and anterior belly of digastric muscles
Nasal, anterior	See *Nasal, external*			
Nasal, external (rami nasales externi nervi infraorbitalis [NA])	Infraorbital	Somatic sensory	Filaments	Skin of side of nose
Nasal, external (rami nasalis externus nervi nasociliaris [NA])	Nasociliary	Somatic sensory	Filaments	Skin of lower half of nose and tip of nose
Nasal, internal	See *Ethmoid, anterior*			
Nasal, lateral (rami nasales laterales nervi nasociliaris [NA])	Nasociliary	Somatic sensory	Filaments	Mucosa of lateral wall of nasal cavity

Name	Central attachment	Components*	Branches	Distribution
Nasal, medial (rami nasales mediales nervi nasociliaris [NA])	Nasociliary	Somatic sensory	Filaments	Mucosa of nasal septum
Nasal, posterior inferior lateral (rami nasales posteriores inferiores laterales [NA])	Greater palatine	Somatic sensory	Filaments	Mucosa of inferior nasal concha
Nasal, posterior superior lateral (rami nasales posteriores superiores laterales [NA])	Maxillary via pterygopalatine ganglion	Somatic sensory	Filaments	Mucosa of superior and middle nasal conchae
Nasociliary (nervus nasociliaris [NA])	Ophthalmic	Somatic sensory	Long ciliary, ethmoid, infratrochlear	Eyeball, skin and mucosa of eyelids and nose, mucosa of ethmoid air cells
Nasopalatine (nervus nasopalatinus [NA])	Maxillary via pterygopalatine ganglion	Somatic sensory	Nasal rami	Mucosa of nose and hard palate
Obturator (nervus obturatorius [NA])	Lumbar plexus	Motor. Somatic sensory	Muscular, cutaneous and articular	Adductor, gracilis, obturator externus muscles, skin of medial aspect of thigh, hip and knee joints
Obturator, accessory (variable)	Lumbar plexus	Motor	Filaments	Pectineus muscle
Obturator internus (variable)	Sacral plexus	Motor	Filaments	Obturator internus and superior gemellus muscles
Occipital, greater (nervus occipitalis major [NA])	Second cervical segment dorsal ramus	Somatic sensory	Filaments	Skin of posterior portion of scalp
Occipital, lesser (nervus occipitalis minor [NA])	Cervical plexus	Somatic sensory	Filaments	Skin of lateral part of scalp and posterior aspect of auricle
Occipital, third (variable) (nervus occipitalis tertius [NA])	Third cervical segment, dorsal ramus	Somatic sensory	Filaments	Skin of posterior aspect of neck and scalp
Octavus (nervus octavus [NA alternative])	See *Vestibulocochlear*			
Oculomotor (third cranial) (nervus oculomotorius [NA])	Brainstem in region of posterior perforated substance	Motor	Filaments	Levator palpebrae superioris, medial, lateral and inferior rectus, inferior oblique muscles
		Parasympathetic	Via ciliary ganglion	Ciliary and sphincter pupillae muscles

Name	Central attachment	Components*	Branches	Distribution
of Andersch	See *Tympanic*			
of Arnold	See *Auricular*			
of Bell	See *Thoracic, long*			
of Eisler	See *Cutaneous, perforating*			
of Jacobson	See *Tympanic*			
of Vidius	See *Pterygoid canal, nerve of*			
of Wrisberg	See *Intermedius*			
Olfactory (first cranial) (nervi olfactorii [NA])	Olfactory bulb	Sensory (smell)	Filaments	Olfactory mucosa
Ophthalmic (nervus ophthalmicus [NA])	Trigeminal	Somatic sensory	Lacrimal, frontal, nasociliary, infratrochlear	Skin of forehead, upper eyelids, anterior part of scalp, orbit and eyeball, meninges, mucosa of nose and air sinuses
Optic (second cranial) (nervus opticus [NA])	Optic tracts	Sensory (vision)	Filaments	Retina
Orbital (rami orbitales [NA])	Maxillary via pterygopalatine ganglion	Somatic sensory	Filaments	Orbit
Orbital	See *Zygomatic*			
Palatine, anterior	See *Palatine, greater*			
Palatine, greater (nervus palatinus major [NA])	Maxillary via pterygopalatine ganglion	Somatic sensory	Filaments	Mucosa of hard and soft palates
Palatine, lesser (nervi palatini minores [NA])	Maxillary via pterygopalatine ganglion	Somatic sensory	Filaments	Mucosa of soft palate, uvula, and palatine tonsil
Palatine, middle	See *Palatine, lesser*			
Palatine, posterior	See *Palatine, lesser*			
Palpebral, inferior (rami palpebrales inferiores [NA])	Infraorbital	Somatic sensory	Filaments	Lower eyelid
Palpebral, superior (rami palpebrales superiores [NA])	Lacrimal, frontal, and nasociliary	Somatic sensory	Filaments	Upper eyelid
Pathetic	See *Trochlear*			

Name	Central attachment	Components*	Branches	Distribution
Pectoral, lateral (nervus pectoralis lateralis [NA])	Brachial plexus	Motor	Filaments	Pectoralis major and minor muscles
Pectoral, medial (nervus pectoralis medialis [NA])	Brachial plexus	Motor	Filaments	Pectoralis major and minor muscles
Pelvic splanchnic	See *Splanchnic, pelvic*			
Perineal (nervi perineales [NA])	Pudendal	Motor. Somatic sensory	Filaments	Muscles of perineum, skin of root of penis and scrotum (labium majus)
Peroneal, anastomotic (variable) (ramus communicans peroneus nervi peronei communis [NA])	Common peroneal	Somatic sensory	Filaments	Skin of lateral aspect of leg
Peroneal, common (nervus peroneus communis [NA])	Sciatic (sacral plexus)	Motor. Somatic sensory	Lateral sural cutaneous, superficial and deep peroneal	Short head of biceps femoris, knee joint
Peroneal, deep (nervus peroneus profundus [NA])	Common peroneal	Motor. Somatic sensory	Dorsal digital, muscular, cutaneous and articular rami	Muscles of anterior compartment of leg, skin between first and second toes
Peroneal, superficial (nervus peroneus superficialis [NA])	Common peroneal	Motor. Somatic sensory	Dorsal cutaneous of foot, muscular and cutaneous rami	Peroneus longus and brevis, skin of lateral aspect of leg and dorsum of foot
Petrosal, deep (nervus petrosus profundus [NA])	Internal carotid plexus	Sympathetic	To nerve of pterygoid canal	
Petrosal, greater (nervus petrosus major [NA])	Geniculate ganglion	Visceral sensory. Parasympathetic	Via nerve of pterygoid canal to pterygopalatine ganglion	Mucosa and glands of palate and nose
Petrosal, greater superficial	See *Petrosal, greater*			
Petrosal, lesser (nervus petrosus minor [NA])	Tympanic plexus	Parasympathetic	To otic ganglion	Parotid gland
Petrosal, lesser superficial	See *Petrosal, lesser*			
Petrosal, small deep	See *Caroticotympanic*			

Name	Central attachment	Components*	Branches	Distribution
Phrenic (nervus phreni-cus [NA])	Cervical plexus	Motor	Filaments	Diaphragm
Phrenic, accessory	See *Accessory phren-ic*			
Piriformis, nerve to	Sacral plexus	Motor	Filaments	Piriformis muscle
Plantar, lateral (nervus plantaris lateralis [NA])	Tibial	Motor. Somatic sensory	Muscular, cuta-neous, and articu-lar rami	Quadratus plantae, adductor hallucis, small muscles of little toe, and lateral 3 lum-brical muscles of foot, skin of lateral aspect of sole, foot joints
Plantar, medial (nervus plantaris medialis [NA])	Tibial	Motor. Somatic sensory	Muscular, cutane-ous, and articular rami	Abductor hallucis, flexor digitorum brevis, flexor hallucis brevis, and first lum-brical of foot, skin of medial aspect of sole, foot joints
Pneumogastric	See *Vagus*			
Popliteal, external	See *Peroneal, com-mon*			
Popliteal, internal	See *Tibial*			
Popliteal, lateral	See *Peroneal, com-mon*			
Popliteal, medial	See *Tibial*			
Presacral (nervus pre-sacralis [NA])	The superior hypo-gastric plexus			
Pterygoid, external	See *Pterygoid, lateral*			
Pterygoid, internal	See *Pterygoid, medial*			
Pterygoid, lateral (nerv-us pterygoideus lateralis [NA])	Mandibular	Motor	Filaments	Lateral pterygoid muscle
Pterygoid, medial (nerv-us pterygoideus medialis [NA])	Mandibular	Motor	Filaments	Medial pterygoid muscle
Pterygoid canal, nerve of (nervus canalis ptery-goidei [NA])	Greater and deep petrosal	Parasympathetic. Sympathetic	Filaments along branches from pterygopalatine ganglion	Glands of nose, palate, and pharynx
Pterygopalatine (nervi pterygopalatini [NA])	Maxillary	Somatic sensory	Filaments	Mucosa of palate and nose

Name	Central attachment	Components*	Branches	Distribution
Pudendal (nervus pudendus [NA])	Pudendal plexus	Motor. Somatic sensory	Rectal, perineal, scrotal (labial)	Muscles and skin of perineal region
Quadratus femoris, nerve to	Sacral plexus	Motor. Somatic sensory	Filaments	Quadratus femoris and inferior gemellus muscles, hip joint
Radial (nervus radialis [NA])	Brachial plexus	Motor. Somatic sensory	Cutaneous, interosseous, muscular, superficial and deep rami	Extensor muscles of forearm and hand, brachioradialis, skin of posterior aspect of arm, forearm and wrist, elbow, carpal, and hand joints
Rectal, inferior (nervi rectales inferiores [NA])	Pudendal	Motor. Somatic sensory	Filaments	External anal sphincter, skin about anus
Recurrent	See *Laryngeal, recurrent*			
Recurrent	See *Spinosal*			
Recurrent	See *Tentorial*			
Rhomboids, nerve to	See *Dorsal scapular*			
Saccular (nervus saccularis [NA])	Vestibular of eighth cranial	Sensory (position of head in space)	Filaments	Macula sacculi
Sacral (5 pairs) (nervi sacrales [NA])	Sacral segments of cord	Motor. Somatic sensory. Visceral sensory. Parasympathetic	Dorsal and ventral rami	Dorsal rami to deep muscles of lower back and overlying skin, ventral rami to sacral and pudendal plexuses, pelvic viscera
Saphenous (nervus saphenus [NA])	Femoral	Somatic sensory	Filaments	Skin of medial aspect of leg and foot, knee joint
Scapular, dorsal	See *Dorsal scapular*			
Scapular, posterior	See *Dorsal scapular*			
Sciatic (nervus ischiadicus [NA])	Sacral plexus	Composed of tibial and common peroneal		
Sciatic, small	See *Cutaneous, femoral posterior*			
Scrotal, anterior (nervi scrotales anteriores [NA])	Ilioinguinal	Somatic sensory	Filaments	Skin of pubic area and scrotum
Scrotal, posterior (nervi scrotales posteriores [NA])	Pudendal	Somatic sensory	Filaments	Skin of scrotum

Name	Central attachment	Components*	Branches	Distribution
Serratus anterior	See *Thoracic, long*			
Spermatic, external (ramus genitalis nervi genitofemoralis [NA])	Genitofemoral	Somatic sensory	Filaments	Skin of scrotum and skin near subcutaneous inguinal ring
Sphenopalatine	See *Pterygopalatine*			
Sphenopalatine, long	See *Nasopalatine*			
Sphenopalatine, short	See *Nasal, posterior superior lateral*			
Spinal accessory	See *Accessory*			
Spinosal (ramus meningeus nervi mandibularis [NA])	Mandibular	Somatic sensory	Filaments	Meninges
Splanchnic, greater (nervus splanchnicus major [NA])	Fifth to ninth or tenth thoracic sympathetic ganglia	Sympathetic. Visceral sensory	Filaments	Cardiac, pulmonary, esophageal, and celiac plexuses
Splanchnic, least (variable) (nervus splanchnicus imus [NA])	Lowest thoracic sympathetic ganglion	Sympathetic. Visceral sensory	Filaments	Renal plexus
Splanchnic, lesser (nervus splanchnicus minor [NA])	Ninth and tenth thoracic sympathetic ganglia	Sympathetic. Visceral sensory	Filaments	Celiac plexus
Splanchnic, lumbar (nervi splanchnici lumbales [NA])	Lumbar sympathetic ganglia	Sympathetic. Visceral sensory	Filaments	Celiac, mesenteric and hypogastric plexuses
Splanchnic, pelvic (nervi splanchnici pelvini [NA])	Second to fourth sacral segments of cord	Parasympathetic. Visceral sensory	Filaments in pelvic plexus	Pelvic viscera
Splanchnic, sacral (nervi splanchnici sacrales [NA])	Sacral sympathetic ganglia	Sympathetic. Visceral sensory	Filaments	Pelvic plexus
Stapedius, nerve to (nervus stapedius [NA])	Facial	Motor	Filaments	Stapedius muscle
Statoacoustic	See *Vestibulocochlear*			
Subclavius, nerve to (nervus subclavius [NA])	Brachial plexus	Motor	Filaments	Subclavius muscle
Subcostal (nervus subcostalis [NA])	Ventral ramus of twelfth thoracic	Motor. Somatic sensory	Muscular and cutaneous rami	Muscles and skin of anterior abdominal wall

Name	Central attachment	Components*	Branches	Distribution
Sublingual (nervus sublingualis [NA])	Lingual	Somatic sensory	Filaments	Area of sublingual gland
Suboccipital (nervus suboccipitalis [NA])	Dorsal ramus of first cervical	Motor	Muscular	Deep muscles of back of neck
Subscapular (nervus subscapularis [NA])	Brachial plexus	Motor	Muscular	Subscapular and teres major muscles
Subscapular, long	See *Thoracodorsal*			
Supraacromial	See *Supraclavicular, lateral*			
Supraclavicular, anterior	See *Supraclavicular, medial*			
Supraclavicular, intermediate (nervi supraclaviculares intermedii [NA])	Cervical plexus	Somatic sensory	Filaments	Skin of lower anterior aspect of neck and anterior chest wall
Supraclavicular, lateral (nervi supraclaviculares laterales [NA])	Cervical plexus	Somatic sensory	Filaments	Skin of lateral aspect of neck and shoulder
Supraclavicular, medial (nervi supraclaviculares mediales [NA])	Cervical plexus	Somatic sensory	Filaments	Skin of lower anterior aspect of neck and anterior chest wall, sternoclavicular joint
Supraclavicular, middle	See *Supraclavicular, intermediate*			
Supraclavicular, posterior	See *Supraclavicular, lateral*			
Supraorbital (nervus supraorbitalis [NA])	Frontal	Somatic sensory	Filaments	Skin of upper eyelid and forehead
Suprascapular (nervus suprascapularis [NA])	Brachial plexus	Motor	Filaments	Supraspinatus and infraspinatus muscles
Suprasternal	See *Supraclavicular, medial*			
Supratrochlear (nervus supratrochlearis [NA])	Frontal	Somatic sensory	Filaments	Skin of medial aspect of forehead, root of nose, and upper eyelid
Sural (variable) (nervus suralis [NA])	Combined medial and lateral sural cutaneous			

Name	Central attachment	Components*	Branches	Distribution
Sural, lateral	See *Cutaneous, sural, lateral*			
Sural, medial	See *Cutaneous, sural, medial*			
Temporal	See *Zygomaticotemporal*			
Temporal, deep (nervi temporales profundi [NA])	Mandibular	Motor	Filaments	Temporal muscle
Temporomalar	See *Zygomatic*			
Tensor tympani, nerve to (nervus tensoris tympani [NA])	Mandibular via otic ganglion	Motor	Filaments	Tensor tympani muscle
Tensor veli palatini, nerve to (nervus tensoris veli palatini [NA])	Mandibular via otic ganglion	Motor	Filaments	Tensor veli palatini muscle
Tentorial (ramus tentorii nervi ophthalmici [NA])	Ophthalmic	Somatic sensory	Filaments	Meninges
Terminal (nervi terminales [NA])	Medial olfactory tract	Not known	Filaments	
Thoracic (12 pairs) (nervi thoracici [NA])	Thoracic segments of cord	Motor. Somatic sensory. Visceral sensory. Sympathetic	Dorsal and ventral rami	Dorsal rami to deep muscles of back and skin of back, ventral rami to brachial plexus and intercostal nerves, sympathetic and visceral sensory to viscera and blood vessels
Thoracic, internal anterior	See *Pectoral, medial*			
Thoracic, lateral anterior	See *Pectoral, lateral*			
Thoracic, long (nervus thoracicus longus [NA])	Brachial plexus	Motor	Filaments	Serratus anterior muscle
Thoracic, medial anterior	See *Pectoral, medial*			
Thoracic, posterior	See *Thoracic, long*			
Thoracodorsal (nervus thoracodorsalis [NA])	Brachial plexus	Motor	Filaments	Latissimus dorsi muscle

Name	Central attachment	Components*	Branches	Distribution
Tibial (nervus tibialis [NA])	Sciatic	Motor. Somatic sensory	Interosseous crural, cutaneous, sural, plantar	Muscles of back of leg and sole of foot, skin of back of leg and sole, knee and foot joints
Tibial, anterior	See *Peroneal, deep*			
Tibial, posterior	Posterior division of tibial			
Tibial, recurrent	Common peroneal	Motor. Somatic sensory	Muscular and articular rami	Tibialis anterior muscle, knee joint
Transverse of neck (nervus transversus colli [NA])	Cervical plexus	Somatic sensory	Filaments	Skin of neck
Trifacial	See *Trigeminal*			
Trigeminal (fifth cranial) (nervus trigeminus [NA])	Brainstem at inferior surface of pons. See *Ophthalmic; Maxillary; Mandibular*			
Trochlear (fourth cranial) (nervus trochlearis [NA])	Dorsal surface of midbrain	Motor	Filaments	Superior oblique muscle of eye
Tympanic (nervus tympanicus [NA])	Glossopharyngeal	Visceral sensory. Parasympathetic	Filaments	Mucosa of middle ear and mastoid air cells, to parotid gland via otic ganglion
Ulnar (nervus ulnaris [NA])	Brachial plexus	Motor. Somatic sensory	Muscular, cutaneous and articular	Flexor carpi ulnaris, flexor digitorum profundus, adductor pollicis, muscles of hypothenar eminence, interossei, medial 2 lumbricals, skin of medial part of hand, joints of hand
Utricular (nervus utricularis [NA])	Vestibular	Somatic sensory (position of head in space—static)	Filaments	Macula utriculi
Utriculoampullary (nervus utriculoampullaris [NA])	Vestibular	Combined utricular and ampullary		
Vaginal (nervi vaginales [NA])	Pelvic plexus	Sympathetic. Parasympathetic	Filaments	Vagina

Name	Central attachment	Components*	Branches	Distribution
Vagus (tenth cranial) (nervus vagus [NA])	Lateral aspect of medulla oblongata	Motor	Pharyngeal and laryngeal	Muscles of pharynx and larynx
		Parasympathetic	Cardiac, esophageal, and abdominal	Heart, smooth muscle of thoracic and abdominal viscera
		Somatic sensory taste	Auricular	Ear, meninges, tongue
		Visceral sensory	Pharyngeal, laryngeal, thoracic, and abdominal (anterior and posterior vagal trunks)	Mucosa of pharynx and larynx; thoracic and abdominal viscera
Vertebral (nervus vertebralis [NA])	First thoracic sympathetic ganglion (cervicothoracic ganglion)	Sympathetic	Vertebral plexus	
Vestibular (vestibular part of eighth cranial)	Brainstem at lower border of pons	Somatic sensory (position of head in space—dynamic)	Ampullary, utricular, saccular	Ampullae of semicircular canals, macula sacculi and macula utriculi
Vestibulocochlear (eighth cranial) (nervus vestibulocochlearis [NA])	See *Cochlear; Vestibular*			
Volar	See *Digital, palmar*			
Zygomatic (nervus zygomaticus [NA])	Maxillary	Somatic sensory	Filaments	Skin over zygoma and temple
Zygomaticofacial (ramus zygomaticofacialis nervi zygomatici [NA])	Zygomatic	Somatic sensory	Filaments	Skin over zygoma
Zygomaticotemporal (ramus zygomaticotemporalis nervi zygomatici [NA])	Zygomatic	Somatic sensory	Filaments	Skin of temple

Name	Type	Named* ligaments

Acromioclavicular (articulatio acromioclavicularis [NA])	Gliding	Articular disk
		Coracoclavicular
		  (1) Conoid
		  (2) Trapezoid
		Acromioclavicular

Ankle (articulatio talocruralis [NA])	Hinge	Medial
		  (1) Anterior tibiotalar
		  (2) Posterior tibiotalar
		  (3) Tibiocalcaneal
		  (4) Tibionavicular
		
		Anterior talofibular
		Posterior talofibular
		Calcaneofibular

Astragalocalcaneal	See *Subtalar*	
Atlantoaxial	See *Lateral atlantoaxial;* *Median atlantoaxial*	
Atlantooccipital (articulatio atlantooccipitalis [NA])	Gliding	Anterior atlantooccipital membrane Posterior atlantooccipital membrane Anterior oblique (lateral) atlantooccipital ligament
Calcaneocuboid (articulatio calcaneocuboidea [NA])	Gliding	Dorsal calcaneocuboid Long plantar Plantar calcaneocuboid Calcaneocuboid
Calcaneonavicular	See *Talocalcaneonavicular*	
Carpal	See *Intercarpal; Mediocarpal; Pisiform*	
Carpometacarpal of thumb (articulatio carpometacarpea pollicis [NA])	Saddle	
Carpometacarpal of fingers (articulationes carpometacarpeae [NA])	Gliding	Dorsal carpometacarpal Interosseous carpometacarpal Palmar carpometacarpal
Central atlantoepistropheal	See *Median atlantoaxial*	
Costotransverse (upper 10 ribs only) (articulatio costotransversaria [NA])	Gliding	Costotransverse Superior costotransverse Lateral costotransverse Lumbocostal
Cuboideometatarsal	Gliding	Dorsal tarsometatarsal Plantar tarsometatarsal

*Each synovial joint has an articular capsule.

Name	Type	Named* ligaments
Cuboideonavicular (inconstant)	Gliding	Dorsal cuboideonavicular Interosseous cuboideonavicular Plantar cuboideonavicular
Cuneocuboid	Gliding	Dorsal cuneocuboid Interosseous cuneocuboid Plantar cuneocuboid
Cuneometatarsal	Gliding	Dorsal tarsometatarsal Interosseous cuneometatarsal Plantar tarsometatarsal
Cuneonavicular (articulatio cuneonavicularis [NA])	Gliding	Dorsal cuneonavicular and plantar cuneonavicular
Distal radioulnar (articulatio radioulnaris distalis [NA])	Gliding	Articular disk
Distal tibiofibular (syndesmosis tibiofibularis [NA])	Frequently contains an extension of the ankle joint	Anterior tibiofibular Posterior tibiofibular Interosseous membrane of the leg
Ear ossicles (articulationes ossiculorum auditus [NA])	See *Incudomalleolar; Incudostapedial*	
Elbow (articulatio cubiti [NA])		Annular radial Quadrate
(1) Humeroradial (articulatio humeroradialis [NA])	Gliding	Oblique cord Radial collateral
(2) Humeroulnar (articulatio humeroulnaris [NA])	Hinge	Ulnar collateral
(3) Proximal radioulnar (articulatio radioulnaris proximalis [NA])	Pivot	Interosseous membrane of forearm
Foot (articulationes pedis [NA])	See *Ankle; Calcaneocuboid; Interphalangeal of toes; Metatarsophalangeal; Subtalar; Talocalcaneonavicular; Tarsometatarsal*	
Hand (articulationes manus [NA])	See *Carpometacarpal of fingers; Carpometacarpal of thumb; Intercarpal; Interphalangeal of fingers; Metacarpophalangeal; Pisiform; Wrist*	
Head of rib (articulatio capitis costae [NA])	Combined hinge and gliding	Intraarticular of head of rib Radiate of head of rib
Hip (articulatio coxae [NA])	Ball-and-socket	Iliofemoral Ischiofemoral Pubofemoral Acetabular Transverse acetabular Ligament of head of femur

Name	Type	Named* ligaments
Humeroradial	See *Elbow* (1)	
Humeroulnar	See *Elbow* (2)	
Incudomalleolar (articulatio incudomallearis [NA])	Gliding	
Incudostapedial (articulatio incudostapedia [NA]	Gliding	
Intercarpal (articulationes intercarpeae [NA]) (1) Distal (between 4 bones of distal row) (2) Proximal (between 3 bones of proximal row excluding pisiform)	Gliding. See also *Mediocarpal, Pisiform*	Interosseous intercarpal Transverse carpal (=flexor retinaculum) Dorsal carpal (=extensor retinaculum) Dorsal intercarpal Palmar intercarpal
Intercuneiform	Gliding	Dorsal intercuneiform Interosseous intercuneiform Plantar intercuneiform
Intermediate tarsometatarsal	See *Cuneometatarsal*	
Intermetacarpal (4 medial metacarpal bases) (articulationes intermetacarpeae [NA])	Gliding	Dorsal metacarpal Interosseous metacarpal Palmar metacarpal
Intermetatarsal (articulationes intermetatarseae [NA])	Gliding	Dorsal metatarsal Interosseous metatarsal Plantar metatarsal Deep transverse metatarsal
Interphalangeal of fingers (articulationes interphalangeae manus [NA])	Hinge	Collateral Palmar
Interphalangeal of toes (articulationes interphalangeae pedis [NA])	Hinge	Collateral Plantar
Intertarsal (articulationes intertarseae [NA])	See *Calcaneocuboid; Cuboideonavicular; Cuneocuboid; Cuneonavicular; Intercuneiform; Subtalar; Talocalcaneonavicular; Transverse tarsal*	
Intervertebral (between articular facets of vertebrae—2 superior and 2 inferior for each) (juncturae zygapophyseales [NA])	Gliding	

Name	Type	Named* ligaments
Knee (articulatio genus [NA])	Combined hinge and gliding	Alar folds Anterior cruciate Anterior meniscofemoral Arcuate popliteal Coronary Fibular collateral Infrapatellar synovial fold Lateral meniscus Lateral patellar retinaculum Medial meniscus Medial patellar retinaculum Oblique popliteal Patellar Posterior cruciate Posterior meniscofemoral Tibial collateral Transverse
Lateral atlantoaxial (articulatio antlantoaxialis lateralis [NA])	Gliding	Accessory atlantoaxial Anterior atlantoaxial Posterior atlantoaxial
Lateral atlantoepistropheal	See *Lateral atlantoaxial*	
Lateral tarsometatarsal	See *Cuboideometatarsal*	
Mandibular	See *Temporomandibular*	
Medial tarsometatarsal	Gliding	Dorsal tarsometatarsal Interosseous tarsometatarsal Plantar tarsometatarsal
Median atlantoaxial (articulatio atlantoaxialis mediana [NA])	Pivot	Alar Apical of dens Cruciform atlantal Transverse atlantal Longitudinal bundles Tectorial membrane
Mediocarpal (articulatio mediocarpea [NA])	Gliding, ball-and-socket	Radiate carpal
Metacarpophalangeal (articulationes metacarpophalangeae [NA])	Ball-and-socket	Collateral Palmar Deep transverse metacarpal
Metatarsophalangeal (articulationes metatarsophalangeae [NA])	Ball-and-socket	Collateral Plantar Deep transverse metatarsal
Midtarsal	See *Transverse tarsal*	
Pisiform (articulatio ossis pisiformis [NA])	Gliding	Pisohamate Pisometacarpal
Pisotriquetral	See *Pisiform*	

Name	Type	Named* ligaments
Proximal radioulnar	See *Elbow* (3)	
Proximal tibiofibular (articulatio tibiofibularis [NA])	Gliding	Anterior of head of fibula Posterior of head of fibula
Radiocarpal	See *Wrist*	
Radioulnar	See *Elbow* (3); *Distal radioulnar*	
Sacroiliac (articulatio sacroiliaca [NA])	Gliding	Ventral sacroiliac Interosseous sacroiliac Dorsal sacroiliac
Shoulder (articulatio humeri [NA])	Ball-and-socket	Coracohumeral Inferior glenohumeral Middle glenohumeral Superior glenohumeral Transverse humeral Glenoid lip
Sternocostal (articulationes sternocostales [NA])	Gliding	Interarticular sternocostal Radiate sternocostal Costoxiphoid Internal and external intercostal membranes
Sternoclavicular (articulatio sternoclavicularis [NA])	Gliding	Articular disk Anterior sternoclavicular Costoclavicular Interclavicular Posterior sternoclavicular
Subtalar (articulatio subtalaris [NA])	Gliding	Interosseous talocalcaneal Lateral talocalcaneal Medial talocalcaneal
Talocalcaneal	See *Subtalar*	
Talocalcaneonavicular (articulatio talocalcaneonavicularis [NA])	Gliding	Calcaneonavicular Talonavicular Plantar calcaneonavicular or spring
Talocrural	See *Ankle*	
Talonavicular	See *Talocalcaneonavicular*	
Tarsal	See *Calcaneocuboid; Cuboideonavicular; Cuneonavicular; Cuneocuboid; Intercuneiform; Subtalar; Talocalcaneonavicular; Transverse tarsal*	

Name	Type	Named* ligaments
Tarsometatarsal (articulationes tarsometatarseae [NA])	See *Cuboideometatarsal; Cuneometatarsal; Medial tarsometatarsal*	
Temporomandibular (articulatio temporomandibularis [NA])	Combined gliding and hinge	Articular disk Sphenomandibular Stylomandibular Lateral
Tibiofibular	See *Distal tibiofibular, Proximal tibiofibular*	
Transverse tarsal (articulatio tarsi transversa [NA])	Combined calcaneocuboid and talocalcaneonavicular	
Wrist (articulatio radiocarpea [NA])	Biaxial	Dorsal radiocarpal Radial collateral of wrist Articular disk of distal radioulnar joint Ulnar collateral of wrist Palmar radiocarpal Palmar ulnocarpal

The following list includes only those veins and venous sinuses and plexuses which have no accompanying artery of the same name, or which differ considerably from the accompanying artery. For all other veins—for example, the deep veins of the upper and lower extremity, or of the body wall—see the Table of Arteries for the accompanying vein of the same name; these veins have tributaries with the same distribution as the branches of the accompanying arteries.

Name	Region or tributary drained	Location	Drains into:
Accessory hemiazygos (vena hemiazygos accessoria [NA])	3 or 4 upper left intercostal spaces	Left side of vertebral column	Either azygos or hemiazygos
Accompanying hypoglossal nerve (vena comitans nervi hypoglossi [NA])	Digastric triangle	Accompanies the hypoglossal nerve	Retromandibular
Anterior cardiac (venae cordis anteriores [NA])	Front of right ventricle	Front of right ventricle	Right atrium
Anterior facial	See *Facial*		
Anterior jugular (vena jugularis anterior [NA])	Anterior part of neck	Near midline of neck	External jugular or subclavian
Ascending lumbar (vena lumbalis ascendens [NA])	Lumbar area	Lumbar spinal column	Azygos on right, hemiazygos on left
Azygos (vena azygos [NA])	Right chest wall; begins from ascending lumbar vein	Right side of vertebral column	Superior vena cava
Basal (vena basalis [NA])	Anterior perforated substance	Base of brain	Internal cerebral
Basilar plexus (plexus basilaris [NA])	Both inferior petrosal sinuses	Basilar part of occipital bone	Anterior part of internal vertebral plexus
Basilic (vena basilica [NA])	Ulnar side of hand and forearm	Medial side of biceps brachii muscle	Joins brachial to form axillary
Basivertebral (venae basivertebrales [NA])	Bodies of vertebrae	Bodies of vertebrae	External vertebral plexuses
Brachiocephalic (venae brachiocephalicae dextra et sinistra [NA])	Internal jugular and subclavian	Root of neck	Superior vena cava
Cavernous sinus (sinus cavernosus [NA])	Superior ophthalmic	Lateral to sella turcica	Superior and inferior petrosal sinuses
Cephalic (vena cephalica [NA])	Radial side of hand and forearm	Lateral side of arm	Axillary
Common facial	See *Facial*		
Confluence of sinuses (confluens sinuum [NA])	Occipital area (inner surface)	Occipital bone	Variable connection between transverse sinuses

Name	Region or tributary drained	Location	Drains into:
Coronary of stomach	Combined right and left gastric veins		
Coronary sinus (sinus coronarius [NA])	Most of the veins of the heart	Posterior part of coronary sulcus	Right atrium
Cubital (vena mediana cubiti [NA])	Palmar forearm	Cubital area	Basilic
Deep cerebral	See *Internal cerebral*		
Diploic (venae diploicae [NA])	Diploë of cranium	Inside the frontal, temporal, parietal, and occipital bones	Either internally into the dural sinuses or externally into superficial veins, such as the occipital or supraorbital
Ductus venosus (ductus venosus [NA])	Embryonic bypass from umbilical vein to inferior vena cava		
Emissary (venae emissariae [NA])	Venous sinuses inside cranium	Small foramens in skull, such as parietal, mastoid, condylar, occipital, and postcondylar	Veins external to the skull, as the posterior auricular or occipital
External jugular (vena jugularis externa [NA])	Posterior auricular and posterior part of facial	Side of neck	Subclavian
External vertebral plexuses, anterior and posterior (plexus venosi vertebrales externi [NA])	Vertebra and surrounding muscles	Anterior and posterior to the vertebral column	Basivertebral and intervertebral veins
Facial (vena facialis [NA])	Continuation of angular	Anterior side of face	Retromandibular or internal jugular
Great cardiac (vena cordis magna [NA])	Anterior aspect of ventricles	Anterior interventricular sulcus of heart	Coronary sinus
Great cerebral (vena cerebri magna [NA])	Internal cerebral veins	Below and behind the splenium of the corpus callosum	Straight sinus
Great saphenous (vena saphena magna [NA])	Medial side of leg and thigh	Medial side of leg and thigh	Femoral
Hemiazygos (vena hemiazygos [NA])	Left ascending lumbar	Left side of vertebral column	Azygos
Hemorrhoidal plexus	See *Rectal plexus*		
Hepatic (venae hepaticae [NA])	Substance of liver	Converge to the sulcus of the inferior vena cava	Inferior vena cava

Name	Region or tributary drained	Location	Drains into:
Inferior anastomotic (venae anastomotica inferior [NA])	Interconnect middle superficial cerebral vein and transverse sinus		
Inferior cerebral (venae cerebri inferiores [NA])	Base of brain	Beneath base of hemispheres	Various sinuses
Inferior ophthalmic (vena ophthalmica inferior [NA])	Lower part of orbit	Floor of orbit	Pterygoid plexus and cavernous sinus
Inferior petrosal sinus (sinus petrosus inferior [NA])	Cavernous sinus	Inferior petrosal sulcus	Internal jugular
Inferior pulmonary, left (vena pulmonalis inferior sinistra [NA])	Apical and basal	Lower lobe of left lung	Left atrium
Inferior pulmonary, right (vena pulmonalis inferior dextra [NA])	Apical and basal	Lower lobe of right lung	Left atrium
Inferior sagittal sinus (sinus sagittalis inferior [NA])	Falx cerebri	Lower edge of falx cerebri	Straight sinus
Inferior vena cava (vena cava inferior [NA])	Common iliac veins, blood from lower extremities and abdomen	In front of vertebral column to the right of the aorta	Right atrium
Innominate	See *Brachiocephalic*		
Intercavernous sinuses, anterior and posterior (sinus intercavernosi [NA])	Connect the cavernous sinuses		
Internal cerebral (venae cerebri internae [NA])	Terminal and choroid veins	Beneath splenium of corpus callosum	Great cerebral
Internal jugular (vena jugularis interna [NA])	Brain, face, and neck; transverse sinus	Side of neck	Brachiocephalic
Internal vertebral plexuses, anterior and posterior (plexus venosi vertebrales interni [NA])	Vertebrae and meninges	Within the vertebral canal, anterior and posterior to the spinal cord	Intervertebral veins
Jugular	See *Anterior jugular; External jugular; Internal jugular*		
Least cardiac (venae cordis minimae [NA])	Walls of heart	Walls of heart	Each chamber of heart

TABLE OF VEINS (Continued)

Name	Region or tributary drained	Location	Drains into:
Long saphenous	See *Great saphenous*		
Median cubital (vena mediana cubiti [NA])	Palmar forearm	Cubital area, between cephalic and basilic	
Middle cardiac (vena cordis media [NA])	Posterior aspect of heart	Posterior interventricular septum	Coronary sinus
Oblique vein of left atrium (vena obliqua atrii sinistri [NA])	Left atrium	Back of left atrium	Coronary sinus
Occipital sinus (sinus occipitalis [NA])	Region around foramen magnum	Attached margin of falx cerebelli	Confluence of sinuses
of Galen	See *Great cerebral*		
of Marshall	See *Oblique vein of left atrium*		
of Sappey	See *Paraumbilical*		
of Vieussens	See *Anterior cardiac*		
Pampiniform plexus (plexus pampiniformis [NA])	Testis or ovary	Surrounding distal part of testicular or ovarian artery	Testicular or ovarian
Paraumbilical (venae paraumbilicales [NA])	Around umbilicus	Round ligament of the liver	Portal
Portal (vena portae [NA])	Superior mesenteric and lienal	Lesser omentum	Sinusoids of liver
Posterior facial	See *Retromandibular*		
Posterior vein of left ventricle (vena posterior ventriculi sinistri [NA])	Left ventricle	Posterior aspect of left ventricle	Coronary sinus
Prepyloric (vena prepylorica [NA])	Pylorus	On ventral surface of junction of stomach and pylorus	Gastric veins
Prostatic plexus (plexus prostaticus [NA])	Prostate	Fascial sheath of prostate	Internal iliac veins
Pterygoid plexus (plexus pterygoideus [NA])	Veins corresponding to branches of maxillary artery	Between pterygoid muscles	Maxillary
Ranine	See *Accompanying hypoglossal nerve*		
Rectal plexus (plexus venosus rectalis)	Rectum	Wall of rectum	Superior, middle, and inferior rectal veins
Retromandibular (vena retromandibularis [NA])	Superficial temporal and maxillary	In parotid gland	Facial

Name	Region or tributary drained	Location	Drains into:
Saphenous	See *Great saphenous; Small saphenous*		
Short saphenous	See *Small saphenous*		
Sigmoid sinus (sinus sigmoideus [NA])	Transverse sinus	Groove on temporal bone	Internal jugular
Small cardiac (vena cordis parva [NA])	Back of right atrium and ventricle	Coronary sulcus	Coronary sinus
Small saphenous (vena saphena parva [NA])	Leg and foot	Back of leg	Popliteal
Sphenoparietal sinus (sinus sphenoparietalis [NA])	Meninges	Small wing of sphenoid	Cavernous sinus
Straight sinus (sinus rectus [NA])	Inferior sagittal sinus and great cerebral vein	Junction of falx cerebri and tentorium cerebelli	Transverse sinus
Superior anastomotic (vena anastomotica superior [NA])	Interconnects middle superficial cerebral vein and superior sagittal sinus		
Superior cerebral (venae cerebri superiores [NA])	Cortex of brain	Surface of brain	Superior sagittal sinus
Superior ophthalmic (vena ophthalmica superior [NA])	Tributaries corresponding to branches of ophthalmic artery	Orbit	Cavernous sinus
Superior petrosal sinus (sinus petrosus superior [NA])	Cavernous sinus	Superior petrosal sulcus of temporal bone	Transverse sinus
Superior pulmonary, left (vena pulmonalis superior sinistra [NA])	Apicoposterior, anterior, and lingual	Upper lobe of left lung	Left atrium
Superior pulmonary, right (vena pulmonalis superior dextra [NA])	Anterior, posterior, and vein from middle lobe	Upper and middle lobes of right lung	Left atrium
Superior sagittal sinus (sinus sagittalis superior [NA])	Superior cerebral veins and diploic veins	Attached margin of falx cerebri	Confluence of sinuses and transverse sinus
Superior vena cava (vena cava superior [NA])	Head, chest wall, and upper extremities	Right upper mediastinum	Right atrium
Thebesian	See *Least cardiac*		
Transverse sinus (sinus transversus durae matris [NA])	Usually the right is a continuation of the superior sagittal and the left of the straight sinus	Attached margin of tentorium cerebelli	Sigmoid sinus

Name	Region or tributary drained	Location	Drains into:
Umbilical (vena umbilicalis sinistra [NA])	Embryonic vein from placenta to fetus		
Vesical plexus (plexus venosus vesicalis [NA])	Pudendal and prostatic plexuses	Around base of urinary bladder	Internal iliac
Vorticose (venae vorticosae [NA])	Veins of eyeball	Eyeball	Superior ophthalmic veins